Rothman-Simeone

THE SPINE

Rothman-Simeone

THE SPINE

Sixth Edition

Volume 1

Harry N. Herkowitz, MD
Chairman, Orthopaedic Surgery
William Beaumont Hospital
Professor and Chairman, Orthopaedic Surgery
Oakland University William Beaumont School of Medicine
Royal Oak, Michigan

Steven R. Garfin, MD
Professor and Chair, Department of Orthopaedic Surgery
University of California
San Diego, California

Frank J. Eismont, MD
Leonard M. Miller Professor and Chairman
Department of Orthopaedic Surgery
University of Miami
Miller School of Medicine
Miami, Florida

Gordon R. Bell, MD
Director, Center for Spine Health
Neurological Institute
Cleveland Clinic
Cleveland, Ohio

Richard A. Balderston, MD
Chief, Spine Service
Pennsylvania Hospital
Clinical Professor, Orthopaedic Surgery
University of Pennsylvania School of Medicine
Philadelphia, Pennsylvania

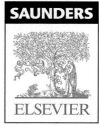
SAUNDERS
ELSEVIER

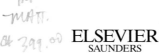

ELSEVIER
SAUNDERS

1600 John F. Kennedy Blvd.
Ste 1800
Philadelphia, PA 19103-2899

ROTHMAN-SIMEONE THE SPINE, SIXTH EDITION   ISBN: 978-1-4160-6726-9
Copyright © 2011, 2006, 1999, 1992, 1982, 1975 by Saunders, an imprint of Elsevier Inc.

Notices

Knowledge and best practice in this field are constantly changing. As new research and experience broaden our understanding, changes in research methods, professional practices, or medical treatment may become necessary.

Practitioners and researchers must always rely on their own experience and knowledge in evaluating and using any information, methods, compounds, or experiments described herein. In using such information or methods they should be mindful of their own safety and the safety of others, including parties for whom they have a professional responsibility.

With respect to any drug or pharmaceutical products identified, readers are advised to check the most current information provided (i) on procedures featured or (ii) by the manufacturer of each product to be administered, to verify the recommended dose or formula, the method and duration of administration, and contraindications. It is the responsibility of practitioners, relying on their own experience and knowledge of their patients, to make diagnoses, to determine dosages and the best treatment for each individual patient, and to take all appropriate safety precautions.

To the fullest extent of the law, neither the Publisher nor the authors, contributors, or editors, assume any liability for any injury and/or damage to persons or property as a matter of products liability, negligence or otherwise, or from any use or operation of any methods, products, instructions, or ideas contained in the material herein.

International Standard Book Number
978-1-4160-6726-9

Acquisitions Editor: Daniel Pepper
Developmental Editor: Beth LoGiudice
Publishing Services Manager: Patricia Tannian
Team Manager: Radhika Pallamparthy
Senior Project Manager: Claire Kramer
Project Manager: Jayavel Radhakrishnan
Designer: Louis Forgione

Printed in the United States of America

Last digit is the print number: 9 8 7 6 5 4 3 2 1

The sixth edition of *The Spine* is based on the principles instilled in us, the Editorial Board, when we were fellows with Drs. Rothman and Simeone. Perhaps the most important are the joys of continually teaching, learning, questioning, and trying to understand the complexities of the spine, including diagnosis and treatment through critical analysis of natural history data and treatment outcomes. These occurred for all of us before the terms evidence-based medicine and comparative effectiveness came into common parlance and are an everyday part of what we do and how we think. As evidenced by this book, other important principles include (1) thorough knowledge of basic science as it relates to the clinical condition, (2) understanding of the natural history of spinal disorders, (3) knowledge and interpretive skills of imaging modalities and laboratory studies, (4) treatment decisions that are based on sound scientific principles, and (5) commitment to education and research to further the knowledge base of spinal disorders. As with all previous editions, this one remains dedicated to Drs. Rothman and Simeone, our teachers and friends.

The Editorial Board also wishes to dedicate this edition of *The Spine* to those giants of spine surgery who have passed on since the last edition was published. These include Leon Wiltse, Allan Levine, and Henry Bohlman. Their contributions have significantly influenced our thought processes and clinical decisions. Their legacies will continue to influence future generations of spine surgeons, as we will always remember the richness of their friendship and their dedication to our profession.

Sincerely,
The Editorial Board

To my wife, Jan, and my children, Seth Adam, Laura, and Rachael Helene, for their love, understanding, and support. To the residents and fellows whose enthusiasm for knowledge and "all the answers" inspires me to continue academic pursuits. To Stanko Stanisavljevic, MD, my chairman, who taught me the meaning of hard work and perseverance. To Richard Rothman, MD, PhD, my mentor and friend, for always being there for me. To Steve Garfin, Frank Eismont, Jim Weinstein, Gordon Bell, Sam Wiesel, and Ed Hanley, whose friendship and camaraderie over the past 30 years have made the journey so special.
HARRY N. HERKOWITZ, MD

As time passes and techniques change, it becomes an increasing challenge to keep this book fresh and updated and to encourage friends and colleagues to write new chapters (for this and other books). It is easier for this one, however, because of the importance this book has attained in the spine world, and the dedication and fondness we have for our mentors. It is also easier for me to do because I am helped by the love and support from my family (Susan, Jessica, Cory, and now Ron) who understand the time it takes to practice medicine, do research, teach, and write. Also, to my friend and colleague Liz Stimson, who is a calm strength and cornerstone of our spine service.
STEVEN R. GARFIN, MD

To my wife, Emily, and my children, Austin, Adam, April, Allison, and Andrew, whose love, encouragement, and tolerance have allowed me to avidly pursue my medical interests, and to Drs. Richard Rothman and Fred Simeone, who have been excellent role models for me to try to emulate regarding medical education and patient care.
FRANK J. EISMONT, MD

To my wife, Kathy, for her love, patience, understanding, and support.
To my children, Gordie, Megan, and Michael, for making efforts such as this worthwhile.
To my parents, Gordon and Ann, for their support in making this possible.
GORDON R. BELL, MD

To my wife, Claudia, for all the help she has given me over the past 35 years.
RICHARD A. BALDERSTON, MD

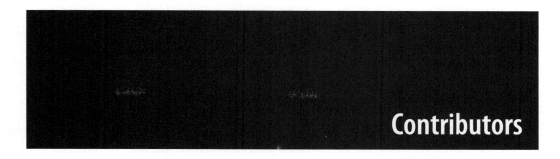

Contributors

Steven S. Agabegi, MD
Assistant Professor, Department of Orthopaedic Surgery, University of Cincinnati College of Medicine; Cincinnati Children's Hospital Medical Center, Cincinnati, Ohio
Pediatric Kyphosis: Scheuermann Disease and Congenital Deformity

Todd J. Albert, MD
Richard Rothman Professor and Chair, Orthopaedics, Thomas Jefferson University and Hospitals, Philadelphia, Pennsylvania
Surgical Management of Lumbar Spinal Stenosis

Howard S. An, MD
The Morton International Endowed Chair, Professor of Orthopaedic Surgery; Director, Division of Spine Surgery and Spine Fellowship Program, Rush University Medical Center, Chicago, Illinois
Cervical Spine: Surgical Approaches

Dheera Ananthakrishnan, MD, MSE
Assistant Professor, Orthopaedic and Spine Center, Emory Healthcare; Assistant Professor, Orthopaedics, Grady Healthcare Systems; Assistant Professor, Orthopaedics, Children's Healthcare of Atlanta; Assistant Professor, Orthopaedics, VA Medical Center, Atlanta, Georgia
Ankylosing Spondylitis

D. Greg Anderson, MD
Associate Professor, Thomas Jefferson University; Spinal Surgeon, Department of Orthopaedic Surgery, Thomas Jefferson University, Rothman Institute, Philadelphia, Pennsylvania
Posterior Minimally Invasive Lumbar Fusion Techniques

Megan E. Anderson, MD
Department of Orthopaedic Surgery, Beth Israel Deaconess Medical Center, Boston, Massachusetts
Tumors of the Spine

Paul A. Anderson, MD
Professor, Department of Orthopedic Surgery and Rehabilitation, University of Wisconsin, Madison, Wisconsin
Injuries of the Lower Cervical Spine

Gunnar B. J. Andersson, MD, PhD
Ronald L. DeWald Professor and Chairman Emeritus, Department of Orthopedic Surgery, Rush University Medical Center, Chicago, Illinois
Lumbar Disc Disease
Annular Repair

Peter D. Angevine, MD, MPH
Assistant Professor, Department of Neurological Surgery, Columbia University College of Physicians and Surgeons, New York, New York
Fixed Sagittal Imbalance
Postoperative Deformity of the Cervical Spine

Joshua D. Auerbach, MD
Chief of Spine Surgery, Bronx-Lebanon Hospital Center; Assistant Professor of Surgery, Albert Einstein College of Medicine, Bronx, New York
Postoperative Deformity of the Cervical Spine

Richard A. Balderston, MD
Chief, Spine Service, Orthopaedics, Pennsylvania Hospital; Clinical Professor, Orthopaedic Surgery, University of Pennsylvania School of Medicine, Philadelphia, Pennsylvania
Anterior Exposure to the Lumbosacral Spine: Anatomy and Techniques
Lumbar Total Disc Replacement

Kresimir Banovac, MD, PhD
Professor, Department of Rehabilitation Medicine, University of Miami; Director of Spinal Cord Division, Jackson Memorial Medical Center, Miami, Florida
Spinal Cord Injury Rehabilitation

Qi-Bin Bao, PhD
Chief Technology Officer, Pioneer Surgical Technology, Marquette, Michigan
Lumbar Nucleus Replacement

Joel A. Bauman, MD
Resident, Neurosurgery, University of Pennsylvania, Philadelphia, Pennsylvania
Congenital Anomalies of the Spinal Cord

Asheesh Bedi, MD
Assistant Professor, Department of Orthopaedic Surgery, University of Michigan Hospitals, Ann Arbor, Michigan
Congenital Anomalies of the Cervical Spine

Gordon R. Bell, MD
Director, Center for Spine Health, Neurological Institute, Cleveland Clinic, Cleveland, Ohio
Spine Imaging
Degenerative Spondylolisthesis

Carlo Bellabarba, MD
Director, Orthopaedic Spine Service, Department of Orthopaedics and Sports Medicine, Harborview Medical Center; Associate Professor, Department of Orthopaedics and Sports Medicine, University of Washington School of Medicine, Seattle, Washington
Sacral Fractures

David M. Benglis, Jr., MD
Resident Physician, Department of Neurosurgery, University of Miami, Miami, Florida
Syringomyelia

Joseph R. Berger, MD
Ruth L. Works Professor and Chairman, Neurology, University of Kentucky, Lexington, Kentucky
Medical Myelopathies

Sigurd Berven, MD
Associate Professor in Residence, Department of Orthopaedic Surgery, University of California San Francisco, San Francisco, California
Adult Scoliosis

Nitin N. Bhatia, MD
Chief, Spine Surgery, University of California Irvine Medical Center; Associate Professor, Orthopaedic Surgery, University of California, Irvine, California
Postoperative Spinal Infections

Ashok Biyani, MD
Associate Professor, Department of Orthopedic Surgery, University of Toledo, Toledo, Ohio
Lumbar Disc Disease

Scott D. Boden, MD
Professor of Orthopaedics and Director, Emory Orthopaedics and Spine Center, Orthopaedic Surgery, Emory University; Staff Physician, Department of Orthopaedic Surgery, Atlanta VA Medical Center, Atlanta, Georgia
Genetic Applications: An Overview

†Henry H. Bohlman, MD
Professor of Orthopaedic Surgery, The Spine Institute, University Hospitals of Cleveland, Case Western Reserve Medical School, Cleveland, Ohio
Late Decompression of Patients with Spinal Cord Injury

Christopher M. Bono, MD
Assistant Professor of Orthopaedic Surgery, Harvard Medical School; Chief, Orthopaedic Spine Service, Brigham and Women's Hospital, Boston, Massachusetts
Development of the Spine
Applied Anatomy of the Spine
Lumbar Disc Herniations

David G. Borenstein, MD
Clinical Professor of Medicine, The George Washington University Medical Center, Washington, DC
Arthritic Disorders

Keith H. Bridwell, MD
Asa C. and Dorothy W. Jones Professor of Orthopaedic Surgery, Washington University in St. Louis; Chief, Adult/Pediatric Spinal Surgery, Orthopaedic Surgery, Barnes Hospital, St. Louis, Missouri
Fixed Sagittal Imbalance

Stephen H. M. Brown, PhD
Assistant Professor, Department of Health and Nutritional Sciences, University of Guelph, Guelph, Ontario, Canada
Anatomy and Mechanics of the Abdominal Muscles

Robert Byers, MD
Mt. Tam Spine Center, Larkspur, California
Surgical Management of Lumbar Spinal Stenosis

Peter G. Campbell, MD
Neurosurgical Resident, Thomas Jefferson University Hospital, Philadelphia, Pennsylvania
Spinal Dural Injuries

Eugene Carragee, MD
Professor and Vice-Chairman, Orthopaedic Surgery, Stanford University School of Medicine; Chief, Division of Spinal Surgery, Stanford University Medical Center, Stanford, California
Discography

Jens R. Chapman, MD
Professor and Acting Chair; Director, Spine Service; Hansjörg Wyss Endowed Chair, Department of Orthopaedics and Sports Medicine; Joint Professor of Neurological Surgery, University of Washington, Seattle, Washington
Sacral Fractures

Kingsley R. Chin, MD
Orthopaedic Spine Surgeon; Founder, The Institute for Minimally Invasive Spine Surgery, West Palm Beach, Florida
Late Decompression for Patients with Spinal Cord Injury

Elisha K. Clouse, RN, BSN, CCRP
Director of Clinical Research, Tristate Orthopaedic Treatment Center; Student, University of Cincinnati, School of Nursing, Cincinnati, Ohio
Vascular Complications in Spinal Surgery

Howard M. Cohen, MD
Adjunct Assistant Professor, Graduate School of Nursing, University of Texas at Arlington, Arlington, Texas; Associate Medical Director, Productive Rehabilitation Institute of Dallas for Ergonomics (P.R.I.D.E.), Dallas, Texas
Functional Restoration

Edward C. Covington, MD
Director, Neurological Center for Pain, Cleveland Clinic Foundation, Cleveland, Ohio
Psychologic Strategies for Chronic Pain

---

†Deceased.

Alvin H. Crawford, MD, FACS
Professor of Pediatric Orthopaedic Surgery, University of Cincinnati Medical Center, University of Cincinnati College of Medicine, Cincinnati, Ohio
Pediatric Kyphosis: Scheuermann Disease and Congenital Deformity

Terrence T. Crowder, MD
Associate, Sonoran Spine Center, Mesa, Arizona
Cervical Radiculopathy: Anterior Surgical Approach

Bryan W. Cunningham, MSc
Director Spinal Research, Orthopaedic Surgery, St. Joseph Medical Center, Baltimore, Maryland
Failed Disc Replacement

Bradford L. Currier, MD
Professor of Orthopaedics; Director of Spine Fellowship Program, Mayo Clinic, Rochester, Minnesota
Infections of the Spine

Scott D. Daffner, MD
Assistant Professor, Department of Orthopaedics, West Virginia University School of Medicine, Morgantown, West Virginia
Surgical Management of Rheumatoid Arthritis

Michael Dahl, PhD
Research Scientist, Disc Dynamics, Inc., Eden Prairie, Minnesota
Lumbar Nucleus Replacement

Clayton L. Dean, MD
The Maryland Spine Center, Baltimore, Maryland
Nonoperative Management of Cervical Disc and Degenerative Disorders

Michael J. DeLeo III, MD
Department of Radiology, University of Massachusetts Medical School, Worcester, Massachusetts
Vascular Anatomy of the Spine, Imaging, and Endovascular Treatment of Spinal Vascular Diseases

Scott L. Delp, PhD
James H. Clark Professor of Bioengineering, Mechanical Engineering, and Orthopaedic Surgery; Co-Director, Stanford Center for Biomedical Computing, Stanford University, Palo Alto, California
Architectural Design and Function of Human Back Muscles

Richard Derby, MD
Medical Director, Spinal Diagnostics and Treatment Center, Daly City, California
Targeting Pain Generators

Clinton J. Devin, MD
Assistant Professor, Orthopaedic Surgery, Vanderbilt University, Nashville, Tennessee
Cervical, Thoracic, and Lumbar Spinal Trauma of the Immature Spine

W. Dalton Dietrich III, PhD
The Miami Project to Cure Paralysis, The Miller School of Medicine, University of Miami, Miami, Florida
Basic Science of Spinal Cord Injury

Jason C. Eck, DO
Assistant Professor of Orthopedics and Physical Rehabilitation, University of Massachusetts Medical School, Worcester, Massachusetts
Thoracic Disc Disease

Robert Eilert, MD
Emeritus Professor of Orthopaedic Surgery and Pediatrics, University of Colorado, Denver, Colorado
The Immature Spine and Athletic Injuries

Frank J. Eismont, MD
Leonard M. Miller Professor and Chairman, Department of Orthopaedic Surgery, University of Miami, Miller School of Medicine, Miami, Florida
Thoracic Disc Disease
Injuries of the Upper Cervical Spine
Infections of the Spine

Sanford E. Emery, MD, MBA
Professor and Chairman, Department of Orthopaedics, West Virginia University, Morgantown, West Virginia
Surgical Management of Rheumatoid Arthritis

Steven T. Ericksen, MD
Resident Physician, Orthopedic Surgery, University of Toledo, Toledo, Ohio
Lumbar Disc Disease

Reginald S. Fayssoux, MD
Fellow in Orthopaedic Spine Surgery; Clinical Instructor, Department of Orthopaedic Surgery, Emory University Spine Center, Atlanta, Georgia
Complications of Spinal Surgery

Catherine J. Fedorka, MD
Orthopaedic Surgery Resident, Drexel University College of Medicine/Hahnemann University Hospital, Philadelphia, Pennsylvania
Cervical, Thoracic, and Lumbar Spinal Trauma of the Immature Spine

Richard G. Fessler, MD
Professor, Department of Neurosurgery, Northwestern University Feinberg School of Medicine, Chicago, Illinois
Rationale of Minimally Invasive Spine Surgery

Jeffrey D. Fischgrund, MD
Fellowship Director, William Beaumont Hospital, Royal Oak, Michigan
Cervical Radiculopathy: Anterior Surgical Approach

Kevin Foley, MD
Department of Neurosurgery, University of Tennessee Health Science Center, Semmes-Murphey Clinic, Memphis, Tennessee
Minimally Invasive Posterior Approaches to the Spine

Winston Fong, MD
Spine Surgeon, Department of Orthopaedic Surgery, McBride Clinic, Oklahoma City, Oklahoma
Bone Substitutes: Basic Science and Clinical Applications

Julie Fritz, PhD, PT, ATC
Associate Professor, The University of Utah; Clinical Outcomes Research Scientist, Intermountain Healthcare, Salt Lake City, Utah
Physical Therapy—The Science

Shyam Gajavelli, PhD
Associate Scientist, The Miami Project to Cure Paralysis, University of Miami, Miami, Florida
Chronic Pain: The Basic Science

Steven R. Garfin, MD
Professor and Chair, Department of Orthopaedic Surgery, University of California, San Diego, California
Development of the Spine
Applied Anatomy of the Spine
Lateral and Posterior Approaches to the Lumbosacral Spine
Lumbar Disc Herniations
Rationale of Minimally Invasive Spine Surgery
Spinal Orthoses for Traumatic and Degenerative Disease
Revision Spine Surgery

Timothy A. Garvey, MD
Staff Surgeon, Twin Cities Spine Center, Minneapolis, Minnesota
Surgical Management of Axial Pain

Alexander J. Ghanayem, MD
Professor, Chief, Division of Spine Surgery, Department of Orthopaedic Surgery and Rehabilitation, Loyola University, Chicago, Illinois
Instrumentation Complications

Brian P. Gladnick, MD
Resident, Department of Orthopedic Surgery, Hospital for Special Surgery, New York, New York
Metabolic Bone Disorders of the Spine

Paul A. Glazer, MD
Assistant Clinical Professor, Orthopedic Surgery, Beth Israel Deaconess Medical Center, Harvard University, Boston, Massachusetts
Electrical Stimulation for Spinal Fusion

Liane Clamen Glazer, MD
Boston, Massachusetts
Electrical Stimulation for Spinal Fusion

Jamieson Glenn, MD
Division of Spine Surgery, CORE Orthopaedic Medical Center, Encinitas, California
Anterior Lumbar Interbody Fusion

David Gloystein, MD
Carl R. Darnell Army Medical Center, Fort Hood, Texas
Failed Disc Replacement

Barth A. Green, MD
Department of Neurological Surgery, University of Miami School of Medicine, Miami, Florida
Thoracic Disc Disease
Intradural Tumors
Syringomyelia

Michael W. Groff, MD
Neurosurgeon-in-Chief; Chief, Neurosurgical Spine Service; Co-Director, Spine Center, Beth Israel Deaconess Medical Center, Boston, Massachusetts
Electrical Stimulation for Spinal Fusion

Richard D. Guyer, MD
Spine Surgeon and Co-Founder, Texas Back Institute, Plano, Texas; Associate Clinical Professor, Orthopedics, University of Texas Southwestern School of Medicine, Dallas, Texas
Anterior Lumbar Interbody Fusion

Aldric Hama, PhD
Scientist, Department of Neurological Surgery, The Miami Project to Cure Paralysis, University of Miami, Miami, Florida
Chronic Pain: The Basic Science

Amgad Hanna, MD
Assistant Professor, Department of Neurological Surgery, University of Wisconsin School of Medicine and Public Health, Madison, Wisconsin
Spinal Dural Injuries

James S. Harrop, MD
Associate Professor of Neurologic and Orthopedic Surgery, Jefferson Medical College, Philadelphia, Pennsylvania
Spinal Dural Injuries

Robert F. Heary, MD
Professor of Neurological Surgery, University of Medicine and Dentistry of New Jersey Medical School; Director, The Spine Center of New Jersey; Director, The Spine Research Laboratory, Newark, New Jersey
Arachnoiditis and Epidural Fibrosis

John G. Heller, MD
Professor of Orthopaedic Surgery, Department of Orthopaedic Surgery, Emory University School of Medicine; Spine Fellowship Director, Emory Spine Center, Atlanta, Georgia
Complications of Spinal Surgery

Robert N. Hensinger, MD
William S. Smith Collegiate Professor of Orthopaedic Surgery, Department of Orthopaedic Surgery, University of Michigan, Ann Arbor, Michigan
Congenital Anomalies of the Cervical Spine

Harry N. Herkowitz, MD
Chairman, Orthopaedic Surgery, William Beaumont Hospital; Professor and Chairman, Orthopaedic Surgery, Oakland University William Beaumont School of Medicine, Royal Oak, Michigan
Thoracic Spine: Surgical Approaches
Cervical Spondylotic Myelopathy: Surgical Management

Stanley A. Herring, MD
Medical Director of Spine Care UW Medicine; Clinical Professor, Department of Rehabilitation Medicine, Department of Orthopaedics and Sports Medicine, and Department of Neurological Surgery, University of Washington, Seattle, Washington
The Patient History and Physical Examination: Cervical, Thoracic, and Lumbar

Alan S. Hilibrand, MD
Professor of Orthopaedic Surgery, Professor of Neurosurgery, Jefferson Medical College, Thomas Jefferson University; Director of Medical Education, Rothman Institute, Philadelphia, Pennsylvania
Transforaminal Lumbar Interbody Fusion

Justin B. Hohl, MD
Resident, Department of Orthopaedic Surgery, University of Pittsburgh Medical Center, Pittsburgh, Pennsylvania
Cervical, Thoracic, and Lumbar Spinal Trauma of the Immature Spine

Eric M. Horn, MD, PhD
Assistant Professor, Neurological Surgery, Indiana University, Indianapolis, Indiana
Acute Treatment of Patients with Spinal Cord Injury

Serena S. Hu, MD
Co-Director, University of California San Francisco Spine Center; Professor and Vice Chair, Department of Orthopaedic Surgery, University of California San Francisco, San Francisco, California
Ankylosing Spondylitis

Motoki Iwasaki, MD, DMSc
Associate Professor, Department of Orthopaedic Surgery; Chief, Spine Surgery, Osaka University Graduate School of Medicine, Osaka, Japan
Ossification of the Posterior Longitudinal Ligament

Ramin J. Javahery, MD
Pediatric Neurosurgery, Miller Children's Hospital, Long Beach, California
Spinal Intradural Infections

Andrew Jea, MD
Assistant Professor, Neurosurgery, Baylor College of Medicine; Staff Neurosurgeon, Pediatric Neurosurgery, Texas Children's Hospital, Houston, Texas
Syringomyelia

Jeremiah N. Johnson, MD
Neurosurgical Resident, Department of Neurological Surgery, University of Miami, Miami, Florida
Intradural Tumors

Sara Jurek, MD
Department of Orthopedic Surgery, Medical College of Wisconsin, Milwaukee, Wisconsin
Cervical Spondylosis: Pathophysiology, Natural History, and Clinical Syndromes of Neck Pain, Radiculopathy, and Myelopathy

James D. Kang, MD
Professor of Orthopaedic and Neurological Surgery; Professor of Physical Medicine and Rehabilitation, UPMC Endowed Chair in Spine Surgery; Vice Chairman of Orthopaedic Surgery; Director of Ferguson Laboratory, University of Pittsburgh School of Medicine, Pittsburgh, Pennsylvania
The Intervertebral Disc: Normal, Aging, and Pathologic Genetic Applications: An Overview

Lori A. Karol, MD
Professor, Orthopaedic Surgery, Texas Scottish Rite Hospital for Children; Professor, Orthopaedic Surgery, University of Texas-Southwestern, Dallas, Texas
Back Pain in Children and Adolescents

Namdar Kazemi, MD
Resident, Orthopaedic Surgery, University of Cincinnati, Cincinnati, Ohio
Pediatric Kyphosis: Scheuermann Disease and Congenital Deformity

Leonard K. Kibuule, MD
Fellow, William Beaumont Hospital, Royal Oak, Michigan; Orthopaedic Spine Surgeon, Spine Team Texas, South Lake, Texas
Thoracic Spine: Surgical Approaches

Shinichi Kikuchi, MD, PhD
Professor and President, Fukushima Medical University, Fukushima City, Japan
Sciatica and Nerve Root Pain in Disc Herniation and Spinal Stenosis: A Basic Science Review and Clinical Perspective

Choll W. Kim, MD, PhD
Spine Institute of San Diego, Center for Minimally Invasive Spine Surgery at Alvarado Hospital; Executive Director, Society for Minimally Invasive Spine Surgery; Associate Clinical Professor of Orthopaedic Surgery, University of California, San Diego, California
Rationale of Minimally Invasive Spine Surgery
Minimally Invasive Posterior Approaches to the Spine
Infections of the Spine

Lawrence T. Kurz, MD
Attending Staff Spine Surgeon, Department of Orthopaedics, William Beaumont Hospital, Royal Oak, Michigan
Techniques and Complications of Bone Graft Harvesting

Joseph M. Lane, MD
Professor of Orthopaedic Surgery, Assistant Dean, Medical Students, Weill Cornell Medical College; Chief, Metabolic Bone Disease Service, Hospital for Special Surgery; Senior Scientist, Hospital for Special Surgery, New York, New York
Metabolic Bone Disorders of the Spine

Nathan H. Lebwohl, MD
Chief of Spinal Deformity Surgery, Department of Orthopaedics, University of Miami Miller School of Medicine, Miami, Florida
Posterior Lumbar Interbody Fusion

Joon Yung Lee, MD
Assistant Professor, Department of Orthopaedic Surgery, Division of Spine Surgery, University of Pittsburgh Medical Center, Pittsburgh, Pennsylvania
Cervical, Thoracic and Lumbar Spinal Trauma of the Immature Spine

Michael J. Lee, MD
Assistant Professor, Sports Medicine and Orthopaedic Surgery, University of Washington Medical Center, Seattle, Washington
Osteoporosis: Surgical Strategies

Yu-Po Lee, MD
Assistant Clinical Professor, University of California San Diego Department of Orthopaedic Surgery, University of California San Diego Medical Center, San Diego, California
Lateral and Posterior Approaches to the Lumbosacral Spine

Ronald A. Lehman, Jr., MD
Chief, Pediatric and Adult Spine, Integrated Department of Orthopaedics and Rehabilitation, Walter Reed AMC and NNMC; Associate Professor, Division of Orthopaedics, USUHS, Washington, DC
Idiopathic Scoliosis

Lawrence G. Lenke, MD
Jerome J. Gilden Professor of Orthopaedic Surgery, Washington University School of Medicine; Co-Chief Adult/Pediatric Scoliosis and Reconstructive Spinal Surgery, Orthopaedic Surgery, Washington University School of Medicine; Chief, Spinal Service, Orthopaedic Surgery, Shriners Hospital for Children, St. Louis Unit; Professor of Neurological Surgery, Washington University School of Medicine, St. Louis, Missouri
Idiopathic Scoliosis

Allan D. Levi, MD, PhD
Professor, University of Miami, Miami, Florida
Spinal Intradural Infections

Kerry H. Levin, MD
Chairman, Department of Neurology, Cleveland Clinic; Director, Neuromuscular Center, Cleveland Clinic; Professor of Medicine (Neurology), Cleveland Clinic Lerner College of Medicine of Case Western Reserve University, Cleveland, Ohio
The Electrodiagnostic Examination

Kai-Uwe Lewandrowski, MD
Center for Advanced Spinal Surgery of Southern Arizona, Tucson, Arizona
Tumors of the Spine

Richard L. Lieber, PhD
Professor and Vice Chair, Department of Orthopaedic Surgery, University of California, San Diego, La Jolla, California; Senior Research Career Scientist, Veterans Affairs San Diego Healthcare System, San Diego, California
Architectural Design and Function of Human Back Muscles
Anatomy and Mechanics of the Abdominal Muscles

Myles Luszczyk, DO
Spine Fellow, Orthopedic Surgery, University of Washington School of Medicine, Seattle, Washington
Cervical Spondylotic Myelopathy: Surgical Management

Michael Mac Millan, MD
Associate Professor of Orthopaedics, Department of Orthopaedics and Rehabilitation, University of Florida, Gainesville, Florida
"Very" Future Directions in Minimally Invasive Spinal Surgery

Gigi R. Madore, MD
Emergency Medicine, New York University School of Medicine, New York, New York
Metabolic Bone Disorders of the Spine

Faisal Mahmood, MD
Spine Fellow, Twin Cities Spine Center, Minneapolis, Minnesota; St. Joseph's Medical Center, Seton Hall University Graduate School of Medical Education, Department of Orthopaedic Surgery, Paterson, New Jersey
Spondylolysis and Spondylolisthesis

Antonios Mammis, MD
Resident in Neurosurgery, Neurological Surgery, University of Medicine and Dentistry–New Jersey Medical School, Newark, New Jersey
Arachnoiditis and Epidural Fibrosis

William S. Marras, PhD
Honda Chair Professor, Biodynamics Laboratory/Integrated Systems Engineering Department, The Ohio State University, Columbus, Ohio
Biomechanics of the Spinal Motion Segment

Lauren E. Matteini, MD
Department of Orthopaedic Surgery, George Washington University, Washington, DC
Late Decompression of Patients with Spinal Cord Injury

Eric A. K. Mayer, MD
Staff Physician, Center for Spine Health, Cleveland Clinic Foundation, Cleveland, Ohio
Lumbar Musculature: Anatomy and Function
Physical Therapy—The Science
Functional Restoration

Tom G. Mayer, MD
Clinical Professor of Orthopedic Surgery, University of Texas Southwestern Medical Center; Medical Director, Productive Rehabilitation Institute of Dallas for Ergonomics (PRIDE), Dallas, Texas
Lumbar Musculature: Anatomy and Function
Functional Restoration

Daniel Mazanec, MD
Associate Professor of Medicine, Cleveland Clinic Lerner College of Medicine at Case Western Reserve University; Associate Director, Center for Spine Health, Cleveland Clinic, Cleveland, Ohio
Nonoperative Management of Lumbar Spinal Stenosis

Paul C. McAfee, MD, MBA
Part-Time Associate Professor of Orthopedic Surgery and Neurosurgery, Johns Hopkins Hospital; Chief of Spinal Surgery, St. Joseph Medical Center, Baltimore, Maryland
Failed Disc Replacement

Paul C. McCormick, MD, MPH
Herbert and Linda Gallen Professor of Neurological Surgery, Neurosurgery, Columbia University College of Physicians and Surgeons, New York, New York
Vascular Malformations of the Spinal Cord

Scott McGovern, MD
Orthopaedic Spine Surgeon, Peninsula Orthopaedic Associates, P.A.; Co-Director, Peninsula Spine Center, Peninsula Regional Medical Center, Salisbury, Maryland
Bone Substitutes: Basic Science and Clinical Applications

Robert McGuire, Jr., MD
Professor and Chairman, Department of Orthopedics and Rehabilitation, University of Mississippi Medical Center, Jackson, Mississippi
Adult Isthmic Spondylolisthesis

Robert F. McLain, MD
Professor of Surgery, Center for Spine Health, Cleveland Clinic Lerner College of Medicine; Associate Staff Surgeon, Department of Orthopaedic Surgery, Cleveland Clinic Foundation; Adjunct Professor, Department of Biomedical Engineering, Cleveland State University, Cleveland, Ohio
Tumors of the Spine

Nagy A. Mekhail, MD, PhD
Director of Evidence-Based Pain Medicine Education and Research, Cleveland Clinic; Professor of Anesthesiology at the Cleveland Clinic Lerner College of Medicine of Case Western Reserve, Cleveland, Ohio
Pharmacologic Strategies in Back Pain and Radiculopathy

Roberto Miki, MD
Assistant Professor, Orthopaedics, University of Miami, Miami, Florida
Metabolic Bone Disorders of the Spine

Andrew Milby, MD
Resident, Orthopaedic Surgery, University of Pennsylvania, Philadelphia, Pennsylvania
Spondylolysis and Spondylolisthesis

Scott J. Mubarak, MD
Clinical Professor, Department of Orthopedics, University of California, San Diego, Medical Center; Director of Orthopedic Clinical Program, Rady Children's Hospital, San Diego, California
Neuromuscular Scoliosis
Thoracoscopic Approach for Spinal Conditions

George F. Muschler, MD
Orthopaedic and Rheumatology Institute and Department of Biomedical Engineering, Cleveland Clinic, Cleveland, Ohio
Principles of Bone Fusion

Robert R. Myers, PhD
Professor of Anesthesiology and Pathology, University of California, San Diego, School of Medicine, La Jolla, California
Sciatica and Nerve Root Pain in Disc Herniation and Spinal Stenosis: A Basic Science Review and Clinical Perspective

K. Durga Nagraju, MD, DNB
Former Pediatric Orthopedic Fellow at A. I. duPont Hospital for Children, Wilmington, Delaware; Consultant Pediatric Orthopedic Surgeon, Anu Hospitals, Vijayawada, India
Spondylolysis and Spondylolisthesis

Dileep R. Nair, MD
Director of Intraoperative Monitoring, Neurology, Cleveland Clinic; Section Head of Adult Epilepsy, Neurology, Cleveland Clinic, Cleveland, Ohio
Intraoperative Neurophysiologic Monitoring of the Spine

Imad M. Najm, MD
Course Director, Neural and Musculoskeletal Sciences, Cleveland Clinic Lerner College of Medicine at Case Western Reserve University; Director, Epilepsy Center, Division of Neurosciences, Cleveland Clinic Neurological Institute, Cleveland, Ohio
Intraoperative Neurophysiologic Monitoring of the Spine

Peter O. Newton, MD
Children's Hospital; University of California, San Diego, California
Neuromuscular Scoliosis
Thoracoscopic Approach for Spinal Conditions

Lokesh B. Ningegowda, MD
Staff, Department of Pain Management, Anesthesiology Institute, Cleveland Clinic, Cleveland, Ohio
Pharmacologic Strategies in Back Pain and Radiculopathy

Patrick T. O'Leary, MD
Midwest Orthopaedic Center, Peoria, Illinois
Fixed Sagittal Imbalance
Instrumentation Complications

Kjell Olmarker, MD, PhD
Professor, Department of Medical Chemistry and Cell Biology, University of Gothenburg, Gothenburg, Sweden
Sciatica and Nerve Root Pain in Disc Herniation and Spinal Stenosis: A Basic Science Review and Clinical Perspective

Douglas G. Orndorff, MD
Orthopaedic Surgery, Spine Colorado, Durango, Colorado
Thoracolumbar Instrumentation: Anterior and Posterior

John E. O'Toole, MD
Assistant Professor, Neurosurgery, Rush University Medical Center, Chicago, Illinois
Vascular Malformations of the Spinal Cord

†Wesley W. Parke, PhD
Professor Emeritus and Former Chairman, Department of Anatomy, University of South Dakota School of Medicine, Vermillion, South Dakota
Development of the Spine
Applied Anatomy of the Spine

Amar A. Patel, BS
Jefferson Medical College, Philadelphia, Pennsylvania
Posterior Minimally Invasive Lumbar Fusion Techniques

Chetan K. Patel, MD
Director of The Spine Center at Altamonte, Orthopaedic Surgery; Global Faculty Member of NCSA, Orthopaedic Surgery, Florida Hospital Altamonte, Altamonte Springs, Florida
Spinal Stenosis: Pathophysiology, Clinical Diagnosis, and Differential Diagnosis

Neil V. Patel, MD
Resident, Diagnostic Radiology–Holman Pathway, Department of Radiology, University of Massachusetts Medical School, Worcester, Massachusetts
Vascular Anatomy of the Spine, Imaging, and Endovascular Treatment of Spinal Vascular Diseases

---

†Deceased.

Adam M. Pearson, MD
Orthopaedic Surgery, Dartmouth-Hitchcock Medical Center, Lebanon, New Hampshire
Outcomes Research for Spinal Disorders

Frank M. Phillips, MD
Professor of Orthopaedic Surgery; Spine Fellowship Co-Director, Rush University Medical Center, Chicago, Illinois
Osteoporosis: Surgical Strategies

Raj D. Rao, MD
Professor of Orthopaedic Surgery and Neurosurgery; Director of Spine Surgery, Department of Orthopaedic Surgery, Medical College of Wisconsin, Milwaukee, Wisconsin
Cervical Spondylosis: Pathophysiology, Natural History, and Clinical Syndromes of Neck Pain, Radiculopathy, and Myelopathy

Alexandre Rasouli, MD
The Spine Center, Cedars-Sinai Medical Center, Beverly Hills, Califormia
Basic Science of Spinal Cord Injury

Arvind Ravinutala, BS
Department of Orthopaedic Surgery, University of California, San Diego, California
Lateral and Posterior Approaches to the Lumbosacral Spine

Dale Reese, BSc, CPed
Project Manager, PTOT, Productive Rehabilitation Institute of Dallas for Ergonomics (PRIDE) Research Foundation, Dallas, Texas
Lumbar Musculature: Anatomy and Function

Mark A. Reiley, MD
Orthopedic Surgeon, Berkeley Orthopedics, Alta Bates Hospital, Berkeley, California
Total Facet Replacement

John M. Rhee, MD
Assistant Professor, Orthopaedic Surgery, Emory Spine Center, Emory University School of Medicine, Atlanta, Georgia
Nonoperative Management of Cervical Disc and Degenerative Disorders

K. Daniel Riew, MD
Mildred B. Simon Distinguished Professor of Orthopedic Surgery, Chief, Cervical Spine Surgery, Professor of Neurosurgery, Co-Director Spine Fellowship, Director of Ortho-Rehab Cervical Spine Institute, Orthopaedic Surgery, Washington University School of Medicine, St. Louis, Missouri
Postoperative Deformity of the Cervical Spine

Jeffrey Rihn, MD
Assistant Professor, Thomas Jefferson University Hospital, The Rothman Institute, Philadelphia, Pennsylvania
Surgical Management of Lumbar Spinal Stenosis

Richard B. Rodgers, MD
Assistant Professor, Department of Neurological Surgery; Director of Neurotrauma and Neurocritical Care, Indiana University School of Medicine, Indianapolis, Indiana
Acute Treatment of Patients with Spinal Cord Injury

Jeffrey S. Ross, MD
Staff Neuroradiologist, Barrow Neurological Institute, St. Joseph's Hospital Medical Center, Phoenix, Arizona
Spine Imaging

Bjorn Rydevik, MD, PhD
Professor, Department of Orthopaedics, University of Gothenburg, Sahlgrenska University, Gothenburg, Sweden
Sciatica and Nerve Root Pain in Disc Herniation and Spinal Stenosis: A Basic Science Review and Clinical Perspective

Jacqueline Sagen, PhD
Professor, Miami Project to Cure Paralysis, University of Miami Miller School of Medicine, Miami, Florida
Chronic Pain: The Basic Science

Rick C. Sasso, MD
Indiana Spine Group; Professor, Clinical Orthopaedic Surgery, Indiana University School of Medicine, Indianapolis, Indiana
Cervical Disc Replacement

Michael Saulino, MD, PhD
Assistant Professor, Thomas Jefferson University, Philadelphia, Pennsylvania; Physiatrist, MossRehab, Elkins Park, Pennsylvania
Surgical Procedures for the Control of Chronic Pain

Judith Scheman, PhD
Director of Psychology, Neurological Center for Pain, Neurological Institute, Cleveland Clinic; Clinical Instructor, Department of Medicine, Cleveland Clinic Lerner College of Medicine of the Case Western Reserve University; Adjunct Graduate Faculty, Psychology, Cleveland State University, Cleveland, Ohio
Psychologic Strategies for Chronic Pain

Thomas A. Schildhauer, MD, PhD
BG-Kliniken Bergmannsheil, Ruhr-Universitat Bochum, Germany
Sacral Fractures

Andrew Schoenfeld, MD
Clinical Fellow, Department of Orthopaedic Surgery, Harvard Medical School/Brigham and Women's Hospital, Boston, Massachusetts
Lumbar Disc Herniations

Daniel M. Schwartz, PhD
President and Chairman, Surgical Monitoring Associates, Springfield, Pennsylvania
Congenital Anomalies of the Spinal Cord

James D. Schwender, MD
Department of Orthopaedic Surgery, University of Minnesota, Twin Cities Spine Center, Minneapolis, Minnesota
Minimally Invasive Posterior Approaches to the Spine
Minimally Invasive Posterior Lumbar Instrumentation

Dilip K. Sengupta, MD, PhD, MCh (Orth), Dr Med
Assistant Professor, Department of Orthopedics, Dartmouth-Hitchcock Medical Center, Lebanon, New Hampshire
Posterior Dynamic Stabilization

Suken A. Shah, MD
Attending Pediatric Orthopaedic Surgeon, Chief, Spine and Scoliosis Division, Director, Clinical Fellowship Program, Nemours/A. I. duPont Hospital for Children, Wilmington, Delaware; Associate Professor of Orthopaedic Surgery, Thomas Jefferson University, Philadelphia, Pennsylvania
Spondylolysis and Spondylolisthesis

Ali Shaibani, MD
Director, Neurointerventional Surgery/Interventional Stroke Program, Northwest Community Hospital, Arlington Heights, Illinois; Director, Pediatric Neurointervention, Children's Memorial Hospital; Associate Professor, Neuroradiology and Interventional Neuroradiology, Departments of Radiology and Neurosurgery, Northwestern University Medical School, Feinberg School of Medicine, Chicago, Illinois
Vascular Anatomy of the Spine, Imaging, and Endovascular Treatment of Spinal Vascular Diseases

Francis H. Shen, MD
Professor of Orthopaedic Surgery; Division Head, Division of Spine Surgery; Director, Spine Fellowship; Co-Director, Spine Center, University of Virginia, Charlottesville, Virginia
Cervical Spine: Surgical Approaches

Andrew L. Sherman, MD
Associate Professor and Vice Chair, Department of Rehabilitation Medicine, University of Miami Leonard M. Miller School of Medicine, Miami, Florida
Spinal Cord Injury Rehabilitation

Pamela J. Sherman, MD
Orthopaedic Surgeon, Piedmont Orthopaedic Center, The Orthopaedic Center of Central Virginia, Lynchburg, Virginia
Metabolic Bone Disorders of the Spine

Adam L. Shimer, MD
Assistant Professor, Department of Orthopaedic Surgery, University of Virginia, Charlottesville, Virginia
Vertebral Artery Injuries Associated with Cervical Spine Trauma

Krzysztof B. Siemionow, MD
Assistant Professor of Orthopaedic Surgery, Department of Orthopaedic Surgery, University of Illinois, Chicago, Illinois
Principles of Bone Fusion

Fernando E. Silva, MD
North Texas Neurosurgical and Spine Center, Fort Worth, Texas
Idiopathic Scoliosis

J. David Sinclair, MD
Independent Consultant for Chronic Pain Management, Seattle, Washington
The Patient History and Physical Examination: Cervical, Thoracic, and Lumbar

Harvey E. Smith, MD
New England Orthopaedic and Spine Surgery, New England Baptist Hospital, Tufts University, Boston, Massachusetts
Transforaminal Lumbar Interbody Fusion

Jeremy Smith, MD
Chief Resident, Orthopaedic Surgery, University of California, Irvine, Orange, California
Postoperative Spinal Infections

Joseph D. Smucker, MD
Assistant Professor, The University of Iowa Department of Orthopaedics and Rehabilitation, Iowa City, Iowa
Cervical Disc Replacement

Volker K. H. Sonntag, MD
Vice Chairman, Emeritus, Barrow Neurological Institute, Phoenix, Arizona
Acute Treatment of Patients with Spinal Cord Injury

Gwendolyn Sowa, MD, PhD
Assistant Professor, Physical Medicine and Rehabilitation; Co-Director, Ferguson Laboratory for Orthopaedic Research, Orthopaedic Surgery, University of Pittsburgh, Pittsburgh, Pennsylvania
The Intervertebral Disc: Normal, Aging, and Pathologic Genetic Applications: An Overview

Jeffrey M. Spivak, MD
Director, New York University Hospital for Joint Diseases Spine Center, Department of Orthopaedic Surgery, New York University Hospital for Joint Diseases; Assistant Professor, Department of Orthopaedic Surgery, New York University School of Medicine, New York, New York
Lumbar Total Disc Replacement

Paul D. Sponseller, MD
Head, Division of Pediatric Orthopaedics, Johns Hopkins Medical Institutions; Professor, Department of Orthopaedic Surgery, Johns Hopkins, Baltimore, Maryland
Congenital Scoliosis

Kevin F. Spratt, PhD
Department of Orthopaedic Surgery, Dartmouth Medical School, Lebanon, New Hampshire
Outcomes Research for Spinal Disorders

Jeffrey L. Stambough, MD, MBA
Adjunct Professor, Department of Engineering, University of Cincinnati; Director and Chief for the Spine Service, Tristate Orthopaedic Treatment Center, Cincinnati, Ohio
Vascular Complications in Spinal Surgery

Christopher J. Standaert, MD
Clinical Associate Professor, Rehabilitation Medicine; Orthopaedic and Sports Medicine; Neurological Surgery, University of Washington, Seattle, Washington
The Patient History and Physical Examination: Cervical, Thoracic, and Lumbar

Tom Stanley, MD, MPH
Midwest Bone and Joint, Chicago, Illinois
Lumbar Total Disc Replacement

David Strothman, MD
Orthopaedic Surgeon, Institute for Low Back and Neck Care, Bloomington, Minnesota
Minimally Invasive Posterior Lumbar Instrumentation

Brian W. Su, MD
Orthopaedic Spine Surgeon, Mt. Tam Orthopedics, The Spine Center, Larkspur, California
Surgical Management of Lumbar Spinal Stenosis

Leslie N. Sutton, MD
Chief, Neurosurgery, Children's Hospital of Philadelphia; Professor, Neurosurgery and Pediatrics, University of Pennsylvania School of Medicine, Philadelphia, Pennsylvania
Congenital Anomalies of the Spinal Cord

Chadi Tannoury, MD
Orthopaedic Academic and Administrative Chief Resident, Thomas Jefferson University Hospital and the Rothman Institute, Philadelphia, Pennsylvania
Posterior Minimally Invasive Lumbar Fusion Techniques

Jinny Tavee, MD
Assistant Professor of Medicine, Neuromuscular Center, Cleveland Clinic Foundation, Cleveland, Ohio
The Electrodiagnostic Examination

Bobby K-B. Tay, MD
Associate Clinical Professor, Orthopaedic Surgery, University of California San Francisco, San Francisco, California
Injuries of the Upper Cervical Spine

Beverlie L. Ting, MD
Department of Orthopaedic Surgery, Johns Hopkins Hospital, Baltimore, Maryland
Congenital Scoliosis

Vernon T. Tolo, MD
John C. Wilson, Jr., Professor of Orthopaedics, Keck School of Medicine at University of Southern California; Chief Emeritus, Children's Orthopaedic Center, Children's Hospital Los Angeles, Los Angeles, California
Spinal Disorders Associated with Skeletal Dysplasias and Metabolic Diseases

Clifford B. Tribus, MD
Associate Professor, University of Wisconsin-Madison, Madison, Wisconsin
Interspinous Process Decompressive Devices

Eeric Truumees, MD
Director of Spinal Research, Seton Spine and Scoliosis Center; Attending Spine Surgeon, Brackenridge University Hospital, Austin, Texas
Spinal Stenosis: Pathophysiology, Clinical Diagnosis, and Differential Diagnosis
Cervical Instrumentation: Anterior and Posterior

Aasis Unnanuntana, MD
Fellow, Orthopaedic Surgery, Hospital for Special Surgery, New York, New York; Clinical Instructor, Orthopaedic Surgery, Siriraj Hospital, Mahidol University, Bangkok, Thailand
Metabolic Bone Disorders of the Spine

Alexander R. Vaccaro, MD, PhD
Professor of Orthopaedic Surgery and Neurosurgery, Thomas Jefferson University/Rothman Institute; Co-Director, Thomas Jefferson University/Rothman Institute; Co-Director, Regional Spinal Cord Injury Center of the Delaware Valley, Philadelphia, Pennsylvania
Injuries of the Lower Cervical Spine
Vertebral Artery Injuries Associated with Cervical Spine Trauma

Steve Vanni, DO
Department of Neurological Surgery, University of Miami School of Medicine, Miami, Florida
Syringomyelia

Eric S. Varley, DO
Postdoctoral Research Fellow, Orthopaedic Surgery, University of California, San Diego, San Diego, California
Neuromuscular Scoliosis
Thoracoscopic Approach for Spinal Conditions

Anita Vasavada, PhD
Associate Professor, The Gene and Linda Voiland School of Chemical Engineering and Bioengineering, Washington State University, Pullman, Washington
Architectural Design and Function of Human Back Muscles

Michael J. Vives, MD
Associate Professor of Orthopaedics, University of Medicine and Dentistry–New Jersey Medical School, Newark, New Jersey
Spinal Orthoses for Traumatic and Degenerative Disease
Revision Spine Surgery

Ajay K. Wakhloo, MD, PhD
Professor and Division Chief, Department of Radiology; Co-Director, Radiology, New England Center for Stroke Research, University of Massachusetts, Worcester, Massachusetts
Vascular Anatomy of the Spine, Imaging, and Endovascular Treatment of Spinal Vascular Diseases

Jeffrey C. Wang, MD
Professor, Orthopaedic Surgery and Neurosurgery, University of California, Los Angeles, Spine Center; University of California, Los Angeles, School of Medicine, Los Angeles, California
Bone Substitutes: Basic Science and Clinical Applications

Samuel R. Ward, PT, PhD
Associate Professor, Radiology, Orthopaedic Surgery, and Bioengineering, University of California San Diego, La Jolla, California
Architectural Design and Function of Human Back Muscles
Anatomy and Mechanics of the Abdominal Muscles

James N. Weinstein, DO
President, Dartmouth-Hitchcock Clinic; Director, The Dartmouth Institute for Health Policy and Clinical Practice; Orthopaedic Surgery, Spine Center, Dartmouth-Hitchcock Medical Center, Lebanon, New Hampshire
Outcomes Research for Spinal Disorders

William C. Welch, MD
Department of Neurosurgery, University of Pennsylvania;
Chief of Neurosurgery, Pennsylvania Hospital, Philadelphia,
Pennsylvania
> *Congenital Anomalies of the Spinal Cord*

Dennis R. Wenger, MD
Director of Pediatric Orthopedic Training Program,
Orthopedic Surgery, Rady Children's Hospital, San
Diego; Clinical Professor, Department of Orthopedic
Surgery, University of California, San Diego, San Diego,
California
> *Neuromuscular Scoliosis*
> *Thoracoscopic Approach for Spinal Conditions*

David S. Wernsing, MD
Clinical Assistant Professor of Surgery, University of
Pennsylvania, Philadelphia, Pennsylvania
> *Anterior Exposure to the Lumbosacral Spine: Anatomy and
> Techniques*

Edward Westrick, MD
Resident Physician, Department of Orthopaedic Surgery,
University of Pittsburgh, Pittsburgh, Pennsylvania
> *The Intervertebral Disc: Normal, Aging, and Pathologic
> Genetic Applications: An Overview*

F. Todd Wetzel, AB, MD
Professor and Vice Chair, Department of Orthopaedic Surgery,
Temple University School of Medicine, Philadelphia,
Pennsylvania
> *Surgical Procedures for the Control of Chronic Pain*

Seth K. Williams, MD
Assistant Professor, Divisions of Spine and Trauma,
Department of Orthopaedics, University of Miami Miller
School of Medicine, Miami, Florida
> *Thoracic and Lumbar Spinal Injuries*

Lee Wolfer, MD
Spinal Diagnostics and Treatment Center, Daly City,
California
> *Targeting Pain Generators*

Praveen K. Yalamanchili, MD
Department of Orthopaedics, University of Medicine and
Dentistry of New Jersey–New Jersey Medical School, Newark,
New Jersey
> *Spinal Orthoses for Traumatic and Degenerative Disease*

Burt Yaszay, MD
Department of Pediatric Orthopaedics, Rady Children's
Hospital, San Diego; Assistant Clinical Professor, Department
of Orthopaedics, University of California, San Diego, San
Diego, California
> *Neuromuscular Scoliosis*
> *Thoracoscopic Approach for Spinal Conditions*

Anthony T. Yeung, MD
Desert Institute for Spine Care, Phoenix, Arizona
> *Lumbar Nucleus Replacement*
> *Posterolateral Endoscopic Lumbar Discectomy*

Christopher A. Yeung, MD
Desert Institute for Spine Care, Phoenix, Arizona
> *Posterolateral Endoscopic Lumbar Discectomy*

Kazuo Yonenobu, MD, DMsc
Director of Hospital, National Hospital Organization, Osaka-
Minami Medical Center, Kawachinagano, Osaka, Japan
> *Ossification of the Posterior Longitudinal Ligament*

Warren D. Yu, MD
Associate Professor; Chief, Spine Section, Orthopaedic Surgery
and Neurosurgery, George Washington University,
Washington, DC
> *Late Decompression of Patients with Spinal Cord Injury*

Hansen A. Yuan, MD
Professor Emeritus, State University of New York Upstate
Medical University, Syracuse, New York
> *Lumbar Nucleus Replacement*

Phillip S. Yuan, MD
Vice Chairman, Department of Orthopedic Surgery, Long
Beach Memorial Medical Center, Memorial Orthopaedic
Surgical Group, Long Beach, California
> *Lumbar Nucleus Replacement*

Thomas A. Zdeblick, MD
Professor and Chairman, Department of Orthopedics and
Rehabilitation; Director, Spine Fellowship; Director, Spine
Center, University of Wisconsin, Madison, Wisconsin
> *Thoracolumbar Instrumentation: Anterior and Posterior*

This edition of *The Spine*, the Sixth, has been assembled under the direction of the same Editorial Board that was responsible for the Fifth edition (2000). The guiding principles taught to us by our mentors, Richard H. Rothman, MD, PhD, and Frederick A. Simeone, MD, permeate the chapters of this Sixth edition. They include (1) understanding of the basic science behind the clinical aspects of spinal disorders, (2) knowledge of natural history and the clinical course, and (3) treatment based on sound science and evidence-based literature.

This new edition of *The Spine* continues the tradition of providing a comprehensive book of spinal disease affecting children and adults. It is dedicated to students of spinal disease regardless of specialty and rank. It is also dedicated to the patients whose care may be influenced by the words contained within its 108 chapters. Because history plays such an important role in furthering scientific knowledge, a review of the previous prefaces will help put this new edition in proper perspective.

The forerunner to *The Spine* was *The Intervertebral Disc* by Drs. Rothman and DePalma. In their preface written in 1970, the authors wrote: "The role of the intervertebral disc in the production of neck and back pain, with or without radiation into one of the extremities, has been the subject of much investigation for many decades. … The disc has been attacked from every conceivable angle, the most important of which is its biochemical nature and its response to physiologic aging and trauma. In spite of the exhaustive studies recorded in the literature, it is alarming to find how little of this knowledge has been acquired by those concerned with neck and back disorders. … This monograph deals with the modern concepts of the biochemical structure of the disc, its functional role, and how different phases of alterations in the disc are related to the presenting clinical syndrome. … We are sure that much that is recorded in this book is still very controversial. Yet, we believe that our approach to this complex problem will be helpful and rewarding to others." This comprehensive monograph on the disc totaled 373 pages. A significant portion of the information it contained was based on the authors' own work and rigorous analysis of their results. The sections on the chemistry and physiology of the disc, though the crux of the book, were limited and reflected the state of knowledge at the time. However, it did crystallize concepts of the disc for spine physicians of the day and served as the forerunner of the books that were to follow.

In the preface to the First edition, Rothman and Simeone stated: "*The Spine* had as its genesis a strong feeling on the part of its editors that a need existed for a comprehensive textbook to include all aspects of diagnosis and treatment of spinal disease. Our goals were to lower the traditional disciplinary barriers and biases and to present a uniform guideline to problem solving in this area. … This book has been designed to include all facets of disease related to the spine, whether orthopedic, neurosurgical, or medical in nature. … An attempt has been made to achieve completeness without exhaustive and burdensome details. The contributing authors have not merely recorded the possibilities in diagnosis and treatment of spinal disorders but have relied on their personal experience to offer concrete recommendations." The success of that effort is legend. The First edition of *The Spine* followed the dictates of the editors, covered the full range of knowledge of spinal disorders known at the time, and became an essential component of the libraries of all medical personnel who dealt with spinal disorders. The authors, one a neurosurgeon (F.A.S.) and one an orthopaedic surgeon (R.H.R.), combined their efforts to teach the world not only diseases of the spine, but also the importance of working together in an attempt to understand and treat the disease processes. Their spinal fellowship, as well as personal fellowship, was (is) based on this team, multidisciplinary, yet regimented approach to the spine, and has been the model that we have sought to achieve in our own clinical and teaching environments. In fact, it may be required in the future that successful spine fellowships be a coordinated effort between multispecialties, as envisioned and taught by Drs. Rothman and Simeone, so that the spine is not broken up into multiple segments (bone, nerves, discs, etc.).

The preface to the Second edition of *The Spine* stated: "Advancements in medicine generally follow broader scientific and even social trends. The treatment of spine diseases is no exception. Consequently, increments of new information have been added to the general body of knowledge in spotty, but predictable areas. These new developments constitute the raison d'etre for this Second edition. The dramatic progress in radiologic imaging stands out as the most useful innovation. … Logic indicates that the next generation of (CT) scanners will delineate all thoracic and cervical disc lesions. Spinal trauma is managed better since the advent of computed tomography. Infections, tumor infiltration, and congenital malformations are being better understood as experience grows. ... Each contributor has demonstrated his commitment to summarizing the most recent information in a manner useful to students and clinicians alike, and for this the editors are proud and appreciative."

The preface to the Third edition included the following: "The current edition has new editorial leadership. Those of us involved in the direction of this project have tried to follow the model previously established by Drs. Rothman and Simeone in finding the best authors for each chapter. We, hopefully, have emphasized, as in past editions, the importance of understanding the basic science in a concise manner, which leads to the ability to make appropriate decisions and manage patients with simple or complex spinal problems. We have attempted to update each section, have eliminated those areas that are not current, and have separated some components of the basic science from the clinical to aid readers in locating pertinent information in the ever-increasing body of knowledge related to the spine."

The current editors have been involved with Dick Rothman and Fred Simeone in various ways. Some have been fellows, some residents, and some partners. Each of us has developed special feelings and interactions with them. Each of us has carried the messages they teach and actively practice to our own clinical and research environments. They have taught us the importance of combining scientific queries with active clinical practices and have fostered in us the desire to succeed clinically and academically in an open and honest fashion.

The Fourth edition of Rothman and Simeone *The Spine* was the largest in terms of physical size and number of pages. The Editorial Board for the Fourth edition carried over from the Third edition.

The Fourth edition provided expanded information on magnetic resonance imaging and laparoscopic and endoscopic surgery. It contained a comprehensive discussion of disc degeneration and its treatment. This edition also introduced a chapter on outcomes research and its importance to our assessment of functional outcome in addition to the more traditional measurements of success, including radiographic parameters. For the first time, the Fourth edition contained a chapter on ossification of the posterior longitudinal ligament and its treatment.

The Fifth edition of *The Spine* added much new information, along with significant updates in content and references. This edition introduced key points, which were four or five important concepts and facts contained at the end of many of the clinical chapters. There was also added a key reference section for each chapter, which highlighted the most significant references. Chapters new to the Fifth edition included surgical management of osteopenic fractures, disc and nuclear replacement, management of flatback deformity, use of transforaminal lumbar interbody fusion, and use of bone graft extenders and bone morphogenetic protein (BMP) in the lumbar spine. Other new chapters included thoracoscopic surgery and its clinical applications and intraoperative monitoring, including motor-evoked potentials. A new chapter on genetic application and its exciting role for future treatments

of degenerative disease was included in the basic science section. Minimally invasive posterior approaches to the lumbar spine were also introduced in that edition.

Significant updating of many of the chapters introduced in the Fourth edition was noted throughout the Fifth edition. These included chapters on spinal instrumentation, adult scoliosis, surgery for rheumatoid arthritis and spondylitis, and cervical myelopathy and its management, including detailed discussions of anterior and posterior approaches, along with the detailed surgical techniques for these approaches.

This new edition, the Sixth, continues under the same Editorial Board as the previous one. The editors were charged with ensuring that the chapters within their sections contained the latest evidence-based information whenever available. This edition also continues the use of key points and key references at the end of each chapter. These have been very useful to highlight the significant information contained within those respective chapters.

New chapters include those devoted to arthroplasty for cervical and lumbar degenerative disorders. In addition, revision strategies for failed disc replacements highlight the potential difficulties in dealing with this complex surgical problem.

The Fifth edition introduced the concepts of minimally invasive surgery. The Sixth edition significantly expands the discussion with six chapters devoted to the rationale for minimally invasive surgery and the surgical techniques, results, and complications. A chapter devoted to soft stabilization for lumbar fixation has also been added.

Also, new to this edition are a chapter devoted to annulus repair, which summarizes the research done in this evolving field, and a chapter devoted to the basic science of spinal cord injury which highlights the advances made in the understanding of this devastating condition. As has been done in previous editions, chapter updates have been incorporated throughout the book whenever appropriate, including updated references. Finally, a video library of surgical techniques and procedures in the cervical and lumbar spine is included in a DVD format for all readers of this new edition.

The editors are confident that readers of this Sixth edition will continue to find the resources and information needed to help care for children and adults with spinal afflictions. The editors are confident that this new edition will continue to serve as a valuable educational resource for all students of *The Spine* from neophytes to experienced practitioners regardless of their chosen specialty.

The Editorial Board remains committed to the broad-based appeal of this book, as demonstrated in the previous editions. The authors include basic scientists, neuroradiologists, neurologists, physiatrists, and rheumatologists, along with orthopaedic surgeons and neurosurgeons. In addition, this book remains unique in providing comprehensive sections on pediatric disorders, as well as adult disease. Its comprehensive content ranges from degenerative disease to deformity to trauma and tumor. Afflictions of the spinal cord along with detailed discussions of complications and their management contribute to this book's broad appeal.

The Editorial Board feels confident that the readers of this Sixth edition will find the information necessary to diagnose and care for pediatric and adult patients afflicted with spinal disease of all types regardless of the complexity.

Finally, the Editorial Board is proud to call *The Spine,* Sixth edition, the continued primary reference resource for all physicians and nonphysicians with an interest in disorders of the spine.

The Editorial Board
HARRY N. HERKOWITZ, MD
STEVEN R. GARFIN, MD
FRANK J. EISMONT, MD
GORDON R. BELL, MD
RICHARD A. BALDERSTON, MD

Acknowledgments

There are many people behind the scenes who helped bring the Sixth edition of *Rothman-Simeone The Spine* to fruition. Each editor relied on individuals in his office to make sure deadlines were met and manuscripts were sent. The Editorial Board thankfully acknowledges Liz Stimson, NP, MS, Nurse Practitioner for Steven R. Garfin, MD, and the UCSD Spine Service; Wendy Hess, Administrative Assistant to Steven R. Garfin, MD; Ivanka Mora and Diana Reconco, Assistants to Frank J. Eismont, MD; and Chris Musich, former Administrator in the Department of Orthopaedic Surgery at Beaumont Hospital, who spent numerous hours making sure deadlines were met.

We also wish to thank Elsevier's Daniel Pepper, Acquisitions Editor; Heather Krehling, Editorial Systems Officer; Claire Kramer, Senior Project Manager; David Dipazo, Producer; Lou Forgione, Designer; and Karen Giacomucci, Art Manager, for their efforts to see this edition published. Thank you to Beth LoGiudice and Rebecca Corradetti, Developmental Editors at Spring Hollow Press. Finally, we want to acknowledge all of the individuals behind the scenes at Elsevier who contributed to the publication of this book.

The Editorial Board

Contents

Volume I

Volume II

Section IX
SPINAL STENOSIS

Section X
SPINAL FUSION AND INSTRUMENTATION

Section XI
ADULT DEFORMITY

Section XII
SPINE TRAUMA

Section XIII
AFFLICTIONS OF THE VERTEBRAE

Rothman-Simeone

THE SPINE

CHAPTER 1

Development of the Spine

Christopher M. Bono, MD
Wesley W. Parke, PhD
Steven R. Garfin, MD

The embryologic development of the human spine is an enormously complex process that is only partially understood. Differentiation of the pluripotent tissues of the embryo leads to early formation of a repetitive segmented vertebral structure. Because the embryo is exquisitely susceptible to malformation and developmental error, each step of formation is critical.[1-4] Familiarity with these various steps can be helpful in understanding not only congenital syndromes, but also the possible developmental role concerning predisposition to some degenerative spinal processes, typically considered "wear and tear" conditions.[5,6] The continuously expanding understanding of the genetic basis of life, with the genetics of spinal development no exception, has aided the understanding of these syndromes.[7-13]

Fundamental to understanding spinal embryology is the concept of metamerism. In principle, *metamerism* is the development of a highly specialized organism, with multifunctional organ systems, from many anatomically similar segments arranged in a linear fashion. This is particularly easy to conceptualize in the spine because the fully developed spine comprises numerous units with similar shape, arrangement, and function. Metamerism also pertains to the development of the appendages from the metameres, however, which do not have such repetitive arrangement of consecutive units.

In embryonic development, the metameric segments are called *somites*. Primitively, all somites have the same developmental potential. Genetic signaling, specific to the species, determines the degree of regional specialization, such as limbs in mammals versus fins in fish or the lack thereof in snakes. Using these comparative examples, one can also understand the concepts of isomerism and anisomerism. *Isomerism* is characteristic of more primitive animals, in which the number of somites is greater but more uniform and not so highly specialized. This is akin to the snake, which has a great number of vertebral units sustaining its long body, but no limbs. In contrast, *anisomerism* is present in more developed species, such as mammals, in which many of the somites have been deleted (resulting in a lesser number of vertebrae), whereas the remaining somites are more highly specialized so that complex, specialized appendages can be developed.

Although the mature vertebral column is composed of numerous similar units, the tissues within each of those units are highly specialized. The vertebrae, discs, nerves, and blood vessels have embryologic precursors that form according to rapidly dynamic interstructural relationships. This chapter provides the essentials of human spinal development as they relate to the fully developed structure to understand its form, function, and various pathologic possibilities better.

Early Embryologic Spine Precursors: Day 17 to Week 4

The development of the human spine begins on the 17th day of gestation. This is within the triploblastic stage of the embryo, during which it is shaped as a disc (Figs. 1–1 and 1–2). On one side of the disc is the amnion cavity, and on the other is the yolk sac. On the dorsal layer (which is in contact with the amnion) of the disc, there are epiblastic cells that converge and invaginate into the disc to form the primitive pit or node. When embedded within the tissue, it forms a tubelike structure that extends craniad, "burrowing" deep to the embryonic disc along its ventral surface. The tube cavity is in continuity with the amniotic fluid. This extension is known as the *notochordal tube*.

At this point, the ventral wall of the notochordal tube is in contact with the yolk sac, which causes disintegration of these cells. A flat remnant of dorsal wall cells from the notochordal tube form the notochordal plate on the 19th day. This plate matures and thickens to form a solid round structure known as the *notochord*. The yolk sac reforms, which obliterates the temporary communication between the amnion and the yolk sac (*note*: persistence of this yolk sac/amnion communication is lethal). The presence of the notochord induces a thickening in the overlying ectodermal cells, which are fated to become neuroectodermal cells. The thickening forms the neural plate. At this time, the neural plate is in continuity with the amniotic cavity. On the 18th day, the sides of the plate begin to curl up to form a tube. When the edges have fused together, it is known as the *neural tube*. The amniotic fluid trapped inside is the precursor to spinal fluid.

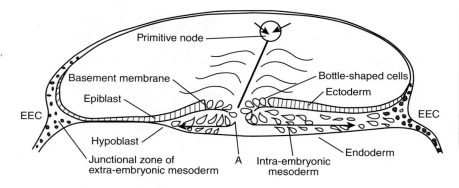

FIGURE 1-1 During triploblastic stage (17th day of gestation), the embryo is shaped as a disc. EEC, extraembryonic coelom. (From Brooks M, Zietman AL: Clinical Embryology: A Color Atlas and Text. Boca Raton, FL, CRC Press, 1998, p 57.)

The notochord lies ventral to the neural tube in the midline. Mesodermal tissues on either side of these structures condense to form longitudinal columns. By the 19th day, there are three distinct columns on either side of the midline: (1) medial paraxial columns, which give rise to the somites; (2) intermediate mesodermal columns, which form the urogenital organs; and (3) lateral mesodermal plates, which form the gut cavities. In considering the development of the spine, attention is focused on the medial paraxial columns. The juxtaposition to the intermediate columns may help explain, however, why abnormalities of the urogenital tract are frequently associated with vertebral anomalies.[1]

The somites are arranged in consecutive fashion along the dorsal aspect of the embryo. They are first formed in the rostral (or cranial) aspect of the embryo, continuing caudad to form 42 to 44 individual segments over a period of days

where the medial paraxial columns previously existed. Because they are close to the dorsal surface, they are visibly apparent as a series of beaded elevations (Fig. 1-3).

Within the somite different regions have specialized fates (Figs. 1-4 and 1-5). The dorsolateral cells become the dermomyotomes. These eventually give rise to the skin (lateral) and muscle (medial) overlying the spine. The ventromedial cells within the somite become the sclerotomes. These are the precursors of the skeletal components (vertebrae) of the spine. The neural tube is fated to become the spinal cord.

From Somites to Spinal Column

The sclerotomes, myotomes, notochord, and neural tube eventually develop into the discoligamentous vertebral complex,

FIGURE 1-2 A, On one side of the disc is the amniotic cavity, and on the other is the yolk sac. The notochordal tube "burrows" deep into the embryonic disc. **B,** When the ventral wall of the notochordal tube contacts the yolk sac, it disintegrates. **C,** Remaining dorsal wall cells thicken to form the notochordal plate; this matures and thickens to become the notochord. (From Brooks M, Zietman AL: Clinical Embryology: A Color Atlas and Text. Boca Raton, FL, CRC Press, 1998, p 57.)

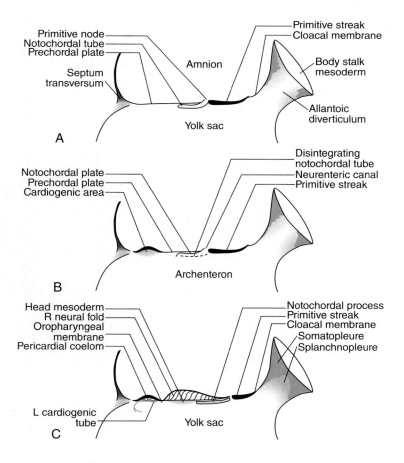

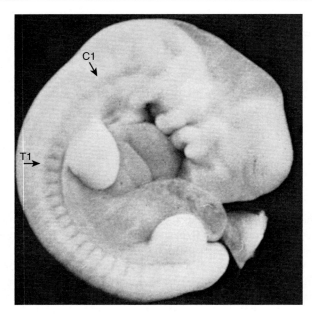

FIGURE 1–3 Somites of the human embryo are externally represented as a series of dorsolateral swellings.

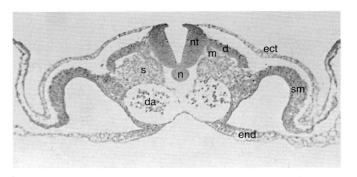

FIGURE 1–4 Cross section of thoracic somite in a chick embryo. The notochord (n) underlies the neural tube (nt). The somite is divided into dermatome (d), myotome (m), and sclerotome (s). Lateral to this, the somatic mesoderm (sm), endoderm (end), and ectoderm (ect) are shown. Ventral to the sclerotomes lie the paired dorsal aortae (da).

paraspinal musculature, nucleus pulposus, and neural elements. This development is achieved through numerous sequential steps and stages.

Precartilaginous (Mesenchymal) Stage: Weeks 4 and 5

The mesenchymal cells within the sclerotome divide into three main regions. One immediately surrounds the notochord. This region is the precursor for the vertebral bodies and the anulus fibrosus portion of the intervertebral discs. A second region surrounds the neural tube; this is destined to develop into the posterior arch of the vertebra. The third

region of cells is within the body wall and is related to extraspinal tissue.

In metameric fashion, the sclerotomes are organized into a consecutively stacked arrangement. The next step in spinal development has been explained by the "resegmentation" theory.[14-18] *Resegmentation* describes the division of each sclerotome into a cranial and caudal half. The cranial half is loosely arranged, whereas the caudal half is composed of densely packed cells. A small portion of the densely packed cells migrate superiorly to form the annular portion of the intervertebral disc, surrounding the notochord. Most of the densely packed cells fuse with the loosely packed cells of the adjacent caudal sclerotome. This fusion creates the centrum, the precursor of the vertebral body. The centrum develops from portions of two neighboring sclerotomes. This has significance on the anatomy of the fully developed spinal column. Initially, the segmental nerve precursors are located at the midportion of each sclerotome, whereas the segmental artery lies at the junction between two adjacent levels. After

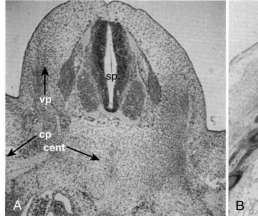
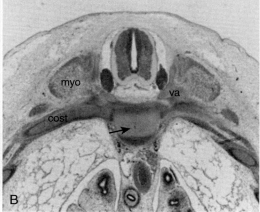

FIGURE 1–5 A, Cross section of pig embryo. *Arrows* indicate the direction of somite cell migration to form the vertebral process (vp), costal process (cp), and centrum (cent). The neural tube shows the anterior horn masses and the dorsal root ganglia. **B,** Cartilaginous vertebral arch (va) and costal process (cost) are evident, as is the myotomic precursor to the spinal muscles (myo). *Arrow* indicates the intracentral vestige of the notochord, called the mucoid streak.

resegmentation, the nerve lies at the level of the disc and the artery lies at the mid-centrum, where one would expect to find them in the fully developed specimen.

Experimental data support the resegmentation theory.[8,19-22] The crux of these experiments includes implanting a quail somite (from a quail embryo) within a chick embryo's native somites. The quail somite is juxtaposed to a chick somite, and they develop together as the embryo grows. The quail tissue can be differentiated from the chick tissue using special staining techniques. Eventually, the somites give rise to sclerotomes that develop into centra. With the use of this model, it has been shown that the centrum does arise from the caudal and cranial halves of adjacent sclerotomes. The posterior arches (i.e., laminae) appear to follow this same pattern of growth.

This process seems to be highly influenced by the *Pax1* and *Pax9* genes.[22] It is unclear whether the spinous process develops from one sclerotome or two adjacent levels.[8,22] Other investigators have produced evidence of resegmentation using genetic labeling techniques.[20] These studies involved injection of retroviral particles containing the lacZ transducing vector BAG into a single somite of a chick embryo. In other words, a single somite was genetically altered so that its cells would produce the lacZ gene product—the protein β-galactosidase. When the investigators evaluated the developed embryo, they detected β-galactosidase in the caudal and cranial halves of two adjacent vertebrae, suggesting that cells from the labeled somite were incorporated into two neighboring vertebrae.

Cartilaginous Stage: Weeks 6 and 7

Before the 6th week, the embryonic spinal precursor is composed of mesenchymal cells. Starting in the 6th week, cartilage-producing centers, or chondrification centers, form within each developing vertebra. Although type II collagen production within the extracellular matrix has been detected in the 5th week, it is most active during the cartilaginous stage; it tapers off during the ossification stage, but its production persists within the notochordal remnants of the nucleus pulposus.[12] Two chondrification centers form in each half of the centrum, which eventually fuse into a solid block of cartilage. A hemivertebra is formed because of a failure of chondrification in one half of the vertebral body. The segmental arteries from either side of the centrum fuse at its middle aspect. Chondrification centers also form within each half of the vertebral arch and eventually fuse with each other in the midline and to the posterior aspect of the centrum.

Next, primitive cartilaginous transverse processes and spinous processes develop from the vertebral arch. More recent evidence has shown that the cartilaginous spinous process is formed from Msx1 and Msx2 (two embryologic proteins), producing mesenchymal cells, which require BMP4 to differentiate.[23] These relationships highlight the important interactions of primordial proteins in governing further development of the spine.

The developing centrum and vertebra have the notochord as a central axis. Intervening segments of loosely packed cells are present between the regions of densely packed cells. The outer disc is formed by these loosely packed cells of the

sclerotome, which are fated to become the anulus fibrosus. The notochord disintegrates within the centrum during resegmentation and chondrification except in the region of the intervertebral disc, where some of its cells remain. The nucleus fibrosus is the replacement of the embryologic notochord.

Ossification Stage: Week 8 and Beyond

Primary ossification centers develop in utero. In the spine, ossification centers form within the cartilaginous template. There are three primary ossification centers in the typical embryonic vertebra: one in the center of the centrum and one in each of the vertebra arch halves. At about the 9th week, the preparation for ossification of the centrum is heralded by anterior and posterior excavations of the cartilaginous centrum produced by the invasion of pericostal vessels.[24] These vessels produce ventral and dorsal vascular lacunae, which support the initial ossification (Fig. 1–6). Ossification of the centra starts first at the lower thoracic spine working craniad and caudad from that point.[25]

Secondary ossification centers develop after birth. In the spine, these appear after puberty. There are five centers: one in the tip of the spinous process, one in each transverse process tip, and one ring epiphysis in the superior and inferior endplates of the vertebral bodies. This development occurs at about 15 or 16 years of age, but eventually these ossification centers fuse in the middle of the 3rd decade (Fig. 1–7).[26] The transverse processes of the lower cervical vertebrae,

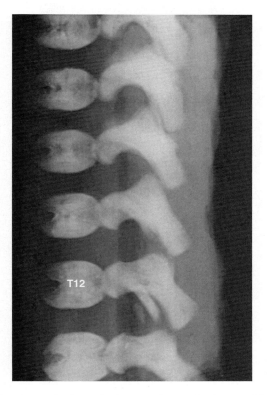

FIGURE 1–6 Lateral radiograph of a 34-week spine. Ossification of the centra starts first at the lower thoracic spine working craniad and caudad from that point.

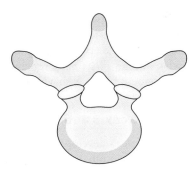

FIGURE 1–7 Secondary centers of ossification of a thoracic vertebra. The centers at the tips of the spinous and transverse processes appear at 16 years and fuse at approximately 25 years. The ring apophysis of the centrum ossifies at around 14 years and fuses at about 25 years.

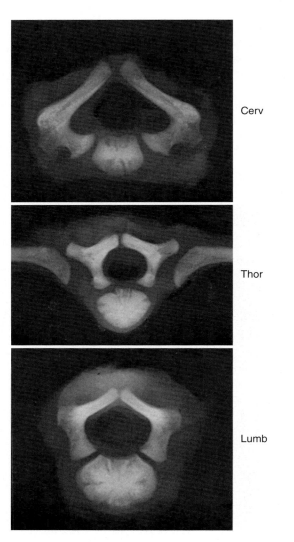

Cerv

Thor

Lumb

FIGURE 1–8 Fusion of the fetal vertebral arches to the centra occurs well anterior to the pedicles, at the site of the neurocentral joints. The contributions of the vertebral arches to the dorsolateral parts of the bodies are apparent. The definitive vertebral body includes more than just the bone derived from the ossification center of the centrum, so that the terms *body* and *centrum* are not accurately interchangeable.

particularly C7, may show an additional costal center of ossification that produces the troublesome cervical rib; this reinforces the concept that all vertebrae primitively had the potential of forming ribs.

A pair of embryologic joints, known as *neurocentral joints*, is not present in the fully developed spine. These are located at the junction of the vertebral arches and the centrum but are anterior to the site of the future pedicle. Although not true "joints," they allow expansion of the vertebral arch and spinal canal along with growth of the vertebral body. This expansion is most rapid between 18 and 36 weeks of gestation.[2] At birth, the spinal canal diameter at L1 through L4 is approximately 70% of adult size, whereas at L5 it is only 50%.[2] This indicates differential growth within regions of the vertebral column during fetal development. Full adult dimensions are reached by 1 year of life at L3 and L4 levels. The neurocentral joints persist until 3 to 6 years of age. The fusion of the fetal vertebral arches to the centra occurs well anterior to the pedicles, at the site of the neurocentral joints. The definitive vertebral body includes more than just the bone derived from the ossification center of the centrum, so the terms *body* and *centrum* are not accurately interchangeable (Figs. 1–8 and 1–9).

It is commonly thought that isthmic spondylolysis occurs because of a stress-type fracture within the pars interarticularis of the lower lumbar vertebrae, most commonly L5. Specific anatomic features of the adult lumbar spine, such as variation of the dimensions of the "lateral buttress" within the lumbar spine, have been described. Prenatal factors have been sought, but with limited success. Sagi and colleagues[5] analyzed histomorphologically the lumbar spines of fetal spines aged 8 to 20 weeks to determine the sequence and location of ossification of the pars interarticularis of the various levels. They reported several findings: First, the pars begins to ossify in the 12th to 13th week of gestation. In the upper lumbar levels, ossification begins at the posterior portion of the pedicle and continues caudad, creating uniform ossification and trabeculation of the pars interarticularis. In contrast, the pars of the lower lumbar levels begins within the center of the pars itself, extending from this point to connect to the neighboring structures. Sagi and colleagues[5] found that this resulted in uneven ossification. This finding may help explain areas of weakness within the pars interarticularis of the lower lumbar levels and may suggest that there is a prenatal predilection for a stress fracture in most individuals.

Fate of the Notochord

In the early embryo, the notochord serves as a rigid template around which the future vertebral column develops. It is a uniform structure that is present throughout the entire length of the primordial spinal column. A sheath exists around the notochord in its early stages. Immunohistochemical staining studies of 4- and 5-week embryos identified that a complex of extracellular matrix molecules is already present within this sheath, including sulfated glycosaminoglycans, hyaluronic acid, fibronectin, laminin, tenascin, and collagen II.[27] Aggrecan, keratan sulfate, and other large aggregating proteoglycans (present in the mature spine) were not detected at this stage, suggesting that these appear later in development. The notochordal cells themselves showed reactivity to transforming growth factor-β, suggesting an early influence of this growth factor on the developing extracellular matrix milieu.[27]

In the 20-mm embryo, the notochord becomes an intrinsically segmented structure in the thoracic and lumbar region; in the 30-mm embryo, this structure is evident in the cervical region as well. Segmentation leads to areas of fusiform enlargements in the region of the intervertebral disc, while the notochord is slowly obliterated in the region of the developing vertebral bodies. Within the developing vertebral body, the notochord is stretched into a "mucoid streak" (see Fig. 1–5B). With continued growth, the mucoid streak disappears, leaving behind only bone.

The notochord expands in the region of the intervertebral disc to form the nucleus pulposus. This was originally described in detail by Luschka.[28] The notochord is a major source of the nucleus pulposus, and it has been shown histochemically and autoradiographically that notochordal cells proliferate and remain vital several years after birth.[29] Although notochordal cells generally do not seem to be demonstrable in the human nucleus pulposus of individuals older than 5 years of age, Schwabe[30] reported their survival in the incarcerated discs of the sacrum in a series of specimens ranging from 22 to 45 years in age. A chordoma is abnormal neoplastic growth of notochord cells that remain within the spine in adult life. This suggests that notochordal rest cells can persist well into middle age in some individuals. These neoplasms may develop at any point along the original notochordal track but are usually in the rostral (basisphenoid or basiocciput) and caudal (sacral) regions.

As a theme of development of the spine, the region of the previous notochord lies anterior to the center of the fully developed vertebral body. This has been verified by Nolting and colleagues,[25] who detected remnants of notochordal tissue anterior to the cartilaginous body center in 13 fetal spines aged 10 to 24 weeks. This finding further reinforces that using the terms *centrum* and *vertebral body* interchangeably is inaccurate.

From Neural Tube to Spinal Cord

On the 20th day, ectodermal tissues on either side of the neural plate become thick and "pucker up." This area is known as the *neural crest*, which contains cells that eventually compose the neural elements. The mesenchymal tissue beneath the neural crest is the neural fold. As the folds grow toward the midline, the two neural crests meet and fuse on day 22. The underlying neural plate forms a tube, known as the *neural tube*, whose walls are composed of the previous neural plate. The neural tube invaginates itself within the dorsum of the embryo. On the 26th day, the fused neural crest cells invaginate into the embryo and divide into right and left globules. They are termed the *dorsal root ganglia*. They are oval and appear before ossification of the spine.[31]

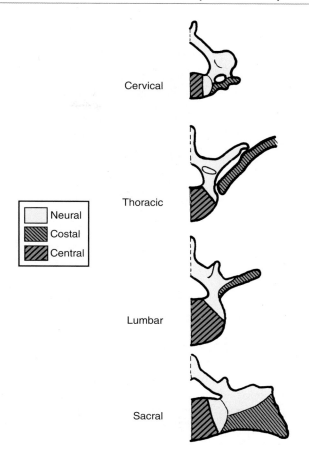

FIGURE 1–9 Neurocentral synchondroses lie well within the vertebral body in all cases. Normally, costovertebral synchondroses develop a true diarthrodial joint only in the thoracic region.

By the 5th week, the neural tube has changed into a diamond shape and is termed the *neural canal*. A sulcus limitans forms between its anterior (basal) and posterior (alar) halves, which are destined to become motor and sensory tracts. The dorsal root ganglion is composed of sensory cells alone. It develops two "arms." One arm is an extension toward the posterior aspect of the neural canal, which eventually joins the future site of the posterior column of the spinal cord. The other arm is a lateral extension that projects from the dorsal ganglion to reach peripheral tissues.

During the 6th week, the sulcus limitans disappears, and the basal and alar halves join together, while keeping their respective motor and sensory functions. Ventral horns form in the basal portion, which appear as gray matter because they are composed of motor cell bodies. Axons grow out from the ventral horns to peripheral structures. These axons join with the dorsal root ganglion to form the spinal nerves, which exit the vertebral column as a single unit.

In the 7th to 8th week, white matter finally develops within the spinal cord, representing myelin formation along axon sheaths; this occurs in ascending and descending tracts. The central part of the spinal cord retains a small cavity lined with ependymal cells that allows the transfer of fluid. This cavity was previously filled with amnion, the early embryologic analogue of cerebrospinal fluid.

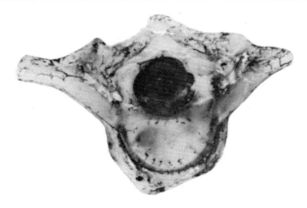

FIGURE 1–10 Section through cartilaginous vertebra of 30 weeks after vascular injection. Note the coronal vascular pattern. Each tuft consists of a central artery entwined by recurrent veins that end in a chondrous lacuna as a terminal arteriovenous anastomotic sinusoid (cul-de-sac). Nutrients diffuse from the sinusoid into the surrounding tissues.

Development of the Costal Elements

The costal elements persist only in the thoracic spine of the fully developed normal spinal column. During the 5th week, costal processes are formed and project from either side of the centrum. By the 7th week, they become sequestrated, or separated, from the centrum, by forming costovertebral and costotransverse joints. The cartilaginous structures begin to ossify in the 8th week, recognizable as ribs. In the cervical spine, the primordial costal processes fuse with transverse processes to form the costotransverse bar. Eventually, the unique cervical transverse processes form, which contain the transverse foramen for the vertebral artery. In the lumbar spine, the costal processes do not fully form. They persist only partially as the transverse processes of the fully developed spine. The embryonic transverse process forms the mammillary process (not the transverse process). The transverse and mammillary processes eventually fuse. In the sacrum, the costal processes fuse with the embryonic transverse processes and merge to become the anlage of bone of the lateral sacral mass.

Development of the Intervertebral Disc

The intervertebral disc warrants special attention because it is the pathologic focus of many spinal conditions. In the early stages of embryonic development, there are an increasing number of cells in the peripheral portion of the disc and a decreasing number adjacent to the notochord. As the embryo grows beyond a crown-rump length of 10 mm, the cells in the peripheral zone become elongated and are arranged in a lamellar pattern. When it reaches a length of 20 to 40 mm, collagen fibers begin to be synthesized and are exported from the cells, forming a collagen-rich extracellular matrix. The collagen fibers follow the pattern of the cells and are arranged in a lamellar pattern as well, giving the peripheral disc (or anulus fibrosus) its characteristic composition of circumferential

bands of tissue. No fully continuous fibers span the entire periphery of the disc, but rather multiple strands interdigitate to create a highly tensile structure. These lamellar bundles appear to be more densely arranged in the anterior anulus and less dense in the posterior anulus of the developing spine, which may explain the propensity for posterior disc rupture in young patients.[6] As the embryo passes into the fetal stage at 2 months, the cells begin to decrease in number, and the production of extracellular matrix is increased.

By the start of the fetal period, the disc has three distinct regions: (1) an external fibrous zone, (2) an internal hyaline zone surrounding the notochord, and (3) a fibrocartilaginous zone. The disc grows by interstitial and appositional growth.[32] *Interstitial growth* refers to growth that occurs at the outer attachment of the anulus to the cartilaginous endplates. *Appositional growth* refers to growth that occurs longitudinally between the vertebra and the disc. Lamellar fibers form attachments to the cartilaginous endplates in the region of the nucleus pulposus, which completely encases the gel-like structure. The outer layers of the anulus become deeply embedded into the peripheral portion of the endplate cartilage.

As the endplate ossifies, forming the ring apophysis, the inserted annular fibers become tightly fixed. The "weak link" in this complex is between the ring apophysis and its corresponding vertebral body, so that apophyseal separation fractures are more common than rupture of the intervertebral disc in the immature spine. The interval between the apophysis and the vertebral ossification center provides an entrance for vessels to supply nutrition to the endplate and to the intervertebral disc by diffusion. This supply is obliterated after union of the ring apophysis to the vertebral body.

There is a lack of agreement regarding the extent of the vascularity of the fetal intervertebral disc. In the fetal disc, the anulus pulposus seems to be vascularized. Taylor and Twomney[33] found that a plexus of vessels around the circumference of the disc sent branches deep within the anulus. In contrast, Whalen and colleagues[34] reported that these vessels entered only the outermost lamellae of the anulus fibrosus. In addition to vessels within the anulus, regularly spaced vascular channels within the cartilage have been shown within the interface between the cartilaginous endplate and the disc (Fig. 1–10). These channels most likely do not act as blood vessels but rather as a sinusoidal "cul-de-sac" system that delivers nutritional factors by diffusion. The deep regions of the disc are probably not vascularized at any point in development. The adult intervertebral disc is avascular, receiving nutrition only through diffusion through the endplates aided by the flux of fluid to and from the nucleus pulposus. This avascularity may be present at 17 to 24 weeks.[24]

Spinal Ligament Development

There is a paucity of literature concerning the development of the spinal ligaments in the human fetus. Misawa and colleagues[35] dissected 25 human fetuses 6 to 24 weeks of age. They found that, at 6 to 7 weeks, "light zones" represented areas of low cell density that correlated with vertebral bodies, whereas "dark zones" were areas of high cell density and corresponded to the intervertebral regions. The posterior longitudinal ligament was first recognized at 10 weeks, whereas the appearance of the ligamentum flavum was concomitant with that of the lamina at 12 weeks. The fibers of the ligamentum flavum became discernible only at 15 weeks.

Influence of Fetal Movement

Development of the human skeleton seems to be strongly influenced by the interaction of its immature moving parts. In the appendicular skeleton, the opposing surfaces of the femoral head and acetabulum are codependent on each other for normal development into a highly mobile, but stable, weight-bearing joint. In the spine, the development of facet joints is thought to be influenced by torsional loading. It is commonly thought, however, that these demands are placed on the spine only postnatally during upright posture.

The importance of fetal spinal movement has been recognized only more recently. Boszczyk and colleagues[36] used ultrasonography to study the movements of 52 normal fetal spines in utero. They found that rotational movements of 4 to 10 degrees were measurable in fetuses at 9 to 36 weeks. These investigators concluded that this amount of rotation influenced the ultimate morphology of the joint and that torsional stresses are present prenatally and postnatally. Functional demands on the spine may begin even before birth.

Development of Specialized Vertebral Regions

Most of the spine develops in a very uniform manner. The more particular mechanical requirements of the cranial and caudal extremes of the spine have led to unique development processes, however, enabling functional transition between the head and lower limbs.

Occipitocervical Complex

Four occipital myotomes can be readily identified in the human embryo of 4-mm crown-rump length.[37] The first is small, the second is of intermediate size, and the third and fourth are equivalent to the succeeding cervical segments. The first cervical nerve and the hypoglossal artery clearly delimit the most caudal occipital segment. Eight rootlets of the hypoglossal nerve can be discerned rostral to the hypoglossal artery, and these usually unite into four, but no less than three, main roots. This confirms the involvement of at least three precervical segments in the formation of the occiput. DeBeer[38] claimed that a total of nine segments might be involved in skull formation. The first four appear very primitive but contribute to the preotic cranium, whereas the fifth is rudimentary, without a myotome. The last four segments are definite precursors of the occipital complex.

The definitive hypoglossal nerve shows some retention of its multisegmental origins. Its rootlets usually coalesce into two distinct fascicles that exit through separate openings in the dura, and occasionally these do not unite until they have left the skull. The formation of the hypoglossal canal may also indicate a multisegmental relationship. The usual single aperture has been regarded in some texts as homologous to the intervertebral foramen between the neural arch equivalents of two occipital somites, but during chondrification a membranous strut that separates the two main fascicles of the nerve may be observed. By further chondrification and ossification, a double hypoglossal canal accommodating both strands of the nerve may result. Most likely, this mesenchymal strut is a representative of the membranous neural arch process of an intervening segment and is a good indicator that at least three somitic levels were involved in forming the part of the occipital bone surrounding the hypoglossal canal.

Atlantoaxial Complex

The axis and atlas, although considered two vertebral levels in the fully developed spine, actually arise from three different centra. Sensenig[39] first described this in detail in 1937, and later O'Rahilly and Meyer[40] provided a description. These three centra have been named the X, Y, and Z components. The apical X component at first projects into the early foramen magnum and forms an occipitoaxial joint. It has come to be known as the *proatlas* and constitutes the main portion of the odontoid process. Although it is commonly written that the odontoid process develops from the centrum of C1, this is probably not entirely true.[41] Remains of the occipitocervical syndesmosis are apparent by the formation of the alar ligaments. The Y component becomes the centrum of the atlas, and the Z component becomes the centrum of the axis (C2). The X, Y, and Z components are related to the first, second, and third cervical nerves, which explains the redundancy of the numbering of the upper cervical nerves. In a more recent study, Muller and O'Rahilly[42] determined that these three components actually develop from only two and a half sclerotomes in the chick embryo.

Considering the segmental complexities involved in the development of the normal human craniocervical articulations, the occasional occurrence of anomalous separations, fusions, and intercalated ossicles should not be surprising. Because the odontoid process develops from its own centrum, it can be better understood how an "os odontoideum" may arise. This anomaly is manifested as a spherule of bone suspended between the two alar ligaments without any apparent bony connection to the C2 body. This embryologic development also helps explain the "watershed" region at the base of the odontoid process that predisposes to nonunion after displaced fractures.

The most frequent manifestation of variant segmentation is the appearance of a third (midline) occipital condyle, also known as a *basilar tubercle*. This structure occurs as a projection on the basion (anterior central point) of the foramen magnum. Sometimes it is expressed as a simple rounded

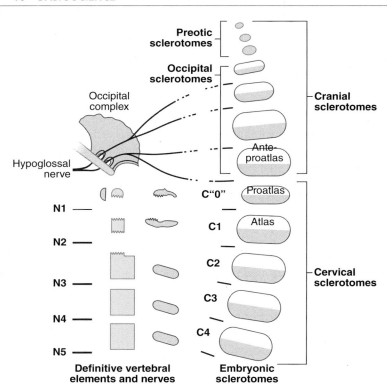

Preotic sclerotomes

Occipital sclerotomes

Occipital complex

Cranial sclerotomes

Hypoglossal nerve

Ante-proatlas

N1 — C"0" Proatlas

N2 — C1 Atlas

N3 — C2

N4 — C3

N5 — C4

Cervical sclerotomes

Definitive vertebral elements and nerves

Embryonic sclerotomes

FIGURE 1–11 Schematic representation of craniocervical sclerotomes and their segmentally related definitive cranial and vertebral elements and nerves. The cranial and cervical sclerotomes originally formed a continuum. The axis incorporates three sclerotomic elements. The caudal four cranial sclerotomes contribute to the occiput, and their nerves coalesce to form the hypoglossal nerve.

tubercle, but in better developed cases there is actually an articular facet that receives the tip of the odontoid process forming a true diarthrosis (joint). Occasionally, accessory facets lateral to the central projection are present. In a series of 600 skulls, some suggestion of a third condyle was present in 14% of specimens.[43]

Toro and Szepe[44] observed that the third condyle often occurs with occipitalization of the atlas. They also thought that it may be the expression of the hypochordal arch of the

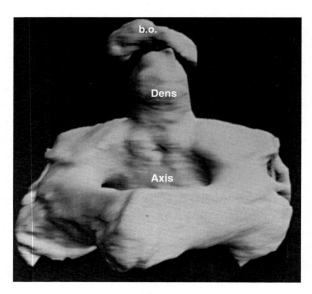

FIGURE 1–12 Nonfused "floating" ossicles may occur within craniocervical syndesmoses. A variably shaped, usually pea-sized, ossification that occurs between the basion and the tip of the odontoid (in the presence of a complete odontoid process) has been labeled Bergmann ossicle.

"ante-proatlas." As they used this term, it seems to designate the most caudal occipital somite (Fig. 1–11). A more complete separation of this ante-proatlas may form a true occipital vertebra. First described by Meckel in 1815, this malformation forms a more or less complete ring inferior to the foramen magnum, and its anterior arch is often fused to the skull, bearing a third condyle. This condition is distinguished from occipitalization of the atlas by the radiologic identification of the true atlas beneath it. Transverse processes of variable relative size may be present in occipital vertebrae, but these do not show a transverse foramen.[45] Because bony eminences on either side of the third condyle are common to these structures, they may encroach on the foramen magnum, causing neurologic sequelae.

Occipitalization of the atlas occurs in 0.1% to 0.8% of the population according to the series of skulls examined. If the occipitalization is complete, there is no movable atlanto-occipital articulation, and the atlas ring is more constricted. Also, the level of the odontoid tip shows a higher relative position, and the fusion is often asymmetrical. Inglemark's[46] series of skulls showed that in 78% of the true congenital cases the posterior arch was fused to the posterior rim of the foramen magnum; the anterior arch was fused in 54%, and lateral fusions occurred in 23%. Toro and Szepe[44] suggested that the variable expressions of fragments of the proatlas arch, which normally form parts of the atlas, may enhance the predilection of this segment to fuse to the skull.

Nonfused "floating" ossicles may occur within the craniocervical syndesmoses. A variably shaped, usually pea-sized, ossification that occurs between the basion and the tip of the odontoid (in the presence of a complete odontoid process) has been labeled Bergmann ossicle (Fig. 1–12)[47] and is most likely a variant derivative of the ante-proatlas mesenchyme. Putz[48] also recorded the incidence of a small ossicle between the anterior lip of the foramen magnum and the anterior arch of the atlas and within the anterior atlanto-occipital membrane. He was convinced that this was a manifestation of the hypochordal potential of the last occipital (ante-proatlas) somite.

Sacrum

Ossification of the bodies of the sacral vertebrae is unique in that, in addition to the single central ossific zone, two true epiphyseal plates later provide accessory ossification to the superior and inferior surfaces of each segment. The central centers for the superior three sacral vertebrae are evident at week 9, whereas these centers for the fourth and fifth segments do not appear until after week 24. Each vertebral arch of the sacrum shows the conventional bilateral centers, but in addition six centers produce the sacral alae. Between weeks 24 and 32, these centers appear anterolateral to the anterior sacral foramina of the upper three sacral vertebrae. They are expressions of the ever-present potential of the vertebral anlagen to produce costal equivalents (Fig. 1–13).

In the early part of the 1st year after birth, the sacral vertebrae are still separated by intervertebral discs, and the lower two are the first to fuse in late adolescence. Before this, the ossific centers for the superior and inferior epiphyseal plates of the bodies appear, and between 18 and 20 years of age, lateral epiphyseal plates form on the auricular surfaces of the sacral alae. By the middle of the 3rd decade, the entire sacrum should be fused, although internal remnants of the intervertebral plates remain throughout life. These may be visualized in a sagittal section or in radiographs taken at the appropriate anteroposterior angle.

The coccygeal segments lack neural arch equivalents and form a single ossific center for their bodies. The first usually appears before 5 years of age, and the succeeding three ossify during consecutive 5-year intervals.

Genetic Control of Spinal Segmentation

In the previous edition, an extensive discussion of the genetic control of segmentation was presented. This discussion focused on the wealth of information provided by studies performed on the fruit fly, *Drosophila*. The most essential concept provided by these studies is the fact that the individual aspects of the advanced stages of development are the result of a sequential action of numerous genes, and the mutation of single-effect genes, whose phenotypic expressions have provided the classic mendelian patterns of heredity, usually show errors in only a single step in this concatenation of events. *Drosophila* development shows that a set of maternal effect genes (so labeled because they are exclusively derived from the maternal genome) initially establishes the axial symmetry of the body within the ovum. A group of approximately 20 segmentation genes guides cellular construction of the defined segments. Mutations of these genes are manifest as

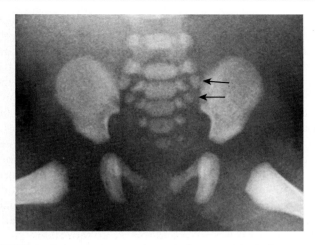

FIGURE 1–13 Anteroposterior radiograph of a 34-week fetal pelvis showing two of the eventual three ossific centers (*arrows*) of the costal contributions to the alae. These form in the cartilage that anchors the fetal sacrum to the auricular processes of the iliac wings.

deletions affecting the normal segment number. Most mutations of the segmentation genes are lethal, and knowledge of them has been obtained from the doomed larval forms. Because they are commonly recessive, however, the mutant strain can be propagated for continuous study. The equivalent genetic effects would not be so readily observable in vertebrates, but comparative evidence strongly indicates that similar genetic mechanisms are operable.

Only after the segmental boundaries have been established can the structures characteristic of each segment be determined. These designations are effected by the homeotic selector genes. The term *homeotic* (from the Latin *homoeos*, meaning "similar") was originally used by Bateson[49] to label the mutant substitution of segment appendages because he surmised that they indicated a similarity (genetic homology) in their underlying developmental mechanisms. In contrast to the segmentation genes whose mutations affect the whole segment, mutations of the homeotic genes are expressed as homologous structures (e.g., legs and wings) grotesquely appearing on inappropriate segments. It is now known that these homeotic genes are closely grouped in two locations on the third chromosome of *Drosophila's* four chromosomes.

Another significant outcome of *Drosophila* genetic research has been the identification of a sequence of nucleotide base pairs that is common to the homeotic selector genes.[10] Intergenetic cross homologies of certain gene regions are not unusual, but the relatively small sequence common to these homeotic genes contained only a 180 base-pair unit that could easily be used as a probe to identify the locations of its homologues. This compact genetic fragment was called the *homeobox* by McGinnis and associates,[50] and the protein it encodes is known as the *homeodomain*.[10]

Links Between Fly and Human

Evolution recognized a fundamental advantage in deriving a body plan from the regional diversification of a series of basically similar modules because virtually all higher organisms develop from some type of segmental organization. Although vertebrate segmentation is not externally obvious in the post-embryonic stages, the sclerotomic contributions to the axial skeleton retain the original metameric organization; the common neurologic examination based on a knowledge of the myotomic and dermatomic distribution of the cranial and spinal nerves pays perpetual homage to the truth that humans and the other vertebrates are segmentally constructed animals.

As would be expected, the homeobox-containing genes discovered in humans[9] do not act in exactly the same manner as they do in *Drosophila* because the types of segmental organization are quite different. Nevertheless, the nucleotide sequence cognates of the *Drosophila* homeobox genes found in mammals seem to have considerable influence in the early establishment of brainstem and spinal cord formation.[13] As in the more primitive forms, malfunctions of the genes controlling the more fundamental aspects of segmentation most likely produce early lethal mutations. Because higher vertebrates do not have an autonomous larval stage, the occurrence of such mutations would be lost to general observation. Nevertheless, some gross errors of segmentation that may reach parturition do show genetic implication.

Congenital Syndromes: Genetic Evidence of Segmentation in Humans

Klippel-Feil Syndrome

In humans, congenital vertebral fusions, most commonly manifest in the various "types" of the Klippel-Feil syndrome, serve as a prime example of segmentation. Many instances of this syndrome seem to result from spontaneous mutations or individual teratogenic accidents in the early developmental sequences because most reports present single case histories without examination of the extended family and the family's pedigree. Gunderson and colleagues[11] provided substantial evidence, however, that many cases of Klippel-Feil syndrome are probands of a familial history of the condition. These authors provided the pedigrees of 11 probands. Of particular interest is their type II of the syndrome, which exhibits fusions limited to the cervical regions at C2-3 and C5-6. Gunderson and colleagues[11] concluded that this disorder, which produced segmentation errors at consistent spine levels through several successive generations, strongly indicated a dominant mutant defect of a gene that controls these specific levels of segmentation.

Caudal Dysplasias

Another class of segmental spinal malformations that indicates genetic import is grouped under the generic term of *caudal dysplasias*.[4] This malformation complex has proved to be heritable and has a marked association with maternal diabetes. From this complex, certain insights into genetic mechanisms of mammalian spinal development may be derived. That some degree of caudal segment regression is a natural phenomenon is shown by the reduction of the original post-sacral somites from eight (±2) to four (±1) in normal human development. In more severe forms of lumbosacral agenesis,

all vertebral elements as far cephalad as the upper lumbar region may fail to develop. The association with maternal diabetes has been attributed to a teratogenic effect of hyperglycemia because experimental elevations of blood glucose have produced varying degrees of caudal deficiencies in animals.[48] Similar effects have been induced by various toxic insults during embryogenesis of the spine.

Because caudal agenesis is not a consistent occurrence in the offspring of diabetic mothers, a more complex genetic association has been suspected, particularly as diabetes mellitus and spine defects have been associated with human leukocyte antigen (HLA)–type histocompatibility genes.[4] This inference has been supported by studies of the T-locus genes in the mouse. This locus apparently is a segment of the mouse chromosomes with a collection of genes that have a profound effect on spine development and other aspects of embryogenesis.[51] There is evidence that a gene complex, functionally similar to the mouse T locus, may be operable in humans because an association between histocompatibility antigens of the HLA type and the inheritance of human spina bifida has been reported.[52]

The HLAs are controlled by a cluster of contiguous genes located on the human chromosome 6. As in the mouse T locus, each gene in this group has several alleles, and numerous serologically discrete forms of cell surface antigens may be coded by the gene complex. The total ensemble of the HLAs produced within an individual determines its HLA "personality."[52] The comparative evidence suggests that the HLA complex, because of its defined chromosomal localization, its coding for the antigen complex, and its effect on spine development, is a reasonable candidate for the human analogue of the mouse T locus.

In vertebrates, as in other forms of segmented animals, a definite sequence of genetically controlled events establishes the basic aspects of segment formation. When this has been accomplished, some analogue of the homeotic system of genes most likely determines the regional specializations of the individual segments. This system provides an early determination within the vertebrate sclerotome because these embryonic cell masses exhibit a marked "position effect" before any regional differentiation of the somite is visibly evident. This effect has been shown in the chick embryo, in which the transplantation of an early thoracic sclerotome into the cervical region results in a rib-bearing thoracic vertebra whose specific character development was not modified by its heterotopic location.[53] This early position identity may be because vertebrate embryonic patterns are mostly established through early cell-to-cell interactions subsequent to cell cleavages, and these involve the antigen-mediated cell surface recognitions and adhesions as shown by the HLAs. Nevertheless, some analogues of the homeotic mechanisms in *Drosophila,* although differing in their modes of expression, must determine whether a given vertebra exhibits cervical, thoracic, or sacral characteristics.

The range of anomalies observed in the human spine well support the concept that regional vertebral specification may be the result of a homeotic type of selective repression. In addition to the obvious articulated ribs of the thoracic region, each human vertebral level shows some expression of the costal element potential, but it is usually incorporated as an immovable projection. Anomalous free or articulated rib components have been observed at virtually every vertebral level, including the sacrum and coccyx.[54] The hypochordal potential may best indicate the existence of early segmental totipotency in the vertebrates, however. This component is normally expressed at only the C1 level in humans and in the caudal region in other mammals. If there is some interference in the normal control mechanisms, it may also arise at other levels because hypochordal elements have been observed to occur below the last normal vertebra in some cases of lumbosacral agenesis.

KEY REFERENCES

1. Aoyama H, Asamoto K: The development fate of the rostral/caudal half of a somite for vertebra and rib formation: Experimental confirmation of the resegmentation theory using chick-quail chimeras. Mech Dev 99:71-82, 2000.
   The theory of resegmentation during the development of the spine has been the focus of numerous more recent studies. This investigation replaced one somite in a developing chicken with a single quail somite. The authors found that the quail somite formed the inferior and superior halves of supracent and infracent vertebral bodies. This finding has been taken as strong evidence that, even in humans, each vertebral body is formed by upper and lower halves of adjacent somites. One intervertebral disc forms from a single somite.

2. David KM, McLachlan JC, Aiton JF, et al: Cartilaginous development of the human craniovertebral junction as visualized by a new three-dimensional computer reconstruction technique. J Anat 192:269-277, 1998.
   In this histologic study of normal human embryos, the development of the cartilaginous template of the upper cervical spine (craniocervical junction) was characterized. The study challenges the well-accepted belief that the odontoid process is derived solely from C1. The odontoid process appeared to develop from a short projection of C2. The authors believed that their findings confirmed that the odontoid process is not derived solely from the centrum of C1. They described that "natural basilar invagination" of the tip of the developing odontoid process may be a normal part of embryonic development.

3. Misawa H, Ohtsuka K, Nakata K, et al: Embryological study of the spinal ligaments in human fetuses. J Spinal Disord 7:495-498, 1994.
   This study characterized a timeline of development of various spinal ligamentous structures. The anterior longitudinal ligament could be identified in an 8-week-old embryo. At 10 weeks, the posterior longitudinal ligament could be delineated. By 12 weeks, the ligamentum flavum could be identified.

REFERENCES

1. Rai AS, Taylor TK, Smith GH, et al: Congenital abnormalities of the urogenital tract in association with congenital vertebral malformations. J Bone Joint Surg Br 84:891-895, 2002.
2. Ursu TR, Porter RW, Navaratnam V: Development of the lumbar and sacral vertebral canal in utero. Spine 21:2705-2708, 1996.
3. Wakimoto BT, Turner FR, Kaufman TC: Defects in embryogenesis in mutants associated with the antennapedia gene complex of Drosophila melanogaster. Dev Biol 102:147-172, 1984.
4. Welch JP, Alterman K: The syndrome of caudal dysplasia. Pediatr Pathol 2:313-327, 1984.
5. Sagi HC, Jarvis JG, Uhtoff HK: Histomorphic analysis of the development of the pars interarticularis and its association with isthmic spondylosis. Spine 23:1635-1639, 1998.
6. Tsuji H, Hirano N, Ohshima H, et al: Structural variation of the anterior and posterior annulus fibrosus in the development of human lumbar intervertebral disc: A risk factor for intervertebral disc rupture. Spine 18:204-210, 1993.
7. Akam ME: The molecular basis for metameric pattern in the Drosophila embryo. Development 101:1-22, 1987.
8. Aoyama H, Asamoto K: The development fate of the rostral/caudal half of a somite for vertebra and rib formation: Experimental confirmation of the resegmentation theory using chick-quail chimeras. Mech Dev 99:71-82, 2000.
9. Cannizzaro LA, Croce CM, Griffin CA, et al: Human homeobox containing genes located at chromosome regions 2q31-2q37 and 12q12-12q13. Am J Hum Genet 41:1-15, 1987.
10. Genring WJ, Hiromi Y: Homeotic genes and the homeobox. Ann Rev Genet 20:147-173, 1986.
11. Gunderson CH, Greenspan RH, Glasner GH, et al: The Klippel-Feil syndrome: Genetic and clinical reevaluation of cervical fusion. Medicine 46:491-511, 1967.
12. Krengel S, Gotz W, Herken R: Expression pattern of type II collagen mRNA during early vertebral development in the human embryo. Anat Embryol (Berl) 193:43-51, 1996.
13. Triboili C, Lufkin T: The murine Bapx1 homeobox gene plays a critical role in embryonic development of the axial skeleton and spleen. Development 126:699-711, 1999.
14. Baur R: Zum Problem der neugliederung der Wirbelsaule. Acta Anat 72:321-356, 1969.
15. Dalgleish AE: A study of the development of the thoracic vertebrae in the mouse assisted by autoradiography. Acta Anat 122:91-98, 1985.
16. Remak R: Untersuchungen uber die entwicklung der Wirbeltiere. Berlin, Riemer, 1855.
17. Verbout AJ: A critical review of the "Neugliederung" concept in relation to the development of the vertebral columns. Acta Biotheoret 25:219-258, 1976.
18. VonEbner V: Urwirbel und Neugliederung der Wirbelsaule. Sitzungber Akad Wiss Wein III/101:235-260, 1889.
19. Bagnall KM, Higgins SJ, Sanders EJ: The contribution made by a single somite to the vertebral column: Experimental evidence in support of resegmentation using the chick-quail chimera model. Development 103:69-85, 1988.
20. Ewan KB, Everett AW: Evidence for resegmentation in the formation of the vertebral column using the novel approach of

retroviral-mediated gene transfer. Exp Cell Res 198:315-320, 1992.

21. Huang R, Zhi Q, Brand-Saberi B, et al: New experimental evidence for somite resegmentation. Anat Embryol 202:195-200, 2000.

22. Huang R, Zhi Q, Neubuser A, et al: Function of somite and somitocele cells in the formation of the vertebral motion segment in avian embryos. Acta Anat 155:231-241, 1996.

23. Monsoro-Burq AH, Duprez D, Watanabe Y, et al: The role of bone morphogenetic proteins in vertebral development. Development 122:3607-3616, 1996.

24. Skawina S, Litwin JA, Gorczyca J, et al: The architecture of internal blood vessels in human fetal vertebral bodies. J Anat 191:259-267, 1997.

25. Nolting D, Hansen BF, Keeling J, et al: Prenatal development of the normal human vertebral corpora in different segments of the spine. Spine 23:2268-2271, 1998.

26. Noback CR, Robertson CC: Sequence of appearance of ossification centers in the human skeleton during the first five prenatal months. Am J Anat 89:1-28, 1951.

27. Gotz W, Osmers R, Herken R: Localisation of extracellular matrix components in the embryonic human notochord and axial mesenchyme. J Anat 186:111-121, 1995.

28. Luschka H: Die Halbgelenke des Menshlichen Korpers. Berlin, Reimer, 1858.

29. Malinski J: Histochemical demonstration of carbohydrates in human intervertebral discs during postnatal development. Acta Histochem 5:120-126, 1958.

30. Schwabe R: Untersuchungen uber die Ruckbildung der Bandscheiben im Menschlichen Kreuzbein. Virchows Arch 287:651-665, 1933.

31. Khorooshi MH, Hansen BF, Keeling J, et al: Prenatal localization of the dorsal root ganglion in different segments of the normal human vertebral column. Spine 26:1-5, 2001.

32. Bohmig R: Die Blutgefassversorg ung der Wirbelbandscheiben das Verhalten des intervertebralen Chordasegments. Arch Klin Chir 158:374-382, 1930.

33. Taylor JR, Twomney LT: The development of the human intervertebral disc. In Ghosh P (ed): The Biology of the Intervertebral Disc. Boca Raton, FL, CRC Press, 1988.

34. Whalen JL, Parke WW, Mazur JM, et al: The intrinsic vasculature of developing vertebral end plates and the nutritive significance to the intervertebral disc. J Pediatr Orthop 5:403-410, 1985.

35. Misawa H, Ohtsuka K, Nakata K, et al: Embryological study of the spinal ligaments in human fetuses. J Spinal Disord 7:495-498, 1994.

36. Boszczyk AA, Boszczyk BM, Putz RV: Prenatal rotation of the lumbar spine and its relevance for the development of the zygapophyseal joints. Spine 27:1094-1101, 2002.

37. Sensenig EC: The early development of the human vertebral column. Contr Embryol Carneg Inst 33:21-51, 1957.

38. DeBeer GR: The Development of the Vertebral Skull. Oxford, Oxford University Press, 1937.

39. Sensenig EC: The origin of the vertebral column in the deer-mouse, Peromyscus maniculatus rufinus. Anat Rec 86:123-141, 1943.

40. O'Rahilly R, Meyer DB: The timing and sequence of events in the development of the vertebral column during the embryonic period proper. Anat Embryol 157:167-176, 1979.

41. David KM, McLachlan JC, Aiton JF, et al: Cartilaginous development of the human craniovertebral junction as visualized by a new three-dimensional computer reconstruction technique. J Anat 192:269-277, 1998.

42. Muller F, O'Rahilly R: Occipitocervical segmentation in staged human embryos. J Anat 185:251-258, 1994.

43. Lang J: Clinical Anatomy of the Head. Wilson R, Winstanley DP (trans). Berlin, Springer-Verlag, 1983.

44. Toro I, Szepe L: Untersuchungen uber die Frage der Assimilation und Manifestation des Atlas. Z Anat Entwickl 111:186-200, 1942.

45. Hadley LA: Atlanto-occipital fusion, ossiculum terminale and occipital vertebra as related to basilar impression with neurological symptoms. Am J Radiol 59:511-524, 1948.

46. Inglemark BE: Uber das Craniovertebrale Grenzgebiet beim Menschen. Acta Anat Suppl VI:1-116, 1947.

47. Bergman E: Die Lehre von den Kopfverletzungen (cited by Lang J). Stuttgart, Enke, 1880.

48. Putz VR: Zur Manifestation der hypochordalen Spangen im cranio-vertebralen Grenzgebiet beim Menschen. Anat Anz 137:65-74, 1975.

49. Bateson W: Materials for the Study of Variation Treated with the Especial Regards to Discontinuity in the Origin of Species. London, Macmillan, 1894.

50. McGinnis W, Garber RL, Wirz J, et al: A homologous protein-coding sequence in Drosophila homeotic genes and its conservation in other metazoans. Cell 37:403-408, 1984.

51. Bennett D: The T-locus of the mouse. Cell 6:441-454, 1975.

52. Check W: First data for human developmental genes. JAMA 238:2253-2254, 1977.

53. Keynes RJ, Stern CD: Mechanisms of vertebrate segmentation. Development 103:413-429, 1988.

54. Kaushal SP: Sacral ribs. Int Surg 62:37-38, 1977.

2 CHAPTER

Applied Anatomy of the Spine

Wesley W. Parke, PhD
Christopher M. Bono, MD
Steven R. Garfin, MD

The spine is a segmental column of similar formed bones that constitutes the major subcranial part of the axial skeleton. Its individual elements are united by a series of intervertebral articulations that form a flexible, although neuroprotective, support to the trunk and limbs. The spinal column typically consists of 33 vertebrae. The mobile section of the spine comprises 7 cervical, 12 thoracic, and 5 lumbar vertebrae; 5 fused vertebrae form the inflexible sacrum that offers a relatively rigid connection to the innominate bones. Caudad to the sacrum, four or five irregular ossicles compose the coccyx.

Vertebrae

The movements of the spine involve 97 diarthroses (i.e., synovial joints, having substantial motion) and an even greater number of amphiarthroses (i.e., fibrocartilaginous joints, having less motion). The individual vertebrae bear multiple processes and surface markings that indicate the attachments of the numerous ligaments that stabilize these articulations. Despite an appreciable degree of regional variation of these characteristics, the embryologically homologous segmental origin of the spine provides a basic uniformity so that a single generalized description can be applied to the basic morphology of all but the most superior and inferior elements.

The typical vertebra consists of two major components: a roughly cylindrical ventral mass of mostly trabecularized cancellous bone, called the *body,* and a denser, more cortical posterior structure, called the *dorsal vertebral arch.* The vertebral bodies vary considerably in size and sectional contour but exhibit no salient processes or unique external features other than the facets for rib articulation in the thoracic region. In contrast, the vertebral arch has a more complex structure. It is attached to the dorsolateral aspects of the body by two stout pillars, called the *pedicles.* These are united dorsally by a pair of arched flat laminae that are surmounted in the midline by a dorsal projection, called the *spinous process.* The pedicles, laminae, and dorsum of the body form the vertebral foramen, a complete osseous ring that encloses the spinal cord.

The transverse processes and the superior and inferior articular processes are found near the junction of the pedicles and the laminae. The transverse processes extend laterally from the sides of the vertebral arches, and because all vertebrae are phyletically and ontogenetically associated with some form of costal element, they either articulate with or incorporate a rib component. In the thoracic spine, the costal process persists as a rib proper. In the cervical spine, the costal process becomes the anterior part of the transverse process that encloses the vertebral artery foramen, and in the lumbar spine it becomes the mature transverse process; the immature posterior (neural arch) component becomes the mammillary process.

The articular processes (zygapophyses) form the paired diarthrodial articulations (facet joints) between the vertebral arches. The superior processes (prezygapophyses) always bear an articulating facet, whose surface is directed dorsally to some degree, whereas the complementary inferior articulating processes (postzygapophyses) direct their articulating surfaces ventrally. Variously shaped bony prominences (mammillary processes or parapophyses) may be found lateral to the articular processes and serve in the multiple origins and insertions of the spinal muscles.

The superoinferior dimensions of the pedicles are roughly half that of their corresponding body, so that in their lateral aspect the pedicles and their articulating processes form the superior and inferior vertebral notches. Because the base of the pedicle arises superiorly from the dorsum of the body, particularly in the lumbar spine, the inferior vertebral notch appears more deeply incised. In the articulated spine, the opposing superior and inferior notches form the intervertebral foramina that transmit the neural and vascular structures between the corresponding levels of the spinal cord and their developmentally related body segments.

Pars Interarticularis

The pars interarticularis defines the parts of the arch that lie between the superior and inferior articular facets of all subatlantal movable vertebral elements (Fig. 2–1). The term *pars interarticularis* arose to designate that area of the arch that is most stressed by translational movement between adjacent

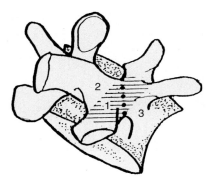

FIGURE 2–1 Graphic rendering of oblique dorsal view of L5 vertebra showing the parts of the vertebral arch: (*1*) pars interarticularis as the *cross-hatched area,* (*2*) pars laminalis, (*3*) pars pedicularis. *Dotted line* indicates most frequent site of mechanical failure of the pars interarticularis.

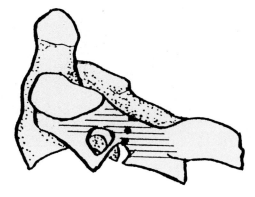

FIGURE 2–2 Graphic depiction of lateral view of C2 (axis) vertebra. The offset relationship of the superior facet to the inferior facet elongates the pars interarticularis (*cross-hatched area*). *Dotted line* indicates most frequent site of failure in upper cervical hyperextension injury (hangman's fracture).

segments, particularly in the second cervical and fifth lumbar vertebrae, which are susceptible to traumatic and stress fractures in this region (i.e., hangman's fracture of C2[1] and isthmic spondylolysis of L5). In sequential alternation with the intervertebral facet joints, it roofs the lateral recesses of the spinal canal and contributes to the dorsal margins of the intervertebral foramina. In the subcervical vertebrae, it also provides the dorsal part of the base of the transverse process.

Biomechanical forces on the pars interarticularis place it in a position to receive the shearing stresses that occur when

translational (spondylolisthetic) forces tend to displace, in a dorsoventral plane, the superior articular processes with respect to their inferior counterparts on the same vertebra. The usual site of failure in the pars interarticularis permits the superior articular facets, pedicles, and vertebral body to be ventrally displaced as a unit, while the inferior articular facets remain attached to the dorsal arch components. These tend to retain their articular relationships with the superior facets of the next lower vertebra.

In the case of the second cervical vertebra (axis) there is a unique anterior relationship of its superior articular facets with the more posteriorly positioned inferior processes that elongates the C2 pars interarticularis. As this offset area receives the greatest leverage between the "cervicocranium" and the lower cervical spine, the indicated line in the illustration in Figure 2–2 shows the common site of mechanical failure in hyperextension injuries to the upper cervical spine.

In the case of the lumbar vertebrae, the pars interarticularis has been subdivided further. McCulloch and Transfelt[2] referred to the "lateral buttress," which they believed offered particular structural support to the intervening structures. They described it as the bony bridge that connects the superolateral edge of the inferior facet to the junction of the transverse process and the pedicle. In a follow-up anatomic study, Weiner and colleagues[3] measured the surface area of the lateral buttress in human cadaveric lumbar spines. They found the greatest areas (about 80 mm^2) from L1 to L3, whereas area averaged 50 mm^2 at L4 and only 15 mm^2 at L5. These investigators thought that the broadness of the buttress in the upper lumbar spine can obscure or confuse landmarks for placement of pedicle screws, and its relative thinness (or nonexistence) in the lower lumbar spine can be a predisposing factor to stress fractures or iatrogenic injury to the pars interarticularis.

Regional Characteristics

Although the 24 vertebrae of the presacral spine are divided into three distinct groups (Fig. 2–3), in which the individual members may be recognized by one or two uniquely regional

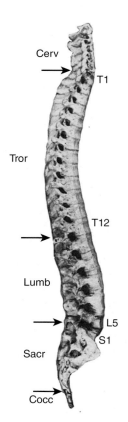

FIGURE 2–3 Lateral view of dried preparation of the spine with anterior longitudinal and supraspinous ligaments intact.

features, there is a gradual craniocaudal progression of morphologic changes. The vertebrae found above and below the point of regional demarcation are transitional and bear some of the characteristics of both areas.

Cervical Vertebrae

Of the seven cervical vertebrae, the first two (Fig. 2–4A to D) and the last require special notation, but the third to the sixth are fairly uniform, and a common description suffices (Fig. 2–4E and F). Because the cervical vertebrae bear the least weight, their bodies are relatively small and thin with respect to the size of the vertebral arch and vertebral foramen. In addition, their diameter is greater transversely than in the anteroposterior direction. The lateral edges of the superior

surface of each body are sharply turned upward to form the uncinate processes that are characteristic of the cervical region. The most obvious diagnostic feature of the cervical vertebrae is the transverse foramina that perforate the transverse processes and transmit the vertebral arteries. The anterior part of the transverse processes represents fused costal elements that arise from the sides of the body. The lateral extremities of the transverse processes bear two projections, the anterior and posterior tubercles. The former serve as origins of anterior cervical muscles; the latter provide origins and insertions for posterior cervical muscles. A deep groove between the upper aspects of the tubercles holds the cervical spinal nerves.

The cervical pedicles connect the posterior vertebral arch to the vertebral body. Anatomic studies have shown that the cervical pedicle height ranges from 5.1 to 9.5 mm, and width

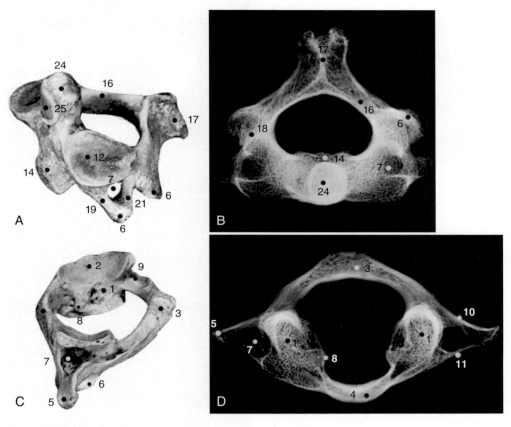

FIGURE 2–4 Atlas, axis, and a typical vertebra of each region are illustrated photographically and radiographically. The following numerical key is applicable to all subdivisions of this figure. **A,** Oblique view of atlas. **B,** Ventral radiographic view of atlas. **C,** Oblique view of axis. **D,** Vertical radiographic view of axis.

1. lateral mass of atlas
2. superior articulating process
3. posterior arch
4. anterior arch
5. transverse process
6. inferior articulating process
7. transverse foramen
8. alar tubercle
9. groove for vertebral artery
10. neural arch element of transverse process
11. costal element of transverse process
12. superior articulating process
13. pedicle

14. body
15. uncinate process
16. lamina
17. spinous process
18. articular pillar
19. anterior tubercle of transverse process
20. neural sulcus
21. posterior tubercle of transverse process
22. superior demifacet for head of rib
23. inferior demifacet for head of rib
24. odontoid process
25. articular facet for anterior arch of atlas

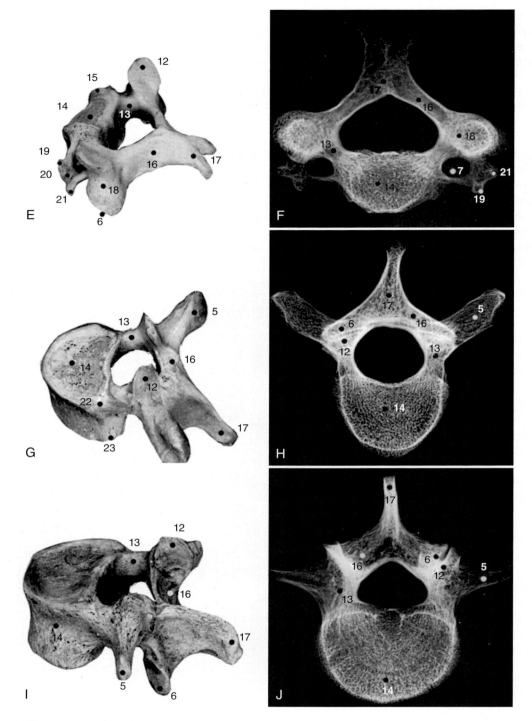

FIGURE 2–4, cont'd E, Oblique view of typical (fourth) cervical vertebra. **F,** Vertical radiographic view of typical cervical vertebra. **G,** Oblique view of typical (fifth) thoracic vertebra. **H,** Vertical radiographic view of thoracic vertebra. The plane of the articular facets would readily permit rotation. **I,** Oblique view of typical (third) lumbar vertebra. **J,** Vertical radiographic view of lumbar vertebra. The plane of the articular facets is situated to lock the lumbar vertebrae against rotation.

ranges from 3 to 7.5 mm.[4,5] The pedicle is angled medially between 90 and 110 degrees.[5]

The superior and inferior articular processes appear as obliquely sectioned surfaces of short cylinders of bone that, when united with the adjacent vertebrae, form two osseous shafts posterolateral to the stacked vertebral bodies. The cervical vertebrae present a tripod of flexible columns for the support of the head. As in the upper cervical spine, the combination of the articular processes and the intervening bone is often referred to as the lateral mass in the subaxial region. It is a common site for screw insertion during internal fixation of the cervical spine.[6]

The laminae are narrow and have a thinner superior edge. At their mid-dorsal junction, they bear a bifid spinous process that receives the insertions of the semispinalis cervicis muscles. The height of the lamina of C4 is 10 to 11 mm, whereas the lamina thickness at C5 is about 2 mm.[7] The lamina is thickest at T2, where it measures an average of 5 mm.

Atlantoaxial Complex

The first two cervical vertebrae are structurally and developmentally different. Together, they form a complex articular system that permits the nutational (i.e., nodding) and rotational movements of the head. The first cervical vertebra, or atlas, is a bony ring consisting of an anterior and a posterior arch, which are connected by the two lateral masses. It has all the homologous features of a typical vertebra with the exception of the body. The lateral masses correspond to the combined pedicles and articular pillars of the lower cervical vertebrae, but the superior and inferior articular facets are concave. The superior articular surfaces face upward and internally to receive the occipital condyles of the skull, whereas the inferior articulating surfaces face downward and internally to rotate on the sloped "shoulders" of the axis. This slope helps prevent lateral translation while permitting rotation.

The posterior arch consists of modified laminae that are more round than flat in their sectional aspect and a posterior tubercle that represents an attenuated spinous process that gives origin to suboccipital muscles. Immediately behind the lateral masses on the superior surface of the posterior arch of C1, two smooth grooves house the vertebral arteries as they penetrate the posterior atlanto-occipital membrane. These arteries take a tortuous course from the transverse processes of the atlas, making an almost 90-degree turn medially as they exit the foramen and a subsequent 90-degree turn superiorly to enter the dura and subsequently the foramen magnum. This second turn occurs more than 1.5 to 2 cm lateral to the midline, risking injury to the structure with surgical dissection beyond this point.

The anterior arch forms a short bridge between the anterior aspects of the lateral masses. It bears an anterior tubercle that is the site of insertion of the longus colli muscle. On the posterior surface of the anterior arch, a semicircular depression marks the synovial articulation of the odontoid process. Internal tubercles on the adjacent lateral masses are the attachment sites of the transverse atlantal ligaments that hold the odontoid against this articular area.

The second cervical vertebra, or axis, provides a bearing surface on which the atlas may rotate. Its most distinctive characteristic is the vertically projecting odontoid process that serves as a pivotal restraint against horizontal displacements of the atlas. This bony prominence represents the phyletically purloined centrum of the first cervical vertebra. It exhibits a slight constriction at its neck and an anterior facet for its articulation with the anterior arch of the atlas. Posteriorly, a groove in the neck of the odontoid marks the position of the strong transverse atlantal ligament.

The apex of the odontoid process is slightly pointed. It is the attachment site of the apical ligament. Posterior to the apex, two lateral roughened prominences indicate the attachments of the alar ligaments. These structures and the apical ligament connect the odontoid process to the base of the skull at the basion, the anterior aspect of the foramen magnum. The superior articulating surfaces of the axis are convex and are directed laterally to receive the lateral masses of the atlas. The inferior articulating surfaces are typical of those of the cervical vertebrae and serve as the start of the articular columns. The transverse processes of the axis are directed downward. Anteriorly, the inferior aspect of the body of the axis forms a liplike process that descends over the first intervertebral disc and the body of the third cervical vertebra.

The seventh cervical vertebra is transitional. The inferior surface of its body is proportionately larger than the superior surface. It has a long, distinct spinous process that is usually easily palpable (the vertebra prominens). The superior and inferior articulating facets are more steeply inclined and presage the form of these structures in the thoracic region. Blunt transverse processes have heavy posterior struts and much lighter anterior struts that surround transverse foramina that are often bilaterally unequal and seldom pass the vertebral arteries. Frequently, one or both of the anterior struts realize their true potential as a costal element and develop into a cervical rib.

Thoracic Vertebrae

All 12 thoracic vertebrae support ribs and have facets for the diarthrodial articulations of these structures. The first and last four have specific peculiarities in the manner of costal articulations, but the second to the eighth are similar (Fig. 2–4G and H).

The body of a mid-thoracic vertebra is heart-shaped. Its length and width are roughly halfway between that of the cervical and lumbar bodies. Often a flattening of the left side of the body indicates its contact with the descending aorta. In the mid-thorax, the heads of the ribs form a joint that spans the intervertebral disc, so that the inferior lip of the body of one vertebra and the corresponding site of the superior lip of the infrajacent element share in the formation of a single articular facet for the costal capitulum. The typical thoracic vertebra bears two demifacets on each side of its body. The thoracic vertebral arch encloses a small, round vertebral foramen that would not admit the tip of an index finger, even when the specimen is from a large adult. This limited space for the spinal cord predisposes to severe spinal cord injury with minimal dimensional compromise.

Because the pedicles arise more superiorly on the dorsum of the body than they do in the cervical region, the inferior vertebral notch forms an even greater contribution to the intervertebral foramen. The pedicle height increases from T1 to T12, but the transverse pedicle width (which is more critical for transpedicular screw containment) does not follow this same craniocaudal pattern.[8] Cinotti and colleagues[9] found that the pedicles in the T4 to T8 region had the smallest transverse diameter. Scoles and colleagues[10] documented similar findings in 50 cadaveric human spines, with the smallest diameters measured at T3 to T6. On average, the transverse pedicle diameter at T3 is 3.4 mm in women and 3.9 mm in men. At T6, it averages 3 mm in women and 3.5 mm in men. At T1, however, the mean diameter is 6.4 mm in women and 7.3 mm in men.

The superior articular facets form a stout shelflike projection from the junction of the laminae and the pedicles. Their ovoid surfaces are slightly convex, are almost vertical, and are coronal in their plane of articulation. They face dorsally and slightly superolaterally, and in bilateral combination they present the segment of an arc whose center of radius lies at the anterior edge of the vertebral body. They permit a slight rotation around the axis of this radius. The inferior articular facets are borne by the inferior edges of the laminae. The geometry of their articular surfaces is complementary to the superior processes.

On the ventral side of the tip of the strong transverse processes, another concave facet receives the tuberculum of the rib whose capitulum articulates with the superior demifacet of the same vertebra. The spinous processes of the thoracic vertebrae are long and triangular in section. The spinous processes of the upper four thoracic vertebrae are more bladelike and are directed downward at an angle of about 40 degrees from the horizontal. The middle four thoracic spinous processes are longer but directed downward at an angle of 60 degrees, so that they completely overlap the adjacent lower

segment. The lower four resemble the upper four in direction and shape.

The first thoracic vertebra has a complete facet on the side of its body for the capitulum of the first rib and an inferior demifacet for the capitulum of the second rib. The costal articulations of the 9th to 12th thoracic vertebrae are confined to the sides of the bodies of their respective segments. On the last two thoracic vertebrae, transitional characteristics are evident in the diminution of the transverse processes and their failure to buttress the last two ribs. Because the ribs are disconnected from the sternum, they are frequently referred to as "floating ribs."

Lumbar Vertebrae

The lumbar vertebrae are the lowest five vertebrae of the presacral column (see Fig. 2–4I and J). All their features are expressed in more massive proportions. They are easily distinguished from other regional elements by their lack of a transverse foramen or costal articular facets. The body is large, having a width greater than its anteroposterior diameter, and is slightly thicker anteriorly than posteriorly. All structures associated with the vertebral arch are blunt and stout. The thick pedicles are widely placed on the dorsolaterosuperior aspects of the body, and with their laminae they enclose a triangular vertebral foramen. Although the inferior vertebral notch is deeper than the superior, both make substantial contributions to the intervertebral foramen. The transverse processes are flat and winglike in the upper three lumbar segments, but in the fifth segment they are thick, rounded stumps. The fourth transverse process is usually the smallest.

Aside from their relative size, the lumbar vertebrae can be recognized by their articular processes. The superior pair arise in the usual manner from the junction of the pedicles and laminae, but their articular facets are concave and directed dorsomedially, so that they almost face each other. The inferior processes are extensions of the laminae that direct the articulating surfaces ventrolaterally and lock themselves between the superior facets of the next inferior vertebra in an almost mortise-and-tenon fashion. This arrangement restricts rotation and translation in the lumbar region. The lumbar segments also have pronounced mammillary processes, which are points of origin and insertion of the thick lower divisions of the deep paraspinal muscles.

Sacral Vertebrae

The sacrum consists of five fused vertebrae that form a single triangular complex of bone that supports the spine and forms the posterior part of the pelvis (Figs. 2–5 and 2–6). It is markedly curved and tilted backward, so that its first element articulates with the fifth lumbar vertebra at a pronounced angle (the sacrovertebral angle).

Close inspection of the flat, concave ventral surface and the rough, ridged convex dorsal surface reveals that, despite their fusion, all the homologous elements of typical vertebrae are

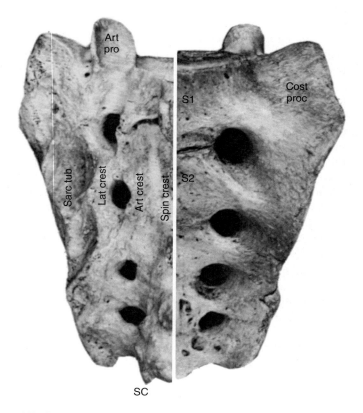

FIGURE 2–5 Composite anteroposterior view of sacrum. The roughened crests on the dorsum (*left side of illustration*) indicate longitudinal fusions of vertebral arch structures. The articular process is directed backward to buttress the vertebral arch of the fifth lumbar vertebra.

still evident in the sacrum. The heavy, laterally projecting alae that bear the articular surfaces for articulation with the pelvis are fused anterior costal and posterior transverse processes of the first three sacral vertebrae. These lateral fusions require that separate dorsal and ventral foramina provide egress for the anterior and posterior divisions of the sacral nerves. The ventral four pairs of sacral foramina are larger than their dorsal counterparts because they must pass the thick sacral contributions to the sciatic nerve. The ventral surface of the sacrum is relatively smooth. There are four transverse ridges that mark the fusions of the vertebral bodies and enclose remnants of the intervertebral discs. Lateral to the bodies of the second, third, and fourth elements, the ridges of bone that separate the anterior sacral foramina are quite prominent and give origin to the piriformis muscle.

The dorsal aspect of the sacrum is convex, rough, and conspicuously marked by five longitudinal ridges. The central one, the middle sacral crest, is formed by the fusion of the spinous processes of the sacral vertebrae. On either side, a sacral groove separates it from the medial sacral articular crest that represents the fused articular process. The superior ends of these crests form the functional superior articular processes of the first sacral vertebra, which articulate with the inferior processes of the fifth lumbar vertebra. They are very strong, and their facets are directed dorsally to resist the tendency of the fifth lumbar vertebra to be displaced forward. Inferiorly, the articular crests terminate as the sacral cornua, two rounded projections that bracket the inferior hiatus where it gives access to the sacral vertebral canal. More laterally, the lateral crests and sacral tuberosities form uneven elevations for the attachments of the dorsal sacroiliac ligaments.

The sacrum and its posterior ligaments lie ventral to the posterior iliac spines and form a deep depression that accommodates, and gives origin to, the inferior parts of the paraspinal muscles. The grooves between the central spinous crest and the articular crests are occupied by the origins of the multifidus muscles. Dorsal and lateral to these are attached the origins of the iliocostal and iliolumbar muscles.

Coccyx

The coccyx is usually composed of four vertebral rudiments, but one fewer or one greater than this number is not uncommon. The coccyx is the vestigial representation of the tail. The first coccygeal segment is larger than the succeeding members and resembles to some extent the inferior sacral element. It has an obvious body that articulates with the homologous component of the inferior sacrum, and it bears two cornua, which may be regarded as vestiges of superior articulating processes. The three inferior coccygeal members are most frequently fused and present a curved profile continuous with that of the sacrum. They incorporate the rudiments of a body and transverse processes but possess no components of the vertebral arch.

The coccyx contributes no supportive function to the spine. It serves as an origin for the gluteus maximus posteriorly and the muscles of the pelvic diaphragm anteriorly.

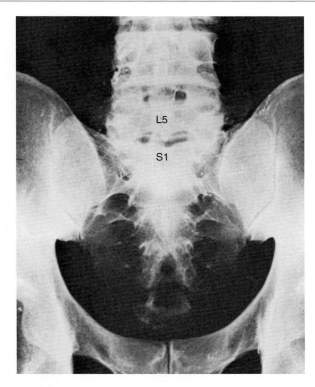

FIGURE 2–6 Anterior radiographic view of lumbosacral and sacroiliac articulations. Load transfer from the lumbar spine to the iliac bones via the costal processes of the first and second sacral segments is obvious.

Arthrology of the Spine

The articulations of the spine include the three major types of joints: synarthroses, diarthroses, and amphiarthroses (Figs. 2–7 to 2–9). The *synarthroses* are found during development and the first decade of life. The best examples are the neurocentral joints of the immature spine, which are the two unions between the centers of ossification for the two halves of the vertebral arch and that of the centrum. Until they are obliterated during the 2nd decade, they possess a thin plate cartilage between the two apposed bony surfaces. Another example is the early union between the articular processes of the sacral vertebrae, known as *ephemeral synchondroses*.

The *diarthroses* are true synovial joints, formed mostly by the facet joints and costovertebral joints, but also include the atlantoaxial and sacroiliac articulations. All the spinal diarthroses are of the arthrodial or gliding type, with the exception of the trochoid or pivot joint of the atlantodens articulation.

The *amphiarthroses* are nonsynovial, slightly movable connective tissue joints. They are of two types: the symphysis, as exemplified by the fibrocartilage of the intervertebral disc, and the syndesmosis, as represented by all the ligamentous connections between the adjacent bodies and the adjacent arches.

Articulations of the Vertebral Arches

The synovial facet joints formed by the articular processes of the vertebral arches possess a true joint capsule and are capable

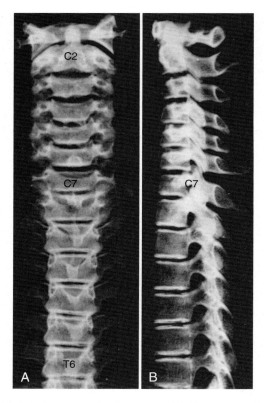

FIGURE 2–7 A, Anteroposterior radiograph of dried preparation of cervical and upper thoracic spine. Note greater relative thickness of cervical discs and more lateral disposition of cervical articular pillars. **B,** Lateral view of preceding specimen. The normal curvatures did not survive the preparation, but the gradual increase in size of the bodies and the intervertebral foramina is well illustrated.

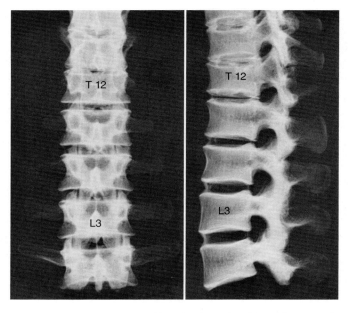

FIGURE 2–8 Anteroposterior and lateral radiographs of lower thoracic and upper lumbar region of articulated dried preparation.

of a limited gliding articulation. The capsules are thin and lax and are attached to the bases of the engaging superior and inferior articulating processes of opposing vertebrae. Because it is mostly the plane of articulation of these joints that determines the types of motion characteristic of the various regions of the spine, it would be expected that the fibers of the articular capsules would be longest and loosest in the cervical region and become increasingly taut in an inferior progression.

The syndesmoses between the vertebral arches are formed by the paired sets of ligamenta flava, the intertransverse ligaments, the interspinous ligaments, and the unpaired

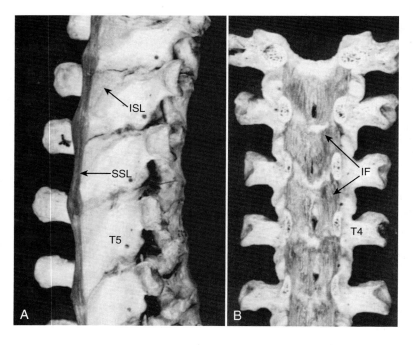

FIGURE 2–9 A, Dried preparation of thoracic vertebrae showing the supraspinous ligament (ssl) and interspinous ligaments (isl). **B,** Anterior view of upper thoracic vertebral arches showing the disposition of the ligamenta flava (lf).

supraspinous ligament. The ligamenta flava bridge the spaces between the laminae of adjacent vertebrae from the second cervical to the lumbosacral interval. The lateral extent of each half of a paired set begins around the bases of the articulating processes and can be traced medially where they nearly join in the midline. This longitudinal central deficiency serves to transmit small vessels and facilitates the passage of a needle during lumbar punctures. The fibers of the ligamenta flava are almost vertical in their disposition, but are attached to the ventral surface of the cephalad lamina and to the superior lip of the suprajacent lamina.

This shinglelike arrangement conceals the true length of the ligaments because of the overlapping of the superior lamina. Their morphology is best appreciated from the ventral aspect as in Figure 2–9B. The yellow elastic fibers that give the ligamenta flava their name maintain their elasticity even in embalmed specimens. It has been stated in some texts that the elasticity of the ligamenta flava serves to assist in the maintenance of the erect posture. A more probable reason for this property is simply to keep the ligament taut during extension, where any laxity would permit redundancy and infolding toward the ventrally related nervous structures, as occurs in degenerative lumbar spinal stenosis.

There are two separable layers of the ligamentum flavum, one superficial and one deep, that have distinct attachments to the inferior lamina.[11] The superficial component inserts at the classically described location along the posterosuperior aspect of the lamina. The deep component inserts along the anterosuperior surface of the lamina.[11] This attachment can have significance during surgical removal of the ligamentum flavum for exposure of the neural elements.

The intertransverse ligaments are fibrous connections between the transverse processes. They are difficult to distinguish from extensions of the tendinous insertions of the segmental muscles and in reality may be just that in some regions. They appear as a few tough, thin fibers between the cervical transverse processes, and in the thoracic area they blend with the intercostal ligaments. Being most distinct between the lumbar transverse processes, the intertransverse ligaments may be isolated here as membranous bands.

The interspinous ligaments (see Fig. 2–9A) are membranous sets of fibers that connect adjoining spinous processes. They are situated medial to the thin pairs of interspinal muscles that bridge the apices of the spine. The fibers of the ligaments are arranged obliquely as they connect the base of the superior spine with the superior ridge and apex of the next most inferior spinous process. These midline ligaments are found in pairs with a distinct dissectible cleft between them.

The supraspinous ligament (see Fig. 2–9A) is a continuous fibrous cord that runs along the apices of the spinous processes from the seventh cervical to the end of the sacral spinous crest. Similar to the longitudinal ligaments of the vertebra, the more superficial fibers of the ligament extend over several spinal segments, whereas the deeper, shorter fibers bridge only two or three segments. In the cervical region the supraspinous ligament assumes a distinctive character and a specific name, the ligamentum nuchae. This structure is bowstrung across the cervical lordosis from the external occipital protuberance to the spine of the seventh cervical vertebra. Its anterior border forms a sagittal fibrous sheet that divides the posterior nuchal muscles and attaches to the spinous processes of all cervical vertebrae. The ligamentum nuchae contains an abundance of elastic fibers. In quadrupeds, it forms a strong truss that supports the cantilevered position of the head.

Special Articulations

The atlanto-occipital articulation consists of the diarthrosis between the lateral masses of the atlas and the occipital condyles of the skull and the syndesmoses formed by the atlanto-occipital membranes. The articular capsules around the condyles are thin and loose and permit a gliding motion between the condylar convexity and the concavity of the lateral masses. The capsules blend laterally with ligaments that connect the transverse processes of the atlas with the jugular processes of the skull. Although the lateral ligaments and the capsules are sufficiently lax to permit nodding, they do not permit rotation.

The anterior atlanto-occipital membrane is a structural extension of the anterior longitudinal ligament that connects the forward rim of the foramen magnum, also known as the *basion*, to the anterior arch of the atlas and blends with the joint capsules laterally. It is dense, tough, and virtually cordlike in its central portion.

The posterior atlanto-occipital membrane is homologous to the ligamenta flava and unites the posterior arch of the atlas. It is deficient laterally where it arches over the groove on the superior surface of the arch. Through this aperture, the vertebral artery enters the neural canal to penetrate the dura. Occasionally, the free edge of this membrane is ossified to form a true bony foramen (called the *ponticulus posticus*) around the artery.

The median atlantoaxial articulation is a pivot (trochoid) joint (Figs. 2–10 and 2–11). The essential features of the articulation are the odontoid process (dens) of the axis and the internal surface of the anterior arch of the atlas. The opposition of the two bones is maintained by the thick, straplike transverse atlantal ligament. The ligament and the arch of the atlas have true synovial cavities intervening between them and the odontoid process. Alar expansions of the transverse ligament attach to tubercles on the lateral rims of the anterior foramen magnum, and a single, unpaired cord, the apical odontoid ligament, attaches the apex of the process to the basion. The entire joint is covered posteriorly by a cranial extension of the posterior longitudinal ligament, which is named *tectorial membrane* in this region. Because the atlas freely glides over the superior articulating facets of C2, the atlantoaxial pivot is essential for preventing horizontal displacements between C1 and C2. Fracture of the odontoid or, less likely, rupture of the transverse ligament produces a very unstable articulation.

Articulations of the Vertebral Bodies

The vertebral bodies are connected by the two forms of amphiarthroses. Symphyses are represented by the intervertebral

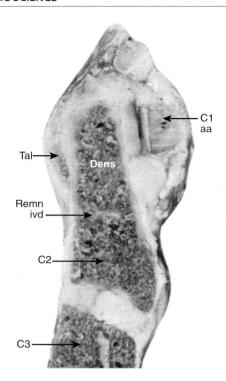

FIGURE 2–10 Sagittal section through adult odontoid process showing articular relationships with anterior arch of the atlas (aa) and transverse atlantal ligament (tal). Despite the fact this patient was older than 50 years, a cartilaginous remnant of the homologue of an intervertebral disc may be discerned. Radiologically, this might be confused with fracture or a nonunion status.

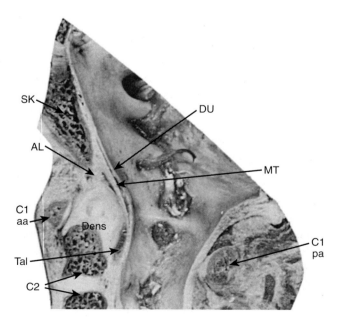

FIGURE 2–11 Sagittal section through atlanto-occipital articulation of a 4-year-old child. The major ossification centers of the odontoid process are still separated from the body of C2 by a well-differentiated disc. The cartilaginous apex of the process shows a condensation marking the apical ossific center. C1 aa and C1 pa mark the anterior and posterior atlantal arches. The dura (du) overlies the membrana tectoria (mt), which is a superior extension of the posterior longitudinal ligament. The transverse atlantal ligament (tal) and apical ligament (al) are also indicated.

discs, and syndesmoses are formed by the anterior and posterior longitudinal ligaments.

Intervertebral Disc

In view of the semiliquid nature of the nucleus pulposus and the vacuities that may be shown in the nucleus of aging specimens, von Luschka[12] attempted to classify the intervertebral disc as a diarthrosis, in which the vertebral chondral plates were the articular cartilages, the anulus provided the articular capsule, and the fluid and ephemeral spaces within the nucleus corresponded to the synovia and the joint cavity. Although the intervertebral disc forms a joint that should be classified in its own exclusive category because its development, structure, and function are generally different from those of any other joint, it most closely conforms to an amphiarthrosis of the symphysis type.

The intervertebral disc is the fibrocartilaginous complex that forms the articulation between the bodies of the vertebrae. Although it provides a very strong union, ensuring the degree of intervertebral fixation that is necessary for effective action and the protective alignment of the neural canal, the summation of the limited movements allowed by each disc imparts to the spinal column as a whole its characteristic mobility. The discs of the various spinal regions may differ considerably in size and in some detail, but they are basically identical in their structural organization. Each consists of two components: the internal semifluid mass, called the *nucleus pulposus,* and its laminar fibrous container, known as the *anulus fibrosus.*

Nucleus Pulposus

Typically, the nucleus pulposus occupies an eccentric position within the confines of the anulus, usually being closer to the posterior margin of the disc. Its most essential character becomes obvious in either transverse or sagittal preparations of the disc in which, as evidence of internal pressure, it bulges beyond the plane of section. Palpation of a dissected nucleus from a young adult shows that it responds as a viscid fluid under applied pressure, but it also exhibits considerable elastic rebound and assumes its original physical state on release. These properties may still be shown in the spine of a cadaver that has been embalmed for many months.

Histologic analysis provides a partial explanation for the characteristics of the nucleus. As the definitive remnant of the embryonic notochord, it is similarly composed of loose, delicate fibrous strands embedded in a gelatinous matrix. In the center of the mass, these fibers show no geometric preference in their arrangement but form a felted mesh of undulating bundles. Only the fibers that are in approximation to the vertebral chondral plates display a definite orientation. These approach the cartilage at an angle and become embedded in its substance to afford an attachment for the nucleus. Numerous cells are suspended in the fibrous network. Many of these are fusiform and resemble typical reticulocytes, but vacuolar and darkly nucleated chondrocytes are also interspersed in the matrix. Even in the absence of vascular elements, the profusion of cells should accentuate the fact that the nucleus pulposus is composed of vital tissue. There is no definite structural interface between the nucleus and the anulus. Rather, the composition of the two tissues blends imperceptibly.

Anulus Fibrosus

The anulus is a concentric series of fibrous lamellae that encase the nucleus and strongly unite the vertebral bodies (Fig. 2–12). The essential function of the nucleus is to resist and redistribute compressive forces within the spine, whereas one of the major functions of the anulus is to withstand tension, whether the tensile forces be from the horizontal extensions of the compressed nucleus, from the torsional stress of the column, or from the separation of the vertebral bodies on the convex side of a spinal flexure. Without optical aid, simple dissection and discernment reveals how well the anulus is constructed for the performance of this function.

On horizontal section, it is noted that an individual lamella encircling the disc is composed of glistening fibers that run an oblique or spiral course in relation to the axis of the vertebral column. Because the disc presents a kidney-shaped or heart-shaped horizontal section, and the nucleus is displaced posteriorly, these lamellae are thinner and more closely packed between the nucleus and the dorsal aspect of the disc. The bands are stoutest and individually more distinct in the anterior third of the disc, and here when transected they may give the impression that they are of varying composition because every other ring presents a difference in color and elevation with reference to the plane of section. Teasing and inspection at an oblique angle shows in the freed lamellae, however, that this difference is due to an abrupt change in the direction of the fibers of adjacent rings. Previous descriptions of the anulus have claimed that the alternating appearance of the banding is the result of the interposition of a chondrous layer between each fibrous ring.[13] In reality, the alternations of glistening white lamellae with translucent rings result from differences in the incidence of light with regard to the direction of the fiber bundles. This repeated reversal of fiber arrangement within the anulus has implications in the biomechanics of the disc, which are discussed later.

The disposition of the lamellae on sagittal section is not consistently vertical. In the regions of the anulus approximating the nucleus pulposus, the first distinct bands curve inward, with their convexity facing the nuclear substance. As one follows the successive layers outward, a true vertical profile is assumed, but as the external laminae of the disc are approached, they may again become bowed, with their convexity facing the periphery of the disc.[14,15]

The attachment of the anulus to its respective vertebral bodies warrants particular mention. This attachment is best understood when a dried preparation of a thoracic or lumbar vertebra is examined first. In the adult, the articular surface of the body presents two aspects: a concave central depression that is quite porous and an elevated ring of compact bone that appears to be rolled over the edge of the vertebral body. Often a demarcating fissure falsely suggests that the ring is a true epiphysis of the body, but postnatal studies of ossification have

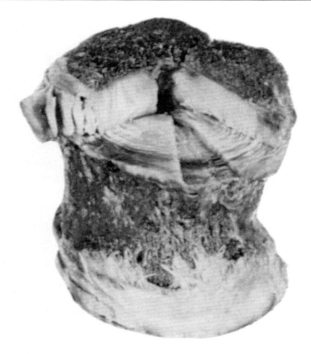

FIGURE 2–12 Photograph of dissected third lumbar disc. Lamellar bands are still visible when the section is cut deep into bony apophyseal ring. A layer of spongiosa was left attached to the superior surface of the disc to show that only a thin chondral plate intervenes between the vascular trabeculae and the disc. The inward buckling of the lamellae near the cavity of the extirpated nuclear material is well shown. The specimen is from a 52-year-old man.

indicated that it is a traction apophysis for the attachment of the anulus and associated longitudinal ligaments.[16]

In life, the depth of the central concavity is filled to the level of the marginal ring by the presence of a cribriform cartilaginous plate. In contrast to other articular surfaces, there is no closing plate of compact osseous material intervening between this cartilage and the cancellous medullary part of the bone. The trabeculations of the spongiosa blend into the internal face of the chondrous plate, whereas fibers from the nucleus and inner lamellae of the anulus penetrate its outer surface. As intimate as this union between the central disc and vertebra may appear, the outer bony ring affords the disc its firmest attachment because the stoutest external lamellar bands of fibers actually penetrate the ring as Sharpey fibers. Scraping the disc to the bone shows the concentric arrangements reflecting the different angles at which the fibers insert (see Fig. 2–12). The fibers of the outermost ring of the anulus have the most extensive range of attachment. They extend beyond the confines of the disc and blend with the vertebral periosteum and the longitudinal ligaments.

Regional Variations of the Disc

The discs in aggregate make up approximately one fourth of the length of the spinal column, exclusive of the sacrum and coccyx. Their degree of contribution is not uniform in the various regions. According to Aeby,[17] the discs provide more than one fifth of the length of the cervical spine, approximately

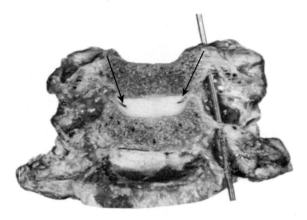

FIGURE 2–13 Frontal section through fourth to fifth cervical vertebrae showing typical cervical disc and its joints of Luschka (*arrows*). A probe has been passed through the vertebral arterial canal to show its relationships to the uncovertebral joints.

one fifth of the length of the thoracic column, and approximately one third of the length of the lumbar region.

The discs are smallest in the cervical spine. Their lateral extent is less than that of the corresponding vertebral body because of the uncinate processes (Fig. 2–13). Here, as in the lumbar region, they are wedge-shaped, the greatest width being anterior, producing lordosis. The thoracic discs are heart-shaped on section, with the nucleus pulposus being more centrally located than in the lumbar region. The thickness and the horizontal dimensions of the thoracic disc increase caudad with the corresponding increase in size of the

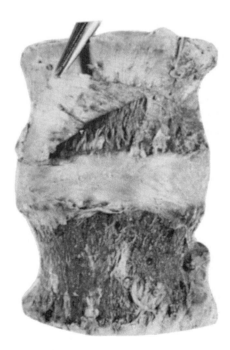

FIGURE 2–14 Bodies of third and fourth lumbar vertebrae from a 58-year-old man. The spiral course of fibers of the outer lamellae is evident. The periosteal attachment of the reflected anterior longitudinal ligament is well shown, in addition to the delineation of the loosely attached area raised from the surface of the disc.

vertebral bodies. The normal thoracic kyphosis results from a disparity between the anterior and posterior heights of the vertebral bodies because the discs are of uniform thickness. The lumbar discs are reniform and are relatively and absolutely the thickest in the spine. The progressive caudal increase in the degree of lumbar lordosis is due to the equivalent increase in the differential between the anterior and posterior thickness of the disc.

The cervical intervertebral discs have been a source of controversy because of the so-called joints of Luschka, or uncovertebral joints. These articular modifications are found on both sides of the cervical discs as oblique, cleftlike cavities between the superior surfaces of the uncinate processes and the corresponding lateral lips of the interior articular surface of the next superior vertebra. Because they initially appear in the latter part of the first decade and are not universally demonstrable in all cervical spines, or even in all subaxial discs of the same cervical spine, it is preferable to call them "accommodative joints" that have developed in response to the shearing stresses of the torsions of cervical mobility (see Fig. 2–13).

Spinal Ligaments

Anterior Longitudinal Ligament

The anterior longitudinal ligament is a strong band of fibers that extends along the ventral surface of the spine from the skull to the sacrum. It is narrowest and cordlike in the upper cervical region, where it is attached to the atlas and axis and their intervening capsular membranes. It widens as it descends the column to the extent, in the lower lumbar region, of covering most of the anterolateral surfaces of the vertebral bodies and discs before it blends into the presacral fibers. The anterior longitudinal ligament is not uniform in its composition or manner of attachment. Its deepest fibers, which span only one intervertebral level, are covered by an intermediate layer that unites two or three vertebrae and a superficial stratum that may connect four or five levels. Where the ligament is adherent to the anterior surface of the vertebra, it also forms its periosteum. It is most firmly attached to the articular lip at the end of each body. It is most readily elevated at the point of its passage over the midsection of the discs, where it is loosely attached to the connective tissue band that encircles the anulus (Fig. 2–14).

Posterior Longitudinal Ligament

The posterior longitudinal ligament differs considerably from its anterior counterpart with respect to the clinical significance of its relationships to the intervertebral disc. Similar to the anterior ligament, it extends from the skull to the sacrum, but it is within the vertebral canal. Its central fiber bundles diminish in breadth as the size of the spinal column increases. The segmental denticulate configuration of the posterior longitudinal ligament is one of its most characteristic features.

Between the pedicles, particularly in the lower thoracic and lumbar regions, it forms a thick band of connective tissue that is not adherent to the posterior surface of the vertebral body. Instead, it is bowstrung across the concavity of the dorsum of the body. The large vascular elements enter and leave the medullary sinus located beneath its fibers.

In approximating the dorsum of the disc, the posterior longitudinal ligament displays two strata of fibers. The superficial, longer strands form a distinct strong strap whose filaments bridge several vertebral elements. A second, deeper stratum spans only two vertebral articulations and forms lateral curving extensions of fibers that pass along the dorsum of the disc and out through the intervertebral foramen. These deeper intervertebral expansions of the ligament have the most significant relationship with the disc.

These fibers are most firmly fixed at the margins of their lateral expansions. This produces a central rhomboidal area of loose attachment, or in some cases an actual fascial cleft of equivalent dimensions, on the dorsolateral aspect of the disc. At dissection, this characteristic may be readily shown by inserting a blunt probe beneath the intervertebral part of the longitudinal ligament and exploring the area to define the margins of the space where the fibers are strongly inserted (Fig. 2–15). This situation is particularly pertinent to problems involving dorsal or dorsolateral prolapse of the nucleus pulposus. With a dorsocentral protrusion of a semifluid mass, the strong midline strap of posterior longitudinal fibers tends to restrain the herniation. If an easily dissectible cleft offers a space for lateral expansion, however, the mass can extend to either side, dissecting the loose attachments.

Trabeculations of connective tissue bind the dura to the dorsal surface of the posterior longitudinal ligament. This attachment is firmest along the lateral edges. Numerous venous cross connections of the epidural sinuses pass between the dura and the ligament. The venous elements are the most ubiquitous structures among the components related to the vertebral articulations.

Although not frequently included in anatomic discussions of the spine, an additional structure travels deep to the posterior longitudinal ligament, extending laterally and posteriorly to surround the dura of the cauda equina. It has been termed the *peridural membrane*, first by Dommissee in 1975[18] and later by Wiltse.[19] The basivertebral veins cross the peridural membrane because it offers no obstruction to vascular communication between the intraosseous vessels of the vertebral body and the epidural space. Its possible clinical significance is that it may provide a containing membrane for herniated discs or hematomas, which may be noted on advanced imaging such as computed tomography (CT) or magnetic resonance imaging (MRI) as a delimiting barrier to the pathology.

Relationships of the Roots of the Spinal Nerves

The dorsal and ventral nerve roots pass through the subarachnoid space and converge to form the spinal nerve at approximately the level of its respective intervertebral foramen. Owing

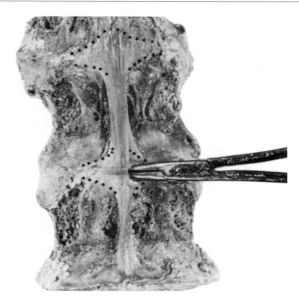

FIGURE 2–15 Photographic illustration of posterior longitudinal ligament traversing the bodies of third and fourth lumbar vertebrae. The central strap of long fibers can be seen passing over the hemostat. The lines of strong attachment of the fibers at the lateral expansions are indicated by the *black dots* as they outline the rhomboid area, where the fibers are readily dissected from the dorsal surface of the disc. In this case, the instrument was inserted into an actual fascial cleft, and the points show the weakest area of the lateral expansion.

to the ascensus spinalis—the apparent cranial migration of the distal end of the spinal cord during development that actually arises from differential growth of the lower parts of the vertebral column—the course of the nerve roots becomes longer and more obliquely directed in the lower lumbar segments. In the cervical region, the nerve root and the spinal nerve are posteriorly related to the same corresponding intervertebral disc; in other words, the nerve root exits the spinal canal at the same level it branches from the spinal cord.

In the lumbar region, a different situation prevails. The nerve roots contributing to the cauda equina travel an almost vertical course over the dorsum of one intervertebral disc to exit with the spinal nerve of the foramen one segment lower. In the cervical and lumbar regions, dorsal or dorsolateral (i.e., paracentral) protrusions of disc material affect the descending rather than exiting nerve root. When the meningeal coverings (dura) blend with the epineurium, the nerve components become extrathecal. The actual point of this transition is variable but usually occurs in relation to the distal aspect of the dorsal root ganglion.

The nerve root is intimately related to the pedicle of the vertebra. Ugur and colleagues[20] found no distance between the upper cervical pedicles and their corresponding nerve roots in 20 cadaveric spines, whereas there was a slight distance in 4 of the 20 specimens in the lower cervical region. For all specimens, the distance from the nerve root to the inferior aspect of the upper pedicle ranged from 1 to 2.5 mm. The distance from the medial aspect of the pedicle to the dural sac ranged from 2.4 to 3.1 mm. A similar relationship between the thoracic nerve roots and pedicle exists.[21] The distance from

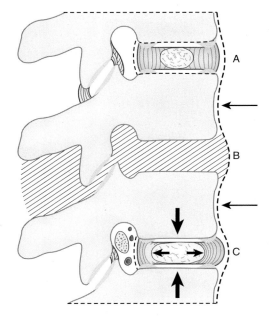

FIGURE 2–16 Schematic representation showing three aspects of the relational anatomy of the disc. **A** shows the topographic arrangement of the normal disc with the apophyseal ring and perforated chondral plate in relation to the nucleus pulposus and the anulus. **B** indicates, in the *cross-hatched area,* the inclusions of the motor segment as originally described by Junghanns. *Arrows* define the limits of the motor segment proposed here. **C** indicates the dissipation by the lateral thrust in a compressed disc. Related anatomy of the intervertebral foramen is also indicated. The two structures passing ventral to the spinal nerve are the sinuvertebral nerve and the artery. The other vessels are veins.

the pedicle to the superior nerve root in the thoracic spine ranges from 1.5 to 6.7 mm, and the distance from the pedicle to the inferior nerve root, 0.8 to 6 mm. Ebraheim and colleagues[22] measured these distances in the lumbar spine, finding a mean distance of 1.5 mm from the pedicle to the inferior nerve root, 5.3 mm from the pedicle to the superior nerve root, and 1.5 mm from the medial pedicle wall to the dura.

Of particular interest is the distribution of epidural fat around and within the intervertebral foramen. This fat has a firm character and forms a mechanically supportive "bushing" for structures entering and leaving the spinal canal. A prominent extension of this fat body also follows the inferior and ventral surfaces of each lumbar nerve. It is interposed between the root and the external surfaces of the pedicle and vertebral body that define the inferior part of the intervertebral foramen. Its amelioration of the downward and ventral distraction of the nerve that accompanies the spine and lower limb motions is obvious. Histologically, it is composed of uniform cells that are contained within a fine membrane (perhaps the elusive peridural membrane).[23] There is no fibrous tissue in normal epidural fat and only tenuous attachments to the dura.

Intervertebral Foramen

The intervertebral foramen is the aperture that gives exit to the segmental spinal nerves and entrance to the vessels and nerve branches that supply the bone and soft tissues of the vertebral canal. It is superiorly and inferiorly bounded by the respective pedicles of the adjacent vertebrae. Its ventral and dorsal components involve the two major intervertebral articulations. The dorsum of the intervertebral disc, covered by the lateral expansion of the posterior longitudinal ligament, provides a large part of its ventral boundary, whereas the joint capsule of the articular facets and the ligamentum flavum contribute the major parts of its dorsal limitation. Along with the root, the remaining space is filled with loose areolar tissue and fat (Fig. 2–16).

However ample the overall dimensions of the intervertebral foramen may be, its elliptical nature is responsible for many of its relational problems. In the lumbar region, the vertical diameter of the foramen ranges from 12 to 19 mm; this undoubtedly accounts for the fact that a complete collapse of the disc may produce little or no evidence of nerve compression. The sagittal diameter may be only 7 mm, however, making this dimension exquisitely sensitive to changes. Because the diameter of the fourth lumbar nerve can be just slightly less than 7 mm, the tolerance for pathologic alteration of the bony or connective tissue relationships is restricted.[24]

The existence of additional ligamentous elements in relation to the intervertebral foramen could limit further the space for the exiting spinal nerve. These structures, known as the *transforaminal ligaments,* are frequently found in the lumbar region.[25,26] The transforaminal ligaments are strong, unyielding cords of fibrous tissue that pass anteriorly from various parts of the neural arch to the body of the same or the adjacent vertebra and may be 5 mm wide. Grimes and colleagues[27] found these ligaments span from the nerve root itself. These investigators noted four different bands, the most significant of which spread from the nerve root to the anterior aspect of the facet capsule. Other bands spanned from the nerve root to the superior pedicle, the inferior pedicle, and the intervertebral disc anteriorly.

In the cervical spine, the space available for the exiting nerve root may be compromised by structures just lateral to the foramen. In 10 adult human cadaveric specimens, Alleyne and colleagues[28] found the dorsal root ganglia of the C3 to C6 spinal nerves to be slightly compressed by the ascending vertebral artery. This compression was most pronounced at the C5 level, which the authors suggested as a possible explanation for the greater susceptibility of this nerve to iatrogenic injury during procedures such as laminoplasty.

Lumbosacral Nerve Root Variations

Numerous anatomic variations in the relationships of the lumbosacral nerve roots can exist. These variations may help explain seemingly anatomically inconsistent neurologic findings with compressive disorders such as herniated discs or lateral stenosis.

The most common variation involves atypical origins, or foraminal exits, of individual lumbosacral roots. Although myelographic studies indicated only a 4% incidence of lumbosacral root anomalies, an anatomic study by Kadish and

Simmons[29] reported an incidence of 14%. The L5-S1 level is the most commonly involved. Observations by these authors provided four types of variations: (1) intradural interconnections between roots at different levels, (2) anomalous levels of origin of nerve roots, (3) extradural connections between roots, and (4) extradural division of nerve roots.

A source of confusing neurologic findings may relate to the variant anatomy of the furcal nerve. The name *furcal nerve* has been applied to the fourth lumbar nerve because it exhibits a prominent bifurcation to contribute to the lumbar plexus (femoral and obturator nerves) and sacral plexus (lumbosacral trunk). Kikuchi and Hasue[30] found that it is often indefinite in its intradural affinities, frequently exhibiting two dorsal root ganglia that have distinct root sources at the conus medullaris. They proposed that when symptoms indicate the involvement of two levels, suspicion should be directed toward four possible causes: (1) two roots compressed by a single lesion, (2) the presence of two lesions, (3) the anomalous emergence of two roots through the same foramen, or (4) the existence of the peculiarly doubled components of the furcal nerve (Fig. 2-17).

Infrequently, variant "fixation" alters the expected sequences of nerve root exit. In a *prefixed* lumbosacral plexus, the furcal nerve (the division between the lumbar and sacral plexuses) exits through the third lumbar foramen, and the preceding and subsequent nerves exit one vertebral level higher than in the conventional distribution. Conversely, in the *postfixed* plexus, the furcal nerve exits the L5-S1 foramen, and the lumbosacral nerve sequence is all one level lower than usually described.[31]

Although Kadish and Simmons[29] noted that the existence of anomalous interconnections between nerve root levels dispels any notion of "absolute innervation," Parke and Watanabe[32] showed that there is a consistent system of intersegmental connections between the roots of the lumbosacral nerves. They described an epispinal system of motor axons that courses among the meningeal fibers of the conus medullaris and virtually ensheathes its ventral and lateral funiculi between the L2 and S2 levels. These nerve fibers apparently arise from motor neuron cells of the ventral horn gray matter

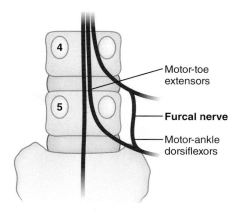

FIGURE 2-17 Schematic representation showing cross connection L4 and L5 nerve roots (spinal nerves) in the extraforaminal region through the furcal nerve. (Adapted from McCulloch JA, Young PH: Essentials of Spinal Microsurgery. Philadelphia, Lippincott-Raven, 1998, p 390.)

and join spinal nerve roots caudal to their level of origin. In all the spinal cords studied, many of these axons commingled at the cord surface to form an irregular group of ectopic rootlets that could be visually traced to join conventional spinal nerve roots at one to several segments inferior to their original segmental level (Figs. 2-18 and 2-19). Occasionally, these ventral ectopic rootlets course dorsocaudad to join a dorsal (sensory) nerve root. Although the function and the clinical significance of this epispinal system of axons have yet to be explained, a given segmental level of motor nerve cells may contribute fibers not only to an adjacent segment, but also to nerve roots of multiple inferior levels.

An additional variant aspect of the lumbosacral nerve roots concerns the relative location of their dorsal root ganglia. Almost all anatomic illustrations depict the lumbosacral dorsal root ganglia in an intraforaminal position, the central part of the ganglion lying between the adjacent pedicles. Hasue and colleagues[33,34] found, however, that the lumbosacral dorsal root ganglia may also be positioned internal or external to their foramina. They designated the internal positions as *subarticular* or *sublaminar,* depending on their relationship to

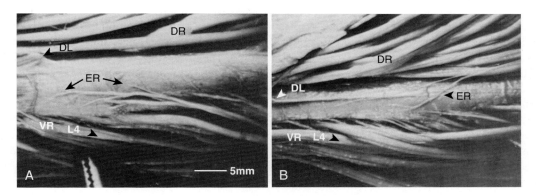

FIGURE 2-18 A, Lateral surface of human conus medullaris showing ectopic rootlets (ER) that receive axons from cells in the ventral horn nuclei. Note origin of some fibers at the level of L4 motor nuclei extends caudad to join S1 root. **B,** Photomicrograph showing ER passing posteriorly to join a dorsal (sensory) nerve root (DR). DL indicates last denticulum of denticulate ligament.

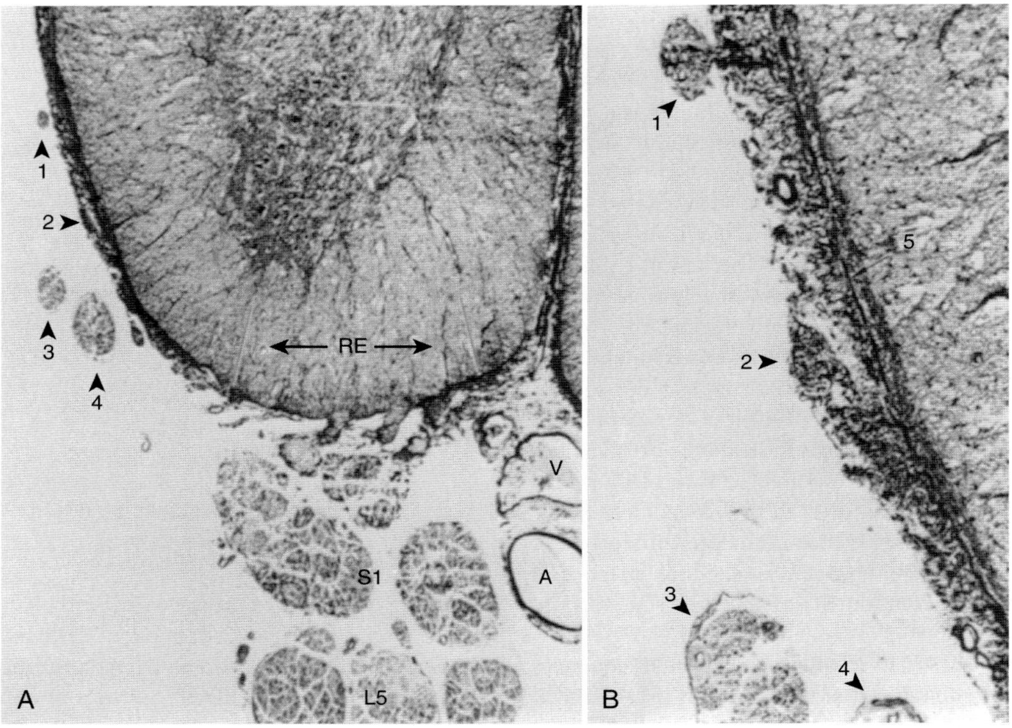

FIGURE 2–19 Photomicrographs of a 5-μm cross section from the conus medullaris at S1 level showing ectopic rootlets in various stages characteristic of their emergence from the ventrolateral surface of the cord. **A,** Rootlets just appearing on the pial surface (*1, 2*) eventually join free rootlets (*3, 4*) that have originated from higher levels. The conventional roots of L5 and S1 nerves have emerged from the typical zone of rootlet emergence (RE). A and V, Anterior spinal artery and vein. **B,** Higher power photomicrograph of preceding section shows greater detail of rootlet emergence. The entire ventrolateral pia is intertwined with epispinal axons, of which only a few form ectopic rootlets. Dense circular band of pial straps (*5*) is characteristic of the region of the epispinal fibers. (**A,** ×33; **B,** ×133.) (From Parke WW, Watanabe R: Lumbosacral intersegmental epispinal axons and ectopic ventral nerve rootlets. J Neurosurg 67:269-277, 1967.)

Innervation of the Spine

The distribution of the medial branches of the dorsal ramus of the spinal nerve to the external periosteum, facet joints, and ligamentous connections of the neural arches (and the general ramification of the "recurrent" sinuvertebral nerve, known as the nerve of Luschka or *ramus meningeus,* to structures related to the spinal canal) has been known for more than a century. The recognition that degenerative disease of the intervertebral disc and its consequences is a major cause of low back pain has stimulated more inquiries, however.

Many investigations have attempted to delineate the origins, terminal ramifications, and nerve ending types of the sinuvertebral nerve, often with contradictory results. More comprehensive works[15,35-42] have agreed on the general source and composition of this nerve and have described it as variously branching from the distal pole of the dorsal root ganglion, the initial part of the spinal nerve, or the dorsal sections of the rami communicantes. It was recognized that a multiple origin is common, especially in the lumbar region, and small autonomic branches often have a separate course, entering the intervertebral foramen independently. The extent and complexity of the relationships of the sinuvertebral nerve within the spinal canal have engendered much argument, however, particularly concerning the segmental range of the individual nerve ramifications.

In illustrations based on dissections, Bogduk and colleagues[35] and Parke[43] agreed that each nerve supplies two intervertebral discs via superiorly and inferiorly directed branches—the inferiorly directed branch ramifying over the dorsum of the disc at the level of entry and the longer, superiorly directed branch coursing along the edge of the posterior longitudinal ligament to reach the disc of the next superior level (Fig. 2–20). Dissections identify mainly the larger ramifications. Smaller fibers are usually localized with staining techniques. Conventional methods of staining using silver or lipotrophic stains have given controversial results, however, because of a lack of specificity.

Groen and colleagues,[44] using a highly specific acetylcholinesterase staining method on large cleared sections of fetal human spines, resolved many conflicts concerning the

these structures roofing the spinal canal, and found that approximately one third of the L4 and L5 ganglia are in the subarticular position. If the ganglion is subarticular, it is in the lateral recess and subject to the direct consequences of a lateral stenosis.

ramifications of the nerves supplying spinal structures. They found that, in contrast to most previous reports, the human sinuvertebral nerves were almost exclusively derivatives of the rami communicantes close to their connections with the spinal nerves. These origins were fairly consistent throughout the length of the thoracolumbar sympathetic trunk, but in the cervical region they were also derived from the perivascular plexus of the vertebral artery.

Five sinuvertebral nerves have been observed passing into one intervertebral foramen. Typically, the group consists of one thick nerve (perhaps the one seen in most conventional dissections) and several fine fibers. The thick, or predominant, sinuvertebral nerve is often absent, however, in the upper cervical and sacral regions. The major sinuvertebral element enters the foramen ventral to the spinal ganglion and gives off some fine branches at this point. As the nerve enters the spinal canal, the major branch usually divides into rami that course in approximation to the distribution of the posterior central branches of the segmental artery, with a long ascending element and a shorter descending one. From these branches, one to three coiled rami supply the ventral dura.

The acetylcholinesterase technique used by Groen and colleagues[44] made it possible to delineate details of the plexus of the posterior longitudinal ligament. The work of these authors supports the idea that the posterior longitudinal ligament is highly innervated by an irregular plexiform distribution of fibers that have a greater density in the ligament expansions dorsal to the discs. These authors were able to note the primary direction, length, and "termination area" of the branches of a single segmental sinuvertebral nerve. They classified the variations of individual nerves as follows: (1) ascending one segment, (2) descending one segment, (3) dichotomizing toward one segment caudal and one segment cranial or horizontal, (4) ascending two or more segments, and (5) descending two or more segments (see Fig. 2–20). The existence of the latter two categories, although they are not as common as the others, shows that the sinuvertebral nerve can supply more than two adjacent segmental levels. A basis for the poor pain localization of an offending disc may be related to the generous distribution possible in the individual sinuvertebral nerve. The large totomounts treated with acetylcholinesterase also showed that the patterns of sinuvertebral nerve distribution to the posterior longitudinal ligament did not display significant regional variations apart from an expected pronounced diminution in the plexus density in the immovable lower sacral region.

The posterior longitudinal ligament is highly innervated with complex encapsulated nerve endings and numerous low-myelinated free nerve endings (Fig. 2–21). The lateral expansion of the posterior longitudinal ligament extends through the intervertebral foramen covering all the dorsal and most of the dorsolateral aspects of the disc. The elevation of this thin, highly innervated strap of connective tissue may provide a significant component of the pain manifest in acute disc protrusions.

The probable range of diverse functions of the sinuvertebral nerve may be indicated by the analysis of its cross-sectional composition. Stained preparations taken from a section near

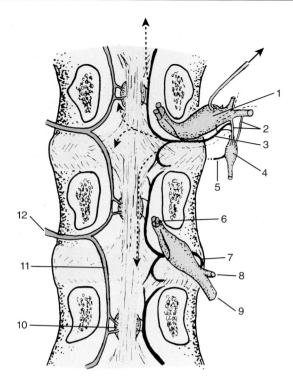

FIGURE 2–20 Schema of major intraspinal distribution of dorsal central branches of segmental vertebromedullary arteries and distribution and source of the sinuvertebral nerves. The pattern of the nerve shown entering the superior foramen is derived from the data provided by Groen and colleagues.[44] *Dotted lines* show a composite of the variant ranges (*arrows* indicate two or more segments) and ramifications tabulated by these authors. The nerve entering the inferior foramen shows the extent and distribution described in previous reports.

1. dorsal root ganglion
2. rami communicantes
3. sinuvertebral nerve and its origin according to Groen and colleagues
4. autonomic ganglion
5. nerve to anterior longitudinal ligament
6. spinal nerve roots
7. sinuvertebral nerve arising from distal pole of ganglion (thought to be its most common source before report of Groen and colleagues)
8. dorsal primary ramus of spinal nerve
9. ventral primary ramus of spinal nerve
10. arteries entering basivertebral sinus to supply cancellous bone
11. descending dorsal central branch of vertebromedullary (spinal) artery
12. ventral branch of vertebromedullary artery

the nerve origin show many small myelinated fibers, although some myelin sheaths are greater than 10 μm in diameter.[45] Many of the smaller fibers are postganglionic efferents from the thoracolumbar autonomic ganglia that mediate the smooth muscle control of the various vascular elements within the spinal canal, and many of the larger fibers are involved in proprioceptive functions. Concerning the latter, Hirsch and colleagues[37,46] found numerous complex encapsulated nerve endings in the posterior longitudinal ligament (see Fig. 2–21B). It is assumed that these may be associated with the larger myelinated fibers whose postganglionic axons enter the cord to mediate postural reflexes because similar fibers in the cervical region of cats have been shown to be important in tonic neck reflexes.[47] It seems, however, that the smaller

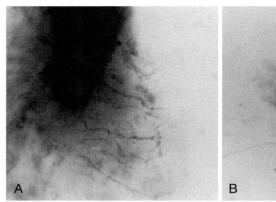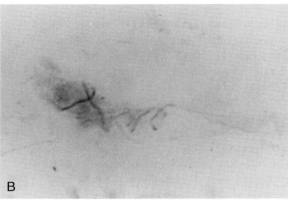

FIGURE 2–21 Photomicrographs of nerve endings in posterior longitudinal ligament of a dog. **A,** Section of ligament dorsal to a lumbar intervertebral disc. The dark area is the central strap of the ligament, and the light area is the thin lateral expansion over the dorsum of the disc. These fine nerve endings are characteristic of those in known nociceptors. **B,** Complex nerve ending from posterior longitudinal ligament. This type of ending is believed to be a transducer of mechanical deformation for postural senses. (Methylene blue vital tissue stain: **A,** ×300; **B,** ×500.)

fibers making up the bulk of the sinuvertebral nerve are afferents, associated with simple, nonencapsulated, or "free" nerve endings that are generally regarded as nociceptive (see Fig. 2–21A).

The fact that the sinuvertebral nerve carries pain fibers has been amply shown by clinical and laboratory experimentation. Direct stimulation of tissues known to be served by the nerve elicits back pain in humans. Pedersen and colleagues[45] showed that stimulation of these tissues in decerebrate cats resulted in blood pressure and respiratory changes similar to those elicited by noxious stimuli to known pain receptors in other areas of the body.

Disagreement exists over whether the anulus itself is innervated and, if so, how extensively. The classic work of Hirsch and colleagues[46] claimed that nerve endings are only in the dorsal aspect of the most superficial layer of the anulus, and these presumably are from branches of the same nerve fibers that innervate the overlying expansions of the posterior longitudinal ligament.

Pedersen and colleagues,[45] Stilwell,[48] and Parke[43] have failed to show nerve endings in the anulus. Because the connective tissue structures intimately related to the disc show a profusion of nerve endings, Parke[43] assumed that their disruption could account for discogenic pain. Inappropriate methodology may account for the failure to show intradiscal nerves. Malinsky,[40] Bogduk and colleagues,[35,36] and Yoshizawa and colleagues[49] published accounts showing nerve fibers in the outer lamina of the anulus. This work has now been supported by the highly specific acetylcholinesterase method of Groen and colleagues.[44]

Most descriptions of the sinuvertebral nerve indicate that the major meningeal fibers to the spinal dura are distributed to its ventral surface.[50] The median dorsal dural surface has been regarded as virtually free of nerve fibers, a convenience that permits its painless penetration during needle puncture. Although Cyriax[51] claimed that irritation of the ventral dura during protrusion of the nucleus may contribute to discogenic pain, a sufficient distortion of the nerve fibers on the movable or unattached dura does not seem likely. The coiled configuration of these dural contributions of the sinuvertebral nerve, noted by Groen and colleagues,[52] may indicate a compensation to permit a degree of dural movement without placing traction on these nerves.

Parke and Watanabe[53] observed that the ventral lower lumbar dura is often fixed to the ventral canal surface by numerous connective tissue fibers, most firmly fixed at the margins of the lower lumbar discs. These apparently acquired adhesions are not to be confused with the ligaments of Hofmann, which are normal straps of tissue connecting the dura to the ventral canal surface that have been obliquely positioned by the developmental cranial traction of the dura and its contents. This observation has been supported by a series of dissections by Blikra,[54] who was seeking a rationale for lower lumbar intradural disc protrusions. His analysis showed that in some cases the dura may be sufficiently fixed to the ventral surface of the canal, particularly at the L4-5 level, for protruding nucleus material to rupture the ventral dura. Parke and Watanabe,[53] by microscopic analysis of sections of the dura that had been forcibly freed from these adhesions overlying the fourth or fifth lumbar disc, showed disruption of the nerve fibers bound in the adhesion. In the numerous cases in which such adhesions are present, the forceful elevation of the dura by a disc protrusion may provide an adjunctive source of the discogenic pain.

Spinal Motion Segment

The inclusion of all articular tissue, the overlying spinal muscles, and the segmental contents of the vertebral canal and intervertebral foramen into a single functional and anatomic unit was first suggested by Junghanns.[55,56] Originally called the "motor" segment, this unit represents a useful concept that stresses the developmental and topographic interdependence between the fibrous structures that surround the intervertebral foramen and the functioning of the structures that pass through it. Although the 23 or 24 individual motion segments must be considered in relation to the spinal column as a whole, no congenital or acquired disorder of a single major component of a unit can exist without affecting first the functions of the other components of the same unit and then the functions of other levels of the spine.

Although Junghanns[55] defined the unit primarily in terms of the movable structures making up the intervertebral articulations, a logical, if not necessary, extension of the motion segment concept should include some aspect of the vertebral elements. DePalma and Rothman[57] included both adjacent vertebrae in their illustration of the unit, but one of us believed that the unit concept would be improved by incorporating only the opposing superior and inferior halves of each vertebra, eliminating redundancy (see Fig. 2–16). In visualizing the motion segment unit as a musculoskeletal complex surrounding a corresponding level of nervous structures, it must be realized that the intervertebral disc and the facets are but two of the articulations involved. The interosseous fibrous connections that include the interspinous, intertransverse, costovertebral, and longitudinal ligaments and the ligamentum flavum are varieties of syndesmoses.

Nutrition of the Intervertebral Disc

Most descriptive accounts of the intervertebral disc dismiss the subject of its vascular nutrition with a brief mention of the general agreement that the normal adult disc is avascular. The demonstrable truth of this statement may give the impression that the substance of the disc is inert biologically. Experimental evidence has indicated that the normal disc tissue is quite vital and has a demonstrable rate of metabolic turnover.[58,59] In contrast to the nonvascular cartilage in the diarthroses, the cellular elements of the disc cannot receive the blood-borne nutrients through the mediation of the synovial fluid but must rely on a diffusional system with the vessels that lie adjacent to the disc.

The qualitative and quantitative aspects of the diffusional nutrition of the disc have been studied.[59-62] The peripheral vascular plexus of the anulus and the vessels adjacent to the hyaline cartilage of the bone-disc interface provide the two sources for the diffusion of metabolites into the disc. Although the interface shows an average permeability of 40%, there is a decreasing centrifugal gradient that starts with an 80% permeability at the center. Because diffusion is the major mechanism that carries small solutes through the disc matrix, the two main parameters affecting this flow are the *partition coefficient,* which defines the equilibrium between the solutes within the plasma and the solutes within the disc, and the *diffusion coefficient,* which characterizes the solute mobility.

The partition coefficient varies with the size and charge of the solute particle. Small uncharged solutes show a near-equilibrium between their plasma and intradiscal concentrations, but because the disc matrix has a predominantly negative charge, anionic solutes have a lower intradiscal concentration in relation to the plasma, whereas the reverse is true for positively charged solutes, whose intradiscal concentration is greater than that of the plasma. Because the range of these effects depends on the concentration of the fixed, negatively charged, larger molecular aggregates (proteoglycans), the partition coefficient is regionally variable within the disc matrix and especially pronounced in the inner annular lamellae and nucleus, where the concentration of proteoglycans is the highest.

Solute mobility (the diffusion coefficient) within the disc is slower than in the plasma because the presence of solids in the form of collagen and proteoglycans impedes diffusional progress. Without regard to charge, the diffusion coefficient within the disc is 40% to 60% of free diffusion within water, and mobility is greatest in the inner anulus and nucleus where the water concentrations are the highest.

Because of the regional differentials in the densities of the fixed charges within the disc, the two vascular sources for disc nutrition vary in their significance in the supply of certain solutes. With respect to the small uncharged particles, there is little difference in the transport potential of either the peripheral or the endplate vascular routes, but because of the greater collective negative charge within the central substances of the disc (from proteoglycans), the interface vasculature is a greater source of cationic solutes, whereas the anions would gain easier access through the peripheral vessels.

The effect of fluid "pumping" under changes in the load applied to the disc is minimal with respect to the transport of small solutes because the matrix has a low hydraulic permeability relative to their higher rates of diffusion. With regard to the larger solutes, however, the pumping may have a more substantial effect.

Metabolic turnover, as indicated by proteoglycan synthesis in discs in dogs, is variable according to age within the range of 2 to 3 years. It is roughly equivalent to that of articular cartilage. The central disc tissues have a low oxygen tension and a high concentration of lactic acid, indicating that the inner disc cell respiration is primarily anaerobic. Because this type of respiration is heavily dependent on glycolytic energy requirements, the interface vasculature must deliver the needed glucose to maintain the central disc cell viability.

Because this interface exchange is precariously dependent on the integrity of the fine vasculature subjacent to the cartilaginous endplate, any change from the optimal state occasioned by age-dependent vagaries in the intrinsic vertebral vasculature may partly explain the marked predisposition to degenerative changes characteristic of the aging disc.

Blood Supply of the Vertebral Column

The descriptions and terminology of the nutritional vessels of the vertebrae vary considerably in anatomy texts. In general, the texts illustrate and discuss the vascularity of a typical thoracic or lumbar vertebra, with a lack of agreement on such basic issues as to whether the vertebral body does[63] or does not[64] receive an anterior supply. In addition, discussions of the vascularization of the atypical (craniocervical, cervical, and sacral) vertebral regions are either superficial or entirely lacking. Much of the information presented here is the result of a de novo investigation by the senior author (W.W.P.) and his colleagues, and the terminology ascribed to the vessels is

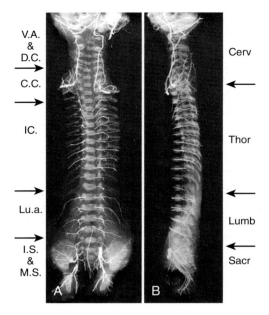

FIGURE 2–22 Anteroposterior and lateral radiographs of spine of an 8-month fetus injected with finely divided barium sulfate. Traditional regional subdivisions of the spine are indicated on the *left*, and regional arteries that provide the segmental branches to the individual vertebrae are shown on the *right*. The upper cervical region is supplied by vertebral and deep cervical arteries (v.a. and d.c.), the lower cervical and upper two thoracic segments are supplied by the costocervical trunk (c.c.), and the remaining thoracic vertebrae receive intercostal vessels (i.c.). The lumbar arteries (lu.a.) supply their regional vertebrae, and the sacral segments are provided with branches from lateral sacral (l.s.) and middle sacral (m.s.) arteries.

elements nevertheless provides a certain constancy. From a segmental artery, or its regional equivalent, each vertebra receives several sets of nutritional vessels, which consist of anterior central, posterior central, prelaminar, and postlaminar branches. The first and last of these are derived from vessels external to the vertebral column, whereas the posterior central and prelaminar branches are derived from spinal branches that enter the intervertebral foramina and supply the neural, meningeal, and epidural tissues as well. In the midspinal region, the internal arteries (i.e., the posterior central and prelaminar branches) provide the greater part of the blood supply to the body and vertebral arch, but reciprocal arrangements may occur, particularly in the cervical region.

This general pattern of the vasculature is best shown in the area between the second thoracic and fifth lumbar vertebrae, where the segments are associated with paired arteries that arise directly from the aorta (Fig. 2–22). Typically, each segmental artery leaves the posterior surface of the aorta and follows a dorsolateral course around the middle of the vertebral body. Near the transverse processes, it divides into a lateral (intercostal or lumbar) and a dorsal branch. The dorsal branch runs lateral to the intervertebral foramen and the articular processes as it continues backward between the transverse processes eventually to reach the spinal muscles. Because the segmental artery is closely applied to the anterolateral surface of the body, its first spinal derivatives are two or more anterior central branches that directly penetrate the cortical bone of the body and that may be traced radiologically into the spongiosa (Figs. 2–23 and 2–24). The same region of

derived from a selection of what seem to be the most descriptive names previously used in other reports and the senior author's reference.[65]

Despite the fact that regional variations may at first seem to thwart the perception of a common pattern of vertebral vascularization, the homologous origin of all vertebral

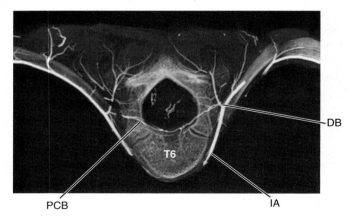

FIGURE 2–23 Ventral radiograph of section through T6 of a specimen from a 6-year-old child injected with barium sulfate. The intercostal arteries (ia) give rise to dorsal branches (db) that provide spinal branches to the vertebral canal and posterior branches to the arch and dorsal musculature. The posterior central branches (pcb) are well shown as they send vessels into the vertebral body. Fine anterior central and anterior laminar and posterior laminar vessels can be seen. Note the neurocentral synchondrosis.

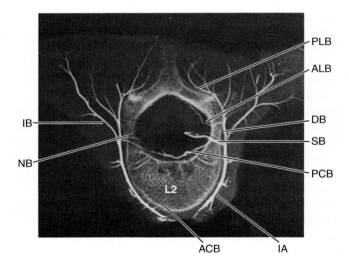

FIGURE 2–24 Vertical radiograph of section through lumbar vertebra of a 6-year-old child. The vascularity of the lumbar vertebra may be regarded as the archetypal pattern from which other regions evolved variations. The segmental lumbar artery (la) gives rise to numerous anterior central branches that penetrate the cortical bone of the body. The spinal branch (sb) sends prominent posterior central branches to the dorsum of the body, whereas the dorsal branch (db) supplies the anterior (alb) and posterior (plb) laminar branches. Neural branches (nb) follow the nerve roots to the cord. In this section, the arteria radicularis magna is seen as a neural branch on the right side. lb, lumbar branches.

the segmental artery also supplies longitudinal arteries to the anterior longitudinal ligament (Fig. 2–25).

After the segmental artery divides into its dorsal and lateral branches, the dorsal component passes lateral to the intervertebral foramen, where it gives off the spinal branch that provides the major vascularity to the bone and contents of the vertebral canal. This branch may enter the foramen as a single vessel, or it may arise from the dorsal segmental branch as numerous independent rami. In either case, it ultimately divides into a triad of posterior central, prelaminar, and intermediate neural branches. The posterior central branch passes over the dorsolateral surface of the intervertebral disc and divides into a caudal and a cranial branch, which supply the two adjacent vertebral bodies.

Coursing in the same plane as the posterior longitudinal ligament, these branches vascularize the ligament and the related dura before entering the large concavity in the central dorsal surface of the vertebral body. The dorsum of each vertebral body is supplied by four arteries derived from two intervertebral levels. As these vessels tend to converge toward the dorsal central concavity, where they are cross-connected with their bilateral counterparts, their connections with other vertebral levels give the appearance of a series of rhomboid anastomotic loops (Fig. 2–26) that illustrate the extent of collateral supply to a single vertebra.

The prelaminar branch of the spinal artery follows the inner surface of the vertebral arch, giving fine penetrating nutrient branches to the laminae and ligamenta flava, while also supplying the regional epidural and dorsal tissue. The neural branches that enter the intervertebral foramen with the above-described vessels supply the pia-arachnoid complex and the spinal cord itself. In the fetus and the adult, the neural or radicular branches are not segmentally uniform in their size or occurrence. Although all spinal nerves receive fine twigs to their ganglia and roots, the major contributions to the cord are found at irregular intervals. Several larger radicular arteries may be discerned in the cervical and upper thoracic regions, but the largest, the arteria radicularis magna (artery of Adamkiewicz[66]), is an asymmetrical contribution from one of the upper lumbar, or lower thoracic, segmental arteries. It travels obliquely upward with a ventral spinal root to join the anterior spinal artery in the region of the conus medullaris. Radicular contributions to the dorsal spinal plexus may usually be distinguished by their more tortuous course (see Figs. 2–25 and 2–26).

After the dorsal branch of the segmental artery has provided the vessels to the intervertebral foramen, it passes between the transverse processes, where it gives off a fine spray of articular branches to the joint capsule of the articular processes. Immediately distal to this point, it divides into dorsal and medial branches; the larger, dorsal branch ramifies in the greater muscle mass of the erector spinae, whereas the medial branch follows the external contours of the lamina and the spinous process. This postlaminar artery supplies the musculature immediately overlying the lamina and sends fine nutrient branches into the bone. The largest of these branches penetrates the lamina through a nutrient foramen located just dorsomedial to the articular capsule.

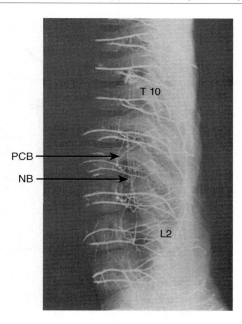

FIGURE 2–25 Lateral view of lumbar vertebra shown in Figure 2–24. Longitudinal anastomoses of posterior central branches (pcb) can be appreciated, and the disposition of neural branches (nb) is clarified. The lumbar arteries also supply small longitudinal branches to the anterior longitudinal ligament.

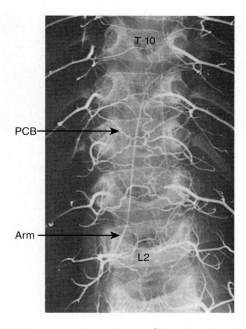

FIGURE 2–26 Anteroposterior arteriogram of lower thoracic and upper lumbar vertebrae in a 6-year-old child. The interlocking anastomotic pattern formed by the posterior central branches (pcb) and the manner in which four branches converge over the center of the dorsum of the body of each vertebra are well shown. The arteria radicularis magna (arm), which forms a major contribution to the anterior spinal artery of the cord, can be seen arising at L2.

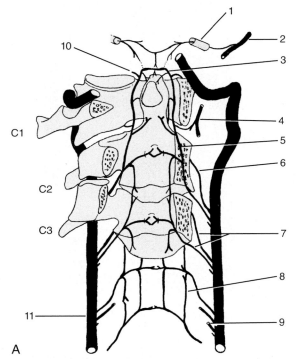

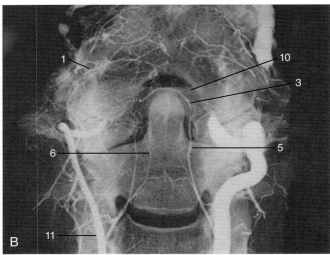

FIGURE 2–27 A, Schema of arterial supply to bodies of the upper cervical vertebrae and the odontoid process. Numerical designations apply to the same structures in **B**.1, Hypoglossal canal passing meningeal artery. 2, Occipital artery. 3, Apical arcade of odontoid process. 4, Ascending pharyngeal artery giving collateral branch beneath anterior arch of atlas. 5, Posterior ascending artery. 6, Anterior ascending artery. 7, Precentral and postcentral arteries to typical cervical vertebral body. 8, Anterior spinal plexus. 9, Medullary branch of vertebral artery; radicular, prelaminar, and meningeal branches are also found at each level. 10, Collateral to ascending pharyngeal artery passing rostral to anterior arch of atlas. 11, Left vertebral artery.

Regional Variations in Spinal Vasculature

Only vertebrae that are related to the aorta have access to direct segmental branches. The cervical, upper thoracic, and sacral regions have different patterns in their segmental supply that affect to various extents the arrangements of the finer vessels. In an arteriogram of the entire fetal spine (see Fig.

2–22), it can be seen that the greater part of the cervical region is supplied by the vertebral arteries and the deep cervical arteries. An intermediate area that usually includes the lower two cervical and upper two thoracic vertebrae is supplied by costocervical branches of the subclavian artery that are of variable pattern and often bilaterally dissimilar. From T2 to L3, the typical segmental arrangement prevails, but in the sacral area lateral sacral branches of the hypogastric artery and middle sacral branches assume the function of supporting the nutritional vasculature to the vertebral elements.

Cervical Region

The general patterns of the arterial supply with respect to the typical cervical vertebrae are schematically represented in Figures 2–27A and 2–28.[67] The vertebral arteries represent a lateral longitudinal fusion of the original segmental vessels and provide a ventrally coursing anterior central artery and a medially directed posterior central artery to each subaxial vertebral element. The anterior spinal plexus is best developed in the cervical region, where it exhibits a rectangular mesh of vessels in which the transverse members (anterior central arteries) run along the upper ventral edges of their respective intervertebral discs. The conspicuousness of this plexus reflects the fact that it also serves the cervical prevertebral musculature. The thyrocervical and costocervical trunks assist in the lower cervical region, and the upper cervical part of the plexus receives contributions from the ascending pharyngeal arteries (Fig. 2–29).

Atlantoaxial Complex

With their complex phyletic and developmental history, the components of the atlantoaxial articulation display the most atypical vascular pattern of all the vertebrae. Although the odontoid process represents the definitive centrum of the first cervical vertebra, it develops and remains as a projecting process of the axis that is almost completely isolated from the

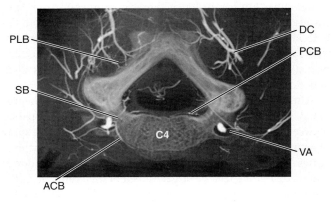

FIGURE 2–28 Vertical radiograph of section through fourth cervical vertebra of a 6-year-old child, showing vascularity. The deep cervical artery (dc) provides the posterior laminar branches (plb). Vertebral arteries show numerous anastomoses with other cervical arteries and send spinal branches (sb) that form posterior central branches (pcb) of the body and anterior lamina branches of the arch. Anterior central branches (acb) may arise independently from the vertebral arteries (va).

rest of the atlas by synovial joint cavities. Its fixed position relative to the rotation of the atlas and the adjacent sections of the vertebral arteries prevents formation of major vascularization by direct branches at its corresponding segmental level.

One might assume that the nutrition of the dens would easily be accomplished by interosseous vessels derived from the spongiosa within the supporting body of the axis. It is axiomatic, however, that the vascular patterns of bones were developmentally established to supply the original ossification centers within the nonvascular cartilage matrices, and despite the eventual obliteration of the separating cartilage, the original patterns of vascularity generally prevail throughout life. The transient cartilaginous plate, which represents an incipient intervertebral disc between the atlas and axis, does not calcify until the latter half of the first decade and effectively prevents the development of any significant vascular communication between the axis centrum and the odontoid process. Occasionally, noncalcified remnants of this plate may persist in adults; although there may be a stable union between the two elements, a radiolucent area may suggest a fracture nonunion or a "false" os odontoideum.

In light of the foregoing facts, it was not unexpected that the investigations of Schiff and Parke[68] revealed that the odontoid process was supplied primarily by pairs of anterior and posterior central branches that coursed upward from the surfaces of the body of the axis and were derived from the vertebral arteries at the level of the foramen of the third cervical nerve. The posterior ascending arteries are the larger members of these two sets of vessels and usually arise independently from the posteromedial sides of their respective vertebral arteries. The individual artery enters the vertebral canal through the foramen between the second and third vertebrae and trifurcates on the dorsum of the axis body. The typical posterior central perforators course medially passing deep to the posterior longitudinal ligament (called the *tectorial membrane* in the craniocervical region) to penetrate into the spongiosa of the axis. A small descending branch anastomoses distally with vessels of the next lower segment.

The major part of the posterior ascending artery crosses the dorsal surface of the transverse ligament of the atlas about 1.5 mm lateral to the neck of the odontoid process (see Fig. 2–27). Dorsal to the alar ligament, it sends an anterior anastomotic branch over the cranial edge of this ligament to form collateral connections with the anterior ascending artery. The posterior ascending artery continues on a medial course to meet its opposite counterpart and forms the apical arcade that arches over the apex of the odontoid process.

The smaller anterior ascending arteries arise from the anteromedial aspect of the vertebral arteries and pass to the ventral surface of the axis body. Fine medial branches send perforators into the substance of the vertebral body and meet in a median anastomosis typical of the anterior central branches of the lower cervical region. The rostral continuance of the anterior ascending arteries brings them dorsal to the anterior arch of the atlas. Here each artery sends numerous fine perforators into the anterolateral surfaces of the neck of the odontoid process and terminates in a spray of vessels that supply the synovial capsule of the median atlantoaxial joint.

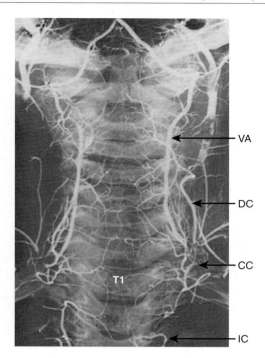

FIGURE 2–29 Arteriogram of cervical and upper thoracic regions of the 6-year-old spine seen in Figures 2–23 and 2–24. The vertebral artery (va) and deep cervical branch (dc) of the costocervical trunk (cc) supply segmental branches to each vertebra. The costocervical artery also typically supplies T1 and T2, but in this case T2 receives a high intercostal (ic) branch on the left side.

Fine branches from the anterior and posterior ascending arteries also assist in the nutrition of the syndesmotic relations of the atlantoaxial and craniovertebral articulations. The main blood supply to the atlanto-occipital joint is provided by a complex of vessels derived from the vertebral and occipital arteries.

Collateral vessels pass over and under the anterior arch of the atlas to anastomose with the apical arcade and ascending arteries.[68] These are derived from some component of the external carotid system. These vessels are branches of the ascending pharyngeal artery, which has a nearly ubiquitous distribution in the upper pharyngeal region and sends a branch along the inner aspect of the carotid sheath that, on reaching the base of the skull, becomes recurrent and descends deep to the prevertebral fascia to supply the upper prevertebral cervical muscles and anastomose with the anterior spinal plexus. Numerous small-bore vessels that descend from the rim of the foramen magnum to anastomose with the apical arcade are derivatives of a meningeal branch of the occipital artery that enters the skull through the hypoglossal canal (see Fig. 2–27). Its descending branches supply the periforaminal dura, the tectorial membrane and alar and apical ligaments, and the fine anastomoses to the arcade.

Sacroiliolumbar Arterial System

From the second thoracic vertebra to the fourth lumbar vertebra, the spine and its regionally related structures are

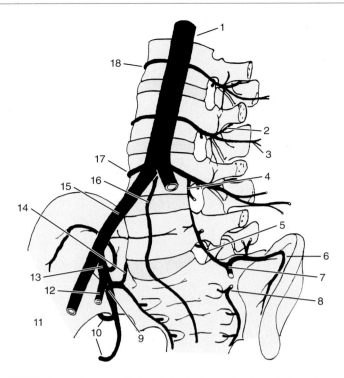

FIGURE 2–30 Graphic rendering of distribution and major variations of sacroiliolumbar system of arteries that supply the vertebrae and their associated structures inferior to the fourth lumbar vertebra. These patterns of the vessels were derived from radiographs of perinatal specimens and dissections of adults and drawn against a tracing of the lumbosacral region taken from a left anterior oblique radiograph of a man. The aorta lies to the left of center as it approaches the bifurcation ventral to the fourth lumbar vertebra. This schema shows the more frequent arrangement of the sacroiliolumbar system on the right side of the illustration, where the iliolumbar vessel (*7*) has a single origin from the dorsum of the posterior division of the (removed) internal iliac artery. The left side shows the common variation where the iliac artery and the lumbar artery (*14*) are derived separately. The middle sacral artery (*16*) is in its typical position, and the anastomotic contribution from the fourth lumbar artery (*4*) shows its most frequent form.

1. aorta
2. musculocutaneous branch of third lumbar artery
3. muscular branch to posterior abdominal wall
4. anastomotic contribution of fourth lumbar artery to sacroiliolumbar system
5. lumbar branch of iliolumbar artery
6. iliac branch of iliolumbar artery
7. iliolumbar artery
8. left lateral sacral artery
9. posterior division of internal iliac artery
10. superior and inferior gluteal arteries
11. external iliac artery
12. anterior (visceral) division of internal iliac artery
13. internal iliac artery
14. variant origin of lumbar branch of iliolumbar artery from lateral sacral artery
15. common iliac artery
16. middle sacral artery
17. left fourth lumbar segmental artery
18. left second lumbar segmental artery

supplied by pairs of segmental arteries that are direct branches of the aorta. Because the aorta terminates in a bifurcation ventral to the fourth lumbar vertebral body, the vertebrae and the associated tissues caudad to this point rely on an arterial complex derived mostly from the internal iliac (hypogastric) arteries. This "sacroiliolumbar system" consists of contributions from the fourth lumbar artery, the iliolumbar artery, and the middle and lateral sacral arteries.

With the increasing use of percutaneous approaches to the lower lumbar discs, this infra-aortic system of vessels has assumed some surgical significance, particularly because, in contrast to the conventional segmental supply to the more superior vertebrae, its major components are longitudinally related to the dorsolateral surfaces of the discs most frequently involved in these procedures.[69]

Fourth Lumbar Arteries

The peculiarities of the sacroiliolumbar system of arteries may best be understood if compared with the pattern of distribution of the typical aortic segmental branches. The ramifications of the fourth lumbar arteries were selected for this purpose because they not only exemplify the conventional segmental distribution, but often are involved in the nutrition of the next lower segments by variable contributions to the iliolumbar vessels. These vessels often may be twice the caliber of their more cephalad homologues because of a greater muscular and intersegmental distribution.

As depicted in Figures 2–30 and 2–31, the distribution of the major ramifications is similar to that of the thoracic segmental vessels, with the exception of additional branches that supply the psoas and quadratus lumborum muscles. The lateral muscular branch (equivalent of the thoracic intercostals) may be quite large at the fourth lumbar level, where, in contrast to the other lumbar laterals, it passes anterior, rather than posterior, to the quadratus lumborum. It then continues to supply the lower posterolateral abdominal wall as it courses superior to the crest of the ilium. As can be seen in Figure 2–30, it may be equivalent in size to the iliac branch of the iliolumbar artery. Its position superior to the crest indicates that it is more likely to be encountered by percutaneous instrumentation than the latter vessel.

The dorsal musculocutaneous branch of the fourth lumbar artery is equivalent in distribution to other thoracolumbar segmental arteries. It usually has a medial branch that supplies the external aspects of the facet joints and neural arch components and the transversospinal group of muscles and a lateral branch to the transversocostal group of the erector spinae. The vertebromedullary (spinal) branches of the fourth lumbar artery are also similar to those of other segmental arteries (see Fig. 2–24). They are a group of vessels of variable caliber that may generally be sorted into three divisions: (1) the ventral periosteal and osseous branches that supply the posterior longitudinal ligament, the periosteum, and the cancellous bone of the vertebral body; (2) the radiculomedullary division that provides the irregularly located medullary arteries of the cord and the constant distal radicular arteries to all the roots; and (3) the dorsal division that supplies fine

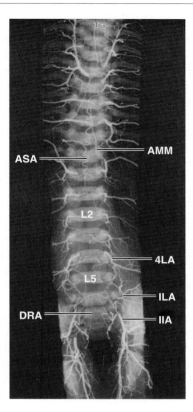

FIGURE 2–31 Anteroposterior radiograph of spine from a perinatal cadaver injected with barium sulfate. The aorta and common iliac vessels have been removed before radiography. This specimen was chosen because it showed considerable variation between the two sides of the sacroiliolumbar system. On the right side of the illustration, a small lumbar branch and a descending branch from the fourth lumbar artery (4LA) enter the L5-S1 intervertebral foramen. On the left side, there is no lumbar branch, and a descending branch of the L4 artery supplies all of the vessels to the L5-S1 foramen. Also, the middle sacral artery is absent, and other branches of the system supply its domain. The radicular branches of the vertebromedullary vessels supply the distal radicular arteries (DRA) and reveal the positions of the lower ends of the lumbosacral nerve roots.

articular branches to the deep aspects of the facet joints and the periosteum of the deep surfaces of the laminae and their associated ligaments. The first two divisions usually originate from a common branch of the segmental artery and enter the intervertebral foramen just rostral to their respective vertebral pedicle and ventral to the dorsal root ganglion, whereas the dorsal division arises from the musculocutaneous branch of the segmental artery and enters the foramen dorsal to the nerve components. All the vertebromedullary branches may provide fine branches to the spinal dura.

The aortic segmental arteries course around their respective vertebral body at its narrowest circumference and are positioned almost equidistant between the adjacent discs. These parts of the arterial distribution are relatively safe from instrumentation properly positioned to enter the discs.

A major peculiarity of the fourth lumbar artery is its proclivity toward providing a relatively large, caudally directed intersegmental branch that arises near the level of the intervertebral foramen and becomes reciprocally involved with the lumbar branch of the iliolumbar artery. When this latter vessel is small or absent, the descending branch of the fourth lumbar

artery may be sufficiently large to provide the predominant nutritional system to two vertebral segments caudad to its origin (see Figs. 2–30 and 2–31).

Iliolumbar Artery

As opposed to the mostly visceral distribution of the anterior division of the internal iliac (hypogastric) artery, the posterior division is essentially a somatic artery giving rise to gluteal, iliolumbar, and lateral sacral branches. The iliolumbar artery most frequently is the first branch of this dorsal division. It is directed dorsosuperiorly, passing close to the ventrolateral surface of the first sacral vertebral segment. It courses superiorly, dorsal to the obturator nerve and ventral to the lumbosacral trunk. Lateral to the inferior margin of the L5-S1 disc, the iliolumbar artery usually divides into a laterally directed iliac artery and an ascending lumbar artery. The first of these crosses the sacroiliac joint to reach the iliac fossa of the pelvis, where it courses inferior to the iliac crest and usually deep to the muscle to provide muscular branches to the iliac muscle and articular twigs to the acetabulum and eventually anastomoses with the deep circumflex branch of the femoral artery.

The lumbar artery ascends posterolateral to the L5-S1 disc, still between the obturator nerve and the lumbosacral trunk, to provide the vertebromedullary vessels to the L5-S1 intervertebral foramen (Fig. 2–32; see Figs. 2–30 and 2–31). In

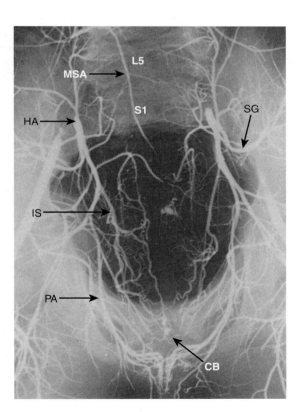

FIGURE 2–32 Anteroposterior arteriogram of sacral region in a 7-year-old child. The lateral sacral arteries (ls) can be seen coming from the hypogastric vessels (ha). The middle sacral artery (msa) is atypical in this specimen because it stops at S1. Just anterior to the coccyx, the coccygeal bodies (cb) are indicated as small knots of arteriovenous anastomoses. Pudendal arteries (pa) are well injected.

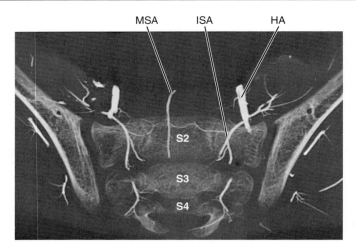

MSA   ISA   HA

S2

S3

S4

FIGURE 2–33 Radiograph of horizontal section through sacroiliac joint. The natural curvature of the sacrum provided oblique sections through segments 2, 3, and 4. The hypogastric artery (ha) gives off the lateral sacral artery (lsa) that sends anastomotic branches to join the middle sacral artery (msa); from these, the sacral segments receive the penetrating anterior central branches. The dorsal branches pass into the anterior sacral foramina to provide posterior, central, neural, and prelaminar branches. The dorsal branches leave through the posterior sacral foramina to supply the muscles and posterior laminar branches.

most cases, a branch of this vessel continues rostrally to anastomose with the descending branch of the fourth lumbar artery. The lumbar branch of the iliolumbar artery provides regional branches to the psoas and quadratus lumborum muscles.

Sacral Arteries

Lateral Sacral Arteries

Lateral sacral arteries usually form the second branch of the dorsal division of the internal iliac arteries and course down the pars lateralis on each side of the sacrum. Opposite the sacral foramina, they give off medial branches that dorsally enter the foramina. After providing the typical vertebromedullary derivatives, their dorsal muscular branches exit through the dorsal sacral foramina to supply the sacral origins of the erector spinae muscles.

Middle Sacral Artery

The middle sacral artery is an unpaired vessel that is the last branch of the aorta, usually derived from its dorsal median surface just above the carina of the bifurcation (Fig. 2–33; see Fig. 2–30). It descends down the ventral surface of the anterior longitudinal ligament over the fourth and fifth lumbar bodies and down the ventral sacrum to terminate at the sacrococcygeal junction in a vascular glomus (sacrococcygeal body) in tail-less mammals or continues ventral to the coccygeal (caudal) vertebrae in tailed mammals as the caudal artery. In humans, this is a variable vessel, being totally absent in some cases or replaced by a branch of one of the lateral sacral arteries. Where

it is a significant component of the sacroiliolumbar system, its first lateral branches on the ventral surface of the fifth lumbar body may entirely replace this segment's contributions from the iliolumbar or fourth lumbar vessels and provide its osseous, muscular, and vertebromedullary requirements.

Where it is conspicuously present in the sacral region, the middle sacral artery may also contribute a vertebromedullary branch to each anterior sacral foramen. When it is absent, these ventral sacral territories are provided with segmental medial branches from the lateral sacral arteries.

Functional Significance

The sacroiliolumbar system, despite its complexity and seemingly endless combinations of reciprocal substitutions, supplies the lower lumbosacral elements of the spine and the inferior half of the lumbosacral spinal nerve roots (cauda equina) and the back musculature inferior to the L4 level. It is also a major contributor to the vasa nervorum of the lumbosacral plexus. The distal radicular arteries define the positions of the lumbosacral roots (see Fig. 2–25). Although significant medullary branches to the spinal cord are seldom found below L4, they do occur, and from the preceding descriptions it is obvious why the ligation of both internal iliac arteries during radical cystoprostatectomy can result in spinal cord ischemia.[70]

Venous System of the Vertebral Column

An external plexus and an internal plexus of veins are associated with the vertebral column. The distribution of the two systems roughly coincides with the areas served by the external and internal arterial supplies. The external venous plexus also consists of an anterior and a posterior set of veins. The small anterior external plexus is coextensive with the anterior central arteries and receives tributaries that perforate the anterior and lateral sides of the vertebral body.

The more extensive posterior external veins drain the regions supplied by posterior (muscular and postlaminar) branches of the segmental artery. The posterior external veins form an essentially paired system, which lies in the two vertebrocostal grooves, but has cross anastomoses between the spinous processes. It is a valveless venous complex that receives the draining segmental tributaries of the internal veins through the intervertebral foramina and communicates ultimately with the lumbar and intercostal tributaries of the caval and azygos system. The posterior external plexus becomes most extensive in the posterior nuchal region, where it receives the intraspinous tributaries via the vertebral veins and drains into the deep cervical and jugular veins.

The internal venous plexus is of more functional and anatomic interest. This plexus is essentially a series of irregular, valveless epidural sinuses that extend from the coccyx to the foramen magnum. Its channels are embedded in the epidural fat and are supported by a network of collagenous fibers, but their walls are so thin that their extent or configuration cannot be discerned by gross dissection. This latter property may

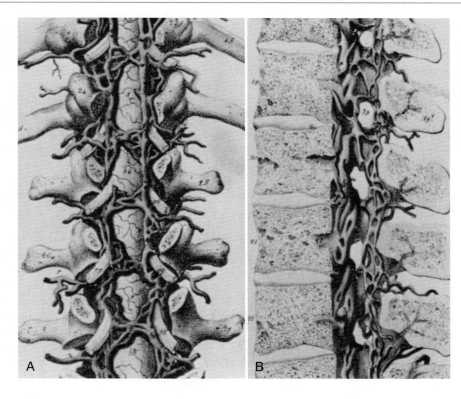

FIGURE 2–34 Posterior (**A**) and lateral (**B**) illustrations of the spinal epidural venous plexus taken from hand-colored copies of Breschet's original work. (ca. 1835, Courtesy of Scott Memorial Library, Jefferson Medical College.)

account for the fact that the epidural venous sinuses have been periodically "rediscovered." The epidural vertebral veins were known to Vesalius and his contemporaries and were described and illustrated in the first part of the 19th century by Breschet.[71] Batson,[72] Clemens,[73] and others made the functional and pathologic significance of these vessels apparent (Fig. 2–34).

The plexus does not entwine the dura in a completely haphazard fashion but is arranged in a series of cross-connected expansions that produce anterior and posterior ladderlike configurations up the vertebral canal. The main anterior components of the epidural plexus consist of two continuous channels that course along the posterior surface of the vertebral bodies just medial to the pedicles. These channels expand medially to create cross anastomoses over the central dorsal area of each vertebral body and are thinnest where they overlie the intervertebral discs. When injected with a contrast medium, the main channels may appear as a segmental chain of rhomboid beads. Chaynes and colleagues[74] studied the internal venous plexus using silicon injection techniques. They found that anterior longitudinal veins were located in a "dehiscence" within the periosteum along the lateral aspect of the spinal canal and that veins of each side communicated with each other through a retrocorporeal vein. In the cervical spine, the retrocorporeal vein was found deep to the posterior longitudinal ligament, whereas it was superficial to the ligament in the thoracic and lumbar regions.

Where the main anterior sinuses cross connect, they receive the large unpaired basivertebral sinus that arises within the dorsal central concavity of the spongiosa and drains the intraosseous labyrinth of sinusoids. Regional visualization of the epidural plexus can be accomplished by

introducing a radiopaque medium directly into the spongiosa or the cancellous bone of the spinous process (intraosseous venography).

The major external connections of the epidural plexus consist of the veins that pass through the intervertebral foramen and eventually empty into the segmentally available intercostal or lumbar veins (Fig. 2–35). Because these sinuses

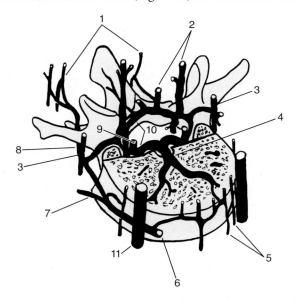

FIGURE 2–35 Schema showing venous relationships of a lumbar vertebra. Engorgement and relative venous hypertension in the epidural vessels exacerbate neuroischemic conditions in the lumbosacral roots. 1, Dorsal external vertebral plexus. 2, Dorsal epidural plexus. 3, Ascending lumbar veins. 4, Basivertebral vein. 5, Ventral external vertebral plexus. 6, Lumbar segmental vein. 7, Muscular vein from posterior abdominal wall. 8, Circumferential channels (sinuses) of epidural plexus.

are valveless, one cannot refer accurately to directions of drainage and flow. The greatest functional significance of these vessels lies in their ability to pass blood in any direction according to the constantly shifting intra-abdominal and intrathoracic pressures. Breschet[71] surmised that the epidural plexus served as a collateral route for the valveless caval and azygos systems. This ability has been shown by experimental ligation of either the superior vena cava or the inferior vena cava. In addition, the Queckenstedt maneuver, which tests the patency of the spinal subarachnoid space by compressing the

jugular or intra-abdominal veins, causes an increase in cerebrospinal fluid pressure through dural compression from the expansion of the collaterally loaded epidural plexus.

The plexus is evidently capable of passing large quantities of blood without developing varices. Clemens claimed that this feature was due to the intricate network of collagenous fibers that supports the thin walls of the sinuses. Also, passive congestion of the spinal cord is prevented by minute valves in the radicular branches draining the spinal cord.[73] This latter fact is anatomically unique because valves exist nowhere else in the venous channels associated with the central nervous system. An ancillary function of the epidural plexus may be to act in a mechanical capacity as a hydraulic shock-absorbing sheath that helps buffer the spinal cord during movements of the vertebral column, similar to the epidural fat.

The vertebral sinuses are largest in the suboccipital and upper cervical region. Here they also receive numerous nerve endings from the sinuvertebral nerves and are associated with glomerular arteriovenous anastomoses, which suggests a possible baroceptive function.[75] The patency of these anastomoses is most easily shown in the fetus, in which arterial injections of a contrast medium may also fill the upper cervical epidural sinuses. Similarly, the coccygeal bodies of the same specimen pass the arterial injection directly into the epidural veins of the lower sacral region.

The detrimental aspects of the vertebral epidural veins have been well stated by Batson.[72] Retrograde flow from venous connections to the lower pelvic organs provides an obvious route of metastasis for pelvic neoplasms to the spine itself and to the regions of the trunk associated with valveless connections to the plexus. Batson[72] claimed that direct metastatic transfer can occur between the pelvic organs and the brain via the vertebral epidural route.

Another extraspinal-intraspinal venous connection implicated in the transfer of pathologic processes involves the pharyngovertebral veins.[76] These vessels constitute a system that drains the superior posterolateral regions of the nasopharynx and coalesces into two to several veins that penetrate the anterior atlanto-occipital membrane to discharge into the venous complex surrounding the median and lateral atlantoaxial joints. Because posterior pharyngeal infections have been linked with the atlantoaxial rotatory subluxations characteristic of Grisel syndrome,[77] it is believed that the pharyngovertebral veins are instrumental in transporting infectious processes that may produce a hyperemic relaxation of the atlantoaxial ligaments. The existence of this venous system also explains the ease in transfer of superior pharyngeal metastatic processes to the upper cervical epidural veins.

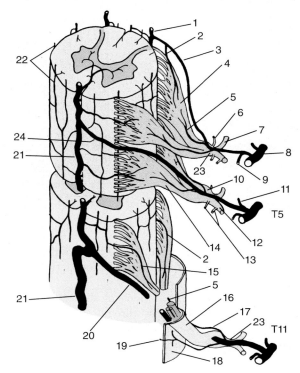

FIGURE 2–36 Composite schema of blood supply to spinal cord and nerve roots showing two regions of the cord. Note the distinction between medullary arteries and true radicular arteries and that the medullary arteries usually run a course that is independent of the roots.

 1. dorsolateral longitudinal artery
 2. proximal radicular artery (of dorsal root)
 3. dorsal medullary artery
 4. dorsal root of thoracic spinal nerve
 5. distal radicular artery (of dorsal root)
 6. sinuvertebral nerve
 7. dorsal ramus of spinal nerve
 8. segmental artery
 9. dorsal central artery
10. dorsal root ganglion
11. anterior laminar artery
12. ventral ramus of spinal nerve
13. rami communicantes
14. ventral root of spinal nerve
15. proximal radicular artery of ventral root
16. periradicular theca of dura
17. dorsal meningeal branch of vertebromedullary artery
18. dura
19. ventral meningeal plexus
20. great ventral medullary artery (great "radicular" artery of Adamkiewicz)
21. anterior (ventral) spinal artery
22. vasa corona of spinal cord
23. spinal nerve
24. ventral medullary artery of thoracic cord

Blood Supply of the Spinal Cord

Throughout the length of the spinal cord, a system of three longitudinal vessels receives blood from the irregularly located medullary branches of the segmental spinal arteries and distributes it to the substance of the cord. This system consists of the single median ventral anterior spinal artery and two smaller dorsolateral spinal arteries (Fig. 2–36).

Anterior Spinal Artery

Despite its great functional significance, the anterior spinal artery remains one of the more inaccurately described and inadequately understood blood vessels. Derived from the fusion of bilateral pairs of ascending and descending anastomotic branches of the original segmental arteries of the developing spinal cord,[78] this median ventral pial vessel supplies approximately 80% of the intrinsic spinal cord vasculature. It is usually depicted in texts as a single continuous artery of nearly uniform caliber that extends from the medulla oblongata to the conus. The anterior spinal artery is actually a longitudinal series of functionally independent vessels that may show wide luminal variations and anatomic discontinuities.[78-80]

Although the investigations of Crock and Yoshizawa[65] have tended to minimize the significance of predominant regional feeders, many functionally oriented reports have claimed that the cord has three major arterial domains along its vertical axis: (1) the cervicothoracic region (C1-T3), (2) the mid-thoracic region (T3-8), and (3) the thoracolumbar (including sacral cord) region (T8-conus). The reports have also claimed that these areas have little anastomotic exchange between their junctions (Fig. 2–37).

Brewer and colleagues[79] and Lazorthes and associates[80] maintained that a series of human anterior spinal arteries consistently show interruptions, or critically narrow zones, in the mid-thoracic region, and these influence the potential collateral blood flow along the longitudinal axis of the cord. It is not only the observed size of the vessel that is of physiologic significance, however. The existence of a marked autoregulatory control of the intrinsic spinal cord blood flow has been independently shown in many mammalian species.[24,81] Microscopic investigation[82] of sections of the descending and ascending contributions of the arteria medullaris magna (artery of Adamkiewicz, also known as the arteria radicularis magna) to the anterior spinal artery showed that these arteries, in addition to their well-developed circumferential muscle of the tunica media, also possess a layer of predominantly longitudinal intimal musculature. Located between the internal elastic lamina and the endothelium, this layer ranges in thickness from one fifth to one half of the tunica media (Fig. 2–38).

In following a series of cranial to caudal sections of the thoracolumbar anterior spinal artery, it was noted that the intimal muscle layer did not extend into any of its branches. At the mouth of the central (sulcal) arteries, which are the largest anterior spinal artery derivatives, the intimal musculature stops abruptly, often forming a liplike projection over the opening of the branch vessel, but no intimal muscle fibers extend into the central arteries. A sphincter-like thickening of the central artery tunica media, seen at the ostium of the vessels, indicates that this muscle layer has a greater contractile influence at this point (see Fig. 2–38). The intimal musculature, in addition to enhancing the luminal control of the anterior spinal artery, also is involved in controlling the blood flow into the central arteries. Where the intimal layer shows the liplike projections, successive serial sections indicate that

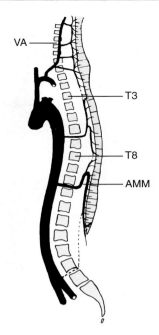

FIGURE 2–37 Schema illustrating sources and relationships of medullary feeder arteries to the spine and the spinal cord. Anterior spinal artery (ASA) is shown to be formed by an anastomotic chain of ascending and descending branches of medullary feeders. Cervicothoracic, mid-thoracic, and thoracolumbar (includes sacral cord) regions are indicated, and their usual boundaries at vertebral levels T3 and T8 are shown. Medullary feeders range from 6 to 14, but the respective domains persist. *Dotted line* indicates frequent position of a smaller accessory medullary feeder to the thoracolumbar area. AMM, arteria medullaris magna; VA, vertebral artery. (From Parke WW, Whalen JL, Bunger PC, et al: Intimal musculature of the lower anterior spinal artery. Spine 20:2074, 1995.)

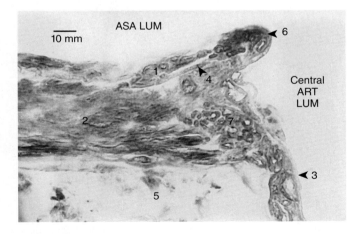

FIGURE 2–38 High-power cross section of thoracolumbar anterior spinal artery (ASA) wall at junction with one side of a central artery. The intimal musculature (*1*) may extend as a liplike projection (*6*) over the central artery orifice. This muscle layer stops at this point and does not extend into branch vessels. A sphincter-like enlargement of the conventional circular muscle of the central artery (*7*) is indicated. Endothelium (*3*) and internal elastic lamina (*4*), tunica media (*2*), and adventitia-pia (*5*) are labeled. (From Parke WW, Whalen JL, Bunger PC, et al: Intimal musculature of the lower anterior spinal artery. Spine 20:2075, 1995.)

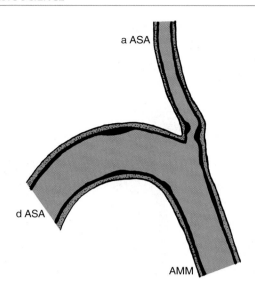

FIGURE 2–39 Schema derived from sections of arteria medullaris magna (AMM)–anterior spinal artery (ASA) junction to show distribution of intimal musculature (*solid black*) in this region. Intimal cushions are shown guarding the orifice of the ascending ASA (aASA) and a typical distribution as found in the arch of the descending ASA (dASA). (From Parke WW, Whalen JL, Bunger PC, et al: Intimal musculature of the lower anterior spinal artery. Spine 20:2076, 1995.)

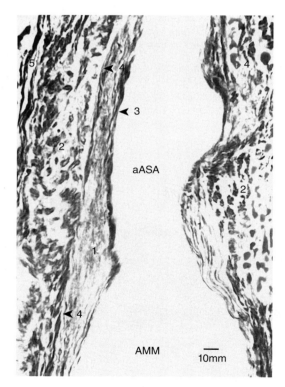

FIGURE 2–40 Sagittal section through junction of arteria medullaris magna (AMM) arch and ascending anterior spinal artery (aASA) showing the intimal cushions guarding the aASA orifice (*1*). These may be reinforced by underlying enhancement of the circular fibers of the tunica media (*2*). Endothelium (*3*) and elastic lamina (*4*) are indicated. The longitudinal disposition of the intimal muscle fibers is apparent, particularly in the intimal cushion on the right side. The contraction of these muscular systems would dramatically alter the radius of the aASA lumen. Adventitia-pia is labeled (*5*). (From Parke WW, Whalen JL, Bunger PC, et al: Intimal musculature of the lower anterior spinal artery. Spine 20:2076, 1995.)

contraction of the longitudinally disposed intimal muscle fibers forms an ellipsoidal buttonhole-shaped orifice whose long axis is parallel to that of the fiber orientation. Such an arrangement permits exquisite muscular control of the blood flow from the anterior spinal artery to its central artery branches.

In addition to the fairly uniform layer of the intimal musculature throughout the walls of the examined sections of the thoracolumbar anterior spinal artery, serial sections cut through the arch-shaped junction of the arteria medullaris magna and the descending anterior spinal artery branches show that this intimal layer, in most cases, is organized into prominent intimal cushions. These muscular thickenings are erratically distributed along the lumen of the hairpin-shaped arterial arch and the initial segment of the ascending branch of the anterior spinal artery (Figs. 2–39 and 2–40). This latter location is of considerable interest because its prominent cushions, with reinforced thickenings of the underlying tunica media, could exert considerable influence over the quantity of blood flow between the thoracolumbar and mid-thoracic vascular domains. This intimal control system, when coupled with the intramedullary arteriovenous anastomoses (described in a subsequent section on intrinsic vascularity), provides an anatomic basis for the dramatic range of spinal cord blood flow autoregulation. The presence of the intimal cushions explains the often-noted failure of the arteria medullaris magna to supply adequately the mid-thoracic cord region above the arteria medullaris magna–anterior spinal artery junction during aortic cross clamping.

The ventral position of the anterior spinal artery and its nutritional importance may have consequence in spinal stenosis. Particularly in the lower cervical region, its compression by dorsal osteophytes and cartilaginous protrusions related to cervical disc degeneration may lead to the neurologically disastrous anterior spinal artery syndrome.[83] The medullary feeder arteries that supply the anterior spinal artery may arise from any spinal segmental artery. Studies by Dommissee[84] showed, however, that there are statistical preferences for certain segmental levels. There are usually three anterior medullary arteries for the cervical region, one or two for the thoracic region, and a conspicuous medullary vessel (the arteria medullaris magna) for the lumbosacral cord region. The levels of origin for all these vessels center around certain "average" locations in each region. The anterior spinal artery is usually of greatest caliber in the lumbosacral part of the cord, where it supplies the considerable tissue mass of the proximal cauda equina in addition to the lumbosacral cord intumescence.

The dorsolateral spinal arteries arise from the posterior inferior cerebellar vessels and are of lesser caliber and nutritional significance. They also are less likely to be longitudinally continuous and often present a more plexiform distribution over the dorsum of the cord. They have a greater frequency of smaller medullary sources.

The larger intradural spinal arteries are unusual in that, similar to the cerebral arteries, they have no significant vasa vasorum. In all other regions of the body, a vessel with an external diameter approaching 1 mm shows a fine vascular plexus (vasa vasorum) on its external surface that supplies nutrients to its outer layers of tissue. Because the cerebral and spinal vessels are bathed in the nutrient-rich cerebrospinal fluid, their external layers presumably derive metabolic exchange from this source.

Lateral Spinal Arteries of the Cervical Cord

The highest three to four segments of the cervical spinal cord receive blood from a unique pair of vessels, the lateral spinal arteries. Although, ontogenetically, these seem to be the most rostral expressions of the dorsolateral spinal arteries, they have a more extensive distribution and are without equivalents in other levels of the cord. They usually arise from the intradural parts of the vertebral arteries near the origins of the posterior inferior cerebellar arteries, or they may arise from the proximal sections of the posterior inferior cerebellar arteries themselves. Their typical course carries them anterior to the posterior roots of the cervical spinal nerves C1 to C4, dorsal to the denticulate ligaments, and parallel to the spinal components of the 11th cranial nerve. Their general distribution is to the dorsolateral and ventrolateral cord regions caudad to the olives.

Although these vessels were observed in the later 19th century, they were usually regarded as variants, and their functional significance was not appreciated. Lasjaunias and colleagues[85] compiled an extensive report on the variations and selective angiography of these important vessels.

Intrinsic Vascularity of the Spinal Cord

The tissues of the spinal cord are supplied by two systems of vessels that enter its substance. The first is a centripetal arrangement of arteries that supplies the superficial tracts of the ventral and lateral funiculi, all of the dorsal funiculus, and the extremities of the dorsal horns. They are radially penetrating branches of the vasa corona and the dorsolateral spinal arteries, which serve only a little more than one fourth of the cord. The greater part of the cord and almost all of its gray matter is supplied by a second centrifugal system of vessels derived from the sulcal (or central) arteries.[86] These arteries are a repetitive series of branches derived from the dorsal aspect of the anterior spinal artery that penetrate the depths of the anterior median fissure. In the mid-sagittal plane, they form a close palisade of vessels that occur with a frequency of 3 to 8 arteries per 1 cm in the cervical region and 2 to 6 per 1 cm in the thoracic cord; they are densest in the lumbar region, where they number 5 to 12 per 1 cm of the anterior spinal artery. The average diameters of the sulcal arteries are greater in the cervical (0.21 mm) and lumbosacral (0.23 mm) regions than in the thoracic cord (0.14 mm).[87]

As these vessels approach the anterior commissure, most turn to either the right or the left and supply only the corresponding side of the cord.[8,63,88,89] This unilateral proclivity reflects their origins in the early embryonic stages when the anterior spinal arteries first condensed from a primitive plexus as a symmetrical pair of longitudinal vessels, each supplying its respective half of the cord. In subsequent development, these two vessels fused in the midline to form the definitive single median anterior spinal artery, but their sulcal branches retained their original unilateral affinities. Bilateral distributions occur in 9%, 7%, and 14% of the cervical, thoracic, and lumbar vessels.[87,90]

Although the sulcal arteries may give infrequent branches to the septomarginal white fibers as they extend into the median anterior fissure, their major distribution is derived after they enter the substance of the cord, just ventral to the anterior white commissure. Here the individual right and left arteries subdivide into dorsal and ventral branches. A group of ventral branches supplies the ventral horns and, through more radial extensions, provides vessels to Clarke column and the deeper fibers of the anterior and lateral funiculi. The smaller, more dorsal group of branches supplies the gray commissure and the ventral one half to two thirds of the dorsal horns. A few second-order or third-order branches form anastomotic arcades with their counterparts of adjacent sulcal artery territories. All these vessels provide the finer arterioles that eventually lead to the spinal capillary beds.

The greater metabolic requirements of the spinal gray matter, in contrast to the funicular tissue, are dramatically reflected in their relative capillary densities. Quantification of the microvascularity in the spinal cord has shown that the capillary density of the gray matter is four to five times as great as the white matter.[91] The capillary distribution within the gray matter is not homogeneous, however, and varies with the regional concentrations of the nuclei. The nuclei of the dorsal horn are fairly uniformly distributed. The ventral horn shows segmental nuclear clusters, which display distinct nerve cell groups.

As noted by Feeney and Watterson,[92] the capillary densities of the white and gray matter of the central nervous system are established at a level that is minimally requisite for the metabolic needs of the given tissue. This situation is in contrast to most other body tissues, which have a capillary "reserve" and normally function with only part of their capillary channels open, varying their intrinsic vascular resistance by dilation of the accessory channels. Nevertheless, despite the lack of this method of control, the spinal cord exhibits a remarkable range of blood flow autoregulation.[1,24,93] The intrinsic cord vasculature maintains a constant blood flow throughout a wide range of systemic blood pressure alterations, although each animal species has a definite upper and lower limit to the systemic blood pressure at which the regulation decompensates. Because transection of the upper cervical cord has no effect on this autoregulatory capacity, it may be assumed that this reflex is local and independent of autonomic nerve control.

Numerous third-order branches of the sulcal arteries communicate directly with veins through convoluted anastomoses. These vascular structures are located primarily in the area that divides the ventral two thirds of the dorsal horn from the dorsal one third and in the more central regions of the ventral horn. They show a paucity of contractile elements and instead exhibit an "epithelioid" type of media that seems capable of swelling and diminishing its thickness. Because this action could rapidly control the caliber of the anastomotic lumina in immediate response to local metabolic changes, these anastomotic convolutions may be the site of the reflex adjustment in the flow resistance of the spinal cord vasculature.[94]

Perhaps the most essential part of knowledge of the vascular supply of the spinal cord is awareness of the ranges of individual variability. The numerous successful surgical cases in which the arteria medullaris magna has been inadvertently interrupted without producing a disastrous spinal cord ischemia give the impression that an adequate collateral vascularity may protect the cord in most individuals when a single major artery is compromised. In procedures involving the interruption of blood flow in numerous consecutive segmental branches of the aorta, such as aortic cross clamping for abdominal vascular surgery, the maintenance of adequate spinal cord blood flow, particularly in the thoracic area, seems to depend more on the regional competence of the anterior spinal artery than on the number of collateral sources to the cord. Spinal cord injury after cross clamping without adjunctive vascular support has been reported to range from 15% to 25%, depending on the series of cases reviewed.[95,96] Proximal-to-distal aortic shunting may alleviate the undesirable hypertension in the aortic distribution proximal to the first clamp and the hypotension in the segments distal to the second clamp. The work of Molina and colleagues[95] on dogs indicated, however, that the shunt capacity should provide more than 60% of the baseline descending aortic flow and have a diameter greater than one half of the descending aorta to be effective.

Of particular significance was the study by Svensson and colleagues[97] on the blood flow in the baboon spinal cord and its implications in aortic cross clamping. This animal was chosen because its spinal vascularity is similar to humans in that its anterior spinal artery is a continuous vessel without the occasional interruptions noted in some quadrupeds. This study indicated that in baboons, as in humans, the caliber of the anterior spinal artery is often critically narrowed where the thoracic anterior spinal artery joins the lumbar segment of this vessel at their common junction with the arteria medullaris magna. The functional implication is that the shunting of the cross-clamped aorta may help maintain an adequate flow in the lumbosacral sections of the cord but is of little help to the supply of the lower sections of the thoracic cord, owing to the marked discrepancy that usually exists between the anterior spinal artery diameters above and below the junction of the arteria medullaris magna.

In accordance with the hemodynamic principles of Poiseuille's equation, the resistance to blood flow upward from the arteria medullaris magna junction was more than 50 times greater than the flow resistance downward into the lumbosacral anterior spinal artery in the baboon. Because a series of direct measurements showed that this discrepancy in the anterior spinal artery diameters was even greater in humans, Svensson and colleagues[97] concluded that even the lowest segments of the thoracic cord were dependent on a blood flow from the superior end of the thoracic anterior spinal artery despite the shunting.

Intrinsic Venous Drainage of the Spinal Cord

Compared with the arterial anatomy, the structural and functional aspects of the venous drainage of the spinal cord have been relatively neglected. In contrast to other organ systems in which the equivalent orders of veins and arteries tend to course in a common vascular bundle, the veins of the central nervous system are generally less numerous than the arteries, they are larger than their corresponding efferent vessels, the larger branches may not show a pattern concurrent with the arterial distribution, and they are not accompanied by lymphatics.

The internal substance of the dorsal half of the cord drains by a centrifugal arrangement of intrinsic vessels that are tributaries, by way of a venous vasa corona, to a large median dorsal longitudinal spinal vein; the ventral half sends tributaries to sulcal veins that empty into a large median ventral longitudinal vein that runs parallel to the anterior spinal artery. Both of these longitudinal vessels are circumferentially connected by a prominent venous vasa corona. This entire system drains into the epidural venous plexus by medullary (previously called *radicular*) veins that are as infrequent in their distribution as the medullary arteries.[98] The proximal sections of the spinal nerve roots drain centripetally into the vasa corona and longitudinal veins of the cord and then to the epidural system via the medullary veins.

Vascularization of the Spinal Nerve Roots

Although it has been generally recognized that much of the pain consequent to degenerative changes in the spinal motion segment is associated with compression or tension on the spinal nerve roots, the mechanisms that initiate the actual nerve discharge have remained obscure. Because experimental studies on peripheral nerves and observations on numerous cases of neurogenic claudication have suggested that much of the pain may have a neuroischemic basis, investigations were undertaken to determine the nature of the intrinsic vascularity of the spinal nerve root and its response to localized compression or tension. The nerve roots had long been regarded as part of the peripheral nervous system and were viewed as histologically and vascularly similar to peripheral nerves. Consequently, research on the latter was often uncritically extrapolated to apply to the nerve roots.

The very long roots of the lumbosacral spinal nerves seemed to be particularly vulnerable because their vascularity was initially believed to be supplied only from their distal ends without the access to the frequent collateral support that is characteristic of peripheral nerves. Because the nerve root fasciculi do not have a strong connective tissue support, it also seemed that the fine vascularity they possessed would be at risk from the repeated tension and relaxation resulting from the flexion and extension of the spine. Parke and colleagues[99] and Parke and Watanabe[100] showed by vascular injection that the roots receive their arterial supply from both ends (Fig. 2–41; see Fig. 2–36), however, a fact physiologically confirmed by Yamamoto.[101]

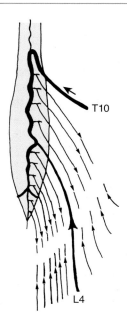

FIGURE 2–41 Schema indicating directions of normal blood flow in cauda equina. The anterior spinal artery of the lumbosacral part of the cord is supplied by medullary arteries and supplies 75% at the cord substance and upper parts of the cauda equina via the proximal radicular arteries. This accounts for enlargement of the anterior spinal artery in the lumbosacral region.

The existence of many redundant coils along the branches of the true radicular arteries ameliorates the stresses that would result from the interfascicular movements that accompany the repeated stretch and relaxation. A significant finding was the occurrence of numerous, relatively large arteriovenous anastomoses throughout the length of the root (Fig. 2–42). These vascular cross connections apparently allow blood flow to be maintained in sections of the root above and below a point of compression. Of particular significance to root nutrition is the work of Rydevik and colleagues[100] who, using isotopically labeled methylglucose, showed that approximately 50% of the root nutrition is derived from the ambient cerebrospinal fluid; this necessitates a gauzelike architecture of the radicular pia-arachnoid sheath (Fig. 2–43; see Fig. 2–42B).

A study by Watanabe and Parke[102,103] of chronically compressed roots indicated that the compressed segment is most likely metabolically deprived. It has been suggested that radicular pain is related to root ischemia because a reduction of oxygen intake in patients with neurogenic claudication exacerbates the symptoms.[104] The arterial side of the vasa radiculorum seems to be well compensated, however, and maintains a continuity despite severe chronic compression. Further study has indicated that the venous side of the radiculomedullary circulation is more vulnerable.[103] Because the roots are part of the central nervous system, the relationships of the arteries to the veins resemble those of the brain more than those of peripheral nerves. The radicular veins do not follow the arterial pattern. They are fewer in number and run a separate and usually deeper (more central) course. Being thin-walled, they are more liable to the spatial restrictions imposed by degenerative changes in the dimensions of the spinal canal

and intervertebral foramina and show complete interruption in the chronically compressed root. The metabolically deprived, or inflamed, nerve root becomes hypersensitive to any mechanical deformation, and any additional insult to such a nerve may initiate ectopic impulses that produce pain.

Impedance of the radiculomedullary venous return can occur without topographically related venous constriction. The exacerbation of neurogenic pain in cases in which spinal stenosis has been associated with venous hypertension has been recorded by clinical investigators. LaBan[105] and LaBan and Wesolowski[106] noted that patients with diminished right-sided heart compliance and spinal stenosis may eventually exhibit neurogenic pain even in static or recumbent situations. They attributed this phenomenon to an increased external

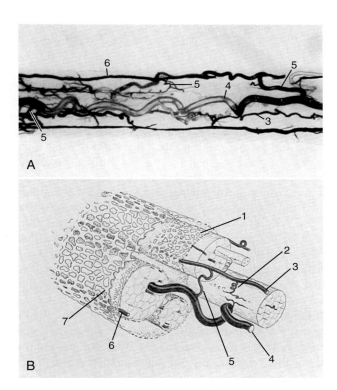

FIGURE 2–42 A, Low-power (×20) transillumination photomicrograph of midsection from part of L4 nerve root that had been treated with hydrogen peroxide after vascular injection with latex–India ink but before clearing in a solution of tributyl-tricresyl phosphates. The peroxidases within the residual blood elements inflated the radicular veins (4) to provide a temporary contrast medium. Note the frequency of the large arteriovenous anastomoses (5) that permitted the latex–India ink to enter the veins.
B, Graphic compilation showing structure of a typical lumbosacral nerve root derived from data obtained by injection studies and scanning electron microscopy (see Fig. 2–38). The gauzelike pia-arachnoid membranes permit the cerebrospinal fluid to percolate into nerve tissues and assist metabolic support. Numbers in **A** and **B** are common to equivalent structures.
1. fascicular pia
2. interfascicular and intrafascicular arteries showing compensating coils to allow interfascicular movement
3. longitudinal radicular artery
4. large radicular vein (does not course with arteries)
5. arteriovenous anastomosis
6. collateral radicular artery
7. gauzelike pia-arachnoid that permits percolation of cerebrospinal fluid to assist in metabolic support

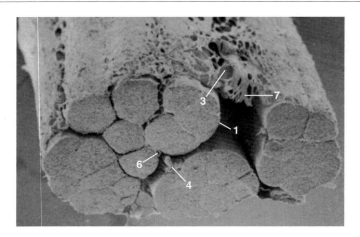

FIGURE 2–43 Scanning electron photomicrograph of section of proximal part of L5 ventral nerve root. The gauzelike pia-arachnoid sheath is very evident. The numbers correspond to the structures labeled in Figure 2–42.

pressure on the already sensitized roots by the engorgement of the epidural venous sinuses (see Fig. 2–35), but the venous hypertension alone may be sufficient to impede the venous return from an already compromised radicular circulation. Madsen and Heros[107] showed that "arterialization" of spinal veins by abnormal arteriovenous shunts in the region of the conus medullaris exacerbates the neurogenic pain in patients with spinal stenosis. Their hypothesis suggested that a variable combination of increased mechanical constriction by dilated epidural veins and the direct increased resistance to the radicular circulation by the venous hypertension could contribute to the elicitation of pain. Aboulker and colleagues[108] also concluded that epidural venous hypertension alone may produce radicular symptoms or cord symptoms or both without adjunctive stenotic compression.

If the intrinsic circulation of the nerve root is impeded in either its arterial input or its venous outflow, the net effect seems to be the same: a neuroischemia of the compressed root segment that may enhance the generation of ectopic nerve impulses. A phenomenon that could be related to radicular venous stasis is the swelling of the disc-distorted nerve root that Takata and colleagues[109] showed in CT myelograms. This phenomenon is difficult to explain because extravasated fluids in the root tissues should have free access to the surrounding cerebrospinal fluid. Nevertheless, the fluid balance of the root tissues seems to be altered, particularly in the segment proximal to the level of the offending disc. The intricacies of the hemodynamic relationships responsible for this change remain unknown.

The role of the ubiquitous arteriovenous anastomosis in autoregulation of the intrinsic radicular vasculature also offers a fertile field for clinical investigations. Because these vascular shunts are mostly without contractile elements but seem instead to control their lumina by the thickening response of an epithelioid endothelium, they probably react to chemical changes in the blood within their lumina and can offer an immediate local reflex to alterations in the nerve root metabolism.

Functional Anatomy of the Spine

The biomechanics of the spine is a very complex and extensive subject. A comprehensive discussion is beyond the scope of this chapter, so the reader is directed to the work of White and Panjabi,[110] which is generally regarded as the major book in this field. Because an appreciation of the essential functional relationships of the spinal components does enhance an understanding of their anatomy, however, a brief overview follows.

The spine is capable of ventroflexion, extension, lateral flexion, and rotation. This remarkable universal mobility may seem at odds with the fact that its most essential function is to provide a firm support for the trunk and appendages. The apparent contradiction may be resolved when one realizes that the total ranges of motion are the result of a summation of limited movements permitted between the individual vertebrae and that the total length of the spine changes very little during its movements. The role of the musculature in the performance of the supportive functions cannot be minimized, as the disastrous scolioses that result from their unilateral loss in a few motor segment units may attest.

The degree and combination of the individual types of motion described earlier vary considerably in the different vertebral regions. Although all subaxial-presacral vertebrae are united in a tripod arrangement consisting of the intervertebral disc and the two zygapophyseal articulations, the relative size and shape of the former and the articular planes of the latter determine the range and types of motion that an individual set of intervertebral articulations contributes to the total mobility of the spine. In general, flexion is the most pronounced movement of the vertebral column as a whole. It requires an anterior compression of the intervertebral disc and a gliding separation of the articular facets, in which the inferior set of an individual vertebra tends to move upward and forward over the opposing superior set of the adjacent inferior vertebra. The movement is checked mainly by the posterior ligaments and epaxial muscles.

Extension tends to be a more limited motion, producing posterior compression of the disc, with the inferior articular process gliding posteriorly and downward over the superior set below. It is checked by the anterior longitudinal ligament and all ventral muscles that directly or indirectly flex the spine. Also, the laminae and spinous processes may sharply limit extension. Lateral flexion is accompanied by some degree of rotation. It involves a rocking of the bodies on their discs, with a sliding separation of the diarthroses on the convex side and an overriding of the diarthroses related to the concavity. The rotational component brings the anterior surface of the bodies toward the convexity of the flexure and the spinous processes toward its concavity. This phenomenon is well illustrated in a dried preparation of a scoliotic spine. Lateral flexion is checked by the intertransverse ligaments and the extensions of the ribs or their costal homologues.

Pure rotation is directly proportional to the relative thickness of the intervertebral disc and is mainly limited by the geometry of the planes of the diarthrodial surfaces. Although the architecture of the disc permits limited rotation between the bodies, it also serves to check this movement by its resistance to compression. The consecutive layers of the anulus fibrosus have their fibers arranged in an alternating helical fashion, and rotation in either direction can be accompanied only by increasing the angularity of the opposing fibers to the horizontal, which requires compression of the disc.

The entire vertebral column rotates approximately 90 degrees to either side of the sagittal plane, but most of this traversion is accomplished in the cervical and thoracic sections. It flexes nearly the same amount, using primarily the cervical and thoracic regions. Approximately 90 degrees of extension is permitted by the cervical and lumbar regions, whereas lateral flexion with rotation is allowed to 60 degrees to both sides, again primarily by the cervical and lumbar areas.

Specific Regional Considerations

The atlanto-occipital joints mostly permit flexion and extension with a limited lateral action, all being checked by the suboccipital musculature and the atlanto-occipital ligaments. The atlantoaxial articulations allow only rotation, the pivoted joint being stabilized and checked by the alar ligaments and the ligaments forming the capsules of the atlantoaxial diarthroses.

One half of the rotational mobility of the entire cervical region takes place between the atlas and the axis, and the remainder is distributed among the joints of the subaxial vertebrae. The atlanto-occipital joint accounts for approximately half of the cervical flexion. The remaining 50% is not evenly distributed among the cervical vertebrae but is greater in the upper section.

The subaxial part of the cervical region shows the ranges of motion that are the most free of all the presacral vertebrae. The discs are quite thick in relation to the heights of the vertebral bodies and contribute about one fourth of the height of this part of the column. In addition, a sagittal section shows the middle part of the cervical disc to be lenticular, so that the anteroinferior lips of the bodies are more capable of sliding slightly forward and overriding one another. The range of spinal flexion is greatest in the cervical region, and although the posterior nuchal ligaments and muscles may tend to resist this motion, it is ultimately checked by the chin coming to rest on the chest.

The cervical spine is normally carried in a moderately extended position and shows a median variation of 91 degrees between extension and flexion. Extension is checked by the anterior longitudinal ligament and the combined resistances of the anterior cervical musculature, fascia, and visceral structures, all three of which may be traumatized in hyperextension injuries.

Cervical lateral flexion is quite limited by the articular pillars and the intertransverse ligaments, and most lateral motion involves considerable rotation. The nearly horizontal position of the planes of the cervical articular facets provides good supportive strength to the articular pillars but increases the lateral rigidity, so that hyperextension injuries may be more disastrous if the head is rotated at the time of impact from the rear.

The mobility of the thoracic region is also not uniform throughout its length. Although the upper segments resemble the cervical vertebrae with respect to the size of the bodies and the discs, the ribs attached to the sternum greatly impair the ranges of motion. The circumferential arc of the plane of the articular facets shows that rotation is the movement least restricted by these structures.

Flexion and extension become freer in the lower thoracic region, where the discs and vertebral bodies progressively increase in size and the more mobile and less restrictive they become. The last few thoracic vertebrae are transitional with respect to the surfaces of the articular facets. These begin to turn more toward the sagittal plane and tend to limit rotation and permit greater extension.

The articulations of the lumbar region permit ventroflexion, lateral flexion, and extension, but the facets of the synovial joints lie in a ventromedial to dorsolateral plane that virtually locks them against rotation. This lumbar nonrotatory rigidity is a feature shared with most mammals and achieves its greatest manifestation in certain quadrupeds in which the inferior articulation fits like a cylindric tenon into the semicircular mortise of the corresponding superior process of the vertebra below. It provides a gliding action that permits the neural arches to separate or approximate each other only during extension and flexion. The morphology of the joints can be well appreciated in an appropriate cut of loin chop or T-bone steak.

The synovial articulations at the lumbosacral junctions are unique. In contrast to the more superior lumbar joints, the facets of the inferior articulating processes of the fifth lumbar vertebra face forward and slightly downward, to engage the reciprocally corresponding articular processes of the sacrum. Because of the position of these joint surfaces, a certain amount of rotation should be possible between the fifth lumbar segment and the sacrum, but the presence of the strong iliolumbar ligaments quite likely restricts much motion of this type.

The most essential function of the synovial lumbosacral articulations involves their role as buttresses against the forward and downward displacement of the fifth lumbar vertebra in relation to the sacrum. When one considers that each region of the spine has its own characteristic curvature, the tracing of the vertical line indicating the center of gravity shows that it intersects the column through the bodies of the transitional vertebrae. The normal cervical lordosis places most of the cervical vertebrae anterior to the center of gravity, and the compensating thoracic kyphosis places the thoracic vertebrae posterior to the center of gravity. The lumbar lordosis brings the middle lumbar vertebrae anterior to the line. The transitional vertebrae between each region intersect the center of gravity and seem to be the most unstable regions of the spine; this is emphasized by the fact that disc problems and fractures most frequently occur in the transitional vertebrae.

Because the sacrovertebral angle produces the most abrupt change of direction in the column, and the center of gravity, which passes through the fifth lumbar body, falls anterior to the sacrum, there is a marked tendency for the thick, wedge-shaped fifth lumbar disc to give way to the shearing vector that the lumbosacral angularity produces. The resulting condition, spondylolisthesis, most frequently reveals a deficiency in the laminae (spondylolysis) that fails to anchor the fifth vertebral body to the sacrum and allows its forward displacement. There has been considerable discussion as to whether spondylolysis is congenital or acquired, but the spondylolisthesis seldom occurs without the laminar deficiencies as a preceding condition.

Biomechanics of the Intervertebral Disc

It is axiomatic in mechanical engineering that a well-designed machine automatically reveals its function through the analysis of its structure. There are few instances in biologic circumstances in which this statement is more applicable than in the case of the intervertebral disc. Even when the disc is simply divided with a knife and examined grossly, it is apparent that one is dealing with an organ that is remarkably constructed simultaneously to alleviate shock and transmit forces from every conceivable combination of vectors. This appreciation of the functional competency of the disc increases as its structure is analyzed at the finer levels of organization.

The internal composition of the disc has evolved to withstand great stresses through the liquid and elastic properties of nucleus and anulus acting in combination. The nucleus is distorted by compression forces, but being liquid it is in itself incompressible. It serves to receive primarily vertical forces from the vertebral bodies and redistribute them radially in a horizontal plane. It is the distortion of the anulus by the internal pressure of the nucleus that gives the disc its compressibility, and its resilience makes possible the recovery from pressure.

Were the nucleus pulposus simply a cavity filled with water, it would momentarily act in the same capacity, but the ability to maintain the appropriate quantity of fluid during the continual compression and recovery cycle would be lacking. This ability to absorb and retain relatively large amounts of water is the unique property of the living tissue of the nucleus.[111] The essential compound involved in this process is a protein-polysaccharide gel, which through a high imbibition pressure binds nearly nine times its volume of water. It is apparent that the hydrophilia is not a form of biochemical bonding because a quantity of water can be expressed from the nucleus by prolonged mechanical pressure. This accounts for the diurnal decrease in the total length of the spine and its recovery in the supine position at night.

The anulus must receive the ultimate effects of most forces transmitted from one vertebral body to another. Because the major loading of the intervertebral disc is in the form of vertical compression, it may seem paradoxical that the anulus is best constructed to resist tension, but the nucleus transforms the vertical thrust into a radial pressure that is resisted by the tensile properties of the lamellae. Although the basic plan of alternating bands of fibers is one of the obvious sources of the tensile strength of the anulus, this arrangement is not uniform with respect to the directions of the fibers or the degrees of resistance and resilience encountered throughout the anulus. The fibers generally become longer, and the angle of their spiral course becomes more horizontal near the circumference of the disc because it is here that the shearing stresses of vertebral torsions would be most effective. Experimental analysis has also shown that various parts of the anulus do not respond equally to the same degree of tension, and the discrepancies were related to the plane of section and the location of the sample.[112] The anulus proved to have the greatest resistance and the greatest recovery in horizontal sections of the peripheral lamellae, whereas vertical and more medial sections were more distensible.

Because the spine acts as a flexible boom to the guidewire actions of the erector spinae muscles, it is essentially the fulcrum of a lever system of the first class, in which the loading has a considerable mechanical advantage. Pure vector analysis has indicated that a theoretical pressure of approximately three fourths of a ton could be applied to a disc when 100 lb is lifted by the hands,[14] but this is considerably in excess of the actual pressures achieved. Increased intrathoracic and intra-abdominal pressures alleviate much of the fulcrum compression of the discs by effectively countering the load of the anterior lever arm.

The actual pressure variations occurring with postural changes have been recorded by inserting transducers into the third lumbar disc.[113,114] This procedure indicated that the internal disc pressure increases from approximately 100 kg in a standing position with the spine erect to 150 kg when the trunk is bent forward and to 220 kg when a 70-kg man lifts a 50-kg weight. It was particularly revealing that the pressure showed a considerable increase when the equivalent maneuvers were repeated in a sitting position, and the weight lifting ultimately created a pressure of 300 kg on the third lumbar disc.

The disc is also "preloaded." The inherent tensions of the intervertebral ligaments and the anulus exert a pressure of about 15 kg because this weight is required to restore the original thickness of the disc after the ligaments have been divided.[100] From a comparative standpoint, this preloading probably offers increased stability to the spine as a functional flexible rod. One is almost induced unconsciously to use teleologic thinking in terms of the vertical thrust resistance when regarding the structure of the disc. In perspective, however, the intervertebral disc shows a consistent morphology in all mammals, yet humans are the only species that truly stand erect. Although analysis of muscular action would most likely show that all mammalian discs must dissipate and transfer axial thrusts, the preloading would enhance the "beam strength" that is obviously necessary in the vertebral column of quadrupeds.

Acknowledgments

The vascular studies presented in this chapter were supported by National Institutes of Health research grant HL-14035.

KEY REFERENCES

1. Bogduk N, Tynan W, Wilson AS: The nerve supply to the human lumbar intervertebral disc. J Anat 132:39-56, 1981.
   In attempts to clarify the nature and source of discogenic back pain, the investigators performed an anatomic study of the microinnervation of the human lumbar intervertebral disc. They found rich innervation of the posterior anulus and posterior longitudinal ligament by penetrating branches of the sinuvertebral nerves from the dorsal root ganglia communicantes.

2. Ebraheim NA, Xu R, Knight T, et al: Morphometric evaluation of lower cervical pedicle and its projection. Spine 22:1-6, 1997.
   Despite being highly technically demanding, insertion of lower cervical pedicle screws has become popular. In this study, the authors assessed various morphometric dimensions of human cervical pedicles, finding significant variations between individuals. They recommended careful preoperative evaluation of CT scans in planning cervical transpedicular screw insertion.

3. Jasani V, Jaffray D: The anatomy of the iliolumbar vein: A cadaver study. J Bone Joint Surg Br 84:1046-1049, 2002.
   The iliolumbar vein can be injured during anterior surgery of the lower lumbar spine and lumbosacral junction. The authors performed a cadaveric study that detailed variations in the path of the vein in relation to the vertebrae and disc spaces.

4. Parke WW, Watanabe R: The intrinsic vasculature of the lumbosacral spinal nerve roots. Spine 10:508-515, 1985.
   This study supports the idea that lumbar spinal nerve roots are structurally, vascularly, and metabolically unique insofar that their intrinsic vasculature and supporting connective tissue may account for suspected "neuroischemic" responses to pathologic mechanical stresses and inflammatory conditions associated with degenerative disease of the lower spine.

5. Scoles PV, Linton AE, Latimer B, et al: Vertebral body and posterior element morphology: The normal spine in middle life. Spine 13:1082-1086, 1988.
   This study was one of the first to examine the variability of pedicle dimensions. The authors recognized that many thoracic pedicles (and some lumbar pedicles) could not safely accommodate a 5-mm diameter screw. In addition, the investigators' data show larger average transverse pedicle widths in the upper thoracic vertebrae than in the middle thoracic vertebrae.

REFERENCES

1. Francis WR, Fielding JW: Traumatic spondylolisthesis of the axis. Orthop Clin North Am 9:1011-1027, 1978.

2. McCulloch JA, Transfelt EE: Macnab's Backache. Baltimore, Williams & Wilkins, 1997.

3. Weiner BK, Walker M, Wiley W, et al: The lateral buttress: An anatomic feature of the lumbar pars interarticularis. Spine 27:E385-E387, 2002.

4. An HS, Wise JJ, Xu R: Anatomy of the cervicothoracic junction: A study of cadaveric dissection, cryomicrotomy and magnetic resonance imaging. J Spinal Disord 12:519-525, 1999.

5. Ebraheim NA, Xu R, Knight T, et al: Morphometric evaluation of lower cervical pedicle and its projection. Spine 22:1-6, 1997.

6. Pait TG, McAllister PV, Kaufman HH: Quadrant anatomy of the articular pillars (lateral cervical mass) of the cervical spine. J Neurosurg 82:1011-1014, 1995.

7. Xu R, Burgar A, Ebraheim NA, et al: The quantitative anatomy of the laminas of the spine. Spine 24:107-113, 1999.

8. Chaynes P, Sol JC, Vaysse P, et al: Vertebral pedicle anatomy in relation to pedicle screw fixation: A cadaver study. Spine 23:85-90, 2001.

9. Cinotti G, Gumina S, Ripani M, et al: Pedicle instrumentation in the thoracic spine: A morphometric and cadaveric study for placement of screws. Spine 24:114-119, 1999.

10. Scoles PV, Linton AE, Latimer B, et al: Vertebral body and posterior element morphology: The normal spine in middle life. Spine 13:1082-1086, 1988.

11. Olszewski AD, Yaszemski MJ, White AA: The anatomy of the human lumbar ligamentum flavum: New observations and their surgical implications. Spine 21:2307-2312, 1996.

12. von Luschka H: Die Halbgelenke des menschlichen Korpers. Berlin, Karpess, 1858.

13. Beadle OA: The Intervertebral Discs. Special Report No. 160. London, Medical Research Council, 1931, pp 6-9.

14. Bradford DL, Spurling RG: The Intervertebral Disc. Springfield, IL, Charles C Thomas, 1945.

15. Humzah MD, Soames RW: Human intervertebral disc: Structure and function. Anat Rec 229:337-356, 1988.

16. Bick EM: The osteohistology of the normal human vertebra. J Mt Sinai Hosp 19:490-527, 1952.

17. Aeby C: Die Alterverschiedenheiten der menschlichen Wirbelsaule. Arch Anat Physiol (Anat Abst) 10:77, 1879.

18. Dommissee G: Morphological aspects of the lumbar spine and lumbosacral regions. Orthop Clin North Am 6:163-175, 1975.

19. Wiltse LL: Anatomy of the extradural compartments of the lumbar spinal canal: Peridural membrane and circumneural sheath. Radiol Clin North Am 38:1177-1206, 2000.

20. Ugur HC, Attar A, Uz A, et al: Surgical anatomic evaluation of the cervical pedicle and adjacent neural structures. Neurosurgery 47:1162-1168, 2000.

21. Ugur HC, Attar A, Uz A, et al: Thoracic pedicle: Surgical anatomic evaluation and relations. J Spinal Disord 14:39-45, 2001.

22. Ebraheim NA, Xu R, Darwich M, et al: Anatomic relations between the lumbar pedicle and the adjacent neural structures. Spine 15:2338-2341, 1997.

23. Hogan Q, Toth J: Anatomy of the soft tissues of the spinal canal. Reg Anesth Pain Med 24:303-310, 1999.

24. Kobrine AI, Doyle DF, Rizzoli HV: Spinal cord blood flow as affected by changes in systemic arterial blood pressure. J Neurosurg 44:12-15, 1976.

25. Golub GS, Silverman B: Transforaminal ligaments of the lumbar spine. J Bone Joint Surg Am 51:947-956, 1969.

26. Park HK, Rudrappa S, Dujovny M, et al: Intervertebral foraminal ligaments of the lumbar spine: Anatomy and biomechanics. Child Nerv Syst 4-5:275-282, 2001.

27. Grimes PF, Massie JB, Garfin SR: Anatomic and biomechanical analysis of the lower lumbar foraminal ligaments. Spine 25:2009-2014, 2000.

28. Alleyne CH, Cawley CM, Barrow DL, et al: Microsurgical anatomy of the dorsal cervical nerve roots and the cervical dorsal root ganglion/ventral root complexes. Surg Neurol 50:213-218, 1998.

29. Kadish LJ, Simmons EH: Anomalies of the lumbosacral nerve roots. J Bone Joint Surg Br 66:411-416, 1984.

30. Kikuchi S, Hasue M: Anatomic features of the furcal nerve and its clinical significance. Spine 11:1002-1007, 1986.

31. Piacsecka-Kacperska A, Gladykowska-Rzeczycka J: The sacral plexus in primates. Folia Morphol (Warsz) 31:21-31, 1972.

32. Parke WW, Watanabe R: Lumbosacral intersegmental epispinal axons and ectopic ventral nerve rootlets. J Neurosurg 67:269-277, 1987.

33. Hasue M, Kunogi J, Konno S, et al: Classification by position of dorsal root ganglia in the lumbosacral region. Spine 14:1261-1264, 1989.

34. Kikuchi S, Hasue M: Combined contrast studies in lumbar spine diseases. Spine 13:1327-1331, 1988.

35. Bogduk N, Tynan W, Wilson AS: The nerve supply to the human lumbar intervertebral disc. J Anat 132:39-56, 1981.

36. Bogduk N, Windsor M, Inglis A: The innervation of the cervical intervertebral discs. Spine 13:2-8, 1988.

37. Hirsch C: Studies on mechanism of low back pain. Acta Orthop Scand 22:184-231, 1953.

38. Jung A, Brunschwig A: Recherches histologiques sur l'innervation des articulations et des corps vertebreaux. Presse Med 40:316-317, 1932.

39. Larmon AW: An anatomic study of the lumbosacral region in relation to low back pain and sciatica. Ann Surg 119:892, 1944.

40. Malinsky J: The ontogenetic development of nerve terminations in the intervertebral discs of man. Acta Anat 38:96-113, 1959.

41. Nade S, Bell S, Wyke BD: The innervation of the lumbar spine joints and its significance. J Bone Joint Surg Br 62:225-261, 1980.

42. Wiberg G: Back pain in relation to nerve supply of intervertebral disc. Acta Orthop Scand 19:211-221, 1949.

43. Parke WW: Applied anatomy of the spine. In Rothman RH, Simeone FA (eds): The Spine. Philadelphia, WB Saunders, 1982, pp 18-51.

44. Groen GJ, Baljet B, Drukker J: The nerves and nerve plexuses of the human vertebral column. Am J Anat 188:282-296, 1990.

45. Pedersen HE, Blunck CFJ, Gardner E: The anatomy of the lumbosacral posterior rami and meningeal branches of spinal nerves (sinuvertebral nerves). J Bone Joint Surg Am 38:377-391, 1956.

46. Hirsch C, Inglemark B, Miller M: The anatomical basis for low back pain. Acta Orthop Scand 33:1-17, 1963.

47. McCouch GP, During ID, Ling TH: Location of receptors for tonic reflexes. J Neurophysiol 14:191-195, 1951.

48. Stilwell DL: The nerve supply of the vertebral column and its associated structures in the monkey. Anat Rec 125:139-169, 1956.

49. Yoshizawa H, O'Brien JP, Thomas-Smith W, et al: The neuropathology of intervertebral discs removed for low back pain. J Pathol 132:95-104, 1980.

50. Kimmel DL: Innervation of the spinal dura and the dura of the posterior cranial fossa. Neurology 11:800-809, 1986.

51. Cyriax J: Dural pain. Lancet 1:919-921, 1978.

52. Groen GJ, Baljet B, Drukker J: The innervation of the spinal dura mater: Anatomy and clinical implications. Acta Neurochir 92:39-46, 1988.

53. Parke WW, Watanabe R: Adhesions of the ventral lumbar dura: An adjunct source of discogenic pain? Spine 15:300-303, 1990.

54. Blikra G: Intradural herniated lumbar disc. J Neurosurg 31:676-679, 1969.

55. Junghanns H: Der Lumboscralwinkel. Dtsch Z Chit 213:332, 1929.

56. Schmorl G, Junghanns H: The Human Spine in Health and Disease. New York, Grune & Stratton, 1959.

57. DePalma AF, Rothman RH: The Intervertebral Disc. Philadelphia, WB Saunders, 1970.

58. Brown MD: The Pathophysiology of the Intervertebral Disc: Anatomical, Physiological and Biomedical Considerations. Philadelphia, Jefferson Medical College, 1969.

59. Maroudas A: Nutrition and metabolism of the intervertebral disc. In Ghosh P (ed): The Biology of the Intervertebral Disc. Boca Raton, FL, CRC Press, 1988.

60. Holm S, Maroudas A, Urban JPG, et al: Nutrition of the intervertebral disc: An in vivo study of solute transport. Clin Orthop 129:104-114, 1977.

61. Holm S, Maroudas A, Urban JPG, et al: Nutrition of the intervertebral disc: Solute transport and metabolism. Connect Tissue Res 8:101-110, 1981.

62. Maroudas A, Nachemson A, Stockwell RA, et al: Factors involved in the nutrition of human lumbar intervertebral disc: Cellularity and diffusion of glucose in vitro. J Anat 120:113-130, 1975.

63. Ferguson WP: Some observations on the circulation in fetal and infant spines. J Bone Joint Surg 32:640-645, 1950.

64. Willis TA: Nutrient arteries of the vertebral bodies. J Bone Joint Surg 31:538-541, 1949.

65. Crock HV, Yoshizawa H: The Blood Supply of the Vertebral Column and Spinal Cord in Man. New York, Springer-Verlag, 1977.

66. Milen MT, Bloom DA, Culligan J, et al: Albert Adamkiewicz (1850-1921)—his artery and its significance for the retroperitoneal surgeon. World J Urol 17:168-170, 1999.

67. Parke WW: The vascular relations of the upper cervical vertebrae. Orthop Clin North Am 9:879-889, 1978.

68. Schiff DCM, Parke WW: The arterial supply of the odontoid process. Anat Rec 172:399-400, 1972.

69. Jasani V, Jaffray D: The anatomy of the iliolumbar vein: a cadaver study. J Bone Joint Surg Br 84:1046-1049, 2002.

70. Kaisary AV, Smith P: Spinal cord ischemia after ligation of both internal iliac arteries during radical cystoprostectomy. Urology 25:395-397, 1985.

71. Breschet G: Essai sur les Veines der Rachis. Paris, Mequigon-Morvith, 1819.

72. Batson OV: The function of the vertebral veins and their role in the spread of metastases. Am Surg 112:138-145, 1940.

73. Clemens HJ: Die Venesysteme der menschlichen Wirbelsaule. Berlin, Walter de Gruyter, 1961.

74. Chaynes P, Verdie JC, Moscovici J, et al: Microsurgical anatomy of the internal vertebral venous plexuses. Surg Radiol Anat 20:47-51, 1998.

75. Parke WW, Valsamis MP: The ampulloglomerular organ: An unusual neurovascular complex in the suboccipital region. Anat Rec 159:193-198, 1967.

76. Parke WW, Rizzoli HV, Brown MD: The pharyngovertebral veins: An anatomic rationale for Grisel's syndrome. J Bone Joint Surg Am 66:568-574, 1984.

77. Wetzel FT, LaRocca H: Grisel's syndrome: A review. Clin Orthop 240:141-152, 1989.

78. Corbib JL: Anatomie et Pathologie Arterielles de la Moelle. Paris, Masson et Cie, 1961, pp 787-796.

79. Brewer LA, Fosburg RG, Mulder GA, et al: Spinal cord complications following surgery for coarctation of the aorta. J Thorac Cardiovasc Surg 64:368-379, 1972.

80. Lazorthes G, Gouaze A, Zadeh JO, et al: Arterial vascularization of the spinal cord. J Neurosurg 35:253-262, 1971.

81. Marcus ML, Heistad DD, Ehrardt JC, et al: Regulation of total and regional spinal cord blood flow. Circ Res 41:128-134, 1977.

82. Parke WW, Whalen JL, Bunger PC, et al: Intimal musculature of the lower anterior spinal artery. Spine 20:2073-2079, 1995.

83. Parke WW: Correlative anatomy of cervical spondylotic myelopathy. Spine 13:831-837, 1988.

84. Dommissee GF: The Arteries and Veins of the Human Spinal Cord from Birth. Edinburgh, Churchill-Livingstone, 1975.

85. Lasjaunias P, Vallee B, Person H, et al: The lateral artery of the upper cervical spinal cord. J Neurosurg 63:235-241, 1985.

86. Gillilan LA: The arterial blood supply of the human spinal cord. J Comp Neurol 110:75-103, 1958.

87. Hassler O: Blood supply to human spinal cord. Arch Neurol 15:302-307, 1966.

88. Herren RY, Alexander L: Sulcal and intrinsic blood vessels of human spinal cord. Arch Neurol Psychiatry 41:678-683, 1939.

89. Kadyi H: Über die Blutgefasse des menschlichen Ruckenmarkes: Nach einer im XV Bande der Denkschriften d. math-naturw. Cl. d. Akad. d. Wissensch. Krakau erschienen Morphology, aus dem Polnischen Ubersaatz vom Verfasser. Lemberg, Grubrnowicz & Schmidt, 1889.

90. Turnbull IM, Brieg A, Hassler O: Blood supply of cervical spinal cord in man. J Neurosurg 24:951-965, 1966.

91. Ireland WP, Fletcher TF, Bingham C: Quantification of microvasculature in the canine spinal cord. Anat Rec 200:103-113, 1981.

92. Feeney JF, Watterson RL: The development of the vascular pattern within the walls of the central nervous system of the chick embryo. J Morphol 78:231-303, 1946.

93. Lobosky JM, Hitchon PW, Torner JC, et al: Spinal cord autoregulation in the sheep. Curr Surg 41:264-267, 1984.

94. Parke WW: Arteriovenous anastomoses in the spinal cord: Probable role in blood flow autoregulation [abstract]. Anat Rec 223:87A, 1989.

95. Molina JE, Cogordon J, Einzig S, et al: Adequacy of ascending-descending aorta shunt during cross-clamping of the thoracic aorta for prevention of spinal cord injury. J Thorac Cardiovasc Surg 90:126-136, 1985.

96. Wadouh F, Arndt CF, Opperman E, et al: The mechanism of spinal cord injury after simple and double aortic cross-clamping. J Thorac Cardiovasc Surg 92:121-127, 1986.

97. Svensson LG, Rickards E, Coull A, et al: Relationship of spinal cord blood flow to vascular anatomy during thoracic aorta cross-clamping and shunting. J Thorac Cardiovasc Surg 91:71-78, 1986.

98. Gillilan LA: Veins of the spinal cord. Neurology 20:860-868, 1970.

99. Parke WW, Gammel K, Rothman RH: Arterial vascularization of the cauda equina. J Bone Joint Surg Am 63:53-62, 1981.

100. Parke WW, Watanabe R: The intrinsic vasculature of the lumbosacral spinal nerve roots. Spine 10:508-515, 1985.

101. Yamamoto H: Quantitative measurements of blood flow in cauda equina in spinal cords of monkeys by using radioactive microspheres. J Jpn Coll Angiol 22:35-42, 1982.

102. Watanabe R, Parke WW: The vascular and neural pathology of lumbosacral spinal stenosis. J Neurosurg 65:64-70, 1986.

103. Watanabe R, Parke WW: Structure of lumbosacral spinal nerve roots: Anatomy and pathology in spinal stenosis. J Clin Orthop Surg (Jpn) 22:529-539, 1987.

104. Evans JG: Neurogenic intermittent claudication. BMJ 2:985-987, 1964.

105. LaBan MM: "Vesper's curse": Night pain, the bane of Hypnos. Arch Phys Med Rehabil 65:501-504, 1984.

106. LaBan MM, Wesolowski DP: Night pain associated with diminished cardiopulmonary compliance. Am J Phys Med Rehabil 67:155-160, 1988.

107. Madsen JR, Heros RC: Spinal arteriovenous malformations and neurogenic claudication. J Neurosurg 68:793-797, 1988.

108. Aboulker J, Bar D, Marsault C, et al: L'hypertension veineuse intra-rachidienne par anomalies multiples du système cave: Une cause majeure de souffrance médullaire. Clin Obstet Gynecol 103:1003-1015, 1977.

109. Takata K, Inoue S, Takashi K, et al: Swelling of the cauda equina in patients who have herniation of a lumbar disc. J Bone Joint Surg Am 70:361-368, 1988.

110. White A, Panjabi M: Clinical Biomechanics of the Spine, 2nd ed. Philadelphia, JB Lippincott, 1990.

111. Puschel J: Der Wassergehalt normaler und degenerierter Zwischenwirbelscheiben. Beitr Pathol Anat 84:123-130, 1930.

112. Galante JO: Tensile properties of the human lumbar annulus fibrosus. Acta Orthop Scand 100(Suppl):1-91, 1967.

113. Nachemson A: The load on lumbar discs in different positions of the body. Clin Orthop 45:107-122, 1966.

114. Petter CK: Methods of measuring the pressure of intervertebral discs. J Bone Joint Surg 15:365, 1933.

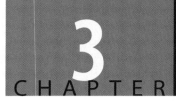

Architectural Design and Function of Human Back Muscles

CHAPTER 3

Anita Vasavada, PhD
Samuel R. Ward, PT, PhD
Scott L. Delp, PhD
Richard L. Lieber, PhD

Spinal muscles generate movements of the spine and provide the stability needed to protect vital anatomic structures. Muscles must work in coordination with the rest of the neuromusculoskeletal system (i.e., vertebrae, tendons, ligaments, and the nervous system) to provide these functions. Large movements of the head require appropriate muscle strength, vertebral geometry (e.g., facet joint orientation), ligament compliance, and neural control. The spinal muscles have been described as one of three subsystems (the others are the passive spinal column and neural control) that must work together to stabilize the spine.[1]

Dysfunction of the spinal musculature is hypothesized to cause various pathologic conditions, such as segmental instability, low back or neck pain, and degenerative disc syndromes. The mechanisms that relate muscle function (or dysfunction) to pathologic processes are unclear, however. Some of the factors that lead to pathologic processes may be elucidated by biomechanical analyses of spine kinematics along with the associated tissue strains and loads. These analyses rely on accurate knowledge of muscle forces, moment arms, and activation patterns to calculate loads and displacements, but such values are frequently unavailable for spinal muscles. Often, spinal muscles are ignored or overly simplified (e.g., modeled as one "lumped" muscle) because the anatomy of these muscles is considered too complex to represent realistically. The complex anatomy and architecture of spinal muscles profoundly influence their function, however, and analyses that incorporate these details are required to provide the information necessary to predict more accurately the role of the muscles in spinal function and dysfunction.

This chapter begins with a description of the important and often neglected principles of skeletal muscle architecture and the way in which architecture determines muscle function. Specific information about the anatomy and architecture of the spinal musculature is provided when such information is available. The chapter concludes with a presentation of the implications of spinal muscle anatomy and architecture for motor control and injury.

Muscle Architecture

Skeletal muscle is highly organized at the microscopic level, as evidenced by classic studies that have elucidated the properties of skeletal muscle fibers. With few exceptions, the arrangement of muscle fibers within and between muscles has received much less attention. The microscopic arrangement of muscle fibers relative to the axis of force generation is known as the architecture of a muscle.[2] Although muscle fiber size (which is directly proportional to force generation) is relatively consistent among muscles of different sizes, architectural differences between muscles show much more variability and more strongly affect function. Muscle architecture is a primary determinant of muscle function, and understanding this structure-function relationship has great practical importance. This understanding not only clarifies the physiologic basis for production of force and movement but also provides a scientific rationale for surgery. Muscle architectural studies also provide guidelines for electrode placement during electromyographic measures of muscle activity, explain the mechanical basis of muscle injury during movement, and aid in the interpretation of histologic specimens obtained from muscle biopsies.

Basic Architectural Definitions

The various types of architectural arrangement are as numerous as the muscles themselves. For discussion purposes, we describe three general classes of muscle fiber architecture. Muscles composed of fibers that extend parallel to the force-generating axis of the muscle are described as having a *parallel* or *longitudinal* architecture (Fig. 3–1A). Muscles with fibers that are oriented at a single angle relative to the force-generating axis are described as having *unipennate* architecture (Fig. 3–1B). The angle between the fiber and the force-generating axis has been measured at resting length in mammalian muscles over different designs and varies from about 0 to 30 degrees. Most muscles fall into the third and most general category, *multipennate* muscles—muscles

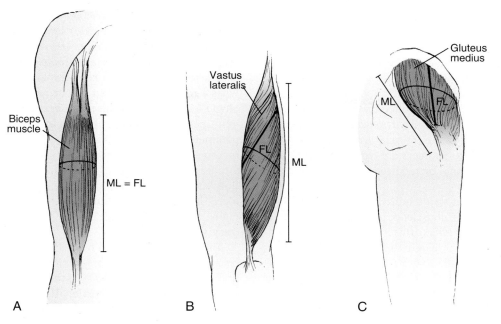

FIGURE 3–1 Artist's conception of three general types of skeletal muscle architecture. **A,** Longitudinal architecture, in which muscle fibers run parallel to the force-generating axis of the muscle. In this case, the natural example is the biceps brachii. **B,** Unipennate architecture, in which muscle fibers run at a fixed angle relative to the force-generating axis of the muscle. Here the example is the vastus lateralis muscle. **C,** Multipennate architecture, in which muscle fibers run at several angles relative to the force-generating axis of the muscle. The example here is the gluteus medius muscle. FL, fiber length; ML, muscle length.

constructed of fibers that are oriented at several angles relative to the axis of force generation (Fig. 3–1C).

These three designations are oversimplified, but they provide a vocabulary with which to describe muscle designs. Because fibers may not be oriented along any of the classic anatomic axes, determination of muscle architecture is impossible from a single biopsy specimen or images obtained by magnetic resonance imaging (MRI), computed tomography (CT), or ultrasonography because these methods cannot account for variations in fiber length and orientation changes that occur along the muscle length. Other methods have been developed to characterize the architectural properties of skeletal muscle.

Experimental Determination of Skeletal Muscle Architecture

Quantitative studies of muscle architecture were pioneered by Gans and colleagues,[2,3] who developed precise methodology for defining muscle architecture based on microdissection of whole muscles. The parameters usually included in an architecture analysis are muscle length, fiber or fascicle length, pennation angle (i.e., the fiber angle relative to the force-generating axis), and physiologic cross-sectional area (PCSA). Typically, muscles are chemically fixed in formalin to maintain fiber integrity during dissection. The muscles should be chemically fixed while attached to the skeleton to preserve their physiologic length, or physiologic length in the skeleton should be noted. After fixation, muscles are dissected from the skeleton, their mass is determined, and their pennation angle and muscle length are measured.

Pennation angle (θ) is measured by determining the average angle of the fibers relative to the axis of force generation of the muscle. Usually only the pennation angle of fibers on the superficial muscle surface is measured; however, this is only an estimate because pennation angles may vary from superficial to deep and from proximal to distal. This superficial to deep variation in pennation has been documented in several spinal muscles (see later). Although more sophisticated methods could be developed for measurement of pennation angle, it is doubtful they would provide a great deal more insight into muscle function because variations in pennation angle may not strongly affect function.[2]

Muscle length is defined as "the distance from the origin of the most proximal muscle fibers to the insertion of the most distal fibers."[4] Fiber length represents the number of sarcomeres in series, and experimental evidence suggests that muscle fiber length is proportional to fiber contraction velocity.[3,5] Muscle length and fiber length are not the same because there is a variable degree of "stagger" seen in muscle fibers as they arise from and insert onto tendon plates (see Fig. 3–1B). Muscle fiber length can be determined only by microdissection of individual fibers from fixed tissues or by laborious identification of fibers by glycogen depletion on serial sections along the length of the muscle.[6] Unless investigators are explicit when they refer to muscle fiber length, they are probably referring to muscle fiber bundle length (also known as fascicle length) because it is extremely difficult to isolate intact fibers, which run from origin to insertion, especially in mammalian tissue.[6,7]

Experimental studies of mammalian muscle suggest that individual muscle fibers do not extend the entire muscle length and may not even extend the entire length of a fascicle.[6,7] Detailed studies of individual muscle fiber length have not been conducted in human spinal muscles, but studies in feline neck muscles illustrate that muscle fibers are often arranged in series, ending in tendinous inscriptions within the muscle or terminating intrafascicularly.[8,9] Although the terms *fiber length* and *fascicle length* are often used interchangeably, technically they are identical only if muscle fibers span the entire length of a fascicle. In muscle architecture studies, bundles consisting of 5 to 50 fibers are typically used to estimate fiber length, which may be reported as either fiber length or fascicle length.

The final experimental step required to perform architectural analysis of a whole muscle is to measure sarcomere length within the isolated fibers. This is necessary to compensate for differences in muscle length that occur during fixation. In other words, to conclude that a muscle has "long fibers," one must ensure that it truly has long fibers and not that it was fixed in a highly stretched position corresponding to a long sarcomere length. Similarly, muscles with "short fibers" must be investigated further to ensure that they were not simply fixed at a short sarcomere length.

To permit such conclusions, fiber length measurements should be normalized to a constant sarcomere length, which eliminates fiber length variability owing to variation in fixation length. Fiber (or fascicle) lengths are usually normalized to the optimal sarcomere length, the length at which a sarcomere generates maximum force. This normalized length is referred to as optimal fiber (or fascicle) length and provides a reference value that can be related back to the physiologic length if the relationship between muscle length and joint position is noted. Based on measured architectural parameters and joint properties, the relationship between sarcomere length and joint angle can be calculated. Because sarcomere length strongly influences muscle force generation, an understanding of the relationship between sarcomere length change and movement has been used in many studies to provide added understanding of muscle design.[10-14]

The PCSA is calculated next. Theoretically, the PCSA represents the sum of the cross-sectional areas of all the muscle fibers within the muscle, and it is the only architectural parameter that is directly proportional to the maximum tetanic tension generated by the muscle. The PCSA is almost never the same as the cross-sectional area of the muscle as measured in any of the traditional anatomic planes, as would be obtained using a noninvasive imaging method such as MRI, CT, or ultrasonography. It is calculated as muscle volume divided by fiber length and has units of area.

Because fibers may be oriented at a pennation angle relative to the axis of force generation, it is believed that not all of the fiber tensile force is transmitted to the tendons. Specifically, if a muscle fiber is pulling with x units of force at a pennation angle θ relative to other muscle axis of force generation, only a *component* of muscle fiber force ($x \cdot \cos\theta$) would actually be transmitted along the muscle axis. The volume/length is often multiplied by cosineθ (pennation angle) and is the calculation of PCSA. In other words, pennation causes a loss of muscle force relative to a muscle with the same mass and fiber length but with a 0-degree pennation angle.

Mechanical Properties of Muscles with Different Architectures

As stated earlier, muscle force is proportional to PCSA, and muscle velocity is proportional to fiber length. By stating that velocity is proportional to fiber length, it is implicit that the total excursion (active range) of a muscle is also proportional to fiber length. It is important to understand how these two architectural parameters, PCSA and fiber length, affect muscle function.

Comparison of Two Muscles with Different Physiologic Cross-Sectional Areas

Suppose that two muscles have identical fiber lengths and pennation angles but one muscle has twice the mass (equivalent to saying that one muscle has twice the number of fibers and twice the PCSA). Also suppose that the two muscles have identical fiber type distributions and that they generate the same force per unit area. The functional difference between these two muscles is shown in Figure 3–2. The muscle with

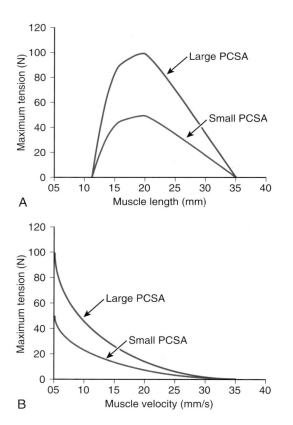

FIGURE 3–2 Schematic drawing of two muscles with different physiologic cross-sectional areas (PCSAs) but identical fiber length. **A,** Comparison of isometric length-tension properties. **B,** Comparison of isotonic force-velocity properties. The effect of increased PCSA with identical fiber length is to shift the absolute length-tension and force-velocity curves to higher values, but with retention of the same range and intrinsic shape.

twice the PCSA has an isometric length-tension curve with the same shape, but it is amplified upward by a factor of 2. The maximal tetanic tension (P_o) of the larger muscle would be twice that of the smaller muscle. Similarly, comparison of isotonic force-velocity curves indicates that the differences between muscles would simply be an upward shift in P_o for the larger muscle.

Comparison of Two Muscles with Different Fiber Lengths

If two muscles have identical PCSAs and pennation angles but fiber lengths that differ, the schematic in Figure 3–3 shows that the effect of increased fiber length is to increase muscle excursion and velocity. Peak force of the length-tension curves is identical between muscles, but the range of lengths over which the muscle generates active force is different. For the same reason that an increased fiber length increases active muscle range of the length-tension relationship, it results in an increase in the maximum velocity (V_{max}) of the muscle. Experimental support for this concept was obtained indirectly through observations of the cat semitendinosus muscle:[4] When the proximal semitendinosus head was activated, its V_{max} was 224 mm/sec, whereas when only the distal semitendinosus head was activated, its V_{max} was 424 mm/sec. When both heads were activated simultaneously, the whole muscle V_{max} was 624 mm/sec, or the sum of the two velocities. The values for V_{max} were proportional to the different lengths of the proximal and distal heads. These data indicate that the longer the fibers in series (equivalent to saying the greater number of sarcomeres in series), the greater the muscle contraction velocity. As expected, maximum isometric tension was essentially the same regardless of which activation pattern was used.

Interplay of Muscle Architecture and Moment Arms

In addition to its architecture, the potential moment generated by a muscle is influenced by its moment arm. Moment arm, the "mechanical advantage" of a muscle, is the distance from the line of action of a muscle to the joint axis of rotation and is directly related to a muscle's change in length with joint rotation.[15] In other words, the amount of muscle fiber length change that occurs as a joint rotates and, consequently, the range of joint angles over which the muscle develops active force depend on the muscle moment arm. This idea can be explained by comparing the situation in which two muscles with identical fiber lengths have different moment arms at a joint (Fig. 3–4). In the case in which the moment arm is greater, the muscle fibers change length much more for a given change in joint angle compared with a muscle with a shorter moment arm. As a result, the range of joint motion over which the muscle develops active force is smaller for the muscle with the larger moment arm despite the fact that the muscular properties of both muscles are identical.

The architectural design of a muscle and its placement in relation to the skeletal geometry are important determinants of its function. Although muscles with longer fibers can generate force over a greater range of lengths than muscles with shorter fibers (see Fig. 3–3A), this does not indicate that muscles with longer fibers are associated with joints that have larger ranges of motion. Muscles that appear to be designed for speed based on their long fibers may not actually produce large joint velocities if they are placed in the skeleton with a very large moment arm because joint excursion and joint angular velocity are inversely related to moment arm. A large moment arm results in a large joint moment, so that the muscle would be highly suited for torque production but at low angular velocities. Similarly, a muscle that appears to be designed for force production because of the large PCSA, if placed in position with a very small moment arm, may actually produce high joint excursions or angular velocities. Differences between muscle-joint systems require complete analysis of joint and muscular properties. These interrelated concepts of architecture and moment arm (gross anatomy) must be considered when examining the design and function of spinal muscles.

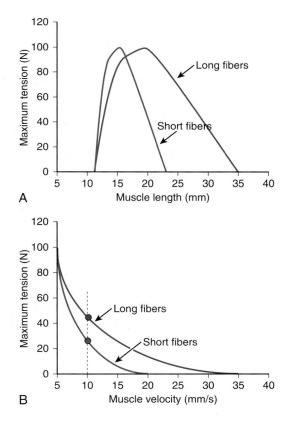

FIGURE 3–3 Schematic drawing of two muscles with different fiber lengths but identical physiologic cross-sectional areas. **A,** Comparison of isometric length-tension properties. **B,** Comparison of isotonic force-velocity properties. The effect of increased fiber length is to increase the absolute range of the length-tension curve and absolute velocity of the force-velocity curve, but with retention of the same peak force and intrinsic shape. *Dotted vertical line* in **B** shows that, for an equivalent absolute velocity, the muscle with longer fibers generates a greater force.

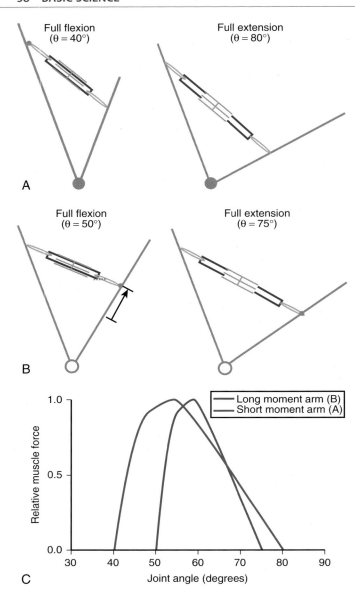

FIGURE 3–4 Effect of changing moment arm on active range of motion. In this example, a schematic muscle (shown as a sarcomere in series with some tendon) is attached with two different moment arms. **A,** 40-degree range of motion for "normal" muscle (from 40 to 80 degrees). **B,** Moment arm increase results in decrease in range of motion to 25-degree muscle (from 50 to 75 degrees). In **B,** the active range of motion is smaller because the moment arm is greater, and more sarcomere length change occurs for a given angular rotation. **C,** Comparison of force versus joint angle (range of motion) for muscles with short (*dotted line*) or long (*solid line*) moment arms.

Anatomy and Architecture of Spinal Musculature

The architecture of spinal muscles is complex and dramatically different from the architecture of limb muscles. Instead of distinct tendinous attachments to bone, many spinal muscles have very little tendon at their ends and have a complex arrangement of internal tendons and aponeuroses. Their attachments are generally broad; many spinal muscles branch and have insertions at multiple vertebral levels. Some spinal muscles have short fascicles and high pennation, whereas others have long, parallel fascicles. All of these factors affect the force-generating and moment-generating capacity of muscles as described earlier, which ultimately influences control and injury mechanisms.

Spinal muscles can be divided into intrinsic muscles, which connect vertebrae with each other, and extrinsic muscles, which attach vertebrae to the limbs. Embryologically, intrinsic muscles originate from the epimere, and extrinsic muscles originate from the hypomere. Intrinsic muscles have innervations from the dorsal rami of spinal nerves, whereas extrinsic muscles are innervated from the ventral rami of spinal nerves and generally have functions related more to the proximal portion of limbs or respiration.

Intrinsic Spinal Muscles Found in the Lumbar, Thoracic, or Cervical Spine

Intrinsic muscles of the spine are dominated by the *erector spinae*, a group of interdigitated muscles that spans the entire length of the spine, from the sacrum and iliac crest to the skull. Another important group of muscles, the *multifidus,* are shorter and deeper and are described in more detail later. In the thoracolumbar region, the erector spinae and multifidus muscles constitute the bulk of the spinal musculature. These two distinct functional units have large differences in innervation that probably result in significant functional differences,[16] although the detailed biomechanical function of these groups remains only partially elucidated.[17] Lying deep to the multifidus are even smaller muscles, the *rotators, interspinales,* and *intertransversarii.* The cervical region is composed of other intrinsic muscles unique to it (see later).

The *erector spinae* are commonly considered to be composed of three muscles; from medial to lateral, they are the *spinalis, longissimus,* and *iliocostalis.* The anatomy and architecture of these muscles vary among different levels of the spine. The words "lumborum," "thoracis," "cervicis," and "capitis" are appended to the muscle name to describe the anatomy more accurately. Although there are varying definitions of the composition of the erector spinae, a study by MacIntosh and Bogduk[17] provides the most comprehensive descriptive anatomy of the lumbar erector spinae, and Delp and colleagues[18] provided the first architectural measurements of these muscles. The continuation of the erector spinae in the cervical region was discussed briefly by Kamibayashi and Richmond.[19]

The *spinalis* muscle is the most medial division of the erector spinae. MacIntosh and Bogduk[17] described the spinalis as mostly aponeurotic in the lumbar region, but Delp and colleagues[18] obtained architecture measurements from the spinalis in the thoracic region (Table 3–1). The spinalis is generally absent in the cervical region.

Caudal to rostral, the *longissimus* consists of the *longissimus thoracis, cervicis,* and *capitis;* the *longissimus thoracis* is divided into lumbar and thoracic portions. The lumbar fascicles of the longissimus thoracis (*longissimus thoracis pars lumborum*) are composed of five bands that arise from the lumbar transverse processes and attach in a caudal fashion onto the iliac crest (Fig. 3–5A). Each band arising from vertebra L1 to L4 is

TABLE 3-1 Architectural Data of Rectus Abdominis and Lumbar Spine Muscles*

Muscle	Musculotendon Length (cm)	Muscle Length (cm)	Fascicle Length (cm)	Pennation Angle (°)	Sarcomere Length (μm)	Optimal Fascicle Length (cm)	Muscle Fiber Mass (g)	PCSA (cm²)
Rectus abdominis	35.9 (1.9)	34.3 (2.7)	28.3 (3.6)	0 (0)	2.83 (0.28)	28 (4.2)	92.5 (30.5)	2.6 (0.9)
Quadratus lumborum (proximal)	11.7 (1.7)	10.7 (1.3)	7.3 (1.3)	7.4 (2.9)	2.39 (0.21)	8.5 (1.5)	13.3 (5.2)	1.6 (0.6)
Quadratus lumborum (distal)	9.3 (1.3)	8.1 (1.2)	4.7 (0.5)	7.4 (6.2)	2.37 (0.20)	5.6 (0.9)	7.3 (2.4)	1.2 (0.4)
Spinalis thoracis	24.7 (1.5)	18.2 (3.2)	5.2 (0.4)	16 (3.8)	2.26 (0.17)	6.4 (0.6)	10.2 (6)	1.6 (0.9)
Longissimus thoracis	42.6 (5.5)	34.7 (4.8)	9.6 (1.2)	12.6 (5.8)	2.31 (0.17)	11.7 (2.1)	73.4 (31)	5.9 (2.5)
Iliocostalis lumborum	43.8 (4.3)	33.1 (9)	12 (1.7)	13.8 (4.5)	2.37 (0.17)	14.2 (2.1)	60.9 (29.9)	4.1(1.9)
Multifidus	NA	NA	4.8 (1.7)	18.4 (4.2)	2.26 (0.18)	5.7 (1.8)	73 (12.4)	23.9 (8.4)

From Delp SL, Suryanarayanan S, Murray WM, et al: Architecture of the rectus abdominis, quadratus lumborum, and erector spine. J Biomech 34:371-375, 2001; Ward, SR, Kim CW, Eng CM, et al: Architectural analysis and intraoperative measurements demonstrate the unique design of the multifidus for lumbar spine stability. J Bone Joint Surg Am 91:176-185, 2009.
NA, not applicable; PCSA, physiologic cross-sectional area.
*Table presents mean values (standard deviation).

actually a small fusiform muscle that has an elongated and flattened caudal tendon of insertion. Bands from more rostral levels attach more medially on the iliac crest. The juxtaposition of these caudally located tendons form the lumbar intermuscular aponeurosis (see LIA in Fig. 3–5B).

Fascicles of the thoracic component of longissimus thoracis (*longissimus thoracis pars thoracis*) arise from all thoracic transverse processes and most ribs and attach to lumbar spinous processes, the sacrum, or the ilium. These are long slender muscles with pronounced caudal tendons that juxtapose to form the strong erector spinae aponeurosis, which bounds the lumbar paraspinal muscles dorsally. In the upper thoracic and cervical region, the *longissimus cervicis* connects transverse processes of thoracic and cervical vertebrae, whereas the *longissimus capitis* originates on transverse processes and inserts on the mastoid process of the skull (Fig. 3–6).

The lumbar fascicles of the *iliocostalis lumborum* (*iliocostalis lumborum pars lumborum*) lie lateral to the longissimus thoracis muscles arising from the tip of the transverse processes of vertebrae L1 to L4 in the lumbar region and are composed of four small, broad bands (see Fig. 3–5C) that attach to the thoracolumbar fascia and the iliac crest. The thoracic fascicles of the iliocostalis lumborum (*iliocostalis lumborum pars thoracis*) arise from ribs and attach to the iliac spine and crest, forming the lateral part of the erector spinae aponeurosis. In contrast to the more medially located longissimus thoracis, the caudal tendons are less prominent, giving the iliocostalis lumborum a much more fleshy appearance. Caudal to rib 10, the iliocostalis lumborum and longissimus thoracis lie side by side, forming the erector spinae aponeurosis. Rostral to rib 9 or 10, the *iliocostalis thoracis* separates the iliocostalis lumborum and longissimus thoracis. In the upper thoracic and cervical region, the *iliocostalis cervicis* connects the ribs to the transverse processes of cervical vertebrae.

MacIntosh and Bogduk[17] measured muscle and tendon lengths in the thoracic portions of the longissimus thoracis and iliocostalis lumborum (Table 3–2). Detailed architecture of the lumbar erector spinae, including muscle tendon and

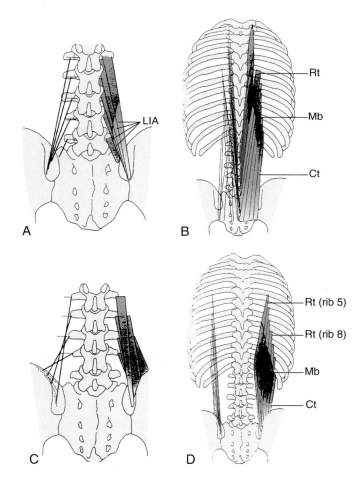

FIGURE 3–5 A-D, Longissimus thoracis (medial division of erector spinae) schematic of lumbar (**A**) and thoracic (**B**) regions and iliocostalis lumborum (lateral division of erector spinae) schematic of lumbar (**C**) and thoracic (**D**) regions. ct, caudal tendon; LIA, lumbar intermuscular aponeurosis; mb, muscle belly; rt, rostral tendon. (From Bogduk N: A reappraisal of the anatomy of the human lumbar erector spinae. J Anat 131:525-540, 1980; MacIntosh JE, Bogduk N: The morphology of the lumbar erector spinae. Spine 12:658-668, 1987.)

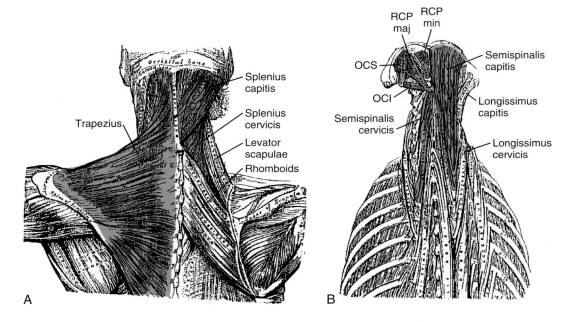

FIGURE 3–6 Posterior view of neck muscles. **A,** Left side shows superficial muscle, the trapezius. Splenius capitis, splenius cervicis, levator scapulae, and rhomboids lie underneath trapezius. **B,** Right side shows semispinalis capitis, longissimus capitis, and longissimus cervicis, which lie deep to splenius capitis. Left side shows semispinalis cervicis and suboccipital muscles, which lie under semispinalis capitis. OCI, obliquus capitis inferior; OCS, obliquus capitis superior; RCP maj, rectus capitis posterior major; RCP min, rectus capitis posterior minor. (Adapted from Gray H: Gray's Anatomy. New York, Gramercy Books, 1977.)

fascicle length, sarcomere lengths, and PCSAs, has been measured (see Table 3–1).[18] Fascicle lengths were found to be approximately 30% of muscle lengths in these muscles, and sarcomere lengths measured from cadavers in the supine position were generally shorter than the optimal length, which may imply that the erector spinae are capable of developing greater force in elongated positions (i.e., in flexion).

The lumbar *multifidus* muscles consist of multiple separate bands arising from each vertebral spinous process and lamina and inserting from two to four segments below the level of origin (Fig. 3–7B). The shortest fascicle of each muscle inserts onto the mammillary process of the vertebra located two segments caudal, whereas longer, more superficial fascicles insert sequentially onto subsequent vertebrae three or more segments lower (see Fig. 3–7). The shortest band of the multifidus arising from L1 inserts on L3, and subsequent bands insert sequentially on L4, L5, and the sacrum. Multifidus muscles

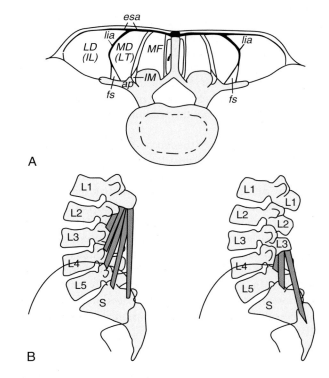

FIGURE 3–7 Schematic arrangement of multifidus muscle in cross section (**A**) and longitudinal section (**B**). (From Bogduk N: A reappraisal of the anatomy of the human lumbar erector spinae. J Anat 131:525-540, 1980.)

TABLE 3–2 Muscle and Tendon Length Data of Lumbar Erector Spinae

Muscle	Muscle Belly Length (cm)	Rostral Tendon Length (cm)	Caudal Tendon Length (cm)
Longissimus thoracis pars thoracis	9-12	3-4	Up to 24
Iliocostalis lumborum pars thoracis	10-13	12-15	18-19

From MacIntosh JE, Bogduk N: The morphology of the lumbar erector spinae. Spine 12:658-668, 1987.

arising from lower lumbar vertebrae consist of fewer fascicles because the number of vertebrae caudal to the origin decreases.

All multifidus muscles that arise from a given level are innervated by the medial branch of the primary dorsal rami of the spinal nerve from a single segment (i.e., each band of multifidus muscle is innervated from a single dorsal ramus). In the cervical region, multifidus fascicles from the spinous processes and laminae of C2, C3, and C4 attach onto facet capsules of two adjacent vertebral articular processes from C4 to C7; fascicles from the spinous processes and laminae of C4 to C7 attach onto transverse processes of upper thoracic vertebrae.[20] The principal action of the multifidus is extension, but the multisegmental nature of the muscle and the complex three-dimensional orientation in the craniocaudal and mediolateral directions renders this statement a gross oversimplification.[21] The multifidus is not considered a prime mover of the spine; rather, its function is likely to produce small vertebral adjustments.

A study of the multifidus muscle revealed three major design factors that suit it well for stabilizing the lumbar spine.[22] First, the architecture of the multifidus is highly pennated with fibers extending only about 20% of the length of the fascicles. Numerous muscle fibers are packed into a small volume, and even though the multifidus has a smaller mass compared with several other lumbar extensors, it is predicted to create the greatest lumbar extension force by a factor of 2 (see Table 3–1). Second, direct mechanical testing of the multifidus muscle cells and extracellular connective tissue revealed that although the multifidus fibers have the same mechanical properties as other limb muscles, the fiber bundles, which include extracellular connective tissue, are about twice as stiff as limb muscles. The multifidus has a high passive elastic capacity that would suit it for passively resisting flexion of the lumbar spine. Third, the multifidus muscle sarcomere length, measured intraoperatively, is relatively short when the spine is extended, suggesting that the muscle gets stronger as it gets longer. In other words, as the spine flexes, multifidus force increases, suiting it to restore spine angles toward neutral or more extended positions.

Deep to the multifidus are smaller muscles that span one or two vertebral segments. The *rotatores* attach from caudal transverse processes to the base of rostral spines one or two segments away. Rotators are prominent in the thoracic region, although some authors claim they exist in the lumbar region.[23,24] MacIntosh and colleagues[25] did not find any muscles deep to the lumbar multifidus. The *interspinalis* and *intertransversarii*, found in the lumbar and cervical regions, connect the spines and transverse processes of adjacent vertebrae.

Intrinsic Spinal Muscles Specific to the Cervical Spine

Because of different functional demands in the cervical spine (e.g., large head movements), this region has additional intrinsic muscles. Kamibayashi and Richmond[19] provided details on neck muscle anatomy and quantitative architecture data of the neck muscles (Table 3–3).

Splenius Capitis and Cervicis

The *splenius capitis* originates at the spinous processes of the lower cervical and upper thoracic vertebrae and inserts on the skull near the mastoid process (see Fig. 3–6A). Contiguous, slightly deeper, and sometimes inseparable is the *splenius cervicis,* which originates on thoracic spinous processes and inserts on cervical transverse processes. Although the splenius capitis and splenius cervicis function in extension, lateral bending, and axial rotation, the splenius capitis is oriented more obliquely than the splenius cervicis, providing more axial rotation capacity for movements of the skull relative to the vertebrae. The fascicle lengths of the splenius capitis and splenius cervicis are similar, but their muscle tendon lengths are not similar; this occurs because the splenius capitis has short aponeuroses, whereas the splenius cervicis has long aponeuroses (Fig. 3–8A).[19]

Semispinalis Capitis and Cervicis

The *semispinalis capitis* originates on the articular processes of the lower cervical vertebrae and transverse processes of the upper thoracic vertebrae and inserts medially on the skull between the inferior and superior nuchal line (see Fig. 3–6A). The semispinalis capitis is characterized by complex patterns of internal tendon and tendinous inscriptions in the medial portion, whereas fascicles in the lateral portion are uninterrupted (see Fig. 3–8B).[19] The *semispinalis cervicis* (deep to the semispinalis capitis) originates on thoracic transverse processes and inserts on cervical spinous processes from C2 to C5, with the bulk of its mass inserting on C2.

Longus Capitis and Colli

On the anterior side of the vertebral column, the *longus capitis* runs from the anterior surface of transverse processes to the baso-occiput (Fig. 3–9). Because it lies close to the vertebral bodies, it has only a small flexion moment arm; the superomedial orientation could provide ipsilateral rotation. Its counterpart, the *longus colli,* has a more complicated structure. Some fibers run vertically along the anterior vertebral bodies, other fibers run superolaterally from thoracic vertebral bodies to lower cervical transverse processes, and others run superomedially from transverse processes to the anterior vertebral bodies (see Fig. 3–9). Although all parts of the longus colli have small flexion moment arms, the superomedial and superolateral portions would have ipsilateral and contralateral rotation moment arms. The longus capitis and longus colli are also characterized by an aponeurosis covering much of the superficial surface, from which fascicles have long tendons that attach to the vertebrae (Fig. 3–10).[19]

Suboccipital Muscles

The suboccipital muscles span the region between C2 and the skull (see Fig. 3–6B). The *rectus capitis posterior major* and *minor* connect the spinous processes of C2 and C1 with the skull. The *obliquus capitis superior* is oriented in a

TABLE 3–3 Morphometric Parameters of Human Neck Muscles

Muscle	N	MASS (G) Range	MASS (G) Mean (SD)	Angle (°) Range	MUSCLE LENGTH (CM) Range	MUSCLE LENGTH (CM) Mean (SD)	NF Length (cm) Mean (SD)	PCSA (CM²) Range	PCSA (CM²) Mean (SD)
Sternocleidomastoideus	9	21-50.5	40.4 (9)	0-20	16.5-21.2	19 (1.6)	10.8 (0.9)	1.81-5.26	3.72 (0.91)
Clavotrapezius		10.7-27.1	18.7 (4.5)	0-30	9-14.8	12 (1.9)	8.4 (2.1)	1.25-2.94	1.96 (0.62)
Acromiotrapezius		68.6-128.4	103.5 (23.5)	0-10	10-14.5	12.6 (1.7)	9.2 (1.8)	7.99-15.26	10.77 (2.38)
Rhomboideus	9	18.8-58.3	40.9 (15.6)	0-5			7.2 (2)	1.76-9.93	5.84 (2.77)
Minor					6.5-12	8.7 (1.9)			
Major					5.3-13	8.2 (2.7)			
Rectus capitis posterior major	9	1.4-5.5	3.5 (1.2)	0-5	3-4.8		3.7 (0.7)	0.44-1.45	0.93 (0.33)
Rectus capitis posterior minor	9	0.6-1.6	1 (0.3)	0-5	2.6-3.1		1.9 (0.2)	0.28-0.83	0.50 (0.19)
Obliquus capitis superior	8	1-3.7	2.5 (0.9)	0-20	4.3-5.7		2.5 (0.5)	0.29-1.69	1.03 (0.46)
Obliquus capitis inferior	9	2.1-8.1	5.1 (1.8)	0-5	3.6-5.4	4.4 (0.6)	3.8 (0.8)	0.69-1.73	1.29 (0.54)
Longus capitis	7	2.4-5.6	3.7 (1.2)	0-10	7.8-11.1	9.2 (1.4)	3.8 (1)	0.54-1.63	0.92 (0.35)
Splenius	9	21.6-59.3	42.9 (13.8)	0-5			9.5 (2.3)	2.57-5.48	4.26 (1.04)
Capitis					9.5-15	12.3 (1.5)			
Cervicis					11.5-18.5	14.7 (2.3)			
Semispinalis capitis	9	21.3-55.8	38.5 (9.4)	0-20	13-20	11.7 (1.9)	6.8 (1.7)	3.93-7.32	5.40 (1.30)
Scalenus anterior	9	5.7-12.4	5.6 (3)	0-20	5.5-7.8	6.8 (0.9)	4.2 (1.3)	0.37-4.51	1.45 (1.23)
Scalenus medius	9	5.6-14.5	10.6 (3.0)	0-30	6.8-9.6	8.1 (1)	5 (0.8)	1.00-3.34	2.00 (0.73)
Scalenus posterior	9	4-23.5	10.6 (7.7)	0-20	7-10	8 (1.1)	6.2 (2.1)	0.59-3.15	1.55 (0.90)
Levator scapulae	8	16.5-38.9	24.6 (8.3)	0-5	13.2-17.5	15.1 (1.6)	11.3 (3.1)	1.39-3.24	2.18 (0.80)

From Kamibayashi LK, Richmond FR: Morphometry of human neck muscles. Spine 23:1314-1323, 1998.
Values in each column represent the range or average of individual values computed on specimen at one time.
NF Length, normalized fascicle length; PCSA, physiologic cross-sectional area.

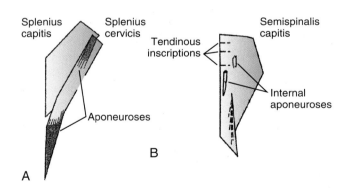

FIGURE 3–8 Architecture of splenius capitis, splenius cervicis, and semispinalis capitis. **A,** Splenius capitis and splenius cervicis. Note aponeuroses at both ends of splenius cervicis. **B,** Semispinalis capitis. Medial portion is characterized by tendinous inscriptions and internal aponeuroses interrupting fascicles. (Adapted from Kamibayashi LK, Richmond FJR: Morphometry of human neck muscles. Spine 23:1314-1323, 1998.)

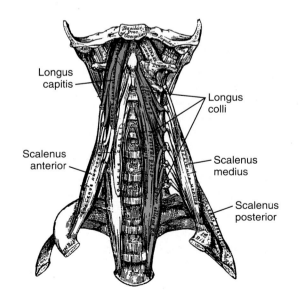

FIGURE 3–9 Anterior view of deep neck muscles: longus capitis, longus colli, and scalenes. Note three parts of longus colli: superior oblique, vertical, and inferior oblique. (Adapted from Gray H: Gray's Anatomy. New York, Gramercy Books, 1977.)

superoinferior direction between the transverse process of C1 and the skull, and the *obliquus capitis inferior* runs primarily mediolaterally from the spinous process of C2 to the transverse process of C1. All four of these muscles can contribute to extension of the head with respect to the neck; in addition, the rectus capitis posterior major and the obliquus capitis inferior are oriented to produce ipsilateral rotation, and the lateral location of the obliquus capitis superior implies a lateral bending function. The obliquus capitis superior has an internal tendon on the deep surface that causes some fascicles to have large pennation angles.[19] On the ventral side, the *rectus capitis anterior* and *rectus capitis lateralis* are very small muscles that connect the skull to C1, presumably with (small) moment arms for flexion and lateral bending.

Extrinsic Muscles Linking Vertebrae to the Pelvis

The *quadratus lumborum* attaches from the iliolumbar ligament and iliac crest onto the 12th rib and transverse processes of L1 to L4. It assists in lateral bending of the lumbar spine. The proximal component of the quadratus lumborum (i.e., the set of fascicles running from the iliac crest to the 12th rib and L1) has a larger moment arm for lateral flexion and has longer fascicles than the distal component of the muscle. Electromyographic evidence shows that the quadratus lumborum has a dominant role in spine stabilization.[26]

The *psoas major* attaches from the anterior surface of the transverse processes, the sides of vertebral bodies, and intervertebral discs of all lumbar vertebrae. Together with the iliacus, which arises from the ilium, they form the iliopsoas, which inserts on the lesser trochanter of the femur and is a major flexor of the thigh and trunk. Fascicles of the psoas generally have the same length, regardless of their level of origin. Because of their attachments to a common tendon, bundles from higher levels are more tendinous, whereas the bundle from L5 remains fleshy until it joins the common tendon.[27]

The psoas is the largest muscle in cross section at the lower levels of the lumbar spine.[28] Biomechanical analysis shows that the psoas has the potential to flex the lumbar spine laterally, generate compressive forces that increase stability, and create large anterior shear forces at L5 to S1.[29] If the psoas were designed for lumbar spine motions, however, one would expect longer fascicles attaching more rostral segments because they would undergo larger excursion. The uniform fascicle lengths suggest that the psoas is actually designed to move the hip,[27] and electromyographic studies confirm that its primary function is hip flexion.[30]

Extrinsic Muscles Linking Vertebrae or Skull to the Shoulder Girdle or Rib Cage

On the anterior and lateral surface of the neck, the *sternocleidomastoid* originates from the sternum and medial clavicle to attach on the skull at the mastoid process and superior nuchal line of the occiput (Fig. 3–11). Kamibayashi and Richmond[19] divided this muscle into three subvolumes: sternomastoid, cleidomastoid, and cleido-occipital. The fascicles on the

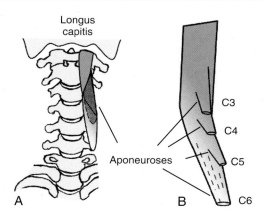

FIGURE 3–10 Architecture of longus capitis. **A,** Superficial surface, with long aponeurosis. **B,** Deep surface, with individual tendons to lower cervical vertebrae. (Adapted from Kamibayashi LK, Richmond FJR: Morphometry of human neck muscles. Spine 23:1314-1323, 1998.)

superficial surface (sternomastoid and cleido-occipital portions) lie in parallel; however, the cleidomastoid portion on the deep surface, which runs from the clavicle to mastoid process, increases the proportion of muscle fascicles exerting force on the mastoid process (Fig. 3–12).[19] Superficial inspection of muscle architecture can neglect the arrangement of these deep fascicles, which would decrease the estimated moment-generating capacity of the sternocleidomastoid in biomechanical models by more than 30%.[31] The sternocleidomastoid has moment arms for flexion, contralateral rotation, and lateral bending and has been found to be active during movements in all three of these directions.

Also on the anterior surface of the neck, the infrahyoid muscles (*sternohyoid, sternothyroid, thyrohyoid*) link the hyoid bone, thyroid cartilage, and sternum, whereas the suprahyoid

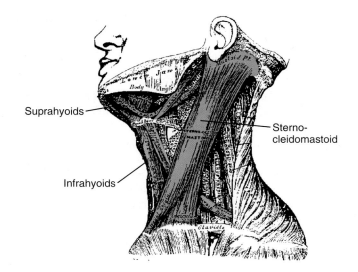

FIGURE 3–11 Lateral view of sternocleidomastoid and hyoid muscles. (Adapted from Gray H: Gray's Anatomy. New York, Gramercy Books, 1977.)

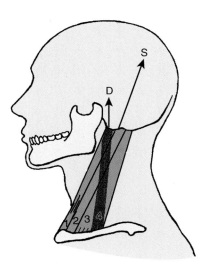

FIGURE 3–12 Lines of action of sternocleidomastoid, including deep cleidomastoid portion. *Arrows* indicate differences in pulling direction of deep (D) and superficial (S) subvolumes. (Adapted from Kamibayashi LK, Richmond FJR: Morphometry of human neck muscles. Spine 23:1314-1323, 1998.)

muscles (*digastric, stylohyoid, mylohyoid,* and *geniohyoid*) connect the hyoid bone to the mastoid process and mandible (see Fig. 3–11). The hyoid muscles are generally considered to maneuver the hyoid bone for deglutition and maintaining airway patency, but these muscles could potentially generate a neck flexion moment if the infrahyoid and suprahyoid muscles were activated in concert.

On the posterior surface of the neck, the *trapezius* is the most superficial muscle (see Fig. 3–6A). It can be divided into three segments: The rostral segment (also called *clavotrapezius* or *trapezius pars descendens*) runs from the lateral part of the clavicle to the occiput or ligamentum nuchae, the middle part (*acromiotrapezius* or *pars transversa*) runs nearly perpendicular to the midline at the lower cervical and upper thoracic levels from the lateral part of the scapular spine, and the caudal part (*spinotrapezius* or *pars ascendens*) attaches to spinous processes of T4 to T12 from the scapula. Its superficial position means that the trapezius has large moment arms for spine and head movements; however, its attachments to the scapula mean that shoulder movements also influence its function. The clavotrapezius (which attaches to the skull) has less than one fifth of the mass of the acromiotrapezius,[19] indicating that the trapezius has less moment-generating potential for movements of the skull than generally believed.

Three other muscles connect the scapula to the cervical and thoracic vertebrae. The *rhomboideus major* and *rhomboideus minor* run from the medial border of the scapula to the midline at upper thoracic levels. Their major function is retraction of the scapula. The *levator scapulae* runs from the superior border of the scapula to the transverse processes of upper cervical vertebrae (see Fig. 3–6A). Similar to the trapezius, the

functions of these muscles are related to movements of the shoulder.

The scalene muscles (*scalenus anterior, medius,* and *posterior*) run from the ribs to transverse processes of cervical vertebrae (see Fig. 3–9). Because of their lateral placement owing to attachments to the ribs, the scalene muscles have substantial moment arms for cervical lateral bending; however, their main function is likely related to respiration. The *serratus posterior superior* and *inferior* also attach the vertebral column to the ribs. The serratus posterior superior arises from the lower part of ligamentum nuchae and the spines of the upper thoracic vertebrae and attaches to ribs 2 to 5. The serratus posterior inferior originates from the spines of the lower thoracic and upper lumbar vertebrae and attaches to ribs 9 to 12. These muscles function to elevate and depress the ribs.

The *latissimus dorsi* arises from the spinous processes of the lower six thoracic and upper two lumbar vertebrae, the thoracolumbar fascia, the iliac crest, and the lower ribs to insert on the humerus. The magnitudes of its potential force and moment on the lumbar spine and sacroiliac joint are small.[32] It is generally considered to move the arm, but if the upper limb were fixed, its activity could move the trunk (e.g., as in wheelchair transfers or crutch locomotion).

The spinal muscles are characterized by complex anatomy and architecture, and important biomechanical features are revealed when the architecture is studied in detail. The architecture and its effects on function of many spinal muscles remain to be determined, however. The function of a muscle also depends on muscle activity, and neural control of a muscle is influenced by its architecture. Understanding biomechanical models and experimental studies is vital to understanding the role of muscles in pain and injury mechanisms.

Implications of Spinal Muscle Anatomy and Architecture for Motor Control

Architectural specialization of muscles means that the nervous system is not the only means available to modify muscular force and excursion. Although neural inputs can change muscle force, the effectiveness of neural input is altered by different muscle architectural features. In other words, the nervous system commands are "interpreted" through the design of muscles to control posture and movement.

Fascicle Length Changes with Posture

In the cervical spine, many extensor muscles undergo large length changes over the flexion-extension range of motion. A biomechanical model showed that the splenius capitis, semispinalis capitis, semispinalis cervicis, rectus capitis posterior major, and rectus capitis posterior minor all experience fascicle length changes greater than 70% of optimal length over the full range of motion.[31] The change in fascicle length depends on the optimal fascicle length of the muscle and the moment arm. The splenius capitis and splenius cervicis have the same optimal fascicle length (see Table 3–3), but the splenius capitis has a much larger moment arm than the splenius

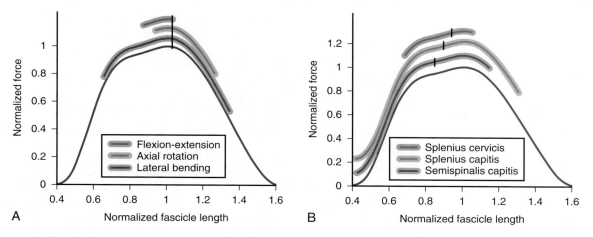

FIGURE 3–13 A, Average range of operation of neck muscles during selected motion. **B,** Range of operation of selected muscles from full flexion to full extension. (Adapted from Vasavada A, Li S, Delp S: Influence of muscle morphometry and moment arms on the moment-generating capacity of human neck muscles. Spine 23:412-421, 1998.)

cervicis. The splenius capitis undergoes larger fascicle length changes than the splenius cervicis over the same range of motion (Fig. 3–13).

The semispinalis capitis has shorter fascicle lengths, but also a smaller moment arm than the splenius capitis. The semispinalis capitis and splenius capitis experience similar, large fascicle length excursions over the range of flexion-extension motion (see Fig. 3–13). In both muscles, fascicle lengths are extremely short in extended postures; this implies that the central nervous system must compensate for the associated decrease in force-generating potential by increasing activation or recruiting other extensors of the neck.

Moment Arm Changes with Posture

Different parts of a muscle may have different moment arms, and the magnitude (and in some cases, direction) of these moment arms changes with posture. Muscles that cross multiple joints (as most spinal muscles do) may have different mechanical functions at different joints. A biomechanical model of the neck muscles[31] showed that the moment arm of the sternocleidomastoid varies dramatically for flexion-extension movements (Fig. 3–14). For motions of the upper cervical joints, the cleido-occipital segment of the sternocleidomastoid actually has an extension moment arm that increases in extended postures (topmost solid line in Fig. 3–14); the other two subvolumes of the sternocleidomastoid (which attach to the mastoid process) have very small moment arms. During flexion of the lower cervical joints, the flexion moment arm of the sternocleidomastoid increases. These results indicate that the function of the sternocleidomastoid depends highly on posture and the joints around which movement occurs. The change in sternocleidomastoid flexion moment arm in the lower cervical region indicates a destabilizing effect because it potentially increases the flexion moment–generating capacity of the muscle in flexed postures.

The same model[31] also showed that for axial rotation of the upper cervical region, many muscles have moment arms that

vary by 2 to 3 cm but remain in the same direction throughout the range of motion (e.g., sternocleidomastoid, splenius capitis) (Fig. 3–15). For other muscles, the direction of moment arm changes with axial rotation. At the neutral position, the right rectus capitis posterior major has a right rotation moment arm; its magnitude increases in left rotated postures. When the head is rotated to the right, the moment arm decreases in magnitude and eventually changes to a left rotation moment arm. These results indicate that the rectus capitis posterior major has an axial rotation moment arm appropriate to restore the head to neutral posture from the most rotated head positions. The moment arms of other muscles such as the semispinalis capitis and longissimus capitis show the same pattern,

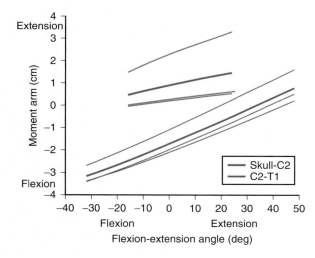

FIGURE 3–14 Sternocleidomastoid flexion-extension moment arms. *Light lines* indicate individual subvolumes (sternomastoid, cleidomastoid, and cleido-occipital), and *dark lines* indicate mass-weighted average. *Solid line* indicates moment arm for upper cervical region; *dashed line* refers to lower cervical region. (Adapted from Vasavada A, Li S, Delp S: Influence of muscle morphometry and moment arms on the moment-generating capacity of human neck muscles. Spine 23:412-421, 1998.)

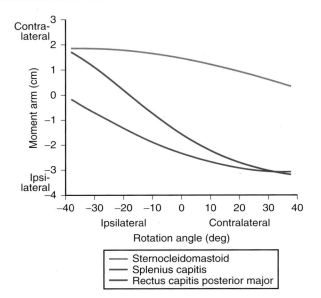

FIGURE 3–15 Axial rotation moment arms for upper cervical region. (Adapted from Vasavada A, Li S, Delp S: Influence of muscle morphometry and moment arms on the moment-generating capacity of human neck muscles. Spine 23:412-421, 1998.)

although their moment arms are smaller. The implication of these findings is that the moment arm provides a "self-stabilizing" function to assist the central nervous system in maintaining neutrally rotated (i.e., eyes forward) head posture. This function is particularly relevant in the upper cervical region because most axial rotation occurs between C1 and C2.

In the lumbar spine, posture also changes the mechanical function of erector spine muscles. McGill and colleagues[33] measured the fiber angles of longissimus thoracic and iliocostalis lumborum with the lumbar spine in neutral and fully flexed using high-resolution ultrasonography. They found that flexion changes the line of action of these muscles, decreasing their capacity to resist anterior shear forces. This finding is important because anterior shear loads are related to the risk of back injury.[34]

Electromyography

Knowledge of the complex spinal muscle anatomy is essential for accurate electromyography studies. These studies may be used to detect abnormal muscle activation patterns or to determine input to biomechanical models. MacIntosh and colleagues[25] showed the medial fibers of the multifidus (i.e., the fibers immediately lateral to a given spinous process) arise from the spinous process directly above, whereas fibers from higher levels are more lateral. All the fibers of the multifidus arising from a particular vertebra are innervated by the same nerve. This unisegmental innervation has implications for diagnosis of zygapophyseal joint pain related to abnormal activity in the multifidus.

The detailed anatomy of the erector spinae provided by MacIntosh and Bogduk[17] also provides important information for electromyography studies. Because thoracic fascicles of the longissimus thoracis and iliocostalis lumborum lie over the lumbar fascicles, electrodes placed at lumbar vertebral levels may not represent activity of fascicles directly attached to lumbar vertebrae. This could result in inaccurate estimation of lumbar joint and tissue loads.

Muscle Injury and Implications for Neck and Back Pain

Neck and back pain frequently begins with an injury, and in many cases muscle injury is involved. Injury to muscle fibers can occur as a result of trauma, disease, application of myotoxic agents (e.g., local anesthetics), inflammatory processes, or intense exercise. The degree to which muscle injury relates to low back or neck pain is unknown. Muscle injury and the pain that accompanies it have been studied extensively, however.

Skeletal muscle injury and soreness frequently occur when a muscle is rapidly lengthened while it is activated. Active lengthening of muscle (also called eccentric contraction) has been used to study injuries in animals and humans for more than 20 years.

Muscle pain accompanying eccentric exercise peaks 24 to 48 hours after the exercise bout. Several studies have reported that eccentric exercise results in a significant increase in serum creatine kinase levels 24 to 48 hours after the exercise bout,[35,36] and the increase may persist for 3 to 6 days, depending on the precise nature of the exercise. The appearance of creatine kinase in the serum is interpreted as an increased permeability or breakdown of the membrane surrounding the muscle cell.

Training prevents or at least attenuates the magnitude of muscle injury that occurs after eccentric exercise. This training effect is produced only after eccentric training of the specific muscle group being tested. In other words, general increased fitness neither prevents nor attenuates eccentric contraction–induced muscle injury.

Based on experimental studies of skeletal muscles directly subjected to eccentric exercise, it is thought that the early events that cause muscle injury are mechanical ones.[37,38] During cyclic eccentric exercise of the rabbit tibialis anterior, significant mechanical changes were observed in the first 5 to 7 minutes of exercise.[39] Other studies have revealed structural disruption of the cytoskeleton within the fibers at these earlier time periods[40,41] that may provide further insights into the damage mechanism.

Animal and human studies have provided evidence for selective damage of fast fiber types after eccentric exercise.[42-44] In human studies, this damage was confined to the type 2 muscle fibers in general; in animal studies, damage has been localized further to the type FG (often equated to type 2B) fast fiber subtype. Because FG fibers are the most highly fatigable muscle fibers,[45] it has been speculated that the high degree of fatigability of these fibers may predispose them to injury. Several clinical studies have proposed that the fatigability of back muscles may be a predisposing factor to injury. It is difficult to test this idea directly, however, because many other differences between FG fibers and other muscle fibers exist. Further studies are required to elucidate the basis for fiber type–specific injury to skeletal muscle and to document the relationship between muscle injury and back and neck pain.

Implications of Spinal Muscle Anatomy and Architecture for Injury

There are at least three ways in which spinal muscles may be implicated in mechanisms of injury and pain. First, as described earlier, the muscle itself may be injured from eccentric contraction during an imposed movement (particularly one in which the kinematics are abnormal). Second, muscle forces may alter the load distribution within anatomic structures that have been clinically linked to pain. Third, muscle activity can alter spinal stiffness and kinematics, which would indirectly affect soft tissue loads and strains. The relationship between muscles and injury can be elucidated by biomechanical models, and accurate modeling of anatomy and architecture can affect the results of those models.

Muscle Injury Resulting from Eccentric Contraction

As noted earlier, rapid lengthening of muscle is an important mechanism of muscle injury. An example of potential muscle injury secondary to imposed lengthening occurs during whiplash. During the retraction phase of whiplash injury, when the head translates rearward with respect to the torso, the sternocleidomastoid muscle can experience lengthening strains of 5% to 10% while it is active.[46,47] During the rebound phase of whiplash injury, when the head translates forward with respect to the torso, the splenius capitis and semispinalis capitis muscles can experience lengthening strains of 10% to 20%. These predictions of muscle strains, based on a biomechanical model that incorporates muscle architecture,[31] are above thresholds for strain that causes injury to active-lengthening muscle.[37,48,49]

Muscles Altering Load Distribution in Other Anatomic Structures

Because muscles are oriented primarily vertically, their activation produces axial compression of the spine. The compressive loads on the discs and facet joints are a function of muscle force, moment arm, and activation. When the detailed anatomy of the lumbar erector spinae was included in a biomechanical model,[50] the predicted disc compression and shear loads were reduced compared with a lumped extensor "muscle equivalent" commonly used in many models. This study highlights the importance of accurate representation of muscle anatomy in biomechanical models.

Compressive loads may severely alter tissue loads, particularly if abnormal vertebral kinematics occur. The synovial fold of the facet joint may become impinged during the abnormal kinematics that occur during whiplash.[51] Muscles may also contribute to injury by directly loading passive structures. The cervical multifidus has attachments directly to facet capsular ligaments[20,52]; the combined loading from joint motion and muscle forces may lead to subcatastrophic injuries in facet capsular ligaments. These observations are important because

the cervical facet joints and ligaments have been clinically isolated as a source of neck pain.[53]

Muscle Effects on Spinal Stiffness and Stability

It has long been recognized that muscles are necessary for spinal stability. It is unclear, however, which muscles contribute most to spinal stability; this question has been addressed in several theoretical and experimental studies. Crisco and Panjabi[54] examined the role of gross muscle architecture (i.e., the number of joints crossed by a muscle) in lateral stabilization of the lumbar spine using a mathematical model. They calculated minimal muscle stiffness necessary for spinal stability and found that muscles spanning only one vertebral body required the highest stiffness (i.e., activation) for stability, whereas muscles that spanned the largest number of vertebrae were most efficient (required the least activation). Efficient stabilization (less muscle activation) is important because it implies lower disc loads.

Electromyographically driven modeling by Cholewicki and McGill[55] suggested that large muscles may provide the bulk of stiffness to the spinal column, as suggested by Crisco and Panjabi,[54] but that the activity of short intrinsic muscles was also necessary to maintain stability. Biomechanical models have shown that buckling (loss of stability) can occur from a temporary reduction in activation to one or more intersegmental muscles.[55] Presumably, small intrinsic muscles are better suited to stabilize displacements at a single joint with a minimum increase in joint loads at other levels. Similarly, Daru[56] and Winters and Peles[57] used computer and physical models of the cervical spine to show that activating only large, long muscles resulted in instability, especially around the upright posture. The authors also concluded that activation of deep muscles was necessary for spinal stability. These types of analyses show the importance of gross anatomy and architecture of spinal muscles on spinal stability. Many important questions remain, however, such as the effect of muscle fatigue on spinal stability and the best muscle activation patterns for stability in the prevention and rehabilitation of low back and neck pain.

Summary

The architecture of a muscle is an important, and often overlooked, determinant of its function. Because muscle architecture interacts with the skeletal and nervous systems in complex ways, all of these factors must be examined together to understand fully the biomechanical function of a muscle and its contribution to any pain or injury mechanisms. Detailed anatomic and architectural studies have yielded insights into spinal muscle functions, but the architecture of many spinal muscles remains to be examined. These data are necessary for accurate biomechanical models, which must be used in conjunction with experimental studies to elucidate the function of spinal muscles and their role in pathologic processes of the spine. This information can ultimately be used in developing improved prevention and rehabilitation strategies.

KEY REFERENCES

1. Burke RE, Levine DN, Tsairis P, et al: Physiological types and histochemical profiles in motor units of the cat gastrocnemius. J Physiol (Lond) 234:723-748, 1973.
   This article is the classic reference that describes the relationship between the anatomic, physiologic, and biochemical properties of the mammalian motor unit. This article helps to explain the orderly recruitment of motor neurons during normal movement.

2. Evans WJ, Meredith CN, Cannon JG, et al: Metabolic changes following eccentric exercise in trained and untrained men. J Appl Physiol 61:1864-1868, 1986.
   This article is one of the earliest demonstrations of the protective effect of training on muscle injury owing to eccentric exercise. It is also a clear demonstration of the delayed nature of the injury that occurs to muscle after eccentric exercise.

3. Fridén J, Sjöström M, Ekblom B: Myofibrillar damage following intense eccentric exercise in man. Int J Sports Med 4:170-176, 1983.
   This article is the seminal demonstration of cytoskeletal damage to muscle after eccentric exercise. It contains classic micrographs showing the "Z band streaming" that occurs when muscles are subjected to high-intensity exercise.

4. Macintosh JE, Bogduk N: The biomechanics of the lumbar multifidus. Clin Biomech 1:205-213, 1986; MacIntosh JE, Bogduk N: The morphology of the lumbar erector spinae. Spine 12:658-668, 1987; MacIntosh JE, Valencia F, Bogduk N, Munro RR: The morphology of the human lumbar multifidus. Clin Biomech 1:196-204, 1986.
   This series of articles describes the complex but highly reproducible anatomy of the lumbar and thoracic spine musculature. Progressing from superficial to deep and thoracic to lumbar, the extraordinary level of organization of this musculature is clearly apparent.

5. Warren GW, Hayes D, Lowe DA, et al: Mechanical factors in the initiation of eccentric contraction-induced injury in rat soleus muscle. J Physiol (Lond) 464:457-475, 1993.
   This article presents a multiple regression experimental model that describes the relationship between muscle stress, muscle strain, and muscle strain rate as mechanical causal factors in muscle injury. The slow mammalian muscle is used as the experimental model.

REFERENCES

1. Panjabi M: The stabilizing system of the spine: I. Function, dysfunction, adaptation, and enhancement. J Spinal Disord 5:383-389, 1992.

2. Gans C, Bock WJ: The functional significance of muscle architecture: A theoretical analysis. Adv Anat Embryol Cell Biol 38:115-142, 1965.

3. Gans C, De Vries F: Functional bases of fiber length and angulation in muscle. J Morphol 192:63-85, 1987.

4. Lieber RL: Skeletal Muscle Structure and Function: Implications for Physical Therapy and Sports Medicine. Baltimore, Lippincott, Williams & Wilkins, 2010.

5. Bodine SC, Roy RR, Meadows DA, et al: Architectural, histochemical, and contractile characteristics of a unique biarticular muscle: The cat semitendinosus. J Neurophysiol 48:192-201, 1982.

6. Ounjian M, Roy RR, Eldred E, et al: Physiological and developmental implications of motor unit anatomy. J Neurobiol 22:547-559, 1991.

7. Loeb GE, Pratt CA, Chanaud CM, et al: Distribution and innervation of short, interdigitated muscle fibers in parallel-fibered muscles of the cat hind limb. J Morphol 1:1-15, 1987.

8. Armstrong JB, Rose PK, Vanner S, et al: Compartmentalization of motor units in the cat neck muscle, biventer cervicis. J Neurophysiol 60:30-45, 1988.

9. Richmond FJR, MacGillis DRR, Scott DA: Muscle-fiber compartmentalization in cat splenius muscles. J Neurophysiol 53:868-885, 1985.

10. Burkholder TJ, Lieber RL: Sarcomere length operating range of muscles during movement. J Exp Biol 204:1529-1536, 2001.

11. Lieber RL, Ljung B-O, Fridén J: Intraoperative sarcomere measurements reveal differential musculoskeletal design of long and short wrist extensors. J Exp Biol 200:19-25, 1997.

12. Lieber RL, Loren GJ, Fridén J: In vivo measurement of human wrist extensor muscle sarcomere length changes. J Neurophysiol 71:874-881, 1994.

13. Rome LC, Choi IH, Lutz G, et al: The influence of temperature on muscle function in the fast swimming scup: I. Shortening velocity and muscle recruitment during swimming. J Exp Biol 163:259-279, 1992.

14. Rome LC, Sosnicki AA: Myofilament overlap in swimming carp: II. Sarcomere length changes during swimming. Am J Physiol 163:281-295, 1991.

15. An KN, Takakashi K, Harrington TP, et al: Determination of muscle orientation and moment arms. J Biomech Eng 106:280-282, 1984.

16. Kalimo H, Rantanen J, Viljanen T, et al: Lumbar muscles: Structure and function. Ann Med 21:353-359, 1989.

17. MacIntosh JE, Bogduk N: The morphology of the lumbar erector spinae. Spine 12:658-668, 1987.

18. Delp SL, Suryanarayanan S, Murray WM, et al: Architecture of the rectus abdominis, quadratus lumborum, and erector spinae. J Biomech 34:371-375, 2001.

19. Kamibayashi LK, Richmond FJR: Morphometry of human neck muscles. Spine 23:1314-1323, 1998.

20. Anderson JS, Hsu AW, Vasavada AN: Morphology, architecture, and biomechanics of human cervical multifidus. Spine 30:86-91, 2005.

21. MacIntosh JE, Bogduk N: The biomechanics of the lumbar multifidus. Clin Biomech 1:205-213, 1986.

22. Ward, SR, Kim CW, Eng CM, et al: Architectural analysis and intraoperative measurements demonstrate the unique design of the multifidus for lumbar spine stability. J Bone Joint Surg Am 91:176-185, 2009.

23. Donisch EW, Basmajian JV: Electromyography of deep back muscles in man. Am J Anat 133:25-36, 1972.

24. Gray H: Gray's Anatomy. New York, Gramercy Books, 1977.

25. MacIntosh JE, Valencia F, Bogduk N, et al: The morphology of the human lumbar multifidus. Clin Biomech 1:196-204, 1986.

26. McGill SM, Juker D, Kropf P: Quantitative intramuscular myoelectric activity of quadratus lumborum during a wide variety of tasks. Clin Biomech 11:170-172, 1996.

27. Bogduk N, Pearcy M, Hadfield G: Anatomy and biomechanics of psoas major. Clin Biomech 7:109-119, 1992.

28. McGill SM, Patt N, Norman RW: Measurement of the trunk musculature of active males using CT scan radiography: Implications for force and moment generating capacity about the L4/L5 joint. J Biomech 21:329-334, 1988.

29. Santaguida PL, McGill SM: The psoas major muscle: A three-dimensional geometric study. J Biomech 28:339-345, 1995.

30. Juker D, McGill SM, Kropf P, et al: Quantitative intramuscular myoelectric activity of lumbar portions of psoas and the abdominal wall during a wide variety of tasks. Med Sci Sports Exerc 30:301-310, 1998.

31. Vasavada A, Li S, Delp S: Influence of muscle morphometry and moment arms on the moment-generating capacity of human neck muscles. Spine 23:412-421, 1998.

32. Bogduk N, Johnson G, Spalding D: The morphology and biomechanics of latissimus dorsi. Clin Biomech 13:377-385, 1998.

33. McGill SM, Hughson RL, Parks K: Changes in lumbar lordosis modify the role of the extensor muscles. Clin Biomech 15:777-780, 2000.

34. Norman RW, Wells P, Neumann P, et al: A comparison of peak vs. cumulative physical work exposure risk factors for the reporting of low back pain in the automotive industry. Clin Biomech 13:561-573, 1998.

35. Clarkson PM, Johnson J, Dextradeur D, et al: The relationships among isokinetic endurance, initial strength level, and fiber type. Res Q Exerc Sport 53:15-19, 1982.

36. Evans WJ, Meredith CN, Cannon JG, et al: Metabolic changes following eccentric exercise in trained and untrained men. J Appl Physiol 61:1864-1868, 1986.

37. Lieber RL, Fridén J: Muscle damage is not a function of muscle force but active muscle strain. J Appl Physiol 74:520-526, 1993.

38. Warren GW, Hayes D, Lowe DA, et al: Mechanical factors in the imitation of eccentric contraction-induced injury in rat soleus muscle. J Physiol (Lond) 464:457-475, 1993.

39. Lieber RL, McKee-Woodburn T, Fridén J: Muscle damage induced by eccentric contraction of 25% strain. J Appl Physiol 70:2498-2507, 1991.

40. Lieber RL, Schmitz MC, Mishra DK, et al: Contractile and cellular remodeling in rabbit skeletal muscle after cyclic eccentric contractions. J Appl Physiol 77:1926-1934, 1994.

41. Lieber RL, Thornell L-E, Fridén J: Muscle cytoskeletal disruption occurs within the first 15 minutes of cyclic eccentric contraction. J Appl Physiol 80:278-284, 1996.

42. Fridén J: Changes in human skeletal muscle induced by long term eccentric exercise. Cell Tissue Res 236:365-372, 1984.

43. Fridén J, Sjöström M, Ekblom B: Myofibrillar damage following intense eccentric exercise in man. Int J Sports Med 4:170-176, 1983.

44. Lieber RL, Fridén J: Selective damage of fast glycolytic muscle fibers with eccentric contraction of the rabbit tibialis anterior. Acta Physiol Scand 133:587-588, 1988.

45. Burke RE, Levine DN, Tsairis P, et al: Physiological types and histochemical profiles in motor units of the cat gastrocnemius. J Physiol (Lond) 234:723-748, 1973.

46. Brault JR, Siegmund GP, Wheeler JB: Cervical muscle response during whiplash: Evidence of a lengthening muscle contraction. Clin Biomech 15:426-435, 2000.

47. Vasavada AN, Brault JR, Siegmund GP: Musculotendon and fascicle strains in anterior and posterior neck muscles during whiplash injury. Spine 32:756-765, 2007.

48. MacPherson PCK, Schork MA, Faulkner JA: Contraction-induced injury in single fiber segments from fast and slow muscles of rats by single stretches. Am J Physiol 271:C1438-C1446, 1996.

49. Patel TJ, Das R, Fridén J, et al: Sarcomere strain and heterogeneity correlate with injury to frog skeletal muscle fiber bundles. J Appl Physiol 97:1803-1813, 2004.

50. McGill SM, Norman RW: Effects of an anatomically detailed erector spinae model of L4/L5 disc compression and shear. J Biomech 20:591-600, 1987.

51. Kaneoka K, Ono K, Inami S, et al: Motion analysis of cervical vertebrae during whiplash loading. Spine 24:763-770, 1999.

52. Winkelstein B, McLendon R, Barbir A, et al: An anatomical investigation of the human cervical facet capsule, quantifying muscle insertion area. J Anat 198:455-461, 2001.

53. Barnsley L, Lord S, Wallis B, et al: The prevalence of chronic cervical zygapophysial joint pain after whiplash. Spine 20:20-26, 1995.

54. Crisco JJ, Panjabi MM: The intersegmental and multisegmental muscles of the lumbar spine: A biomechanical model comparing lateral stabilizing potential. Spine 16:793-797, 1991.

55. Cholewicki J, McGill SM: Mechanical stability of the in vivo lumbar spine: Implications for injury and chronic low back pain. Clin Biomech 11:1-15, 1996.

56. Daru KR: Computer simulation and static analysis of the human head, neck and upper torso. MS thesis, Arizona State University, 1989.

57. Winters JM, Peles JD: Neck muscle activity and 3-D head kinematics during quasi-static and dynamic tracking movements. In Winters JM, Woo SL (eds): Multiple Muscle Systems: Biomechanics and Movement Organization. New York, Springer-Verlag, 1990, pp 461-480.

SECTION

I

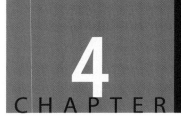

4
CHAPTER

Anatomy and Mechanics of the Abdominal Muscles

Stephen H. M. Brown, PhD
Samuel R. Ward, PT, PhD
Richard L. Lieber, PhD

Relatively little is known about the mechanics of the abdominal muscles. It is clear, however, that abdominal wall muscles are morphologically unique and are responsible for an array of mechanical roles, including the production and control of spine movement, stabilization of the spinal column, generation of intra-abdominal pressure (IAP), and respiration. The four muscles of the abdominal wall consist of three broad, sheetlike muscles that overlay one another (*external oblique, internal oblique, transverse abdominis*) and the more anterior *rectus abdominis,* across which the sheetlike muscles are linked (Fig. 4–1). This chapter discusses abdominal muscular anatomy, characteristics and considerations that affect the force-generating and moment-generating capabilities of the muscles, novel data regarding the architectural properties of the muscles, mechanical roles and consequences of the muscles, and finally possible relationships between abdominal muscle function and low back pain and injury.

Gross Morphologic Anatomy

Rectus Abdominis

The rectus abdominis runs longitudinally down the anterior trunk and is divided into two separate muscles (right and left) by the linea alba. The muscle originates from the lower sternum and costal cartilage of the fifth to seventh ribs,[1] and it inserts into the pubic symphysis (Fig. 4–2A). It is divided transversely along its length by tendinous intersections (normally three) that separate the muscle into four regions (in-series with one another) of muscle fibers. These intersections often do not span the complete mediolateral distance across the muscle, with some fibers therefore extending extra length.[2,3]

The mechanical role of the septa of the tendinous intersections is unclear, but two main hypotheses have been proposed. The first purports that these tendons provide bending locations within the muscle, allowing it to fold effectively as the trunk flexes forward, preventing muscle fiber bunching that could occur with extreme shortening of long fibers.[4] The second hypothesis pertains to the transverse mechanical strength of the rectus abdominis; the oblique and transverse abdominis muscles can apply substantial forces transversely across or, via anchoring on the rectus sheath, through the rectus abdominis.[5] The tendinous intersections may provide transverse strength to rectus abdominis fibers, preventing them being pulled apart by the forces transmitted by the external oblique, internal oblique, and transverse abdominis.

External Oblique

The external oblique is a large sheetlike muscle, the most superficial of the abdominal wall, with fibers spanning from the rib cage (5th to 12th ribs),[1] running inferomedially, and attaching across two main anatomic regions: the rectus sheath (covering the rectus abdominis) and the iliac crest (Fig. 4–2B). Muscle fiber orientations have been described for the external oblique, internal oblique, and transverse abdominis relative to a line connecting left and right anterior superior iliac spines (ASIS)[6] and are described here as such. External oblique fibers originating superior to the base of the rib cage are oriented approximately 50 degrees (standard deviation [SD] 7 degrees) inferomedially[6] and terminate to form the most superficial layers of the rectus sheath. Fibers originating between the base of the rib cage and iliac crest run approximately 59 degrees (SD 11 degrees) inferomedially (slightly more vertically).[6] The most inferior fibers originating from the rib cage that do not terminate on the iliac crest become aponeurotic superior to the ASIS,[6] form the lower-most superficial portions of the rectus sheath, and insert into the pubic symphysis. Some authors report that a small proportion of posterior fibers run from the mid-posterior of the iliac crest and terminate as part of the middle[7] and posterior[8] layers of the lumbar fascia, although this is not a universal finding.

Internal Oblique

The internal oblique is a large sheetlike muscle that lies deep to the external oblique and superficial to the transverse abdominis. Within different regions of the muscle, its fibers run at angles highly oblique to one another, creating a fanlike appearance (Fig. 4–2C). Fibers originating from the base of the rib cage run from the costal margins of the 10th to 12th ribs[1] to the iliac crest at an angle of approximately 48 degrees

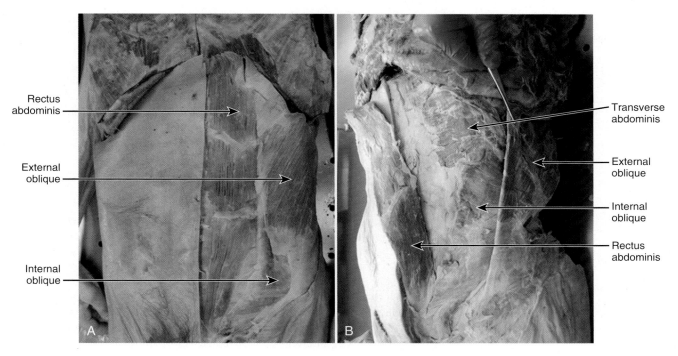

FIGURE 4–1 A, Cadaveric dissection of abdominal wall from anterior view. Part of inferior external oblique aponeurosis has been cut away to uncover internal oblique deep to it. **B,** Cadaveric dissection of abdominal wall from anterolateral view. Rectus abdominis was cut and external oblique folded back to uncover deep internal oblique and transverse abdominis. Note dissimilar fiber orientations in different muscles.

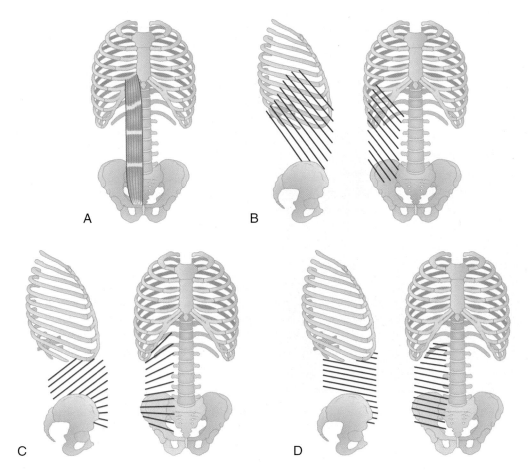

FIGURE 4–2 A-D, Schematic representations of muscle fiber lines of action for rectus abdominis (**A**), external oblique (**B**), internal oblique (**C**), and transverse abdominis (**D**).

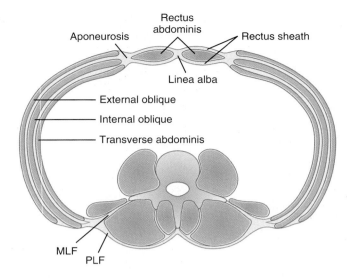

FIGURE 4–3 Transverse cross section of abdomen at mid–lumbar spine level. Internal oblique, external oblique, and transverse abdominis come together at anterior of abdominal wall to form a common aponeurosis, which continues to form the rectus sheath surrounding rectus abdominis. At posterior of abdominal wall, internal oblique and transverse abdominis terminate into middle (MLF) and posterior (PLF) layers of lumbar fascia.

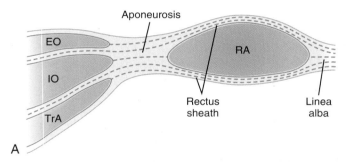

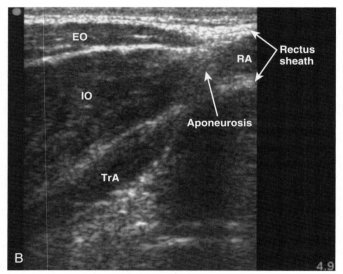

FIGURE 4–4 A, Schematic transverse cross section of anterior abdominal aponeurosis and rectus sheath. Note trilaminar nature of superficial and deep layers of rectus sheath. Fascial sheets arise from superficial and deep layers of each of external oblique, internal oblique, and transverse abdominis to form aponeurosis and rectus sheath and terminate across midline of the body through the linea alba. **B,** Ultrasound image of transverse cross section of anterior abdominal wall.

(SD 13 degrees) superomedially.[6] These fibers terminate across the rectus abdominis to create deep and superficial layers of the rectus sheath. Fibers spanning the region between the base of the rib cage and the iliac crest run at an angle of approximately 35 degrees (SD 10 degrees) superomedially.[6]

All of the fibers in this region attach to the iliac crest but can terminate at one of three anatomic locations: (1) medial fibers terminating as deep and superficial layers of the rectus sheath; (2) more lateral fibers terminating on the costal margin of the base of the rib cage; (3) and the most posterior fibers terminating to form a fascial layer deep to the erector spinae (middle layer of lumbar fascia), which ends at the transverse processes,[7-9] with some fibers adjoining a superficial fascial layer overlying the erector spinae (posterior layer of lumbar fascia), which attaches to the spinous processes (Fig. 4–3).[8,9] In the final functional region of the abdominal wall, fibers originate from the anterior of the iliac crest, terminate as deep and superficial layers of the rectus sheath, and are oriented at completely different angles to the more superior fibers. The fibers originating between the iliac crest and the ASIS run approximately horizontally and become continually more inferomedially oriented below the ASIS (up to an angle of approximately 16 degrees [SD 10 degrees] inferomedially).[6]

Transverse Abdominis

The transverse abdominis is the deepest of the sheetlike abdominal wall muscles. Its fibers above the base of the rib cage originate from the costal margins of the ribs and terminate as the deepest layers of the rectus sheath (Fig. 4–2D). These fibers run almost horizontally, with only a slight inferomedial orientation of 3 degrees (SD 9 degrees).[6] The fibers between the base of the rib cage and iliac crest run from the posterior fascia (terminating as the same fascial layers as the internal oblique [discussed earlier; see Fig. 4–3]) to the rectus sheath and are oriented at approximately 13 degrees inferomedially. Fibers originating from the anterior iliac crest and ASIS run approximately 21 degrees (SD 11 degrees) inferomedially and terminate again as the deepest slips of the rectus sheath.[6]

Rectus Sheath

Each of the abdominal wall muscles attaches at the anterior margin of the torso through an aponeurosis that ultimately leads to the formation of the rectus sheath (Fig. 4–4). Detailed investigations of the morphology of the abdominal wall aponeuroses reveal a bilayered arrangement stemming from each muscle. Specifically, the aponeurosis of each of the external oblique, internal oblique, and transverse abdominis can be anatomically separated into two layers, one arising from the superficial fascial layer of the muscle and the other arising from the deep fascial layer of the muscle.[10,11] The superficial and deep layers of the rectus sheath comprise three fascial layers (superficial—two from external and one from internal oblique, and deep—one from internal oblique and two from transverse abdominis). It is thought that the functional or mechanical purpose of this structural arrangement is to enable transfer of forces generated by the abdominal wall muscles (external oblique, internal oblique, transverse abdominis) around the torso, creating a pressurized abdominal cavity that assists in stiffening the spinal column.[4,12] Although highly variable and inferior to the umbilicus, most individuals display a gradual movement of deep internal oblique and transverse abdominis aponeurotic fibers from the posterior to the anterior of the rectus sheath; this may be due to the need for increased resistance to bulging of the anterior wall in the lower abdomen.

The connective tissue networks overlying each of the three abdominal wall muscles, giving way to the formation of the rectus sheath, also provide a strong mechanical shear linkage between the muscle layers. This linkage has been shown to transmit forces mechanically among the muscle layers in a rat preparation[13] and has been hypothesized to afford composite laminate structural properties that assist in strengthening the abdominal wall and stiffening the spinal column. Additional study of mechanical interactions between the muscle layers is needed to further understanding of abdominal muscle function, in particular related to deformation during contraction or movement and force generation and transmission around the abdomen.

Mechanical Properties of the Abdominal Muscles

Muscle force–generating capacities depend on architectural characteristics.[14,15] Specifically, the number, length, and orientation of fibers acting in parallel with the axis of force generation, together with the moment arms around the joints the muscle crosses, determine the functional capabilities of a muscle.

Most information regarding the physiologic cross-sectional area (PCSA) of the abdominal muscles comes from various imaging modalities, including computed tomography (CT), magnetic resonance imaging (MRI), and ultrasonography. More recent work in the authors' laboratory has further documented the PCSA of the abdominal muscles from cadaveric dissections of 11 donors ranging in age from 52 to 94 years (mean age 77.7 years [SD 16.3 years]).[16] McGill and colleagues[17] and Marras and colleagues,[18] measuring young healthy men using CT and MRI, measured a rectus abdominis PCSA of approximately 8 cm^2 at the level of the L4-L5 disc. This value is much larger than the mean 3.3 cm^2 measured from the elderly cadavers.[16] Similarly, the overall force-generating capacities of the internal and external oblique muscles, documented in McGill[19] measuring healthy young men, were much larger than in the cadaveric dissections of Brown and colleagues[16] (approximately 16 cm^2 and 19 cm^2 vs. 6.6 cm^2 and 8.6 cm^2 for the external oblique and internal oblique). This discrepancy between the data from cadavers and imaging data from young men likely points to an aging-related atrophy of the muscles. Similar measures of transverse abdominis PCSA have been reported, however, between the two modalities (approximately 5 cm^2 in the studies by McGill[19] and Brown and colleagues[16]). In addition, Marras and colleagues[18] reported PCSA gender differences (males greater than females) for external oblique and internal oblique in young individuals and reported an increasing rectus abdominis PCSA toward lower vertebral levels; these findings were not apparent in the cadaveric analyses.[16]

Although lines of action in the external oblique, the transverse abdominis, and in particular the internal oblique run at various angles in different regions of the muscles, all fibers act directly in line with connective tissue attachments through which they apply force. It is inappropriate to consider these muscles as pennate to a force line of action but more appropriately as applying force to the body across a wide span of fiber angles and attachments.

The ability of a muscle to generate force also depends on the instantaneous length and velocity of muscle fibers or, more specifically, of the sarcomeres that make up the muscle fibers.[20] The more recent study by Brown and colleagues[16] reported fixed sarcomere lengths of the abdominal muscles in the approximate neutral spine posture. Sarcomere lengths of the rectus abdominis and external oblique (mean 3.29 μm [SD 0.22 μm] and 3.18 μm [SD 0.37 μm] for the rectus abdominis and external oblique) in this position were well above optimal (optimal approximately 2.70 μm in human muscle[21]), whereas the lengths of the internal oblique and transverse abdominis (mean 2.61 μm [SD 0.21 μm] and 2.58 μm [SD 0.16 μm] for the internal oblique and transverse abdominis) were slightly below optimal. Because anteriorly acting fibers of the internal oblique shorten during flexion, whereas more laterally acting fibers lengthen, biomechanical modeling predicts the muscle, as a whole, to produce maximum force near the neutral spine posture. The rectus abdominis and external oblique (which shorten during spine flexion) and the transverse abdominis (which primarily lengthens during spine flexion) act together at optimal force-generating length in the mid-range of lumbar flexion, where the internal oblique can still generate in the range of 90% or greater of its maximum force.

Normalized fiber lengths were also calculated for the muscles to provide an indication of their excursion capabilities (Fig. 4–5).[16] A muscle with longer fibers can produce force over a greater range of lengths because a greater number of sarcomeres act to produce this overall length change effectively. This also has direct implications for the velocities at which a muscle can produce force because in a longer muscle each sarcomere experiences a lower relative velocity compared with a shorter muscle-changing length at the same rate. The data in Figure 4–5 imply that the rectus abdominis and external oblique have the potential to undergo greater length changes and produce force at higher absolute velocities compared with the internal oblique and transverse abdominis. How these muscles adapt to changes in body shape (e.g., to chronic visceral weight gain or loss) has yet to be explored, and any potential adaptations (or lack thereof) can have important implications for abdominal muscle function related to obesity.

Similar to the PCSA literature, functional moment arms of the abdominal muscles have been reported based on imaging data. Caution is needed, however, when examining this literature because McGill and colleagues[22] and Jorgensen and colleagues[23] have detailed large underestimations of the moment

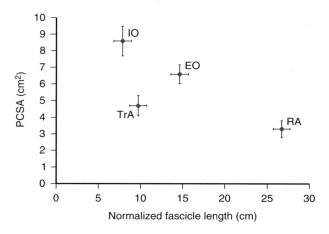

FIGURE 4–5 Plot of physiologic cross-sectional area (PCSA) and normalized fascicle lengths of abdominal muscles. Rectus abdominis fascicle length represents total in-series length across all regions. Standard error bars are shown. Large PCSA indicates large isometric force–generating ability, and long optimal fascicle length indicates ability to generate force across a wide range of lengths and at high velocities. (From Brown SHM, Ward SR, Cook M, et al: Architectural analysis of human abdominal muscles: Implications for mechanical function. Spine [in press].)

action acting between rigid locations on a movable skeleton. The moment-generating potential of a muscle depends on the amount of force that it can generate and its moment arm about a given joint. The abdominal muscles cross numerous individual spinal joints, including the entire lumbar spine. Spinal disc centers, representing rotational and translational joint centers, are also reported in these models, and using the knowledge of the muscle lines of action and these joint centers, moment arms around all three of the functional orthopaedic spine axes (flexion-extension, lateral bend, axial twist) can be computed (Table 4–1).

Two very important points need to be made about the moment-generating capabilities of the external oblique, internal oblique, and transverse abdominis. Because of their broad attachments across the rib cage, iliac crest, and rectus sheath, different fiber regions can have opposing moment-generating capabilities. For example, McGill,[28] Stokes and Gardner-Morse,[25] Dumas and colleagues,[29] and Marras and Sommerich[30] recognized that the posterior fibers of the internal oblique, attaching to the posterior elements of the spine, produce an extensor moment in the neutral posture, whereas the remaining bulk of the fibers produce flexor moments. Inferior fibers of the transverse abdominis produce a contralateral rotation of an unfixed pelvis (producing a relative ipsilateral rotation of the spine), whereas the more superior fibers attaching to the posterior elements of the spine and rib cage may generate contralateral rotation of the spine.

The second major point that needs to be understood is that the moment-generating capabilities of these muscles and muscle fiber regions are highly dependent on spine and trunk orientation (see Table 4–1). Examining these models, it becomes apparent that the moment arms and moment-generating capabilities of the abdominal muscles can change

arms when subjects are positioned supine compared with upright standing, owing to the depression of the abdominal cavity. Anatomically detailed biomechanical models of the abdominal muscles, in relation to skeletal attachments and specific spinal joints, can provide a more justified assessment of the moment-generating capacity of these muscles.

In particular, Cholewicki and McGill[24] and Stokes and Gardner-Morse[25] reported anatomically detailed representations of the spine skeletal and muscle geometry. Both of these models represented muscles as a series of straight lines of

TABLE 4–1 Moment Arms*

	RECTUS ABDOMINIS			EXTERNAL OBLIQUE			INTERNAL OBLIQUE		
	Flex	LB	AT	Flex	LB	AT	Flex	LB	AT
Neutral	**8.1**	**5.1**	**1†**	**4**	**8.1**	**4.7†**	**1.9**	**7.4**	**6.4**
	10.8	3.8	0.4†	6.2	8.8	6.9†	3.3	10.6	4.1
Flexion	**11.9**	**5.2**	**0.6**	**1.6**	**9.9**	**1.4**	**0.7**	**2.4†**	**9.5**
	13.6	3.2	2.9	0	6.1	6	0.7	2†	11
Extension	**6.4**	**5**	**1.5†**	**3.8**	**6.8**	**6†**	**2.4**	**9**	**3.3**
	8.7	3.4	1.1†	5.9	7.2	8.8†	3	10.9	0.2
Ipsilateral LB	**7.3**	**8.2**	**3.6†**	**3.1**	**5.6**	**6.7†**	**2.1**	**4.7**	**8.6**
	9.5	5.6	5.1†	1.8	0.1†	11†	3.6	3.5	4.4
Contralateral LB	**8**	**2.5**	**1.2**	**4.4**	**8.5**	**3.2†**	**1.5**	**7.9**	**5.3**
	10.2	1.9	3.8	6.1	12.8	2.1†	2.9	11.8	3.4
Ipsilateral twist	**7.9**	**5.6**	**1.6†**	**3.8†**	**8**	**5.6†**	**2.3**	**8.4**	**5.3**
	10.5	4.2	1.2†	6	7.7	8.1†	2.9	11.4	0.9
Contralateral twist	**8**	**4.5**	**0.4†**	**4.1**	**8.1**	**3.5†**	**1.4**	**6.6**	**6.5**
	11	3.5	0.4	6.4	10.1	5.1†	3.3	9.3	6.6

*Moment arms (cm) estimated by the biomechanical models of Cholewicki and McGill[24] (*upper bold values*) and Stokes and Gardner-Morse[25] (*lower values*), about each of the flexion-extension (flex), lateral bend (LB), and axial twist (AT) axes, for the following lumbar spine postures: neutral, maximum flexion (52 degrees[26]), maximum extension (16 degrees[26]), maximum ipsilateral and contralateral bend (29 degrees each[27]), maximum ipsilateral and contralateral twist (9 degrees each[27]).

†Moment arm in the direction contralateral to the muscle side (e.g., right external oblique would produce a left axial twist in the neutral posture).

greatly as the spine rotates into various postures (see Table 4–1). In the neutral posture, the external oblique can produce fairly substantial spine flexion (moment arm 4 to 6.2 cm), lateral bend (moment arm 8.1 to 8.8 cm), and contralateral axial twist (moment arm contralateral 4.7 to 6.9 cm) moments. When the lumbar spine is fully flexed, the external oblique loses its ability to produce a flexor moment (moment arm 0 to 1.6 cm), however, and becomes an ipsilateral twister of the lumbar spine (moment arm now ipsilateral 1.4 to 6 cm). Attributing gross mechanical roles to the abdominal muscles without consideration of spine orientation and position is folly and can lead to erroneous functional interpretations of actions and roles. This has additional importance in understanding the roles of each of these muscles in stabilizing the lumbar spine, which are discussed later.

The transverse abdominis has been less frequently modeled in biomechanical representations of the spine and is absent from the published models of Cholewicki and McGill,[24] Marras and Sommerich,[30] and Stokes and Gardner-Morse.[25] The recent focus on this muscle in the clinical literature, to be discussed later, indicates that consideration and study of its action is warranted. McGill,[19] using ultrasonography and CT, modeled the force action of the transverse abdominis as projected along the anterior of the torso through the rectus abdominis and rectus sheath complex. This consideration produced an average flexor moment arm of approximately 0.8 cm in a neutral spine posture. Alternatively, modeling its force action as pulling laterally through its attachments to the transverse and spinous processes, the muscle would act with a small extension moment arm (approximately 1 cm) in the neutral spine posture. Considering either or both of these actions of this muscle, it is clear that the transverse abdominis produces little moment about the flexion-extension axis.

The transverse abdominis does produce more substantial lateral bend and twist moments; however, its net relationship to ipsilateral versus contralateral twist is unclear. Although most of the fiber attachments suggest a possible contralateral twist moment similar to the external oblique,[29] its neural activation is much higher during ipsilateral twist efforts.[31,32] As mentioned earlier, how the transverse abdominis moment arm and moment-generating potential change as the spine rotates around each of its functional axes needs to be considered.

Neural Control of Abdominal Muscles

Force and moment generation are also highly dependent on neural signals received by muscles from the central nervous system. Each of the four abdominal muscles receives efferent nerve supply from multiple spinal levels: rectus abdominis, lower six thoracic nerves[33]; external oblique, lateral cutaneous branches of lower eight thoracic nerves[34]; internal oblique and transverse abdominis, lower six thoracic nerves and first lumbar nerve.[33] Woodley and colleagues[3] also showed that some longer fascicles within each of the four abdominal muscles contain multiple motor endplate bands, suggesting that individual fascicles may receive multiple nerve supplies.

Innervation from a wide span of spinal nerves across different regions of the muscles seems to enable specific regional activation of these muscles. For example, Mirka and colleagues[35] and Urquhart and Hodges[32] showed regionally different activation magnitudes in the external oblique and transverse abdominis. More convincingly, Moreside and colleagues[36] revealed activation timing differences with regions of the rectus abdominis and external oblique, reporting antiphasic patterns of activation between anterior and lateral regions of the external oblique and between upper and lower regions of the rectus abdominis in Middle Eastern style–trained dancers.

Corresponding to their mechanical orientation, the abdominal muscles are most active in loading scenarios that require the generation of flexion, lateral bend, and twist moments. The abdominal muscles, having a postural and stabilizing role, display consistent levels of low tonic activation during even minimal loading upright tasks. Masani and colleagues[37] and Gregory and colleagues,[38] both during sitting, and Gregory,[39] during standing, found average abdominal muscle activations never to exceed 3% of their maximum voluntary capability. Gregory and colleagues[38,39] indicated similar low levels of activation during seated work on an unstable surface (exercise ball) designed to challenge the maintenance of spine stability. More dynamic tasks such as walking rarely involve abdominal muscle activation greater than 5% of maximum.[40] Although these activation levels are seemingly modest, they are probably crucial for maintenance of a stable spine, discussed later.

Mechanical Consequences: Compression Force, Shear Force, and Stability

Contraction of trunk muscles exerts forces onto and stabilizes the spinal column. The consideration and study of spinal forces cannot be separated from stability because they are inextricably linked. The spinal column is a highly unstable structure that, in the absence of muscular attachments, would buckle at loads far below the weight of the upper body.[41,42] The bulk of the loading experienced by the lumbar spine is developed and imposed by the spinal musculature.[43,44] The predominant reason for the extreme loading imparted by the muscles onto the spine is the large relative amounts of coactivation that occur during trunk muscle recruitment.[44-46] This coactivation serves to stabilize the spine[47-49] and as a secondary consequence imparts additional load on the spine.[49-51]

Because most spine-loading events produce net extensor moments (the spine extensors generate the dominant loading moment), the abdominal muscles most often serve the role of coactivators. It has further been definitively established that some coactivation is necessary to ensure a stable spine.[24,49] Coordinated contraction of the abdominal muscles plays a vital role in maintaining the mechanical integrity of the spinal column during light and heavy loading scenarios. Finally, abdominal muscles are mechanically well equipped to stabilize the spine owing to their relatively large moment arms[52-54] around the three anatomic axes in various postures (Table 4–1).

Despite this information, it is important to consider that activation and contraction of the abdominal muscles do not ensure stability and that poorly balanced patterns of contraction can compromise stability.[55] Finally, based on the differing demands under which the spine can be placed (e.g., different anatomic loading axes, spine orientation and position), it is likely that no abdominal muscle, or no muscle in general, should be considered *the* most important spine stabilizer.[56,57]

Biomechanical models can be used to estimate forces applied by individual muscles to the intervertebral discs and vertebral bodies and to estimate whether, under a given loading scenario, the spine is considered stable or unstable. With the exception of the transverse abdominis, the abdominal muscles are oriented such that they have potential to apply significant compressive loads to the lumbar spine. Because of the large role that the abdominal muscles play in generating twisting moments, actions that involve twisting or twisted postures often carry substantial compressive penalties.[58] Exercises and work-related tasks (e.g., lifting while twisted or twisting) that substantially recruit the abdominal muscles have the potential to impart tremendous compressive loads on the lumbar spine and must be employed with care. Anteroposterior shear forces are more difficult to interpret because the line of action of the fibers in different regions of the muscles, the relative angle of the endplates at each vertebral level, and the changes in these variables as the spine rotates all must be considered.[59] The general thought is that the rectus abdominis, external oblique, and transverse abdominis produce a net anterior shear load, and the internal oblique produces a net posterior shear load on the lumbar spine.

IAP is often discussed relative to abdominal muscles, and its effects on spine mechanics are often debated. The contraction of the abdominal wall muscles and IAP are directly linked.[60] Specifically, IAP is generated and controlled by abdominal wall muscle contraction. As discussed earlier, abdominal muscles often contract as part of a coactivation strategy in response to a physical exertion of the back muscles, resulting in a concomitant increase in IAP. Early biomechanical models suggested that IAP acted to unload the spinal column during back loading tasks, by creating a net trunk extensor moment through the diaphragm.[61] This theory has since been negated based on an understanding of the exact mechanism of abdominal muscle contraction coinciding with the increase in IAP—this imposes compressive forces on the spine that negate unloading owing to an IAP-induced extensor moment.[62-64] Correlations have been shown between IAP generation and spine stability,[60,64-66] but it is difficult to isolate the level of the stabilizing effect that results from the IAP, the abdominal muscle contraction, or a combination thereof.

Finally, it has been hypothesized that IAP, which creates a firm abdomen around which the abdominal muscles can contract, acts to improve their ability to generate moments through an increased mechanical advantage.[67] This final effect is likely saturated at low levels of tonic activation; McGill and colleagues[22] found no discernible change in moment arms with conscious abdominal activation in the neutral standing posture. The hypothesized benefits of contracting around a pressurized abdomen may also extend to neural factors because individuals seem better able to recruit the abdominal muscles isometrically in an upright, as opposed to supine, posture.[68,69]

Abdominal muscles are also involved in respiration, particularly during conscious forceful breathing and cardiovascular challenge.[70-72] Evidence shows that the four abdominal muscles contract cyclically to assist with active expiration, as ventilatory demand increases. Although phasic activation (expiration) and relaxation (inspiration) patterns become quite clear during challenged breathing, peak abdominal activation levels (related to breathing alone) rarely exceed 5% of maximum capability. This finding suggests that the phasic activation patterns become apparent because of slight increases in activation (during expiration to push air from the lungs) and improved relaxation (during inspiration to ease airflow into the lungs). Wang[73] showed that patients with chronic obstructive pulmonary disease display phasic abdominal muscle activation and relaxation patterns at baseline breathing levels to assist with their increased ventilatory difficulty.

Abdominal Muscles and Low Back Pain

More recent research and clinical focus have highlighted a link between abdominal muscle dysfunction and low back pain and injury.[74-77] The most compelling evidence for this association comes from the large prospective study conducted by Cholewicki and colleagues,[74] who showed that athletes who displayed delayed activation onsets of the abdominal muscles, in response to spine perturbations, were more likely to sustain a low back injury in the future. These delayed abdominal muscle onsets were not a predictor of past low back incidents. This finding led the authors to conclude that altered abdominal muscle function, at least in response to rapid spine perturbations, is more a cause of than an adaptation to low back pain and injury. The underlying culprit for this type of low back injury would seem to be insufficient stiffening of the spine. Based on this evidence, numerous abdominal muscle training and rehabilitation techniques have been and are currently being developed and prescribed. When properly administered, these programs have been shown to have the potential for success.[78,79] Clinical interventions designed to activate the abdominal wall to stabilize the spine need to be considered carefully,[4] however, because increased abdominal activation has the potential to stabilize and destabilize the lumbar spine.[55]

The transverse abdominis has received special clinical consideration more recently, based on a series of articles (e.g., Hodges and Richardson[75,80]) that showed that transverse abdominis activation timing, in preparation for rapid limb movement, often precedes (by 10 to 40 msec) the activation of the other spine muscles. These authors also noted an exacerbated delay in the activation of this muscle in patients with low back pain. The mechanical consequences of these findings are unclear. First, the early activation of this muscle has been uncovered predominantly during very specialized actions, specifically rapid isolated limb movements. These actions do not readily replicate functional scenarios. Second, the other abdominal muscles also show delayed firing in patients with low back pain, albeit to a lesser degree than the transverse abdominis. Finally, Mannion and colleagues[81] determined that it was difficult to detect clearly a difference in the mechanical contraction of these muscles via ultrasonography, despite an apparent difference in electromyography activation; it is unclear whether this is a methodologic limitation of ultrasonography or whether the mechanical effects of the muscles are actually synchronized owing to differing delays between the electrical stimulation of the muscle layers and the resultant contraction dynamics.

The transverse abdominis is a small muscle with relatively small moment arms and has little ability to affect spine loading and stability directly. It may play a stabilizing role elsewhere, however, such as through the rapid development of IAP.[82] Regardless, because of the composite laminate-like nature of the abdominal wall, it is unlikely that the mechanical effects of the transverse abdominis, or any other abdominal muscle, can be effectively isolated. Attempting to do so can lead to aberrant muscle activation patterns that can compromise the stability of the spine[55,83,84] in functional situations. Isolated focus on the transverse abdominis, or any single spine muscle, is not recommended for spine injury prevention or rehabilitation.[57,85]

KEY REFERENCES

1. Urquhart DM, Barker PJ, Hodges PW, et al: Regional morphology of the transversus abdominis and obliquus internus and externus abdominis muscles. Clin Biomech 20:233-241, 2005.
   This article explores the regionalized anatomy of the abdominal wall muscles.

2. Brown SHM, Ward SR, Cook M, et al: Architectural analysis of human abdominal muscles: Implications for mechanical function. Spine (in press).
   Functional capabilities of abdominal muscles are uncovered and interpreted based on architectural analyses.

3. McGill SM: A revised anatomical model of the abdominal musculature for torso flexion efforts. J Biomech 29:973-977, 1996.
   This article discusses mechanical considerations and functions of the abdominal muscles.

4. Cholewicki J, Silfies SP, Shah RA, et al: Delayed trunk muscle reflex responses increase the risk of low back injuries. Spine 30:2614-2620, 2005.
   A causative link between abdominal muscle dysfunction and low back injury is examined.

5. Granata KP, Marras WS: Cost-benefit of muscle cocontraction in protecting against spinal instability. Spine 25:1398-1404, 2000.
   The relationship between trunk muscle coactivation, spine loading, and spine stability is investigated.

REFERENCES

1. Agur AMR, Dalley AF: Grant's Atlas of Anatomy. Philadelphia, Lippincott Williams & Wilkins, 2005.

2. Whetzel TP, Huang V: The vascular anatomy of the tendinous intersections of the rectus abdominis muscle. Plast Reconstr Surg 98:83-89, 1996.

3. Woodley SJ, Duxson MJ, Mercer SR: Preliminary observations on the microarchitecture of the human abdominal muscles. Clin Anat 20:808-813, 1997.

4. McGill SM: Low Back Disorders: Evidence-Based Prevention and Rehabilitation. Champaign, IL, Human Kinetics Publishers, 2002.

5. Brown SHM, McGill SM: An ultrasound investigation into the morphology of the human abdominal wall uncovers complex deformation patterns during contraction. Eur J Appl Physiol 104:1021-1030, 2008.

6. Urquhart DM, Barker PJ, Hodges PW, et al. Regional morphology of the transversus abdominis and obliquus internus and externus abdominis muscles. Clin Biomech 20:233-241, 2005.

7. Barker PJ, Urquhart DM, Story IH, et al: The middle layer of lumbar fascia and attachments to lumbar transverse processes: Implications for segmental control and fracture. Eur Spine J 16:2232-2237, 2007.

8. Vleeming A, Pool-Goudzwaard AL, Stoeckart R, et al: The posterior layer of the thoracolumbar fascia: Its function in load transfer from spine to legs. Spine 20:753-758, 1995.

9. Bogduk N, Macintosh JE: The applied anatomy of the thoracolumbar fascia. Spine 9:164-170, 1984.

10. Askar OM: Surgical anatomy of the aponeurotic expansions of the anterior abdominal wall. Ann R Coll Surg Engl 59:313-321, 1977.

11. Rizk NN: A new description of the anterior abdominal wall in man and mammals. J Anat 131:373-385, 1980.

12. Daggfeldt K, Thorstensson A: The role of intra-abdominal pressure in spinal unloading. J Biomech 30:1149-1155, 1997.

13. Brown SHM, McGill SM: Transmission of muscularly generated force and stiffness between layers of the rat abdominal wall. Spine 34:E70-E75, 2009.

14. Powell PL, Roy RR, Kanim P, et al: Predictability of skeletal muscle tension from architectural determinations in guinea pig hindlimbs. J Appl Physiol 57:1715-1721, 1984.

15. Lieber RL, Friden J: Functional and clinical significance of skeletal muscle architecture. Muscle Nerve 23:1647-1666, 2000.

16. Brown SHM, Ward SR, Cook M, et al: Architectural analysis of human abdominal muscles: Implications for mechanical function. Spine (in press).

17. McGill SM, Patt N, Norman RW: Measurement of the trunk musculature of active males using CT scan radiography: Implications for force and moment generating capacity about the L4/L5 joint. J Biomech 21:329-341, 1988.

18. Marras WS, Jorgensen MJ, Granata KP, et al: Female and male trunk geometry: Size and prediction of the spine loading trunk muscles derived from MRI. Clin Biomech 16:38-46, 2001.

19. McGill SM: A revised anatomical model of the abdominal musculature for torso flexion efforts. J Biomech 29:973-977, 1996.

20. Lieber RL: Skeletal Muscle Structure, Function and Plasticity: The Physiological Basis of Rehabilitation. Philadelphia, Lippincott Williams & Wilkins, 2002.

21. Lieber RL, Loren GJ, Fridén J: In vivo measurement of human wrist extensor muscle sarcomere length changes. J Neurophysiol 71:874-881, 1994.

22. McGill SM, Juker D, Axler C: Correcting trunk muscle geometry obtained from MRI and CT scans of supine postures for use in standing postures. J Biomech 29:643-646, 1996.

23. Jorgensen MJ, Marras WS, Smith FW, et al. Sagittal plane moment arms of the female lumbar region rectus abdominis in an upright neutral torso posture. Clin Biomech 20:242-246, 2005.

24. Cholewicki J, McGill SM: Mechanical stability of the in vivo lumbar spine: Implications for injury and chronic low back pain. Clin Biomech 11:1-15, 1996.

25. Stokes IAF, Gardner-Morse M: Quantitative anatomy of the lumbar musculature. J Biomech 32:311-316, 1999.

26. Pearcy M, Portek I, Shepherd J: 3-dimensional x-ray analysis of normal movement in the lumbar spine. Spine 9:294-297, 1984.

27. White AA, Panjabi MM: Clinical Biomechanics of the Spine, 2nd ed, Philadelphia, JB Lippincott, 1990.

28. McGill SM: A myoelectrically based dynamic three-dimensional model to predict loads on lumbar spine tissues during lateral bending. J Biomech 25:395-414, 1992.

29. Dumas GA, Poulin MJ, Roy B, et al: Orientation and moment arms of some trunk muscles. Spine 16:293-303, 1991.

30. Marras WS, Sommerich CM: A 3-dimensional motion model of loads on the lumbar spine: 1. Model structure. Human Factors 33:123-137, 1991.

31. Juker D, McGill S, Kropf P, et al: Quantitative intramuscular myoelectric activity of lumbar portions of psoas and the abdominal wall during a wide variety of tasks. Med Sci Sports Exerc 30:301-310, 1998.

32. Urquhart DM, Hodges PW: Differential activity of regions of transversus abdominis during trunk rotation. Eur Spine J 14:393-400, 2005.

33. Iscoe S: Control of abdominal muscles. Prog Neurobiol 56:433-506, 1998.

34. Schlenz I, Burggasser G, Kuzbari, R, et al. External oblique abdominal muscle: A new look on its blood supply and innervations. Anat Rec 255:388-395, 1999.

35. Mirka G, Kelaher D, Baker A, et al: Selective activation of the external oblique musculature during axial torque production. Clin Biomech 12:172-180, 1997.

36. Moreside JM, Vera-Garcia FJ, McGill SM: Neuromuscular independence of abdominal wall muscles as demonstrated by Middle-Eastern style dancers. J Electromyogr Kinesiol 18:527-537, 2008.

37. Masani K, Sin VW, Vette AH, et al: Postural reactions of the trunk muscles to multi-directional perturbations in sitting. Clin Biomech 24:176-182, 2009.

38. Gregory DE, Dunk NM, Callaghan JP: Stability ball versus office chair: Comparison of muscle activation and lumbar spine posture during prolonged sitting. Human Factors 48:142-153, 2006.

39. Gregory DE: Prolonged standing as a precursor for the development of low back discomfort: An investigation of possible mechanisms. Masters Thesis; Waterloo, ON, University of Waterloo, 2005.

40. Callaghan JP, Patla AE, McGill SM: Low back three-dimensional joint forces, kinematics, and kinetics during walking. Clin Biomech 14:203-216, 1999.

41. Lucas D, Bresler B: Stability of the Ligamentous Lumbar Spine. Technical Report No. 40. San Francisco, University of California, San Francisco, Biomechanics Laboratory, 1961.

42. Crisco JJ, Panjabi MM, Yamamoto I, et al: Euler stability of the human ligamentous lumbar spine: 2. Experiment. Clin Biomech 7:27-32, 1992.

43. McGill SM, Norman RW: Partitioning of the L4-L5 dynamic moment into disc, ligamentous, and muscular components during lifting. Spine 11:666-678, 1986.

44. Granata KP, Marras WS: The influence of trunk muscle coactivity on dynamic spinal loads. Spine 20:913-919, 1995.

45. Pope MH, Andersson GBJ, Broman H, et al: Electromyographic studies of lumbar trunk musculature during the development of axial torques. J Orthop Res 4:288-297, 1986.

46. Brown SHM, McGill SM: Co-activation alters the linear versus non-linear impression of the EMG-torque relationship of trunk muscles. J Biomech 41:491-497, 2008.

47. Gardner-Morse MG, Stokes IAF: The effects of abdominal muscle coactivation on lumbar spine stability. Spine 23:86-91, 1998.

48. Granata KP, Marras WS: Cost-benefit of muscle cocontraction in protecting against spinal instability. Spine 25:1398-1404, 2000.

49. Brown SHM, Potvin JR: Constraining spine stability levels in an optimization model leads to the prediction of trunk muscle cocontraction and improved spine compression force estimates. J Biomech 38:745-754, 2005.

50. van Dieën JH, Kingma I, van der Bug P: Evidence for a role of antagonistic cocontraction in controlling trunk stiffness during lifting. J Biomech 36:1829-1836, 2003.

51. El-Rich M, Shirazi-Adl A, Arjmand N: Muscle activity, internal loads, and stability of the human spine in standing postures: Combined model and in vivo studies. Spine 29:2633-2642, 2004.

52. Potvin JR, Brown SHM: An equation to calculate individual muscle contributions to joint stability. J Biomech 38:973-980, 2005.

53. Brown SHM, Potvin JR: Exploring the geometric and mechanical characteristics of the spine musculature to provide rotational stiffness to two spine joints in the neutral posture. Hum Mov Sci 26:113-123, 2007.

54. Howarth SJ, Beach TA, Callaghan JP: Abdominal muscles dominate contributions to vertebral joint stiffness during the push-up. J Appl Biomech 24:130-139, 2008.

55. Brown SHM, Vera-Garcia FJ, McGill SM: Effects of abdominal muscle co-activation on the externally preloaded trunk: Variations in motor control and its effect on spine stability. Spine 31:E387-E393, 2006.

56. Cholewicki J, VanVliet JJ: Relative contribution of trunk muscles to the stability of the lumbar spine during isometric exertions. Clin Biomech 17:99-105, 2002.

57. Kavcic N, Grenier S, McGill SM: Determining the stabilizing role of individual torso muscles during rehabilitation exercises. Spine 29:1254-1265, 2004.

58. Marras WS, Ferguson SA, Burr D, et al: Functional impairment as a predictor of spine loading. Spine 30:729-737, 2005.

59. Kingma I, Staudenmann D, van Dieën JH: Trunk muscle activation and associated lumbar spine joint shear forces under different levels of external forward force applied to the trunk. J Electromyogr Kinesiol 17:14-24, 2007.

60. Cholewicki J, Ivancic PC, Radebold A: Can increased intra-abdominal pressure in humans be decoupled from trunk muscle co-contraction during steady state isometric exertions? Eur J Appl Physiol 87:127-133, 2002.

61. Morris JM, Lucas DB, Bresler B: Role of the trunk in stability of the spine. J Bone Joint Surg Am 43:327-351, 1961.

62. McGill SM, Norman RW: Reassessment of the role of intra-abdominal pressure in spinal compression. Ergonomics 30:1565-1588, 1987.

63. Ivancic PC, Cholewicki J, Radebold A: Effects of the abdominal belt on muscle-generated spinal stability and L4/L5 joint compression force. Ergonomics 45:501-513, 2002.

64. Arjmand N, Shirazi-Adl A: Role of intra-abdominal pressure in the unloading and stabilization of the human spine during static lifting tasks. Eur Spine J 15:1265-1275, 2006.

65. Cholewicki J, Juluru K, McGill SM: Intra-abdominal pressure mechanism for stabilizing the lumbar spine. J Biomech 32:13-17, 1999.

66. Hodges PW, Eriksson AE, Shirley D, et al: Intra-abdominal pressure increases stiffness of the lumbar spine. J Biomech 38:1873-1880, 2005.

67. Cresswell AG, Thorstensson A: The role of the abdominal musculature in the elevation of the intra-abdominal pressure during specified tasks. Ergonomics 32:1237-1246, 1989.

68. Brown SHM, McGill SM: How the inherent stiffness of the in-vivo human trunk varies with changing magnitudes of muscular activation. Clin Biomech 23:15-22, 2008.

69. Brown SHM, McGill SM: The intrinsic stiffness of the in vivo lumbar spine in response to quick releases: Implications for reflexive requirements. J Electromyogr Kinesiol 19:727-736, 2009.

70. Campbell EJM, Green JH: The variations in intra-abdominal pressure and the activity of the abdominal muscles during breathing: A study in man. J Physiol 122:282-290, 1953.

71. Gandevia SC, McKenzie DK, Plassman BL: Activation of human respiratory muscles during different voluntary manoeuvres. J Physiol 428:387-403, 1990.

72. Wang S, McGill SM: Links between the mechanics of ventilation and spine stability. J Appl Biomech 24:166-174, 2008.

73. Wang S: The links between ventilation mechanics, spine mechanics and stability. Masters Thesis; Waterloo, ON, University of Waterloo, 2004.

74. Cholewicki J, Silfies SP, Shah RA, et al: Delayed trunk muscle reflex responses increase the risk of low back injuries. Spine 30:2614-2620, 2005.

75. Hodges PW, Richardson CA: Inefficient muscular stabilization of the lumbar spine associated with low back pain: A motor control evaluation of transversus abdominis. Spine 21:2640-2650, 1996.

76. Ferreira PH, Ferreira ML, Hodges PW: Changes in recruitment of the abdominal muscles in people with low back pain: Ultrasound measurement of muscle activity. Spine 29:2560-2566, 2004.

77. Silfies SP, Squillante D, Maurer P, et al: Trunk muscle recruitment patterns in specific chronic low back pain populations. Clin Biomech 20:465-473, 2005.

78. O'Sullivan PB, Phyty GD, Twomey LT, et al: Evaluation of specific stabilizing exercise in the treatment of chronic low back pain with radiologic diagnosis of spondylolysis or spondylolisthesis. Spine 15:2959-2967, 1997.

79. Hicks GE, Fritz JM, Delitto A, et al: Preliminary development of a clinical prediction rule for determining which patients with low back pain will respond to a stabilization exercise program. Arch Phys Med Rehabil 86:1753-1762, 2005.

80. Hodges PW, Richardson CA: Delayed postural contraction of transversus abdominis in low back pain associated with movement of the lower limb. J Spinal Disord 11:46-56, 1998.

81. Mannion AF, Pulkovski N, Schenk P, et al: A new method for the noninvasive determination of abdominal muscle feedforward activity based on tissue velocity information from tissue Doppler imaging. J Appl Physiol 104:1192-1201, 2008.

82. Cresswell AG: Responses of intra-abdominal pressure and abdominal muscle activity during trunk loading in man. Eur J Appl Physiol 66:315-320, 1993.

83. Vera-Garcia FJ, Elvira JL, Brown SH, et al: Effects of abdominal stabilization maneuvers on the control of spine motion and stability against sudden trunk perturbations. J Electromyogr Kinesiol 17:556-567, 2007.

84. Grenier SG, McGill SM: Quantification of lumbar stability by using 2 different abdominal activation strategies. Arch Phys Med Rehabil 88:54-62, 2007.

85. Hodges P: Transversus abdominis: A different view of the elephant. Br J Sports Med 42:941-944, 2008.

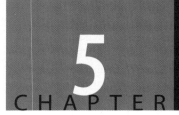

5
CHAPTER

Lumbar Musculature: Anatomy and Function

Tom G. Mayer, MD
Eric A. K. Mayer, MD
Dale Reese BSc, CPed

Muscles are the dynamic stabilizers of the spine, with functions similar to those performed in other parts of the musculoskeletal system. In their ability to control movement and provide stability, muscles must be seen not as isolated structures, but as part of a system including ligaments, joints and their capsules, and an intricate neurologic feedback mechanism to coordinate system efficiency. Much understanding about the importance of this entire system, and specifically of the muscular component, comes from the extremities, where the structures are accessible, easily visualized, and accompanied by a contralateral side for comparison. Spinal musculature is considerably more complex, but new technology involving quantitative assessment, electromyography (EMG), and mathematical modeling has incrementally increased the level of knowledge about the spinal musculoligamentous system.

Physiology

Muscle, the dynamic control mechanism of the skeletal system, consists of long, overlapping cells specifically adapted for shortening. Voluntary muscle, or skeletal muscle, is the most voluminous muscle type in humans. Muscles controlling spinal movement are the largest aggregation of skeletal muscles in the body. The axial muscle fibers may be only a few millimeters in diameter but can extend 5 cm or more in length. Many fibers are bound together by perimysium collagen to form organized fascicles, which are bundled together to form what is known as muscle. The contractile elements of muscles are called *myofibrils* and are so numerous that the cell nuclei and organelles are relegated to the periphery. Surrounding the myofibrils, nuclei, and organelles is a fluid called *sarcoplasm* that has a fluctuating electrolyte concentration controlled by an external, semipermeable lipid bilayer known as the *sarcolemma*.

The myofibrils attach to the sarcolemma at two ends, which connects one cell to its neighbor in the fiber structure. The myofibrils are highly organized, aligning longitudinally within the sarcolemma, which itself is indented by a motor axon at its myoneural junction. By convention, the smallest contractile subunit within the myofibrils is called the *sarcomere*. The sarcomere is composed of smaller subunits called *myofilaments*. The myofilaments are organized longitudinally with alternating light and dark striations (hence skeletal muscles are known as "striated muscle") when visualized microscopically. The myofilaments within the sarcomere (smallest contractile subunit) are composed predominantly of two protein varieties: myosin and actin.[1]

Under normal circumstances, contraction of striated muscle does not occur without a neural stimulus, whereas contraction of cardiac and most smooth muscle fibers can trigger adjacent fibers to contract without neural stimulation. The cellular mechanics of contractions are relatively simple: Actin filaments (occupying the light-colored I-band at rest) slide over the myosin filaments (found in the A-band and interdigitating with I-band at rest) until, with complete contraction, they completely overlap and eliminate the light H-band under microscopic visualization. The biochemical reactions are far more complex (Fig. 5–1). Contraction is initiated by release of acetylcholine at the myoneural junction, depolarizing the sarcolemma by changing its permeability to sodium and potassium ions. This sarcolemma stimulates release of calcium ions, sequestered in the sarcoplasmic reticulum, that bind to the troponin complex (C, T, and I). Calcium ions binding troponin induce a conformational change, which uncovers the binding portion of the actin filament. Myosin binds and unbinds actin, in concert with adenosine phosphate molecules (adenosine triphosphate [ATP] and adenosine diphosphate [ADP]), to induce the "racheting" of the myosin along the length of the actin filament.

Acetylcholine is rapidly hydrolyzed by acetylcholine esterase and calcium is rapidly resequestered so that each nerve firing in skeletal muscle is a discrete, "pulsed" event, rather than a sustained spasm. In large spine muscles, an alpha motor neuron in the spinal cord innervates and simultaneously controls a few hundred to a few thousand muscle fibers. Discrete, independent fiber control of only a few motor units by multiple motor neurons permits a gradation of contraction that enables conscious choice to employ refined control or rapid, maximal contraction depending on the situational necessity. The strength of a single contraction or "twitch" depends on the number of fibers that contract. The ability to sustain the contraction (endurance) depends on the ability to recruit more muscle fibers with increasingly repeated firing frequency so that *just* enough fibers are recruited to do the minimum necessary to complete a task (muscle efficiency). Other factors, such as muscle fiber type, independently affect endurance (ability to sustain a contraction), but recruitment can be altered by training and motivational factors.

The contraction that follows nerve firing is powered by conversion of ATP to ADP, which is recycled to produce ATP again by the hydrolysis of glucose into water and carbon dioxide or by the citric acid cycle (Krebs cycle), which uses fatty acids as efficiently as glucose. The Krebs cycle requires oxygen. When adequate oxygen cannot be supplied (e.g., vigorous exercise exceeding an oxygen replacement threshold), glucose is converted to lactic acid, producing less energy per unit substrate while an "oxygen debt" ensues in "anaerobic metabolism."

A growing body of research shows that lactate is not a "dead-end metabolite," and it is not the "mediator" of fatigue and inefficiency as widely published in the 1960s through the 1980s.[2] On the contrary, current research implicates the hydrogen ion excess as the primary agent of diminished contractile power. The lactate ion may serve multiple roles in maintaining constant energy; recruiting new energy sources (gluconeogenesis); recruiting new vascularity (angiogenesis); and promoting a local cascade of healing, plasticity, and hyperplasia.[2-4] A growing body of research based on the experimental work of Brooks,[4] termed *lactate shuttle theory*, suggests that higher concentrations of lactic acid produced in the skeletal muscles stressed by exercise have significant increased benefit in remote tissue such as brain, liver, heart, peripheral nerves, and peripheral vasculature over baseline metabolism.[2]

The ATPase work of Engel[5] in 1962 established a body of research showing the presence of distinctly different motor units within skeletal muscle. There are many myotype classification schemes based on histology, morphology, or function. In brief, the interaction between the type of myosin heavy chain (ATP binding site) and actin within individual sarcomeres is probably the greatest contributor to functional differences within myofibrils. The functional difference is related to the rate that the myosin heavy chains can repetitively bind ATP and release ADP under conditions of physiologic stress.[6]

Roughly divided, sarcomeres fall into one of three broad functional categories. Type I fibers have a slower "twitch" response with good fatigue resistance and lower tension development.[7] Structurally, these groups of sarcomeres (known collectively as *fibers*) have rich capillary beds and high concentrations of mitochondrial enzymes with relatively low concentrations of glycogen and myosin ATPase. They seem ideally suited for aerobic activity with good fatigue resistance. These type I muscles predominate in areas that require aerobic or endurance demands. Type II muscle displays a fast twitch with good strength but relatively poor endurance compared with type I muscle fibers. Type II fibers can be subdivided further into type IIA, which still show a fast twitch response but a fatigue threshold between type I and type IIB, and type IIB, which show the fastest contractions, the highest tension

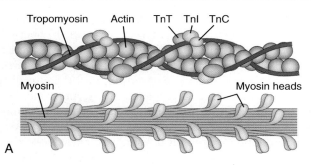

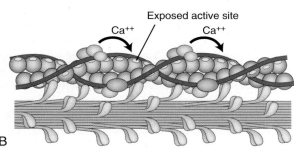

FIGURE 5–1 Regulatory function of troponin and tropomyosin. Troponin is a small globular protein with three subunits (TnT, TnI, TnC). **A,** Resting condition: Tropomyosin under resting condition blocks the active site of actin, preventing actin and myosin from binding. **B,** Contraction: When troponin binds with Ca^{2+}, it undergoes a conformational change and pulls tropomyosin from the blocking position on the actin filament, allowing myosin heads to form cross-bridges with actin. (From Plowman SA, Smith DL: Exercise Physiology for Health, Fitness, and Performance. Boston, MA, Allyn & Bacon, 1997, p 433. Copyright 1997 by Allyn & Bacon.)

development, and the most rapid onset of fatigue.[7,8] Although other fiber subtypes continue to be identified, type I, type IIA, and type IIB show the major functional categories of voluntary skeletal muscles.[7] Whether individual fibers have biochemical characteristics for high-intensity, short-duration contractile bursts or more sustained activity, each muscle is a heterogeneous, woven tapestry of *all* of the above-mentioned fiber subtypes. Any relative predominance of one particular fiber type is based on genetics, anatomic location of the muscle, demand on the muscle, age of the individual, nutrition, and multiple other external factors.[9]

Although the contribution to parental lineage to phenotypic expression may remain paramount in predicting functional potential, the actual fiber composition of muscle groups has great capacity for plasticity in response to environmental stress. Multiple studies show fiber conversion within major groups from type IIB to type IIA to be common.[10] Other conversions, such as type I to either type IIA or type IIB, are less common and seen most often with denervation, immobilization, and profound deconditioning.[8] There is emerging evidence of conversion of type II to type I in the electrical stimulation literature, but data remain sparse and confounded by the fact that type II muscle tends to atrophy with age. The relative absence of type II muscle may confound data trying to analyze conversion.[11]

A human infant is normally born with a full complement of muscle fibers that may continue to differentiate in childhood. Muscle fiber genesis seems to be biphasic. Myoblasts fuse to form fibrils at 8 to 10 weeks of gestation—primarily resulting in the formation of type I (slow-twitch) fibers. The second wave of fiber formation occurs at 15 to 18 weeks of gestation creating fast-twitch, type II fibers, which differentiate and change with early postpartum use.[7] The growth and change in muscle size after adolescence seems to be due to increase in size of the fibers rather than increase in numbers (although controversial studies still contend that extreme muscle exertion may result in some new fiber development) that accompanies increased neuronal innervation and finer control of contractile force.

Although animal data suggest that hyperplasia and genesis of new muscle fibers may be possible with training and endogenous, hormonal feedback, these data have not been replicated in humans. Instead, increasing strength of contraction with training seems to be related not only to muscular factors, such as muscle size, fiber type, and fiber number, but also (and perhaps to a greater extent) to neural factors.[12] The specific neural characteristics that change with training include frequency, extent, order, and synchrony of motor unit firing, with feedback to the spinal pyramidal tracts to control system efficiency—maximal force at minimal energy expenditure. Training, age, and certain anabolic hormones (either endogenous or exogenous) seem to exert the greatest effect on muscle plasticity—the characteristic rapid increase in strength and muscle diameter under the hormonal influence of puberty is a specific example.

Muscle hypertrophy seems to occur through two processes that may proceed simultaneously: myofibrillar hypertrophy and splitting. The degree and sequence to maximize muscle size and function remain under study, but it seems clear that isometric contraction (in which the contracting muscle is not permitted to shorten) is far more effective in increasing muscle bulk than concentric (isotonic or isokinetic) contractions. Nevertheless, this increased bulk may come at a price of increased injury risk and lower dynamic function with very poor correlation to strength gains (isotonic and isokinetic training correlate better than isometric with dynamic strength). By contrast, various pathologic factors, such as denervation, starvation, and immobilization and disuse, produce muscle atrophy. Multiple factors, including a functional nerve supply, good nutrition, hormonal input, and periodic muscle activity, are necessary to maintain, or increase, muscle function and fibrillar "bulk."

Anatomy

The spine consists of a series of bilaterally symmetrical joints phylogenetically adapted for protection of the neural communications network linking brain to periphery.[13] The critical role of the spine musculature in dynamically protecting and vitalizing these articulations with their passive ligamentous supports and accompanying neural transmission lines is infrequently acknowledged in biomechanical modeling. For this reason, a perspective based in evolutionary theory aids in understanding the complexity of lumbar spine musculature.[14] From an evolutionary standpoint, it seems that all land-dwelling vertebrates (including mammals) evolved from ocean-dwelling cousins; in the ocean, gravitational force acted differently when contributing to function and form. Large paravertebral spine muscles likely developed to provide lateral (coronal plane) flexion-extension to propel bodies through water, as shown by the lateral tail motion of the fish. This form of locomotion was initially preserved in amphibians and land reptiles (even after the development of extremities), as seen in the *Crocodylia* species including the modern alligator and crocodile. Reptiles with legs (currently living) all propel themselves through lateral spinal motion in which propulsion is achieved by contracting spine muscles to create alternating coronal convexities on one side of the spine that allow the ipsilateral foreleg to move forward while the contralateral hindfoot (on the concave side) is brought closer to the contralateral foreleg in preparation for the next reciprocal lateral movement that repeats the motion-event.

Mammalian adaptations resulted in a 90-degree evolutionary shift to the sagittal spinal motion characteristic of all four-legged mammals (the platypus and echidna being partial exceptions), which presumably provides an advantage during land locomotion, allowing for explosive growth of the class Mammalia. Land mammals that subsequently retreated to the sea (e.g., whales, porpoises, seals) maintain the sagittal orientation of spinal locomotion resulting in the 90-degree rotation of the tail fluke (when compared with fish), even after adaptive pressure resulted in other changes to their extremities. The later adaptation of humans to full bipedal stance and locomotion presumably necessitated a lordotic lumbar spine, kyphotic thoracic spine, and lordotic cervical spine for balance and ambulation (Fig. 5–2).

It is further theorized that the lordotic curve converts lateral bending to produce torsion at the hips, adding propulsion efficiency to the balanced human gait that would be impossible without lumbar lordosis. Ambulation without lumbar lordosis leads to the shuffling strides of the upright apes, whose gait is clearly dissimilar to that of humans. Laboratory modeling strongly suggests that cocontraction of spinal and abdominal muscles is the primary generator of the curvilinear structure of the spine that sustains logarithmically more force than "straight" models of spine motion (>1200 N vs. 100 N). The theory holds that instantaneous, axial-rotational forces between segments in "straight-spine" models lead to rapid failure when the spine is progressively loaded.[15]

This model focuses on the dynamic contribution of spine muscles to create a compressive-stabilizing force through bony and ligamentous structures that withstands physiologic forces modeled in sagittal motion. Similar to taut "guy wires" or tensioned cables adding structural stability to allow gauzy tent material to withstand 90 mph winds, muscle tension is hypothesized by the "follower-load" theory to provide a stabilizing force (in at least one plane of motion—sagittal) that directs the force vector to pure compression of the motion segment, minimizing shear (shear force being implicated in degenerative cascade).[16]

Another unique human evolutionary adaptation for manipulation of objects near the ground from a bipedal stance involves the ability to bend efficiently from the waist

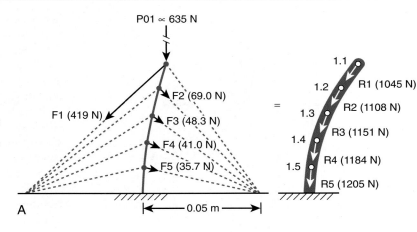

FIGURE 5–2 A, Muscle activation pattern needed to maintain lumbar spine model under compressive follower loads. The resultant force acting on the spine approximates the tangents to the deformed shape of the spine. **B,** Response of spine model to a compressive vertical load applied at L1 and to compressive follower load. Lumbar spine model could support substantially larger compressive loads when load path approximated the tangent to curve of lumbar spine. (Borrowed with permission from Patwardhan AG, Meade KP, Lee B: A frontal plane model of the lumbar spine subjected to a follower load: implications for the role of muscles. J Biomech Eng 123:212-217, 2001.)

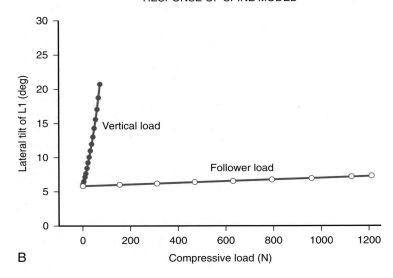

in combination with squatting and hunkering. A stable "biomechanical chain," transferring force efficiently from hands through arms, shoulder girdle, spine, pelvis, legs, and feet to make ground contact, is necessary (Fig. 5–3). In this functional concept, the muscle acts as a dynamic stabilizer of the biomechanical chain in several ways. During flexion-extension of the lumbar spine, the co-tensioning abdominal muscles at a distance (force plus lever arm) allows maintenance of a "balance point" at each individual motion segment. Next, coupled anterior and posterior forces have a net compressive (downward) force, which balances motion at the instantaneous axis of rotation for each motion segment—maintaining compression at the disc and minimizing angular change. The net muscle tension force downward serves to offset any other forces, maintaining the force vector perpendicular to the disc's plane similar to the tent "guy-wires" explained previously.[16,17] Muscles supply dynamic and static downward force to create a form that allows maximal load bearing (for bipedal carrying and lifting) capacity, while maintaining function that allows maximal efficiency of muscle energy output—maintaining a plumb line (not working against gravity to maintain posture), sharing tension bands to distribute loads, coupling forces

when motion is required, and distributing load/work among the other osteoligamentous static structures.

As stated previously, controlling forward flexion with muscles alone is inefficient, and the space required for the abdominal and thoracic contents imposes size constraints on spine muscles. The evolutionary solution is twofold: (1) strong, elastic posterior spinal ligaments (midline ligaments, joint capsules, and lumbodorsal fascia) that (a) produce passive constraint, particularly to lumbar spine flexion, and (b) allow static "hanging on the ligaments" subject only to slow, plastic "creep" but without muscular effort; (2) a manipulation of the lever arm advantage from quadrupeds through use of posterior pelvic muscles as "motors" and "stabilizers" of lumbar extension and abduction motion. This combination of a posterior ligamentous complex and powerful muscles of the buttocks and posterior thighs (along with the psoas muscle controlling degree of lordosis) permits the spine to function in a way not generally recognized: as a crane, whose boom is the ligament-stabilized flexed spine, whose fulcrum is the hips, and whose engine is the pelvic extensor musculature.

These observations lead to multiple functional inferences, one of which is the tendency of the spine to "hang on its

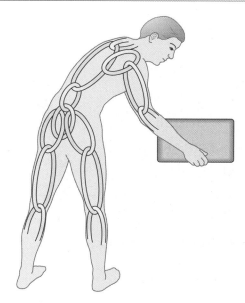

FIGURE 5–3 Biomechanical chain for permitting manual handling of objects while maintaining balance over bipedal base, transmitting forces through four functional units: (1) upper extremities, (2) shoulder girdle and thoracic spine, (3) lumbar spine and pelvic unit, and (4) lower extremities. (From Mayer TG, Gatchel RJ: Functional Restoration for Spinal Disorders: The Sports Medicine Approach. Philadelphia, Lea & Febiger, 1988.)

ligaments" in an efficient, muscle-sparing manner frequently observed in "stooped laborers." Efficiency of motion is documented by the way most normal subjects make the universal unconscious choice of allowing spine flexion to precede hip flexion when bending forward at the waist, eventually resulting in an EMG "silent period" when the spine is fully flexed and stabilized by posterior ligaments.[14,18,19]

It is beyond the scope of this chapter to discuss these concepts in greater depth; however, one quickly develops an appreciation of the spinal musculature as an efficiently evolved functional unit, improved on from earlier iterations, that encompasses paravertebral, abdominal, buttock, pelvic floor, and hamstring muscles to exert specific force vectors that combine with gravity and the constraint of the passive structures to allow bipedal stance, locomotion, and balance. This spine and pelvis functional module links the carrying and manipulation capacity of the cervicothoracic, shoulder girdle, and upper extremity functional modules with the propulsion capability of the lower extremity functional module. This relationship provides a complete biomechanical chain that allows manual handling tasks by the upper extremities to be performed while maintaining stable foot-to-ground contact for maximal evolutionary advantage in virtually any environmental context.

The small interconnecting vertebrae motion segments with the multiplanar motions of the three-joint complex produce difficulties when assigning specific uniaxial functions to individual groups of muscles. The erector spinae group of muscles are generally thought of as extensors of the spine. Functioning unilaterally, they may also be powerful abductors or lateral stabilizers (assisting with locomotion) and have been shown to function to some extent in spine derotation.[18] Similarly,

lateral abdominal musculature (internal and external oblique and transversus abdominis) may act as spine flexors and extensors (working through the lumbosacral fascia).[14] The "girdling" abdominal muscles are also powerful spine rotators and assist in abduction and lateral stabilization.[20] As noted previously in this chapter, the force-coupling of spinal, pelvic, and abdominal muscles acting in concert increases compressive load through the disc and vertebral bodies to minimize shear force and imbalance axially across the three-joint complex.

In describing the gross anatomy of the spinal muscular functional unit, the extreme importance of the posterior stabilizing structures cannot be overemphasized in spinal functional integrity. The intrinsic lumbar musculature is only a part of the functional unit. The lumbodorsal fascia, interspinous ligaments, and facet joint capsules are crucial structures providing constraint and fulcrum points.[21] There is growing appreciation among some surgeons to maintain the integrity of these collagenous and elastic structures, which may decrease adjacent segment shear, dysfunction, or instability.

Mammals as a class share many characteristics, including those of the spine musculature, that may account for the evolutionary success of the class. The most superficial layers of spine musculature, extensions of the functional unit of the shoulder girdle, include muscles such as the serratus posterior and latissimus dorsi. In contrast to other spinal musculature, the modified proximal function of these muscles is matched by innervation from the proximal spinal cord. The true lumbar spinal muscles, by contrast, have segmental innervations that arise from the posterior rami of the contiguous spinal nerves (the same nerves that perceive proprioceptive input from facet capsules, posterior ligaments, and peripheral anulus). Although true spinal muscles function together, their most characteristic differentiating factor is span length. The deepest muscles, such as the interspinalis, span only a single segment. The most superficial muscles may traverse a large portion of the entire spinal column. Controlled, coordinated action of individual vertebrae is a critical part of spine function, whereas loss of appropriate musculoligamentous control may contribute to various pathologic syndromes, such as segmental instability, segmental rigidity, facet syndromes, and perhaps even discogenic pain.[22]

Musculature of the Lumbar Spinal Functional Unit

Intrinsic Muscles

Erector Spinae

The erector spinae is a large and superficial muscle that lies just deep to the lumbodorsal fascia and arises from an aponeurosis on the sacrum, iliac crest, and thoracolumbar spinous processes.[13] The muscle mass is poorly differentiated, but divides into three sections in the upper lumbar area: (1) The iliocostalis is most lateral and inserts into the angles of the rib; (2) the longissimus, the intermediate column, inserts into the tips of the spinous processes of thoracic and cervical vertebrae;

FIGURE 5–4 Cross section of body musculature and fascia through L3 showing intrinsic spinal musculature. Abdominal muscles also function in containing viscera and respiration. (From Finneson B: Low Back Pain, 2nd ed. Philadelphia, JB Lippincott, 1977.)

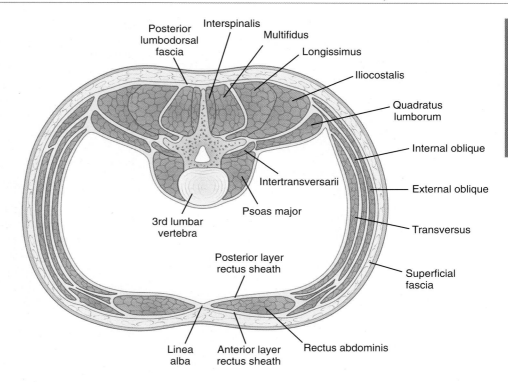

(3) the spinalis is most medial and inserts into spinous processes of the cervical and thoracic vertebrae (Fig. 5–4). The innervation of all the lumbar paraspinal muscles is from the dorsal rami of the nerve root as it exits at the most approximate level and overlaps proximally and distally along the muscle length.

The importance of the lumbar musculature is inferred by the intricate redundancy of the paraspinal innervation. Each area of these long muscles has overlapping innervation that may include up to two segments craniad and two segments caudal of coinnervation. This redundancy allows maintenance of function even if a particular level is affected by injury to its respective neural structure.

Multifidi

Multifidi are a series of small muscles, best developed in the lumbar spine, that originate on the mammillary processes of the superior facets and run upward and medially for two to four segments, inserting on the spinous processes (Fig. 5–5). This orientation produces greater capacity for rotation and abduction, in addition to extension. They also share a multilevel innervation (similar to the erector spinae bundle or group) where function is maintained even with injury to the proximate dorsal rami.

Quadratus Lumborum

The quadratus lumborum is the most lateral of the lumbar muscles (see Fig. 5–4); it originates on the iliac crest and iliolumbar ligament and runs obliquely to insert into the lowest rib and transverse processes of the upper four lumbar

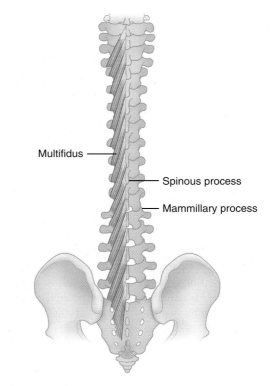

FIGURE 5–5 Multifidi consist of numerous small muscle slips that arise from small bony prominences on the articular facet. (From Finneson B: Low Back Pain, 2nd ed. Philadelphia, JB Lippincott, 1977.)

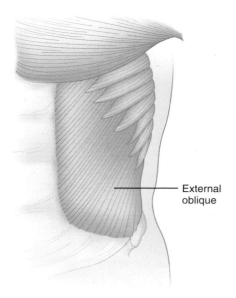

External oblique

FIGURE 5–6 External oblique muscle. (From Finneson B: Low Back Pain, 2nd ed. Philadelphia, JB Lippincott, 1977.)

vertebrae. Its orientation provides strong abduction motor and stabilizer properties. The innervation is from the ventral rami of T12-L1-L2-L3 roots.

Deep Muscles

The interspinalis muscles are pairs of deep muscles spanning one segment on either side of the strong and elastic interspinous ligaments. In the lumbar spine, the intertransversarii consist of a pair of muscles on each side, spanning the transverse processes of adjacent vertebrae. Each side has dorsal and ventral slips.

Psoas and Iliacus Muscles

The psoas major, although usually thought of primarily as a hip flexor, has a direct effect on the vertebral column because it originates bilaterally from the vertebral bodies and posterior aspects of the transverse processes, providing the only intrinsic spinal muscle acting anterior to the sagittal axis. Yet, paradoxically, the psoas is usually an intersegmental extensor in the mid-lumbar spine, even as it flexes at the lumbosacral junction in the process of increasing the lumbar lordosis. It is an important spine stabilizer in sitting and standing.[23] Acting asymmetrically, the psoas may produce abduction or abduction-resistance to maintain coronal balance. Pathophysiologically, low back or pelvic pain may result from contracture or spasm of the iliopsoas producing combined hip and lumbosacral junction flexion. As in other situations, appropriately targeted stretches, followed by strengthening, may produce dramatic improvement.

The psoas major and iliacus muscles are innervated by the femoral nerve and lie in close proximity to the lumbosacral plexus. The primary innervation of this group is from the L2

and L3 root segments with minor contribution of L4 in some individuals. Proximal weakness and pain is occasionally a consequence of surgical approaches with susceptibility to denervation or devascularization injury from aggressive retraction. Care should be taken by surgeons because injury to this muscle can be a harbinger of occult lumbosacral plexus injury. The iliopsoas complex as the floor of Scarpa fascia serves as an important surgical landmark.

Extrinsic Muscles

Abdominal Musculature

There are four important abdominal girdling muscles in spine function.[24] The rectus abdominis is primarily a flexor, spanning the anterior abdomen from its origin on the pubic crest to its insertion on the anterior rib cage between the fifth and seventh ribs. The obliquely oriented abdominal muscles are, from superficial to deep, the external oblique, internal oblique, and transversalis abdominis. They all may act to produce rotation or abduction and assist flexion and extension under different circumstances.[14]

The fibers of the external oblique run in an anteroinferior direction from attachments on the lower eight ribs to insert along the anterior rectus sheath and anterior wall of the iliac crest (Fig. 5–6). The external oblique fibers are almost perpendicular in direction to those of the internal oblique fibers. This muscle courses transversely only in its lowermost portion, with most of the muscle running anteriorly and proximally from its origins on the lumbodorsal fascia and anterior two thirds of the iliac crest. It inserts on the lower three ribs and rectus sheath anteriorly. The transversalis abdominis, the deepest muscle of the group, runs transversely like a horizontal girdle from the lumbodorsal fascia, anterior iliac crest, and inner surface of the lower six ribs. The main mass of the muscle inserts into the linea alba in the midline. In the act of flexion, it is probable that the abdominal muscles act not only to create a ventral moment, but also to stabilize the spine posteriorly through their action on the lumbodorsal fascia. The innervation of the abdominal muscles is shared via intercostal nerves from root levels T7-T12. The thoracic nature of the innervation means that these muscles are spared from radicular-type injuries.

Gluteal Muscles

The large muscles of the buttocks, chiefly the gluteus maximus, gluteus medius, and gluteus minimus, act variously as hip extensors and abductors. As such, they act as motors to the spinal "crane" in forward bending and twisting movements. They also provide the "spinal engine" for locomotion (Fig. 5–7).[13,14] The gluteus maximus receives innervation via the inferior gluteal nerve and is primarily an S1 muscle, although it receives contributions from L5 and S2 root levels. The superior gluteal nerve innervates the gluteus medius primarily with L5 contribution. Although it receives contributions from L4 and S1 root segments, it is often an important "internal verifier" of a true L5 radiculopathy when combined with clinical or electrodiagnostic abnormalities in distal L5 muscles.

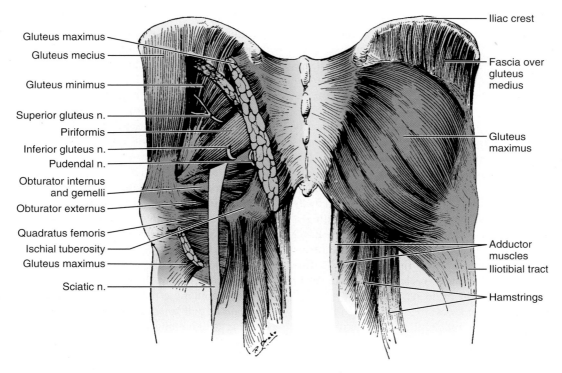

FIGURE 5–7 Musculature of buttocks and proximal thigh. (From Hollinshead WH: Anatomy for Surgeons, 3rd ed. Hagerstown, MD, Harper & Row, 1982.)

Posterior Thigh Musculature

Muscles attached to the ischial tuberosity, such as the hamstrings, are also strong pelvic extensors acting around the hip fulcrum. They provide powerful assistance to the buttocks musculature in raising or resisting lowering of the pelvis. Additionally, the hamstrings provide efficient passive restraint on pelvic flexion when the knees are locked in extension. The hamstrings are the inferior restraint providing the most efficient forward flexion by controlled forward rotation of the pelvis around the hips. These muscles, which include the two heads (long and short) of the biceps femoris and semimembranosus and semitendinosus, are innervated by the tibial portion of the sciatic nerve (except the short head of the biceps from the peroneal division of the sciatic nerve) and confirm lower root dysfunction (L5, S1, and S2).

Rectus Femoris

The rectus femoris serves a similar but weaker role than the iliopsoas complex in transmitting force from the spine to hip and pelvis motion segments. The rectus femoris crosses the hip and knee joint and has a primary role in creating a more efficient and synchronized gait. Intrinsic spinal muscle limit the sagittal motion transmitting forces to the lower limbs. Coordination of these muscle groups is fundamental to the spine and pelvis functional unit to supporting bipedal function and efficiency. Patients with cerebral palsy are exemplars of the importance of spine and pelvis coordination insofar as hip flexor spasticity and contracture create a kyphotic imbalance that prevents or extinguishes gait. The rectus femoris is innervated by the femoral nerve and L2 and L3 root segments with minor L4 contribution.

Electrophysiology

A great deal of energy has been devoted clinically to the use of the EMG signal for detecting radiculopathy in the lower extremity musculature associated with lumbar disc derangements. EMG needle electrodes have been used in the extremities to detect characteristic denervation, reinnervation, and muscle changes to muscle fibers within a discrete motor unit that is seen with nerve injury or muscle injury. These tests are often accompanied by nerve conduction velocity studies to assess peripheral nerve function, serving as a check to rule out other pathologic conditions, such as peripheral nerve disease, motor neuron disease, or myopathies that may mimic intracanal spinal lesions.

EMG employed to analyze normal function, as opposed to pathologic conditions, of the spine musculature is less well understood. There has not been a concerted research effort to document the natural history of adaptive electrodiagnostic findings as patients evolve from symptomatic to asymptomatic. This section discusses the clinical utility and limitations of electrodiagnostics further. In assessing low back pain without corresponding neurologic sequelae in the extremities, EMG and nerve conduction velocity remain investigational. Biomechanical studies have often relied on use of the raw, integrated EMG or root mean square EMG signals to estimate muscle loads in studies involving lifting performance in normal subjects. Trunk stabilization and initiation of motion are two particular patterns of EMG activity that have been identified in trunk movements.[25-27] Different movements recruit muscles in varying patterns of activity. Intrinsic spine musculature supplies a net sum of movement using various lever arms to initiate and arrest motion by combining concentric and eccentric contraction in either movement or maintenance of posture.

Longissimus and other paravertebral muscles are frequently silent in the "flexion-relaxation" position, in which the maximally flexed spine is "hanging on its posterior ligaments." It is also relatively quiet in gentle extension of the spine, but with full extension, lateral bend, or torsion, the role of the intrinsic musculature is as a "balancer" of spinal motion—shown by its prominent activity.[26] Subsequently, it was found that loading of the flexed spine in the posture normally producing EMG silence leads to an increase in myoelectric activity in the intrinsic spine musculature proportional to the load applied. This proportion of increased EMG and muscle activity is similar to the changes seen in loading the spine in the upright position.[28] Presumably, these increasing loads stress and stretch the posterior ligamentous structures sufficiently to require compensatory muscle firing. The multifidus and rotatores muscles have similar activity in sagittal plane movements. They are active in rotation to the contralateral side, however, in conjunction with bilateral abdominal muscular contraction.[20]

These muscles also achieve flexion-relaxation silence when the spine is in the ligamentous support phase. Early investigators discovered that the slouching or full flexion seated posture (often considered "bad posture") is, in reality, quite comfortable for prolonged periods and that EMG silence is generally maintained in the erector spinae.[29] Issues of posture, movement, load, and speed have usually been studied through surface EMG measurements.[30] This "silent period" is also known as the flexion-relaxation phenomenon.[31] The phenomenon represents an EMG pattern seen in most normal subjects but frequently absent in subjects with chronic low back pain. These patients show elevated muscle activity during full voluntary trunk flexion and fail to achieve flexion-relaxation.[32-36] The phenomenon is noted with needle and surface EMG measurements, which has led many researchers to use surface EMG in studying the phenomenon.[37]

More recent research suggests that the hypothesis of a dichotomous pattern (muscles either "on" or "off") is likely misleading. Physiologically, lumbar muscles show electrical activity because they are contracting, and the degree of electrical activity is roughly proportional to the rate and amplitude of muscle fiber firing. Lumbar muscle activity is almost never "completely silent" during trunk flexion maneuvers. More recent descriptions of the phenomenon suggest a significant contractile force associated with high surface EMG activity during flexion, followed by a relaxation phase associated with low surface EMG activity.[38,39]

Several researchers have also proposed quantitative formulas for defining the presence or absence of flexion-relaxation.[36,40,41] More recent work has compared inclinometric range of motion and surface EMG measures, with several interesting findings.[19] Using this quantified approach, almost all normal subjects can achieve flexion-relaxation, even if they lack completely normal spine motion. Even in patients with chronic low back pain who are symptomatic and completely disabled, approximately 30% can achieve flexion-relaxation before rehabilitation. After a functional restoration program that stressed improved lumbar mobility with pain management techniques aimed at the lumbar musculature, however, 94% of the patients completing treatment achieved flexion-relaxation. Larger studies performed subsequently show that quantified lumbar flexion-relaxation phenomenon can be an objective tool for measuring improvement in a functional restoration program, correlated to improvements in lumbar range of motion measurements.[42] Almost all the improvement in achieving flexion-relaxation is directly attributable to a component of the interdisciplinary program that involves surface EMG biofeedback involving surface EMG–assisted stretching training.[43]

Contractions of the abdominal musculature, particularly muscles attaching to the lumbosacral fascia, are also important in maintaining flexed postures and initiating extension. The lateral pull on the lumbodorsal fascia has two effects: creating a tightening of the craniocaudal dimension in the lumbar spine ("guy-wire model" discussed earlier) and "encapsulating" the intrinsic spine musculature to provide greater efficiency. In so doing, the abdominal mechanism also serves as a force-coupling mechanism: eccentrically controlling extension of the flexed spine while resisting flexion loads.[14]

Some groups have tried to correlate functional tasks and training, EMG data, and computed tomography (CT) and magnetic resonance imaging (MRI).[44] Small studies have shown correlations between postoperative strength deficits, imaging of muscle atrophy (decreased cross-sectional area or fatty infiltration), and changes in EMG characteristics.[18,45,46] CT seems to provide reliable measurements of paraspinal muscle cross-sectional area and density in normal subjects and patients with chronic low back pain.[47-49] Although some early pilot work at several institutions is intriguing, serial imaging remains cost prohibitive and is of little value for altering treatment outcomes. More recently, needle EMG sampling of the multifidus has been described in the diagnosis of lumbar spinal stenosis.

Trunk Muscle Strength

The obvious relationship between extremity joints and strength of the contiguous musculature in athletic and pathologic (traumatic, arthritic, or deconditioned) situations has stimulated many investigators to study similar relationships in the spine.[29,50] Early investigators were limited to the use of cable tensiometers and isometric and isotonic machines. Work began 30 years ago using individually modified isokinetic dynamometers in various positions.[51-53] Later technology provided computerized isokinetic devices for separately measuring isolated lumbar trunk strength in the sagittal and axial planes concentrically and eccentrically that also allowed measurements isometrically and isotonically.[20,41,54-56]

Isokinetics has been deemed a safe way to measure muscular output.[57-59] Studies have shown a diversity of normative

FIGURE 5–8 Modern-day test isokinetic equipment for back extension and flexion in semistanding position and lift analysis.

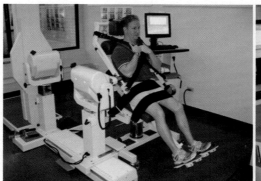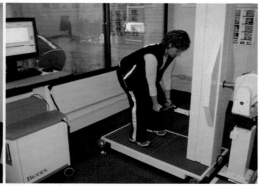

data owing to factors such as different protocols, positioning (reclined, sitting, or standing), instrument, study samples, gravity correction, and axis of rotation. The normative data are specific to instrumentation, protocol, and positioning.[60-63] The development and availability of isokinetic dynamometers or attachments specifically for back testing increased beginning around 1980. The number of manufacturers of isokinetic dynamometers available to test the back has decreased since then as a result of a combination of managed care reimbursement issues and lack of training for physical or occupational therapists likely to use such devices. At the present time, only Biodex (Shirley, NY), CSMi (formerly Cybex; Stoughton, MA), and Technogym (Gambettola, Italy) remain, limiting the development in the field of quantitative functional measurement of the spine (Fig. 5–8).

Cady and colleagues[64] showed a relationship between physical fitness and back injury rates that has been confirmed through isometric lifting testing in several industrial environments. Blay and colleagues[65] supported the use of isokinetic measurements for the assessment of trunk muscle strength in scoliotic patients. Results indicate that the reliability of trunk testing was satisfactory (Fig. 5–9). These results are in accordance with other studies of trunk testing relating to healthy subjects and patients with low back pain.[66] Although joint range of motion seems to be an independent variable in trunk

function, muscular factors such as trunk strength, endurance, and neuromuscular coordination seem to be critical factors in maintaining the integrity of the lumbar spine. Tests of isokinetic trunk strength in the sagittal plane have revealed a typical gaussian distribution of strength in the normal population. Normalizing strength by body weight narrows the width of the distribution curve. Using other normalizing factors, men seem to be 10% to 20% stronger than women and have greater ability to sustain strength at high speeds. The variety of test methods used to examine trunk muscles makes it difficult to compare results. The assessment requires an understanding of the force relationship throughout the defined range of motion (work).[67]

Another challenge is the absence of a contralateral measurement within the same person to provide a "gold standard." Comparison with a normative database stratified by age (past the 5th decade), weight, and gender has emerged as the standard for quantifying strength. Patient inhibition by pain or reduced voluntary effort is often a major factor in low torque output (Fig. 5–10), a pattern that had been identified in sports medicine testing of limbs but not as well documented in patients with chronic low back pain. Age through the 5th decade does not seem to be a critical variable.

Similar findings are noted when measuring isolated axial strength.[20,68,69] Ability to generate trunk rotational torques

FIGURE 5–9 Isokinetic torque measurement of isolated thoracolumbar motion segment during dynamic flexion-extension in a normal subject.

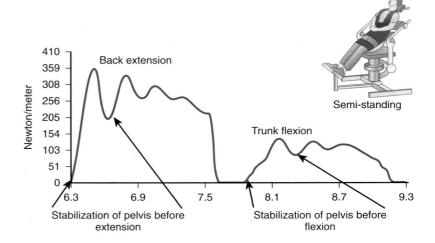

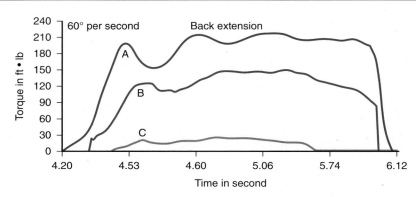

FIGURE 5–10 Torque production in dynamic thoraco-lumbar motion between 90 degrees of extension and 10 degrees of flexion in three different populations. **A,** Normal force production. Note rapid increase in torque and ability to maintain strength throughout motion. **B,** Postrehabilitation force production. Note similarity to normal force production in shape, although the amount of work (area under the curve) is less than normal. **C,** Before rehabilitation, force production exhibits a slow increase in force and inability to sustain force through the motion.

within the same individual is generally symmetrical, although there is a trend toward slightly greater strength rotating to the dominant side in men, which may be due to training in pulling activities. There seems to be a greater tolerance for applying loads at high speeds in the axial plane. This tolerance may be due to the greater fast-twitch fiber type composition of the lateral abdominal musculature, which is primarily responsible for axial plane lumbar spine movements. Rotational strength depends on the direction; for men and women the force produced from the rotated position toward the neutral position is stronger than the neutral position rotating outward.[70]

In the pathologic state, significant decrements of muscle strength are frequently noted. Patients with chronic back pain show a selective loss of extensor strength compared with flexors and an inability to maintain strength at high speeds.[59,71-74] In rotation, there is also a substantial decrement in strength, but it seems to be relatively symmetrical in the chronic state and less subject to high-speed variation.[54] Although most early work was based on peak torque measurements, advances in computerization made measurements of work performed, power consumed, and curve analysis possible, while allowing variability determination to assess "effort." Because only maximal muscular effort is truly reproducible, variability of curve shape and height becomes a potential measure of effort. In the absence of visual feedback of trunk muscle function to the clinician, these measures become exceedingly important in documenting optimal functional capacity and effort.[75,76] Some controversy exists regarding

clinical utility and discriminating power of trunk strength testing, partly because of normal human variability and partly because of unrecognized sources of error related to testing procedures.[59,73,77] The discriminating power of a test depends not only on the ability to distinguish the "normal" from the pathologic state, but also on distinguishing prerehabilitation and postrehabilitation performance. Many such longitudinal studies have been performed, including some that correlate spinal strength performance to imaging (e.g., CT and MRI) findings.[18,45,78-81]

By contrast, supernormal or athletic individuals who have been studied (Fig. 5–11), such as female gymnasts, male soccer players, male tennis players, and male wrestlers, seem to exceed mean torque-to-body weight strength ratios for the normal population by 15% to 40%.[82] In contrast to pathologic and normal populations, supernormal or athletic individuals show almost no "high-speed drop-off"—that is, decreased torque output at high speeds. They also maintain a very stable ratio of extensor to flexor strength (well-balanced, efficient use of coupled forces).

The factors that contribute to decreased strength in the pathologic state are not entirely understood. Although muscle atrophy undoubtedly occurs with prolonged disuse and deconditioning, pain may inhibit neuromuscular function through nociceptive reflex feedback mechanisms. Similarly, various psychosocially induced phenomena, such as anxiety, fear of reinjury, or depression, may unconsciously attenuate effort, producing submaximal measurements. At this time,

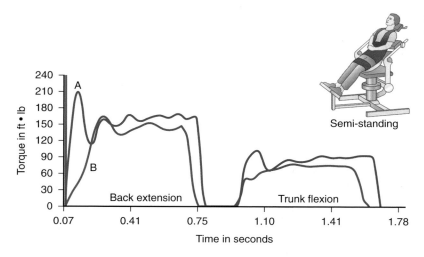

FIGURE 5–11 Normal force production at two different speeds for an athlete. **A,** 60 degrees/sec. **B,** 120 degrees/sec.

techniques for assessing subject motivation do not seem to be available, although curve variability and ratio of work to peak torque seem to be promising tools for identifying attempts to produce submaximal output consciously.[76,83]

Myofascial Pain

In recent years, there has been an increase in the diagnosis of myofascial pain syndromes. Often, there is overlap, with lumbar axial "mechanical" pain (without concurrent extremity pain) having a strong or occasionally predominant myofascial component. Frequently, patients are referred to spine specialists with simultaneous diagnoses of back pain and myofascial pain that do not correlate with radiologic or other diagnostic information. Aggressive use of invasive options often yields poor outcomes. Marginal benefit from pills often leaves the spine specialist at a loss for how to treat this poorly characterized cluster of symptoms that seem to center on primary muscle "dysfunction" generating pain with concomitant patient fear-inhibition creating disability.

A highly used but poorly understood treatment for lumbar myofascial or "back muscle pain" is "trigger point" management. Trigger points themselves are fairly well described, hyperirritable, isolated, focal areas in a "taut band" of multiple fibers of skeletal muscle that produce sustained contraction that fails to relax or release fully, which creates local and referred pain in discrete, predetermined patterns.[84] Although numerous authors have described the diagnosis and treatment of trigger points, many others have questioned the interphysician reliability of judging trigger points and the more slippery generalized diagnosis of myofascial pain.[85-88] Although by no means definitive, a growing number of physicians diagnose the widespread, painful summation of multiple areas of hyperirritability nonspecifically as myofascial pain or fibromyalgia—which is treated partially with trigger point injection and pharmacologic intervention.

Although trigger points are a *clinical* diagnosis, some academicians believe that the presence of a local twitch response (identified most reliably with EMG) is a prerequisite to treatment.[84,85] Nevertheless, many patients find relief from interventions aimed at modifying trigger points, even if present in multiple body regions. Treatments directed toward trigger points are widespread among many different physician fields and alternative medicine specialists. Although many practitioners have a favorite "needling" technique, multiple studies have found no statistical difference between "dry needling," saline injection, or medication.[89] The preeminence of needle injection as the most effective way to inactivate a trigger point has been questioned in several published articles.[90,91] Other modalities for refractory myofascial or trigger point pain include ultrasound, manipulation, massage, acupressure, acupuncture, and "spray and stretch" techniques.

Within the last decade, use of botulinum toxin (Botox) has become popular, first to inactivate refractory trigger points and then more generally for use in muscle spasticity associated with back pain. Botulinum toxin, one of the most potent biologic poisons known, is created by a gram-positive, rod-shaped

bacillus, *Clostridium botulinum,* first identified in the 1820s. The toxin is a heat-labile, zinc-dependent, metalloprotease polypeptide composed of a heavy chain and a light chain about 150 kDa in size (too large to cross the blood-brain barrier) that denatures at 80° C.[92-94] There are currently eight classified toxin types: A, B, C1, C2, D, E, F, and G. The presynaptic, cholinergic neuromuscular junctions are the target of botulinum toxin. The toxin inhibits the release of acetylcholine, which results in blockage of muscle activation and paralysis.[95,96] The toxin targets zinc-dependent endoproteases of the SNARE complex—SNAP-25, synaptobrevin II, and syntaxin I—each involved in the packaging and release of acetylcholine at the postsynaptic nerve terminal.[97] Each toxin type (A to G) acts slightly differently on the three SNARE proteins, leading to speculation, without clinical evidence, that different toxins may have different clinical uses and safety profiles.

A Medline search reveals 230 publications in the last 10 years that describe direct or indirect reduction of pain as one of the sequelae of Botox/Myobloc use. Despite the sheer number of publications, most of these are pilot or open-label studies and fail to show convincingly a discrete mechanism of action for additional analgesia beyond that of muscle fiber paralysis. At the time of this writing, two types of toxins, A and B, enjoy widespread, off-label use. Their safety profiles seem to be equal. Both inactivate neuromuscular junctions at roughly equal concentrations, "weakening" the muscle, for 70 to 120 days, with a mean peak occurring around 90 days. Over time, the body builds an immunologic response to the toxin, which may eventually render some individuals nonresponders after multiple exposures. This tolerance seems to have a heterogeneous distribution with no clear prognostic data as to who will fail to respond over time. Some reported side effects include respiratory distress, dysphagia, dysphonia, autonomic instability, and temporary impotence. The temporary nature of the muscular dysfunction and the emerging evidence of additional analgesic effects has made this medication extremely popular not only for muscular back pain, but also in a wide assortment of medical fields and for cosmetic indications.

Muscle-Sparing Surgery

In the last decade, improvements in technology, visualization, technique, material innovation, and device performance have led to greater use of lumbar surgical approaches that claim to be "muscle sparing." These techniques are discussed in greater detail in the rest of the book, but it is worth examining the claims of muscle sparing. As noted earlier, the lumbar spine is a finely balanced biomechanical mechanism that relies on the integration of intervertebral height, joint mobility and proprioception, muscle balance, and osseoligamentous constraint to allow people to function without pain. Although ample redundancy is undoubtedly built into the system, it is hoped that minimizing disruption of biomechanical integrity will lead to better functional outcomes for all spine specialists.

Lumbar surgery has classically involved extensive dissection of the posterior muscle, fascia, ligamentous structures, and occasionally joints that is even more extensive when fusion (with or without instrumentation) is attempted. Additionally, unintended consequences of denervation, compression, retraction, and vascular injury have led to other biomechanical sequelae.[18,98] Decreased morbidity by sparing vulnerable structures may serve to maintain mobility and function, improving outcomes.

The posterior lateral approach first described by Cloward[99] in 1953 has been controversial.[100] The improved tubular retractor combined with fluoroscopy and improved implantable devices have allowed for a repopularization of this approach, although denervation and devascularization of the deep muscles is still a likely possibility. The more lateral approach first described in 1968 by Wiltse and colleagues[101] for fusion allows paraspinal muscles to be bluntly divided along their aponeurosis sparing the muscle, fascia, and some of the ligamentous structures. Adequate decompression of far lateral or foraminal disc herniations can be achieved, but more centrally located pathology is difficult to access from this approach. Good fusion rates are reportedly achieved with marginally increased operative time and conflicting length of stay comparisons as a tradeoff for "sparing" devascularization and denervation injury to muscle.[102] Multiple sources advocate percutaneous or open supplementary instrumentation to the contralateral side to achieve a consistently high fusion rate.

The anterior transperitoneal approach has been described since the 1930s in various iterations.[103] A spine surgeon can achieve (indirect) decompression, stabilization, fusion (at a variable rate), and now motion preservation through this approach. Often these surgeries lose the benefit of posterior muscle preservation when surgeons later elect for additional posterior stabilization. Additionally, retraction can damage abdominal and anterior lumbar musculature that play a key role in maintenance of proper spine balance. The anterior approach has been modified to go retroperitoneally with laparoscopic devices that allow perceived (unconfirmed) benefit of splitting of the abdominal musculature to allow for more rapid postoperative healing and less perturbation of the abdominal viscera but often at the cost of crossing and possibly injuring the psoas muscle, which may have a very important role in lumbar pelvic coordination of functional tasks. Keeping in mind the advantages of protecting lumbar musculature and maintaining mobility, there is hope that the functional outcomes of spine specialists will continue to improve.

Summary

The trunk is one of the most complex musculoligamentous regions in the body. Great strides have been made in the past 2 decades in analyzing the relationship between structure and function, but difficulties with model development, oversensitive diagnostics, and disagreement over discrete "pain generators" versus multifactorial system breakdown continue to make the area of spine biomechanics a hotbed of research. Since this chapter was last written, newer diagnostic and treatment capabilities have been developed, accelerating our rate of knowledge acquisition. Nevertheless, morbidity from spine-related injury continues to increase as does the cost of treatment, both of which continue to be disassociated from significantly improved functional outcomes. By inference, many of the treatment protocols used in the limbs can be applied to the low back, with the knowledge that similar to the knee, hip, and shoulder, muscle strength, balance, and integrity play the greatest role in postinterventional recovery. Potential implications of trunk muscle strength and integrity to surgery, rehabilitation, and the industrial setting must continue to be studied and analyzed aggressively to improve on today's functional outcomes.

KEY POINTS

1. Lumbar muscles are the dynamic stabilizers of the spine, with similar functions to the muscles of the periphery. The spine muscles move the functional unit around the three-joint complex, maintain upright posture that is the evolutionary advantage of *Homo sapiens,* and maintain efficient upright motion while lifting and carrying. The muscles also serve an additional role in the spine not seen in the limbs—proprioceptive and elastic restraint to protect the neural elements within the spinal canal.

2. Emerging research shows that lactate and lactic acid generated by muscle activity may have local and distant benefits to cardiac, vascular, and nerve tissue. Instead of a dead-end waste product, lactate may be the cell-to-cell mediator of the observed beneficial effects of exercise.

3. The biomechanics of the spinal musculature are poorly understood. In addition to motion, static downward force, termed *follower load* by some authors, may provide protection to the discs from extraneous shear forces that may hasten degenerative changes in physically unfit individuals.

4. Muscles that are allowed to atrophy through disuse may themselves be a pain generator through the poorly characterized and poorly understood mode of myofascial pain.

5. The ability to achieve good range of motion and EMG silence at the lumbar flexion end point may be an objective goal of therapy that improves function and reduces pain. Additionally, strength and endurance of the deep lumbar muscles, superficial lumbar muscles, and abdominal muscles seems to be important for improving function and decreasing pain.

KEY REFERENCES

1. Brooks GA: Intra- and extra-cellular lactate shuttles. Med Sci Sports Exerc 32:790-799, 2003.
   The article discusses the changing conception of lactate and lactic acid. Instead of being a "dead-end" metabolite, research over the last 10 years shows that lactate is an important messenger via the "lactate shuttle" to signal for cellular repair and improved metabolic efficiency in a host of local and distant tissue that may receive benefit from aerobic and anaerobic exercise.

2. Antonio JA, Gonyea WJ: Skeletal muscle fiber hyperplasia. Med Sci Sports Exerc 25:1333-1345, 1993.

This article provides a summary of changes to muscle, in human and animal models, resulting from exercise overload and stretch overload. Models provide direct and indirect evidence of fiber hypertrophy and hyperplasia in both overload scenarios (10% to 82%), although the presence of "embryonic" myosin isoforms may imply new fiber formation from cells that resemble satellite cells but are stem cells that respond to exercise and stretch overload.

3. Patwardhan AG, Havey RM, Carandang G, et al: Effect of compressive follower preload on the flexion-extension response of the human lumbar spine. J Orthop Res 21:540-546, 2003.

This article presents an optimized experimental model analyzing the effects of combined muscle vectors in minimizing shear force and artifact moment during flexion and extension of the lumbar spine. This model takes into account the muscle vector contribution to decreasing shear force and allowing physiologic support during lumbar motion—particularly flexion and extension.

4. Mayer T, Vanharanta H, Gatchel R, et al: Comparison of CT scan muscle measurements and isokinetic trunk strength in postoperative patients. Spine 14:33-36, 1989.

This study shows that in patients after lumbar fusion, strength deficits on isokinetic trunk strength testing correlate to dramatically reduced muscle density on CT axial cross-sectional images. This loss of visible muscle density and strength is greater in postfusion patients than postdiscectomy patients.

5. Neblett R, Mayer T, Gatchel R, et al: Quantifying the lumbar flexion-relaxation phenomenon: Theory, normative data and clinical applications. Spine 28:1435-1446, 2003.

Lumbar flexion-relaxation is a term applied to the point at maximal flexion range of motion where the muscles relax and achieve "electrical silence" to maximize their efficiency during task performance. This relaxation is thought to represent a point at which the lumbar spine is "hanging off its ligaments" at end range of the normal subject true lumbar active range of motion and does not need the contribution of muscle for stability. Additionally, the study found that full lumbar range of motion always precedes maximal hip-gluteal-hamstring range of motion in asymptomatic individuals. Third, this study shows that absent flexion-relaxation phenomenon in symptomatic patients with chronic low back pain can be retrained. Finally, training to achieve flexion-relaxation in symptomatic patients correlates with a reduction in symptoms.

6. Newton M, Waddell G: Trunk strength testing with iso-machines: I. Review of a decade of scientific evidence. Spine 18:801-811, 1993.

This study concludes that testing still provides some contradictory evidence and needs refining and more study before being employed for policy, employment, or indemnity purposes. Despite the shortcomings of testing, it is clear that patients with chronic back pain lose extension strength in greater proportion than flexion strength compared with normal subjects. This effect may be ameliorable with training and exercise, although effects on pain and patient morbidity are uncertain.

7. Styf JR, Willen J: The effects of external compression by three different retractors on pressure in the erector spine muscles during and after posterior lumbar spine surgery in humans. Spine 23:354-358, 1998.

Compression of muscles by retractors during surgery reaches pressures (61 to 158 mm Hg) in human spine surgeries that likely result in ischemia and muscle injury compared with other studies compressing human musculature. Injury may be reduced by several methods, but the degree of injury needs further study.

8. Wiltse LL, Spencer CW: New uses and refinements of the paraspinal approach to the lumbar spine. Spine 13:696-706, 1988.

This article describes and refines the surgical technique described in 1968 to spare incisional and retractor injury to the lumbar musculature during spine surgery approaches.

REFERENCES

1. McComas A: Neuromuscular Function and Disorders. Boston, Butterworth, 1977.
2. Gladden LB: Lactate metabolism: A new paradigm for the third millennium. J Physiol 558:5-30. 2004.
3. Favero T, Zable AC, Bowman M, et al: Metabolic end products inhibit sarcoplasmic reticulum Ca^{2+} release and [^{3}H]ryanodine binding. J Appl Physiol 78:1665-1672, 1995.
4. Brooks GA: Intra- and extra-cellular lactate shuttles. Med Sci Sports Exerc 32:790-799, 2003.
5. Engel WK: The essentiality of histo- and cytochemical studies of skeletal muscle in the investigation of neuromuscular disease. Neurology 12:778-784, 1962.
6. Brook MH, Engel WK: The histographic analysis of human muscle biopsies with regard to fiber types: Adult male and female. Neurology 19:221-233, 1969.
7. Staron R: Human skeletal muscle fiber types: Delineation, development, and distribution. Can J Appl Physiol 22:307-327, 1997.
8. Scott W, Stevens J, Binder-Macleod SA: Human skeletal muscle fiber type classifications. Phys Ther 81:1810-1816, 2001.
9. Antonio JA, Gonyea WJ: Skeletal muscle fiber hyperplasia. Med Sci Sports Exerc 25:1333-1345, 1993.
10. Staron RS, Malicky ES, Leonardi MJ, et al: Muscle hypertrophy and fast fiber type conversions in heavy resistance-trained women. Eur J Appl Physiol Occup Physiol 60:71-79, 1990.
11. Roy RR, Talmadge RJ, Hodgson J, et al: Differential response of fast hindlimb extensor and flexor muscles to exercise in adult spinalized cats. Muscle Nerve 22:230-241, 1999.
12. McArdle WD, Katch FI, Katch VL: Essentials of Exercise Physiology. Philadelphia, Lea & Febiger, 1994.
13. Hollinshead W: Anatomy for Surgeons, 3rd ed. Hagerstown, MD, Harper & Row, 1982.

14. Gracovetsky S, Farfan H: The optimum spine. Spine 11:543-573, 1986.

15. Patwardhan AG, Havey R, Meade K, et al: A follower load increases the load-carrying capacity of the lumbar spine in compression. Spine 24:1003-1009, 1999.

16. Stanley SK, Ghanayem A, Voronov L, et al: Flexion-extension response of the thoracolumbar spine under compressive follower preload. Spine 29:E510-E514, 2004.

17. Patwardhan AG, Havey RM, Carandang G, et al: Effect of compressive follower preload on the flexion-extension response of the human lumbar spine. J Orthop Res 21:540-546, 2003.

18. Mayer T, Vanharanta H, Gatchel R, et al: Comparison of CT scan muscle measurements and isokinetic trunk strength in postoperative patients. Spine 14:33-36, 1989.

19. Nachemson A: The possible importance of the psoas muscle for stabilization of the lumbar spine. Acta Orthop Scand 39:47-57, 1968.

20. Mayer T, Smith S, Kondraske G, et al: Quantification of lumbar function: III. Preliminary data on isokinetic torso rotation testing with myoelectric spectral analysis in normal and low back pain subjects. Spine 10:912-920, 1985.

21. Bogduk N, Macintosh J: The applied anatomy of the thoracolumbar fascia. Spine 9:165-170, 1984.

22. Macintosh J, Bogduk N, Gracovetsky S: The biomechanics of the thoracolumbar fascia. Clin Biomech 2:78-83, 1987.

23. Mayer T, Robinson R, Pegues P, et al: Lumbar segmental rigidity: Can its identification with facet injections and stretching exercises be useful? Arch Phys Med Rehabil 81:1143-1150, 2000.

24. Tesh K, Dunn J, Evans J: The abdominal muscles and vertebral stability. Spine 12:501-508, 1987.

25. Basmajian J: Muscles Alive: Their Functions Revealed by Electromyography, 4th ed. Baltimore, Williams & Wilkins, 1978.

26. Floyd W, Silver P: The function of the erector spinae muscles in certain movements and postures in man. J Physiol (Lond) 129:184-203, 1955.

27. Morris J, Benner G, Lucas D: An electromyographic study of the intrinsic muscles of the back in man. J Anat 196:509-512, 1962.

28. Neblett R, Mayer T, Gatchel R, et al: Quantifying the lumbar flexion-relaxation phenomenon: Theory, normative data and clinical applications. Spine 28:1435-1446, 2003.

29. Flint M: Effect of increasing back and abdominal muscle strength on low back pain. Res Q 29:160-171, 1955.

30. Sarti M, Lison J, Monfort M, et al: Response of the flexion-relaxation phenomenon relative to the lumbar motion to load and speed. Spine 26:E421-E426, 2001.

31. Floyd W, Silver P: The function of the erector spinae muscles in flexion of the trunk. Lancet 133-143, 1951.

32. Ahern D, Follick M, Council J, et al: Comparison of lumbar paravertebral EMG patterns in chronic low back pain patients and non-patient controls. Pain 34:153-160, 1988.

33. Golding JS: Electromyography of the erector spinae in low back pain. Postgrad Med J 28:401-406, 1951.

34. Paquet N, Malouin F, Richards C: Hip-spine movement interaction and muscle activation patterns during sagittal trunk movements in low back patients. Spine 19:596-603, 1994.

35. Sihvonen T: Averaged (RMS) surface EMG in testing back function. Electromyogr Clin Neurophysiol 28:335-339, 1988.

36. Wolf SL, Basmajian JV, Russe CTC, et al: Normative data on low back mobility and activity levels: Implications for neuromuscular reeducation. Am J Phys Med 58:217-229, 1979.

37. Sihvonen T: Flexion-relaxation of the hamstring muscles during lumbar-pelvic rhythm. Arch Phys Med Rehabil 78:486-490, 1977.

38. Ng J, Vaughan K, Richardson C, et al: Range of motion and lordosis of the lumbar spine: Reliability of measurement and normative values. Spine 26:53-60, 2001.

39. Triano JJ, Schultz AB: Correlation of objective measure of trunk motion and muscle function with low back disability ratings. Spine 12:561-565, 1987.

40. Haig A, Weismann G, Haugh L, et al: Prospective evidence for change in paraspinal muscle activity after herniated nucleus pulposus. Spine 18:926-930, 1993.

41. Mayer T, Gatchel R: Functional Restoration for Spinal Disorders: The Sports Medicine Approach. Philadelphia, Lea & Febiger, 1988.

42. Mayer T, Neblett R, Brede E, et al: The quantified lumbar flexion-relaxation phenomenon (QLFRP) is a useful measurement of improvement in a functional restoration program. Spine 34:2458-2465, 2009.

43. Neblett R, Mayer T, Brede E, et al: Effectiveness of a clinical protocol for correcting abnormal lumbar flexion-relaxation in chronic lumbar pain. Spine. In press.

44. Mooney V, Gulick J, Perlman M, et al: Relationships between myoelectric activity, strength, and MRI of lumbar extensor muscles in back pain patients and normal subjects. J Spinal Disord 10:348-356, 1997.

45. Flicker P, Fleckenstein J, Ferry K, et al: Lumbar muscle usage in chronic low back pain: MRI evaluation. Spine 18:582-586, 1993.

46. Yoshihara K, Nakayama Y, Fujii N, et al: Atrophy of the multifidus muscle in patients with lumbar disc herniation: Histochemical and electromyographic study. Orthopedics 26:493-495. 2003.

47. Cooper R, St. Clair Forbes W, Jayson M: Radiographic demonstration of paraspinal muscle wasting in patients with chronic low back pain. Br J Rheumatol 31:389-394, 1992.

48. Damneels L, Vanderstraeten G, Gambier D, et al: CT imaging of trunk muscles in chronic low back pain patients and healthy control subjects. Eur Spine J 9:266-272, 2000.

49. Keller A, Gunderson R, Reikeras O, et al: Reliability of computed tomography measurements of paraspinal muscle cross-sectional area and density in patients with chronic low back pain. Spine 28:1455-1460, 2003.

50. Mayer L, Greenberg B: Measurement of the strength of trunk muscles. J Bone Joint Surg 24:842-856, 1942.

51. Langrana N, Lee C: Isokinetic evaluation of trunk muscles. Spine 9:171-175, 1984.

52. Smidt G, Herring T, Amundsen L, et al: Assessment of abdominal and back extensor function: A quantitative approach and results for chronic low-back patients. Spine 8:211-219, 1983.

53. Suzuki N, Endo S: A quantitative study of trunk muscle strength and fatigability in the low-back pain syndrome. Spine 8:69-74, 1983.

54. Mayer T, Smith S, Keeley J, et al: Quantification of lumbar function: II. Sagittal plane trunk strength in chronic low back pain patients. Spine 10:765-772, 1985.

55. Smith S, Mayer T, Gatchel R, et al: Quantification of lumbar function: I. Isometric and multispeed isokinetic trunk strength measures in sagittal and axial planes in normal subjects. Spine 10:757-764, 1985.

56. Mayer T, Gatchel R, Betancur J, et al: Lumbar trunk muscle endurance measurement: Isometric contrasted to isokinetic testing in normal subjects. Spine 20:920-927, 1995.

57. Dueker I, Ritchie S, Knox T, Rose S: Isokinetic trunk testing and employment. ACOEM 46:42-48, 1994.

58. Dvir Z: lsokinetics: Muscle Testing, Interpretation and Clinical Applications, 2nd ed. Philadelphia, Churchill Livingstone, 2004.

59. Newton M, Thow N, Somerville D, et al: Trunk strength testing with iso-machines: II. Experimental evaluation of the Cybex II back testing system in normal subjects and patients with chronic low back pain. Spine 7:812-824, 1993.

60. Benjamin S, Flood J, Bechtel R: Isokinetic testing prior to and following anterior lumbar interbody fusion surgery: A pilot study. IES 13:159-162, 2005.

61. Dervisevica E, Hadzica V, Burger H: Reproducibility of trunk isokinetic strength findings in healthy individuals. IES 15:99-109, 2007.

62. Skrzek A, Anwajler J, Mraz M, et al: Evaluation of force-speed parameters of the trunk muscles in idiopathic scoliosis. IES 11:197-203, 2003.

63. Palmer K: Reliability and typical isokinetic values as measured by the Biodex. IES 4:20-29, 1994.

64. Cady L, Bischoff D, O'Connell E, et al: Strength and fitness and subsequent back injuries in firefighters. J Occup Med 21:269-272, 1979.

65. Blay G, Atamaz F, Biot B, et al: Isokinetic findings in scoliosis: Their relationship to clinical measurements and reliability studies. IES 15:23-28, 2007.

66. Keller A, Hellesnes J, Brox J: Reliability of the isokinetic trunk extensor test, Biering-Sorensen test, and Astrand bicycle test. Spine 26:771-777, 2001.

67. Andersson E, Oddsson L, Grundstrom H, et al: The role of the psoas and iliacus muscles for stability and movement of the lumbar spine, pelvis and hip. Scand J Med Sci Sports 5:10-16, 1995.

68. Kumar S, Dufresne R, Schoor T: Human trunk strength profile in lateral flexion and axial rotation. Spine 20:169-177, 1995.

69. Ng J, Richardson C, Parnianpour M, et al: EMG activity of trunk muscles and torque output during isometric axial rotation exertion: a comparison between back pain patients and matched controls. J Orthop Res 20:112-121, 2002.

70. McIntire K, Asher M, Burton D, et al: Development of a protocol for isometric trunk rotational strength testing and strength asymmetry assessment. IES 15:183-194, 2007.

71. Beimborn D, Morrissey M: A review of the literature related to trunk muscle performance. Spine 13:655-660, 1988.

72. Malchaire J, Masset D: Isometric and dynamic performances of the trunk and associated factors. Spine 20:1649-1656, 1995.

73. Newton M, Waddell G: Trunk strength testing with iso-machines: I. Review of a decade of scientific evidence. Spine 7:801-811, 1993.

74. Sapega A: Current concepts review: Muscle performance evaluation in orthopaedic practice. J Bone Joint Surg Am 72:1562-1574, 1990.

75. Dvir Z, Keating J: Identifying feigned isokinetic trunk extension effort in normal subjects: An efficiency study of the DEC. Spine 26:1046-1051, 2001.

76. Hazard R, Reid S, Fenwick J, et al: Isokinetic trunk and lifting strength measurements: Variability as an indicator of effort. Spine 13:54-57, 1988.

77. Mooney V, Andersson G: Controversies: Trunk strength testing in patient evaluation and treatment. Spine 19:2483-2485, 1994.

78. Brady S, Mayer T, Gatchel R: Physical progress and residual impairment quantification after functional restoration: II. Isokinetic trunk strength. Spine 18:395-400, 1994.

79. Curtis L, Mayer T, Gatchel R: Physical progress and residual impairment after functional restoration: III. Isokinetic and isoinertial lifting capacity. Spine 18:401-415, 1994.

80. Kohles S, Barnes D, Gatchel R, et al: Improved physical performance outcomes following functional restoration treatment in patient with chronic low back pain: Early versus recent training results. Spine 15:1321-1324, 1990.

81. Rissanen A, Kalimo H, Alaranta H: Effect of intensive training on the isokinetic strength and structure of lumbar muscles in patients with chronic low back pain. Spine 20:333-340, 1995.

82. Andersson E, Sward L, Torstensson A: Trunk muscle strength in athletes. Med Sci Sports Exerc 20:587-593, 1988.

83. Mayer T, Gatchel R, Kishino N, et al: Objective assessment of spine function following industrial injury: A prospective study with comparison group and one-year follow-up. 1985 Volvo Award in Clinical Sciences. Spine 10:482-493, 1985.

84. Fricton JR, Auvinen MD, Dykstra D, et al: Myofascial pain syndrome: Electromyographic changes associated with local twitch response. Arch Phys Med Rehabil 66:314-317, 1985.

85. Gerwin RD, Shannon S, Hong CZ, et al: Interrater reliability in myofascial trigger point examination. Pain 69:65-73, 1997.

86. Hsieh CY, Hong CZ, Adams AH, et al: Inter-examiner reliability in the palpation of trigger points in the trunk and lower limb muscles. Arch Phys Med Rehabil 81:1257-1258, 2000.

87. Nice DA, Riddle DL, Lamb RL, et al: Intertester reliability of judgments of the presence of trigger points in patients with low back pain. Arch Phys Med Rehabil 73:893-898, 1992.

88. Simons DG, Travell JG: Myofascial origins of low back pain. Postgrad Med 73:65-70, 81-92, 99-105, 108, 1983.

89. Cummings TM, White AR: Needling therapies in the management of myofascial trigger point pain: A systematic review. Arch Phys Med Rehabil 82:986-992, 2000.

90. Han SC, Harrison P: Myofascial pain syndrome and trigger-point management. Reg Anesth 22:89-101, 1997.

91. Irnich D, Behrens N, et al: Immediate effects of dry needling and acupuncture at distant points in chronic neck pain: Results of a randomized, double-blinded, sham-controlled crossover trial. Pain 99:83-89, 2002.

92. Simpson LL: Ammonium chloride and methylamine hydrochloride antagonize clostridial neurotoxins. J Pharmacol Exp Ther 225:546-552, 1983.

93. Simpson LL, Coffield JA, Bakry N: Chelation of zinc antagonizes the neuromuscular blocking properties of the seven serotypes of botulinum neurotoxin as well as tetanus toxin. J Pharmacol Exp Ther 267:720-727, 1993.

94. Simpson LL, Coffield JA, Bakry N: Inhibition of vacuolar adenosine triphosphate antagonizes the effects of clostridial neurotoxins but not phospholipase A2 neurotoxins. J Pharmacol Exp Ther 269:256-262, 1994.

95. Simpson LL: Kinetic studies on the interaction between botulinum toxin type A and the cholinergic neuromuscular junction. J Pharmacol Exp Ther 212:16-21, 1980.

96. Simpson LL: The origin, structure, and pharmacological activity of botulinum toxin. Pharmacol Rev 33:155-188, 1981

97. Kalandakanond S, Coffield JA: Cleavage of intracellular substrates of botulinum toxins A, C, and D in a mammalian target tissue. J Pharmacol Exp Ther 296:749-755, 2001.

98. Styf JR, Willen J: The effects of external compression by three different retractors on pressure in the erector spine muscles during and after posterior lumbar spine surgery in humans. Spine 23:354-358, 1998.

99. Cloward RB: The treatment of ruptured intervertebral discs by vertebral body fusion. Indications, operative technique, after care. J Neurosurg 10:154, 1953.

100. Steffee AD, Sitkowski DJ: Posterior lumbar interbody fusion and plates. Clin Orthop 227:99-102, 1988.

101. Wiltse LL, Bateman J, Hutchinson RH, et al: The paraspinal sacrospinalis-splitting approach to the lumbar spine. J Bone Joint Surg 50:919-926, 1968.

102. Wiltse LL, Spencer CW: New uses and refinements of the paraspinal approach to the lumbar spine. Spine 13:696-706, 1988.

103. Carpenter N: Spondylolisthesis. Br J Surg 19:374-386, 1932.

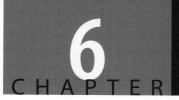

The Intervertebral Disc: Normal, Aging, and Pathologic

Edward Westrick, MD

Gwendolyn Sowa, MD, PhD

James D. Kang, MD

The intervertebral disc is a fibrocartilaginous structure whose principal function is to act as a shock absorber, transmitting compressive loads between vertebral bodies. Degeneration of the disc is associated with several clinical conditions, including herniation of the nucleus pulposus, mechanical back pain, spinal stenosis, and other spinal deformities such as scoliosis. The human intervertebral disc is considered to undergo more dramatic degenerative changes than any other musculoskeletal tissue in the body[1] and to undergo these changes at an earlier age.[2]

This chapter discusses the normal intervertebral disc anatomy, the morphologic and biochemical processes known to occur in the degenerative process, and the consequences of degeneration on the function of the disc and surrounding structures. Although the exact mechanism of intervertebral disc degeneration has not been elucidated, it is known to involve a complex interaction of biologic, genetic, and biomechanical factors. Understanding the disease process is imperative for spine researchers to develop potential therapies to slow or reverse the degenerative cascade and for spine surgeons to select appropriate treatments.

Normal Disc

Disc Anatomy

The intervertebral disc is composed of three main structures: the cartilaginous endplates, the central nucleus pulposus, and the peripherally located anulus fibrosus (Fig. 6–1).

Cartilaginous Endplates

The intervertebral disc is separated from adjacent vertebral bodies by a cartilaginous endplate superiorly and inferiorly. In humans, the endplate serves as the growth plate for the vertebral bodies, having the typical structure of an epiphyseal growth plate.[3] In infancy, this growth plate is thick and occupies a substantial fraction of the disc. The endplates thin as growth progresses and eventually consist of only a 1-mm-thick, avascular layer of hyaline cartilage in adults.[3] Similar to hyaline

cartilage elsewhere in the body, the cartilaginous endplates are composed of rounded chondrocytes.[4] Biomechanically, most compressive forces are transmitted through the superior vertebral body to the endplate, to the nucleus pulposus, and to the inferior endplate and vertebral body. The endplates and adjacent trabecular bone can undergo temporary deformation when a load is applied.

Nucleus Pulposus

The nucleus lies between adjacent endplates and forms the gel-like core of the disc. The nucleus consists of a proteoglycan and water matrix held together by an irregular network of collagen type II and elastin fibers. Proteoglycans have numerous highly anionic glycosaminoglycan (GAG) side chains (i.e., chondroitan sulfate and keratan sulfate), which allows the nucleus to imbibe water. This composition is similar to articular cartilage, and the ability of the matrix to imbibe and release water in relation to applied stresses allows the disc to cushion against compressive loads. The primary proteoglycan is aggrecan, and the high concentration of this hydrophilic molecule provides the osmotic properties needed to resist compression.[5]

Cells in the nucleus are initially notochordal, but their number declines after birth and they eventually become undetectable at about age 4 to 10 years.[6] The nucleus is gradually replaced during growth by rounded cells resembling the chondrocytes of articular cartilage.[7] These chondrocyte-like cells synthesize mostly proteoglycans and collagen type II in response to changes in hydrostatic pressure. The nucleus functions as a shock absorber, acting as a pressurized, deformable sphere that dissipates compressive forces to the anulus and the adjacent vertebral bodies. As compressive forces on the spine increase, hydrostatic pressure within the nucleus pushes outward from its center in all directions.

Anulus Fibrosus

The anulus fibrosus surrounds the nucleus and is composed of approximately 20 concentric rings (lamellae) of highly organized collagen fibers, primarily collagen type I. The

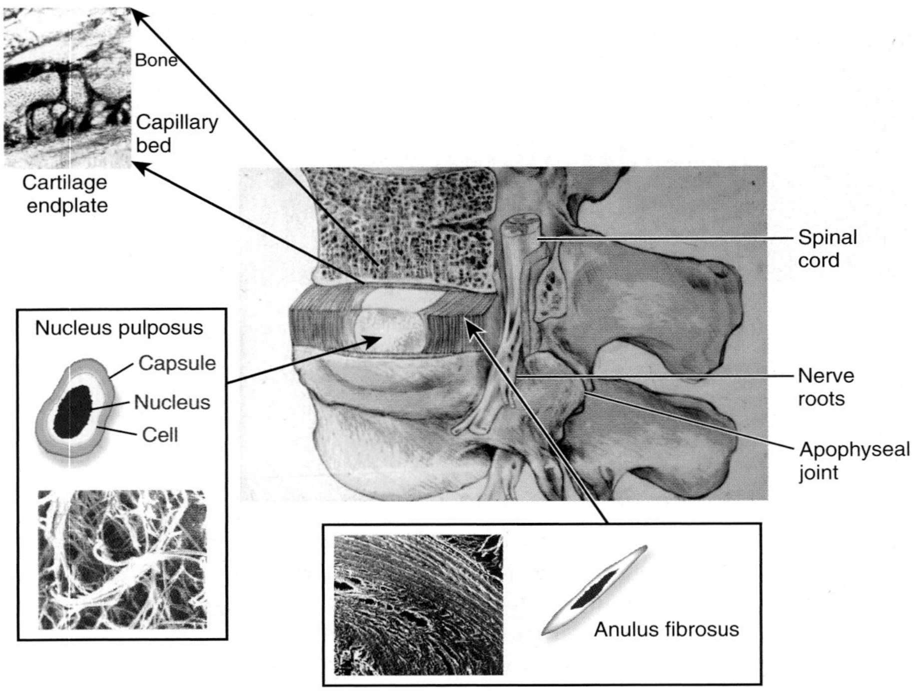

FIGURE 6–1 The intervertebral disc is a pivotal part of the spinal column, and its properties influence behavior of adjacent tissues. There is great variation in matrix organization, composition, and cell morphology and activity in different regions of the disc.

collagen fibers are orientated approximately 60 degrees to the vertical axis of the spine and run parallel within each lamella but perpendicular between adjacent lamellae allowing for maximal tensile strength.[8] Fibers of the outer anulus attach to the periphery of the vertebral bodies, whereas inner fibers pass from one endplate to another. Cells in the anulus are found between lamellae, arranged in parallel to the collagen fibers. Outer anulus cells are thin and elongated and phenotypically similar to fibroblasts, whereas cells of the innermost anulus are more spheroid similar to articular chondrocytes.[1,9] The anulus contains the nucleus pulposus and maintains its pressurization under compressive loads. The tensile properties of the anulus allow the nucleus to recover its original shape and position when the compressive load is reduced.

Blood Supply, Nutrition, and Innervation

Blood Supply

In early fetal life, vascular channels traverse the endplates, but they diminish in size starting at birth until complete disappearance by approximately 5 years of age. In adults, the blood supply of the disc arises from two capillary plexuses. One plexus penetrates 1 to 2 mm into the outer anulus, supplying only the periphery of the anulus. The other capillary plexus begins in the vertebral body and penetrates the subchondral bone (see Fig. 6–1), terminating in capillary loops at the bone-cartilage junction.[10] The density of this capillary network varies in location across the endplate, being greatest in the center and lowest at the periphery. Cells in the center of the adult nucleus pulposus are 8 mm from the nearest blood source, making the disc one of the largest avascular structures in the body.

Nutrition

The limited vascularity of the intervertebral disc has important physiologic implications—mainly that nutrition depends almost entirely on diffusion (Fig. 6–2).[11-13] The nutritional environment of the cells varies throughout the disc because of its size; cells in the nucleus are 6 to 8 mm from the nearest blood vessel. Small molecules necessary to maintain cellular function (i.e., glucose and oxygen) readily leave vertebral capillaries and diffuse across the thin cartilaginous endplate and the outermost layers of the anulus into the ECM. Concentration gradients of glucose, oxygen, and other nutrients and metabolites exist across the disc, regulated by the rates of nutrient supply and consumption. The low oxygen tension in the nucleus leads to anaerobic metabolism (i.e., glycolysis), resulting in a high concentration of lactic acid and a lower pH in the nucleus compared with the periphery of the disc.[13] Metabolic by-products such as lactic acid are removed from the disc by diffusion in the opposite direction of nutrient entry.

Innervation

Under normal conditions, only the outer 1 to 2 mm of the anulus fibrosus is innervated in nondegenerated human discs. The remainder of the anulus and nucleus are uniquely avascular and lacking neurons under normal, nondegenerated conditions. Several studies have described further nerve ingrowth into degenerated lumbar discs, however, which is discussed later in this chapter.

Disc Composition

The function of the intervertebral disc depends greatly on the properties of the extracellular matrix (ECM). The ECM

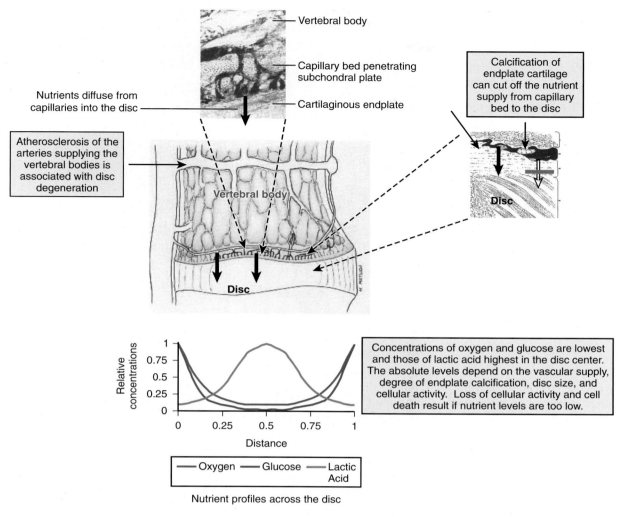

Vertebral body

Capillary bed penetrating
subchondral plate

Nutrients diffuse from
capillaries into the disc

Cartilaginous endplate

Calcification of
endplate cartilage
can cut off the nutrient
supply from capillary
bed to the disc

Atherosclerosis of the
arteries supplying the
vertebral bodies is
associated with disc
degeneration

Vertebral body

Disc

Disc

Concentrations of oxygen and glucose are lowest
and those of lactic acid highest in the disc center.
The absolute levels depend on the vascular supply,
degree of endplate calcification, disc size, and
cellular activity. Loss of cellular activity and cell
death result if nutrient levels are too low.

Nutrient profiles across the disc

FIGURE 6–2 Schematic view of routes for nutrient transport into avascular disc and resulting nutrient profiles. Diagram also shows possible regions of disturbance. (Adapted from Crock HV, Goldwasser M, Yoshizawa H: Vascular anatomy related to the intervertebral disc. In Ghosh P [ed]: Biology of the Intervertebral Disc. Boca Raton, FL, CRC Press, 1991, pp 109-133.)

provides the biomechanical properties and acts as a filter to regulate the extracellular fluid composition and the rate at which nutrients and metabolites are exchanged. The ECM consists of a complex network of macromolecules whose composition varies in different regions of the disc (Fig. 6–3).[4,14] ECM macromolecules are synthesized and maintained by a small population of cells (9000 cells/mm^3 in the anulus and 5000 cells/mm^3 in the nucleus) occupying less than 1% of the disc volume.[4] Disc cells also produce a complex array of cytokines, growth factors, and proteases to maintain equilibrium between the rates of synthesis and degradation of ECM components.[15,16]

Water

The major component of the intervertebral disc is water, and its concentration is regulated by the GAG side chains of proteoglycans. The concentration of water varies with age, location within the disc, and body position.[17] The nucleus pulposus is most highly hydrated, and the water concentration may be 90% in an infant, declining to approximately 80% in nondegenerated young adult discs.[18] The water content of the anulus is lower than the nucleus, declining to 65% in the outer anulus in adult discs.

Water content varies with load, leading to diurnal changes in disc hydration.[19] During the diurnal cycle in young, highly hydrated lumbar discs, 25% of the disc's water can be lost and regained.[20] Water is expressed from the disc during the day because of the increased forces of body weight and muscle contractions, and it is reimbibed at night when the compressive forces are removed. This diurnal cycle results in changes in disc height and affects the disc's mechanical properties.

Macromolecules

Collagen is one major macromolecular component of the disc. The collagen content of the disc is highest in the outer anulus, and the dry weight decreases significantly in the nucleus of adult discs.[21] The concentration of collagen type I is highest in the outer anulus and decreases toward the nucleus, where

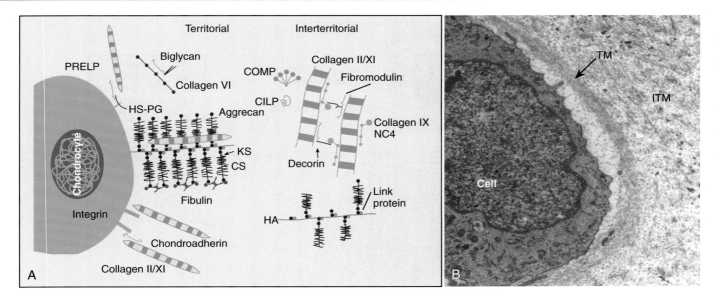

FIGURE 6–3 A, Schematic view of different matrix macromolecules, their interactions with the cell and with other matrix molecules, and their distribution within territorial matrix (TM) and interterritorial matrix (ITM). **B,** Transmission electron micrograph of section through disc cell and its surrounding matrix. TM and ITM not only have different molecular compositions but also a different morphology. (**A,** Adapted from Heinegard D, Aspberg A, Morgelin M, et al: Extracellular matrix of cartilage. Section for Connective Tissue Biology, University of Lund, 2003. Available at http://www.cmb.lu.se/ctb.)

virtually none is present.[21] Collagen type II follows the opposite gradient, with the highest concentration located in the nucleus. Along with collagen types I and II, the ECM contains many other collagens, including types III, V, VI, IX, and XI.

The other major macromolecule of the disc is aggrecan,[22] which consists of a protein core with approximately 100 anionic GAG side chains. Many aggrecan molecules covalently attach to hyaluronan chains forming large aggregates. These aggregates are trapped by the surrounding collagen network, imparting a net negative charge to the ECM. The interstitial water contains an excess of cations, which is directly related to the concentration of negative charge (i.e., GAG concentration). The high concentration of cations imparts a high osmotic pressure in the nucleus, which consequently leads to imbibition of water. Changes in proteoglycan concentration and GAG concentration lead to changes in osmotic pressure, affecting the ability of the disc to maintain hydration and turgor when loaded.[23]

In addition to collagens and aggrecan, the disc contains lower concentrations of numerous other macromolecules,[14] including elastin, the smaller proteoglycans decorin and fibromodulin, cartilage oligomeric matrix protein, and cartilage intermediate layer protein. These molecules function either structurally or biomechanically and are important for normal disc function.

Intervertebral Disc: Aging and Degeneration

Aging

Human intervertebral discs undergo very early aging and degeneration, resulting in histomorphologic and functional changes (Fig. 6–4).[24] Endplate permeability and vascular

supply decrease throughout growth and aging, leading to altered metabolite transport.[24] Proteoglycans begin to fragment during childhood, and the overall proteoglycan content decreases with age, especially in the nucleus. There is a corresponding increase in collagen content, with collagen type I fibers replacing collagen type II fibers in the inner anulus and nucleus. In addition, reduced matrix turnover in older discs enables collagen fibrils to become increasingly cross-linked,[25] leading to retention of damaged fibers and reduced tissue strength. Synthesis of ECM components decreases steadily throughout life, and this is partly attributable to decreased cell density, although synthesis rates per cell also decrease.

In infants, the nucleus contains approximately 90% water and appears translucent.[18] The disc dehydrates slowly with aging, with water content of the nucleus declining to around 80% in young adults.[24] The nucleus also accumulates yellow pigmentation and becomes less distinguishable from the surrounding anulus.[18,24] As the disc water content decreases, the nucleus becomes smaller and decompressed, often condensing into several fibrous lumps. Dehydration of the nucleus leads to altered biomechanical properties of the disc, forcing the anulus to act as a fibrous solid to resist compression directly. The proteoglycan content of the anulus also decreases with aging, and the anulus becomes stiffer and weaker, resisting compressive loads in a haphazard manner.

Degeneration

Intervertebral disc degeneration mimics age-related changes of the disc, but the process occurs prematurely or at an accelerated rate[26,27] and usually results in symptoms. There are no widely accepted definitions of disc degeneration in the literature, reflecting the difficulty in distinguishing degeneration from the physiologic processes of growth, aging, and remodeling. More recent definitions describe degeneration as an aberrant, cell-mediated response to progressive damage, with combined structural failure and accelerated or advanced signs of aging. These proposed definitions also suggest that structurally intact discs with accelerated age-related changes be classified as *early degenerative discs,* whereas the term *degenerative disc disease* should be applied if the disc is also painful.[26]

Although the exact mechanism of disc degeneration has not been determined, it is known to involve a complex interaction of factors, including ECM macromolecule changes, decreased water content, altered enzyme activity, decreased endplate permeability, impaired metabolite transport, structural failure, cell senescence and death, and genetic factors. These biologic and biomechanical factors cause extensive histomorphologic changes of the disc leading to disorganization of the anulus, solidification of the nucleus, and thinning and calcification of the cartilaginous endplates.

Matrix Macromolecule Changes

The most physiologically important changes of disc degeneration start in the nucleus.[18] Early changes include increased degradation of aggrecan and other aggregating proteoglycans coupled with an increased concentration of nonaggregating proteoglycans. The accumulation of degraded proteoglycans further impairs diffusion of nutrients and oxygen through the disc. A change in the proportions of the GAGs chondroitan sulfate, heparan sulfate, and keratan sulfate also occurs, with increasing amounts of heparan sulfate and keratan sulfate as degeneration progresses. These changes diminish the hydroscopic properties of the ECM further, resulting in decreased water content and decreased ability to imbibe water. Loss of proteoglycans and GAGs leads to decreased swelling pressure,[23] loss of hydration, and loss of disc height. The changes result in altered responses to applied biomechanical loads, ultimately leading to the structural features of degeneration.

Intervertebral disc degeneration also results in disorganization and destruction of the collagen network.[28] As the overall proteoglycan and water content decreases, there is a corresponding increase in collagen content. Collagen type I replaces collagen type II in the inner anulus and nucleus, and there is a tendency for collagen type I fibrils throughout the disc to become coarser. The highly organized collagen fiber arrangements of the anulus are also disrupted, and collagen and elastin networks become more haphazard. When the collagen network has been damaged, disc biomechanics are markedly altered, and the potential for structural damage increases.

Increased levels of cytokines, as discussed subsequently, leads to increased production of proteinases, causing alterations in other collagens such as types VI, IX, and X. Collagen type IX is degraded in the pericellular microenvironment, allowing for local expansion of this microenvironment during degeneration. Collagen type IX decreases similarly to collagen type II, implying advanced stages of degeneration and fibrosis of the nucleus. The synthesis of collagen type VI increases as degeneration progresses and functions to hold proliferating cells together.

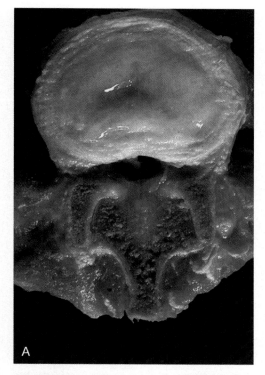

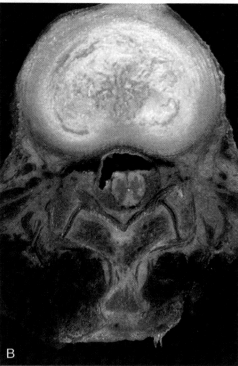

FIGURE 6–4 Transverse sections of lumbar discs and apophyseal joints showing decrease in nucleus hydration, loss of demarcation between anulus and nucleus with age, and appearance of circumferential fissures by the 3rd decade. **A,** Adolescent. **B,** At age 28 years. (Courtesy of Bullough PG, Vigorita VJ: Bullough's and Vigorita's Atlas of Orthopaedic Pathology, Baltimore, University Park Press–Gower Medical Publishing, 1995.)

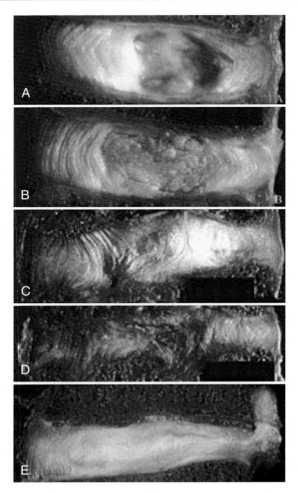

FIGURE 6–5 Cadaveric lumbar intervertebral discs sectioned in mid-sagittal plane (anterior on left). **A,** Young disc (35-year-old man). **B,** Mature disc (47-year-old man). **C,** Disrupted young disc (31-year-old man). Note endplate damage and inward collapse of inner anulus. **D,** Severely disrupted young disc (31-year-old man). Note collapse of disc height. **E,** Disc induced to prolapse in the laboratory (40-year-old man). Some nucleus pulposus has herniated through radial fissure in posterior anulus (right). (From Adams MA, Bogduk N, Burton K, et al: The Biomechanics of Back Pain. Edinburgh, Churchill Livingstone, 2002.)

The overall ECM content in the nucleus is a well-controlled equilibrium between degradative and synthetic pathways involving numerous proteins. In disc degeneration, there is an imbalance between degradative and synthetic pathways and a predominance of catabolic enzyme activity. Proteinases of the matrix metalloproteinase (MMP) and ADAMTS families cleave collagens and other macromolecules and have been implicated in the breakdown of the ECM.[29] The degradative enzymes MMP-3 and MMP-13 (also known as stromelysin-1 [MMP-3] and collagenase 3 [MMP-13]) have been found at increased levels in degenerated human discs.

The regulation of MMP and ADAMTS production and ECM macromolecule production is achieved by numerous cytokines and growth factors. Of particular importance in disc ECM homeostasis are members of the interleukin (IL) family (catabolism) and transforming growth factor-β (anabolism) superfamily.[30,31] Mediators of inflammation such as nitric oxide and prostaglandin E_2 and the cytokines IL-1 and IL-6

are found at increased levels in degenerated discs.[30-32] The synthetic capabilities of nucleus cells are unable to sustain appropriate levels of aggrecan and collagen production in the face of this increased catabolism, which contributes to further degeneration of the disc.

Cellular Changes

It has long been recognized that there is a slowly progressive loss of cells during disc degeneration,[33] leading to further loss of the ECM. An increasing body of literature has shown that apoptosis, or programmed cell death, may be responsible for many of the features of degeneration.[34-36] More recent literature has also shown an increase in lacunae containing cell clusters,[37,38] possibly causing an overall increased number of cells as disc degeneration progresses. This increased cell proliferation may be an attempt to offset the progressive destruction and loss of the ECM. One reason for increased cellularity may be the focal increase in nutrient supply owing to the ingrowth of blood vessels in degenerating discs, as discussed elsewhere in this chapter.

Cell clusters have been discovered in areas adjacent to the newly formed blood vessels within degenerated discs. Cells in these areas have access to nutrient supply and growth factors and undergo proliferation. The cellular changes in degenerated discs resemble osteoarthritis, where remodeling of the pericellular microenvironment with chondrocyte proliferation and cluster formation have also been found. Ultimately, cellular attempts at repair become ineffective as disc degeneration progresses because the local mechanical environment of the cells has become abnormal.

Structural Changes

As disc hydration decreases, the distinction between anulus and nucleus becomes less defined and disc height decreases (Fig. 6–5).[24] In later stages, gross tissue changes become increasingly apparent, including loss of lamellae organization, fissuring of the anulus,[39] and discoloration and solidification of the nucleus.[40,41] Radial and circumferential annular tears are often evident, sometimes extending to the disc periphery.[39] These changes are accompanied by ingrowth of nerves and blood vessels into the disc and deposition of granulation tissue and calcification within the endplates. These structural changes ultimately lead to altered, abnormal biomechanical properties of the disc. Damage to one area of the disc increases load bearing by adjacent tissues, making it more likely for damage to spread. Although a healthy intervertebral disc equalizes pressure within it, the decreased shock-absorbing capacity of the decompressed nucleus leads to high compressive stresses in the anulus.[42] Other gross morphologic changes of degeneration include disc bulging, disc space narrowing, endplate irregularities, and osteophyte formation and arthritis.

Neovascularization and Ingrowth of Sensory Nerves

As stated previously, the disc is largely avascular in adults with blood vessels normally restricted to only the outermost layers of the anulus. Likewise, only the outer 1 to 2 mm of the anulus is innervated in the normal human disc. The ingrowth of blood vessels and sensory nerves is an important feature of degenerated discs, however, and seems to be associated with pain.[43] Ingrowth of capillaries is facilitated by the loss of hydrostatic pressure in the inner regions of the disc, which would normally collapse small vessels. These newly formed microvessels release neurotrophic growth factors such as nerve growth factor, allowing the ingrowth of small, nonmyelinated nerve fibers.[44-46] It has been hypothesized that discogenic pain arises because these nociceptive nerve fibers grow into areas of the disc that previously had no neurons.

Etiology of Intervertebral Disc Degeneration

The incidence of intervertebral disc degeneration increases with age and is most common in the lumbar spine.[47,48] Multiple risk factors have been hypothesized as the underlying cause, including age-related factors, genetic predisposition, and numerous environmental factors. Biomechanical studies have shown that excessive mechanical loading causes disruption of disc structure including endplate defects, fissures, bulging, disc prolapse, and annular collapse.[49] Further experiments have confirmed that structural damage precipitates a cascade of cell-mediated responses, leading to further damage. Although mechanical loading may precipitate degeneration, the most important cause may be processes that weaken the disc before structural damage or processes that impair the healing response. The combined effects of aging, unfavorable genetics, altered nutrition and metabolite transport, excessive or repetitive loading, and the resulting cascade of cellular events all contribute to the process of degeneration.

Aging

Aging causes progressive changes in disc nutrient supply and ECM composition, and these changes decrease tissue strength and alter cell metabolism. The alterations of proteoglycans and GAGs, decreased hydration, and changes in collagen distribution and cross-linking make the disc physically more vulnerable to injury. The altered vascular supply to the disc has been hypothesized as the primary cause of disc degeneration. Experimental endplate damage leads to degeneration[33] despite enhanced metabolite transport into the disc, however, suggesting that structural damage more strongly influences the degenerative process. Inadequate nutrition likely predisposes the disc to degeneration by compromising its ability to respond to increased loading or injury.

Genetic Predisposition

Some authors suggest that genetic predisposition is the greatest risk factor for disc degeneration, accounting for approximately 50% to 70% of the variability in identical twin studies.[50-52] Individual gene polymorphisms associated with disc degeneration include aggrecan,[53] cartilage intermediate layer protein,[54] collagen type IX,[55,56] MMP-3,[57] and vitamin D receptor.[58,59] The products of these genes alter the ECM

composition, decrease tissue strength, impair regenerative capability, and undoubtedly influence disc cell function. Degeneration develops after many decades, however, and preferentially affects the lumbar spine, even though the unfavorable genetic predisposition is present since birth. This suggests that genetic inheritance and polymorphic variations in susceptibility genes predispose the disc toward degeneration, but further insults such as excessive loading or structural damage are necessary to trigger the cascade of degenerative events.

Nutrition

The failure of nutrient supply is hypothesized to be a primary cause of disc degeneration.[60] The metabolic activity of disc cells in vitro is sensitive to extracellular oxygen and pH, with matrix synthesis rates decreasing at acidic pH and low oxygen concentrations.[61,62] A decrease in nutrient supply causing decreased oxygen concentration or pH could negatively affect the ability of disc cells to synthesize and maintain the ECM, ultimately leading to disc degeneration.

A relationship between loss of cell viability and a decrease in nutrient transport in scoliotic discs has been found,[63] and there is evidence that nutrient transport is affected in disc degeneration in vivo.[64,65] Likewise, the transport of solutes from bone to disc measured in vitro was significantly lower in degenerated discs compared with normal discs.[60] Other factors affecting the blood supply to the vertebral body that may lead to an increased incidence of disc degeneration include atherosclerosis,[66,67] sickle cell anemia, caisson disease (decompression sickness), and Gaucher disease. In addition, calcification of the cartilaginous endplates can cause decreased nutritional supply even if the blood supply remains undisturbed, as seen in scoliotic discs.[60,68] This evidence supports the hypothesis that a decrease in nutrient supply ultimately leads to degeneration of the disc.

Environmental Factors

Environmental risk factors hypothesized to influence disc degeneration include heavy or repetitive mechanical loading (i.e., occupational physical loading and whole-body vibration),[51,69] obesity, and cigarette smoking.[70] Heavy physical loading, particularly related to occupation, was previously suspected to be a major risk factor for degeneration and commonly viewed as a "wear and tear" phenomenon. Results of identical twin studies on physical loading specific to occupation or sport suggest, however, that repetitive physical loading plays a relatively minor role in disc degeneration.[69]

Obesity has often been implicated as a risk factor for degeneration, but epidemiologic studies have reported mixed findings. More recently, obesity was found to be a risk factor for marked reduction of the nucleus pulposus magnetic resonance imaging (MRI) signal intensity of lumbar discs. The mechanism by which obesity contributes to degeneration is thought to be a combination of mechanical and systemic factors. Some authors suggest that atherosclerosis and cardiovascular disease associated with obesity parallel

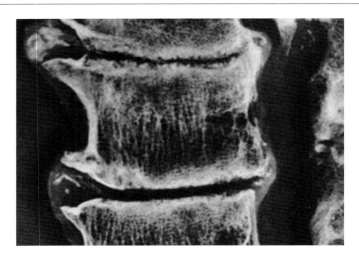

FIGURE 6–6 Radiograph of old cadaveric lumbar spine (anterior on left). Radiograph depicts how severe disc narrowing can be associated with vertebral osteophytes, sclerosis of vertebral endplates, and selective loss of horizontal trabeculae from vertebral body. (From Adams MA, Bogduk N, Burton K, et al: The Biomechanics of Back Pain. Edinburgh, Churchill Livingstone, 2002.)

atherosclerosis of the spinal vessels, with decreased blood and nutrient supply leading to increased risk of degeneration.

The only chemical exposure associated with disc degeneration is cigarette smoking, which explains only 2% of the variance in lumbar disc MRI changes between identical twins with highly discordant lifetime exposures. In other studies of monozygotic twins in whom the mean of cotwin discordance was less, no significant association between disc degeneration and cigarette smoking was found. Cigarette smoke is presumed to alter blood flow to disc capillaries and nutrient transport, possibly as a result of the presence of muscarinic receptors in blood vessels of the vertebral endplate.

Facet Joints, Ligaments, and Vertebral Bodies

No discussion of intervertebral disc degeneration would be complete without consideration of the other elements of the spine. Degeneration of the spine has an impact not only on the disc, but also the surrounding structures, such as the facet joints, ligaments, and vertebral bodies. Degenerative changes occur simultaneously in each of these components, altering the ability of the spine to respond to normal physiologic loads. In addition, degeneration of the surrounding structures may cause pain and reduced mobility of the spine.

Facet Joints

Degeneration of the facet joints resembles osteoarthritic changes occurring at other synovial joints, starting with synovitis and progressing to articular cartilage loss, capsular redundancy, and eventually degenerative spondylolisthesis. Hypertrophic osteophytes at the joint margins and periarticular fibrosis can also result in reduced mobility and pain at the facet joint. Osteoarthritis of the facet joints parallels degenerative changes of the disc, possibly resulting from abnormal loading and narrowing of the disc in the early stages of degeneration.[71]

Ligaments

The anterior longitudinal ligament and posterior longitudinal ligament contribute to the overall stability of the spine. The strong anterior longitudinal ligament buttresses the anulus anteriorly, whereas the posterior longitudinal ligament offers only weak reinforcement to the posterior anulus. Information regarding degenerative changes of these ligaments is minimal, but the anterior longitudinal ligament and the posterior longitudinal ligament become more redundant as disc height decreases, and ossification occurs in later stages. These changes may contribute to pain and reduced mobility of the spine.

Vertebral Bodies

Osteoarthritic changes of the vertebral body are also associated with intervertebral disc degeneration.[72] The cartilaginous endplates are normally the weakest structure under compressive loads, and thinning and calcification with aging further compromise endplate strength. The endplates accumulate trabecular microdamage[73] and undergo remodeling in response to altered loads, and the nucleus bulges into the vertebral body as degeneration progresses. Endplate damage decompresses the nucleus further, and loss of disc height transfers forces onto the anulus, causing it to bulge into the nucleus.[49,74] The nucleus may eventually herniate through a damaged endplate, and subsequent calcification of the herniated nucleus is called a Schmorl node. The loss of disc height and annular laxity leads to formation of osteophytes at the vertebral body margins, decreased separation of the posterior neural arches, and eventual bony ankylosis (Fig. 6–6).

Intervertebral Disc Disorders and Treatment

Disc Herniation

The most common intervertebral disc disorder spinal surgeons encounter is a herniated or prolapsed nucleus pulposus, resulting in nerve root compression and radiculopathic pain. Although herniation is often thought to result from a mechanically induced rupture, it can be induced in vitro only in healthy discs by forces greater than normally encountered in vivo.[75] Examination of postmortem and surgical disc specimens suggests sequestration or herniation results from the migration of isolated, degenerated fragments of the normally central nucleus pulposus through preexisting tears in the anulus fibrosus.[76]

Herniation-induced pressure of the nerve root alone may not account for pain associated with this condition because more than 70% of asymptomatic people have disc prolapses but no pain.[77,78] Researchers have hypothesized that the nerves in symptomatic patients are sensitized to pressure,[79] possibly by molecules such as prostaglandin E_2, thromboxane, phospholipase A_2, tumor necrosis factor-α, ILs, and MMPs. These molecules are produced by cells of herniated discs[30] and may sensitize the affected nerve root because of the close proximity between the nerve and herniated disc material.[80]

Spinal Stenosis

Spinal stenosis is a narrowing of the spinal canal that results in mechanical compression of the spinal nerve roots, causing radicular pain, paresthesias, weakness, and neurogenic claudication. Degeneration of the intervertebral disc, combined with degenerative changes of the vertebral bodies and hypertrophy of the facet joints, contributes to narrowing of the spinal canal.

Spinal Deformities

With scoliosis and kyphosis, whether congenital, neuromuscular, or idiopathic, there is wedging of the intervertebral discs and vertebral bodies. Several biochemical changes have been identified in scoliotic discs, which have been shown to differ from discs without scoliosis.[25] These alterations include alterations in collagen production and cross-linking patterns,[81] marked endplate calcification,[82] and alterations in nutrient pathways.[63]

Treatment

Currently, no treatment is available to prevent, slow, or reverse intervertebral disc degeneration. The conservative and surgical treatments currently offered to patients are aimed at treating the end-stage manifestations of the disease rather than altering the course. The major surgical treatments available to spine surgeons include discectomy, spinal arthrodesis, and disc replacement. These procedures can produce pain relief, but they also change the biomechanics of the spine, possibly accelerating degeneration at adjacent levels.[83,84]

Alternatively, several biologic treatment strategies, including gene therapy and stem cell therapy, are currently under investigation for spinal applications. The aim of these biologic treatments is to prevent, slow, or reverse the degenerative cascade at the cellular or molecular level to restore normal tissue properties and biomechanical function. At present, experimental work shows the potential of these biologic therapies, but several barriers prevent their use clinically, including the correct choice of therapeutic genes and proper patient selection. Several of these therapies are discussed in detail in later chapters.

KEY REFERENCES

1. Boos N, Weissbach S, Rohrback H, et al: Classification of age-related changes in lumbar intervertebral discs. 2002 Volvo Award in basic science. Spine 27:2631-2644, 2002.
    This article presents a detailed study of the changes in discs with age and pathology at the morphologic and immunohistochemical levels.

2. Battié MC, Videman T, Gibbons LE, et al: 1995 Volvo Award in clinical sciences. Determinants of lumbar disc degeneration: A study relating lifetime exposures and magnetic resonance imaging findings in identical twins. Spine 20:2601-2612, 1995.
    This study shows that genetic factors have an overriding influence in determining disc degeneration; environmental risk factors such as mechanical stress or smoking play only a minor role.

3. Boden SD, Davis DO, Dina TS, et al: Abnormal magnetic-resonance scans of the lumbar spine in asymptomatic subjects: A prospective investigation. J Bone Joint Surg Am 72:403-408, 1990.
    This study confirms that a significant number of pain-free subjects have herniated discs.

4. Le Maitre CL, Freemont AJ, Hoyland JA: Localization of degradative enzymes and their inhibitors in the degenerate human intervertebral disc. J Pathol 204:47-54, 2004.
    This study reported on a survey of degenerative and nondegenerative discs from surgical and postmortem samples. Immunohistochemistry was used to quantify the production of anabolic enzymes and their inhibitors.

5. Kang JD, Stefanovic-Racic M, McIntyre LA, et al: Toward a biochemical understanding of human intervertebral disc degeneration and herniation: Contributions of nitric oxide, interleukins, prostaglandin E2, and matrix metalloproteinases. Spine 22:1065-1073, 1997.
    Intervertebral disc cells increased their production of MMPs, nitric oxide, IL-6, and prostaglandin E_2 when stimulated by IL-1β. The effect was more dramatic in nondegenerated discs, but cells of herniated degenerated discs were capable of further increasing their synthesis of several of these biochemical agents in response to IL-1β.

REFERENCES

1. Buckwalter JA: Aging and degeneration of the human intervertebral disc. Spine 20:1307-1314, 1995.
2. Miller JA, Schmatz C, Schultz AB: Lumbar disc degeneration: Correlation with age, sex, and spine level in 600 autopsy specimens. Spine 13:173-178, 1988.
3. Bernick S, Cailliet R: Vertebral end-plate changes with aging of human vertebrae. Spine 7:97-102, 1982.
4. Maroudas A, Stockwell RA, Nachemson A, et al: Factors involved in the nutrition of the human lumbar intervertebral disc: Cellularity and diffusion of glucose in vitro. J Anat 120(Pt 1):113-130, 1975.
5. Watanabe H, Yamada Y, Kimata K: Roles of aggrecan, a large chondroitin sulfate proteoglycan, in cartilage structure and function. J Biochem 124:687-693, 1998.
6. Pazzaglia UE, Salisbury JR, Byers PD: Development and involution of the notochord in the human spine. J R Soc Med 82:413-415, 1989.
7. Sive JI, Baird P, Jeziorsk M, et al: Expression of chondrocyte markers by cells of normal and degenerate intervertebral discs. Mol Pathol 55:91-97, 2002.

8. Inoue H: Three-dimensional architecture of lumbar intervertebral discs. Spine 6:139-146, 1981.

9. Errington RJ, Puustjarvi K, White IR, et al: Characterisation of cytoplasm-filled processes in cells of the intervertebral disc. J Anat 192(Pt 3):369-378, 1998.

10. Urban JP, Holm S, Maroudas A: Diffusion of small solutes into the intervertebral disc: As in vivo study. Biorheology 15:203-221, 1978.

11. Holm S, Maroudas A, Urban JP, et al: Nutrition of the intervertebral disc: Solute transport and metabolism. Connect Tissue Res 8:101-119, 1981.

12. Ferguson SJ, Ito K, Nolte LP: Fluid flow and convective transport of solutes within the intervertebral disc. J Biomech 37:213-221, 2004.

13. Urban JP, Smith S, Fairbank JC: Nutrition of the intervertebral disc. Spine 29:2700-2709, 2004.

14. Feng H, Danfelter M, Strömqvist B, et al: Extracellular matrix in disc degeneration. J Bone Joint Surg Am 88(Suppl 2):25-29, 2006.

15. Roberts S, Caterson B, Menage J, et al: Matrix metalloproteinases and aggrecanase: Their role in disorders of the human intervertebral disc. Spine 25:3005-3013, 2000.

16. Melrose J, Ghosh P, Taylor TK: Neutral proteinases of the human intervertebral disc. Biochim Biophys Acta 923:483-495, 1987.

17. Roberts S, Menage J, Urban JP: Biochemical and structural properties of the cartilage end-plate and its relation to the intervertebral disc. Spine 14:166-174, 1989.

18. Antoniou J, Steffen T, Nelson F, et al: The human lumbar intervertebral disc: Evidence for changes in the biosynthesis and denaturation of the extracellular matrix with growth, maturation, ageing, and degeneration. J Clin Invest 98:996-1003, 1996.

19. Nachemson A, Elfstrom G: Intravital dynamic pressure measurements in lumbar discs: A study of common movements, maneuvers and exercises. Scand J Rehabil Med Suppl 1:1-40, 1970.

20. Boos N, Wallin A, Gbedegbegnon T, et al: Quantitative MR imaging of lumbar intervertebral disks and vertebral bodies: Influence of diurnal water content variations. Radiology 188:351-354, 1993.

21. Eyre DR, Muir H: Quantitative analysis of types I and II collagens in human intervertebral discs at various ages. Biochim Biophys Acta 492:29-42, 1977.

22. Johnstone B, Bayliss MT: The large proteoglycans of the human intervertebral disc: Changes in their biosynthesis and structure with age, topography, and pathology. Spine 20:674-684, 1995.

23. Urban JP, McMullin JF: Swelling pressure of the intervertebral disc: Influence of proteoglycan and collagen contents. Biorheology 22:145-157, 1985.

24. Boos N, Weissbach S, Rohrbach H, et al: Classification of age-related changes in lumbar intervertebral discs. 2002 Volvo Award in basic science. Spine 27:2631-2644, 2002.

25. Duance VC, Crean JK, Sims TJ, et al: Changes in collagen cross-linking in degenerative disc disease and scoliosis. Spine 23:2545-2551, 1998.

26. Adams MA, Roughley PJ: What is intervertebral disc degeneration, and what causes it? Spine 31:2151-2161, 2006.

27. Le Maitre CL, Pockert A, Buttle DJ, et al: Matrix synthesis and degradation in human intervertebral disc degeneration. Biochem Soc Trans 35(Pt 4):652-655, 2007.

28. Roberts S, Evans H, Trivedi J, et al: Histology and pathology of the human intervertebral disc. J Bone Joint Surg Am 88(Suppl 2):10-14, 2006.

29. Le Maitre CL, Freemont AJ, Hoyland JA: Localization of degradative enzymes and their inhibitors in the degenerate human intervertebral disc. J Pathol 204:47-54, 2004.

30. Kang JD, Georgescu HI, McIntyre-Larkin L, et al: Herniated lumbar intervertebral discs spontaneously produce matrix metalloproteinases, nitric oxide, interleukin-6, and prostaglandin E2. Spine 21:271-277, 1996.

31. Kang JD, Stefanovic-Racic M, McIntyre LA, et al: Toward a biochemical understanding of human intervertebral disc degeneration and herniation: Contributions of nitric oxide, interleukins, prostaglandin E2, and matrix metalloproteinases. Spine 22:1065-1073, 1997.

32. Le Maitre CL, Freemont AJ, Hoyland JA: The role of interleukin-1 in the pathogenesis of human intervertebral disc degeneration. Arthritis Res Ther 7:R732-R745, 2005.

33. Holm S, Holm AK, Ekström L, et al: Experimental disc degeneration due to endplate injury. J Spinal Disord Tech 17:64-71, 2004.

34. Gruber HE, Hanley EN Jr: Analysis of aging and degeneration of the human intervertebral disc: Comparison of surgical specimens with normal controls. Spine 23:751-757, 1998.

35. Trout JJ, Buckwalter JA, Moore KC: Ultrastructure of the human intervertebral disc: II. Cells of the nucleus pulposus. Anat Rec 204:307-314, 1982.

36. Zhao CQ, Wang LM, Jiang LS, et al: The cell biology of intervertebral disc aging and degeneration. Ageing Res Rev 6:247-261, 2007.

37. Hastreiter D, Ozuna RM, Spector M: Regional variations in certain cellular characteristics in human lumbar intervertebral discs, including the presence of alpha-smooth muscle actin. J Orthop Res 19:597-604, 2001.

38. Johnson WE, Eisenstein SM, Roberts S: Cell cluster formation in degenerate lumbar intervertebral discs is associated with increased disc cell proliferation. Connect Tissue Res 42:197-207, 2001.

39. Osti OL, Vernon-Roberts B, Fraser RD: 1990 Volvo Award in experimental studies. Annulus tears and intervertebral disc degeneration: An experimental study using an animal model. Spine 15:762-767, 1990.

40. Thompson JP, Pearce RH, Schechter MT, et al: Preliminary evaluation of a scheme for grading the gross morphology of the human intervertebral disc. Spine 15:411-415, 1990.

41. Yasuma T, Koh S, Okamura T, et al: Histological changes in aging lumbar intervertebral discs: Their role in protrusions and prolapses. J Bone Joint Surg Am 72:220-229, 1990.

42. Adams MA, McMillan DW, Green TP, et al: Sustained loading generates stress concentrations in lumbar intervertebral discs. Spine 21:434-438, 1996.

43. Roberts S, Eisenstein SM, Menage J, et al: Mechanoreceptors in intervertebral discs: Morphology, distribution, and neuropeptides. Spine 20:2645-2651, 1995.

44. Freemont AJ, Peacock TE, Goupille P, et al: Nerve ingrowth into diseased intervertebral disc in chronic back pain. Lancet 350:178-181, 1997.

45. Freemont AJ, Watkins A, Le Maitre C, et al: Nerve growth factor expression and innervation of the painful intervertebral disc. J Pathol 197:286-292, 2002.

46. Kauppila LI: Ingrowth of blood vessels in disc degeneration: Angiographic and histological studies of cadaveric spines. J Bone Joint Surg Am 77:26-31, 1995.

47. Luoma K, Riihimäki H, Luukkonen R, et al: Low back pain in relation to lumbar disc degeneration. Spine 25:487-492, 2000.

48. Videman T, Battié MC, Gill K, et al: Magnetic resonance imaging findings and their relationships in the thoracic and lumbar spine: Insights into the etiopathogenesis of spinal degeneration. Spine 20:928-935, 1995.

49. Adams MA, Freeman BJ, Morrison HP, et al: Mechanical initiation of intervertebral disc degeneration. Spine 25:1625-1636, 2000.

50. Battié MC, Videman T, Gibbons LE, et al: 1995 Volvo Award in clinical sciences. Determinants of lumbar disc degeneration: A study relating lifetime exposures and magnetic resonance imaging findings in identical twins. Spine 20:2601-2612, 1995.

51. Battie MC, Videman T, Parent E: Lumbar disc degeneration: Epidemiology and genetic influences. Spine 29:2679-2690, 2004.

52. Sambrook PN, MacGregor AJ, Spector TD: Genetic influences on cervical and lumbar disc degeneration: A magnetic resonance imaging study in twins. Arthritis Rheum 42:366-372, 1999.

53. Kawaguchi Y, Osada R, Kanamori M, et al: Association between an aggrecan gene polymorphism and lumbar disc degeneration. Spine 24:2456-2460, 1999.

54. Seki S, Kawaguchi Y, Chiba K, et al: A functional SNP in CILP, encoding cartilage intermediate layer protein, is associated with susceptibility to lumbar disc disease. Nat Genet 37:607-612, 2005.

55. Ala-Kokko L. Genetic risk factors for lumbar disc disease. Ann Med 34:42-47, 2002.

56. Paassilta P, Lohiniva J, Göring HH, et al: Identification of a novel common genetic risk factor for lumbar disk disease. JAMA 285:1843-1849, 2001.

57. Takahashi M, Haro H, Wakabayashi Y, et al: The association of degeneration of the intervertebral disc with 5a/6a polymorphism in the promoter of the human matrix metalloproteinase-3 gene. J Bone Joint Surg Br 83:491-495, 2001.

58. Kawaguchi Y,Kanamori M, Ishihara H, et al: The association of lumbar disc disease with vitamin-D receptor gene polymorphism. J Bone Joint Surg Am 84:2022-2028, 2002.

59. Videman T, Gibbons LE, Battié MC, et al: The relative roles of intragenic polymorphisms of the vitamin D receptor gene in lumbar spine degeneration and bone density. Spine 26:E7-E12, 2001.

60. Nachemson A, Lewin T, Maroudas A, et al: In vitro diffusion of dye through the end-plates and the annulus fibrosus of human lumbar inter-vertebral discs. Acta Orthop Scand 41:589-607, 1970.

61. Ishihara H, Urban JP: Effects of low oxygen concentrations and metabolic inhibitors on proteoglycan and protein synthesis rates in the intervertebral disc. J Orthop Res 17:829-835, 1999.

62. Ohshima H, Urban JP: The effect of lactate and pH on proteoglycan and protein synthesis rates in the intervertebral disc. Spine 17:1079-1082, 1992.

63. Urban MR, Fairbank JC, Bibby SR, et al: Intervertebral disc composition in neuromuscular scoliosis: Changes in cell density and glycosaminoglycan concentration at the curve apex. Spine 26:610-617, 2001.

64. Bartels EM, Fairbank JC, Winlove CP, et al: Oxygen and lactate concentrations measured in vivo in the intervertebral discs of patients with scoliosis and back pain. Spine 23:1-7; discussion 8, 1998.

65. Rajasekaran S, Babu JN, Arun R, et al: ISSLS prize winner. A study of diffusion in human lumbar discs: A serial magnetic resonance imaging study documenting the influence of the endplate on diffusion in normal and degenerate discs. Spine 29:2654-2667, 2004.

66. Kauppila LI: Prevalence of stenotic changes in arteries supplying the lumbar spine: A postmortem angiographic study on 140 subjects. Ann Rheum Dis 56:591-595, 1997.

67. Kauppila LI, McAlindon T, Evans S, et al: Disc degeneration/back pain and calcification of the abdominal aorta: A 25-year follow-up study in Framingham. Spine 22:1642-1647; discussion 1648-1649, 1997.

68. Roberts S, Urban JP, Evans H, et al: Transport properties of the human cartilage endplate in relation to its composition and calcification. Spine 21:415-420, 1996.

69. Videman T, Sarna S, Battié MC, et al: The long-term effects of physical loading and exercise lifestyles on back-related symptoms, disability, and spinal pathology among men. Spine 20:699-709, 1995.

70. Battié MC, Videman T, Gill K, et al: 1991 Volvo Award in clinical sciences. Smoking and lumbar intervertebral disc degeneration: An MRI study of identical twins. Spine 16:1015-1021, 1991.

71. Boden SD, Riew KD, Yamaguchi K, et al: Orientation of the lumbar facet joints: Association with degenerative disc disease. J Bone Joint Surg Am 78:403-411, 1996.

72. Simpson EK, Parkinson IH, Manthey B, et al: Intervertebral disc disorganization is related to trabecular bone architecture in the lumbar spine. J Bone Miner Res 16:681-687, 2001.

73. Vernon-Roberts B, Pirie CJ: Healing trabecular microfractures in the bodies of lumbar vertebrae. Ann Rheum Dis 32:406-412, 1973.

74. Urban JP, Roberts S: Degeneration of the intervertebral disc. Arthritis Res Ther 5:120-130, 2003.

75. Adams MA, Hutton WC: Prolapsed intervertebral disc: A hyperflexion injury. 1981 Volvo Award in Basic Science. Spine 7:184-191, 1982.

76. Moore RJ, Vernon-Roberts B, Fraser RD, et al: The origin and fate of herniated lumbar intervertebral disc tissue. Spine 21:2149-2155, 1996.

77. Boden SD, Davis DO, Dina TS, et al: Abnormal magnetic-resonance scans of the lumbar spine in asymptomatic subjects: A prospective investigation. J Bone Joint Surg Am 72:403-408, 1990.

78. Boos N, Rieder R, Schade V, et al: 1995 Volvo Award in clinical sciences. The diagnostic accuracy of magnetic resonance imaging, work perception, and psychosocial factors in identifying symptomatic disc herniations. Spine 20:2613-2625, 1995.

79. Cavanaugh JM: Neural mechanisms of lumbar pain. Spine 20:1804-1809, 1995.

80. Kawakami M, Tamaki T, Weinstein JN, et al: Pathomechanism of pain-related behavior produced by allografts of intervertebral disc in the rat. Spine 21:2101-2107, 1996.

81. Crean JK, Roberts S, Jaffray DC, et al: Matrix metalloproteinases in the human intervertebral disc: Role in disc degeneration and scoliosis. Spine 22:2877-2884, 1997.

82. Roberts S, Menage J, Eisenstein SM: The cartilage end-plate and intervertebral disc in scoliosis: calcification and other sequelae. J Orthop Res 11:747-757, 1993.

83. Bao QB, McCullen GM, Higham PA, et al: The artificial disc: Theory, design and materials. Biomaterials 17:1157-1167, 1996.

84. Eck JC, Humphreys SC, Hodges SD: Adjacent-segment degeneration after lumbar fusion: A review of clinical, biomechanical, and radiologic studies. Am J Orthop 28:336-340, 1999.

7

CHAPTER

Biomechanics of the Spinal Motion Segment

William S. Marras, PhD

In biomechanics, information from the biologic sciences and engineering mechanics is integrated for the purpose of analyzing and quantifying the function of and forces occurring on tissue under various conditions. With an understanding of the natural behavior mechanics of the spinal motion segment, it can be possible to understand better the limitations of the system and the conditions under which tissue damage occurs and subsequent pain would be likely. Biomechanical assessments provide a quantitative means by which to accomplish this goal.

From a biomechanical standpoint, the spine seems to accomplish three major functions.[1] First, the spine provides a structure by which loads can be transmitted through the body. Second, the spine permits motion in multidimensional space. Third, the spine provides a structure to protect the spinal cord. To appreciate the ability of the spine to accomplish these functions, we need to understand the natural movements of the spine and the ability of the spine to withstand forces or loads that are transmitted through the structure.

With these goals in mind, this chapter (1) considers the physical characteristics of the spinal tissues that could influence function, (2) assesses the motion characteristics (kinematics) of the different portions of the spine, and (3) summarizes the ability of the spine to withstand forces that it is supporting (load tolerance). Collectively, this chapter shows, from a biomechanical perspective, how the spine functions and how it breaks down.

Assessing the Biomechanics of the Spinal Motion Segment

Ideally, it would be desirable to measure directly the forces imposed on the various tissues within the spine. With current technology, invasive measures would be required, however, to understand the loading imposed on the various spinal tissues. Such invasive measures would disrupt the tissues of interest and would most likely alter the very factors that one is attempting to measure. Direct biomechanical measurements of the spine in vivo are rare and currently difficult in live humans. Subsequently, much of the biomechanical information about the human spinal motion segment is based on in vitro studies. This information must be considered with caution because the

properties of the spine derived from cadaveric studies are understood to be different in many respects from those of a live individual.

An alternative to direct measurement of spine tissue loading is the prediction of tissue loads based on biomechanical models. A biomechanical model is a conceptual representation and prediction of how the forces within the biomechanical system interact ultimately to impose force on a particular tissue of interest. Biomechanical analyses assume that the body behaves according to the laws of newtonian mechanics that must govern the distribution of forces within the musculoskeletal system. The object of interest in spinal biomechanics is a precise quantitative assessment of the movement behavior and mechanical loading occurring within the tissue of the musculoskeletal system. Biomechanical modeling permits one to estimate the direction and magnitude of forces acting on the spinal motion segment and allows one to estimate when natural motion tolerances have been exceeded and when damage or degeneration would be expected to occur. Biomechanical assessments help one understand potential pathways of low back disorders and can potentially help surgeons understand how contemplated surgical interventions might affect the health of the spine. Biomechanical modeling is outside the scope of this chapter, however.

Ultimately, biomechanical assessments are intended to determine "how much loading of the tissues within the spinal motion segment is too much loading?" This high degree of precision and quantification is the characteristic that distinguishes biomechanical analyses from other types of analyses.

Physical Characteristics of Spine Structures

The spine is composed of four types of vertebrae classified according to their regional location along the spinal column—cervical, thoracic, lumbar, and sacral. There are 7 cervical vertebrae, 12 thoracic vertebrae, and 5 lumbar vertebrae. In addition, the sacrum consists of five immobile or "fused" vertebrae, and the coccyx (often referred to as the tailbone) is a fusion of four coccygeal vertebrae at the very base of the spine. Each vertebra is referenced according to a nomenclature system wherein the spine region (e.g., cervical, thoracic) is followed by a numbering system that refers to the vertical

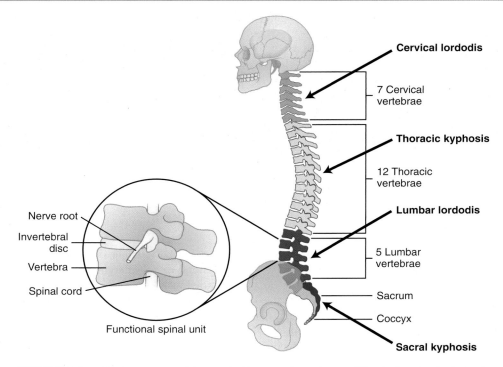

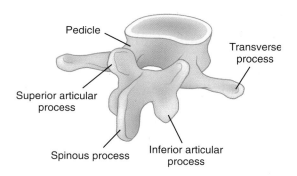

FIGURE 7–1 A and **B,** Arrangement of the vertebral bones and spinal curves (**A**) and a functional spinal unit or spinal motion segment (**B**). (Adapted from Marras WS: The Working Back: A Systems View. Hoboken, John Wiley & Sons, 2008.)

position of the vertebral body along the spine (beginning with the vertebra closest to the head) (e.g., first cervical vertebra, or C1). Disc levels are referenced relative to the vertebral levels surrounding the disc. The lowest lumbar vertebra (fifth lumbar vertebra, or L5) is adjacent to the first sacral vertebra (S1), and the disc between these vertebrae is referred to as L5-S1.

The shape of the vertebrae changes from level to level in the spine. The vertebral body shape and the orientation of the posterior elements change. In particular, the orientation of the bony structures that compose the posterior elements change in their shapes and contact angles. These subtle changes permit or restrict motions in different directions along the human spine.

Several physiologic curves are also characteristic of the upright spine (Fig. 7–1A). The curves within the cervical and lumbar regions of the spine are referred to as *cervical lordosis* and *lumbar lordosis,* whereas the thoracic and sacral curves are referred to as *thoracic kyphosis* and *sacral kyphosis* because these curves bow in the opposite direction of the lordotic curves. These curves work collectively to accommodate pelvic orientation under different conditions. When sitting, the pelvis rotates backward and the lumbar curve flattens. When the pelvis is rotated forward, the lumbar curve is accentuated. Collectively, the spinal curves balance each other and form a stable system that maintains the center of gravity in a balanced state.

The "building blocks" of the spine are the spinal motion segments (Fig. 7–1B), also known as the *functional spinal unit.* This unit consists of two vertebrae and the disc in between them. This unit represents the central focus of biomechanical functioning and clinical assessment. This chapter explores the spinal motion segment from a biomechanical perspective with the intent of understanding the significance of features that may influence status.

Support Structures

The spine is constructed of a series of vertebral bones that are stacked on one another to form the spinal column that runs from the pelvis to the head. A vertebral bone, or vertebra, is shown in Figure 7–2. The large round portion of the bone is the vertebral body and represents the major load-bearing structure of the spinal column. The outer portion of this bone is composed of a thin yet very strong layer of cortical bone. Cortical bone, also known as *compact bone,* forms a protective

FIGURE 7–2 Lumbar vertebra and its posterior elements. (Adapted from Marras WS: The Working Back: A Systems View. Hoboken, John Wiley & Sons, 2008.)

outer shell, has a high resistance to bending and torsion, and provides strength in situations where bending would be undesirable. The inner portion of the bone consists of a spongy matrix of cancellous bone. This type of bone is less dense and more elastic than cortical bone. Cancellous bone forms the interior scaffolding of the structure and helps the bone to maintain its shape despite compressive forces. This structure is composed of bundles of short and parallel strands of bone fused together.

Posterior of the vertebral body are bony structures that constitute the posterior elements and form a protective channel or tunnel for the spinal cord (see Fig. 7–1B). The biomechanical role of the posterior elements is to control the position of the vertebral bodies. These elements provide attachment points for muscles to control the position of the vertebra and supply lever arms to provide the system with mechanical advantage. In addition, these structures control motion and provide mechanical "stops" to prevent excessive movement of the vertebral body. A significant portion of the mechanical load is borne by the posterior elements, relieving the disc of excessive loading.

As shown in Figure 7–2, toward the top of the posterior surface of each vertebra are pedicles. The pedicles provide a robust support structure (a type of pillar) to transmit force between the posterior elements and the vertebral body. Projecting out from each pedicle are the lamina structures that come together at the midline of the body and form a neural arch. This arch is a strong structure that provides protection to the spinal cord in the form of a channel (vertebral foramen).

Emanating out from the junction of the two laminae at the midline of the body is a bony protrusion called the *spinous process*. Projecting laterally on each side of the structure at the junction of the pedicle and the laminae is another bony structure called the *transverse process*. These processes provide muscle attachment surfaces and mechanical advantage for control of the spinal column.

Two sets of articulating surfaces are also present in the posterior elements. Projecting out from each of the cephalic lateral corners of the lamina is a bony extension called the *superior articular process*. A portion of this surface is covered by articular cartilage. Emanating from the caudal lateral corner of the lamina on each side are the *inferior articular processes*. The superior articular process from the lower vertebra interacts with the inferior articular process of the vertebra above it to form a synovial joint known as the *zygapophyseal joint*. This joint is also referred to as the *facet joint*. The inclination of the facet joint changes from the cervical spine to the thoracic spine to the lumbar spine. This joint is defined as a plane surface in the cervical and thoracic joints, but becomes a curved surface in the lumbar spine. In the lumbar spine, the inferior facets are convex in shape, whereas the superior facets have a concave shape. In addition, the angle of these surfaces relative to the sagittal plane changes (increases) as one moves down the lumbar spine. The differences in orientation of these facet joints restrict movement in different planes of motion. They serve an important function in that they permit certain motions and limit other motions of the spine. They can be thought of as the guidance system of the spine.

Collectively, the posterior elements can provide a significant load path for the forces running through the spinal column. Approximately one third of a spinal load is carried through the posterior elements in the upright posture. The nature of the load transmission can be altered when spine degeneration occurs by altering the vector of force and magnitude of force transmitted through these posterior elements. This load path can be disengaged, however, when the spine is in a flexed posture, and the load can be entirely passed through the disc.

Disc

The vertebral bodies are connected by discs that serve several biomechanical purposes. First, the discs act as shock absorbers between the vertebrae, absorbing a portion of the mechanical forces transmitted through the spine. Second, they can transmit a portion of the mechanical load between vertebrae. Third, the discs are able to permit and govern motion between the vertebral bodies. Functionally, the discs are intended to provide a separation between consecutive vertebrae. This separation provides space between vertebrae so that the vertebral bodies can independently change their orientation and execute bending movements. With this arrangement, a pliable and deformable spinal structure is possible.

The disc consists of two distinct portions, each of which is associated with a distinct mechanical function. The outer portion of the disc, called the *anulus fibrosus,* consists of alternating layers of fibers that are oriented at a 60- to 65-degree angle relative to the vertical. The anulus fibrosus consists of about 10 to 20 concentric, circumferential sheets of collagen called *lamellae* that are nestled together around the periphery of the disc (Fig. 7–3). The lamellae are stiff and can withstand significant compression loading. Given the collagenous nature of these lamellae, they are pliable and can also permit bending of the spinal column. If the structure were to buckle, however, it would lose its stiffness and would be unable to support compression. The second portion of the disc (nucleus pulposus) is designed to overcome this potential problem.

Within the anulus fibrosus is a gelatinous core referred to as the *nucleus pulposus* (see Fig. 7–3). When compressed, this core expands radially and places the anulus fibrosus in tension,

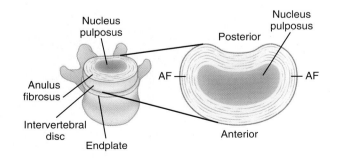

FIGURE 7–3 A, Disc, vertebral endplate, and vertebral body. **B,** Construction of intervertebral disc. (Adapted from Marras WS: The Working Back: A Systems View. Hoboken, John Wiley & Sons, 2008; Bogduk N: Clinical Anatomy of the Lumbar Spine and Sacrum, 4th ed. Edinburgh, Churchill Livingstone, 2005.)

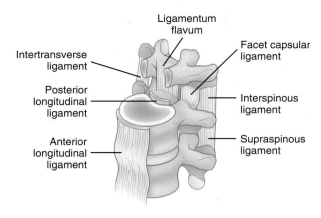

FIGURE 7–4 Ligaments of the spine. (From White AA III, Panjabi MM: Clinical Biomechanics of the Spine, 2nd ed. Philadelphia, JB Lippincott, 1990.)

providing stiffness. The integrity of the system changes throughout the day. The disc absorbs water while one is recumbent, which makes the system stiffer than when one is upright. Conversely, when one is upright, water is squeezed out of the disc, and the structure becomes more lax.

Finally, the endplate is located at the intersection of the disc and the vertebral body. The endplates are composed of cartilage and cover the superior and inferior portions of the disc. These structures bind the disc fibers to the vertebral bones and play a significant role in disc nutritional transport.

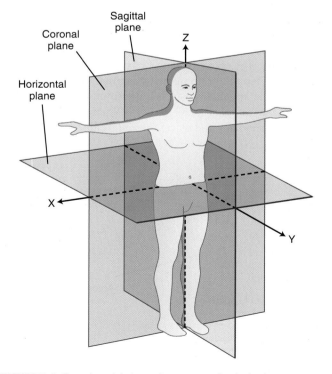

FIGURE 7–5 Central or global coordinate system for the body.

Spinal Ligaments

The spinal ligaments play a significant role from a biomechanical standpoint. Ligaments are most effective in supporting loads in the direction in which their fibers run. They support loads under tension and can buckle under compression. These structures can store energy and act much like a rubber band in that they can provide resistance to loads by developing tension.

The ligaments serve three roles. First, they permit motion and help orient the vertebrae without muscle recruitment. Second, ligaments protect the spinal cord by restricting spinal motion segment movement to within specific ranges. Third, they absorb energy and protect the spinal cord during rapid motions.

The spinal ligaments are shown in Figure 7–4. The arrangement of these structures provides support for the spine in different dimensions of loading. Because support is offered in the different directions of motion, these structures provide stability when the spinal system is intact.

Coordinate System and Force and Movement Definitions

A biomechanical assessment of the spine is concerned with the assessment of movements and forces developing within the spine as it is exposed to activities of daily living and other work or environmental conditions. Movements or motions are compared with the natural limits of movement, and forces imposed on a tissue (also called *tissue loading*) are compared with the tissue tolerances (magnitude of load at which damage occurs). To describe movement and force transmission through tissue accurately, it is necessary to describe precisely direction of movement and direction and magnitude of the force application on the tissue. Direction is defined relative to a coordinate system or reference frame. The central (global) coordinate system of the body is shown in Figure 7–5. The origin or center of this coordinate system is located at the base of the spine. Figure 7–5 describes the coordinate system (used in this chapter) as a traditional three-dimensional cartesian coordinate system with three mutually perpendicular axes oriented with a vertical Z-axis. Some references have adopted the ISB coordinate convention, where the Y-axis is defined as the vertical axis.

All movements of the spine are described relative to the origin of the central coordinate system. Flexion and extension are typically described in the sagittal plane, lateral bending occurs in the coronal plane, and twisting occurs along the horizontal or transverse plane. In reality, most activities are combinations of movements in these planes.

Within the spinal motion segment or functional spinal unit, a local coordinate system can also be defined. The convention that defines this local coordinate system is shown in Figure 7–6. Movement of the spinal motion segments is defined relative to the subjacent vertebrae. Movements of the motion segment can be either translations (indicating straight line movements in any direction) or rotations (indicating movement around a point as when bending).

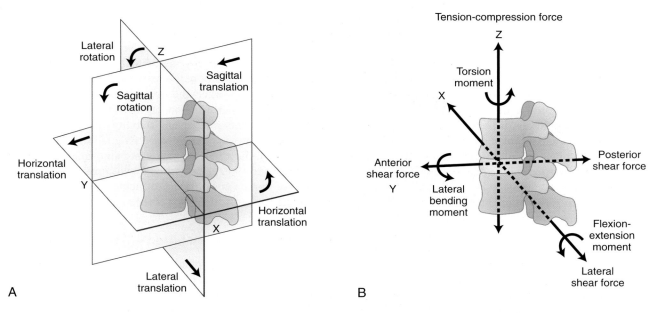

FIGURE 7–6 A and **B,** Spinal motion segment planes and directions of motion (**A**) and biomechanical coordinate system and direction of forces and moments (**B**). Motions and forces are described relative to this coordinate system. (From Bogduk N: Clinical Anatomy of the Lumbar Spine and Sacrum, 4th ed. Edinburgh, Churchill Livingstone, 2005.)

Figure 7–6 indicates that forces and moments (torques) can develop along each dimension of the reference frame. Forces along the Z dimension are either compression or tension depending on whether they compress the spinal motions segment or pull on the tissues. These are typically the forces one is concerned about when lifting an object in the sagittal plane. Two types of shear forces are also of concern when evaluating the biomechanics of the spine. Anteroposterior shear force describes the forward or backward force in the Y-axis that can result from pushing or pulling activities. The lateral shear forces refer to the sideways forces acting along the X-axis and represent the forces that develop in the spinal motion segment when one pushes an object to the side of the body.

Compression of the disc causes pressure within the nucleus pulposus in all directions, and this pressure places the anulus fibrosus under tension. As shown in Figure 7–7, the nucleus pressure can lead to deformation near the center of the endplate with this form of loading.

Figure 7–8 illustrates how shear, torsion, and tension influence the fibers of the anulus. Shear forces tense the fibers in the direction of movement and relax the fibers in the opposite direction. Similarly, torsion or twisting tenses the fibers that are lengthened by the movement and relaxes the remaining fibers. This differential of force among the fibers is believed to result in tissue damage. Finally, lengthening of the spine places the fibers under tension. This action increases the force on all the fibers regardless of their orientation.

Bending moments refer to forces acting around an axis in Figure 7–6. The curved arrows in this figure show the direction in which moments act around a spinal segment. A bending moment can be defined around the X-axis resulting in a movement in the sagittal plane (forward bending moment), or it can be defined around the Y-axis indicating a

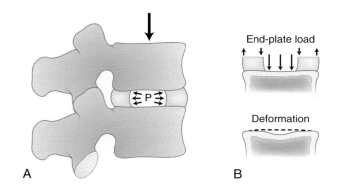

FIGURE 7–7 Compression of disc leading to increased pressure in disc nucleus and deformation of endplate. (From White AA III, Panjabi MM: Clinical Biomechanics of the Spine, 2nd ed. Philadelphia, JB Lippincott, 1990.)

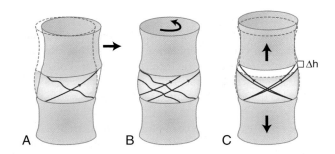

FIGURE 7–8 The effects of shear (**A**), torsion (**B**), and tension (**C**) on the fibers of the anulus fibrosus. (From Adams MA, Bogduk N, Burton AK, et al: The Biomechanics of Back Pain, 2nd ed. Edinburgh, Churchill Livingstone, 2006.)

sideways or lateral bend. In either of these situations, the moment or toque around the central axis defines the loading of the segment. Twisting of the spine can result when forces are applied around the Z-axis of the spine. This situation results in what is typically referred to as *torsional moment.*

The forces and moment can be defined around each vertebra along the spine resulting in a very large number of forces and moments and numerous degrees of freedom. For practical purposes, the forces and moment are typically defined in most situations around one particular vertebra or disc (e.g., L5-S1) depending on the purpose of the study.

Movements between vertebral bodies can also be coupled. Coupling refers to the motion relationship of one vertebra around an axis relative to another vertebra around a different axis. In other words, coupling refers to the motion in different planes that occurs simultaneously. The spine can bend forward and twist at the same time: This is a coupled motion.

The amount of displacement between the neutral position of the vertebra and the point at which resistance to physiologic motion is experienced is referred to as a *neutral zone.*[2] Neutral zones can be defined for translational and rotational movements. The neutral zone can be described for each of 6 degrees of freedom.

Tissue Load Characteristics

The forces represented in Figure 7–6 define the direction of load application and the magnitude of the force. The nature and temporal characteristics of the loading situation also define the probability that the load application will result in tissue damage. It is believed that tissue damage can result from several different "types" of trauma to the tissue. Each type of trauma is believed to be associated with very different tolerance levels. First, acute trauma is the most familiar type of loading. *Acute trauma* refers to a single application of force that exceeds the tolerance level of the tissue. This would be the case if a large load were imposed on the spinal motion segment and a rupture of the disc occurred. In this case, the magnitude of the force applied in a particular direction would far exceed the tissue strength of the disc resulting in a rupture.

Another well-recognized mechanism of tissue disruption involves repeated cumulative loading of the tissues. With *cumulative trauma,* moderate repetitive loads are applied to the tissues, and this repeated loading is believed to weaken the structure so that the tolerance of the tissue is reduced. Although moderate loading can cause the tissues to strengthen and adapt to load, repetitive loading without proper rest (adaptation) time can cause degeneration of the tissues. Repetitive application of force to a structure is believed to cause microtrauma, which weakens the structure and leads to failure at lower levels than would expected with an acute trauma to the tissue.

More recently, a third type of biomechanical trauma (instability) has received much attention in the literature.[3-8] Stability is the ability of a system to respond to a perturbation and reestablish a state of equilibrium.[2] *Instability* of the spine refers to the abnormal displacement of spine under physiologic loading. The abnormal displacement can occur in translation or rotation, but most likely would be some combination of these two types of motions. These abnormal motions are often small in magnitude, but the displacement may be enough to stimulate pain in sensitive tissue. Stability is significant because it is often the initiator of tissue damage when the system is out of alignment or when the musculoskeletal system overcompensates for a perturbation.[2] When the supporting musculature cannot offer adequate stability to a joint (owing to improper muscle recruitment, fatigue, structure laxity, or weakness), the structure may move abnormally and result in sudden and unexpected force applications on a tissue. This type of trauma is similar to the acute trauma pathway, but is initiated by a miscalculation of the muscle recruitment pattern.

Mechanical Degeneration—Tissues at Risk

Many tissues in the spinal motion segment can be influenced by structure loading. These tissues include bones, discs, ligaments, tendons, and nerves. Tissue loading can result in a disruption of the tissue integrity. Bones can be cracked or broken, disc endplates can sustain microfractures, the disc can bulge or rupture, muscle can experience fiber tears, and blood flow to the tissues can be disrupted. All of these events are believed to be capable of initiating a sequence of events leading to back pain. The tolerance of many of these structures within the spine is reviewed in detail.

Clinicians are beginning to understand that low back disorders can occur before tissue damage. Biochemical studies have shown that these types of tissue insults can result in an upregulation of proinflammatory cytokines. This upregulation may result in tissue inflammation at much lower levels of load than would occur under normal conditions. This inflammation makes nociceptive tissues more sensitive to pain and may initiate back pain.[9]

Much attention in spine biomechanics and clinical care has been focused on the intervertebral disc because disc disruption has been associated with pain. Over the past several decades, clinicians have also begun to understand how spine loading can initiate the degeneration process within the disc. To appreciate this process, the system behavior of the disc, vertebral body, and endplate must be considered in response to cumulative trauma. The disc receives no direct blood supply for nourishment. It relies heavily on nutrient flow and diffusion from surrounding vascularized tissue for disc viability. The nourishment is transported from the vertebral body through the endplate to the disc. The endplate is very thin (about 1 mm thick) and facilitates nutrient transport to the disc.

When endplate loading exceeds its tolerance limit, microfractures can occur in the structure. Microfracture of the endplate itself usually does not initiate pain because few pain receptors reside within the disc and endplate. Repeated microfracture of this vertebral endplate can lead to the formation of scar tissue and calcification that can interfere with nutrient flow to the disc fibers. Because scar tissue is thicker and denser than endplate tissue, the scar tissue interferes with nutrient delivery to the disc. This reduced nutrient flow can lead to atrophy and weakening of the disc fibers and disc degeneration. Because the disc has relatively few nociceptors except at the outer layers, this degenerative process is usually not noticed by the individual until the disc is weakened to the point where bulging or rupture occurs, and surrounding tissues that are rich in nociceptors are stimulated. Figure 7–9 describes this sequence of events that are believed to lead to disc degeneration.[9]

The literature also provides some evidence that excessive motion within the spinal segment can lead to degeneration. Excessive motion at a joint is believed to increase the cumulative trauma on the spinal structures and potentially initiate either tissue degeneration or an upregulation of proinflammatory cytokines. This has become apparent in studies that have examined the degeneration of segments adjacent to spinal fusions.[10] If two spinal levels are fused, trunk motion usually results in exacerbated movement especially at the facet joints within spinal levels adjacent to the fusion. One study noted hypertrophic degenerative arthritis of the facet joints in motion segments adjacent to a fusion typically following a symptom-free period (8.5 years on average).[10] Another study found significant evidence of degeneration at levels adjacent to a fusion with the rate of symptomatic degeneration at the adjacent segment warranting either decompression or arthrodesis to be 16.4% at 5 years after fusion and 36.1% at 10 years after the surgery.[11] In addition, more recent studies examining artificial discs have reported facet arthrosis.[12] Facet load forces have been shown to depend on artificial disc placement and the subsequent load transferred to the facets.[13]

The application of damaging compressive forces on the vertebral body can result in several different types of failures of vertebrae. The failure characteristics have been described in the literature[14] and are shown graphically in Figure 7–10. This figure indicates that seven types of failures are typically seen as a result of compression. These consist of stellate fracture, step fracture, intrusion fracture, depression of the endplate, Y-shaped fracture, edge fracture, and transverse fracture. Many of these fractures suggest weakness of the endplate. This weakness is a result of the thinness of the endplate necessary for nutrient transport to the disc. These fractures are believed to result from the nucleus pulposus of the adjacent disc bulging into the vertebra.[15]

Motion Characteristics (Kinematics) of the Spinal Motion Segments

Spine Kinematics

To appreciate the differences involved in spine impairment, it is important to understand the normal motion or kinematics of the spine. It has been observed that people with low back pain move more slowly.[16-18] Motion reduction is assumed to be a result of the "guarding" that occurs in an attempt to minimize the stimulation of pain-producing nociceptors. Abnormal coupling of movement has also been shown to be associated with low back pain.[19]

Spine kinematic profiles associated with asymptomatic individuals and people with low back pain have been reported

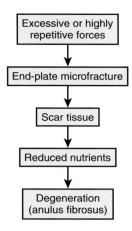

FIGURE 7–9 Sequence of events associated with cumulative or repeated trauma leading to disc degeneration.

in the literature at least for the lumbar spine. Figure 7–11 summarizes how trunk range of motion, velocity, and acceleration change as a function of low back pain in the sagittal, lateral and transverse planes of the body. There seem to be no differences in range of motion between the low back pain group and the asymptomatic group. Significant differences are apparent, however, when trunk velocity and acceleration are considered. This seems to be the case in all motion planes of the body. More recent studies have shown that kinematic ability can be used to document the extent of a low back disorder.[16,17] These differences in velocity and acceleration are believed to be a result of protective "guarding" employed in patients with low back pain through the excessive coactive recruitment of the trunk muscles. This coactivity is believed to slow the motions of the torso.

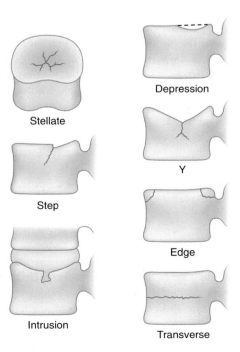

FIGURE 7–10 Seven types of fractures identified by Brinkmann and colleagues.[14] (From Adams MA, Bogduk N, Burton AK, et al: The Biomechanics of Back Pain, 2nd ed. Edinburgh, Churchill Livingstone, 2006.)

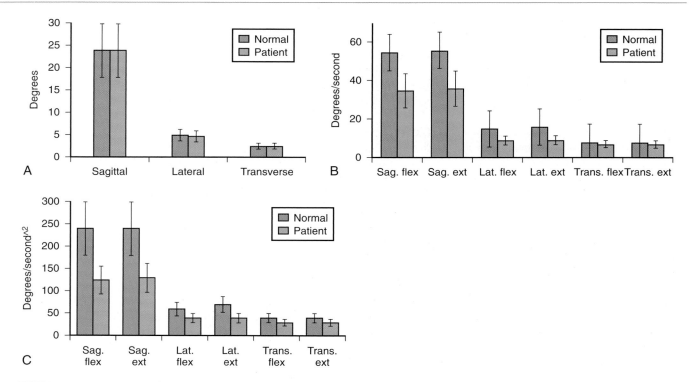

FIGURE 7–11 A, Spine range of motion characteristics (mean and standard deviation [SD]) associated with asymptomatic patients versus patients with low back pain in sagittal, lateral, and transverse planes of the body. **B,** Spine velocity characteristics (mean and SD) associated with asymptomatic patients versus patients with low back pain in sagittal, lateral, and transverse planes of the body. **C,** Spine acceleration characteristics (mean and SD) associated with asymptomatic patients versus patients with low back pain in sagittal, lateral, and transverse planes of the body.

Segment Kinematics

The typical ranges of motion associated with cervical, thoracic, and lumbar motion segments have been well described in the literature[4] and are summarized in Table 7–1. In addition, a graphic estimate of spinal segment range of motion associated with the entire spine is presented in Figure 7–12.[2] Table 7–1 shows the vast differences in motion capacity for the various vertebrae as a function of the spine region and the vertebral level. Each region of the spine allows or limits motion in a particular motion direction compared with other regions of the spine. This information shows that in the sagittal plane the most range of motion occurs in the cervical spine followed by the lumbar spine. Lateral directed motions, although much smaller in magnitude than motions in the sagittal plane, occur freely in the cervical spine, with much less movement available in the thoracic and lumbar spine. Finally, very little axial rotation is possible in the lumbar spine, with most motion occurring in the thoracic vertebrae except for C1-C2.

Collectively, the body of work described in Table 7–1 and Figure 7–12 represents the summary of expected movement characteristics derived in vitro. To the extent that in vitro characteristics are indicative of in vivo characteristics, they can provide a baseline for movement expectations for the various vertebrae along the spinal column.

Several studies have also attempted to document the motion of the spinal motion segments in vivo. Figure 7–13 illustrates the estimated normal movement characteristics of the lumbar spine measured in living subjects. This figure indicates significantly different normal movements, particularly in flexion-extension, between in vivo and in vitro observations.[20] Figure 7–14 highlights this difference between the in vitro and in vivo observations in the sagittal plane.[20] There is a general overestimation of extension movement range in vitro and a general underestimation of flexion range in vitro. In addition, significant differences can be seen between levels between the two states.

It is also possible that abnormal movement of the motion segment can indicate disc damage. Studies have also shown that tears in the anulus fibrosus change the movement characteristics of the motion segments. Specifically, tears in the anulus increase the amount of motion in the motion segment when torque is applied to the segment.[21]

Axis of Rotation

To understand and describe better how motion occurs among vertebrae, an axis (or center) of rotation is often defined. When bones move relative to one another in a single plane, there is a point around which the object rotates. If a hypothetical line is extended from the constant point within a vertebra, the point at which these two lines meet when the vertebra moves between two different positions is called the *instantaneous axis of rotation*. This concept can be extended to three-dimensional space; however, identifying the axis of rotation becomes more complex. Understanding of the axis of rotation helps one understand how kinematics are altered because of

TABLE 7–1 Limits and Representative Values of Ranges of Rotation for Cervical, Thoracic, and Lumbar Spine

Interspace	COMBINED FLEXION-EXTENSION (± Y-AXIS ROTATION)		ONE SIDE LATERAL BENDING (X-AXIS ROTATION)		ONE SIDE AXIAL ROTATION (Z-AXIS ROTATION)	
	Limits of Ranges (degrees)	Representative Angle (degrees)	Limits of Ranges (degrees)	Representative Angle (degrees)	Limits of Ranges (degrees)	Representative Angle (degrees)
C0-C1		25		5		5
C1-C2		20		5		40
Middle						
C2-3	5-16	10	11-20	10	0-10	3
C3-4	7-26	15	9-15	11	3-10	7
C4-5	13-29	20	0-16	11	1-12	7
Lower						
C5-6	13-29	20	0-16	8	2-12	7
C6-7	6-26	17	0-17	7	2-10	6
C7-T1	4-7	9	0-17	4	0-7	2
T1-T2	3-5	4	5	5	14	9
T2-T3	3-5	4	5-7	6	4-12	8
T3-T4	2-5	4	3-7	5	5-11	8
T4-T5	2-5	4	5-6	6	5-11	8
T5-T6	3-5	4	5-6	6	5-11	8
T6-T7	2-7	5	6	6	4-11	7
T7-T8	3-8	6	3-8	6	4-11	7
T8-T9	3-8	6	4-7	6	6-7	6
T9-T10	3-8	6	4-7	6	3-5	4
T10-T11	4-14	9	3-10	7	2-3	2
T11-T12	6-20	12	4-13	9	2-3	2
T12-L1	6-20	12	5-10	8	2-3	2
L1-L2	5-16	12	3-8	6	1-3	2
L2-L3	8-18	14	3-10	6	1-3	2
L3-L4	6-17	15	4-12	8	1-3	2
L4-L5	9-21	16	3-9	6	1-3	2
L5-S1	10-24	17	2-6	3	0-2	1

From White AA III, Panjabi MM: Clinical Biomechanics of the Spine, 2nd ed. Philadelphia, JB Lippincott, 1990.

degeneration or surgical intervention. Identification of this point also has implications for how forces are transmitted through the spine.

Relative movement of a vertebra can be divided into translational movement (sliding motions) and rotational movement. During physiologic movements, the components of compression force and bending moment acting on the spine vary along with the translational and bending movements. This action results in a varying axis of rotation position. The axis of rotation is defined as a "locus" or path the axis of rotation takes.[20]

During sagittal and frontal plane motions, the axis of rotation in the cervical spine is believed to be located in the anterior portion of the subjacent vertebra.[2] Coupling also occurs with cervical motions, however. In the thoracic spine, loads applied during flexion and extension motions result in an axis of rotation located at the inferior endplate of the lower

vertebra. This axis of rotation moves further down the vertebra when posterior shear force occurs during extension motions.[2] During flexion and extension motions, the axis of rotation occurs in the superior endplate of the inferior vertebra of the spinal motion segment.

During sagittal plane bending, the axis of rotation varies according to whether forward or backward bending is occurring. Because much of the flexion and extension in the sagittal plane occurs in the lumbar spine, much of the interest in the axis of rotation has also been focused on the lumbar spine. The superior vertebra translates anteriorly and posteriorly relative to the inferior vertebra as the vertebral body rotates around the nucleus. After degeneration of the disc, the axis of rotation can change dramatically[22] and result in marked changes in spine loading. Under these degenerative conditions, the axis of rotation has been reported to migrate toward the zygapophyseal joint during extension motions.[23] During

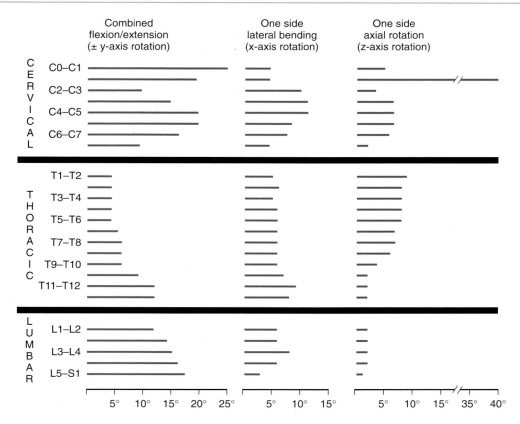

FIGURE 7–12 Composite estimate of representative values for ranges of motion at different levels of the spine in sagittal, lateral, and transverse planes of the body. (From White AA III, Panjabi MM: Clinical Biomechanics of the Spine, 2nd ed. Philadelphia, JB Lippincott, 1990.)

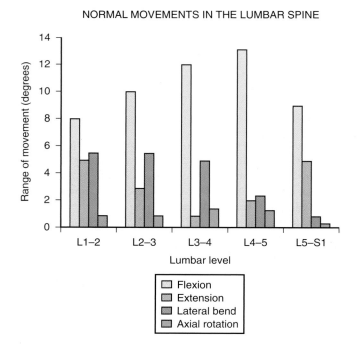

FIGURE 7–13 Ranges of motion in lumbar spine during flexion, extension, lateral bending, and rotation.[29,31] (From Adams MA, Bogduk N, Burton AK, et al: The Biomechanics of Back Pain, 2nd ed. Edinburgh, Churchill Livingstone, 2006.)

flexion, the axis of rotation seems to move and is dependent on coupling patterns during the flexion movement.

During lateral motions, the axis of rotation in the lumbar spine lies at the opposite side of the disc from the direction of motion. In other words, when bending to the right, the left side of the disc is where the axis of rotation is located.[2]

The axis of rotation for axial (torsion) movements has been difficult to locate. This axis of rotation is believed to lie within the posterior anulus fibrosus when exposed to torque.[24] Even small axial motion can create compression at one facet surface and tension at the opposite facet surface.[5] With disc degeneration, the axis of rotation becomes far less apparent, however, in the lumbar spine.[4] Under degenerative conditions, the locus of the axis of rotation has been reported to be significantly spread out over an extended area.[25]

Collectively, the literature has described the locations of the axis of rotation for various "normal" motions. It is apparent, however, that these axes change dramatically with degeneration and should be considered when considering load bearing through the spine and motion profiles.

Motion Coupling

A significant amount of coupling has been observed along the spinal column. Coupling is a function of the geometric characteristics of specific vertebrae, limitations in tissue properties of the disc and ligaments, and spine curvature. Movements are considered coupled when one motion is accompanied by motion in a different plane.[2] The motion in the primary or intended plane of movement is referred to as the main motion, and the accompanying motions are referred to as coupled motions.

Because coupling can have profound implications on the transmission of forces through the spine, it is important that the nature of coupling in the different regions of the spine be understood. From a clinical perspective, coupling is important in understanding the impact of various pathologies such as scoliosis and different types of spine trauma. In addition, an appreciation for coupling is important for understanding the impact of surgical interventions, such as the impact of fusion.

Coupling is most common in the cervical and lumbar spine, but can also occur in the thoracic spine. Coupling in the cervical and lumbar spine involves axial rotation coupled with lateral bending. Lumbar motion can involve cross-coupling in all three rotation directions. Motions in the lumbar spine are rarely unaccompanied by coupled movements. Coupled motions of the lumbar spine vary as a function of the spine level and a function of spine posture.[2]

Coupling patterns within the spine differ depending on the region of the spine. The cervical spine exhibits a striking degree of coupling in that lateral bending of the head is accompanied by significant amounts of cervical rotation; this is evident by observing the position of the spinous processes as lateral bending occurs. When lateral bend to the left occurs, the spinous processes point to the right, and when lateral bending to the right occurs, the spinous processes go to the left. It is generally thought that the angle of incline of the facet joints in the sagittal plane increases from the head toward the lower spine.[2] Generally, the average ratio of the coupled lateral bending compared with axial rotation is 0.51.[26]

The coupling of lateral bending and spine rotation can also occur in the thoracic spine. As with the cervical spine, lateral bending is coupled with axial rotation in such a way that the spinous process moves toward the convexity of the lateral curve. The vertebrae in the upper portion of the thoracic spine have motions that are strongly coupled, but not to the same degree as in the cervical spine. In the middle segments of the thoracic spine, the coupling motions are far less apparent. Coupled motions in this portion of the thoracic spine are inconsistent and can result in rotations opposite of those in the upper thoracic spine. Coupling patterns in the lower portion of the thoracic spine are weak. Although the patterns of coupling between axial rotation and lateral bending have been described in the literature, most likely owing to a desire to understand scoliosis, Panjabi and colleagues[27] have shown that coupling can occur in all 6 degrees of freedom.

Coupling patterns in the lumbar spine seem to differ from those of the cervical and thoracic spine. The most dominant coupling pattern of the lumbar spine seems to be lateral bending coupled with axial rotation (Table 7–2).[28] In this case, the spinous process moves in the same direction as lateral

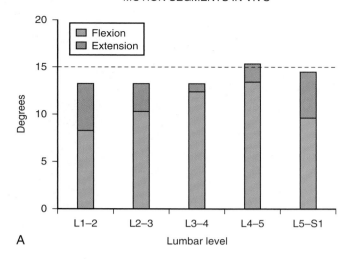

A

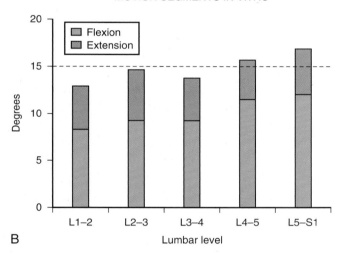

B

FIGURE 7–14 A and **B,** Range of flexion and extension motion in lumbar spine measured in vivo (**A**) and in vitro (**B**).[20,31] (From Adams MA, Bogduk N, Burton AK, et al: The Biomechanics of Back Pain, 2nd ed. Edinburgh, Churchill Livingstone, 2006.)

bending. This is exactly opposite the pattern in the cervical and upper thoracic spine. One group of researchers[29] reported, however, that coupling at L5-S1 occurs in a fashion similar to that of the lower cervical spine and opposite to that of the rest of the lumbar spine.

In vivo studies of the lumbar spine have shown the importance of muscular involvement in determining coupling patterns of the lumbar spine.[29] In vitro studies have reported that lateral bending motion was coupled with flexion motions between L1-L3, whereas in vivo studies reported that lateral motions are coupled with extension movements in these vertebrae. In addition, biomechanical analyses have shown that coupling in the lumbar spine can be influenced by posture of the spine.[29,30] One would expect that muscle control can also play an important role in coupling patterns.

TABLE 7-2 Coupled Motions of the Lumbar Spine

Primary Movement and Level	COUPLED MOVEMENTS					
	AXIAL ROTATION, DEGREES (+ TO LEFT)		FLEXION-EXTENSION, DEGREES (+ FLEXION)		LATERAL FLEXION, DEGREES (+ TO LEFT)	
	Mean	Range	Mean	Range	Mean	Range
Right Rotation						
L1	−1	−2 to 1	0	−3 to 3	3	−1 to 5
L2	−1	−2 to 1	0	−2 to 2	4	1 to 9
L3	−1	−3 to 1	0	−2 to 2	3	1 to 6
L4	−1	−2 to 1	0	−9 to 6	1	−3 to 3
L5	−1	−2 to 1	0	−5 to 3	−2	−7 to 0
Left Rotation						
L1	1	−1 to 1	0	−4 to 4	−3	−7 to −1
L2	1	−1 to 1	0	−4 to 4	−3	−5 to 0
L3	2	0 to 1	0	−3 to 2	−3	−6 to 0
L4	2	0 to 1	0	−7 to 2	−2	−5 to 1
L5	0	−2 to 1	0	−5 to 3	1	0 to 2
Right Lateral Flexion						
L1	0	−3 to 1	−2	−5 to 1	−5	−8 to −2
L2	1	−1 to 1	−1	−3 to 1	−5	−8 to −4
L3	1	−1 to 1	−1	−3 to 1	−5	−11 to 2
L4	1	0 to 1	0	−1 to 4	−3	−5 to 1
L5	0	−1 to 1	2	−3 to 8	0	−2 to 3
Left Lateral Flexion						
L1	0	−2 to 1)	−2	−9 to 0	6	4 to 10
L2	−1	−3 to 1)	−3	−4 to −1	6	2 to 10
L3	−1	−4 to 1)	−2	−4 to 3	6	−3 to 8
L4	−1	−4 to 1)	−1	−4 to 2	3	−3 to 6
L5	−2	−3 to 1)	0	−5 to 5	−3	−6 to 1

From Adams MA, Bogduk N, Burton AK, et al: The Biomechanics of Back Pain, 2nd ed. Edinburgh, Churchill Livingstone, 2006 (as reported by Pearcy and Tiberwall, 1984[23]).

TABLE 7-3 Average Neutral Zone (Degrees of Motion) for Different Spinal Motion Segments in Different Motion Planes

Vertebral Segments	Flexion-Extension	Lateral Bending	Axial Rotation
C0-C1	1.1	1.6	1.5
C1-C2	3.2	1.2	29.6
C3-C6	4.9	4	3.8
C7-T1 and T11-T1	1.5	2.2	1.2
L1-L2 and L3-L4	1.5	1.6	0.7
L5-S1	3	1.8	0.4

From White AA III, Panjabi MM: Clinical Biomechanics of the Spine, 2nd ed. Philadelphia, JB Lippincott, 1990.

Neutral Zone Limits

As discussed earlier, the neutral zone is important for understanding when tissues first experience resistance to movement. Low intersegmental resistance to motion can be an indication of biomechanical problems. The neutral zones for the different planes of motion have been extensively described by Panjabi and colleagues.[31-33] Table 7-3 shows estimates for the neutral zones for rotary motions as a function of the plane of motion and the spine level.[2] For the most part, the neutral zone is limited in range except for certain vertebrae in certain axes of rotation. From a clinical perspective, one must be sensitive to the fact that normal and abnormal neutral zones can be very different for different vertebrae.

A large neutral zone can be an indication of several biomechanical factors. First, the neutral zone has been observed to increase with age.[34] Second, a larger than expected neutral zone can indicate injury to the tissue.[35] Third, some clinicians contend that low resistance to movement is an indication of clinical instability.[36] There are several reasons to consider carefully the range of movement within the neutral zone.

Load Tolerance of Spinal Motion Segments

The precise tolerance characteristics of human spinal tissues, such as muscles, ligaments, tendons, and bones, loaded under various conditions has been difficult to establish. Structure tolerances have been observed to vary greatly even under similar loading conditions because of their dependence on many factors, such as strain rate (rate of loading), age of the structure, frequency of loading, physiologic influences, heredity, conditioning, and other unknown factors. In addition, it has been impossible to measure these tolerances under in vivo conditions. Many of the estimates of tissue tolerance have been derived from various animal or theoretical constructs.

Tolerance data limits have been derived primarily from cadaveric tissue. The obvious compromise in this approach is that in vitro tissue when tested does not have the ability to adapt or recover (and potentially increase tolerance) as does a live human. The material properties of cadaveric tissue vary depending on the manner in which the specimen was prepared for testing. At least one study suggests that living tissue failure might occur at magnitudes below those observed in cadaveric specimens.[37]

Muscle and Tendon Strain

Muscle has the lowest tolerance among the tissues of the spine. The ultimate strength of a muscle has been estimated at 32 MPa.[38] Muscle often ruptures before a (healthy) tendon.[39] Tendon stress has been estimated to be between 60 MPa and 100 MPa.[38,39] There seems to be a safety margin between the muscle failure point and the failure point of the tendon by a factor of about twofold[39] to threefold.[38]

Ligament and Bone Tolerance

Ultimate ligament stress has been estimated at approximately 20 MPa. The ultimate stress of bone has been found to depend on the direction of loading. Bone tolerance can range from 51 MPa in transverse tension to 190 MPa in longitudinal compression.

A temporal component to ligament recovery has also been reported. One study found that ligaments required extended periods to regain structural integrity. During the recovery period, compensatory muscle activities have been observed.[40-47] Recovery time has been observed to be several times the loading duration.

Because the spinal ligaments often are the structure that protects the spinal system, it is important to appreciate the failure limits of the various spinal ligaments; these are shown in Table 7–4. Note that the load tolerance of these ligaments and the deformation characteristics of the ligaments vary

markedly according to the region of the spine and the specific ligament involved. Generally, the lower the level of the spinal ligament, the greater is the tolerance of the ligament. There are notable exceptions to this trend, however. Spinal ligaments are viscoelastic and can increase their length under load. They can be responsible for an increase in the neutral zone; excessive movement can also initiate muscle activities intended to regain stability.[40,48]

Contact Force Tolerance

Contemporary logic suggests that pain secondary to biomechanical loading of the spine may result from direct stimulation to the facet joints, pressure on the anulus, or pressure on the longitudinal ligaments.[9] At these sites, inflammatory responses and analgesic responses are thought to be involved in the development of pressure and pain. It is much more difficult to specify load tolerance thresholds for contact pressures because the body's individual responses to the imposed loads collectively define the pressure imposed on the spinal structure. The tolerance limits for these structures has not been well defined at this time.

Tolerance of Specific Spine Structures

The general structure tolerance, or failure, limits in response to loading of the lumbar spine have been well investigated. Table 7–5 provides a summary of these tolerances reported as a function of the nature of the loading for the spinal motion segment structures and the disc and vertebral body structures.[20]

Compression

The compression dimension of spine tolerance has been widely examined. Of all the structures in the spinal motion segment, the endplate is considered to be the "weak point of the system," or the structure with the lowest tolerance to force. Compression failure limits are a function of age, with older endplates failing at lower levels of force, and gender, with female tolerances lower than male tolerances.[49,50] Figure 7–15 shows a summary of the compression strength for much of the spine. The magnitude of force required for endplate tissue failure follows a normal distribution that ranges from 2000 to greater than 14,000 N. When compression forces increase on a spinal motion segment, the first signs of damage usually occur at the endplate or the trabeculae that support the endplate. The endplate must be a thin structure to serve its nutrition transport function. Because it is thin, it is also a very weak structure, however, and subject to early failure when load is applied.

Failure is believed to be initiated by the nucleus pulposus of the adjacent disc. This nucleus causes the endplate to bulge and compromise the vertebral body. The superior endplate is damaged more often than the lower endplate. In some cases, it is possible for a portion of the nucleus pulposus to make its way vertically through a herniation of the endplate into the bone.[20] This herniation can calcify and form a Schmorl node.

TABLE 7–4 Failure Strength of Spinal Ligaments

	LOAD (N)		DEFORMATION (mm)		STRESS (MPa)		STRAIN (%)	
	Average	Range	Average	Range	Average	Range	Average	Range
Upper Cervical								
C0-C1								
Anterior atlanto-occipital membrane	233		18.9					
Posterior atlanto-occipital membrane	83		18.1					
C1-C2								
ALL	281	170-700	12.3					
Atlanto-axial membrane	113		8.7					
CL	157		11.4					
Transverse ligament	354							
C0-C2								
Apical	214		11.5					
Alar	286	215-357	14.1					
Vertical cruciate	436		25.2					
Tectorial membrane	76		11.9					
Lower Cervical								
ALL	111.5	47-176	8.95	4.2-13.7				
PLL	74.5	47-102	6.4	3.4-9.4				
LF	138.5	56-221	8.3	3.7-12.9				
CL	204	144-264	8.4	6.8-10				
ISL	35.5	26-45	7.35	5.5-9.2				
SSL								
Thoracic								
ALL	295.5	123-468	10.25	6.3-14.2				
PLL	106	74-138	5.25	3.2-7.3				
LF	200	135-265	8.65	6.3-11				
CL	168	63-273	6.75	3.9-9.6				
ISL	75.5	31-120	5.25	3.8-6.7				
SSL	319.5	101-538	14.1	7.2-21				
Lumbar								
ALL	450	390-510	15.2	7-20	11.6	2.4-21	36.5	16-57
PLL	324	264-384	5.1	4.2-7	11.5	2.9-20	26	8-44
LF	285	230-340	12.7	12-14.5	8.7	2.4-15	26	10-46
CL	222	160-284	11.3	9.8-12.8	7.6	7.6	12	12
ISL	125	120-130	13	7.4-17.8	3.2	1.8-4.6	13	13
SSL	150	100-200	25.9	22.1-28.1	5.4	2-8.7	32.5	26-39

ALL, anterior longitudinal ligament; CL, capsular ligament; ISL, interspinous ligament; LF, ligamentum flavum; PLL, posterior longitudinal ligament; SSL, supraspinous ligament.
From White AA III, Panjabi MM: Clinical Biomechanics of the Spine, 2nd ed. Philadelphia, JB Lippincott, 1990 (data from Chazal et al, Dvorak et al, Goel et al, Myklebust et al, Nachemson and Evans, Panjabi et al, and Tkaczuk).

Endplate fractures are difficult to detect via routine radiographs; however, magnetic resonance imaging (MRI) can indicate biologic (modic) changes that are characteristic of vertical displacement of the nucleus pulposus.[20]

When the endplate experiences excessive compressive load, the endplate can bulge into the vertebral body, increasing the volume available to the nucleus. This decompression of the nucleus means that it cannot resist compression well, and more of the load is borne by the anulus fibrosus. The anulus can become unstable and the lamellae can become compressed and cannot be supported any longer by the nucleus. It is believed that this form of disc loading can result in internal derangement of the disc and, potentially, reverse bulging of the inner lamellae.

As noted earlier, endplate tolerance seems to be a function of gender and age.[49,50] Tolerance estimates based on a review of the literature are shown in Figure 7–16. Although great variability is evident, women generally have lower compression tolerance by an average of almost 2 kN compared with men. In addition, tolerance reduces significantly with age. Age

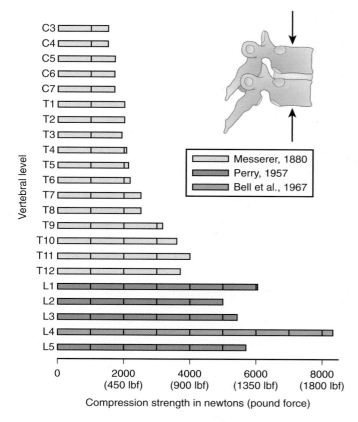

FIGURE 7–15 Estimates of vertebral compression tolerance (strength) under slow load rates for the various vertebrae from C3 to L5.[75-77] (From White AA III, Panjabi MM: Clinical Biomechanics of the Spine, 2nd ed. Philadelphia, JB Lippincott, 1990.)

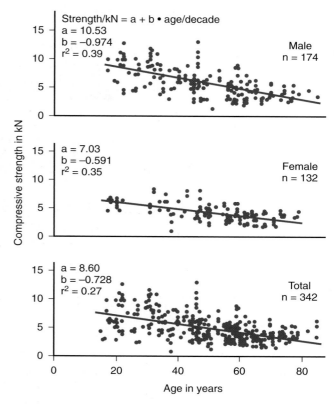

FIGURE 7–16 Strength tolerance to static lumbar compression derived from the literature as a function of age and gender. (From Jager M, Luttmann A, Laurig W: Lumbar load during one-hand bricklaying. Int J Indust Ergo 8:261-277, 1991.)

influences endplate tolerance differently between men and women, however. The decrease in tolerance with age is nearly two times greater for men compared with women.[49,50] In addition, the strength of the vertebrae is nearly 0.8 kN lower than that of the disc.[50] Finally, strength increases as one moves down the lumbar spine by approximately 0.3 kN per lumbar level.[51]

Repetitive loading also seems to influence the tolerance to load of the motion segment. Figure 7–17 shows how the number of load repetitions and the relative magnitude of the load collectively have a dramatic impact on probability of failure of the segment. As can be seen in this figure, when the relative load becomes greater, the chances of failure increase the risk significantly when the number of loading cycles increase.[51] Studies have also shown that as the flexion angle increases, the number of cycles required for failure is dramatically reduced.[52,53]

Shear

The disc fibers and intervertebral ligaments are inadequately oriented to resist shear forces. Shear causes the disc to creep during repetitive loading.[54] Under many situations, the neural arch resists shear force, however. The articular process resists on average 2 kN of load before failure; however, this can range from 0.6 to 2.8 kN.[55] The specific point of load application can

TABLE 7–5 Tolerance of Lumbar Motion Segment and Disc Structures as a Function Load and Motion Characteristics

	Failure Site	**Average Tolerance**
Motion Segments		
Compression	Endplate	5.2 (± 1.8) kN all specimens
		6.1 (± 1.8) kN men (20-50 yr old)
Shear	Neural arch	2 kN
Flexion	Posterior ligaments	73 (± 18) N-m with compressive load of 0.5-1 kN
Extension	Neural arch	26-45 N-m
Torsion	Neural arch	25-88 N-m
Flexion and compression	Disc or vertebra	5.4 kN
Disc plus Vertebral Bodies		
Shear	Anulus	0.5 kN
Flexion	Posterior anulus	33(± 13 N-m)
Torsion	Anulus	10-31 N-m

From Adams MA, Bogduk N, Burton AK, et al: The Biomechanics of Back Pain, 2nd ed. Edinburgh, Churchill Livingstone, 2006.

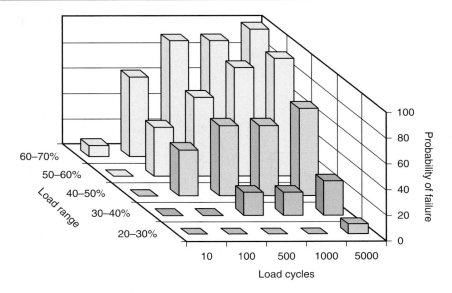

FIGURE 7–17 Probability of vertebrae failure as a function of load magnitude and number of cycles of loading.[51] (Adapted from Marras WS: The Working Back: A Systems View. Hoboken, John Wiley & Sons, 2008.)

also greatly affect tolerance of the neural arch to shear. Figure 7–18 shows how differing methods of shear force application can result in dramatically different neural arch load tolerances.[56,57]

Repetitive shear loading can also reduce the tolerance to 380 N.[55] Some authors have concluded that the limit at which shear begins to increase risk is 750 to 1000 N,[58-60] although this is also known to vary according to load rate.[61,62] In addition, studies have reported failure occurring at the pars under these conditions.

Torsion

The motion segments offer little resistance to small angles of axial rotation. Torsion is first resisted by collagen fibers

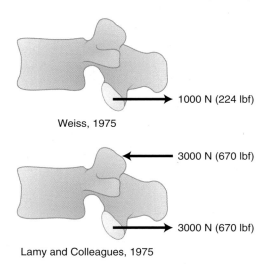

FIGURE 7–18 Force tolerance of neural arch varies greatly as a function of shear force application method.[26,57] (From White AA III, Panjabi MM: Clinical Biomechanics of the Spine, 2nd ed. Philadelphia, JB Lippincott, 1990.)

in the anulus that simply stretch slightly.[20,63] With further axial motion, the articular surfaces make contact at one of the zygapophyseal joints, and motion is limited to 1 or 2 degrees.[24] This range of motion increases, however, with greater disc degeneration.[64-66] Under typical loading conditions (involving torsion and compression), the loads imposed on the spine are shared by several structures. At the limit of the natural range of movement, 30% to 70% of the applied torque is resisted by the zygapophyseal joint as a compressive load, 20% to 50% is resisted by the disc, and less than 15% is resisted by all of the intervertebral ligaments collectively.[20,24]

The lower limit for initiation of damage owing to torque application seems to begin at about 10 to 30 N-m.[24] Many clinicians believe that damage owing to torsional movements occurs at the zygapophyseal joint before damage occurs to the discs.[20]

Flexion and Extension

Significant repositioning of the spine occurs when flexion and extension of the spine occurs. Different structures are responsible for resisting force, and the tolerance of the spine can change. During extension of the spine, 60% to 70% of the applied load is resisted by the neural arch. Studies have reported damage resulting from 3 to 8 degrees of extension under bending moments of 28 to 45 N-m.[67,68] Resistance to extension is offered by the disc and the anterior longitudinal ligament.[20] Of particular concern is the risk of the anulus bulging into the vertebral canal and compromising canal space.

It is hypothesized that the zygapophyseal joint would be the structure damaged first owing to extension; however, it is also believed that the interspinous ligament may be at risk because it would be compressed by opposing spinous processes. Rapid load rates, possibly resulting from athletic endeavors, are also thought potentially to increase risk.

Flexion can lead to injury when imposed moments reach 50 to 80 N-m.[69-71] Damage occurs when the spinal motion segment reaches 5 to 9 degrees per motion segment in the upper lumbar spine and 10 to 16 degrees per segment in the lower lumbar spine. The first structures to sustain damage are the interspinous and supraspinous ligaments.[71] During complex motions involving flexion and lateral bending, the capsular ligaments can also be compromised. The final tissue to fail is the outer posterior anulus fibrosus. In isolation (without the ligaments), the disc can fail when flexed at 18 degrees with an application of 15 to 50 N-m of load.[72] As with most structures, load rate also plays a role in tolerance. Resistance to flexion can increase by more than 10% when rapid motions (10 seconds) are compared with slow (1 second) motions.[73] Static postures seem to reduce resistance to bending by very large amounts, probably owing to the interrelationship between the ligamentous system and muscular control.[42]

Lateral Motion

Less has been reported about the tolerance associated with lateral bending moment exposure. Some studies have reported that a lateral bending moment of 10 N-m results in 4 to 6 degrees of lateral bending in the lumbar spine with most of the resistance occurring at the disc.[65,74] If the disc experiences degeneration, the range of motion is greatly reduced to 3 to 4 degrees, however, practically eliminating the neutral zone.[65]

System

As can be seen through this review, the spine performs several important functions: It transmits force, allows motion, and protects the spinal cord. Although these functions have been considered independently here, it is important to develop an appreciation for the systematic nature of these spine functions. Although these functions have been described independently, these functions interact in such a way that the inability to perform one of these functions can also affect the ability to perform other functions.

If the disc becomes compromised in its mechanical integrity, and disc space is reduced, it can alter the load transmission between vertebrae. With less disc space, more of the load may be transmitted through the posterior elements, and this repeated loading may change the biochemical behavior of the system. This change may result in an upregulation of pro-inflammatory biochemical activity and increased pain transmission. Similarly, reduced disc space height may alter the motion characteristics of the spinal motion segments. With less disc space, the stability of the joint can be compromised, and the contact points of the posterior elements can be altered. This alteration could change the kinematic signature of the spine.

Finally, a narrowed disc space could compromise the protection of the nerve root because there is less space for the nerve root to pass through the intervertebral foramen. A compromise of the disc could lead to load transmission irregularities, instability, motion restrictions, and a compromise of the nerve root. This is just one example of how interrelated the components of the spine are from a biomechanical perspective.

As can be seen from this discussion, biomechanics of the spine not only can influence the various dimensions of the biomechanical system, but it also can influence the biochemical behavior of the system. Because biomechanical considerations provide an understanding of the forces that are generated on the system, some authors are beginning to consider the spine as a mechanobiologic system.

Summary

By nature, the spine is a complex structure that provides protection for the spinal cord and a structure to support loads in numerous postures and positions. In addition, the healthy spine limits physiologic movement to conditions that protect the structures of the spine. With trauma and degeneration, the spine loses its ability to achieve these functions adequately.

Biomechanics provides a means to characterize and assess the status of the spine quantitatively and precisely. Quantification provides a rationale for one to determine "how much is too much" exposure to the physical conditions that might damage the spinal system. This chapter has systematically summarized and characterized the capacity of the spinal motion segments in terms of kinematic capacity and load tolerance.

The spinal structures themselves are physiologically unique and have evolved in such a manner that their functions are unique. Although this chapter has examined the capacity of the individual motion segments, this evaluation should make it clear that the spine is truly a system of components that act collectively and interactively to achieve the functions of motion and load support. The kinematic and load support capacities of the motion segment vary significantly as a function of spinal level, direction of motion, direction of load application, and temporal exposure characteristics.

Although presented as basic information, this information should be considered the fundamental scientific foundation for understanding how the spine functions, how disorders and pain might occur in the spine, how exposure to activities of daily living and occupational conditions might affect the spine status, and what functions need to be restored clinically. Biomechanical features and function change throughout life. Aging alone alters the biomechanical properties of the spine. It has also been well established, however, that various exposures can greatly accelerate the degenerative process and the biomechanical functioning of the spine.

As knowledge of the spine increases, it is clear that a biomechanical foundation is essential for prevention and treatment of spinal disorders. A better understanding of spine function can be achieved through a better quantification of physical attributes, yielding improved sensitivity and specificity of functional understanding and interventions.

KEY REFERENCES

1. Adams MA, Bogduk N, Burton AK, et al: The Biomechanics of Back Pain, 2nd ed. Edinburgh, Churchill Livingstone, 2006.
   This book incorporates scientific evidence into a mechanistic review of low back pain pathology.

2. White AA 3rd, Panjabi MM: Clinical Biomechanics of the Spine. Philadelphia, Lippincott-Raven, 1990.
   This classic reference reviews how pure biomechanical principles relate to clinical thinking regarding the spine.

3. Marras WS: The Working Back: A Systems View. Hoboken, NJ, John Wiley & Sons, 2008.
   This book shows how scientific findings related to physical exposure, psychosocial exposures, and individual findings interact to influence spine tissue loading that may initiate potential pain pathways.

4. McGill S: Ultimate Back Fitness and Performance. Waterloo, Canada, Wabuno Publishers, 2004.
   This reference shows how biomechanical principles relate to function and rehabilitation of the back.

5. National Research Council (NRC)/Institute of Medicine (IOM): Musculoskeletal Disorders and the Workplace: Low Back and Upper Extremities. Washington, DC, National Academy of Sciences, National Research Council, National Academy Press, 2001.
   This is a scientific review of the available evidence relating personal, physical, and psychological exposures to risk of low back pain.

REFERENCES

1. Bernhardt M, White AA 3rd, Panjabi MM: Biomechanical considerations of spinal stability. In Herkowitz HN, Garfin SR, Eismont FJ, et al (eds): Rothman-Simeone The Spine. Philadelphia, WB Saunders, 2006.

2. White AA 3rd, Panjabi MM: Clinical Biomechanics of the Spine. Philadelphia, Lippincott-Raven, 1990.

3. Quint U, Wilke HJ, Shirazi-Adl A, et al: Importance of the intersegmental trunk muscles for the stability of the lumbar spine: A biomechanical study in vitro. Spine 23:1937-1945, 1998.

4. Cholewicki J, McGill S: Mechanical stability of the in vivo lumbar spine: Implications of injury and chronic low back pain. Clin Biomech (Bristol, Avon) 11:1-15, 1996.

5. Farfan HF, Gracovetsky S: The nature of instability. Spine 9:714-719, 1984.

6. Granata KP, Marras WS: Cost-benefit of muscle cocontraction in protecting against spinal instability. Spine 25:1398-1404, 2000.

7. Panjabi MM: Clinical spinal instability and low back pain. J Electromyogr Kinesiol 13:371-379, 2003.

8. Reeves NP, Narendra KS, Cholewicki J: Spine stability: The six blind men and the elephant. Clin Biomech (Bristol, Avon) 22:266-274, 2007.

9. Marras WS: The Working Back: A Systems View. Hoboken, NJ, John Wiley & Sons, 2008.

10. Lee CK: Accelerated degeneration of the segment adjacent to a lumbar fusion. Spine 13:375-377, 1988.

11. Ghiselli G, Wang JC, Bhatia NN, et al: Adjacent segment degeneration in the lumbar spine. J Bone Joint Surg Am 86:1497-1503, 2004.

12. van Ooij A, Oner FC, Verbout AJ: Complications of artificial disc replacement: A report of 27 patients with the SB Charite disc. J Spinal Disord Tech 16:369-383, 2003.

13. Dooris AP, Goel VK, Grosland NM, et al: Load-sharing between anterior and posterior elements in a lumbar motion segment implanted with an artificial disc. Spine 26:E122-E129, 2001.

14. Brinkmann P, Biggermann M, Hilweg D: Prediction of the compressive strength of human lumbar vertebrae. Clin Biomech (Bristol, Avon) 4:S1-S27, 1989.

15. Yoganandan N, Larson SJ, Gallagher M, et al: Correlation of microtrauma in the lumbar spine with intraosseous pressures. Spine 19:435-440, 1994.

16. Marras WS, et al: The quantification of low back disorder using motion measures: Methodology and validation. Spine 24:2091-2100, 1999.

17. Marras WS, et al: The classification of anatomic- and symptom-based low back disorders using motion measure models. Spine 20:2531-2546, 1995.

18. Marras WS, Wongsam PE: Flexibility and velocity of the normal and impaired lumbar spine. Arch Phys Med Rehabil 67:213-217, 1986.

19. Stokes IA, Wilder DG, Frymoyer JW, et al: 1980 Volvo award in clinical sciences. Assessment of patients with low-back pain by biplanar radiographic measurement of intervertebral motion. Spine 6:233-240, 1981.

20. Adams MA, Bogduk N, Burton AK, et al: The Biomechanics of Back Pain, 2nd ed. Edinburgh, Churchill Livingstone, 2006.

21. Haughton VM, Schmidt TA, Keele K, et al: Flexibility of lumbar spinal motion segments correlated to type of tears in the annulus fibrosus. J Neurosurg 92:81-86, 2000.

22. Gertzbein SD, et al: Centrode patterns and segmental instability in degenerative disc disease. Spine 10:257-261, 1985.

23. Zhao F, Pollintine P, Hole BD, et al: Discogenic origins of spinal instability. Spine 30:2621-2630, 2005.

24. Adams MA, Hutton WC: The relevance of torsion to the mechanical derangement of the lumbar spine. Spine 6:241-248, 1981.

25. Rolander SD: Motion of the lumbar spine with special reference to the stabilizing effect of posterior fusion: An experimental study on autopsy specimens. Acta Orthop Scand Suppl 90:1-144, 1966.

26. Moroney SP, Schultz AB, Miller JA, et al: Load-displacement properties of lower cervical spine motion segments. J Biomech 21:769-779, 1988.

27. Panjabi MM, Brand RA Jr, White AA 3rd: Three-dimensional flexibility and stiffness properties of the human thoracic spine. J Biomech 9:185-192, 1976.

28. Bogduk N: Clinical Anatomy of the Lumbar Spine and Sacrum. Edinburgh, Churchill Livingstone, 2005.

29. Pearcy MJ, Tibrewal SB: Axial rotation and lateral bending in the normal lumbar spine measured by three-dimensional radiography. Spine 9:582-587, 1984.

30. Cholewicki J, Crisco JJ 3rd, Oxland TR, et al: Effects of posture and structure on three-dimensional coupled rotations in the lumbar spine: A biomechanical analysis. Spine 21:2421-2428, 1996.

31. Pearcy M, Portek I, Shepherd J: Three-dimensional x-ray analysis of normal movement in the lumbar spine. Spine 9:294-297, 1984.

32. Panjabi M, et al: Three-dimensional movements of the upper cervical spine. Spine 13:726-730, 1988.

33. Yamamoto I, Panjabi MM, Crisco T, et al: Three-dimensional movements of the whole lumbar spine and lumbosacral joint. Spine 14:1256-1260, 1989.

34. Mimura M, et al: Disc degeneration affects the multidirectional flexibility of the lumbar spine. Spine 19:1371-1380, 1994.

35. Oxland TR, Panjabi MM: The onset and progression of spinal injury: A demonstration of neutral zone sensitivity. J Biomech 25:1165-1172, 1992.

36. Panjabi MM: The stabilizing system of the spine. Part II: Neutral zone and instability hypothesis. J Spinal Disord 5:390-396; discussion 397, 1992.

37. Yoganandan N: Biomechanical identification of injury to an intervertebral joint. Clin Biomech 1:149, 1986.

38. Hoy MG, Zajac FE, Gordon ME: A musculoskeletal model of the human lower extremity: The effect of muscle, tendon, and moment arm on the moment-angle relationship of musculotendon actuators at the hip, knee, and ankle. J Biomech 23:157-169, 1990.

39. Nordin M, Frankel V: Basic Biomechanics of the Musculoskeletal System. Philadelphia, Lea & Febiger, 1989.

40. Solomonow M: Ligaments: A source of work-related musculoskeletal disorders. J Electromyogr Kinesiol 14:49-60, 2004.

41. Solomonow M, Zhou BH, Baratta RV, et al: Biomechanics of increased exposure to lumbar injury caused by cyclic loading. Part 1: Loss of reflexive muscular stabilization. Spine 24:2426-2434, 1999.

42. Solomonow M, Zhou BH, Harris M, et al: The ligamento-muscular stabilizing system of the spine. Spine 23:2552-2562, 1998.

43. Stubbs M, et al: Ligamento-muscular protective reflex in the lumbar spine of the feline. J Electromyogr Kinesiol 8:197-204, 1998.

44. Gedalia U, et al: Biomechanics of increased exposure to lumbar injury caused by cyclic loading. Part 2: Recovery of reflexive muscular stability with rest. Spine 24:2461-2467, 1999.

45. Wang JL, Parnianpour M, Shirazi-Adl A, et al: Viscoelastic finite-element analysis of a lumbar motion segment in combined compression and sagittal flexion: Effect of loading rate. Spine 25:310-318, 2000.

46. Solomonow M, Zhou B, Baratta RV, et al: Neuromuscular disorders associated with static lumbar flexion: A feline model. J Electromyogr Kinesiol 12:81-90, 2002.

47. Solomonow M, et al: Biexponential recovery model of lumbar viscoelastic laxity and reflexive muscular activity after prolonged cyclic loading. Clin Biomech (Bristol, Avon) 15:167-175, 2000.

48. Solomonow M, Eversull E, He Zhou B, et al: Neuromuscular neutral zones associated with viscoelastic hysteresis during cyclic lumbar flexion. Spine 26:E314-E324, 2001.

49. Jager M, Luttmann A: Compressive strength of lumbar spine elements related to age, gender, and other influences. J Electromyogr Kinesiol 1:291-294, 1991.

50. Jager M, Luttmann A, Laurig W: Lumbar load during one-hand bricklaying. Int J Indust Ergo 8:261-277, 1991.

51. Brinkmann P, Biggermann M, Hilweg D: Fatigue fracture of human lumbar vertebrae. Clin Biomech (Bristol, Avon) 3:S1-S23, 1988.

52. Gallagher S, Marras WS, Litsky AS, et al: Torso flexion loads and the fatigue failure of human lumbosacral motion segments. Spine 30:2265-2273, 2005.

53. Gallagher S, Marras WS, Litsky AS, et al: An exploratory study of loading and morphometric factors associated with specific failure modes in fatigue testing of lumbar motion segments. Clin Biomech (Bristol, Avon) 21:228-234, 2006.

54. Cyron BM, Hutton WC: The behaviour of the lumbar intervertebral disc under repetitive forces. Int Orthop 5:203-207, 1981.

55. Cyron BM, Hutton WC, Troup JD: Spondylolytic fractures. J Bone Joint Surg Br 58:462-466, 1976.

56. Lamy C, Bazergui A, Kraus H, et al: The strength of the neural arch and the etiology of spondylolysis. Orthop Clin North Am 6:215-231, 1975.

57. Weiss EB: Stress at the lumbosacral junction. Orthop Clin North Am 66:83, 1975.

58. McGill S: Low Back Disorders: Evidence-Based Prevention and Rehabilitation. Champaign, IL, Human Kinetics, 2002.

59. Marras WS: Occupational low back disorder causation and control. Ergonomics 43:880-902, 2000.

60. NRC/IOM: Musculoskeletal disorders and the workplace: low back and upper extremity. Washington, DC, National Academy of Sciences, National Research Council, National Academy Press, 2001.

61. Yingling VR, McGill SM: Anterior shear of spinal motion segments: Kinematics, kinetics, and resultant injuries observed in a porcine model. Spine 24:1882-1889, 1999.

62. Yingling VR, McGill SM: Mechanical properties and failure mechanics of the spine under posterior shear load: Observations from a porcine model. J Spinal Disord 12:501-508, 1999.

63. Adams MA, Dolan P: Spine biomechanics. J Biomech 38:1972-1983, 2005.

64. Oxland TR, Crisco JJ 3rd, Panjabi MM, et al: The effect of injury on rotational coupling at the lumbosacral joint: A biomechanical investigation. Spine 17:74-80, 1992.

65. Oxland TR, et al: The relative importance of vertebral bone density and disc degeneration in spinal flexibility and interbody implant performance: An in vitro study. Spine 21:2558-2569, 1996.

66. Oxland TR, Grant JP, Dvorak MF, et al: Effects of endplate removal on the structural properties of the lower lumbar vertebral bodies. Spine 28:771-777, 2003.

67. Adams MA, Dolan P, Hutton WC: The lumbar spine in backward bending. Spine 13:1019-1026, 1988.

68. Green TP, Allvey JC, Adams MA: Spondylolysis: Bending of the inferior articular processes of lumbar vertebrae during simulated spinal movements. Spine 19:2683-2691, 1994.

69. Adams MA, Dolan P: A technique for quantifying the bending moment acting on the lumbar spine in vivo. J Biomech 24:117-126, 1991.

70. Adams MA, Hutton WC: The effect of posture on diffusion into lumbar intervertebral discs. J Anat 147:121-134, 1986.

71. Adams MA, Hutton WC, Stott JR: The resistance to flexion of the lumbar intervertebral joint. Spine 5:245-253, 1980.

72. Adams MA, Green TP, Dolan P: The strength in anterior bending of lumbar intervertebral discs. Spine 19:2197-2203, 1994.

73. Adams MA, Dolan P: Time-dependent changes in the lumbar spine's resistance to bending. Clin Biomech (Bristol, Avon) 11:194-200, 1996.

74. Peng B, et al: Possible pathogenesis of painful intervertebral disc degeneration. Spine 31:560-566, 2006.

75. Bell GH, Dunbar O, Beck JS, et al: Variations in strength of vertebrae with age and their relation to osteoporosis. Calcif Tissue Res 1:75-86, 1967.

76. Messerer O: In: Gottaschen Buchhandling. JG Stutgart, 1880.

77. Perry O: In: Encyclopedia of Medical Radiology. New York, Springer-Verlag, 1974.

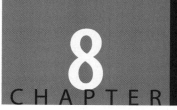

8
CHAPTER

Sciatica and Nerve Root Pain in Disc Herniation and Spinal Stenosis: A Basic Science Review and Clinical Perspective

Kjell Olmarker, MD, PhD
Björn Rydevik, MD, PhD
Shinichi Kikuchi, MD, PhD
Robert R. Myers, PhD

The clinical symptoms seen in association with lumbar disc herniation and spinal stenosis[1,2] are based on pathophysiologic involvement of spinal nerve roots. There has been an increasing interest in this topic during the past decade, and more recent research has been aimed at defining basic pathophysiologic events at the tissue, cellular, or subcellular level that are involved in the generation of sciatica and nerve root pain. This chapter reviews the current knowledge about these mechanisms and discusses these mechanisms in relation to the clinical features of lumbar disc herniation and spinal stenosis.

Pathophysiologic Mechanisms in Relation to Clinical Symptoms

The symptoms of nerve root pathophysiology may be divided into two main categories: pain and nerve dysfunction.[2] Nerve root pain is typically radiating in nature and is usually related to a specific nerve root or roots. Nerve dysfunction may be present in motor and sensory modalities, producing motor weakness and sensory disturbances. One may assume that pain and nerve dysfunction are due to different pathophysiologic events, but they are tightly linked through mechanisms that are discussed in this chapter.

Two specific mechanisms at the "tissue level" may be defined: (1) mechanical deformation of the nerve roots and (2) biologic or biochemical activity of the disc tissue with effects on the roots. The mechanical deformation theory is the oldest concept of nerve root injury induced by herniated disc tissue and dates back to the turn of the 20th century with clinical observations on injuries in the lumbosacral junction with subsequent leg pain and includes the more recent seminal observations of Mixter and Barr.[1-5] The theory that biologic activity of the disc tissue may injure the nerve roots was demonstrated experimentally in 1993.[6] The experimental knowledge regarding these two mechanisms is discussed separately.

Mechanical Effects on Nerve Roots

Enclosed by the vertebral bones, the spinal nerve roots are relatively well protected from external trauma. The nerve roots do not possess the same amounts and organization of protective connective tissue sheaths as do the peripheral nerves, however. The spinal nerve roots may be particularly sensitive to mechanical deformation secondary to intraspinal disorders, such as disc herniations and protrusions, spinal stenosis, degenerative disorders, and tumors.[7-9] There has been moderate research interest in the past regarding nerve root compression. Gelfan and Tarlov[10] in 1956 and Sharpless[11] in 1975 performed some initial experiments on the effects of compression on nerve impulse conduction. Although no calibration was performed on the compression devices used, the results of both studies indicated that nerve roots were more susceptible to compression than peripheral nerves. Interest in nerve root pathophysiology has increased considerably more recently, and numerous studies are reviewed here.

Experimental Compression of Nerve Roots

In 1991, a model was presented that for the first time allowed for experimental, graded compression of cauda equina nerve roots at known pressure levels.[7,8] In this model, the cauda equina of pigs was compressed by an inflatable balloon that was fixed to the spine (Fig. 8–1). The cauda equina could also be observed through the translucent balloon. This model made it possible to study the flow in the intrinsic nerve root blood vessels at various pressure levels[12] because the blood flow and vessel diameters of the intrinsic vessels could be observed simultaneously through the balloon with the use of a vital microscope. The average occlusion pressure for the arterioles was found to be slightly below and directly related to the systolic blood pressure. The blood flow in the capillary networks was intimately dependent on the blood flow of the adjacent venules. This finding corroborates the assumption that venular stasis may induce capillary stasis and changes in the microcirculation of the nerve tissue, which has been

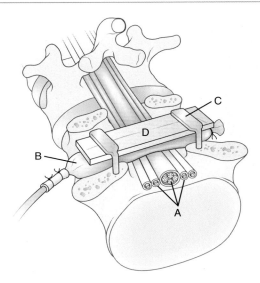

FIGURE 8–1 Schematic drawing of experimental nerve root compression model. Cauda equina (*A*) is compressed by inflatable balloon (*B*) that is fixed to spine by two L-shaped pins (*C*) and Plexiglas plate (*D*). (From Olmarker K, Holm S, Rosenqvist A-L, et al: Experimental nerve root compression: A model of acute, graded compression of the porcine cauda equina and an analysis of neural and vascular anatomy. Spine [Phila Pa 1976] 16:61-69, 1991.)

suggested as one mechanism in carpal tunnel syndrome.[13] The mean occlusion pressures for the venules showed large variations. A pressure of 5 to 10 mm Hg was found to be sufficient for inducing venular occlusion. Because of retrograde stasis, it is assumed that the capillary blood flow also would be affected in such situations.

In the same experimental setup, the effects of gradual decompression, after initial acute compression maintained for only a short while, were studied.[14] The average pressure for starting the blood flow was seen to be slightly lower at decompression than at compression for arterioles, capillaries, and venules. With this protocol, there was not a full restoration of the blood flow, however, until the compression was reduced from 5 to 0 mm Hg. This observation stresses further the previous impression that vascular impairment is present even at low pressure levels.

Because the nutrition of the nerve root is affected, a compression-induced impairment of the vasculature may be one mechanism for nerve root dysfunction. The nerve roots also have a considerable nutritional supply, however, via diffusion from the cerebrospinal fluid.[15] To assess the compression-induced effects on the total contribution to the nerve roots, an experiment was designed in which ^{3}H-labeled methylglucose was allowed to be transported to the nerve tissue in the compressed segment via the blood vessels and via the cerebrospinal fluid diffusion after systemic injection.[16] The results showed that no compensatory mechanism from cerebrospinal fluid diffusion could be expected at the low pressure levels. On the contrary, 10 mm Hg compression was sufficient to induce a 20% to 30% reduction of the transport of methylglucose to the nerve roots compared with control.

It is known from experimental studies on peripheral nerves that compression also may induce an increase in the vascular permeability, leading to intraneural edema formation.[17] Such edema may increase the endoneurial fluid pressure, which may impair the endoneurial capillary blood flow and jeopardize the nutrition of the nerve roots.[18-20] Because the edema usually persists for some time after the removal of a compressive agent, edema may negatively affect the nerve root for a longer period than the compression itself. The presence of intraneural edema is also related to subsequent formation of intraneural fibrosis[21] and may contribute to the slow recovery seen in some patients with nerve compression disorders. To assess if intraneural edema also may form in nerve roots as the result of compression, the distribution of Evans blue–labeled albumin in the nerve tissue was analyzed after compression at various pressures and at various durations.[22] The study showed that edema was formed even at low-pressure levels. The predominant location was at the edges of the compression zone.

The function of the nerve roots has been studied by direct electrical stimulation and recordings either on the nerve itself or in the corresponding muscular segments.[23-26] During a 2-hour compression period, a critical pressure level for inducing a reduction of minimal alveolar pressure or amplitude was between 50 mm Hg and 75 mm Hg. Higher pressure levels (100 to 200 mm Hg) induced a total conduction block with varying degrees of recovery after compression release. To study the effects of compression on sensory nerve fibers, the electrodes in the sacrum were instead used to record a compound nerve action potential after stimulating the sensory nerves in the tail (i.e., distal to the compression zone). The results showed that the sensory fibers were slightly more susceptible to compression than the motor fibers.[25,26] Also, the nerve roots were more susceptible to compression injury if the blood pressure was reduced pharmacologically.[24] This finding further implies the importance of the blood supply to maintain the functional properties of the nerve roots.

Onset Rate of Compression

One factor that has not been fully recognized in compression trauma of nerve tissue is the onset rate of the compression. The onset rate (i.e., the time from compression start until full compression) may vary clinically from fractions of seconds in traumatic conditions to months or years in association with degenerative processes.

A rapid onset rate of less than 1 second has been found to induce more pronounced edema formation,[22] methylglucose transport,[16] and impulse propagation[23] than a slow onset rate of approximately 20 seconds. Regarding methylglucose transport, the results show that the levels within the compression zone are more pronounced at a rapid onset rate than at a slow onset rate at corresponding pressure levels. There was also a striking difference between the two onset rates when considering the segments outside the compression zones. In the slow onset series, the levels approached baseline values closer to the compression zone than in the rapid onset series; this may indicate the presence of a more pronounced edge-zone edema in the rapid onset series, with a subsequent reduction of the

8 Sciatica and Nerve Root Pain in Disc Herniation and Spinal Stenosis: A Basic Science Review and Clinical Perspective   131

SECTION

I

nutritional transport also in the nerve tissue adjacent to the compression zone.

For the rapid onset compression, which is likely to be more closely related to spine trauma or disc herniation than to spinal stenosis, it has been seen that a pressure of 600 mm Hg maintained only for 1 second is sufficient to induce a gradual impairment of nerve conduction during the 2 hours studied after the compression was ended.[27] Overall, the mechanisms for these pronounced differences between the different onset rates are unclear, but they may be related to differences in displacement rates of the compressed nerve tissue toward the uncompressed parts, owing to the viscoelastic properties of the nerve tissue.[9] Such phenomena may lead not only to structural damage to the nerve fibers but also to structural changes in the blood vessels with subsequent edema formation. The gradual formation of intraneural edema may also be closely related to the described observations of a gradually increasing difference in nerve conduction impairment between the two onset rates.[22,23] In the case of spinal stenosis, the rate may be a great deal slower, and pain or nerve dysfunction may not be seen until after considerable ischemic injury.

Double or Multiple Levels of Nerve Root Compression

Patients with double or multiple levels of spinal stenosis seem to have more pronounced symptoms than patients with stenosis only at one level.[28] The presented model was modified to address this clinical issue. Using two balloons at two adjacent disc levels, which resulted in a 10-mm uncompressed nerve segment between the balloons, induced a much more pronounced impairment of nerve impulse conduction than had been previously found at corresponding pressure levels.[29] A pressure of 10 mm Hg in two balloons induced a 60% reduction of nerve impulse amplitude during 2 hours of compression, whereas 50 mm Hg in one balloon showed no reduction.

The mechanism for the difference between single and double compression may not simply be based on the fact that the nerve impulses have to pass more than one compression zone at double level compression. There may also be a mechanism based on the local vascular anatomy of the nerve roots. In contrast to peripheral nerves, there are no regional nutritive arteries from surrounding structures to the intraneural vascular system in spinal nerve roots.[7,30-33] Compression at two levels might induce a nutritionally impaired region between the two compression sites. In this way the segment affected by the compression would be widened from one balloon diameter (10 mm) to two balloon diameters, including the nerve segment (30 mm) in between. This hypothesis was partly confirmed in an experiment on continuous analyses of the total blood flow in the uncompressed nerve segment located between two compression balloons. The results showed that a 64% reduction of total blood flow in the uncompressed segment was induced when both balloons were inflated to 10 mm Hg.[34] At a pressure close to the systemic blood pressure, there was complete ischemia in the nerve segment. Data from a study on the nutritional transport to the nerve tissue

in double-level compression showed that there is a reduction of this transport to the uncompressed nerve segment located between the two compression balloons that was similar to the reduction within the two compression sites.[35] There is experimental evidence that the nutrition to the nerve segment located between two compression sites in nerve roots is severely impaired, although this nerve segment itself is uncompressed.

Regarding nerve conduction, it was also evident that the effects were enhanced if the distance between the compression balloons was increased from one vertebral segment to two vertebral segments.[29] This was not the case, however, in the nutritional transport study where the methylglucose levels in the compression zones and in the uncompressed intermediate segment were similar between double compression over one and two vertebral segments.[35] This similarity indicates that the nutrition to the uncompressed nerve segment located between two compression sites is affected almost to the same extent as at the compression sites, regardless of the distance between the compression sites but that functional impairment may be directly related to the distance between the two compression sites. The impairment of the nutrition to the nerve segment between the two compression balloons seems to be a more important mechanism than the fact that the nerve impulses have to overcome two compression sites in double-level compression.

By using electrical nerve root stimulation to increase metabolic rate and simulate a walking situation in the double-level compression model, an initial short-term increase in cauda equina blood flow was seen that rapidly decreased.[36] Such observations further support the pathophysiologic significance of double-level cauda equina compression in spinal stenosis.

Chronic Experimental Nerve Root Compression

To mimic various clinical situations, compression must be applied for long periods. In clinical syndromes with nerve root compression, the onset time may be quite slow and the duration may be quite long. A gradual development of degenerative changes that induce spinal stenosis leads to an onset time that can be many years. It is difficult to mimic such a situation in an experimental model. It also would be impossible to have absolute control over the pressure acting on the nerve roots in chronic models owing to the remodeling and adaptation of the nerve tissue to the applied pressure. Knowledge of the exact pressures is probably less important, however, in chronic than in acute compression situations. Instead, chronic models should induce a controlled compression with a slow onset time that is easily reproducible. Such models may be well suited for studies on pathophysiologic events and intervention by surgery or drugs. Some attempts have been made to induce such compression.

Delamarter and colleagues[37] presented a model on the dog cauda equina in which they applied a constricting plastic band. The band was tightened around the thecal sac to induce a 25%, 50%, or 75% reduction of the cross-sectional area. The band was left in its place for various times. Analyses were performed and showed structural and functional changes that were proportional to the degree of constriction.

To induce a slower onset and more controlled compression, Cornefjord and colleagues[38] used a constrictor to compress the nerve roots in the pig. The constrictor was initially intended for inducing vascular occlusion in experimental ischemic conditions in dogs. The constrictor consists of an outer metal shell that on the inside is covered with a material called *ameroid* that expands when in contact with fluids. Because of the metal shell, the ameroid expands inward with a maximum of expansion after 2 weeks, resulting in a compression of a nerve root placed in the central opening of the constrictor. Compression of the first sacral nerve root in the pig resulted in a significant reduction of nerve conduction velocity and axonal injuries.[38] It has also been found that there is an increase in substance P in the nerve root and the dorsal root ganglion after such compression.[39] Substance P is a neurotransmitter that is related to pain transmission. The study may provide experimental evidence that compression of nerve roots produces pain. The constrictor model has also been used to study blood flow changes in the nerve root vasculature.[40] It could be observed that the blood flow is not reduced just outside the compression zone but significantly reduced in parts of the nerve roots located inside the constrictor.

One important aspect in clinical nerve root compression conditions is that the compression level is probably unstable and varies as the result of changes in posture and movements.[41,42] In 1995, Konno and colleagues[43] introduced a model in which the pressure could be changed after some time of initial chronic compression. An inflatable balloon was introduced under the lamina of the seventh lumbar vertebrae in the dog. The normal anatomy and the effects of acute compression using compressed air were first evaluated in previous studies.[44] By inflating the balloon at a known pressure slowly over 1 hour with a viscous substance that would harden in the balloon, a compression of the cauda equina could be induced with a known initial pressure level. The compression was verified by myelography. Because the balloon under the lamina comprised a twin set of balloons, the second balloon component could be connected to a compressed air device and could be used to add compression to the already chronically compressed cauda equina.

Acute nerve root compression experiments have established critical pressure levels for interference with various physiologic parameters in the spinal nerve roots. Studies on chronic compression may provide knowledge that would be more applicable to the clinical situation, however.

Spinal Stenosis: Experimental-Clinical Correlation

If nerve compression is of an extremely low onset rate as in spinal stenosis, there may be an adaptation of the nerve tissue to the applied pressure. In cadaveric experiments, Schönström and colleagues[45] found that when a hose clamp was tightened around a human cadaveric cauda equina specimen there was a critical cross-sectional area of the dural sac when the first signs of pressure increase among nerve roots were recorded by a catheter placed in the compression zone. This cross-sectional area was approximately 75 mm², which was also found to correlate with a corresponding measurement on computed tomography (CT) in patients with spinal stenosis.[46] When the hose clamp was tightened further, the pressure increased. Owing to creep phenomena in the nerve tissue, the pressure decreased with time, however. When the pressure did not normalize within 10 minutes, the "sustained size" was registered and was found to be in the range of 45 to 50 mm².[45] This study indicates that even in acute compression there is an adaptation of the nerve tissue to the applied pressure. From a longer perspective, this probably means that the nerve may also be reorganized in its microstructural elements, which would result in a nerve with a smaller diameter. Under such circumstances, with gradually decreasing nerve diameter, the nerve pressure acting on the nerve would be reduced to some degree.

There is a correlation between the animal experimental observations regarding critical pressures for functional and nutritional changes in nerve roots under compression on one side and the measurements of pressure levels among nerve roots in human cadaveric lumbar spines after experimental constriction of the dural sac. An acute pressure increase among cauda equina nerve roots to 50 mm Hg was induced when the cross-sectional area of the dural sac was reduced to 63 mm², and a pressure of 100 mm Hg was induced at a cross-sectional area of 57 mm².[45] Such pressure levels correlate with in vivo observations regarding physiologic changes in cauda equina nerve roots after experimental compression.[7,12,22]

Epidural pressure measurements have been performed, evaluating the relationship between epidural pressure and posture.[42] It was found that the local epidural pressure at the stenotic level was low in lying and sitting postures and high in standing postures. Pressure was increased with extension but decreased with flexion of the spine. The highest epidural pressure, 117 mm Hg, was found in standing with extension. Measurements have also been reported regarding changes in epidural pressure during walking in patients with lumbar spinal stenosis.[47] The pressure changed during walking with a wave pattern of increase and decrease. Such observations correlate with the previously mentioned experimental observations regarding intermittent cauda equina compression.[41]

Mechanical Nerve Root Deformation and Pain

Some experimental observations indicate that mechanical nerve root deformation per se may induce impulses that cause pain. Howe and colleagues[48] found that mechanical stimulation of nerve roots or peripheral nerves resulted in nerve impulses of short duration and that these impulses were prolonged if the nerve tissue had been exposed to mechanical irritation by a chromic gut ligature for 2 to 4 weeks. Corresponding results were obtained in an in vitro system using rabbit nerve roots.[49] In this setup, it was also evident that the dorsal root ganglion was more susceptible to mechanical stimulation than the nerve roots. The dorsal root ganglion has elicited special interest in this regard, and an increase in the level of neurotransmitters related to pain transmission has

8 Sciatica and Nerve Root Pain in Disc Herniation and Spinal Stenosis: A Basic Science Review and Clinical Perspective   133

SECTION

I

been found in the dorsal root ganglion in response to whole-body vibration of rabbits.[50] A similar increase has been seen in the dorsal root ganglion and nerve root after local constriction of the same nerve root.[39] In vivo models of pain behavior have shown that mechanical nerve deformation superimposed on inflammation is painful, whereas either factor alone might not cause severe pain.[51-56] The magnitude of nerve root compression pressure (measured intraoperatively) correlates with neurologic deficit but not with degree of straight-leg raising test.[57]

Neuropathologic Changes and Pain

There is considerable research evidence regarding the relationship of pain to neuropathologic changes.[58] Much of what is known has been studied in relationship to mechanical and inflammatory injury of the sciatic nerve in the rat. Entrapment of a peripheral nerve produces pathologic change in proportion to the degree of compression and its duration,[59] as is known to be the case for nerve root compression. In an electron microscopic study,[59] minor degrees of nerve compression were associated with ischemic injury to Schwann cells, resulting in their necrosis and in demyelination. Severe nerve compression was associated with injury to the axon, resulting in wallerian degeneration.

Subsequent experiments established the relationship of pain to these forms of neuropathologic change.[60] These studies established that mild levels of ischemia producing demyelination were generally not painful, whereas severe ischemia-producing wallerian degeneration resulted in hyperalgesia. The pathology of the chronic constriction injury model of neuropathic pain is based on this relationship and the added insult of inflammation caused by the chromic gut ligatures used to compress the nerve.[61] It is now recognized that the cytokine-driven processes of wallerian degeneration are the dominant neuropathologic factors linking nerve injury and pain[60,62,63] and that the degree and extent of wallerian degeneration relate directly to the magnitude and duration of hyperalgesia.[64]

Biologic and Biochemical Effects on Nerve Roots

The clinical picture of sciatica with a characteristic distribution of pain and nerve dysfunction but in the absence of herniated disc material at radiologic examination and at surgery has indicated that mechanical nerve root compression may not be the only factor that is responsible for sciatic pain. It has been suggested that the disc tissue per se may have some injurious properties.[9] Not until 1993 was it confirmed experimentally, however, that local, epidural application of autologous nucleus pulposus with no mechanical deformation induces significant changes in structure and function of the adjacent nerve roots.[6]

Biologic Effects of Nucleus Pulposus

In 1993, Olmarker and colleagues[6] published a study that showed that autologous nucleus pulposus can induce a

reduction in nerve conduction velocity and light microscopic structural changes in a pig cauda equina model of nerve root injury. These axonal changes had a focal distribution, however, and the quantity of injured axons was too low to be responsible for the significant neurophysiologic dysfunction observed. A follow-up study of areas of the nerve roots exposed to nucleus pulposus that appeared to be normal by light microscopy revealed that there were significant injuries of Schwann cells with vacuolization and disintegration of Schmidt-Lanterman incisures (Fig. 8–2).[65] Schmidt-Lanterman incisures are essential for the normal exchange of ions between the axon and the surrounding tissues. An injury to this structure would be likely to interfere with the normal impulse conduction properties of the axons, although these models' changes may not fully explain the neurophysiologic dysfunction observed.

The pathophysiologic potential of the nucleus pulposus was emphasized further in an experiment using a dog model in which it was seen that a surgical incision of the anulus fibrosus, with minimal leakage of nucleus pulposus, was enough to induce significant changes in structure and function of the adjacent nerve root.[66] It has also been seen that epidural application of the autologous nucleus pulposus within 2 hours induces an intraneural edema[67,68] that leads to a reduction of

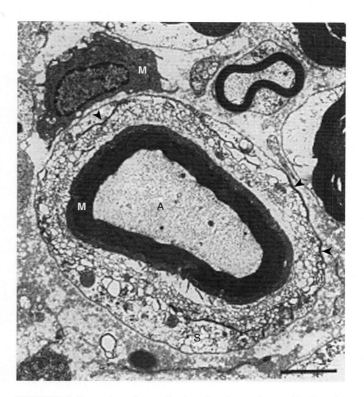

FIGURE 8–2 Seven days after application of nucleus pulposus. Myelinated nerve fiber with prominent vesicular swelling of Schmidt-Lanterman incisure. Note mononuclear cell (*black M*) in close contact with nerve fiber. *Arrowheads* indicate myelin sheath layers outside Schmidt-Lanterman incisure. A, well-preserved axon; white M, myelin sheath; S, outer Schwann cell cytoplasm. (*Bar* = 2.5 μm.) (From Olmarker K, Nordborg C, Larsson K, et al: Ultrastructural changes in spinal nerve roots induced by autologous nucleus pulposus. Spine [Phila Pa 1976] 21:411-414, 1996.)

the intraneural blood flow.[68] Histologic changes of the nerve roots are present after 3 hours,[69] and a subsequent reduction of the nerve conduction velocity starts 3 to 24 hours after application.[6,69] The nucleus pulposus may also interfere with the nutrition to the intraspinal nerve tissue. After application to the dorsal root ganglion, it was found that the intraneural blood flow was dramatically decreased and that there was a simultaneous increase of the tissue fluid pressure.[68]

Methylprednisolone reduces the pathophysiologic events of the nucleus pulposus–induced nerve root injury if given within 24 hours. To establish if the presence of autologous nucleus pulposus could initiate a leukotactic response from the surrounding tissues, a study was initiated that assessed the potential inflammatogenic properties of the nucleus pulposus.[70] Autologous nucleus pulposus and autologous retroperitoneal fat were placed in separate perforated titanium chambers and placed subcutaneously, together with a sham chamber, in the pig. The number of leukocytes was assessed 7 days later for the chambers. The nucleus pulposus–containing chambers had a number of leukocytes that exceeded the two others by 150%. In another experiment, autologous nucleus pulposus and muscle were placed in Gore-Tex tubes subcutaneously in rabbits.[71] After 2 weeks, there was an accumulation of macrophages and T-helper and T-suppresser cells in the tube with nucleus pulposus that persisted the full observation time of 4 weeks.

Kawakami and colleagues[72] showed that neuropathic pain in an experimental setting seems to be mediated by infiltrating leukocytes, a finding consistent with the previous observations of neuroimmunologic inflammatory changes and pain.[73] In rats made leukopenic by using nitrogen mustard, the pain response was absent after application of nucleus pulposus, whereas normal rats with nucleus pulposus application displayed a pathologic response to stimulation. The same group also showed that inhibition of cyclooxygenase-2 might reduce nucleus pulposus–induced pain behavior.[74] Taken together, these data further support the impression that autologous nucleus pulposus may elicit inflammatory reactions when outside the intervertebral disc space and that such reactions may not be restricted to resorption of the herniated tissue but also may be intimately involved in the pathophysiology of sciatica.

Nucleus Pulposus and Sciatic Pain

Pain is much more difficult to assess than nerve conduction in controlled experimental studies. The available literature indicates that pain may be induced by mechanical factors and nucleus pulposus–mediated factors. The role of the nucleus pulposus in this context is interesting in view of patients with obvious symptoms of disc herniation but with no visible herniation at radiologic examination or surgery.[75,76] The potential of nucleus pulposus material to induce pain has also been indicated in clinical studies that showed that noncontained herniations (the nucleus pulposus was in contact with the epidural space) were much more painful and had a more pronounced straight-leg raising test result than contained herniations.[77-79]

Studies on rats using pain behavior assessment indicated that the nucleus pulposus is involved in pain production. Pain behavior in this context refers to response thresholds to thermal and mechanical stimulation. Kawakami and colleagues[52,53] showed that a three-level laminectomy and application of homologous nucleus pulposus or anulus fibrosus taken from three intervertebral discs in another rat, applied at three nerve roots, produces pain behavior. Other studies[54] suggest a dose-response relationship between pain behavior and the amount of nucleus pulposus material in the epidural space. The combination of nucleus pulposus herniation and mechanical injury produces pain.[54] This observation is consistent with the neuropathologic understanding of pain and the consequences of combined mechanical and inflammatory injury to nerve fibers that are superimposed to increase the number of fibers injured and the corresponding increase in proinflammatory cytokines.[63,64] The same pathophysiologic response was observed in a study assessing walking patterns, in which it was seen that only the combination of displacement and disc incision produced detectable changes.[56] Also, a pain behavior study assessing changes in spontaneous behavior showed that only the combined action of displacement and disc incision produced changes, whereas displacement or disc incision per se did not produce changes.[80]

These experimental studies on pain behavior suggest that the presence of nucleus pulposus has sensitized the nerve tissue. Minor compression of peripheral nerves is not painful, and touching of a normal nerve root during local anesthesia is not painful.[81] Touching of a nerve root exposed to a disc herniation often reproduces the sciatic pain, however.[81] Although the combination of a mechanical component and the presence of nucleus pulposus seems to be a prerequisite to produce changes in the in vivo situation, more recent neurophysiologic studies have shown that the mere application of nucleus pulposus may induce increased neuronal pain transmission.[82] This finding reflects that pain behavior assessment is a gross instrument to detect pain and that nucleus pulposus may induce pain in the absence of a mechanical component as well.

The spinal dura mater is known to contain nerve endings, and stimulation of the dura has been suggested as a mechanism for sciatic pain.[9,81,83,84] Irritation or stimulation of the dura as one important factor for sciatica is an interesting theory that could explain many clinical features. One may assume that the dura is segmentally innervated, the sensory nerves travel in a caudal-lateral direction, and the dura is drained to the corresponding nerve root by the nerve of Luschka.[85-88] Stimulation of the dura at a point where the dorsolateral herniations appear (*I* in Fig. 8–3) should be recorded by the corresponding nerve root.[89] At this location, the irritation may spread medially to the contralateral segment, however, producing bilateral symptoms, or laterally, producing symptoms from levels above. Similarly, a lateral disc herniation (*II* in Fig. 8–3) could produce symptoms in the lower level.

If the pain of the straight-leg raising test is the result of dura irritation owing to friction to the herniated mass, one may consider the phenomenon of crossed straight-leg raising to be

8 Sciatica and Nerve Root Pain in Disc Herniation and Spinal Stenosis: A Basic Science Review and Clinical Perspective   135

SECTION

I

based on simultaneous stimulation of the contralateral dura. Such a "radiculitis" or "local meningitis" probably could be regarded as similar to peritonitis. When there is peritonitis, there is usually a reflectory muscle contraction present over the affected area. An analogue for this local meningitis could be the reflectory ipsilateral contraction of the spinal muscles, producing the "sciatic scoliosis" or lateral bending of the spine at the level of herniation.

To speculate further, one could elaborate the idea that the deep visceral pain manifested earlier as "referred pain" may be related to painful conditions in the nerve, such as neuroischemia, and that the sharp, distinct pain manifesting as "radicular pain" may be related to dural irritation. Although these proposed mechanisms are subject to speculation, perceived mechanisms of spinal pain may change dramatically over the coming years based on new ideas and concepts and on the rapidly increasing knowledge of the molecular events active in the pathophysiology of sciatica.

Other Consequences of Herniated Nucleus Pulposus

Histologic observations have indicated that nerve root changes caused by nucleus pulposus are focal and mainly found in the center of the nerve roots, resembling a mononeuritis simplex that is induced by nerve infarction secondary to embolism of the intraneural vessels.[6,65,90] Particularly in view of the work of Jayson and colleagues[91-94] indicating an impairment of the venous outflow from the nerve roots owing to periradicular vascular changes, one must consider vascular impairment as one factor. Large molecules deposited in the epidural space can be found in the intraneural vessels of the adjacent nerve roots within seconds after application.[95] Epidurally placed substances can penetrate the relatively impermeable dura, cross over the cerebrospinal fluid, and diffuse through the root sheath and into the axons.

The inflammatory components of nucleus pulposus may be involved in vascular and rheologic phenomena, such as coagulation, and may be involved in nerve root vascular embolism. It has been observed that the presence of nucleus pulposus may induce thrombus formation in microvessels.[70] Inflammatory mediators may also exert a direct effect on the myelin sheaths, as indicated by an electron microscopic study of nerve roots exposed to autologous nucleus pulposus in the pig.[65] There were significant injuries of Schwann cells with vacuolization and disintegration of Schmidt-Lanterman incisures, which closely resembles the injury pattern of inflammatory nerve disease.[96,97] As previously described, results from studies have also indicated that epidural application of nucleus pulposus induces an increase of the vascular permeability and a subsequent reduction of the blood flow in the adjacent nerve roots, which suggests vascular impairment as being of pathophysiologic importance.

It has also been suggested that because the nucleus pulposus is avascular and "hidden" from the systemic circulation, a presentation of the nucleus pulposus could result in an autoimmune reaction directed to antigens present in the nucleus pulposus and that bioactive substances from this reaction may injure the nerve tissue.[98-105] One may also hypothesize that

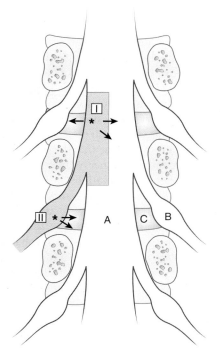

FIGURE 8–3 Suggested area of innervation by one recurrent sinuvertebral nerve (nerve of Luschka). Disc herniation at location I may be recorded by the same nerve and by the nearby innervation areas, laterally and contralaterally, as indicated by *arrows*. At location II, lateral disc herniation of disc one level below may affect same nerve root but also root one level below, located medial to this root, as indicated by *arrows*. **A,** Thecal sac. **B,** Dorsal root ganglion. **C,** Intervertebral disc. (From Olmarker K: The experimental basis of sciatica. J Orthop Sci 1:230-242, 1996.)

there could be autoimmune reactions not only to the disc but also to components from the nerve tissue that are released as the result of injury, such as basic myelin proteins. A study also assessed the possible presence of immune complexes in herniated disc tissue obtained at surgery as an indicator of immunoactivation.[106] IgG was found in close relation to the disc cells in herniated disc material. No IgG was found, however, in the residual disc that was evacuated at the time of surgery. No immune complexes were found in control disc material obtained at spine surgery for other causes than pain. Although inconclusive, this study may indicate that immunologic activation may be present in some cases of sciatica.

Chemical Components of Nucleus Pulposus

The nucleus pulposus is composed mainly of proteoglycans, collagen, and cells.[107,108] The proteoglycan component has gained the most attention and has been suggested to have a direct irritating effect on nerve tissue.[104,109,110] Neither the collagen nor the cells have previously been suggested to be of pathophysiologic importance. More recent studies of the cells of the nucleus pulposus have shown, however, that these cells are capable of producing metalloproteinases such as collagenase or gelatinase and interleukin (IL)-6 and prostaglandin E_2 and do so spontaneously in culture. Using the same pig model previously described, the possible role of the nucleus pulposus cells for the nucleus pulposus–induced nerve injury has been assessed.[111] In a blinded fashion, autologous nucleus pulposus was subjected to 24 hours of freezing at −20°C, digestion by hyaluronidase, or just heating the box at 37°C for 24 hours. The treated nucleus pulposus was reapplied after 24 hours, and analyses were performed 7 days later. In animals in which the nucleus pulposus had been frozen and the cells killed, there were no changes in nerve conduction velocity, whereas in the other two series the results were similar to application of unaltered nucleus pulposus.

It seems reasonable to believe that the cells are responsible in some way for inducing the nerve injury. This assumption was supported further by observations indicating that application of cultured pig disc cells to the cauda equina reproduced the reduction in nerve conduction velocity.[111] Application of disc cell membranes also reproduced this reduction, however, indicating that the responsible substances probably are membrane bound.

Substances such as IgG, hydrogen ions, nitric oxide, and phospholipase A$_2$ have previously been suggested to be responsible for the pathophysiologic reactions.[104,112-116] Another substance produced by the disc cells that has similar pathophysiologic effects as nucleus pulposus is tumor necrosis factor (TNF)-α.[117]

Cytokines as Mediators of Nerve Dysfunction and Pain

TNF is known to be a regulatory proinflammatory cytokine that has specific biologic effects and the ability to upregulate and act synergistically with other cytokines such as IL-1β and IL-6.[118-127] Immediately after nerve injury, TNF is released and upregulated by Schwann cells at the site of nerve injury[124]; this is followed by release and upregulation of TNF in many other endoneurial cells, including endothelial cells, fibroblasts, and mast cells. TNF is also produced by chondrocytes and disc cells.[117,125-128] This local production of TNF is the stimulus that results in macrophage attraction to the injury site,[62] which contributes massively to the concentration of proinflammatory cytokines in the injured tissue. Several studies have shown that blocking TNF production or delaying the invasion of macrophages to the site of nerve injury results in reduced or delayed neuropathologic change and reduced hyperalgesia.[73,129]

When performing a meta-analysis on the biologic and pathophysiologic effects induced by TNF and by nucleus pulposus, one may find that there is almost a perfect match. TNF is known to induce axonal and myelin injury similar to that observed after nucleus pulposus application,[130-136] intravascular coagulation,[137-139] and increased vascular permeability.[139] TNF is also known to be neurotoxic[133,135,140,141] and to induce painful behavioral changes[130,142] and ectopic nerve activity when applied locally.[131,143] TNF is sequestered in a membrane-bound form and is activated after shedding by certain enzymes. Matrix metalloproteinases (MMPs) are particularly important in this regard. MMP-9 and MMP-2 are upregulated immediately after a nerve injury.[144] MMPs process the inactive, membrane-bound form of TNF and its receptors to

the biologically active form and are directly associated with breakdown of the blood-brain and blood-nerve barriers. MMP-9 and TNF receptors are also retrogradely transported from the site of nerve injury to the corresponding dorsal root ganglion and spinal cord,[145] where they may have a direct role in gene regulation. This may relate to the observation that cell membranes of disc cells are sufficient to mediate the nucleus pulposus–induced effects.[111]

TNF induces activation of endothelial adhesion molecules such as intercellular and vascular cell adhesion molecules, adhering circulating immune cells to the vessel walls (Fig. 8–4).[121,146,147] As a consequence of the TNF-induced increased vascular permeability, these cells migrate into the endoneurial space where the axons are located.[148-150] The cells release their content of TNF and other cytokines, which may induce accumulation of ion channels locally in the axonal membranes.[151-153] The channels may allow for an increased passage of sodium and potassium, which may result in spontaneous discharges and in discharges of ectopic impulses after mechanical stimulation. TNF by itself can cause spontaneous electrical activity in A-delta and C nociceptors.[143] Such discharges, whether they come from a pain fiber or a nerve fiber transmitting other sensory information, are interpreted as pain by the brain.[154-157] Such a mechanism may relate to the sensitization of the nerve roots seen in the experimental and clinical studies just discussed and to motion-evoked sciatic pain, such as the straight-leg raising test.

Previous studies have also indicated that local application of nucleus pulposus may disintegrate the myelin sheath[65,66]; this is also a known effect of TNF.[130,148,158-160] In particular, this injury seems to affect Schmidt-Lanterman incisures, which are responsible for the ion exchange between the axon and the surrounding tissues.[161-164] This injury could also contribute to the formation of ectopic impulses and to the sensitization to mechanical stimulus. Experimental and clinical studies have shown that nerve root compression and disc herniation can induce increased concentrations of neurofilament in the cerebrospinal fluid.[165,166] Increased levels of serum antibodies against one or more nervous system–associated glycosphingolipids have been shown in patients with sciatica and disc herniation, indicating a possible autoimmune response.[167]

More recent work regarding molecular events in the pathophysiology of neuropathic pain has suggested a potential role of TNF for inducing allodynia.[131,168-173] TNF may mediate the formation of allodynia in the dorsal root ganglion and at the spinal cord level because of its local upregulation, which occurs via a positive feedback loop caused by TNF itself. This cycle seems to be broken by a direct effect of TNF on the upregulation of anti-inflammatory cytokines such as IL-10, which eventually leads to a reduction of TNF and the physiologic balance of proinflammatory and anti-inflammatory cytokines. Such regulation seems to be induced by mechanical injury to peripheral parts of the axons and by a direct effect of TNF exposure and further enhances the impression that TNF may be an important mediator of neuropathic pain. TNF is a potent activator of cells; because it is retrogradely transported from the site of nerve injury to the dorsal root ganglion

8 Sciatica and Nerve Root Pain in Disc Herniation and Spinal Stenosis: A Basic Science Review and Clinical Perspective   137

SECTION

I

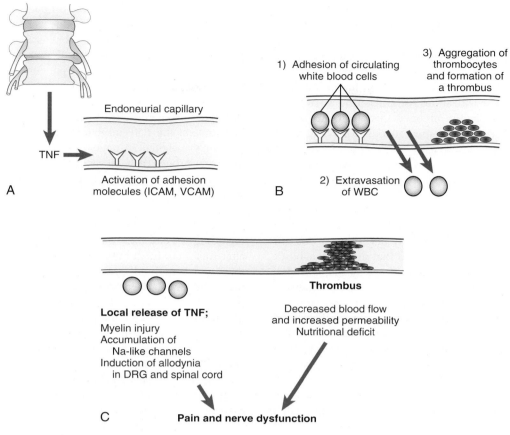

FIGURE 8–4 Suggested mechanism of action for tumor necrosis factor (TNF). **A,** TNF from cells of herniated nucleus pulposus enters endoneurial capillaries and activates endothelial adhesion molecules. **B,** Circulating white blood cells adhere to vessel walls (*1*) and extravasate from capillaries out among axons owing to TNF-induced increase in vascular permeability (*2*). TNF also induces accumulation of thrombocytes that form intravascular thrombus (*3*). **C,** There is local release of TNF from extravasated white blood cells (WBC) among axons that induce myelin injury, accumulation of sodium channels, and allodynia in dorsal root ganglion (DRG) and at spinal cord level. Thrombus, together with edema owing to increased permeability, induces nutritional deficit in nerve root. Local effects of TNF and nutritional deficit may induce pain and nerve dysfunction. CAM, cell adhesion molecule; VCAM, vascular cell adhesion molecule. (From Olmarker K, Myers R, Kikuchi S, et al: Pathophysiology of nerve root pain in disc herniation and spinal stenosis. In Herkowitz H, Dvorak J, Bell G, et al [eds]: The Lumbar Spine, 3rd ed. Philadelphia, Lippincott Williams & Wilkins, 2004, pp 11-30.)

and spinal cord, it may be this proinflammatory stimulus that activates central glia and neurons.[145]

Apart from directly affecting the endoneurially located axons, TNF may also indirectly interfere with the axons by compromising the nutritional transport. TNF may induce intravascular coagulation, similar to nucleus pulposus, after local application[137,174-176]; this reduces the local blood flow in the intraneural capillaries.[75] A nutritional reduction induces ischemia in the nerve root, which may induce neuroischemic pain.

There is much evidence that TNF may be an important mediator of nerve dysfunction and pain. The circumstance of TNF being produced and released from cells in the nucleus pulposus, when displaced from its natural environment in the center of the intervertebral disc out into the spinal canal in close contact to the nervous structures, may be one key event for the onset of nerve dysfunction and sciatic pain.

TNF was found in disc cells; when TNF was inhibited with a nonspecific cytokine inhibitor, the nucleus pulposus–induced reduction in nerve conduction velocity after experimental application of nucleus pulposus in a pig model was completely blocked.[117] When using more specific TNF inhibitors, such as a monoclonal antibody to TNF (infliximab) and a soluble TNF receptor (etanercept), the inhibition was equally effective.[174] Investigations have shown that infliximab may attenuate immunoreactivity of brain-derived neurotrophic factor and may prevent neurologic and histologic changes in dorsal root ganglion in rats after experimental disc herniation.[177-179] Application of selected cytokines in the pig model showed that TNF reduced the nerve conduction velocity per se.[180] IL-1β and interferon-γ induced only a slight reduction of nerve conduction velocity.

Application of certain cytokines to intraspinal nerves may also increase the somatosensory neural response.[181] Discharges from wide-dynamic-range neurons after stimulation of a receptor field of a dorsal root ganglion exposed to nucleus pulposus increased significantly after application.[182] This increase may be related to the sensitization of the sensory system caused by proinflammatory cytokines and the production of low-grade spontaneous electrophysiologic activity in nociceptors by TNF,[143] which by itself is an important factor that contributes to sensitization. Administering an antibody specific for TNF efficiently inhibited this effect. An in vivo study assessing changes in spontaneous behavior clearly showed that changes induced by the combined action of mechanical deformation and disc incision were markedly inhibited by intraperitoneal injection of a monoclonal antibody specific for TNF.[55]

TNF seems to be an important mediator for the observed effects on nerve function and for pain induced by local application of nucleus pulposus. Additional support for this hypothesis comes from previous work that showed that blockade of TNF upregulation in macrophages by thalidomide[129] and downregulation of TNF by IL-10 administration[183] reduced the magnitude and duration of hyperalgesia after nerve injury. Because cytokine interactions are complex, other cytokines such as IL-1β and IL-6 may be involved as well.[180,181,184,185] Because these cytokines are induced by TNF, as well as inducing TNF, their exact role has not been completely evaluated.

The possible role of brain-derived neurotrophic factor in nerve root pathophysiology and experimental disc herniation has been analyzed.[186] The appearance and distribution of macrophages and TNF in the dorsal root ganglion of rats after experimental disc herniation[187,188] and the relationship between nerve growth factor and pain behavioral changes have been described.[189] It has also been shown that disc-related cytokines can inhibit axonal outgrowth from dorsal root ganglion cells in vitro.[190]

Clinical Use of Cytokine Inhibitors for Treatment of Sciatica

On the basis of the experimental findings that TNF may mimic nucleus pulposus–induced nerve dysfunction and pain, pilot clinical trials regarding the possible use of TNF inhibition for the treatment of sciatica have been initiated. Karppinen and colleagues[191] administered a monoclonal antibody specific for TNF (infliximab [Remicade]) to 10 volunteers waiting for surgery for radiologically verified disc herniations with severe sciatica. In this open-label study, infliximab reduced pain assessed by visual analog scale by 50% at 1 hour after infusion. After 2 weeks, 60% of the patients were pain-free. At 3 months after the single infusion, 90% were pain-free. No adverse drug reactions were noted, and no patients required surgery. A 1-year follow-up[192] of the 10 patients treated with infliximab showed that the beneficial effect of a single infusion of 3 mg/kg of infliximab for disc herniation–induced sciatica was sustained in most patients. The study authors also noted that infliximab did not seem to interfere with spontaneous resorption of disc herniations.

Genevay and colleagues[193] administered a TNF inhibitor in the form of a soluble TNF receptor (etanercept [Enbrel]) by three subcutaneous injections to 10 patients with severe sciatica. The patients had a 70% reduction of leg pain assessed by visual analog scale 10 days after starting the treatment. At 6 weeks, the reduction was 83%. The results were statistically significantly better than for 10 patients treated with three intravenous injections of methylprednisolone.

There is one randomized study published by Cohen and colleagues[194] regarding treatment of sciatica by local epidural injections of the TNF inhibitor etanercept. The investigators randomly assigned 24 patients with subacute radiculopathy into three groups each consisting of 8 patients. The patients in each group received either 2 mg, 4 mg, or 6 mg on two occasions, and two of the eight patients were saline controls. All etanercept-treated patients had significant improvement 1 month after treatment compared with saline-treated patients regarding leg and back pain. The effects persisted 6 months after treatment in all but one patient. The authors concluded that "etanercept holds promise as a treatment for lumbosacral radiculopathy."[194] Genevay and colleagues[195] published the results of a multicenter, double-blind, placebo-controlled trial on the use of the TNF inhibitor adalimumab (Humira) subcutaneously injected in 31 patients with severe, acute sciatica caused by disc herniation. Two injections were given 7 days apart; 30 control patients received placebo injections in the same manner. The results showed that there was a significantly more favorable evolution of leg pain in the adalimumab group than in the placebo group, but the effect size was relatively small. There were twice as many patients in the adalimumab group who fulfilled the criteria for "responders," and there were significantly fewer surgical discectomies in this group compared with the placebo-treated controls.

Taken together, these observations indicate a potential clinical effect of TNF inhibition for the treatment of sciatica. It may be surprising that TNF inhibition seems to be so much superior to anti-inflammatory treatment by nonsteroidal anti-inflammatory drugs or methylprednisolone or even morphine. One may conclude that it is more efficient to act at the responsible mediators directly than aiming at general anti-inflammatory effects. This clinical comparison strongly supports the TNF hypothesis of neuropathic pain.[63,117,174] Sciatica has a neuropathic pain component, and nonspecific anti-inflammatory medication and morphine are less efficient in such conditions. Nevertheless, further studies must be undertaken before any definite conclusions regarding its efficacy for the treatment of sciatica may be drawn.[196,197]

Summary

The pathophysiology of sciatica is complex with numerous substances and mechanisms acting at various levels of the neural axis. These mechanisms more recently have attracted attention of basic scientists, and numerous studies looking into neuroimmunologic events have provided important insights into the pathophysiologic mechanisms of the human disease state. The intervertebral disc has certain biologic effects that contribute directly to these pathophysiologic processes. Epidural application of nucleus pulposus induces structural and functional changes that relate closely to sciatica. The nucleus pulposus also sensitizes nerve roots, producing a painful condition. These experimental observations correlate with the clinical impression that preoperative touching of nerve roots that have been exposed to disc herniation under local anesthesia reproduces the sciatic pain and that surgical removal of the mechanical compression of the nerve root often relieves symptoms.

The biologic substance of importance in the pathogenesis of painful radiculopathy seems clearly at this stage of understanding to be TNF-α. The activation and upregulation of this ubiquitous proinflammatory cytokine produces acute pain and neuropathologic changes associated with chronic pain states. TNF stimulates fibroblast scar formation in a vicious cycle whereby the local presence of TNF stimulates other cells to upregulate this cytokine. Initiation of this cycle by the leakage of TNF from herniated nucleus pulposus produces a cascade of tissue injury, scar formation, and local pain. Superimposition of mechanical injury to the nerve root in this environment exacerbates the neural immune insult, causing macrophage-mediated wallerian degeneration with significant increases in TNF concentrations. The authors suggest that these combined events explain the problem of sciatica. Although the pathophysiology of sciatica is far more complex than one might first suspect, future research is certain to reveal substances and mechanisms of importance to the induction of symptoms in sciatica, and such research would provide a basis for improved diagnosis and treatment of this common disorder.

Acknowledgments

This chapter is partly based on research supported by grants from the Swedish Medical Research Council (521-2007-2956), Fukushima Society for Promotion of Medicine, National Institutes of Health (No. NS18715), and Department of Veterans Affairs.

KEY REFERENCES

1. Mixter WJ, Barr JS: Rupture of the intervertebral disc with involvement of the spinal canal. N Engl J Med 211:210-215, 1934.
    This article is about the discovery of the herniated disc.

2. Olmarker K, Holm S, Rosenqvist AL, Rydevik B: Experimental nerve root compression. A model of acute, graded compression of the porcine cauda equina and an analysis of neural and vascular anatomy. Spine (Phila Pa 1976) 16:61-69, 1991.
    This articles discusses the first time a model for graded compression of nerve roots was introduced.

3. Olmarker K, Rydevik B, Nordborg C: Autologous nucleus pulposus induces neurophysiologic and histologic changes in porcine cauda equina nerve roots. Spine 1;18:1425-1432, 1993.
    This study demonstrated for the first time the injurious effects of autologous nucleus puposus.

4. Kawakami M, Weinstein JN, Chatani K, et al: Experimental lumbar radiculopathy. Behavioral and histologic changes in a model of radicular pain after spinal nerve root irritation with chromic gut ligatures in the rat. Spine 15;19:1795-1802, 1994.
    This study was the first to examine nerve root pain in an experimental model.

5. Olmarker K, Myers RR: Pathogenesis of sciatic pain: role of herniated nucleus pulposus and deformation of spinal nerve root and dorsal root ganglion. Pain 78:99-105, 1998.
    This study was the first to examine nerve root pain induced by nucleus pulposus in a autologous system.

6. Olmarker K, Larsson K: Tumor necrosis factor alpha and nucleus-pulposus-induced nerve root injury. Spine 23:2538-2544, 1998.
    This was the first study to link a specific molecule to the pathophysiology of sciatica.

7. Cohen SP, Bogduk N, Dragovich A, et al: Randomized, double-blind, placebo-controlled, dose-response, and preclinical safety study of transforaminal epidural etanercept for the treatment of sciatica. Anesthesiology 110:1116-1126, 2009.
    This was the first placebo randomized study to indicate that pharmacological inhibition of a specific molecule may be an alternative treatment of sciatica.

REFERENCES

1. Mixter WJ, Barr JS: Rupture of the intervertebral disc with involvement of the spinal canal. N Engl J Med 211:210-215, 1934.

2. Olmarker K, Hasue M: Classification and pathophysiology of spinal pain syndromes. In Weinstein JN, Rydevik B, Sonntag VKH (eds): Essentials of the Spine. New York, Raven Press, 1995, pp 11-25.

3. Bailey P, Casamajor L: Osteo-arthritis of the spine as a cause of compression of the spinal cord and its roots. J Nerv Ment Dis 38:588-609, 1911.

4. Goldthwait JE: The lumbo-sacral articulation: An explanation of many cases of "lumbago" and "sciatica" and paraplegia. Boston Med Surg J 164:365-372, 1911.

5. Sachs B, Fraenkel J: Progressive ankylotic rigidity of the spine. J Nerv Ment Dis 27:1-15, 1900.

6. Olmarker K, Rydevik B, Nordborg C: Autologous nucleus pulposus induces neurophysiologic and histologic changes in porcine cauda equina nerve roots. Spine (Phila Pa 1976) 18:1425-1432, 1993.

7. Olmarker K: Spinal nerve root compression: Nutrition and function of the porcine cauda equina compressed in vivo. Acta Orthop Scand Suppl 242:1-27, 1991.

8. Olmarker K, Holm S, Rosenqvist AL, et al: Experimental nerve root compression: A model of acute, graded compression of the porcine cauda equina and an analysis of neural and vascular anatomy. Spine (Phila Pa 1976) 16:61-69, 1991.

9. Rydevik B, Brown MD, Lundborg G: Pathoanatomy and pathophysiology of nerve root compression. Spine (Phila Pa 1976) 9:7-15, 1984.

10. Gelfan S, Tarlov IM: Physiology of spinal cord, nerve root and peripheral nerve compression. Am J Physiol 185:217-229, 1956.

11. Sharpless SK: Susceptibility of spinal nerve roots to compression block: The research status of spinal manipulative therapy. In Goldstein M (ed): NIH-Workshop: NINCDS Monograph. 1975, pp 155-161.

12. Olmarker K, Rydevik B, Holm S, et al: Effects of experimental graded compression on blood flow in spinal nerve roots: A vital microscopic study on the porcine cauda equina. J Orthop Res 7:817-823, 1989.

13. Sunderland S: The nerve lesion in the carpal tunnel. J Neurol Neurosurg Psychiatry 39:615-626, 1976.

14. Olmarker K, Holm S, Rydevik B, et al: Restoration of blood flow during gradual decompression of a compressed segment of the porcine cauda equina: A vital microscopic study. Neuroorthopaedics 10:83-87, 1991.

15. Rydevik B, Holm S, Brown MD, et al: Diffusion from the cerebrospinal fluid as a nutritional pathway for spinal nerve roots. Acta Physiol Scand 138:247-248, 1990.

16. Olmarker K, Rydevik B, Hansson T, et al: Compression-induced changes of the nutritional supply to the porcine cauda equina. J Spinal Disord 3:25-29, 1990.

17. Rydevik B, Lundborg G: Permeability of intraneural microvessels and perineurium following acute, graded experimental nerve compression. Scand J Plast Reconstr Surg 11:179-187, 1977.

18. Myers RR, Murakami H, Powell HC: Reduced nerve blood flow in edematous neuropathies: A biomechanical mechanism. Microvasc Res 32:145-151, 1986.

19. Myers RR, Mizisin AP, Powell HC, et al: Reduced nerve blood flow in hexachlorophene neuropathy: Relationship to elevated endoneurial fluid pressure. J Neuropathol Exp Neurol 41:391-399, 1982.

20. Myers R, Powell H: Galactose neuropathy: Impact of chronic endoneurial edema on nerve blood flow. Ann Neurol 16:587-594, 1984.

21. Rydevik B, Lundborg G, Nordborg C: Intraneural tissue reactions induced by internal neurolysis: An experimental study on the blood-nerve barrier, connective tissues and nerve fibres of rabbit tibial nerve. Scand J Plast Reconstr Surg 10:3-8, 1976.

22. Olmarker K, Rydevik B, Holm S: Edema formation in spinal nerve roots induced by experimental, graded compression: An experimental study on the pig cauda equina with special reference to differences in effects between rapid and slow onset of compression. Spine (Phila Pa 1976) 14:569-573, 1989.

23. Olmarker K, Holm S, Rydevik B: Importance of compression onset rate for the degree of impairment of impulse propagation in experimental compression injury of the porcine cauda equina. Spine (Phila Pa 1976) 15:416-419, 1990.

24. Garfin SR, Cohen MS, Massie JB, et al: Nerve-roots of the cauda equina: The effect of hypotension and acute graded compression on function. J Bone Joint Surg Am 72:1185-1192, 1990.

25. Pedowitz RA, Garfin SR, Massie JB, et al: Effects of magnitude and duration of compression on spinal nerve root conduction. Spine (Phila Pa 1976) 17:194-199, 1992.

26. Rydevik BL, Pedowitz RA, Hargens AR, et al: Effects of acute, graded compression on spinal nerve root function and structure: An experimental study of the pig cauda equina. Spine (Phila Pa 1976) 16:487-493, 1991.

27. Olmarker K, Lind B, Holm S, et al: Continued compression increases impairment of impulse propagation in experimental compression of the porcine cauda equina. Neuroorthopaedics 11:75-81, 1991.

28. Porter RW, Ward D: Cauda equina dysfunction: The significance of two-level pathology. Spine (Phila Pa 1976) 17:9-15, 1992.

29. Olmarker K, Rydevik B: Single- versus double-level nerve root compression: An experimental study on the porcine cauda equina with analyses of nerve impulse conduction properties. Clin Orthop Relat Res 279:35-39, 1992.

30. Lundborg G: Structure and function of the intraneural microvessels as related to trauma, edema formation, and nerve function. J Bone Joint Surg Am 57:938-948, 1975.

31. Parke WW, Watanabe R: The intrinsic vasculature of the lumbosacral spinal nerve roots. Spine (Phila Pa 1976) 10:508-515, 1985.

32. Parke WW, Gammell K, Rothman RH: Arterial vascularization of the cauda equina. J Bone Joint Surg Am 63:53-62, 1981.

33. Petterson CA, Olsson Y: Blood supply of spinal nerve roots: An experimental study in the rat. Acta Neuropathol (Berl) 78:455-461, 1989.

34. Takahashi K, Olmarker K, Holm S, et al: Double-level cauda equina compression: An experimental study with continuous monitoring of intraneural blood flow in the porcine cauda equina. J Orthop Res 11:104-109, 1993.

35. Cornefjord M, Takahashi K, Matsui Y, et al: Impairment of nutritional transport at double-level cauda equina compression: An experimental study. Neuroorthopaedics 13:107-112, 1992.

36. Baker AR, Collins TA, Porter RW, et al: Laser Doppler study of porcine cauda equina blood flow: The effect of electrical stimulation of the rootlets during single and double site, low pressure compression of the cauda equina. Spine (Phila Pa 1976) 20:660-664, 1995.

37. Delamarter RB, Bohlman HH, Dodge LD, et al: Experimental lumbar spinal stenosis: Analysis of the cortical evoked potentials, microvasculature, and histopathology. J Bone Joint Surg Am 72:110-120, 1990.

38. Cornefjord M, Sato K, Olmarker K, et al: A model for chronic nerve root compression studies: Presentation of a porcine model for controlled, slow-onset compression with analyses of anatomic aspects, compression onset rate, and morphologic and neurophysiologic effects. Spine (Phila Pa 1976) 22:946-957, 1997.

39. Cornefjord M, Olmarker K, Farley DB, et al: Neuropeptide changes in compressed spinal nerve roots. Spine (Phila Pa 1976) 20:670-673, 1995.

40. Sato K, Olmarker K, Cornefjord M, et al: Changes of intraradicular blood flow in chronic nerve root compression: An experimental study on pigs. Neuroorthopaedics 16:1-7, 1994.

41. Konno S, Olmarker K, Byrod G, et al: Intermittent cauda equina compression: An experimental study of the porcine cauda equina with analyses of nerve impulse conduction properties. Spine (Phila Pa 1976) 20:1223-1226, 1995.

8 Sciatica and Nerve Root Pain in Disc Herniation and Spinal Stenosis: A Basic Science Review and Clinical Perspective   141

SECTION

I

42. Takahashi K, Miyazaki T, Takino T, et al: Epidural pressure measurements: Relationship between epidural pressure and posture in patients with lumbar spinal stenosis. Spine (Phila Pa 1976) 20:650-653, 1995.

43. Konno S, Yabuki S, Sato K, et al: A model for acute, chronic, and delayed graded compression of the dog cauda equina: Presentation of the gross, microscopic, and vascular anatomy of the dog cauda equina and accuracy in pressure transmission of the compression model. Spine (Phila Pa 1976) 20:2758-2764, 1995.

44. Sato K, Konno S, Yabuki S, et al: A model for acute, chronic, and delayed graded compression of the dog cauda equina: Neurophysiologic and histologic changes induced by acute, graded compression. Spine (Phila Pa 1976) 20:2386-2391, 1995.

45. Schönström N, Bolender NF, Spengler DM, et al: Pressure changes within the cauda equina following constriction of the dural sac: An in vitro experimental study. Spine (Phila Pa 1976) 9:604-607, 1984.

46. Schönström NS, Bolender NF, Spengler DM: The pathomorphology of spinal stenosis as seen on CT scans of the lumbar spine. Spine (Phila Pa 1976) 10:806-811, 1985.

47. Takahashi K, Kagechika K, Takino T, et al: Changes in epidural pressure during walking in patients with lumbar spinal stenosis. Spine (Phila Pa 1976) 20:2746-2749, 1995.

48. Howe JF, Loeser JD, Calvin WH: Mechanosensitivity of dorsal root ganglia and chronically injured axons: A physiological basis for the radicular pain of nerve root compression. Pain 3:25-41, 1977.

49. Cavanaugh JM, Ozaktay AC, Yamashita T, et al: Mechanisms of low back pain: A neurophysiologic and neuroanatomic study. Clin Orthop Relat Res 335:166-180, 1997.

50. Weinstein J, Pope M, Schmidt R, et al: Neuropharmacologic effects of vibration on the dorsal root ganglion: An animal model. Spine (Phila Pa 1976) 13:521-525, 1988.

51. Chatani K, Kawakami M, Weinstein JN, et al: Characterization of thermal hyperalgesia, c-fos expression, and alterations in neuropeptides after mechanical irritation of the dorsal root ganglion. Spine (Phila Pa 1976) 20:277-289; discussion 290, 1995.

52. Kawakami M, Weinstein JN, Spratt KF, et al: Experimental lumbar radiculopathy: Immunohistochemical and quantitative demonstrations of pain induced by lumbar nerve root irritation of the rat. Spine (Phila Pa 1976) 19:1780-1794, 1994.

53. Kawakami M, Weinstein JN, Chatani K, et al: Experimental lumbar radiculopathy: Behavioral and histologic changes in a model of radicular pain after spinal nerve root irritation with chromic gut ligatures in the rat. Spine (Phila Pa 1976) 19:1795-1802, 1994.

54. Olmarker K, Myers RR: Pathogenesis of sciatic pain: Role of herniated nucleus pulposus and deformation of spinal nerve root and dorsal root ganglion. Pain 78:99-105, 1998.

55. Olmarker K, Nutu M, Storkson R: Changes in spontaneous behavior in rats exposed to experimental disc herniation are blocked by selective TNF-alpha inhibition. Spine (Phila Pa 1976) 28:1635-1641, 2003.

56. Olmarker K, Iwabuchi M, Larsson K, et al: Walking analysis of rats subjected to experimental disc herniation. Eur Spine J 7:394-399, 1998.

57. Takahashi K, Shima I, Porter RW: Nerve root pressure in lumbar disc herniation. Spine (Phila Pa 1976) 24:2003-2006, 1999.

58. Myers R, Shubayev VI, Campana WM: Neuropathology of painful neuropathies. In Sommer C (ed): Pain in Peripheral Nerve Disease. Basel, Karger, 2001, pp 8-30.

59. Powell HC, Myers RR: Pathology of experimental nerve compression. Lab Invest 55:91-100, 1986.

60. Myers RR, Yamamoto T, Yaksh TL, et al: The role of focal nerve ischemia and Wallerian degeneration in peripheral nerve injury producing hyperesthesia. Anesthesiology 78:308-316, 1993.

61. Sommer C, Galbraith JA, Heckman HM, et al: Pathology of experimental compression neuropathy producing hyperesthesia. J Neuropathol Exp Neurol 52:223-233, 1993.

62. Stoll G, Jander S, Myers RR: Degeneration and regeneration of the peripheral nervous system: From Augustus Waller's observations to neuroinflammation. J Peripher Nerv Syst 7:13-27, 2002.

63. Myers R, Wagner R, Sorkin LS: Hyperalgesic action of cytokines on peripheral nerves. In Watkins LR, Maier SF (eds): Cytokines and Pain. Basel, Birkhäuser Verlag, 1999, pp 133-157.

64. Myers RR, Heckman HM, Powell HC: Axonal viability and the persistence of thermal hyperalgesia after partial freeze lesions of nerve. J Neurol Sci 139:28-38, 1996.

65. Olmarker K, Nordborg C, Larsson K, et al: Ultrastructural changes in spinal nerve roots induced by autologous nucleus pulposus. Spine (Phila Pa 1976) 21:411-414, 1996.

66. Kayama S, Konno S, Olmarker K, et al: Incision of the anulus fibrosus induces nerve root morphologic, vascular, and functional changes: An experimental study. Spine (Phila Pa 1976) 21:2539-2543, 1996.

67. Byrod G, Otani K, Brisby H, et al: Methylprednisolone reduces the early vascular permeability increase in spinal nerve roots induced by epidural nucleus pulposus application. J Orthop Res 18:983-987, 2000.

68. Yabuki S, Kikuchi S, Olmarker K, et al: Acute effects of nucleus pulposus on blood flow and endoneurial fluid pressure in rat dorsal root ganglia. Spine (Phila Pa 1976) 23:2517-2523, 1998.

69. Byrod G, Rydevik B, Nordborg C, et al: Early effects of nucleus pulposus application on spinal nerve root morphology and function. Eur Spine J 7:445-449, 1998.

70. Olmarker K, Blomquist J, Stromberg J, et al: Inflammatogenic properties of nucleus pulposus. Spine (Phila Pa 1976) 20:665-669, 1995.

71. Takino T, Takahashi K, Miyazaki T, et al: Immunoreactivity of nucleus pulposus. Presented at International Society for the Study of the Lumbar Spine, Helsinki, Finland, 1995.

72. Kawakami M, Tamaki T, Matsumoto T, et al: Role of leukocytes in radicular pain secondary to herniated nucleus pulposus. Clin Orthop Relat Res 376:268-277, 2000.

73. Myers RR, Heckman HM, Rodriguez M: Reduced hyperalgesia in nerve-injured WLD mice: Relationship to nerve fiber phagocytosis, axonal degeneration, and regeneration in normal mice. Exp Neurol 141:94-101, 1996.

74. Kawakami M, Matsumoto T, Hashizume H, et al: Epidural injection of cyclooxygenase-2 inhibitor attenuates pain-related

behavior following application of nucleus pulposus to the nerve root in the rat. J Orthop Res 20:376-381, 2002.

75. Macnab I: Negative disc exploration: An analysis of the causes of nerve-root involvement in sixty-eight patients. J Bone Joint Surg Am 53:891-903, 1971.

76. Crock HV: Observations on the management of failed spinal operations. J Bone Joint Surg Br 58:193-199, 1976.

77. Jonsson B, Stromqvist B: Clinical appearance of contained and noncontained lumbar disc herniation. J Spinal Disord 9:32-38, 1996.

78. Ito T, Takano Y, Yuasa N: Types of lumbar herniated disc and clinical course. Spine (Phila Pa 1976) 26:648-651, 2001.

79. Nygaard OP, Mellgren SI, Osterud B: The inflammatory properties of contained and noncontained lumbar disc herniation. Spine (Phila Pa 1976) 22:2484-2488, 1997.

80. Olmarker K, Storkson R, Berge OG: Pathogenesis of sciatic pain: A study of spontaneous behavior in rats exposed to experimental disc herniation. Spine (Phila Pa 1976) 27:1312-1317, 2002.

81. Kuslich SD, Ulstrom CL, Michael CJ: The tissue origin of low back pain and sciatica: A report of pain response to tissue stimulation during operations on the lumbar spine using local anesthesia. Orthop Clin North Am 22:181-187, 1991.

82. Anzai H, Hamba M, Onda A, et al: Epidural application of nucleus pulposus enhances nociresponses of rat dorsal horn neurons. Spine (Phila Pa 1976) 27:E50-E55, 2002.

83. Olmarker K, Rydevik B: Pathophysiology of sciatica. Orthop Clin North Am 22:223-234, 1991.

84. El-Mahdi MA, Abdel Latif FY, Janko M: The spinal nerve root "innervation," and a new concept of the clinicopathological interrelations in back pain and sciatica. Neurochirurgia (Stuttg) 24:137-141, 1981.

85. Edgar MA, Nundy S: Innervation of the spinal dura. J Neurol Neurosurg Psychiatry 29:530-534, 1966.

86. Kaplan EB: Recurrent meningeal branch of the spinal nerve. Bull Hosp Joint Dis 1947.

87. von Luschka H: Die Nerven des Menschen, 1850.

88. Rudinger N: Die Gelenkennerven des menschlichen Körpers. Erlangen, Ferdinand Enke, 1857.

89. Olmarker K: Experimental basis of sciatica. J Orthop Sci 1:230-242, 1996.

90. Dyck PJ, Karnes J, Lais A, et al: Pathologic alterations of the peripheral nervous system of humans. In Dyck PJ, Thomas PK, Lambert EH, et al (eds): Peripheral Neuropathy. Philadelphia, WB Saunders, 1984, pp 828-930.

91. Hoyland JA, Freemont AJ, Jayson MI: Intervertebral foramen venous obstruction: A cause of periradicular fibrosis? Spine (Phila Pa 1976) 14:558-568, 1989.

92. Cooper RG, Freemont AJ, Hoyland JA, et al: Herniated intervertebral disc-associated periradicular fibrosis and vascular abnormalities occur without inflammatory cell infiltration. Spine (Phila Pa 1976) 20:591-598, 1995.

93. Jayson MI, Keegan A, Million R, et al: A fibrinolytic defect in chronic back pain syndromes. Lancet 2:1186-1187, 1984.

94. Klimiuk PS, Pountain GD, Keegan AL, et al: Serial measurements of fibrinolytic activity in acute low back pain and sciatica. Spine (Phila Pa 1976) 12:925-928, 1987.

95. Byrod G, Olmarker K, Konno S, et al: A rapid transport route between the epidural space and the intraneural capillaries of the nerve roots. Spine (Phila Pa 1976) 20:138-143, 1995.

96. Dalcanto MC, Wisniewski HM, Johnson AB, et al: Vesicular disruption of myelin in autoimmune demyelination. J Neurol Sci 24:313-319, 1975.

97. Hahn AF, Gilbert JJ, Feasby TE: Passive transfer of demyelination by experimental allergic neuritis serum. Acta Neuropathol (Berl) 49:169-176, 1980.

98. Bisla RS, Marchisello PJ, Lockshin MD, et al: Auto-immunological basis of disk degeneration. Clin Orthop Relat Res 121:205-211, 1976.

99. Bobechko WP, Hirsch C: Auto-immune response to nucleus pulposus in the rabbit. J Bone Joint Surg Br 47:574-580, 1965.

100. Gertzbein SD, Tile M, Gross A, Falk R: Autoimmunity in degenerative disc disease of the lumbar spine. Orthop Clin North Am 6:67-73, 1975.

101. Gertzbein SD: Degenerative disk disease of the lumbar spine: Immunological implications. Clin Orthop Relat Res 129:68-71, 1977.

102. Gertzbein SD, Tait JH, Devlin SR: The stimulation of lymphocytes by nucleus pulposus in patients with degenerative disk disease of the lumbar spine. Clin Orthop Relat Res 123:149-154, 1977.

103. LaRocca H: New horizons in research on disc disease. Orthop Clin North Am 2:521-531, 1971.

104. Naylor A: The biophysical and biochemical aspects of intervertebral disc herniation and degeneration. Ann R Coll Surg Engl 31:91-114, 1962.

105. Geiss A, Larsson K, Rydevik B, et al: Autoimmune properties of nucleus pulposus: An experimental study in pigs. Spine (Phila Pa 1976) 32:168-173, 2007

106. Satoh K, Konno S, Nishiyama K, et al: Presence and distribution of antigen-antibody complexes in the herniated nucleus pulposus. Spine (Phila Pa 1976) 24:1980-1984, 1999.

107. Bayliss MT, Johnstone B: Biochemistry of the intervertebral disc. In Jayson MIV (ed): The Lumbar Spine and Back Pain. Edinburgh, Churchill-Livingstone, 1992, pp 111-131.

108. Eyre D, Benya P, Buckwalter J: Intervertebral disc. In Frymoyer JW, Gordon SL (eds): New Perspectives on Low Back Pain. Rosemont, American Academy of Orthopaedic Surgeons, 1988, pp 149-207.

109. Marshall LL, Trethewie ER: Chemical irritation of nerve-root in disc prolapse. Lancet 2:320, 1973.

110. Marshall LL, Trethewie ER, Curtain CC: Chemical radiculitis: A clinical, physiological and immunological study. Clin Orthop Relat Res 129:61-67, 1977.

111. Kayama S, Olmarker K, Larsson K, et al: Cultured, autologous nucleus pulposus cells induce structural and functional changes in spinal nerve roots. Spine (Phila Pa 1976) 23:2155-2158, 1998.

112. Brisby H, Byrod G, Olmarker K, et al: Nitric oxide as a mediator of nucleus pulposus-induced effects on spinal nerve roots. J Orthop Res 18:815-820, 2000.

113. Diamant B, Karlsson J, Nachemson A: Correlation between lactate levels and pH in discs of patients with lumbar rhizopathies. Experientia 24:1195-1196, 1968.

114. Nachemson A: Intradiscal measurements of pH in patients with lumbar rhizopathies. Acta Orthop Scand 40:23-42, 1969.

115. Pennington JB, McCarron RF, Laros GS: Identification of IgG in the canine intervertebral disc. Spine (Phila Pa 1976) 13:909-912, 1988.

116. Saal JS, Franson RC, Dobrow R, et al: High levels of inflammatory phospholipase A2 activity in lumbar disc herniations. Spine (Phila Pa 1976) 15:674-678, 1990.

117. Olmarker K, Larsson K: Tumor necrosis factor alpha and nucleus-pulposus-induced nerve root injury. Spine (Phila Pa 1976) 23:2538-2544, 1998.

118. Chao CC, Hu S, Ehrlich L, et al: Interleukin-1 and tumor necrosis factor-alpha synergistically mediate neurotoxicity: Involvement of nitric oxide and of N-methyl-D-aspartate receptors. Brain Behav Immun 9:355-365, 1995.

119. Gadient RA, Cron KC, Otten U: Interleukin-1 beta and tumor necrosis factor-alpha synergistically stimulate nerve growth factor (NGF) release from cultured rat astrocytes. Neurosci Lett 117:335-340, 1990.

120. Bluthe RM, Dantzer R, Kelley KW: Interleukin-1 mediates behavioural but not metabolic effects of tumor necrosis factor alpha in mice. Eur J Pharmacol 209:281-283, 1991.

121. McHale JF, Harari OA, Marshall D, et al: TNF-alpha and IL-1 sequentially induce endothelial ICAM-1 and VCAM-1 expression in MRL/lpr lupus-prone mice. J Immunol 163:3993-4000, 1999.

122. Siwik DA, Chang DL, Colucci WS: Interleukin-1beta and tumor necrosis factor-alpha decrease collagen synthesis and increase matrix metalloproteinase activity in cardiac fibroblasts in vitro. Circ Res 86:1259-1265, 2000.

123. McGee DW, Bamberg T, Vitkus SJ, et al: A synergistic relationship between TNF-alpha, IL-1 beta, and TGF-beta 1 on IL-6 secretion by the IEC-6 intestinal epithelial cell line. Immunology 86:6-11, 1995.

124. Wagner R, Myers RR: Schwann cells produce tumor necrosis factor alpha: Expression in injured and non-injured nerves. Neuroscience 73:625-629, 1996.

125. Satomi N, Haranaka K, Kunii O: Research on the production site of tumor necrosis factor (TNF). Jpn J Exp Med 51:317-322, 1981.

126. Bachwich PR, Lynch JP 3rd, Larrick J, et al: Tumor necrosis factor production by human sarcoid alveolar macrophages. Am J Pathol 125:421-425, 1986.

127. Robbins DS, Shirazi Y, Drysdale BE, et al: Production of cytotoxic factor for oligodendrocytes by stimulated astrocytes. J Immunol 139:2593-2597, 1987.

128. Sayers TJ, Macher I, Chung J, et al: The production of tumor necrosis factor by mouse bone marrow-derived macrophages in response to bacterial lipopolysaccharide and a chemically synthesized monosaccharide precursor. J Immunol 138:2935-2940, 1987.

129. Sommer C, Marziniak M, Myers RR: The effect of thalidomide treatment on vascular pathology and hyperalgesia caused by chronic constriction injury of rat nerve. Pain 74:83-91, 1998.

130. Wagner R, Myers RR: Endoneurial injection of TNF-alpha produces neuropathic pain behaviors. Neuroreport 7:2897-2901, 1996.

131. Igarashi T, Kikuchi S, Shubayev V, et al: 2000 Volvo Award winner in basic science studies: Exogenous tumor necrosis factor-alpha mimics nucleus pulposus-induced neuropathology: Molecular, histologic, and behavioral comparisons in rats. Spine (Phila Pa 1976) 25:2975-2980, 2000.

132. Liberski PP, Yanagihara R, Nerurkar V, et al: Further ultrastructural studies of lesions produced in the optic nerve by tumor necrosis factor alpha (TNF-alpha): A comparison with experimental Creutzfeldt-Jakob disease. Acta Neurobiol Exp (Warsz) 54:209-218, 1994.

133. Madigan MC, Sadun AA, Rao NS, et al: Tumor necrosis factor-alpha (TNF-alpha)-induced optic neuropathy in rabbits. Neurol Res 18:176-184, 1996.

134. Redford EJ, Hall SM, Smith KJ: Vascular changes and demyelination induced by the intraneural injection of tumour necrosis factor. Brain 118(Pt 4):869-878, 1995.

135. Selmaj K, Raine CS: Tumor necrosis factor mediates myelin damage in organotypic cultures of nervous tissue. Ann N Y Acad Sci 540:568-570, 1988.

136. Stoll G, Jung S, Jander S, et al: Tumor necrosis factor-alpha in immune-mediated demyelination and Wallerian degeneration of the rat peripheral nervous system. J Neuroimmunol 45:175-182, 1993.

137. Nawroth P, Handley D, Matsueda G, et al: Tumor necrosis factor/cachectin-induced intravascular fibrin formation in meth A fibrosarcomas. J Exp Med 168:637-647, 1988.

138. van der Poll T, Jansen PM, Van Zee KJ, et al: Tumor necrosis factor-alpha induces activation of coagulation and fibrinolysis in baboons through an exclusive effect on the p55 receptor. Blood 88:922-927, 1996.

139. Watts ME, Arnold S, Chaplin DJ: Changes in coagulation and permeability properties of human endothelial cells in vitro induced by TNF-alpha or 5,6 MeXAA. Br J Cancer 74(Suppl 27):S164-S167, 1996.

140. Viviani B, Corsini E, Galli CL, et al: Glia increase degeneration of hippocampal neurons through release of tumor necrosis factor-alpha. Toxicol Appl Pharmacol 150:271-276, 1998.

141. Wuthrich RP, Jevnikar AM, Takei F, et al: Intercellular adhesion molecule-1 (ICAM-1) expression is upregulated in autoimmune murine lupus nephritis. Am J Pathol 136:441-450, 1990.

142. Sommer C, Schmidt C, George A, et al: A metalloprotease-inhibitor reduces pain associated behavior in mice with experimental neuropathy. Neurosci Lett 237:45-48, 1997.

143. Sorkin LS, Xiao WH, Wagner R, et al: Tumour necrosis factor-alpha induces ectopic activity in nociceptive primary afferent fibres. Neuroscience 81:255-262, 1997.

144. Shubayev VI, Myers RR: Upregulation and interaction of TNFalpha and gelatinases A and B in painful peripheral nerve injury. Brain Res 855:83-89, 2000.

145. Shubayev VI, Myers RR: Axonal transport of TNF-alpha in painful neuropathy: Distribution of ligand tracer and TNF receptors. J Neuroimmunol 114:48-56, 2001.

146. Mattila P, Majuri ML, Mattila PS, et al: TNF alpha-induced expression of endothelial adhesion molecules, ICAM-1 and VCAM-1, is linked to protein kinase C activation. Scand J Immunol 36:159-165, 1992.

147. Pober JS: Effects of tumour necrosis factor and related cytokines on vascular endothelial cells. Ciba Found Symp 131:170-184, 1987.

148. Creange A, Barlovatz-Meimon G, Gherardi RK: Cytokines and peripheral nerve disorders. Eur Cytokine Netw 8:145-151, 1997.

149. Munro JM, Pober JS, Cotran RS: Tumor necrosis factor and interferon-gamma induce distinct patterns of endothelial activation and associated leukocyte accumulation in skin of *Papio anubis*. Am J Pathol 135:121-133, 1989.

150. Oku N, Araki R, Araki H, et al: Tumor necrosis factor-induced permeability increase of negatively charged phospholipid vesicles. J Biochem (Tokyo) 102:1303-1310, 1987.

151. Kagan BL, Baldwin RL, Munoz D, et al: Formation of ion-permeable channels by tumor necrosis factor-alpha. Science 255:1427-1430, 1992.

152. Baldwin RL, Stolowitz ML, Hood L, et al: Structural changes of tumor necrosis factor alpha associated with membrane insertion and channel formation. Proc Natl Acad Sci U S A 93:1021-1026, 1996.

153. Wei Y, Babilonia E, Pedraza PL, et al: Acute application of TNF stimulates apical 70-pS K+ channels in the thick ascending limb of rat kidney. Am J Physiol Renal Physiol 285:F491-F497, 2003.

154. Woolf CJ: The pathophysiology of peripheral neuropathic pain-abnormal peripheral input and abnormal central processing. Acta Neurochir Suppl (Wien) 58:125-130, 1993.

155. Attal N, Bouhassira D: Mechanisms of pain in peripheral neuropathy. Acta Neurol Scand Suppl 173:12-24; discussion 48-52, 1999.

156. Zimmermann M: Pathobiology of neuropathic pain. Eur J Pharmacol 429:23-37, 2001.

157. Wall PD: Neuropathic pain and injured nerve: central mechanisms. Br Med Bull 47:631-643, 1991.

158. Selmaj K, Raine CS, Cross AH: Anti-tumor necrosis factor therapy abrogates autoimmune demyelination. Ann Neurol 30:694-700, 1991.

159. Selmaj KW, Raine CS: Tumor necrosis factor mediates myelin and oligodendrocyte damage in vitro. Ann Neurol 23:339-346, 1988.

160. Villarroya H, Violleau K, Ben Younes-Chennoufi A, et al: Myelin-induced experimental allergic encephalomyelitis in Lewis rats: Tumor necrosis factor alpha levels in serum and cerebrospinal fluid immunohistochemical expression in glial cells and macrophages of optic nerve and spinal cord. J Neuroimmunol 64:55-61, 1996.

161. Ghabriel MN, Allt G: Schmidt-Lanterman incisures: I. A quantitative teased fibre study of remyelinating peripheral nerve fibres. Acta Neuropathol (Berl) 52:85-95, 1980.

162. Shanklin WM, Azzam NA: Histological and histochemical studies on the incisures of Schmidt-Lanterman. J Comp Neurol 123:5-10, 1964.

163. Robertson JD: The ultrastructure of Schmidt-Lanterman clefts and related shearing defects of the myelin sheath. J Biophys Biochem Cytol 4:39-46, 1958.

164. Todd BA, Inman C, Sedgwick EM, et al: Ionic permeability of the frog sciatic nerve perineurium: Parallel studies of potassium and lanthanum penetration using electrophysiological and electron microscopic techniques. J Neurocytol 29:551-567, 2000.

165. Brisby H, Olmarker K, Rosengren L, et al: Markers of nerve tissue injury in the cerebrospinal fluid in patients with lumbar disc herniation and sciatica. Spine (Phila Pa 1976) 24:742-746, 1999.

166. Cornefjord M, Nyberg F, Rosengren L, et al: Cerebrospinal fluid biomarkers in experimental spinal nerve root injury. Spine (Phila Pa 1976) 29:1862-1868, 2004.

167. Brisby H, Balague F, Schafer D, et al: Glycosphingolipid antibodies in serum in patients with sciatica. Spine (Phila Pa 1976) 27:380-386, 2002.

168. Schafers M, Sorkin LS, Geis C, et al: Spinal nerve ligation induces transient upregulation of tumor necrosis factor receptors 1 and 2 in injured and adjacent uninjured dorsal root ganglia in the rat. Neurosci Lett 347:179-182, 2003.

169. Schafers M, Lee DH, Brors D, et al: Increased sensitivity of injured and adjacent uninjured rat primary sensory neurons to exogenous tumor necrosis factor-alpha after spinal nerve ligation. J Neurosci 23:3028-3038, 2003.

170. Schafers M, Svensson CI, Sommer C, et al: Tumor necrosis factor-alpha induces mechanical allodynia after spinal nerve ligation by activation of p38 MAPK in primary sensory neurons. J Neurosci 23:2517-2521, 2003.

171. Winkelstein BA, Rutkowski MD, Sweitzer SM, et al: Nerve injury proximal or distal to the DRG induces similar spinal glial activation and selective cytokine expression but differential behavioral responses to pharmacologic treatment. J Comp Neurol 439:127-139, 2001.

172. Raghavendra V, Rutkowski MD, DeLeo JA: The role of spinal neuroimmune activation in morphine tolerance/hyperalgesia in neuropathic and sham-operated rats. J Neurosci 22:9980-9989, 2002.

173. DeLeo JA, Rutkowski MD, Stalder AK, et al: Transgenic expression of TNF by astrocytes increases mechanical allodynia in a mouse neuropathy model. Neuroreport 11:599-602, 2000.

174. Olmarker K, Rydevik B: Selective inhibition of tumor necrosis factor-alpha prevents nucleus pulposus-induced thrombus formation, intraneural edema, and reduction of nerve conduction velocity: Possible implications for future pharmacologic treatment strategies of sciatica. Spine (Phila Pa 1976) 26:863-869, 2001.

175. Spillert CR, Sun S, Ponnudurai R, et al: Tumor necrosis factor-induced necrosis: A monocyte-mediated hypercoagulable effect. J Natl Med Assoc 87:508-509, 1995.

176. Aderka D: Role of tumor necrosis factor in the pathogenesis of intravascular coagulopathy of sepsis: Potential new therapeutic implications. Isr J Med Sci 27:52-60, 1991.

177. Onda A, Murata Y, Rydevik B, et al: Infliximab attenuates immunoreactivity of brain-derived neurotrophic factor in a rat model of herniated nucleus pulposus. Spine (Phila Pa 1976) 29:1857-1861, 2004.

178. Murata Y, Onda A, Rydevik B, et al: Selective inhibition of tumor necrosis factor-alpha prevents nucleus pulposus-induced histologic changes in the dorsal root ganglion. Spine (Phila Pa 1976) 29:2477-2484, 2004.

179. Murata Y, Olmarker K, Takahashi I, et al: Effects of selective tumor necrosis factor-alpha inhibition to pain-behavioral changes caused by nucleus pulposus-induced damage to the spinal nerve in rats. Neurosci Lett 382:148-152, 2005.

180. Aoki Y, Rydevik B, Kikuchi S, et al: Local application of disc-related cytokines on spinal nerve roots. Spine (Phila Pa 1976) 27:1614-1617, 2002.

181. Ozaktay AC, Cavanaugh JM, Asik I, et al: Dorsal root sensitivity to interleukin-1 beta, interleukin-6 and tumor necrosis factor in rats. Eur Spine J 11:467-475, 2002.

182. Onda A, Yabuki S, Kikuchi S: Effects of neutralizing antibodies to tumor necrosis factor-alpha on nucleus pulposus-induced abnormal nociresponses in rat dorsal horn neurons. Spine (Phila Pa 1976) 28:967-972, 2003.

183. Wagner R, Janjigian M, Myers RR: Anti-inflammatory interleukin-10 therapy in CCI neuropathy decreases thermal hyperalgesia, macrophage recruitment, and endoneurial TNF-alpha expression. Pain 74:35-42, 1998.

184. Wehling P, Cleveland SJ, Heininger K, et al: Neurophysiologic changes in lumbar nerve root inflammation in the rat after treatment with cytokine inhibitors: Evidence for a role of interleukin-1. Spine (Phila Pa 1976) 21:931-935, 1996.

185. Brisby H, Olmarker K, Larsson K, et al: Proinflammatory cytokines in cerebrospinal fluid and serum in patients with disc herniation and sciatica. Eur Spine J 11:62-66, 2002.

186. Onda A, Murata Y, Rydevik B, et al: Immunoreactivity of brain-derived neurotrophic factor in rat dorsal root ganglion and spinal cord dorsal horn following exposure to herniated nucleus pulposus. Neurosci Lett 352:49-52, 2003.

187. Murata Y, Onda A, Rydevik B, et al: Distribution and appearance of tumor necrosis factor-alpha in the dorsal root ganglion exposed to experimental disc herniation in rats. Spine (Phila Pa 1976) 29:2235-2241, 2004.

188. Murata Y, Rydevik B, Takahashi K, et al: Macrophage appearance in the epineurium and endoneurium of dorsal root ganglion exposed to nucleus pulposus. J Peripher Nerv Syst 9:158-164, 2004.

189. Onda A, Murata Y, Rydevik B, et al: Nerve growth factor content in dorsal root ganglion as related to changes in pain behavior in a rat model of experimental lumbar disc herniation. Spine (Phila Pa 1976) 30:188-193, 2005.

190. Larsson K, Rydevik B, Olmarker K: Disc related cytokines inhibit axonal outgrowth from dorsal root ganglion cells in vitro. Spine (Phila Pa 1976) 30:621-624, 2005.

191. Karppinen J, Korhonen T, Malmivaara A, et al: Tumor necrosis factor-alpha monoclonal antibody, infliximab, used to manage severe sciatica. Spine (Phila Pa 1976) 28:750-753, 2003.

192. Korhonen T, Karppinen J, Malmivaara A, et al: Efficacy of infliximab for disc herniation-induced sciatica: One-year follow-up. Spine (Phila Pa 1976) 29:2115-2119, 2004.

193. Genevay S, Stingelin S, Gabay C: Efficacy of etanercept in the treatment of acute severe sciatica. Ann Rheum Dis 63:1120-1123, 2004.

194. Cohen SP, Bogduk N, Dragovich A, et al: Randomized, double-blind, placebo-controlled, dose-response, and preclinical safety of transforaminal epidural etanercept for the treatment of sciatica. Anesthesiology 110:1116-1126, 2009.

195. Genevay S, Viatte S, Finck A, et al: Adalimumab in severe and acute sciatica: A multicentre, randomised, double-blind, placebo controlled trial. Arthritis Rheum April 6, 2010 [E-pub ahead of print].

196. Cooper RG, Freemont AJ: TNF-alpha blockade for herniated intervertebral disc-induced sciatica: A way forward at last? [editorial]. Rheumatology 43:119-121, 2004.

197. Genevay S, Gabay C: Is disk-related sciatica a TNFα-dependent inflammatory disease? Joint Bone Spine 72:4-6, 2005.

Genetic Applications: An Overview

Edward Westrick, MD
Gwendolyn Sowa, MD, PhD
Scott D. Boden, MD
James D. Kang, MD

Exciting developments in biomedical technology, molecular biology, and genetics have opened avenues into novel approaches for treating musculoskeletal disorders at the molecular level. These advances have catalyzed intense investigations into biologic therapies for bone healing, intervertebral disc degeneration, arthritides, muscle injuries, and genetic disorders such as muscular dystrophy and osteogenesis imperfecta. In particular, gene therapy (the process by which therapeutic genes are delivered to target cells to alter disease course) has exhibited much promise as a biologic therapy. Gene therapy is an elegant way to deliver sustained levels of growth factors to musculoskeletal tissues by introducing therapeutic proteins via the injection of a viral vector carrying the genetic blueprint, allowing cells to release therapeutic levels of the desired growth factor continuously. Investigators have shown successful gene transfer to several tissues within the musculoskeletal system, including synovial cells, chondrocytes, tendons, ligaments, muscles, intervertebral discs, and bone. It is apparent from the growing literature that gene therapy has the potential of becoming a valuable treatment modality.

Investigations into the potential applications of gene therapy for spinal disorders have been similarly promising. Most of these studies have focused on developing gene therapy strategies for treating intervertebral disc degeneration and for improving spinal fusion rates. A multitude of issues dealing with vector choice, growth factor biology, method of delivery, and safety considerations must be resolved before clinical translation. Despite these obstacles, gene therapy for spinal disorders holds much clinical promise for the future. Spine surgeons should have a fundamental understanding of this new technology. This chapter discusses the pertinent terminology and concepts involved and gives an overview of the literature on gene therapy for intervertebral disc pathology and spinal fusion.

Basics

Definition

The term *gene therapy* was previously used to describe replacement of a defective gene with a functional copy by means of gene transfer. The diseases originally targeted for gene therapy were classic, heritable genetic disorders. The term now broadly defines therapy involving the transfer of exogenous genes (complementary DNA [cDNA]) encoding therapeutic proteins into cells to treat disease.[1] The genetically altered cells are made into protein-producing "factories" churning out disease-altering gene products. Specifically, the host cell transcribes the exogenous gene (or transgene) into messenger RNA (mRNA); cytoplasmic ribosomes translate mRNA into the protein product. These products can affect not only the metabolism of cells from which they were made but also the metabolism of adjacent non–genetically altered cells via paracrine mechanisms (Fig. 9–1).

Exogenous genes are produced and packaged in the laboratory in the following manner. First, cDNA of a gene of interest is constructed by the enzyme reverse transcriptase from mRNA. The cDNA is incorporated into a plasmid, a circular piece of DNA that is self-replicating and capable of delivering exogenous genes into cells, albeit at an inefficient rate. The cDNA plasmid is next integrated into a larger plasmid with a promoter sequence, assembling an expression plasmid. The promoter sequence initiates transcription of the gene of interest by target cells after gene transfer has occurred. The cytomegalovirus promoter is commonly used in gene transfer experiments. This promoter is constitutive, meaning it consistently initiates transcription throughout the life of the gene. The expression plasmid is integrated into either a viral or nonviral molecular vehicle that facilitates transfer of the exogenous gene to cells. These *vectors* are discussed in the following section.

There are two basic strategies for delivering exogenous genes to target cells. The first is the in vivo method, in which a gene-carrying vector is directly transferred to an intended population of cells within the host. The second approach, known as ex vivo gene therapy, involves removing target cells from the body, genetically altering them in vitro, and reimplanting them in the body (Fig. 9–2). Ex vivo methods are more complex and involve multiple, time-intensive steps. This approach is relatively safer, however, because the genetically altered cells may be observed for abnormal behavior before implantation. The ex vivo strategy allows the opportunity for in vitro selection of cells that express the gene of interest at high levels. Gene transfer via the in vivo method is technically simpler. There are relative advantages and disadvantages to both approaches that depend on the anatomy and physiology of the target organs, the pathophysiology of the disease being treated, the vector of choice, and safety considerations.[2]

Overview of Vectors

Successful gene therapy generally depends on the efficient transfer of genes to target cells with subsequent expression. Generally, the duration of transgene production to treat disease successfully depends on the disease being targeted. Sustained expression is necessary for chronic conditions such as disc degeneration, whereas brief expression may be sufficient for acute conditions such as bone healing. With few exceptions, naked plasmid DNA is not taken up and expressed by cells effectively. Consequently, vectors are often necessary to package and insert genes into cells in such a way that the genetic information can be expressed. There are two broad categories of vectors, viral and nonviral. Gene delivery involving viral vectors is termed *transduction,* whereas transfer using nonviral vectors is termed *transfection.*

Nonviral Vectors

Nonviral vectors include liposomes, DNA-ligand complexes, gene guns, and microbubble-enhanced ultrasound. Liposomes are phospholipid vesicles that deliver genetic material into a cell by fusing with the cell membrane. Liposome vectors are simple, inexpensive, and safe, but drawbacks include transient expression of the transgene, cytotoxicity at higher concentrations, and low efficiency of transfection. DNA-ligand complexes and gene gun are nonpathogenic and relatively inexpensive to construct, but there is concern with lower transfer efficiencies and limited persistence of gene expression. Nishida and colleagues[3] showed that ultrasound transfection with microbubbles significantly enhanced the transfection efficiency of plasmid DNA into the nucleus pulposus cells of rats in vivo, observing transgene expression up to 24 weeks. The overall transfection efficiency and level of gene expression of these nonviral vectors are generally inferior, however, to that of viral-mediated gene transfer. Consequently, most current studies involving gene therapy employ viral vectors.[4]

Viral Vectors

Viral vectors take advantage of the natural ability of viruses to infect and deliver genetic information efficiently to specific cell populations. The most commonly used viral vectors are derived from retroviruses, herpes simplex viruses (HSV), adenoviruses, and adeno-associated viruses (AAV). These viruses are often rendered *incapable of replication* before gene therapy application in an effort to make them less pathogenic. There are inherent merits and drawbacks associated with each viral vector, which are discussed in the following section. The choice of viral vector for gene transfer experiments is based

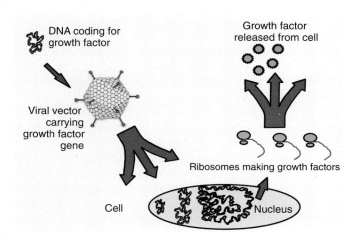

FIGURE 9–1 DNA encoding the gene of interest is constructed into a viral vector that is rendered incapable of replication. The vector is exposed to host cells, attaches to their surface, and is internalized. The released genetic information can either travel to the nucleus, where it may become integrated into the host genome, or remain episomal. It commandeers the normal protein-making machinery of the cell and produces large quantities of transgene.

on multiple considerations, including the gene to be delivered, the disease to be treated, and safety considerations.

Retroviruses are small RNA viruses that replicate their genomic RNA into double-stranded DNA (dsDNA) via the action of reverse transcriptase. The dsDNA is integrated into the host genome at a random location where it is able to express transgene for the life of the cell. Exogenous dsDNA is replicated by the transduced cell and passed on to all progeny cells during cell division. Gene delivery with retroviral vectors results in stable, long-term expression because the gene is integrated into the cell's genome. Because the integration is at a random site, however, the risk of potential mutagenesis of oncogenes exists. Until more recently, this risk was considered only a theoretical possibility, but preliminary reports from a gene therapy trial involving retroviral vectors suggest one of the enrolled subjects developed leukemia as a result

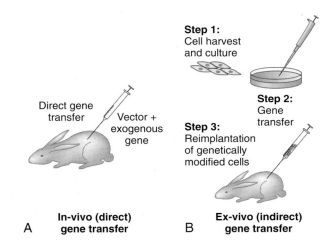

FIGURE 9–2 A, In vivo gene therapy involves direct injection of vector-gene constructs into target tissues within the host. **B,** In ex vivo method, target cells are harvested from the host and then transduced, expanded, and propagated before reimplantation.

of oncogene mutation.[5] Another disadvantage of the most commonly used retroviral vector, the murine leukemia virus (MLV), is that it infects and transduces only actively dividing cells. For these reasons, MLV is most suited for ex vivo applications. Lentiviruses, another class of retroviruses, are capable of infecting nondividing cells. Their drawbacks lie in their wild-type pathogenicity and complex genomic configuration, which make molecular processing for gene transfer much more intricate.

HSV vectors are dsDNA viruses, and the wild-type virus is a human pathogen that is trophic for sensory neurons. The replication-deficient vectors can infect dividing and nondividing cells of almost all types in vitro and in vivo. In addition, HSV vectors have the capacity to carry large amounts of exogenous DNA. This large carrying capacity allows for the production of HSV vectors that are capable of expressing multiple transgenes, which may be highly desirable for gene therapy applications involving complex disease pathophysiology, as in cancer or arthritis. HSV vectors do not integrate the genes they are carrying into the genome of the target cell. A disadvantage of HSV vectors is that they result in transient expression of the transgene despite efficient transduction. Consequently, these vectors would be insufficient for chronic conditions, such as intervertebral disc degeneration.

Adenoviruses are dsDNA viruses capable of infecting many cell types, including nondividing cells. There are 47 known human serotypes of adenoviruses, with serotypes 2 and 5 most commonly used for gene therapy studies. Wild-type adenoviral infections result in mild respiratory and gastrointestinal illnesses. The ability of adenoviral vectors to transfer genes to target cells is particularly efficient. Consequently, the adenovirus is an appealing option for in vivo gene delivery to quiescent, nondividing cell populations. The adenovirus genome exists as an episome within the nucleus of the infected cell and is not integrated into the genome of the host cell, so the risk of insertional mutagenesis does not exist.

The vectors are relatively easy to engineer in very high titers, in contrast to the HSV vector. A major disadvantage with the adenoviral vector is its short duration of transgene expression in most tissues. The transient expression of gene product is thought to occur because of low-level production of adenoviral antigens by the infected cell, resulting in an immune response directed against these cells. The episomal location of the vector genome is also thought to contribute to the short duration of expression. During cell division, the viral episome is not replicated and instead ultimately is degraded. Research is ongoing to engineer adenoviral vectors to minimize viral protein expression and consequently be less immunogenic.

AAV is a parvovirus with a 4.7-kb single-stranded DNA genome. Wild-type AAV lacks the viral machinery to self-replicate and can reproduce only in association with concomitant viral infection, usually adenovirus. AAV is also capable of infecting many different cell types, dividing and nondividing, but its level of infection efficiency is varied. The wild type is not known to cause disease.

The AAV vector differs from the adenoviral vector in several important ways. First, the AAV vector integrates reliably into a specific site on chromosome 19 in a nonpathogenic manner. Second, AAV does not provoke a significant immune response because the vector fails to express viral gene products after infection of target cells. Wild-type AAV has only two genes, *Rep* and *Cap*, which cannot be replicated without the presence of a helper virus. There is no expression of AAV gene products after transduction, theoretically leading to minimal host cell–mediated immune reaction. Although nearly 80% of the population has circulating antibodies against AAV2 (serotype 2) as a result of silent infections, titers of these neutralizing antibodies are usually low. For these reasons, sustained transgene expression can be achieved for 1 year in an immunocompetent host. The main shortcoming of AAV vectors is that they are capable of carrying only small amounts of foreign DNA. In addition, these vectors are difficult to construct and purify in the laboratory without helper virus contamination. There are multiple serotypes of AAV, but AAV2 has been most thoroughly studied for musculoskeletal applications, including degenerative disc disease.

There is a wide range of vector systems with different profiles for delivery efficiency, duration of expression, technical feasibility, and safety. Ongoing investigations are attempting to improve these profiles, and this research is likely to result in enhanced vectors with inducible promoters, tissue-specific promoters, or tissue-specific tropism. As mentioned, the appropriate vector system for a gene therapy application depends on multiple factors, including the method of delivery, pathophysiology of the disease targeted, and the gene selected for transfer.

Spinal Application: Fusion

Clinical Problem

Disorders of the spine often necessitate intervertebral fusion. Although internal fixation devices can successfully achieve temporary stabilization at practically all levels, long-term stability requires osseous consolidation. In contrast to fracture healing, spinal arthrodesis involves deposition of new bone in intersegmental locations that are not biologically structured for bone formation. Consequently, the nonunion rate is 40%[6,7] with single-level fusions and higher when multiple levels are attempted. Although instrumentation has improved the rate of bony union, pseudarthrosis remains a considerable clinical problem. Autogenous bone graft may be scarce in volume in cases such as pediatric fusions and revision surgery. It is associated with substantial donor site morbidity. Owing to these significant obstacles to clinical success, extensive research has been directed at developing molecular therapies to facilitate intersegmental fusion.

Augmentation of Spinal Fusion with Bone Morphogenetic Proteins

Bone morphogenetic proteins (BMPs) are a group of osteoinductive cytokines that play an essential role in the formation and maturation of osseous tissues. Urist and colleagues[8,9] originally recognized these proteins for their ability to form ectopic bone by inducing mesenchymal stem cell differentiation into chondrocytes and osteoblasts. Numerous subsequent animal studies have shown the ability of BMPs to enhance bone deposition at fusion sites.[10-19] This was followed by several clinical trials that validated these preclinical findings. In a study by Patel and colleagues,[20] patients undergoing posterolateral lumbar fusion augmented with iliac crest autograft and recombinant human BMP-7 (rhBMP-7) had better outcomes as measured by the Oswestry score and radiographic analysis than patients who received iliac crest autograft alone. In another human trial using rhBMP-2 in interbody fusion cages for single-level lumbar degenerative disc disease, patients who received cages filled with collagen sponge–delivered rhBMP-2 had superior clinical and radiographic results compared with control patients who received cages filled with autogenous bone graft.[21] Various other clinical trials have similarly shown the efficacy of BMPs to enhance spinal arthrodesis.[22,23]

Gene Therapy for Spinal Fusion

Gene therapy represents a potential next step in the evolution of therapies directed at promoting a spinal fusion. Gene therapy techniques to deliver various BMP genes could overcome the barriers of high dosing and complex carrier systems and achieve long-term, controllable BMP expression. The transduced cells would secrete the BMP extracellularly, delivering it to the environment at physiologically appropriate doses for a sustained period, maximizing the osteoinductive potential of these growth factors. In addition, BMP expression could be regulated in a temporal fashion by using vectors with inducible promoters, which would allow the ability to control the activity of the protein tightly to the clinical setting. Another potential advantage is the capacity to deliver gene therapy for spine arthrodesis in a minimally invasive procedure with percutaneous injections to the spine. Lieberman and colleagues[24] found an increase in the total volume of new bone with improved histologic quality when the gene for BMP-2 was delivered compared with rhBMP-2 protein alone.

Several studies have shown the feasibility of using gene therapy to enhance spinal fusion. Alden and colleagues[25] showed new enchondral bone formation in paraspinal muscles injected with adenoviral BMP-2 constructs (Ad-BMP-2). Important observations made by this study included the absence of bone deposition distant from the injection site and the absence of neural compromise, suggesting that this approach may be safe for the clinical setting. In addition, Helm and colleagues[26] documented that the direct injection of Ad-BMP-9 resulted in fusion in a rodent model without the development of nerve root compression or systemic side effects. In a rabbit model, Riew and associates[27] showed that mesenchymal cells transduced with BMP-2 can promote spinal arthrodesis.

Many of these studies used first-generation adenoviral vectors for gene delivery to immunocompromised animals, allowing for sustained expression. Gene therapy experiments with immunocompetent animals have led to a relative paucity of bone formation,[27] however, owing to the immune response elicited by adenoviral vectors. Further studies using second-generation adenoviral vectors or other vectors such as lentivirus could minimize these responses and maximize gene expression.

Another molecular avenue for bypassing the limitation of adenoviral immunogenicity is to deliver a gene for a factor that is "upstream" from the actions of BMP cytokines. In this way, neither efficient transduction nor sustained duration would be necessary because this factor would start a cascade of BMP activity after only a short period of expression. This intriguing strategy has been developed by Boden and colleagues,[28,29] who showed that a novel intracellular transcription factor, LIM mineralization protein-1 (LMP-1), could be used to upregulate the expression of BMPs and their receptors. LMP-1 initiates a cascade of events intracellularly, which stimulates the secretion of osteoinductive factors, which increases BMP activity. All of the study animals that were implanted with peripheral blood buffy coat cells genetically modified with Ad-LMP-1 showed successful lumbar fusion.[28] None of the 10 controlled rabbits had evidence of any bone formation, and the investigators concluded that local gene therapy could reliably induce spinal fusion in an immunocompetent animal.

Future Directions

With further development, gene therapy techniques will likely be able to induce bony union between vertebral bodies, transverse processes, facets, laminae, and spinous processes in a minimally invasive fashion. Although the studies mentioned earlier establish the potential of gene therapy for enhancing spinal fusion, many issues related to safety, efficacy, and cost remain to be resolved before translation into clinical success.

Spinal Application: Intervertebral Disc Degeneration

Clinical Problem

Degenerative disc disease is a chronic process that can clinically manifest in multiple disorders, such as idiopathic low back pain, disc herniation, radiculopathy, myelopathy, and spinal stenosis. It is a significant source of patient pain and morbidity, using a large portion of health care resources.[30] Available treatment options include conservative measures such as bed rest, anti-inflammatory agents, analgesic medications, and physical therapy. When conservative measures fail, invasive surgical procedures such as discectomy, instrumentation, or fusion, with their inherent risks and expenses, are often required. Conservative and surgical treatment modalities focus on the clinical symptoms of intervertebral disc degeneration without addressing the underlying pathologic processes occurring throughout the course of degeneration.

Although the precise pathophysiology of degenerative disc disease remains to be delineated, it is known to involve a complex interaction of biologic, genetic, and biomechanical factors. The progressive decline in aggrecan, the primary proteoglycan of the nucleus pulposus, is known to be a significant and characteristic factor.[31-33] At the biochemical level, aggrecan homeostasis is altered by various combinations of decreased synthesis and increased breakdown. With reductions in proteoglycan content, the nucleus pulposus dehydrates, decreasing disc height and its load-bearing capacity.[34-36] This situation may directly affect biomechanical function by altering the loads experienced by the facet joints, leading to degenerative changes. Although disc degeneration most probably evolves in response to a complex interplay of multiple biochemical and biomechanical factors,[37] the ability to restore proteoglycan content may have therapeutic benefit by increasing disc hydration and potentially improving biomechanics.

The development of newer biologic therapies may allow for the treatment of intervertebral disc degeneration on a molecular level, without the need for disc excision or fusion surgery. In the last decade, numerous biologic factors involved in the regulation of disc extracellular matrix production, cell proliferation, and cell death have been identified. Many of these growth factors and cytokines have been shown to be present or involved in the degenerating intervertebral disc, and such growth factors may have therapeutic potential for regulating matrix production. The goal of gene therapy for disc degeneration is to transfer the gene of interest to the cells of the nucleus pulposus, allowing sustained transgene expression and upregulation of proteoglycan synthesis or inhibition of catabolic activity, increasing water content and maintaining or improving disc biology and biomechanics.

Growth Factors

The ability to increase proteoglycan synthesis in the intervertebral disc was shown by Thompson and colleagues,[38] who showed that the exogenous application of human transforming growth factor (TGF)-β1 to canine disc tissue in culture stimulated in vitro proteoglycan synthesis. The authors suggested that growth factors may be useful for the treatment of disc degeneration. Subsequent studies with other growth factors, such as insulinlike growth factor (IGF)-I, BMP-2, and osteogenic protein (OP)-1 (OP-1) also exhibited the ability to upregulate proteoglycan content in intervertebral disc cells.[39,40] Owing to the relatively brief half-life of these factors, however, practical application of growth factor therapy to chronic conditions such as degenerative disc disease would necessitate repeated administrations. Consequently, efforts were directed at developing approaches to induce endogenous synthesis of growth factors via gene therapy such that genetically modified disc cells manufacture the desired growth factors on a continuous basis, enabling long-term regulation of matrix synthesis with the potential to prevent or delay degenerative disc disease.

Previous Studies of Intradiscal Gene Therapy

The notion of using gene transfer for intervertebral disc applications was initially introduced by Wehling and colleagues.[41] In an in vitro study, these investigators reported on a retroviral mediated transfer of two different genes to cultured chondrocytic cells from bovine intervertebral endplates: (1) the bacterial β-galactosidase marker gene (LacZ) and (2) the cDNA of the human interleukin-1 receptor antagonist (IL-1Ra). Transfer of LacZ resulted in transduction of approximately 1% of the cell population. Transfer of the IL-1Ra cDNA resulted in significant levels of IL-1Ra protein by 48 hours. The authors concluded that this ex vivo approach, involving harvesting of endplate tissue from a degenerating disc, transducing these cultured cells with therapeutic genes, and reimplanting the genetically modified cells into the disc, could provide a novel strategy for treating degenerative diseases of the spine.

Nishida and colleagues[42] reported the first successful in vivo gene transfer to the intervertebral disc using an adenoviral vector to deliver the LacZ marker gene to the rabbit lumbar disc. The authors were able to show sustained transgene production with no significant reduction in expression 3 months after transduction (Fig. 9–3). The rabbits used in these studies showed no signs of systemic illness in response to the adenoviral vector and its transgene synthesis. In addition, no histologic changes suggesting a cellular immune response were observed.

Encouraged by these results with a marker gene, the successful in vivo transduction of the intervertebral disc with a therapeutic gene, human TGF-β1, was soon accomplished.[43] This study showed a 30-fold increase in active TGF-β1 synthesis and a 5-fold increase in total TGF-β1 production in discs injected with the adenoviral–growth factor construct (Fig. 9–4). Biologic modulation was also documented by a 100% increase in proteoglycan synthesis (Fig. 9–5). As in the previous studies, no signs of local or systemic immune response were noted.

Additional in vitro studies with cultured human nucleus pulposus cells yielded similar promising results. Successful transduction of the LacZ marker gene delivered with adenoviral vectors was achieved in human cells from degenerated discs.[44] The response of human cells from degenerated discs to adenoviral-mediated delivery of TGF-β1 was subsequently assessed.[45] Increased production of TGF-β1, proteoglycan, and collagen was shown in cells receiving gene therapy compared with controls. Cells receiving the adenovirus–TGF-β1 construct showed increased proteoglycan and collagen synthesis compared with cells receiving exogenous TGF-β1 protein, presumably in response to the sustained expression of this growth factor with gene transfer.

The viral load required to increase proteoglycan synthesis was significantly less than the load necessary for transduction of the entire cell population, perhaps highlighting the ability of a transduced cell to influence the biologic activity of non–genetically altered neighboring cells. The concept that successfully transduced cells exert a paracrinelike effect on their nontransduced neighboring cells implies that significant alteration in protein synthesis can be achieved with only a few transduced cells.[2] A better understanding of this paracrine effect may enable the use of decreased viral loads to achieve a therapeutic effect, minimizing potential viral toxicity.

Additional in vitro studies with other promising growth factors such as BMP-2 and IGF-I documented the potential of

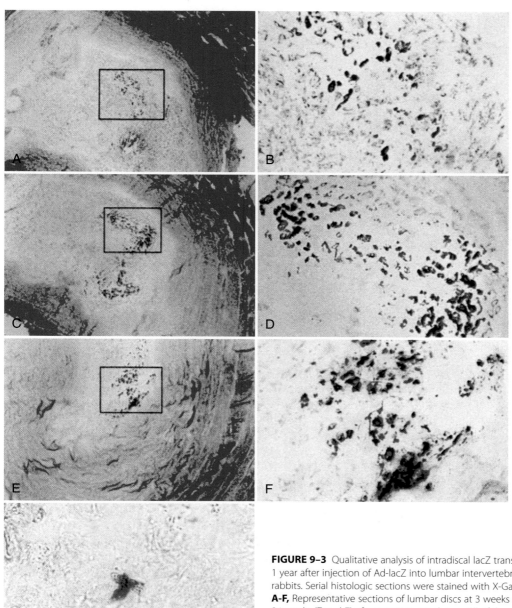

FIGURE 9–3 Qualitative analysis of intradiscal lacZ transgene expression up to and including 1 year after injection of Ad-lacZ into lumbar intervertebral discs of adult New Zealand White rabbits. Serial histologic sections were stained with X-Gal and counterstained with eosin. **A-F,** Representative sections of lumbar discs at 3 weeks (**A** and **B**), 6 weeks (**C** and **D**), and 24 weeks (**E** and **F**) after injection are shown. All of the discs injected with Ad-LacZ exhibited positive X-Gal staining. **G,** At 52 weeks after injection, positive X-Gal staining was observed in the discs from two of three rabbits. The intensity of positive staining was less than in discs from the other time periods, however. (Original magnifications 40× [A, C, E], 200× [B, D, F], and 600× [G].)

adenoviral delivery of these factors to increase proteoglycan synthesis in a viral dose–dependent manner.[46,47] Adenoviral delivery of tissue inhibitor of metalloproteinase (TIMP)-1 showed the same ability.[47] TIMP-1 is an endogenous inhibitor of matrix metalloproteinases, enzymes capable of degrading the extracellular matrix of the intervertebral disc. This finding established a second gene therapy strategy to modify the disrupted balance of synthesis and catabolism occurring in the degenerated intervertebral disc: inhibition of matrix degradation with ensuing net increase in proteoglycan content.

Considering the potential adverse effects of viral vectors, studies have been undertaken to develop strategies to minimize viral loads while maintaining the same biologic effects. Experiments with combination gene therapy involving TGF-β1, IGF-I, and BMP-2 suggested that these growth factors are synergistic in amplifying matrix synthesis.[46] Adenoviral delivery of a single growth factor increased proteoglycan synthesis by a range of 180% to 295%, whereas combination gene therapy with two agents resulted in increases of 322% to 398%. When all three growth factors were combined, proteoglycan synthesis was increased by 471% (Fig. 9–6). It remains to be determined if combination gene therapy with an anabolic growth factor and a catabolic inhibitor such as TIMP-1 would have a similar synergistic effect.

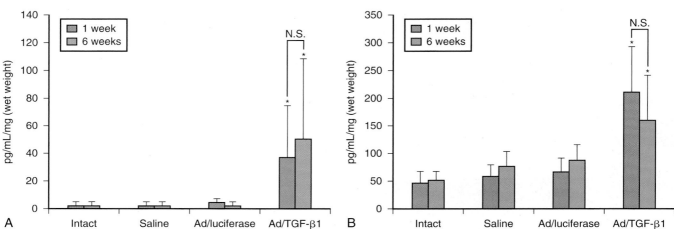

FIGURE 9–4 A, Active transforming growth factor (TGF)-β1 production in rabbit nucleus pulposus tissue 1 and 6 weeks after in vivo injection of Ad-TGF-β1 compared with intact control discs and discs injected with saline and Ad-luciferase. **B,** Total (active and latent) TGF-β1 production in rabbit disc tissue 1 and 6 weeks after in vivo injection. There were no significant differences in either active or total TGF-β1 production at 1 week and 6 weeks, indicating that the therapeutic gene expression was sustained. *Asterisk* denotes significant increase over corresponding intact, saline, and viral (Ad-luciferase) control groups ($P < .05$).

Lattermann and colleagues[48] investigated the transduction efficiency of the AAV vector on nucleus pulposus cells compared with an adenoviral vector in vitro and in vivo. This study showed that the transduction efficacy of the AAV vector on human nucleus pulposus cells in vitro was high, but 48% lower than adenovirus (Fig. 9–7). Next, in vivo gene expression in rabbits after transduction with an AAV vector carrying the luciferase marker gene was achieved at all time points up to 6 weeks (Fig. 9–8). Similar to the in vitro results, the maximum transgene expression using the AAV-luciferase was approximately 50% of the maximum obtained after transduction with the adenoviral vector. Although transgene expression in vivo was decreased compared with levels achieved after adenoviral vector transduction, the overall amount of luciferase was high, likely exceeding any potential therapeutic dose. The authors concluded these experiments showed the feasibility of the AAV vector, as these levels of gene expression may be sufficient for the sustained delivery of a growth factor gene to the nucleus pulposus.

Other studies have focused on the role of LIM mineralization protein (LMP)-1 and Sox9 in the intervertebral disc. LMP-1 is an intracellular regulatory protein that upregulates expression and enhances anabolic activity of the BMP family of proteins. Yoon and colleagues[49] showed an increase in total proteoglycan and aggrecan synthesis in vitro and in vivo after transduction of rat intervertebral disc cells with an adenoviral vector construct containing LMP-1. They found significant increases in expression of BMP-2 and BMP-7 mRNA after in vitro transduction with LMP-1. Sox9 is a transcription factor responsible for chondrogenesis and type II collagen expression. Paul and colleagues[50] treated human intervertebral disc cells with an adenoviral vector construct containing Sox9 and found an increase in type II collagen production compared with controls. These studies make LMP-1 and Sox9 attractive candidates for further investigation as effective tools for intervertebral disc degeneration gene therapy.

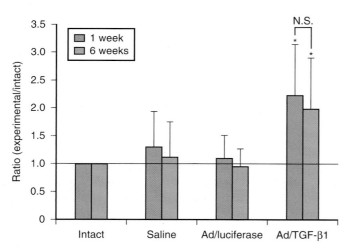

FIGURE 9–5 Proteoglycan synthesis in rabbit nucleus pulposus tissue 1 and 6 weeks after in vivo injection of Ad-TGF-β1 compared with intact control discs and discs injected with saline and Ad-luciferase. There were no significant differences in proteoglycan synthesis at 1 week and 6 weeks, indicating that the biologic effect of transgene synthesis was sustained. *Asterisk* denotes significant increase over corresponding intact, saline, and viral (Ad-luciferase) control groups ($P < .05$).

Gene Expression Time Frame

Adenoviral vectors have been frequently used in gene therapy studies for the intervertebral disc owing to their ability to transduce efficiently highly differentiated, nondividing cells such as the cells of the nucleus pulposus. Successful gene

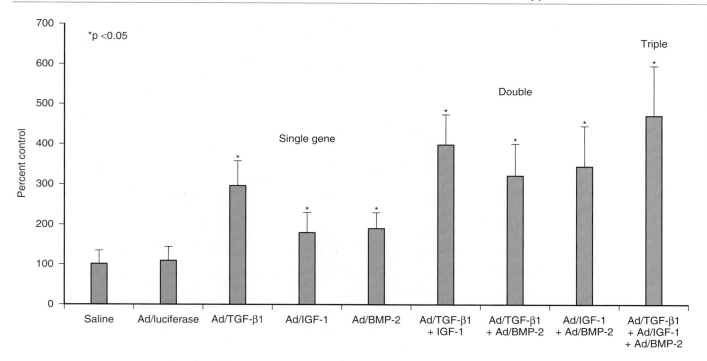

*p <0.05

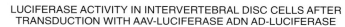

FIGURE 9-6 Proteoglycan synthesis in human intervertebral disc cells treated with different combinations of therapeutic adenoviral vectors (Ad-TGF-β1, Ad-IGF-I, Ad-BMP-2). All groups showed significant increase in synthesis compared with saline and viral (Ad-luciferase) control groups. *Asterisk* indicates P < .05.

FIGURE 9-7 A, Luciferase activity in human nucleus pulposus cells after transfection with AAV-luc and Ad-luc after 8 days. Transduction with 100,000 particles/cell AAV-luc yields 23.74 ± 4.62 ng (SEM) luciferase protein. This is exactly 52% of 45.23 ± 9.34 ng (SEM) luciferase protein measured for 100,000 particles of Ad-luc. With decreasing virus concentrations, gene expression decreases in a linear fashion in both groups. *Asterisk* refers to *t* test with Bonferroni correction. **B,** Human nucleus pulposus (hNP) cells show very high transgene expression after transduction with AAV viral vectors compared with other orthopaedically relevant cell types. Although human synovial fibroblasts (HIG82) generally show low transgene expression with both vector systems, human bone marrow–derived (hBMDC) cells show comparable response to human nucleus pulposus cells after transduction with adenoviral vectors. This may make hNP cells an ideal target for AAV viral vectors. (From Lattermann C, Oxner W, Ixiao X, et al: The adeno-associated viral vector as a strategy for intradiscal gene transfer in immune competent and pre-exposed rabbits. Spine 30:500, 2005.)

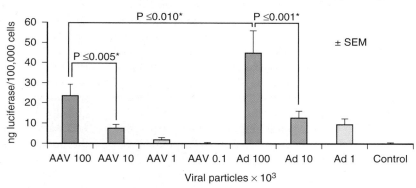

LUCIFERASE ACTIVITY IN INTERVERTEBRAL DISC CELLS AFTER TRANSDUCTION WITH AAV-LUCIFERASE ADN AD-LUCIFERASE

A   * = T-test with Bonferoni correction

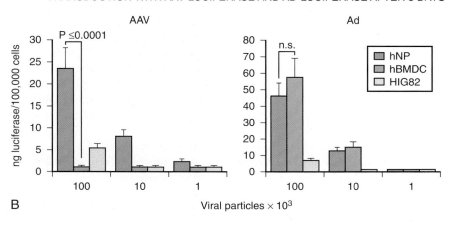

LUCIFERASE PRODUCTION IN DIFFERENT CELL TYPES AFTER TRANSDUCTION WITH AAV-LUCIFERASE AND AD-LUCIFERASE AFTER 8 DAYS

B

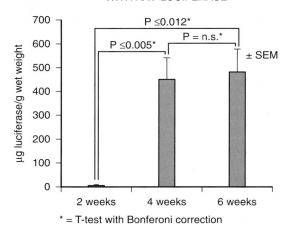

FIGURE 9–8 Luciferase expression after in vivo gene delivery of luciferase gene using AAV-luc vector. At 2 weeks, there is very little gene expression in intervertebral discs. At 4 weeks, there is a significant increase in gene expression. This sustained level is maintained through 6 weeks. *Asterisk* refers to *t* test with Bonferroni correction. (From Lattermann C, Oxner W, Ixiao X, et al: The adeno-associated viral vector as a strategy for intradiscal gene transfer in immune competent and pre-exposed rabbits. Spine 30:501, 2005.)

therapy for the degenerated disc depends not only on efficient gene transfer but also on the expression of transgene for sufficiently long periods. The duration of gene expression after adenoviral transfer to an immunocompetent animal is limited in most organs and tissues by immune reactions to viral proteins and to foreign proteins encoded by the transgene. Specifically, expression for longer than 12 weeks has been difficult to achieve in most musculoskeletal tissues after adenoviral delivery, owing to brisk immune responses. Gene expression can occur for longer periods, however, in an "immune privileged" site. In studies by Nishida and colleagues,[42,43] intradiscal marker gene expression was achieved in the rabbit lumbar disc for 1 year after transduction by adenovirus. Because the intervertebral disc is well encapsulated and avascular, it seems to act as an "immune privileged" organ, permitting longer durations of transgene expression compared with other musculoskeletal tissues.

Compared with the adenoviral vector, the AAV vector has a relatively slower initial gene expression after transduction, likely attributable to an increased latency period. This delay in gene expression was also observed in the previously described in vivo experiments involving the intervertebral disc.[48] At 2 weeks, transgene expression was present but low compared with the adenovirus. At 4 weeks, transgene expression increased 60-fold, however, and that level was maintained at 6 weeks. This characteristic delay in gene expression could potentially preclude the use of AAV vectors in acute processes such as fracture healing, but there is no theoretical disadvantage when treating more chronic diseases such as degenerative disc disease.

Future Directions

The aforementioned studies documented the feasibility of in vivo gene transfer to the intact intervertebral disc. There are reasonable concerns, however, regarding the feasibility of efficient gene transfer to a degenerated disc in which the cell population and extracellular environment are distorted. More recent studies have identified possible genetic causes for disc degeneration.[47-49] Gene transfer to replace the defective gene with a normal copy may have great therapeutic benefit in susceptible populations. Although the intervertebral disc seems to be an "immune privileged" organ, the issue of viral vector immunogenicity is still crucial in light of a reported death of a patient undergoing a clinical trial with the adenovirus. Consequently, other vectors, such as the AAV vector, have been rigorously investigated because of their decreased side-effect profile.

To address the issue of transgene product toxicity, regulatory control systems may be necessary to control transgene expression, including the ability to turn on or off expression in the event of an errant injection or leakage of the injection contents into surrounding tissues.[51] The ability to turn the transgene on or off based on the application of an externally applied stimulus (i.e., oral pharmaceutical) is an advantageous safety feature and a method to modify treatment by titrating transgene expression. Numerous inducible gene expression systems have been investigated, including systems using heat shock proteins, metallothionein, steroid regulatory promoters, tetracycline, and, most recently, the EcR insect receptor. Regulation systems with tissue-specific promoters would further optimize efficacy and minimize treatment side effects.

The length of transgene expression that is necessary for the treatment of a chronic condition such as intervertebral disc degeneration also requires further investigation. The persistence of gene expression after transduction has not been adequately defined in animal models, and the time course necessary for continued treatment is unknown. In addition, the possibility remains that the host immune response will eventually detect and destroy cells that have been transduced.

Another strategy for gene modulation that has emerged is RNA interference (RNAi). RNAi is mediated by small interfering RNA (siRNA) molecules that bind in a sequence-specific manner to target mRNAs, marking them for degradation and preventing translation of the target gene. The efficacy of RNAi mediated by siRNAs has been reported in nucleus pulposus cells in vitro using an exogenous reporter gene and an endogenous gene.[52] To overcome the short half-life of the siRNA, Nishida and colleagues[53] used DNA vector–based RNAi and showed a stable downregulation of specific gene expression. RNAi has potential use as a novel strategy of gene therapy for treatment of degenerative disc disease by silencing expression of catabolic genes.

Summary

The potential of gene therapy to alleviate the biologic challenges of spinal fusion and disc degeneration has been clearly established, yet significant work remains before human clinical trials can be considered. Detailed safety profiles of vectors and therapeutic genes must be thoroughly established in preclinical studies before clinical efficacy is sought. In addition, the basic science of the various candidate genes and their biologic effects must be delineated. Pharmacology studies detailing the relationship of viral concentration, transgene synthesis, and biologic effect are essential before clinical use. Finally, regulation systems with tissue-specific vectors, tissue-specific promoters, or inducible promoters must be developed to optimize efficacy and to minimize side effects. Despite the hurdles that remain, the potential of gene therapy to alter the course of spinal disorders holds much clinical promise and will continue to stimulate future investigations. Ideally, spine surgeons in the future will have the ability to tailor genetic therapies for individual patients from an assortment of safe and efficacious vector-gene constructs.

KEY REFERENCES

1. Evans CH, Robbins PD: Possible orthopaedic applications of gene therapy. J Bone Joint Surg Am 77:1103-1114, 1995.
    This comprehensive review defined the terminology and concepts pertinent to the new field of gene therapy and gave an overview of potential applications for orthopaedic conditions.

2. Thompson JP, Oegema TR Jr, Bradford DS: Stimulation of mature canine intervertebral disc by growth factors. Spine 16:253-260, 1991.
    The authors showed exogenous application of growth factors (TGF-β1 and epidermal growth factor) to canine disc tissue in culture-stimulated proteoglycan synthesis. They suggested the novel concept that growth factors may be used for the treatment of disc degeneration.

3. Wehling P, Schulitz KP, Robbins PD, et al: Transfer of genes to chondrocytic cells of the lumbar spine: Proposal for a treatment strategy of spinal disorders by local gene therapy. Spine 22:1092-1097, 1997.
    The authors reported successful retroviral-mediated transfer of two different genes to cultured chondrocytic cells from bovine intervertebral endplates. By doing so, they introduced the notion of using gene transfer for treating degenerative diseases of the spine.

4. Boden SD, Titus L, Hair G, et al: Lumbar spine fusion by local gene therapy with a cDNA encoding a novel osteoinductive protein (LMP-1). Spine 23:2486-2492, 1998.
    These authors showed in vivo gene therapy with LMP-1 led to successful fusion in nine of nine (100%) of the sites receiving marrow cells transfected with the active LMP-1 cDNA and in zero of nine (0%) of the sites receiving marrow cells transfected with the inactive LMP-1 cDNA (control group). This study established the in vivo feasibility of gene therapy with LMP-1 for spinal fusion.

5. Nishida K, Kang JD, Suh JK, et al: Adenovirus-mediated gene transfer to nucleus pulposus cells: Implications for the treatment of intervertebral disc degeneration. Spine 23:2437-2442; discussion 2443, 1998.
    This article reports the first successful in vivo gene transfer to the intervertebral disc using an adenoviral vector. The authors were able to show sustained transgene production with no significant reduction in expression up to 3 months. The rabbits used in these studies showed no signs of systemic illness in response to the adenoviral vector and its transgene synthesis.

REFERENCES

1. Robbins PD, Ghivizzani SC. Viral vectors for gene therapy. Pharmacol Ther 80:35-47, 1998.

2. Evans CH, Robbins PD. Possible orthopaedic applications of gene therapy. J Bone Joint Surg Am 77:1103-1114, 1995.

3. Nishida K, Doita M, Takada T,et al: Sustained transgene expression in intervertebral disc cells in vivo mediated by microbubble-enhanced ultrasound gene therapy. Spine 31:1415-1419, 2006.

4. Sobajima S, Kim JS, Gilbertson LG, et al: Gene therapy for degenerative disc disease. Gene Ther 11:390-401, 2004.

5. Hacein-Bey-Abina S, von Kalle C, Schmidt M, et al: A serious adverse event after successful gene therapy for X-linked severe combined immunodeficiency. N Engl J Med 348:255-256, 2003.

6. DePalma AF, Rothman RH: The nature of pseudarthrosis. Clin Orthop Relat Res 59:113-118, 1968.

7. Steinmann JC, Herkowitz HN: Pseudarthrosis of the spine. Clin Orthop Relat Res (284):80-90, 1992.

8. Urist MR: Bone: Formation by autoinduction. Science 150:893-899, 1965.

9. Urist MR, Sato K, Brownell AG, et al: Human bone morphogenetic protein (hBMP). Proc Soc Exp Biol Med 173:194-199, 1983.

10. Boden SD, Martin GJ Jr, Morone MA, et al: Posterolateral lumbar intertransverse process spine arthrodesis with recombinant human bone morphogenetic protein 2/hydroxyapatite-tricalcium phosphate after laminectomy in the nonhuman primate. Spine 24:1179-1185, 1999.

11. Cheung KMC, Leong JCY, Liu SL. Augmentation of intertransverse spinal fusion in primates using OP-1. Annual Meeting of the International Society for the Study of the Lumbar Spine, Kona, HI, 1999.

12. Cook SD, Dalton JE, Tan EH, et al: In vivo evaluation of recombinant human osteogenic protein (rhOP-1) implants as a bone graft substitute for spinal fusions. Spine 19:1655-1663, 1994.

13. Frenkel SR, Moskovich R, Spivak J, et al: Demineralized bone matrix: Enhancement of spinal fusion. Spine 18:1634-1639, 1993.

14. Holliger EH, Trawick RH, Boden SD, et al: Morphology of the lumbar intertransverse process fusion mass in the rabbit model: A comparison between two bone graft materials—rhBMP-2 and autograft. J Spinal Disord 9:125-128, 1996.

15. Lovell TP, Dawson EG, Nilsson OS, et al: Augmentation of spinal fusion with bone morphogenetic protein in dogs. Clin Orthop Relat Res (243):266-274, 1989.

16. Magin M: BMP-7 (rhOP-1) is able to enhance lumbar vertebral interbody fusion: Results of a sheep trial and clinical impact. Annual Meeting of the International Society for the Study of the Lumbar Spine, Kona, HI, 1999.

17. Oikarinen J: Experimental spinal fusion with decalcified bone matrix and deep-frozen allogeneic bone in rabbits. Clin Orthop Relat Res (162):210-218, 1982.

18. Schimandle JH, Boden SD, Hutton WC: Experimental spinal fusion with recombinant human bone morphogenetic protein-2. Spine 20:1326-1337, 1995.

19. Sheehan JP, Kallmes DF, Sheehan JM, et al: Molecular methods of enhancing lumbar spine fusion. Neurosurgery 39:548-554, 1996.

20. Patel TC, Vaccaro AR, Truumees E: A safety and efficacy study of OP-1 (rhBMP-7) as an adjunct to posterolateral lumbar fusion. Annual Meeting of the North American Spine Society, New Orleans, 2000.

21. Boden SD, et al: The use of rhBMP-2 in interbody fusion cages: Definitive evidence of osteoinduction in humans: A preliminary report. Spine 25:376-381, 2000.

22. Burkus KJ, Transfeldt EE, Kitchel SH: A prospective and randomized study assessing the clinical and radiographic outcomes of patients treated with RhBMP-2 and threaded cortical bone dowels in the lumbar spine. Annual Meeting of the North American Spine Society, New Orleans, 2000.

23. Kleeman TJ, Talbot-Kleeman A: Laparoscopic ALIF: rhBMP-2 with titanium cages vs autograft with bone dowels. Annual Meeting of the North American Spine Society, New Orleans, 2000.

24. Lieberman JR, Le LQ, Wu L, et al: Regional gene therapy with a BMP-2-producing murine stromal cell line induces heterotopic and orthotopic bone formation in rodents. J Orthop Res 16:330-339, 1998.

25. Alden TD, Pittman DD, Beres EJ, et al: Percutaneous spinal fusion using bone morphogenetic protein-2 gene therapy. J Neurosurg 90(1 Suppl):109-114, 1999.

26. Helm GA, Alden TD, Beres EJ, et al: Use of bone morphogenetic protein-9 gene therapy to induce spinal arthrodesis in the rodent. J Neurosurg 92(2 Suppl):191-196, 2000.

27. Riew KD, Wright NM, Cheng S, et al: Induction of bone formation using a recombinant adenoviral vector carrying the human BMP-2 gene in a rabbit spinal fusion model. Calcif Tissue Int 63:357-360, 1998.

28. Boden SD, Titus L, Hair G, et al: Lumbar spine fusion by local gene therapy with a cDNA encoding a novel osteoinductive protein (LMP-1). Spine 23:2486-2492, 1998.

29. Viggeswarapu M, Boden SD, Liu Y, et al: Adenoviral delivery of LIM mineralization protein-1 induces new-bone formation in vitro and in vivo. J Bone Joint Surg Am 83:364-376, 2001.

30. Conrad DA: Cost of low back pain problems: An economic analysis. In Weinstein JN, Gordon SL (eds): Low Back Pain: A Clinical and Scientific Overview. Rosemont, IL, American Association of Orthopedic Surgeons, 1996.

31. Adler JH, Schoenbaum M, Silberberg R: Early onset of disk degeneration and spondylosis in sand rats (*Psammomys obesus*). Vet Pathol 20:13-22, 1983.

32. Buckwalter JA: Aging and degeneration of the human intervertebral disc. Spine 20:1307-1314, 1995.

33. Pearce RH, Grimmer BJ, Adams ME: Degeneration and the chemical composition of the human lumbar intervertebral disc. J Orthop Res 5:198-205, 1987.

34. Butler D, Trafimow JH, Andersson GB, et al: Discs degenerate before facets. Spine 15:111-113, 1990.

35. Urban JP, McMullin JF: Swelling pressure of the intervertebral disc: Influence of proteoglycan and collagen contents. Biorheology 22:145-157, 1985.

36. Urban JP, McMullin JF: Swelling pressure of the lumbar intervertebral discs: Influence of age, spinal level, composition, and degeneration. Spine 13:179-187, 1988.

37. Garfin SR: The intervertebral disc disease—does it exist? In Weinstein WJN (ed): The Lumbar Spine. Philadelphia, WB Saunders, 1990, pp 369-380.

38. Thompson JP, Oegema TR Jr, Bradford DS: Stimulation of mature canine intervertebral disc by growth factors. Spine 16:253-260, 1991.

39. Osada R, Ohshima H, Ishihara H, et al: Autocrine/paracrine mechanism of insulin-like growth factor-1 secretion, and the effect of insulin-like growth factor-1 on proteoglycan synthesis in bovine intervertebral discs. J Orthop Res 14:690-699, 1996.

40. Takegami K, Thonar EJ, An HS, et al: Osteogenic protein-1 enhances matrix replenishment by intervertebral disc cells previously exposed to interleukin-1. Spine 27:1318-1325, 2002.

41. Wehling P, Schulitz KP, Robbins PD, et al: Transfer of genes to chondrocytic cells of the lumbar spine: Proposal for a treatment strategy of spinal disorders by local gene therapy. Spine 22:1092-1097, 1997.

42. Nishida K, Kang JD, Suh JK, et al: Adenovirus-mediated gene transfer to nucleus pulposus cells: Implications for the treatment of intervertebral disc degeneration. Spine 23:2437-2442; discussion 2443, 1998.

43. Nishida K, Kang JD, Gilbertson LG, et al: Modulation of the biologic activity of the rabbit intervertebral disc by gene therapy: An in vivo study of adenovirus-mediated transfer of the human transforming growth factor beta 1 encoding gene. Spine 24:2419-2425, 1999.

44. Moon SH, Gilbertson LG, Nishida K, et al: Human intervertebral disc cells are genetically modifiable by adenovirus-mediated gene transfer: Implications for the clinical management of intervertebral disc disorders. Spine 25:2573-2579, 2000.

45. Moon SH: Proteoglycan synthesis in human intervertebral disc cells cultured in alginate beads; exogenous TGF-beta1 vs. adenovirus-mediated gene transfer of TGF beta1 cDNA. Orthopaedic Research Society, Orlando, FL, 2000.

46. Moon SH, Nishida K, Gilbertson LG, et al: Biologic response of human intervertebral disc cells to gene therapy cocktail. Spine 33:1850-1855, 2008.

47. Wallach CJ, Sobajima S, Watanabe Y, et al: Gene transfer of the catabolic inhibitor TIMP-1 increases measured proteoglycans in cells from degenerated human intervertebral discs. Spine 28:2331-2337, 2003.

48. Lattermann C, Oxner WM, Xiao X, et al: The adeno associated viral vector as a strategy for intradiscal gene transfer in immune competent and pre-exposed rabbits. Spine 30:497-504, 2005.

49. Yoon ST, Park JS, Kim KS, et al: ISSLS prize winner: LMP-1 upregulates intervertebral disc cell production of proteoglycans and BMPs in vitro and in vivo. Spine 29:2603-2611, 2004.

Outcomes Research for Spinal Disorders

Adam M. Pearson, MD
Kevin Spratt, PhD
James N. Weinstein, DO

Need for Outcomes Research

Outcomes research can be defined simply as "the measurement of the value of a particular course of therapy."[1] It is based on the principle that every clinical intervention produces a change in the health status of a patient that *can be measured*. The motivation for outcomes research varies depending on one's perspective, but all parties involved in health care have a vested interest in defining outcomes related to medical interventions. Health care providers have a responsibility to provide the highest level of care to their patients, and this can be done only if the best treatment for a given condition has been determined through research. Patients need to be well informed about their prognosis, treatment options, and expected outcomes associated with each treatment option so that they can make a well-informed decision with their physician. Private and government payers have the right to demand evidence that the interventions for which they are paying yield improvement in the health of the patients they cover.

The United States has the highest gross domestic product (GDP) in the world and spends a higher proportion of its GDP on health care than any other country in the world, with little evidence to suggest that the level of public health is better than other developed countries.[2,3] Wennberg and Gittelsohn[4] developed the method of small area analysis in which variations in practice patterns, spending, and outcomes could be compared across hospital referral regions. They showed markedly different rates of hospital use between Boston, Massachusetts, and New Haven, Connecticut, for conditions without defined treatment protocols such as back pain, with no discernible differences in outcomes.[5] Using the technique of small area analysis, Fisher and colleagues[6,7] studied the relationship between Medicare expenditures and outcomes in hospital referral regions across the United States and found no relationship between the level of health care spending and outcomes. The substantial geographic variation in rates of lumbar surgery in the Medicare population was documented by Weinstein and colleagues (Fig. 10–1).[8] These studies have shown that practice patterns vary substantially across different regions, indicating that the "best" practice for many

conditions is unknown. The wide variation in the rates of health care use suggests that many regions are not practicing in the optimal zone of use, indicating that health services are likely underused in some regions and overused in others.

In the past, health care providers have assumed that increased use of health care services was associated with higher quality outcomes, a relationship that is shown by the upward-sloping portion of the curve shown in Figure 10–2. Economists have theorized, however, that eventually this curve flattens out such that additional expenditures yield increasingly fewer benefits until there is no marginal benefit (law of diminishing marginal returns).[9] Although it has not been explicitly shown, it is possible that the curve eventually starts sloping downward, indicating that outcomes worsen with increasing use. Such a phenomenon could occur if patients were being inappropriately selected for treatment from which they were unlikely to benefit but might still experience treatment side effects. The Maine Lumbar Spine Study suggested that such a down-sloping portion of the curve might exist as outcomes for lumbar intervertebral disc herniation and spinal stenosis were worst in the regions where the rates of surgery were the greatest.[10,11]

Given the wide variation in practice across all of medicine and spine surgery in particular, policymakers have demanded that the research community perform outcome studies to determine the best practices for treating various conditions. In 2007, a Medicare Evidence Development and Coverage Advisory Committee (MedCAC) questioned the role of fusion for degenerative lumbar conditions in patients older than 65 years and suggested that Medicare could discontinue reimbursement for the procedure unless it could be shown to be effective.[12] In response, Glassman and colleagues[13] analyzed their results of lumbar fusion in this population and found that older patients had equivalent or better outcomes compared with younger patients. Although it is unclear how these data will be acted on, the MedCAC study and response to it provide an example of how researchers can respond effectively to policymakers who are looking for evidence to justify health care expenditures. As part of the 2009 economic stimulus package, more than 1 billion dollars was allocated for comparative health research, suggesting that outcomes and

RATIO OF RATES OF LUMBAR FUSION TO THE U.S AVERAGE BY HOSPITAL
REFERRAL REGION (2002–03)

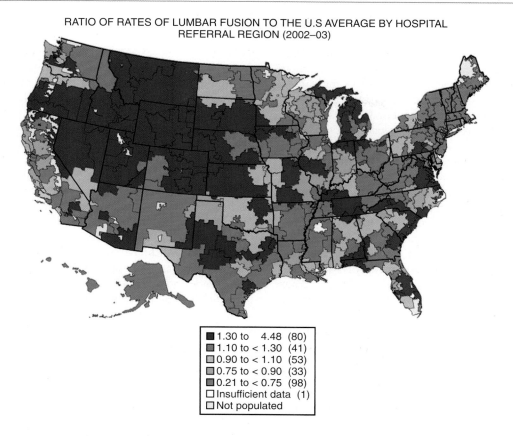

■ 1.30 to   4.48 (80)
■ 1.10 to < 1.30 (41)
■ 0.90 to < 1.10 (53)
■ 0.75 to < 0.90 (33)
■ 0.21 to < 0.75 (98)
□ Insufficient data (1)
□ Not populated

FIGURE 10–1 Rates of lumbar fusion in hospital referral regions across the United States in 2002-2003, normalized to average rate. (From Weinstein JN, Lurie JD, Olson PR, et al: United States' trends and regional variations in lumbar spine surgery: 1992-2003. Spine 31:2707-2714, 2006.)

cost-effectiveness research are likely to play an increasingly important role in guiding health policy. This chapter introduces the spine surgeon to some methods of outcomes research, including outcomes measurement, study design, and cost-effectiveness analysis.

Measuring Outcomes in Spinal Disorders

One of the first principles of science is that you have to measure something, and a cornerstone of outcomes research is that any change in health status is *measurable*. Measuring subjective qualities such as pain and function, two important outcomes in patients with spinal disorders, can be quite challenging, however. In the classic literature, outcomes were often physiologic (i.e., motor function), radiographic (i.e., fusion), or subjectively defined by the treating physician (i.e., "poor," "fair," or "good").[14,15] Over the last 30 years, clinical studies have adopted patient-based outcome measures. Outcome measures can be classified as global measures of health (i.e., SF-36 Health Survey,[16] EuroQoL,[17] Sickness Impact Profile [SIP][18]) or condition-specific measures (i.e., Oswestry Disability Index [ODI],[19] Roland-Morris Disability Questionnaire [RDQ][20]). High-quality outcome measures need to be practical, precise (reliable), accurate (valid), and responsive.[21]

Practical surveys are of an acceptable length and include easily answered questions so that patients are willing and able to complete them. *Precision,* or reliability, refers to the reproducibility of a survey—will a patient in the same state of health score the same on the outcome measure on different occasions? *Validity* is the ability of the survey to measure the quality it aims to measure. Assessing the validity of a tool often requires multiple approaches. The score on a new instrument can be compared with a "gold standard" outcome measure to

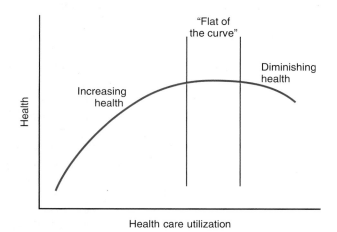

FIGURE 10–2 Theoretical relationship between health and resource use. At low levels of use, health increases with use. As use increases, the marginal return decreases until there is no marginal return ("flat of the curve"). In some cases, increasing use further could lead to worse health outcomes.

assess its convergent validity. Additionally, the ability of the measure to discriminate between patients in different health states can be evaluated to determine its discriminate validity. Ironically, "face" validity, the concept that the instrument appears to be measuring what it is designed to measure, is fundamental to instrument development and often the weakest form of validity evidence. This is especially true when the group that designed the instrument is evaluating its face validity. Responsive outcome measures are able to detect health status changes in an individual patient before and after successful treatment of low back pain.

In the medical literature, it is commonly held that many of the well-known generic and back-specific outcome measures have been shown to be practical, precise, valid, and responsive and can be considered "validated" outcome measures.[22] From a psychometric perspective, much of this evidence is post-hoc, however, meaning that the instrument's validity is based on its use in a study where the results showed that one group improved more than another by some statistically significant amount. By this logic, the fact that the tool "worked" (i.e., allowed for a statistically significant difference to be observed) is taken as de facto evidence that (1) the tool is practical because the patients completed it, (2) the tool is reliable because a significant difference between groups was observed, (3) the tool is valid because the goal of the instrument is to document the magnitude of an outcome that was expected to be different for the various treatment groups, and (4) the tool is responsive because the difference in outcomes was detectable. Subsequent studies use these same tools, often for different populations, justifying their use because the instrument has been "validated" in a previous study.

The Spine Patient Outcomes Research Trial (SPORT) intervertebral discs herniation (IDH) study serves as a good example to examine the selection of outcome measures. The primary outcome measures were the SF-36 bodily pain and physical function scales and the ODI (American Academy of Orthopaedic Surgeons MODEMS version), and secondary outcome measures included work status, satisfaction, and the Sciatica Bothersomeness Index.[23] The distinction between the primary and secondary outcome measures was that the study was powered to detect a prespecified difference in the primary outcome measures (i.e., a 10-point difference on the SF-36 scales or ODI), whereas the secondary outcome measures did not factor into the power analysis. As has been recommended, SPORT included a generic (SF-36) and condition-specific (ODI) primary outcome measure.[24] Given the extensive use of the SF-36, ODI, and RDQ in the spine literature, we examine these questionnaires in greater detail.

The SF-36 is among the most commonly used generic health questionnaires and has been extensively validated across many medical conditions.[25] It consists of 36 questions and can be completed in less than 10 minutes. Responses are scored on eight nonoverlapping scales (physical functioning, role-physical, bodily pain, general health, vitality, social functioning, role-emotional, and mental health), which are summarized as a physical and mental component summary score. All scales range from 0-100 (lower scores represent worse symptoms), with the component summary scores transformed

to have means of 50 and standard deviations of 10. In looking at the specific scales used in SPORT, the physical function scale is based on ratings of activity limitation (i.e., carrying groceries, climbing stairs, walking), and the bodily pain scale is based on two questions about the severity of pain and the degree to which pain interferes with work. At baseline, the patients in the SPORT IDH randomized controlled trial (RCT) had a mean baseline physical function score of 39.4 (age-adjusted and sex-adjusted norm of 89) and bodily pain score of 26.9 (age-adjusted and sex-adjusted norm of 81), suggesting they were markedly affected by their disc herniation.

The ODI was designed specifically for use in a back pain clinic and asks one question about the intensity of pain and nine questions about the degree to which pain limits specific activities (i.e., lifting, walking, traveling). Scores can range from 0-100, with higher scores indicating more severe disability. The mean score among "normals" is about 10, with mean scores in the 30s for patients with neurogenic claudication and 40s for patients with metastatic disease.[26] In the SPORT IDH RCT, the average baseline ODI score was 46.9, indicating substantial pain-related disability.[27] The ODI has been extensively validated and used in the spine literature and has been recommended to be used as a back pain–specific questionnaire (the Roland-Morris Disability Questionnaire is the other outcome measure recommended for this purpose).[26]

The RDQ is a 24-item survey developed from the 136-item SIP, with the phrase "because of my back" added to the end of the SIP statements to focus the survey on back-related problems.[20,26] The questions focus primarily on function and pain, with only one question asking about the psychological effects of back pain and none inquiring about social function. Each question is a statement about the effect of back pain on function on the day the survey is taken (i.e., walking, bending, sitting, lying down, dressing, sleeping, self-care), with which the respondent must agree or disagree. The number of positive responses is the score (0-24), with median scores of 11 in a population with back pain presenting to a primary care clinic.[28] The RDQ has been shown to be valid and responsive, although reproducibility has been difficult to show because it refers to symptoms only over a 24-hour period. In comparing the RDQ and the ODI, it has been suggested that the RDQ may be better able to detect changes in function in patients with a mild to moderate degree of disability, whereas the ODI may be better suited to patients with a more severe degree of disability.[26]

Experts have recommended using global health and back-specific outcomes questionnaires.[29] The SF-36 or EuroQoL are recommended for measuring global health in spine patients, whereas the ODI or RDQ are the recommended back-specific instruments. In addition to these formal outcome measures, measuring work status and overall satisfaction with treatment is recommended.

Importance of Study Design in Outcomes Research

The goal of any outcomes research study is to measure results from a study sample and extrapolate those results to understand health outcomes in the real world. The results of research studies are highly dependent on the details of study design, however. Reviewing three RCTs comparing lumbar fusion with nonoperative treatment for chronic low back pain reveals one study that showed a clear advantage for surgery,[30] one that showed only a minor benefit to surgery,[31] and one that reported no benefit for surgery.[32] How can three RCTs asking the same essential question come to three contradictory conclusions? The answer may reflect differences in research methods and details of study design. In designing or evaluating a research study, one must consider the research question, the target population and study sample, the interventions being compared, the outcome measures employed, and the specific study design.

A well-posed *research question* is the foundation of the entire research project. No elaborate study methodology, new data collection technique, or statistical expertise can make up for a poorly chosen research question. For this reason, sufficient time and energy should be devoted to developing, critically evaluating, and refining the research question. In evaluating the results of a study, one must determine what question was really answered because it may be different than what was suggested by the authors.

When the research question has been specified, the next step is to define the target population and study sample. The *target population* is the group of people to whom the results of the study should be generalizable, whereas the *study sample* is the group of patients actually available for study.[33] The target population is defined by the inclusion and exclusion criteria. There is an inherent struggle between having inclusion and exclusion criteria that are very restrictive yet provide a homogeneous study population (i.e., 34-year-old women with left-sided posterolateral L4-L5 disc extrusions and extensor hallucis longus weakness) and criteria that are less restrictive and yield a more diverse study population (i.e., anyone with a disk herniation). More restrictive studies can specifically evaluate the effect of treatment on specific patient subgroups, whereas less restrictive studies are inherently more generalizable. Defining subgroups that have different outcomes is important to determine the best treatment for individual patients, although it is not usually possible to perform separate trials for each subgroup.[34] Understanding the actual target population is essential to interpreting and acting on the findings of a study.

Most clinical studies evaluate the effect of an intervention on an outcome.[35] Similar to the study participants and outcome measures, the intervention also needs to be clearly defined. The intervention for the control or comparative group also needs to be specified. Differences in the experimental and control interventions may explain some of the differences among the aforementioned studies comparing fusion with nonoperative treatment for the treatment of chronic low back pain. Fritzell and colleagues[30] compared three types of fusion techniques with nonspecific physical therapy and showed a clear benefit to fusion. In contrast, Brox and colleagues[32] compared instrumented posterolateral fusion with a very specific program of cognitive therapy and 3 weeks of intensive physical therapy and reported no differences in results. These two studies did not compare the same interventions, and this may be one reason for the discrepant results.

The specific study design used by a research project can have profound effects on the interpretation of the results. Each study design has inherent advantages and disadvantages that must be weighed when planning an investigation. Although the RCT is considered the "gold standard" of clinical research designs, it is often the case that mounting an RCT before the preliminary case series, case-control, and cohort studies have been performed would be counterproductive. The high cost in terms of researcher and clinical time often greatly outweigh the results obtained from a poorly planned RCT. Before launching a large RCT, observational pilot studies should be performed to generate hypotheses and reveal challenges (e.g., adequate assessment, compliance with treatment, treatment harms and side effects) that are difficult to anticipate. A unique aspect of the study design of SPORT was its concurrent use of an RCT and observational cohort study that allowed patients to choose enrollment in the randomized or observational arms.[36] Before discussion about the merits and problems associated with each specific study design, we consider the general threats to the validity of a study.

Understanding Threats to Study Validity

Generally, threats to study validity have been classified as internal and external (Table 10–1). *Internal validity* is related to the validity of the conclusions of a study within the study sample—was the observed difference between the treatment groups real? *External validity* refers to whether or not the findings of the study can be generalized to populations and settings outside of the study sample—would the difference observed in the trial be observed in the real world?

Clinical studies generally aim to determine if a specific intervention results in a certain outcome. Although a study may show an association between an intervention and an outcome, this association may be spurious (i.e., the association exists in the study but not in the real world), or the association may not represent a cause-effect relationship (i.e., the intervention was associated with but was not the cause of the observed outcome). The two main causes of spurious associations are chance (random measurement errors) and bias.[37] Confounding is another threat to validity that can obscure the cause-effect relationship between the intervention and outcome being studied. Different types of study designs are prone to different types of inferential errors, and this is discussed in detail when each study design is considered.

Chance

When an association is observed between an intervention and an outcome, it is possible that this observation is due to chance rather than to the intervention causing the outcome. Fritzell and colleagues[30] reported that fusion for chronic back pain reduced ODI scores by 11 points, whereas nonoperative treatment resulted in only a 2-point decrease. Although surgery effectiveness may have been responsible for the difference, it

TABLE 10-1 Internal and External Validity Threats

Internal Validity Threats	External Validity Threats
History: Specific events occurring between first and second assessment in addition to experimental variable	**Selection bias:** To the extent that patients presenting at study sites are not representative of patients in general
Maturation: Processes within patient operating as a function of time (e.g., favorable natural history)	**Reactive or interactive effects:** Screening process (informed consent, extra attention, additional procedures to identify inclusion/exclusion criteria) is not done with nonstudy patients
Testing: Effects that testing itself has on subsequent scores	**Reactive effects of experimental procedures:** Just being in a study may affect patient responses
Instrumentation: Changes in obtained measurements owing to changes in instrument calibration, observers, or raters	**Multiple treatment effects:** When treatments have multiple components (i.e., surgery, postsurgical rehabilitation) or when patient has multiple treatments (i.e., nonoperative treatment followed by surgery), possible effects of former treatment on latter may influence efficacy
Statistical regression: Lack of reliability in tools, which is especially problematic when patients are selected on basis of extreme scores	
Selection: Biases resulting from differential selection of patients into treatment arms	
Patient attrition: Differential loss of patients from treatment groups (e.g., loss to follow-up, crossover)	
Interactions of above effects: Interactions among above variables may have effects that are mistakenly attributed to treatment	

is also possible that surgery had no beneficial effect and that the observed differences were due to chance alone. Statistical tests are used to evaluate the possibility that an observed relationship between an intervention and outcome was due to chance. In the case of the study by Fritzell and colleagues,[30]

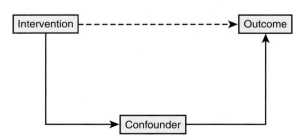

FIGURE 10-3 Relationship between intervention, outcome, and a confounder is shown. Although there may be an association between the intervention and the outcome, there may be a third variable, or confounder, that is associated with the intervention but is the actual cause of the outcome observed.

statistical testing showed a statistically significant difference ($P = .015$), indicating that the association between surgery and symptom improvement was probably real. Details about the theories underlying probability testing are beyond the scope of this chapter and can be found in standard biostatistics textbooks.[38]

Bias

Bias is the other major cause of spurious associations. Bias has been defined as "the non-random-systematic error in the design or conduct of a study."[35] Although numerous types of biases have been identified, most bias is related to patient selection, treatment, attrition, and outcome detection. If the patients enrolled in a study differ from the target population, an association observed in the study may not exist in the target population. If the patients who enrolled in the SPORT IDH RCT had less severe symptoms than the target population, the benefit of surgery could be understated if the treatment effect is less among this group. Performance bias exists when patients are treated differently in ways other than the intervention being studied, with a "cointervention" being the true driver of the association. If patients undergoing discectomy were more likely to be treated with long-term narcotics postoperatively, the association observed between surgery and outcome could actually be due to narcotics.

Attrition bias results when patients drop out of a study in a nonrandom manner that is associated with the group assignment. If patients who failed nonoperative treatment dropped out of the study to receive surgical treatment elsewhere, the outcomes for the nonoperative patients remaining in the study would be spuriously inflated. Bias in outcome detection can occur if outcome assessors are nonsystematic in their evaluation of patients and tend to change their procedures depending on the assigned treatment. Generally, if the outcomes assessor is not blinded to the treatment received, the assessor is liable to be biased (consciously or not) in his or her assessment. Similarly, patients who are not blinded to their treatment may also be biased in self-reported outcomes.

Bias tends to be insidious, and investigators should attempt to prevent it in the planning stages and detect it during the analysis. Efforts should be made to ensure that the patients enrolling in the study are similar to the target population to eliminate selection bias. Blinding can eliminate many forms of bias related to treatment and outcomes assessment because patients cannot be treated or assessed differently if the patient and the assessor are unaware of the treatment group. Blinding (shams) can often be difficult, however, or potentially unethical in surgical studies.[39] The best way to combat attrition bias is to limit attrition through aggressive efforts to ensure follow-up. After a study has been completed, the authors should consider the role bias could have played in their findings and address these limitations transparently.

Confounding

Confounders are variables that are associated with the exposure (i.e., the intervention) and affect the outcome (Fig. 10-3).

If patients undergoing discectomy are less likely to be depressed than patients undergoing nonoperative treatment, and depression is associated with worse outcomes, the relationship between treatment and outcome is confounded by depression. Although the association between better outcomes with surgery is real (i.e., greater than would be expected by chance) in this case, the true cause of the difference may be the better psychological state of the surgical patients rather than the surgery itself. The only way to eliminate confounding is to ensure that the treatment groups are equivalent. True equivalence is never achievable, however, given the vast number of potential differences in patients. The best method to minimize group differences is to randomize.

Depending on the nature of the particular study, randomization might be simple (i.e., each subject has an equal chance of being placed in any of the available treatments) or stratified on specific variables of interest given the context of the problem. It is common to stratify patients by gender and age group, ensuring that the various treatment groups are "reasonably" equivalent with respect to these factors before randomly assigning these subgroups to treatment. Randomization does not ensure equivalence for any given finite sample, however. With small samples (i.e., ≤20), randomization often can fail to produce reasonably equivalent groups. If an investigator randomizes 20 patients, 10 males (M) and 10 females (F), and defines a "fair" split of males to females as 6M4F, 5M5F, or 4M6F, this result is likely to occur 82.1% of the time. More extreme splits occur 17.9% of the time. Thus, with smaller sample sizes, stratification should be considered. Confounding can be a major threat to the validity of observational studies. Strategies to eliminate confounding in observational studies can be used in either the design or the analysis phase; however, potential confounders must be anticipated and measured to be addressed.[37] Specification and matching are techniques that can be used when designing the study. *Specification* involves stipulating a certain level of the confounder as an inclusion criterion. In an observational study comparing discectomy with nonoperative treatment, the investigator could specify that only patients without depression be included to eliminate depression as a potential confounder. The disadvantage of this strategy would be that the results would apply only to patients without depression. Attempting to use this strategy for many confounders would soon become quite limiting. *Matching* is another technique that is often used in case-control studies, in which a control is found for each case that is matched on numerous potential confounders. Although this approach can eliminate the effects of confounding, it also makes it impossible to evaluate the association between potential confounders and the outcome. In addition, matching can be difficult and require a large sample of potential controls to match successfully on many variables.

Analytic techniques are used more commonly than design techniques to address potential confounding. The most straightforward approach is a stratified analysis with a stratum defined for each level of confounder. If many confounders and their interactions are being considered, the individual strata soon contain too few subjects, however, to make meaningful estimates. The most common statistical method used to control for potential confounders is adjustment using multiple regression. The details of multiple regression analysis and analysis of covariance are beyond the scope of this chapter, and readers should consult a biostatistics text for further information.[38]

Randomized Controlled Trials

The "gold standard" for evaluating the effect of an intervention on an outcome is the prospective, double-blinded RCT. Most providers are familiar with the basic design of an RCT: A group of patients that have met selection criteria are randomly assigned to either the intervention or the control treatment and followed prospectively to compare outcomes between the two groups (Fig. 10–4). The main advantage to an RCT is that successful randomization minimizes baseline differences between the two groups. To the extent that randomization is successful, the potential for confounding by either measured or unmeasured variables is reduced. As mentioned previously, successful blinding of study participants and investigators should eliminate the effects of observer and reporting biases. The double-blinded RCT is the design that most convincingly shows the cause-effect relationship between an intervention and an outcome because it provides the best defenses against confounding and bias.

RCTs can have substantial limitations and disadvantages. They tend to be prospective studies with large sample sizes and can be very expensive and time-consuming to perform. By design, they usually address only one primary research question. The generalizability of the study can be limited if the patients who are willing to be randomly assigned are markedly different from the target population. The effects of potentially harmful exposures cannot easily be studied ethically using an experimental design, although some trials involving cessation of exposures presumed to be harmful may be possible. Studies of certain interventions, especially surgery, are difficult to blind, and RCTs that not blinded are subject to observer and detection bias. Prospective trials where definitive treatment is not performed at the time of randomization are potentially subject to crossover between treatment groups.

To maintain the benefits of randomization, results should be analyzed using an intention-to-treat (ITT) analysis. An ITT

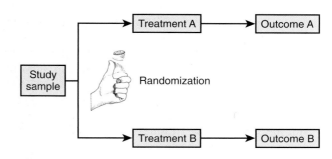

FIGURE 10–4 Diagram showing basic design of randomized controlled trial. Study sample is randomized to different treatments, and outcomes are prospectively determined.

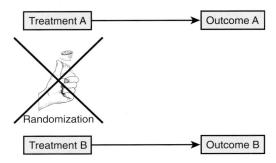

FIGURE 10–5 Diagram showing basic design of observational cohort study. Treatment is chosen by patient and physician rather than through randomization. Study groups are defined by treatment, and outcomes are compared. Cohort studies can be prospective or retrospective.

analysis compares the outcomes between the groups based on the treatment assigned rather than actual treatment received. Patients who crossover are analyzed as part of their assigned treatment group despite receiving the alternate treatment. Crossover typically results in an underestimation of the treatment effect of the intervention. Researchers studying treatments where crossover is likely, such as surgical versus nonoperative care in patients with back pain, are encouraged to develop recruitment, consent, and treatment procedures to minimize crossover, within the obvious constraint that patients ultimately have the right to change their course of treatment. Finally, RCTs are also subject to attrition bias if patients are lost to follow-up.

To illustrate how these principles affect the interpretation of an RCT, we consider how these issues apply to the SPORT IDH RCT. Inspection of Table 1 from the RCT reveals that there were no significant differences between the surgery and nonoperative groups at baseline on more than 25 variables, suggesting that randomization was effective.[27] Given that patients were randomly assigned to either surgery or nonoperative treatment, blinding was considered inappropriate because it would have required a sham surgery with significant risks.[36,39] As such, the possibility of treatment and detection bias must be considered. Greater than 80% of patients in both groups completed the 1-year follow-up, although follow-up decreased to around 75% in both groups at 2 years. The role of attrition bias should be considered for the 2-year data.

The most striking aspect of the SPORT IDH RCT was the high rate of crossover between the treatment groups in both directions, attributable to the elective nature of the procedure and the generous period allowed per protocol for receiving assigned surgery. In the first 2 years of follow-up, 40% of patients assigned to surgery did not have surgery, and 45% of patients assigned to nonoperative treatment did have surgery.[27] As a result, the surgery and nonoperative groups ended up receiving nearly the same treatment, and the ITT analysis revealed no significant differences on the primary outcome measures. Given the high rate of crossover, the ITT analysis alone does not allow one to make strong conclusions based on the RCT.

Observational Cohort Studies

The key difference between randomized and observational studies is that the determination of treatment is not randomized. In a study evaluating an intervention, the patient and physician determine the patient's treatment. The study groups are defined by the exposure or intervention, and the outcomes are compared (Fig. 10–5). Cohort studies can be prospective or retrospective, but the group assignment is determined by the exposure in both types of cohort study. The main advantage of a cohort study is that the temporal relationship between exposure and outcome is known, making it unlikely that the outcome was actually the cause of the exposure (this is known as "effect-cause"). This type of study may also have better generalizability to the target population because the patient treatment is determined in the same manner as for a nonstudy patient. Prospective observational cohort studies are also a very powerful design when randomization is impossible (i.e., studying a harmful exposure).

Observational studies have many potential disadvantages. Because randomization and blinding are impossible in an observational design, confounding and bias must be taken into account. The two groups being compared often have important baseline differences, some of which can be responsible for confounding. Methods for addressing confounding were discussed earlier. The lack of blinding makes treatment and detection bias possible, and these issues are much more difficult to address. Blinding is often impossible in RCTs comparing surgery with nonoperative treatment, however, so the RCT does not always offer an advantage in this regard. Prospective cohort studies tend to require large numbers of patients and can take many years to perform. On the other hand, retrospective cohort studies tend to be much less resource intensive, but evaluation of the exposures and outcomes is limited by what was recorded in the medical record.

Comparison of the SPORT IDH RCT[27] and observational cohort study[40] helps to illustrate the differences in the two study designs. Whereas the ITT analysis of the RCT showed no significant differences between the surgery and nonoperative groups on the primary outcome measures, the observational study (and the as-treated analysis of the RCT) showed clinically and statistically significant advantages for surgery on all outcome measures. How should these differences be interpreted? Longitudinal regression was used in the observational analysis to account for potential confounding and attrition related to the baseline variables that were measured. Such an analysis cannot control for potential confounding by unmeasured variables, however. Baseline differences on unmeasured variables could act as confounders and be responsible for some of the differences observed between the surgery and nonoperative groups. Similar to the RCT, the lack of blinding in the observational study limits the control of observer biases. Attrition rates were lower in the observational cohort than the RCT (<20% for both groups at 2 years), so the potential for attrition bias is less. Given these considerations, are the results of the observational study valid?

In 2000, Benson and Hartz[41] compared findings between modern randomized and observational studies on various medical questions and found that the results were similar for most studies. In the two instances where there were different findings between the study designs, the RCTs reported a greater treatment effect than the observational studies. These findings strongly support the validity of well-designed observational studies. Although confounding by unmeasured variables and bias may have resulted in some overstatement or understatement of the treatment effect of surgery for IDH in SPORT, with the numerous potential confounders measured and used to adjust the analysis and the strong effects observed, it seems likely that there was a benefit to surgery.

Case-Control Studies

The case-control study is another commonly used observational design, although it has not been used frequently in the spine literature. In this study design, the groups are defined by their outcomes, and the rates of exposure are compared between the two groups (Fig. 10–6). Typically, cases are identified, a matching control group is assembled, and the rates of exposure to the risk factor of interest are compared between the two groups. The main advantage of a case-control study is its ability to assess risk factors for a rare outcome with a relatively small group of cases in a retrospective fashion.

There are many potential pitfalls with case-control studies, however, with sampling and recall bias being the two most difficult to overcome.[42] *Sampling bias* results when the cases and controls are not drawn from the same population. *Recall bias* results when cases are more likely to report exposure to the risk factor of interest. Although case-control studies have rarely been used in the spine literature, a hypothetical example would be the comparison of the rate of exposure to nonsteroidal anti-inflammatory drugs (NSAIDs) between patients with a lumbar pseudarthrosis (the cases) and patients with a successful fusion (controls). This approach might prove useful in evaluating the hypothesis that NSAID use might affect the likelihood of successful fusion. Sampling bias (i.e., differential rates of smoking, diabetes, and other risk factors for nonunion between the cases and controls) and recall bias (patients with pseudarthroses might be more likely to report exposure to NSAIDs) would have to be taken into account.

Case Series

Case series are reports of outcomes for patients undergoing a treatment without any control group. The spine literature is replete with this type of study. No inferential conclusions can be made from case series because there is no control group with which to compare outcomes. Case series should be based on a consecutive series of patients to avoid selection bias in which the investigator includes only patients with desirable outcomes. These studies are useful for hypothesis generating or reporting outcomes on rare conditions. They should not be used to develop treatment guidelines because they lack a

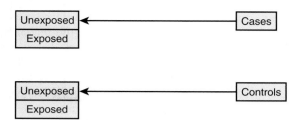

FIGURE 10–6 Diagram showing basic design of case-control study. Study groups are determined by outcomes: Patients with a particular outcome are cases, whereas patients without the outcome are controls. This study design looks retrospectively to determine if there is a difference in rate of exposure to a particular variable between cases and controls.

control group and do not allow for the assessment of effectiveness of a treatment.

Levels of Evidence

Investigators have created a hierarchy of study designs based on the quality of causal inference one can make with each study design (Fig. 10–7). Well-controlled RCTs and meta-analyses of such studies are at the pinnacle of the hierarchy. These studies have been labeled level 1 evidence.[43] Observational cohort studies or RCTs with methodologic shortcomings are level 2 evidence. Case-control studies are considered level 3 evidence. Descriptive studies such as case series and case reports are level 4 evidence. Expert opinion is considered level 5 evidence. As shown by the SPORT IDH RCT, all questions are not best answered with a randomized design. In addition, when modern observational studies are compared with RCTs, it has been shown that they do not usually overstate the treatment effect of an intervention.[41,44] Whereas the hierarchy of evidence is useful for comparing study designs in general, the merits of each individual study should be assessed, and high-quality, observational studies should not be discounted.

Cost-Effectiveness Analysis

Given the ever-increasing costs of health care, policymakers have recommended that medical interventions be evaluated

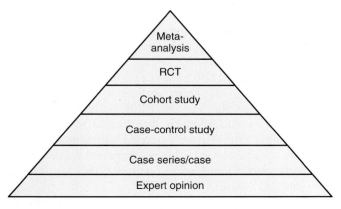

FIGURE 10–7 Hierarchy of research designs in evidence-based medicine.

for their cost-effectiveness.[45] Cost-effectiveness analysis aims to determine the cost to society for the incremental health benefit derived from an intervention that is more costly than an alternative, less effective treatment. Although an RCT can show the efficacy of a treatment, further economic analysis can be performed alongside the RCT to evaluate how much society must pay for the treatment effect. To compare the cost-effectiveness of a wide variety of treatments across many medical specialties, a universal scale of health must be used to measure preference for health outcomes. In cost-effectiveness analysis, the *quality-adjusted life-year* (QALY), which combines length and quality of life in a single number, is the recommended measure of health benefit.

To estimate QALYs, a *utility*, which is a numeric preference rating of health ranging from 0 (equivalent to death) to 1 (perfect health) is used to value the health states associated with a treatment. Classically, utilities have been derived using techniques such as the time trade-off, which essentially determines how much time in a state of suboptimal health people would be willing to trade for a lesser amount of time in perfect health.[45] More recently, techniques have been developed to determine utilities based on standard questionnaires such as the SF-36.[46] QALYs are determined by multiplying utility for each health state by the length of time in each health state and summing up over time. For example, 2 years spent in a poor health state with a utility of 0.5 followed by 10 years in a good health state with a utility of 0.8 would be equivalent to 9 QALYs ($2 \times 5 + 10 \times 8$). To compare the benefits of various interventions, cost-effectiveness analysis determines the gain in QALYs associated with an intervention. The advantage of QALYs is that they allow for the comparison of very different health states across medical disciplines.

The other half of the cost-effectiveness equation is the cost. Although an intervention typically produces a health benefit, that benefit comes at a cost to society. Determining the cost of an intervention is challenging, so many cost-effectiveness analyses use gross costing based on average reimbursements for various procedures. After determining the costs and benefits associated with an intervention, these must be compared with another treatment. This is done by determining the *incremental cost-effectiveness ratio* (ICER). The ICER is defined as the difference in cost between the two treatments divided by the difference in utility. Tosteson and colleagues[47] reported that discectomy resulted in a gain of 0.21 QALYs compared with nonoperative treatment at an additional cost of $14,137, which yielded an ICER of $69,403/QALY ($14,137/0.21 QALY). Traditionally, an ICER of $50,000/QALY has been used as a cost-effectiveness threshold because this was the ICER for hemodialysis, an intervention for which society has decided to pay.[48] More recently, some authors have suggested that $100,000/QALY is a more realistic cost-effectiveness threshold because many frequently used interventions fall in the $50,000 to $100,000/QALY range.[47,49,50]

Theoretically, cost-effectiveness analysis should allow societies to maximize the value of their health care expenditures,

and Great Britain has set ICER thresholds to determine which services should be provided by their National Health Service.[51] There is little evidence, however, that health care systems, including systems that currently ration care, have been consistently using cost-effectiveness analysis to guide rational treatment guidelines.[52] As health care spending comes under greater scrutiny and decisions regarding which treatments to provide are made, evaluating the cost-effectiveness of an intervention will be essential.

Future of Outcomes Research: Patient-Specific Recommendations

Since the prior edition of this textbook, the quality of spine outcomes research has improved markedly alongside a more sophisticated understanding of the issues surrounding outcomes research within the spine community. A study of spine-related clinical trials published in 2007 reported 60% were performed and reported in an acceptable fashion, a result that is better than seen in a general orthopaedic journal.[53] Although this percentage is likely an improvement from years prior, there is further work to be done on the quality of the spine literature. The 4-year outcome data from the SPORT IDH study, the largest scale outcomes research study ever performed in the field of spinal disorders, have been published more recently.[54] Although this and most large-scale trials are able to determine the treatment effect of an intervention for the "average" patient, it can be difficult to apply the results to clinical practice, in which no patient is "average."

In the case of IDH, there are clearly patients who fail surgical treatment and others who are very successful with nonoperative treatment. Blind application of the results of SPORT to all patients who met the inclusion criteria (symptoms lasting at least 6 weeks, the presence of neurologic findings, and imaging consistent with their symptoms) would result in surgery for all such patients. Although this approach would result in greater clinical improvement than nonoperative treatment on average, surgery would be performed on some patients who would have improved to an acceptable, and even to a greater, degree with nonoperative treatment, and other patients would fail to improve with surgery and perhaps experience additional lessening in their quality of life.

To avoid unnecessary surgery on these two groups of patients, models that take individual characteristics and values into account when predicting outcomes are needed. When sufficiently powerful models are developed, individual baseline characteristics, physical findings, and results from imaging studies can be entered into such models to determine the likelihood of success with surgery or nonoperative treatment. Individual patient values should also be considered in defining success and assigning utilities to the various possible outcomes. Such an approach represents the true integration of evidence-based medicine with shared decision making at the level of the individual patient and should be the next step in spine outcomes research.

KEY POINTS

1. With constantly increasing health care costs, policymakers are demanding outcomes research to show the effectiveness of treatments, especially in fields that require expensive technology such as spine surgery.

2. There is substantial geographic variation in the rates of spine surgery across the United States, indicating that further research is needed to determine which patients are served best with surgery.

3. Chance, bias, and confounding all threaten the validity of conclusions based on clinical research and need to be addressed in study design and data analysis.

4. RCTs can yield the highest level of evidence, although many surgical questions are not amenable to this type of study design. In these cases, well-designed observational studies may be more appropriate.

5. Cost-effectiveness analysis will become more important as decisions need to be made about the use of scarce health care resources.

KEY REFERENCES

1. Fisher ES, Wennberg DE, Stukel TA, et al: The implications of regional variations in Medicare spending. Part 2: Health outcomes and satisfaction with care. Ann Intern Med 138:288-298, 2003.
   This study showed wide variation in Medicare spending across hospital referral regions with no measurable improvement in outcomes in areas with the highest levels of spending.

2. Weinstein JN, Lurie JD, Olson PR, et al: United States' trends and regional variations in lumbar spine surgery: 1992-2003. Spine 31:2707-2714, 2006.
   This small area analysis showed the increase in the rate of lumbar fusion in the Medicare population throughout the 1990s and the wide geographic variation in fusion rates in this population.

3. Bombardier C: Outcome assessments in the evaluation of treatment of spinal disorders. Introduction. Spine 25:3097-3099, 2000.
   This article reviews the differences between different outcome measures used in the spine literature and introduces an issue dedicated to this topic.

4. Kocher MS, Zurakowski D: Clinical epidemiology and biostatistics: A primer for orthopaedic surgeons. J Bone Joint Surg Am 86:607-620, 2004.
   This is a good review of basic epidemiology and biostatistics as it applies to orthopaedics.

5. Benson K, Hartz AJ: A comparison of observational studies and randomized, controlled trials. N Engl J Med 342:1878-1886, 2000.
   This article shows convincingly that well-designed observational trials yield similar results to RCTs.

REFERENCES

1. Webster's New World Medical Dictionary, 3rd ed. Hoboken, NJ, Wiley Publishing, 2008.

2. Musgrove P, Zeramdini R, Carrin G: Basic patterns in national health expenditure. Bull World Health Organ 80:134-142, 2002.

3. Wilkinson RG, Pickett KE: Income inequality and population health: A review and explanation of the evidence. Soc Sci Med 62:1768-1784, 2006.

4. Wennberg JE, Gittelsohn A: Health care delivery in Maine, I: Patterns of use of common surgical procedures. J Maine Med Assoc 66:123-130, 149, 1975.

5. Wennberg JE, Freeman JL, Culp WJ: Are hospital services rationed in New Haven or over-utilised in Boston? Lancet 1:1185-1189, 1987.

6. Fisher ES, Wennberg DE, Stukel TA, et al: The implications of regional variations in Medicare spending. Part 1: The content, quality, and accessibility of care. Ann Intern Med 138:273-287, 2003.

7. Fisher ES, Wennberg DE, Stukel TA, et al: The implications of regional variations in Medicare spending. Part 2: Health outcomes and satisfaction with care. Ann Intern Med 138:288-298, 2003.

8. Weinstein JN, Lurie JD, Olson PR, et al: United States' trends and regional variations in lumbar spine surgery: 1992-2003. Spine 31:2707-2714, 2006.

9. Fuchs VR: More variation in use of care, more flat-of-the-curve medicine. Health Aff (Millwood) Suppl Web Exclusives: VAR104-7, 2004.

10. Atlas SJ, Deyo RA, Keller RB, et al: The Maine Lumbar Spine Study, Part II: 1-year outcomes of surgical and nonsurgical management of sciatica. Spine 21:1777-1786, 1996.

11. Atlas SJ, Deyo RA, Keller RB, et al: The Maine Lumbar Spine Study, Part III: 1-year outcomes of surgical and nonsurgical management of lumbar spinal stenosis. Spine 21:1787-1794; discussion 1794-1795, 1996.

12. Schafer J, O'Connor D, Feinglass S, et al: Medicare Evidence Development and Coverage Advisory Committee Meeting on lumbar fusion surgery for treatment of chronic back pain from degenerative disc disease. Spine 32:2403-2404, 2007.

13. Glassman SD, Polly DW, Bono C, et al: Outcome of lumbar fusion in patients over 65 years old. American Academy of Orthopaedic Surgeons Annual Meeting, Las Vegas, NV, 2009.

14. Bombardier C: Outcome assessments in the evaluation of treatment of spinal disorders. Introduction. Spine 25:3097-3099, 2000.

15. Weber H: Lumbar disc herniation: A controlled, prospective study with ten years of observation. Spine 8:131-140, 1983

16. Ware JE Jr, Sherbourne CD: The MOS 36-item short-form health survey (SF-36): I. Conceptual framework and item selection. Med Care 30:473-483, 1992.

17. Brooks R: EuroQol: the current state of play. Health Policy 37:53-72, 1996.

18. Bergner M, Bobbitt RA, Carter WB, et al: The Sickness Impact Profile: Development and final revision of a health status measure. Med Care 19:787-805, 1981.

19. Fairbank JC, Couper J, Davies JB, et al: The Oswestry low back pain disability questionnaire. Physiotherapy 66:271-273, 1980.

20. Roland M, Morris R: A study of the natural history of back pain. Part I: Development of a reliable and sensitive measure of disability in low-back pain. Spine 8:141-144, 1983.

21. Lurie J: A review of generic health status measures in patients with low back pain. Spine 25:3125-3129, 2000.

22. Zanoli G, Stromqvist B, Padua R, et al: Lessons learned searching for a HRQoL instrument to assess the results of treatment in persons with lumbar disorders. Spine 25:3178-3185, 2000.

23. Atlas SJ, Deyo RA, Patrick DL, et al: The Quebec Task Force Classification for Spinal Disorders and the severity, treatment, and outcomes of sciatica and lumbar spinal stenosis. Spine 21:2885-2892, 1996.

24. Deyo RA, Battie M, Beurskens AJ, et al: Outcome measures for low back pain research: A proposal for standardized use. Spine 23:2003-2013, 1998.

25. Ware JE Jr: SF-36 health survey update. Spine 25:3130-3139, 2000.

26. Roland M, Fairbank J: The Roland-Morris Disability Questionnaire and the Oswestry Disability Questionnaire. Spine 25:3115-3124, 2000.

27. Weinstein JN, Tosteson TD, Lurie JD, et al: Surgical vs nonoperative treatment for lumbar disk herniation. The Spine Patient Outcomes Research Trial (SPORT): A randomized trial. JAMA 296:2441-2450, 2006.

28. Roland M, Morris R: A study of the natural history of low-back pain. Part II: Development of guidelines for trials of treatment in primary care. Spine 8:145-150, 1983.

29. Kopec JA: Measuring functional outcomes in persons with back pain: A review of back-specific questionnaires. Spine 25:3110-3114, 2000.

30. Fritzell P, Hagg O, Wessberg P, et al: 2001 Volvo Award Winner in Clinical Studies. Lumbar fusion versus nonsurgical treatment for chronic low back pain: A multicenter randomized controlled trial from the Swedish Lumbar Spine Study Group. Spine 26:2521-2532; discussion 2532-2534, 2001.

31. Fairbank J, Frost H, Wilson-MacDonald J, et al: Randomised controlled trial to compare surgical stabilisation of the lumbar spine with an intensive rehabilitation programme for patients with chronic low back pain: The MRC spine stabilisation trial. BMJ 330:1233, 2005.

32. Brox JI, Sorensen R, Friis A, et al: Randomized clinical trial of lumbar instrumented fusion and cognitive intervention and exercises in patients with chronic low back pain and disc degeneration. Spine 28:1913-1921, 2003.

33. Hulley SB, Newman TB, Cummings SR: Choosing the study subjects: Specification, sampling, and recruitment. In: Designing Clinical Research, 2nd ed. Philadelphia, Lippincott Williams & Wilkins, 2001, pp 25-35.

34. Spratt K: Statistical relevance. In Garfin S, Abitbolet J (eds): Orthopaedic Knowledge Update: Spine. Rosemont, IL, American Academy of Orthopaedic Surgeons, 2002, pp 497-505.

35. Kocher MS, Zurakowski D: Clinical epidemiology and biostatistics: A primer for orthopaedic surgeons. J Bone Joint Surg Am 86:607-620, 2004.

36. Birkmeyer NJ, Weinstein JN, Tosteson AN, et al: Design of the Spine Patient Outcomes Research Trial (SPORT). Spine 27:1361-1372, 2002.

37. Newman TB, Browner WS, Hulley SB: Enhancing causal inference in observational studies. In: Designing Clinical Research, 2nd ed. Philadelphia, Lippincott Williams & Wilkins, 2001, pp 125-137.

38. Dawson B, Trapp RG: Basic and Clinical Biostatistics, 4th ed. New York, McGraw-Hill, 2004.

39. Flum DR: Interpreting surgical trials with subjective outcomes: Avoiding UnSPORTsmanlike conduct. JAMA 296:2483-2485, 2006.

40. Weinstein JN, Lurie JD, Tosteson TD, et al: Surgical vs nonoperative treatment for lumbar disk herniation: The Spine Patient Outcomes Research Trial (SPORT) observational cohort. JAMA 296:2451-2459, 2006.

41. Benson K, Hartz AJ: A comparison of observational studies and randomized, controlled trials. N Engl J Med 342:1878-1886, 2000.

42. Newman TB, Browner WS, Cummings SR, et al: Designing an observational study: Cross-sectional and case-control studies. In: Designing Clinical Research, 2nd ed. Philadelphia: Lippincott Williams & Wilkins, 2001, pp 107-123.

43. Brighton B, Bhandari M, Tornetta P 3rd, et al: Hierarchy of evidence: From case reports to randomized controlled trials. Clin Orthop Relat Res 19-24, 2003.

44. Concato J, Shah N, Horwitz RI: Randomized, controlled trials, observational studies, and the hierarchy of research designs. N Engl J Med 342:1887-1892, 2000.

45. Gold MG, Siegel JE, Russell LB, et al: Cost-Effectiveness in Health and Medicine. New York, Oxford University Press, 1996.

46. Brazier J, Roberts J, Deverill M: The estimation of a preference-based measure of health from the SF-36. J Health Econ 21:271-292, 2002.

47. Tosteson AN, Skinner JS, Tosteson TD, et al: The cost effectiveness of surgical versus nonoperative treatment for lumbar disc herniation over two years: Evidence from the Spine Patient Outcomes Research Trial (SPORT). Spine 33:2108-2115, 2008.

48. Winkelmayer WC, Weinstein MC, Mittleman MA, et al: Health economic evaluations: The special case of end-stage renal disease treatment. Med Decis Making 22:417-430, 2002.

49. Laupacis A, Feeny D, Detsky AS, et al: How attractive does a new technology have to be to warrant adoption and utilization? Tentative guidelines for using clinical and economic evaluations. Can Med Assoc J 146:473-481, 1992.

50. Tosteson AN, Lurie JD, Tosteson TD, et al: Surgical treatment of spinal stenosis with and without degenerative spondylolisthesis: cost-effectiveness after 2 years. Ann Intern Med 149:845-853, 2008.

51. Rawlins MD, Culyer AJ: National Institute for Clinical Excellence and its value judgments. BMJ 329:224-227, 2004.

52. Appleby J, Devlin N, Parkin D, et al: Searching for cost effectiveness thresholds in the NHS. Health Policy 91:239-245, 2009.

53. Dodwell E, Fischer CG, Reilly CW, et al: A quality assessment of randomized controlled trials in the spine literature. American Academy of Orthopaedic Surgeons Annual Meeting, Las Vegas, NV, 2009.

54. Weinstein JN, Lurie JD, Tosteson TD, et al: Surgical versus nonoperative treatment for lumbar disc herniation: Four-year results for the Spine Patient Outcomes Research Trial (SPORT). Spine 33:2789-2800, 2008.

The Patient History and Physical Examination: Cervical, Thoracic, and Lumbar

Christopher J. Standaert, MD
Stanley A. Herring, MD
J. David Sinclair, MD

Caring for patients with spine disorders can be extremely challenging for clinicians because of the complexities of spinal anatomy and pathophysiology and the multifactorial nature of pain. Despite extensive advances in imaging of and interventions for the spine, a massive medical and social problem related to spinal pain and disability remains. To address the needs of patients with spine disorders and to select appropriately patients for whom specific care may be beneficial, clinicians need to identify the true nature of a patient's problem. Frequently, the patient's problem may extend well beyond any anatomic derangement that can be identified on imaging studies and involve numerous psychosocial factors in the patient's life. Through the history and physical examination, clinicians are able to identify not only the physical manifestations of a spine disorder but also the root causes of a patient's distress, suffering, and disability, all of which ultimately need to be addressed if a successful outcome is to be achieved.

A thorough history and physical examination of a patient with a spine disorder has several aims. From a strictly medical perspective, the examiner must be aware of the full medical context of the patient's complaints and how the complaints may relate to the overall health of the patient. It is imperative to ascertain the presence of an emergent medical problem promptly and to identify patients who need more urgent (or emergent) assessment and care. Clinicians must also identify any secondary medical issues that may directly affect the care of spine-related problems or be associated with broader health concerns. In a more focused sense, the history and physical examination should allow an examiner to identify relevant spine problems that have led to the issue for which the patient is seeking care (e.g., the source of pain or neurologic loss, anatomic derangements). The history and physical examination also allow the practitioner to understand the level of function and impairment that is associated with the patient's presentation.

Moving beyond the strictly medical context, identification of the factors associated with the patient's pain and disability that pose the dominant barriers to optimal functional recovery is an important goal of the history and physical examination. To decide on the appropriate intervention for a patient, it is imperative to understand what exactly is being treated.

Despite all the attention paid to pain, frequently the patient's sense of suffering is the real problem, particularly in patients with chronic pain. The only way to identify the issues behind the presentation of many patients is by asking the right questions. This chapter addresses relevant issues in the history and physical examination in patients with spine disorders, particularly as these issues relate to the assessment of patients seen commonly in clinical practice, and provides information on how to identify patients at risk for ongoing pain despite what seems to be appropriate care for their structural problems.

Differential Diagnosis

The differential diagnosis of spinal pain or related symptoms is enormous when considered in a general sense. Numerous anatomic structures may be associated with pain, multiple local or systemic disease processes can affect the spine, and numerous non–spine-related structures or conditions can result in back or neck pain or mimic syndromes related to spine disorders.[1-5] In addition, numerous psychosocial factors can produce ongoing pain and disability. The ability to process all of the available possibilities and to develop a relatively short list of diagnostic options depends heavily on the ability to obtain a thorough history and physical examination. It is helpful to begin with an understanding of structures in the spine that can be associated with pain and their patterns of pain referral.

From an anatomic perspective, a structure must be innervated to cause pain. In the spine, the list of discrete anatomic structures with sensory innervation (i.e., potential pain generators) includes muscles, tendons, ligaments, fascia, anulus of the intervertebral discs, bone, zygapophyseal joints, dura mater, nerve roots and dorsal root ganglia, and vascular elements.[1,2] All structures of common embryologic segmental origin tend to refer pain in very similar patterns, and the pattern of pain is determined by the nerve supply to the structure.[1] The end result is that there is substantial overlap between the referral patterns for anatomic structures of the same spinal level, such as intervertebral discs and zygapophyseal joints, and dermatomal, myotomal, and sclerotomal referral patterns at many spinal levels (Fig. 11–1). The location of pain or radiating symptoms can often be a useful feature in the identification of an affected spinal level, although the location of pain alone does not indicate which particular anatomic structure is the source of the specific symptom.

The zygapophyseal joints are one of the best-studied structures in terms of pain referral patterns and relative prevalence

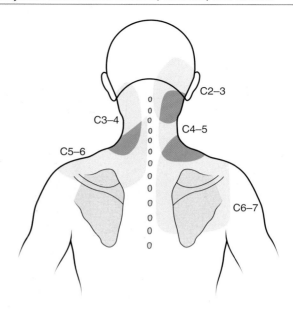

FIGURE 11–2 Map of characteristic areas of pain referred from cervical zygapophyseal joints (C2-3 to C6-7). (From Dwyer A, Aprill C, Bogduk N: Cervical zygapophyseal joint pain patterns I: A study in normal volunteers. Spine 15:453-457, 1990.)

in patients with spinal pain. In the cervical spine, the pattern of pain distribution from the stimulation of specific zygapophyseal joints has been described (Fig. 11–2).[6] Those results were subsequently validated in a study of patients with cervical complaints based on pain distribution and response to diagnostic blocks.[7] Another study using a double-block protocol on patients with persisting symptoms after whiplash injury found that the prevalence of C2-3 zygapophyseal joint pain in patients with headache was 50%; in patients without C2-3 zygapophyseal joint pain, the prevalence of symptoms related to the lower cervical zygapophyseal joints was 49%.[8] Although there is far less clinical information on pain associated with thoracic zygapophyseal joints, a similar map of referral patterns has been identified (Fig. 11–3).[9]

In the lumbar spine, there has also been a great deal of attention directed to the zygapophyseal joints as potential sources of pain, although the relative frequency with which they seem to be primary pain generators is less than for cervical zygapophyseal joints causing pain in patients with chronic whiplash. A more recent study noted a 15% overall prevalence of zygapophyseal pain in a group of 176 patients with chronic low back pain using a diagnostic double-block protocol.[10] Although pain associated with lumbar zygapophyseal joints is generally described as occurring with lumbar extension and rotation, the authors of that study did not find any consistent clinical features that were associated with the presence of a positive diagnostic response to injections.[10] Stimulation of lumbar zygapophyseal joints can result in either local axial or, far less frequently, radiating pain, and pain referral patterns have been documented.[11]

Multiple authors have addressed the distribution of pain associated with intervertebral discs. Cloward[12] first described cervical discography and noted that pain that seemed to be emanating from irritation of the anulus resulted in radiating

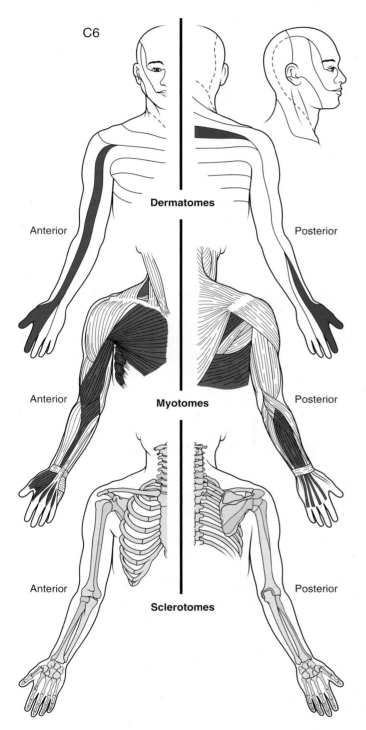

FIGURE 11–1 Drawing of dermatome, myotome, and sclerotome of C6 level showing substantial overlap in distribution. (From Bland JH: Disorders of the Cervical Spine: Diagnosis and Medical Management, 2nd ed. Philadelphia, WB Saunders, 1994.)

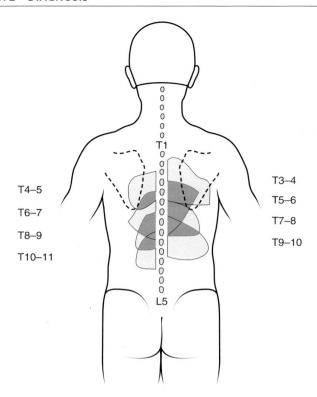

FIGURE 11-3 Map of characteristic areas of pain referred from thoracic zygapophyseal joints (T3-4 to T10-11). (From Dreyfuss P, Tibiletti C, Dreyer S: Thoracic zygapophyseal joint pain patterns: A study in normal volunteers. Spine 19:807-811, 1994.)

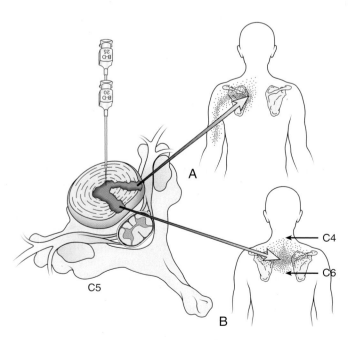

FIGURE 11-4 A and **B,** Pain referral pattern from posterolateral (**A**) and central (**B**) discs. (From Cloward RB: Cervical discography: A contribution to the etiology and mechanism of neck, shoulder and arm pain. Ann Surg 150:1052-1064, 1959.)

pain into the thoracic or scapular regions in distinct patterns (Fig. 11-4). Similar findings were more recently described by others.[13] As mentioned previously, pain referral patterns are similar to patterns noted for cervical zygapophyseal joints, with the level of spine pathology, rather than the actual structure involved, affecting the pain referral pattern.

Other pain referral patterns that should be recognized by all physicians treating patients with spine disorders include patterns related to neurologic injury. These patterns are discussed further later in the section on the neurologic examination, but identifying the dermatomal pattern of pain is central to the assessment of individuals with potential nerve root pathology (Fig. 11-5). Nerve root symptoms include paresthesias, burning, hyperalgesia, aching, analgesia, or pain. The ability to identify a dermatomal pattern to the symptoms can help localize the area of spine involvement.

The clinical utility of pain provocation is uncertain because there are inherent problems with this approach owing to the complex nature of pain perception.[1,14-18] The identification of a "pain generator" in individuals with chronic spinal pain can be difficult. In contrast to cutaneous sensation, nociceptive signals from deep somatic structures such as joint capsules, fascia, and periosteum are carried by relatively few primary afferent fibers, resulting in only vague localization of pain.[16] Additionally, there is the issue of convergence, in which a single dorsal horn cell may receive synaptic input from afferent fibers that innervate many structures and can result in multiple structures producing similar patterns of pain perception. This convergence makes it extremely difficult to validate a single entity as "the cause" of an individual's pain because the stimulation of any one of numerous structures may result in identical perceptions of pain.[16] These issues become even more complex when additional potential neurologic and psychological changes that can occur with chronic pain are involved.

Biomedical Factors and the Medical History

It is essential to obtain a thorough and appropriate medical history from patients presenting with spine disorders or related complaints. The identification of potentially serious problems is one of the most important functions of obtaining a good medical history. Ideally, the medical history also should help the clinician establish a reasonable differential diagnosis that can direct further diagnostic or therapeutic steps. Given the scope and complexities of spine disorders, it can be useful to break down some aspects of the clinical presentation into broad categories. This categorization may allow clinicians to focus their thought process and subsequent efforts more effectively. Useful categories to consider relate to the presence or absence of radiating pain and specific demographic factors. The following categories can help in obtaining a concise medical history.

"Red Flags"—What Not to Miss

It is essential to identify all conditions that pose a substantial, imminent risk for further harm to the patient. Many authors

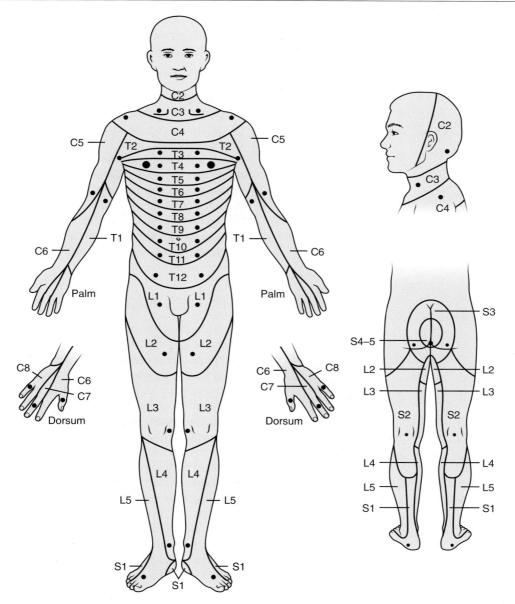

FIGURE 11–5 Dermatomal distribution and key sensory points. (From American Spinal Injury Association: International Standards for Neurological Classification of Spinal Cord Injury [reprint]. Chicago, American Spinal Injury Association, 2008.)

have identified specific "red flags" in the history of patients with low back complaints that indicate the presence of such a condition; these include infection, tumor, fracture, cauda equina injury, and progressive neurologic injury such as motor loss or myelopathy (Table 11–1).[19-22] "Red flags" for the possibility of *cancer* include age older than 50 years, previous cancer history, unexplained weight loss, pain not relieved by bed rest, duration of pain for more than 1 month, and failure of conservative therapy after 1 month.[22] The combined sensitivity of age older than 50 years, history of cancer, unexplained weight loss, and failure of conservative therapy is nearly 100%.[22] A history of smoking also increases a patient's risk for cancer.[21] Although similar data are unavailable for cervical and thoracic pain, the same factors seem relevant.

Spine infections, including discitis, osteomyelitis, and epidural abscess, are usually blood-borne from other regions.[22] Important risk factors for infection include the use of illicit intravenous drugs, active or recent infection elsewhere (e.g., urinary tract, pulmonary, skin, dental), and immunosuppression (owing to either medications or illness affecting the immune system).[19,22] Additional risk factors for infection include diabetes and history of tuberculosis or exposure to a region endemic for tuberculosis.

The risk of *fracture* is elevated in patients older than 50 years, particularly patients older than 70 years.[22] Patients with a history of corticosteroid use or known osteopenia or osteoporosis are also at increased risk for fracture. A history of fracture in a younger individual after major trauma, in an

TABLE 11–1 "Red Flags": Emergent or Urgent Medical Conditions That Need to Be Identified Promptly in All Patients Presenting with Possible Issues Related to the Spine

Symptom or Finding	Possible Significance
History of cancer	Cancer
Unexplained weight loss	
Age >50 yr	
Failure to respond to >1 mo of conservative care	
Duration of pain >1 mo	
No pain relief with bed rest	
Night pain	
History of smoking	
Known osteopenia or osteoporosis	Fracture
History of corticosteroid use	
Age >50 yr	
DISH or ankylosing spondylitis	
Trauma (major in younger individual, minor in older individual)	
Fever	Infection
Illicit use of intravenous or percutaneously injected drugs	
Recent or known infection	
Immunosuppressive illness	
Use of immunosuppressive medications	
Tuberculosis exposure	
Progressive weakness in limbs	Cauda equina or spinal cord injury
Progressive balance deficit or loss of coordination	
Bowel or bladder dysfunction or urinary retention	
Sexual dysfunction	
Numbness or paresthesias in perineum or saddle anesthesia	
Significant weakness of major muscle group or progressive motor loss in limb	Severe or progressive radiculopathy

DISH, diffuse idiopathic skeletal hyperostosis.

older individual after minor trauma, or in anyone with the potential for reduced bone density should also be considered a risk factor. Trauma and fracture risk are discussed further elsewhere in this book.

Significant *neurologic* injuries include cauda equina syndrome, progressive radiculopathy, or myelopathy. Cauda equina syndrome should be considered in a patient with saddle anesthesia; bowel, bladder, or sexual dysfunction; or significant lower extremity pain and weakness, particularly if bilateral.[19,22] Progressive neurologic loss from nerve root compression is an indication for urgent surgical intervention and needs to be identified promptly. Myelopathy can present in various ways, including hand paresthesias or decreased fine motor control; lower extremity weakness or gait instability; sensory alterations in the trunk or extremities; or changes in bowel, bladder, or sexual function.[23]

Historical Features of the Presenting Complaint

Specifying the exact nature of the patient's chief complaint and provocative and palliative factors is an extremely important part of the diagnostic assessment. The examiner must identify the nature, onset, duration, and course of the primary complaint; history of previous injury; character and distribution of symptoms; prior diagnostic testing and treatment; other circumstances surrounding an injury (e.g., perceived fault, the presence of workers' compensation or litigation status); and the degree of pain and disability perceived by the patient. All of these factors are important in establishing an appropriate differential diagnosis and identifying some of the potential barriers to recovery.

Axial Versus Radicular Pain

The distinction between axial and radicular pain is fundamental in assessing a patient with a potentially neurogenic problem. *Axial* pain in the cervical, thoracic, or lumbar region suggests a different etiology, evaluation, diagnosis, and potentially treatment than radicular pain. For all levels of the spine, pathology involving the musculotendinous and ligamentous structures, zygapophyseal joints, vertebrae, and anulus of the intervertebral discs tends to cause axial pain. Other structures in the cervical and thoracic regions that can result in axial pain include soft tissue structures in the neck; vascular structures (e.g., aorta or carotid arteries); portions of the brachial plexus such as the long thoracic or suprascapular nerves; the proximal portion of ribs; costovertebral or costotransverse articulations; various structures within the shoulder; and various visceral structures, including the pancreas, gallbladder, lung and pleura, and stomach or duodenum (Fig. 11–6).

Radicular pain radiating into the upper extremities generally has a different etiology. If related to spine pathology, radicular pain implies neural compression from many potential causes, including disc herniation, spinal canal or neuroforaminal stenosis, or intrinsic disease of the spinal cord or nerve roots (e.g., herpes zoster). Radicular pain in the thoracic region can result in a bandlike distribution on one or both sides of the chest wall or abdominal region. Additional structures that can result in radiating upper extremity pain include peripheral nerves such as the median nerve (e.g., carpal tunnel syndrome); ulnar nerve; portions of the brachial plexus (e.g., lower trunk plexopathies related to true neurogenic thoracic outlet syndrome or a Pancoast tumor); vascular structures; the shoulder; the heart; and musculotendinous, ligamentous, or bony structures in the upper extremities.

For the lumbar spine, the hip and pelvic structures must be considered as potential sources of low back, buttocks, or posterolateral hip pain. Particular sources of low back or buttock pain related to the bony pelvis include the sacroiliac joints, the sacrum (e.g., stress fractures), the ilia, and the hip joints. Other structures and processes that can result in low back pain include the kidneys and ureters; the pancreas; gastric ulcers;

FIGURE 11–6 Posterior referral sites from distant visceral or somatic structures. (From Nakano KK: Neck pain. In Kelley WN, Harris ED Jr, Ruddy S, et al [eds]: Textbook of Rheumatology, 4th ed. Philadelphia, WB Saunders, 1993.)

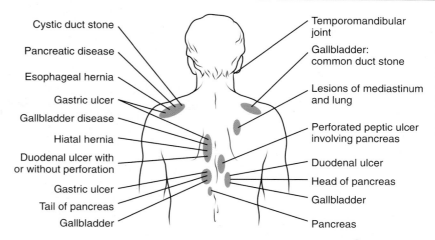

Cystic duct stone
Pancreatic disease
Esophageal hernia
Gastric ulcer
Gallbladder disease
Hiatal hernia
Duodenal ulcer with or without perforation
Gastric ulcer
Tail of pancreas
Gallbladder

Temporomandibular joint
Gallbladder: common duct stone
Lesions of mediastinum and lung
Perforated peptic ulcer involving pancreas
Duodenal ulcer
Head of pancreas
Gallbladder
Pancreas

vascular abnormalities (e.g., aortic aneurysm); and retroperitoneal processes such as hematoma, endometriosis, or lymphadenopathy associated with malignancy.[24]

As with upper extremity pain, lower extremity radicular pain often has different etiologies and generally implies involvement of the lumbosacral nerve roots, the conus medullaris, or the spine. The lumbar zygapophyseal joints and the sacroiliac joints also may occasionally be associated with radicular leg pain.[11,25] Distal lower extremity symptoms also may arise from intra-articular hip pathology; greater trochanteric bursitis; vascular pathology (e.g., vascular claudication); peripheral nerve injuries; compartment syndrome; local musculotendinous, ligamentous, or bony structures; and pelvic causes such as endometriosis.

Patient Demographics

Demographic characteristics such as age, gender, educational background, occupation, and cultural milieu are important factors that must be considered in the history of a patient with a spine problem. Age is a primary determinant in establishing a differential diagnosis. Different spine problems appear at different frequencies at different ages. The social and psychological issues of individuals can also be quite distinct at different ages. In children and adolescents, there are different issues than are seen in adults.

Growth and development have a profound impact on the development and approach to various processes, such as spondylolisthesis, scoliosis, and Scheuermann kyphosis. In contrast to the adult spine, the developing bony spine is relatively more prone to injury than some soft tissue structures. In a study by Micheli and Wood,[26] 47% of adolescents presenting to a pediatric sports medicine clinic were diagnosed with spondylolysis and only 11% had disc abnormalities compared with 48% of adults presenting to a low back pain clinic who were thought to have disc pathology. Generally, symptomatic isthmic spondylolysis is almost entirely seen in older children, adolescents, or young adults, although the rate of pars defects identified in the general population does not change substantially between the ages of 20 and 80.[27,28] Although 50% or more of children may be affected by low back pain by age 15,[29,30] significant spinal pain in children is uncommon and should raise concern for the presence of serious medical

pathology.[31,32] Infection, neoplasm, rheumatologic conditions such as ankylosing spondylitis and juvenile rheumatoid arthritis, and other nonspine sources of pain may be more common in children and adolescents than in adults.[31,32]

In adults, the frequency of certain spine conditions varies by age group. Disc herniations are most frequent during the 4th and 5th decades, although they can affect individuals in their 50s and 60s or children and young adults.[33] Degenerative spinal stenosis and degenerative spondylolisthesis tend to present later in life. As mentioned previously, some medical conditions, including ankylosing spondylitis, spondylitis associated with inflammatory bowel disease, and tumors such as osteoid osteoma and osteoblastoma, tend to manifest in younger adults (20s and 30s). Other conditions, such as osteoporosis, polymyalgia rheumatica, metastatic cancer, or multiple myeloma, tend to occur in older adults (40s and 50s or older) (Fig. 11–7).[3,34]

Gender is a factor in many spine pathologies. Osteoporosis is more common in women than in men, and osteoporotic fractures are more common in women. Neck pain also has been noted to be more prevalent in women than in men.[35,36] Rheumatoid arthritis, polymyalgia rheumatica, and endocrine disorders also tend to occur more frequently in women.[34] Spondyloarthropathies; infections; and various spine tumors, such as multiple myeloma, lymphoma, osteoblastoma, and eosinophilic granuloma, occur more frequently in men.

Demographic factors such as race, ethnicity, and cultural milieu may also play a role in the prevalence of some spine disorders but are less well studied. Whites tend to have higher rates of osteoporosis than some other races, and metabolic conditions such as Gaucher disease can be associated with certain ethnic groups.[3] Whites have a higher rate of spondylolysis than African Americans.[27] The prevalence of low back pain also varies in different parts of the world, with industrialized regions reporting a higher prevalence of low back complaints than rural, low-income areas.[37] Pain perception, disability, and other effects of pain on individuals vary widely and depend on many cultural and social factors.

Past Medical History

In addition to identifying prior surgical procedures, it is important to identify all past and current medical conditions

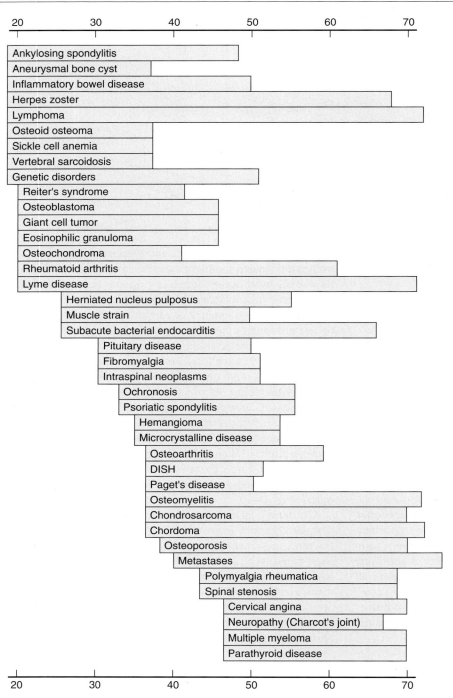

FIGURE 11–7 Age at peak incidence of neck pain associated with various disorders. (From Borenstein DG, Wiesel SW, Boden SD: Neck Pain: Medical Diagnosis and Comprehensive Management. Philadelphia, WB Saunders, 1996.)

because many medical problems can be associated with spine issues and can affect care of a patient with a spine disorder. As noted previously, a history of cancer, recent infection, or disease processes that affect the immune system or may require immunosuppressive medications can be associated with significant spine problems. Other medical conditions, such as osteoporosis, ankylosing spondylitis, and diffuse idiopathic skeletal hyperostosis, may place patients at increased risk for spine fracture.[38] Some congenital or genetic syndromes, such as Marfan syndrome and Down syndrome, can be associated with spine anomalies that must be identified. Vascular disease, such as vascular claudication or aortic aneurysm, can produce

symptoms that mimic spine pathology. Other disorders, including cardiac or pulmonary disease, renal disorders, skin conditions, gastric ulcers, diabetes, and hepatic disorders, may have an impact on potential treatment options and may preclude certain therapies. Clinicians need to be aware of all facets of a patient's medical history and the potential influence that medical issues may have on the care of the patient.

An additional aspect that must be considered in a patient with a spine disorder is a history of prior injury. Previous spine problems, trauma, and surgery may have important implications for the care of the patient. Details about the type and severity of injury and the type of treatment (including surgery) and the patient's response to it are important historical features. Whenever possible, prior operative reports should be obtained. Short-term and long-term problems potentially can develop after surgery, and it is important to understand the nature of any prior surgery. Such adverse events include adjacent segment degeneration or instability after a fusion, epidural fibrosis, infection, hardware-related problems such as loosening, and recurrent disc herniation. A history of multiple or prolonged periods of pain or disability after prior treatments should raise concerns about the chances for success with future treatments.

Family History

The family history is a necessary component of a complete medical history. Although back pain and many other spinal conditions are common in the general population, data suggest possible genetic risk factors for lumbar degenerative disc disease.[39] A family history of rheumatologic diseases, particularly conditions associated with HLA B-27 such as ankylosing spondylitis, Reiter syndrome, and inflammatory bowel disease, can suggest a tendency for, or risk of, developing a similar process.[3,40] Other inheritable diseases, including certain neuromuscular diseases, may be associated with progressive spinal deformity, and patients with a genetic predisposition for certain medical conditions (e.g., vascular disease, specific cancers) may also present additional diagnostic considerations.

Obtaining a thorough family history may also allow a clinician to understand potentially complicated or delicate psychosocial aspects of a patient's life. Identifying significant disability in a family member or altered family dynamics from a spine issue may provide useful insight into a patient's expectations, fears, or other psychological features that could have a strong bearing on outcome. By asking about family members and parents, one can begin to understand the nature of family dynamics that may be influencing the presentation of a patient with spinal pain. A history of abuse, the presence of a disruptive home environment, and a history of poor parenting or alcoholism in the family may have a significant future impact on the psychological makeup of an individual. Anger, unmet dependency needs, and problems with trust in authority figures are some of the issues that could result in chronic pain issues. Probing these issues in taking a family history may provide valuable insight into potential barriers to recovery.

"Yellow Flags"—Predictors of Poor Outcome in the Patient's History

Numerous factors in a patient's history have been identified as potential predictors of poor outcome in the treatment of spinal pain. These factors are known as "yellow flags" (Table 11-2).[41] The presence of more than one of these factors in a patient is a strong predictor of poor outcome and chronic pain and disability.[41] These "yellow flags" include issues related to the nature of the patient's injury and general medical health, occupational and social issues, and psychological factors. It is imperative to identify these factors, if present, early in the

TABLE 11-2 "Yellow Flags": Potential Predictors of Poor Outcomes or Persisting Pain and Disability, Particularly When More than One Is Present

Biomedical Factors
Widespread pain
High levels of comorbidity
Prior episodes of spinal pain (particularly if associated with disability)
Severe radiating limb pain
Poor sleep
Occupational Factors
Poor job satisfaction
Perceived poor-quality work environment
Absence of light duty alternatives
Short time at current position
Low level of education
Physically demanding work
Extensive time off of work
Psychosocial or Cognitive Factors
Fear avoidance beliefs
Catastrophizing
Passive coping style
Depression
Anxiety
Somatization
Psychological distress
History of abuse
Self-perceived poor health
Social withdrawal
History of substance abuse

From Gaunt AM: Caring for patients who have acute and subacute low back pain. CME Bull 7:1-7, 2008.

course of evaluation and treatment of patients with spinal pain because they have been shown to be more powerful predictors of outcome than other biomedical issues.[42-44]

Patients who report more widespread symptoms of neck or back pain, who have more severe pain or disability at the onset of their injury, or who have higher rates of concurrent comorbidities tend to have a higher risk of developing protracted pain complaints or disability.[43-46] For low back pain specifically, dominant medical factors associated with the development of protracted pain or disability seem to be the presence of severe leg pain and a history of prior episodes of low back pain.[43,45,47] Some distinct occupational factors that have been shown to be related to the development of chronic pain include heavy physical workload, unavailability of light duties on return to work, perceived poor working environment or job dissatisfaction, a low level of education, and a short time of employment on the job.[43-45,47,48] The amount of time off work from an injury also has a negative correlation with return to work rates.[49,50]

As noted previously, psychological factors seem to play a substantial role in the development of chronic spinal pain. In a review on this topic, Linton[42] noted that psychological variables are clearly linked to the transition from acute to chronic pain and generally have a stronger impact on chronicity than medical or biomechanical factors. Pertinent emotional factors cited include depression, anxiety, distress, and self-perceived poor health. Cognitive and behavioral factors also apparently play a key role in the development of a chronic pain state; these include a passive coping style, "catastrophizing," and fear-avoidance beliefs (beliefs that certain activities should be avoided owing to fear of injury). A history of sexual or physical abuse also may be related to chronic pain and disability.[42] A systematic review of psychosocial factors found that psychological distress, depressed mood, and somatization were associated with the transition to chronic low back pain.[51]

Despite the high prevalence of psychopathology in patients with chronic pain, there does not seem to be a premorbid "pain-prone" personality; the depressive features of chronic spinal pain generally seem to arise more as a consequence, rather than a cause, of the pain state.[42,52,53] One study did identify premorbid depression, however, as an independent, robust risk factor for the onset of an episode of troublesome neck or low back pain.[54]

From a strictly surgical perspective, the outcomes of lumbar surgical procedures are influenced by numerous factors completely unrelated to the anatomy or pathophysiology of the spine. The results of lumbar discography are influenced by psychosocial variables to such a large degree that there are concerns about the validity of the procedure.[15] Factors identified as predictors of poor outcome from surgical intervention in the lumbar spine include low level of education, low income at the time of injury, the presence of pending litigation, the presence of an industrial injury, and depression.[55-58] Surgical outcomes have also been found to be worse in geographic regions with higher rates of surgical intervention.[59] From a clinical standpoint, it is important to identify predictors of poor outcome or chronicity to provide appropriate care to address these issues and to *avoid* invasive care that is highly unlikely to be helpful and could contribute to the perpetuation of chronic pain and disability.

Obtaining a Psychosocial History

Although a thorough review of the psychological factors that can influence pain is beyond the scope of this chapter and is provided elsewhere in the book, a few observations are in order. Obtaining information necessary for successful decisions about care requires the spine specialist to evaluate a patient with chronic pain differently from a patient with an acute injury. It is particularly true in treating the patient with chronic pain that the foundation for good decision making is having a good knowledge of the *person* with a back disorder; the spine itself is less important. In other words, it is more important to know about the patient who has the disease than to know about the disease the patient has.

It is dangerous to assume that a patient's presenting symptoms are solely the result of the injury that led to the consultation. Patients in whom disability greatly exceeds that expected on the basis of objective findings have been shown to be much more likely to have encountered childhood abuse and conflict, parental job stress, or a difficult divorce. Pain is an experience that is influenced by everything that is currently occurring in the life of the patient. Equally or sometimes more important is everything that has gone on in the patient's life in the past. In a study of more than 25,000 subjects in 14 countries, the World Health Organization found that physical disability is more closely associated with psychological factors than with medical diagnosis.[60] An appreciation of the power of this observation is extremely valuable.

Regardless of the presence of anatomic pathology, it is important to understand that a family member, a stressful circumstance, regular use of opioid analgesics, money issues related to compensation or litigation, and other factors can be contributors to a patient's ongoing pain and disability. This comment should not be construed as indicating that the pain is "all in the patient's head," and it is not intended to suggest that the patient is malingering or that the patient's pain is invalid or trivial. Pain and the disability it may produce are complex and multidimensional.

It has been estimated that approximately 50% of patients with chronic pain in rehabilitation and family practice settings have a personality disorder, as documented through structured interviews and psychological testing.[61] Thorough evaluation of patients with back pain needs to include some form of psychological testing because psychological factors play a critical role in patient recovery from illness or injury. Ignoring either the physical or the psychological components of pain in diagnosis and treatment is a prescription for failure, disappointment, and dissatisfaction. Several psychological test instruments are available for this purpose.

Additional Assessment Tools

Although there is no substitute for a concise, yet thorough, history, there are some tools that can improve efficiency. Pre-printed questionnaires can be used to obtain details of a patient's history. Including some questions about the psychological issues noted previously can facilitate the efficient acquisition of a large pool of information. Other vehicles, such as pain drawings, pain scales, and functional outcome measures, can also be used.

Pain drawings have been used since the 1940s, and research into their significance has provided mixed results.[62] Although there are data supporting an association between psychological distress and widespread, nonanatomic markings on the pain drawing, there is contradictory evidence in other studies. Data are also contradictory on the usefulness of pain drawings in predicting surgical outcomes.[62] Pain drawings have been assessed using various means and have been shown to have relatively high repeatability.[62,63] Intraobserver reliability is relatively good, although interobserver reliability is more questionable, particularly for qualitative assessments.[62,63] Although the presence of widespread or nonanatomic patterns of pain on these drawings may be of some use in identifying pain intensity and the presence of depression or psychological distress, one systematic review did not find evidence to support their use as a formal psychological assessment tool (Fig 11–8).[62,64,65]

A variety of pain scales may be used in patient assessment. Various visual analog scales have been reported. The Million Visual Analog Scale has been shown to have good reliability, validity, and responsiveness.[66] The McGill Pain Questionnaire has also been widely used and is well validated. This questionnaire provides a quantitative assessment using numerous descriptors of pain over three separate domains that are identified by the test taker and scored.[34,66] Other scales identifying the "bothersomeness" of pain and the bodily pain item in the Medical Outcomes Study 36-item Short Form Health Survey (SF-36) have also been applied in the assessment of patients with spine disorders.[67]

Numerous functional scales exist, including the Oswestry Low Back Pain Disability Questionnaire, the modified Roland scale, the Neck Disability Index, the Sickness Impact Profile and the related Disability Questionnaire, and the SF-36.[66-70] The Oswestry questionnaire, which uses self-rated functional impairment in numerous activities of daily living, has been shown to be valid and responsive and is generally easy to administer and score.[66,68] The modified Roland scale, which consists of 24 "yes" or "no" questions regarding the functional impact of back pain, was originally derived from the Sickness Impact Profile, has been well validated, has a high responsiveness, and is very easy to score.[66,67]

Several brief psychological scales are also useful. The presence of fear-avoidance beliefs and catastrophizing are particularly important in the development and maintenance of chronic pain and disability. The Fear-Avoidance Beliefs Questionnaire[71] and the Pain Catastrophizing Scale[72] are validated assessment tools that can be used to quantify these factors.

The Battery for Health Improvement (BHI-2) is a self-report multiple-choice instrument designed for assessment of medical patients. It is intended to provide one source of clinical hypotheses that professionals can use to explore the interrelationships between a patient's psychological and medical conditions. The information can be particularly useful in helping to determine factors that may be influencing an inexplicable delay in recovery of an injured patient. The Opioid Risk Tool is clinically relevant and easily employed during the interview.[73]

Physical Examination

After obtaining a complete history, a focused examination can be performed to establish a baseline functional and neurologic assessment, identify pertinent positive and negative findings that can help narrow the differential diagnosis, and define further issues that may need to be addressed through additional testing. Although a thorough discussion is beyond the scope of this chapter, appropriate portions of a general medical examination need to be included in the assessment of a spinal patient depending on the nature of the presenting issues. Neurologic and orthopaedic examinations of varying degree and complexity are also necessary. This chapter follows a more focused approach to the examination of the spine

with a discussion of basic neurologic assessment and relevant provocative maneuvers appropriate to a patient's presenting problem.

Observation

The physical examination begins with observation, which begins when the physician first sees the patient. Movement patterns, preferred postures, inconsistencies, and gait abnormalities should be noted by the clinician and staff members throughout the patient's visit. This observation needs to be done casually during office or facility interactions and during the medical history and in a more formal manner during the examination. Formal observation should include an examination from the feet to the head. Trunk and appendicular

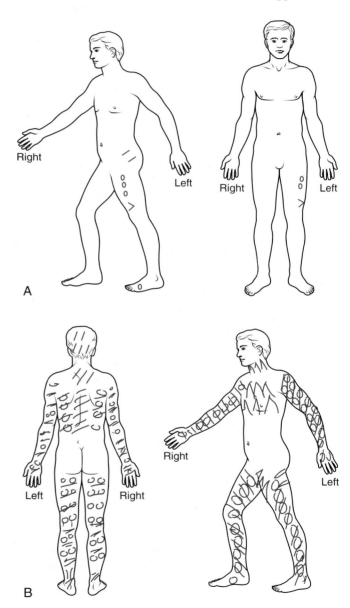

FIGURE 11–8 A and **B,** Pain drawings by patients. The patient in **A** had radiating pain in an L3 pattern related to intraforaminal disc herniation at L3-4, and the patient in **B** had long-standing, widespread pain in nonanatomic distribution.

alignment should be noted, paying particular attention to hip and knee alignment. The spine should be assessed for alterations from normal alignment or resting curvature, including scoliosis, kyphosis, alterations in lumbar or cervical lordosis, a lumbar shift, and head and neck alignment with the trunk. Symmetry of shoulder height and scapular positioning should also be noted.

Gait assessment can be done after initial observation, looking specifically for gait patterns suggestive of neurologic deficits, such as a steppage gait associated with footdrop or a wide-based gait suggestive of proprioceptive, cerebellar, or myelopathic pathology. Gait can be tested further by tandem gait testing (heel-to-toe walking). Balance can be assessed by simple observation and performing a single-leg stance with various postural challenges (e.g., crouching on one leg). If a patient has an antalgic gait (i.e., shortened stance phase of the gait cycle), consideration should be given to a musculoskeletal problem involving the hips, knees, or foot and ankle. Generally, patients with a lumbar radiculopathy do not exhibit an antalgic gait pattern.

Spine range of motion should be assessed for all relevant spine segments. There is debate as to what constitutes "normal" range of spine motion and the significance of any perceived restriction of motion. In the lumbar spine, range of motion has been variably reported by using inclinometry, measuring the distance from the fingertips to the floor, assessing segmental motion, measuring dynamic motion, measuring motion with the pelvis restrained, radiographic measurement, and using variations of the Schober test (measuring the change in distance between a mark over the S1 spinous process and one made 10 cm above this in standing that occurs between standing and flexion).[74-77]

The value of range of motion measurements is questionable, however, because some data do indicate that there is no consistent relationship between range of motion and physical or functional impairment in subjects with chronic low back pain.[75] Range of motion generally seems to decline with age, further complicating attempts at establishing normative data.[74] Gross lumbar motions generally include motion from the hips and lower extremities, and any lateral flexion or rotation involves coupled motion at multiple levels, making it difficult to assess these reliably. It is important to examine hip motion, however, because painful and restricted hip motion, particularly in flexion with internal rotation, that mimics the patient's usual pain would generally implicate the hip as the source of pain.

Despite these substantial limitations, it is still important to assess active spine motion in flexion, extension, rotation, and lateral flexion. Along with absolute degrees of movement, the examiner can assess symmetry of motion, preferred movement patterns, pain or symptom reproduction associated with motion, the relative contributions of associated body segments to motion (e.g., hips), motor control, and inconsistencies between movement noted on formal examination and that seen during casual observation or while the patient is otherwise distracted. Generally, patient motion should be assessed actively within the patient's range of comfort. There is little or no role for passive range of motion because this adds little to the clinical assessment and may place the patient at risk for further injury.[34]

For cervical and thoracic complaints, it is also important to assess shoulder and scapular motion. Shoulder range of motion can be assessed actively by flexion and abduction along with passive motion of the glenohumeral joint. Scapular position at rest and with various arm positions can reveal abnormal movement patterns and may indicate problems with scapulothoracic function, other shoulder joint complex disorders, or neurologic injury affecting the parascapular musculature (e.g., a long thoracic or spinal accessory nerve injury). Scapulothoracic dysfunction of various kinds may also be a source of pain in patients with thoracic complaints.[78] Reproduction of a patient's shoulder region pain by passive shoulder motion, particularly if it is restricted, would generally implicate the shoulder rather than the neck as the source of pain. Patients with a cervical radiculopathy obtain relief with ipsilateral shoulder abduction (the shoulder abduction relief maneuver); patients with intrinsic shoulder pathology often have reproduction of pain with shoulder abduction.

Observation should also include looking for atrophy, edema, vasomotor changes, skin lesions, limb or joint deformity, contracture, and other signs that may have an impact on a patient's care.

Palpation

The relevant areas of the patient's spine and related structures should be palpated with the patient standing or, when appropriate, in side-lying or prone position. Palpation may aid in the localization of the patient's symptoms, the identification of an injured structure, or the identification of associated soft tissue or bony abnormalities. It should be noted whether tenderness is elicited in the midline or to either side of midline, potentially differentiating between spinal pain and pain from an adjacent soft tissue source.[34] Localized tenderness should be distinguished from diffuse tenderness, the latter being less consistent with a focal injury.

In the cervical spine, palpation should include the occipital region; the anterior neck; the clavicular, supraclavicular, and scapular regions; and the areas of the associated cervicothoracic musculature.[34] In the thoracic region, palpation should also extend across the posterior ribs to identify focal bony tenderness that may suggest rib pathology rather than spine pathology. Pain with palpation or percussion of the costovertebral angle may suggest renal pathology.[79] Spondylolisthesis can frequently be appreciated by a palpable step-off of the spinous processes in the lumbar spine. In the lumbar region, palpation should include not only the lumbar spine but also the iliac crests, sacrum, sacroiliac joints, ischial tuberosities, proximal hamstring, and greater trochanteric areas, as indicated, to assess for the possibility of contributing problems from these regions. Trochanteric pain may mimic pain from a spine etiology.

Neurologic Examination

As with the general medical examination, the neurologic examination may cover a wide range of factors, depending on the particular presenting problem. The most common neurologic manifestations of spine pathology generally involve the spinal nerve roots or the spinal cord, resulting in radicular or myelopathic findings on examination. The symptoms resulting from spine pathology may frequently overlap, however, with symptoms of various peripheral nerve processes, central nervous system disease, or anterior horn cell disease. An examiner needs to be aware of the clinical presentations and neurologic findings associated with these disorders. A full discussion of all relevant examination techniques and neurologic pathology is beyond the scope of this chapter but can be found in general neurology texts.[80,81] This section focuses on findings more directly related to spine pathology.

A thorough understanding of dermatomal patterns is essential for all clinicians examining spine patients. As a reference, the key sensory points identified by the American Spinal Injury Association (ASIA)[82] can be helpful in assessing or screening patients with spine pathology (see Fig. 11–5). Soft touch and pin-prick sensation can be assessed well in most patients, and the examiner should distinguish between a dermatomal distribution suggesting nerve root pathology, a stocking or stocking-and-glove distribution suggesting peripheral polyneuropathy, multiple nerve distribution suggesting alternative peripheral nerve pathology, or a nonorganic distribution. Proprioception, vibration, position sense, and temperature sensation may also be tested, particularly when there is concern for a spinal cord or central nervous system process or a peripheral neuropathy.

Motor examination consists of several parts, including strength, tone, coordination, muscle bulk, and involuntary movements.[79] Strength is the modality most generally assessed by clinicians, but all portions of the motor examination may be important in some patients with spine disorders. Involuntary movements may be noted in patients with cervical dystonia or in various neurologic diseases that may affect function, such as Parkinson disease. The presence or absence of focal muscle atrophy should be noted in all patients. The mere presence of focal atrophy implies neurologic injury or disease, and the distribution of atrophic muscles can be helpful in defining the type of pathology present. Fasciculations associated with atrophic muscles imply the presence of lower motor neuron injury. Muscle tone can be affected by many neurologic processes. Reduced tone suggests lower motor neuron involvement, whereas increased tone or spasticity is seen with upper motor neuron disease. Coordination may be disrupted by numerous pathways, generally involving the cerebellum or its pathways, but weakness, proprioceptive loss, and cognitive disturbance may also affect motor performance on tests of coordination. Clinical methods to assess coordination include rapid alternating hand and foot movements and finger-to-nose testing.[79]

Strength testing is generally done isometrically, but sometimes weakness can be better appreciated through dynamic or repetitive movements that address endurance (e.g., multiple single-leg toe raises to assess plantar flexor strength). It is essential to be aware of key muscle groups by myotome and the peripheral nerve origin of those muscles. Important

muscle groups and motions associated with cervical and lumbar myotomes are as follows:

C5—elbow flexors, shoulder abductors and external rotators

C6—elbow flexors, wrist extensors and pronators, shoulder external rotators

C7—elbow extensors, wrist pronators

C8—extension of index finger, finger abduction and flexion, abduction of thumb

T1—finger abduction

L2—hip flexion

L3—hip flexion, hip adduction, knee extension

L4—knee extension, ankle dorsiflexion

L5—ankle dorsiflexion, great toe extension, ankle eversion, hip abduction and internal rotation

S1—ankle plantar flexion, toe flexion

Strength is generally graded on a scale of 1 to 5 as follows:[79]

5—active movement against full resistance (normal strength)

4—active movement against gravity and some resistance

3—active movement against gravity

2—active movement with gravity eliminated

1—trace movement or barely detectable contraction

0—no muscular contraction identified

Active movement is generally meant to imply joint motion through the full available range of motion. For some muscle groups, patients can often have significant loss of strength that is not detectable by providing manual resistance with the examiner's arms, and other test maneuvers may be necessary to identify more subtle weakness. Examples of such maneuvers would be having the patient do a partial squat or arise from sitting without using the upper extremities to assess for weakness in the knee extensors. Beevor sign (in which the umbilicus moves craniad during contraction of the abdominal muscles with supine neck flexion) indicates weakness of the lower abdominal muscles.[23]

Reflex testing can further aid in the localization of neurologic injury and help distinguish upper motor neuron from lower motor neuron disease. In lower motor neuron injuries, deep tendon reflexes of affected regions are generally reduced, whereas they are brisk in upper motor neuron injuries. Babinski response to appropriate plantar stimulation, Hoffman sign in the hand, and clonus all can indicate the presence of upper motor neuron injury. As with other physical examination findings, the sensitivity and specificity of these findings are limited for any particular condition. In a study assessing the prevalence of physical examination findings in cervical myelopathy treated surgically, it was noted that 21% of the patients had no myelopathic findings on examination. Of the findings just mentioned, Hoffman sign was the most sensitive (59%), whereas Babinski response had very low sensitivity (13%) but was highly specific.[83] Various other reflexes, including abdominal, cremasteric, and palmomental, can also be used as part of the neurologic examination where appropriate.

Although a neurologic injury often manifests as either an upper or a lower motor neuron lesion, it can also manifest with a mixed pattern of upper and lower motor neuron features, as can be seen with amyotrophic lateral sclerosis. The segmental distribution of commonly tested deep tendon reflexes is as follows:[79]

Biceps reflex—C5, C6

Brachioradialis reflex—C5, C6

Triceps reflex—C6, C7

Patellar tendon reflex—L2, L3, L4

Medial hamstring reflex—L5, S1

Ankle jerk reflex (Achilles tendon)—S1

For the most part, the sensitivity and specificity of isolated tests for sensation, strength, and reflexes are relatively limited in the assessment of spine conditions, particularly when any one single test is considered.[22,77,84] There may be more utility in combining a variety of findings across multiple modalities, especially when the findings are consistently reproducible. The degree of consistency between examination findings, history, imaging results, and self-reported levels of pain and disability for affected patients should always be considered when clinical decisions on care are made.

Special Tests and Provocative Maneuvers

In addition to the standard examination techniques described earlier, various provocative maneuvers and other tests have been used to aid in the diagnosis of patients with spine conditions. The sensitivity and specificity of many of these tests are either unclear or suboptimal, but a working knowledge of their applicability is useful in the diagnosis and management of patients with spine conditions.

Lhermitte sign, although more technically a symptom, is the presence of an electric shock–type sensation radiating into the limbs with cervical flexion. Although first described in a patient with multiple sclerosis, this sign is associated with various spinal cord lesions.[23,34] If elicited with neck flexion, this sign should raise concern for the presence of a cervical cord lesion. If elicited with trunk flexion, this may indicate a thoracic cord lesion.[23]

Spurling maneuver is a test for cervical nerve root compression or irritation. A positive test is elicited by extending, rotating, and laterally bending the head to one side with reproduction of radicular pain into the affected ipsilateral extremity.[23,34] One study comparing Spurling maneuver with the results of electrodiagnostic testing found that the maneuver had poor sensitivity (30%) but good specificity (93%) in the diagnosis of electrodiagnostically confirmed cervical radiculopathy.[85]

Valsalva maneuver is performed by having a patient hold his or her breath and bear down. A reproduction of the patient's radicular symptoms or spinal pain with this maneuver is believed to indicate a space-occupying lesion, such as a disc herniation, in the spinal canal.[23,34]

Dural tension signs are frequently used to assess lumbar spine pathology. Many different maneuvers have been described. A supine *straight-leg raise* is performed by elevating the leg with knee extended and assessing for the reproduction of pain into the leg. The test is considered positive if pain occurs between 30 degrees and 70 degrees of elevation because no true change in tension on the nerve roots is believed to occur outside of this range.[3,77] Variations on this test include *Lasègue sign* or *Bragard sign,* which involves raising the leg to the point of symptom reproduction and then lowering the leg slightly and dorsiflexing the foot passively; a positive test results in reproduction of the patient's radiating leg pain.[3,86] Other variants include internally rotating the leg to increase "dural tension," raising the leg with knee flexed and then slowly extending the knee to the point of reproduction of leg pain (also sometimes referred to as *Lasègue sign*), and either relieving pain by flexing the already extended knee at the point of symptom reproduction or eliciting pain by pressing on the popliteal fossa of the elevated leg with the knee partially flexed (both varyingly called the *bowstring sign*).[3,77,84,86]

Additional tests include the *crossed straight-leg raise,* in which symptoms are reproduced in the symptomatic leg by performing a supine straight-leg raise on the contralateral leg, and the *femoral nerve stretch test* or *reverse straight-leg raise,* in which the patient is prone and the knee is passively flexed, with a positive test reproducing pain into the anterior thigh. A positive straight-leg raise test and its variations indicates tension on the lower lumbar roots and upper sacral root (L4, L5, and S1 nerve roots). A positive femoral nerve stretch test is the equivalent tension sign for the upper lumbar (L2-4) nerve roots.[3,77,84]

Numerous studies have looked at the sensitivity and specificity of some of the above-mentioned maneuvers. As might be surmised by the varying descriptions and terminology, there are some difficulties with consistency in the literature. Overall, the ipsilateral straight-leg raise test has a good sensitivity of 72% to 97% but a poorer specificity of 11% to 66%.[84] The crossed straight-leg raise test is less sensitive (23% to 42%) but more specific (85% to 100%) than the ipsilateral straight-leg raise.[77,84]

Tests proposed for assessing the sacroiliac joint include *Gillet, Patrick,* and *Gaenslen tests.* Although the sacroiliac joint can be a source of pain, the diagnosis of "sacroiliac joint dysfunction" is debated as a true pathologic entity. Dreyfuss and colleagues[25] studied numerous supposedly diagnostic tests for this condition, including the Gillet, Patrick, and Gaenslen tests, and compared the responses on these test maneuvers with the results of fluoroscopically guided sacroiliac joint blocks. They found that no historical feature, none of the diagnostic tests performed, and no combination of these tests showed any significant and reliable diagnostic value.

Nonorganic Signs

Chronic pain behavior is often believed to display common physical examination findings suggesting symptom magnification and psychological distress, possibly an expression of suffering.[87,88] Waddell and colleagues[87] defined and studied a group of five findings on physical examination, commonly known as *Waddell signs*. These findings consist of a superficial or nonanatomic distribution of tenderness; a nonanatomic motor or sensory impairment (regional disturbance); excessive verbalization of pain or gesturing (overreaction); production of pain complaints by tests that simulate only a specific movement, such as low back pain that occurs with axial loading on the crown of the head (simulation); and inconsistent reports of pain when the same movement is performed in different positions, such as a straight-leg raise in a seated versus supine position (distraction).[87]

The presence of three or more of these signs indicates a nonorganic component to an individual's pain complaints. The presence of Waddell signs does not mean, however, that there is no significant organic pathology present or that the patient is malingering, and objective clinical signs may be present as well. Although some studies have found these maneuvers to be reproducible, an evidence-based review by Fishbain and colleagues[89] noted that these findings do not correlate with psychological distress or secondary gain, and they do not discriminate nonorganic from organic problems. They are associated with poorer treatment outcomes and higher pain levels. Although these maneuvers may be useful, the clinician should be wary of placing too much emphasis on any one part of the physical examination.

Additional Orthopaedic Assessment

Depending on the area of the spine involved, it is frequently important to cover additional areas of the orthopaedic examination. As was previously mentioned, examination of the shoulder complex is often necessary in evaluating the cervical and thoracic spine. Following the concept of the *kinetic chain*, it is also often helpful to assess multiple other joint structures and movement patterns from the feet up through the trunk to the neck, depending on the individual patient's situation.[90] For the lumbar spine, examination of the hip is also generally important, although examination of more distal lower extremity structures and more cranial regions of the spine and upper extremities may be necessary as well. Because other conditions such as carpal tunnel syndrome, ulnar neuropathy, brachial plexopathy, peroneal neuropathy, and femoral nerve injury (among others) can masquerade as radiculopathies, examination for these entities is also often indicated. As noted previously, an appropriate history can help greatly in defining the scope of examination necessary to evaluate a particular patient.

There is a large body of literature on manual orthopaedic examination.[91,92] These techniques generally are poorly validated and of uncertain correlation to some of the more "objective" findings noted earlier. A systematic review of the literature on the reliability of palpatory examination maneuvers found that most procedures have moderate or strong evidence for low reliability.[93] The authors noted that "a consistent finding from work in this field is the generally low reliability of palpation-based assessment."[93] These techniques may be

helpful in certain treatment paradigms, however, and they may be more useful when symptom response with repeated movements is considered.[93] Another systematic review assessed the literature on chiropractic tests of the lumbar spine and found insufficient evidence on the reliability and validity of these tests to support their clinical role.[94]

Conclusions

The history and physical examination of a spine patient is a complex undertaking. The nature of the patient's presenting complaints and relevant aspects of the history have a strong bearing on the nature and extent of assessment required. Clinicians caring for patients with spine disorders need to be aware of all of the issues that may affect the presentation of a patient and how these issues can affect the delivery of care. As noted previously, it is of paramount importance to realize that the person presenting with the spine problem is the primary concern, and the problem with the spine is only secondary. Only by speaking with and directly examining a patient can clinicians truly understand the nature of the problem that they are being asked to address.

KEY POINTS

1. A thorough and appropriate history and physical examination are essential in the assessment of patients with spine disorders to identify the physical manifestations of a spine disorder and the root causes of the patient's distress, suffering, and disability.

2. It is crucial to identify "red flags" and "yellow flags" in a patient's clinical presentation. "Red flags" are factors suggestive of the presence of an urgent or emergent medical issue (e.g., infection, tumor, fracture, cauda equina injury, progressive neurologic loss), whereas "yellow flags" are factors associated with poor outcomes and persisting pain and disability.

3. The medical history can be used to narrow down the differential diagnosis and direct further diagnostic efforts through physical examination and other tools.

4. The value of isolated findings on physical examination is limited, although physical examination findings become much more significant in the context of correlating history and imaging.

5. Despite the importance of a thorough medical history, clinicians need to realize that psychosocial factors are a more important predictor of outcome in patients with spinal pain than biomedical factors.

6. Pain is not a "thing" that can be excised. Pain is an experience, and it is influenced by everything that is currently occurring in the life of the patient. In addition to anatomic factors, it is important to look for psychosocial factors that can affect a patient's pain and distress.

KEY REFERENCES

1. Bogduk N: The anatomy and pathophysiology of neck pain. Phys Med Rehabil Clin N Am 14:455-472, 2003.
   This is a concise overview of some important issues in assessing patients with neck pain.

2. Deyo RA, Rainville J, Kent DL: What can the history and physical examination tell us about low back pain? JAMA 268:760-765, 1992.
   This article provides detailed analyses of commonly used approaches in the assessment of patients with low back pain.

3. Linton SJ: A review of psychosocial risk factors in back and neck pain. Spine 25:1148-1156, 2000.
   This is a useful and well-executed review of the role of psychosocial risk factors in the development of chronic spinal pain.

4. Gatchel RJ (ed): Compendium of Outcome Instruments for Assessment and Research of Spinal Disorders. La Grange, IL, North American Spine Society, 2001.
   This text addresses the reliability, validity, and relevance of numerous outcome scales commonly used in the medical literature and in the clinical management of patients with spine disorders.

5. Solomon J, Nadler SF, Press J: Physical examination: Of the lumbar spine. In Malanga G, Nadler SF (eds): Musculoskeletal Physical Examination: An Evidence-based Approach. Philadelphia, Hanley & Belfus, 2006, pp 189-226.
   This is one of many useful chapters in a well-prepared text assessing the literature on musculoskeletal physical examination.

6. American Spinal Injury Association: International Standards for Neurological Classification of Spinal Cord Injury (reprint). Chicago, American Spinal Injury Association, 2008.
   ASIA has a wide range of materials available on the assessment and management of patients with spinal cord injury.

REFERENCES

1. Bogduk N: The anatomy and pathophysiology of neck pain. Phys Med Rehabil Clin N Am 14:455-472, 2003.

2. Bogduk N: Clinical Anatomy of the Lumbar Spine and Sacrum, 3rd ed. New York, Churchill-Livingstone, 1997.

3. Borenstein DG, Wiesel SW: Low Back Pain: Medical Diagnosis and Comprehensive Management. Philadelphia, WB Saunders, 1989.

4. Liss H, Liss D, Pavell J: History and past medical history. In Cole AJ, Herring SA (eds): The Low Back Pain Handbook, 2nd ed. Philadelphia, Hanley & Belfus, 2003, pp 49-67.

5. Weinstein SM, Herring SA, Standaert CJ: Low back pain. In Delisa JA, Gans BM, Walsh NE (eds): Physical Medicine and Rehabilitation: Principles and Practice, 4th ed. Philadelphia, Lippincott-Williams & Wilkins, 2005, pp 653-678.

6. Dwyer A, Aprill C, Bogduk N: Cervical zygapophyseal joint pain patterns I: A study in normal volunteers. Spine 15:453-457, 1990.

7. Aprill C, Dwyer A, Bogdul N: Cervical zygapophyseal joint pain patterns II: A clinical evaluation. Spine 15:458-461, 1990.

8. Lord SM, Barnsley L, Wallis BJ, et al: Chronic cervical zygapophyseal joint pain after whiplash: A placebo-controlled prevalence study. Spine 21:1737-1745, 1996.

9. Dreyfuss P, Tibiletti C, Dreyer S: Thoracic zygapophyseal joint pain patterns: A study in normal volunteers. Spine 19:807-811, 1994.

10. Schwarzer AC, Aprill CN, Derby R, et al: Clinical features of patients with pain stemming from the lumbar zygapophysial joints: Is the lumbar facet syndrome a clinical entity? Spine 19:1132-1137, 1994.

11. Marks R: Distribution of pain provoked from lumbar facet joints and related structures during diagnostic spinal infiltration. Pain 39:37-40, 1989.

12. Cloward RB: Cervical discography: A contribution to the etiology and mechanism of neck, shoulder and arm pain. Ann Surg 150:1052-1064, 1959.

13. Grubb SA, Kelly CK: Cervical discography: Clinical implications from 12 years of experience. Spine 25:1382-1389, 2000.

14. Campbell JN: Nerve lesions and the generation of pain. Muscle Nerve 24:1261-1273, 2001.

15. Carragee EJ, Alamin TF: Discography: A review. Spine J 1:364-372, 2001.

16. Hogan Q: Back pain: Beguiling physiology (and politics). Reg Anesth 22:395-399, 1997.

17. Sinclair JD: Chronic noncancer pain basics for the primary care physician. Primary Care Rep 8:63-73, 2002.

18. Sheather-Reid RB, Cohen ML: Psychophysiological evidence for a neuropathic component of chronic neck pain. Pain 75:341-347, 1998.

19. Agency for Health Care Policy and Research: Acute Low Back Problems in Adults: Assessment and Treatment. Washington, DC: US Department of Health and Human Services, 1994.

20. Akuthota V, Willick SE, Harden RN: The adult spine: A practical approach to low back pain. In Rucker KS, Cole AJ, Weinstein SM (eds): Low Back Pain: A Symptom-based Approach to Diagnosis and Treatment. Boston, Butterworth-Heinemann, 2001, pp 15-41.

21. Carragee EJ, Hannibal M: Diagnostic evaluation of low back pain. Orthop Clin North Am 35:7-16, 2004.

22. Deyo RA, Rainville J, Kent DL: What can the history and physical examination tell us about low back pain? JAMA 268:760-765, 1992.

23. Bland JH: Disorders of the Cervical Spine: Diagnosis and Medical Management, 2nd ed. Philadelphia, WB Saunders, 1994.

24. Mazanec D: Pseudospine pain: Conditions that mimic spine pain. In Cole AJ, Herring SA (eds): The Low Back Pain Handbook, 2nd ed. Philadelphia, Hanley & Belfus, 2003, pp 117-131.

25. Dreyfuss P, Michaelsen M, Pauza K, et al: The value of medical history and physical examination in diagnosing sacroiliac joint pain. Spine 21:2594-2602, 1996.

26. Micheli LJ, Wood R: Back pain in young athletes: Significant differences from adults in causes and patterns. Arch Pediatr Adolesc Med 149:15-18, 1995.

27. Roche MA, Rowe GG: The incidence of separate neural arch and coincident bone variations: A survey of 4,200 skeletons. Anat Rec 109:233-252, 1951.

28. Standaert CJ, Herring SA: Spondylolysis: A critical review. Br J Sports Med 34:415-422, 2000.

29. Burton AK, Clarke RD, McClune TD, et al: The natural history of low back pain in adolescents. Spine 21:2323-2328, 1996.

30. Kovacs FM, Gestoso M, Gil del Real MT, et al: Risk factors for non-specific low back pain in schoolchildren and their parents: A population based study. Pain 103:259-268, 2003.

31. Andersen SJ: Adolescent lumbar spine disorders. In Rucker KS, Cole AJ, Weinstein SM (eds): Low Back Pain: A Symptom-based Approach to Diagnosis and Treatment. Boston, Butterworth-Heinemann, 2001, pp 3-14.

32. Hosalkar H, Dormans J: Back pain in children requires extensive workup. Biomechanics 10:51-58, 2003.

33. Malanga GA, Nadler SF, Ageson T: Epidemiology. In Cole AJ, Herring SA (eds): The Low Back Pain Handbook, 2nd ed. Philadelphia, Hanley & Belfus, 2003, pp 1-7.

34. Borenstein DG, Wiesel SW, Boden SD: Neck Pain: Medical Diagnosis and Comprehensive Management. Philadelphia, WB Saunders, 1996.

35. Bovim G, Schrader H, Sand T: Neck pain in the general population. Spine 19:1307-1309, 1994.

36. Makela M, Heliovaara M, Sievers K, et al: Prevalence, determinants, and consequences of chronic neck pain in Finland. Am J Epidemiol 134:1356-1367, 1991.

37. Volinn E: The epidemiology of low back pain in the rest of the world: A review of surveys in low- and middle-income countries. Spine 22:1747-1754, 1997.

38. Belanger TA, Rowe DE: Diffuse idiopathic skeletal hyperostosis: Musculoskeletal manifestations. J Am Acad Orthop Surg 9:258-267, 2001.

39. Paassilta P, Lohiniva J, Goring HH, et al: Identification of a novel common genetic risk factor for lumbar disk disease. JAMA 285:1843-1849, 2001.

40. Canoso JJ: Rheumatology in Primary Care. Philadelphia, WB Saunders, 1997.

41. Gaunt AM: Caring for patients who have acute and subacute low back pain. CME Bull 7:1-7, 2008.

42. Linton SJ: A review of psychosocial risk factors in back and neck pain. Spine 25:1148-1156, 2000.

43. Valat JP, Goupille P, Vedere V: Low back pain: risk factors for chronicity. Rev Rheum [Engl Ed] 64:189-194, 1997.

44. van der Giezen AM, Bouter LM, Nijhuis FJN: Prediction of return-to-work of low back pain patients sicklisted 3-4 months. Pain 87:285-294, 2000.

45. Fransen M, Woodward M, Norton R, et al: Risk factors associated with the transition from acute to chronic occupational back pain. Spine 27:92-98, 2002.

46. Radanov BP, Sturzenegger M: The effect of accident mechanisms and initial findings on the long-term outcome of whiplash injury. J Musculoskelet Pain 4:47-59, 1996.

47. McIntosh G, Frank J, Hogg-Johnson S, et al: Prognostic factors for time receiving workers' compensation benefits in a cohort of patients with low back pain. Spine 25:147-157, 2000.

48. Krause N, Ragland DR, Greiner BA, et al: Physical workload and ergonomic factors associated with prevalence of back and neck pain in urban transit operators. Spine 22:2117-2126, 1997.

49. McGill CM: Industrial back problems: A control program. J Occup Med 10:174-178, 1968.

50. Waddell G: Epidemiology: A new clinical model for the treatment of low back pain. In Weinstein JN, Wiesel SW (eds): The Lumbar Spine: The International Society for the Study of the Lumbar Spine. Philadelphia, Saunders, 1990, pp 38-56.

51. Pincus T, Burton AK, Vogel S, et al: A systematic review of psychosocial factors as predictors of chronicity/disability in prospective cohorts of low back pain. Spine 27:E109-E120, 2002.

52. Gatchel RJ, Polatin PB, Mayer TG: The dominant role of psychosocial risk factors in the development of chronic low back pain disability. Spine 20:2702-2709, 1995.

53. Wallis BJ, Lord SM, Bogduk N: Resolution of psychological distress of whiplash patients following treatment by radiofrequency neurotomy: A randomized, double-blind, placebo-controlled trial. Pain 73:15-22, 1997.

54. Carroll LJ, Cassidy JD. Cote P: Depression as a risk factor for onset of an episode of troublesome neck and low back pain. Pain 107:134-139, 2004.

55. DeBerard MS, Masters KS, Colledge AL, et al: Outcomes of posterolateral lumbar fusion in Utah patients receiving workers' compensation: A retrospective cohort study. Spine 26:738-747, 2001.

56. Junge A, Dvorak J, Ahrens S: Predictors of bad and good outcomes of lumbar disc surgery: A prospective clinical study with recommendations for screening to avoid bad outcomes. Spine 20:460-468, 1995.

57. Loupasis GA, Stamos K, Katonis PG, et al: Seven to 20-year outcome of lumbar discectomy. Spine 24:2313-2317, 1999.

58. Pappas CTE, Harrington T, Sonntag VK: Outcome analysis in 654 surgically treated lumbar disc herniations. Neurosurgery 30:862-866, 1992.

59. Keller RB, Atlas SJ, Soule DN, et al: Relationship between rates and outcomes of operative treatment for lumbar disc herniation and spinal stenosis. J Bone Joint Surg Am 81:752-762, 1999.

60. Fishbain DA, Goldberg M, Meagher BR, et al: Male and female chronic pain patients categorized by DSN-III psychiatric diagnostic criteria. Pain 26:181-197, 1986.

61. Ormel J, VonKorff M, Ustun TB, et al: Common mental disorders and disability across cultures: Results from the WHO Collaborative Study on Psychological Problems in General Health Care. JAMA 272:1741-1748, 1994.

62. Hagg O, Fritzell P, Hedlund R, et al: Pain-drawing does not predict the outcome of fusion surgery for chronic low-back pain: A report from the Swedish Lumbar Spine Study. Eur Spine J 12:2-11, 2003.

63. Ohnmeiss DD: Repeatability of pain drawings in a low back pain population. Spine 25:980-988, 2000.

64. Dahl B, Gehrchen PM, Kiaer T, et al: Nonorganic pain drawings are associated with low psychological scores on the preoperative SF-36 questionnaire in patients with chronic low back pain. Eur Spine J 10:211-214, 2001.

65. Carnes D, Ashbey D, Underwood M. A systematic review of pain drawing literature: Should pain drawings be used for psychologic screening? Clin J Pain 22:449-457, 2006.

66. Gatchel RJ (ed): Compendium of Outcome Instruments for Assessment and Research of Spinal Disorders. La Grange, IL, North American Spine Society, 2001.

67. Patrick DL, Deyo RA, Atlas SJ, et al: Assessing health-related quality of life in patients with sciatica. Spine 20:1899-1908, 1995.

68. Fairbank JCT, Couper J, Davies JB, et al: The Oswestry low back pain disability questionnaire. Physiotherapy 66:271-273, 1980.

69. Millard RW: A critical review of questionnaires for assessing pain-related disability. J Occup Rehabil 1:289-302, 1991.

70. Vernon H, Mior S: The neck disability index: A study of reliability and validity. J Manipulative Physiol Ther 14:409-415, 1991.

71. Waddell G, Newton M, Henderson I, et al: A fear-avoidance beliefs questionnaire (FABQ) and the role of fear-avoidance beliefs in chronic back pain and disability. Pain 52:157-168, 1993.

72. Sullivan MJL, Bishop SR, Pivik J: The pain catastrophizing scale: Development and validation. Psychol Assess 7:524-532, 1995.

73. Webster LR, Webster RM: Predicting aberrant behaviours in opioid treated patients: Preliminary validation of the opioid risk tool. Pain Med 6:432-442, 2005.

74. McGregor AH, McCarthy ID, Hughes SP: Motion characteristics of the lumbar spine in the normal population. Spine 20:2421-2428, 1995.

75. Nattrass CL, Nitschke JE, Disler PB, et al: Lumbar spine range of motion as a measure of physical and functional impairment: An investigation of validity. Clin Rehabil 13:211-218, 1999.

76. Ng JKF, Kippers V, Richardson CA, et al: Range of motion and lordosis of the lumbar spine: Reliability and measurement of normative values. Spine 26:53-60, 2001.

77. Solomon J, Nadler SF, Press J: Physical examination: Of the lumbar spine. In Malanga G, Nadler SF (eds): Musculoskeletal Physical Examination: An Evidence-based Approach. Philadelphia, Hanley & Belfus, 2006, pp 189-226.

78. Burkhart SS, Morgan CD, Kibler WB: The disabled throwing shoulder: Spectrum of pathology part III: The SICK scapula, scapular dyskinesis, the kinetic chain, and rehabilitation. Arthroscopy 19:641-661, 2003.

79. Bates B: A Guide to Physical Examination and History Taking, 5th ed. Philadelphia, JB Lippincott, 1991.

80. Bradley WG, Daroff RB, Fenichel GM, et al (eds): Neurology in Clinical Practice: Principles of Diagnosis and Management, 5th ed. Boston, Butterworth Heinemann, 2007.

81. Goetz CG (ed): Textbook of Clinical Neurology, 3rd ed. Philadelphia, WB Saunders, 2007.

82. American Spinal Injury Association: International Standards for Neurological Classification of Spinal Cord Injury (reprint). Chicago, American Spinal Injury Association, 2008.

83. Rhee JM, Heflin JA, Hamasaki T, et al: Prevalence of physical signs in cervical myelopathy: A prospective, controlled study. Spine 34:890-895, 2009.

84. Andersson GBJ, Deyo RA: History and physical examination in patients with herniated lumbar discs. Spine 21:10S-18S, 1996.

85. Tong HC, Haig AJ, Yamakawa K: The Spurling test and cervical radiculopathy. Spine 27:156-159, 2002.

86. Supik LF, Broom MJ: Sciatic tension signs and lumbar disc herniation. Spine 19:1066-1069, 1994.

87. Waddell G, McCulloch JA, Kummel E, et al: Nonorganic physical signs in low-back pain. Spine 5:117-125, 1980.

88. Maruta T, Goldman S, Chan CW, et al: Waddell's nonorganic signs and Minnesota Multiphasic Personality Inventory profiles in patients with chronic low back pain. Spine 22:72-75, 1997.

89. Fishbain DA, Cole B, Cutler RB, et al: A structured evidence-based review on the meaning of nonorganic physical signs: Waddell signs. Pain Med 4:141-181, 2003.

90. Kibler WB: Determining the extent of the functional deficit. In Kibler WB, Herring SA, Press JM, et al (eds): Functional Rehabilitation of Sports and Musculoskeletal Injuries. Gaithersburg, MD, Aspen, 1998, pp 1-8.

91. Basmajian JV, Nyberg R (eds): Rational Manual Therapies. Baltimore, William & Wilkins, 1993.

92. Brieve GP: Mobilization of the Spine, 4th ed. New York, Churchill-Livingstone, 1984.

93. May S, Littlewood C, Bishop A: Reliability of procedures used in the physical examination of non-specific low back pain: A systematic review. Aust J Physiother 52:91-102, 2006.

94. Hestbaek L, Leboeuf-Yde C: Are chiropractic tests for the lumbo-pelvic spine reliable and valid? A systematic critical literature review. J Manipulative Physiol Ther 23:258-275, 2000.

12

CHAPTER

Spine Imaging

Jeffrey S. Ross, MD
Gordon R. Bell, MD

Multiple imaging methods with tremendous technologic complexity and sophistication can be used to evaluate spinal pathology. Magnetic resonance imaging (MRI) quickly emerged as the study of choice for many disorders of the spine, with computed tomography (CT) continuing to play a key role, bolstered by newer innovations such as helical scanning and multidetector arrays allowing isotropic voxels and multiplanar reformatting without loss of resolution. This chapter reviews the basic imaging approaches to the spine and their usefulness in specific disease states.

Techniques

Plain Films

Routine plain films are universally available and inexpensive, but are limited by an inability to visualize directly neural structures and nerve root or cord compression. The presence of degenerative changes within the cervical and lumbar spine has been shown to be age related and equally present in asymptomatic and symptomatic individuals.[1] By the 5th decade of life, 25% of asymptomatic patients have degenerative changes in the intervertebral disc spaces. By the 7th decade, 75% have degenerative changes. Routine spine radiographs are of little value in determining the degree and clinical severity of cervical or lumbar degenerative disc disease.

In the instrumented spine, conventional radiography remains the first line of imaging because it is convenient, inexpensive, sometimes able to show motion with changes in position, and not degraded by the presence of implants. It is limited to single planar imaging and is less suitable for postprocessing and unable to provide the bone and soft tissue discrimination that is possible with MRI and CT.

Orthogonal conventional radiography is the first line of evaluation in an instrumented postoperative patient, and plain radiographs are usually obtained at 6 weeks and 3, 6, and 12 months postoperatively.[2] Regardless of which fusion approach is taken, the presence or absence of demonstrable motion or evidence of hardware failure or loosening is a key factor in the evaluation. In the case of posterolateral fusion, arthrodesis is deemed successful if follow-up radiographs show continuity in the fusion mass between the cephalad and the caudal transverse processes. Instrumented interbody fusion is considered fused if:

1. There is increased or maintained bony density within the cage implant because of the presence of mature bony trabeculae bridging the interbody space.

2. There is an absence of a halo or a periprosthetic lucency around the implant.

3. There is a sclerotic line between the cage and the vertebral bone because of bone remodeling and new bone formation.

4. There is resorption of anterior vertebral traction spurs or the presence of bone graft anterior to an intervertebral implant (sentinel sign).

5. There is lack of motion on flexion-extension views.

Pseudarthrosis or failure of fusion is indicated by progressive loss of disc height, vertebral displacement, broken or loose hardware, and loss of position of the implant or resorption of the bone graft. Flexion and extension views are useful for assessing stability or functional fusion, but the central x-ray beam should pass through the same area in both views.[3]

Myelography

The diagnosis of extradural neural compression by myelography is inferred indirectly by changes in the contour of normal contrast agent–filled thecal sac and root sleeves rather than by direct visualization of the lesion.[4] Multiple water-soluble agents are available that provide excellent contrast and lower rates of side effects, such as iohexol (Omnipaque) and iopamidol (Isovue). Current water-soluble agents are associated with less toxicity, and their absorption through the theca and arachnoid villi makes their removal unnecessary.[5] Newer nonionic water-soluble agents generally produce mild side effects, although significant adverse reactions can still rarely occur, such as hallucinations, confusion, or seizures.

The major disadvantage of myelography is its invasive nature and lack of diagnostic specificity.[6] The use of less toxic second-generation, water-soluble nonionic agents has obviated the need for overnight hospitalization after the procedure. Routine postprocedural monitoring of 2 to 4 hours is usually sufficient. The technique of myelography involves instillation of the contrast agent through either lumbar puncture (midline or oblique approaches) or lateral C1-2 puncture. Adequate visualization depends on pooling of sufficient contrast agent in the region of interest to provide enough electron density to stop the x-ray beam. Absence of a significant cervical lordosis can make it difficult to concentrate the dye in the cervical region, resulting in dilution of the dye and suboptimal image quality.[7] Dilution of contrast agent also occurs when attempting to visualize more than one spine region, such as lumbar and cervical. The plain film image quality of the second region studied invariably is markedly diminished (although most of these cases are diagnostically adequate by CT myelography).

Accuracy rates for water-soluble nonionic cervical myelography in the diagnosis of nerve root compression range from 67% to 92%.[1,6,8,9] In a study of 53 patients with surgical confirmation of pathologic entities, myelography was associated with no false-positive findings and a 15% false-negative rate for an overall accuracy of 85%.[8] Because the diagnosis of extradural neural compression is inferred indirectly by changes in the contour of the contrast agent–filled subarachnoid space, the exact nature of the compressing lesion may be uncertain. Central indentation of the dye column at the level of the disc space may be due to either compression by the disc itself or compression by a marginal osteophyte. Similarly, incomplete filling of a nerve root sleeve may be due to either a lateral disc herniation or foraminal narrowing; the distinction is sometimes difficult by myelography. There is currently almost no role for conventional myelography alone, without postmyelographic CT. The exception is the presence of stainless steel spinal implants, where CT image quality is degraded by the presence of the spinal instrumentation.

Computed Tomography

CT permits direct visualization of potential neural compressing structures and provides better visualization of lateral pathology, such as foraminal stenosis.[10-12] An important benefit from a surgical perspective is the ability of CT to distinguish neural compression owing to soft tissue from compression owing to bone.[9,11,13,14] CT is still limited compared with MRI in visualization of the neural structures below a complete myelographic block. What often appears as a complete myelographic block may permit passage, however, of enough contrast agent past the block to allow CT myelographic distinction.

Disadvantages of CT include radiation exposure, the effects of partial volume averaging, the time involved in performing multiple thin (1.5 to 3 mm) sections over multiple vertebral bodies and intervening discs, streak artifacts in the cervical spine caused by the dense bone of the shoulder girdle, and changes in configuration of the spine that occur between successive motion segments.[15] Many of the limitations can be obviated by obtaining multiple thin sections (1.5 to 3 mm) with the gantry tilted to permit imaging parallel to the plane of the disc. Further accuracy is obtained by routinely imaging the spine by CT after the introduction of water-soluble contrast agents (intrathecal contrast medium–enhanced CT).

Reported accuracy rates for CT range from 72% to 91%.[6,9,11,14] Agreement rates between contrast medium–enhanced CT and myelography have been reported to range from 75% to 96%.[11,14] When a discrepancy exists between myelographic and CT findings, postcontrast CT is invariably the more accurate study (Fig. 12–1). New multirow detector

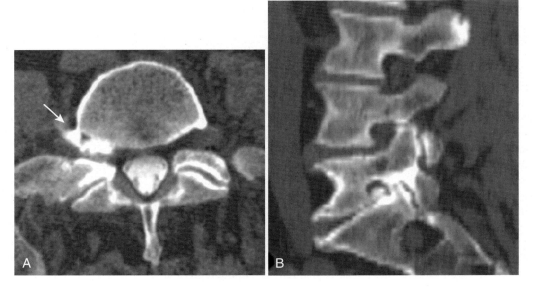

FIGURE 12–1 Foraminal stenosis. **A,** Axial CT scan after myelography shows severe right bony foraminal stenosis, with no evidence of central stenosis or herniations (*arrow*). **B,** Sagittal reformat of CT data also shows severe foraminal narrowing, in contrast to more normal superior foramen.

technology is becoming available that allows for extremely rapid thin-slice acquisitions over long body segments. With this new technology, contiguous 3-mm slices can be obtained from L1 to S1 in less than 30 seconds. The acquisition of isotropic voxels allows for multiplanar reformation of the CT data with no loss in spatial resolution.

Magnetic Resonance Imaging

For most patients who present for evaluation of suspected degenerative disease, spin-echo (SE) T1-weighted and fast spin-echo (FSE) T2-weighted sagittal images and T1-weighted axial images suffice. This examination can be completed in approximately 20 minutes. If contrast between the disc and cerebrospinal fluid (CSF) is inadequate on axial images, FSE T2-weighted axial study may be useful. If there is a history of prior low back surgery, gadolinium-based intravenous contrast medium is administered, and T1-weighted sagittal and axial images are included. Patients with possible vertebral osteomyelitis can undergo this routine study. If the study shows an area that suggests a disc space infection, post–gadolinium-enhanced T1-weighted sagittal and axial sequences are often very helpful in defining disease extent and in characterizing epidural inflammatory disease.[16-24]

For axially oriented images, low flip angle, two-dimensional or three-dimensional, gradient-echo (GE) sequences producing "myelographic" contrast are a reasonable baseline standard of comparison, acknowledging that these sequences were developed for detecting disc herniations and are not the "gold standard" for detecting intramedullary cord lesions.[17,25,26] Short tau inversion recovery (STIR) has shown a high sensitivity for musculoskeletal pathology (Fig. 12–2).[27-29] STIR has been favorably compared with T1-weighted and T2-weighted FSE, conventional SE, and fat-saturated FSE in the detection of vertebral metastatic disease.[30-32] STIR may also be used for intramedullary cord lesions.

For disc disease, bright CSF-type images are preferred because of the problem of visualizing low signal intensity ligaments or osteophytes against the dark CSF images on T1-weighted images.[33-37] The major problem of two-dimensional MRI techniques for cervical disease is the failure to identify foraminal disease accurately owing to long echo times, relatively thick image slices (3 to 5 mm), and the inability to view the course of the exiting nerve roots in planes other than axial.[38] Three-dimensional imaging allows an increase in signal-to-noise ratio over two-dimensional imaging with thin contiguous slices with a more accurate slice thickness that can be obtained without the problem of crosstalk.[39,40]

Artifacts

Stainless steel implants are known to generate substantial metal artifact with MRI and CT. On CT, metal causes severe x-ray attenuation (missing data) in selected planes. These missing data or hollow projections cause classic "starburst" or streak artifacts during image reconstruction. The resulting distortions often render these studies useless. Materials with lower x-ray attenuation coefficients (plastic < titanium

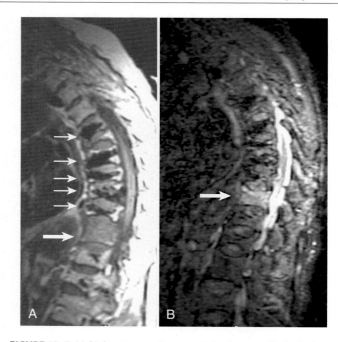

FIGURE 12–2 Multiple osteoporotic compression fractures. **A,** Sagittal T1-weighted MR image through thoracic spine shows multiple collapsed bodies with central low signal reflecting prior vertebroplasties (*small arrows*). The marrow adjacent to methacrylate shows normal fatty signal intensity. **B,** T12 body (*large arrow*) shows low signal on T1-weighted image and increased signal on sagittal STIR image consistent with acute age.

< tantalum < stainless steel < cobalt chrome) produce less distortions. Metal composition, mass, orientation, and position of the implant in the body all are important factors that determine the magnitude of image artifact. Titanium wires exhibit the least artifact on CT and MRI compared with cobalt chrome or stainless steel.

MRI studies may be severely compromised in the presence of spinal instrumentation, and there can be potential safety and biologic considerations (Fig. 12–3). There are many strategies one can employ to reduce susceptibility artifacts on MRI, including the use of SE techniques, especially FSE variants over GE; larger fields of view; higher readout bandwidths; smaller voxel sizes; and appropriate geometric orientation of the frequency-encoded direction in relationship to metallic objects. Geometric orientation is especially important in the case of pedicle screws.[41] There is less apparent widening of the short axis of screws when the direction of the frequency-encoded gradient is parallel, as opposed to perpendicular to the long axis of the screw.

Spinal Angiography

Spinal angiography is extremely useful for spinal vascular malformations for the delineation of the vascular supply and for therapeutic treatment.[42,43] Spinal angiography is also used in the pretherapeutic workup of suspected vascular neoplasms involving the vertebral bodies, posterior elements, and spinal canal and is coupled with preoperative or palliative embolization. Spinal angiography should address three areas for the surgeon or interventionalist: (1) the exact location and

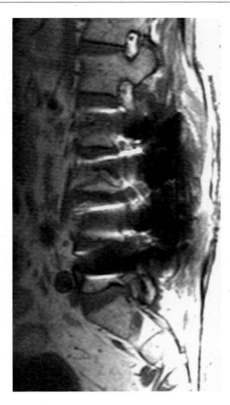

FIGURE 12–3 Metal artifact. Sagittal T1-weighted MR image is severely degraded by fixation hardware (four-level pedicle screws) that does not allow adequate evaluation of neural foramen.

configuration of the lesion, (2) vascularity of the lesion including feeding and draining vessels, and (3) regional vascular anatomy.[44]

Spinal vascular malformations are a very heterogeneous group of lesions that have had a wide variety of classification schemes applied to them. One common classification system is from Anson and Spetzler,[45] who classify them as types 1 to 4:

Type 1—spinal dural arteriovenous fistula, between the dural branch of the spinal ramus of the radicular artery and intradural medullary vein

Type 2—spinal cord arteriovenous malformation with shunting across an interposed vascular nidus (intramedullary glomus malformation)

Type 3—complex spinal arteriovenous malformation with metameric extension (juvenile malformation)

Type 4—direct arteriovenous fistula (intradural perimedullary fistula)

The most common spinal vascular lesion is a dural arteriovenous fistula (Fig. 12–4). These lesions are thought to be acquired and are particularly present in the thoracic and lower lumbar spine. Spinal dural arteriovenous fistulas are more common in men (3.4 : 1) older than 60 years. There is often a delay from symptom onset to time of diagnosis, averaging 27 months. Clinical findings include weakness (55%), a progressive clinical course (100%), and a myelopathy on examination

(84%). The nidus of the fistula is most often located between T6 and T12 and in the sacrum and intracranially in 8% to 9% each. In 1977, Kendall and Logue[46] definitively identified the site of the arteriovenous shunting within the root sleeve. The symptoms are a result of intramedullary edema and ischemia secondary to increased venous backpressure within the varicose coronal veins. Gilbertson and colleagues[47,48] identified increased signal intensity on T2-weighted images within the cord as the most sensitive imaging finding in spinal dural fistula.

Although imaging, in particular MRI, has become a mainstay for the evaluation of vascular malformations, spinal angiography remains a crucial technique for precise definition of the type of lesion, the overall morphology, the flow characteristics, and the identification of specific feeding vessels.[49] Selective intercostal or lumbar injection using digital subtraction angiography typically uses 2 to 4 mL of nonionic contrast agent per injection, diluted with heparinized saline. Arterial and delayed venous imaging may be necessary to appreciate fully the venous drainage of the vascular pathology, particularly in arteriovenous malformations and dural fistulas. Arterial films allow examination of abnormal blush or arteriovenous shunting. The normal vascular supply to the cord, in particular, the artery of Adamkiewicz, should be defined. In addition to the usual general complications of angiography, embolization to the anterior spinal artery could occur after angiography, which may lead to an ascending paralysis. Generally, given the small catheters used, nonionic contrast medium, and an improved speed of the examination with digital subtraction angiography, complications are rare.

Spinal Angiography Using Magnetic Resonance Imaging and Computed Tomography

Technologic advances have allowed high-resolution, high-contrast discrimination imaging for evaluation of the spinal arteries, with the goal of minimizing the need for conventional catheter angiography for identification of spinal vascular disease.[50-52] The size of the anterior spinal artery (0.2 to 0.8 mm) and the close approximation of the spinal veins necessitate a sophisticated MRI sequence with bolus gadolinium–based intravenous contrast medium administration. Although various techniques may be used, the three main requirements are a large field of view, high spatial resolution, and high temporal resolution.

The large field of view should be 30 to 50 cm, which would allow visualization of the mid-thoracic and lower thoracic spine and the upper lumbar spine covering the major sources of the anterior spinal artery (70% arise from T8-L1). The high spatial resolution is required because of the small target vessel size and should employ a voxel size on the order of 1 mm or less. Temporal resolution is required to try to separate the anterior spinal artery from the adjacent vein, which is larger (0.4 to 1.5 mm). Simply trying to define the artery and vein based on morphology is extremely difficult. Temporal resolution is often in a tradeoff with spatial resolution for MRI, and time frames vary with the particular sequence and hardware, but is generally 40 to 60 seconds per acquisition to 2 to 4

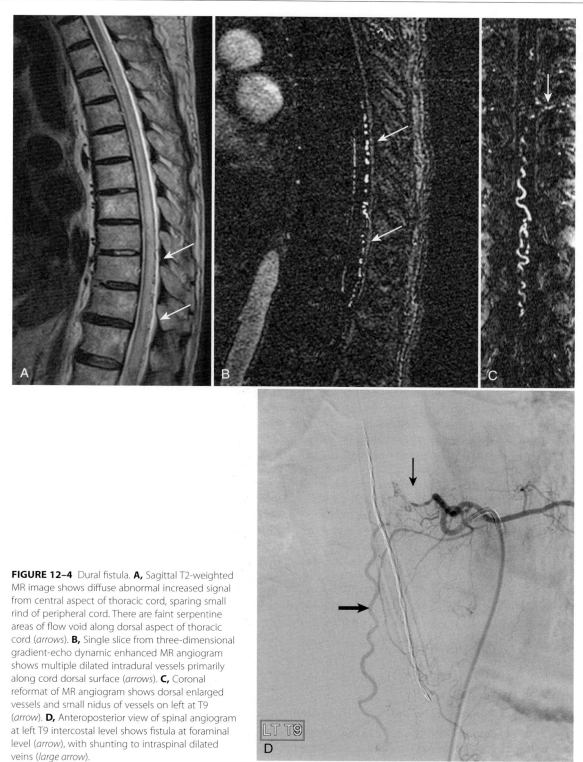

FIGURE 12–4 Dural fistula. **A,** Sagittal T2-weighted MR image shows diffuse abnormal increased signal from central aspect of thoracic cord, sparing small rind of peripheral cord. There are faint serpentine areas of flow void along dorsal aspect of thoracic cord (*arrows*). **B,** Single slice from three-dimensional gradient-echo dynamic enhanced MR angiogram shows multiple dilated intradural vessels primarily along cord dorsal surface (*arrows*). **C,** Coronal reformat of MR angiogram shows dorsal enlarged vessels and small nidus of vessels on left at T9 (*arrow*). **D,** Anteroposterior view of spinal angiogram at left T9 intercostal level shows fistula at foraminal level (*arrow*), with shunting to intraspinal dilated veins (*large arrow*).

minutes. Mull and colleagues[52] in a series of 34 patients showed that contrast-enhanced spinal magnetic resonance angiography (MRA) could reliably detect or exclude spinal cord arteriovenous abnormalities, with a 100% predictive value. The main arterial feeder can be reliably defined by MRA, but small secondary feeders may be missed. The main reasons for obtaining MRA would be for primary identification of a vascular abnormality and to pinpoint the likely site of a feeder for conventional catheter angiography.

CT angiography can also define normal and abnormal spinal vasculature.[53,54] The technique requires a multidetector row CT scanner (generally ≥16) and 1-mm section thickness. Given the tremendous speed of current CT scanners, the thoracic and upper lumbar spine can be covered in 30 seconds.

As with MRA, the examination relies on a bolus of intravenous contrast medium and precise triggering of the contrast bolus at its maximum density within the thoracic aorta. Contrast injection rates are on the order of 2 to 3 mL/sec for a total of 50 to 75 mL. Considerable postprocessing is required to segment the target vessel and to connect the intraspinal vessel with the appropriate intercostal vessel to define the arterial side of the vasculature. CT angiography does not have the ability to separate out the artery and vein based on temporal resolution, as does MRA.

Discography

Discography was originally conceived as a morphologic study of disc herniation but then morphed into a useful but limited test relying on pain provocation through disc pressurization.[55,56] Although discography can accurately define disc degeneration, this procedure is now seen as a physiologic evaluation of the disc consisting of volumetric, manometric, radiographic, and pain provocative challenge.[57,58] This procedure remains quite controversial; it has enthusiastic supporters and detractors and has generated a voluminous literature. Some authors see discography as helpful in identifying internal disc disruption and in verifying painful disc levels before surgery (particularly fusion), whereas others see it as unproven and of questionable benefit.[59-66]

Discography is an invasive procedure and is not performed as a screening technique. Discography is most accurate when the diagnosis of discogenic pain is probable based on appropriate history, physical examination, and imaging.[56] This test is always limited in sensitivity and specificity owing to the subjective report of pain type and location by the patient. According to Tehranzadeh and others,[67-69] indications for discography include the following:

1. Negative MRI, CT, or myelography with equivocal findings for disc disease
2. Cases with positive MRI, CT, or myelography with disc disease at multiple levels
3. Presence of equivocal MRI, CT, or myelography
4. Recurrent back pain in postsurgical patients with difficulty in evaluating scar versus disc
5. Cases of failed back surgery to evaluate painful pseudarthrosis or symptomatic disc
6. Evaluation of spinal fusion disc above or below the fusion level
7. Therapeutic injection of corticosteroid or anesthetic into the disc itself

Generally, small-gauge needles (22-gauge) are placed with fluoroscopic guidance into the nucleus pulposus of one or more discs. With proper placement of the needles confirmed under fluoroscopy, contrast medium is injected into the nucleus pulposus centrally. A normal disc takes 1 to 2 mL of contrast agent. A normal disc is painless, with the contrast agent remaining centrally within the nucleus pulposus. Abnormal discs are associated with pain on injection, which simulates the patient's symptoms and which may or may not be referred to the legs. Videotaping of the patient's pain response and the fluoroscopic display may be performed.[66] After injection of contrast agent, anteroposterior and lateral plain radiographs are obtained, followed by axial CT images through the level of the discograms. Different grading of radial pairs can be performed accurately only on the axial CT projections. The main complication for this invasive technique is a disc space infection. The main risk of discitis is 0.1% to 0.2%.[70-72] A prophylactic broad-spectrum antibiotic is often used.

Magnetic Resonance Imaging Safety

The specific and important aspects of MRI safety are widely available on multiple websites, and the interested reader is referred to them for detailed answers.[73-75] One more recent aspect of MRI safety that is perhaps less widely recognized outside of radiology is nephrogenic systemic fibrosis (NSF), previously called nephrogenic fibrosing dermopathy. NSF is a systemic disorder of widespread fibrosis that has been tied to prior administration of gadolinium-based contrast agents in the setting of renal disease. The incidence of NSF in the setting of severe renal dysfunction is approximately 1% to 7% after exposure to gadolinium-based contrast material. The U.S. Food and Drug Administration (FDA) has asked manufacturers to include a new boxed warning on the product labeling of all gadolinium-based contrast agents that are used to enhance the quality of MRI. The warning states that patients with severe kidney insufficiency who receive gadolinium-based agents are at risk for developing NSF, a debilitating and potentially fatal disease.[74] Also, patients just before or just after liver transplantation and patients with chronic liver disease are at risk for developing NSF if they are experiencing kidney insufficiency of any severity.

The risk of a patient developing NSF may be minimized by the following steps:[76-80]

1. Identify patients with glomerular filtration rate less than 30 mL/min/1.73 m^2 as at risk.
2. Administer contrast medium to a patient at risk for developing NSF only when the expected benefit clearly outweighs the risk of administration.
3. Perform unenhanced MRI first with proper monitoring so that unnecessary contrast medium administration is avoided.
4. Use the lowest dose of gadolinium-based contrast medium that is feasible for the examination.

Patients at risk for NSF should receive gadolinium-based contrast medium only after informed consent by the radiologist.

Degenerative Disc Disease

Multiple authors suggest that an imaging study is indicated in the evaluation of a patient with sciatica when (1) true radicular symptoms are present, (2) there is objective evidence of nerve root irritation on physical examination (i.e., positive straight-leg raise test), and (3) the patient has failed "conservative management" of 4 to 6 weeks' duration.[81-83] Earlier imaging is considered appropriate if clinical features raise concern regarding malignant or infectious causes or if neurologic findings worsen during observation. These recommendations are based on several studies of successful nonoperative treatment of sciatica.[84-89] Imaging is recommended only for the remaining minority of patients with persistent signs and symptoms who are believed to be surgical candidates or in whom diagnostic uncertainty remains.

Regardless of the various theories proposed to explain its cause, degeneration of the intervertebral disc initiates a complex cascade of morphologic and biochemical changes. These changes may ultimately lead to one or a combination of four morphologic abnormalities: disc degeneration and its sequelae, spinal stenosis, facet arthrosis, and malalignment-instability.

Because of its inherent contrast sensitivity, MRI not only reveals morphologic abnormalities well, but also provides insight into the biochemical changes of the degenerating disc. With aging and degeneration, there is gradual narrowing of the disc space and loss of the normal high intradiscal signal intensity on T2-weighted images. The latter is believed to be secondary to changes in proteoglycan composition within the disc rather than to absolute changes in water content. As degeneration progresses, small fluid-filled fissures or cracks may develop that manifest as intradiscal areas of linear high signal on T2-weighted images. Gas and calcification can also develop within a degenerating disc.

In addition to these observed changes within the degenerating disc, vertebral marrow signal abnormalities adjacent to the degenerating disc are common.[90] Type I endplate change manifests as decreased marrow signal paralleling the endplates on T1-weighted images and increased signal on T2-weighted images. These changes reflect replacement of normal fatty marrow with fibrovascular marrow, which has greater water content. Type II endplate changes are slightly more common than type I changes, showing increased signal on T1-weighted images and isointense to slightly increased signal on T2-weighted images. Histologically, these changes correlate with fatty marrow replacement. These changes may be preceded by type I changes, and often these changes exist in combination at the same level or different levels. Type III endplate changes show decreased marrow signal on T1-weighted and T2-weighted images, a finding that correlates with endplate sclerosis seen radiographically.[90]

Fissures (tears) of the anulus fibrosus can also be visualized with MRI. They appear as small areas of increased signal on T2-weighted images and can enhance after contrast agent administration, presumably secondary to the ingrowth of granulation tissue into the fissure as a consequence of healing.[91] Three types of annular fissures have been described, depending on their orientation relative to the concentric annular fibers.[92] The high frequency of annular fissures seen in association with large disc bulges challenges the concept that the anulus fibrosis is intact in bulging discs but ruptured in herniated discs. The clinical significance of annular fissures is

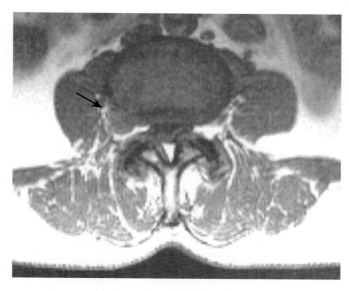

FIGURE 12-5 Lateral disc herniation. Axial T1-weighted MR image shows well-defined right lateral herniation with no thecal sac compromise (*arrow*).

unknown. In patients without nerve root compression, back pain may be secondary to irritation of the nerve endings in the peripheral anulus either from scar tissue within an annular fissure or from a disc herniation; this is what is referred to as *discogenic pain*. Although this concept is often used to ascribe clinical significance to these lesions, many asymptomatic patients harbor annular fissures.

There is no universally accepted classification system describing degenerative disc disease. A multispecialty task force released recommendations for disc nomenclature spanning the orthopaedic, neurosurgical, and radiologic communities.[93] This group has defined a *protrusion* as a herniation that maintains contact with the disc of origin by a bridge as wide as, or wider than, any diameter of the displaced material (Fig. 12-5). An *extruded* disc is a larger herniation where the diameter of the disc material beyond the interspace is wider than the bridge, if any, that connects it to the disc of origin (Fig. 12-6). A *sequestered (free)* disc fragment is an extrusion that is no longer contiguous with the parent disc. It may reside either anterior or posterior to the posterior longitudinal ligament or rarely may be intradural (Figs. 12-7 and 12-8). A free fragment may be located at the disc level or may migrate superiorly or inferiorly, often lateralized by the thin, sagittally oriented midline septum seen in the lower anterior epidural space.

Lumbar Stenosis

As an anatomic entity, spinal stenosis refers to narrowing of the central spinal canal, neural foramina, or lateral recesses. Most commonly, it is acquired secondary to degenerative disease of the intervertebral disc or facets or both, although developmentally shortened pedicles are an important component of symptomatic spinal stenosis in patients with otherwise mild degenerative changes (Figs. 12-9 and 12-10).[94] Before the development of MRI, plain films and CT were used to

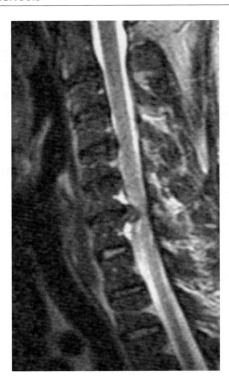

FIGURE 12–6 Cervical disc extrusion. Sagittal T2-weighted MR image shows large disc extrusion at C6-7 severely effacing anterior thecal sac and cord. Signal intensity of cord is normal.

diagnose spinal stenosis by measuring the dimensions of the bony canal. At present, such measurements are not commonly performed. These measurements do not take into account the normal anatomic variation between patients or the role of the disc and ligamentum flavum in spinal stenosis and are inaccurate predictors of clinical symptoms. MRI accurately depicts the degree and cause of thecal sac narrowing in patients with central canal stenosis. Such narrowing is most commonly due to bony and ligamentous hypertrophy.

In addition to central canal stenosis, stenosis of the lateral recess is an important cause of lower extremity pain and paresthesias. The lateral recess is bordered anteriorly by the posterior aspect of the vertebral body and disc, laterally by the pedicle, and posteriorly by the superior articular facet. The root sleeve within the lateral recess is often compressed by bony hypertrophy of the superior facet, often in combination with disc bulging and osteophyte along the anterior border of the lateral recess. Lateral recess pathology can clinically mimic disc herniation. MRI allows differentiation between central and lateral recess stenosis and provides important information for presurgical planning.

Facet Disease

Degenerative disease of the facet joints typically occurs in combination with degenerative disc disease, although facet disease alone may be responsible for symptoms of back pain and radiculopathy. As with any synovial-lined joint, facet joints are susceptible to the development of joint space loss, subchondral sclerosis and cyst formation, osteophytosis, and subluxation. Because of the richly innervated synovium and joint capsule, these changes alone can be a source of pain, or alternatively they can contribute to nerve root impingement by causing spinal stenosis or foraminal compromise. On MRI, degenerated facets appear hypertrophied, sclerotic, and irregular. Enlarged ligamentum flavum is commonly present. Facet degeneration can lead to the formation of synovial cysts that can compress the thecal sac and roots from a posterior direction. Synovial cysts are best depicted on axial images and appear as posterolateral epidural masses adjacent to a degenerated facet, most commonly at the L4-5 level. Synovial cysts have variable signal characteristics secondary to varying cyst fluid composition and associated hemorrhage, calcification, or gas within the cyst (Fig. 12–11).[95] A peripheral hypointense rim on T2-weighted images related to calcification may be seen. Intravenous contrast medium is useful in suspected cases to define better the lesion and its relationship to the adjacent facet joint and thecal sac.

Instability

The most frequently seen alignment abnormality is spondylolisthesis, which is defined as ventral slippage of a vertebra relative to the vertebrae below. The two most common causes of spondylolisthesis are bilateral defects in the pars interarticularis (isthmic spondylolisthesis) and facet disease (degenerative spondylolisthesis). The degenerative variety is the most common in older adults.

Because of its ability to obtain direct sagittal images free of overlapping structures and patient rotation, MRI is an accurate method of diagnosing spondylolisthesis. MRI is nearly always performed with the patient supine, however. In that position, a vertebra with subluxation can be normally aligned. A more accurate method of detecting listhesis is by weight-bearing lateral lumbar radiographs. The detection of spondylolysis (pars interarticularis defect without ventral slippage) by MRI can be problematic, and it is generally agreed that plain films and CT are more reliable for its diagnosis. Because MRI is being increasingly used as the first and only imaging modality in evaluating patients with low back pain and radicular symptoms, many cases of spondylolysis are imaged without the benefit of correlative plain films or CT studies.[96] Using MRI, sagittal T1-weighted images are best for showing the pars interarticularis owing to their higher signal-to-noise ratio, the depiction of the pars marrow as hyperintense, and the minimal obliquity of the pars in this imaging plane (Fig. 12–12). If the pars appears normal (i.e., contiguous normal marrow signal), one can be certain that it is intact.[97] The presence of abnormal pars signal is not specific for spondylolysis, however, because benign sclerosis, partial volume averaging with an adjacent degenerative facet, and osteoblastic metastases can also give this appearance.

Cervical Radiculopathy and Myelopathy

Various studies have shown that canal size is reduced in patients with cervical spondylotic myelopathy. The normal

FIGURE 12–7 Disc extrusion with free fragment. **A** and **B,** Sagittal (**A**) and axial (**B**) T1-weighted MR images show large central extrusion at L5-S1 extending dorsally and inferiorly, suggesting a free fragment. There is severe effacement of caudal thecal sac. **C** and **D,** Sagittal (**C**) and axial (**D**) T2-weighted MR images show extrusion as intermediate signal and confirm mass effect on sac.

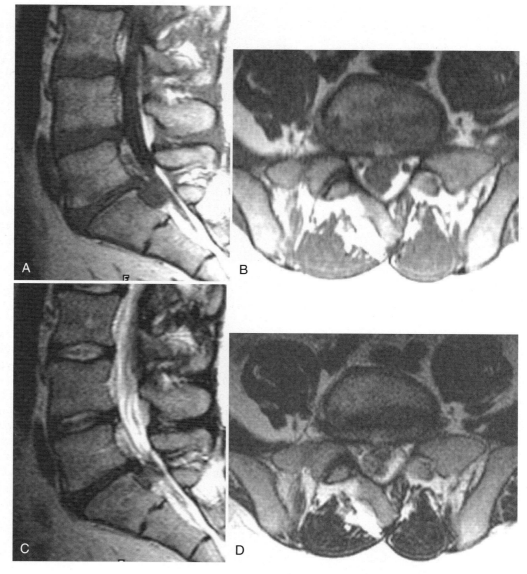

FIGURE 12–8 Cervical disc herniation. **A** and **B,** Axial CT scan (**A**) and sagittal reformat (**B**) after myelography show well-defined extradural lesion at C4-5 effacing anterior thecal sac and touching cord. Small osteophyte is present at C5-6 with no cord compromise.

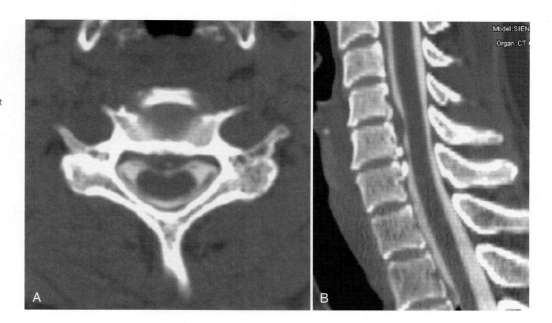

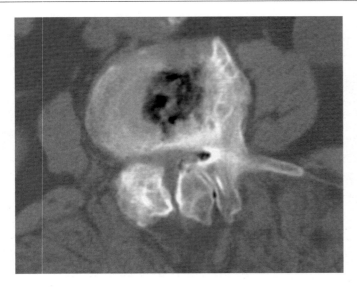

FIGURE 12–9 Lumbar canal stenosis. Axial CT scan at L4-5 shows marked bony central canal stenosis with mild anterior osteophyte and marked facet hypertropic degenerative change. Disc is degenerated with vacuum phenomenon.

diameter of the canal from C3 to C7 is approximately 17 mm and can be decreased to 12 mm or less in cervical spondylotic myelopathy. The size that is associated with myelopathy has ranged, however, from less than 10 mm to 14 mm. Additionally, myelopathic symptoms tend to occur when the canal cross-sectional area is less than 60 mm². The ratio of the anteroposterior canal diameter to the vertebral body diameter has been used to assess cervical stenosis. This Pavlov ratio (sometimes referred to as the Torg ratio) is normal if it is 1 or greater.[98] A ratio of 0.8 or less is considered abnormal. As a ratio, however, it can be abnormal not only because of an abnormally small canal diameter (small numerator), but also because of an abnormally large vertebral body (large denominator). This ratio method also does not take into account the size of the spinal cord itself. As an isolated tool, this method is of historical interest only and is useless in evaluating cervical spinal cord compression.

Takahashi and colleagues[99] and others have described areas of increased signal intensity on T2-weighted images within the cervical cord owing to extradural compression, which variously reflects myelomalacia, gliosis, and demyelination and edema (Fig. 12–13). Patients who show areas of abnormal signal within the cord tend to have a worse clinical condition than patients with normal cord signal intensity. These abnormal signal changes can disappear or diminish after surgery to relieve the cord compression.

Ossification of Posterior Longitudinal Ligament

Ossification of the posterior longitudinal ligament (OPLL) begins with calcification followed by frank ossification of the posterior longitudinal ligament in the upper cervical spine (C3-4 or C4-5). It may progress inferiorly to the upper thoracic spine (Figs. 12–14 and 12–15).[100] Patients tend to present in the 6th decade, are generally older than the usual patients with disc disease, and are younger than patients with cervical spondylosis. Presenting complaints include neck pain, dysesthesias, and upper and lower extremity weakness. Hirabayashi and Satomi[101] divided OPLL into four types based on CT: (1) *Continuous* OPLL extends between vertebral bodies and crosses multiple disc spaces (27% of cases), (2) *segmental* OPLL is limited to the posterior vertebral body margins (39%

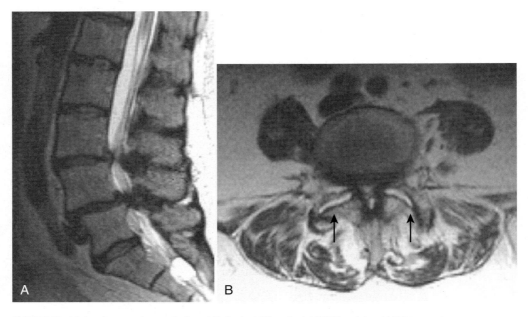

FIGURE 12–10 Lumbar canal stenosis. **A** and **B,** Sagittal (**A**) and axial (**B**) T2-weighted MR images show severe central canal stenosis at L3-4 and L4-5 with marked compression of thecal sac owing to anterior bulge of anulus fibrosus and facet hypertrophic degenerative change. There are small bilateral facet effusions (*arrows*).

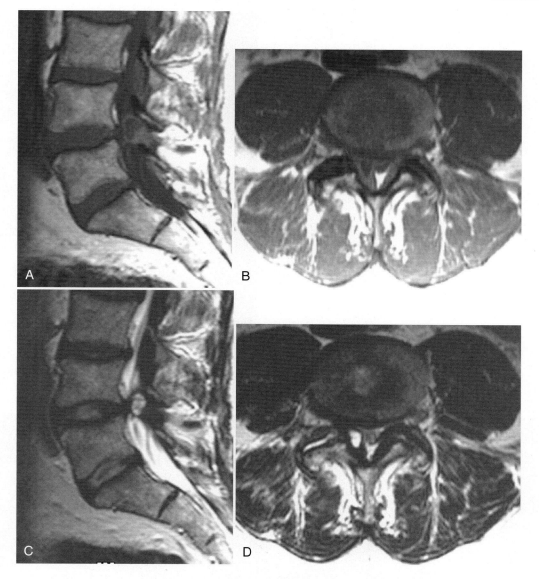

FIGURE 12–11 Synovial cyst. **A** and **B,** Sagittal (**A**) and axial (**B**) T1-weighted MR images show mass with central low signal centered on right anterior facet that effaces right dorsal aspect of thecal sac. **C** and **D,** Sagittal (**C**) and axial (**D**) T2-weighted MR images show central high signal of fluid, consistent with synovial cyst.

of cases), (3) *mixed* OPLL is continuous and segmental (29% of cases), and (4) the remaining 5% of OPLL is restricted to the disc space level.

Circumferential compression of the cord may result from combined OPLL and ossification of the ligamentum flavum. In continuous OPLL, MRI shows a thick band of decreased signal on T1-weighted and T2-weighted images. The segmental type is more difficult to discern on MRI and shows a thin area of decreased signal intensity, without signal from within the ossification region.

Postoperative Issues

Causes of early and delayed failure of surgery are listed in Tables 12–1 and 12–2. Caution must be used in interpretation of CT, CT myelography, and MRI within the first 6 weeks after surgery owing to the large amount of tissue disruption and edema that may be present producing a mass effect on the anterior thecal sac, even in the absence of any clinical symptoms. MRI may be used in the immediate postoperative period for a more gross view of the thecal sac and epidural space, to exclude significant postoperative hemorrhage, pseudomeningocele, or disc space infection at the laminectomy site. CT myelography is also a direct way to define a pseudomeningocele and to image the spine when hardware is present (Fig. 12–16).

Small fluid collections are commonly seen in the posterior tissues after laminectomy. The signal intensities can vary depending on whether the collections are serous (follow CSF signal intensity) or serosanguineous (increased signal on T1-weighted images owing to hemoglobin breakdown

FIGURE 12–12 Spondylolysis. Sagittal T1-weighted MR image shows disruption of cortical margin of pars interarticularis at L5-S1, consistent with spondylolysis. There is severe foraminal stenosis at L5-S1.

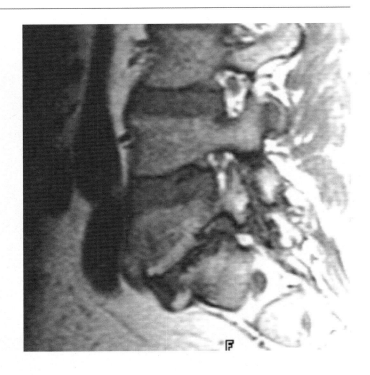

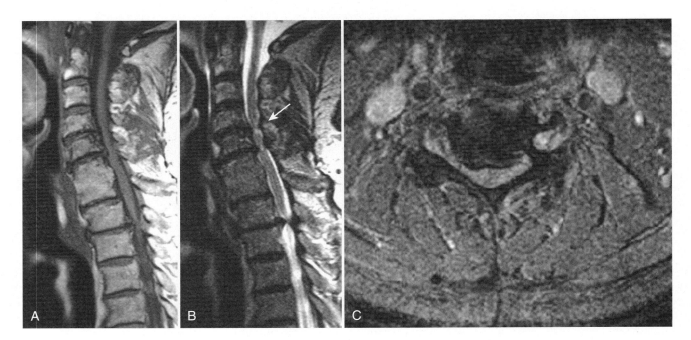

FIGURE 12–13 Cervical spondylosis. **A** and **B,** Sagittal T1-weighted (**A**) and T2-weighted (**B**) MR images show solid fusion at C6-7 level with small osteophyte. There is severe central stenosis of the disc and osteophyte complex and posterior ligamentous hypertrophy at C4-5, C5-6, and T1-2 levels. There is myelomalacia within cord seen as high signal intensity on T2-weighted image at C4-5 (*arrow*). **C,** Axial gradient-echo image at C4-5 confirms severity of central stenosis owing to broad-based disc and osteophyte.

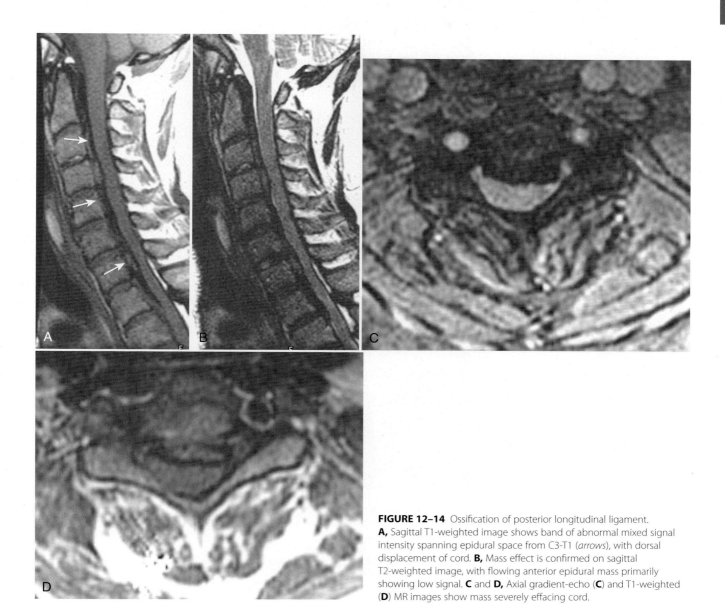

FIGURE 12–14 Ossification of posterior longitudinal ligament.
A, Sagittal T1-weighted image shows band of abnormal mixed signal
intensity spanning epidural space from C3-T1 (*arrows*), with dorsal
displacement of cord. **B,** Mass effect is confirmed on sagittal
T2-weighted image, with flowing anterior epidural mass primarily
showing low signal. **C** and **D,** Axial gradient-echo (**C**) and T1-weighted
(**D**) MR images show mass severely effacing cord.

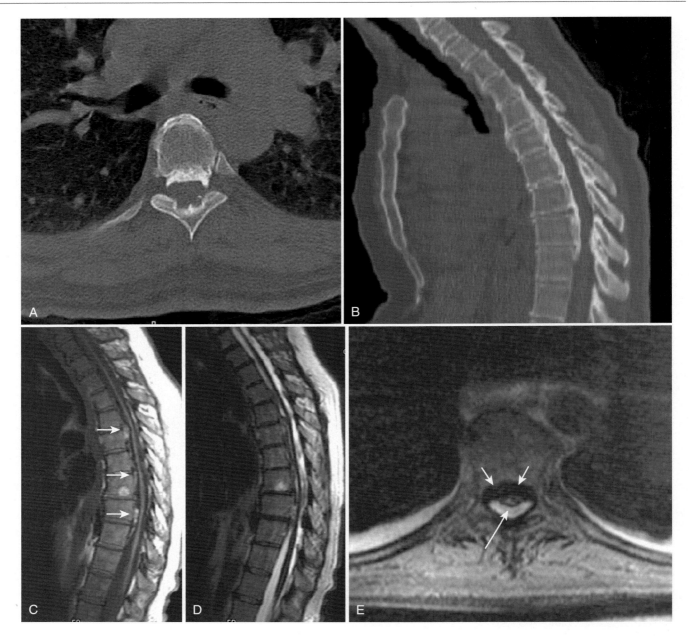

FIGURE 12–15 Thoracic ossification of posterior longitudinal ligament. **A** and **B,** Axial CT scan (**A**) with sagittal reformat (**B**) shows large flowing bony mass encompassing anterior epidural space throughout mid-thoracic spine. **C** and **D,** Sagittal T1-weighted and T2-weighted images (**C** and **D**) are more difficult to interpret without CT guidance because the heterogeneous anterior epidural signal could reflect blood or fatty marrow (*arrows*). MR images do show the degree of mass effect on the thecal sac and cord. **E,** On axial gradient-echo image, cord is atrophic, and there is diffuse hemosiderosis of cord surface seen as linear low signal (*single arrow*), with ossification of posterior longitudinal ligament mass of very low signal within anterior epidural space (*small arrows*). There are small bilateral pleural effusions.

TABLE 12–1 Technical Causes of Early Spine Surgery Failure

Hematoma
Infection
Inadequate decompression of bony foraminal or central stenosis
Insufficient removal of herniation
Neural trauma
Unrecognized free disc fragment
Wrong level surgery

TABLE 12–2 Technical Causes of Delayed Recurrence of Low Back Pain or Radiculopathy

Arachnoiditis
Epidural fibrosis
Facet arthropathy with foraminal stenosis
Instability
New or recurrent herniation
Pseudomeningocele
Central canal stenosis
Infection

products). The distinction between small postoperative fluid collections and infected collections cannot be made by MRI morphology or signal intensity. Acute hemorrhage typically shows isointense to increased signal in the epidural space on T1-weighted images and should show diminished signal on GE or T2-weighted images. Very acute blood collections may be isointense, however, on T1-weighted and T2-weighted images (Fig. 12–17).

Epidural Fibrosis and Disc Herniations

The use of contrast medium–enhanced MRI in the evaluation of scar versus disc has been examined by several authors, with reported accuracy rates of 96% to 100% for distinguishing scar from disc.[102] Lumbar epidural fibrosis (scar) is a replacement of the normal epidural fat with postoperative fibrotic tissue, which is capable of binding the dura and nerve roots to the surrounding structures anteriorly and posteriorly. Epidural fibrosis is seen to enhance consistently immediately after injection of contrast material (Fig. 12–18). This enhancement occurs regardless of the time since surgery. Disc material does not enhance on the early postinjection images owing to its lack of vascularity (Fig. 12–19). In cases with a mixture of scar and disc material, scar enhances, and the disc material does not enhance on early postinjection images.

Selective fat suppression on T1-weighted images has been used in the evaluation of postoperative patients. Georgy[103] examined 25 patients with recurrent pain after lumbar disc surgery with MRI to evaluate the usefulness of gadolinium-enhanced fat suppression imaging in patients with failed

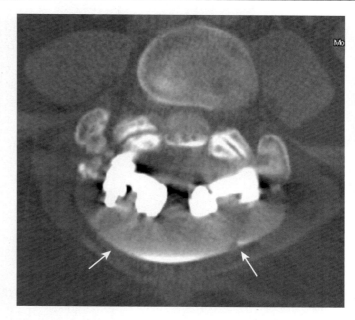

FIGURE 12–16 Pseudomeningocele. Axial CT scan after myelography shows metal artifact from prior pedicle screw fixation. There is pooling of contrast medium around and dorsal to hardware owing to large pseudomeningocele (*arrows*).

back surgery. The addition of fat suppression to enhanced T1-weighted images improved the visualization of enhancing scar in all of their cases, helped distinguish scar from recurrent herniated disc, and showed more clearly the relationship of scar to the nerve roots and thecal sac.

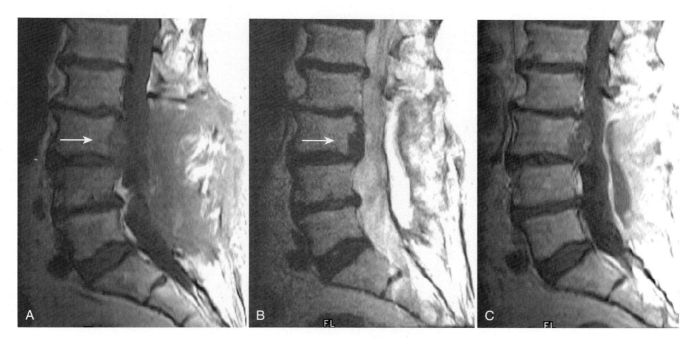

FIGURE 12–17 Recurrent herniation mimicking blood. The patient underwent multilevel laminectomy and L3-4 discectomy 3 weeks before examination. **A,** Sagittal T1-weighted MR image shows vague anterior epidural mass at L3 and extensive postoperative changes in dorsal epidural soft tissues. **B,** Sagittal T2-weighted MR image shows L3 epidural mass to be of low signal, with effacement of anterior thecal sac. **C,** After contrast material is instilled, sagittal T1-weighted MR image shows slight peripheral enhancement. Differential diagnosis included acute blood (deoxyhemoglobin) and large recurrent herniation. Because of homogeneity of low signal and contiguity with disc space at L3-4, recurrent herniation was favored. This was found to be a large herniation at reoperation.

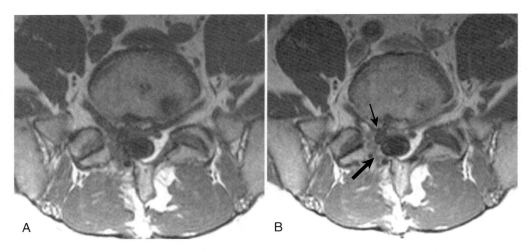

FIGURE 12–18 Postoperative epidural scar. **A** and **B,** Axial T1-weighted MR images before (**A**) and after (**B**) contrast medium instillation show diffuse enhancement of tissue surrounding right lateral aspect of thecal sac (*long arrow*) and exiting right S1 root (*short arrow*).

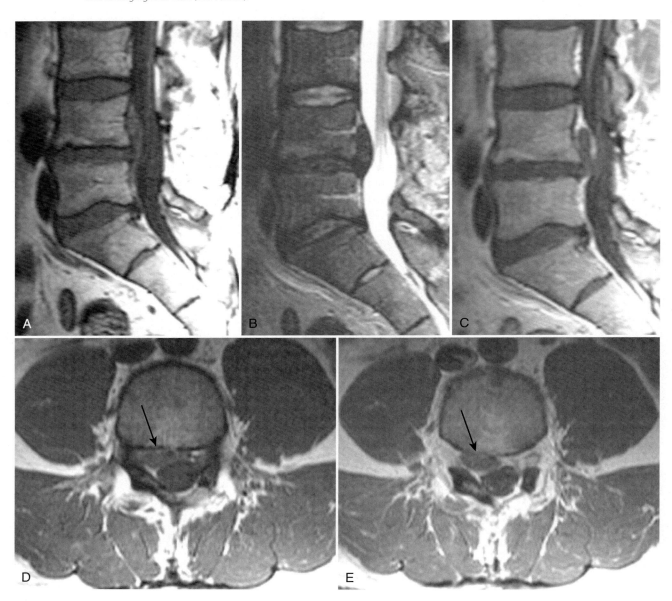

FIGURE 12–19 Recurrent herniation. **A,** Sagittal T1-weighted MR image shows large anterior epidural mass extending dorsal to L4 body from L4-5 disc space. The patient previously underwent L4 laminectomy and discectomy. **B,** Sagittal T2-weighted MR image shows large disc extrusion migrating superiorly from disc space level reflecting free fragment. **C,** After contrast medium administration, sagittal T1-weighted MR image shows typical peripheral enhancement of large herniation. **D** and **E,** Axial T1-weighted MR images before (**D**) and after (**E**) contrast medium instillation show peripheral enhancement of disc component at mid-L4 level (*arrow*).

Stenosis

Bony stenosis has been implicated as a cause of failed back surgery in 60% of cases. Various mechanisms can lead to stenotic changes in the canal or foramina. Their significance may vary, and many of these stenoses are not symptomatic. Examples of mechanisms are as follows:

1. Bony overgrowth after facetectomy may compromise a lateral recess.
2. After posterior fusion, there may be late overgrowth of bone into the posterior or lateral canals.
3. After anterior fusion, bone may extend into the canal or foramen.
4. The narrowing of the interspace after discectomy may allow sufficient facet overriding to produce a decreased size of the lateral recesses or foramina.
5. Postoperative spondylolisthesis can produce focal stenosis.

Arachnoiditis

Spinal MRI can identify the varied patterns of lumbar arachnoiditis, as can CT and myelography.[104-106] These patterns may be classified into three categories or patterns, which can be applied to MRI, CT, or myelography, although a mixture of patterns can occur in any one patient.[107]

The first pattern is central adhesion of the nerve roots within the thecal sac into a central clump of soft tissue signal. Instead of showing their normal feathery pattern, the nerve roots are clumped into one or more cords. This pattern is most easily identified on axial CT myelography or T1-weighted MRI. The second pattern is adhesion of the nerve roots to the meninges, giving rise to an "empty thecal sac" sign. On MRI, only the homogeneous signal of the CSF is present within the thecal sac, and the nerve roots are peripherally attached to the meninges. On CT myelography, only the high-attenuation contrast agent within the thecal sac is visualized, without the nerve roots. In the third pattern, which can be viewed as an end stage of the inflammatory response, the arachnoid becomes an inflammatory mass that fills the thecal sac. On myelography, this type of arachnoiditis gives rise to a block, with an irregular "candle-dripping" appearance. MRI shows a nonspecific soft tissue mass, as does CT myelography.

Infection

Infection may not be considered in the differential diagnosis for back pain because it is an uncommon disorder (<1% of all cases of osteomyelitis). When infection is considered, accurate imaging is a necessary prelude for microbiologic diagnosis or surgical drainage. Because abnormalities that appear on plain radiographs usually take days to weeks to become apparent, radionuclide studies have been the primary imaging modalities for diagnosis of vertebral osteomyelitis.

Radionuclides most commonly used for detecting inflammatory changes of the spine are technetium 99m (^{99m}Tc) phosphate complexes, gallium (^{67}Ga) citrate, and indium-111 (^{111}In)–labeled white blood cells. Although scintigraphy with ^{99m}Tc and ^{67}Ga compounds is sensitive to infection, it is also nonspecific. Healing fractures, degenerative arthritis, sterile inflammatory reactions, tumors, and loosened prosthetic devices can show increased uptake.[108-110]

^{111}In has several advantages compared with other radionuclides, including higher target-to-background ratios, better image quality (compared with ^{67}Ga), and more intense uptake by abscesses. Its main disadvantage is its accumulation within any inflammatory lesion, whether infectious or not.[111] The radionuclide study also takes time to perform—hours to days. CT has played a minor diagnostic role in cases with bony or soft tissue components and is not considered a mainstay for the diagnosis of disc space infection.[112,113] In appropriate situations, the sensitivity of MRI for detecting vertebral osteomyelitis seems to exceed the sensitivity of plain films and CT, and it approaches or equals the sensitivity of radionuclide studies (Figs. 12–20 and 12–21).[114,115]

It is imperative to obtain T1-weighted and T2-weighted images in the sagittal plane for optimal sensitivity to detect disease. The T1-weighted SE image allows detection of the increased water content or marrow fluid seen with inflammatory exudate or edema. Similar to most pathologic processes, disc space infection or vertebral osteomyelitis results in increased signal intensity on T2-weighted images. The diagnostic specificity of MRI is provided by the signal intensity changes on T1-weighted and T2-weighted images and by the anatomic pattern of disease involvement and the appropriate clinical situation.

On T2-weighted images, the normal intervertebral disc usually shows increased signal intensity within its central portion that is bisected by a thin horizontal line of decreased signal, termed the *intranuclear cleft*. After the age of 30 years, the cleft is almost a constant feature of normal intervertebral discs. Disc space infections on MRI typically produce confluent decreased signal intensity of the adjacent vertebral bodies and the involved intervertebral disc space on T1-weighted images compared with the normal vertebral body marrow. A poorly defined endplate margin exists between the disc and adjacent vertebral bodies. T2-weighted images show increased signal intensity of the vertebral bodies adjacent to the involved disc and an abnormal morphology and increased signal intensity from the disc itself, with absence of the normal intranuclear cleft. These MRI findings are much more typical of pyogenic than of tuberculous spondylitis.[116] In a comparative study of patients with suspected vertebral osteomyelitis, MRI had a sensitivity of 96%, a specificity of 92%, and an overall accuracy of 94%.[114] Scintigraphy with ^{67}Ga and ^{99m}Tc bone scintigraphy had a sensitivity of 90%, specificity of 100%, and accuracy of 94% when combined. In this study, MRI was as accurate and sensitive as radionuclide scanning for the detection of osteomyelitis.

Dagirmanjian and colleagues[117] investigated the sensitivity of MRI findings for vertebral osteomyelitis. They considered

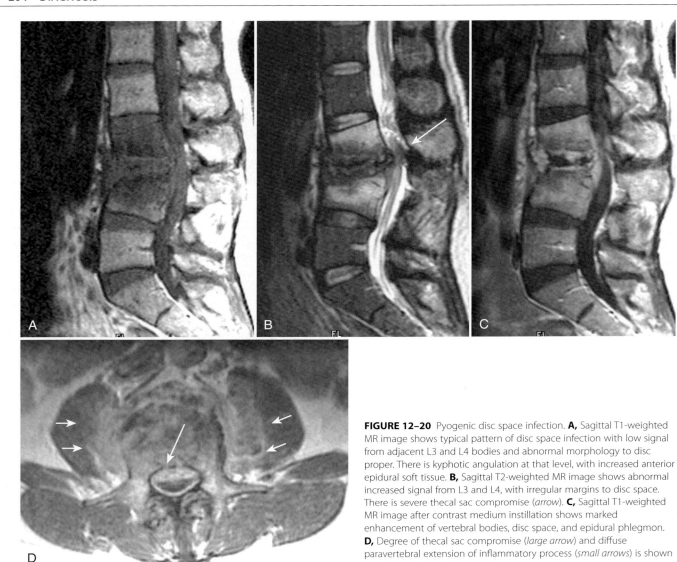

FIGURE 12–20 Pyogenic disc space infection. **A,** Sagittal T1-weighted MR image shows typical pattern of disc space infection with low signal from adjacent L3 and L4 bodies and abnormal morphology to disc proper. There is kyphotic angulation at that level, with increased anterior epidural soft tissue. **B,** Sagittal T2-weighted MR image shows abnormal increased signal from L3 and L4, with irregular margins to disc space. There is severe thecal sac compromise (*arrow*). **C,** Sagittal T1-weighted MR image after contrast medium instillation shows marked enhancement of vertebral bodies, disc space, and epidural phlegmon. **D,** Degree of thecal sac compromise (*large arrow*) and diffuse paravertebral extension of inflammatory process (*small arrows*) is shown on axial T1-weighted MR image.

the "classic" MRI changes of vertebral osteomyelitis to include decreased signal of disc and adjacent vertebral bodies on T1-weighted images, increased nonanatomic signal of the disc on T2-weighted images, increased signal of the adjacent vertebral bodies on T2-weighted images, and enhancement of the disc and adjacent vertebral bodies. These investigators found 95% of disc space infection levels had typical T1-weighted vertebral body changes, and 90% had increased nonanatomic signal of the disc on T2-weighted images. Only 54% of the abnormal levels showed increased signal of the vertebral bodies on T2-weighted images, however. Although 84% of patients showed the typical T1-weighted vertebral body and T1-weighted and T2-weighted disc changes, only 49% of cases showed the typical T1-weighted and T2-weighted vertebral body and disc findings as originally described. T1-weighted vertebral body, disc, and endplate changes and T2-weighted disc changes are the most reliable findings of disc space infection and vertebral osteomyelitis. In the initial stages of

vertebral osteomyelitis, when the disc space is not yet involved, it may be difficult to exclude neoplastic disease or compression fracture from the differential diagnosis using only MRI. Follow-up studies are usually necessary to define the nature of the lesion further.

Boden and colleagues[118] suggested that in the postoperative spine the triad of intervertebral disc space enhancement, annular enhancement, and vertebral body enhancement leads to the diagnosis of disc space infection, with the appropriate laboratory findings, such as an elevated sedimentation rate. There is a group of normal postoperative patients, however, with anulus enhancement (at the surgical site), intervertebral disc enhancement, and vertebral endplate enhancement without evidence of disc space infection. In these cases, the intervertebral disc enhancement is typically seen as thin bands paralleling the adjacent endplates, and the vertebral body enhancement is associated with type I degenerative endplate changes. This pattern should be distinguished from the

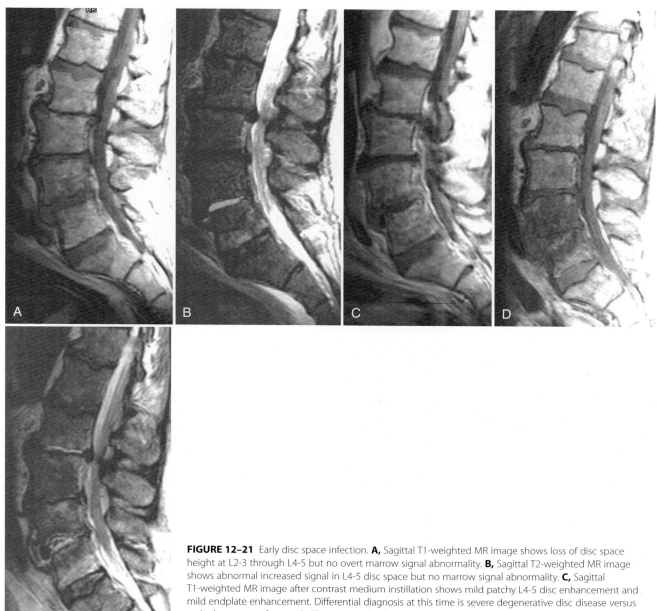

FIGURE 12–21 Early disc space infection. **A,** Sagittal T1-weighted MR image shows loss of disc space height at L2-3 through L4-5 but no overt marrow signal abnormality. **B,** Sagittal T2-weighted MR image shows abnormal increased signal in L4-5 disc space but no marrow signal abnormality. **C,** Sagittal T1-weighted MR image after contrast medium instillation shows mild patchy L4-5 disc enhancement and mild endplate enhancement. Differential diagnosis at this time is severe degenerative disc disease versus early disc space infection. **D,** There is grossly abnormal signal involving L4 and L5 bodies with loss of disc margin 5 weeks later on T1-weighted MR image. **E,** L4-5 disc now shows more marked increased signal on T2-weighted MR image.

amorphous enhancement seen within the intervertebral disc with disc space infection.

Staphylococcus aureus is the organism most commonly associated with vertebral osteomyelitis and epidural abscess, accounting for approximately 60% of the cases (Fig. 12–22). *S. aureus* is ubiquitous, tends to form abscesses, and can infect compromised and normal hosts. Other gram-positive cocci account for approximately 13% of cases, and gram-negative organisms account for approximately 15%. Clinical acute symptoms classically include back pain, fever, obtundation in severe cases, and neurologic deficits. Chronic cases may have less pain and no elevated temperature. Rankin and Flothow[119] described the classic course of epidural abscess in four stages:

spinal ache, root pain, weakness, and paralysis. Acute deterioration from spinal epidural abscess remains unpredictable, however. Patients may present with abrupt paraplegia and anesthesia. The cause for this precipitous course is unknown, but it is thought to be related to a vascular mechanism (e.g., epidural thrombosis and thrombophlebitis, venous infarction).[120,121]

The primary diagnostic modality in the evaluation of epidural abscess is MRI. MRI is as sensitive as CT myelography for diagnosing epidural infection, but it also allows the exclusion of other entities, such as herniation, syrinx, tumor, and cord infarction.[122,123] MRI of epidural abscess shows a soft tissue mass in the epidural space with tapered

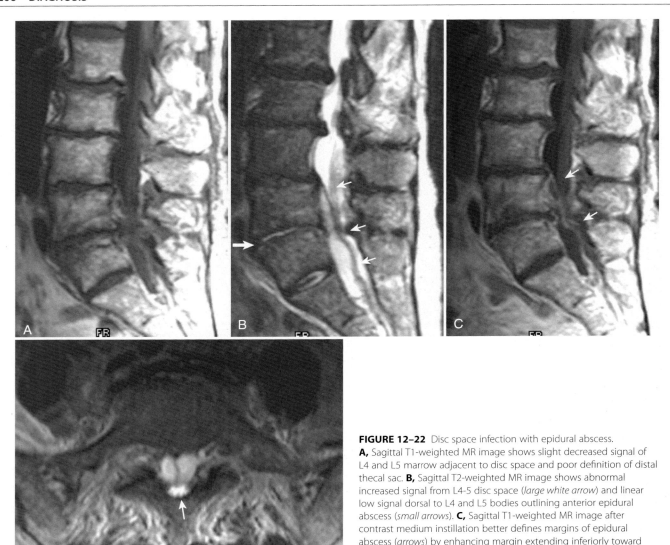

FIGURE 12–22 Disc space infection with epidural abscess. **A,** Sagittal T1-weighted MR image shows slight decreased signal of L4 and L5 marrow adjacent to disc space and poor definition of distal thecal sac. **B,** Sagittal T2-weighted MR image shows abnormal increased signal from L4-5 disc space (*large white arrow*) and linear low signal dorsal to L4 and L5 bodies outlining anterior epidural abscess (*small arrows*). **C,** Sagittal T1-weighted MR image after contrast medium instillation better defines margins of epidural abscess (*arrows*) by enhancing margin extending inferiorly toward S1 level. Slight abnormal enhancement is present within disc itself. **D,** Axial T2-weighted MR image shows loculated abscess as foci of high signal, displacing caudal thecal sac dorsally (*arrow*).

edges and an associated mass effect on the thecal sac and cord. The epidural masses are usually isointense to the cord on T1-weighted images and of increased signal on T2-weighted images. Post and colleagues[124,125] recommended that in ambiguous cases either CT myelography or contrast medium–enhanced MRI is necessary for full elucidation of the abscess (Fig. 12–23).

The patterns of MRI contrast medium enhancement of epidural abscess include (1) diffuse and homogeneous, (2) heterogeneous, and (3) thin peripheral. Post and colleagues[125] found that enhancement was a very useful adjunct for identifying the extent of a lesion when the plain MR image was equivocal, for showing activity of an infection, and for directing needle biopsy and follow-up treatment. Successful therapy should cause a progressive decrease in enhancement of the paraspinal soft tissues, disc, and vertebral bodies.

Tumors

The most critical piece of imaging information regarding spinal neoplasms used in forming a differential diagnosis involves determination of whether the lesion is intramedullary, intradural extramedullary, or extradural.

Intramedullary Lesions

The most common intramedullary neoplasms are *gliomas,* principally astrocytomas and ependymomas. *Ependymomas* are cited as the most frequent intramedullary tumors in adults (Fig. 12–24). Although ependymomas may involve any portion of the cord, they most commonly involve the conus medullaris and filum terminale and are the most common primary tumor of the lower spinal cord. Patients with these tumors present in

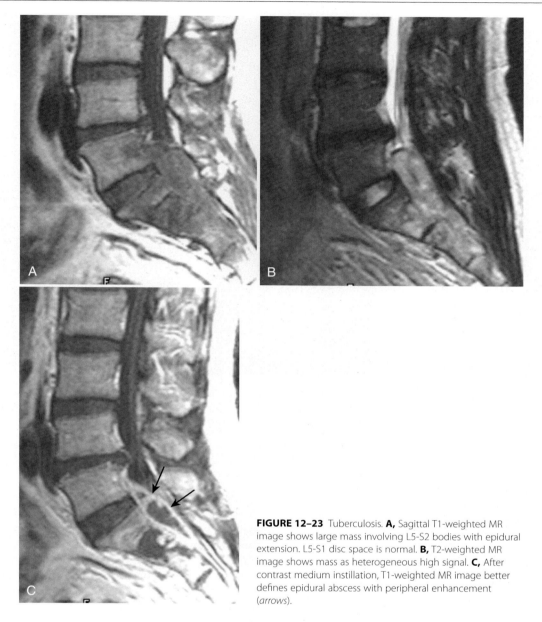

FIGURE 12–23 Tuberculosis. **A,** Sagittal T1-weighted MR image shows large mass involving L5-S2 bodies with epidural extension. L5-S1 disc space is normal. **B,** T2-weighted MR image shows mass as heterogeneous high signal. **C,** After contrast medium instillation, T1-weighted MR image better defines epidural abscess with peripheral enhancement (*arrows*).

the 4th to 5th decades, often with back pain.[126,127] A typical appearance would be an intradural extramedullary mass involving the filum terminale and cauda equina, although it can appear as fusiform enlargement of the cord itself.[128] Cervical intramedullary tumors may be seen in patients with neurofibromatosis type 2 (Fig. 12–25). These tumors typically enhance and may have intratumoral cysts. The myxopapillary subtype is particularly common in the lumbosacral region, typically appearing as a large, intensely enhancing mass spanning several vertebral levels. In most cases, the tumors appear as intradural extramedullary lesions because of their bulky exophytic growth, which fills the spinal canal. Overall signal intensities are nonspecific, but because of their highly vascular nature, ependymomas often show areas of T2-weighted shortening secondary to the presence of hemosiderin and ferritin,

which is strongly suggestive of the diagnosis.[129] They also may manifest as subarachnoid hemorrhage.[130]

Intramedullary astrocytomas constitute 6% to 8% of primary spine tumors, with a peak incidence in the 3rd to 4th decades of life. Astrocytomas produce focal enlargement and occasionally exophytic growth involving the cord. Of these tumors, 75% to 92% are relatively benign, such as grades 1 and 2. Imaging shows fusiform enlargement of the cord over several segments, whereas T2-weighted MRI shows increased signal intensity reflecting tumor and edematous cord. Cysts are often associated with these intramedullary tumors. These cysts may be benign, syringomyelic type of cavities or actual cysts associated with the tumor.

Hemangioblastomas are unusual cord tumors and usually manifest in the 3rd to 4th decades of life. They are frequently

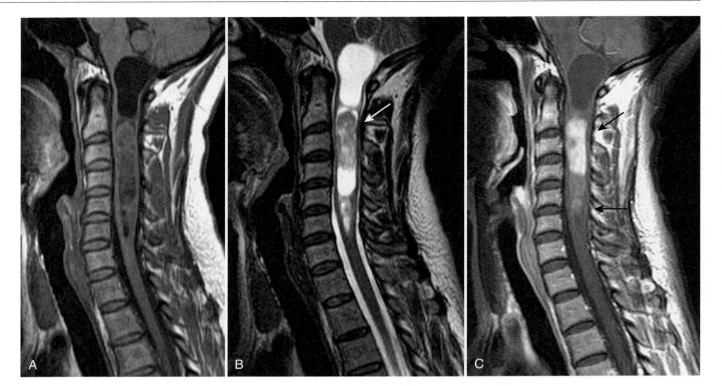

FIGURE 12-24 Ependymoma. **A,** Sagittal T1-weighted image shows large cystic and solid intramedullary mass within cervical cord. Tumor-associated cyst extends to medulla. **B,** Sagittal T2-weighted image shows central solid component (*arrow*) with cephalad and caudad cystic components. **C,** Sagittal T1-weighted image after contrast medium instillation shows large enhancing solid component extending down to C5-6 (*black arrows*).

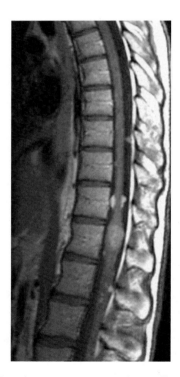

FIGURE 12-25 Ependymoma in a patient with neurofibromatosis type 2. Sagittal T1-weighted MR image after contrast medium instillation shows multiple intradural extramedullary enhancing masses (schwannomas or meningiomas), combined with less intensely enhancing mass within conus (ependymoma).

multiple and seen in association with von Hippel–Lindau disease.[131-136] These lesions most often manifest as dorsal intramedullary masses containing a nodule that enhances, although these vary between the amount of cyst component and solid component. There may be extensive widening of the cord showing increased signal intensity on T2-weighted images related to cord edema, extending several segments away from the nidus itself. Occasionally, metastatic disease may manifest as an intramedullary enhancing mass. Carcinoma of the lung and breast are the most common, with melanoma, lymphoma, and renal cell carcinoma also being reported.[137,138] Spread of intracranial neoplasms such as ependymoma and glioma may also seed the leptomeninges and produce direct involvement of the cord.[139-141] Benign intramedullary tumors are uncommon, but *cavernous angiomas* can occur in the cord with typical signal characteristics of speckled increased and decreased signal on T1-weighted images and evidence of hemosiderin deposition on T2-weighted images (Fig. 12–26).

The various causes of inflammatory myelopathies include multiple sclerosis, postviral demyelinating disease, viral infection, pyogenic infection, and granulomatous disease. The archetypal inflammatory lesion is *multiple sclerosis* (Fig. 12–27). The spinal cord is the site of much clinical involvement in patients with multiple sclerosis; however, imaging of the spinal cord has always been subordinate to brain imaging in radiologic investigations of multiple sclerosis. Because some

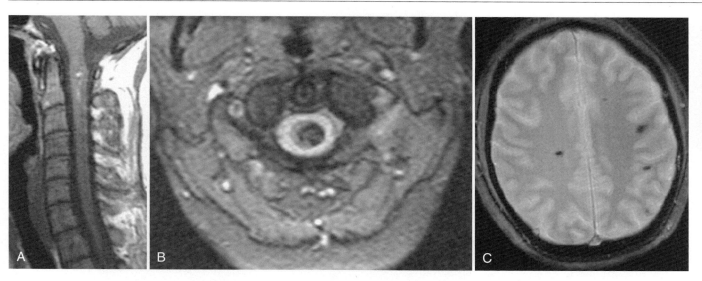

FIGURE 12–26 Cavernous angioma. **A,** Sagittal T1-weighted MR image shows linear focus of high signal reflecting hemorrhage within cord at C2 level. **B,** Axial gradient-echo MR image confirms blood as focal low signal within substance of cord. **C,** Axial gradient-echo MR image through brain shows multiple areas of low signal reflecting hemosiderin deposition owing to multiple cavernous angiomas.

of the clinical disease activity in multiple sclerosis is related to the spinal cord, it is important to correlate cord disease activity to gain further insights into the nature of disability in these patients and to correlate objective improvements in brain and cord lesion burden with changes in clinical disability scoring. Most focal plaques are less than two vertebral body lengths in size, occupy less than half the cross-sectional diameter of the cord, and are characteristically peripherally located with respect to a transverse, cross-sectional reference. Of spinal cord multiple sclerosis lesions, 60% to 75% are present in the cervical region, and more than half of multiple sclerosis patients with cord plaques have multiple plaques. Of patients with cord plaques, 90% have intracranial multiple sclerosis plaques.

Intradural Extramedullary Lesions

Intradural extramedullary neoplasms constitute the largest single group of primary spine neoplasms, accounting for approximately 55% of all primary spine tumors. Most of these

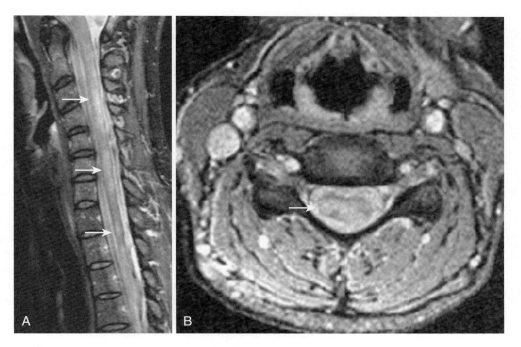

FIGURE 12–27 STIR imaging for intramedullary inflammatory disease. **A** and **B,** Sagittal (**A**) and axial (**B**) images show multiple foci of abnormal increased signal throughout cervical cord without expansion reflecting demyelinating disease (*arrows*).

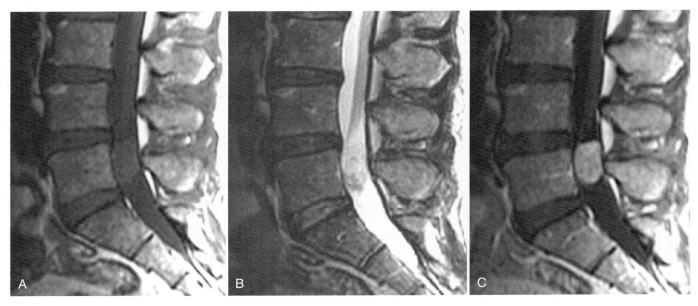

FIGURE 12–28 Schwannoma. **A-C,** Sagittal T1-weighted (**A**), T2-weighted (**B**), and T1-weighted enhanced (**C**) MR images show round, intensely enhancing intradural mass at L4 level, displacing adjacent cauda equina.

tumors are benign, with *nerve sheath tumors* and *meningiomas* representing the most common lesions.[141] *Nerve sheath tumors* are the most common intraspinal tumors and are divided histologically into two types: *schwannomas* (i.e., neuromas, neurinomas, neurilemmomas) and *neurofibromas* (Fig. 12–28). Solitary schwannomas constitute most intraspinal nerve sheath tumors, whereas neurofibromas are almost

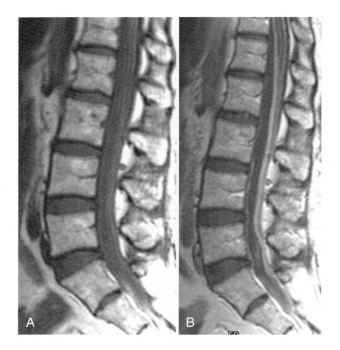

FIGURE 12–29 Leptomeningeal enhancement. **A** and **B,** Sagittal T1-weighted MR images before (**A**) and after (**B**) contrast medium instillation show extensive leptomeningeal enhancement of cauda equina and distal cord surface in a patient with *Staphylococcus aureus* meningitis.

always associated with neurofibromatosis type 1. Patients with neurofibromatosis type 2 more commonly have multiple schwannomas rather than neurofibromas, however.[142] Isolated nerve sheath tumors can arise anywhere in the spine.[143]

Nerve sheath tumors are easily recognized on MRI as typically isolated, well-circumscribed, solid masses of soft tissue signal intensity on T1-weighted images surrounded by low signal CSF. On T2-weighted images, they are of variable signal intensity. Schwannomas are more vascular and include cystic degeneration, necrosis, and hemorrhage more commonly than neurofibromas. Various local osseous changes, consisting mainly of smooth bony remodeling or foraminal enlargement, are common. Enhancement is almost always present, but the pattern is variable.

Meningiomas most commonly occur in the thoracic spine.[144] As is the case intracranially, there is a female sex predilection, and these lesions occur in a slightly older age group than nerve sheath tumors. Most are entirely intradural and typically are isointense to the neural elements on T1-weighted and T2-weighted images. Meningiomas enhance intensely after gadolinium–diethylenetetraminepentaacetic acid (DTPA) administration, which may allow demonstration of the typical broad dural base.[145,146]

The last category of intradural extramedullary lesions is the so-called *leptomeningeal* pattern, which includes leptomeningeal metastatic disease, inflammation, and benign granulomatous processes such as sarcoid and tuberculosis (Fig. 12–29).[147] The list of tumors that may seed the CSF is long, but the most common offenders are cranial ependymomas, glioblastomas, and medulloblastomas (especially in pediatric patients). Additional malignancies that can spread less commonly are ependymoma, pineoblastoma, germinoma, and retinoblastoma. Lesions outside the central nervous system that are capable of spreading along the leptomeninges include carcinoma of the

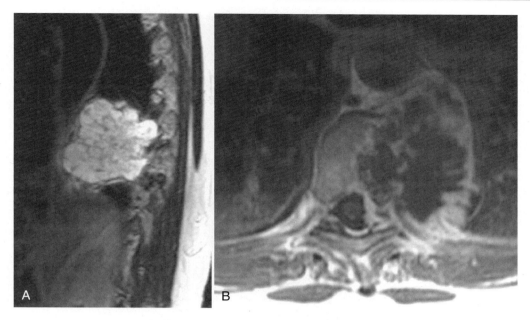

FIGURE 12-30 Chondroblastic osteosarcoma. **A,** Sagittal T2-weighted MR image shows large paraspinal mass with well-defined margins and heterogeneous internal signal typical of cartilaginous lesions, including chordoma. **B,** Axial T1-weighted MR image after contrast medium instillation shows large, irregularly enhancing mass involving left lateral aspect of thoracic body with extension into paravertebral region. There is left lateral epidural extension of tumor with mild mass effect on cord.

lung and breast, lymphoma, leukemia, and melanoma. Administration of contrast material with T1-weighted images is mandatory and shows a linear and nodular enhancement pattern along the leptomeninges. The overall sensitivity of MRI examinations is low in patients with proven histologic evidence of neoplastic seeding, so examination of the CSF remains the "gold standard."

Extradural Lesions

Primary and secondary tumors to the extradural space are well evaluated by MRI and CT (Fig. 12–30). *Metastatic disease to the spine is the most common type of extradural tumor.* Because of its high contrast sensitivity and spatial resolution, MRI is the examination of choice in the detection of osseous metastases (Fig. 12–31).[148-150] Because many metastatic tumors enhance, the routine use of contrast medium–enhanced studies alone is not recommended because the distinction between metastases and normal marrow fat is diminished, occasionally to the point of masking even large lesions (Fig. 12–32). Although diffuse osseous metastases can appear as homogeneous diffuse low marrow signal on T1-weighted images, this appearance is not specific.

Cysts

Nabors and colleagues[151-153] have clarified the confusing array of terms for spinal meningeal cysts. *Spinal meningeal cysts* are congenital diverticula of the dural sac, root sheaths, or arachnoid that may be classified into three major groups. The first group includes extradural cysts without spinal nerve roots (type I), the second includes extradural cysts with spinal nerve

roots (type II), and the third includes intradural cysts (type III) (Fig. 12–33). Type I are diverticula that maintain contact with the thecal sac by a narrow ostium. Type I cysts include extradural cysts, pouches, and diverticula and the so-called occult intrasacral meningoceles. Sacral type I cysts are found

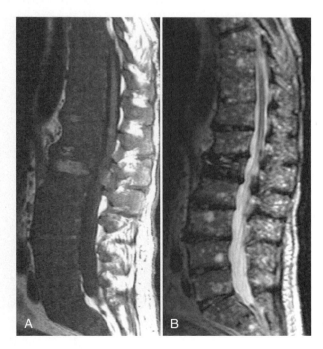

FIGURE 12-31 Multiple myeloma. **A,** Sagittal T1-weighted MR image shows markedly diminished signal from all the visualized marrow of thoracolumbar spine. There is severe compression deformity at L1. **B,** Sagittal T2-weighted MR image shows typical "salt and pepper" pattern of multiple myeloma. No epidural tumor is identified.

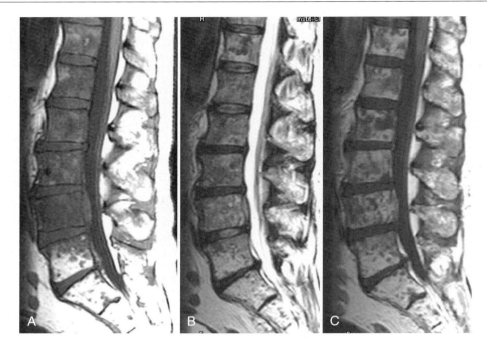

FIGURE 12–32 Diffuse metastatic disease. **A,** Sagittal T1-weighted MR image shows diffuse abnormal decreased marrow signal from L4 through L1 bodies. There is residual fatty marrow replacement involving L5 and sacrum from prior radiation therapy. There is mild anterior epidural extension of tumor at L4. **B,** T2-weighted MR image shows mass effect of epidural tumor but tends to minimize marrow signal abnormality. **C,** Likewise, after contrast material is instilled, T1-weighted MR image now shows less marrow abnormality, owing to enhancing tumor mimicking fatty marrow signal.

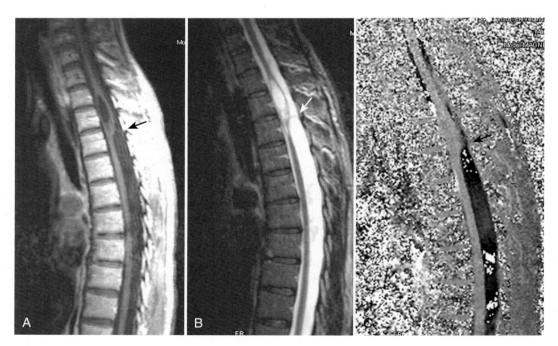

FIGURE 12–33 Arachnoid cyst and syrinx. **A,** Sagittal T1-weighted MR image through thoracic spine shows ventrally displaced cord with abruptly expanding dorsal margin at T4 level (*arrow*), with small syrinx seen as linear low signal within cord. **B,** Sagittal T2-weighted MR image shows thin line of low signal at cephalad margin of dorsally expanded cerebrospinal fluid (CSF) (*arrow*) space with "windsock" pattern reflecting arachnoid cyst margin. **C,** Single sagittal MR image from cine CSF flow series is encoded to show upward motion as dark areas. This technique outlines abrupt change in CSF flow pattern at top of cyst (*arrow*).

in adults and are connected to the tip of the caudal thecal sac by a pedicle. Type II meningeal cysts with contained nerve roots are extradural lesions previously called Tarlov cysts, perineural cysts, or nerve root diverticula. These are generally seen as multiple incidental lesions, but are occasionally associated with radiculopathy or incontinence. Type III meningeal cysts are intradural lesions most commonly found on the posterior subarachnoid space and have been called arachnoid diverticula or arachnoid cysts. These are lined by a single layer of normal arachnoid cells and filled with CSF.

Trauma

Plain films are the initial study for screening or "clearing" the cervical spine in trauma. Three to five views are considered adequate for a trauma series: anteroposterior, lateral, open mouth odontoid, with or without supine right and left obliques. A single lateral view is inadequate, and all seven cervical vertebral bodies must be visualized. Plain films are also of primary importance in defining instability in patients with persistent pain or soft tissue swelling without a definite fracture on the initial plain film evaluation.

Studies have shown that if strict criteria are followed, patients who arrive at the emergency department with a collar in place can be clinically evaluated as to whether or not plain films are required.[154,155] Patients with cervical fractures typically have at least one of the following: intoxication, neck tenderness, altered level of consciousness, or a painful injury elsewhere. Indications for CT in evaluation of the cervical spine include further evaluation of known or questioned fracture on plain films and evaluation of areas inadequately seen on plain films.[156,157] Techniques vary from institution to institution, but slice thickness is generally 1.5 to 3 mm, soft tissue and bone windows, with no intravenous contrast material. The sensitivity of CT to detect fracture is 78% to 100%.[158,159] CT is particularly useful in diagnosing posterior element (laminar) fractures. The use of spiral thin-section techniques (1 to 1.5 mm) with multiplanar reformats should enable sensitivity approaching 100%. Some institutions and studies use CT as the primary screening study in patients with multiple areas of trauma, bypassing plain films.[160,161]

MRI allows direct visualization of cord abnormalities, which cannot be identified by any other imaging modality. MRI can define intramedullary hematoma, intramedullary edema and contusion, disc herniations, ligamentous injury, and epidural hemorrhage (Fig. 12–34).[162-165] Hemorrhage within the 1st week is seen as low signal on T2-weighted images related to deoxyhemoglobin. Contusion without hemorrhage is identified as high signal on T2-weighted images and as isointense or decreased signal on T1-weighted images. Ligamentous disruption is seen as loss of the usual low signal from the anterior and posterior longitudinal ligaments, with increased signal on T2-weighted images in the adjacent tissues.[166,167]

The most common area of traumatic involvement in the lumbar spine is the thoracolumbar junction, which acts as a fulcrum for spine motion and is susceptible to unstable traumatic injury. The thick, sagittally oriented lumbar facets minimize rotational injury, but flexion and axial loading injuries often occur. The forces may combine to produce flexion-compression injuries or the so-called burst fracture. Burst fractures are notable for instability and a predisposition for displacing fracture fragments and causing spinal cord compression.[168,169] CT remains the method of choice for the detection of retropulsed bony fragments and for the demonstration of fractures of the posterior elements.[170]

A hyperflexion injury occurring in the lumbar spine is the seat belt or Chance fracture, which is associated with rapid deceleration motor vehicle accidents. This type of trauma produces a horizontal fracture through anterior and posterior elements.[171,172] The anterior component may be through the vertebral body or through the disc itself. Although CT is more sensitive than MRI for detecting bony abnormalities, MRI is often superior for evaluating soft tissue structures. In particular, the spinal ligaments show focal discontinuity on T1-weighted images and areas of increased signal intensity on T2-weighted images.

Hemorrhage

Epidural spinal hematomas occur most frequently in elderly adults but can occur at any age.[173-176] Epidural spinal hematomas are broadly classified into two groups: nonspontaneous and spontaneous. Nonspontaneous epidural spinal hematomas may result from spinal taps, spinal anesthesia, trauma, pregnancy, bleeding diathesis, anticoagulant therapy, spinal hemangiomas, vascular malformations, hypertension, and neoplasms. The history can often be revealing, yet these tumors commonly occur merely from an episode of sneezing, bending, voiding, turning in bed, or other mild trauma. Epidural spinal hematomas can be localized or can spread anywhere along the spinal column. Blood more commonly accumulates posterolaterally.

Subdural hemorrhage is capable of producing severe and irreversible neurologic deficits, and acute surgical intervention may be needed. Spinal subdural hematomas can have a typical configuration (Fig. 12–35).[177-179] As opposed to epidural hematomas, which tend to be capped by fat, subdural hematomas are located within the thecal sac and are separate from the adjacent extradural fat, the vertebral bodies, and the posterior elements. Axial images are useful in defining the epidural fat surrounding the thecal sac and in defining the blood relating to the interior of the sac with subdural hematomas. These may be loculated anteriorly and posteriorly within the thecal sac. The loculation can take the form of a "Mercedes Benz" sign, showing a trefoil configuration (see Fig. 12–35B).

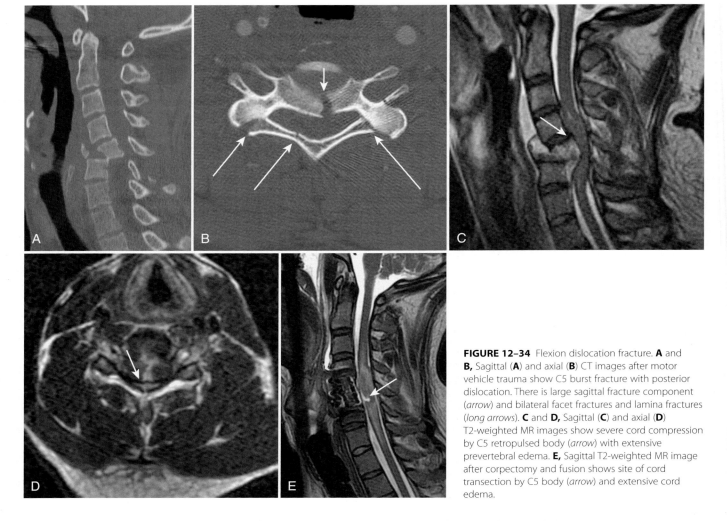

FIGURE 12–34 Flexion dislocation fracture. **A** and **B,** Sagittal (**A**) and axial (**B**) CT images after motor vehicle trauma show C5 burst fracture with posterior dislocation. There is large sagittal fracture component (*arrow*) and bilateral facet fractures and lamina fractures (*long arrows*). **C** and **D,** Sagittal (**C**) and axial (**D**) T2-weighted MR images show severe cord compression by C5 retropulsed body (*arrow*) with extensive prevertebral edema. **E,** Sagittal T2-weighted MR image after corpectomy and fusion shows site of cord transection by C5 body (*arrow*) and extensive cord edema.

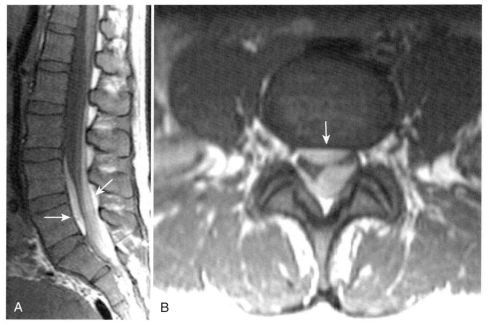

FIGURE 12–35 Subdural hemorrhage. **A** and **B,** Sagittal (**A**) and axial (**B**) T1-weighted MR images show high signal blood along dural margin from L3 to S1 (*arrows*). Axial image shows that exterior margin of blood is delimited by dura, so it must be either subarachnoid or subdural in location. Loculation on axial view is typical for subdural location.

KEY POINTS

1. Metal artifact on MRI can be reduced with use of FSE, larger fields of view, higher readout bandwidths, smaller voxel sizes, and appropriate geometric orientation of the frequency-encoded direction in relationship to the metal.

2. The most common spinal vascular lesion is the dural fistula, and the most sensitive MRI finding is increased signal on T2-weighted images within the cord.

3. The most critical imaging information regarding spinal neoplasms used in forming a differential diagnosis involves determining whether the lesion is intramedullary, intradural extramedullary, or extradural.

4. CT remains the method of choice for detecting retropulsed bony fragments and for showing fractures of the posterior elements.

5. MRI is useful in the immediate postoperative period for evaluating fluid collections including hemorrhage and for showing mass effect on the thecal sac, cord, and cauda equina but not for defining residual disc material.

6. Paravertebral enhancement on fat-suppressed axial T1-weighted images is very helpful in defining early disc space infection.

7. The apparent size of neural foramina on axial gradient MR images is critically dependent on the sequence echo time; longer echo times give susceptibility artifact, which may give the false appearance of stenosis.

8. Synovial cysts are very difficult to identify on T1-weighted images and require T2-weighted images or intravenous contrast medium enhancement, or both, for definition.

9. Early disc space infection and degenerative disc disease with type I endplate change can be indistinguishable by MRI alone.

10. Acute spinal hemorrhage may show no characteristics of "blood" on MRI owing to the lack of susceptibility effect of oxyhemoglobin.

11. OPLL may be missed on T1-weighted images by merging into the low signal of CSF.

12. Use of contrast medium may mask spinal bony metastatic disease by causing the enhancing tumor signal to match that of adjacent normal fatty marrow.

KEY REFERENCES

1. Fardon DF, Milette PC: Nomenclature and classification of lumbar disc pathology: Recommendations of the combined task forces of the North American Spine Society, American Society of Spine Radiology, and American Society of Neuroradiology. Spine 26:E93-E113, 2001.
   This is "must reading" for standardization of this Tower of Babel.

2. Mehta RC, Marks MP, Hinks RS, et al: MR evaluation of vertebral metastases: T1-weighted, short-inversion-time inversion recovery, fast spin-echo, and inversion-recovery fast spin-echo sequences. AJNR Am J Neuroradiol 16:281-288, 1995.
   T1-weighted images, FSE, and fat-saturated FSE are superior for detecting epidural metastatic disease.

3. Modic MT, Feiglin DH, Piraino DW, et al: Vertebral osteomyelitis: Assessment using MR. Radiology 157:157-166, 1985.
   This classic definition of MRI changes still applies today.

4. Nabors MW, Pait TG, Byrd EB, et al: Updated assessment and current classification of spinal meningeal cysts. J Neurosurg 68:366-377, 1988.
   A cogent classification of a confusing area is presented.

5. Russell EJ: Cervical disk disease. Radiology 177:313-325, 1990.
   The author provides an excellent summary of a broad subject.

REFERENCES

1. Hitselberger WE, Witten RM: Abnormal myelograms in asymptomatic patients. J Neurosurg 28:204-206, 1968.

2. Slone RM, McEnery KW, Bridwell KH, et al: Principles and imaging of spinal instrumentation. Radiol Clin North Am 33:189-211, 1995.

3. Hanley SD, Gun MT, Osti O, et al: Radiology of intervertebral cages in spinal surgery. Clin Radiol 54:201-206, 1999.

4. Bell GR, Modic MT: Radiology of the lumbar spine. In Rothman RH, Simeone FA (eds): The Spine, 3rd ed. Philadelphia, WB Saunders, 1992, pp 125-153.

5. Olsen NK, Madsen HH, Eriksen FB, et al: Intracranial iohexol-distribution following cervical myelography: Postmyelographic registration of adverse effects, psychometric assessment and electroencephalographic recording. Acta Neurol Scand 82:321-328, 1990.

6. Modic MT, Ross JS, Masaryk TJ: Imaging of degenerative disease of the cervical spine. Clin Orthop 239:109-120, 1989.

7. Fon GT, Sage MR: Computed tomography in cervical disc disease when myelography is unsatisfactory. Clin Radiol 35:47-50, 1984.

8. Coin CG: Cervical disk degeneration and herniation: Diagnosis by computerized tomography. South Med J 77:979-982, 1984.

9. Sobel DF, Barkovich AJ, Munderloh SH: Metrizamide myelography and postmyelographic computed tomography: Comparative adequacy in the cervical spine. AJNR Am J Neuroradiol 45:385-390, 1984.

10. Jahnke RW, Hart BL: Cervical stenosis, spondylosis and herniated disc disease. Radiol Clin North Am 29:777-791, 1991.

11. Landman JA, Hoffman JC, Braun IF, et al: Value of computed tomographic myelography in the recognition of cervical herniated disk. AJNR Am J Neuroradiol 5:391-394, 1984.

12. Simon JE, Lukin RR: Diskogenic disease of the cervical spine. Semin Roentgenol 23:118-124, 1988.

13. Vassilouthis J, Kalovithouris A, Papandreou A, et al: The symptomatic incompetent cervical intervertebral disk. Neurosurgery 25:232-239, 1989.

14. Nakagawa H, Okumura T, Sugiyama T, et al: Discrepancy between metrizamide CT and myelography in diagnosis of cervical disk protrusions. AJNR Am J Neuroradiol 4:604-606, 1983.

15. Dorwart RH, LaMasters DL: Applications of computed tomographic scanning of the cervical spine. Orthop Clin North Am 16:381-393, 1985.

16. Filippi M, Yousry T, Baratti C, et al: Quantitative assessment of MRI lesion load in multiple sclerosis: A comparison of conventional spin echo with fast fluid-attenuated inversion recovery. Brain 119:1349-1355, 1996.

17. Finelli DA, Hurst GC, Karaman B, et al: Use of magnetization transfer for improved contrast on gradient echo images of the cervical spine. Radiology 193:165-171, 1994.

18. Kidd D, Thorpe JW, Thompson AJ, et al: Spinal cord MRI using multi-array coils and fast spin echo: Findings in multiple sclerosis. Neurology 43:2632-2637, 1993.

19. Lyclama A, Nijeholt GJ, Barkof F, et al: Comparison of two MR sequences for the detection of multiple sclerosis lesions in the spinal cord. AJNR Am J Neuroradiol 17:1533-1538, 1996.

20. Ross JS, Ruggieri P, Tkach J, et al: Lumbar degenerative disk disease: Prospective comparison of conventional T2-weighted spin echo imaging and T2-weighted RARE. AJNR Am J Neuroradiol 14:1215-1223, 1993.

21. Rocca MA, Mastronardo G, Horsfield MA, et al: Comparison of three MR sequences for the detection of cervical cord lesions in patients with multiple sclerosis. AJNR Am J Neuroradiol 20:1710-1716, 1999.

22. Sze G, Merriam M, Oshio K, et al: Fast spin echo imaging in the evaluation of intradural disease of the spine. AJNR Am J Neuroradiol 13:1383-1392, 1992.

23. Tartaglino LM, Friedman DP, Flanders AE, et al: Multiple sclerosis in the spinal cord: MR appearance and correlation with clinical parameters. Radiology 195:725-732, 1995.

24. Thorpe JW, Halpin SF, MacManus DG, et al: A comparison between fast and conventional spin echo in the detection of multiple sclerosis lesions. Neuroradiology 36:388-392, 1994.

25. Melhem ER, Caruthers SD, Jara H: Cervical spine: Three-dimensional MR imaging with magnetization transfer prepulsed turbo field echo techniques. Radiology 207:815-821, 1998.

26. Melhem ER, Benson ML, Beauchamp NJ, et al: Cervical spondylosis: Three dimensional gradient echo MR with magnetization transfer. AJNR Am J Neuroradiol 17:705-711, 1996.

27. Dwyer AJ, Frank JA, Sank VJ, et al: Short-tau inversion-recovery pulse sequence: Analysis and initial experience in cancer imaging. Radiology 168:827-836, 1988.

28. Mehta RC, Marks MP, Hinks RS, et al: MR evaluation of vertebral metastases: T1-weighted, short-inversion-time inversion recovery, fast spin-echo, and inversion-recovery fast spin-echo sequences. AJNR Am J Neuroradiol 16:281-288, 1995.

29. Weinberger E, Shaw DW, White KS, et al: Nontraumatic pediatric musculoskeletal MR imaging: Comparison of conventional and fast-spin-echo short inversion time inversion-recovery technique. Radiology 194:721-726, 1995.

30. Hilfiker P, Zanetti M, Debatin JF, et al: Fast spin-echo inversion-recovery imaging versus fast T2-weighted spin-echo imaging in bone marrow abnormalities. Invest Radiol 30:110-114, 1995.

31. Baker LL, Goodman SB, Perkash I, et al: Benign versus pathologic compression fractures of vertebral bodies: Assessment with conventional spin-echo, chemical-shift, and STIR MR imaging. Radiology 174:495-502, 1990.

32. Jones KM, Schwartz RB, Mantello MT, et al: Fast spin-echo MR in the detection of vertebral metastases: Comparison of three sequences. AJNR Am J Neuroradiol 15:401-407, 1994.

33. Enzmann DR, Rubin JB: Cervical spine: MR imaging with a partial flip angle, gradient-refocused pulse sequence: I. General considerations and disk disease. Radiology 166:467-472, 1988.

34. Enzmann DR, Rubin JB: Cervical spine: MR imaging with a partial flip angle, gradient-refocused pulse sequence: II. Spinal cord disease. Radiology 166:473-478, 1988.

35. Hedberg MC, Drayer BP, Flom RA, et al: Gradient echo (GRASS) MR imaging in cervical radiculopathy. AJR Am J Roentgenol 150: 683-689, 1988.

36. Kulkarni MV, Narayana PA, McArdle CB, et al: Cervical spine MR imaging using multislice gradient echo imaging: Comparison with cardiac gated spin echo. Magn Reson Imaging 6:517-525, 1988.

37. Tsuruda JS, Norman D, Dillon W, et al: Three-dimensional gradient-recalled MR imaging as a screening tool for the diagnosis of cervical radiculopathy. AJNR Am J Neuroradiol 10:1263-1271, 1989.

38. Russell EJ: Cervical disk disease. Radiology 177:313-325, 1990.

39. Carlson J, Crooks L, Ortendahl D, et al: Signal-to-noise ratio and section thickness in two-dimensional versus three-dimensional Fourier transform MR imaging. Radiology 166:266-270, 1988.

40. Frahm J, Haase A, Matthaei D: Rapid three-dimensional MR imaging using the FLASH technique. J Comput Assist Tomogr 10:363-368, 1986.

41. Frazzini VI, Kegetsu NJ, Johnson CE, et al: Internally stabilized spine: Optimal choice of frequency-encoding gradient direction during MR imaging minimizes susceptibility artifact from titanium vertebral body screws. Radiology 204:268-272, 1997.

42. Choi IS, Berenstein A: Surgical neuroangiography of the spine and spinal cord. Radiol Clin North Am 26:1131-1141, 1988.

43. Di Chiro G, Wener L: Angiography of the spinal cord: A review of contemporary techniques and applications. J Neurosurg 39:1-29, 1973.

44. Nelson PK, Setton A, Berenstein A: Vertebrospinal angiography in the evaluation of vertebral and spinal cord disease. Neuroimaging Clin North Am 6:589-605, 1996.

45. Anson JA, Spetzler RF: Interventional neuroradiology for spinal pathology. Clin Neurosurg 39:388-417, 1992.

46. Kendall BE, Logue V: Spinal epidural angiomatous malformations draining into intrathecal veins. Neuroradiology 13:181-189, 1977.

47. Gilbertson JR, Miller GM, Goldman MS, et al: Spinal dural arteriovenous fistulas: MR and myelographic findings. AJNR Am J Neuroradiol 16:2049-2057, 1995.

48. Masaryk T, Ross JS, Modic MT, et al: Radiculomeningeal vascular malformations of the spine: MR imaging. Radiology 164:845-849, 1987.

49. Merland JJ, Riche MC, Chiras J: Intraspinal extramedullary arteriovenous fistulae draining into the medullary veins. J Neuroradiol 7:271-320, 1980.

50. Backes WH, Nijenhuis RJ: Advances in spinal cord MR angiography. AJNR Am J Neuroradiol 29:619, 2008.

51. Bowen BC, Fraser K, Kochan JP, et al: Spinal dural arteriovenous fistulas: Evaluation with MR angiography. AJNR Am J Neuroradiol 16:2029, 1995.

52. Mull M, Nijenhuis RJ, Backes WH, et al: Value and limitations of contrast-enhanced MR angiography in spinal arteriovenous malformations and dural arteriovenous fistulas. AJNR Am J Neuroradiol 28:1249, 2007.

53. Lai PH, Weng MJ, Lee KW, et al: Multidetector CT angiography in diagnosing type I and IVA spinal vascular malformations. AJNR Am J Neuroradiol 27:813, 2006.

54. Yoshioka K, Niinuma H, Ohira A, et al: MR angiography and CT angiography of the artery of Adamkiewicz: Noninvasive preoperative assessment of thoracoabdominal aortic aneurysm. RadioGraphics 23:1215, 2003.

55. Guyer RD, Ohnmeiss DD: Lumbar discography. Position statement from the North American Spine Society Diagnostic and Therapeutic Committee. Spine 20:2048-2059, 1995.

56. Saal JS: General principles of diagnostic testing as related to painful lumbar spine disorders. Spine 27:2538-2545, 2002.

57. Bernard TN Jr: Don't discard discography. Radiology 162:285, 1987.

58. Milette P, Fontaine S, Lepanto L: Differentiating lumbar disc protrusions, disc bulges, and discs with normal contour but abnormal signal intensity: Magnetic resonance imaging with discographic correlations. Spine 24:44-53, 1999.

59. Bernard TNJ: Repeat lumbar spine surgery: Factors influencing outcome. Spine 18:2196-2200, 1993.

60. Bogduk N, Modic MT: Lumbar discography. Spine 21:402-404, 1996.

61. Holt EPJ: The question of lumbar discography. J Bone Joint Surg Am 50:720-726, 1968.

62. Modic MT: Diskography: Science and the ad hoc hypothesis. AJNR Am J Neuroradiol 21:241-242, 2000.

63. Mooney V: Lumbar discography. Spine 21:1479, 1996.

64. Simmons JW, Aprill CN, Dwyer AP, et al: A reassessment of Holt's data on: "The question of lumbar discography." Clin Orthop 237:120-124, 1988.

65. Smith SE, Darden BV, Rhyne AL, et al: Outcome of unoperated discogram-positive low back pain. Spine 20:1997-2000, 1995.

66. Walsh T, Weinstein J, Spratt K, et al: Lumbar discography in normal subjects. J Bone Joint Surg Am 72:1081-1088, 1990.

67. Tehranzadeh J: Discography 2000. Radiol Clin North Am 36:463-495, 1998.

68. Bosacco SJ: Lumbar discography: Redefining its role with intradiscal therapy. Orthopedics 9:399-401, 1986.

69. Simmons JW, McMillin JN, Emery SF, et al: Intradiscal steroids: A prospective double-blind clinical trial. Spine 17(Suppl):S172-S175, 1992.

70. Smith MD, Kim SS: A herniated cervical disc resulting from discography: An unusual complication. J Spinal Disord 3:392-394, 1990.

71. Schreck RI, Manion WL, Kambin P, et al: Nucleus pulposus pulmonary embolism: A case report. Spine 20:2463-2466, 1995.

72. Zeidman SM, Thompson K, Ducker TB: Complications of cervical discography: Analysis of 4400 diagnostic disc injections. Neurosurgery 37:414-417, 1995.

73. The International Center for Nephrogenic Fibrosing Dermopathy Research. Available at http://www.icnfdr.org/. Accessed January 19, 2008.

74. U.S. Food and Drug Administration. Available at http://www.fda.gov/cder/drug/InfoSheets/HCP/gcca_200705.htm. Accessed January 19, 2008.

75. Institute for Magnetic Resonance Safety, Education and Research. Available at http://www.imrser.org/. Accessed January 19, 2008.

76. Shellock FG, Spinazzi A: MRI safety update 2008: Part I. AJR Am J Roentgenol 191:1129, 2008.

77. Sadowski EA, Bennett LK, Chan MR, et al: Nephrogenic systemic fibrosis: Risk factors and incidence estimation. Radiology 243:148, 2007.

78. Kuo PH, Kanal E, Abu-Alfa AK, et al: Gadolinium-based MR contrast agents and nephrogenic systemic fibrosis. Radiology 242:647, 2007.

79. Broome DR, Girguis MS, Baron PW, et al: Gadodiamide-associated nephrogenic systemic fibrosis: Why radiologists should be concerned. AJR Am J Roentgenol 188:586, 2007.

80. Prince MR, Zhang H, Morris M, et al: Incidence of nephrogenic systemic fibrosis at two large medical centers. Radiology 248:807, 2008.

81. Deyo RA, Bigos SJ, Maravilla KR: Diagnostic imaging procedures for the lumbar spine. Ann Intern Med 111:865-867, 1989.

82. Long DM: Decision making in lumbar disc disease. Clin Neurosurg 39:36-51, 1992.

83. Fager CA: Identification and management of radiculopathy. Neurosurg Clin North Am 4:1-12, 1993.

84. Bell GR, Rothman RH: The conservative treatment of sciatica. Spine 9:54-56, 1984.

85. Bozzao A, Gallucci M, Masciocchi C, et al: Lumbar disc herniation: MR imaging assessment of natural history in patients treated without surgery. Radiology 185:135-141, 1992.

86. Bush K, Cowan N, Katz DE, et al: The natural history of sciatica associated with disc pathology. Spine 17:1205-1212, 1992.

87. Cowan N, Bush K, Katz D, et al: The natural history of sciatica: A prospective radiological study. Clin Radiol 46:7-12, 1992.

88. Delauche-Cavallier MC, Budet C, Laredo JD, et al: Lumbar disc herniation. Spine 17:927-933, 1992.

89. Saal JA, Saal JS: Nonoperative treatment of lumbar intervertebral disc with radiculopathy: An outcome study. Spine 14:431-437, 1989.

90. Modic MT, Steinberg PM, Ross JS, et al: Degenerative disk disease: Assessment of changes in vertebral body marrow with MRI. Radiology 166:193-199, 1988.

91. Ross JS, Modic MT, Masaryk TJ: Tears of the annulus fibrosus: Assessment with Gd-DTPA-enhanced MR imaging. AJNR Am J Neuroradiol 10:1251-1254, 1989.

92. Yu S, Sether LA, Ho SP, et al: Tears of the annulus fibrosus: Correlation between MR and pathologic findings in cadavers. AJNR Am J Neuroradiol 9:367-370, 1988.

93. Fardon DF, Milette PC; Combined Task Forces of the North American Spine Society, American Society of Spine Radiology,

and American Society of Neuroradiology: Nomenclature and classification of lumbar disc pathology. Recommendations of the Combined Task Forces of the North American Spine Society, American Society of Spine Radiology and American Society of Neuroradiology. Spine 26:E93-E113, 2001.

94. Amunosen T, Weber H, Lilleas F, et al: Lumbar spinal stenosis: Clinical and radiologic features. Spine 20:1178-1186, 1995.

95. Silbergleit R, Gebarski SS, Brungerg JA, et al: Lumbar synovial cysts: Correlation of myelographic, CT, MR and pathologic findings. AJNR Am J Neuroradiol 11:777-779, 1990.

96. Ulmer JL, Elster AD, Mathews VP, et al: Distinction between degenerative and isthmic spondylolisthesis on sagittal MR images: Importance of increased anteroposterior diameter of the spinal canal ("wide canal sign"). AJR Am J Roentgenol 163:411, 1994.

97. Jinkins JR, Matthes JC, Sener RN, et al: Spondylolysis, spondylolisthesis, and associated nerve root entrapment in the lumbosacral spine: MR evaluation. AJR Am J Roentgenol 159:799, 1992.

98. Pavlov H, Torg JS, Robie B, et al: Cervical spinal stenosis: Determination with vertebral body ratio method. Radiology 164:771-775, 1987.

99. Takahashi M, Yamashita Y, Sakamoto Y, et al: Chronic cervical cord compression: Clinical significance of increased signal intensity on MR images. Radiology 173:219-224, 1989.

100. Epstein NE: Ossification of the posterior longitudinal ligament: Diagnosis and surgical management. Neurosurg Q 2:223-241, 1992.

101. Hirabayashi K, Satomi K: Operative procedure and results of expansive open-door laminoplasty. Spine 13:870-876, 1988.

102. Hueftle MG, Modic MT, Ross JS, et al: Lumbar spine: Postoperative MR imaging with Gd-DTPA. Radiology 167:817-824, 1988.

103. Georgy BA, Hesselink JR, Middleton MS: Fat suppression contrast-enhanced MRI in the failed back surgery syndrome: A prospective study. Neuroradiology 37:51-57, 1995.

104. Burton CV: Causes of failure of surgery on the lumbar spine: Ten-year follow-up. Mt Sinai J Med 58:183-187, 1991.

105. Djukic S, Genant HK, Helms CA, et al: Magnetic resonance imaging of the postoperative lumbar spine. Radiol Clin North Am 28:341-360, 1990.

106. Johnson CE, Sze G: Benign lumbar arachnoiditis: MR imaging with gadopentetate dimeglumine. AJR Am J Roentgenol 155:873-880, 1990.

107. Ross JS, Masaryk TJ, Modic MT, et al: MR imaging of lumbar arachnoiditis. AJNR Am J Neuroradiol 8:885-892, 1987.

108. Lisbona R, Rosenthal L: Observations on the sequential use of Tc-99m phosphate complex and Ga-67 imaging in osteomyelitis, cellulitis, and septic arthritis. Radiology 123:123-129, 1977.

109. Gelman MI, Coleman RE, Stevens PM, et al: Radiography, radionuclide imaging, and arthrography in the evaluation of total hip and knee replacement. Radiology 128:677-682, 1978.

110. Weiss PPE, Mall JC, Hoffer PB, et al: Tc-99m methylene diphosphonate bone imaging in the evaluation of total hip prosthesis. Radiology 133:727-729, 1979.

111. McAfee JG, Samin A: In-111 labeled leukocytes: A review of problems in image interpretation. Radiology 155:221-229, 1985.

112. Golimbu C, Firooznia H, Rafii M: CT of osteomyelitis of the spine. AJR Am J Roentgenol 142:159-163, 1984.

113. Jeffrey RB, Callen PW, Federle MP: Computed tomography of psoas abscesses. J Comput Assist Tomogr 4:639-641, 1980.

114. Modic MT, Feiglin DH, Piraino DW, et al: Vertebral osteomyelitis: assessment using MR. Radiology 157:157-166, 1985.

115. Modic MT, Weinstein MA, Pavlicek W, et al: Nuclear magnetic resonance imaging of the spine. Radiology 148:757-762, 1983.

116. deRoos A, Van Meerten EL, Bloem JL, et al: MRI of tuberculosis spondylitis. AJR Am J Roentgenol 146:79-82, 1986.

117. Dagirmanjian A, Schils J, Modic MT: Vertebral osteomyelitis revisited. Radiology 189(Suppl P):193, 1993.

118. Boden SD, Davis DO, Dina TS, et al: Postoperative diskitis: Distinguishing early MR imaging findings from normal postoperative disk space changes. Radiology 184:765-771, 1992.

119. Rankin RM, Flothow PG: Pyogenic infection of the spinal epidural space. West J Surg Obstet Gynecol 54:320-323, 1946.

120. Baker AS, Ojemann RG, Swartz MN, et al: Spinal epidural abscess. N Engl J Med 293:463-468, 1975.

121. Browder J, Meyers R: Pyogenic infections of the spinal epidural space. Surgery 10:296-308, 1941.

122. Angtuaco EJC, McConnell JR, Chadduck WM, et al: MR imaging of spinal epidural sepsis. AJNR Am J Neuroradiol 8:879-883, 1987.

123. Tins BJ, Cassar-Pullicino VN, Lalam RK: Magnetic resonance imaging of spinal infection. Top Magn Reson Imaging 18:213-222, 2007.

124. Post MJD, Quencer RM, Montalvo BM, et al: Spinal infection: Evaluation with MR imaging and intraoperative US. Radiology 169:765-771, 1988.

125. Post MJD, Sze G, Quencer RM, et al: Gadolinium-enhanced MR in spinal infection. J Comput Assist Tomogr 14:721-729, 1990.

126. Rawlings CE, Giangaspero F, Burger PC, et al: Ependymomas: A clinicopathologic study. Surg Neurol 29:271, 1988.

127. Kahan H, Sklar EM, Post MJ, et al: MR characteristics of histopathologic subtypes of spinal ependymoma. AJNR Am J Neuroradiol 17:143-150, 1996.

128. Wippold FJ II, Smirniotopoulos JG, Moran CJ, et al: MR Imaging of myxopapillary ependymoma: Findings and value of determining extent of tumor and its relation to intraspinal structures. AJR Am J Roentgenol 165:1263-1267, 1995.

129. Nemoto Y, Inove Y, Tashiro T, et al: Intramedullary spinal cord tumors: Significance of associated hemorrhage at MR imaging. Radiology 82:793, 1992.

130. Shen W-C, Ho Y-J, Lee S-K, et al: Ependymoma of the cauda equina presenting with subarachnoid hemorrhage. AJNR Am J Neuroradiol 14:399, 1993.

131. Choyke PL, Glenn GM, Walther MM, et al: von Hippel-Lindau disease: Genetic, clinical, and imaging features. Radiology 194:629-642, 1995.

132. Ho VB, Smirniotopoulos JG, Murphy FM, et al: Radiologic-pathologic correlation: Hemangioblastoma. AJNR Am J Neuroradiol 13:1343-1352, 1992.

133. Hoff DJ, Tampieri D, Just N: Imaging of spinal cord hemangioblastomas. Can Assoc Radiol J 44:377-383, 1993.

134. Murota T, Symon L: Surgical management of hemangioblastoma of the spinal cord: A report of 18 cases. Neurosurgery 25:699-707, 1989.

135. Sze G, Krol G, Zimmerman RD, et al: Intramedullary disease of the spine: Diagnosis using gadolinium-DTPA-enhanced MR imaging. AJR Am J Roentgenol 151:1193-1204, 1988.

136. Yu JS, Short MP, Schumacher J, et al: Intramedullary hemorrhage in spinal cord hemangioblastoma: Report of two cases. J Neurosurg 81:937-940, 1994.

137. Tognetti F, Lanzino G, Calbucci F: Metastases of the spinal cord from remote neoplasms: Study of five cases. Surg Neurol 30:220-227, 1988.

138. Winkelman MD, Adelstein DJ, Karlins NL: Intramedullary spinal cord metastasis: Diagnostic and therapeutic considerations. Arch Neurol 44:526-531, 1987.

139. Hamilton MG, Tranmer BI, Hagen NA: Supratentorial glioblastoma with spinal cord intramedullary metastasis. Can J Neurol Sci 20:65-68, 1993.

140. DeAngelis LM: Current diagnosis and treatment of leptomeningeal metastasis. J Neurooncol 38:245-252, 1998.

141. McCormick PC, Post KD, Stein BM: Intradural extramedullary tumors in adults. Neurosurg Clin North Am 1:591, 1990.

142. Halliday AL, Sobel RA, Martuza RL: Benign spinal nerve sheath tumors: Their occurrence sporadically and in neurofibromatosis types 1 and 2. J Neurosurg 74:248, 1991.

143. Edelhoff JC, Bates DJ, Ross JS, et al: Spinal MR findings in neurofibromatosis type 1 and 2. AJNR Am J Neuroradiol 13:1071, 1992.

144. Levy WJ, Bay J, Donn D: Spinal cord meningioma. J Neurosurg 57:804, 1982.

145. Roux FX, Nataf F, Pinaudeau M, et al: Intraspinal meningiomas: Review of 54 cases with discussion of poor prognosis factors and modern therapeutic management. Surg Neurol 46:458-463, 1996.

146. Sevick RJ: Cervical spine tumors. Neuroimaging Clin North Am 5:385-400, 1995.

147. Yousem DM, Patrone PM, Grossman RI: Leptomeningeal metastases: MR evaluation. J Comput Assist Tomogr 14:255, 1990.

148. Sze G, Abramson A, Krol G, et al: Gadolinium-DTPA: Malignant extradural spinal tumors. Radiology 67:217, 1988.

149. Smolen WR, Godersky JC, Knutzon RK, et al: The role of MR imaging in evaluating metastatic spinal disease. AJNR Am J Neuroradiol 8:901, 1987.

150. Carmody RF, Yang PJ, Seeley GW, et al: Spinal cord compression due to metastatic disease: Diagnosis with MR imaging versus myelography. Radiology 173:225, 1989.

151. Nabors MW, Pait TG, Byrd EB, et al: Updated assessment and current classification of spinal meningeal cysts. J Neurosurg 68:366-377, 1988.

152. Kronborg O: Extradural spinal cysts: A literature survey and a case of multiple extradural cysts. Dan Med Bull 14:46-48, 1967.

153. Rothman RH, Jacobs SR, Appleman W: Spinal extradural cysts: A report of five cases. Clin Orthop 71:186-192, 1970.

154. Hoffman J, Schriger D, Mower W, et al: Low risk criteria for cervical spine radiography in blunt trauma: A prospective study. Ann Emerg Med 21:1454, 1992.

155. Roberge R, Wears R, Kelly M: Selective application of cervical spine radiography in alert victims of blunt trauma: A prospective study. J Trauma 28:784, 1988.

156. Cornelius RS, Leach JL: Imaging evaluation of cervical spine trauma. Neuroimaging Clin North Am 5:451-463, 1995.

157. Schwartz ED, Flanders AE (eds): Spinal Trauma: Imaging, Diagnosis, and Management. Philadelphia, Lippincott Williams & Wilkins, 2007.

158. Kaye J, Nance E: Cervical spine trauma. Orthop Clin North Am 21:449, 1990.

159. Schleehauf K, Ross S, Civil I, et al: Computed tomography in the initial evaluation of the cervical spine. Ann Emerg Med 18:815, 1989.

160. Kirshenbaum K, Nadimpalli S, Fantus R, et al: Unsuspected upper cervical spine fractures associated with significant head trauma: Role of CT. J Emerg Med 8:183, 1990.

161. Lindsey R, Diliberti T, Doherty B, et al: Efficacy of radiographic evaluation of the cervical spine in emergency situations. South Med J 86:1253, 1993.

162. Schaefer D, Flanders A, Osterholm J, et al: Prognostic significance of magnetic resonance imaging in the acute phase of cervical spine injury. J Neurosurg 76:218, 1992.

163. Flanders AE, Spettell CM, Tartaglino LM, et al: Forecasting motor recovery after cervical spinal cord injury: Value of MR imaging. Radiology 201:649-655, 1996.

164. Kulkarni M, Bondurant F, Rose S, et al: 1.5T Magnetic resonance imaging of acute spinal trauma. RadioGraphics 8:1059, 1988.

165. Davis S, Teresi L, Bradley W, et al: Cervical spine hyperextension injuries: MR findings. Radiology 180:245, 1991.

166. Hall A, Wagle V, Raycroft J, et al: Magnetic resonance imaging in cervical spine trauma. J Trauma 34:21, 1993.

167. Silberstein M, Tress B, Hennessy O: Prevertebral swelling in cervical spine injury: Identification of ligament injury with magnetic resonance imaging. Clin Radiol 46:318, 1992.

168. Roab R: International classification of spine injuries. Paraplegia 10:78, 1972.

169. Holdsworth F: Fractures, dislocations, and fracture-dislocations of the spine. J Bone Joint Surg Am 52:1534, 1970.

170. Tarr RW, Drolshagen LF, Kerner TC, et al: MR imaging of recent spinal trauma. J Comput Assist Tomogr 11:412, 1987.

171. Chance GQ: Note on a type of flexion fracture of the spine. Br J Radiol 21:452, 1948.

172. Smith WS, Kaufer H: Patterns and mechanisms of lumbar injuries associated with lap seat belts. J Bone Joint Surg Am 52:239, 1969.

173. Foo D, Rossier AB: Preoperative neurological status in predicting surgical outcome of spinal epidural hematomas. Surg Neurol 15:389-401, 1981.

174. Beatty RM, Winston KR: Spontaneous epidural hematoma. J Neurosurg 61:143-148, 1984.

SECTION II

175. Avrahami E, Tadmor R, Ram Z, et al: MR demonstration of spontaneous acute epidural hematoma of the thoracic spine. Neuroradiology 31:90-92, 1989.

176. Goldman P, Kulkarni M, MacDugall DJ, et al: Traumatic epidural hematoma of the cervical spine: Diagnosis with magnetic resonance imaging. Radiology 170:589-591, 1989.

177. Donovan-Post MJ, Becerra JL, Madsen PW, et al: Acute spinal subdural hematoma: MR and CT findings with pathologic correlates. AJNR Am J Neuroradiol 15:1895-1905, 1994.

178. Johnson PJ, Hahn F, McConnell J, et al: The importance of MRI findings for the diagnosis of nontraumatic lumbar subacute subdural haematomas. Acta Neurochir 113:186-188, 1991.

179. Levy JM: Spontaneous lumbar subdural hematoma. AJNR Am J Neuroradiol 11:780-781, 1990.

13 CHAPTER

The Electrodiagnostic Examination

Jinny Tavee, MD
Kerry H. Levin, MD

The electrodiagnostic examination comprises two parts: nerve conduction studies (NCS) and needle electrode examination (NEE). Together, they assess the peripheral sensory and motor nervous system. Sensory NCS assess the integrity of dorsal root ganglion (DRG) cells (usually residing within the intervertebral foramina), their axonal projections within mixed sensory and motor nerve trunks, and arborizations into individual nerve fibers innervating sensory organs subserving primarily vibration and proprioception. Motor NCS assess the integrity of anterior horn cells (in the anterior region of the spinal cord), their axonal projections within pure motor or mixed nerve trunks, arborizations into individual motor nerve fibers, the neuromuscular junctions, and attached muscle fibers.

The electrodiagnostic examination is best conceptualized as an extension of the neurologic examination of the peripheral nervous system. In the setting of abnormalities identified in the neurologic history and examination, the electrodiagnostic examination can be valuable in (1) confirming the clinical impression, (2) investigating the presence of other conditions in the differential diagnosis, and (3) localizing the precise site of a focal nerve trunk lesion not clearly defined on clinical examination.

The electrodiagnostic examination can discriminate between the two main types of pathologic responses that can affect nerve fibers: axon loss (neurotmesis and axonotmesis) and demyelinating conduction block (neurapraxia). In cases of axon loss, the electrodiagnostic examination has the potential of discriminating acute, subacute, and chronic nerve lesions. It can identify early evidence of reinnervation and can quantitatively track the reinnervation process over weeks to months. In the setting of diffuse signs and symptoms, the electrodiagnostic examination can discriminate among generalized sensory and motor peripheral polyneuropathy, myopathy, and diffuse motor axon loss processes such as motor neuron disease.

A well-executed electrodiagnostic examination can confirm or refute the presumptive diagnosis and can provide a screening assessment for other peripheral nerve and muscle conditions that could reasonably be the cause of the patient's symptoms. In that way, the electrodiagnostic examination should be thought of as an electrodiagnostic consultation and not solely a test to rule in a specific diagnosis. Qualified electrodiagnostic consultants usually are board certified in electrodiagnosis, clinical neurophysiology, or neuromuscular medicine, having completed an approved training program and having shown competence by examination. The electrodiagnostic examination must be interpreted by the individual performing the study because there is no single machine-generated tracing (as would be the case for an electrocardiogram or electroencephalogram) that can be interpreted simply by reviewing data collected elsewhere.

Pathophysiology

The clinical practice of electrodiagnosis is based on numerous precepts that are derived from the pathophysiology of nerve and muscle function. These provide the basic principles that define the clinical utility and limits of this procedure.

Regardless of etiology, most focal nerve lesions—including lesions at the root level—result in either *axon loss* or *demyelination*. Axon loss produces nerve transmission failure along the affected fibers, whereas focal demyelination causes either conduction block or conduction slowing at the lesion site, depending on its severity. One fundamental difference between these two types of lesions is that focal demyelination remains localized and does not materially affect the segments of the axon proximal or distal to the lesion. In contrast, an axon loss lesion results in wallerian degeneration that eventually involves the entire course of the nerve affected.

Because axon loss and demyelinating conduction block stop nerve impulse transmission across the lesion site rather than merely slowing it, both can result in clinical weakness and sensory abnormalities whenever they affect a sufficient number of motor and sensory axons. Demyelinating conduction slowing does not affect muscle strength, however. This is because all of the nerve impulses ultimately reach their destination, although slightly later in time than they normally would.[1]

The electrodiagnostic examination assesses the integrity of large sensory and motor nerve fibers because the electrical

TYPES OF NCS

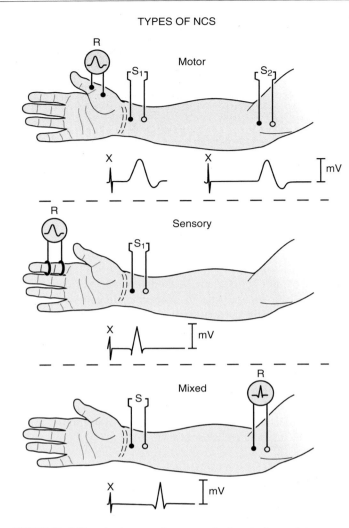

FIGURE 13–1 Three basic types of nerve conduction studies: motor, sensory, and mixed (S_1 and S_2 are stimulation sites, whereas R is the recording site; X overlies the shock artifact.) (Modified from Isle M, Krauss G, Levin K, et al: Electromyography/Electroencephalography. Redford, WA, Spacelabs Medical, 1993, p 4.)

fields generated by small nerve fibers are too small to reach the recording electrodes in routine studies. For this reason, pain alone cannot be assessed because that sensory modality is mediated through small C-type nerve fibers. When pain is associated with large nerve fiber dysfunction, such as weakness, electrodiagnostic testing is more valuable.

General Concepts of Electrodiagnostic Examination

Nerve Conduction Studies

NCS are the first component of the electrodiagnostic examination. During NCS, a peripheral nerve is stimulated resulting in an electrical response generated directly by the nerve itself (as in a sensory response) or the muscle it innervates (as in a motor response). The duration and intensity of the stimulus are gradually increased until a maximal response is generated.

These responses are recorded using surface electrodes placed over the skin and then analyzed. During each study, valuable information is produced regarding the number of functioning nerve fibers, the speed of conduction along those fibers, and their relative rates of conduction.

Three basic types of NCS are available: motor, sensory, and mixed (Fig. 13–1). Motor and sensory NCS are generally performed on every patient. Mixed NCS are typically used in the evaluation of specific disorders, such as carpal tunnel syndrome, and are of limited value in the evaluation of spine-related nerve pathology. NCS protocols vary depending on the diagnosis in question and can be tailored to help exclude other diagnoses in the differential. Most electrodiagnostic laboratories have a routine protocol, however, for a general study of the upper extremity (Table 13–1) and lower extremity (Table 13–2).

Motor Nerve Conduction Studies

For motor NCS, the recording electrode is placed over the muscle belly, and the reference electrode is affixed over the tendon. The nerve supplying that muscle is stimulated, and the resulting motor nerve response is a compound muscle action potential (CMAP), a biphasic waveform that represents summated muscle fiber action potentials (Fig. 13–2). In routine motor NCS, small muscles of the hand and feet serve as recording muscles, and the nerves supplying them are stimulated at two separate points along their course. For the upper extremity, the wrist (distal) and elbow (proximal) are used as stimulation sites, and for the lower extremity, the ankle (distal) and knee (proximal) are used as stimulation sites.

Numerous parameters are assessed with each CMAP obtained, including amplitude, latency, and conduction velocity (Fig. 13–3). The CMAP *amplitude* represents the number of nerve fibers that responded to the stimulus and are capable of conducting impulses to the recorded muscle.[1,2] It is measured from baseline to negative peak (negative being up) and reported in millivolts. The *latency* is the time interval between the instant the nerve was stimulated and the onset of CMAPs; these are reported in milliseconds. The *conduction velocity* is the speed of transmission over the fastest conducting nerve fibers assessed and is reported in meters per second. Conduction velocities are calculated by dividing the distance traveled along a nerve segment (as determined by surface measurements) by the latency difference between the responses to proximal and distal stimulation. Normal conduction velocity in the upper limb is greater than 50 m/sec; in the lower limb, it is greater than 40 m/sec.

Sensory Nerve Conduction Studies

For sensory NCS, a sensory nerve or the sensory component of a mixed nerve is stimulated at one point with recording electrodes placed distally, usually on the fingers or on the ankle with routine studies. This stimulation results in a sensory nerve action potential (SNAP), which is a biphasic or triphasic waveform that represents summated nerve action potentials. In contrast to CMAPs, which are generated by muscle fibers

$$\frac{\text{Distance (cm)}}{\text{Proxi. lat.} - \text{Dist. lat. (ms)}} = \text{CV (m/s)}$$

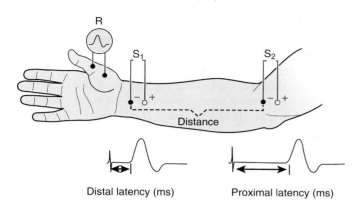

Distal latency (ms)   Proximal latency (ms)

FIGURE 13–2 Various components of motor nerve conduction study. (The median nerve is being assessed.) (Modified from Isley M, Krauss G, Levin K, et al: Electromyography/Electroencephalography. Redford, WA, Spacelabs Medical, 1993, p 40.)

MOTOR NERVE CONDUCTION STUDY

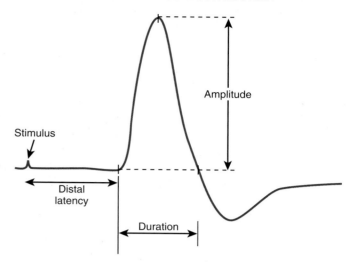

FIGURE 13–3 Compound muscle action potential (CMAP). Distal latency is measured from stimulus to onset of negative response. Amplitude is measured from baseline to negative peak.

and are measured in millivolts, SNAPs are generated directly by the nerve fibers. SNAPs are 100 times smaller and are measured in microvolts. Generally, only two sensory NCS measurements are reported: (1) the *amplitude,* which is the height of the response measured from baseline to negative peak and represents the number of sensory axons that depolarize, and (2) the *peak latency,* which is the time interval between the moment the nerve was stimulated and the negative peak of the response, reported in milliseconds (see Fig. 13–3).[1]

Late Responses (H Responses and F Waves)

Two special studies, the H response and the F wave, are NCS used to measure the time in which nerve impulses travel proximally to the spinal cord along the peripheral nerve trunk and then back down the limb to the recorded muscle after distal stimulation of the nerve. Because the potentials seen with both of these techniques are much delayed after nerve stimulation

compared with potentials seen with standard NCS, they are referred to as late responses.

The *H response* is the electrophysiologic correlate of the Achilles tendon reflex and is named after Hoffmann, who first described it in 1918. To obtain the H response, the tibial nerve is stimulated in the popliteal fossa using low voltage to activate sensory fibers (as opposed to motor fibers), which carry the nerve impulse proximally to the spinal cord (Fig. 13–4). The fibers synapse there with motor neuron cells to complete a monosynaptic reflex arc. The nerve impulse travels down the motor efferent nerve to the gastrocnemius where the recording electrode captures the response. Although the amplitude and the latency of the H response are analyzed, the amplitude is more reliable for diagnostic purposes in the authors' laboratory.

The *F wave* was first described by Magladery and McDougall in 1950 and was named the F wave because it

TABLE 13–1 Nerve Conduction Studies in the Upper Limb	
Motor	**Sensory**
Standard	
Median: thenar (C8, <u>T1</u>)	Median: index (C6, <u>C7</u>)
Ulnar: hypothenar (<u>C8</u>, T1)	Ulnar: fifth (C8)
Nonstandard	
Ulnar: first dorsal interosseus (*C8*, T1)	Median: thumb (C6)
Radial: extensor indicis proprius (C8)	Median: middle (C7)
Radial: brachioradialis (<u>C5</u>, <u>C6</u>)	Ulnar: hand dorsum (C8)
Musculocutaneous: biceps (C5, <u>C6</u>)	Radial: thumb base (<u>C6</u>, <u>C7</u>)
Axillary: deltoid (<u>C5</u>, C6)	Lateral antebrachial cutaneous: forearm (C6)
	Medial antebrachial cutaneous: forearm (T1)

Note: On each line, the nerve being studied is listed first, followed after the colon by the recording site and then, in parentheses, the root innervation (motor) or derivation (sensory). <u>Underlined root</u> provides major innervation.

TABLE 13–2 Nerve Conduction Studies in the Lower Limb	
Motor	**Sensory**
Standard	
Peroneal: extensor digitorum brevis (L5-S1)	Sural: lateral ankle (S1)
Tibial: abductor hallucis (S1)	
Nonstandard	
Peroneal: tibialis anterior (L5)	Superficial peroneal sensory: dorsum ankle (L5)
Tibial: abductor digiti quinti pedis (S1)	Saphenous: medial ankle (L4)†
Tibial: gastrocnemii (S1)*	Lateral femoral cutaneous: lateral thigh (L3, L4)†
Femoral: quadriceps (L3, L4)	

Note: On each line, the nerve being studied is listed first, followed after the colon by the recording site and then, in parentheses, the root innervation (motor) or derivation (sensory).
*M component of H response.
†Studies technically difficult to perform.

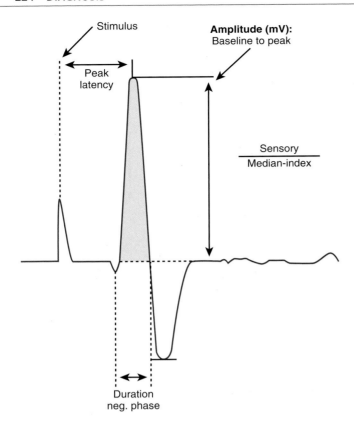

FIGURE 13–4 Sensory nerve action potential (SNAP). Peak latency is measured to onset of negative phase. Amplitude is measured from baseline to negative peak.

was first recorded from muscles in the foot. In contrast to H responses, F waves are not a component of a reflex arc because the nerve impulses recorded travel only along motor axons. F waves are produced when, after distal motor nerve stimulation, some of the impulses passing antidromically up the motor axons cause a few of the motor cell bodies in the anterior horns to backfire; the resulting nerve impulses travel back down the motor axons to produce submaximal muscle activations that are recorded several milliseconds after the initial CMAP as F waves. Several consecutive responses from the same muscle are elicited, and the shortest latency time usually is used for diagnosis. Also in contrast to H responses, F waves can be elicited with any of the standard motor NCS with consistency.

Needle Electrode Examination

NEE is the second and oldest component of the basic electrodiagnostic examination. During this procedure, a recording needle electrode is inserted into various muscles, and the electrical activity being generated in them is evaluated on a visual and audio display system via a differential amplifier. NEE records activity in muscle (1) at rest during needle insertion, (2) at rest without needle movement, and (3) during voluntary muscle activation.

Insertional Phase

During the *insertional phase,* the electrical activity resulting from needle movement in a relaxed muscle is evaluated. In a normal muscle, each needle insertion and advancement injures a few individual muscle fibers, which generate a small burst of electrical potentials called *insertional activity.* These electrical potentials prove that the needle electrode is in a viable muscle because they are not seen if it is in subcutaneous tissue, fat, or severely fibrotic muscle. In the context of peripheral nerve fiber lesions, if the NEE is performed on a partially denervated muscle a few days before spontaneous fibrillation potentials appear (see later), the insertional activity becomes abnormal, in that unsustained trains of positive sharp waves, called *insertional positive sharp waves,* are seen.

At-Rest Phase

During the *at-rest phase,* electrical silence ordinarily is noted. Various types of spontaneous activity may appear, however, with neuromuscular pathology. Only three of these are relevant to spine-related nerve disease: fibrillation potentials, fasciculation potentials, and complex repetitive discharges.[2-4]

Fibrillation potentials are spontaneous, usually regularly firing action potentials of individual muscle fibers. Although nonspecific in that they can be seen with neuropathic and myopathic disorders, their presence indicates denervation. Fibrillation potentials typically appear in the form of a biphasic spike if the tip of the recording needle electrode is near the denervated muscle fiber; alternatively, they may appear as a positive sharp wave if the needle has injured the abnormal muscle fiber. In the setting of nerve lesions, fibrillation potentials are not present at the onset of motor axon loss. Instead, they are first seen 14 to 35 days after axon degeneration has been initiated; the most widely cited average time is 21 days. When established, fibrillation potentials persist until the denervated muscle fibers generating them either reinnervate or degenerate for lack of a nerve supply; the latter usually occurs 18 to 24 months after the initial nerve fiber injury.

Fibrillation potentials are the most reliable and objective manifestation of active or recent motor axon loss. They can be neither produced nor abolished voluntarily by the patient. They are very sensitive indicators of such loss because the degeneration of a single motor axon can result in hundreds of individual muscle fibers fibrillating within a given muscle, depending on the innervation ratio of the latter. Fibrillation potentials objectively can show that motor axon loss has occurred, when the lesion is far too mild in degree to produce clinical muscle weakness, atrophy, or loss of CMAP amplitude on motor NCS.[3] Showing fibrillation potentials in a myotome distribution has been the principal method of identifying root lesions in the electrodiagnostic laboratory for more than half a century.[5,6]

Fasciculation potentials are spontaneous action potentials of an individual motor unit. In contrast to fibrillation potentials, they are indicative of motor unit *irritation,* rather than denervation; only intact motor unit potentials (MUPs) can generate them. They are encountered far less often than fibrillation potentials, being restricted essentially to radiculopathies, anterior horn cell disorders, radiation-induced plexopathies, a few entrapment neuropathies, polyneuropathies, and, most often, the syndrome of generalized benign fasciculations.

Complex repetitive discharges are produced when a single muscle fiber is depolarized and that depolarization is spread by ephaptic transmission to adjacent muscle fibers, which reactivate the initial muscle fiber. A recurrent cycle of firing is established. These potentials have a bizarre configuration and fire at high frequency. For many years, they were known as *bizarre high-frequency discharges*. Although they are abnormal, they are nonspecific, being seen with neuropathic and myopathic disorders. Generally, they appear when there is grouped atrophy (i.e., denervation, reinnervation, and subsequent denervation) and are evidence of chronicity. Although these potentials are not helpful in localization, they are frequently encountered on NEE of the cervical paraspinal muscles in patients with chronic cervical root lesions.[3]

Activation Phase

After the muscle is evaluated at rest, the patient is asked to contract the muscle. This contraction results in the generation of MUPs, which represent the summated electrical activity produced by contracting muscle fibers of a single motor unit. MUPs are assessed in regard to their recruitment pattern and appearance.

Recruitment

Recruitment of MUPs refers to the orderly increase in number and firing rate of activated motor units as force is increased during contraction of muscle. On initial activation of the muscle with minimal force, a single motor unit fires at its basal rate of 5 to 10 Hz. As the force is increased, additional units are recruited, and the firing rate gradually increases by 5 Hz with each additional unit—up to 20 to 30 Hz. With progressively increasing force, spatial and temporal recruitment occurs, resulting in a full interference pattern in which the screen is obscured by the firing patterns of several MUPs.

Reduced MUP recruitment, also known as a *neurogenic MUP firing pattern,* is observed whenever numerous motor units in the muscle being sampled cannot be activated on maximal effort because either conduction block or axon loss affects their axons. The fewer MUPs seen on maximal effort, the weaker the muscle is clinically. MUPs that are capable of firing are noted to do so in decreased numbers and often faster than their basal firing rate of 5 to 10 Hz.[3,7] The rapid rate of firing of the still functioning motor units is important because, similar to fibrillation potentials, it is unequivocal evidence of involuntary interruption of motor axon impulse transmission. Conversely, if the muscle was weak because of an upper motor neuron lesion or because voluntary effort was simply submaximal (e.g., because of malingering or pain on activation), incomplete MUP activation would be seen—that is, MUPs would fire in equally decreased numbers but at a *slow to moderate rate.*

Morphology

The amplitude, duration, and configuration of MUPs are important morphologic characteristics that are assessed during the activation phase. Together, these features reflect the number and size of muscle fibers within a motor unit and their ability to fire in synchrony. Patient age, technical details (e.g., filter setting, type of needle used), and the specific muscle being examined are some of the factors that affect the appearance of MUPs. Based on quantitative analyses, normal ranges for MUP morphology are available for comparison, which vary depending on the patient age and proximity of the muscle to the trunk. A normal MUP has a triphasic waveform appearance.

With chronic nerve lesions, the process of reinnervation of denervated muscle fibers can occur as the result of regeneration of the nerve trunk from the point of nerve transection or (when the nerve transection is not total) by collateral nerve branch sprouting from remaining intact nerve fibers close to the denervated muscle fibers. The latter process is much faster because nerve fiber regeneration occurs at the rate of about 1 mm/day. On NEE, manifestations of reinnervation include resolution of fibrillation potentials; return of activation of motor unit action potentials with voluntary muscle contraction; and appearance of polyphasic, enlarged (so-called neurogenic) motor unit action potentials, reflecting the increased number of muscle fibers attached to surviving nerve fibers owing to collateral sprouting.

Chronic neurogenic MUP changes generally develop about 4 to 6 months after an axon loss injury has occurred because it takes this much time for such configurational remodeling to occur. After chronic neurogenic MUP changes develop, they can persist indefinitely. With many remote, proximal neurogenic lesions (e.g., radiculopathies and particularly poliomyelitis), they are the sole electrical residuals detected during the entire electrodiagnostic examination.[3,7,8]

Electrodiagnostic Findings in Radiculopathy

The electrodiagnostic examination has been used to assess patients with possible radiculopathies for more than 50 years. Root lesions were one of the first focal peripheral nerve fiber disorders for which the diagnostic utility of NEE was shown.[5,6] For many years, lumbosacral radiculopathies were the most common reason for referral to the electrodiagnostic laboratory.[9,10] Although several other electrodiagnostic procedures have been introduced over the past half-century, NEE remains the mainstay for diagnosing radiculopathies. The amplitudes of motor NCS are also helpful when root damage is severe, extensive, or both.[8,9]

Radiculopathies are most commonly caused by nerve root compression secondary to degenerative spine changes, disc herniation, or rupture. The type of nerve pathology at the lesion site depends on the nature of the injury and degree of nerve compression. When the injury results in significant

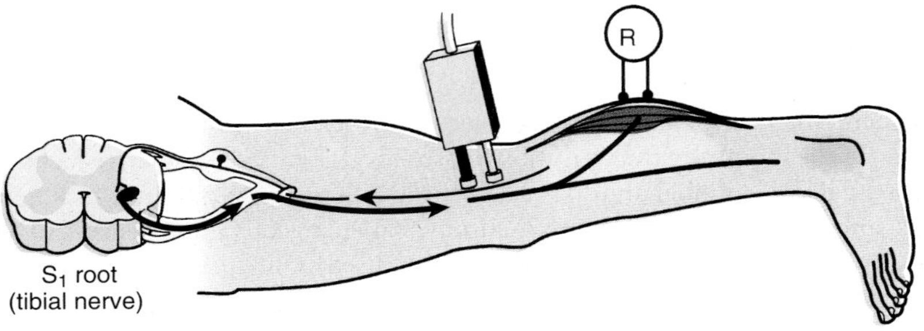

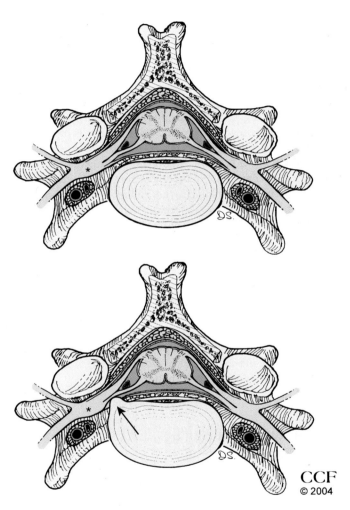

S₁ root
(tibial nerve)

FIGURE 13–5 Standard lower limb H response. **A,** With minimal stimulus strength, only the H wave is elicited. **B,** As stimulation strength increases, the M wave appears and becomes progressively larger, while the H wave progressively loses amplitude.

FIGURE 13–6 A and **B,** Cross-sectional views of cervical region, showing relationship of dorsal root ganglia (*asterisk*) to surrounding structures (**A**) and usual site of disc herniation (*arrow*) (**B**). Preganglionic sensory root fibers usually are compromised (**B**).

motor axon loss, NEE shows numerous abnormalities, including the presence of fibrillation potentials in corresponding myotomes. Demyelinating conduction block may also be inferred by findings on the electrodiagnostic examination. In many cases of nerve root disease, the electrodiagnostic examination can provide invaluable information regarding localization, severity, age of the lesion, and nerve pathophysiology.

Nerve Conduction Studies

Routine Studies

Axon loss occurs when the axon is disconnected from its cell body. The motor cell body (anterior horn cell) resides in the anterior zone of the spinal cord; the sensory cell body (DRG) resides outside the spinal cord, either within individual intervertebral foramina or within the spinal canal (intradural and intra-arachnoid) (Fig. 13–5). A disc protrusion causing severe compression of a motor and sensory nerve root within the spinal canal disconnects the anterior horn cell from its motor axon, but if the DRG is distal to the point of compression, the extra spinal sensory axons remain connected to their DRG and do not undergo degeneration (Fig. 13–6). In that setting, motor NCS show amplitude loss, but sensory NCS are normal despite marked clinical sensory impairment with few exceptions.

One exception is seen with nerve root pathology that extends beyond the intraspinal canal. A mass lesion (e.g., meningioma) or infiltrative process (e.g., malignancy, inflammatory cause, or infection) that progresses distally along the nerve root to involve the DRG can result in decreased SNAP amplitudes. The other exception is when the DRG resides inside the intraspinal canal, proximal to the intervertebral foramina; this has been found to occur in the lumbosacral region. Based on cadaveric, radiographic, and magnetic resonance imaging (MRI) studies, 3% of L3 and L4 DRG are intraspinal, about 11% to 38% of L5 DRG are intraspinal, and 71% of S1 DRG are intraspinal.[11] As a result, root lesions in the lower spine, particularly lesions involving the L5 root, can affect the corresponding SNAP amplitude, which in the case of an L5 lesion is the superficial peroneal SNAP (see later). SNAP peak latency and nerve conduction velocity are never involved in radiculopathy, however.

The CMAP amplitude is the only portion of motor NCS that may be significantly affected in radiculopathy. Because it is a measure of the number of viable, conducting nerve fibers, the CMAP amplitude can be decreased with severe motor axon loss lesions. The ulnar CMAP amplitude would be reduced in a severe C8 radiculopathy. In chronic lesions, reinnervation changes such as collateral sprouting can contribute to the CMAP amplitude and may lead to normal or near-normal values over time.

In many cases, motor NCS remain relatively unaffected in radiculopathies for two reasons. First, most radiculopathies result in only partial nerve injuries. For the CMAP amplitude to be significantly reduced on motor NCS, about half of the motor axons within the peripheral nerve trunk need to be lost or injured. Second, the myotomes of the affected nerve root must be accessible to stimulation and recording. The ulnar-innervated hand muscles may be examined for a C8 radiculopathy, and the biceps and deltoids are available for assessing a C5 radiculopathy. Muscles innervated by C6 and C7 nerve roots cannot be reliably examined with routine motor NCS, however, owing to technical factors and overlap in innervation.

Late Responses

Although the H response and F wave are theoretically helpful in the evaluation of the damaged proximal nerve root segment, there are technical limitations to each procedure that can hamper their utility in the evaluation of a radiculopathy.[7,9] Because the H response is elicited by stimulating the tibial nerve in the popliteal fossa while recording from the gastrocnemius/soleus muscle group as described previously, it is highly sensitive and very useful in the evaluation of S1 radiculopathy. In axon loss lesions affecting the S1 nerve root, the amplitude may be either reduced or absent. The normal value of the H amplitude as defined by the authors' electrodiagnostic laboratory is 1 mV, with abnormal values being either less than 1 mV or reduced by 50% compared with the contralateral response. Additionally, the H response may become abnormal at the onset of nerve root injury and remain so until the injury is resolved or may remain abnormal despite resolution of clinical symptoms.[7]

A major limitation of the H responses is that they are frequently absent bilaterally in patients older than 60 years; in patients with polyneuropathies; and in patients who have had lumbar laminectomies, even when the S1 roots reportedly were not within the operative field. Also, when the H responses are abnormal, they do not localize to the S1 root because the lesion could be at many other points along the extended neural pathway that the impulses traverse (e.g., S1 spinal cord segment, sacral plexus, sciatic nerve, and proximal tibial nerve). When H responses are abnormal, they remain so indefinitely in many cases.[8,9]

Despite these limiting and confounding factors, H responses are very helpful in the evaluation of a possible lumbosacral radiculopathy because they are seldom normal with S1 root lesions. Part of their high sensitivity may be because, in contrast to all other constituents of the electrodiagnostic examination, they evaluate the preganglionic components of the S1 sensory root fibers.[8,9] Although most electrodiagnostic physicians agree on the value of H responses, they disagree regarding which component (amplitude or latency) of the H response is likely to be abnormal.[9,12-14]

Ideally, F waves should be able to detect demyelinating conduction slowing along the motor fibers at the root level.[9,15,16] This is not the case, however, in practical application. They are often normal in unequivocal cases of radiculopathy, and even when abnormal, they do not provide any additional information because the abnormalities are already clearly seen on NEE.[4,7] F waves are of no significant value in the evaluation of root lesions.

Needle Electrode Examination

Because NCS and the late responses generally are normal with isolated root lesions (except for the H response with S1 radiculopathies), NEE usually is the sole component of the electrodiagnostic examination that is beneficial in detecting a radiculopathy. The diagnosis depends on finding abnormalities on NEE in a root, or *myotome* (all the muscles that receive innervation from a single spinal cord segment or root). These abnormalities include insertional positive sharp waves, fibrillation potentials, a reduced or neurogenic recruitment of motor units, and changes in the motor unit morphology (e.g., increased duration, amplitude, and polyphasia).

The most widely used criterion for diagnosing radiculopathies by NEE is that abnormalities should be found in two, and preferably more, limb muscles innervated by the same root but different peripheral nerves. In addition, muscles in the limb not innervated by the damaged root, but by the roots contiguous to it, should appear normal. A patient with a C7 radiculopathy should have fibrillation potentials or other signs of denervation in the triceps (radial nerve) and pronator teres (medial nerve), but not the abductor digiti minimi or deltoid muscles. Needle electromyography (EMG) not only should be tailored to the clinical question and the patient's symptoms, but it also should include a comprehensive survey of a sufficient number of muscles (proximal and distal when possible) to make a reliable diagnosis of a radiculopathy.

Numerous myotome charts derived from radiographic, cadaveric, and electrodiagnostic studies have been established to help guide the electrodiagnostic physician in choosing the best muscles to examine for each patient (Figs. 13–7 through 13–9). A radiculopathy screen in the authors' laboratory consists of an examination of at least seven muscles, including the paraspinals to help with localization in the upper extremity (Table 13–3) and lower extremity (Table 13–4). The presence of fibrillation potentials in the paraspinals is typically indicative of an axon loss lesion localized to or near the intraspinal canal, excluding the possibility of a plexopathy or more distal lesion. Paraspinal fibrillation potentials are most valuable for the support of radiculopathy when they are present at only one or two contiguous segmental levels and absent at levels above, below, and contralaterally.

TABLE 13–3 Screening Needle Electrode Examination for the Arm

Muscle	Root Level	Nerve Trunk
First dorsal interosseus	C8	Ulnar
Extensor indicis proprius	C8	Posterior interosseous (radial)
Flexor pollicis longus	C8	Anterior interosseous (median)
Pronator teres	C6-7	Median
Triceps	C6-7	Radial
Biceps	C5-6	Musculocutaneous
Deltoids	C5-6	Axillary
C7 paraspinal	Overlap	

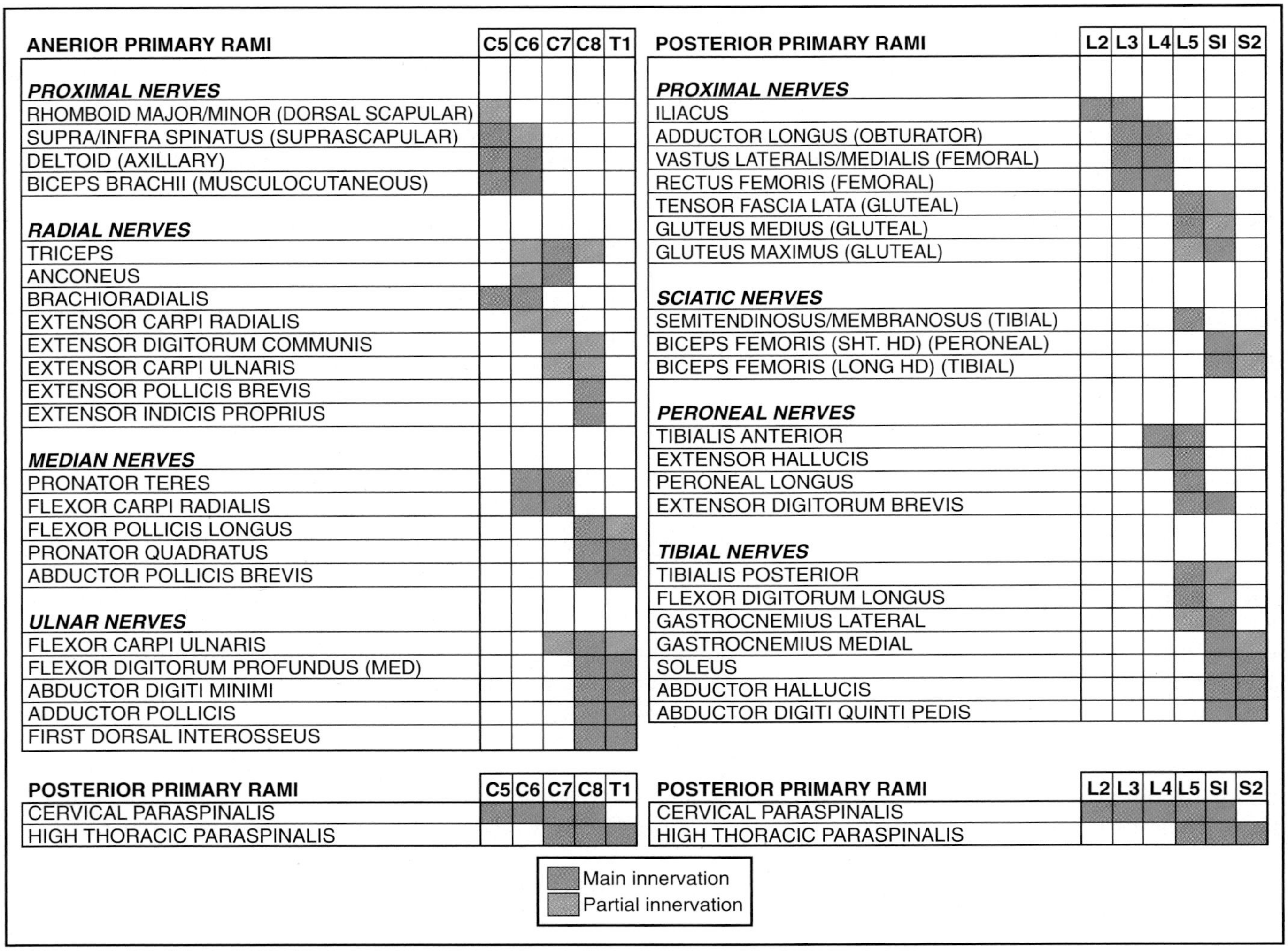

ANTERIOR PRIMARY RAMI

	C5	C6	C7	C8	T1
PROXIMAL NERVES					
RHOMBOID MAJOR/MINOR (DORSAL SCAPULAR)	■				
SUPRA/INFRA SPINATUS (SUPRASCAPULAR)	■	■			
DELTOID (AXILLARY)	■	■			
BICEPS BRACHII (MUSCULOCUTANEOUS)	■	■			
RADIAL NERVES					
TRICEPS		□	■	■	
ANCONEUS			■	■	
BRACHIORADIALIS	□	■			
EXTENSOR CARPI RADIALIS		■	■		
EXTENSOR DIGITORUM COMMUNIS			■	■	
EXTENSOR CARPI ULNARIS			■	■	
EXTENSOR POLLICIS BREVIS			■	■	
EXTENSOR INDICIS PROPRIUS			■	■	
MEDIAN NERVES					
PRONATOR TERES		■	■		
FLEXOR CARPI RADIALIS		■	■		
FLEXOR POLLICIS LONGUS			■	■	■
PRONATOR QUADRATUS			■	■	■
ABDUCTOR POLLICIS BREVIS				■	■
ULNAR NERVES					
FLEXOR CARPI ULNARIS			■	■	■
FLEXOR DIGITORUM PROFUNDUS (MED)				■	■
ABDUCTOR DIGITI MINIMI				■	■
ADDUCTOR POLLICIS				■	■
FIRST DORSAL INTEROSSEUS				■	■

POSTERIOR PRIMARY RAMI

	C5	C6	C7	C8	T1
CERVICAL PARASPINALIS	■	■	■	■	
HIGH THORACIC PARASPINALIS					■

POSTERIOR PRIMARY RAMI

	L2	L3	L4	L5	S1	S2
PROXIMAL NERVES						
ILIACUS	■	■	■			
ADDUCTOR LONGUS (OBTURATOR)	■	■	■			
VASTUS LATERALIS/MEDIALIS (FEMORAL)		■	■			
RECTUS FEMORIS (FEMORAL)		■	■			
TENSOR FASCIA LATA (GLUTEAL)				■	■	
GLUTEUS MEDIUS (GLUTEAL)				■	■	
GLUTEUS MAXIMUS (GLUTEAL)				■	■	■
SCIATIC NERVES						
SEMITENDINOSUS/MEMBRANOSUS (TIBIAL)				■	■	
BICEPS FEMORIS (SHT. HD) (PERONEAL)				■	■	■
BICEPS FEMORIS (LONG HD) (TIBIAL)				■	■	■
PERONEAL NERVES						
TIBIALIS ANTERIOR			■	■		
EXTENSOR HALLUCIS				■	■	
PERONEAL LONGUS				■	■	
EXTENSOR DIGITORUM BREVIS				■	■	
TIBIAL NERVES						
TIBIALIS POSTERIOR				■	■	
FLEXOR DIGITORUM LONGUS				■	■	
GASTROCNEMIUS LATERAL					■	■
GASTROCNEMIUS MEDIAL					■	■
SOLEUS					■	■
ABDUCTOR HALLUCIS					■	■
ABDUCTOR DIGITI QUINTI PEDIS					■	■

POSTERIOR PRIMARY RAMI

	L2	L3	L4	L5	S1	S2
CERVICAL PARASPINALIS	■	■	■	■	■	■
HIGH THORACIC PARASPINALIS						

■ Main innervation □ Partial innervation

FIGURE 13–7 Traditional myotome chart. (From Wilbourn AJ, Aminoff MF: Radiculopathies. In Brown WF, Bolton CF [eds]: Clinical Electromyography, 2nd ed. Boston, Butterworth-Heinemnann, 1993, p 192.)

TABLE 13–4 Screening Needle Electrode Examination for the Leg

Muscle	Root Level	Nerve Trunk
Abductor hallucis	S1	Tibial
Medial gastrocnemius	S1	Tibial
Biceps femoris (short head)	S1	Peroneal
Extensor digitorum brevis	L5–S1	Peroneal
Flexor digitorum longus	L5	Tibial
Gluteus medius	L5	Superior gluteal
Tibialis anterior	L4–5	Peroneal
Rectus femoris	L2, L3, L4	Femoral
S1 paraspinal	Overlap	

Many limitations can reduce the value of the paraspinal examination. First, there is overlapping innervation of most paraspinals, which prevents accurate localization of fibrillation potentials to one specific segment or root. Second, even in proven radiculopathies, fibrillation potentials may be absent owing to reinnervation or sampling error. Third, paraspinal fibrillation potentials may be seen in diabetic patients, in patients with a prior history of spine surgery, or in some asymptomatic elderly patients. Finally, paraspinal denervation is not specific to radiculopathy and is seen in other disorders, including diseases of the muscle (e.g., inflammatory myopathy) and the anterior horn cell (e.g., amyotrophic lateral sclerosis). Nonetheless, NEE of the paraspinal muscles is an integral portion of the electrodiagnostic examination and should be routinely performed in all patients with suspected nerve root disease.

The timing of needle EMG is also crucial. Fibrillation potentials do not appear in a denervated muscle until 2 to 3 weeks after the onset of the initial injury and in some patients may require 4 to 6 weeks to develop.[11] Consequently, the findings on NEE performed earlier than 3 weeks after onset of a radiculopathy are likely to be false-negative or, at best, indeterminate, even if subsequently they would be positive for a root lesion. It is optimal to wait at least 3 weeks after the onset of symptoms before performing NEE. Guidelines that help the

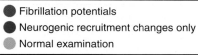

FIGURE 13–8 Lower limb myotome chart. Needle electrode examination results grouped by surgically defined root level of involvement. Numbers in the left column represent patients. AD, abductor digiti quinti; AH, abductor hallucis; AL, adductor longus; BFLH, biceps femoris long head; BFSH, biceps femoris short head; EDB, extensor digitorum brevis; EHL, extensor hallucis longus; GM, gluteus maximus; GMED, gluteus medius; IL, iliacus; LG, lateral gastrocnemius; MG, medial gastrocnemius; PL, peroneus longus; PSP, paraspinal; PT, posterior tibialis/flexor digitorum longus; RF, rectus femoris; ST, semitendinosus; TA, tibialis anterior; TFL, tensor fascia lata; VL, vastus lateralis; VM, vastus medialis. (From Tsao BE, Levin KH, Bodner RA: Comparison of surgical and electrodiagnostic findings in single root lumbosacral radiculopathies. Muscle Nerve 27:61, 2003.)

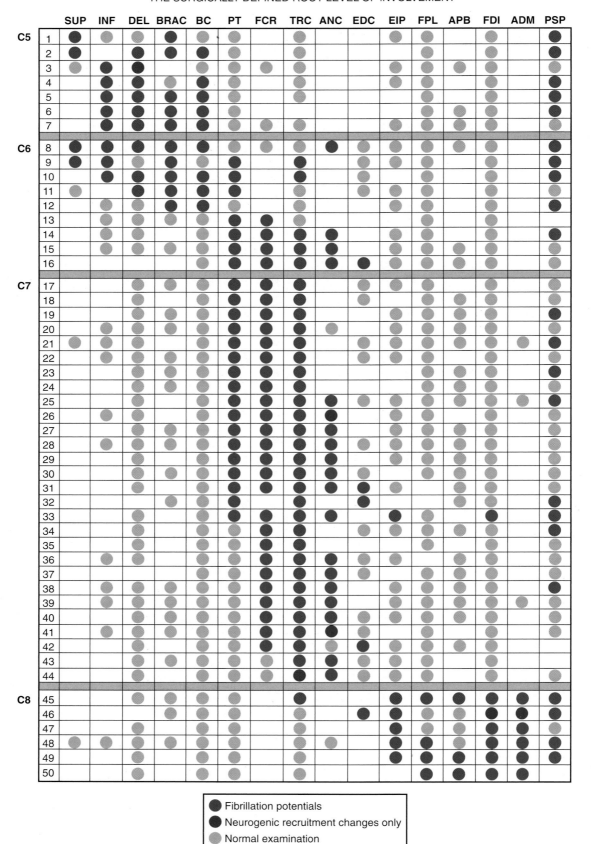

FIGURE 13–9 Upper limb myotome chart. Needle electrode examination results grouped by surgically defined root level of involvement. *Blue circle*, positive waves or fibrillation, with or without neurogenic recruitment and motor unit changes; *red circle*, neurogenic recruitment changes only; *green circle*, normal examination. ADM, abductor digiti minimi; ANC, anconeus; APB, abductor pollicis brevis; BIC, biceps; BRAC, brachioradialis; DEL, deltoid; EDC, extensor digitorum communis; EIP, extensor indicis proprius; FCR, flexor carpi radialis; FDI, first dorsal interosseus; FPL, flexor pollicis longus; INF, infraspinatus; SUP, supraspinatus; PSP, paraspinal; PT, pronator teres; TRIC, triceps. (From Levin KH, Maggiano HJ, Wilbourn AJ: Cervical radiculopathies: Comparison of surgical and EMG localization of single-root lesions. Neurology 46:1023, 1996.)

clinician decide the best timing of a study to obtain maximal information are provided in Table 13–5. These are based on the neurophysiologic concepts of axon loss as described in Table 13–6.

Determining Duration of Radiculopathy: Acute versus Chronic

Information regarding the duration of a radiculopathy is often derived by findings on NEE. Whenever evidence of an isolated compressive root disorder of recent onset is detected on the electrodiagnostic examination, the typical combination of findings is as follows: (1) motor NCS are normal (unless the degree of axon loss is severe); (2) sensory NCS are normal; (3) with S1 root involvement, the H response usually is abnormal; and (4) NEE discloses fibrillation potentials in several muscles that are innervated by the compromised root unaccompanied by changes in the size and configuration of the MUP.

In contrast, when chronic neurogenic MUP changes (poly-phasic configuration with increased duration and amplitude) are the prominent finding on NEE with only a few fibrillation potentials, the lesion is likely to be chronic. When the chronic neurogenic MUP changes are limited to distal muscles within a myotome in the absence of fibrillation potentials, the radiculopathy is likely to be static and remote.

Finally, when fibrillation potentials and chronic neurogenic MUP changes are found in a myotome distribution, the diagnostic possibilities include a chronic, progressive radiculopathy or an acute root lesion superimposed on a remote lesion. The latter possibility is the more likely choice if fibrillation potentials are found in proximal muscles (e.g., the glutei and hamstrings with L5 or S1 root lesions), in addition to more distal muscles in the same myotome.[7-9]

When the previous factors are considered, it is apparent that whenever the classic NEE presentation of a radiculopathy is encountered—fibrillation potentials in most or all of the muscles constituting the myotome—the root lesion in question usually is of more recent onset, and motor root axon loss has been substantial. Whenever other circumstances prevail, as is far more commonly the case, fibrillation potentials usually are found in only some, if any, of the muscles of the myotome. They are typically seen in the more distal muscles. Fibrillation potentials generally are important only if they are present; their absence in any specific muscle does not exclude the diagnosis.[8,9]

Determining Severity of Radiculopathy

The severity of a nerve root lesion is based on motor NCS and NEE. The degree of reduced MUP recruitment seen on NEE correlates with the degree of muscle weakness and, in combination with the CMAP amplitude reduction (in muscles that can be assessed with NCS), the degree of axon loss. The amount of fibrillation potentials seen in a muscle is a subjective measure and does not correlate as well with the degree of axon loss.

TABLE 13–5 Appropriate Timing of the Electrodiagnostic Examination

When aiming for single comprehensive study, reliable interpretations can be made from NCS and NEE obtained any time after 3 wk from onset of symptoms

For earliest possible information about axon loss lesion, reliable interpretations can be made from NCS obtained after 10 days from onset of symptoms

For earliest possible information about demyelinating conduction block lesion (neurapraxia), such as might be the case for perioperative peroneal or ulnar neuropathy owing to positioning on operating table, reliable interpretations can be made from NCS obtained any time after onset of symptoms

In setting of preexisting symptoms of peripheral nerve disease, such as diabetic polyneuropathy, it is reasonable to consider baseline electrodiagnostic examination (NCS and NEE) immediately after onset of new symptoms of potential iatrogenic cause. This study is to assess the nature of preexisting abnormalities, before acute changes from new symptoms are visible on electrodiagnostic examination. This is especially useful if a medicolegal issue may arise from new symptoms because it would be valuable to differentiate preexisting nerve pathology from any procedure-related changes. A second study is necessary when sufficient time has elapsed to assess new lesion

NCS, nerve conduction studies; NEE, needle electrode examination.

TABLE 13–6 Timing of Nerve Pathology: Neurophysiologic Concepts

After transection of motor nerve trunk, nerve conduction response amplitude from electrical stimulation distal to transection point decreases from day 3 through day 5-8 after transection. For sensory nerve fibers, response amplitude decreases progressively from day 5 through day 9-11, coinciding with evolution of wallerian degeneration of nerve fibers. For this reason, identifying maximum axon degeneration cannot be assessed by nerve conduction studies until at least 11 days have elapsed since date of nerve injury or onset of symptoms

As wallerian degeneration of motor nerve fiber reaches completion, attached muscle fiber becomes denervated, leading to breakdown of neuromuscular junction. Over 2-3 wk, membrane changes occur along muscle fiber, resulting in spontaneous, continuous action potential propagation along muscle fiber, recognized during NEE as fibrillation potentials. About 3 wk must elapse after acute axon loss event before fibrillation potentials can be reliably visualized on NEE

Process of reinnervation of denervated muscle fibers can occur as the result of regeneration of nerve trunk from point of nerve transection, or (when nerve transection is not total) by collateral nerve branch sprouting from remaining intact nerve fibers close to denervated muscle fibers. The latter process is much faster because nerve fiber regeneration occurs at rate of about 1 mm/day. On NEE, manifestations of reinnervation include resolution of fibrillation potentials, return of activation of motor unit action potentials with voluntary muscle contraction, and appearance of polyphasic motor unit potential changes.

NEE, needle electrode examination.

Electrodiagnostic Findings at Specific Root Levels

Cervical Radiculopathy

Lesions of the cervical nerve roots account for 36% of all radiculopathies.[9] In clinical and radiographic studies, the most common root affected is at the C7 level (70% of the time) followed by C6 (19% to 25%), C8 (4% to 10%), and C5 (2%).[9,16-18] The electrodiagnostic examination presentations with C5

TABLE 13–7 Disorders Commonly Confused with Compressive Radiculopathies

Roots	Entity
Cervical	
C5, C6	Upper trunk brachial plexopathy
	Neuralgic amyotrophy
	Axillary/suprascapular neuropathies
	Motor neuron disease
	Rotator cuff tear
C6, C7	Carpal tunnel syndrome
C8, T1	Lower trunk brachial plexopathy
	Ulnar neuropathy
	Motor neuron disease
Thoracic	
T1	Neurogenic thoracic outlet syndrome
Lumbosacral	
L2-4	Diabetic amyotrophy
	Lumbar plexopathy
	Femoral neuropathy
L5	Sacral plexopathy
	Peroneal neuropathy
	Motor neuron disease
S1, S2	Sacral plexopathy
	Sciatic neuropathy
	Tibial neuropathy
Bilateral (L5), S1, S2	Polyneuropathy

radiculopathies are typically manifested as abnormalities in the spinati, deltoid, biceps, and brachioradialis muscles. NCS are typically unhelpful because proximal muscles are not assessed during routine studies, although the biceps and deltoid muscles are amenable to NCS and may show reduced CMAP amplitudes when axon loss is sufficiently severe.

C6 radiculopathies do not have a single, discrete appearance. Rather, they have two very different ones, which imitate those of C5 and C7 root lesions. Manifestations of C5 root lesions may also be seen with some C6 radiculopathies.[19] C7 lesions are diagnosed by the presence of abnormalities in some muscles innervated by radial and median nerves: the triceps and anconeus (radial) and the pronator teres and flexor carpi radialis (median). As stated before, NEE abnormalities sometimes are seen in the same combination of upper limb muscles with C6 root lesions as well.

In contrast, C8 radiculopathies have a very characteristic electrodiagnostic presentation, manifesting as abnormalities in ulnar-innervated muscles, the extensor indicis proprius, and the flexor pollicis longus.[19] Nonetheless, they can sometimes be confused with combined axon loss lesions of the posterior interosseous nerve and the ulnar nerve whenever the ipsilateral ulnar SNAP is of low amplitude or cannot be elicited (e.g., because of advanced age or a coexisting polyneuropathy). For uncertain reasons, the axon loss that occurs with many C8 radiculopathies is exceptionally severe, so much so that the CMAPs recorded from the ulnar nerve–innervated hand muscles, particularly the hypothenar, are low in amplitude. Some of these patients never regain normal hand strength.

Differential Diagnoses

Findings on NEE of cervical radiculopathies can look identical to brachial plexopathies (Table 13–7). In particular, lesions affecting the C5 and C6 roots may resemble upper trunk plexus lesions, whereas lesions of the C8 and T1 roots can mimic lower trunk lesions. There are two critical parameters on the electrodiagnostic examination that can discern the two types of lesions. The first parameter is NEE findings in the paraspinals. With nerve root lesions, the paraspinal muscles show fibrillation potentials but are spared in a lesion of the brachial plexus. The second parameter is the assessment of the SNAPs. In radiculopathies, the lesion is located within the intraspinal canal and proximal to the DRG, which results in normal SNAPs. In plexopathies, the lesion is distal to the DRG, producing reduced amplitude or absent SNAPs.

Clinically, this second parameter is especially important when distinguishing a radiculopathy from neuralgic amyotrophy, which commonly affects proximal shoulder girdle muscles (e.g., the spinati and the deltoids) derived from C5 and C6 roots. Abnormally reduced or absent SNAP amplitudes of the lateral antebrachial cutaneous sensory nerve and median sensory branch recording from the thumb and index finger point toward a plexus lesion.

Likewise, carpal tunnel syndrome can resemble C6 and C7 radiculopathies clinically but are easily distinguished by the presence of abnormalities seen in the triceps and pronator teres and other muscles proximal to the hand or outside of the median nerve territory. In contrast, C8 radiculopathies may be difficult to discern from an ulnar mononeuropathy, especially in the setting of partial lesions in which the ulnar SNAP is unaffected. Finding abnormalities in C8 innervated radial muscles is important in this setting. Finally, unless a rotator cuff injury results in entrapment of a nerve innervating proximal muscles located in the shoulder girdle (e.g., suprascapular nerve), the electrodiagnostic examination would show no abnormalities.

Thoracic Radiculopathy

Radiculopathies in this region are difficult to assess by electrodiagnostic examination because there are relatively few muscles in each myotome, and only some of them can be sampled. With suspected thoracic radiculopathies, only the paraspinal and abdominal muscles are sampled routinely; the intercostal muscles are typically not studied for fear of entering the pleural space. Generally, if NEE abnormalities are seen, no attempt is made to identify a specific root lesion. Instead, the localization is limited to upper thoracic, mid-thoracic, or lower thoracic root involvement. Most patients found to have thoracic radiculopathies have diabetes mellitus, and the pathology is probably root infarction or ischemia rather than compression. In any case, these radiculopathies often produce very severe axon loss and frequently apparently involve two or more adjacent roots.[9,20,21] T1 radiculopathies are quite rare and typically produce changes only in the lateral thenar muscles.[22]

Differential Diagnoses

Although neurogenic thoracic outlet syndrome may technically be considered an extraspinal radiculopathy affecting the T1 nerve root and to a lesser extent C8, it has classically been categorized as a lower trunk brachial plexopathy (see Table 13–7). The preferential involvement of the T1 nerve root leads to prominent abnormalities of the abductor pollicis brevis muscle and the medial antebrachial cutaneous sensory response, both of which are heavily innervated by T1. In contrast, the ulnar innervated segments, which are predominantly innervated by C8, are sometimes spared or only mildly affected. Abnormalities in the abductor pollicis brevis are evident on motor NCS (manifested as decreased CMAP amplitude) and NEE (fibrillation potentials or neurogenic recruitment pattern), whereas the medial antebrachial cutaneous SNAP is reduced or absent. The latter abnormality is helpful in distinguishing this syndrome from a typical T1 radiculopathy.

Lumbosacral Radiculopathy

Nerve root lesions are most commonly seen in the lumbosacral spine: More than two thirds of all radiculopathies occur in this region.[7] In contrast to lesions involving the cervical roots, it is difficult sometimes to localize lumbosacral radiculopathies accurately to a vertebral level with the electrodiagnostic examination. This difficulty is primarily due to anatomic reasons. Given their long intraspinal course, lumbosacral nerve roots may be injured anywhere along their tract from the T12-L1 vertebral level where they are formed, down through the canal into the cauda equina, and the site where they exit from their respective foramina. The L5 nerve root can be compressed by a central disc herniation at the L3-4 level, a posterolateral disc herniation at the L4-5 level, or foraminal stenosis at the L5-S1 level. Additionally, when nerves are affected at the level of the cauda equina where the fibers are compact, a single lesion in this location can result in injury to multiple roots bilaterally. It is important to perform comparison NEE of the contralateral limb when any abnormalities are seen to exclude the possibility of subclinical nerve root involvement.

L2, L3, and L4 radiculopathies are generally considered together because of the myotome overlap of the thigh muscles and the paucity of muscles that are innervated solely by one individual nerve root. Localization of an L2 root lesion is difficult because only the iliacus muscle may show abnormalities on NEE. Lesions at these levels typically produce denervation changes in the quadriceps, thigh adductors, and iliacus. With L4 lesions, abnormalities may also be seen in the tibialis anterior occasionally.

The most common lumbosacral radiculopathies involve the L5 and S1 roots. Lesions of these two roots are most amenable to recognition on electrodiagnostic examination. In addition, the L5 nerve root is the most common single radiculopathy seen.[3] L5 radiculopathies produce abnormalities in the tibialis anterior, flexor digitorum longus, and posterior tibialis in greater than 75% of surgically proven cases.[23] In a more recent study, 100% of patients with L5 radiculopathies, which were also surgically proven, showed abnormalities in the peroneus longus and tensor fascia lata.[24] Changes may also be seen in the extensor digitorum brevis, gluteus medius, and semitendinosis.

An exception to the rule that SNAPs are not affected in radiculopathies has been found to occur with some L5 root lesions. As stated before, SNAPs are typically spared in radiculopathies because the lesion is situated proximal to sensory cell bodies (DRG), which lie in the intervertebral foramina *outside* of the intraspinal canal. At the level of the lumbosacral spine, the DRG is sometimes found proximal to the intervertebral foramina, however, *within* the intraspinal canal, leaving them vulnerable to injury from a herniated disc or other degenerative spine condition. Based on cadaveric, radiographic, and MRI studies, 3% of L3 and L4 DRG are intraspinal, 11% to 38% of L5 DRG are intraspinal, and up to 71% of S1 DRG are intraspinal.[24-26]

The L5 nerve root in some cases may be affected distal to the DRG, resulting in an abnormal superficial peroneal SNAP. In one retrospective study, six patients with clinical and radiographic evidence of an L5 radiculopathy were found to have reduced amplitude of the ipsilateral superficial peroneal SNAP along with denervation changes in the L5 myotome.[27] This condition has not been found with S1 nerve root lesions, in which the sural SNAP remains normal despite the higher percentage of DRG located within the intraspinal canal.

S1 radiculopathies are the second most common root lesion encountered. Needle EMG may show abnormalities in the gastrocnemii, abductor hallucis, abductor digit quinti pedis, glutei, and biceps femoris short head. In addition, the H response is either absent or reduced in amplitude.

Differential Diagnoses

As seen in the cervical spine, it is often difficult to distinguish clinically lesions of the lumbosacral nerve roots from lesions of the lumbar and sacral plexuses (see Table 13–7). L2-4 radiculopathies can look identical to lumbar plexopathies, whereas L5-S1 nerve root lesions closely resemble lesions of the sacral plexus. In both cases, the combination of fibrillation potentials in the lumbosacral paraspinals and normal sensory nerve conduction responses (lateral femoral cutaneous and saphenous SNAPs for L2-4 lesions and sural and superficial peroneal SNAPs for L5-S1 lesions) points toward the diagnosis of radiculopathy.

A major limitation is encountered when SNAPs are absent bilaterally. In the workup of a lesion in the lumbar plexus versus an L2-4 nerve root lesion, the sensory nerve conduction responses are not consistently obtainable from a technical standpoint even in normal individuals. Likewise, in the evaluation of a sacral plexus versus an L5-S1 lesion, SNAPs may be absent in elderly patients or patients with a history of a polyneuropathy. In both instances, the diagnosis rests on a single crucial finding: the absence or presence of denervation in the paraspinals. This finding in itself is unreliable as noted earlier, in that paraspinal fibrillation potentials may be present rarely in normal individuals older than age 60, in patients with a

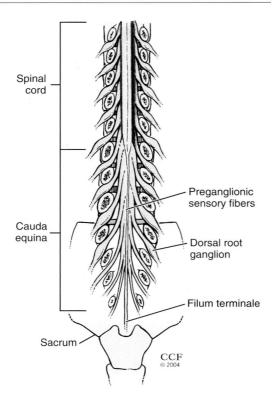

Spinal cord

Preganglionic sensory fibers

Cauda equina

Dorsal root ganglion

Filum terminale

Sacrum

CCF
© 2004

FIGURE 13–10 Coronal view of inferior spinal cord, cauda equina, and surrounding structures. Dorsal root ganglia are located in intervertebral foramina so that all the sensory fibers composing the cauda equina are "preganglionic." Axon loss lesion of cauda equina generally has no effect on lower limb sensory nerve conduction studies, regardless of its severity.

history of prior spine surgery, and in patients with diabetes. Denervation changes may be absent because of early reinnervation or sampling error. As a result, in patients with bilaterally absent SNAPs (owing to technical or other reasons), the final electrodiagnostic impression may be inconclusive.

For similar reasons, bilateral S1 radiculopathies, particularly when chronic, may be confused with distal axon loss polyneuropathies. In younger patients (<60 years old), an absent sural response combined with abnormalities seen in the intrinsic foot muscles on NEE typically indicate the presence of a polyneuropathy rather than S1 radiculopathy.

Electrodiagnostic Findings of Other Spine-Related Disorders

Cauda Equina Syndrome

Multiple lumbosacral radiculopathies are encountered with some frequency. Typically, the involvement is bilateral and often asymmetrical.[10,20] Most of these lesions are attributable to midline lumbar disc protrusions or lumbar canal stenosis. Characteristically, S1 and S2 roots, being the most medial of the roots supplying the lower limbs, are affected. In many patients, more extensive lumbosacral root involvement occurs; a common combination is bilateral S1 and S2 root compromise accompanied by unilateral or bilateral L5 root involvement.

The electrodiagnostic findings most commonly seen consist of a mixture of low-amplitude CMAPs and normal SNAPs on NCS, along with fibrillation potentials and MUP dropout on needle EMG (Fig. 13–10). On NEE, the abnormalities often are more severe in muscles located distal to the knees. With some substantial lesions of recent onset, they are just as prominent in the more proximal muscles. Whenever the disorder is subacute or chronic, fibrillation potentials usually are accompanied by chronic neurogenic MUP changes. Low lumbar or high sacral paraspinal fibrillation potentials often are found bilaterally with more acute lesions, but are undetectable with many chronic ones. Typically, the H responses cannot be elicited, and even the M components of the H responses, recorded from the gastrocnemius/soleus muscles, are quite low in amplitude.

Lumbar Canal Stenosis

Lumbar canal stenosis has no single characteristic electrodiagnostic presentation. Rather, the findings are extremely variable, depending on the degree of axon loss affecting the lumbosacral motor roots. At one extreme are patients who experience only intermittent, short-lived symptoms that often can be relieved completely by various maneuvers (e.g., sitting, flexing at the waist). In these patients, the electrodiagnostic examination often is completely normal. At the opposite end of the spectrum are patients who have substantial cauda equina lesions with severe, bilateral, fixed motor and sensory deficits. These lesions produce the electrodiagnostic presentation described previously.

Between these two extremes are numerous different electrodiagnostic patterns: (1) two or more radiculopathies, far more often bilateral than strictly unilateral; (2) a single radiculopathy, typically S1, that is sometimes detected in the less symptomatic or asymptomatic limb; (3) unilateral or bilateral absent H responses alone; (4) NEE changes restricted to just one or two limb muscles, most commonly those innervated by the S1 roots; or (5) fibrillation potentials limited to the paraspinal muscles.[9,19]

Myelopathy

The effect that a focal myelopathy has on the electrodiagnostic examination depends principally on whether the anterior horn cells or their existing fibers are compromised at the level of the lesion. If only the descending corticospinal tracts of the spinal cord are affected (upper motor neuron lesion), the only abnormality found on the electrodiagnostic examination concerns the MUP firing pattern of muscles receiving innervation from spinal cord segments caudal to the lesion; in these muscles, the MUPs show no or incomplete activation (i.e., they fire in decreased numbers at a slow to moderate rate).

In contrast, if the anterior horn cells or the intramedullary fibers derived from them are involved, the electrodiagnostic findings are those of a focal intraspinal canal lesion that are characteristically bilateral, but often asymmetric. How prominent the electrodiagnostic changes are with such focal disorders depends mainly on where the lesions are located along the spinal cord. Lesions situated in C5-T1 segments and

L4-S2 segments produce substantial abnormalities on motor NCS and NEE and generally are readily recognized as intraspinal canal lesions. All such disorders result in low-amplitude CMAPs or CMAPs that cannot be elicited and normal SNAPs on NCS, accompanied by fibrillation potentials, MUP dropout, and, depending on lesion duration, chronic neurogenic MUP changes on needle EMG. Conversely, lesions involving T2 through L3 segments result only in NEE changes (i.e., motor NCS using various limb muscles as recording sites are normal). Finally, lesions involving the upper cervical cord segments (C1-4) have essentially no electrodiagnostic manifestations because that region of the spinal cord cannot be assessed.[27]

Postlaminectomy Electrodiagnostic Findings

Electrodiagnostic examinations are obtained frequently on patients who have undergone neck or back surgery. The specific diagnostic benefit derived from such assessments varies considerably, depending on the reason for referral and the time that has elapsed since operation. Overall, such postoperative studies are of limited value, however, unless they are obtained after very remote surgery to diagnose a recent-onset lesion. In the immediate postoperative period (first 10 to 14 days after surgery), the electrodiagnostic examination can reveal preexisting abnormalities because any NEE changes observed during that period, with the exception of a reduced MUP recruitment, are caused by a lesion that predated the operation.

During the early postoperative period (3 weeks to 3 to 4 months after surgery), the electrodiagnostic examination is of considerable benefit in assessing patients with postoperative weakness, principally because a normal CMAP amplitude recorded from a weak muscle (e.g., the tibialis anterior, resulting in footdrop) 7 or more days after onset of symptoms virtually excludes motor axon loss as the cause. The remaining possibilities include a proximal conduction block (neurapraxia), an upper motor neuron lesion, or hysteria or malingering. In the rare patient who develops nonorganic weakness postoperatively, the electrodiagnostic examination can prove that the symptoms are not the result of significant nerve fiber damage.

The electrodiagnostic examination usually cannot answer reliably the early postoperative question: "Was the root adequately decompressed?" Axon loss features of radiculopathy persist for weeks to months or indefinitely. Even an electrodiagnostic examination performed 2 to 3 months postoperatively is not likely to show significant improvement compared with a preoperative study. An exception is radiculopathy resulting from conduction block at the root level, which may resolve rapidly after the pressure is relieved. With an S1 radiculopathy, an H response that could not be elicited preoperatively may reappear in the early postoperative period. Similarly, on NEE, reduced MUP recruitment (and clinical weakness) could resolve rapidly in the affected muscles postoperatively.

An electrodiagnostic examination can be valuable in identifying root damage as the cause of new or worsening weakness in the postoperative period. The extent, amount, and distribution of fibrillation potentials provide information when compared with the preoperative study.

Cervical Root Avulsion

Root avulsions, which are usually restricted to the cervical region, differ from the typical single compressive radiculopathy principally in the degree of axon loss that results. Because the entire motor supply from one or both roots innervating the particular muscle has been disrupted, that muscle is severely or totally denervated. If it is used as a recorded muscle during motor NCS, the CMAP obtained is of very low amplitude, if it can be elicited. Similarly, during needle EMG of that muscle, fibrillation potentials are abundant, and MUPs are either absent or, if present, quite sparse and show reduced recruitment. Sensory NCS responses derived from the same roots are normal because the sensory roots are interrupted proximal to their DRG. Fibrillation potentials are not found in the appropriate paraspinal muscles in patients with cervical avulsion injuries, so their absence does not exclude this diagnosis.[9]

Acknowledgments

The authors acknowledge the late Dr. Asa J. Wilbourn for his contribution to the original version of this chapter.

KEY POINTS

1. The electrodiagnostic examination is an essential tool in the evaluation of radiculopathy. When performed by an experienced electrodiagnostic consultant, the electrodiagnostic examination can confirm the diagnosis and determine the localization, lesion duration, and severity.

2. For a comprehensive study, the electrodiagnostic examination should be performed at least 3 weeks after the onset of symptoms.

3. The most widely used criteria for diagnosing radiculopathies by NEE is that abnormalities (e.g., fibrillation potentials or neurogenic MUP changes) should be found in at least two limb muscles within the same myotome that are innervated by different peripheral nerves.

4. Sensory nerve conduction responses are typically normal in radiculopathy owing to the location of the DRG outside of the intraspinal canal, distal to the site of the nerve lesion. In contrast, amplitudes of the motor NCS may be decreased when root damage is severe, extensive, or both.

KEY REFERENCES

1. Wilbourn AJ, Aminoff MJ: AAEM Minimonograph #32: The electrodiagnostic examination in patients with radiculopathies. Muscle Nerve 21:1612-1631, 1998.
   This review article describes and critically analyzes the various neurophysiologic techniques used in assessment of radiculopathy and details the findings with root lesions at various levels.

2. Wilbourn AJ: Nerve conduction studies: Types, components, abnormalities, and value in localization. Neurol Clin North Am 20:305-338, 2002.
This article reviews the types of pathophysiology manifested by focal nerve fiber lesions and what effect each has on NCS; it also describes the types of localization possible with the electrodiagnostic examination and the major sources of error.

3. Shea PA, Woods WW, Werden DH: Electromyography in diagnosis of nerve root compression syndrome. Arch Neurol Psychiatry 64:93-104, 1950.
This article and the article by Woods and Shea were the first to discuss the methodology used for diagnosing radiculopathies in the clinical EMG laboratory (which is still used currently).

4. Woods WW, Shea PA: The value of electromyography in neurology and neurosurgery. J Neurosurg 8:595-607, 1951.
This article and the one by Shea and colleagues were the first to discuss the methodology used for diagnosing radiculopathies in the clinical EMG laboratory (which is still used currently).

5. Yoss RE, Corbin KB, MacCarty CS, et al: Significance of symptoms and signs in localization of involved root in cervical disc protrusion. Neurology 7:673-683, 1957.
This unique article remains the best source regarding the specific symptoms and clinical findings with lesions of each of the cervical roots (C5 through C8).

REFERENCES

1. Wilbourn AJ: Nerve conduction studies: Types, components, abnormalities, and value in localization. Neurol Clin North Am 20:305-338, 2002.

2. Preston DC, Shapiro BE: Electromyography and Neuromuscular Disorders. Boston, Butterworth-Heinemann, 1998.

3. Wilbourn AJ, Ferrante MA: Clinical electromyography. In Joynt RJ, Greggs RC (eds): Baker's Clinical Neurology on CD-Rom. Philadelphia, Lippincott Williams & Wilkins, 2000.

4. Dimitru D, Amato AA, Awarts MJ: Electrodiagnostic Medicine, 2nd ed. Philadelphia, Hanley & Belfus, 2002.

5. Shea PA, Woods WW, Werden DH: Electromyography in diagnosis of nerve root compression syndrome. Arch Neurol Psychiatry 64:93-104, 1950.

6. Woods WW, Shea PA: The value of electromyography in neurology and neurosurgery. J Neurosurg 8:595-607, 1951.

7. Wilbourn AJ, Aminoff MJ: Radiculopathies. In Brown WF, Bolton CF (eds): Clinical Electromyography, 2nd ed. Boston, Butterworth-Heinemann, 1993, pp 177-209.

8. Wilbourn AJ: The value and limitations of the electromyographic examination in the diagnosis of lumbosacral radiculopathy. In Hardy RW (ed): Lumbar Disc Disease. New York, Raven Press, 1982, pp 65-109.

9. Wilbourn AJ, Aminoff MJ: AAEM Minimonograph #32: The electrodiagnostic examination in patients with radiculopathies. Muscle Nerve 21:1612-1631, 1998.

10. Raynor EM, Kleiner-Fisman G, Nardin RA: Lumbosacral and thoracic radiculopathies. In Kitirji B, Kaminski HJ, Preston DC, et al (eds): Neuromuscular Disorders in Clinical Practice. Boston, Butterworth-Heinemann, 2002, pp 859-883.

11. Levin KH: Radiculopathy. In Levin KH, Luders HO (eds): Comprehensive Clinical Neurophysiology. Philadelphia, WB Saunders, 2000, pp 189-200.

12. Johnson EW: Electrodiagnosis of radiculopathy. In Johnson EW (ed): Practical Electromyography, 2nd ed. Baltimore, Williams & Wilkins, 1988, pp 229-245.

13. Braddom RI, Johnson EW: Standardization of "H" reflex and diagnostic use in S1 radiculopathies. Arch Phys Med Rehabil 55:161-164, 1974.

14. Schuchmann J: H-reflex latency in radiculopathy. Arch Phys Med Rehabil 59:185-187, 1978.

15. Eisen A, Schomer D, Melmad C: An electrophysiological method for examining lumbosacral root compression. Can J Neurol Sci 4:117-123, 1977.

16. Fisher MN, Shidve AJ, Terxera C, et al: The F response—a clinically useful physiological parameter for the evaluation of radicular injury. Electromyogr Clin Neurophysiol 19:65-75, 1979.

17. Yoss RE, Corbin KB, MacCarty CS, et al: Significance of symptoms and signs in localization of involved root in cervical disc protrusion. Neurology 7:673-683, 1957.

18. Marinacci AA: A correlation between operative findings in cervical herniated disc with the EMGs and opaxuq myelograms. EMG 6:5-20, 1966.

19. Levin KH, Maggiano HJ, Wilbourn AJ: Cervical radiculopathies: Comparison of surgical and EMG localization of single-root lesions. Neurology 46:1022-1025, 1996.

20. Wilbourn AJ: The electrodiagnostic examination. In Herkowitz HN, Garfin SR, Barlderston RA, et al (eds): The Spine, 4th ed. Philadelphia, WB Saunders, 1999, pp 135-150.

21. Wilbourn AJ: Diabetic neuropathies. In Brown WF, Bolton CF (eds): Clinical Electromyography, 2nd ed. Boston, Butterworth-Heinemann, 1993, pp 447-515.

22. Levin KH: Neurological manifestations of compressive radiculopathy of the first thoracic root. Neurology 53:1149-1151, 1999.

23. Bodner RA, Levin KH, Wilbourn AJ: Lumbosacral radiculopathies: comparison of surgical and EMG localization. Muscle Nerve 18:1071, 1995.

24. Tsao BE, Levin KH, Bodner RA: Comparison of surgical and electrodiagnostic findings in single root lumbosacral radiculopathies. Muscle Nerve 27:60-64, 2003.

25. Hamanishi C, Tanaka S: Dorsal root ganglia in the lumbosacral region observed from the axial view of MIR. Spine 18:1753-1756, 1993.

26. Sato K, Kikuchi S: An anatomic study of foraminal nerve root lesions in the lumbar spine. Spine 18:2246-2251, 1993

27. Levin KH: L5 radiculopathy with reduced superficial peroneal sensory responses: Intraspinal and extraspinal causes. Muscle Nerve 21:3-7, 1998.

14 CHAPTER

Intraoperative Neurophysiologic Monitoring of the Spine

Dileep R. Nair, MD
Imad M. Najm, MD

The primary objective in intraoperative neurophysiologic monitoring is to identify and prevent the development of a new neurologic deficit or worsening of a preexisting neurologic injury in a patient who is undergoing surgery. The aim of most spinal cord monitoring is to prevent intraoperative injury that results in irreversible paraplegia or quadriplegia. Because a neurologic examination cannot be performed in an anesthetized patient, intraoperative neurophysiologic monitoring is used to determine the patient's neurologic status during surgery. By evaluating the responses that are produced by the patient's nervous system to various stimulations, the integrity of that neural pathway can be monitored.

These recordings are started before surgery, referred to as *baseline recordings,* and continued throughout the surgery. Any significant changes or fluctuations from these baseline values are used to determine whether significant neurologic injury has occurred. In using this strategy, the patient's own response serves as the control for the detection of any abnormalities that may occur during the surgery. The term *significant change* is used to refer to the degree of changes seen in the neurophysiologic recordings. Changes that are termed significant have been shown to correlate well with intraoperative injury to the nervous system.

It is also possible that some of these significant changes may arise from other changes in physiologic parameters, anesthetic parameters, or technical issues. It is the responsibility of the intraoperative neurophysiologic monitoring team to determine whether or not the significant changes noted in the neurophysiologic responses are truly related to the surgical procedure at hand. The challenge to the intraoperative neurophysiologist and the monitoring team is to alert the surgeon of these changes as early as possible so that changes can be instituted to reverse the electrophysiologic changes and to avert neurologic catastrophe.

Key to the success of intraoperative neurophysiologic monitoring is a good understanding of the capabilities and limitations of the neurophysiologic tests being monitored. These limitations should be understood not only by the intraoperative neurophysiologist, but also by the anesthesiologist and surgeon. For seamless integration of intraoperative neurophysiologic monitoring into the intraoperative team, it is imperative that a good established working relationship eventually develops between the intraoperative neurophysiology team, anesthesiologist, and surgeon. This relationship allows for rapid communication between teams and a quick resolution of issues, optimizing the benefits of intraoperative neurophysiologic monitoring for the patient.

One of the first issues to address when planning for intraoperative neurophysiologic monitoring is to determine the types of neurophysiologic tests to perform on a particular patient undergoing surgery. This decision is made based on an understanding of the type of surgery the patient is to undergo, the types of intraoperative injuries that may occur, and the mechanisms of how these injuries occur in surgery. By planning ahead with these issues in mind, the team can also attempt to anticipate the type of changes that might be expected to occur and the risky periods during surgery when these changes would likely occur. Ideally, the team would prospectively plan for interventions to reduce intraoperative neurologic injury.

Intraoperative Monitoring of the Spinal Cord

Somatosensory-evoked potential (SEP) monitoring has been used for many years to monitor spinal function intraoperatively during various surgeries involving the spine, such as corrective surgery for scoliosis or other congenital deformities and removal of intraspinal tumors or arteriovenous malformations. SEP monitoring has been shown to reduce the incidence of neurologic damage in large studies of experienced monitoring teams.[1] SEPs monitor only sensory transmission through the dorsal column pathways, however; SEPs do not provide a direct measure of motor function. In addition, the dorsal columns receive their blood supply from the posterior spinal arteries, whereas the anterior spinal arteries supply the motor pathways. Ischemic damage to the spinal cord from the anterior spinal artery may be undetectable with SEP monitoring.[2,3]

A significant change in SEP monitoring might mandate further assessment of the patient's motor function by waking the patient up during surgery to evaluate leg and arm motor function (this has been called the "wake-up" test). The disadvantages of this strategy include the lack of real-time intraoperative motor function assessment and the anesthesia risks associated with performing the "wake-up" test. An alternative is monitoring of the motor pathway through the recording of motor-evoked potentials (MEPs).

MEPs are a more direct technique that evaluates the motor pathway. Monitoring has been previously performed by relying on stimulation of the spinal cord directly.[4] Spinal cord stimulation can be done with the use of epidural electrodes inserted after a laminectomy has been performed or by percutaneous intraspinous needle electrodes. The epidural electrodes are invasive and often require placement by a skilled anesthesiologist. Percutaneous intraspinous needles are difficult to place accurately and may not achieve adequate or consistent stimulation of the spinal cord. In addition, there is the question of whether MEPs generated through spinal cord stimulation arise solely from propagation through the motor pathway or if multiple pathways are involved in their generation.[5,6] There are reports of MEP monitoring in which spinal cord stimulation resulted in no significant intraoperative changes despite postoperative neurologic motor deficits (so-called false-negative result).[7] It is now believed that motor cortex stimulation with transcranial electrical stimulation provides a more reliable method for monitoring of the motor pathways. This technique is now routinely used in spinal cord monitoring together with SEPs.

Somatosensory-Evoked Potential Monitoring

The use of SEPs in intraoperative monitoring of complex spine surgeries began in the early 1970s.[8] Although SEP monitoring evaluates primarily the integrity of the posterior columns, it is often used to give an overall assessment of the spinal cord based on the assumption that many intraoperative mechanisms of injury would affect the spinal cord diffusely. An example of such an injury is spine distraction during scoliosis surgery. In addition, ischemic injury may initially result in a more diffuse dysfunction of the spinal cord that could be detected by SEPs (Fig. 14–1). SEP responses are thought to pass through large fiber somatosensory pathways of the dorsal column and possibly through the anterior spinothalamic tract, and this may be another reason why anterior spinal artery ischemia could be detected using this technique.

Generators of Somatosensory-Evoked Potential Responses

The cortical response for the lower extremity is called the *P37 potential*. The generator of this response arises from the primary somatosensory cortex of the leg, which is located in the mesial parietal cortex. The cortical response for the upper extremity, which is generated from the primary somatosensory cortex of the hand, is called the *N20 potential* (Fig. 14–2). Two important characteristics of these waveforms are (1) *amplitude*, which is recorded in microvolts and determined by either a baseline-to-peak or a peak-to-trough measure of the

waveform, and (2) *latency*, which is recorded in milliseconds and is the time interval from the stimulus to the occurrence of the potential. An amplitude change from the initial baseline measure to a decrease of more than 50% is often considered a significant change in SEP amplitudes.[9]

Significant latency changes in SEP monitoring consist of a 10% prolongation beyond the baseline latency value (Table 14–1).[10] Although these deviations from the baseline measures are thought to be significant, they should be interpreted with caution, taking into account various factors, including the evolution of the changes (e.g., a trend toward worsening is an ominous sign) and other intraoperative factors such as length of the surgery, type of anesthetic agent, and temperature effects. Also, significant latency and amplitude changes can occur in isolation. It is quite common to see a significant amplitude change without any associated latency changes. The most significant change is a complete loss of the cortical potential.

Another measurement made in posterior tibial or peroneal nerve SEP monitoring is the popliteal fossa potential. This is a nerve action potential that is recorded as the impulses pass within the popliteal fossa in the peripheral nervous system. The reason for this measurement is to ensure that an adequate stimulus has been applied. If there is an absence of the popliteal fossa response in addition to an absence of the leg cortical (P37) response, it suggests that the changes seen are not a result of a lesion at the level of the spinal cord. In this case, the change may be technical (e.g., the stimulating needles may have dislodged) or may be seen when the leg is ischemic (e.g., with femoral artery catheterization during thoracoabdominal aneurysm surgery or with direct compression of the peripheral nerve) (Fig. 14–3).

The other posterior tibial stimulation SEP response that can be monitored (besides the P37 response) is the P31/N34 complex, often termed the *subcortical response* because the generator for this response is at the level of medulla and midbrain. The benefit in recording these responses is that they are relatively more resistant to the effects of anesthesia compared with the cortical P37 response (see Fig. 14–3). The same is true for the subcortical potentials from median nerve stimulation (P14/N18) potential. In pediatric cases, the subcortical potentials may also be better formed and more easily monitored than cortical responses. Some of this effect may be the result of the variation of myelination in the younger age groups and the more significant effects of anesthetics on these patients. These differences from the adult morphology can persist into the early teenage years. Other factors affecting the responses include core body temperature changes. The core body temperature commonly decreases more than 1° C. The cooling affects the limbs more than the core body temperature, which can result in slowing of conduction.

Motor-Evoked Potential Monitoring

As mentioned earlier, various methods have been used to monitor spinal motor pathways during surgery. Most of these methods involve recording of electromyography (EMG) readings from appropriate muscles in response to stimulation of a

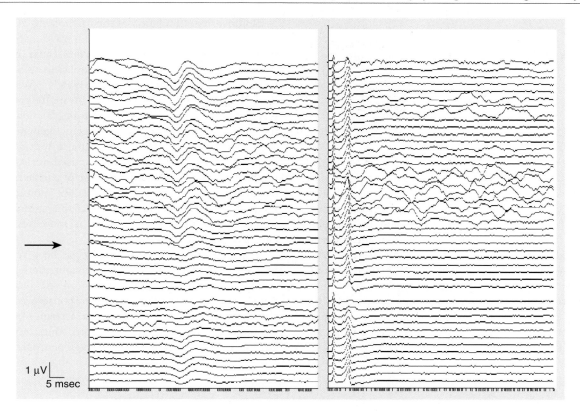

FIGURE 14–1 Significant amplitude change in cortical response owing to ischemic etiology. Stack on the left shows leg cortical response, and stack on the right shows popliteal fossa response. Both were obtained after left posterior tibial stimulation. Responses are represented with baseline responses shown at the top of the stack and end of monitoring shown at the bottom of the stack. Decrease in leg cortical amplitude can be appreciated at point depicted by *arrow*. Popliteal fossa responses are intact during this time. There is a return of response by the end of surgery seen at the bottom of the stack. This change was attributed to ischemic change to cord with retractor placed over left iliac artery. Responses returned when retractor was adjusted away from artery.

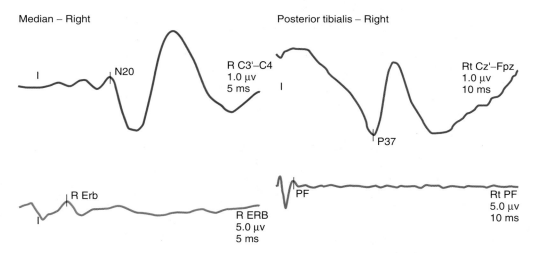

FIGURE 14–2 Typical morphology of cortical generators of median nerve and posterior tibial nerve somatosensory-evoked potential (SEP) waveforms are shown. Display time is different between two modalities. Median nerve SEP is shown in 5 msec per division display, and posterior tibial nerve SEP is shown in 10 msec per division display.

TABLE 14-1 Significant Changes in Different Monitoring Modalities

Type of Study	Significant Changes	Highly Significant Changes
Somatosensory-evoked potentials	Amplitude <50%; latency >10%	Complete loss of amplitude
Motor-evoked potentials	Increase threshold voltage >50-100 V	Complete loss of amplitude
Pedicle screw stimulation	Current intensity <7-10 mA	

motor pathway rostral to the operative site. The difference between the various methods is the nature of the stimulation. There are three basic categories of stimulation: rostral spinal stimulation, transcranial magnetic stimulation, and transcranial electrical stimulation (TCES). Magnetic stimulation is effective in nonanesthetized patients for evaluation of motor pathways, but the suppression of cortical responsiveness under anesthesia (mainly inhalational anesthetics) renders this method less effective for surgical use. In addition, the equipment used for magnetic stimulation is expensive, is bulky, and has a tendency to overheat.

Noninvasive stimulation of the brain using TCES was first reported in 1980.[11] Single-pulse TCES was subsequently used in monitoring motor pathways.[12-17] Because of effects of general anesthesia, single-pulse stimulation was found to be less effective in reliably recording MEPs.[18-22] With the introduction of the multipulse technique for motor pathway monitoring, reliable and robust MEP recording can now be obtained in most patients using some specific general anesthesia protocols.[23-27] The use of the multipulse technique requires that neuromuscular blockade not be used during this part of the monitoring. Occasionally, the use of partial neuromuscular blockade may still allow for TCES monitoring.[28] This method reportedly achieves more reliable stimulation of the motor cortex intraoperatively and is more resilient to the effects of general anesthesia.

The method of MEP monitoring has been revolutionized by the use of multipulse TCES. Previous methods for MEP recording used a variety of stimulation and recording techniques. Spinally elicited neurogenic responses were used in the past and were putatively stated to be a result of activation of the motor pathways in the spinal cord. More recent evidence has suggested that these spinally elicited neurogenic responses

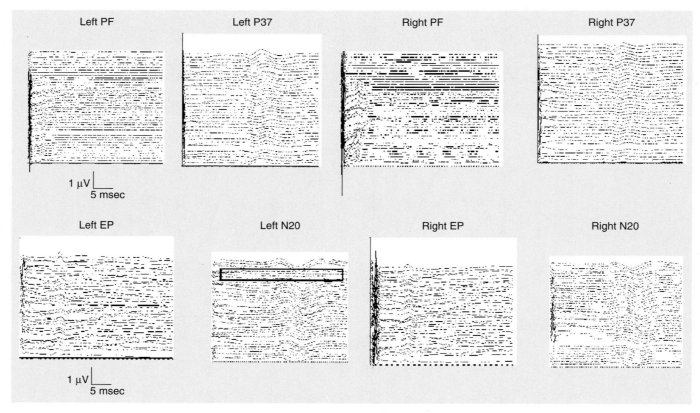

FIGURE 14-3 Significant change in left N20 cortical amplitude owing to arm positioning and nonsignificant latency prolongation of all cortical responses owing to anesthetic effect. Top row of stacks shows popliteal fossa (PF) and leg cortical (P37) responses from posterior tibial stimulation first from left-side stimulation and then from right-side stimulation. Bottom row of stacks shows Erb point (EP) and arm cortical (N20) response from median nerve stimulation with left side shown first followed by right side. There is a decrease in left N20 amplitude. This is highlighted with rectangular box in figure. At this point, there is also loss of left EP response. This change was attributed to malpositioning of left arm. When left arm was repositioned, response returned to baseline. Also noticeable in all leg and arm cortical responses from left and right sides is mild prolongation of latencies in the stacks, but these latencies all return to baseline by end of surgery. These changes are likely from anesthetic effect because they are bilateral, affecting arm and leg responses in a spine operation, which was performed at L3-S1 level.

are generated through activation of the sensory pathways and retrograde activation of alpha motor neurons. In a collision experiment using stimulation of the spinal cord followed by stimulation of the posterior tibial nerve at various inter-stimulus intervals, the neurogenic responses were abolished, suggesting that the potentials were colliding in the spinal cord.[6]

At the beginning of TCES-MEP monitoring, threshold voltages for each side of the body and MEP amplitudes are calculated.[23] The motor cortex on the side of the brain receiving the anodal stimulus is typically the first region to activate at the lowest stimulus threshold. The initial current used is typically 100 V, with a train of stimuli delivered to the cortex. After the stimulation, an MEP response is monitored in the muscles contralateral to the side receiving the anodal stimulus. If no response is seen, the voltage is increased typically by 50-V increments, and the process is repeated until an MEP response is seen in all the muscles contralateral to the anodal stimulus. This voltage is called the *threshold voltage* for that side.

The highest amplitude of the myogenic response below the level of surgery is also noted. Typically, amplitude measures for myogenic responses are best recorded as the area-under-the-curve measurements or simply by just documenting either presence or absence of the myogenic response. This procedure is repeated after reversing the anodal-cathodal configuration using a switch box. The voltage used for TCES-MEP record-ings typically does not exceed 500 V. The anticipated latency of the EMG responses ranges from 20 to 40 msec or more, depending on the patient's height, owing to the conduction time in the descending motor pathways. Latency values have not always been found to be reliable indicators of significant change in TCES monitoring in clinical practice. Another advantage of the multipulse technique is that it elicits a train of pulses that is of sufficient amplitude that it does not require averaging.

Two different methods of recording MEPs can be used. In myogenic MEPs, responses can be recorded directly from the muscle (either a surface electrode or needle electrodes placed within the muscle). In spinal cord MEPs, responses may be recorded directly from the spinal cord with use of an epidural catheter electrode that records a direct "D" wave and a volley of indirect "I" waves. Using single-pulse TCES, recording "D" and "I" waves is frequently required, meaning a "D" wave could be recorded when a myogenic MEP is not yet seen. This is because a series of "D" and "I" waves is required for alpha motor neurons to generate a myogenic response. The spinal recorded responses can also be recorded with full muscle relaxation, whereas myogenic responses require either no or very little muscle relaxation, even with the multipulse technique.

Determining significant changes during the course of surgery typically is most reliable if there is an absolute loss of myogenic responses to stimulation (Fig. 14–4). Some authors have also suggested that reduction of MEP amplitude to 25% of baseline amplitude values is predictive of motor pathway impairments.[29] Significant changes can also be determined by the change of voltage required to obtain MEPs of greater than 50 V beyond baseline thresholds used in obtaining MEPs at the beginning of monitoring (see Table 14–1).[30]

Clinical Use of Intraoperative Monitoring

SEPs have become a useful modality in monitoring scoliosis surgery and have been shown to reduce the risk of neurologic deficit. The occurrence of definite neurologic deficits in the presence of unchanged SEP recordings has been estimated to be approximately 0.063%.[31] Intraoperative neurophysiology can play a neuroprotective role (through the detection of early changes) and an educational role during surgery.[32] Surgeons who use intraoperative neurophysiologic monitoring regu-larly can learn which surgical techniques and maneuvers have a risk for producing a neurologic deficit and avoid those methods.

TCES-evoked MEP monitoring during spinal surgery is a safe and reliable method of monitoring corticospinal tract activity and is indispensable for high-risk surgeries.[33] There is no evidence that TCES has resulted in the development of epilepsy or brain damage. Some other risks are associated with TCES monitoring, including tongue or lip laceration and rarely mandibular fractures. The use of a soft bite-block may prevent these injuries. Relative contraindications to TCES include epilepsy, cortical lesions, convexity skull deficits, increased intracranial pressure, cardiac disease, intracranial electrodes or shunts, cardiac pacemakers, or other implantable biomedical devices.[34]

One study that looked at the reproducibility of various methods that could be monitored during scoliosis surgery found that MEPs could be obtained in 80% of patients and SEPs could be obtained in 93% of patients.[35] In spinal surgery, MEPs obtained from upper and lower extremities were con-sistently recorded in 22 patients with multipulse stimulation using trains of three to six pulses separated by 2 msec, with responses measuring more than 100 µV in all but 1 patient. These responses persisted with nitrous oxide concentration of up to 74%. One patient had loss of responses from one lower limb in which increased weakness was noted for a few days after surgery; in 3 patients, there was an increase in weakness or spasticity without any accompanying intraoperative MEP changes.[36] In another study,[37] MEPs during TCES were repro-ducibly recorded during spinal surgery in 40 patients with partial neuromuscular blockade. In two patients, there were some significant changes in the motor potentials that corre-lated with postoperative neurologic deficits. No postoperative neurologic deficits were observed in nine patients in whom MEP amplitudes decreased to less than 20% of baseline values.[37]

TCES-induced MEPs have been used to monitor cases of intramedullary spinal cord tumor resection. In 32 consecutive patients, MEPs were elicited in 19 patients before myelotomy, and 3 of these patients had MEP amplitude decrease less than 50% from baseline; all of these patients had postoperative neurologic deficits.[38]

In a review of 160 patients undergoing scoliosis surgery, a combination of SEP and transcranial MEP monitoring was successfully recorded in 81% of the patients, with changes seen

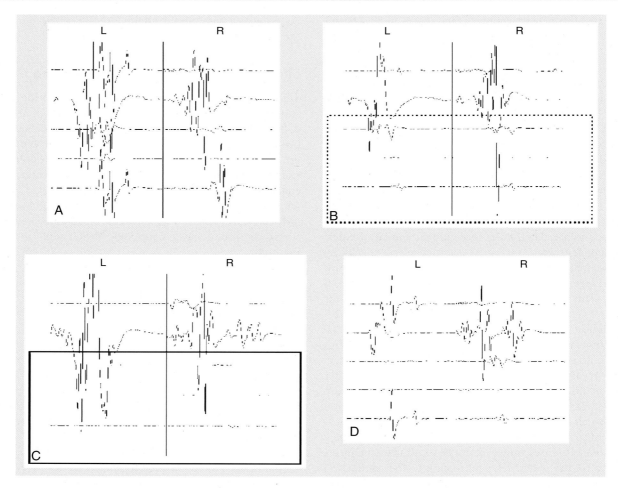

FIGURE 14–4 Significant change in transcranial electrical motor-evoked potential (MEP) response during spinal instrumentation. Figure shows transcranial MEP responses at four points during surgery. Each set of responses shows response from left (L) and right (R) sides of body. First two rows are responses from muscles of upper extremity (biceps and first dorsal interosseous muscle), and bottom three rows are from muscles of lower extremity (anterior tibialis, medial gastrocnemius, and adductor hallucis longus). **A,** This set is MEPs at baseline or beginning of monitoring obtained at intensity of 300-V train-of-four with interstimulus interval of 2 msec. **B,** This set depicts decrease in amplitude of leg responses obtained at 500 V at one point during instrumentation. **C,** These responses are obtained soon after initial change in **B** with total loss of amplitude in leg MEPs (*in box*). MEPs from arms are still intact. This suggests a lesion in cord below level of C8-T1. **D,** With some release of degree of distraction of spine, responses are shown to return in lower extremity.

in 5% of monitored cases that were reversible after taking appropriate surgical corrective measures. None of these patients had new postoperative deficits or worsening of pre-existing deficits. This combination of techniques was considered safe, reliable, and accurate and obviated the need for the "wake-up" test.[39]

Use of TCES-evoked MEPs has been easily accomplished with an anesthetic combination of narcotic drip accompanied by nitrous oxide. The use of isoflurane in addition to this combination resulted in a tendency for deterioration of MEP amplitude responses.[40] MEPs elicited by TCES are more feasible with total intravenous anesthesia compared with balanced anesthesia using nitrous oxide, isoflurane, and fentanyl. Some of the suppressant effects of balanced anesthesia can be overcome with higher stimulation intensities and repetitive stimulation.[41]

Pedicle Screw Stimulation

Intraoperative assessment during pedicle screw insertion can be used to minimize the risk of nerve root trauma from a misdirected screw. The integrity of pedicle screw placement can be assessed by directly stimulating the screw and by simultaneously recording myogenic responses from the appropriate myotomes. Using a direct monopolar nerve stimulator, with serial increments of the level of current intensity from 1 to 20 mA, triggered EMG recordings can be performed (Fig. 14–5). Absence of a myogenic response up to 10 mA is thought to indicate an intact pedicle. The presence of a pedicle breach is suspected by a stimulation-induced myogenic response at less than 7 to 10 mA (see Table 14–1).[7]

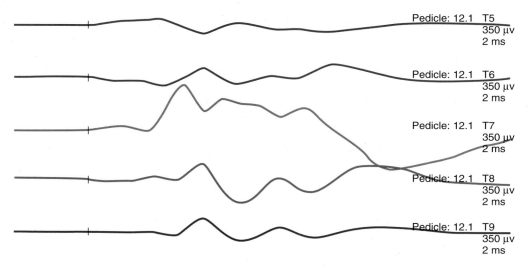

FIGURE 14–5 Nonsignificant triggered electromyography (EMG) response with pedicle screw stimulation. Pedicle screw stimulation of T7 screw shows threshold of triggered EMG response at intensity of 12 mA.

Summary

Intraoperative neurophysiologic monitoring of the spinal cord can be used to help detect early occurrence of neurophysiologic changes, allowing corrective action to reduce the incidence of neurologic injury to patients undergoing spine surgery. In the authors' opinion, the most important aspects of successful intraoperative monitoring include the following:

1. Availability of the right equipment to allow multimodality recordings (e.g., combinations of EMG, SEP, or MEPs)

2. Presence of a highly skilled and experienced technical and neurophysiologic team that ensures optimal technical recordings and accurate interpretation of any changes that may occur

3. Rapid communication between the neurophysiologic team and the surgical and anesthesia teams

4. Knowledge of the functional anatomy of the structures to be monitored and the limitations of the techniques to be used

The combination of different monitoring techniques, such as SEP and transcranial MEP monitoring, has enabled better interpretations of the neurologic status of the spinal cord. The newer technique of MEPs with TCES has gained widespread acceptance as a standard clinical intraoperative neurophysiologic application. MEPs have allowed for a more accurate assessment and interpretation of the functional status of the motor pathways at various levels of the neuraxis.

PEARLS

1. Key to the success of intraoperative neurophysiologic monitoring is a good understanding of the capabilities and limitations of the neurophysiologic tests being monitored.

2. One of the first issues to address when planning for intraoperative neurophysiologic monitoring is to determine the types of neurophysiologic tests to perform on a particular patient undergoing surgery.

3. SEPs monitor only sensory transmission through the dorsal column pathways. SEPs do not provide a direct measure of motor function.

4. In SEP monitoring, an amplitude decrease of greater than 50% and latency prolongation of more than 10% are considered significant. The most significant change is a complete loss of the cortical potential.

5. MEPs are a more direct technique that evaluates the motor pathway. Motor cortex stimulation with transcranial electrical stimulation provides a more reliable method for monitoring of the motor pathways.

PITFALLS

1. Significant changes in SEP monitoring can involve significant latency and amplitude changes that can occur in isolation.

2. If the peripheral response in SEP monitoring is absent, a technical cause for the change must be ruled out.

3. More recent evidence suggests that these spinally elicited neurogenic responses are generated through activation of the sensory pathways and retrograde activation of the alpha motor neurons.

4. Latency values have not always been found to be reliable indicators of significant change in TCES monitoring in clinical practice.

5. The use of fluorinated inhalational agents tends to lead to deterioration of MEP amplitudes.

KEY POINTS

1. The aim of most spinal cord monitoring is to prevent intraoperative injury that results in irreversible paraplegia or quadriplegia. Because a neurologic examination cannot be performed in an anesthetized patient, intraoperative neurophysiologic monitoring is used to determine the patient's neurologic status during surgery.

2. The term *significant change* is used to refer to the degree of changes seen in the neurophysiologic recordings. Changes that are termed significant have been shown to correlate well with intraoperative injury to the nervous system.

3. SEP monitoring has been used for many years to monitor spinal function intraoperatively during various surgeries involving the spine, such as corrective surgery for scoliosis or other congenital deformities and removal of intraspinal tumors or arteriovenous malformations. SEPs monitor only sensory transmission through the dorsal column pathways.

4. Various methods have been used to monitor spinal motor pathways during surgery. The methodology of MEP monitoring has been revolutionized by the use of multipulse TCES. Two different methods of recording MEPs can be used. In myogenic MEPs, responses can be recorded directly from the muscle. The second method involves recording responses directly from the spinal cord with use of an epidural catheter electrode that records a direct "D" wave and a volley of indirect "I" waves.

5. A combination of SEP and transcranial MEP monitoring can be used to monitor the spinal cord successfully. This combination of techniques is considered safe, reliable, and accurate and may obviate the need for the "wake-up" test.

6. Intraoperative assessment during pedicle screw insertion can be used to minimize the risk of nerve root trauma from a misdirected screw. The integrity of pedicle screw placement can be assessed by directly stimulating the screw and by simultaneously recording myogenic responses from the appropriate myotomes.

KEY REFERENCES

1. Nuwer MR, Dawson EG, Carlson LG, et al: Somatosensory evoked potential spinal cord monitoring reduces neurologic deficits after scoliosis surgery: Results of a large multicenter survey. Electroencephalogr Clin Neurophysiol 96:6-11, 1995.

2. Toleikis JR, Skelly JP, Carlvin AO, et al: Spinally elicited peripheral nerve responses are sensory rather than motor. Clin Neurophysiol 111:736-742, 2000.

3. Calancie B, Harris W, Broton JG, et al: "Threshold-level" multipulse transcranial electrical stimulation of motor cortex for intraoperative monitoring of spinal motor tracts: Description of method and comparison to somatosensory evoked potential monitoring. J Neurosurg 88:457-470, 1998.

4. Deletis V, Sala F: The role of intraoperative neurophysiology in the protection or documentation of surgically induced injury to the spinal cord. Ann N Y Acad Sci 939:137-144, 2001.

5. MacDonal DB: Safety of intraoperative transcranial electrical stimulation motor evoked potential monitoring. J Clin Neurophysiol 19:416-429, 2002.

REFERENCES

1. Nuwer MR, Dawson EG, Carlson LG, et al: Somatosensory evoked potential spinal cord monitoring reduces neurologic deficits after scoliosis surgery: Results of a large multicenter survey. Electroencephalogr Clin Neurophysiol 96:6-11, 1995.

2. Lesser RP, Raudzens P, Luders H, et al: Postoperative neurological deficits may occur despite unchanged intraoperative somatosensory evoked potentials. Ann Neurol 19:22-25, 1986.

3. Zornow MH, Grafe MR, Tybor C, et al: Preservation of evoked potentials in a case of anterior spinal artery syndrome. Electroencephalogr Clin Neurophysiol 77:137-139, 1990.

4. Lueders H, Gurd A, Hahn J, et al: A new technique for intraoperative monitoring of spinal cord function: Multichannel recording of spinal cord and subcortical evoked potentials. Spine 7:110-115, 1982.

5. Su CF, Haghighi SS, Oro JJ, et al: "Backfiring" in spinal cord monitoring: High thoracic spinal cord stimulation evokes sciatic response by antidromic sensory pathway conduction, not motor tract conduction. Spine 17:504-508, 1992.

6. Toleikis JR, Skelly JP, Carlvin AO, et al: Spinally elicited peripheral nerve responses are sensory rather than motor. Clin Neurophysiol 111:736-742, 2000.

7. Minahan RE, Sepkuty JP, Lesser RP, et al: Anterior spinal cord injury with preserved neurogenic "motor" evoked potentials. Clin Neurophysiol 112:1442-1450, 2001.

8. Nash CL Jr, Lorig RA, Schatzinger LA, et al: Spinal cord monitoring during operative treatment of the spine. Clin Orthop 126:100-105, 1977.

9. Jones SJ, Edgar MA, Ransford AO: Sensory nerve conduction in the human spinal cord: Epidural recordings made during scoliosis surgery. J Neurol Neurosurg Psychiatry 45:446-451, 1982.

10. Nuwer MR, Daube J, Fischer C, et al: Neuromonitoring during surgery. Report of an IFCN Committee. Electroencephalogr Clin Neurophysiol 87:263-276, 1993.

11. Merton PA, Morton HB: Stimulation of the cerebral cortex in the intact human subject. Nature 285:227, 1980.

12. Agnew WF, McCreery DB: Considerations for safety in the use of extracranial stimulation for motor evoked potentials. Neurosurgery 20:143-147, 1987.

13. Amassian VE, Cracco RQ: Human cerebral cortical responses to contralateral transcranial stimulation. Neurosurgery 20:148-155, 1987.

14. Amassian VE, Stewart M, Quirk GJ, et al: Physiological basis of motor effects of a transient stimulus to cerebral cortex. Neurosurgery 20:74-93, 1987.

15. Cracco RQ: Evaluation of conduction in central motor pathways: Techniques, pathophysiology, and clinical interpretation. Neurosurgery 20:199-203, 1987.

16. Cracco RQ, Amassian VE, Maccabee PJ, et al: Comparison of human transcallosal responses evoked by magnetic coil and electrical stimulation. Electroencephalogr Clin Neurophysiol 74:417-424, 1989.

17. Day BL, Rothwell JC, Thompson PD, et al: Motor cortex stimulation in intact man: II. Multiple descending volleys. Brain 110:1191-1209, 1987.

18. Jellinek D, Jewkes D, Symon L: Noninvasive intraoperative monitoring of motor evoked potentials under propofol anesthesia: Effects of spinal surgery on the amplitude and latency of motor evoked potentials. Neurosurgery 29:551-557, 1991.

19. Jellinek D, Platt M, Jewkes D, et al: Effects of nitrous oxide on motor evoked potentials recorded from skeletal muscle in patients under total anesthesia with intravenously administered propofol. Neurosurgery 29:558-562, 1991.

20. Kalkman CJ, Drummond JC, Ribberink AA: Low concentrations of isoflurane abolish motor evoked responses to transcranial electrical stimulation during nitrous oxide/opioid anesthesia in humans. Anesth Analg 73:410-415, 1991.

21. Hicks R, Burke D, Stephen J, et al: Corticospinal volleys evoked by electrical stimulation of human motor cortex after withdrawal of volatile anaesthetics. J Physiol 456:393-404, 1992.

22. Hicks RG, Woodforth IJ, Crawford MR, et al: Some effects of isoflurane on I waves of the motor evoked potential. Br J Anaesth 69:130-136, 1992.

23. Calancie B, Harris W, Broton JG, et al: "Threshold-level" multipulse transcranial electrical stimulation of motor cortex for intraoperative monitoring of spinal motor tracts: Description of method and comparison to somatosensory evoked potential monitoring. J Neurosurg 88:457-470, 1998.

24. Jones SJ, Harrison R, Koh KF, et al: Motor evoked potential monitoring during spinal surgery: Responses of distal limb muscles to transcranial cortical stimulation with pulse trains. Electroencephalogr Clin Neurophysiol 100:375-383, 1996.

25. Rodi Z, Deletis V, Morota N, et al: Motor evoked potentials during brain surgery. Pflugers Arch 431:R291-R292, 1996.

26. van Dongen EP, ter Beek HT, Schepens MA, et al: Effect of nitrous oxide on myogenic motor potentials evoked by a six pulse train of transcranial electrical stimuli: A possible monitor for aortic surgery. Br J Anaesth 82:323-328, 1999.

27. van Dongen EP, ter Beek HT, Schepens MA, et al: The influence of nitrous oxide to supplement fentanyl/low-dose propofol anesthesia on transcranial myogenic motor-evoked potentials during thoracic aortic surgery. J Cardiothorac Vasc Anesth 13:30-34, 1999.

28. van Dongen EP, ter Beek HT, Schepens MA, et al: Within-patient variability of myogenic motor-evoked potentials to multipulse transcranial electrical stimulation during two levels of partial neuromuscular blockade in aortic surgery. Anesth Analg 88:22-27, 1999.

29. Meylaerts SA, Jacobs MJ, van Iterson V, et al: Comparison of transcranial motor evoked potentials and somatosensory evoked potentials during thoracoabdominal aortic aneurysm repair. Ann Surg 230:742-749, 1999.

30. Calancie B, Harris W, Broton JG, et al: "Threshold-level" multipulse transcranial electrical stimulation of motor cortex for intraoperative monitoring of spinal motor tracts: Description of method and comparison to somatosensory evoked potential monitoring. J Neurosurg 88:457-470, 1998.

31. Nuwer MR, Dawson EG, Carlson LG, et al: Somatosensory evoked potential spinal cord monitoring reduces neurologic deficits after scoliosis surgery: Results of a large multicenter survey. Electroencephalogr Clin Neurophysiol 96:6-11, 1995.

32. Deletis V, Sala F: The role of intraoperative neurophysiology in the protection or documentation of surgically induced injury to the spinal cord. Ann N Y Acad Sci 939:137-144, 2001.

33. Cioni B, Meglio M, Rossi GF: Intraoperative motor evoked potentials monitoring in spinal neurosurgery. Arch Ital Biol 137:115-126, 1999.

34. MacDonal DB: Safety of intraoperative transcranial electrical stimulation motor evoked potential monitoring. J Clin Neurophysiol 19:416-429, 2002.

35. Luk KD, Hu Y, Wong YW, et al: Evaluation of various evoked potential techniques for spinal cord monitoring during scoliosis surgery. Spine 26:1772-1777, 2001.

36. Jones SJ, Harrison R, Koh KF, et al: Motor evoked potential monitoring during spinal surgery: Responses of distal limb muscles to transcranial cortical stimulation with pulse trains. Electroencephalogr Clin Neurophysiol 100:375-383, 1996.

37. Lang EW, Beutler AS, Chesnut RM, et al: Myogenic motor-evoked potential monitoring using partial neuromuscular blockade in surgery of the spine. Spine 21:1676-1686, 1996.

38. Morota N, Deletis V, Constantini S, et al: The role of motor evoked potentials during surgery for intramedullary spinal cord tumors. Neurosurgery 41:1327-1336, 1997.

39. Stephen JP, Sullivan MR, Hicks RG, et al: Cotrel-Dubousset instrumentation in children using simultaneous motor and somatosensory evoked potential monitoring. Spine 21:2450-2457, 1996.

40. Calancie B, Klose KJ, Baier S, et al: Isoflurane-induced attenuation of motor evoked potentials caused by electrical motor cortex stimulation during surgery. J Neurosurg 74:897-904, 1991.

41. Pechstein U, Nadstawek J, Zentner J, et al: Isoflurane plus nitrous oxide versus propofol for recording of motor evoked potentials after high frequency repetitive electrical stimulation. Electroencephalogr Clin Neurophysiol 108:175-181, 1998.

15 CHAPTER

Targeting Pain Generators

Richard Derby, MD
Lee Wolfer, MD

Spinal pain is very common and exacts a significant toll for the individual and society. Low back pain has a lifetime prevalence from 54% to 80%, an annual prevalence of 15% to 45%, and a point prevalence of 30%.[1] Low back pain is the second most common reason for disability among adults in the United States with approximately 150 million work days lost per year.[2,3] Spinal pain is the second most common reason for outpatient generalist physician visits, the third most common reason for surgical interventions, and the fifth most common reason for hospitalization.[4,5] The cost to care for patients with low back pain is more than $100 billion per year.[6] The prevalence of individuals seeking care for low back pain also seems to be increasing significantly. From 1992-2006, the prevalence of patients presenting with chronic impairing low back pain increased from 4% to 10%.[7] Cervical pain exacts a significant toll in terms of individual morbidity and socioeconomic burden. Targeting pain generators through precision diagnostic methods is the first step toward appropriate and effective treatments for chronic spinal pain.

Much of the epidemiologic data on low back pain are nonspecific, meaning that a cause cannot be found in most cases. Despite evidence to the contrary in the 21st century, these older, inaccurate epidemiologic studies continue to be quoted by current authors. One of the oldest epidemiologic studies commonly quoted was published more than 40 years ago by Dillane and colleagues[8] and was based on a retrospective practice audit of data gathered more than *50 years ago.* Dillane and colleagues[8] reported that they could not detect a cause for low back pain in approximately 80% of female and 90% of male patients with acute back syndrome. These authors did not report the use of any x-ray studies and apparently relied solely on history and physical examination.[8] They diagnosed approximately 11% of male patients and approximately 4% of female patients with low back "strain." Until more recently, the only tools to diagnose the etiology of low back pain have been history, physical examination, and sometimes x-ray or computed tomography (CT) scan.

In 1982, Nachemson[9] reviewed the literature on chronic low back pain. In perhaps the most frequently quoted epidemiologic study on the cause of chronic low back pain,

Nachemson[9] reported that in only 15% of cases could a pathoanatomic explanation be found for patients with chronic low back pain (>3 months). Nachemson[9] stated, "probably very little can be done at our present state of ignorance to treat these patients and to improve their natural histories." Low back pain is a symptom, not a diagnosis, in the same way that abdominal pain is a symptom and not a diagnosis. In acute cases of low back pain, this nonspecific diagnosis usually suffices because most cases of acute, first-time low back pain resolve with minimal intervention; however, when low back pain becomes chronic, recurrent, and disabling, the clinician must diagnose the source of the pain so that an appropriate treatment plan may be devised.

When a source of pain is not obvious, diagnosis often depends on who makes the diagnosis and sets the reference standards by which the diagnosis is "proven." Who is right? For that matter, can anyone reliably diagnose the cause of chronic benign spinal pain? Many authors argue that chronic benign spinal pain is largely due to exaggerated functional complaints and irreversible central nervous system sensitization,[10] making pain self-perpetuating and diagnosis all but impossible. These contentions are not often supported by primary studies,[11] however, and authors and clinicians question this diagnosis.[12,13]

Interventionalists developed and refined precision, fluoroscopically guided diagnostic interventional spine procedures in the 1980s and 1990s[14] to diagnose and treat nonspecific spinal pain better. Fluoroscopically guided block procedures are now considered the reference standard to confirm a tissue diagnosis. Out of the previous era of "ignorance," many diagnostic protocols have been validated and standardized.[15,16] Using the results of precision-guided diagnostic procedures, surgeons identify spinal segments for fusion at various stages of the degenerative cascade.[17] Most surgeons still depend on an accurate diagnosis of a specific pain generator to select appropriate therapy[18] because surgical results for chronic benign pain syndromes without a reversible anatomic cause are generally poor.[19]

The debate continues regarding diagnostic injections as new research emerges, along with better treatment options.

Spinal pain is a complex interaction of many biopsychosocial factors. Chronic spinal pain may originate from one or more spinal levels and different anatomic structures in the anterior, middle, and posterior columns. Spinal pain also varies over time. Pain can be caused by abnormal mechanical stress on normal tissue affected by structural deformity, normal mechanical stress on injured tissues, minor stress on chronically inflamed and sensitized tissues, damaged nerves, and a varying combination of all of these. Chronic pain causes a greater or lesser degree of central sensitization and together with a multitude of functional factors, including the requirement for copious amounts of opiates, often makes accurate diagnosis difficult. Nevertheless, it can be argued that most chronic axial spinal pain is due to accumulated repetitive strain or low-grade trauma,[20] acute injuries to the major underlying structures and their supporting ligaments, or both. Ongoing stimulation from these peripheral structures to a greater or lesser extent maintains a state of peripheral and central sensitization. In time, adaptive responses within the posterior, middle, and anterior columns may attenuate, exacerbate, or cause new sources of pain.

Despite this complexity, specific tissue pain generators can be hypothesized based on history, physical examination, imaging studies, and response to directed treatment. Interventional procedures are used to test the hypothesis that pain is related to a structural abnormality hypothesized by clinical and imaging findings. (The word *hypothesis* is used loosely here; arguably one only can confirm a *clinical impression* using diagnostic blocks. A hypothesis is confirmed using a study protocol that can show approximately <5% probability that the findings are due to chance). Foremost, interventional procedures are perhaps best used to refute one's hypothesis that a particular structure is painful. That is, diagnosis is made through the process of systematically excluding various tissue causes of axial and extremity pain in the posterior, middle, and anterior columns.[19]

This chapter presents primarily evidenced-based standards and some expert opinions for confirming or refuting one's hypothesis that a particular structure, structures, or segments are a source of spinal pain.[15] A discussion of pain resulting from "red flag" conditions, such as fracture, tumor, infection, systemic diseases, or referred from nonspinal structures, is not included; likewise, "yellow flag" conditions (psychosocial factors) are not discussed in detail. Evaluation of the anterior column using provocative discography is discussed elsewhere, so the discussion in this chapter is focused on diagnosis of pain originating from the posterior and middle columns, in particular, pain originating from the zygapophyseal joint and sacroiliac joint in the posterior column and from the nerve root, dorsal root ganglion, and dura in the middle column. The diagnostic use of injection procedures is explored and not their therapeutic value other than the diagnostic value of response or nonresponse to treatment. Finally and most importantly, this chapter is not a systematic review, and the interested reader is referred to numerous systematic reviews on the diagnostic value of spine injections.[1,15,16,20-26]

Diagnostic Analgesic Injections as Reference Standard

The belief that chronic benign spinal pain is difficult to diagnose is supported by the low specificity and sensitivity of the history, physical examination, and various imaging modalities as the reference standard for diagnosing chronic benign spinal pain[11,27,28] and a bias that chronic pain is to a greater rather than lesser extent a neuropathic process with central sensitization.[19] If one uses interventional diagnosis with precision fluoroscopically guided procedures as a reference standard for identifying pain, however, one can arrive at a tissue diagnosis in approximately 70% to 80% of cases.[29,30] Which approach is right? Truth usually lies somewhere in between.

The primary treating physician or consultant needs to formulate the diagnosis based on the available information and be prepared to defend the diagnosis to contracted physician reviewers. Understanding the strengths and weaknesses of diagnostic analgesic data may help the practitioner decide whether the risk-to-benefit ratio of obtaining such information is appropriate for any given circumstance. Perhaps more important, the process of investigation itself may lead to a better understanding of the patient's capacity to respond appropriately to a technically successful surgical or interventional procedure.

The rationale for facet blocks is based on the anatomic fact that the innervation of facet joints (medial branches) is known and that zygapophyseal joints are capable of causing pain.[15] Local anesthetic blocks rely on the specificity of anesthetizing a single or limited number of structures or nerves and on the patient's capacity to distinguish clearly a reduction in preblock pain after anesthetizing one or more structures. Injection of a limited volume of local anesthetic into a zygapophyseal joint or its nerve supply is relatively specific for anesthetizing a joint and its capsule. Similarly, local anesthetic injected into the disc should anesthetize nociceptors within radial annular fissures that communicate with the nucleus. When anesthetizing the nerve root within the middle column, the block is less specific for axial pain relief because several structures may be partially blocked (e.g., dorsal root ganglion, ventral rami, sinuvertebral nerve, posterior longitudinal ligament).

Anesthetizing a structure does not reveal the cause of pain; anesthetizing the nerve supply simply relieves pain. This is an important concept. The cause of pain should dictate the type of treatment, and the treatment is only as good or bad as its success in eliminating or modulating the cause. If the cause of pain in the case of a specific zygapophyseal joint is synovial inflammation, one would expect short-term to intermediate pain relief after the intra-articular injection of corticosteroids. If a patient's pain is due to mechanical or neuropathic causes, there is no reason that corticosteroids would be effective other than the expected duration of the local anesthetic. There is no reason that there should be longer term pain relief except for the expected rate of placebo response or reported pain relief secondary to spontaneous pain regression.[31] That is, relief of pain during the local anesthetic phase does not distinguish irreversible neuropathic pain from reversible nociceptive pain.

In the case of chronic radicular pain, significant relief of pain for several weeks after the injection of corticosteroids would suggest that there is a reversible structural cause.[32]

Testing Protocols for Diagnostic Injections

As essential as precision technique is in the performance of diagnostic blocks, so is standardized assessment. Standardized diagnostic block evaluation sheets should be filled out for each patient; detailed postprocedure assessment protocols and sample evaluation instruments are available in the International Spine Intervention Society Practice Guidelines.[15] Preprocedural and postprocedural evaluation should be performed by unbiased personnel and checked by the physician. It is recommended that the patient fill out a body pain diagram with pain scores (visual analog scale [VAS]) before and after the procedure. Additionally, the patient should rate current pain levels with various movements (e.g., lumbar flexion, extension, side-bending, sitting, and standing).

Evaluation after the procedure includes VAS scores with the same positions and maneuvers and a subjective report of percent relief of pain. The patient's narrative response should corroborate with VAS score, and any discrepancies should be explained. With medial branch blocks, relief of pain may vary according to the mass of drug reaching the nerve, and one may not reliably achieve a long-acting block; however, relief for less than 1 hour is unconvincing. In the case of selective nerve root blocks, it is often useful to have the patient distinguish between axial, proximal (shoulder or buttock), and extremity pain, the caveat being that a diagnostic block may not significantly reduce axial pain, but that does not mean that the block was unsuccessful. Some patients also need to be counseled to ignore injection site pain. Specific provoking maneuvers should also be evaluated, such as the Spurling test for cervical radiculopathy and three or more sacroiliac joint provocative maneuvers before and after the procedure. Ideally, the patient would be tested at approximately 15 minutes after a lidocaine block and approximately 30 minutes after a bupivacaine block. Additional evaluations at 1 and 2 hours after block are useful but may depend on availability of staff.

The patient may be sent home with a pain diary to keep for 4 to 6 hours after the procedure. For any diagnostic injection, a patient should have at least approximately 5/10 intensity of pain to be able to judge the degree of relief reliably. A subject should have at least 50% relief for a positive response to be considered; at least 70% relief is more convincing. In regard to selective nerve root blocks, no more than two levels should be checked on one session. Depending on the importance of refuting or confirming whether a particular nerve is symptomatic, one may choose to inject the most probable source of pain or a level that it is hoped can be proven nonpainful.

Confounding Factors

Sedation

An important, potentially confounding factor when performing diagnostic blocks concerns the use of sedation. Logically, one would assume that administration of opiates and sedatives before a diagnostic block would increase the false-positive rate; however, Manchikanti and colleagues[33] found that this proportion of patients was relatively small, and there was no difference with use of saline, opiate, or sedative. In a randomized study of 60 patients, Manchikanti and colleagues[33] titrated medication to relaxation using saline, midazolam, or fentanyl. They found that only 50% of patients receiving sodium were relaxed, whereas 100% of patients receiving either fentanyl or midazolam were relaxed. In all groups, 10% of the patients reported greater than 80% pain relief with active motion testing. Even so, typically, one limits or omits sedation before a diagnostic injection, however.

Another method to mitigate false-positive results is to administer a short-acting sedative such as propofol and delay testing to 30 minutes after the procedure to minimize the sedative effects. If the patient is anxious or especially if the patient routinely takes significant doses of opiates and may be in early opiate withdrawal owing to NPO status, the patient could be sedated and tested after the administration of a judicious dose of opiate.

Biopsychosocial Factors

More recently, authors have reiterated the importance of shifting the concept of "backache." Kikuchi[34] recommended changing the term *spinal disorder* to *biopsychosocial pain syndrome* and the term *morphologic abnormality* to *mechanical, functional disorder*. According to Kikuchi,[34] morphologic and structural abnormalities do not always explain all of a patient's pain, and chronic backache should not be seen as an isolated spinal disease. A significant amount of scholarship has been devoted to enumerating the psychosocial factors associated with spinal pain. In a classic study comparing workers with symptomatic disc herniation (requiring surgery) versus asymptomatic workers, significant differences were found in three areas: presence of nerve root compromise, psychosocial factors (depression, anxiety, marital status, self-control), and work perception (satisfaction, job loss, occupational stress, intensity of concentration).[35] Of the risk factors, two of three were functional, not morphologic.

The authors agree with this model and acknowledge that psychosocial factors have a significant impact on spinal pain; the authors also acknowledge the importance of treating the "bio" component of the *biopsychosocial syndrome*. Today's spine specialists readily acknowledge that patients often benefit from a multidisciplinary approach to treatment. Research continues to investigate the best way to treat patients with chronic spinal pain and significant psychosocial comorbidities.

Although the long-term results of treatment for chronic axial back pain may be influenced by various psychosocial factors,[36,37] the possible effect of psychosocial factors in determining the patient's tested perception of pain and functional improvement with treatment does not indicate that the diagnosis was incorrect. In many cases, when a "biologic" pain generator can be correctly identified and treated, the psychosocial distress resolves. If it is true that psychological variables determine whether a patient admits relief on various testing instruments, does the evidence of physiologic distress noted on test scores reverse when the patient's chronic pain is relieved?

Wallis and colleagues[38] studied 17 patients after whiplash injury with a single symptomatic cervical zygapophyseal joint who were enrolled in a randomized controlled trial of percutaneous radiofrequency neurotomy. At 3 months after the procedure, all patients whose pain was relieved had complete resolution of preoperative psychological distress; in contrast, all but one of the patients who did not experience pain relief continued to experience psychological distress. Manchikanti and colleagues[39] found no correlation between somatization disorder and inappropriate Waddell signs and symptoms to response in pain relief after a comparative double block protocol for diagnosing facet pain. Derby and colleagues[40] found no difference in response to pressure-controlled disc stimulation between patients with abnormal psychometric Distress Risk Assessment Method scores and asymptomatic volunteers.

Posterior Compartment: Zygapophyseal Joint and Sacroiliac Joint

The zygapophyseal joint and sacroiliac joint are the two primary structures within the posterior compartment that are sources of chronic spinal pain. In addition, hip and shoulder pain may cause symptoms similar to spinal structures and localized injections into these joints with preblock and postblock active examination can help differentiate hip and shoulder pain from spinal pain. Although soft tissues may be painful, for the purpose and brevity of this chapter these structures are considered a secondary source of pain in most chronic spinal conditions.

Zygapophyseal Joint

Each spinal segment is composed of a three-joint complex: the intervertebral discs and two posterolateral facet joints.[41] Facet joints can also be called *zygapophyseal joints*. The word *apophysis* is Greek, meaning an "offshoot" or a "bony protuberance."[42] Anatomically, the zygapophyseal joint is an outgrowth of the vertebral body. The zygapophyseal or facet joints are formed by the articulation of the inferior articular process of one vertebra with the superior articular process of the adjoining vertebra. Zygapophyseal joints have classic synovial joint features: hyaline cartilage surfaces, a synovial membrane, and a surrounding joint capsule.[43] Facet joints have varied morphology and function based on their location within the spine. Although the intervertebral disc is loaded primarily in flexion, the zygapophyseal joints are loaded in extension and lumbar rotation.[44,45] The orientation of the facet joint varies based on the requirements of regional spine function. Lumbar facets are situated sagittally to limit axial rotation and loading, whereas the cervical and thoracic facets are oriented coronally to limit shearing forces on the disc. Innervation is via the medial branches of the dorsal ramus in most locations.

Pathophysiology of Facet Pain

Traumatic injury to lumbar and cervical zygapophyseal joints is common and probably occurs to a lesser extent to the thoracic joints. In the setting of trauma, there is a clear pathophysiologic difference between facet joints and nontraumatic controls. Zygapophyseal joint sections from autopsy specimens of individuals with a past history of trauma but dying of natural causes show significant age-related, gender-related, and trauma-related changes in the bone, cartilage, and soft tissues, including subchondral sclerosis, fibrillation and splitting of cartilage, and cartilage length differences, versus subjects with no history of trauma.[46] Histologic sections of the lumbar zygapophyseal joints of mostly motor vehicle accident victims revealed fractures of the superior articular process, central infarctions of the subchondral bone plate, and capsule tears including the ligamentum flavum.[47,48] Most tissue sections (77%) show soft tissue injuries, and approximately 30% (11 of 33) show fractures and infarctions. Sections from the cervical spine in trauma victims show similar injuries to the zygapophyseal joint articular cartilage and annular lesions in the intervertebral discs and cartilaginous endplates (Fig. 15–1).[49] In the lumbar and cervical spines, lesions were found exclusively in the trauma patients and in none of the patients in the control group.[46,49,50]

Many of these pathoanatomic findings are occult on routine x-ray, CT scan, and magnetic resonance imaging (MRI) but may be the cause of ongoing neck pain in survivors of motor vehicle accidents or other significant trauma. In a small study with short-term follow-up (approximately 3 months), Eisenstein and Parry[51] examined zygapophyseal joints in 12 patients who underwent successful fusion for zygapophyseal joint mediated pain (diagnosed by provocation arthrography, intra-articular blocks, and negative discography) versus controls and found histologic changes similar to changes of chondromalacia patellae and osteoarthritis of large joints. The most frequent finding was focal full-thickness cartilage necrosis or loss of cartilage with exposure of subchondral

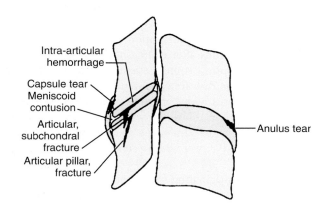

FIGURE 15–1 Postmortem studies of motor vehicle victims reveal the following sites of injury; many of these injuries may not be visible on routine MRI. (From Bogduk N, McGuirk B: Management of Acute and Chronic Neck Pain: An Evidence-based Approach. Philadelphia, Elsevier, 2006.)

bone; osteophyte formation was absent in all specimens.[51] Degenerative histologic findings alone do not make a definitive diagnosis of facet syndrome, however. Ziv and colleagues[52] reported a high proportion of coarsely fibrillated or ulcerated (or both) facets in fresh cadaveric spines from young adults (30 to 50 years old); such degeneration remains constant throughout adulthood.

Traumatic and repetitive injury leading to painful "facet arthritis"[48] may cause pain because zygapophyseal joints and their capsules are heavily innervated structures subject to high stress and strain during spinal loading.[53] Joints comprise free and encapsulated nerve endings containing substance P and calcitonin gene-related peptide.[54-56] Substance P, calcitonin gene-related peptide, and immunoreactive sensory and autonomic nerves are found in zygapophyseal joint synovial membranes.[57] Facet capsules contain low-threshold mechanoreceptors, mechanically sensitive nociceptors, and silent nociceptors.[58] These low-threshold and high-threshold mechanoreceptors fire when the joint capsule is stretched or compressed, and their firing can be suppressed by injected lidocaine and hydrocortisone.[59] In animal models, induced inflammation decreases the threshold of nerves within the joint capsules and causes elevated baseline discharge rates.[59] In animal models of knee arthritis, acute inflammation sensitizes fine articular afferents, which become active at rest and respond more vigorously to routine painless joint range of motion.[60]

Excessive stretching damages the zygapophyseal joint capsules and causes axonal swelling, retraction balls, and inflammation.[58] The result is hyperexcitability and spontaneous firing, which are synonymous with neuropathic pain. Capsular injury during a whiplash injury may cause persistent neck pain secondary to chronic capsular overstretching. Animal studies suggest that facet capsule strains comparable to strains previously reported for whiplash kinematics and subcatastrophic failures of this ligament activate nociceptors within the capsule.[61-65] In addition, chronic capsular loading in animals may cause central inflammation resulting in mechanical hyperalgesia and in some cases centrally maintained pain.[56,63,66,67]

Animal studies showing central sensitization are consistent with the widespread hypersensitivity documented in whiplash patients. Although focal sensitization to mechanical stimuli may be found 3 months after whiplash injury, which mostly resolves by 6 months, some patients develop persistent pain with symptoms that are consistent with chronic neuropathic pain.[68] Patients with persistent pain at approximately 6 months show signs of more widespread hyperalgesia[69] and hypersensitivity to cutaneous and muscular stimulation in neck and lower limb consistent with central hypersensitivity.[10,70]

If chronic pain originating from injury to the zygapophyseal joints is due to capsular stretch and maintained by central hypersensitivity, local anesthetic with or without corticosteroid should suppress nociceptive input for the duration of the local anesthetic effect and in some cases (e.g., similar to a sympathetically maintained pain state) for days to weeks.[71] If most of a patient's pain is due to mechanical and central causes, there would be no reason why local anesthetic and corticosteroid would be more effective than local anesthetic alone.[72-74] Former and latter logical outcomes are supported in prospective and randomized controlled trials,[74] although alleviating pain with medial branch blocks was shown in one study to relieve pain for an average of several months.[75,76]

Decreasing peripheral input 6 months or longer by heat ablation of medial branches relieves pain[77]; the pain typically returns within the expected time it takes for the medial branches to regenerate. Such prolonged relief of pain, if accompanied by resolution of widespread hypersensitivity, would imply that central hypersensitivity is reversible when the peripheral source of input is interrupted. That is, if there is a concern that persistent central hypersensitivity would lead to failure of a proposed localized or segmental stabilization procedure, resolution of widespread and local hypersensitivity after medial branch neurotomy might predict that decrease in nociceptive input by surgical stabilization would be successful. Zygapophyseal joint pain often occurs at more than one segment, however, and one must identify adjacent or skipped level sources of zygapophyseal joint pain, especially if one is considering surgical fusion or arthroplasty.

When cadaveric lumbar spines are anteriorly fixated at one level, motion is transferred to adjacent segments causing increased capsular stretch in the adjacent facet joints.[78] In extension, cervical arthroplasty models exhibit significant increases of facet force at the treated level. In the fusion model, the facet forces decrease at the treated segment and increase at the adjacent segment.[79] Failure to recognize symptomatic pathology at an adjacent level or the same level may lead to early or late return of pain. This is not a failure of the diagnostic blocks; it is a failure to obtain a thorough diagnosis.

Rationale for Control Blocks in Diagnostic Facet Intra-articular and Medial Branch Blocks

Can a diagnosis of facet syndrome be made without injections? The diagnosis of zygapophyseal joint pain is typically hypothesized based on clinical findings and imaging studies. Most clinicians rely on a variety of favorite criteria, such as localized unilateral pain that is worse in extension, pain worse in the morning and better with gentle movement, concordant pain provoked with palpation approximately 1 cm lateral to the midline over the zygapophyseal joints, and imaging studies showing signs of facet degeneration. A "facet syndrome"[80] diagnosed by clinical findings has not been substantiated, however, if one uses as a reference standard the relief of pain after placebo-controlled anesthetic blocks.[23,27,81] The current best evidence has not found any individual clinical finding or cluster of findings that can predict response to the reference standard of pain relief after local anesthetic block of the medial branches or intra-articular zygapophyseal joint block.

The purpose of diagnostic facet blocks is to establish the diagnosis or rule it out, similar to a liver biopsy of a suspicious lesion. Diagnostic facet blocks are a tertiary intervention in patients with chronic pain that has not resolved with time and conservative care. The current standard for the diagnosis of facet mediated pain is the use of controlled differential (double) blocks to confirm or refute one's hypothesis that the facet joint is a pain generator. Because of the high false-positive rates of single diagnostic blocks, a single block does not constitute a diagnosis, and control blocks are essential to decrease the incidence of false-positive responses.[82] The reported false-positive rate of a single diagnostic block ranges from 17% to 63%.[83] In a retrospective review of 438 patients using a double block paradigm requiring 80% relief, the false-positive rates for a single diagnostic block were 45%, 42%, and 45% for the cervical, thoracic, and lumbar regions.[83]

Although Cohen and colleagues[84] showed that treatment results after medial branch neurotomies were not changed by requiring a placebo control, the current published standard of interventional societies requires a confirmatory block before making a diagnosis of zygapophyseal joint mediated pain. The best-studied double block protocol requires a difference in pain relief duration based on a shorter or longer acting medication—typically, greater than 1 hour for lidocaine and greater than 2 hours for bupivacaine.[85,86] Because the goal is to have a placebo control and because consent and patient compliance issues hinder using a saline block control, one may argue that any prior diagnostic injection in which the patient reports no relief is a valid control block, especially because the patient and the physician were anticipating relief. Because many insurance companies in the United States no longer authorize or consider double blocks medically necessary, the occurrence of a previous "negative" block evaluation could be the negative control.

When the treatment is relatively benign, convincing relief with physician and staff testing after facet or medial branch injections in an older patient with clinical symptoms consistent with zygapophyseal joint pain may not justify confirmatory injections.[84] A young patient who has little or no facet abnormalities, who is on a significant dose of narcotics, and who reports less than convincing approximately 80% relief should undergo a second confirmatory injection before considering interventional or surgical treatment based on the block results.

The rationale for how many and which levels to test is debated. Levels are typically chosen based on known pain referral patterns, prevalence studies, and localized manual palpation. Using a comparative double block control, Manchukonda and colleagues[83] found that most often two joints were symptomatic in the lumbar spine and three adjacent joints were symptomatic in the thoracic and cervical spine. The most logistically efficient and least costly method is to rule out facet pain globally on the side or sides of the patient's pain and at the proximity of approximately two to three adjacent levels. One would inject (in the case of lumbar spine) the L2-5 medial branches to block the L3-4, L4-5, and L5-S1 zygapophyseal joints (Fig. 15–2 shows medial branch anatomy of the lumbar spine; Fig. 15–3 shows a lumbar medial branch block). If no relief occurred and there was no evidence that the higher joints were involved, and if one is confident that the facets were denervated, one can eliminate facet pain from the

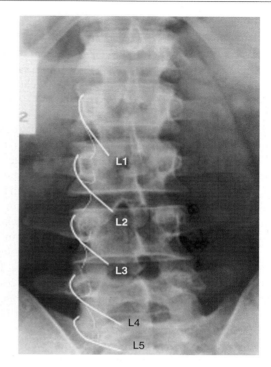

FIGURE 15–2 Anteroposterior radiograph of lumbar spine showing course of medial branches of L1-4 dorsal rami, L5 dorsal ramus, and their articular branches to lumbar zygapophyseal joints. Medial branches are blocked at junction of superior articular process and transverse process. (From Bogduk N [ed]: Practice Guidelines for Spinal Diagnostic and Treatment Procedures. San Francisco, International Spine Intervention Society, 2004.)

diagnosis. If the result is positive, one can perform more selected denervation on a confirmatory injection. Although this could be argued to be the most efficient method, many third-party payers in the United States limit injections to two levels per session.

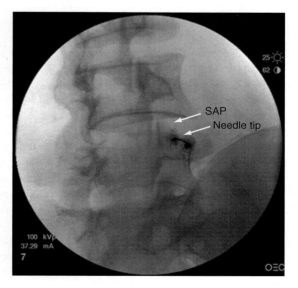

FIGURE 15–3 Oblique view of right L4 medial branch block. A 3.5-inch 25-gauge needle is placed at junction of L5 superior articular process and transverse process. A total of 0.5 mL of contrast dye is injected along medial branch. SAP, superior articular process. (Courtesy Richard Derby, MD.)

Diagnostic Accuracy

The features of a test that indicate its diagnostic accuracy are sensitivity and specificity. From these measures, the false-positive and false-negative rates and predictive value can be derived. *Sensitivity* refers to the ability of the test to identify correctly patients with the disease. Several factors that affect sensitivity should be discussed. Vessels accompany the medial branch as they course around the waist of the superior articular pillar, and injecting local anesthetic into a vessel rather than around the nerve may cause a false-negative response.

Kaplan and colleagues[87] reported that medial branch blocks may fail because of venous uptake. Venous uptake occurred in 7 of 20 (35%) medial branch blocks. If venous uptake was encountered, repositioning of the needle resulted in joint anesthesia only 50% of the time. When venous uptake was encountered, the subjects were brought back for a later injection. These findings stress the importance of using contrast medium for medial branch blocks and carefully observing the flow pattern. Kaplan and colleagues[87] also found that in 11% of cases they were unable to anesthetize the joint, even in the absence of venous uptake. Medial branch blocks in the lumbar spine would have an 11% false-negative rate; this may have been due to anomalous or collateral facet innervation or insufficient volume of local anesthetic reaching the target nerve.

Rarely discussed is the consistency with which one may expect a longer duration of action of bupivacaine versus lidocaine. Although bupivacaine has a longer duration of action than lidocaine, the mass of drug reaching the nerve is the most important variable, and one cannot guarantee that the same amount will be available on consecutive sessions. In addition, most patients are not kept in the recovery area for the duration of local anesthetic to be evaluated, and the duration depends on a patient's self-reporting, which may or may not be consistent between injections. Lord and colleagues[86] showed that using a double block comparative standard, 65% of patients failed to recognize the difference in duration of pain relief but did accurately distinguish a separate placebo-controlled block with saline.

The crucial factors for specificity of the diagnosis of zygapophyseal joint pain are accurate targeting of the intended structure under fluoroscopy, confirmed by contrast medium, and the delivery of the appropriate volume of local anesthetic. Intra-articular joint blocks are specific, unless there is a medial capsular tear or injection of excessive volumes (>1 mL injected into a lumbar zygapophyseal joint or 0.3 mL injected into a cervical zygapophyseal joint), which may rupture the capsule and spread medially into the epidural space.[88,89] Many early studies of facet intra-articular blocks used 2 to 8 mL per injection. When reviewing negative studies regarding facet injections and the systematic reviews that still quote these studies, the discerning reader should check the total volume of injectant used.[89,90] Destouet and colleagues[89] found that volumes of injectant of 0.5 to 1.5 mL commonly ruptured the superior recess of the capsule and extravasated; in later studies, Destouet and Murphy[91] aspirated the 0.5 to 1.5 mL of contrast dye before adding local anesthetic and steroid. Cadaveric studies performed with variable volumes of methylene blue injected into facet joint (1 to 4 mL) showed that the dye extended not as expected into the paraspinal tissues but rather into the epidural space and around the spinal nerves.[92] Moran and colleagues[92] described the facet capsule as thick dorsally, whereas anteriorly the facet synovial membrane is contiguous with the ligamentum flavum, and the adipose tissue in the superior recess is in direct contact with the adipose tissue around the spinal nerve. Randomized controlled studies validate the specificity of medial branch blocks for relief of zygapophyseal joint mediated pain.[93]

To maintain the specificity of medial branch block, a low volume of local anesthetic is used to anesthetize a specific cervical[93] or lumbar medial branch.[87,88] If volumes greater than 0.5 mL are used, the close proximity of the lumbar lateral and intermediate branch to the medial branch potentially might increase false-positive rates by blocking paraspinal soft tissues (ligaments or muscles or both).[20,94] In addition, volumes greater than 0.5 mL on the superior edge of the lumbar transverse process may spread onto the dorsal and ventral spinal nerves.[88] Decreasing input into the central nervous system by anesthetizing any structure or nerve could relieve pain by decreasing or modulating central input. Although this is a probable confounding factor, the reference typically cited is the study by North and colleagues,[95] which reported an unacceptably high false-positive rate for diagnostic blocks in patients with low back pain. The conclusion reached by North and colleagues[95] was that diagnostic blocks had limited specificity, however. Their protocol clearly lacked diagnostic specificity, however. They used an excessive 3 mL volume of bupivacaine for the medial branch blocks. Because 0.5 mL of local anesthetic placed too close to the superior edge flows onto the exiting root, the reported decrease in sciatic pain was more likely due to anesthetizing the spinal nerve and not a false-positive effect of neuromodulation.[88]

Because patients in the study by North and colleagues[95] reported an average relief of 75% to 80% after anesthetizing the sciatic nerve, operators must be aware that blocking this nerve anywhere along its course may result in the report of pain relief. As previously mentioned, relief of pain for the duration of the local anesthetic effect cannot distinguish between reversible inflammatory or compressive causes of pain and nonreversible neuropathic causes of pain.

Although North and colleagues[95] found that 3 mL of local anesthetic placed into muscles at several levels has relatively minimal effect on sciatic pain, some authors question whether anesthetizing the needle track increases false-positive responses.[20] Patients probably report more pain relief when the needle track is anesthetized. Rather than a false-positive response, one would expect better pain relief when patients are not experiencing lingering needle-related pain at the same time as pain relief resulting from anesthetizing the zygapophyseal joints.

Lumbar Spine: Facet Syndrome

History

In 1911, Goldthwait[96] reported that facet joint asymmetry could cause lumbago, sciatica, and paraplegia. Ghormley[97] first coined the term *facet syndrome* as a cause of referred pain and the sciatica resulting from direct nerve root compression by the facet. Badgley[97a] first described the facet joint as an independent source of referred pain in greater detail. Mooney and Robertson[80] described "facet syndrome" referral patterns by injection of hypertonic saline into the lumbar facets of patients with positive diagnostic blocks. Subsequently, Mooney and Robertson[80] were the first to use x-ray–guided intra-articular injections with local anesthetic and corticosteroid; they reported complete pain relief in approximately one fifth of patients presenting with low back and leg pain. Dreyfuss and colleagues[88] were the first to describe an effective lumbar medial branch block technique. Using this technique, Kaplan and colleagues[87] showed that pain resulting from facet capsular distention could be successfully blocked in approximately 90% of cases by a medial branch block with 2% lidocaine versus saline.

Lumbar Zygapophyseal Joint Pain

Lumbar zygapophyseal joint pain is common and seems to become more prevalent as patients age and as the duration of chronic back pain increases. The prevalence is directly inversely correlated, however, to the stringency of the reference standard. Prevalence studies consistently find the zygapophyseal joint as a common source of pain, but diagnosis using a single anesthetic block has a potential high placebo rate versus a double comparative block control requiring a longer duration of relief after lidocaine versus bupivacaine.

Studies reporting the prevalence of zygapophyseal joint pain report figures ranging from 15% to 52%. In 1994, Schwarzer and colleagues[98] established the prevalence of zygapophyseal joint pain using a double block comparative protocol in 96 patients with a mean age of 38 years and mean duration of low back pain of 16 months mostly secondary to work-related injuries and trauma presenting to two tertiary U.S. clinics. (Fig. 15–4 shows a lumbar intra-articular zygapophyseal joint block.) Schwarzer and colleagues[98] found that the combination of discogenic pain and zygapophyseal joint pain is uncommon. In a group of 176 patients, 47% had initial relief with a screening lidocaine block, but only 15% had 50% or greater relief with a confirmatory block.

Manchikanti and colleagues,[99] also using a double block protocol but requiring 75% pain relief and a differential response, reported an even higher initial response of 81 of 120 (67.5%) to lidocaine medial branch blocks and a much greater percentage (45%) of the total reporting longer 75% relief after confirmatory bupivacaine medial branch blocks. This patient group was older, however, than Schwarzer's group with a mean age of 47 years and with a longer mean duration of low back pain of 47 months. The false-positive rate for one block was 41%. In a later study, Manchikanti and colleagues[100] revised the prevalence of zygapophyseal joint pain downward from 45% to 27% (95% confidence interval 22% to 32%). Schwarzer and colleagues[101] studied an older group of patients with a mean age of 57 years referred to an Australian rheumatology clinic with low back pain for an average of 7 years. A diagnosis of zygapophyseal joint pain was made in 40% (95% confidence

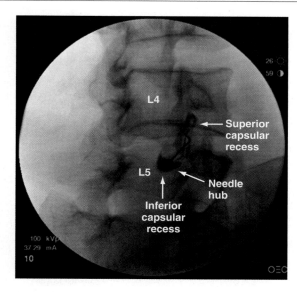

FIGURE 15–4 Right L4-5 zygapophyseal joint intra-articular injection. Note filling of superior and inferior subcapsular capsular recesses with contrast dye (*arrow*). Needle hub partially overlies inferior capsular recess. (Courtesy of Richard Derby, MD.)

interval 27% to 53%). Requiring 90% relief of original pain, the prevalence was 32%, and requiring 100% relief, the prevalence was 11%. Manchikanti and colleagues[100] reported an even higher prevalence of 52% zygapophyseal joint pain in a group of patients 65 years old or older.

No consistent history, physical examination, or imaging findings correlated to positive block responses have been found. In the early 1980s, uncontrolled single, variable injectant volume, intra-articular zygapophyseal joint injections were used as the reference standard for identifying lumbar zygapophyseal joint pain, and these authors reported correlations with various history or physical examination findings.[51,102] Some studies[103,104] reported that a cluster of five of seven features (*Revel criteria*) could predict a 75% decrease in pain after a single intra-articular block. The seven items in the cluster are age older than 65 years, pain well relieved by recumbency, no exacerbation of pain with coughing and sneezing, no exacerbation of pain with forward flexion, no exacerbation of pain with extension, no exacerbation of pain with rising from flexion, and no exacerbation of pain with the extension-rotation test. Subsequent well-conducted studies did not replicate these studies.[28,105] As mentioned, most of these earlier studies used single medial branch blocks, which have been reported to have 25% and 38% false-positive rates for the diagnosis of zygapophyseal joint pain.[106,107]

Newer studies of clinical correlations refined the technique with an appropriate injectant volume and a confirmatory double block paradigm with either a second intra-articular injection or a medial branch confirmatory injection with bupivacaine lasting longer than the pain relief after a prior lidocaine block.[28,92,101,106,108,109] These studies did not find any clinical correlates with history or physical examination. In particular, extension and rotation were not predictive of response. A systematic review of all published studies

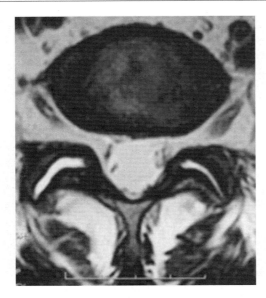

FIGURE 15–5 L5-S1 axial T2-weighted MRI showing facet edema (right greater than left), suggestive of instability. In upright weight-bearing position, anterolisthesis was noted; in unloaded supine position, anterolisthesis reduced, and zygapophyseal joints gapped and filled with fluid. (Courtesy of Richard Derby, MD.)

comparing clinical outcome after local anesthetic blocks and clinical signs and symptoms found no consistent clinical features with a high specificity.[11] The review found several clinical features with a high sensitivity, however, and these features may be cautiously used to *exclude* the diagnosis of facet mediated pain. These features include pain not increased with cough, pain not relieved with recumbency, and pain that can be centralized.[11] There are no consistent reproducible history or physical examination criteria that predict a positive response to a facet block. History and physical examination are better at ruling out facet mediated pain than diagnosing facet pain.

The current best evidence also shows that radiologic imaging, with a few more recent exceptions, does not correlate with response to zygapophyseal joint blocks. The conflicting evidence that radiologic imaging may predict outcome from uncontrolled lumbar zygapophyseal joint blocks may be partially due to lack of rigor in the reference standard used to define a positive response in earlier studies.[20] In 1979, Carrera[110] reported that 73% (*n* = 63) of patients describing pain relief after uncontrolled intra-articular injection of 2 to 4 mL of local anesthetic had CT evidence of lumbar facet disease versus 13% who had no evidence of disease. It is well accepted, however, that injectant volume should not exceed 1 mL; otherwise, the injection loses specificity, with a leak of local anesthetic around the nerve root and along vertebral levels within the epidural space.[92]

A large study by Jackson and colleagues[111] of 390 patients found no relationship between imaging and pain relief after uncontrolled intra-articular lumbar zygapophyseal joint injections. Supporting the findings by Jackson and colleagues,[111] Schwarzer and colleagues,[112] in the only study using placebo-controlled injection, found no correlation between CT findings and a positive response comparing local anesthetic with saline blocks in 63 patients when more stringent criteria of controlled injections were used as the reference standard. Similarly, Cohen and colleagues[113] found no relationship in 192 patients between MRI findings of zygapophyseal joint hypertrophy or degeneration and response to medial branch neurotomies based on positive response to a single medial branch block. Kawaguchi and colleagues[114] likewise found no significant relationship between low back pain symptoms and radiographic abnormalities in a group of 106 patients with rheumatoid arthritis.

The intriguing bright spot on the horizon is the finding that where MRI or single photon emission computed tomography (SPECT) shows imaging findings consistent with either "inflammation" or "edema," a stronger correlation emerges (Fig. 15–5). Although not confirming the diagnosis of zygapophyseal joint pain with a reference standard, Friedrich and colleagues[115] more recently found that an estimated 14% (21 of 145) of patients with low back pain had MRI evidence of facet joint edema, and follow-up MRI scan showed "almost perfect" agreement between change in pain and a reduction in intensity of edema on sagittal short tau inversion recovery (STIR) images. Radionuclide bone scintigraphy detects bone areas with synovial changes (inflammation or hyperemia) or increased osteoblast activity and degenerative regions with a high degree of remodeling. Osteophytes in process of growing show a high degree of bone scan activity. As mentioned earlier, a positive lumbar SPECT scan predicts a statistically significant reduction in pain after facet blocks.[31]

Zygapophyseal Joint Pain Referral Maps

Pain referral patterns have been studied using stimulation of patients during provocative diagnostic injections[116] by injection of hypertonic solutions into normal and abnormal subjects[80] or by electrical stimulation of medial branches.[80,117] Most studies showed distinct but overlapping referral areas; it is likely that the pain referral patterns obtained in normal volunteers are smaller because of less sensitization. There are also limits to the referral maps; Mooney and Robertson[80] reported on lumbar facet referral maps in normal volunteers and subjects with a positive diagnostic facet block (Fig. 15–6). Under fluoroscopic guidance, they injected contrast dye (unspecified volume) followed by 3 to 5 mL of hypertonic saline. Some of the distal extremity pain seen in the diagrams may be due to excessive volume of saline with irritation of the sciatic nerve roots. Given the lack of sensitivity and specificity of history, physical examination, and imaging and until more research is performed with finite injectant volumes (in patients with confirmed dual positive blocks), these referral maps can be used as a starting point to guide selection of levels to be injected.

Predictive Value

How useful are diagnostic facet injections? The predictive value of any spinal diagnostic test directly varies with the rigorousness of test standards and the inherent ability of that treatment to alleviate the source of pain without creating new sources unrelated to the original cause or causes. A positive test is valuable if it can guide treatment and obtain better outcomes than not using the diagnostic test at all. A systematic review of the evidence for treatment of zygapophyseal joint pain is beyond the scope of this chapter; however, a case is made for the therapeutic utility of zygapophyseal joint blocks.

Historically, lacking robust studies, guideline and systematic review articles have been relegated to quoting studies with methodologic flaws as implied evidence that one need not diagnose facet mediated pain before surgery.[22,94] There is no reason that a variable amount of relief after uncontrolled, variable volume, intra-articular zygapophyseal joint blocks should predict fusion outcomes using surgical fusion techniques from the 1980s in a group of patients being operated on for various unknown or unstated reasons. Jackson[118] correlated relief after spinal fusion in 36 patients from 1980-1988 to results of a single intra-articular facet injection with 1.5 mL of local anesthetic and an unknown volume of contrast dye. Of patients, 85% had "some improvement" with an average relief after injection of 29%. The authors found no relationship between fusion surgery performed for unstated reasons and a "favorable response" to facet injection. The surgeries were presumably performed not because the authors believed the patients' symptoms were due to their zygapophyseal joints. The surgical results based on their "mean pain and functional assessment scores" also seemed to improve by significantly less than 50%, suggesting poor patient selection.

An important historical study, published by Esses and Moro in 1993,[119] is often quoted to refute the therapeutic utility of zygapophyseal joint blocks; however, it warrants a careful, critical review. Esses and Moro[119] concluded that single intra-articular diagnostic facet joint injections "should not be used in determining treatment because they are not predictive of either surgical or nonsurgical success." This study had significant methodologic shortcomings, which limit the validity of the authors' conclusions. First, the study was retrospective with patients surveyed by telephone approximately 5 years after surgery. Second, 1.5 mL of local anesthetic was injected into the facets, and no mention is made of the volume of contrast dye needed to confirm needle position; the injections likely were nonspecific because of facet capsule rupture from excessive volume (>1 mL). Third, the patient population was markedly heterogeneous with significant confounding factors: an average duration of back pain of 8 years and approximately 40% of patients with a history of prior surgeries, including failed fusions. More than 50% of patients underwent three-level, four-level, or five-level fusions, which are known to have a poorer outcome than single-level or two-level fusions.

Fourth, of the 82 patients who underwent surgery, 36 (44%) had 0% relief from facet injections. Almost one half of the patients undergoing surgery had no relief from diagnostic blocks. Eight of 19 (42%) of the patients with complete relief after facet injections declined surgery, leaving only 11 of 82 (13%) patients who underwent surgery who had 100% relief from facet blocks. The remaining 35 of 82 patients (43%) had "partial but significant relief" (the exact percentage relief is

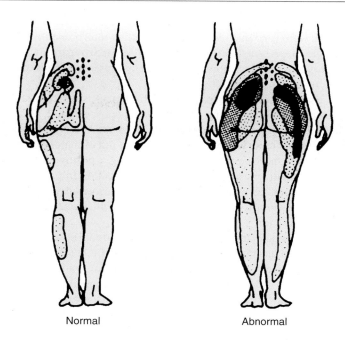

Normal   Abnormal

FIGURE 15–6 Pain referral patterns for asymptomatic (normal) and symptomatic (abnormal) subjects obtained by intra-articular zygapophyseal joint injection of contrast dye followed by 3 to 5 mL of hypertonic saline. (From Mooney V, Robertson J: The facet syndrome. Clin Orthop Relat Res [115]:149-156, 1976.)

not reported). Fifth, 30 of 82 (37%) patients had prior surgeries (laminectomy, discectomy, and fusion). It is well known that patients with failed back surgery syndrome often fare poorly with repeat surgery. Also, during the 1980s, diagnosis of the etiology of failed back surgery syndrome was elusive and might not be corrected by a posterior arthrodesis. For failed back surgery syndrome, facet joint pain comprises only 3% of cases; the most common diagnoses are foraminal stenosis (25% to 29%), painful disc (20% to 22%), pseudarthrosis (14%), neuropathic pain (10%), recurrent disc herniation (7% to 12%), and sacroiliac joint pain (2%).[120]

Next, Esses and Moro[119] did not match the surgery to specific facet levels blocked. Patients had either one-level or two-level facet blocks, yet the following posterior fusions were performed: 20, single-level; 3, two-level; 10, three-level; 4, four-level; and 12, five-level or greater, including thoracic spine (wherein facets were never blocked). Finally, significant questions arise regarding the efficacy of the surgical intervention because there was no significant difference between surgical and nonsurgical outcomes. As reported, only approximately one third of patients in either the surgical or the nonsurgical group had a good outcome. Because of methodologic flaws and limitations of the Esses and Moro study,[119] facet intra-articular injections cannot be impugned as either predictive or nonpredictive of surgical success.

In another observational study, Lovely and Rastogi[121] required a "positive response" to intra-articular injection of greater than 70% relief after bupivacaine facet block for 6 hours and required a confirmatory response on two subsequent injections. Of 28 patients, 23 had a good to excellent outcome after fusion surgery; however, large volumes of 3 to 5 mL were used during the blocks, making interpretation difficult. At present (2008), there is no research regarding the utility of cervical or thoracic facet blocks as presurgical screening tests.

By comparison, when a specific treatment is directed at a cause of pain originating from the zygapophyseal joint, accurate diagnostic testing does matter. In a more recent study, researchers reported that when a putative inflammatory cause of lumbar facet pain was confirmed using a positive SPECT scan, a positive response (a significant reduction in pain) was clearly predicted with intra-articular and pericapsular steroids at 1 and 3 months compared with subjects with negative scans or routine care.[31]

In regard to the therapeutic utility of double, controlled differential facet blocks, there is a clear and direct relationship between relief of pain after controlled medial branch blocks with a well-validated treatment for zygapophyseal joint pain, medial branch neurotomies. In a study by Dreyfuss and colleagues,[122] patients who obtained greater than or equal to 80% relief from medial branch blocks were selected to undergo lumbar radiofrequency neurotomy. At 12 months, 60% of the patients obtained at least 90% relief of pain, and 87% obtained at least 60% relief. Dreyfuss and colleagues[122] concluded that lumbar medial branch neurotomy is an effective means of reducing pain in patients carefully selected on the basis of controlled diagnostic blocks. The most recent, high-quality study available on radiofrequency is a randomized controlled trial evaluating radiofrequency neurotomy in patients with chronic low back pain.[123] The trial used three positive blocks in the inclusion criteria and a "sham radiofrequency" procedure for comparison; statistically significant reduction in pain and improvement in various quality of life variables were obtained. In another study, when the diagnosis is confirmed by relief of pain for greater than 3 months after medial branch neurotomies, repeat neurotomies are successful in greater than 75% in lumbar and cervical spine.[124,125]

In regard to newer surgical treatments, the development and perfection of procedures such as minimally invasive facet fusions or various types of total and subtotal arthroplasties require accurate diagnosis along with stringent criteria for success. The many confounding variables and often reported weak results of current spinal fusion and arthroplasty techniques make disproving these results relatively easy. The diagnosis of zygapophyseal joint pain employing strict double block or placebo-controlled standards should perhaps be used to restrain a surgeon from offering a circumferential (360 degrees or 280 degrees) segmental fusion or arthroplasty. The failure to confirm zygapophyseal joint pain is perhaps even more important because so doing leaves other sources of pain that may be better suited to a particular surgical technique or limits the number of levels needing stabilization.

Cervical Spine Facet Syndrome

History

The cervical facet joints are known to be sources of neck and extremity pain and headache. In 1940, Hadden[126] described pain from zygapophyseal joints causing headache. In the 1970s, Macnab[127] described pain arising from the facet joints after whiplash injury. Bogduk and Marsland[128] devised a technique to block the third occipital nerve, which relieved neck pain and headache stemming from the C2-3 facet joint in 70% of patients. Headache arising from C0-1 or C1-2 joints has also been described.[129,130] Bogduk and Marsland[131] were also the first to describe medial branch blocks for all cervical spine levels. They studied patients presenting with idiopathic neck pain and reported that medial branch block and intra-articular blocks provided complete, temporary relief of pain for 70% of patients.

Cervical Zygapophyseal Joint Pain

Based on the confirmatory block paradigm, the cervical facet joints are a common source of chronic neck pain; the prevalence of cervical facet syndrome is greater than the prevalence of lumbar facet syndrome. Cervical discogenic pain shares referral patterns with facet pain, but it is far less common.[132] Based on comparative blocks of cervical facet joints causing chronic neck pain with either associated headache or shoulder pain, the C2-3 (36%) and C5-6 facet joints (35%) were the most common pain generators.[133] After whiplash injury, Level I prospective clinical studies provide evidence that facet joints are the most common source of chronic pain.[134,135] Cervicogenic headache stemming from the C2-3 facet after whiplash has a 53% prevalence.[134]

Often neglected are C0-1 and C1-2 joints in evaluation of upper neck pain and headache. Dreyfuss and colleagues[129] studied the referral patterns for the atlantoaxial and lateral atlantoaxial joints. In 2002, Aprill and colleagues[136] failed to confirm the null hypothesis that lateral atlantoaxial joints are *not* a common source of occipital headache. These investigators found that of 34 patients presenting with symptoms and signs of atlantoaxial joint pain, 21 obtained complete relief of headache after diagnostic injection of local anesthetic. Pain referral patterns have been defined in C2-3 through C7-T1 facets (Fig. 15–7).[15] Innervation of the cervical facet joints is well described (Fig. 15–8).[15] The cervical zygapophyseal joints can be blocked either by medial branch blocks or with intra-articular injections (Fig. 15–9).

Prevalence rates for pain originating from cervical facets range from 36% to 60%. The false-positive rate for a single, uncontrolled block is 27% (95% confidence interval 15% to 38%).[137] The following prevalence rates (mean [95% confidence interval]) are reported from studies using either a double block or a triple block paradigm (normal saline as a placebo): 54% (40% to 68%),[134] 36% (27% to 45%),[138] 60% (33% to 64%),[135] and 60% (50% to 70%).[139] Manchikanti and colleagues[100] restudied the prevalence of cervical zygapophyseal joint pain in a larger group of patients and found a similar 55% (95% confidence interval 49% to 61%) prevalence. The most recent study by Manchikanti's group in 2007,[83] of 438 patients requiring 80% relief of pain for 2 hours' duration with lidocaine and 3 hours' duration with bupivacaine, reported a prevalence of 39%. Corroborating the high prevalence of cervical zygapophyseal joint pain, Yin and Bogduk[139a] in a private practice clinic audit found a 55% prevalence of cervical

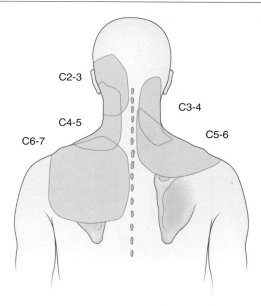

FIGURE 15–7 Patterns of referred pain from cervical zygapophyseal joints in normal volunteers from Dwyer A, Aprill C, Bogduk N: Cervical zygapophyseal joint pain patterns. 1:A study in normal volunteers. Spine 15:453-457, 1990. (From Bogduk N [ed]: Practice Guidelines for Spinal Diagnostic and Treatment Procedures. San Francisco, International Spine Intervention Society, 2004.)

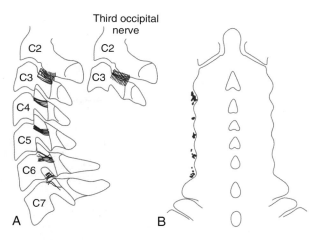

FIGURE 15–8 A, Lateral view of cervical spine showing variable locations of medial branches. At C3, location of C3 deep medial branch is shown. *Inset* shows location of third occipital nerve (TON). *Shaded area* shows where C3 deep branches and TON overlap. C5 medial branch is located in the middle of the articular pillar; at C6 and C7, medial branches are located progressively higher. **B,** Anteroposterior view of cervical medial branches. (From Bogduk N [ed]: Practice Guidelines for Spinal Diagnostic and Treatment Procedures. San Francisco, International Spine Intervention Society, 2004.)

zygapophyseal joint pain using a strict double comparative block protocol.

Similar to lumbar zygapophyseal joint pain, there are no high-quality studies showing a particular set of clinical features that can predict results of diagnostic cervical facet or medial branch blocks.[140] With diagnosis by medial branch blocks, one exceptionally skilled manipulative therapist was able to identify all 15 subjects with diagnostic block–proven symptomatic zygapophyseal joints and specify the correct symptomatic segment. None of the five patients with asymptomatic joints was misdiagnosed as having symptomatic zygapophyseal joints.[141] A later follow-up study by the same group failed to confirm the apparent high specificity and sensitivity, however, and reported a high sensitivity but low specificity and concluded that manual examination of the cervical spine lacks validity for the diagnosis of cervical zygapophyseal joint pain. In the study by Aprill and colleagues[136] of C1-2 facet pain as a source of occipital headache, only 60% of the patients shared clinical criteria that predicted a positive response to the block.

Advanced imaging has not been correlated with positive responses to diagnostic blocks. Hechelhammer and colleagues[142] found no relationship between short-term pain relief after cervical intra-articular and pericapsular injection of local anesthetic and corticosteroid and the degree of osteoarthritis graded on a CT scan.

Thoracic Spine

The prevalence of patients who complain of chronic upper back or mid-back pain ranges from 3% to 22%.[30,143,144] One survey study of 35- to 45-year-olds estimated the prevalence of thoracic pain to be 15%.[145] Thoracic zygapophyseal joint

pain referral patterns have been reported (Fig. 15–10).[146,147] Thoracic medial branch anatomy has also been described (Fig. 15–11).[148]

There are no pathognomonic clinical or radiographic findings by which thoracic zygapophyseal joint pain may be diagnosed.[149] As with the cervical and thoracic spine, diagnosis is by suspicion and, at a minimum, the pain pattern should correlate with established pain referral maps.[15] The methods physicians apply clinically to the diagnosis and treatment of thoracic facet joint pain rest largely on research done in the lumbar and cervical spine. This is not an entirely unreasonable

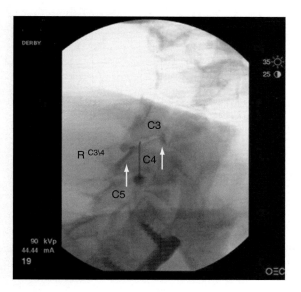

FIGURE 15–9 Lateral fluoroscopic view of C3-4 zygapophyseal joint injection using 3.5-inch 25-gauge needle. Note contrast dye in posterior and anterior capsular folds (*arrows*). (Courtesy Richard Derby, MD.)

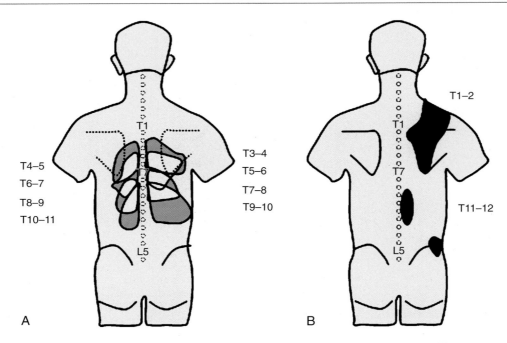

FIGURE 15–10 Maps of referred pain patterns in segments indicated. **A,** Based on Dreyfuss et al[146] in normal volunteers. **B,** Based on Fukui et al[147] in patients with single positive facet block. (From Bogduk N [ed]: Practice Guidelines for Spinal Diagnostic and Treatment Procedures. San Francisco, International Spine Intervention Society, 2004.)

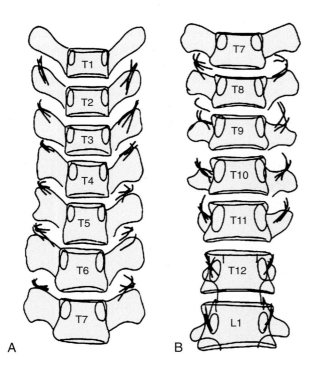

FIGURE 15–11 A and **B,** Composite sketch of work by Chua and Bogduk[148] with radiographs of cadaveric thoracic spines. Medial branches of thoracic dorsal rami marked with wires to depict location with respect to transverse processes. Note middle thoracic levels, where medial branches are within intertransverse space versus crossing transverse process. (From Bogduk N [ed]: Practice Guidelines for Spinal Diagnostic and Treatment Procedures. San Francisco, International Spine Intervention Society, 2004.)

approach based on what clinicians know in general regarding facet anatomy and innervation; however, more research is needed.

Investigators have mapped out the referral patterns for the thoracic joints. These findings are often used as a starting point to select which thoracic facets to block.[146,147] Dreyfuss and colleagues[146] mapped out thoracic facet joint referral patterns in normal volunteers and found that capsular distention did not provoke pain in 27.5% of volunteers. Fukui and colleagues[147] mapped out referral patterns in patients with suspected thoracic zygapophyseal joint pain who had a positive response to local anesthetic in C7-T1 to T2-3 and T11-12 facet joints. There was considerable overlap between the C7-T1 and T2-3 thoracic joints, and pain maps from these joints are not considered reliable enough to identify the symptomatic segmental level. Dreyfuss and colleagues[146] studied nine asymptomatic volunteers who underwent 40 provocative thoracic facet injections from T3-4 to T10-11. Referral patterns were consistently unilateral. The area of the most intense pain for segments from T2-3 to T11-12 was one level inferior and lateral. Significant overlap occurred over three to five levels. The researchers found that needle position can be confirmed with 0.1 to 0.3 mL of contrast dye, and adequate blocks can be achieved with a volume of 0.5 to 0.6 mL. Normally, thoracic zygapophyseal joints cannot hold more than 0.75 mL (Fig. 15–12 shows a typical thoracic zygapophyseal joint block).[15]

One research group has performed the three studies in the literature using a controlled, double block paradigm, requiring 75% to 80% relief based on the duration of the local anesthetic used.[150-152] Combining all three studies with patients presenting with chronic middle or upper spinal pain ($n = 183$), using dual blocks obtains a 40% prevalence of thoracic facet syndrome, with a false-positive rate of 42% if using a single block paradigm.[26]

What is the predictive value of a positive dual block? In other words, how well do patients fare who have positive dual blocks and undergo therapeutic intervention? Research is limited in this regard. One systematic review[26] reported that only therapeutic thoracic medial branch blocks received a 1A or 1B/strong recommendation. Manchikanti and colleagues[153,154] performed two studies. In the first study, 55 consecutive patients were studied; greater than 70% of patients had statistically significant relief (defined as >50% relief) at 3, 6, and 12 months. Most patients received four injections of bupivacaine with or without 1 mL of sarapin and 1 mg of methylprednisolone per milliliter of solution with 1 to 1.5 mL of solution injected per nerve. In the second study of 48 patients with positive dual blocks, 24 patients received bupivacaine, and 20 patients received bupivacaine plus betamethasone. Statistically significant (>50%) pain relief was reported in both groups at all time points up to 1 year. In the systematic review of radiofrequency neurotomy, only two studies were on thoracic medial branch neurotomy; however, both were of low quality and failed to meet inclusion criteria for the review because of lack of diagnosis by controlled blocks, small patient sample, and other methodologic shortcomings.[26] More research is needed in regard to diagnosis and treatment of thoracic pain so that the evidence can be graded and systematically reviewed, the caveat being that a lack of evidence is not equivalent to no evidence.

Summary

Chronic disabling spinal pain in a patient suggestive of facet syndrome that is unresponsive to usual care may be considered for diagnostic comparative facet intra-articular or medial branch blocks. The levels to be investigated are typically chosen by pain referral patterns described by the patient, which are correlated with validated zygapophyseal joint pain referral patterns. Upper neck pain and headache are most commonly caused by the C2-3 zygapophyseal joint, and neck pain with shoulder girdle pain is most commonly caused by the C5-6 zygapophyseal joint. The clinician should not neglect C0-1 and C1-2 as potential pain generators. Evaluation of the exact level of thoracic facet pain can be more challenging because pain may be referred over more than three segments. Lumbar zygapophyseal joint referral patterns are also reported in the literature; zygapophyseal joint pain may be localized or referred to the lower extremity.

Although comparative double blocks are considered the reference standard for diagnosis, routine history, physical examination, x-rays, and advanced imaging should be obtained for completeness. The clinician often finds elements that rule out facet syndrome and are more suggestive of disc pathology, radiculopathy, or "red flag" conditions that require different diagnostic and treatment methods. There are also cases where a history of trauma, particularly whiplash, is highly suggestive

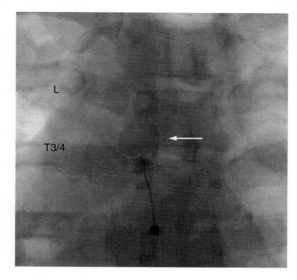

FIGURE 15–12 Left T3-4 zygapophyseal joint intra-articular injection. Note circular zygapophyseal joint arthrogram (*arrow*). (Courtesy of Richard Derby, MD.)

of pain of zygapophyseal joint origin, with a known greater than 50% prevalence in the cervical spine. Certain specific imaging findings, if present, also may suggest facet syndrome, such as a positive SPECT scan, approximately 2 mm edema on axial MRI of lumbar zygapophyseal joints, or a single zygapophyseal joint with markedly deforming arthropathy compared with other joints.

In terms of testing protocol, one's preference to perform medial branch blocks, intra-articular zygapophyseal joint injections, or both varies depending on the situation and preference of the physician. If one is confirming zygapophyseal joint mediated pain in preparation for possible medial branch neurotomy, one could argue that medial branch block should be the method of choice. Because one medial branch innervates adjacent joints, if one is considering one of the current or emerging stabilization or intra-articular spacer facet devices, diagnosis should include or be limited to a specific intra-articular block. In addition, the medial branches innervate the multifidus muscle and supply branches to the supraspinous and interspinous ligaments and fascia. In the case of C0-1 and C1-2, intra-articular injections are the only practical method of diagnosing facet pain.

As noted earlier, preprocedural and postprocedural evaluation should be performed by unbiased personnel and checked by the physician using standardized instruments. Evaluation after the procedure includes VAS of standard provocative maneuvers and positions and a report of subjective percent relief of pain. Ideally, the patient would be tested at approximately 15 minutes after lidocaine block and approximately 30 minutes after bupivacaine block. A subject should have at least 50% relief for a positive response to be considered; at least 70% relief is more convincing. Usually, two to three levels are evaluated per session. Depending on the importance of refuting or confirming whether a particular zygapophyseal joint is symptomatic, one may select fewer joints if needed.

Several technical parameters must be met to obtain useful diagnostic information. Diagnostic volumes must be

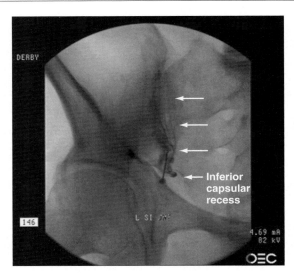

FIGURE 15-13 Anteroposterior view of left sacroiliac joint injection. Note contrast dye filling capsule, including inferior capsular recess (*arrows*). (Courtesy Richard Derby, MD.)

appropriate. Contrast medium must always be used to confirm accurate target identification. For intra-articular zygapophyseal joints blocks, injectant volumes should be limited to 0.3 mL, 0.75 mL, and 1 mL in the cervical, thoracic, and lumbar spine. For medial branch blocks, needle position must be confirmed with injection of a small volume (0.3 to 0.5 mL) of contrast dye and the same volume of local anesthetic. The interventionalist should observe for venous uptake or undesirable flow patterns. If there is venous uptake, there is only a 50% chance of successfully anesthetizing the joint, so the interventionalist may consider bringing the patient back at a later date or interpreting the results of the block accordingly.

Infection may occur after any interventional procedure. Various infections are reported after zygapophyseal joint

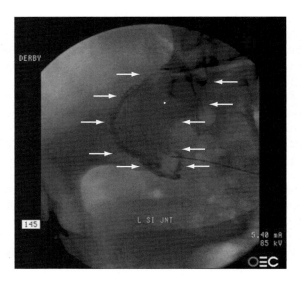

FIGURE 15-14 Lateral view of sacroiliac joint injection. Note contrast dye filling joint space. Also note C shape of joint facing anteriorly. (Courtesy Richard Derby, MD.)

injections, including paraspinal abscess,[155] facet abscess,[156] osteomyelitis,[157] and epidural abscess.[158] In addition to infections, subdural injections or injection into the spinal cord may occur. A case of transient tetraplegia[159] was reported during a cervical facet injection performed without fluoroscopy and most likely was an accidental subdural injection of local anesthetic. Even when using fluoroscopy there is a risk of accidental subdural injection or potential spinal cord injection. The danger is especially real when performing cervical intra-articular injection using a lateral technique. Using this technique, the needle is passed laterally using a lateral fluoroscopy view. If the anteroposterior view is not periodically checked, one may not recognize passage of the needle through the facet and dura and then into the cord. In a thin individual, the cord may be reached with a 1-inch needle. Keeping the needle directly over the inferior or superior facet and touching the bone before entering the joint helps the interventionalist avoid accidentally entering the spinal canal.

Sacroiliac Joint

With the gradual acceptance of local anesthetic block relief after fluoroscopy-guided sacroiliac joint blocks as the reference standard for diagnosis, there is a renewed interest in the sacroiliac joint as a legitimate source of chronic pain.[160] The degree of impact on health is the same as that of radiculopathy as evidenced by statistically similar scores in health-related quality of life testing instruments between patients with a diagnosis of sacroiliac joint pain and patients with a diagnosis of radiculopathy.[161]

Similar to zygapophyseal joint and discogenic pain, the diagnosis of sacroiliac joint pain depends on the reference standard used (and the particular population studied) to confirm the diagnosis. Society guidelines most often require a placebo control or differential blockade with 50% to 90% relief.[1,15,162] Typically, a differential duration of reported pain relief of lidocaine (approximately 1 hour) compared with bupivacaine (approximately 4 hours) is required. Although concordant provocation of pain during joint arthrography has been used as an additional requirement, the high percentage of asymptomatic patients reporting pain during sacroiliac joint injection implies that provocation has a high false-positive potential. Currently, using the dual block paradigm, the best estimates of prevalence of sacroiliac joint pain range from 10% to 38%. For single, uncontrolled sacroiliac joint injections, the false-positive rate is 20% to 54%.[163-167]

Pathophysiology

The sacroiliac joint has long been recognized as a synovial, fluid-filled diarthrodial joint between the sacrum and ilia with thick 6-mm sacral cartilage and thinner, approximately 1-mm iliac cartilage (Fig. 15-13). The joint is auricular or C-shaped with the convex side of the "C" facing anteriorly and inferiorly (Fig. 15-14).[168] Although the anterior portion is no more than a thickened capsule, the posterior capsule blends into the extensive, thick posterior ligamentous structures, which bind the sacrum to the spine and bilaterally to the ilia. After puberty, the iliac surface develops a convex ridge, and the sacral surface develops a corresponding concave depression. These articular surfaces allow slight movement between the contiguous bony surfaces.

Although early in life gliding motions in all directions are permitted, by the middle of the 2nd decade of life the joints develop prominent ridges centrally along the entire length of the iliac surface and a corresponding groove along the sacral surface. Bowen and Cassidy[168] believed that this interdigitation of the joint surfaces restricts motion to a sagittal rotation or posterosuperior-anteroinferior "nodding" along the crest of the interdigitations. The motion is complex, however, and usually limited to less than 4 degrees of rotation and less than 1.6 mm of translation. Significant motion occurs only after severing the interosseous ligament.[169] It is unclear whether a type or degree of sacroiliac joint motion causes pain in older individuals. Beyond the 6th decade, cadaveric specimens commonly show a central region of ossification of the interosseous sacroiliac ligament and the presence of ridges and depressions, which likely result in little to no movement of the sacroiliac joint in these older individuals.[170] Although restricted by para-articular osteophyte formation, intra-articular bony ankylosis may be rare.[168]

Several investigators have studied the innervation of the sacroiliac joint. Nakagawa[171] reported innervation from the ventral rami of L4 and L5; the superior gluteal nerve; and the dorsal rami of L5, S1, and S2. An anatomic dissection of the innervation of the sacroiliac joint was performed by Yin and colleagues[172] for the purpose of defining the exact position of the nerves for "sensory stimulation–guided sacroiliac joint radiofrequency neurotomy." These authors dissected cadavers and placed small-gauge wires adjacent to the lateral branch nerves entering the joint and over the dorsal sacrum to the dorsal sacral foramen from S1 to S3. In 1998, Willard[173] reported dissection of 10 cadavers that revealed that the S1 and S2 lateral branches provide the primary innervation of the sacroiliac joint and associated dorsal ligaments. Occasional contribution was found by S3 but not S4. Predominant innervation from lateral branches of S1 was also reported by Grob and colleagues.[174] These authors found dorsal nerves derived from S1-4 exclusively innervated the sacroiliac joint and associated ligaments. Nerves were distributed to superficial and deep dorsal sacroiliac ligaments and to the sacrotuberous and sacrospinous ligaments. Emerging from the sacral foramen, the nerves course laterally, sandwiched between superficial and deep portions of the sacroiliac ligaments. There is a great variability in the location and number of lateral branch nerves side to side and between individuals.[172] Currently, the standard for blocking the sacroiliac joint is to block the L5 dorsal ramus and S1-3 lateral branches.

Berthelot and colleagues[174a] used the term *sacroiliac joint lato-sensu* to describe pain from the sacroiliac joint that may be emanating from adjoining ligaments rather than simply the synovial joint. These ligaments include the iliolumbar ligaments, dorsal and ventral sacroiliac ligaments, and sacrospinous and sacrotuberous ligaments. The prevalence of pain originating from these structures has received little formal study, and there is no validated technique to diagnose

ligamentous pain. Nevertheless, sacroiliac joint ligamentous pain is proclaimed as a frequent primary source of low back and buttock pain by orthopaedists.[175] More importantly, a negative response to a sacroiliac joint injection does not mean that pain does not originate from the iliolumbar ligament and sacroiliac joint ligaments. A more recent histologic study found calcitonin gene-related peptide and substance P immunoreactive nerve fibers in the normal sacroiliac joint anterior capsular ligament and interosseous ligament. The authors of the study opined that diagnostic infiltration techniques for sacroiliac joint pain should employ extra-articular and intra-articular approaches.[176]

In contrast to the zygapophyseal joints, the sacroiliac joint supporting ligaments are thick, and intra-articular injected local anesthetic may not adequately diffuse into the sacroiliac ligaments. Using a single or comparative block protocol, one can investigate sacroiliac joint ligaments by fluoroscopically guided injections of local anesthetics into the ligaments. Ligamentous injections have not undergone rigorous academic inquiry, however, and because the injections are rarely or poorly reimbursed by third-party payers and treatment of ligamentous laxity typically involves unreimbursed "prolotherapy," there is little incentive for expensive investigations. The information is important, however, and differential pain arising from the sacroiliac joint versus sacroiliac joint ligaments is reported.

In a comparative study, Murakami and colleagues[177] performed periarticular injections in 25 patients and intra-articular injections in another 25 patients. Periarticular injections relieved on average 92% pain in 100% of the injected patients compared with only 9 of 25 patients receiving intra-articular injections. All 16 patients not receiving relief by intra-articular injections were improved after periarticular injections. The presence of other structural abnormalities does not rule out the sacroiliac joint as a primary source of pain. Weksler and colleagues[178] studied 55 patients with herniated discs with axial and referred leg pain, without objective neurologic deficits but with positive sacroiliac provocation tests. Using intra-articular injection of local anesthetic as the reference standard, the mean baseline VAS pain score decreased 30 minutes after injection from 7.8 to 1.3. In 46 patients 8 weeks after injection, VAS scores ranged from 0 to 3.

The question of whether fusion surgery leads to increased stress on the sacroiliac joint and may be a cause of failed back surgery syndrome was first raised by Frymoyer and colleagues,[179] although their method of assessing sacroiliac joint pathology yielded a negative result; in 1978, Frymoyer and colleagues[179] evaluated patients with radiographs (no diagnostic blocks) 10 years after posterior fusion versus postdiscectomy and found no significant difference in radiographic abnormalities; they opined that sacroiliac pain was "noncontributory" to persistent low back pain after surgery. In their subject population, they believed that the graft donor site was a more common pain generator. Fusion to the sacrum might be expected to stress the sacroiliac joints and lead to late failures or to early failures owing to undiagnosed sacroiliac joint pain. Ha and colleagues[180] prospectively examined 37 patients undergoing posterolateral lumbar and lumbosacral fusions; 22

patients had a floating fusion, and 10 patients had a lumbosacral fusion. CT scans of the sacroiliac joint were performed before surgery and at 2 weeks, 1 year, and 5 years after surgery and compared with 34 matched controls. The incidence of sacroiliac joint degeneration was 75% in the fusion group versus 38.2% in the control group and greater in patients fused to the sacrum. Both groups reported significant improvements in VAS and Oswestry Disability Index scores, and there was no difference in scores between the two groups.

More recent research has shown that the sacroiliac joint can be a significant source of pain after fusion. Biomechanical models seem to support these conclusions. Ivanov and colleagues[181] performed a finite element study with lumbosacral models and fusion constructs and found that fusion to the sacrum increased motion and stresses at the sacroiliac joint. Cadaveric studies show that disruption of the ventral band of the iliolumbar ligament significantly increases sacroiliac joint mobility.[182] Ebraheim and colleagues[183] evaluated the prevalence of sacroiliac joint disruption by CT scan in 24 patients after fusion with persistent "donor site pain" after posterior superior iliac crest graft harvesting. They found a high prevalence of persistent sacroiliac joint pain in patients with inner table disruption. Patients with violation of the synovial portion of the sacroiliac joint had severe degenerative changes on CT versus mild to moderate degeneration with inner table disruption only. It seems that the original hypothesis by Frymoyer and colleagues[179] that sacroiliac joint dysfunction was the cause of donor site pain may have been correct.

What is the evidence for using diagnostic blocks as the reference standard? Diagnosis of sacroiliac joint pain has been reported by researchers using single and dual blocks; with these methods, prevalence rates of sacroiliac joint pain after lumbar fusion range from 27% to 35%. Maigne and Planchon[184] studied 40 patients after fusion with continued pain using 75% pain relief after a single sacroiliac joint intra-articular injection as the "gold standard." They reported a 35% rate of positive blocks. The only characteristic that distinguished the positive from the negative responders was a different distribution of postoperative pain compared with preoperative pain. A pain-free interval of 3 months after surgery was significant; however, increased uptake in the sacroiliac joint on bone scintigraphy or posterior iliac bone graft harvesting was not significant.

Katz and colleagues[185] studied 34 patients after lumbosacral fusion with continued pain thought to be due to sacroiliac joint with intra-articular injections of local anesthetic and corticosteroids. Eleven patients (32%) had greater than 75% pain relief with local anesthetic and a minimum of 10 days' continued pain relief (with steroid) and were considered to have definite sacroiliac joint pain. Another 10 patients (29%) had greater than 75% relief with local anesthetic but no long-term relief. There was no correlation between the donor site and pain side. Irwin and colleagues[163] used dual comparative sacroiliac joint blocks as the reference standard to define sacroiliac joint pain and found that the 27% positive responders tended to be older. They found no statistical relationship between age, body mass index, and gender.

Diagnostic Accuracy of Clinical History and Physical Examination for Sacroiliac Pain

The diagnostic utility of history and accepted sacroiliac joint physical examination tests was first rigorously examined by Dreyfuss and colleagues in 1996.[186] Their study was designed to determine if any single or combination of 12 history and physical examination findings could predict intra-articular sacroiliac joint pain as judged against a single positive intra-articular sacroiliac joint block with greater than 90% pain relief. In 85 patients, there were 45 positive blocks. None of the 12 physical examination tests or the presence of 5 to 12 positive tests or any combination of these 12 tests correlated with the presence of sacroiliac joint pain. One important historical feature was notable, however: only 2 of 45 patients drew pain above the L5 level, suggesting that pain below L5 is more likely to be of sacroiliac joint origin. Maigne and colleagues[187] reached a similar conclusion using dual comparative blocks: no single provocation test reached statistical significance in the 10 patients (18.5%) who had temporary pain relief on the confirmatory injection.

Although no single provocative maneuver has been shown to be of diagnostic value, using the dual block paradigm, several studies have obtained highly acceptable sensitivity (85% to 91%) and specificity (78% to 79%) rates by combining three or more sacroiliac joint pain provocation tests for diagnosis by physical examination.[11,164,165,167,188] There is some slight variation in the tests used by various authors, but in summary they include the following provocation tests: thigh thrust, distraction test, Gaenslen test, Patrick sign, compression test, midline sacral thrust test, and heel drop test. Specificity increased to 87% if the patient's pain did not centralize or could not be made to move toward the spinal midline (which is typical of discogenic pain).[189] When three or more provocation tests (distraction, compression, thigh thrust, Patrick sign, Gaenslen test) are negative, the likelihood of sacroiliac joint pain is very low (6% to 15%); when all provocation tests are negative, the sacroiliac joint was never the source of pain.[164,165,167,189]

In terms of pain referral maps, Slipman and colleagues[190] and Dreyfuss and colleagues[186] concluded that of all alleged signs of sacroiliac joint pain, maximum pain below L5 coupled with pointing to the posterior superior iliac spine or tenderness just medial to the posterior superior iliac spine (sacral sulcus tenderness) has the highest positive predictive value of 60%; if these do not exist, the likelihood of sacroiliac joint pain is less than 10%. Although the maximal sacroiliac joint pain is below L5, pain can be referred into the entire lower extremity, with 94% of patients reporting buttock pain, 48% reporting thigh pain, and 28% reporting lower leg pain (Fig. 15-15).[187,191,192] Referral to the lower extremity is possible from sacroiliac joint pain and cannot reliably be distinguished from other pain sources (e.g., S1 radiculopathy).[191,193]

Lastly, although pain referral patterns between responders and nonresponders are similar, Fortin and colleagues[194] described an area of pain approximately 3 × 10 cm just inferior to the posterior superior iliac spine that was common in all their subjects with sacroiliac joint pain. More recently, Murakami and colleagues[195] studied the specificity and sensitivity of the "Fortin" point with periarticular injections. Labeled the *one finger test*, 18 of 38 patients pointed to a location of pain at the posterior superior iliac spine or within 2 cm of the posterior superior iliac spine, which had a positive effect with periarticular sacroiliac joint block. The authors recommended that sacroiliac joint pain should be considered in patients who can point to their pain using one finger in the vicinity of the posterior superior iliac spine.

Systematic reviews report various conclusions regarding the specificity of the physical examination and sacroiliac joint block to diagnose sacroiliac joint pain based on the authors' assessment of the diagnostic accuracy of diagnostic sacroiliac joint blocks. The review by Berthelot and colleagues[196] concluded that sacroiliac joint blocks and sacroiliac joint maneuvers were unreliable for diagnosing sacroiliac joint pain. In contrast, Hansen and colleagues[197] concluded in their review that there was moderate evidence for the specificity and validity of diagnostic sacroiliac joint injection and limited evidence for the accuracy of provocative maneuvers. Using a comparative double block reference standard, the most recent meta-analysis and systematic review concluded that the pooled data of the thigh thrust test, compression test, and three or more positive stress tests showed discriminative power for diagnosing sacroiliac joint pain.[198]

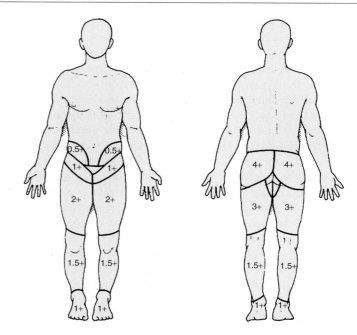

FIGURE 15–15 Density of referral zones for sacroiliac joint pain. 0.5+ is the least common referral zone; 4+ is the most common referral zone. (From Dreyfuss P, Dreyer S: Sacroiliac joint pain. J Am Acad Orthop Surg 12:255-265, 2004.)

Diagnostic Accuracy of Imaging

No imaging studies consistently provide findings that are helpful to diagnose primary sacroiliac joint pain. CT, MRI, and bone scan are done predominantly to exclude other causes of pain rather than to diagnose mechanical sacroiliac joint pain. Among patients referred to a low back pain clinic with a variety of pathologies, Hodge and Bessette[199] found a high percentage (75%) of patients with sacroiliac joint arthritis shown on CT scan. Although these authors did not confirm the diagnosis with sacroiliac joint injections, they opined that sacroiliac joint arthritis should be considered a possible diagnosis.

There is limited diagnostic value of CT scan in mechanical sacroiliac joint disease as defined by pain relief after sacroiliac joint blocks under CT scan guidance. Comparing the CT scans of patients diagnosed with sacroiliac joint pain using image-guided analgesic sacroiliac joint blocks with a matched control group of asymptomatic patients, Elgafy and colleagues[200] reported that an abnormal sacroiliac joint CT scan had a sensitivity of 57% and a specificity of 69%. Although sacroiliac joint scintigraphy can detect early sacroiliitis,[201] stress fractures, infection, and tumors, the sensitivity of bone scans for detecting mechanical sacroiliac joint pain is poor (range 12% to 46%).[202,203] Patients with a positive bone scan are likely to have mechanical or arthritic sacroiliac joint pain with a reported specificity of 90% to 100%.[190,203]

Diagnostic Accuracy of Sacroiliac Joint Injections

The current standard for diagnosing sacroiliac joint pain is pain relief after dual controlled sacroiliac joint injections, owing to the high false-positive rate of single blocks.[162] When blocking the sacroiliac joint or lateral branches of the sacroiliac joint, imaging guidance must be used. The success of "blind" intra-articular injection is only 22%.[204] A positive response should include approximately 70% relief for 1 to 2 hours of relief after a lidocaine block and 3 to 4 hours of relief after a confirmatory block with bupivacaine. Although the reference standard is reasonable, there are several caveats for the diagnosis of mechanical pain originating within the sacroiliac joint. Patients may exhibit extra-articular or periarticular sacroiliac joint pain or perhaps both. As noted earlier, Murakami and colleagues[177] relieved a significant amount of sacroiliac joint pain with periarticular injections. In a retrospective review of 120 patients, subjects who received intra-articular and periarticular injections had superior pain relief compared with subjects receiving intra-articular injections alone.[205]

False-positive results may occur secondary to leak of contrast dye through capsular tears, which may be present even in asymptomatic individuals. Extracapsular flow is present in 61% of sacroiliac joint intra-articular injections in patients.[206] Of sacroiliac joint intra-articular injections, 27% show extravasation that communicates with nearby neural structures, including dorsal sacral foramina extravasation, superior recess extravasation at the sacral ala level to the fifth lumbar epiradicular sheath, and ventral extravasation to the lumbosacral plexus.[206] Patients who have postblock extremity numbness are usually considered to have a leak, and the block is typically repeated at a different session.

More important is the potentially significant false-negative response rate because of a failure to anesthetize extracapsular pain sources mentioned previously. Block of the sacroiliac joint dorsal innervations may offer a solution because the block would potentially denervate intra-articular and extra-articular pain sources. Because the sacroiliac joint and ligaments are innervated, similar to the zygapophyseal joint, the joint and capsules are regarded as the same structure. In contrast to the zygapophyseal joint, the sacroiliac joint is surrounded by thick supporting ligaments, and intra-articular injected local anesthetic may not anesthetize the ligaments.

Dreyfuss and colleagues[193] used a double-blind randomized controlled trial to assess ability of single-site, single-depth L5 dorsal ramus and S1-3 lateral branch blocks to anesthetize the sacroiliac joint in 19 volunteers, using sacroiliac joint fluid distraction before and after blocks to determine effectiveness. The authors reported that only 40% of the volunteers did not feel distention after the blocks. The poor results prompted a cadaveric study of multisite, multidepth blocks to anesthetize the joint. L5 dorsal ramus block was performed at the standard location of the S1 superior articular process and the sacral ala; S1-2 lateral branches were blocked (right side) at the 2:30 o'clock, 4:00 o'clock, and 5:30 o'clock positions; and S3 lateral branch was blocked at the right 2:30 o'clock and 4:00 o'clock positions. The lateral branch blocks were performed 8 to 10 mm lateral to the posterior sacral foramen. A 0.2 mL volume of green dye was injected on the dorsal sacral plate, and an additional 0.2 mL was injected 2 to 3 mm above the sacral plate.

Dissection revealed S1-3 lateral branch nerves were stained in 91% (31 of 34) of cases. Employing the same protocol on 20 volunteer subjects using intraosseous ligament probing and capsular distention, Dreyfuss and colleagues[193] found that 86% of the sham local anesthetic injection subjects retained the ability to feel capsular distention, leading the authors to conclude that lateral branch blocks do not reliably block the intra-articular portion of the joint and that intra-articular blocks do not reliably block the extra-articular ligaments. One may conclude that to evaluate fully intra-articular and extra-articular pain sources, dorsal ramus and lateral branch blocks and intra-articular injections should be done. The caveat is the nerve blocks were successful in 70% of cases leaving a potential 30% false-negative cases. Injecting larger volumes or injecting the ligaments directly may potentially reduce the false-negative results with the risk of increasing false-positive results secondary to leak of local anesthetic through the posterior foramen.

Predictive Value

Surgical fusion outcomes for mechanical sacroiliac joint pain are reported for only a few small case series audits of initial outcomes after several "new" techniques for fusing the sacroiliac joint.[207-210] Published case series use pain relief after image-guided analgesic sacroiliac joint injections as the reference standard for diagnosing sacroiliac joint pain. Although Schutz and Grob[208] reported an 82% unacceptable outcome after bilateral sacroiliac joint fusion in 17 patients based on results from sacroiliac joint anesthetic block, three other studies using novel techniques reported more favorable results for mostly unilateral fusions. Al-Khayer and colleagues[209] reported an approximate 50% decrease in VAS and a 14-point decrease in Oswestry Disability Index in nine patients at 2 years after percutaneous sacroiliac joint arthrodesis using a Hollow Modular Anchorage screw (Aesculap, Sheffield, UK). Using percutaneously inserted fusion cages and bone morphogenetic protein, Wise and Dall[207] reported an average back pain VAS improvement of 4.9 and leg pain VAS improvement of 2.4 in 13 patients at 6 months. Finally, Ziran and colleagues,[210] using CT-guided sacroiliac joint blocks as a reference standard, percutaneously fused 17 patients with recalcitrant sacroiliac joint pain and found a statistically significant correlation ($P < .02$) between final postoperative pain scores and preinjection and postinjection pain scores.

Evidence has been limited based on observation studies assessing the outcome of various treatments for sacroiliac joint pain. Cohen and colleagues[211] selected patients for various types of radiofrequency neurotomy of the L4 medial branch, L5 dorsal branch, and S1-3 lateral branches using the reference standard of a single sacroiliac joint intra-articular block with greater than or equal to 75% relief of pain for 2 hours after injection of 2 mL of bupivacaine. Of 18 patients, 13 obtained satisfactory relief of pain with average scores reduced by 60%, 50%, and 57% at 1 month, 3 months, and 6 months. Only two patients in the placebo group obtained relief; pain scores of the placebo subjects were unchanged from baseline. Yin and colleagues[172] used dual injection into the sacroiliac joint intraosseous ligament to diagnose sacroiliac joint pain. Of patients, 64% reported a minimum of 60% subjective pain relief for a minimum of 6 months after sensory stimulation–guided sacral lateral branch radiofrequency neurotomy.

Summary

Sacroiliac joint pain is a significant cause of chronic low back pain that is diagnosable and treatable with precision injection techniques. Prevalence of sacroiliac joint pain, based on a dual differential block protocol, ranges from 10% to 38%; for single, uncontrolled blocks, the false-positive rate is 54%.[163-167] The sacroiliac joint as a pain generator is no longer disputed. Current research also suggests that the sacroiliac joint is a significant source of persistent pain after lumbar fusion and may be a cause of graft donor site pain.[183-185] Although motion is limited and complex, the joint is known to rotate less than 4 degrees and to translate less than 1.6 mm. Anatomic studies have elucidated the innervation to the joint, with most practitioners directing diagnostic and therapeutic interventions to the L5 dorsal ramus and S1-3 lateral branches.[171,173] Sacroiliac joint pain is now thought to emanate from the joint itself and extra-articular ligamentous sources. Interventionalists are just beginning to diagnose and treat putative extra-articular pain generators.

In contrast to the history and physical examination for zygapophyseal joint pain, certain diagnostic features for sacroiliac joint pain have been validated by controlled blocks. Maximal pain below L5 coupled with pointing to the posterior superior iliac spine has a predictive value of 60%.[186,190] Although no single physical examination test has been shown to be of diagnostic value, using the dual block paradigm, several studies have shown high sensitivity (85% to 91%) and specificity (78% to 79%) by combining three or more provocative sacroiliac joint maneuvers.[165,167] Specificity increases to 87% if the patient's pain cannot be centralized.[212] Diagnostic imaging of sacroiliac joint pain has not been shown to be helpful, other than excluding nonmechanical causes of sacroiliac joint pain. The sensitivity of bone scans for detecting sacroiliac joint pain is poor (range 12% to 46%).[202,203] CT scan of the sacrum in a patient with persistent low back or buttock pain after lumbar fusion may be useful, particularly if the synovial joint has been violated. In these patients, severe degenerative changes were found on CT scan.[183]

The current standard for diagnosis of sacroiliac joint pain is approximately 70% relief of pain for 1 to 2 hours after lidocaine block and 3 to 4 hours after bupivacaine block. Total volume should be limited to 1.5 mL. The interventionalist should carefully study the joint arthrogram for any evidence of extravasation via the dorsal sacral foramina, superior joint recess and fifth lumbar epiradicular sheath, or ventral capsule to the lumbosacral plexus because this can cause false-positive responses. Not all patients obtain relief from intra-articular joint injections, and extra-articular sources of pain must be evaluated as well. Other techniques for diagnosis and treatment of the sacroiliac joint include targeting the L5 dorsal ramus and S1-3 lateral branches.

If pain persists, new techniques have also been described for blocking the interosseous sacral ligaments.[205] Regarding the predictive value of diagnostic sacroiliac joint injection for sacroiliac joint arthrodesis, some case studies show poor results for arthrodesis; other studies using novel techniques report better results.[207-210] Neurotomy of sacroiliac joint lateral branches after diagnostic block has shown promising results in an observational study.[213] Other researchers have also shown promising results with periarticular blockade.[177]

Middle Compartment: Selective Nerve Root Blocks

Despite the growing sophistication of modern imaging, the source of extremity pain is not always clearly apparent. Extremity pain may also be referred from the hip, buttock, or shoulder secondary to intrinsic pathology in these structures. Radicular pain can be secondary to entrapment by bone, ligament, or disc or result from leakage of noxious cytokines from either the disc or an inflamed zygapophyseal joint without evidence of compression. *Segmental instability,* albeit difficult to detect or prove, may cause repetitive dynamic irritation of the dorsal root ganglion leading to chronic dorsal root ganglion hypersensitivity. Advanced MRI often shows multilevel degenerative pathology, abnormalities on the side opposite the patient's symptoms, or abnormalities that are asymptomatic.[214-216] Except for the most profound structural abnormalities, MRI provides morphologic information only; significant correlations must be made by the clinician.[217] Confounding the diagnosis further, pain patterns often do not follow classic referral pain distributions.[218,219]

Before considering surgical interventions, one should have a clear diagnosis with concordant imaging studies that show a surgically correctable lesion compressing the root, dorsal root ganglion, or ventral ramus. Pain referral patterns and physical examination findings should also be consistent with the suspected level of pathology. Most single-level entrapments are obvious. If not, further diagnostic information may be considered, such as selective nerve root blocks. Some interventionalists and surgeons still find myelography useful because MRI may miss a sequestered fragment, or the MRI cuts may not be fine enough to detect the pathologic lesion.

Selective injection of local anesthetic around the spinal nerve within or near the intervertebral foramen has long been used to help surgeons confirm or refute their hypothesis that a particular root is the source of pain. Selective nerve root blocks are distinguished from transforaminal epidural steroid injections. With a selective nerve root block, a small volume of contrast medium, approximately 0.5 mL, is injected just to outline the exiting spinal nerve and ventral and dorsal roots (Figs. 15–16 through 15–18); then the same volume of local anesthetic is injected to maintain specificity. Greater volumes of local anesthetic spread to adjacent levels. With selective nerve root blocks, relief of pain does not determine the cause of pain. Greater or lesser relief of pain may occur even if the cause of pain is peripheral entrapment or if the blocked nerve innervates a painful structure such as the hip. Relief of pain for the duration of the local anesthetic may occur even if the root has irreversible damage.

Diagnostic Accuracy of Selective Nerve Root Blocks

Diagnostic accuracy and ultimately utility depend on the degree to which a technically satisfactory block of a nerve stops the nociceptive input into the spinal canal and the degree that pain caused by any lesion within the nerve at or distal to the injection site is relieved. A greater or lesser degree of pain relief caused by a lesion affecting the nerve proximal to the

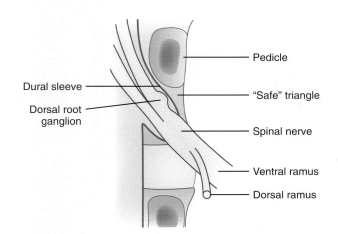

FIGURE 15–16 Drawing of spinal nerve within intervertebral foramen. The spinal nerve is a short segmental structure that quickly divides into ventral and dorsal rami. A selective nerve root block places local anesthetic no further than 6:00 o'clock position on pedicle. (From Bogduk N, Aprill C, Derby R: Epidural steroid injections. In White AH [ed]: Spine Care. Volume 1: Diagnosis and Conservative Treatment. St Louis, Mosby, 1995, pp 322-343.)

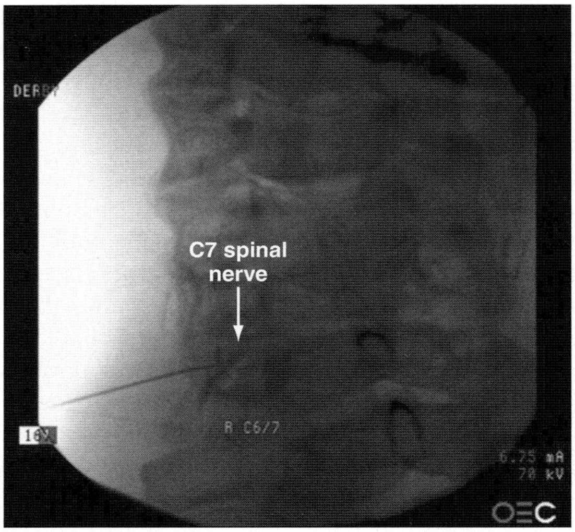

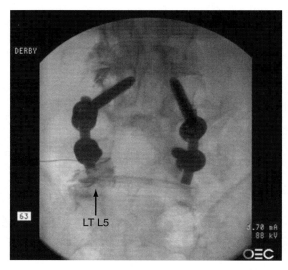

FIGURE 15–17 Anteroposterior view of right C7 selective nerve root block (*arrow*). C7 nerve root is outlined by contrast dye and is located in C6-7 foramen. A 1.5-inch 25-gauge needle was used to inject 0.3 mL of contrast dye. There is no spread of contrast dye around pedicle and into epidural space. (Courtesy Richard Derby, MD.)

injection site should also be taken into account when determining value.[95] Ideally, blocking an unaffected nerve would not relieve any pain. The degree to which these goals are accomplished constitutes the diagnostic accuracy as measured by sensitivity, specificity, and predictive value. Understanding these variables guides the clinician in terms of either accepting or discarding the block results or whether even to consider obtaining the information.

To study the diagnostic accuracy, one would select cases of acute or subacute monoradiculopathy caused by an obvious single-level lesion verified by imaging studies, intraoperative findings, and relief after surgical intervention. The most common "gold standard" lesion would be L4-5 paracentral

FIGURE 15–18 Left L5 selective nerve root block. Note how 0.5 mL of injected contrast dye surrounds and outlines root and dorsal root ganglion. There is a cutoff of contrast dye at lower and medial border of pedicle because of scar tissue from prior surgery (*arrow*).

herniation irritating the traversing L5 root.[220] Blinding the patient, the symptomatic root and presumably at least one unaffected root would be blocked at different sessions, and the data would be prospectively collected. The lesion would be confirmed at surgery and by postsurgical pain relief.

Although many prior studies retrospectively studied the ability of provocation and relief of pain to predict structural nerve entrapment and surgical outcome, only two studies examined injections performed on symptomatic roots and presumed asymptomatic roots with the expressed goal of defining sensitivity and specificity, and both studied only the value of lumbar injections.[220,221] From these two studies, particularly the more recent study by Yeom and colleagues,[220] one may estimate the diagnostic value of lumbar diagnostic root blocks.

Assessment of Effect

Only the study by Yeom and colleagues[220] determined the optimal cutoff level in the percent relief of pain reported by a patient after a procedure needed to qualify for a positive response. Using receiver operator curves, Yeom and colleagues[220] chose a cutoff of 70% subjective relief of pain after a lumbar transforaminal block as the best value to provide optimal accuracy but stated that this level could be adjusted depending on the importance of avoiding false-negative versus false-positive results.

The authors recommend adjusting the cutoff criteria between 50% and 90% depending on the importance of avoiding false-negative versus false-positive blocks. In the authors' opinion, it is probably best not to treat results as a dichotomous variable but rather as a data point that is more or less likely to indicate the root is a source of pain. If a discrete cutoff is required, 70% is a good compromise. One might also consider requiring a similar degree in change of VAS improvement or, if inconsistent with the patient's subjective report of pain relief, asking the patient why the discrepancy exists or performing a confirmatory injection. The patient often reports a global relief of pain, whereas diagnostically one is interested only in the degree of pain relief of the particular extremity distribution being evaluated. Relief or nonrelief of axial pain is important information but not pertinent to the location of the patient's extremity pain and to surgical outcomes.

Although provocation of concordant pain was frequently used in the past and perhaps is useful information, more recent studies use techniques to avoid creating pain during injection.[220,222] Pain referral patterns obtained by electrical stimulation may be considered as supplementary proof or nonproof.[222]

Sensitivity

The most likely causes of low sensitivity or a high rate of false-negative injections are inadequate blocks owing to poor spread around the root, failure to reach pathologic site, dilutional effects with inadequate mass of anesthetic reaching the root, or poor diffusion because of scarring.[220] van Akkerveeken[221] calculated 100% sensitivity in 46 patients using 0.2 to 0.5 mL of 0.5% bupivacaine (with provocation) and reported 100% of pain relief at 1 hour. Yeom and colleagues,[220] using 1 mL of 2% lidocaine without considering provocation, calculated a lower sensitivity of 57% (27 of 47) in all patients, increasing to 71% (25 of 35) when injections with inadequate spread were excluded. The causes of the inadequate blocks were spread of injectant into adjacent tissues in 4 of 10 patients, block by huge herniation in 4 of 10 patients, and intraepiradicular sheath injection in 2 of 10 patients. Although Yeom and colleagues[220] had no explanation in the remaining 10 cases, these false-negative results might be explained by a paracentral herniated disc, which, although affecting primarily the traversing root, may also cause chemical irritation of the exiting root.

In addition, Dooley and colleagues[223] found that the most common reason for typical pain provocation during lumbar block with incomplete pain relief is multilevel pathology. The most probable cause in obvious cases is an inadequate block performed at a location distal to the structural entrapment. Diagnostic injections are often performed in patients with long-standing chronic pain and patients with prior surgery who may have intraneural and extraneural scarring. In such cases, local anesthetic may not penetrate the nerve effectively, and incomplete relief would be expected. Using a more concentrated anesthetic or an anesthetic that preferentially blocks nociceptors (e.g., bupivacaine) may reduce these false-negative responses.

Specificity

Because surgery is often less effective in patients with equivocal structural pathology, in patients with atypical, long-standing pain or prior surgery, one would ideally want to have minimal or no pain relief after the block of an asymptomatic root. van Akkerveeken[221] used a 0.2- to 0.5-mL volume of 0.5% bupivacaine and required 100% pain relief for 1 hour. He reported a specificity of "around" 90%.[221] In the lumbar spine, using 1 mL of 2% lidocaine and a cutoff value of equal or greater than 70% pain relief, Yeom and colleagues[220] calculated 86% (50 of 58) specificity, which increased to 91% (43 of 47) specificity after excluding 7 patients with overflow of local anesthetic. Although this overflow was thought to be a probable cause of false-positive blocks in 4 of 11 cases, 7 of 11 cases were true-negatives, indicating that the estimated overflow when using 1 mL is about 20% (10 of 47) and with a potentially clinically observable effect in less than 10%.

Furman and colleagues[224] showed that even after injecting only 0.5 mL, the contrast pattern indicated nonselective flow in 30% of lumbar injections. The mass of drug overflowing at these low volumes may not be significant and is consistent with van Akkerveeken's higher, approximately 90% specificity. North and colleagues[95] reported an average 50% relief of sciatic pain when blocking the medial branches at several levels using a 3-mL volume, which would spread into the neuroforamen and epidural space, making the putative medial branch block nonspecific.[88] Nevertheless, convergence may be an alternative explanation of less than 50% pain relief in some cases, and a nonspecific "placebo" response may explain some or most false-positive responses.

Predictive Value

Many, mostly retrospective, observational studies describe in variable levels of detail the predictive value of lumbar root blocks. One retrospective study included the surgical predictive value of cervical and lumbar injections.[222] Another prospective, diagnostic cervical selective root block study compared the diagnostic value of imaging with the short-term surgical predictive value of the test.[225] No studies to date support the use of diagnostic thoracic selective root injections, although this is primarily because the thoracic spine is not often studied because of the low prevalence of herniated thoracic discs.

In the only prospective outcome study, van Akkerveeken,[221] in his doctoral thesis, presented a series of studies correlating the value of selective root blocks to diagnosis of various lumbar entrapment syndromes and later summarized the data in a journal publication in 1993. A positive response was provocation of concordant pain and "disappearance" of leg pain after 0.2 to 0.5 mL of 0.5% bupivacaine. He studied patients with radiologic signs of nerve root entrapment but without localizing neurologic signs who subsequently underwent surgical decompression. Excluding the patients who had positive blocks and refused surgery, van Akkerveeken[221] reported a positive predictive value of 95% with a 95% confidence interval of 77% to 100%.

History

Spine surgeons began using diagnostic root blocks in the late 1960s to help locate sources of radicular pain not well visualized with myelography.[219,226-229] Provocation of symptoms, pattern of the neurogram, and relief of pain were used to identify hidden pathology that was later confirmed or refuted during surgical exploration. A high degree of correlation was found between "positive" blocks and surgical findings. In addition, some early studies began reporting the surgical outcome based on selective nerve root block findings.[227] The routine use of CT and MRI improved the identification of structural causes of root compression, and some surgeons began using root blocks in difficult cases where provocation and relief of pain helped to determine the operated level.[223,230-232] Surgeons noted that although MRI and CT improved visualization of pathology, imaging did not correlate with cause of pain, and it did not correlate the abnormal anatomy with actual symptoms.[223]

Structural confirmation of suspected pathology and subsequent pain relief after surgery were reported in mostly retrospective case series. These studies also reported selective nerve root blocks were better able to identify a symptomatic root compared with CT and MRI in "difficult" cases.[217,222,230,231,233] Of particular note was a finding that although outcome of patients diagnosed with various nerve root entrapment syndromes was excellent, patients diagnosed with scarring or arachnoiditis had very poor outcomes.[223,231] All studies reported "successful" surgery to a greater or lesser extent in approximately 90% to 95% of patients following pain relief after selective nerve injections, if patients having prior surgery, scarring, and arachnoiditis were excluded. In the two studies that evaluated surgical outcome on patients with less than approximately 95% relief after injection, surgical results were modest to poor.[222,223]

In an observational study in 1971, Macnab[226] analyzed the causes of nerve root involvement in 68 patients who had undergone a "negative exploration" for presumed radicular pain caused by a herniated disc. Various pathologies were described, including migration of a disc fragment into the intervertebral foramen, nerve root kinking by the pedicle, articular process impingement, and extraforaminal lateral disc herniation. In the case of pedicular kinking, Macnab[226] described a technique of placing a 25-gauge needle into the intervertebral foramen and injecting 0.5 to 1 mL of oil-soluble contrast material. The provocation of concordant pain by striking the nerve with the needle, the characteristic contrast outline of the "kinked" nerve root within the foramen, and subsequent relief of pain after injection of 1 mL of 2% lidocaine were used to establish the diagnosis and led to "excellent results" in the six studied patients. Macnab[226] also described two patients with an undiscovered extraforaminal lateral disc herniation who underwent successful operation after relief of pain with a selective nerve root block. Likewise, Schutz and colleagues[228] in 1973 described the use of selective root blocks in 23 patients. In 13 of 15 patients who underwent surgery, the positive results of the selective nerve root blocks were confirmed.

Using a selective nerve root block technique similar to Macnab, Tajima and colleagues[229] in 1977 described various contrast patterns after injection of 2 mL of water-soluble contrast media, including cutoff patterns of contrast flow within the foramen and lateral recess indicating stenosis or block by a herniated disc. Provocation and pain relief after injection of 3 mL of 1% lidocaine confirmed the diagnosis, which was later proven during surgical exploration in this small case series. Kikuchi and colleagues[219] published a larger case series comprising 332 patients in 1982, in which they performed nerve root infiltration in all patients and correlated the resulting neurogram with anatomic findings of cadaveric dissections. In most patients, pain was relieved by injection at a single level. The cadaveric studies revealed the following causes of atypical pain: congenital or acquired abnormalities of nerve and nerve roots, sensory rootlets communicating with adjacent nerves, conjoined nerves, and the common occurrence of the furcal nerve exiting much more commonly at L4 than L5 level and giving branches to the lumbosacral trunk and femoral and obturator nerves. Kikuchi and colleagues[219] also described the descent of the vertebral pedicle associated with disc collapse, degenerative changes of the articular facet, and compression of nerve at different sites.

Krempen and Smith[227] in 1974 were the first to report surgical outcomes based on provocation and pain relief after injection of the nerve root with 1 mL of 1% lidocaine. They also described and included radiographs of neurogram patterns of extraforaminal disc herniations, pedicle kinking, articular process impingement, and scar tissue. These authors used the injections to diagnose pain in 21 patients with prior lumbar laminectomies and commented that most patients were able to pinpoint the level of the lesion to either of two injected levels. Of the 16 operated patients, 3 had excellent results, 9 had good results, and 4 had moderate results. The technique involved inserting an 18-gauge spinal needle 4 cm above the transverse process and approximately 6 cm from midline, directed downward and medially to strike the nerve. In the 1980s, Haueisen and colleagues[233] used Krempen and Smith's technique of spinal nerve injections to diagnose pain in difficult-to-diagnose patients, including 57% who had previous lumbar surgery. Of 63 operated patients, Haueisen and colleagues[233] confirmed compression of the suspected nerve root in 93% of the cases; at an average follow-up of 20 months, 73% of patients had no pain, slight pain, or some pain. Myelography and electromyelography aided in correct diagnosis of the lesion in only 24% and 38% of the cases.

Dooley and colleagues[223] used provocation and relief of pain after selective nerve root block to review retrospectively the results of 63 patients undergoing operations based on positive pain reproduction and pain relief after injection of 1 mL of 1% lidocaine correlated with surgical findings and outcome. The authors presented results according to whether the patients had full or incomplete pain relief and whether pain was reproduced. Of patients with reproduction and full pain relief, 45 of 46 had an anatomic diagnosis made at the time of surgery. Eight patients had herniated nucleus pulposus, and all were relieved of leg pain at follow-up. At follow-up, 17 patients had bony entrapment, and 14 (82%) were asymptomatic. Only 1 of 11 patients found to have arachnoiditis was pain-free at follow-up, although 5 of 7 patients found to have periradicular adhesions but without intraneural scarring were asymptomatic at follow-up. Patients with reproduction but incomplete relief included one patient who was diabetic with probable neuropathy causing failed surgery; the other three patients had pathology at other levels, and only one of the three had a satisfactory surgical outcome. In patients who had no reproduction and incomplete relief, only 5 of 14 cases were relieved of symptoms, and the authors recommended that patients with this group of responses should undergo careful reevaluation.

In 1988, Jonsson and colleagues[225] reported total relief of pain in 51% of patients undergoing diagnostic lumbar "root anesthesia" in 100 cases of sciatic pain with normal findings on myelography or CT or MRI or minor inconsistent abnormalities ($n = 40$) or multilevel involvement ($n = 9$). The patients experiencing pain relief underwent surgical root decompression with short-term surgical outcome comparable to conventional surgery in more obvious cases.

In 1990, Stanley and colleagues[230] likewise reported outcome based on response to injection in which they included only positive and negative responses. Positive responses required pain provocation and relief of pain with 1 mL of 1% lidocaine; a negative response was defined as nonconcordant pain and only partial relief or no relief of pain. At least two roots were studied in every patient. Of 20 patients with positive responses, 19 underwent operation, and Stanley and colleagues[230] found that "nerve root infiltration" identified the symptomatic level in 18 of 19 cases compared with CT scan and myelogram, which identified the correct level in 14 of 19 cases and 12 of 19 cases. Patients with negative blocks were not offered operation. The 2 of 16 patients with prior spinal surgery who had a "positive" response underwent successful surgery.

In 1989, Herron[231] reported the use of root blocks with pain provocation and pain relief after 1 mL of 0.5% bupivacaine. A positive response included reproduction of pain and at least 75% pain relief. Herron[231] divided outcomes into good, fair, and poor. For a good outcome, he required 75% pain relief and return to previous work status with minimal medications and minimal or no restrictions of physical activities. In the previously unoperated disc herniation group, 15 of 18 patients had good results, and 3 had fair results. In nine patients, the imaging studies were positive at two levels, but surgery was performed only at one symptomatic level identified with a root block. There were seven good results and two fair results. In patients with previous unoperated spinal stenosis, 19% had a poor outcome versus 52% poor outcomes in patients with prior stenosis surgery. Herron[231] noted that in most patients with radiculopathy, selective nerve root blocks are not needed because the level was readily apparent on clinical examination and imaging studies; however, root blocks were useful for patients with equivocal findings, previous surgery, and multilevel structural pathology.

Porter and colleagues[232] used CT-guided root blocks employing a two-needle technique to place an inner needle adjacent to the target nerve. In contrast to previous authors, these authors did not include provocation and injected 1.5 mL of 0.5% bupivacaine. Porter and colleagues[232] reported that of the 18 patients undergoing surgery, 78% had a good outcome; 2 patients had unsuccessful surgeries.

The study in 2005 by Sasso and colleagues[222] is the most comprehensive, albeit retrospective, evaluation of the value of selective nerve root injections to predict lumbar and cervical surgical outcomes. Sasso and colleagues[222] studied 101 patients culled from an institutional database from 1996-1999. Injections were performed by placing the needle tip just below the superior pedicle without intentional pain provocation. Additionally, a stimulating electrode to locate the needle close to the exiting nerve was employed. The authors noted the neurogram. A volume of 0.5 to 0.75 mL of 2% lidocaine was injected requiring greater than 95% pain relief during postblock provocative testing for a positive result. Confirmatory injections were performed when pain relief was 80% to 95%. Surgical follow-up was at a mean of 16.2 months with 18 patients undergoing cervical surgery and 83 patients undergoing lumbar surgery.

Of patients with positive selective nerve root injections, 91% had a good surgical outcome defined as a follow-up VAS of 2 or less and a positive patient satisfaction score. In 10 patients with negative selective nerve root injections, only 60% obtained a good surgical outcome. Patients undergoing surgery at a level with a positive block were 9.1 times more likely to have good outcomes than patients who had surgery

at negative selective nerve root injection levels. When the findings between selective nerve root injection and MRI differed ($n = 20$), surgery at a level consistent with the selective nerve root injection was more strongly associated with a good surgical outcome than surgery based on MRI. For selective nerve root injection, the positive predictive value was 91.2% with a negative predictive value of 40% compared with 88.4% positive predictive value of MRI. A breakdown between lumbar and cervical results was not reported.

Finally, Derby and colleagues[32] in 1992 reported the correlation between immediate leg pain relief after lumbar block and 1-year surgical outcomes. The authors segregated 78 patients undergoing epidural injections with a minimum of 80% immediate postblock leg pain relief into two dichotomous groups including patients with 50% or greater subjective leg pain relief lasting for 1 week or longer and patients with duration of extremity pain lasting 1 year or longer. Regardless of immediate pain relief, 85% of patients who had pain for less than 1 year had a positive surgical result defined as 50% or greater pain relief at 1 year regardless of immediate pain relief. More importantly, and by far the largest group (38 of 71), 95% of the patients who did not respond to the block had a poor surgical outcome. Derby and colleagues[32] opined that the poor outcome might be explained in some cases by an inadequate structural correction, inadequate stabilization, or functional reasons, but most failures probably represented irreversible changes in the neural structures. Although unstudied and so unconfirmed, the results by Derby and colleagues[32] are consistent with findings reported by Kumar and colleagues[234] that outcome after spinal cord stimulation in patients with failed back surgery syndrome was superior to revision surgery.

Technical Considerations

Techniques used by diagnostic lumbar studies place a needle varying in size from 18-gauge to 25-gauge into the foramen. Although older studies located the root by producing paresthesias,[219,223,226,229,231-233] more recent studies use a standard International Spine Intervention Society technique of placing the needle tip just below the pedicle at the approximate 6:00 o'clock position without purposefully provoking pain.[15] The transforaminal lumbar technique used by Macnab in the 1960s is similar to the current technique and the technique often used by many "older" interventionalists, including the senior author.[32,235] The needle is first advanced to contact the transverse process beginning approximately 6 cm from the midline, parallel to the transverse process and at an angle of approximately 30 degrees. The needle is advanced into the foramen at a position that would be approximately 6:00 o'clock below the pedicle.[223,226]

Another older described selective nerve root block technique used in the lumbar spine starts with needle insertion approximately 6 cm from the midline and approximately 2 to 3 cm above the transverse process and directs the needle into the foramen at a cephalad-caudad angle to contact the ventral root at approximately the midpoint between the upper and lower pedicles and slightly lateral to the foramen.[219,229,233] A stimulating electrode can also be used to verify close proximity of the needle tip to the nerve.[222] Although this technique has been referred to as a selective nerve root block, it is actually a selective ventral ramus block or, if the dorsal root ganglion is outside the foramen, a dorsal root ganglion block.

All prior lumbar studies except one[232] used approximately 1 mL of contrast dye to outline the nerve. Most studies and guidelines recommend visualizing contrast spread using live fluoroscopy during injection. In the cervical spine, some authors advocate observing contrast flow in an anteroposterior view using digital subtraction fluoroscopy to be better able to recognize potential injection into an artery coursing medially toward the spinal cord.[236,237]

Some prior studies used a volume varying from 0.3 to 0.5 mL of 0.5% bupivacaine[221] to 1.5 mL of 0.5% bupivacaine in the lumbar spine,[232] but most injected 1 mL of either 1% or 2% lidocaine. In the only diagnostic article that evaluated cervical injections, Sasso and colleagues[222] used 0.5 to 0.75 mL of 2% lidocaine but varied their volume depending on the observed contrast dye distribution. No studies have evaluated the diagnostic value of thoracic injections.

The authors recommend limiting the volume to 0.3 to 1 mL in the lumbar spine and 0.3 to 0.5 mL in cervical and thoracic spine. Although many prior studies used 1% to 2% lidocaine, the authors recommend a higher concentration to ensure adequate block.[220,222] At a minimum, 2% lidocaine should be used; however, an equal combination of 4% lidocaine with 0.75% bupivacaine or 0.5% bupivacaine alone can be used. The volume can be adjusted between the lower and upper limit depending on the contrast flow pattern.

Confounding Factors

Blocking the exiting spinal nerve blocks several important neural elements. Receiving branches from the sympathetic system, the sinuvertebral nerve emerges lateral to the foramen and courses back through the foramen to innervate the posterior longitudinal ligament, the disc anulus at that level and one or two levels above. The sinuvertebral nerve can also innervate the contralateral side. In addition, lateral to the dorsal root ganglion, the dorsal root branches and innervates posterior structures including branches to the zygapophyseal joint at the same level and level below and the interspinous and supraspinous ligaments. Relief of pain may be due to blocking structures not typically considered. The furcal nerve typically exits the L4 foramen; is a separate nerve with its own dorsal root ganglion; and sends branches to the lumbosacral trunk, femoral, and obturator nerves. Irritation of this nerve causes seemingly aberrant pain distribution to the hip, groin, and inner thigh. Nerve root scarring is a barrier to diffusion. A scarred nerve root may have insufficient penetration of local anesthetic to effect an adequate block. Postblock subjective pain relief would probably be less than approximately 50% and not meet qualification for a positive block. Although such a response decreases the sensitivity, such a response is desired clinically because repeat unsuccessful surgery may be avoided.

Summary

Patients with clinically significant radicular pain unresponsive to conservative care and medications may be offered a therapeutic injection including local anesthetic and corticosteroids. The injection can be performed using an interlaminar, transforaminal, or combined approach and can be performed at all suspected levels using volumes of injectant that cover all suspected symptomatic levels. If the patient has convincing pain relief for 1 week or longer, it is likely that the cause of pain is reversible and secondary to inflammation.[32] More importantly, if the patient reports minimal or very short-term relief of extremity pain, the pain has been present for greater than 1 year, and the offending pathology is unconvincing, the pain may be neuropathic or referred somatic pain.[32] If pain relief is satisfactory and lasts several weeks or longer, one may use additional therapeutic injections to facilitate conservative care, and there may be no need to proceed with exactly identifying the symptomatic level. When pain is recurring or poorly responsive to therapeutic injections and the clinical and imaging studies are inconclusive or indicate more than one potential pain level, diagnostic transforaminal injections may be considered. Table 15–1 summarizes indications for diagnostic selective nerve root blocks.

As with all diagnostic spine injections, preprocedural and postprocedural evaluation should be performed with a standardized protocol by unbiased personnel and checked by the physician. Using the same testing protocol, the patient is tested at approximately 15 to 20 minutes after block with lidocaine and approximately 30 minutes after block with bupivacaine or ropivacaine. The block should last at least 1 hour if lidocaine is used and about 2 hours or longer if bupivacaine or ropivacaine is used. If the pain relief is less than 70%, one can return the patient to the interventional suite and block one more additional suspected level. Diagnostic injection should be performed using one of the standard transforaminal approaches, preferably performed by an experienced interventionalist or surgeon. The patient should be no more than lightly sedated or sedated with a low dose of propofol with a very short half-life.

A standard needle, blunt tip needle, or a polytef (Teflon)-coated (e.g., approximately 3.5-inch, 22-gauge) radiofrequency

---

TABLE 15–1 Indications for Diagnostic Selective Nerve Root Blocks

1. Patients with radicular pain without localizing signs to indicate which level is involved
2. Patients without obvious nerve root entrapment on high-quality imaging studies
3. Patients with chronic radicular pain present for ≥1 year, resistant to usual care and being considered for surgery
4. Patients with persistent pain after surgery or status post multiple surgeries
5. Patients with radicular symptoms in more than one distribution with multilevel structure impingement
6. Patients with atypical extremity pain
7. Imaging studies, discography, or electromyography nondiagnostic or conflicting

needle may be used to position the needle tip within approximately 1 to 2 mm of the nerve, which in many cases is adjacent to the dorsal root ganglion. If a stimulating needle is used, observing motor stimulation at 2 Hz and approximately 2 V helps position the needle, and pain referral patterns can be noted using sensory stimulation at 50 Hz at approximately 0.2 to 0.5 V. Using live fluoroscopic monitoring, one injects a volume of contrast medium equal to that used for local anesthesia. One should record the presence or absence of axial, buttock-hip, and extremity provocation and the location of contrast dye when provocation occurs (e.g., within the foramen or more proximal or distal to the foramen). The pattern and extent of contrast flow is recorded on digital "hard copy." Flow of contrast dye should show a negative outline of the dorsal root ganglion, spinal nerve, and ventral ramus. If spread of contrast dye is clearly outside the foramen and does not surround the nerve, the needle can be repositioned and reinjected.

A low volume of a concentrated anesthetic solution should be used that is limited to 0.3 mL or less in the cervical spine, 0.5 mL or less in the thoracic spine, and 1 mL or less in the lumbar spine.[224] One might consider using an equal mixture of 4% lidocaine and 0.75% bupivacaine or 0.5% bupivacaine alone. If performing a therapeutic injection, 0.5 mL of nonparticulate corticosteroid (e.g., 5 mg dexamethasone) may be injected in the cervical and thoracic spine approximately 1 to 2 minutes after local anesthetic injection, and either nonparticulate or a longer acting depot preparation may be injected in the lumbar spine (e.g., approximately 20 mg of triamcinolone acetonide or 3 mg of betamethasone).

The immediate results and the patient's longer term pain relief are used to counsel the patient on his or her chances of obtaining relief of extremity pain after a surgical procedure. Patients who have immediate pain relief after one level block of approximately 70% or greater and pain less than 1 year's duration have an 85% or greater chance of a satisfactory result.[220-223,230,235] If the patient has had prior surgery, one might want to lower the patient's expectation from 85% to perhaps approximately 70% or less depending on how convincing the structural pathology appears on MRI or CT.[231,233] Patients who have unconvincing structural pathology, radicular pain greater than 1 year's duration, relief of less than approximately 70% of pain after block, less than approximately 1 week of therapeutic pain relief, and especially evidence of intraradicular or extraradicular scarring should be referred for possible spinal cord stimulation or other nonoperative treatment.[32,220,221,223,231]

Patients with clear structural nerve entrapment with radicular pain less than approximately 1 year's duration, with no immediate or delayed longer duration relief, may be offered surgery, but the patient should be counseled that there is an approximately 60% chance of a good outcome.[222] If the duration of the patient's pain is greater than 1 year, perhaps the patient should be told that there is an approximately 60% chance of having partial pain relief but that the pain relief would likely be less than 50%.[32,222] Even if the same patient with more chronic radicular pain had immediate pain relief but no longer term relief, and especially if there was suspected

neuropathic pain and a prior surgery, the patient should be counseled that the chances of a good outcome are no greater than approximately 50%.[231] Finally, the authors emphasize that relief of pain does not determine the cause of the pain, and if a patient's root pain is neuropathic, decompression with or without stabilization would most likely not provide satisfactory relief of pain.[238]

Pitfalls regarding selective nerve root blocks include complications of the procedure. Although complications after transforaminal injections are mostly minor,[239-241] there are growing concerns regarding the safety of cervical transforaminal injections[242,243] and to a lesser extent thoracic and lumbar injections based on published and unpublished cases of neurologic damage after the injection of local anesthetic and depot corticosteroids into the neuroforamen.[244-248] Reported and unreported complications mostly involve the use of particulate corticosteroids that are alleged to have been injected into the vertebral or radicular artery. Some unpublished legal cases are, however, consistent with direct injection into the cord. Although legal cases claim injury was secondary to injection of particulate corticosteroids into a lumbar or thoracic radicular artery, to the authors' knowledge there has been no reported case of neurologic damage secondary to arterial injection using nonparticulate corticosteroids; nonparticulate corticosteroids are now recommended when performing cervical transforaminal injections.[249] Spinal cord injection is rare and is easily preventable by using a shorter needle, always advancing the needle over bone (superior articular process), checking an anteroposterior fluoroscopy view before injection, and titrating patient sedation appropriately.

Although current techniques strive to avoid contacting the nerve, contact does occasionally occur, and probing for paresthesias was a common technique in the past. Lasting effects are probably uncommon, and none of the prior reviewed diagnostic block studies reported any complications. Injecting local anesthetic or contrast dye directly into the dorsal root ganglion, nerve, or epiradicular sheath may cause a flare in pain, however, lasting several days to several weeks.[220] Permanent injury is probably rare and to the authors' knowledge unreported.

A needle placed too far medially can pierce the nerve root sleeve surrounded by the dura contiguous with the subarachnoid space. Injection may cause a high spinal block, which may necessitate resuscitation if injected in the cervical spine and may potentially lead to some degree of cord or root irritation secondary to added preservatives if depot steroids are injected. Puncture of the dura may also cause a low-pressure cerebrospinal fluid headache, which usually resolves spontaneously or can be treated with a routine blood patch. Slipman and colleagues[218] reported a case of recalcitrant headache cured after transforaminal blood patch. Infection may occur, but is rare. If the patient has a foraminal disc protrusion, inadvertently passing a needle into the disc may occasionally occur and could lead to a disc space infection.[250] If the operator knows that disc injection has occurred, use of a small amount of intradiscal and intravenous antibiotics should be considered (as would be the routine with discography).

PEARLS AND PITFALLS

1. Much is learned during the process of diagnosis, especially if the process includes unpleasant diagnostic interventional procedures.

2. Diagnosis is the process of elimination. Patients should be counseled that negative responses are useful and important information.

3. Beware of patients with chronic pain without convincing structural pathology who consistently complain that they are no better or worse after appropriate therapeutic interventional procedures. Your reconstructive spine is likely to suffer the same fate.

4. Indeterminate and negative diagnostic block results are more common than clearly positive results.

5. Chronic spinal pain is often caused by structures in different columns and levels. Treating one source of pain often unmasks pain from a different source. Failure to relieve other sources of pain does not necessarily mean one's surgery failed, but the possibility of failure due to other sources is best identified before surgery.

6. When the diagnosis is not obvious and most of the pain is axial and referred extremity pain, consider first evaluating the posterior elements. Blocking the medial and/or lateral branches of the dorsal ramus will denervate most structures in the posterior column.

7. Do not neglect to rule out shoulder and hip pathology.

8. Convincing relief of pain for several weeks or longer is consistent with a reversible cause of pain.

9. Fusing to a painful SI joint is best avoided. Investigate and discuss the possibility before surgery rather than after.

10. Chronic dynamic irritation of neuroaxial structures can cause buttock and axial pain in addition to referred extremity pain. Relief of axial pain following selective epidural block(s) that lasts several weeks or longer is consistent with pain due to static or dynamic stenosis. If in doubt, diagnosis can be confirmed by a *negative* response to medial branch block and a *negative* response to pressure-controlled discography, analgesic discography, or both.

KEY POINTS

1. Image-guided, precision injections (with local anesthetic and a dual block paradigm) are the current reference standard for diagnosis of chronic spinal pain emanating from the middle and posterior column. Current research shows that history, physical examination, and advanced imaging findings have insufficient sensitivity and specificity for identifying the pain generator. Ideally, as with sacroiliac pain, the reference standard will evolve to include validated and accurate historical and physical examination features; however, with radicular pain and zygapophyseal joint pain, this is not yet the case.

2. Diagnostic injections are typically reserved as a tertiary intervention for patients with chronic, disabling spinal pain that is nonresponsive to conservative care and for patients with atypical presentations, in whom the history, physical examination, and electrodiagnostic and imaging studies are unrevealing or nondiagnostic.

3. During a diagnostic block, relief of pain is more convincing than provocation of pain. The standard for percent relief is, at a minimum, greater than 50%; however, greater than 70% is more convincing.

4. Patients with psychosocial distress can have legitimate pain. Often the psychosocial distress resolves with appropriate diagnosis and treatment of the pain generator.

5. Negative diagnostic blocks also provide useful information. If the diagnostic blocks do not relieve the pain, this can suggest many possible explanations: first, that the structure evaluated is not the source of pain and additional structures must be evaluated. Lack of relief may also be due to the development of irreversible local damage (e.g., intraneural fibrosis) or neuropathic pain with significant peripheral and central sensitization.

6. If rigorous technical and procedural performance standards are adhered to, the response to diagnostic blocks has been shown to predict good to excellent surgical and interventional treatment outcomes. Fair or poor response to diagnostic blocks can be used to counsel patients appropriately in terms of surgical outcomes.

KEY REFERENCES

1. Hancock MJ, Maher CG, Latimer J, et al: Systematic review of tests to identify the disc, SIJ or facet joint as the source of low back pain. Eur Spine J 16:1539-1550, 2007.
   This is a systematic review of the evidence for identifying the source of chronic low back pain.

2. Cohen SP, Raja SN: Pathogenesis, diagnosis, and treatment of lumbar zygapophysial (facet) joint pain. Anesthesiology 106:591-614, 2007.
   This article provides a comprehensive review of zygapophyseal joint anatomy, biomechanics, and function and a systematic review of diagnosis and treatment of zygapophyseal joint pain.

3. Manchukonda R, Manchikanti KN, Cash KA, et al: Facet joint pain in chronic spinal pain: An evaluation of prevalence and false-positive rate of diagnostic blocks. J Spinal Disord Tech 20:539-545, 2007.
   This study of prevalence of facet joint pain based on dual block paradigm reported a high false-positive rate with single diagnostic blocks.

4. Dreyfuss P, Dreyer, SJ, Cole A, et al: Sacroiliac pain. J Am Acad Orthop Surg 12:255-265, 2004.
   This excellent review of the anatomy, pathophysiology, history, physical examination, and imaging findings associated with sacroiliac joint pain discusses the standards for diagnosis of sacroiliac joint pain with controlled blocks and treatment.

5. Bogduk N: Practice Guidelines: Spinal Diagnostic and Treatment Procedures. San Francisco, International Spine Intervention Society, 2004.
State-of-the-art guidelines for the performance of diagnostic and therapeutic spinal injections are presented.

REFERENCES

1. Boswell MV, Trescot AM, Datta S, et al: Interventional techniques: Evidence-based practice guidelines in the management of chronic spinal pain. Pain Physician 10:7-111, 2007.

2. CDC: Prevalence of disabilities and associated health conditions among adults—United States 1999. MMWR Morb Mortal Wkly Rep 50:120-125, 2001.

3. Guo HR, Tanaka S, Halperin WE, et al: Back pain prevalence in US industry and estimates of lost workdays. Am J Public Health (1971) 89:1029-1035, 1999.

4. Cypress BK: Characteristics of physician visits for back symptoms: A national perspective. Am J Public Health (1971) 73:389-395, 1983.

5. Shekelle PG, Markovich M, Louie R: An epidemiologic study of episodes of back pain care. Spine (Phila Pa 1976) 20:1668-1673, 1995.

6. Katz JN: Lumbar disc disorders and low-back pain: Socioeconomic factors and consequences. J Bone Joint Surg Am 88(Suppl 2):21-24, 2006.

7. Freburger JK, Holmes GM, Agans RP, et al: The rising prevalence of chronic low back pain. Arch Intern Med 169:251-258, 2009.

8. Dillane JB, Fry J, Kalton G: Acute back syndrome: A study from general practice. BMJ 2:82-84, 1966.

9. Nachemson AL: The natural course of low back pain. In White A, Gordon SL (eds): Symposium on Idiopathic Low Back Pain. St Louis, Mosby, 1982, pp 46-51.

10. Sheather-Reid RB, Cohen ML: Psychophysical evidence for a neuropathic component of chronic neck pain. Pain 75:341-347, 1998.

11. Hancock MJ, Maher CG, Latimer J, et al: Systematic review of tests to identify the disc, SIJ or facet joint as the source of low back pain. Eur Spine J 16:1539-1550, 2007.

12. Fritz JM, George S: The use of a classification approach to identify subgroups of patients with acute low back pain: Interrater reliability and short-term treatment outcomes. Spine (Phila Pa 1976) 25:106-114, 2000.

13. Kent P, Keating J: Do primary-care clinicians think that nonspecific low back pain is one condition? Spine (Phila Pa 1976) 29:1022-1031, 2004.

14. Derby R: Diagnostic block procedures. Spine (Phila Pa 1976) 1:47-64, 1986.

15. Bogduk N: Practice Guidelines: Spinal Diagnostic and Treatment Procedures. San Francisco, International Spine Intervention Society, 2004.

16. Boswell MV, Colson JD, Sehgal N, et al: A systematic review of therapeutic facet joint interventions in chronic spinal pain. Pain Physician 10:229-253, 2007.

17. Boden S, Wiesel SW, Laws ER, et al: The Aging Spine. Philadelphia, WB Saunders, 1991.

18. Berven S, Tay BB, Colman W, et al: The lumbar zygapophyseal (facet) joints: A role in the pathogenesis of spinal pain syndromes and degenerative spondylolisthesis. Semin Neurol 22:187-196, 2002.

19. Wetzel FT: Chronic benign cervical pain syndromes: Surgical considerations. Spine (Phila Pa 1976) 17(10 Suppl):S367-S374, 1992.

20. Cohen SP, Raja SN: Pathogenesis, diagnosis, and treatment of lumbar zygapophysial (facet) joint pain. Anesthesiology 106:591-614, 2007.

21. Cohen SP: Sacroiliac joint pain: A comprehensive review of anatomy, diagnosis and treatment. Anesth Analg 101:1440-1453, 2005.

22. Resnick DK, Choudhri TF, Dailey AT, et al: Guidelines for the performance of fusion procedures for degenerative disease of the lumbar spine. Part 13: Injection therapies, low-back pain, and lumbar fusion. J Neurosurg Spine 2:707-715, 2005.

23. Boswell MV, Singh V, Staats PS, et al: Accuracy of precision diagnostic blocks in the diagnosis of chronic spinal pain of facet or zygapophysial joint origin. Pain Physician 6:449-456, 2003.

24. Dreyfuss P, Dreyer SJ, Cole A, et al: Sacroiliac joint pain. J Am Acad Orthop Surg 12:255-265, 2004.

25. Dutta S, Lee M, Falco FJ, et al: Systematic assessment of diagnostic accuracy therapeutic utility of lumbar facet interventions. Pain Physician 12:437-460, 2009.

26. Atluri S, Datta S, Falco FJ, et al: Systematic review of diagnostic utility and therapeutic effectiveness of thoracic facet joint interventions. Pain Physician 11:611-629, 2008.

27. Sehgal N, Dunbar EE, Shah RV, et al: Systematic review of diagnostic utility of facet (zygapophysial) joint injections in chronic spinal pain: An update. Pain Physician 10:213-228, 2007.

28. Manchikanti L, Pampati V, Fellows B, et al: The inability of the clinical picture to characterize pain from facet joints. Pain Physician 3:158-166, 2000.

29. Yin W, Bogduk N: The nature of neck pain in a private pain clinic in the United States. Pain Med 9:196-203, 2008.

30. Manchikanti L, Pampati V, Rivera J, et al: Role of facet joints in chronic low back pain in the elderly: A controlled comparative prevalence study. Pain Pract 1:332-337, 2001.

31. Pneumaticos SG, Chatziioannou SN, Hipp JA, et al: Low back pain: Prediction of short-term outcome of facet joint injection with bone scintigraphy. Radiology 238:693-698, 2006.

32. Derby R, Kine G, Saal JA, et al: Response to steroid and duration of radicular pain as predictors of surgical outcome. Spine (Phila Pa 1976) 17(6 Suppl):S176-S183, 1992.

33. Manchikanti L, Boswell MV, Manchukonda R, et al: Influence of prior opioid exposure on diagnostic facet joint nerve blocks. J Opioid Manag 4:351-360, 2008.

34. Kikuchi S: New concept for backache: Biopsychosocial pain syndrome. Eur Spine J 17(Suppl 4):421-427, 2008.

35. Boos N, Rieder R, Schade V, et al: 1995 Volvo Award in clinical sciences: The diagnostic accuracy of magnetic resonance imaging, work perception, and psychosocial factors in identifying symptomatic disc herniations. Spine (Phila Pa 1976) 20:2613-2625, 1995.

36. Lilius G, Laasonen EM, Myllynen P, et al: Lumbar facet joint syndrome: A randomised clinical trial. J Bone Joint Surg Br 71:681-684, 1989.

SECTION II

37. Lilius G, Harilainen A, Laasonen EM, et al: Chronic unilateral low-back pain: Predictors of outcome of facet joint injections. Spine (Phila Pa 1976) 15:780-782, 1990.

38. Wallis BJ, Lord SM, Bogduk N: Resolution of psychological distress of whiplash patients following treatment by radiofrequency neurotomy: A randomised, double-blind, placebo-controlled trial. Pain 73:15-22, 1997.

39. Manchikanti L, Pampati V, Fellows B, et al: Influence of psychological factors on the ability to diagnose chronic low back pain of facet joint origin. Pain Physician 4:349-357, 2001.

40. Derby R, Lee S-H, Chen Y, et al: The influence of psychologic factors on diskography in patients with chronic axial low back pain. Arch Phys Med Rehabil 89:1300-1304, 2008.

41. Kirkaldy-Willis WH, Farfan FH: Instability of the lumbar spine. Clin Orthop Relat Res 165:110-123, 1982.

42. Apophysis. Available at http://en.wikipedia.org/wiki/Apophysis. Accessed April 13, 2009.

43. Bogduk N: Clinical Anatomy of the Lumbar Spine, 4th ed. London, Elsevier, 2005.

44. Andersson GB, Ortengren R, Nachemson AL: Intradiskal pressure, intra-abdominal pressure and myoelectric back muscle activity related to posture and loading. Clin Orthop Relat Res 129:156-164, 1977.

45. Adams MA, Hutton WC: The mechanical function of the lumbar apophyseal joints. Spine (Phila Pa 1976) 8:327-330, 1983.

46. Uhrenholt L, Hauge E, Charles AV, et al: Degenerative and traumatic changes in the lower cervical spine facet joints. Scand J Rheumatol 37:375-384, 2008.

47. Taylor JR, Twomey LT, Corker M: Bone and soft tissue injuries in post-mortem lumbar spines. Paraplegia 28:119-129, 1990.

48. Twomey LT, Taylor JR, Taylor MM: Unsuspected damage to lumbar zygapophyseal (facet) joints after motor-vehicle accidents. Med J Aust 151:210-212, 215, 1989.

49. Taylor JR, Twomey LT: Acute injuries to cervical joints: An autopsy study of neck sprain. Spine (Phila Pa 1976) 18:1115-1122, 1993.

50. Uhrenholt L, Grunnet-Nilsson N, Hartvigsen J: Cervical spine lesions after road traffic accidents: A systematic review. Spine (Phila Pa 1976) 27:1934-1941; discussion 1940, 2002.

51. Eisenstein SM, Parry CR: The lumbar facet arthrosis syndrome: Clinical presentation and articular surface changes. J Bone Joint Surg Br 69:3-7, 1987.

52. Ziv I, Maroudas C, Robin G, et al: Human facet cartilage: Swelling and some physicochemical characteristics as a function of age. Part 2: Age changes in some biophysical parameters of human facet joint cartilage. Spine (Phila Pa 1976) 18:136-146, 1993.

53. Kallakuri S, Singh A, Chen C, et al: Demonstration of substance P, calcitonin gene-related peptide, and protein gene product 9.5 containing nerve fibers in human cervical facet joint capsules. Spine (Phila Pa 1976) 29:1182-1186, 2004.

54. Giles LG, Taylor JR: Innervation of lumbar zygapophyseal joint synovial folds. Acta Orthop Scand 58:43-46, 1987.

55. Giles LG, Taylor JR: Human zygapophyseal joint capsule and synovial fold innervation. Br J Rheumatol 26:93-98, 1987.

56. Kallakuri S, Singh A, Lu Y, et al: Tensile stretching of cervical facet joint capsule and related axonal changes. Eur Spine J 17:556-563, 2008.

57. Ahmed M, Bjurholm A, Kreicbergs A, et al: Sensory and autonomic innervation of the facet joint in the rat lumbar spine. Spine (Phila Pa 1976) 18:2121-2126, 1993.

58. Cavanaugh JM, Lu Y, Chen C, et al: Pain generation in lumbar and cervical facet joints. J Bone Joint Surg Am 88(Suppl 2): 63-67, 2006.

59. Cavanaugh JM, Ozaktay AC, Yamashita HT, et al: Lumbar facet pain: Biomechanics, neuroanatomy and neurophysiology. J Biomech 29:1117-1129, 1996.

60. Schaible HG, Schmidt RF: Effects of an experimental arthritis on the sensory properties of fine articular afferent units. J Neurophysiol 54:1109-1122, 1985.

61. Lu Y, Chen C, Kallakuri S, et al: Neural response of cervical facet joint capsule to stretch: A study of whiplash pain mechanism. Stapp Car Crash J 49:49-65, 2005.

62. Lu Y, Chen C, Kallakuri S, et al: Neurophysiological and biomechanical characterization of goat cervical facet joint capsules. J Orthop Res 23:779-787, 2005.

63. Lee KE, Davis MB, Winkelstein BA: Capsular ligament involvement in the development of mechanical hyperalgesia after facet joint loading: Behavioral and inflammatory outcomes in a rodent model of pain. J Neurotrauma 25:1383-1393, 2008.

64. Lee KE, Davis MB, Mejilla RM, et al: In vivo cervical facet capsule distraction: Mechanical implications for whiplash and neck pain. Stapp Car Crash J 48:373-395, 2004.

65. Winkelstein BA, Santos DG: An intact facet capsular ligament modulates behavioral sensitivity and spinal glial activation produced by cervical facet joint tension. Spine (Phila Pa 1976) 33:856-862, 2008.

66. Woolf CJ: Evidence for a central component of post-injury pain hypersensitivity. Nature 306:686-688, 1983.

67. Quinn KP, Lee KE, Ahaghotu CC, et al: Structural changes in the cervical facet capsular ligament: Potential contributions to pain following subfailure loading. Stapp Car Crash J 51:169-187, 2007.

68. Kasch H, Stengaard-Pedersen K, Arendt-Nielsen L, et al: Pain thresholds and tenderness in neck and head following acute whiplash injury: A prospective study. Cephalalgia 21:189-197, 2001.

69. Sterling M, Jull G, Vicenzino B, et al: Sensory hypersensitivity occurs soon after whiplash injury and is associated with poor recovery. Pain 104:509-517, 2003.

70. Curatolo M, Petersen-Felix S, Arendt-Nielsen L, et al: Central hypersensitivity in chronic pain after whiplash injury. Clin J Pain 17:306-315, 2001.

71. Manchikanti L, Manchikanti KN, Manchukonda R, et al: Evaluation of lumbar facet joint nerve blocks in the management of chronic low back pain: Preliminary report of a randomized, double-blind controlled trial: Clinical trial NCT00355914. Pain Physician 10:425-440, 2007.

72. Bogduk N: A narrative review of intra-articular corticosteroid injections for low back pain. Pain Med 6:287-296, 2005.

73. Barnsley L, Lord SM, Wallis BJ, et al: Lack of effect of intraarticular corticosteroids for chronic pain in the cervical zygapophyseal joints. N Engl J Med 330:1047-1050, 1994.

74. Carette S, Marcoux S, Truchon R, et al: A controlled trial of corticosteroid injections into facet joints for chronic low back pain. N Engl J Med 325:1002-1007, 1991.

75. Manchikanti L, Singh V, Falco FJ, et al: Cervical medial branch blocks for chronic cervical facet joint pain: A randomized, double-blind, controlled trial with one-year follow-up. Spine (Phila Pa 1976) 33:1813-1820, 2008.

76. Manchikanti L, Singh V, Falco FJ, et al: Lumbar facet joint nerve blocks in managing chronic facet joint pain: One-year follow-up of a randomized, double-blind controlled trial: Clinical Trial NCT00355914. Pain Physician 11:121-132, 2008.

77. Manchikanti L, Singh V, Vilims BD, et al: Medial branch neurotomy in management of chronic spinal pain: Systematic review of the evidence. Pain Physician 5:405-418, 2002.

78. Little JS, Ianuzzi A, Chiu JB, et al: Human lumbar facet joint capsule strains: II. Alteration of strains subsequent to anterior interbody fixation. Spine J 4:153-162, 2004.

79. Chang UK, Kim DH, Lee MC, et al: Changes in adjacent-level disc pressure and facet joint force after cervical arthroplasty compared with cervical discectomy and fusion. J Neurosurg Spine 7:33-39, 2007.

80. Mooney V, Robertson J: The facet syndrome. Clin Orthop Relat Res (115):149-156, 1976.

81. Sehgal N, Shah RV, McKenzie-Brown AM, et al: Diagnostic utility of facet (zygapophysial) joint injections in chronic spinal pain: A systematic review of evidence. Pain Physician 8:211-224, 2005.

82. Bogduk N: Evidence-informed management of chronic low back pain with facet injections and radiofrequency neurotomy. Spine J 8:56-64, 2008.

83. Manchukonda R, Manchikanti KN, Cash KA, et al: Facet joint pain in chronic spinal pain: An evaluation of prevalence and false-positive rate of diagnostic blocks. J Spinal Disord Tech 20:539-545, 2007.

84. Cohen SP, Stojanovic MP, Crooks M, et al: Lumbar zygapophysial (facet) joint radiofrequency denervation success as a function of pain relief during diagnostic medial branch blocks: A multicenter analysis. Spine J 8:498-504, 2008.

85. Barnsley L, Lord S, Bogduk N: Comparative local anaesthetic blocks in the diagnosis of cervical zygapophysial joint pain. Pain 55:99-106, 1993.

86. Lord SM, Barnsley L, Bogduk N: The utility of comparative local anesthetic blocks versus placebo-controlled blocks for the diagnosis of cervical zygapophysial joint pain. Clin J Pain 11:208-213, 1995.

87. Kaplan M, Dreyfuss P, Halbrook B, et al: The ability of lumbar medial branch blocks to anesthetize the zygapophysial joint: A physiologic challenge. Spine (Phila Pa 1976) 23:1847-1852, 1998.

88. Dreyfuss P, Schwarzer AC, Lau P, et al: Specificity of lumbar medial branch and L5 dorsal ramus blocks: A computed tomography study. Spine (Phila Pa 1976) 22:895-902, 1997.

89. Destouet JM, Gilula LA, Murphy WA, et al: Lumbar facet joint injection: Indication, technique, clinical correlation, and preliminary results. Radiology 145:321-325, 1982.

90. Carrera GF: Lumbar facet joint injection in low back pain and sciatica: Description of technique. Radiology 137:661-664, 1980.

91. Destouet JM, Murphy WA: Lumbar facet block indications and technique. Orthop Rev 14, 1985.

92. Moran R, O'Connell D, Walsh MG: The diagnostic value of facet joint injections. Spine (Phila Pa 1976) 13:1407-1410, 1988.

93. Barnsley L, Bogduk N: Medial branch blocks are specific for the diagnosis of cervical zygapophyseal joint pain. Reg Anesth 18:343-350, 1993.

94. Cohen SP, Hurley RW: The ability of diagnostic spinal injections to predict surgical outcomes. Anesth Analg 105:1756-1775, 2007.

95. North RB, Kidd DH, Zahurak M, et al: Specificity of diagnostic nerve blocks: A prospective, randomized study of sciatica due to lumbosacral spine disease. Pain 65:77-85, 1996.

96. Goldthwait JE: The lumbosacral articulation: An explanation of many cases of lumbago, sciatica and paraplegia. Boston Med Surg J 164:356-372, 1911.

97. Ghormley RK: Low back pain with special reference to the articular facets, with presentation of an operative procedure. JAMA 101:1773-1777, 1933.

97a. Badgley CE: Pain of spinal origin. J Mich State Med Soc 46:812, 1947.

98. Schwarzer AC, Aprill CN, Derby R, et al: The relative contributions of the disc and zygapophyseal joint in chronic low back pain. Spine (Phila Pa 1976) 19:801-806, 1994.

99. Manchikanti L, Pampati V, Fellows B, et al: Prevalence of lumbar facet joint pain in chronic low back pain. Pain Physician 2:59-64, 1999.

100. Manchikanti L, Boswell MV, Singh V, et al: Prevalence of facet joint pain in chronic spinal pain of cervical, thoracic, and lumbar regions. BMC Musculoskelet Disord 5:15, 2004.

101. Schwarzer AC, Wang SC, Bogduk N, et al: Prevalence and clinical features of lumbar zygapophysial joint pain: A study in an Australian population with chronic low back pain. Ann Rheum Dis 54:100-106, 1995.

102. Fairbank JC, Park WM, McCall IW, et al: Apophyseal injection of local anesthetic as a diagnostic aid in primary low-back pain syndromes. Spine (Phila Pa 1976) 6:598-605, 1981.

103. Revel ME, Listrat VM, Chevalier XJ, et al: Facet joint block for low back pain: Identifying predictors of a good response. Arch Phys Med Rehabil 73:824-828, 1992.

104. Revel M, Poiraudeau S, Auleley GR, et al: Capacity of the clinical picture to characterize low back pain relieved by facet joint anesthesia: Proposed criteria to identify patients with painful facet joints. Spine (Phila Pa 1976) 23:1972-1976; discussion 1977, 1998.

105. Laslett M, Oberg B, Aprill CN, et al: Zygapophysial joint blocks in chronic low back pain: A test of Revel's model as a screening test. BMC Musculoskelet Disord 5:43, 2004.

106. Schwarzer AC, Aprill CN, Derby R, et al: The false-positive rate of uncontrolled diagnostic blocks of the lumbar zygapophysial joints. Pain 58:195-200, 1994.

107. Manchikanti L, Pampati V, Fellows B, et al: The diagnostic validity and therapeutic value of lumbar facet joint nerve blocks with or without adjuvant agents. Curr Rev Pain 4:337-344, 2000.

108. Schwarzer AC, Derby R, Aprill CN, et al: Pain from the lumbar zygapophysial joints: A test of two models. J Spinal Disord 7:331-336, 1994.

109. Anand S, Butt MS: Patients' response to facet joint injection. Acta Orthop Belg 73:230-233, 2007.

110. Carrera GF: Lumbar facet arthrography and injection in low back pain. Wisc Med J 78:35-37, 1979.

111. Jackson RP, Jacobs RR, Montesano PX: 1988 Volvo award in clinical sciences: Facet joint injection in low-back pain: A prospective statistical study. Spine (Phila Pa 1976) 13:966-971, 1988.

112. Schwarzer AC, Wang SC, O'Driscoll D, et al: The ability of computed tomography to identify a painful zygapophysial joint in patients with chronic low back pain. Spine (Phila Pa 1976) 20:907-912, 1995.

113. Cohen SP, Hurley RW, Christo PJ, et al: Clinical predictors of success and failure for lumbar facet radiofrequency denervation. Clin J Pain 23:45-52, 2007.

114. Kawaguchi Y, Matsuno H, Kanamori M, et al: Radiologic findings of the lumbar spine in patients with rheumatoid arthritis, and a review of pathologic mechanisms. J Spinal Disord Tech 16:38-43, 2003.

115. Friedrich KM, Nemec S, Peloschek P, et al: The prevalence of lumbar facet joint edema in patients with low back pain. Skeletal Radiol 36:755-760, 2007.

116. Marks R: Distribution of pain provoked from lumbar facet joints and related structures during diagnostic spinal infiltration. Pain 39:37-40, 1989.

117. Windsor RE, King FJ, Roman SJ, et al: Electrical stimulation induced lumbar medial branch referral patterns. Pain Physician 5:347-353, 2002.

118. Jackson RP: The facet syndrome: Myth or reality? Clin Orthop Relat Res (279):110-121, 1992.

119. Esses SI, Moro JK: The value of facet joint blocks in patient selection for lumbar fusion. Spine (Phila Pa 1976) 18:185-190, 1993.

120. Schofferman J, Reynolds J, Herzog R, et al: Failed back surgery: Etiology and diagnostic evaluation. Spine J 3:400-403, 2003.

121. Lovely TJ, Rastogi P: The value of provocative facet blocking as a predictor of success in lumbar spine fusion. J Spinal Disord 10:512-517, 1997.

122. Dreyfuss P, Halbrook B, Pauza K, et al: Efficacy and validity of radiofrequency neurotomy for chronic lumbar zygapophysial joint pain. Spine (Phila Pa 1976) 25:1270-1277, 2000.

123. Nath S, Nath CA, Pettersson K: Percutaneous lumbar zygapophysial (facet) joint neurotomy using radiofrequency current, in the management of chronic low back pain: A randomized double-blind trial. Spine (Phila Pa 1976) 33:1291-1297; discussion 1298, 2008.

124. Husted DS, Orton D, Schofferman J, et al: Effectiveness of repeated radiofrequency neurotomy for cervical facet joint pain. J Spinal Disord Tech 21:406-408, 2008.

125. Schofferman J, Kine G: Effectiveness of repeated radiofrequency neurotomy for lumbar facet pain. Spine (Phila Pa 1976) 29:2471-2473, 2004.

126. Hadden SB: Neurologic headache and facial pain. Arch Neurol 43:405, 1940.

127. Macnab I: The whiplash syndrome. Clin Neurosurg 20:232-241, 1973.

128. Bogduk N, Marsland A: On the concept of third occipital headache. J Neurol Neurosurg Psychiatry 49:775-780, 1986.

129. Dreyfuss P, Michaelsen M, Fletcher D: Atlanto-occipital and lateral atlanto-axial joint pain patterns. Spine (Phila Pa 1976) 19:1125-1131, 1994.

130. Dreyfuss P, Rogers J, Dreyer S, et al: Atlanto-occipital joint pain: A report of three cases and description of an intraarticular joint block technique. Reg Anesth 19:344-351, 1994.

131. Bogduk N, Marsland A: The cervical zygapophysial joints as a source of neck pain. Spine (Phila Pa 1976) 13:610-617, 1988.

132. Bogduk N, Aprill C: On the nature of neck pain, discography and cervical zygapophysial joint blocks. Pain 54:213-217, 1993.

133. Cooper G, Bailey B, Bogduk N: Cervical zygapophysial joint pain maps. Pain Med 8:344-353, 2007.

134. Barnsley L, Lord SM, Wallis BJ, et al: The prevalence of chronic cervical zygapophysial joint pain after whiplash. Spine (Phila Pa 1976) 20:20-25; discussion 26, 1995.

135. Lord SM, Barnsley L, Wallis BJ, et al: Chronic cervical zygapophysial joint pain after whiplash: A placebo-controlled prevalence study. Spine (Phila Pa 1976) 21:1737-1744; discussion 1744, 1996.

136. Aprill C, Axinn MJ, Bogduk N: Occipital headaches stemming from the lateral atlanto-axial (C1-2) joint. Cephalalgia 22:15-22, 2002.

137. Barnsley L, Lord S, Wallis B, et al: False-positive rates of cervical zygapophysial joint blocks. Clin J Pain 9:124-130, 1993.

138. Speldewinde GC, Bashford GM, Davidson IR: Diagnostic cervical zygapophyseal joint blocks for chronic cervical pain. Med J Aust 174:174-176, 2001.

139. Manchikanti L, Singh V, Rivera J, et al: Prevalence of cervical facet joint pain in chronic neck pain. Pain Physician 5:243-249, 2002.

139a. Yin W, Bogduk N: The nature of neck pain in a private pain clinic in the United States. Pain Med 9:196-203, 2008.

140. Kirpalani D, Mitra R: Cervical facet joint dysfunction: A review. Arch Phys Med Rehabil 89:770-774, 2008.

141. Jull G, Bogduk N, Marsland A: The accuracy of manual diagnosis for cervical zygapophysial joint pain syndromes. Med J Aust 148:233-236, 1988.

142. Hechelhammer L, Pfirrmann CW, Zanetti M, et al: Imaging findings predicting the outcome of cervical facet joint blocks. Eur Radiol 17:959-964, 2007.

143. Manchikanti L, Pampati V: Research designs in interventional pain management: Is randomization superior, desirable or essential? Pain Physician 5:275-284, 2002.

144. Stolker RJ, Vervest AC, Groen GJ: Percutaneous facet denervation in chronic thoracic spinal pain. Acta Neurochir 122:82-90, 1993.

145. Linton SJ, Hellsing AL, Halldan K: A population-based study of spinal pain among 35-45-year-old individuals: Prevalence, sick leave, and health care use. Spine (Phila Pa 1976) 23:1457-1463, 1998.

146. Dreyfuss P, Tibiletti C, Dreyer SJ: Thoracic zygapophyseal joint pain patterns: A study in normal volunteers. Spine (Phila Pa 1976) 19:807-811, 1994.

147. Fukui S, Ohseto K, Shiotani M: Patterns of pain induced by distending the thoracic zygapophyseal joints. Reg Anesth 22:332-336, 1997.

148. Chua WH, Bogduk N: The surgical anatomy of thoracic facet denervation. Acta Neurochir (Wien) 136:140-144, 1995.

149. Dreyfuss P, Tibiletti C, Dreyer S, et al: Thoracic zygapophyseal joint pain: A review and description of an intra-articular block technique. Pain Digest 4:46-54, 1994.

150. Manchikanti L, Boswell MV, Singh V, et al: Prevalence of facet joint pain in chronic spinal pain of cervical, thoracic and lumbar regions. BMC Musculoskelet Disord 5:15, 2004.

151. Manchikanti L, Singh V, Pampati V, et al: Evaluation of the prevalence of facet joint pain in chronic thoracic pain. Pain Physician 5:354-359, 2002.

152. Manchukonda R, Manchikanti KN, Cash KA, et al: Facet joint pain in chronic spinal pain: An evaluation of prevalence and false-positive rate of diagnostic blocks. J Spinal Disord Tech 20:539-545, 2007.

153. Manchikanti L, Manchikanti KN, Manchukonda R, et al: Evaluation of therapeutic thoracic medial branch block effectiveness in chronic thoracic pain: A prospective outcome study with minimum 1-year follow-up. Pain Physician 9:97-105, 2006.

154. Manchikanti L, Singh V, Falco FJ, et al: Effectiveness of thoracic medial branch blocks in managing chronic pain: A preliminary report of a randomized, double-blind controlled trial: Clinical Trial NCT00355706. Pain Physician 11:491-504, 2008.

155. Cook NJ, Hanrahan P, Song S: Paraspinal abscess following facet joint injection. Clin Rheumatol 18:52-53, 1999.

156. Coscia MF, Trammell TR: Pyogenic lumbar facet joint arthritis with intradural extension: A case report. J Spinal Disord Tech 15:526-528, 2002.

157. Arun R, Al-Nammari SS, Mehdian SM: Multilevel vertebral osteomyelitis and facet joint infection following epidural catheterisation. Acta Orthop Belg 73:665-669, 2007.

158. Alcock E, Regaard A, Browne J: Facet joint injection: A rare form cause of epidural abscess formation. Pain 103:209-210, 2003.

159. Heckmann JG, Maihafner C, Lanz S, et al: Transient tetraplegia after cervical facet joint injection for chronic neck pain administered without imaging guidance. Clin Neurol Neurosurg 108:709-711, 2006.

160. Dreyfuss P, Dreyer SJ, Cole A, et al: Sacroiliac joint pain. J Am Acad Orthop Surg 12:255-265, 2004.

161. Cheng MB, Ferrante FM: Health-related quality of life in sacroiliac syndrome: A comparison to lumbosacral radiculopathy. Reg Anesth Pain Med 31:422-427, 2006.

162. Rupert MP, Lee M, Manchikanti L, et al: Evaluation of sacroiliac joint interventions: A systematic appraisal of the literature. Pain Physician 12:399-418, 2009.

163. Irwin RW, Watson T, Minick RP, et al: Age, body mass index, and gender differences in sacroiliac joint pathology. Am J Phys Med Rehabil 86:37-44, 2007.

164. Laslett M, April CN, McDonald B, et al: Diagnosis of sacroiliac joint pain: Validity of individual provocation tests and composites of tests. Manual Ther 10:207-218, 2005.

165. Laslett M, Young SB, April CN, et al: Diagnosing painful sacroiliac joints: A validity study of a McKenzie evaluation and sacroiliac provocation tests. Aust J Physiother 49:89-97, 2003.

166. Manchikanti L, Singh V, Pampati V, et al: Evaluation of the relative contributions of various structures in chronic low back pain. Pain Physician 4:308-316, 2001.

167. van der Wurff P, Buijs EJ, Groen GJ: A multitest regimen of pain provocation tests as an aid to reduce unnecessary minimally invasive sacroiliac joint procedures. Arch Phys Med Rehabil 87:10-14, 2006.

168. Bowen V, Cassidy JD: Macroscopic and microscopic anatomy of the sacroiliac joint from embryonic life until the eighth decade. Spine (Phila Pa 1976) 6:620-628, 1981.

169. Simonian PT, Routt ML Jr, Harrington RM, et al: Anterior versus posterior provisional fixation in the unstable pelvis: A biomechanical comparison. Clin Orthop Relat Res (310): 245-251, 1995.

170. Rosatelli AL, Agur AM, Chhaya S: Anatomy of the interosseous region of the sacroiliac joint. J Orthop Sports Phys Ther 36:200-208, 2006.

171. Nakagawa T: [Study on the distribution of nerve filaments over the iliosacral joint and its adjacent region in the Japanese]. Nippon Seikeigeka Gakkai Zasshi 40:419-430, 1966.

172. Yin W, Willard F, Carreiro J, et al: Sensory stimulation-guided sacroiliac joint radiofrequency neurotomy: Technique based on neuroanatomy of the dorsal sacral plexus. Spine (Phila Pa 1976) 28:2419-2425, 2003.

173. Willard F: S1-S4 dorsal rami and divisions. Presented at Third World Conference on Low Back and Pelvic Pain, Vienna, Austria, 1998.

174. Grob KR, Neuhuber WL, Kissling RO: [Innervation of the sacroiliac joint of the human]. Z Rheumatol 54:117-122, 1995.

174a. Berthelot JM, Labat JJ, Le Gorff B, et al: Provocative sacroiliac joint maneuvers and sacroiliac joint block are unreliable for diagnosing sacroiliac joint pain. Joint Bone Spine 73:17-23, 2006.

175. Dorman T, Ravin T: Diagnosis and Injection Techniques in Orthopedic Medicine. Baltimore, Williams & Wilkins, 1999.

176. Szadek KM, Hoogland PV, Zuurmond WW, et al: Nociceptive nerve fibers in the sacroiliac joint in humans. Reg Anesth Pain Med 33:36-43, 2008.

177. Murakami E, Tanaka Y, Aizawa T, et al: Effect of periarticular and intraarticular lidocaine injections for sacroiliac joint pain: Prospective comparative study. J Orthop Sci 12:274-280, 2007.

178. Weksler N, Velan GJ, Semionov M, et al: The role of sacroiliac joint dysfunction in the genesis of low back pain: The obvious is not always right. Arch Orthop Trauma Surg 127:885-888, 2007.

179. Frymoyer JW, Howe J, Kuhlmann D: The longterm effects of fusion on the sacroiliac joints and ilium. Clin Orthop Relat Res 134:196-201, 1978.

180. Ha KY, Lee JS, Kim KW: Degeneration of sacroiliac joint after instrumented lumbar or lumbosacral fusion: A prospective cohort study over five-year follow-up. Spine (Phila Pa 1976) 33:1192-1198, 2008.

181. Ivanov AA, Kiapour A, Ebraheim NA, et al: Lumbar fusion leads to increases in angular motion and stress across sacroiliac joint: A finite element study. Spine (Phila Pa 1976) 34:E162-E169, 2009.

182. Pool-Goudzwaard A, Hoek van Dijke G, Mulder P, et al: The iliolumbar ligament: Its influence on stability of the sacroiliac joint. Clin Biomech (Bristol, Avon) 18:99-105, 2003.

183. Ebraheim NA, Elgafy H, Semaan HB: Computed tomographic findings in patients with persistent sacroiliac pain after posterior iliac graft harvesting. Spine (Phila Pa 1976) 25:2047-2051, 2000.

184. Maigne JY, Planchon CA: Sacroiliac joint pain after lumbar fusion: A study with anesthetic blocks. Eur Spine J 14:654-658, 2005.

185. Katz V, Schofferman J, Reynolds J: The sacroiliac joint: A potential cause of pain after lumbar fusion to the sacrum. J Spinal Disord Tech 16:96-99, 2003.

186. Dreyfuss P, Michaelsen M, Pauza K, et al: The value of medical history and physical examination in diagnosing sacroiliac joint pain. Spine (Phila Pa 1976) 21:2594-2602, 1996.

187. Maigne JY, Aivaliklis A, Pfefer F: Results of sacroiliac joint double block and value of sacroiliac pain provocation tests in 54 patients with low back pain. Spine (Phila Pa 1976) 21:1889-1892, 1996.

188. Young S, Aprill C, Laslett M: Correlation of clinical examination characteristics with three sources of chronic low back pain. Spine J 3:460-465, 2003.

189. Laslett M: Evidence-based diagnosis and treatment of the painful sacroiliac joint. J Man Manip Ther 16:142-152, 2008.

190. Slipman CW, Sterenfeld EB, Chou LH, et al: The predictive value of provocative sacroiliac joint stress maneuvers in the diagnosis of sacroiliac joint syndrome. Arch Phys Med Rehabil 79:288-292, 1998.

191. Schwarzer AC, Aprill CN, Bogduk N: The sacroiliac joint in chronic low back pain. Spine (Phila Pa 1976) 20:31-37, 1995.

192. Slipman CW, Jackson HB, Lipetz JS, et al: Sacroiliac joint pain referral zones. Arch Phys Med Rehabil 81:334-338, 2000.

193. Dreyfuss P, Snyder BD, Park K, et al: The ability of single site, single depth sacral lateral branch blocks to anesthetize the sacroiliac joint complex. Pain Med 9:844-850, 2008.

194. Fortin JD, Dwyer AP, West S, et al: Sacroiliac joint: Pain referral maps upon applying a new injection/arthrography technique. Part I: Asymptomatic volunteers. Spine (Phila Pa 1976) 19:1475-1482, 1994.

195. Murakami E, Aizawa T, Noguchi K, et al: Diagram specific to sacroiliac joint pain site indicated by one-finger test. J Orthop Sci 13:492-497, 2008.

196. Berthelot J-M, Labat J-J, Le Goff BT, et al: Provocative sacroiliac joint maneuvers and sacroiliac joint block are unreliable for diagnosing sacroiliac joint pain. Joint Bone Spine 73:17-23, 2006.

197. Hansen HC, McKenzie-Brown AM, Cohen SP, et al: Sacroiliac joint interventions: A systematic review. Pain Physician 10:165-184, 2007.

198. Szadek KM, van der Wurff P, van Tulder MW, et al: Diagnostic validity of criteria for sacroiliac joint pain: A systematic review. J Pain 10:354-368, 2009.

199. Hodge JC, Bessette B: The incidence of sacroiliac joint disease in patients with low-back pain. Can Assoc Radiol J 50:321-323, 1999.

200. Elgafy H, Semaan HB, Ebraheim NA, et al: Computed tomography findings in patients with sacroiliac pain. Clin Orthop Relat Res (382):112-118, 2001.

201. Kacar G, Kacar C, Karayalcin B, et al: Quantitative sacroiliac joint scintigraphy in normal subjects and patients with sacroiliitis. Ann Nucl Med 12:169-173, 1998.

202. Slipman CW, Sterenfeld EB, Chou LH, et al: The value of radionuclide imaging in the diagnosis of sacroiliac joint syndrome. Spine (Phila Pa 1976) 21:2251-2254, 1996.

203. Maigne JY, Boulahdour H, Chatellier G: Value of quantitative radionuclide bone scanning in the diagnosis of sacroiliac joint syndrome in 32 patients with low back pain. Eur Spine J 7:328-331, 1998.

204. Rosenberg JM, Quint TJ, de Rosayro AM: Computerized tomographic localization of clinically-guided sacroiliac joint injections. Clin J Pain 16:18-21, 2000.

205. Borowsky CD, Fagen G: Sources of sacroiliac region pain: Insights gained from a study comparing standard intra-articular injection with a technique combining intra- and peri-articular injection. Arch Phys Med Rehabil 89:2048-2056, 2008.

206. Fortin JD, Washington WJ, Falco FJ: Three pathways between the sacroiliac joint and neural structures. AJNR Am J Neuroradiol 20:1429-1434, 1999.

207. Wise CL, Dall BE: Minimally invasive sacroiliac arthrodesis: Outcomes of a new technique. J Spinal Disord Tech 21:579-584, 2008.

208. Schutz U, Grob D: Poor outcome following bilateral sacroiliac joint fusion for degenerative sacroiliac joint syndrome. Acta Orthop Belg 72:296-308, 2006.

209. Al-Khayer A, Hegarty J, Hahn D, et al: Percutaneous sacroiliac joint arthrodesis: A novel technique. J Spinal Disord Tech 21:359-363, 2008.

210. Ziran BH, Heckman D, Smith WR: CT-guided stabilization for chronic sacroiliac pain: A preliminary report. J Trauma 63:90-96, 2007.

211. Cohen SP, Hurley RW, Buckenmaier CC 3rd, et al: Randomized placebo-controlled study evaluating lateral branch radiofrequency denervation for sacroiliac joint pain. Anesthesiology 109:279-288, 2008.

212. Laslett M: Evidence-based diagnosis and treatment of the painful sacroiliac joint. J Man Manip Ther 16:142-152, 2008.

213. Cohen SP, Abdi S: Lateral branch blocks as a treatment for sacroiliac joint pain: A pilot study. Reg Anesth Pain Med 28:113-119, 2003.

214. Benzel EC, Hart BL, Ball PA, et al: Magnetic resonance imaging for the evaluation of patients with occult cervical spine injury. J Neurosurg 85:824-829, 1996.

215. Lehto IJ, Tertti MO, Komu ME, et al: Age-related MRI changes at 0.1 T in cervical discs in asymptomatic subjects. Neuroradiology 36:49-53, 1994.

216. Siivola SM, Levoska S, Tervonen O, et al: MRI changes of cervical spine in asymptomatic and symptomatic young adults. Eur Spine J 11:358-363, 2002.

217. Anderberg L, Annertz M, Brandt L, et al: Selective diagnostic cervical nerve root block—correlation with clinical symptoms and MRI-pathology. Acta Neurochir (Wien) 146:559-565; discussion 565, 2004.

218. Slipman CW, Plastaras CT, Palmitier RA, et al: Symptom provocation of fluoroscopically guided cervical nerve root stimulation: Are dynatomal maps identical to dermatomal maps? Spine (Phila Pa 1976) 23:2235-2242, 1998.

219. Kikuchi S, Hasue M, Nishiyama K, et al: Anatomic and clinical studies of radicular symptoms. Spine (Phila Pa 1976) 9:23-30, 1984.

220. Yeom JS, Lee JW, Park KW, et al: Value of diagnostic lumbar selective nerve root block: A prospective controlled study. AJNR Am J Neuroradiol 29:1017-1023, 2008.

221. van Akkerveeken PF: The diagnostic value of nerve root sheath infiltration. Acta Orthop Scand Suppl 251:61-63, 1993.

222. Sasso RC, Macadaeg K, Nordmann D, et al: Selective nerve root injections can predict surgical outcome for lumbar and cervical radiculopathy: Comparison to magnetic resonance imaging. J Spinal Disord Tech 18:471-478, 2005.

223. Dooley JF, McBroom RJ, Taguchi T, et al: Nerve root infiltration in the diagnosis of radicular pain. Spine (Phila Pa 1976) 13:79-83, 1988.

224. Furman MB, Lee TS, Mehta A, et al: Contrast flow selectivity during transforaminal lumbosacral epidural steroid injections. Pain Physician 11:855-861, 2008.

225. Jonsson B, Stromqvist B, Annertz M, et al: Diagnostic lumbar nerve root block. J Spinal Disord 1:232-235, 1988.

226. Macnab I: Negative disc exploration: An analysis of the causes of nerve-root involvement in sixty-eight patients. J Bone Joint Surg Am 53:891-903, 1971.

227. Krempen JF, Smith BS: Nerve-root injection: A method for evaluating the etiology of sciatica. J Bone Joint Surg Am 56:1435-1444, 1974.

228. Schutz H, Lougheed WM, Wortzman G, et al: Intervertebral nerve-root in the investigation of chronic lumbar disc disease. Can J Surg 16:217-221, 1973.

229. Tajima T, Furukawa K, Kuramochi E: Selective lumbosacral radiculography and block. Spine (Phila Pa 1976) 5:68-77, 1980.

230. Stanley D, McLaren MI, Euinton HA, et al: A prospective study of nerve root infiltration in the diagnosis of sciatica: A comparison with radiculography, computed tomography, and operative findings. Spine (Phila Pa 1976) 15:540-543, 1990.

231. Herron LD: Selective nerve root block in patient selection for lumbar surgery: Surgical results. J Spinal Disord 2:75-79, 1989.

232. Porter DG, Valentine AR, Bradford R: A retrospective study to assess the results of CT-directed peri-neural root infiltration in a cohort of 56 patients with low back pain and sciatica. Br J Neurosurg 13:290-293, 1999.

233. Haueisen DC, Smith BS, Myers SR, et al: The diagnostic accuracy of spinal nerve injection studies: Their role in the evaluation of recurrent sciatica. Clin Orthop Relat Res (198):179-183, 1985.

234. Kumar K, Taylor RS, Jacques L, et al: Spinal cord stimulation versus conventional medical management for neuropathic pain: A multicentre randomised controlled trial in patients with failed back surgery syndrome. Pain 132:179-188, 2007.

235. White AH, Derby R, Wynne G: Epidural injections for the diagnosis and treatment of low-back pain. Spine (Phila Pa 1976) 5:78-86, 1980.

236. Jasper JF: Role of digital subtraction fluoroscopic imaging in detecting intravascular injections. Pain Physician 6:369-372, 2003.

237. Baker R, Dreyfuss P, Mercer S, et al: Cervical transforaminal injection of corticosteroids into a radicular artery: A possible mechanism for spinal cord injury. Pain 103:211-215, 2003.

238. North RB, Kidd DH, Campbell JN, et al: Dorsal root ganglionectomy for failed back surgery syndrome: A 5-year follow-up study. J Neurosurg 74:236-242, 1991.

239. Derby R, Lee SH, Kim BJ, et al: Complications following cervical epidural steroid injections by expert interventionalists in 2003. Pain Physician 7:445-449, 2004.

240. Pobiel RS, Schellhas KP, Eklund JA, et al: Selective cervical nerve root blockade: Prospective study of immediate and longer term complications. AJNR Am J Neuroradiol 30:507-511, 2009.

241. Huston CW, Slipman CW, Garvin C: Complications and side effects of cervical and lumbosacral selective nerve root injections. Arch Phys Med Rehabil 86:277-283, 2005.

242. Scanlon GC, Moeller-Bertram T, Romanowsky SM, et al: Cervical transforaminal epidural steroid injections: More dangerous than we think? Spine (Phila Pa 1976) 32:1249-1256, 2007.

243. Provenzano DA, Fanciullo G: Cervical transforaminal epidural steroid injections: Should we be performing them? Reg Anesth Pain Med 32:168; author reply 169-170, 2007.

244. Lee JH, Lee JK, Seo BR, et al: Spinal cord injury produced by direct damage during cervical transforaminal epidural injection. Reg Anesth Pain Med 33:377-379, 2008.

245. Ruppen W, Hugli R, Reuss S, et al: Neurological symptoms after cervical transforaminal injection with steroids in a patient with hypoplasia of the vertebral artery. Acta Anaesthesiol Scand 52:165-166, 2008.

246. Muro K, O'Shaughnessy B, Ganju A: Infarction of the cervical spinal cord following multilevel transforaminal epidural steroid injection: Case report and review of the literature. J Spinal Cord Med 30:385-388, 2007.

247. Suresh S, Berman J, Connell DA: Cerebellar and brainstem infarction as a complication of CT-guided transforaminal cervical nerve root block. Skeletal Radiol 36:449-452, 2007.

248. Tiso RL, Cutler T, Catania JA, et al: Adverse central nervous system sequelae after selective transforaminal block: The role of corticosteroids. Spine J 4:468-474, 2004.

249. Derby R, Lee SH, Date ES, et al: Size and aggregation of corticosteroids used for epidural injections. Pain Med 9:227-234, 2008.

250. Hooten WM, Mizerak A, Carns PE, et al: Discitis after lumbar epidural corticosteroid injection: A case report and analysis of the case report literature. Pain Med 7:46-51, 2006.

Eugene Carragee, MD

Provocative discography is a diagnostic test sometimes used to evaluate the disc as a potential source of persistent back and neck pain syndromes. In its simplest form, provocative discography is an injection into the nucleus of an intervertebral disc, and the test result is determined by the pain response to this injection. If the injection reproduces the patient's usual pain, some authors have proposed that the "cause" of the axial pain syndrome can be ascribed to that disc—that is, *primary discogenic pain.*

In 1948, Lindblom[1] originally reported discography as a method to identify herniated discs in the lumbar spine by injecting contrast medium into the disc and following the outline of contrast medium into the spinal canal. It was noted as only a secondary consideration of the test that reproduction of the patient's usual sciatica sometimes occurred during the disc injection. It was observed later that back pain was sometimes reproduced during the injection, as opposed to sciatica. Eventually some clinicians began using the test to evaluate discs as the source of axial pain in patients without radicular symptoms.

Since the early use of discography, it has been unclear whether reproduction of pain with injection indicated that the injected disc is the true primary source of clinical back pain, or whether the injection had simulated the usual pain in an artificial manner. Over time, attempts have been made to determine the specificity of the test and to refine the technique to reduce the risk of false-positive or false-negative results. Still this test remains highly controversial. Even the staunchest proponents of the procedure state that "discography is a test that is easily abused."[2] Basic diagnostic test assessment has found fundamental problems with test reliability (i.e., does the test give the same result on repeated testing?) and validity (i.e., does the test prove what it purports to prove?). Also, it has not been shown that using the test improves the outcomes in patients receiving the test compared with patients not receiving the test. More recently, the long-term safety of disc puncture and injection has also been questioned. This chapter discusses the rationale and technique of provocative discography when used in patients with primary axial pain syndromes.

Clinical Context

Back and neck pain are very common, and in most cases determining the "cause" of a specific episode of back or neck pain is unimportant because these symptoms frequently resolve in a short time or do not seriously interfere with function.[1] Provocative discography may be described as representing a *tertiary diagnostic* evaluation, which should be considered only in a select group of patients.

A *primary diagnostic* evaluation usually involves screening for serious underlying disease ("red flags") by history and physical examination aimed at detecting systemic disease, spinal deformity, and neurologic loss. In most patients, these examinations are negative, and nonspecific treatment alone is recommended.

In a patient who does not recover good function in 6 to 12 weeks, a *secondary diagnostic* survey may be indicated. This follow-up evaluation should identify serious psychosocial barriers to recovery ("yellow flags") and definitively "rule out" serious conditions that may result in neurologic injury; structural failure; or progression of a visceral disease, systemic infection, or malignant process. Diagnostic tests for serious structural disease, including blood tests and imaging studies, have become so sensitive that these serious conditions are usually identified in the early stages.

Establishing a more specific pathoanatomic diagnosis than "nonspecific back pain syndrome" or "persistent back pain illness" becomes important only if specific therapy directed to common age-related structural changes is considered because of continued serious symptoms and functional loss. At this point, if the primary and secondary evaluations have revealed neither serious structural pathology nor significant confounding psychosocial or neurophysiologic factors, a tertiary diagnostic evaluation may be undertaken. This evaluation may occasionally uncover a clear degenerative cause of symptoms, such as unstable spondylolisthesis or progressive degenerative deformity such as an unstable degenerative scoliosis.

The most common structural degenerative changes (e.g., loss of disc height, loss of nuclear signal, minor facet arthrosis, annular fissures) may be very difficult to reconcile with the severity of apparent symptoms and pain behavior, however, because many people with minimal or no spinal symptoms have similar mild degenerative findings. The question is why do individuals with such benign findings sometimes report severe and persistent pain and impairment? The rationale of provocative discography in the tertiary evaluation is to separate anatomic spinal changes causing serious primary pain illnesses from similarly appearing common degenerative changes that do not cause serious illness. As this chapter shows, it is unclear that this goal is routinely achievable with provocative discography.

Discography Technique

Discography is performed using local anesthetic and mild sedation. The objective is percutaneous injection of a nonirritating radiopaque dye, under fluoroscopic guidance, into one or more intervertebral discs. Ideally, the central portion of the disc, the nucleus, is penetrated by a long fine-gauge needle; this is usually done from a posterolateral approach in the thoracolumbar spine and anterolaterally in the cervical spine. In the lumbar spine, the needle passes posterior to the exiting nerve root and anterolateral to the traversing root. Sometimes a bend of the needle or introducer is required to place the needle accurately, especially at L5-S1.

The passage of the needle in skilled hands should be quick and atraumatic. When the position is verified in two planes using fluoroscopy, the dye is slowly injected into the nucleus of several lumbar discs with the patient blinded to the timing and site of injection. The spread of the dye in the disc is noted on the images, and the patient's response to injection is documented. The patient is queried at each injection, or at random intervals, whether or not the procedure is painful and is asked to rate the pain against some standardized scale (e.g., 0-5, 0-10, none-to-unbearable). If the injection is painful, the patient is asked to describe the discomfort provoked qualitatively: The injection is usually rated as exactly the same as, or similar to (concordant), or dissimilar to the patient's usual back or neck pain.

Criteria for Positive Test

In an effort to improve the specificity of discography in diagnosing so-called discogenic pain, some investigators have used additional criteria beyond pain reproduction on injection. The criteria for establishing a positive discogram are controversial. The primary criteria for a "positive" disc injection are pain of "significant" intensity on disc injections (usually defined as ≥6 out of 10 pain scale) and a reported similarity of that pain to the patient's usual, clinical discomfort (concordant pain). These basic criteria were proposed in the experimental work by Walsh and colleagues in 1990,[29] which proposed "significant pain" be defined as 3 out of 5 (or 6 out of 10) on an arbitrary pain thermometer. "Bad pain" was

defined as 3 out of 5 pain, and "moderate pain" was described as 2 out of 5 pain. The authors did not stringently define concordance of pain reproduction. Some investigators have proposed additional and sometimes idiosyncratic criteria for positive injections (Table 16–1).

Pain Generator Concept and Provocative Discography

The diagnosis made by a "positive provocative discogram" should indicate that the disc identified is the primary or only cause of the patient's back pain illness, or the *pain generator*. This term has proven problematic, however. In a patient with persistent symptoms and a secondary workup with only degenerative findings, the task of identifying a specific isolated pain generator may be formidable. Most patients have multiple findings of disc changes and facet arthrosis, often at different levels. To distinguish which, if any, "degenerative" findings may be definitively established as causing severe back pain illness is a complex problem. Many people have occasional back or neck ache with common activities or episodic axial pain without impairment. The question is not whether any previous or possible future back or neck pain may be coming from a certain spinal structure. Rather, it may be assumed that most people with degenerative change of the axial skeleton may have occasional discomfort from several sites alone or at the same time.

The pertinent question is whether or not a suspected local anatomic structure (e.g., disc, facet, sacroiliac joint) is causing serious, disabling axial pain illness or is only a minor contributor to a generalized pain-sensitivity syndrome (e.g., fibromyalgia), a central pain-processing syndrome, an overuse syndrome related to posture or activity, or other conditions. It is hoped that some diagnostic test can identify whether or not a specific *local* spinal pathoanatomic structure adequately explains the severity of clinical symptoms. As a matter of practical definition, for a pathoanatomic diagnosis to be *clinically relevant* requires that the identified *pain generator* not only be capable of causing some discomfort under any circumstances (e.g., puncture and injection of a disc), but also that this structure is a primary independent cause of the patient's apparent severe illness.

When only degenerative changes are found, it is controversial whether or not a discrete local pain generator as the cause of serious back pain illness can be commonly identified. Some clinicians believe that serious axial pain and disability can be so multifactorial (mechanical, psychological, social, and neurophysiologic contributors) that it is unreasonable to expect specific diagnostic studies to confirm an anatomic "diagnosis" for axial pain illness in every patient.[3-5] Even if a pain generator is suspected, it is unclear how this can be reliably confirmed to be the cause of the patient's perceived pain, impairment, and disability in the face of complex social, emotional, and neurophysiologic confounders.

Other clinicians believe that identifying a pain generator is central to spine evaluations, is an expectation of patients, and

TABLE 16–1 Suggested Criteria for Positive Provocative Discographic Injection

Test Criteria for Positive Result	Positive Test Threshold	Comments
Pain response (intensity)	≥6/10 or 3/5	Subjective and arbitrary scale. No data on reliability. Data on validity in small groups of asymptomatic subjects without psychosocial comorbidity are good (specificity >90%). Data in several studies of subjects with increased psychosocial or chronic pain comorbidity indicate validity in these subgroups is poor (specificity 20%-60%)
	"Bad" pain or worse on pain thermometer ≥7/10	
Qualitative pain assessment (concordant pain)	"Concordant pain" usually including "similar" but not exact pain	Subjective response. Data on reliability are unknown. Data on validity in small study of experimental nondiscogenic low back pain indicate validity is questionable
	"Exact" pain only	
Annular disruption	Dye must show fissure to or through outer anulus	Tested only in clinical studies without follow-up to confirm outcome or other "gold standard." Radiologic reliability best with computed tomography scan after disc injection compared with x-ray alone. Validity of additional criteria as confirming true-positive test unknown; positive injection in discs without annular disruption more common in psychologically disturbed subjects
Control disc injections	"Negative" injection (minimal or discordant pain) required adjacent to proposed "positive" disc	Injections in morphologically normal discs seem to be reliably negative even in subjects with serious psychological distress and no back pain. Reliability in other disc morphology unknown. Validity of this additional criterion as confirming true-positive test unknown
	"Normal" injection (i.e., no pain) Some authors insist that adjacent "control disc" must also have grade 3 annular fissure, which is "relatively painless" at equal or higher pressures than "positive disc"	
Demonstration of pain behavior	Facial expressions of pain must be observed to confirm verbal pain report	Reliability and validity of this criterion as confirming true-positive test unknown
Pressure-controlled injection	Disc injections should be classified into low (<15 psi or <20 psi) or high (>50 psi) pressures at time of significant pain response; responses at pressures in between are indeterminate	Small outcomes series suggest low pressure sensitive discs are better treated with interbody fusion techniques. Reliability and validity unknown
Volume-controlled injections	"Excessive volume" or speed to injection invalidated injection	Unvalidated concept based on anecdotal evidence. Primary data unavailable to analyze
Maximum one or two positive disc injections	More than one or two positive disc injections invalidates study (all are indeterminate)	Assumption is made that generalized hyperalgesic effect may lead to multiple positive discs around single pain generator
Quantify pain tolerance by response to buffered anesthetic injection	Subjects with poor pain tolerance may not be "ideal" candidates for discography; this feature needs to be detected	It is unclear that pain tolerance to intradermal anesthetic injection is valid test to determine "pain tolerance" in patients with long-standing axial pain
Needles should be inserted from asymptomatic or least symptomatic side	Theoretically this may decrease confusion between injection and insertion pain	Some data suggest this is not an important technique. No "gold standard" confirmation was applied
Any positive disc injection must be repeated with similar outcomes before accepting result as "positive"	Intraprocedure reliability test	No data available on whether this improved or decreased test accuracy

determines the choice of treatments by focusing on the anatomic structure deemed responsible for the pain. In this model, social issues such as disability, litigation, psychological distress, and pain intolerance are believed to be *secondary* issues to the structural pathology.[1,6-12] These clinicians generally believe that although the history and physical examination may be helpful in suggesting serious underlying pathology such as infection and tumor, these methods are not helpful in determining the true pain generator among many degenerative structures.

Diagnostic Injections and Modulation of Pain Perception in Axial Pain Syndromes

Provocative discography relies on a patient's subjective perception and report of pain after a progressive pressurization injection of a disc. Alternatively, a disc may be injected with an anesthetic agent with subsequent documentation of the patient's subjective pain relief after activities that usually provoke pain. These diagnostic injections seek to identify a primary pain generator by provocative testing (stimulating a potential site of pain as in discography) or by temporary local anesthetic relief. These are subjective tests of pain perception and are subject to the effects of volitional and neurophysiologic modulation at multiple points along the neuraxis.

Many common factors are known to have potential dampening or amplifying effects on the perception of back and neck pain. These factors must be considered when evaluating the validity of diagnoses determined by diagnostic injections.[13-18]

Adjacent Tissue Injury

Injury to adjacent tissues may increase the perception of pain in surrounding structures by a local *hyperalgesic effect*. This is a well-known phenomenon that occurs with any tissue damage; it may amplify pain perception by increasing local inflammatory processes with secondary neurologic sensitization in areas not directly injured, such as the area surrounding a burn or a fracture that is sensitive but without any thermal or mechanical injury. This is an important phenomenon in patients with low back pain with serious disease at one or more levels, which may sensitize the adjacent segments to provocative testing (e.g., a spine that has undergone multiple operations).[13,19]

Local Anesthetic

Local anesthetic injections may decrease the perception of pain at a local site. This is the specific, active effect used in diagnostic blocks. This decrease in pain perception can also be a source of confounding effects if the exact placement of the agent is not well controlled. In addition to this direct local effect, a nonspecific placebo effect and a neurophysiologic modulation effect may occur. A relevant example is the effect of local anesthetic blockade on the perception of painful stimulus along the neuraxis proximal to the injection. A local anesthetic injection in the lower extremity may be perceived as relieving sciatica owing to disc herniation.[20] This is not a placebo effect (i.e., the phenomenon is seen only with an active anesthetic agent) but rather an effect on neuromodulation. This effect is important in diagnostic anesthetic blockade as a source of false-positive and false-negative findings.[21]

Tissue Injury and Nociception in Adjacent or Same Sclerotome

Tissue injury having the same or adjacent sclerotomal afferents as lower spinal elements may increase pain sensitivity at any given site. This effect is thought to be due to physiologic and anatomic changes at the level of the dorsal root ganglion or spinal cord ascending tracts. In animal models, single afferent neurons from a dorsal root ganglion may innervate three adjacent discs and a wide range of adjacent structures. This effect is important in considering the specificity of discography at sites of similar embryonic derivation to a known pathologic structure (e.g., nonunion, spondylolisthesis, painful iliac crest bone graft site). The confounding effect of this phenomenon in discography has been experimentally and empirically shown (see later).[13,22]

Chronic Pain Syndromes

Chronic pain syndromes may complicate the evaluation of low back pain syndromes. Chronic pain from regional sites near the lumbar spine (chronic pelvic pain, irritable bowel syndrome, failed hip arthroplasty) or distant to the lumbar spine (chronic neck pain, chronic headache, temporomandibular joint syndrome) may increase pain sensitivity at lower spinal elements. This effect may be regional or global and may be related to neurophysiologic changes at multiple levels along the neuraxis. Preexisting chronic pain syndromes are also associated with depression, narcotic use, and habituation, which have independent pain perception effects. This effect has been shown to have an impact on the intensity of pain intensity from discography in experimental subjects.[13,22]

Narcotic Analgesia

Narcotic medications act at multiple levels to decrease pain sensitivity thresholds, intensity, and affective response. Administration of a narcotic medication may act as a common confounder of diagnostic techniques of any type requiring accurate feedback of pain perception from a patient.[13,23,24]

Narcotic Habituation

Chronic narcotic habituation may act to decrease pain tolerance in the absence of increased narcotic intake. Narcotic habituation decreases endogenous abilities to modulate peripheral nociceptive input. This effect is multifactorial. Chronic narcotic habituation is also associated with depression and sleep disturbances.

Depression, Anxiety, and Somatic Distress

Clinical depression, anxiety disorders, and increased somatic awareness may be seen as predisposing factors to chronic low back pain syndromes or reactions to the pain and disability of chronic low back pain illness or both. In either event, psychological distress usually decreases the pain threshold perception and increases perceived pain intensity and affective response.[5,23,25] These effects are likely due to central neurochemical changes and systemic effects and have been shown to affect pain responses in discographic evaluation.

Social Imperatives

Overriding social imperatives may result in a decreased pain perception or a dissociation of pain perception and functional loss. A decreased pain perception or even an absence of pain perception despite injury can be seen during some short-term stressful events, such as in accident victims, soldiers in combat, or individuals in certain training environments. Even over long periods, social and cultural factors reinforce low pain reporting and muted or absent pain behaviors.

Social Disincentive

Secondary gain issues may exaggerate pain responses of all types. When the intensity of pain behavior and report is correlated with a real or perceived social benefit or monetary compensation, the reported pain perception and pain behavior may be increased. This situation can have direct effects on provocative testing (e.g., discography) and the need for a specific anatomic diagnosis to establish social validity of an ongoing "sick role."

Summary

When considering the diagnostic certainty of a possible pain generator in chronic axial pain illness, it is necessary to view the aforementioned confounding factors for contribution to the illness behavior observed (Table 16–2). An injured soldier with facial trauma, after narcotic administration and in the heat of combat, may mask the perception of a significant low back pain injury, which otherwise could be clearly symptomatic. In this case, a bona fide local pain generator results in little pain perception. Conversely, a very minor nociceptive input (common backache) from a disc can be amplified in the case of a patient with multiple chronic pain syndromes, narcotic habituation, depression, and compensation issues (social disincentives). In this case, a common mild backache pain generator is amplified to become a catastrophic illness.

Evidence for Validity and Usefulness of Provocative Discography

The criteria for an evidence-based evaluation of the validity of diagnostic tests have been described by Sackett and Haynes.[26] Four phases of scientific scrutiny and evidence in discography research are shown in Table 16–3. These phases of evidence progress from the simple comparison of testing in subjects known to have a disease with subjects who are completely normal without any signs, symptoms, or morbidity associated with the disease (phase I) to the blinded study of a diagnostic test in determining outcomes in actual clinical therapeutic intervention (phase IV).

An example of a phase I diagnostic study is the classic study of discography by Walsh and colleagues[29] in asymptomatic healthy young men without significant degenerative disease or comorbidities associated with chronic low back pain illness (e.g., depression, chronic pain behavior, compensation issues). Discography seemed to perform well in this phase I study, with little pain provocation in the subjects known to have no evidence of disease (1 of 10 subjects [10%, 95% confidence interval 0, 40%] had pain intensity rated "bad"). Phase II and III studies, comparing subjects without low back pain illness but with significant comorbidities, were more problematical, however.[14,15]

Generally, there has been limited high-quality evidence supporting provocative disc injections. Despite the limited evidence, some authors believe that primary discogenic pain is the most common cause of chronic low back pain illness.[11,12,27,28] As is shown subsequently, a major constraint in this research has been a failure to use a bona fide "gold standard" for primary discogenic pain causing low back pain

TABLE 16–2 Neurophysiologic Factors Influencing Result of Diagnostic Injections

Modulator of Diagnostic Injection Effect	Type of Effect on Pain Perception at Site of Injection	Diagnostic Effect
Adjacent tissue injury	Increased regional pain perception	Decreased specificity in provocative injection
Local anesthetic	Decreased pain perception at depot site and sometimes in sclerotomal or referral pattern	Decreased specificity in provocative injection
Tissue injury in adjacent or same sclerotome	Increased regional pain perception	Decreased specificity in provocative injection
Chronic pain syndrome	Increased generalized pain perception	Decreased specificity in provocative injection
Narcotic analgesia	Decreased generalized pain perception and affective response	Decreased sensitivity and increased specificity of provocative injections
Narcotic habituation	Increased pain perception and exaggerated affective response	Decreased specificity in provocative injection
Depression, anxiety, and somatic distress	Decreased generalized pain perception and unpredictable affective response	Decreased specificity in provocative injection
Social imperatives	Decreased pain perception, suppressed affective response	Decreased sensitivity and increased specificity of provocative injections
Social disincentives	Specific increased pain reporting and demonstration of pain behavior	Decreased specificity in provocative injection

TABLE 16–3 Four Phases of Evidence-Based Criteria for Evaluation Diagnostic Tests

Phase of Study	Strategy	Discography Evidence
Phase 1	Diagnostic test compared in subjects with index disease vs. results in complete normals (experimental setting)	Few painful disc injections in completely normal asymptomatic subjects (e.g., normal psychometric testing, normal disc morphology, no chronic pain issues, no compensation issues) Phase 1 study examples: Walsh et al, 1990[29]; Carragee et al, 2000[15]
Phase 2	Evaluation of range of test results in subjects with disease (establishes positive result guidelines) compared with known normals	Wide range of pain reactions to injections in asymptomatic subjects depending on psychological status, disc morphology, chronic pain issues, compensation issues. Wide overlap between asymptomatic subjects and patients with presumed discogenic pain. Phase 2 study examples: Carragee et al, 2000[15]; O'Neill and Kurgansky, 2004[22]; Carragee et al, 2006[38]
Phase 3	Diagnostic test applied in clinical subjects likely to have disease (clinical setting of test application in subjects with similar presentation signs, symptoms, and risk factors)	Poor validity testing subjects with persistent low back pain with known nondiscogenic pain syndromes (e.g., iliac crest pain) or asymptomatic disc pathology (i.e., previous disc surgery). PPV approximately 50% in ideal patient, PPV ≪50% in typical discography patient (outcome findings) Phase 3 study examples: Carragee et al, 1999[14]; Carragee et al, 2000[35]; Derby et al, 2005[36]; Carragee et al, 2002[37]; Carragee et al, 2006[43]
Phase 4	Does having the diagnostic test result improve outcomes compared with management without test result (controlled trial)	Little to no evidence of provocative discography improving outcomes compared with modern diagnostic techniques.[40] Substantial evidence provocative discography is worse than anesthetic injection alone.[42] Substantial evidence discography may worsen outcomes in certain at-risk groups[44-46]

PPV, positive predictive value.

After Sackett D, Haynes R: Evidence base of clinical diagnosis: The architecture of diagnostic research. BMJ 324:539-541, 2002.

illness against which investigators document that the diagnosis suggested by discography is correct.

Validity of Discography

Discography purports to diagnose the presence or absence of a disc lesion responsible for the syndrome of chronic low back pain illness caused by primary discogenic pain. There is no commonly used "gold standard" or criterion to determine who actually has chronic low back pain illness from primary discogenic pain. There are well-accepted standards, however, for who does not—someone with no evidence of significant low back pain. Similarly, someone with new pain resulting from another process (pelvic fracture) does not have "chronic low back pain illness caused by primary discogenic pain." Provocative discography can be assessed by the results of disc injections in subjects who definitively do not have chronic low back pain illness caused by primary discogenic pain.

Alternatively, a patient's response to treatment may be considered a surrogate "gold standard" if the treatment definitively removes the pain generator (the disc) and adjustments can be made for surgical and nonspecific limitations of the treatment. The following section describes a series of clinical and experimental studies that have attempted to define the specificity of discography in different at-risk subgroups.

Specificity of Positive Discography: Testing on Subjects with No Axial Pain History

Careful technique and the standardization of discography were believed by many discographers to have reduced the

false-positive rate to a negligible level in experienced hands. In 1990, Walsh and colleagues[29] performed a carefully controlled set of discographic lumbar injections in 10 paid volunteers, all asymptomatic young men (mean age 22) with little disc degeneration. Of 30 discs injected in this asymptomatic group, 5 produced "minimum" pain (16.7%), 2 produced "moderate" pain (6.7%), and 1 produced "bad" pain (3.3%). Based on these data, the authors believed the risk of false-positive injections was very low. This study is frequently, and incorrectly, cited to confirm a 0% false-positive rate.

In 1997, a review of one discography practice[25] found cases that seemed to be clinically apparent false-positive cases. These injections were believed to meet full criteria for discogenic pain, with concordant, painful injections and negative control injections. Clinical follow-up revealed other causes of the patients' back pain illness, however, including spinal tumor, sacroiliac joint disease, and emotional problems. Block and colleagues[30] related abnormal Minnesota Multiphasic Personality Inventory (MMPI) testing and Ohnmeiss and colleagues[31] related abnormal pain drawings with "nonorganic" features, suggesting possible false-positive discographic injections. Other authors performed thoracic[32] and cervical[33] injections in subjects asymptomatic for pain in those areas. Significantly painful injections were found to occur in approximately 30% of these volunteers.

Following the Walsh protocol, Carragee and colleagues[15] examined 30 volunteer subjects with no history of low back pain who were recruited to undergo a physical examination, magnetic resonance imaging (MRI), psychometric testing, and provocative discography. The results showed that little pain was elicited by injection of any anatomically normal disc. Discs with advanced degenerative annular fissuring with dye leakage to the outer (innervated) annular margins were more commonly painful after discography than less degenerative or normal discs. The intensity of the pain reported by the subjects with annular disruption was predicted by the presence of chronic nonlumbar pain and abnormal psychological scores. Only 10% of subjects without any other pain processes had a positive disc injection by the Walsh criteria, but 50% of subjects with nonback chronic pain had at least one positive disc injection.

The interaction between pending compensation claim and discographic pain was also significant in this select group of volunteers. Of the 10 subjects with positive injections, 8 had had contested workers' compensation or personal injury claims with resulting litigation. Conversely, of 9 subjects with disputed litigation claims, 8 had positive injections ($P < .0001$).[15] It was not found, however, that all subjects involved in previous work injury claims had similar rates of positive disc injection. A history of an uncontested claim from a past compensation injury and no pending legal action did not predict significant pain on disc injection. Given that no subject in this study stood to have any secondary gain from positive discography, the increased pain reporting in subjects with unrelated but contested compensation claims is intriguing. It is possible that the effect of the prolonged social turmoil associated with a litigation dispute has the effect of diminishing one's resilience to irritative stimuli. Another explanation could be that persons with abnormally low pain tolerance are more likely to have a legal dispute regarding the significance and damages associated with previous minor injury.

Discographic Injections in Previously Operated Discs

Provocative discography is frequently used to evaluate persistent or recurrent low back pain syndromes in patients who had undergone posterior discectomy. The validity of interpreting painful injections after herniation is unknown despite its common usage. Heggeness and colleagues[34] reported on 83 postdiscectomy patients and found that 72% had a positive concordant pain response on injection of the previously operated disc. This study did not address the possibility of false-positive injections. All positive injections were assumed to be true-positive injections for identifying the source of the patient's pain.

Using the same methodology developed by Walsh and colleagues,[29] a large study of discography in asymptomatic patients after discectomy for sciatica was performed.[35] Painful disc injections were frequently seen in the asymptomatic postdiscectomy group. As in previous studies, a higher rate of painful injections was seen in patients with abnormal psychological profiles.

Validity of Concordance Report

Provocative discography is considered positive only when injection elicits the patient's usual pain in quality and in location. The reliability of the test would be substantially supported *if* patients could identify the quality of pain coming from a particular disc and differentially compare that sensation with their usual pain.

It is unclear to what extent similar neurologic and behavioral factors may influence the results in provocative discography. It is possible that the disc stimulation in discography may also provoke a "concordant" pain response without actually having located a true pain source. As discussed earlier, there have been reported cases of individuals undergoing discography who were diagnosed as having discogenic pain as the source of their illness on the basis of positive concordant disc injections, but who were subsequently shown to have nonspinal sources for their pain.[25]

This issue was investigated using an experimental model to determine the response to disc injection in patients known to have nonspinal back pain.[14] Subjects with no history of back pain were recruited who were scheduled to undergo posterior iliac crest bone graft harvesting for nonspinal problems, mainly fracture nonunions or bone tumors. Most of these patients experienced low back and buttock pain from the bone grafting for several months postoperatively, and this pain was in a similar distribution to what is normally considered discogenic lumbar pain. Discography was performed several months after the bone graft harvesting, and subjects were asked to compare the quality and location of disc injection pain with their usual iliac crest pain.

Eight volunteer subjects were studied using the same protocol as the Walsh and colleagues study.[29] All subjects had some disc degeneration on MRI, and 24 of the discs were injected. Of the 14 disc injections causing some pain response, 5 were believed to be "different" (nonconcordant) pains (35.7%), 7 were "similar" (50%), and 2 were "exact" pain reproductions (14.3%). The presence of annular disruption was correlated with concordant pain reproduction ($P < .05$). Of 10 discs with annular tears, injection of 7 elicited "similar" or "exact" pain reproduction to the pain at iliac crest bone graft harvest sites. By the strict criteria for positive discography, four of the eight patients (50%) had positive injections: The pain on a single disc injection was "bad" or "very bad," and the pain quality was noted to be exact or similar to the usual discomfort. All subjects had a negative control disc. All positive disc injections had annular fissures. Half of the positive disc injections occurred at low pressures (<20 psi).[14]

Discography in Subjects with Minimal Low Back Symptoms

The ability of a test such as discography to discriminate a true pain generator disc responsible for causing serious disabling low back pain illness from another disc that causes only trivial or clinically inconsequential backache is critical to the test's validity in clinical practice. Derby and colleagues[36] performed discography in a group of 16 subjects with occasional or minimal low back pain, none of whom required current medical care or were experiencing disability because of low back pain. Of the 16 subjects, 5 (31%) had a pain response at 5 out of 10 or greater, and 2 (12.5%) had a pain response at 6 out of 10 or greater. The subjects with more frequent benign low back pain had more painful injections. None of these subjects had abnormal psychological profiles, compensation issues, or chronic pain syndromes or had significant secondary gain motivation to underreport pain. This study was confounded by potentially significant methodologic issues making the results open to criticism. These issues include using the investigators' employees and staff as the subjects of the study.

In another study, the Stanford group performed experimental discography on 25 volunteer subjects with no clinical back pain illness; these volunteers had persistent low backache unassociated with any physical restrictions that was not bad enough to seek medical care.[37] All subjects had normal psychological profiles, but half had other chronic pain syndromes that are risk factors for positive injections. In 36% of these subjects with common backache, discographic injection of one or more discs was significantly painful and concordant. All positive discs had annular disruption, and all had negative control discs. By the usual proposed criteria, these were positive disc injections for clinically significant discogenic pain illness. Discs sensitive to low pressure injections were found in 28% of subjects.

Pressure-Sensitive Injections and Discography Validity

In some cases, dye injected at low pressures may cause significant pain. Derby and colleagues[8] labeled these "chemically" sensitive discs, as opposed to discs that are painful only on injection with high pressures. These authors theorized that "chemically" sensitive discs are painful because of the exposure of annular nerve endings or nearby neural structures to the leakage of some irritating substances. It is postulated that this pain is incited by chemical leakage from the disc during daily activities. This leakage is thought to be simulated by the disc injections. Low-pressure–positive discs are arbitrarily defined as discs found to be painful at pressures less than 15 psi or 22 psi greater than opening pressures.[8,22] Derby and colleagues[8] postulated further that disc injections eliciting pain at higher pressures (>50 psi), called "mechanically" sensitive discs, physically distend the anulus and simulate mechanical loading. In these discs, it is presumed that a mechanical deformation of the anulus is the inciting painful event.

The use of pressure measurements has been postulated as a means to decrease the risk of false-positive injections. This assertion would be true if injections were rarely, if ever, positive at low pressures in subjects without true low back pain illness. Previous neurophysiologic considerations suggest that a pain and pressure profile for a given disc lesion may depend on individual pain sensitivity and local pain processes not related to the disc. Hypothetically, the pain and pressure profile may be depicted as shown in Figure 16–1. The presence of the factors enumerated in Table 16–2 thought to have a desensitizing effect would move the curve down and to the right, whereas factors that increase pain sensitivity may move the pain and pressure curve up and to the left.

Experimental work has corroborated this hypothetical pain response. Discographic injections have been performed with pressure measurements in asymptomatic or minimally symptomatic volunteers.[15,29,35-37] Figure 16–2 shows the proportion

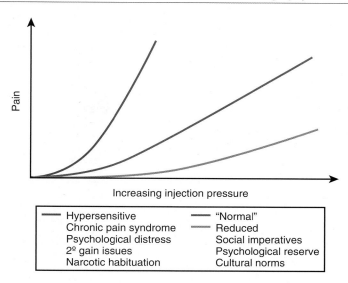

FIGURE 16–1 Hypothetical responses to pressurization of degenerative disc depending on "pain sensitivity" and "reporting biases" of the patient.

of painful injections at low pressures in volunteers with varying risk factors for increased pain sensitization. It seems from these and other data[38] that low-pressure injections are more likely positive in subjects with some type of chronic pain state, psychological distress, and, presumably, a generalized sensitization to irritable stimuli. An increased perception of pain at low-pressure injections seems to affect the pain response even when the chronic pain state is not in the low back region.

Evidence That Discography in Clinical Practice May Improve Outcomes

Many case series report that provocative discography is helpful in management of patients with chronic low back pain illness.

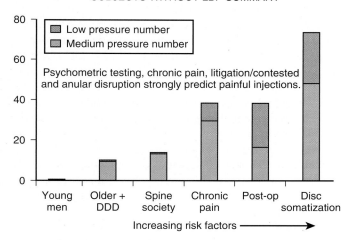

FIGURE 16–2 Discography testing in asymptomatic subjects with varying risk factors. Proportion of painful disc injections and painful injections at low pressures seems to increase with increasing risk factors. (Data from references 15, 20, 29, and 36.)

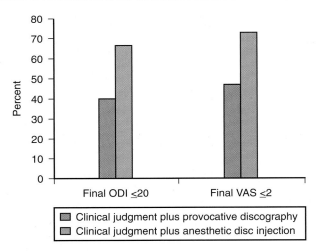

FIGURE 16–3 Randomized clinical trial by Ohtori and colleagues comparing the proportion of good outcomes for pain and function after single-level spinal fusion in patients selected by best clinical judgment and provocative discography with best clinical judgment plus anesthetic disc injection. These were "best-case" scenario subjects in many respects: no workers' compensation cases, no road traffic accident litigation cases, no high somatic distress cases, no depression cases, all selected by very experienced spinal surgeons in Japan. Outcomes are clearly inferior when discography is used to select patients for fusion. (Data from Ohtori S, Kinoshita T, Yamashita M, et al: Results of surgery for discogenic low back pain: A randomized study using discography versus discoblock for diagnosis. Spine 34:1345-1348, 2009.)

These are uncontrolled studies, however, and the relationship of discography findings to clinical outcome after surgery is speculative: Good outcomes when encountered may be the result of nonspecific effects, natural history of the condition independent of diagnosis or treatment, scrupulous patient selection, or confounding findings on standard imaging studies. In a retrospective literature review, Cohen and Hurley[39] compared outcomes of spinal fusions in studies that included discography with fusion outcomes without preoperative discography. The outcomes were not significantly different.

In the era before routine MRI use, Colhoun and colleagues[40] retrospectively compared a series of fusions planned with and without preoperative discography. Evaluation methods of these patients having surgery in the 1970s and early 1980s did not include dynamic radiographs, MRI, or computed tomography (CT). The authors reported better results in the discography group. The two groups were not similar at baseline, however, and potential biases resulting in some patients having preoperative discography and others not having it were not examined. In the era before contemporary imaging techniques, this study suggested that discography may assist in the evaluation of patients before surgery. This is an extremely rare clinical scenario today and has little applicability to current evaluation protocols.

Madan and colleagues[41] did a retrospective review of consecutive patients undergoing spinal fusion performed by the same surgeons, with and without preoperative discography. The two groups seemed well matched for demographic, psychometric, and radiographic features. At a minimum of 2-year

follow-up, there was no significant difference in outcome between the two groups. The addition of discography to radiographs and MRI did not improve outcomes compared with radiographs and MRI alone.

A more recent randomized clinical trial compared outcomes of subjects having single-level fusion based on preoperative evaluation using provocative discography with subjects having an anesthetic disc injection.[42] These were in some respects subjects with best-case scenarios (no psychological distress, no depression, no workers' compensation cases, and no traffic accident litigants). The discography was performed using low-pressure injections. The outcomes in the discography group were uniformly worse than the group using an anesthetic block to determine fusion (Fig. 16–3). A phase IV evaluation (based on evidence-based criteria as described by Sackett and Haynes[26]) of discography has not been performed to date (see Table 16–3).

Clinical Outcome as a "Gold Standard" in Provocative Discography

From the evidence reviewed in this chapter, discography has been shown to be frequently positive in asymptomatic subjects and in subjects with pelvic pain owing to iliac crest harvesting and has been shown to be frequently fully concordant in subjects with clinically insignificant backache. These findings suggest there is limited experimental evidence to support the premise that discography can accurately identify clinically significant lesions responsible for a patient's chronic low back pain illness. Direct assessment of a positive test against an accepted "gold standard," confirming a true-positive result, has not been performed.

A common empirical "gold standard" would involve comparing the test results with clinical surgical outcomes, assuming an excellent clinical outcome would confirm a true-positive test. There is concern, however, that an excellent clinical result may overestimate the number of true-positive results because of a placebo or nonspecific effect of spinal fusion or other intervention. There is also concern that clinical outcomes may underestimate the number of true-positive tests because the ability to achieve outstanding results is limited by patient-specific variables (psychological distress or social issues preventing recovery despite surgical cure of the lesion) or by operative morbidity or technical limitations, which, even in the best of cases, cannot achieve 100% success even with an accurate diagnosis.

An attempt was made to control these variables (patient-specific variables and operative comorbidities) in a prospective controlled study of spinal fusion for presumed diagnoses of unstable spondylolisthesis versus discogenic pain diagnosed by discography. Identical operative techniques were used, and patients had no psychosocial comorbidities.[43] Both groups included only highly selected patients with 6 to 18 months of severe low back pain, normal psychological testing, no previous or concomitant pain syndromes, and no workers' compensation or personal injury claims. All patients had either positive discography at one level only and at low pressures (<20 psi) or unstable spondylolisthesis by strict radiographic criteria. All patients had been working full-time before their back problem, and no patient was taking daily narcotic medications.

Both groups underwent an anterior spinal fusion with posterior instrumentation and fusion. Two years after surgery, only 27% of patients in the discography group met stringent criteria for clinical success compared with 71% of the spondylolisthesis group. Success was defined as full return to work and recreational activities, pain scores on a visual analog pain scale (VAS) less than 2, Oswestry Disability Index score less than 15, and no daily medications for back pain. Even using less rigorous outcome measures, 43% of the discography group compared with 91% of the spondylolisthesis group reported at least moderate improvement. Even after controlling for operative morbidity, the maximum proportion of true-positive discograms in a best-case scenario (i.e., assuming normal psychometric testing, no other chronic pain history, no compensation issues or litigation, and single-level degeneration) was 40% to 60%, with a false-positive rate of approximately 50%.

For less "ideal" patients, provocative discography may be an extremely poor tool to select appropriate operative candidates. Freedman and colleagues,[44] using CT and provocative discography to select a wide range of typical low back pain subjects for an intradiscal electrothermal therapy trial (including patients with psychometric distress and compensation claims), found no improvement at all compared with control subjects. Pauza and colleagues,[45] in a similar intradiscal electrothermal therapy trial but excluding subjects with psychological abnormality, workers' compensation claims, or litigation claims, found only slightly better outcomes: Most subjects did not have improvement better than expected by placebo.

Even more striking, Derby and colleagues[46] found such poor outcomes of spinal fusion after provocative discography in patients with abnormal mental component scores (MCS) on the SF-36 that the discography seemed to preselect patients who were extremely unlikely to have a satisfactory outcome. These results, illustrated in Figure 16–4, may be substantially worse than using alternative patient selection strategies without discography (e.g., radiographs, MRI, patient interview, or psychological screening).

Complications

Although there are many potential complications of any invasive procedure, several potential complications of discography warrant specific discussion, as follows:

1. *Infection*: There is a small but definite risk of discitis after percutaneous puncture and injection. The absolute risk is difficult to calculate, but modern methods likely limit this risk to much less than 1%. Double needle techniques for insertion, less irritating dye, and intravenous or injectate antibiotics all have been postulated to decrease the infection risk.

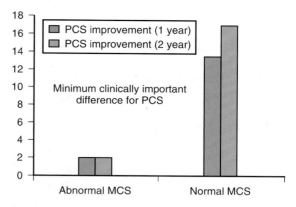

FIGURE 16–4 Outcomes of spinal fusion when discography was used in patient selection. Subjects with positive discogram in setting of abnormal mental component scores in SF-36 were highly unlikely to improve or reach even minimum clinically important change in physical outcomes. In contrast, subjects with more normalized mental component scores had significantly better improvement in outcomes (*P* < .005). In this study, positive provocative discography result in clinical subset of psychologically distressed patients seems to select patients unlikely to improve with surgical treatment.

2. *Prolonged pain episode*: Occasionally, patients may experience a prolonged episode of pain after a disc injection. One reason given for this phenomenon is the hypothetical displacement of fibrous repair over annular fissures owing to disc pressurization.[2] Other work has shown that 40% of subjects with psychological distress at the time of injection can have markedly increased back pain for 1 year after discography. This effect was not seen in subjects with normal psychological profiles.[47]

3. *Misleading diagnosis resulting in inappropriate or nonproductive invasive treatments*: As discussed previously, subjects with one or more risk factors for false-positive testing may be misdiagnosed as having primary discogenic pain as the cause of their persistent low back pain illness. Patients with abnormal psychometric testing undergoing surgery based on this test are extremely unlikely to have substantial benefit from disc-directed interventions (see Fig. 16–4) and are exposed to the hazards and morbidity of these procedures.[46]

4. *Accelerated disc degeneration*: In animal models, disc puncture with a needle has provided a reliable model to initiate rapid disc injury with structural changes similar in some respects to naturally occurring disc degeneration. Working with a large animal model, Korecki and colleagues[48] showed that relatively minor disruption in the disc from even a 25-gauge needle puncture injury had "immediate and progressive mechanical and biologic consequences with important implications for the use of discography…." Similarly, Nassr and colleagues[49] showed that needle puncture in cervical discs during cervical spinal surgery localization radiographs was apparently associated with a threefold risk of rapid disc degeneration.

Carragee and colleagues[50] performed a prospective, match-cohort study of disc degeneration progression over 10 years with and without baseline discography. The investigators performed a protocol MRI and L3-4, L4-5, and L5-S1 discography examination at baseline in 75 subjects without serious low back pain illness. The investigators enrolled a matched group at the same time and performed the same protocol MRI examination. Subjects were followed for 10 years. At 7 to 10 years after baseline assessment, eligible discography and control subjects underwent another protocol MRI examination. MRI examinations were scored for qualitative findings (Pfirrmann grade, herniations, endplate changes, and high-intensity zone). Loss of disc height and loss of disc signal were measured by quantitative methods (Fig. 16–5). The investigators found that modern discography techniques with small-gauge needle and limited pressurization resulted in accelerated disc degeneration, disc herniation, loss of disc height and signal, and development of reactive endplate changes compared with matched controls.

Conclusions Regarding Provocative Discography

As for most diagnostic tests, the usefulness of discography is affected by the characteristics of the population being studied.

As a provocative test depending on the subjective reporting of pain with injection, the central factors influencing reliability and validity have to do with the neurophysiologic, psychological, and social factors that affect pain perception and expression. In the subset of patients without significant confounding factors, the test may be more likely to identify accurately a local pain generator as a primary cause of disabling axial pain illness. In subjects with significant psychosocial risk factors or confounding neurophysiologic factors, even the theoretical basis of the test is in doubt. Finally, the ability of the test to improve clinical outcomes has not been proven, and studies so far have been disappointing. Serious risks of accelerated disc degeneration are also suspected after disc puncture and injection. The risk and benefits of this procedure must be carefully weighed.

PEARLS

1. Patient selection for discography is of primary importance in determining the accuracy and utility of the test.

2. Results need to be interpreted in the context of the patient's entire medical history, including other chronic pain issues.

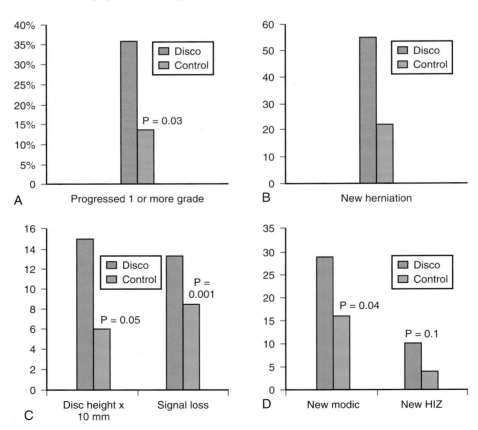

FIGURE 16–5 A-D, Progression of disc degeneration in matched cohorts of subjects, discography (Disco) versus nondiscography controls. Baseline versus 10-year follow-up MRI studies were compared for progression of Pfirrmann grade (**A**), development of new disc herniations (**B**), loss of disc height and nuclear signal (**C**), and development of new Modic findings or high-intensity zones (**D**). In all parameters, degeneration was greater in discography group. (Data from Carragee EJ, Don AS, Hurwitz EL, et al: 2009 ISSLS Prize Winner. Does discography cause accelerated progression of degeneration changes in the lumbar disc: A ten-year matched cohort study. Spine 34:2338-2345, 2009.)

3. It is extremely unlikely that a disc with a negative injection, normal morphology, and no pain with the injection would be a primary cause of serious low back pain illness.

4. In the best-case scenario of a patient with no known risk factors for a false-positive test, the positive predictive value of the test is not greater than 50%.

5. Most low back pain syndromes are multifactorial.

PITFALLS

1. During injection, it is important to avoid high-pressure injections (<100 psi) because these may cause gross mechanical motion of the segment or injure the endplate directly.

2. In patients with psychological distress, disputed compensation claims, or multiple chronic pain syndromes, the reported pain responses to disc injection have not been shown to be reliable or valid.

3. There is a small risk of accelerated disc degeneration with discographic injections.

4. Disc injections in patients with psychological distress may result in an increase in back pain for weeks or months.

KEY POINTS

1. Provocative discography is a diagnostic test that may identify primary "discogenic" pain if present in psychologically normal patients without confounding pain or compensation issues.

2. Patient responses to disc injection are subjective and strongly influenced by pain sensitivity and reporting variables, including psychological factors, chronic pain behavior, regional or central pain syndromes, and compensation issues.

3. Provocative discography has not been proven to improve outcomes of treatment for low back pain syndromes. In patients with emotional distress issues or compensation issues, there is some evidence that using discography may result in poorer outcomes and inappropriate invasive procedures.

4. Risks of provocative discography include false and misleading diagnoses in patients with high pain-sensitive risk factors, increased axial pain for weeks or months after injection, pyogenic discitis, and accelerated disc degeneration over many years.

KEY REFERENCES

1. Sackett D, Haynes R: Evidence base of clinical diagnosis: The architecture of diagnostic research. BMJ 324:539-541, 2002.
   This article defines the necessary conditions to establish validity and clinical usefulness of a diagnostic test. The "gold standard" necessary to compare diagnostic test results is of prime importance, as is a careful assessment of the study population. These conditions are problematic in the evaluation of provocative discography.

2. Carragee EJ, Tanner CM, Yang B, et al: False-positive findings on lumbar discography: Reliability of subjective concordance assessment during provocative disc injection. Spine 24:2542-2547, 1999.
   This study looks at the reliability of the concordance response during discography. The authors found that volunteer subjects with known pelvic area pain cannot reliably distinguish the sensation coming from a pelvic pain generator from the sensation caused by the injection of an asymptomatic disc. The implications for validity of provocative injections are discussed.

3. Ohtori S, Kinoshita T, Yamashita M, et al: Results of surgery for discogenic low back pain: A randomized study using discography versus discoblock for diagnosis. Spine (Phila Pa 1976) 34:1345-1348, 2009.
   The authors performed a randomized clinical trial comparing outcomes of subjects having single-level fusion based on an evaluation using provocative discography with subjects having an anesthetic disc injection. These were in some respects best-case scenario subjects (no psychological distress, no depression, no workers' compensation cases, and no traffic accident litigants). The discography was performed using low-pressure injections. The outcomes in the discography group (reported pain, function, pain medications) were uniformly worse than the group using an anesthetic block to determine fusion.

4. Carragee EJ, Don AS, Hurwitz EJ, et al: The 2009 ISSLS Prize Winner. Does discography cause accelerated progression of degeneration changes in the lumbar disc: A ten-year matched cohort study. Spine 34:2338-2345, 2009.
   Matched asymptomatic cohorts with and without baseline pressure-limited provocative discography were followed with a detailed MRI protocol compared against baseline MRI findings. The discography group had greater progression of disc degeneration scores, more new disc herniations, greater loss of disc height, and greater loss of disc signal compared with the control group. In the discography cohort, new disc herniations were disproportionately found near the puncture site.

5. Chou R, Loesser JD, Owens DK: Interventional therapies, surgery, and interdisciplinary rehabilitation for low back pain: An evidence-based clinical practice guideline from the American Pain Society. Spine 34:1066-1077, 2009.
   In a comprehensive multidisciplinary review, the authors concluded: "In patients with chronic nonradicular low back pain, provocative discography is not recommended as a procedure for diagnosing discogenic low back pain (strong recommendation, moderate-quality evidence)."

REFERENCES

1. Lindblom L: Diagnostic puncture of intervertebral disks in sciatica. Acta Orthop Scand 17:231-239, 1948.

2. Derby R, Guyer R, Lee S-H, et al: The rational use and limitations of provocative discography. ISIS Scientific News Letter 5:6-20, 2005.

3. Allan DB, Waddell G: An historical perspective on low back pain and disability. Acta Orthop Scand Suppl 234:1-23, 1989.

4. Burton A: Spine update: Back injury and work loss: Biomechanical and psychosocial influences. Spine 22:2575-2580, 1997.

5. Burton A, Tillotson K, Main C, et al: Psychosocial predictors of outcome in acute and subacute low back trouble. Spine 20:722-728, 1995.

6. Aprill C, Bogduk N: High-intensity zone: A diagnostic sign of painful lumbar disc on magnetic resonance imaging. Br J Radiol 65:361-369, 1992.

7. Crock H: Internal disc disruption. Med J Aust 1:983-990, 1970.

8. Derby R, Howard MW, Grant JM, et al: The ability of pressure-controlled discography to predict surgical and nonsurgical outcomes. Spine 24:364-371; discussion 371-372, 1999.

9. O'Neill C, Derby R, Kanderes L: Precision injection techniques for diagnosis and treatment of lumbar disc disease. Semin Spine Surg 11:104-118, 1999.

10. Schwarzer A, Aprill C, Derby R, et al: The prevalence and clinical features of internal disc disruption in patients with chronic LBP. Spine 20:1878-1883, 1995.

11. Schwarzer A, Aprill C, Fortin J, et al: The relative contribution of the zygapophyseal joint in chronic low back pain. Spine 19:801-806, 1994.

12. Schwarzer A, Bogduk N: Letter to Editor. The prevalence and clinical features of internal disk disruption in patients with low back pain. Spine 21:776, 1996.

13. Siddle P, Cousins M: Spinal pain mechanisms. Spine 22:98-104, 1997.

14. Carragee EJ, Tanner CM, Yang B, et al: False-positive findings on lumbar discography: Reliability of subjective concordance assessment during provocative disc injection. Spine 24:2542-2547, 1999.

15. Carragee EJ, Tanner CM, Khurana S, et al: The rates of false-positive lumbar discography in select patients without low back symptoms. Spine 25:1373-1380; discussion 1381, 2000.

16. Gracely R, Dubner R, McGrath P: Narcotic analgesia: Fentanyl reduces the intensity but not the unpleasantness of painful tooth pulp stimulation. Science 203:1261-1263, 1979.

17. Lenz F, Gracely R, Romanoski A, et al: Stimulation in the somatosensory thalamus can reproduce both the affective and sensory dimensions of previously experienced pain. Nat Med 1:910-913, 1995.

18. Lenz FA, Gracely RH, Hope EJ, et al: The sensation of angina can be evoked by stimulation of the human thalamus. Pain 59:119-125, 1994.

19. Saal JSM: General principles of diagnostic testing as related to painful lumbar spine disorders—a critical appraisal of current diagnostic techniques. Spine 27:2538-2545, 2002.

20. Carragee EJ: Psychological screening in the surgical treatment of lumbar disc herniation. Clin J Pain 17:215-219, 2001.

21. North R, Kidd D, Zahurak M, et al: Specificity of diagnostic nerve blocks: A prospective, randomized study of sciatica due to lumbosacral spine disease. Pain 65:77-85, 1996.

22. O'Neill C, Kurgansky M: Subgroups of positive discs on discography. Spine 29:2134-2139, 2004.

23. Handwerker HO, Kobal G: Psychophysiology of experimentally induced pain. Physiol Rev 73:639-671, 1993.

24. Rhudy JL, Meagher MW: Fear and anxiety: Divergent effects on human pain thresholds. Pain 84:65-75, 2000.

25. Carragee E, Tanner C, Vittum D, et al: Positive provocative discography as a misleading finding in the evaluation of low back pain. NASS Proceedings, 1997, p 388.

26. Sackett D, Haynes R: Evidence base of clinical diagnosis: The architecture of diagnostic research. BMJ 324:539-541, 2002.

27. Schwarzer A, Wang S, Bogduk N, et al: Prevalence and clinical features of lumbar zygapophysial joint pain: A study in an Australian population with chronic low back pain. Ann Rheum Dis 54:100-106, 1995.

28. Schwarzer AC, Aprill CN, Derby R, et al: The false-positive rate of uncontrolled diagnostic blocks of the lumbar zygapophysial joints. Pain 58:195-200, 1994.

29. Walsh T, Weinstein J, Spratt K, et al: Lumbar discography in normal subjects: A controlled prospective study. J Bone Joint Surg Am 72:1081-1088, 1990.

30. Block A, Vanharanta H, Ohnmeiss D, et al: Discographic pain report: Influence of psychological factors. Spine 21:334-338, 1996.

31. Ohnmeiss DD, Vanharanta H, Guyer RD: The association between pain drawings and computed tomographic/discographic pain responses. Spine 20:729-733, 1995.

32. Schellhas KP, Pollei SR, Dorwart RH: Thoracic discography: A safe and reliable technique. Spine 19:2103-2109, 1994.

33. Nordin M, Carragee EJ, Hogg-Johnson S, et al: Assessment of neck pain and its associated disorders. Results of the Bone and Joint Decade 2000-2010 Task Force on Neck Pain and Its Associated Disorders. Spine 33:S101-S122, 2008.

34. Heggeness MH, Watters WC III, Gray PM Jr: Discography of lumbar discs after surgical treatment for disc herniation. Spine 22:1606-1609, 1997.

35. Carragee EJ, Chen Y, Tanner CM, et al: Provocative discography in patients after limited lumbar discectomy: A controlled, randomized study of pain response in symptomatic and asymptomatic subjects. Spine 25:3065-3071, 2000.

36. Derby R, Kim B-J, Lee S-H, et al: Comparison of discographic findings in asymptomatic subject discs and the negative discs of chronic LBP patients: Can discography distinguish asymptomatic discs among morphologically abnormal discs? Spine J 5:389-394, 2005.

37. Carragee EJ, Alamin TF, Miller J, et al: Provocative discography in volunteer subjects with mild persistent low back pain. Spine J 2:25-34, 2002.

38. Carragee EJ, Alamin TF, Parmar V, et al: Low pressure positive discography in subjects asymptomatic of significant LBP illness. Spine 31:505-509, 2006.

39. Cohen SP, Hurley RW: The ability of diagnostic spinal injections to predict surgical outcomes. Anesth Analg 105:1756-1775, 2007.

40. Colhoun E, McCall IW, Williams L, et al: Provocation discography as a guide to planning operations on the spine. J Bone Joint Surg Br 70:267-271, 1988.

41. Madan S, Gundanna M, Harley JM, et al: Does provocative discography screening of discogenic back pain improve surgical outcome? J Spinal Disord Tech 15:245-251, 2002.

42. Ohtori S, Kinoshita T, Yamashita M, et al: Results of surgery for discogenic low back pain: A randomized study using discography versus discoblock for diagnosis. Spine 34:1345-1348, 2009.

43. Carragee EJ, Lincoln T, Parmar VS, et al: A gold standard evaluation of the "discogenic pain" diagnosis as determined by provocative discography. Spine 31:2115-2123, 2006.

44. Freeman BJ, Fraser RD, Cain CM, et al: A randomized, double-blind, controlled trial: Intradiscal electrothermal therapy versus placebo for the treatment of chronic discogenic low back pain. Spine 30:2369-2377; discussion 2378, 2005.

45. Pauza KJ, Howell S, Dreyfuss P, et al: A randomized, placebo-controlled trial of intradiscal electrothermal therapy for the treatment of discogenic low back pain. Spine 4:27-35, 2004.

46. Derby R, Lettice JJ, Kula TA, et al: Single-level lumbar fusion in chronic discogenic low-back pain: Psychological and emotional status as a predictor of outcome measured using the 36-item Short Form. J Neurosurg Spine 3:255-261, 2005.

47. Carragee EJ, Chen Y, Tanner CM, et al: Can discography cause long-term back symptoms in previously asymptomatic subjects? Spine 25:1803-1808, 2000.

48. Korecki CL, Costi JJ, Iatridis JC: Needle puncture injury affects intervertebral disc mechanics and biology in an organ culture model. Spine 33:235-241, 2008.

49. Nassr A, Lee JY, Bashir RS, et al: Does incorrect level needle localization during anterior cervical discectomy and fusion lead to accelerated disc degeneration? Spine 34:189-192, 2009.

50. Carragee EJ, Don AS, Hurwitz EL, et al: 2009 ISSLS Prize Winner. Does discography cause accelerated progression of degeneration changes in the lumbar disc: A ten-year matched cohort study. Spine 34:2338-2345, 2009.

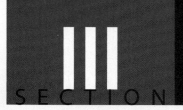

SECTION III

SURGICAL ANATOMY AND APPROACHES

Cervical Spine: Surgical Approaches

Francis H. Shen, MD
Howard S. An, MD

Successful surgery in the cervical spine depends not only on understanding normal anatomy in the neck, but also on appreciating the complex relationship these structures have to one another. Thorough understanding of these relationships allows for safe access to the cervical spine while minimizing complications. The first section of this chapter discusses the surface anatomy, osseous anatomy, bony articulations, ligaments, intervertebral discs, neurovascular structures, musculature, and triangles of the cervical spine. In the second section, the focus is on the applied surgical anatomy for successful anterior and posterior cervical approaches.

Surgical Anatomy

Surface Anatomy and Skin

An understanding of the relationship of surface landmarks to anatomic structures in the neck is useful for localizing vertebral levels. The hyoid bone lies at the level of C3, the thyroid cartilage lies at the level of C4, and the cricoid cartilage lies opposite C6.[1] Gentle but firm palpation laterally allows inspection of the transverse processes. Superiorly, the transverse process of the atlas is most prominent and is found just anterior and inferior to the mastoid process. To help differentiate it from the skull, rotation of the head shows the atlas moving independently from the skull. The anterior tubercle of the transverse process of the sixth cervical vertebra, Chassaignac tubercle, is an important palpable landmark. Posteriorly, in the midline, the first bony prominence palpated inferior to the occiput is the spinous process of the second vertebra. The next palpable spinous processes are typically from the sixth and the seventh vertebrae, with the seventh being the most prominent.

Anteriorly in the cervical spine, every attempt should be made to place the surgical incision in line with the skin creases. These incisions heal more easily and with a less noticeable scar than incisions that cross these lines. Anteriorly in the lower neck, the skin lines are transverse, but superiorly near the mandible they tend to run obliquely. The skin in the anterior neck tends to be more mobile, soft, and well vascularized, whereas the skin in the back of the neck is thicker and less mobile. As a result, the common extensile longitudinal midline skin incision used posteriorly often creates more prominent scars that tend to spread because of tension from the trapezius muscle.

Osseous Anatomy and Bony Articulation

The cervical spine comprises the first seven vertebrae in the spinal column. The bony anatomy and articulations of the upper cervical spine (occiput-C1-C2) are unique and distinct from the remaining lower five cervical vertebrae (C3-7).

The atlas, or C1, is a ringlike structure lacking a body and a spinous process. It consists of two thick lateral masses plus an anterior and posterior arch. The longus colli muscle and anterior longitudinal ligament attach to the anterior tubercle of the atlas, whereas the posterior tubercle serves as the bony attachments for the rectus minor muscle and suboccipital membrane. The superior and inferior oblique muscles attach to the large transverse processes. The vertebral artery passes through the foramen transversarium located within the transverse process and courses posteriorly within a sulcus on the superior aspect of the posterior arch of the atlas. In 15% of the population, the sulcus for the vertebral artery can be completely covered by an anomalous ossification, which has been called the *ponticulus posticus* and may have surgical implications when identifying anatomic landmarks for bony fixation of C1.

The axis, or C2, is characterized by an odontoid process or dens that projects upward anteriorly, articulating with the posterior aspect of the anterior arch of the atlas as a synovial joint. At its narrowest portion, at the base of the dens, the coronal and sagittal plane diameters are 8 to 10 mm and 10 to 11 mm.[2,3] Posteriorly, the axis has a large lamina and a bifid spinous process, which serve as attachments for the rectus major and inferior oblique muscles. The zone between the lamina and the lateral mass of the axis is indistinct, and posteriorly the neural arch connects to the body by large pedicles that are 8 mm wide and 10 mm long.[4] Lying directly anterolateral to the pedicle is the vertebral artery, which runs through the foramen transversarium. The pedicle of the axis projects 30 degrees medially and 20 degrees superiorly from a posterior-to-anterior direction.[3]

The bony articulations of the upper cervical spine (occiput-C1-C2) are unique and warrant special attention (Fig. 17–1). The atlanto-occipital articulation is a shallow ball-and-socket joint allowing for considerable motion mostly in flexion, extension, and lateral bending. The greatest degree of flexion and extension of any cervical articulation occurs at this level (25 degrees).[5] Lateral displacement is minimized because the lateral wall of the cup-shaped articulation of the atlas is higher than the medial wall. The superior articular surface of the atlas projects cephalad and medially, articulating with the occipital condyle, which projects caudad and laterally. Conversely, the inferior articular surface of the atlas projects caudad and medially and articulates with the laterally projecting superior facet of the axis. As a result of this bony configuration, axial loads on the atlas tend to result in horizontal displacement of the lateral masses.[6]

The atlantoaxial articulation provides about 50% of rotatory motion of the cervical spine.[5,7] The transverse ligament, which spans across the arch of the atlas, holds the odontoid process against the anterior arch of the atlas, creating a pivot joint with a synovial membrane and capsular ligaments anteriorly and posteriorly to the dens. This transverse ligament is the principal stabilizing structure for the atlantoaxial articulation and averages 21.9 mm in length.[8] The transverse ligament has superior and inferior extensions, which form the cruciform ligament of the atlas, connecting it to the anterior edge of the foramen magnum and posterior aspect of the C2 body. To allow more rotatory motion, the inferior facets of the atlas are flatter and more circular than the superior facets and face inferiorly to articulate with the axis.

The lower cervical vertebrae are morphologically similar and increase in dimension as they proceed inferiorly from C3 to C6, with C7 as the transitional vertebra into the thoracic spine. The vertebral bodies are small and oval, with the medio-lateral diameter greater than the anteroposterior diameter.

The inferior surface of the vertebral body is convex in the coronal plane and concave in the sagittal plane, with the anterior lip occasionally overlapping the inferior vertebra.[8] Conversely, the superior surface of the vertebral body is convex or straight in the sagittal plane and concave in the coronal plane, creating projections on either side of the lateral superior surface, called the *uncus,* or hook. These processes project upward and conform to small grooves in the inferolateral border of the cephalad vertebra, forming the uncovertebral joints, or joints of Luschka. The width and depth of the vertebral surfaces average 17 mm and 15 mm from C2 to C6 and increase to about 20 mm and 17 mm at C7. Vertebral heights on the posterior wall in the mid-sagittal plane range from 11 to 13 mm.[9]

The pedicles project posterolaterally from the vertebral body and join the lamina to form the vertebral arch. From C3 to C7, the angulation of the pedicles varies from 8 degrees below to 11 degrees above the transverse plane and decreases from 45 degrees to 30 degrees in relation to the sagittal plane.[9] The width and height of the pedicles increase slightly in size from C3 to C7, and average diameters are 5 to 6 mm and

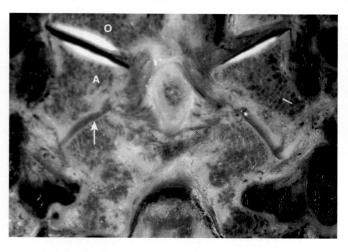

FIGURE 17–1 Coronal cryomicrotome section of upper cervical spine. Note articulation between occiput (O) and atlas (A). Atlantoaxial joint is identified by *white arrow.*

7 mm. The lateral wall of the pedicle is thinner than the medial wall and should be taken into consideration if attempts at pedicle fixation are considered in this region.[10-12]

At the junction of the pedicle and lamina, the anterior tubercle of the transverse process projects laterally and is connected to the posterior tubercle by the costotransverse lamella (bar), creating the foramen transversarium. Passing through the foramen transversarium is the vertebral artery and venous system. The transverse processes increase significantly in size at C6 and C7. The C6 anterior tubercle, also known as the carotid tubercle or Chassaignac tubercle, is a prominent surgical landmark.

In the lower cervical spine, the neural foramina are bounded anteriorly by the uncinate process, the posterolateral aspect of the intervertebral disc, and the inferior portion of the vertebral body; posteriorly by the facet joint and superior articular process of the vertebral body below; and superiorly and inferiorly by adjacent pedicles. Vertebral notches located on the superior and inferior aspect of each pedicle contribute to the size of the neural foramina, which are 9 to 12 mm in height, 4 to 6 mm in width, and 4 to 6 mm in length and are aligned 45 degrees to the sagittal plane.[13,14] They can be visualized radiographically with oblique views, with the right neural foramina outlined on the left posterior oblique view and the left neural foramina outlined on the right posterior oblique view.

The spinal canal is triangular and at all levels in the cervical spine is significantly greater in the medial-to-lateral dimension than in the anterior-to-posterior dimension. The cross-sectional area of the spinal canal is largest at C2 and smallest at C7, with a sagittal diameter of about 23 mm at C1 and 20 mm at C2, decreasing to 17 to 18 mm at C3-6 and to 15 mm at C7.[7] This is one reason that the passage of sublaminar wires is safer in the upper cervical spine than in the lower cervical spine.

The lateral mass, an important structure for posterior cervical plate-screw systems, forms at the junction of the lamina and the pedicle and gives rise to the superior and inferior articular processes. These processes project upward and

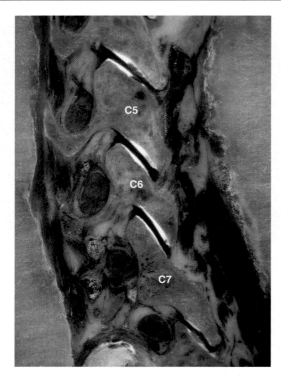

FIGURE 17–2 Parasagittal cryomicrotome section of facet joints. Lateral mass of C7 is more elongated from superior to inferior and thinner from anterior to posterior. Facet joint angle is roughly 45 degrees from transverse plane and assumes more vertical position distally.

downward and are angled approximately 45 degrees cephalad from the transverse plane and gradually assume a more vertical position as they descend into the thoracic region (Fig. 17–2). The articular process of the superior facet faces posteriorly, whereas the inferior facet of the upper vertebra faces anteriorly, and the facets oppose one another to form a zygapophyseal joint. The facet joints are true diarthrodial joints with articular cartilage and menisci surrounded by a fibrous

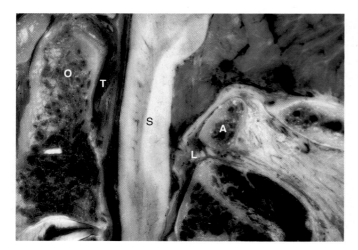

FIGURE 17–3 Midsagittal microtome section at upper cervical spine. Transverse ligament (T) acts as stabilizer of atlantoaxial joint by helping to restrain odontoid (O) from posterior translation. Spinal cord (S), ligamentum flavum (L), and posterior arch of atlas (A) are also identified.

capsule lined by a synovial membrane. The interfacet distances are relatively constant between levels, with individual variations ranging from 9 to 16 mm (average 13 mm).[4,15]

Posteriorly, the spinous processes project inferiorly and are bifid from C3 to C6; the C7 spinous process is large and not bifid and is often called the *vertebra prominens*. The junction between the spinous process and lamina, the spinolaminar line, is an important anatomic landmark during spinous process wiring. Inadvertent penetration of the wire anterior to this line may result in spinal cord impingement.

The cervicothoracic junction is a transition region, with C7 having similar anatomic characteristics at T1 and T2. The dimensions of the vertebral body and the sizes of the transverse processes and spinous processes are larger at C6 and C7. Additionally, dimensions of the spinal canal decrease at C6 and C7, representing a distinct transition to the thoracic region. The articulating facet joint between C7 and T1 resembles the thoracic facet joint, and the lateral mass of C7 is thinner than that of upper levels. Morphologic characteristics of pedicles of C7, T1, and T2 were obtained with respect to diameters, depths, and medial angulations. Inner diameters of the pedicles at C7, T1, and T2 from medial to lateral plane averaged 5.2 mm, 6.3 mm, and 5.5 mm. Medial angulations were 34 degrees, 30 degrees, and 26 degrees at C7, T1, and T2.[9,16] These morphologic characteristics should be remembered when performing transpedicular procedures in the cervicothoracic region.

Ligaments

In addition to the bony anatomy, the ligamentous attachments provide support to the cervical spine and associated articulations. In the atlanto-occipital complex, two membranous attachments, the anterior and posterior atlanto-occipital membranes, connect the anterior and posterior arch of C1 to the margins of the foramen magnum. The anterior atlanto-occipital membrane is the superior continuation of the anterior longitudinal ligament, whereas the posterior membrane is the superior continuation of the ligamentum flavum.

The transverse ligament is the major stabilizer of the atlantoaxial complex (Fig. 17–3). It attaches laterally to tubercles located on the posterior aspect of the anterior arch of C1, where it blends with the lateral mass. Secondary stabilizers include the thick alar ligament, which arises from the sides of the dens to the medial aspects of the condyles of the occipital bone, and the apical ligament, which arises from the apex of the dens to the anterior edge of the foramen magnum. In some individuals, an anterior atlantodental ligament exists connecting the base of the dens to the anterior arch of the atlas.[17] The tectorial membrane, the superior continuation of the posterior longitudinal ligament, covers the dens and all the occipitoaxial ligaments and extends from the posterior body of C2 to the basilar portion of the occipital bone and the anterior aspect of the foramen magnum.

The bodies of the lower cervical vertebrae (C3-7) are connected by two longitudinal ligaments and the intervertebral discs. The anterior longitudinal ligament is a strong band that attaches from the skull, as the anterior atlanto-occipital membrane, and continues caudad over the entire length of the spine down to the sacrum. The anterior longitudinal ligament is thinner and more closely attached at the intervertebral disc margins than at the anterior vertebral surfaces.[18] The anterior longitudinal ligament also sweeps around and envelops the lateral aspect of the vertebral bodies under the longus collis muscle, and the lateral extension is continuous with the deep layer of the posterior longitudinal ligament in the region of the intervertebral foramina.

The posterior longitudinal ligament, lying within the vertebral canal on the posterior aspect of the vertebral body and intervertebral disc, is wider in the upper cervical spine than the lower cervical spine.[18] Superiorly, it is continuous with the tectorial membrane, and as it descends it widens over the intervertebral discs and narrows behind each vertebral body. The posterior longitudinal ligament supplies additional strength and stability to the posteromedial fibers of the anulus. There is an area of relative weakness in the posterolateral corners of the disc, however, at the junction of the posterior longitudinal ligament and uncinate process; as a result, it is the site of most cervical disc herniations.[19] According to Hayashi and colleagues,[20] the posterior longitudinal ligament is double-layered, and the deep layer sends fibers to the anulus fibrosus and continues laterally to the region of the intervertebral foramina. The superficial or more dorsal layer of the posterior longitudinal ligament is adjacent to the dura mater and continues as a connective tissue membrane, which envelops the dura mater, nerve roots, and vertebral artery, suggesting that this membrane may serve as a protective barrier.

The ligamentum flavum of the cervical spine attaches to the anterior surface of the lamina above and to the superior margin of the lamina below and extends laterally to the articular processes, contributing to the boundary of the intervertebral foramen. The ligamentum flavum consists primarily of elastic fibers, whose numbers lessen with aging, resulting in anterior buckling that can contribute to symptoms of spinal cord compression. A gap in the midline of the ligamentum flavum allows for the exit of veins.

The interspinous ligament of the cervical spine is thin and less well developed than in the lumbar region. It attaches in an oblique orientation from the posterosuperior aspect to the anteroinferior aspect of the spinous process. There is no separate supraspinous ligament in the cervical region. The ligamentum nuchae, a fibroelastic septum, is the superior continuation of the supraspinous ligament of the thoracolumbar spine and extends from the external occipital protuberance to C7.

Intervertebral Discs

Intervertebral discs are present between vertebrae except at the atlantoaxial level. Each intervertebral disc is an avascular structure that consists of the nucleus pulposus at the interior of the disc, the outer anulus fibrosus, and the cartilaginous endplates adjacent to the vertebral surfaces. The nucleus pulposus functions as a shock absorber, and the anulus fibrosus maintains the stability of the motion segment. With increasing age, the margin between the nucleus pulposus and anulus

fibrosus becomes less distinct, and often by age 50 the nucleus pulposus has become a fibrocartilaginous mass similar to the inner zone of the anulus fibrosus.[21]

The anulus has an outer collagenous layer, in which the fibers are arranged in oblique layers of lamellae. The outermost fibers of the anulus fibrosus are contiguous with the anterior and posterior longitudinal ligaments and are firmly attached to the adjacent vertebral endplates. The fibers of the lamella run perpendicular to the fibers of the adjacent lamella. The collagen fibers in the posterior portion of the disc run more vertical than oblique, and this may account for the relative frequency of radial tears seen clinically. The discs are shaped to conform to the surface of the bodies; the superior surface of the disc is concave, and the inferior surface of the disc is correspondingly convex in the coronal plane. The discs are also slightly thicker anteriorly than posteriorly, which contributes to the lordotic posture of the cervical spine. The cervical intervertebral discs allow some translational movement in the sagittal plane, but the uncinate processes resist lateral movement. The uncinate process, located in the posterolateral aspect of the disc, also helps prevent disc herniations in this area. Degeneration of the anulus fibrosus (Fig. 17–4) in the cervical region is similar to the lumbar region in that concentric, transverse, and radial tears of the anulus occur, and the radial tear in the posterior aspect of the disc may be more clinically significant.

The cartilaginous endplate is a layer of hyaline cartilage resting on the subchondral bone and serves as a barrier between the pressure of the nucleus pulposus and the adjacent

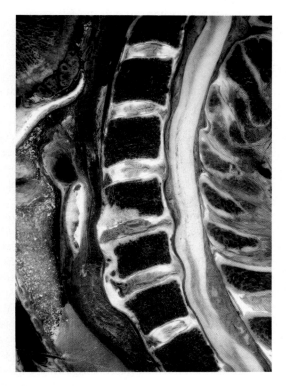

FIGURE 17–4 Mid-sagittal cryomicrotome section of degenerative cervical spine showing degeneration of anulus fibrosus and herniation of nucleus pulposus posteriorly with impingement of spinal cord.

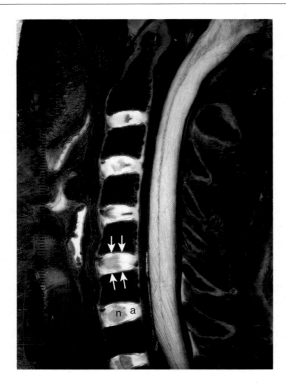

FIGURE 17–5 Mid-sagittal microtome section of cervical spine showing nucleus pulposus (n) and outer anulus fibrosus (a) of intervertebral disc. *White arrows* identify cartilaginous endplate.

vertebral bodies. This cartilage is a growth plate and responsible for endochondral ossification during growth (Fig. 17–5). The cartilaginous endplates also allow the insertion of the inner fibers of the anulus fibrosus and the diffusion of nutrients from the subchondral bone to the disc.

Neural Elements

The cervical cord emerges from the foramen magnum as a continuation of the medulla oblongata. There is considerable variation in size of the spinal cord; however, in general, owing to the increased nerve supply to the upper limbs, the cervical cord enlarges from C3 and becomes maximal at C6. Maximal transverse diameters of 13 to 14 mm have been reported,[22] with transverse areas ranging from 58.3 ± 6.7 mm^2 at C6[23] to 85.8 ± 7.2 mm^2 at C4-5.[24]

The spinal cord includes the outer white matter and the inner gray matter. The white matter of the spinal cord contains nerve fibers and glia and is divided into the posterior, lateral, and anterior columns. The posterior column includes the fasciculus cuneatus laterally and fasciculus gracilis medially, mediating proprioceptive, vibratory, and tactile sensations. The lateral column contains the descending motor lateral corticospinal and lateral spinothalamic fasciculi, and the anterior funiculus contains the ascending anterior spinothalamic tract and other descending tracts. The lateral spinothalamic tracts cross through the ventral commissure to the contralateral side of the cord, conveying pain and temperature sensations. The anterior spinothalamic tract conveys the crude touch sensation.

The gray matter of the spinal cord contains cell bodies of efferent and internuncial neurons. The somatosensory neurons are located in the posterior horn, and the somatomotor neurons are found in the anterior horn of the gray matter. The visceral center of the gray matter is found in the intermediolateral horn. In the center of the spinal cord is the central ependymal canal for the passage of cerebrospinal fluid.

The spinal cord is covered by the pia mater, which is the outer lining of the cord, and transparent arachnoid membrane that contains the cerebrospinal fluid. The dura mater is the outer covering of the spinal cord and becomes the inner layer of the cranial dura at the level of the foramen magnum. The cervical cord is anchored to the dura by the dentate ligaments that project laterally from the lateral side of the cord to the arachnoid and dura at points midway between exiting spinal nerves. By suspending the spinal cord in the cerebrospinal fluid, the dentate ligaments cushion and protect the cord, while minimizing the movement of the cord during ranges of motion. The epidural space contains fat, internal vertebral venous plexus, and loose connective tissue. This venous plexus may be involved in spreading infection or neoplasm. There is a potential space between the dura and the arachnoid, and the subarachnoid space is between the arachnoid and the pia. The subarachnoid space contains the cerebrospinal fluid, spinal blood vessels, and nerve rootlets from the spinal cord.

The dorsal sensory rootlets enter the cord through the lateral longitudinal sulcus, and the ventral motor rootlets exit the cord through the ventral lateral sulcus. The six or eight rootlets at each level leave the spinal cord laterally to lie in the lateral subarachnoid space bathed in the cerebrospinal fluid. The rootlets join to form the dorsal and ventral root, which together enter a narrow sleeve of arachnoid and pass through the dura to become a nerve root at each level. The cervical nerve roots that form from the ventral and dorsal nerve rootlet extend anterolaterally at a 45-degree angle to the coronal plane and inferiorly at about 10 degrees to the axial plane.[14] The nerve roots enter the intervertebral foramina by passing directly laterally from the spinal canal adjacent to the corresponding disc and over the top of the corresponding pedicle. The anterior root lies anteroinferiorly adjacent to the uncovertebral joint, and the posterior root is close to the superior articular process. The nerve root is positioned at the tip of the superior articular process in the medial aspect of the neural foramen, and it courses more inferiorly to position over the pedicle in the lateral aspect of the neural foramen (Fig. 17–6).

The roots occupy about one third of the foraminal space in the normal spine but much more in the degenerative spine. The roots are located in the inferior half of the neural foramen normally, but the nerve roots occupy a more cranial part of the foramina, and the size of the foramen is diminished if the neck is fully extended.[25] The upper half of the neural foramen contains fat and small veins.[26] The nerve root is enlarged in the distal aspect of the intervertebral foramen, and the dorsal root ganglion is located just distal to the foramen.[27] The dorsal root ganglion is located between the vertebral artery and a small concavity in the superior articular process. Just distal to the ganglion and outside the intervertebral foramen, the anterior and posterior roots join to form the spinal nerve. The spinal nerve divides into dorsal and ventral primary rami branches.

The gray rami from the sympathetic cervical ganglion join the ventral primary rami. There are interconnections between gray rami, the perivascular plexus around the vertebral artery, and the sympathetic trunk, all of which give contributions to the ventral nerve plexus to innervate the anterior longitudinal ligament, outer anulus fibrosus, and anterior vertebral body.[28,29] The dorsal nerve plexus receives contributions from the sinuvertebral nerves, which originate from the gray rami and perivascular plexus of the vertebral artery. The dorsal nerve plexus innervates the posterior longitudinal ligament, and the sinuvertebral nerves give branches to the posterior part of the anulus and the ventral part of the dura. The sinuvertebral nerves innervate two or more discs or motion segments.

The first cervical nerve or suboccipital nerve exits the vertebral canal above the posterior arch of the atlas and posteromedial to the lateral mass and lies between the vertebral artery and the posterior arch. The posterior primary ramus of the first cervical nerve enters the suboccipital triangle and sends motor fibers to the deep muscles. The anterior primary ramus of the first cervical nerve forms a loop with the second anterior primary ramus and sends fibers to the hypoglossal nerve. The cervical plexus receives fibers from anterior primary rami of C1-4. The cervical plexus is located opposite C1-3, ventral and lateral to the levator scapulae and middle scalene muscles. The cervical plexus has distributions to the skin and muscles, such as rectus capitis anterior and lateralis, longus capitis and cervicis, levator scapulae, and middle scalene. The cervical plexus forms loops and branches to supply the sternocleidomastoid and trapezius muscles. It has communications with the hypoglossal nerve from C1 and C2 and leaves this trunk as the superior root of the *ansa cervicalis*, which is a nerve loop that is formed with the inferior root from C2 and C3.

The second cervical nerve lies on the lamina of the axis posterior to the lateral mass, and the posterior primary ramus or the greater occipital nerve pierces the trapezius about 2 cm below the external occipital protuberance and 2 to 4 cm from the midline. Trauma or irritation to any of the three terminal nerves (the greater and lesser occipital nerve and the greater auricular nerve) can produce pain, headache, or hyperesthesia in their dermal distribution over the occiput and around the ear.

Cutaneous branches of the posterior primary rami of C2-5 are consistently present in the skin of the nuchal region, and the largest cutaneous nerve in this region is the greater occipital nerve. The lesser occipital nerve is a branch from the anterior cervical plexus and runs upward and lateral to the greater occipital nerve. The posterior primary ramus of C3 or the third occipital nerve pierces the trapezius more inferiorly and about 1 cm medial from the midline. The cervical nerve exits over the pedicle that bears the same number except the C8 cervical nerve lies between the C7 and T1 vertebrae. The posterior primary rami of cervical nerves send motor fibers to the deep muscles and sensory fibers to the skin, but the first cervical nerve has no cutaneous branches. The anterior primary rami of C1-4 form the cervical plexus, and the rami of C5-T1 form the brachial plexus.

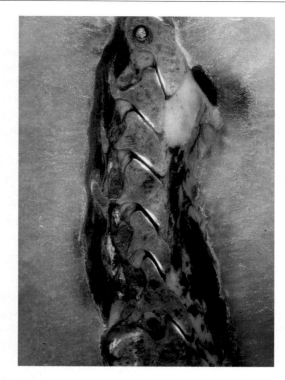

FIGURE 17–6 Parasagittal cryomicrotome section of lateral aspect of neural foramen shows nerve root coursing more inferiorly lying over pedicle as it begins to exit foramen.

Vascular Structures

The major blood supply of the cervical cord and the cervical spine is the vertebral artery. Variations of the course of the vertebral artery have been reported.[30] In most cases, the vertebral artery originates from the first part of the subclavian artery and begins its ascent behind the common carotid artery between the longus colli and the anterior scalene. In the lower cervical spine, the vertebral arteries are crossed by the inferior thyroid artery and on the left by the thoracic duct. The vertebral arteries course anterior to the ventral rami of the seventh and eighth cervical nerves and the C7 transverse process before entering the C6 transverse foramen, where they ascend within the transverse foramen of C6-C2.

The surgeon should remember that the vertebral artery is located lateral to the uncinate process and in line with the middle one third of the vertebral body just anterior to the nerve root. During anterior exposure of the vertebral body and intervertebral discs, too far lateral dissection on the inferior half of the vertebral body and uncovertebral joints would endanger the vertebral artery and spinal nerve around the intervertebral foramen. The vertebral artery may also be involved in patients with severe cervical spondylosis when it may be impinged by the osteophyte. At the level of the atlas, the artery winds posteromedially around the lateral mass and over the posterior arch of the atlas before passing through the posterior atlanto-occipital membrane into the foramen magnum, joining the other vertebral artery to form the basilar artery.

In the foramen magnum region, the vertebral artery gives branches anteriorly that join together to form the single anterior spinal artery, whereas the paired posterior spinal arteries are branches from the posterior inferior cerebellar arteries. The anterior and posterior spinal arteries are the major blood supplies of the spinal cord. The posterior spinal arteries give rise to plexiform channels that are arranged transversely on the dorsum of the cord. The anterior spinal artery supplies most of the spinal cord except the posterior columns.[31] The spinal cord also receives blood supplies from radicular arteries or medullary feeders from the vertebral arteries and ascending cervical arteries.[31] The segmental arteries that are branches of the vertebral artery are present at each level to supply the vertebrae and surrounding tissues, but only a few segmental vessels give rise to radicular arteries or medullary feeders to the spinal cord. These vessels have a variable distribution, but medullary feeders are more commonly present at C6 and C3 from the left and C5 and T1 from the right.[18]

Venous blood returns from the cord through three veins posteriorly and three veins anteriorly. The venous system within the spinal canal consists of valveless sinuses in the epidural space. The venous plexus is most apparent anteriorly just medial to the pedicles over the mid-portion of the vertebral bodies and anastomoses with the veins from the opposite side and with the basivertebral sinus, which is located in the space between the posterior longitudinal ligament and the posterior aspect of the vertebral body.

Musculature

The musculature of the cervical spine can be grouped into the anterolateral and posterior muscle groups. The anterolateral muscles of the neck include platysma muscle, sternocleidomastoid muscle, hyoid muscles, strap muscles of the larynx, scalene muscles, longus colli muscle, and longus capitis muscle. The posterior musculature is subdivided into superficial, intermediate, and deep muscle groups.[32]

The platysma is a thin muscle underneath the subcutaneous tissue that spans from the deltoid and upper pectoral fascia and crosses over the clavicle and passes obliquely upward and medially to insert to the mandible, muscles of the lip, and skin of the lower part of the face. The platysma depresses the lower jaw and the lip and tenses and ridges the skin of the neck.

The sternocleidomastoid originates from the sternum and the medial clavicle to the mastoid process and the lateral half of the superior nuchal line of the occipital bone. The second cervical nerve and the spinal accessory nerve innervate the sternocleidomastoid, which functions to draw the head toward the ipsilateral shoulder and rotate it and point the chin craniad toward the contralateral side. The sternocleidomastoid muscles together flex the head and raise the thorax when the head is fixed.

Muscles that attach to the hyoid bone include the digastric, stylohyoid, mylohyoid, geniohyoid, and omohyoid muscles; the strap muscles of the larynx include the sternohyoid and sternothyroid muscles. These muscles do not control the cervical spine but are important in controlling the movement of the hyoid and larynx and are important landmarks in the anterior approach to the cervical spine.

The longus colli and longus capitis are the prevertebral muscles of the neck. The longus colli spans from C1 to T3 and extends laterally to attach to the anterior tubercles of the transverse processes of C3-6. The longus capitis originates from the anterior tubercles of the transverse processes of C3-6 and attaches on the inferior surface of the basilar part of the occipital bone. Underneath the longus capitis, the rectus capitis anterior spans from the lateral mass of the atlas to the base of the occipital bone, and the rectus capitis lateralis runs laterally from the transverse process of the atlas to the inferior surface of the jugular process of the occipital bone.

The scalenus anterior originates from the anterior tubercles of the transverse processes of C3-6 and inserts on the first rib, and the scalenus medius originates from the posterior tubercles of the transverse processes of C2-7 and inserts on the first rib. A vascular impingement of the subclavian artery may occur as it runs between the scalenus anterior and scalenus medius as seen in the thoracic outlet syndrome. The scalenus posterior originates from the posterior tubercles of the transverse processes of C4-6 and inserts on the second rib.

The posterior muscles of the neck are divided into superficial, intermediate, and deep groups.[32] The most superficial muscle is the trapezius, which originates from the external occipital protuberance and the medial nuchal line of C7-T12 spinous processes and inserts on the spine of the scapula, the acromion, and the lateral aspect of the clavicle. The trapezius is innervated by the 11th cranial nerve and functions to extend the head. The intermediate muscles beneath the trapezius muscle are the splenius capitis and splenius cervicis, which originate from the spinous processes of the lower cervical and upper thoracic spines and insert on the transverse processes of the upper cervical spine and the mastoid process. In the deep layer, the erector spinal muscles continue into the cervical region, which includes the iliocostalis laterally; the longissimus cervicis and longissimus capitis centrally; and the spinalis cervicis, semispinalis capitis, and semispinalis cervicis medially. Beneath the semispinalis muscles lie the multifidus from C4-7 and rotatores muscles, which cross only one segment from the transverse processes to the spinous processes.

In the upper cervical spine, suboccipital muscles attach at the occiput to the second vertebra. The rectus capitis posterior major originates from the C2 spinous process and inserts to the inferior nuchal line of the occiput, and the rectus capitis posterior minor originates from the posterior tubercle of the atlas and inserts to the occiput. The obliquus capitis inferior originates from the C2 spinous process and inserts on the transverse process of the atlas, and the obliquus capitis superior originates from the transverse process of the atlas and inserts on the occiput between the superior and inferior nuchal lines. Most posterior muscles are involved in producing extension of the neck and head, and some muscles produce rotation and lateral flexion. The posterior deep muscles are innervated by the posterior primary rami, and the blood supply is by the deep cervical vessels.

Fascial Layers

The key to understanding the anterior approach to the cervical spine lies in recognizing the fascial layers of the neck, which invest the muscles and viscera and separate them into different compartments.[19] Anteriorly, the cervical fascia is divided into one superficial and four deep layers. The superficial fascia contains fat and areolar tissue, including the platysma muscle, external jugular vein, and cutaneous sensory nerves. The deep cervical fascia, including the outer investing layer of deep fascia, middle cervical fascia, and prevertebral fascia, compartmentalizes the structures deep to the superficial fascia. The superficial layer of the deep fascia extends from the trapezius muscle over the posterior triangle and splits to enclose the sternocleidomastoid muscle. The middle layers of the deep cervical fascia enclose the strap muscles and omohyoid and extend as far laterally as the scapula. The deeper middle layer is the visceral fascia that surrounds the thyroid gland, larynx, trachea, pharynx, and esophagus. The alar fascia spreads behind the esophagus and surrounds the carotid sheath structures laterally. The carotid sheath encloses the carotid artery, internal jugular vein, and vagus nerve. The deepest layer of the deep fascia is the prevertebral fascia, which covers the scaleni muscles, longus colli muscles, and anterior longitudinal ligament.

Understanding these fascial planes also helps localize the source of cervical infections. Abscesses originating from either the vertebral body or the intervertebral disc generally start in the midline, whereas abscesses that are pharyngeal in origin tend to occur lateral to the midline. This is because the prevertebral fascia and alar fascia are fused laterally over the transverse processes but not in the midline. If this infection breaks through the prevertebral fascia, it can spread inferiorly between the alar fascia and prevertebral fascia into the posterior mediastinum. With pharyngeal infections, the opposite occurs because the visceral fascia and alar fascia are fused in the midline; these abscesses tend to occur laterally, on either side of the midline.

Triangles of the Neck

The cervical region is divided into two anatomic compartments, the anterior and posterior triangles, by the sternocleidomastoid. The anterior triangle is formed by the midline anteriorly, the anterior border of the sternocleidomastoid posteriorly, and the inferior border of the mandible superiorly. The posterior triangle is bound anteriorly by the posterior border of the sternocleidomastoid, posteriorly by the anterior border of the trapezius, and inferiorly by the middle third of the clavicle. Understanding the structures within the triangles and their complex relationship helps the surgeon to learn these important landmarks during surgical approaches to the neck.[5]

The anterior triangle is subdivided further into the digastric (submandibular), carotid, and muscular triangles. The digastric triangle, so called because it is bound by the two bellies of the digastric muscle and inferior border of the mandible, contains the submandibular gland; facial artery and vein; mylohyoid artery and nerve; and, posteriorly, a portion of the parotid gland and external carotid artery. Lying deeper in the digastric triangle is the internal carotid artery, jugular vein, and glossopharyngeal and vagus nerves. The carotid and muscular triangles are separated by the superior belly of the omohyoid muscle. The carotid triangle contains the carotid artery and its bifurcation; the superior thyroid, lingual, and facial branches of the external carotid artery; and the internal jugular vein. It also contains the ansa cervicalis; portions of cranial nerves X, XI, and XII; and the larynx, pharynx, and superior laryngeal nerve.

The posterior triangle is subdivided into the occipital and supraclavicular triangles by the inferior belly of the omohyoid muscle. The posterior triangle contains the accessory nerve, the brachial plexus, the third part of the subclavian artery, the dorsal scapular nerve, the long thoracic nerve, the nerve to the subclavius, the suprascapular nerve, and the transverse cervical artery.[18]

The brachial plexus travels behind the inferior belly of the omohyoid, crossing between the anterior and middle scalene muscles and over the first rib and beneath the clavicle. Its location in the posterior triangle can be identified by drawing a line from the posterior margin of the sternocleidomastoid at the level of the cricoid cartilage to the midpoint of the clavicle. The accessory nerve lies on the levator scapula on the floor of the posterior triangle. Emerging from behind the posterior border of the sternocleidomastoid muscle are the lesser occipital, greater auricular, and supraclavicular nerves. The subclavian artery lies inferior to the inferior belly of the omohyoid in the subclavian triangle and courses behind the anterior scalene laterally toward the border of the first rib.

Surgical Approaches

Although surgical approaches to the cervical spine are well described in the literature, certain approaches are more commonly used than others. A decision to use a particular approach should take into account the site of the pathologic process, the health of the patient, and the skill and comfort level of the surgeon with that specific exposure. An understanding of the advantages and limitations of each surgical exposure can help improve patient outcome and reduce complications. In this section, anterior and posterior operative approaches from the occiput to the cervicothoracic junction are described with their associated complications.

Anterior Approaches to Upper Cervical Spine

The complex anatomy of the upper neck makes adequate and safe exposure of the upper cervical spine challenging. The two main techniques are transoral and retropharyngeal exposures. If necessary, both techniques can be combined with a mandibulotomy or dislocation of the temporomandibular joint to gain additional local exposure.

The transoral approach provides anterior exposure to the atlantoaxial complex. Inferior exposure down to C3-4 can be obtained with the addition of a lip-splitting approach with mandibulotomy, whereas superior exposure up to the clivus of the occiput can be obtained by splitting the uvula, soft palate, and posterior pharyngeal wall.[33,34] If necessary, a portion of the hard palate can also be cut with a rongeur. Thoughtful placement of a self-retaining retractor system also facilitates exposure by retraction of the hard and soft palate and tongue.

Several variations to the retropharyngeal exposure have been described and can be divided into anteromedial and anterolateral approaches depending on the relationship of the dissection to the carotid sheath.[35-37] The anteromedial retropharyngeal approach uses the interval medial (anterior) to the carotid sheath, whereas the anterolateral approach uses the plane lateral (posterior) to the carotid sheath. In both cases, a thorough understanding of the local anatomy is imperative. For right-handed surgeons, the approach is typically from the patient's right side. At this level, above C5 the recurrent laryngeal nerve has already crossed the surgical field from lateral to medial and runs safely within the tracheoesophageal groove.

Transoral Technique

For the transoral technique, prophylactic antibiotics are given immediately preoperatively and 72 hours postoperatively based on preoperative nasopharyngeal culture and sensitivity studies. Care must be exercised during this approach to stay in the midline and develop full-thickness pharyngomucosal flaps. A vertical incision is made through the posterior pharyngeal mucosa, the constrictors, and the longus colli muscle with the anterior arch of the atlas as the landmark. After adequate superior and inferior exposure is obtained, subperiosteal lateral dissection is done to expose the medial edge of the C1-2 facet joint. Dissection beyond the lateral edge of the C1-2 facet risks injury to the vertebral artery, which usually lies at a minimum of 20 mm from the midline.[38]

In a pure transoral approach, exposure is limited by the amount that the retractors can open the oral cavity. The addition of a mandibulotomy can increase exposure significantly. The mandibulotomy is achieved with a midline incision of the lower lip around the chin in a C-shaped fashion and then straight down to the hyoid bone to expose the mandible subperiosteally.[39] When this is done, a reconstruction plate is bent, and the screw holes in the mandible are drilled before the mandibular osteotomy is done; this decreases the risk of postoperative malocclusion. The plate should be placed low on the mandible to decrease the risk of injuring the dental roots by the drill. The mandibulotomy is performed between the central incisors. If the decision is made also to split the tongue, this should be done in the midline, with care taken not to injure the epiglottis.[39]

Complications

Reported results with this exposure are variable. Although access to the upper cervical vertebra through this approach is relatively direct, the potential for significant morbidity and mortality exists owing to the risk of infection by pharyngeal flora, the confined working area, and the lack of extensile exposure.[40] Complications can be minimized with careful patient selection and proper surgical technique.

Infection is a frequently reported complication with the transoral approach,[41] particularly with extensive resections and use of bone graft. Direct contamination and septic encephalomeningitis can occur through direct exposure or opening of the dura. In a series reported by Fang and Ong[41] in six patients who underwent extensive vertebral body resection and bone grafting, four developed wound infections, and one developed encephalomeningitis. Using perioperative antibiotics, limiting the use of bone graft when possible, and minimizing the exposure and resection can help decrease these risks. The use of a nasogastric tube postoperatively for 5 days until evidence of mucosal healing may decrease wound contamination.

Difficulty with wound closure may occur, especially if the incision is extended inferiorly to C3. At this level, the overlying tissues can be thin and intimately adherent to the underlying vertebral body. Difficulty with wound closure can also occur if bone grafting is excessive or placed improperly. This difficulty can be managed by ensuring that the grafts are recessed beyond the anterior margin of the vertebral body or by creating lateral flaps to help provide additional tissue length to assist in coverage.

Venous hemorrhage from epidural veins can typically be controlled with the use of cellulose and cottonoid patties. Arterial hemorrhage owing to injury to the vertebral artery or its branches can be more problematic. Excessive or uncontrolled bleeding can occur if the dissection is not performed subperiosteally or strays too lateral into the vertebral arteries. Life-threatening hemorrhage or basilar artery ischemia, especially in elderly patients, can result. Tamponade of the bleeding with hemostatic agents and bone wax may result in a false aneurysm or late bleeding requiring urgent surgery or balloon embolization.[38] Uncontrolled bleeding often requires emergent balloon embolization or immediate surgical exposure of the vertebral artery in the foramen transversarium for ligation.

After surgery, the airway remains at risk from edema, hemorrhage, or continued drainage. Careful intraoperative placement of retractors to ensure that the tongue and lips are not trapped and the application of topical hydrocortisone can help decrease postoperative oropharyngeal edema. If a tongue-splitting approach is planned, a tracheotomy should be considered. Care is taken postoperatively not to extubate these patients prematurely. Studying the soft tissue shadow for swelling on the lateral cervical radiographs may help assist in the decision to extubate postoperatively.

Anteromedial Retropharyngeal Technique

Described by deAndrade and McNab in 1969[36] and later by McAfee and colleagues in 1987,[35] the anteromedial retropharyngeal approach is the superior extension of the anteromedial approach to the lower cervical spine as described by Southwick and Robinson.[42] Similar to the anteromedial approach to the lower cervical spine, familiarity with the fascial planes is vital to understanding the approach. These planes include (1) the superficial fascia containing the platysma; (2) the superficial layer of the deep fascia extending from the sternocleidomastoid anteriorly and enclosing the trapezius posteriorly; (3) the middle layer of the deep fascia covering the strap muscles and omohyoid and visceral fascia surrounding the thyroid gland, larynx, trachea, pharynx, and esophagus; and (4) the deep layer of the cervical fascia, which includes the alar fascia connecting the two carotid sheaths laterally and fusing in the midline to the visceral fascia and the prevertebral fascia covering the scaleni and longus colli muscles and the anterior longitudinal ligament (Fig. 17–7).

A transverse submandibular incision is used in this approach, or, alternatively, an incision is made along the anterior aspect of the sternocleidomastoid muscle and curved toward the mastoid process (Fig. 17–8A). The platysma and the superficial layer of the deep cervical fascia are divided in line with the incision to expose the anterior border of the sternocleidomastoid (Fig. 17–8B). With the help of a nerve stimulator, the marginal mandibular branch of the facial nerve (cranial nerve VII) is isolated and protected. Because the branches of the mandibular nerve are superficial to the lateral crossing veins, ligating the retromandibular vein as it joins the internal jugular vein and keeping the dissection deep and inferior to the vein during the exposure help protect the superficial branch of the facial nerve.

Next, the superficial layer of the deep cervical fascia is incised anterior to the sternocleidomastoid, and the carotid sheath is identified by palpating for the carotid pulse. The digastric lymph nodes and salivary gland are resected, and the salivary duct is sutured to prevent a fistula. The stylohyoid and digastric muscle are identified and ligated to help mobilize the hyoid bone to improve exposure. Injury to the facial nerve may occur with excessive superior traction of the stylohyoid muscle. The nerve stimulator is used to identify and completely mobilize the hypoglossal nerve, which is retracted superiorly.

The retropharyngeal space is entered by using blunt dissection to develop the plane between the carotid sheath laterally and the visceral fascia containing the larynx and pharynx medially. Exposure can be improved by sequentially ligating tethering branches of the carotid artery and jugular vein, which may include the superior thyroid artery and vein, lingual artery and vein, ascending pharyngeal artery and vein, and facial artery and vein (Fig. 17–8C). The superior laryngeal nerve is identified, protected, and mobilized as it travels from its origin near the nodose ganglion into the larynx.

The prevertebral fascia overlying the vertebral body, intervertebral disc, and longus colli are now visible (Fig. 17–8D). The two longus colli converge in the midline on the anterior tubercle of the atlas. Because the hypoglossal, glossopharyngeal, vagus, and accessory nerves and the internal carotid artery and jugular vein are tethered to the occiput as they exit their respective foramina, they can be injured with vigorous retraction or greater than 2 cm lateral dissection from the midline. Additionally, excess anterior retraction of the pharynx can result in injury to the pharyngeal and laryngeal branches of the vagus nerve. At this point, a midline incision over the basiocciput, atlas, and axis can be performed, and the anterior longitudinal ligament and longus colli muscle can be dissected subperiosteally to obtain lateral exposure to the cervical spine.

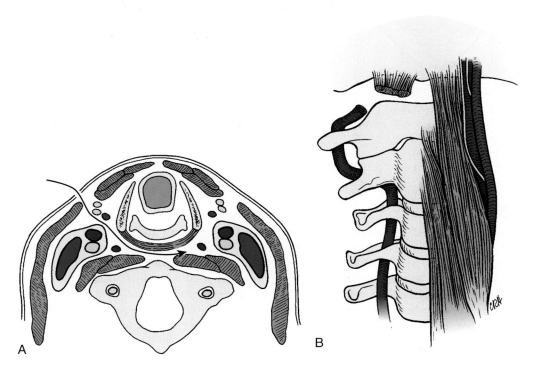

FIGURE 17–7 Anteromedial approach to upper cervical spine. **A,** Dissection is done through retropharyngeal approach as extension of Southwick-Robinson approach to lower cervical spine. **B,** Longus colli muscle is retracted to expose anterior tubercle of atlas and body of axis.

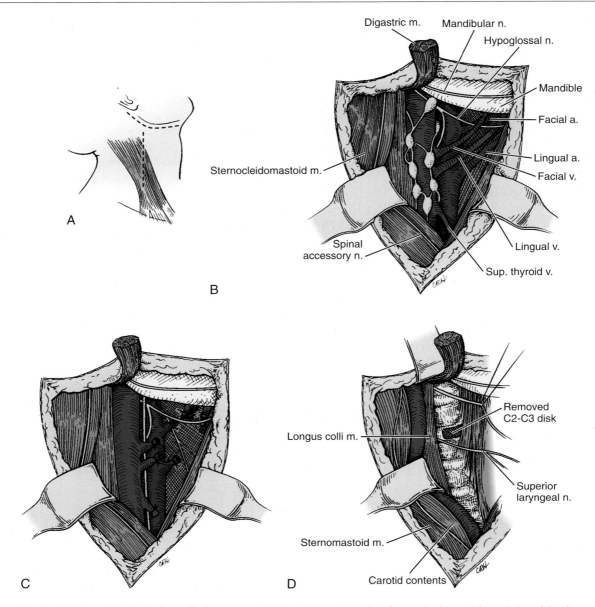

FIGURE 17-8 A, Right-sided submandibular transverse incision. **B,** Anterior border of sternocleidomastoid muscle is mobilized, and digastric tendon is divided. Submandibular salivary gland and jugular digastric lymph nodes are resected. Hypoglossal nerve is identified and mobilized. **C,** Carotid sheath is opened, and arterial and venous branches are ligated. **D,** Superior laryngeal nerve is identified and protected.

Anterolateral Retropharyngeal Technique

Described by Whitesides and Kelly,[43] the anterolateral retropharyngeal approach provides exposure of the upper cervical spine by partially transecting the sternocleidomastoid and proceeding laterally and posterior to the carotid sheath (Fig. 17–9). As a result, the major branches of the external carotid and laryngeal nerves are not disturbed. Although this exposure allows for distal extension to include T1, its superior extension is limited to the ring of the atlas. Because the internal carotid artery; jugular vein; and vagus, accessory, and hypoglossal nerves are tethered to the skull, adequate retraction necessary to expose the basiocciput would result in injury to these structures.

A longitudinal skin incision is made from the mastoid extending distally and anteriorly along the anterior aspect of the sternocleidomastoid muscle. The external jugular vein is identified and ligated, and the greater auricular nerve running parallel to the external jugular vein is spared if possible. The sternocleidomastoid now is prominent; if only a limited exposure (C1-2) is required, consideration can be given to preserving the sternocleidomastoid. In most cases, the sternocleidomastoid and splenius capitis muscles are detached from the mastoid, leaving a fascial edge for later repair. The spinal accessory nerve enters the sternocleidomastoid approximately 3 cm distal to the mastoid tip and should be identified and protected.[43]

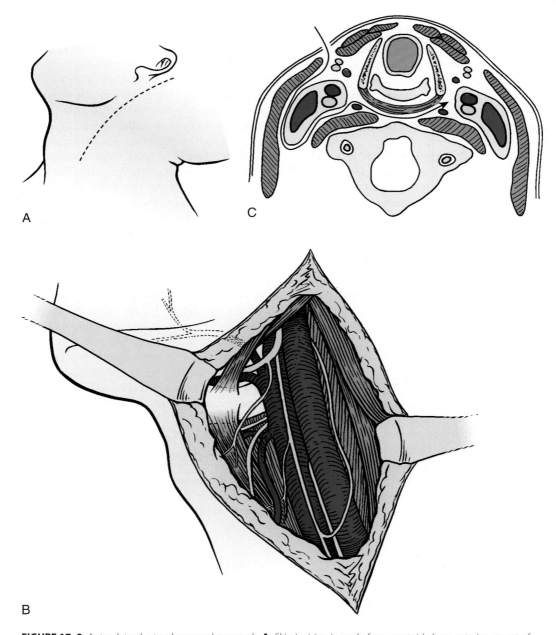

FIGURE 17–9 Anterolateral retropharyngeal approach. **A,** Skin incision is made from mastoid along anterior aspect of sternocleidomastoid. **B,** This approach involves dissection anterior to sternocleidomastoid but posterior to carotid sheath. **C,** Neurovascular structures that are encountered in this approach include carotid contents and branches, superior laryngeal nerves, hypoglossal nerve, and ansa cervicalis.

Next, one can proceed laterally and posterior to the carotid sheath and dissect it free from the sternocleidomastoid. The carotid contents are retracted along with the hypoglossal nerve anteriorly and the sternocleidomastoid muscle and accessory nerve posteriorly. The plane between the alar and prevertebral fascia is developed with blunt dissection to expose the transverse processes and anterior aspect of C1-3. The most pronounced bony prominence laterally is the transverse process of C1. Although the basiocciput, clivus, and sphenoid may be palpated through this approach, they are poorly visualized.

When the appropriate level is identified, a midline longitudinal incision is made in the middle of the vertebral body, and the ligament and overlying muscles are dissected subperiosteally and laterally. Alternatively, if more lateral exposure is needed, the longus colli and capitis muscles can be separated from their bony insertion on the transverse process and retracted anteriorly. This provides direct exposure to the nerve roots, transverse processes, and vertebral artery but disturbs the sympathetic rami communicantes and may cause Horner syndrome.

Complications

Complications common to the anterolateral and the anteromedial retropharyngeal approaches include airway obstruction, hemorrhage, and nerve injury. Airway obstruction and difficulty swallowing secondary to hematoma or edema of the pharynx and larynx can be an immediate life-threatening complication. Typically, nasotracheal intubation is adequate; however, a tracheostomy can be considered either preoperatively or postoperatively for airway management if this complication is expected or encountered. Hemorrhage from the carotid artery, jugular vein, or their branches can occur and can be difficult to control.

Laryngeal and pharyngeal dysfunction can result from retraction of the laryngeal nerves. Patients should be advised preoperatively to expect difficulty with phonation and swallowing, especially in the early postoperative course. Problems can persist if the external branch of the superior laryngeal nerve is sacrificed or is transected. In three of five cases reported by deAndrade and McNab,[36] persistent postoperative hoarseness, laryngeal fatigue, and inability to produce high tones persisted. Nerve injury to the spinal accessory nerve can occur particularly with the anterolateral retropharyngeal approach. Care should be taken to identify and protect this nerve intraoperatively because weakness to the sternocleidomastoid and trapezius muscle can result.

Anterior Exposure of Lower Cervical Spine

Similar to approaches to the upper cervical spine, anterior exposures to the lower cervical spine can be divided into anterolateral and anteromedial approaches based on their relationship to the carotid sheath. First described by Southwick and Robinson,[42] the anteromedial approach employs the interval between the sternocleidomastoid laterally and the strap muscles and tracheoesophageal complex medially and is used in most cases. In special circumstances, the anterolateral approach described by Henry[44] and Hogson[45] may be used. Hogson[45] described an approach to the lower cervical spine in which dissection was done posterior to the carotid sheath to expose the anterior and lateral aspects. Verbiest[46] described a modification of the original approach for the exposure of the vertebral artery. Dissection anterior to the carotid sheath, as in the anteromedial Smith-Robinson technique, provides more lateral exposure to the cervical spine and may be better in cases in which the lesion is localized more laterally or if the vertebral artery must be exposed. The spinal nerve can also be identified posterior to the vertebral artery (Fig. 17–10).

To minimize injury to the recurrent laryngeal nerve, the cervical spine is often approached from the left, particularly at the C6-T1 region. Although a right-handed surgeon may prefer the right-sided approach, the recurrent laryngeal nerve is at greater risk of injury because it may leave the carotid sheath at a higher level on the right side. The hyoid bone overlies the third vertebra, the thyroid cartilage overlies the C4-5 intervertebral disc space, and the cricoid ring is at the C6 vertebra (Fig. 17–11).[5] In many cases, when the neck is in a significantly extended position, these landmarks may be displaced inferior in relationship to the vertebral bodies, and moving the incision slightly higher can help accommodate for the shift. A horizontal incision is used in most cases, but a vertical incision anterior to the sternocleidomastoid may be necessary in cases in which multiple levels need to be exposed.

Anteromedial Approach

For the anteromedial approach, a transverse incision in line with the skin crease is made from the midline beyond the anterior aspect of the sternocleidomastoid muscle. The skin

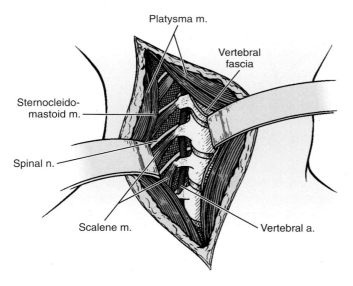

FIGURE 17–10 Verbiest's approach. Sternocleidomastoid and carotid sheath are identified and retracted laterally, and visceral structures are retracted medially. Anterior tubercle of transverse process is identified by palpation. Muscular insertions of longus colli, longus capitis, and anterior scalene are dissected sharply to bone, and anterior tubercle is cleared of soft tissues. Costotransverse lamellae can be resected to provide exposure to vertebral artery and spinal nerve lying posteriorly.

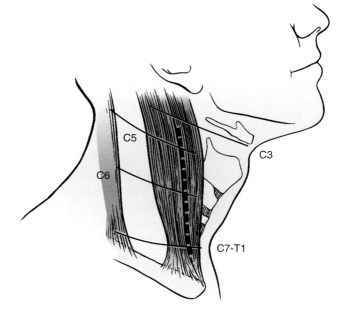

FIGURE 17–11 Surface anatomy can help identify approximate level of vertebral bodies in cervical spine. Hyoid bone overlies C3, thyroid cartilage overlies C5, cricoid ring is at C6, and supraclavicular level is in C7-T1 region.

and subcutaneous tissue are undermined slightly, and division of the platysma muscle is completed. The platysma muscle may be divided either horizontally or vertically. Retraction of the divided muscle exposes the sternocleidomastoid muscle laterally and strap muscles medially. The anterior and external jugular veins may be encountered and can be ligated to improve exposure. The deep cervical fascia is divided between the sternocleidomastoid muscle and strap muscles, and blunt finger dissection is done through the pretracheal fascia while palpating and retracting the carotid sheath laterally.

A self-retaining retractor is positioned to expose the prevertebral fascia and longus colli muscles. One must be careful not to enter the carotid sheath laterally to avoid injury to the carotid artery, internal jugular vein, or vagus nerve. Great caution should also be exercised medially because the strap muscles surround the thyroid gland, trachea, and esophagus. The surgical dissection should not enter the plane between the trachea and esophagus because the recurrent laryngeal nerve is at risk. A sharp self-retaining retractor should be avoided to prevent perforation of the esophagus medially. It is also important to check for the temporal arterial pulse when the retractor is spread because prolonged occlusion of the carotid artery may cause brain ischemia and stroke. The superior thyroid artery is encountered above C4, and the inferior thyroid artery is seen below C6. These vessels should be identified and ligated as necessary. One should also be aware of the thoracic duct below C7 during the left-sided approach. Further dissection is performed by palpating the prominent disc margins ("hills") and concave anterior vertebral bodies ("valleys").

An 18-gauge needle with two 90-degree bends to prevent spinal canal penetration is placed in the disc space, and a lateral radiograph is taken. When the correct level is confirmed, the exposure is completed by dividing the pretracheal fascia and anterior longitudinal ligament in the midline to minimize bleeding and prevent injury to the sympathetic chain and subperiosteal mobilization of the longus colli laterally. Too vigorous lateral dissection may damage the vertebral artery or nerve roots, especially at the level of the intervertebral disc space.[19] At the level of the vertebral body, the anterior aspect of the foramen transversarium offers some protection to the vertebral artery.

Anterolateral Approach

By performing the dissection posterior to the carotid sheath, the anterolateral approach avoids the thyroid vessel, vagus nerve, and superior laryngeal nerve and provides access to the anterior and lateral aspect of the cervical spine. Superior extension of this approach allows access to the upper cervical spine as described by Whitesides and Kelly[43] (see anterior retropharyngeal approach to upper cervical spine). A transverse or oblique skin incision is made from the right side. The subcutaneous tissue and the platysma muscle are divided, and the branches of the external jugular vein are ligated, but the cutaneous nerves should be protected if possible. The posterior border of the sternocleidomastoid muscle is identified, and blunt dissection should follow the fat pad through the posterior triangle of the cervical spine. The dissection should

stay anterior to the anterior scalene muscle and anterior to the anterior tubercle of the transverse process to avoid injuries to the vertebral artery or nerve root. If retraction of the sternocleidomastoid muscle is difficult, the posterior third and the omohyoid muscle can be divided to enhance exposure. The cervical sympathetic plexus on the lateral aspect of the prevertebral musculature should be identified and protected. The prevertebral fascia and longus colli muscle are incised in the midline for subperiosteal exposure of the cervical spine. After palpation of the anterior tubercle of the transverse process, the anterior tubercle can be removed to gain access to the vertebral artery and venous plexus.

Complications

The most devastating complication is neurologic deterioration. Most spinal cord or nerve root injuries are associated with technical mishaps. In myelopathic patients, attention should be paid to proper positioning of the neck, fiberoptic nasotracheal awake intubation, and intraoperative monitoring of the spinal cord function. Utmost care should be taken when removing osteophytes and disc material in the lateral corner near the uncovertebral joint to avoid nerve root injury. If removal of the posterior longitudinal ligament or osteophytes is necessary because of perforating disc fragments or large osteophytes, an operating microscope should be used. If neurologic complications are discovered postoperatively, one should administer dexamethasone and obtain a lateral radiograph to determine the position of the bone graft. Computed tomography (CT) or magnetic resonance imaging (MRI) may be valuable in determining hematoma or cord contusion. If hematoma or bone graft is suspected to be the cause of postoperative myelopathy, expeditious re-exploration is required.

Airway obstruction after extubation may occur in the postoperative period. One must be certain that the patient can exchange air before extubation. In cases in which multiple vertebrectomy has been performed with retraction of soft tissues for a prolonged period, intubation should continue for a few days until retropharyngeal edema subsides. Corticosteroids may be used to decrease edema in these cases. Postoperatively, a patient who underwent a prolonged operation for decompression of the spinal cord should be intubated for 2 to 3 days until retropharyngeal edema subsides. Corticosteroids may decrease severe edema in the postoperative period. Airway obstruction and difficulty with swallowing because of retropharyngeal edema may require reintubation or tracheostomy.

Serious bleeding complications after anterior cervical surgery are rare, but hematoma-related wound complications are common, with an incidence of 9% in one series. Arterial bleeding from the superior or inferior thyroid artery can be prevented by careful identification and ligation during surgery. Care should be taken not to dissect too far laterally because the vertebral artery is in danger along with the nerve roots. Tears on the vertebral artery should be repaired by direct exposure of the vessel in the foramen rather than merely packing the bleeding site. Injuries to the carotid artery or internal jugular vein are exceedingly rare. A hematoma rarely may be responsible for airway obstruction or spinal cord compression. The patient should have the head elevated in the immediate postoperative period because the source of bleeding is frequently venous. Meticulous hemostasis and placement of a drain should be routine to prevent these complications.

Esophageal perforation is a rare but serious complication of anterior cervical spine fusion, occurring in about 1 of 500 procedures. Sharp retractors must be avoided, and gentle handling of the medial soft structures is mandatory. In revision cases, the use of a nasogastric tube may help identify the esophagus intraoperatively. If perforation is suspected during surgery, methylene blue can be injected for better visualization. The perforation is frequently not recognized until the patient develops an abscess, tracheoesophageal fistula, or mediastinitis in the postoperative period.[47] The usual treatment consists of intravenous antibiotics, nasogastric feeding, drainage, débridement, and repair. Early consultation with head and neck surgeons is recommended.

Minor hoarseness or sore throat after anterior cervical fusion may be due to edema or endotracheal intubation and occurs in nearly half of the patients. Recurrent laryngeal nerve palsy may be the cause of persistent hoarseness, however, in a few patients. The incidence is about 1%, but in one report it was 11%. The superior laryngeal nerve is a branch of the inferior ganglion of the vagus nerve and travels along with the superior thyroid artery to innervate the cricothyroid muscle. Damage to this nerve may result in hoarseness but often produces symptoms such as easy fatiguing of the voice. The inferior laryngeal nerve is a recurrent branch of the vagus nerve that innervates all laryngeal muscles except the cricothyroid.

On the left side, the recurrent laryngeal nerve loops under the arch of the aorta and is protected in the left tracheoesophageal groove. On the right side, the recurrent nerve travels around the subclavian artery, passing dorsomedial to the side of the trachea and esophagus. It is vulnerable as it passes from the subclavian artery to the right tracheoesophageal groove. The recurrent laryngeal nerve should be located when working from C6 downward. The best guideline to its location is the inferior thyroid artery. The nerve usually enters the tracheoesophageal groove where the inferior thyroid artery enters the lower pole of the thyroid. It is also more common for the right inferior laryngeal nerve to be nonrecurrent where it travels directly from the vagus nerve and carotid sheath to the larynx. The incidence of nonrecurrent laryngeal nerve on the right side is reported as 1%.

If hoarseness persists for more than 6 weeks after anterior cervical surgery, laryngoscopy should be done to evaluate the vocal cord and laryngeal muscles. Treatment of inferior laryngeal nerve should include waiting at least 6 months for spontaneous recovery of function to occur. Further treatment or surgery by the otolaryngologist may be necessary in persistent cases.

Injury to the sympathetic chain may result in Horner syndrome. The cervical sympathetic chain lies on the anterior surface of the longus colli muscles posterior to the carotid sheath. Subperiosteal dissection is important to prevent damage to these nerves. Horner syndrome is usually temporary but may be permanent in some cases. The incidence of permanent Horner syndrome is less than 1%. Ophthalmologic consultation may be needed for treatment of ptosis.

Anterior Approach to Cervicothoracic Junction

Anterior approaches to the cervicothoracic junction are challenging because of the proximity of the great vessels and overlying sternum and clavicle (Fig. 17–12). Three main approaches have been described to address access in this region: the modified anterior approach, the sternal-splitting approach, and the transthoracic approach.[48-50] Each approach has its own advantages and disadvantages and should be chosen accordingly. Theoretically, the modified anterior approach can provide visualization and access to the anterior spinal structures from C4 to T4 but requires resection of the medial clavicle and sternoclavicular joint. Similarly, the sternal-splitting approach when combined with the anteromedial approach to the neck offers access from C4 to T4 through retraction of the great vessels. Although the transthoracic approach provides adequate exposure to the upper thoracic spine, access to the cervical spine is limited to C7 at best. This approach generally provides limited access to the cervical spine.

Modified Anterior Approach

The patient is positioned supine on the operating table with a bump between the scapula. Typically, an angled incision is used for this approach. The transverse limb is made 2 to 5 cm proximal to and parallel to the left clavicle extending from the midline to the lateral border of the sternocleidomastoid. The vertical limb runs from the medial aspect of the transverse incision and extends just distally past the manubriosternal junction. The platysma is divided in line with the skin incision and undermined proximally and distally to mobilize the muscle. The superficial veins and external jugular vein are cauterized as necessary for exposure.

The strap muscles and sternocleidomastoid are dissected and divided subperiosteally off the medial clavicle and manubrium and retracted proximally. With care taken to avoid the subclavian vein, the clavicle is osteotomized at the junction of the middle and medial third and disarticulated from the manubrium. In some cases, the inferior thyroid vein may lie medially in the surgical field and require ligation for exposure.

Next, the interval is developed between the carotid sheath laterally and the strap muscles, esophagus, and trachea medially. The recurrent laryngeal nerve muscle must be identified from the right-sided approach, whereas the thoracic duct must be protected and spared with the left-sided approach. At this level, the recurrent laryngeal nerve already lies safely within the tracheoesophageal groove with a left-sided approach.

With the use of hand-held retractors, the cervicothoracic junction can now be accessed by carefully mobilizing the esophagus, trachea, and right brachiocephalic artery and vein toward the patient's right, while the left carotid sheath and brachiocephalic and subclavian veins are retracted to the left.

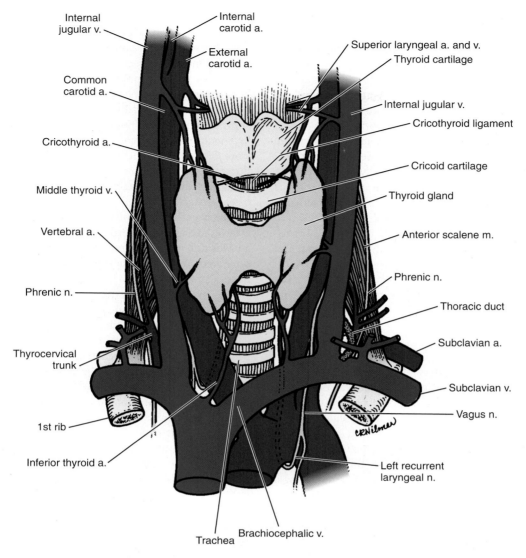

FIGURE 17–12 Anterior access to cervicothoracic junction is complicated by proximity of great vessels and associated neural structures.

The prevertebral fascia overlying the anterior aspect of the vertebrae from C4 to T4 can now be visualized.

Sternal-Splitting Approach

Combined with the anteromedial approach to the cervical spine, the sternal-splitting approach provides access to the cervicothoracic junction from C4 to T4, particularly in obese or muscular patients. A vertical skin incision is made anterior to the left sternocleidomastoid muscle and extended along the midline from the suprasternal notch proximally to the xiphoid process distally. Proximally, after division of the platysma muscle and superficial cervical fascia, blunt dissection is performed between the laterally situated carotid sheath and medial visceral structures. Distally, the subcutaneous soft tissue over the sternum is divided in line with the skin incision, and the retrosternal space is developed with blunt finger dissection; this helps reflect the parietal pleura from the posterior surface of the sternum and costal cartilage. The sternum

is cut longitudinally with an oscillating saw. The inferior thyroid vein located just proximal to the suprasternal notch must be avoided. A self-retainer is inserted to split the sternum.

Blunt dissection is performed from the cranial toward the caudal portion until the left brachiocephalic vein is exposed. As in the modified anterior approach to the cervicothoracic junction (see earlier), the esophagus, trachea, left carotid sheath, left subclavian artery, and brachiocephalic vein are retracted to the patient's left, whereas the esophagus, trachea, and right brachiocephalic artery and vein are mobilized to the right. The prevertebral fascia can now be divided in the midline to provide access to the C4-T4 vertebral bodies.

Transthoracic Approach

With the patient positioned in the left lateral decubitus position, the right chest is prepared and draped. The bony prominences are padded accordingly, and a left roll is placed in the axilla to prevent neurovascular compromise to the left upper extremity. A right-sided approach is preferred because of the location of the great vessels and heart in the left-sided approach. A standard thoracotomy centered on the third rib provides access to the upper thoracic vertebra, but exposure to the low cervical region is restricted. A first or second rib level entry does not improve access because these ribs are much shorter, and the scapula interferes posteriorly.

The incision is made beginning at the anterior axillary line and extending posteriorly to the lateral border of the paraspinal muscles. The scapula is retracted laterally by dividing the trapezius and latissimus dorsi muscles. The subscapular space is developed with blunt dissection, and the third rib is identified by counting down from the thoracic inlet.

While the neurovascular bundle of the intercostals is protected, the appropriate rib is subperiosteally dissected out and resected anteriorly and posteriorly as far as possible. A rib spreader is inserted, and the lung is retracted anteriorly. The parietal pleura is incised overlying the vertebral artery, making sure to identify the segmental vessels.

Complications

Postoperative weakness secondary to weakness of the shoulder girdle musculature from the joint resection can occur. The thoracic duct should be identified if approached from the left. If damaged, the thoracic duct should be doubly ligated proximally and distally to prevent chylothorax. Great caution should be taken to avoid injuries to the sympathetic nerves, the cupola of the pleura at the level of T1, the great vessels, and the thoracic duct, which passes into the left venous angle between the subclavian artery and the common carotid artery. Potential complications of this approach include restriction of scapular movement and paralysis of intercostal muscles owing to the muscle-splitting aspects of this dissection. We recommend use of this approach in older patients and perhaps in patients with malignant conditions.

Posterior Approaches

Posterior exposures to the cervical spine are among the safest and most used exposures for management of cervical spine disorders, allowing direct access to the posterior elements from the occiput to the thoracic spine.[5,51] The particular anatomy of the upper cervical spine and the transitional anatomy of the cervicothoracic junction should also be understood when approaching these regions posteriorly.

Posterior Approach to Upper Cervical Spine

The posterior approach to the upper cervical spine uses an internervous plane in the midline that separates the muscles from the segmental innervation supplied by the right and left posterior rami of the cervical nerves. Staying in the midline, within the plane of the ligamentum nuchae, a relatively avascular structure, minimizes bleeding and the risk of injury to surrounding neurovascular structures, while providing a stout tissue layer for tissue closure at the end of the case.

The approach to the occipitocervical junction is not commonly used, but may be the primary procedure for stabilization of basilar impression, tumor, or fractures of the odontoid with a concurrent fracture of C1. Bony landmarks can help determine the appropriate level. The external occipital protuberance and the spinous process of C2 can typically be easily palpated, and the incision can be made from the inion caudad approximately 8 cm. The dissection is continued through the ligamentum nuchae, and the paraspinal muscles are stripped from C3 to the occiput. The surgeon should be cautious when dissecting at the inferior edge of the foramen magnum because uncontrollable bleeding may be encountered. Sharp subperiosteal dissection of the external occipital protuberance and lamina is performed, and care is taken to protect the vertebral arteries at the lateral border of the atlas. With a fine curet or an elevator, the posterior atlanto-occipital ligament can be separated from the posterior lip of the foramen magnum if necessary.

The greater occipital nerve (C2) and the third occipital nerve cross the field and course laterally in the paracervical muscles. Subperiosteal dissection and avoidance of vigorous lateral dissection should prevent injury to these nerves. If occipital fixation is required, the inion is thickest at its prominence near the ridge, and the passage of wires is possible without violating both tables of the occiput. If screw fixation is being used, bicortical purchase is recommended for the occiput, and screw lengths of typically 10 to 12 mm can be accepted in this region.[52]

If access to the posterior elements of C1-2 is necessary, the incision can be extended inferiorly. Palpation of the large C2 spinous process and the posterior C1 ring confirms the correct level. The posterior arch of the atlas is deeper anteriorly than the occiput and C2 spinous process, and the facet joint of C1-2 lies about 2.5 cm anterior to the C2-3 joint. A large broad elevator is used to dissect the posterior paracervical muscles from the arches of C1 and C2, and caution should be taken to avoid plunging instruments into the spinal canal. A small curet can be helpful to remove the muscular attachments on the bifid spinous process of C2 while stabilizing the arch of C2. Capsular ligaments of the facets should be preserved to maintain stability.

The passage of sublaminar wires at the C1-2 level is common because the spinal canal at this level is capacious, but passage at lower cervical levels is associated with increased risk of neurologic injury. The removal of the atlantoaxial ligament or atlanto-occipital membrane is not required except for laminectomy cases. Careful separation of the membrane or ligament from the bone is all that is usually needed to pass sublaminar wires. This separation can be performed with a small-angled curet or a small Freer elevator. Slight head flexion can also help by opening the space between the ring of C1 and the occiput. The mean thickness of the posterior ring is 8 mm, and the cortical bone is thin[53]; great care must be taken not to fracture the posterior ring of C1 while dissecting the ligamentum flavum.

An additional technique to expose the lateral aspect of C1 or C2 is to elevate the periosteum with a small Freer elevator. This allows the vertebral artery to be protected at the lateral aspect of the C1 arch. To avoid injury to the vertebral artery, lateral dissection should not exceed greater than 1.5 cm from the midline in an adult and 1 cm in a child. The vertebral artery is at risk during posterior exposures and lateral decompressions of C1 if the dissection is performed more than 15 mm from the midline of the posterior tubercle in adults or 10 mm in children.[54,55] The vertebral artery courses over the arch of the atlas and pierces the lateral angle of the posterior atlanto-occipital membrane.

Brief consideration is given here to the regional anatomy for the C1-2 transarticular screw fixation (Magerl) technique,[56-58] C1 lateral mass and C2 pedicle screw (Harms) technique,[58,59] and C2 translaminar screw.[58,60] A preoperative thin-cut CT scan with sagittal reconstructions should be obtained to evaluate the course of the vertebral artery. This imaging is especially important to obtain in rheumatoid patients in whom an anomalous or enlarged foramen transversarium is common, which may place the vertebral arteries at increased risk with this technique. Attention should be paid to the presence of a ponticulus posticus, an anomalous ossification overlying the vertebral artery as it runs in the superior sulcus of C1, which can occur in 15% of the population. Regardless of the technique used, the intraoperative use of anteroposterior and lateral fluoroscopy can provide screw inclination in the coronal and parasagittal plane.

Because of the amount of cephalad angulation required to place the C1-2 transarticular screw, subperiosteal exposure should extend down to C4.[54] The main landmark is the medial part of the isthmus of the axis, which can be visualized directly by subperiosteal dissection of the C2 lamina proceeding along the bony contour around the spinal canal until the maximum width in the coronal plane is reached. A Kirschner wire can be used to retract the soft tissues containing the greater occipital nerve and accompanying the venous plexus. The drilling for the screw is strictly sagittal, 2 to 3 mm lateral to the inner border of the isthmus. The screw should perforate the atlantoaxial joint approximately in the posteromedial part entering the lateral mass of the atlas.[61]

In the case of placement of a C1 lateral mass screw, the C1-2 joint is the key anatomic landmark to be identified.[59] This identification can be facilitated by caudal retraction of the C2 nerve, which exposes the posterior aspect of the lateral mass of C1.[58] The starting point of the C1 lateral mass screw lies directly in the mid-portion in the lateral mass. The C2 pedicle screw is identified by delineating the medial border of the isthmus and pars of the axis as in the C1-2 transarticular screw; however, the trajectory of the C2 pedicle screw is more medial and follows the path of the pedicle as would be expected.[58,59]

Technical challenges associated with the C1-2 transarticular screw and C2 pedicle screw placement led to the development of the C2 translaminar screw. Use of this screw is possible because of the predictably large size of the C2 lamina combined with the fact that the use of this screw eliminates the possibility for vertebral artery injury.[58,60] The starting point is identified as the junction of the C2 spinous process and the lamina, and the trajectory of the screw parallels the down slope of the dorsal aspect of the contralateral lamina. Care

should be taken not to breach the ventral aspect of the lamina resulting in placement of the screw within the spinal canal and to ensure that the C2-3 facet joint is not violated by placement of a screw that is too long.[60]

Posterior Approach to Lower Cervical Spine

A reverse Trendelenburg position minimizes venous bleeding and reduces cerebrospinal fluid pressure (Fig. 17–13). The posterior approach uses a longitudinal midline incision that extends above and below the segments required for the procedure. This extension of the skin and subcutaneous tissues is necessary because the skin of the posterior neck is less mobile and thicker for retraction. The skin is incised sharply, and electrocautery is used to incise the ligamentum nuchae in the midline. With a wide flat periosteal elevator such as a Cobb, the dissection is carried subperiosteally down the spinous processes. Inadvertent penetration of instruments into the spinal canal can be minimized by examining preoperative films for evidence of spina bifida and other bony defects and by realizing that, in the cervical spine, the laminae do not override each other as much as in the thoracic spine, resulting in wider interlaminar spaces. Care should be taken to stay subperiosteal because the bifid nature of the spinous processes may result in a bulbous expanse, and the dissection may err into the paraspinal musculature. A superficial plexus of veins may be encountered and should be cauterized as needed.

Subperiosteal dissection of muscles is performed to expose the spinous processes, lamina, lateral mass, and facet joints. The capsules of the facet joints should be left intact except for fusion cases. Extreme caution is needed during the exposure of the lamina and the interlaminar space to prevent dural tear and cerebrospinal fluid leakage. Care should be taken at the lateral edge of the joint because the nerve root and vertebral artery lie anterior to the spinolamellar membrane of the adjoining transverse processes. Vigorous decortication or stripping may damage the thin bone and subsequently the nerve root and vertebral artery. The segmental artery at the

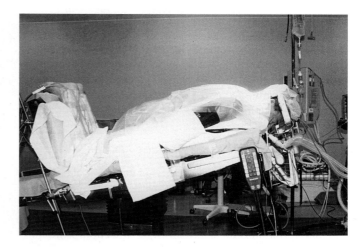

FIGURE 17–13 Standard prone positioning for posterior cervical procedures. Reverse Trendelenburg position minimizes venous bleeding and reduces cerebrospinal fluid pressure.

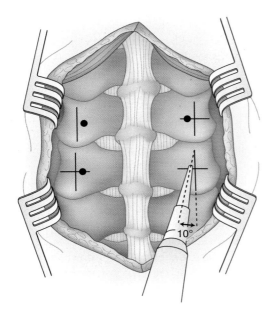

FIGURE 17–14 Roy-Camille technique for lateral mass screws. Entry point is at or near anatomic center of lateral mass and directed 10 degrees laterally.

lateral edge of the facet joints may be cauterized as it exits between the transverse processes. Various retractors may be used to facilitate exposure. The capsule is a stabilizing structure that can be damaged easily during dissection and should be preserved except in cases of fusion. For fusion cases, one should expose only the levels to be fused because creeping fusion extension is common. Supplementation of the fusion with posterior lateral mass plating may obviate the need for a halo vest postoperatively.

First popularized by Roy-Camille and colleagues,[62] placement of posterior cervical screws requires a thorough understanding of the lateral mass anatomy to minimize injury to associated neurovascular structures. Different entry points and screw orientations have been recommended. In the original description by Roy-Camille and colleagues,[62] the entry point was the center of the lateral mass with the screw angled 10 degrees laterally (Fig. 17–14), whereas Magerl recommended the drilling angle to be 25 degrees laterally and 45 degrees superiorly. An and colleagues[4] found that by orienting the screw 15 degrees cephalad and 30 degrees laterally with an entry point 1 mm medial to the anatomic center of the lateral mass, the facet joint and nerve root are avoided.

Posterior Approach to Cervicothoracic Junction

Lesions of the cervicothoracic junction are generally anterior, and extensive anterior approaches with or without posterior fixation are usually required. Lesions that may require posterior stabilization include lesions resulting from tumors, trauma, postlaminectomy instability, or infection. If the posterior elements are intact, the simple triple-wiring procedure can be done for a short fusion, or rods may be used for a longer fusion. Pedicle screw fixation is an alternative technique if the

posterior elements are deficient. The transpedicular technique at the cervicothoracic junction is an exacting procedure with very little margin for error. Through cadaveric studies, the pedicle landmarks and anatomic characteristics of the cervicothoracic region were found. A standard posterior approach is used with the dissection performed to expose the lateral mass and to the tips of the transverse processes of the upper thoracic vertebrae. The facet joint to be fused is cleaned of its capsule, and the articular margins are identified. The entry point of the pedicle lies at the intersection of a horizontal line at the mid-portion of the transverse processes and a vertical line at the lamina–transverse process junction. This pedicle entrance point is 1 mm inferior to the facet joint and the middle point from the medial to the lateral margins of the facet joint. The outer cortex is decorticated at this point with a small bur, and a small Penfield elevator or straight curet is used to probe bluntly and enter the pedicle. A 2.5-mm drill may be used to enter the pedicle when it is identified. Medial angulation is required for entry of the pedicle into the vertebral body; it averages 34 degrees at T1, 31.8 degrees at T1, and 26.5 degrees at T2. Compared with the pedicles of the lumbar spine, the superoinferior diameter of the thoracic pedicle is relatively greater than its mediolateral diameter, which leaves little margin for error in the mediolateral plane.

Complications

Complications associated with posterior approaches to the upper and lower cervical spine are uncommon but can be catastrophic. Bleeding can be minimized by staying subperiosteal and within the midline to prevent entering into the paraspinous musculature. The arch of the atlas should be dissected laterally only approximately 1.5 cm because the vertebral artery is at risk. One should minimize dissecting at the inferior edge of the foramen magnum to prevent uncontrollable venous bleeding.

Neurologic injury is a devastating complication of spine surgery, and care is required during passage of sublaminar wires or application of the screws to prevent injury to the brain or spinal cord. Dissection on the ring of the atlas must be done in a gentle manner because the direct pressure may result in fracture or slippage of an instrument into the spinal canal. A thorough understanding of the size, orientation, and relationship of the pedicles and lateral masses to surrounding neurovascular structures is imperative before the use of spinal instrumentation is undertaken. Posterior fusion without decompressive laminectomy tends to compress the spinal canal.

PEARLS
1. The anterior tubercle of the transverse process of C6 is an important palpable surface landmark for anterior cervical approaches.
2. The key to understanding the anterior approach to the cervical spine lies in recognizing the various investing fascial layers of the neck.

3. Placement of the deep retractors anteriorly should be deep to the longus colli to reduce the risk of injury to the sympathetic chain.

4. Posteriorly, the first bony prominence palpated inferior to the occiput is the spinous process of C2.

5. Reformatted fine-cut CT scans of the cervical spine help to improve understanding of the bony anatomy.

PITFALLS

1. The variable course of the vertebral artery as it ascends through the cervical spine places it at risk for injury during the anterior and the posterior cervical approach.

2. Careful review of preoperative radiographs, MRI, and CT scan helps identify the location of the pathology to be addressed.

3. Anterior exposures to the upper cervical spine may require a modified approach to reduce injury to structures in this area.

4. Subperiosteal midline dissection helps to reduce bleeding during the posterior cervical approach.

5. Airway obstruction after extubation may occur in the postoperative period after anterior and posterior cervical procedures.

KEY POINTS

1. Understanding the surgical anatomy of the cervical spine requires knowledge of the bony, ligamentous, muscular, and neurovascular anatomy of the neck and the complex relationship these structures have to one another.

2. The surgical approach selected should take into account the site of the pathologic process, the health of the patient, and the skill and comfort level of the surgeon with each particular exposure.

3. Understanding the advantages and limitation of each surgical exposure improves patient outcome and reduces complications.

4. Anatomic and surgical considerations at the occipitocervical and cervicothoracic junction are particularly challenging and should be thoroughly understood before approaching pathologic processes in these regions.

5. Complications of the cervical spine are infrequent but potentially devastating; careful preoperative planning, precise surgical technique, and a high index of suspicion should be maintained to minimize and identify complications.

KEY REFERENCES

1. An HS, Cotler JM (eds): Spinal Instrumentation, 2nd ed. Philadelphia, Lippincott Williams & Wilkins, 1990.
   This text compiles the knowledge of multiple contributing authors to provide valuable information on surgical indications, principles, and techniques of new and classic spinal instrumentation.

2. Graham JJ: Complications of cervical spine surgery: A five-year report on a survey of the membership of the Cervical Spine Research Society by the Morbidity and Mortality Committee. Spine 14:1046, 1989.
   A compilation of annual reports collected, at the time, by the newly formed Morbidity and Mortality Committee headed by Graham, this article analyzed 5 years of data submitted to the Cervical Spine Research Society from its members.

3. Heller JG, Pedlow FX: Anatomy of the cervical spine. In Clark CR (ed): The Cervical Spine, 3rd ed. Philadelphia, Lippincott-Raven, 1998, pp 3-36.
   Edited and reviewed by the Cervical Spine Research Society Editorial Committee, this chapter provides the pertinent anatomy necessary to understand the complex relationship of the structures in the cervical spine.

4. Miller MD, Chhabra AB, Hurwitz SR, et al (eds): Orthopaedic Surgical Approaches. Philadelphia, WB Saunders, 2008, pp 211-329.
   This updated text of orthopaedic exposures not only focuses on applied surgical anatomy and intraoperative photographs, but also provides valuable insight into patient positioning, bony and topical landmarks, and planes of surgical dissection.

5. Southwick WO, Robinson RA: Surgical approaches to the vertebral bodies in the cervical and lumbar regions. J Bone Joint Surg Am 39:631-644, 1957.
   This article provides the original description of the classic anteromedial approach to the cervical spine that popularized anterior cervical surgery.

REFERENCES

1. Albert TJ: Anterior, middle, and lower cervical exposures. In Albert TJ, Balderston RA, Northrup BE (eds): Surgical Approaches to the Spine. Philadelphia, WB Saunders, 1997, pp 9-24.

2. Schaffler MB, Alson MD, Heller JG, et al: Morphology of the dens. Spine 17:738-743, 1992.

3. Xu R, Naduad MC, Ebraheim NA, et al: Morphology of the second cervical vertebra and the posterior projection of the cervical pedicle axis. Spine 20:259-263, 1995.

4. An H, Gordin R, Renner K: Anatomic considerations for plate-screw fixation of the cervical spine. Spine 16(Suppl):S548-S551, 1991.

5. Johnson RM, Murphy MJ, Southwick WO: Surgical approaches to the spine: Function and surgical anatomy of the neck. In Herkowitz HN, Garfin SR, Balderston RA, et al (eds): Rothman-Simeone the Spine, 4th ed. Philadelphia, WB Saunders, 1999, pp 1463-1571.

6. Jefferson G: Fracture of atlas vertebra: Report of four cases and review of those previously reported. Br J Surg 7:407, 1920.

7. An HS: Anatomy of the spine. In An HS (ed): Principles and Techniques of Spine Surgery. Philadelphia, Lippincott Williams & Wilkins, 1998, pp 1-30.

8. Heller JG, Pedlow FX: Anatomy of the cervical spine. In Clark CR (ed): The Cervical Spine, 3rd ed. Philadelphia, Lippincott-Raven, 1998, pp 3-36.

9. Panjabi MM, Duranceau J, Goel V, et al: Cervical human vertebrae: Quantitative three-dimensional anatomy of the middle and lower regions. Spine 16:861-874, 1993.

10. Karaikovic EE, Kunakornsawat S, Daubs MD, et al: Surgical anatomy of the cervical pedicles: Landmarks for posterior cervical pedicle entrance localization. J Spinal Disord 13:63-72, 2000.

11. Karaikovic EE, Yingsakmongkol W, Gaines RW Jr: Accuracy of cervical pedicle screw placement using the funnel technique. Spine 26:2456-2462, 2001.

12. Karaikovic EE, Yingsakmongko LW, Griffiths HJ, et al: Possible complications of anterior perforation of the vertebral body using cervical pedicle screws. J Spinal Disord Tech 15:75-78, 2002.

13. Czervionke LF, Daniels DL, Ho PSP, et al: Cervical neural foramina: Correlative anatomic and MR imaging study. AJNR Am J Neuroradiol 169:753-759, 1988.

14. Daniels DL, Hyde JS, Kneeland JB, et al: The cervical nerves and foramina: Local-coil MR imaging. AJNR Am J Neuroradiol 7:129-133, 1986.

15. Aebi M, Thalgott JS, Webb JK: Stabilization techniques: Lower cervical spine. In Aebi M, Thalgott JS, Webb JK (eds): AO/ASIF Principles in Spine Surgery. New York, Springer, 1998, pp 54-79.

16. Ebraheim NA, Xu R, Knight T, et al: Morphometric evaluation of the lower cervical pedicle and its projection. Spine 22:1-6, 1997.

17. Dvorak JPM: Functional anatomy of the alar ligaments. Spine 12:183-189, 1987.

18. Parke WW, Sherk HH: Normal adult anatomy. In Sherk HH, Dunn EJ, Eismont FJ (eds): The Cervical Spine. Philadelphia, JB Lippincott, 1988, pp 11-32.

19. An HS: Anatomy of the cervical spine. In An HS, Simpson MJ (eds): Surgery of the Cervical Spine. London, Martin Dunitz, 1994, pp 1-40.

20. Hayashi K, Yabuki T, Kurokawa T, et al: The anterior and posterior longitudinal ligaments of the lower cervical spine. J Anat 124:633-636, 1977.

21. Bland JH, Boushey DR: Anatomy and physiology of the cervical spine. Semin Arthritis Rheumatol 20:1-20, 1990.

22. Lang J: Clinical Anatomy of the Cervical Spine. New York, Thieme, 1993.

23. Kameyama T, Hashizume Y, Ando T, et al: Morphometry of the normal cadaveric cervical spinal cord. Spine 19:2077-2081, 1994.

24. Okada Y, Ikata T, Katoh S, et al: Morphologic analysis of the cervical spinal cord, dural tube and spinal canal by magnetic resonance imaging in normal adults and patients with cervical spondylotic myelopathy. Spine 19:2231-2235, 1994.

25. Rauschning W: Anatomy and pathology of the cervical spine. In Frymoyer JW (ed): The Adult Spine. New York, Raven Press, 1991, pp 907-929.

26. Flannigan BD, Lufkin RB, McGlade C, et al: MR imaging of the cervical spine: Neurovascular anatomy. AJR Am J Roentgenol 148:785-790, 1987.

27. Pech P, Daniels DL, Williams AL, et al: The cervical neural foramina: Correlation of microtomy and CT anatomy. Radiology 155:143-146, 1985.

28. Bogduk N: The clinical anatomy of the cervical dorsal rami. Spine 7:319-320, 1982.

29. Gerbrand JG, Baljet B, Drukker J: Nerves and nerve plexuses of the human vertebral column. Am J Anat 188:282-296, 1990.

30. Rickenbacher J, Landolt AM, Theiler K: Applied Anatomy of the Back. Berlin, Springer-Verlag, 1982.

31. Dommisse GF: The blood supply of the spinal cord. J Bone Joint Surg Br 56:225, 1974.

32. Hoppenfeld S, deBoer P: The spine. In Hoppenfeld S, deBoer P (eds): Surgical Exposures in Orthopaedics: The Anatomic Approach, 2nd ed. Philadelphia, JB Lippincott, 1994, pp 215-301.

33. Arbit E, Patterson RH Jr: Combined transoral and median labio-mandibular glossotomy approach to the upper cervical spine. Neurosurgery 8:672-674, 1981.

34. Ashraf J, Crockard HA: Transoral fusion for high cervical fractures. J Bone Joint Surg Br 72:76, 1990.

35. McAfee PC, Bohlman HH, Riley LH III, et al: The anterior retropharyngeal approach to the upper part of the cervical spine. J Bone Joint Surg Am 69:1371, 1987.

36. deAndrade J, McNab I: Anterior occipitocervical fusion using extrapharyngeal approach. J Bone Joint Surg Am 51:1621, 1969.

37. Whitesides TE, McDonald P: Lateral retropharyngeal approach to the upper cervical spine. Orthop Clin North Am 9:115, 1978.

38. Mendoza N, Crockard HA: Anterior transoral procedures. In An HS, Riley LH III (eds): An Atlas of Surgery of the Spine. Philadelphia, Lippincott-Raven, 1998, pp 55-69.

39. Rosen MR, Keane WM, Rosen D: Anterior upper cervical exposures. In Albert TJ, Balderston RA, Northrup BE (eds): Surgical Approaches to the Spine. Philadelphia, WB Saunders, 1997, pp 25-52.

40. Menezes AH: Complications of surgery at the craniovertebral junction: Avoidance and management. Pediatr Neurosurg 17:254, 1992.

41. Fang H, Ong G: Direct anterior approach to the upper cervical spine. J Bone Joint Surg Am 44:1588-1604, 1962.

42. Southwick WO, Robinson RA: Surgical approaches to the vertebral bodies in the cervical and lumbar regions. J Bone Joint Surg Am 39:631-644, 1957.

43. Whitesides TE, Kelly RP: Lateral approach to the upper cervical spine for anterior fusion. South Med J 59:879, 1966.

44. Henry AK: Extensile Exposure. Baltimore, Williams & Wilkins, 1959, p 53.

45. Hogson AR: An approach to the cervical spine (C3-C7). Clin Orthop 39:129, 1965.

46. Verbiest H: Anterolateral operations for fractures and dislocations in the middle and lower parts of the cervical spine. J Bone Joint Surg 51:1489-1530, 1969.

47. Whitehill R: Late esophageal perforation from an autogenous bone graft: Report of a case. J Bone Joint Surg Am 67:644-645, 1985.

48. Kurz LT, Herkowitz HN: Anterior exposures of the cervicothoracic junction and upper thoracic spine. In Albert TJ, Balderston RA, Northrup BE (eds): Surgical Approaches to the Spine. Philadelphia, WB Saunders, 1997, pp 61-80.

49. Sundaresan N, Shah J, Foley KM, et al: An anterior surgical approach to the upper thoracic vertebrae. J Neurosurg 61:686-690, 1984.

50. Vaccaro AR, An HS: Anterior exposures of the cervicothoracic junction. In An HS, Riley LH III (eds): An Atlas of Surgery of the Spine. Philadelphia, Martin Dunitz, 1998, pp 113-130.

51. Andreshak TG, An HS: Posterior cervical exposures. In Albert TJ, Balderston RA, Northrup BE (eds): Surgical Approaches to the Spine. Philadelphia, WB Saunders, 1997, pp 81-114.

52. Winter RB, Lonstein JW, Denis F, et al: Posterior upper cervical procedures. In Winter RB, Lonstein JW, Denis F, et al (eds): Atlas of Spine Surgery. Philadelphia, WB Saunders, 1995, pp 19-33.

53. Doherty B, Heggeness MH: The quantitative anatomy of the atlas. Spine 19:2497-2500, 1994.

54. An H, Xu R: Posterior cervical spine procedures. In An H, Riley L III (eds): An Atlas of Surgery of the Spine. Philadelphia, Lippincott-Raven, 1998, pp 13-14.

55. Ebraheim N, Xu R, Ahmad M, et al: The quantitative anatomy of the vertebral artery groove of the atlas and its relation to the posterior atlantoaxial approach. Spine 23:320-323, 1998.

56. Magerl F, Seemann P: Stable posterior fusion of the atlas and axis by transarticular screw fixation. In Kehr P, Weidner A (eds): Cervical Spine. New York, Springer-Verlag, 1987, p 322.

57. Grob D, Crisco J, Panjabi MM, et al: Biomechanical evaluation of four different posterior atlantoaxial fixation techniques. Spine 17:480-490, 1991.

58. Shen FH: Spine. In Miller MD, Chhabra AB, Hurwitz SR, et al (eds): Orthopaedic Surgical Approaches. Philadelphia, WB Saunders, 2008, pp 211-329.

59. Harms J, Melcher RP: Posterior C1-C2 fusion with polyaxial screw and rod fixation. Spine 26:2467-2471, 2001.

60. Wright NM: Posterior C2 fixation using bilateral, crossing C2 laminar screws. J Spinal Disord Tech 17:158-162, 2004.

61. Grob D, An HS: Posterior occipital and C1/C2 instrumentation. In An HS, Cotler JS (eds): Spinal Instrumentation, 2nd ed. Philadelphia, Lippincott Williams & Wilkins, 1999, pp 191-201.

62. Roy-Camille RR, Sailant G, Mazel C: Internal fixation of the unstable cervical spine by posterior osteosynthesis with plate and screws. In Cervical Spine Research Society (ed): The Cervical Spine, 2nd ed. Philadelphia, JB Lippincott, 1989, pp 390-404.

Thoracic Spine: Surgical Approaches

Leonard K. Kibuule, MD
Harry N. Herkowitz, MD

Anatomy of Anterior Cervicothoracic Spine

The cervicothoracic junction corresponds to the area just superior to the mediastinum and extends into the sternum and T4-5 intervertebral discs. The left brachiocephalic vein, formed by the confluence of the left internal jugular and subclavian veins, lies immediately posterior to the upper sternum. The thymus gland lies just anterior to this structure. The left and right brachiocephalic veins combine to form the superior vena cava at the right first intercostal space. The superior vena cava enters the left atrium posterior to the third costal cartilage. The vagus and phrenic nerves lie anterior to the arch of aorta (Fig. 18–1). The recurrent laryngeal nerve branches off the vagus nerve between T1 and T3 on the left side and reliably loops around the aorta to ascend into the tracheoesophageal groove. The right recurrent laryngeal nerve branches off the vagus nerve in the upper cervical region and loops around the right subclavian artery. On this side, it may also leave the carotid sheath at a higher level and course anteriorly behind the thyroid before entering the groove.

Injury to the recurrent laryngeal nerve may occur with indiscriminant dissection to the cervicothoracic junction. C5-T1 levels are especially vulnerable. Controversy exists regarding which approach (left-sided vs. right-sided) minimizes the risk of injury to the recurrent laryngeal nerve. Tew and Mayfield[1] described the asymmetry between the right and left laryngeal nerves and described the anatomic loop of the nerve around the aortic arch on the left side as longer, more predictable, and more protected than the right-sided nerve. These authors believed that the anatomic loop on the left side rendered the recurrent laryngeal nerve less susceptible to contusion and stretch injury when a left-sided surgical approach was used. Other authors have reported that there is no statistical difference between the rate of injury and the side of the surgical approach.[2] It is acknowledged that injury to this structure can cause mild dysphagia and dysphonia. The reported incidence of dysphagia after anterior surgery ranges from 28% to 57%, and the incidence of dysphonia is 2% to 30%.[3]

The phrenic nerve, another neural structure, descends anterior to the pulmonary hilum to innervate the diaphragm. Lastly, the thoracic duct enters the superior mediastinum on the left side behind the arch of the aorta and ascends between the left subclavian artery and the esophagus before draining into the angle at the junction of the left subclavian vein and the left internal jugular vein.

Surgical Approaches to Anterior Spine

Cervicothoracic Junction

Low Anterior Cervical and High Transsternal Approach

The cervicothoracic junction is unique because this is the transitional area between cervical lordosis and thoracic kyphosis. This area is subject to a great deal of mechanical stress and is at risk for kyphotic deformities if these forces are not clearly understood and respected. Exposure in this region of the spine allows access to much of the lower cervical spine and proximal thoracic region. Although entry into this area involves navigating around and through numerous neurovascular structures as described earlier, when this area is exposed, it provides the surgeon full access to the spine for various procedures, including corpectomy, discectomy, débridement, deformity correction, and fracture reduction.

Indications for the anterior cervicothoracic approach include the following:

- Anterior exposure of vertebral bodies C7-T4
- Débridement of vertebral osteomyelitis or discitis
- Anterior vertebral body tumor excision
- Decompression and fusion of upper thoracic fractures

Operative Procedure

The patient is positioned supine on the operating table after general endotracheal anesthesia has been instituted. The arms should be tucked at the side, and the hands and wrist should be checked to ensure that they are positioned without undue pressure. Typically, a towel roll or other bolster is placed between the scapulae. This towel roll allows the head to be placed in a slight amount of extension and the shoulders to lie slightly extended at the side for adequate exposure of the junction. The head should also be turned either slightly right or slightly left depending on the surgeon's preferred approach. A left-sided approach to a virgin neck is preferable because the laryngeal nerve has a more reliable course into the tracheo-esophageal groove on this side.[4,5]

If possible, the head section of the operating table should be lowered to allow further extension of the neck. The shoulders are pulled distally at the side with adhesive tape and secured to the bed frame so that if a lateral intraoperative image is obtained, it is relatively unimpeded by the overlying shoulder osseous structures. Care should be taken not to over-pull the shoulders and risk a traction neurapraxia of the brachial plexus. Patients may be placed in slight Trendelenburg position to decrease venous pooling and engorgement. Next, the area of the neck from the angle of the jaw and mastoid process to the xiphoid is prepared. Enough room should be left distal on the chest so that if the incision needs to be extended, it is still within a sterile field.

The surgical incision is typically made from the left anterior border of the sternocleidomastoid muscle to the notch and can be continued distally along the middle of the manubrium (Fig. 18–2A). The first portion of the approach is an extension of the standard Smith-Robinson approach. Other authors have described a transverse incision that parallels the medial half of the clavicle. The vertical extension of the incision depends on the overall exposure required by the treating surgeon. If exposure from C7 to T4 is needed in its entirety, the vertical portion of the incision is made with the distal portion terminating just distal to the suprasternal notch. The extent of the incision is typically to the third costal cartilage.

After marking the incision, a No. 10 blade scalpel is used to incise down to the subcutaneous layer. Dissection is done through the platysma, creating flaps on either side for easier closure at the end of the case. Care should be taken not to injure the jugular veins, but they may be sacrificed if further exposure is needed. The strap muscles including the sternocleidomastoid are identified as they insert into the clavicle (Fig. 18–2B and C). Next, the clavicular and manubrial insertions of the sternocleidomastoid muscle are elevated subperiosteally proximally and laterally. The remaining strap muscles should be elevated in a similar manner and taken medially.

When visualized, subperiosteal stripping of the medial third of the clavicle and ipsilateral half of the manubrium should be performed. This stripping exposes the osseous structures for distal exposure to the lower cervical thoracic junction. The clavicle can be sectioned at the middle to medial third junction with an oscillating saw or osteotome (Fig. 18–2D). Care should be taken not to injure the underlying subclavian vein that is in close proximity. When freed laterally, the clavicle can be disarticulated from the manubrium providing exposure to the proximal cervicothoracic junction.

For a more extensive distal exposure, an alternative to clavicular resection and disarticulation involves a sternum-splitting approach. After performing the proximal incision, the skin incision can be extended further distally for added exposure (see Fig. 18–2A). Next, the sternocleidomastoid and

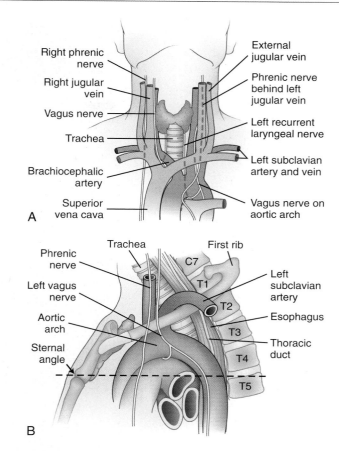

FIGURE 18–1 A, Anteroposterior view of cervicothoracic junction. **B,** Lateral view of cervicothoracic junction.

strap muscles are dissected subperiosteally from the manubrium and sternum to expose the midline to the anticipated level desired. One is usually able to use this dissection to visualize down to the T4 vertebral level. The manubrium is split longitudinally in the midline with an oscillating or Gigli saw and retracted with self-retaining retractors. Care should be taken not to injure the structures in the retropleural fascia with the saw. This area is protected by dissecting the thymus and surrounding fat from behind the manubrium. Also, care should be taken to avoid injuring the thoracic duct because it ascends to the left of the esophagus from the level of T4 to its junction with the left internal jugular and subclavian veins. A Kerrison rongeur can be used to complete the osteotomy on the posterior aspect of the manubrium. The innominate vein and inferior thyroid vein may also be encountered and can be ligated if necessary for exposure.

When adequate exposure from overlying osseous structures is obtained, dissection proceeds by finding an interval between the trachea and esophagus medially and the carotid sheath laterally. This is a relatively avascular plane, and one should encounter minimal bleeding in this zone. The surgeon should palpate for the carotid pulse laterally before dissection to ensure that the approach stays medial to the sheath. The laryngeal nerve reliably runs between the trachea and esophagus on the left side after looping around the aorta. If retractors are used in this area, the surgeon should ensure that they

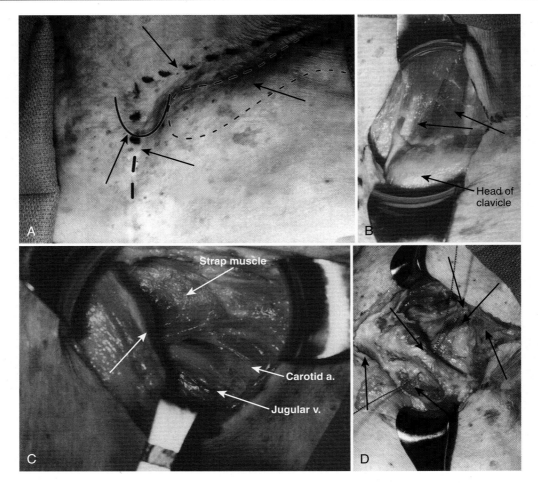

FIGURE 18–2 A, Inverted L-shaped incision for cervicothoracic junction. Mid-sternal extension of incision can be extended further vertically for more exposure distally. **B,** Insertion of sternocleidomastoid muscle into clavicular head. **C,** Sternocleidomastoid muscle retracted laterally revealing underlying strap muscle. Carotid sheath and jugular vein should be mobilized laterally as well. **D,** Skin incision extended in preparation for resection of clavicle.

remain outside this tissue; otherwise, injury to the nerve may occur. After placing the retractors and developing the interval, distally the right brachiocephalic artery can be taken laterally to the patient's right along with the trachea and esophagus. The left brachiocephalic and subclavian veins can be retracted inferolaterally to the patient's left. When approaching the prevertebral fascia, a kitner can be used to thin the fascia in a longitudinal manner. This thinning allows the surgeon to visualize the longus colli muscles, which run on either side of the cervicothoracic spine. With the junction fully exposed, the surgeon can proceed with the primary operative objective (i.e., corpectomy, fusion, discectomy, débridement).

Finally, closure should be performed in a stepwise manner.[6] If a sternal split was performed, wiring of the sternum and manubrium should be employed to reapproximate the two halves. If the clavicle is disarticulated, it should be reintroduced and fixed into place. Next, strap muscles should be repaired with absorbable sutures, and the sternocleidomastoid should be reattached to its insertion in a similar manner. The platysma can be reapproximated with running or interrupted absorbable sutures, and a suction drain can be placed just underneath this muscle before its closure.

KEY POINTS

1. The patient is positioned with the head extended, and the operative area is draped distal to the manubrium in case the incision needs to be extended for adequate exposure.

2. Approaching the cervicothoracic junction from the left is preferred because the recurrent laryngeal nerve has a more reliable course on this side.

3. The surgeon should palpate for the carotid pulse to ensure that he or she stays medial with the dissection in the avascular plane between the artery and the trachea and esophagus.

Transthoracic (Third Rib Resection)

When exposure of the anterolateral thoracic spine is needed, a transthoracic third rib resection can be employed. This approach provides excellent exposure of upper thoracic spine and may provide autologous bone graft from the resected rib. Transthoracic third rib resection provides access to T1-4 vertebral areas.

Disadvantages to using this approach include the need to mobilize the scapula and violation of chest wall muscles during dissection. This approach also requires violating the pleural space and necessitates placement of a chest tube at the end of the procedure.[7]

The indication for the transthoracic approach is as follows:

- Anterior exposure of vertebral bodies T1-4 anterolateral region

Operative Procedure

Before positioning the patient, it is recommended that a double-lumen endotracheal tube with lung isolation be used.[8] The patient is placed in the lateral decubitus position with the desired operative side up (Fig. 18–3A). Positioning the patient in this manner can be accomplished using a deflatable beanbag or foam-type bolster. The surgeon should ensure that all bony prominences are well padded. A soft roll is placed just distal to the axilla to prevent pressure on the brachial plexus. The arms are abducted, and the elbows and knees are slightly flexed in a position of comfort. The ipsilateral arm may be positioned comfortably by keeping it abducted on stacked pillows or blankets just under the arm and forearm. The surgeon should ensure that the head is also positioned comfortably and that no undue stress is placed on the head-neck junction. Preparation and draping is done in the usual sterile fashion from the shoulder to just above the iliac crest and from below the mid-spine posteriorly to below the umbilicus anteriorly.

The incision is drawn from the T1 spinous process, following the curvature of the medial-to-inferior border of the scapula. The incision is continued anteriorly along the seventh rib and ends on the costal cartilage of the third rib. This same trajectory is followed by incising through skin and subcutaneous tissue with a No. 10 blade knife. Next, the muscles of the trapezius and latissimus dorsi are identified and divided in a layered fashion with electrocautery. Any bleeders that are encountered in the muscle during this approach are cauterized. Rarely, the rhomboid major and serratus posterior also need to be divided in a similar manner.[7] As the muscle layers are divided further, using a retractor, the scapula is retracted proximally; doing this makes it easier to cut the muscles.

When exposure of the chest wall is accomplished, the surgeon counts down the ribs to the operative level. The second rib is often the highest easily palpated rib, and the first rib is situated inside the second (Fig. 18–3B). At this stage, the lung on the operative side can be selectively deflated. When

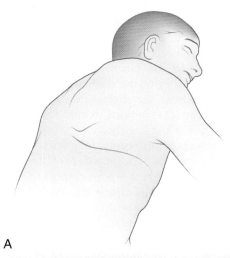

FIGURE 18–3 A, Patient in lateral decubitus position with left side up. Positioning of patient in this manner can be accomplished using deflatable beanbag or foam-type bolster. All bony prominences must be well padded as well. **B,** Second rib is often highest easily palpated rib, whereas first rib is situated inside the second. **C,** Parietal pleura is resected back from vertebral column exposing intervertebral discs. It is safer to begin dissection over disc where it is relatively avascular.

A

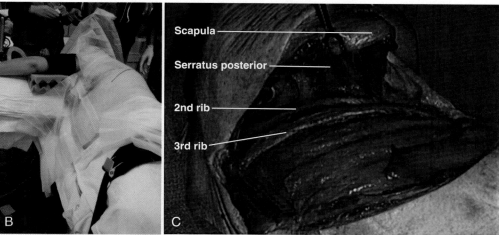

Scapula
Serratus posterior
2nd rib
3rd rib

B

C

the operative level (the third rib in this case) has been confirmed and the lung has been deflated, the intercostal muscles are stripped off of the rib extraperiosteally using a periosteal elevator. A Doyen rib elevator is an excellent dissection tool to strip the muscle circumferentially from the rib while preserving the underlying intercostal nerve and vessels. When exposed, the rib can be resected using a rib cutter. The rib is cut as far posterolaterally and anteromedially as possible. This rib can be used as bone graft if desired. The remaining rib bed can be transected, and the pleural cavity can be entered; this can be done safely with the lung selectively deflated on this side. A chest spreader can be used to provide retraction for entry into the chest cavity. A second spreader can be placed at a right angle in the surrounding soft tissue to allow for maximal exposure. The lung can be protected further with a malleable retractor shielded with a sponge.

With the lung deflated, the spine can be visualized at the base of the incision. At this time, it is important to identify clearly the neurovascular structures in the area. The aorta, the spine, parietal pleura, veins, and sympathetic plexus should be recognized. The parietal pleura is incised over the desired disc space with atraumatic pickups and Metzenbaum scissors in a longitudinal fashion with the spine. This area is typically relatively avascular and a safer plane for initial dissection than the vertebral body (Fig. 18–3C). When the vertebral body is exposed, the intercostal arteries and veins are visualized, ligated, and cut appropriately. Further exposure of the adjacent vertebral bodies and intervertebral discs can be obtained by extending the incision of the pleura proximally or distally or both, but with each level, ligature of the intercostal artery and vein may be required.

Closure of the approach and incision should be performed in a stepwise fashion. The parietal pleura should be reapproximated if possible. Reinflation of the lung should be visualized before closure of the remaining ribs. A rib reapproximator can assist with closing the defect of the resected rib with nonabsorbable suture or wire in a figure-of-eight fashion. Care should be taken not to encompass the inferior neurovascular bundle. Also, the lung should be protected during closure. A chest tube drain should be placed through a separate aperture inferiorly, preferably the ninth intercostal space, and set to water seal. The wound is dressed appropriately with sterile dressings.

KEY POINTS

1. A double-lumen endotracheal tube should be used to help with selective lung deflation during the case.

2. When identifying the rib level, the second rib is often the highest palpable rib, and the first rib is encompassed in the second.

3. The initial incision is made into the parietal pleura at the disc space, where it is relatively safer.

4. The wound is closed in a stepwise fashion, and a chest tube is placed before complete closure.

Thoracic Spine

Thoracotomy

A traditional thoracotomy provides access to the anterior spine from T6 to T12. In addition to these levels, further manipulation of the thoracolumbar junction of T12-L1 can be performed if the diaphragm is taken down. Access to T4 and T5 can also be accomplished, but one frequently has to elevate the scapula to do so.[7] The thoracotomy provides a versatile tool for exposure of much of the thoracic spine for manipulation and instrumentation.

The indication for thoracotomy is as follows:

- Anterior exposure of vertebral bodies of T4-L1

Operative Procedure

A double-lumen endotracheal tube with lung isolation is used.[8] The patient is placed in the lateral decubitus position with the desired operative side up. Approaching from the left side may require one to manipulate the aorta and segmental vessels on the left. When possible, a right-sided approach allows more spinal surface area exposure from behind the azygos vein than behind the aorta. Exposure from T10 to T12 is more easily accomplished from the left, however, because the liver causes the diaphragm to ride higher on the right; limiting the visibility of the spine on this side.

Selective positioning can be accomplished by using a deflatable beanbag or foam-type bolster placed underneath the patient's right torso. The surgeon should ensure that all bony prominences are well padded. An intravenous fluid bag or other soft roll can be placed just distal to the axilla to prevent pressure on the brachial plexus. The arms are abducted and the elbows are slightly flexed in a position of comfort using blankets or pillows to hold them in position (Fig. 18–4A). The hip and knee nearest the bed are slightly flexed, and the contralateral extremity is allowed to remain more extended and slightly adducted. The weight of the contralateral leg helps open the rib interspace when exposure is accomplished. The surgeon also should ensure that the head is positioned comfortably in a neutral position.

To localize the operative level, a fluoroscopic image can be obtained preoperatively before the incision. Otherwise, the desired rib level can be confirmed by counting the ribs by palpating from proximal to distal. One may also count from the 12th rib proximally. Typically, the numbered rib that is resected is considered to be two levels above the expected working area because of the oblique orientation of the ribs. When the numbered rib is identified, the incision is drawn from the posterior angle of the corresponding rib following its curvature anteriorly (Fig. 18–4B). The incision should be made through skin and subcutaneous tissue with a No. 10 blade knife. The incision is deepened with electrocautery, and any bleeders that are encountered are coagulated. Care should be taken not to injure the neurovascular bundle that runs on the undersurface of the rib.

Next, the muscles of the latissimus dorsi are identified and divided in a layered fashion in line with the incision and overlying the rib with the electrocautery. It should not be necessary

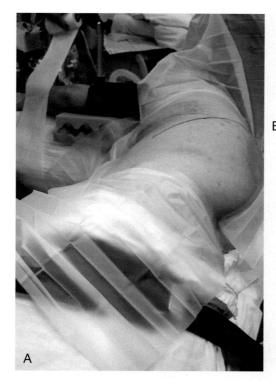

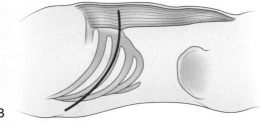

B

A

FIGURE 18–4 A, Patient is placed in lateral decubitus position. Arms are abducted and elbows are slightly flexed in a position of comfort using blankets or pillows to hold their position. **B,** Thoracotomy incision is centered over rib to be resected. Incision is drawn from posterior angle of corresponding rib and following its curvature anteriorly. Typically, numbered rib that is resected is considered to be two levels above expected working level.

to separate this muscle from the surrounding tissue. A portion of the posterior margin of the serratus anterior lies on the undersurface of the latissimus and may be divided. As the muscle is divided anteriorly, any bleeders that are encountered are cauterized. When the superficial surface of the rib is exposed, the intercostal muscles are separated from the periosteum with a periosteal elevator, such as an Alexander-Farabeuf periosteotome. Also, the undersurface of tissue is released from the rib; this can be done circumferentially with a Doyen dissector (Fig. 18–4C). Dissection should be far posteriorly and anteriorly for adequate exposure. Next, a rib cutter is used to cut the rib anteriorly at the costal junction and posteriorly at the costotransverse junction for sufficient surgical access (Fig. 18–4D). This rib can be used as bone graft if desired. The cut edges are smoothed with a rasp, and bone wax is applied if active bleeding is present.

The ipsilateral lung is selectively deflated, and the pleural cavity is entered with a pickup and Metzenbaum scissors (Fig. 18–4E). A rib spreader can be used to provide retraction for entry into the chest cavity. A second spreader can be placed at a right angle in the surrounding soft tissue to allow for maximal exposure. The lung can be protected further with a malleable retractor shielded with a sponge.

With the lung deflated, the spine can be clearly visualized. The neurovascular structures in the area are identified (Fig. 18–4F). The parietal pleura is incised over the desired disc space with atraumatic pickups and Metzenbaum scissors in a longitudinal fashion, and the pleura is retracted laterally. Care should be taken not to injure the segmental vessels, which may bleed incessantly if not tied or clipped in a controlled fashion. The vessels close to the middle of the vertebral body are dissected and ligated, and the arteries are clamped away from the aorta. If the segmental arteries are tied too close to the aorta,

the tie can loosen, and bleeding can resume. A right-angle clamp is used to free the vessel, and a 2-0 tie is passed around the vessel (Fig. 18–4G). Further exposure of the adjacent vertebral bodies and intervertebral discs can be obtained by extending the incision of the pleura proximally or distally or both, but with each level ligature of the segmental vessels may be required. With adequate exposure, the disc interspace and pedicle can be identified by following the head of the rib to its base. The disc is the more prominent, white, soft structure flanking the larger recessed vertebral bodies.

Closure of the incision should be performed in a stepwise fashion. The parietal pleura should be reapproximated, and reinflation of the lung should be visualized before closure of the incision. A chest tube drain is placed through a separate aperture inferiorly, preferably the ninth intercostal space, and set to water seal. A rib reapproximator is used to assist with closing the defect of the resected rib with nonabsorbable suture or wire in a figure-of-eight fashion. The lung should be protected during closure. The wound should be dressed appropriately with sterile dressings.

KEY POINTS
1. A double-lumen endotracheal tube is used to help with selective lung deflation during the case.
2. To identify the rib level, one may count proximally from the 12th rib up.
3. The initial incision is made into the parietal pleura at the disc space in this relatively safer, avascular area.
4. The segmental arteries are tied over the vertebral arteries away from the aorta.

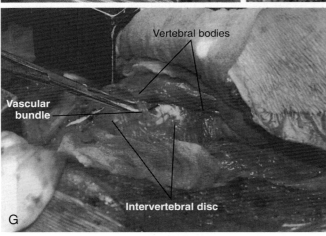

Cephalad

Costal cartilage

Periosteum removed from undersurface of rib

C

Posterior

D

Lung

Anterior

Parietal pleura covering aorta and spine

Edge of pleura

Pleural cacity

Inner periosteum of rib bed

Aorta

Spine

E

F

Vertebral bodies

Vascular bundle

Intervertebral disc

G

FIGURE 18–4, cont'd C, Doyen elevator can be used to remove muscle subperiosteally from undersurface of rib. **D,** Rib cutter is used to cut rib posteriorly from costotransverse joint and angle of rib and anteriorly at costal junction. **E,** Edge of pleura can be picked up with Adson forceps, and rib bed can be opened with semiclosed scissors. Rib spreader is used to provide retraction during entry into chest cavity. **F,** Parietal pleura covers spine and adjacent neurovascular structures. Dissection is begun over disc space to avoid injury to these structures. **G,** Intercostal vessels are dissected and isolated with right-angle clamp; 2-0 sutures or clips are used to tie off each vessel before being cut in center between ties.

Thoracolumbar Junction

Exposure of the thoracolumbar spine may be necessary to gain access to T10-L2 of the spine. The key to this approach is exposure and partial mobilization of the diaphragm and entry into the thorax and retroperitoneum.[9]

Indications for approaching the thoracolumbar junction include the following:

- Treatment of pathology (tumor, trauma, osteomyelitis or discitis, pseudarthrosis) between T10 and L2
- Correction of deformity (scoliosis, kyphosis) at these levels
- Failed posterior fusion

This approach may not be advantageous for patients with previous retroperitoneal surgery with suspected adhesions or severe respiratory conditions. There is also risk of injury to abdominal viscera, risk of postoperative ileus, and other risks associated with entry into the thorax. Otherwise, this approach is considered very versatile with minimal disruption of retroperitoneal structures.

Anatomy of Thoracolumbar Junction

The thoracolumbar junction constitutes the lower three thoracic and upper two lumbar vertebrae. This region is a transition zone from a stiffer and less mobile kyphotic thoracic spine to a more mobile, lordotic lumbar spine. It is this characteristic that lends this region to a higher incidence of trauma.[10]

When examining the thoracolumbar junction, the aorta lies to the left of midline in the lower chest, and the azygos vein, splanchnic nerves, and thoracic duct lie to the right of midline. From T10 to L2, the segmental arteries run in a horizontal direction from the posterior aortic midline. The L2-4 arteries run in a descending direction from the midline aorta and horizontally toward their corresponding vertebral body.

Understanding the orientation of the diaphragm is one of the most important concepts of this approach. This dome-shaped organ marks the junction between the thoracic and abdominal cavities. It is composed of two parts—a clover-shaped central tendon and a fleshier peripheral portion that has parietal attachments. The diaphragm attaches to L1, through the crura, and through the arcuate ligaments and four lower ribs. Anteriorly, it attaches to the six lower costal cartilages and the posterior surface of the xiphoid process. Posteriorly, it attaches to the spine via the medial arcuate ligaments, which arise from the crura, bridge the psoas muscle, and insert onto the transverse process of L1. The lateral arcuate ligament leaves the same transverse process and bridges over the quadratus lumborum to attach to the tips of the 12th rib. The left and right crura continue with the anterior longitudinal ligament to surround the aorta and the esophagus.

The psoas muscle remains in a retroperitoneal space where it attaches to the transverse process of the lumbar vertebrae before inserting into the lesser trochanter of the femur. Other structures include the ureter that runs between the peritoneum and the psoas fascia, which normally falls forward away from the operative field.

Operative Procedure

Either a left-sided or a right-sided surgical approach can be undertaken; a left-sided dissection is preferred. A left-sided approach avoids being obscured by the liver or having to mobilize the vena cava. If injured, the vena cava can bleed profusely, and the thin-walled vessel can often be difficult to suture. A right-sided approach may be necessary, however, to treat some pathology or may be the required approach in accessing the convexity in a scoliotic spine.[11]

A double-lumen endotracheal tube is recommended to deflate the lung selectively on the operative side. Placement of a Foley catheter and nasogastric tube may be done before positioning the patient. The patient is placed in the lateral decubitus position with the desired operative side up. The preferable position is with the left side up. If there is a break in the operative table, the operative level must be centered over this break. Positioning may be accomplished using a deflatable beanbag or foam-type bolster. The surgeon should ensure all bony prominences are well padded. An intravenous fluid bag or other soft roll is placed just distal to the axilla to prevent pressure on the brachial plexus. The arms are abducted, and the elbows are slightly flexed in a position of comfort using blankets or pillows to hold their position. The hip and knee nearest the operating table are flexed, and the contralateral extremity is allowed to remain more extended and slightly adducted. The surgeon should ensure that the head is also positioned comfortably in a neutral position on a small cushion.

The patient is secured to the operating room table with 3-inch tape over the shoulders and over the distal hip. When the patient is secured, a brief preoperative image with fluoroscopy can be obtained to ensure adequate visualization of the intended level. When visualization is satisfactory, the surgical site can be isolated with ten-ten drapes, and the skin can be sterilely draped.

The operative level is reconfirmed with a fluoroscopic image before incision. The desired rib level also can be isolated by counting the ribs; this can be accomplished by counting from the 12th rib proximally. The incision is typically made at the 9th, 10th, or 11th rib depending on the operative level and amount of exposure required (Fig. 18–5A). After the site of the incision is identified, the surgeon draws the incision from the posterior angle of the corresponding rib, following its curvature anteriorly and ending distally to the level just lateral of the pubic symphysis if needed. The curvilinear incision allows for exposure of the distal thoracic and lumbar spine. The incision should be made through skin with a No. 10 blade knife and deepened with the electrocautery. Any bleeders are coagulated as they are encountered. Care is taken not to injure the neurovascular bundle that runs on the undersurface of the rib during its exposure.

Next, the muscles of the latissimus dorsi and the external oblique muscle are identified and divided above the desired rib in a layered fashion with the electrocautery. As the muscle is divided anteriorly, any bleeders that are encountered are cauterized. The superficial surface of the rib is exposed to the costal cartilage, and the intercostal muscles are separated from the periosteum with a periosteal elevator. The release can also be performed with a Doyen dissector. Dissection should occur far posteriorly and anteriorly for adequate exposure. A rib cutter is used to cut the rib anteriorly at the costal junction and posteriorly at the costotransverse junction for sufficient surgical access. The rib bed is left intact at this junction of the exposure. This rib can be used as bone graft if desired (Fig. 18–5B). The cut edges are smoothed with a rasp, and bone wax is applied if actively bleeding.

The ipsilateral lung is selectively deflated, and the pleura is identified; this can be accomplished by splitting the undersurface of the costal cartilage anteriorly. Care is taken to avoid injuring the pleura. The retroperitoneal space is entered through the cartilaginous portion of the rib with blunt dissection (Fig. 18–5C). If resecting the 12th rib, the diaphragm attaches to it superiorly and the transverse abdominis muscle inferiorly. Retracing the diaphragm proximal and the abdominal muscle distal allows entrance into the retroperitoneum. The peritoneum should be swept off the abdominal muscles and diaphragm (Fig. 18–5D). The peritoneum occasionally extends to the tip of the 11th rib, but it usually extends to the mid-portion of the 12th rib. The surgeon can use a sponge gauze wrapped on his or her fingertip or a sponge stick to sweep off the peritoneum.

The internal and external oblique and transversus abdominis muscles are incised in a layered fashion as needed for exposure. With the pleura dissected, the rib bed can be opened with scissors. A rib spreader can be used to provide retraction for entry into the chest cavity. A second spreader can be placed at a right angle in the surrounding soft tissue to allow for maximal exposure. The lung is

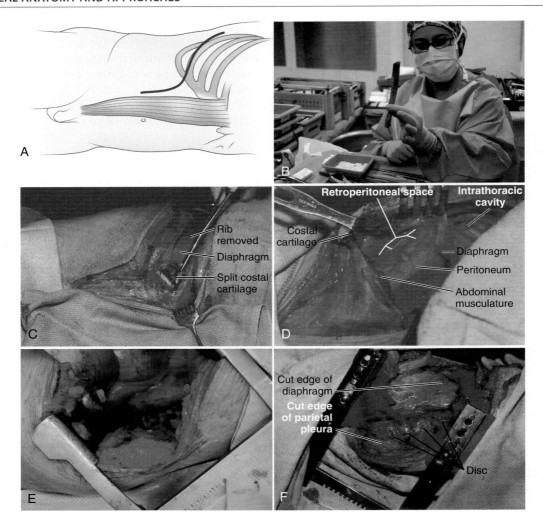

FIGURE 18–5 A, Patient is placed in lateral decubitus position with desired operative side up. Incision is typically made at 9th, 10th, or 11th rib depending on operative level and amount of exposure required. **B,** Resected rib can be used as bone graft during procedure. **C,** Costal cartilage is split allowing entrance into retroperitoneal space. **D,** Peritoneum should be swept off abdominal muscles and diaphragm. **E,** Rib spreader can be used to provide retraction for entry into chest cavity. Lung is further protected with malleable retractor shielded with sponge. **F,** Diaphragm is incised exposing discs of spine.

protected further with a malleable retractor shielded with a sponge (Fig. 18–5E).

When exposure into the thoracoabdominal cavity has been achieved, the peritoneum should be bluntly swept off the psoas muscle and the undersurface of the diaphragm to expose the retroperitoneal space further. This allows the diaphragm to be clearly visualized for release. The diaphragm is incised from the inside chest wall for a circumferential release (Fig. 18–5F). A 1-cm cuff of muscle must be left for later reapproximation during closure. It is beneficial to tag the ends of the muscle and diaphragm for anatomic positioning during the repair. The crus of the diaphragm may need to be taken down from L1 to L2 for further exposure; this allows access to vertebral bodies T12-L1.

In the thoracic spine, the parietal pleura is opened in the usual fashion to expose the vertebral body. The intercostal vessels are tied and ligated before mobilizing the major vessels for access to the vertebral bodies. The vessels should be tied at least 1 cm from the intervertebral foramen. The sympathetic plexus should be avoided when exposing the intercostal vessels. In the lumbar spine, if the psoas muscle needs to be mobilized, this should be done subperiosteally to prevent any injury to the lumbar roots. Any bleeding that may occur with electrocautery must be controlled.

Closure should be performed in a layered fashion. An appropriately sized chest tube is placed. The diaphragm should be reapproximated and repaired with nonabsorbable sutures. The pleura over the spine and rib head should be closed if possible. The intra-abdominal muscles should be closed in a layered fashion, and the lung should be visualized while reinflated. A malleable retractor is used to protect the viscera while repairing the muscles. The surgeon needs to pay close attention to the junction of the diaphragm and abdominal muscles. Lack of appropriate closure risks the development of a hernia. Finally, the skin is closed with suture or staples, and sterile dressings are applied.

KEY POINTS

1. A double-lumen endotracheal tube is used to help with selective lung deflation during the case.

2. The surgeon dissects the parietal pleura of the diaphragm and abdominal musculature carefully with gauze and his or her finger.

3. The psoas muscle is elevated subperiosteally to protect the lumbar roots from injury.

4. The surgeon needs to pay careful attention to the diaphragm and abdominal muscle closure to help minimize risk of a hernia.

Additional Anterior Approaches

Endoscopic Approach to Anterior Thoracic Spine

Endoscopic approaches to the thorax have been used to treat many pathologic conditions in the chest and mediastinum.[12] Thoracoscopic techniques have been used to perform anterior decompression, reconstruction, and instrumentation of the entire thoracic spine and its junction. This alternative to traditional open techniques has been shown to reduce postoperative pain, improve recovery time, and minimize some associated complications of open procedures.[13,14] Over several decades, many surgeons have attempted to improve and expand the use of video-assisted thoracoscopic surgery (VATS), also known as thoracoscopic surgery. Mack, Regan, Rosenthal, and colleagues were the first to report the application of VATS principles to an anterior approach to the thoracic and lumbar spine.[15] Since then, numerous authors have described their experiences with video-assisted spine surgery for various operative indications, including treatment of fractures, correction of deformity, and decompression.

Advantages of VATS for spine procedures are as follows:

- Small incisions into the intercostal space allow access for instruments without the need for rib resection.
- High-resolution video allows the surgeon to see pathology in great detail.
- Postoperative pain and morbidity are reduced, leading to decreased recovery time.
- Less postoperative pulmonary dysfunction is present.[7]

Surgical Procedure

Intraoperative monitoring for thoracic procedures may be used, including an arterial pressure catheter, pulse oximeter, and end-tidal carbon dioxide measurement. Neurologic monitoring may be beneficial to monitor patients undergoing spinal deformity correction or corpectomy. A thoracic surgeon should be available in the event of any vascular complication or need to convert to an open thoracotomy procedure.

The patient should be positioned in a similar manner as for an open thoracotomy. The patient is placed in a lateral decubitus position on a beanbag with the table flexed maximally to widen the intercostal spaces. General endotracheal anesthesia should be administered with the use of a double-lumen or Univent tube to allow selective ventilation of the contralateral lung. Collapse of the ipsilateral lung allows clearer visualization of the operative field. After positioning the patient, the surgeon needs to ensure the patient is appropriately secured to the operative table and that all bony prominences are well padded. Securing the patient allows the surgeon to rotate or maneuver the table for more comfortable instrument positioning and to use gravity for better visualization of the operative field as the lung falls forward; this can be accomplished by rolling the patient forward by 10 to 15 degrees.

Mark the portal positions and check with intraoperative imaging to ensure they are in accordance to the desired operative level. These portals are placed in a manner to triangulate directly over the level of the pathology. There are numerous portal configurations ranging from T-shaped to L-shaped.[7] Typically, two to three working portals are used, and two others are used for instrumentation (Fig. 18–6A and B). One portal may be placed directly over the pathology posterior to the midaxillary line. Another portal is placed two levels superiorly at the midaxillary line, and one is placed at the level of pathology or more distal. The fourth portal may be placed anterior to the midaxillary line also near the operative level.

A 1-inch oblique incision is made into the skin with the ipsilateral lung deflated. An anterosuperior portal is typically placed to minimize injury of the diaphragm. Sharp dissection is performed down to the intercostal muscles. The fascia may be taken down with electrocautery. The chest cavity is entered with a blunt clamp or thoracoscopic introducer. The surgeon should enter on the superior surface of the rib to protect the intercostal neurovascular bundle.

A 10-mm, 30-degree angled rigid telescope is placed through a 10-mm trocar. A 0-degree end-viewing scope and a 30-degree scope are used for direct vision of the intervertebral disc space to avoid impeding surgical instrumentation or obscuring the operative field. Subsequent portals should be placed under direct thoracoscopic visualization. The portals are used for placement of surgical instruments. The patient is rotated anteriorly 10 to 15 degrees and placed in a Trendelenburg position for the lower thoracic spine or reverse Trendelenburg for the upper thoracic spine. The lung usually falls away from the operative field when completely collapsed, obviating the need for retraction instruments. Otherwise, a fan retractor can be used to retract the lung further.

In contrast to other VATS procedures in which the surgeon and assistant are positioned on opposite sides of the operating table, the surgeon and assistant for spine surgery are positioned on the anterior side of the patient viewing a monitor on the opposite side. In addition, the camera and the viewing field are rotated 90 degrees from the standard VATS approach so that the spine is viewed horizontally.

An initial exploratory thoracoscopy is performed to determine the correct spinal level for operative intervention. If any pleural adhesions are encountered, these can be taken down with monopolar cautery scissors. The ribs are counted by "palpation" with a blunt grasping instrument. When the target level has been defined, a 20-gauge long needle or Kirschner

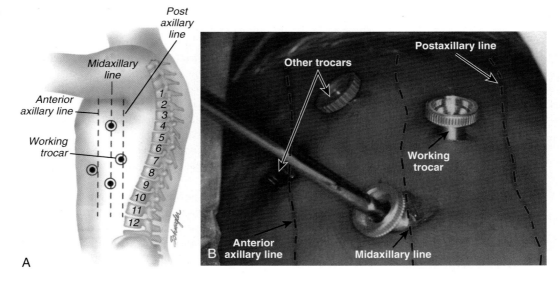

FIGURE 18–6 A, Diagram for trocar positions for T7-8 pathology. **B,** Actual trocar positions.

wire is placed percutaneously into the disc space from the lateral aspect and confirmed radiographically.

When the correct level is determined, the parietal pleura is incised over the rib head with cautery and monopolar scissors. The edge of the pleura is grasped, and the incision is extended cephalad and caudad with a hook dissector to expose the desired levels. Care is taken not to injure the segmental vessels as exposure proceeds. If a discectomy is planned, exposure of the adjacent vertebral bodies may be sufficient without the need to ligate the segmental vessels. If more extensive exposure is necessary, the segmental vessels need to be clipped and ligated.

The rib head is exposed and mobilized by dividing the costovertebral ligaments. Division of the rib is done 2 to 3 cm from the spine with the use of a Kerrison rib cutter or high-speed drill. The disc space, pedicle, and posterior margins of the vertebral body are revealed after the rib head is removed. Further exposure of the exiting nerve root and orientation of the spinal canal are accomplished by resecting the pedicle and superior vertebra.

After completion of the intended thoracoscopic procedure, the surgeon should recheck to ensure adequate hemostasis is present. Any visceral pleural tears should be repaired using standard thoracoscopic methods. The wound is irrigated copiously, and a chest tube is placed through the most caudad trocar site with the tip near the apex. The lung is allowed to expand under direct vision to ensure all segments reinflate appropriately. All trocar sites are closed with absorbable 2-0 sutures for the fascia and staples for the skin. The chest tube is secured with 2-0 silk and placed to underwater seal and suction.

Postoperative x-rays are obtained to ensure re-expansion of the lung, and serial x-rays are done each day until it is determined this follow-up imaging can be discontinued. Typically, this occurs when drainage is less than 150 mL in a 24-hour period and no air leak has been present.

KEY POINTS

1. A double-lumen endotracheal tube is used to deflate the lung selectively on the ipsilateral side.

2. The initial trocar is inserted using blunt dissection over the superior intercostal space, and an additional trocar is placed under direct vision.

3. The patient is rotated 15 to 20 degrees anteriorly to allow the ipsilateral lung to fall away from the operative field.

4. A postoperative x-ray is obtained to ensure complete expansion of the lung and to visualize its expansion before complete closure of the wound.

Anatomy of Thoracic Spine

The thoracic spine is the largest part of the spinal column. It consists of 12 vertebral bodies, which diminish in size from T1 to T3 and increase in size to T12, with intervening intervertebral discs.[16] The spinous processes of the posterior thoracic spine can often be palpated in most individuals despite their posteroinferior angulations. As one follows their projection from inferior to superior, the tip of the spinous process overlays the vertebral body that precedes it. At the midline, a layer of subcutaneous fat separates the skin from the thoracic fascia and supraspinous ligament. Deep to this fat on either side of midline are the muscles of the thoracolumbar spine.

The muscles can be grouped into three layers: superficial, intermediate, and deep layer (Fig. 18–7A). These layers are not distinct during the exposure, but grouping them in this manner helps to visualize their arrangement around the osseoligamentous spine. In the superficial layer, mooring muscles are located that attach the upper extremity to the spine. This layer contains the trapezius and the latissimus dorsi muscle. Deeper to this are the rhomboid major and minor muscles.[17]

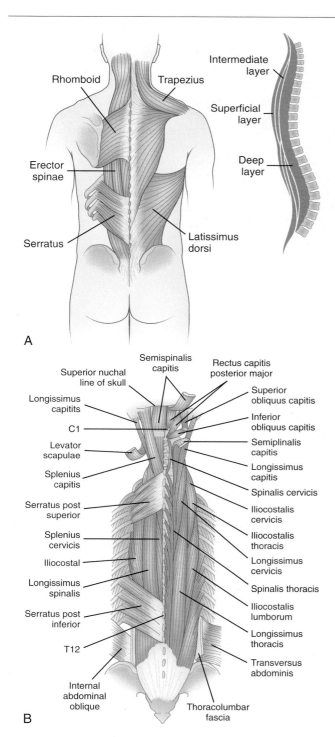

FIGURE 18–7 A, Muscles of thoracic spine. **B,** Intermediate and deep muscles of thoracic spine. (**B,** From An HS: Principles and Techniques of Thoracic Surgery. Baltimore, Williams & Wilkins, 1998.)

continuous with the aponeurosis of the transverse abdominis muscle.[7]

Dissection in the posterior spine typically occurs through an area that minimizes risk to nerves innervating the muscles. Peripheral nerves innervate the trapezius, latissimus, and rhomboids. Dissection in the midline avoids the spinal accessory and thoracodorsal muscles and C5 nerve that innervates these muscles. The same applies to the intermediate muscles, which are innervated by the anterior primary rami, and the muscles of the deep layer, which are innervated by the posterior rami of the thoracic nerves. Even the facet joints are covered by the dorsal branches of the nerve roots as they exit the neural foramina.

The ribs and facets of the thoracic spine help provide stability to the region. Care must be taken to recognize and respect their relationship to the surrounding soft tissue and exiting nerve roots. It is relatively easy to identify the C7 and T1 spinous processes with simple palpation. These two landmarks are usually the largest processes in the cervicothoracic junction. Distally, the gluteal cleft should be inline with the large L5 spinous process if there is no deformity. If there is no significant scoliosis or other deformity within the thoracic or lumbar spine, other spinous processes should fall underneath a line intersecting these two points. Because the thoracic spine is smaller than the lumbar spine and has more variability in its anatomy from proximal to distal, surgical planning is imperative, especially in the face of any associated misalignment disorder. On either side of the spinous processes, the lamina forms the dorsal roof of the spinal canal.

The ligaments of the spine from superficial to deep include the supraspinous ligament, interspinous ligament, ligamentum flavum, facet capsule, posterior longitudinal ligament, and anterior longitudinal ligament (Fig. 18–8). The supraspinous ligament attaches the tips of the spinous processes. The interspinous ligament attaches to the adjacent spinous processes with the fibers running in an oblique fashion. The ligamentum flavum inserts on the top of each inferior lamina and

The intermediate layer contains the serratus posterior inferior and superior muscles. These smaller muscles attach from the midline of the spinous process to the middle of the inferiormost and superiormost ribs. Deeper still is the last layer, which houses the erector spinae muscle column (Fig. 18–7B). These muscles, which consist of the semispinalis, multifidus, and rotator muscles, have an investing fascia whose dorsal layer constitutes the thoracolumbar fascia. This fascia becomes

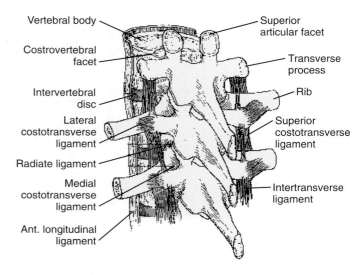

FIGURE 18–8 Ligaments of thoracic spine. (From An HS: Principles and Techniques of Thoracic Surgery. Baltimore, Williams & Wilkins, 1998.)

to the undersurface of each cephalad lamina. This is the strongest and most well developed of the spinous ligaments and functions to maintain extension of adjacent vertebrae. The posterior longitudinal ligament traverses the dorsal aspect of the vertebral bodies and intervertebral disc spaces, whereas the anterior longitudinal ligament runs on the ventral surface.

The par interarticularis emerges where the inferior and superior facets meet. In most instances, the pars should be preserved during surgery unless fusion is preplanned.

The facet joints are uniquely oriented throughout the thoracic spine. The superior facet of T1 is similar to the cervical facet in its orientation. It faces up and back, whereas the inferior facet faces down and forward. Moving from T2 to T11,

this orientation changes slightly. The superior facet begins to face up, back, and slightly lateral; the inferior facet faces down, forward, and more medial. This shift in orientation allows the thoracic spine the ability to rotate a bit more.

At the base of each facet is the pedicle of each vertebral body (Fig. 18–9A). Pedicle morphometry has been extensively studied and characterized by numerous authors in the past.[18-23] With the development of more powerful reduction tools and robust fixation devices, pedicle screw fixation in the thoracic spine is becoming more and more popular as a method of instrumentation.[21,24,25] A clear understanding of pedicle anatomy is essential for successful instrumentation at this level.[26] The sagittal and axial angulation changes relatively

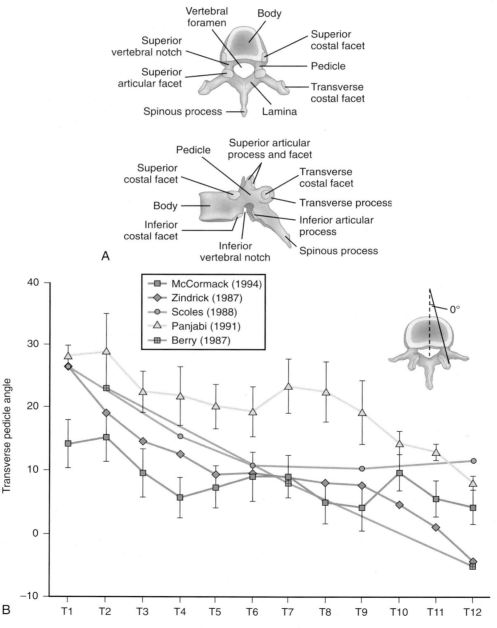

FIGURE 18–9 A, Osseous structure of thoracic spine and thoracic vertebra. **B,** Transverse pedicle angles found in five different studies.

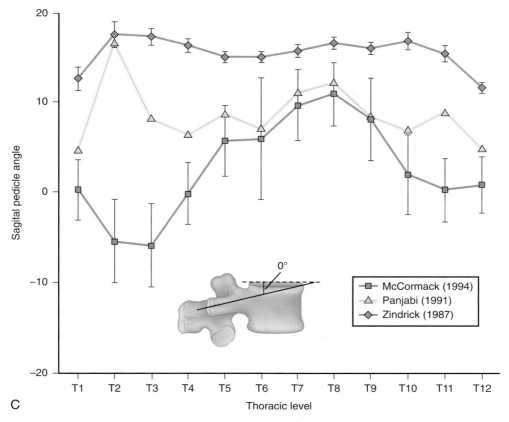

C

FIGURE 18–9, cont'd C, Sagittal pedicle angles found in five different studies. (A, From Netter FH: Atlas of Human Anatomy, 2nd ed. 1998; B and C, from McCormack BM, Benzel EC, Adams MS, et al: Anatomy of the thoracic pedicle. Neurosurgery 37:303-308, 1995.)

reliably with each subsequent thoracic level (Fig. 18–9B and C).[27] The pedicles are typically angled in a posterior lateral fashion from their respective vertebrae. As one moves distally from T1 to T12, the medial angulation of the pedicle decreases, however. The superoinferior pedicle diameter is consistently larger than the mediolateral pedicle diameter.[18] Of all the thoracic pedicles, the T4 pedicle is usually the narrowest. The pedicle wall is also two to three times thicker medially than laterally.[18]

The thoracic facets arise from above and below the pedicle. The superior facet has its articular surface on the dorsal aspect, whereas the inferior facet has its articular orientation on the ventral aspect. Generally, the thoracic facets are oriented in a more coronal direction. As one moves from the thoracic to the lumbar spine, the facets change from a coronal to a more sagittal orientation.

The thoracic ribs articulate with the vertebral bodies beginning with T1 via a costal facet. The first rib articulates with the vertebral body of only T1. Ribs 1 through 7 also intersect the sternum and are classified as true ribs. Ribs 8 through 10 connect through costal cartilage to the rib above and are termed false ribs. Ribs 11 and 12 are classified as floating ribs because they do not attach to either the sternum or the costal cartilage, only their corresponding vertebral bodies.[16] The other rib heads overlie adjoining intervertebral disc space via two types of articulations. The costovertebral articulation is

between the head of the rib and the vertebral body (Fig. 18–10). The articular capsule, radiate ligament, and intra-articular ligaments stabilize this articulation. The costotransverse articulation is between the neck and the tubercle of the rib and the transverse process. The superior and lateral costotransverse ligaments stabilize this junction. The T11 and T12 transverse processes do not articulate with their ribs.

The transverse process is at the junction of the facet and the par interarticularis. The nerve roots are anterior and superior to the transverse process, whereas the branches of the dorsal rami are found anteroinferiorly.[7] The nerve roots run immediately ventral to the transverse process of the next lower

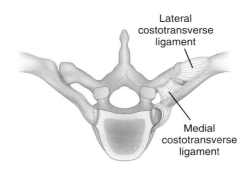

FIGURE 18–10 Costovertebral articulations. (From Netter FH: Atlas of Human Anatomy, 2nd ed. 1998.)

spinal level. An intertransverse aponeurosis bridges between adjacent processes, and if dissection remains dorsal to this aponeurosis, the nerve roots remain relatively safe and protected.

Posterior Approaches to Thoracic Spine

The posterior approach to the thoracic spine is the workhorse of most spine surgeons. It is a versatile approach that allows access to the osseoligamentous portions of the posterior spine to treat various conditions that affect this area. The posterior approach can be used for managing trauma, accessing neoplasms, correcting deformity, and eradicating infection. Knowledge of this approach and the anatomy allows the surgeon to address pathologies of the posterior spine comfortably.

Posterior Approach for Decompressive Laminectomy

Dorsal decompressive laminectomy can sometimes be indicated and advantageous in treating pathology in the thoracic spine. The exposure of the spine is typically very direct and avoids any major neurovascular structures. Laminectomy is often performed to decompress the thoracic spine and allow additional space for the spinal cord, but surgeons should be careful in using this approach alone in patients whose stability in this region may be compromised. The approach involves stripping the soft tissue of the posterior elements, which normally act as a tension band on the spine, off the osseous structures. Patients who have perioperative instability or anterior column incompetence may not benefit from isolated posterior thoracic decompression because of risk of secondary kyphosis.[28] Additional augmented stability may be necessary, such as fusion with or without instrumentation.

Indications for laminectomy include the following:

- Decompression of the thoracic spine because of stenosis or spondylosis or other mechanical impingement
- Evacuation of epidural abscess or hematoma
- Treatment of traumatic spine injuries
- Removal of bony neoplasms of the posterior elements
- Access to intradural and extradural tumors

From the time when laminectomy was first described by Smith in 1828[29] to its promotion by Hibb and Albee in the early 1900s and its use today, this surgical procedure has been used for a wide variety of applications. It provides access to the spinal canal for posterior decompression, posterior fusion, thoracic discectomy, access to intradural lesions, and stabilization procedures.[30] The relative contraindications for each case and the surgeon's expertise should be carefully reviewed with each preoperative plan.

Preoperative images should be reviewed and made available for the case before proceeding. Choice of anesthesia depends on the patient's comorbidities, the preference of the treating surgeon, and experience of the anesthesiologist.

Most patients receive a general anesthetic at the start of the case.

After anesthesia is administered, the patient is positioned in a prone position on the Jackson frame or on chest rolls on the operative table. It is important to provide sufficient space for the abdomen to prevent venous engorgement of the epidural venous plexus. Doing so minimizes excessive bleeding; aids with exposure; and minimizes use of electrocautery, which may place the surrounding nerve roots at risk for injury.

The surgeon should determine the levels to be decompressed and plan for sufficient exposure of the thoracic spine by isolating the region with ten-ten drapes before preparing the skin. Surface landmarks of the thoracic spine that can reasonably be palpated include the C7 spinous process and T7 spinous process, which typically lies at the inferior margin of the scapula. Intraoperative imaging can also be obtained before the incision to confirm the location of the operative level.

After localizing the area to be treated, a longitudinal line is drawn directly over the spinous processes of the levels desired. It is reasonable to extend the incision up to one level proximal and distal to obtain adequate exposure. The initial incision should be made with a No. 10 knife. The incision is deepened through the subcutaneous tissue with electrocautery, and any bleeders that are encountered along the way are coagulated. Care is taken not to devascularize the skin during the approach; otherwise, there is a risk of wound healing challenges.

After cutting through the subcutaneous tissue, the muscles of the back are encountered. The muscles are separated subperiosteally from either side of the spinous process and retracted laterally. The trapezius and rhomboid muscle aponeurosis is located in the upper thoracic spine, and the latissimus dorsi is located in the lower thoracic spine. Deeper still, the intrinsic muscles of the erector spinae and the transversospinal group are separated subperiosteally from the spinous processes and laminae.[31] Staying subperiosteal helps to minimize bleeding.

Self-retaining retractors are used to hold the paraspinal muscle aside during the exposure. Care is taken not to dissect deep to the ribs or too far lateral to the pars, or there is risk of injuring the pleura. The facet joint is exposed without stripping the capsule, unless fusion is planned at the operative levels. Also, care is taken not to injure the neurovascular bundle that runs on the undersurface of the ribs.

When adequate exposure of the laminae is obtained, the formal laminectomy can be started. This can be accomplished by one of several ways. A high-speed bur or drill can be used to create a trough bilaterally at the junction of the lamina and facet. When thinned, a small or medium Kerrison rongeur should be used to complete the laminectomy (Fig. 18–11). The ligamentum flavum on the undersurface should also be cut sharply with the rongeur with complete visualization of the dura to keep it protected. Further decompression should be performed where appropriate by removing the facet or pedicle without destabilizing the spine.

Closure of the wound should be performed in a sequential fashion. The surgeon should ensure that hemostasis is obtained and that there is no evidence of cerebrospinal fluid leak. Any bleeder should be controlled with electrocautery, and thrombin-soaked absorbable gelatin sponge (Gelfoam) should be used if bony bleeding is noted from the laminectomy site. An epidural drain can be used for a few days postoperatively to limit the buildup of epidural fluid. The aponeurosis of the paraspinal muscles should be reapproximated with absorbable suture, and the subcutaneous skin and tissue should be brought together. The surgeon staples the skin or uses a running Monocryl suture and applies sterile dressings to the incision.

KEY POINTS

1. A high-speed bur is used to create a trough at the laminae and facet junction to help create the start point of the laminectomy.

2. A small or medium-sized Kerrison rongeur with a small footplate is used to complete the resection of the laminae and to minimize pressure on the cord.

3. Dissection should be performed subperiosteally under the paraspinal muscles to limit bleeding of this tissue.

Transpedicular Approach

The transpedicular approach of thoracic decompression is often used to debulk tumors, to treat herniated soft discs, or mainly to decompress the associated nerve root. Symptomatic thoracic discs occur in about 1% of patients requiring an operation. Wood and colleagues[32] prospectively followed 20 patients with 48 thoracic disc herniations and performed serial magnetic resonance imaging (MRI) and clinical follow-up examinations. All patients remained asymptomatic during a median follow-up of 26 months. Most protruding discs occur below T8, and a common patient presentation is pain.[9] About one third of patients complain of radiating pain in the distribution of the intercostal nerve, but paracentral and central disc protrusion causes compression of the spinal cord and clinical symptoms of myelopathy.

Multiple surgical approaches have been proposed over several decades to treat these rare lesions in this area of the spine. In 1978, Patterson and Arbit[33] first published the posterior transpedicular approach to treatment of herniated thoracic discs, and it has gained acceptance as a reasonable way to access other pathology in the area. This approach evolved as other proposed procedures were discovered to have disappointing results and especially risked injury to the spinal cord.[32,34,35]

In approaching a lesion using the transpedicular approach, the patient is intubated and placed in a supine position on the Jackson table or a radiolucent table on chest supporters. The desired area to be treated is prepared and draped in a sterile fashion. An image intensifier may be used to localize the area that is to be treated before incision, or one may estimate by counting ribs.

When the level is established, an incision is made midline over the spinous process with a No. 10 blade knife. Subperiosteal dissection is continued laterally underneath the

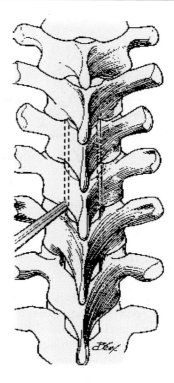

FIGURE 18–11 Laminectomy approach.

paraspinal muscles until one has exposed the laminae and facet joint. Patterson and Arbit[33] described a unilateral approach. Either a unilateral or a bilateral transpedicular approach can be accomplished depending on the goals of treatment. A unilateral approach may be less destabilizing to the spine but limits exposure to the posterolateral aspect of the vertebral body. A bilateral approach may allow one to perform almost a complete discectomy or even vertebrectomy.

Next, the thoracic pedicle overlying the disc herniations or level to be treated is identified. The caudal pedicle is just adjacent to the intervertebral discs (i.e., the T9-10 disc is next to the T10 pedicle.). Removal of the superior and inferior facets may allow better exposure of the intended pedicle; this may be accomplished with a bur or a rongeur. It may be necessary to remove the facets, costovertebral joint, and pars completely if a vertebrectomy is intended and an interbody graft is going to be placed.

The surgeon enters and removes the cancellous, central portion of the pedicle with a high-speed bur. An image intensifier helps one reach the appropriate depth and stop short of the vertebral body. When the depth of the resection is established, the cortical bone adjacent to the spinal canal medially and superiorly is removed using small down-biting curets. The lateral and inferior portions of the pedicle do not need to be violated. The fasciae of the psoas and the quadratus lumborum muscles make up the lateral borders of this approach. Disc material is removed through this opening, and care is taken not to injure the cord or nerve roots during this process (Fig. 18–12).

Performing a laminectomy before this stage allows for clear identification of the exiting nerve root before removing the

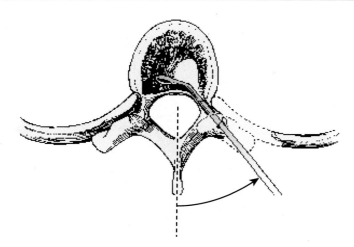

FIGURE 18–12 Transpedicular approach.

pedicle. The lateral disc space is incised, and a large cavity is created in the disc space by using curets and pituitary rongeurs, working in a lateral-to-medial direction beneath the spinal dura. The disc fragments causing cord compression can be removed using down-biting curets. When decompression of the ventral surface of the cord is accomplished through either simple discectomy or partial vertebrectomy, additional space for the cord can be created by performing a standard laminectomy if desired.

KEY POINTS

1. Because of the angle of the approach, this approach may not be well suited for lesions centrally located in the spinal column.

2. The spinal cord must always be protected and should never be retracted. The surgeon should remove bone as required to improve exposure.

3. Intraoperative imaging is helpful for localizing the level and determining depth of resection.

Costotransversectomy

Costotransversectomy can be performed in either a prone position or with a classic posterolateral approach. In 1984, Menard provided the first known description of costotransversectomy in the treatment of a spinal abscess.[36] This surgical procedure was traditionally performed to drain tuberculosis abscesses while avoiding the major risks associated with an anterior surgery. The utility of this procedure to treat other conditions of the posterior thoracic spine has grown as other surgeons have modified and expanded on the original technique over the years. The costotransversectomy approach has also been used for excising disc herniations, removing nonincarcerated hemivertebra, and accessing intraspinal lesions. Other authors have gone a step further and used this approach to treat congenital and acquired kyphoscoliosis.[36]

Generally, costotransversectomy allows access to the posterior vertebral body, intervertebral disc, anterior and lateral epidural space, and intervertebral foramen. One shortfall of this approach is that the surgeon has a limited view of the anterior spinal canal. It is frequently better tolerated, however, than a formal thoracotomy in patients with high morbidity and allows for exposure of the entire length of the spine.

Indications for costotransversectomy include the following:

- Abscess drainage
- Partial vertebral body resection
- Treatment of traumatic spine injuries
- Anterolateral decompression of the cord
- Biopsy and decompression of neoplasms

Anesthesia is administered to the patient before positioning. Traditionally, the patient is placed in a prone position on the Jackson frame or on chest rolls on the operative table. The patient may also be placed in a semiprone or modified lateral decubitus position if desired. When positioning, the surgeon should double check and ensure that all bony prominences are well padded and if in a lateral position that the axilla is padded distally and leaving sufficient clearance.

The patient is prepared and draped widely to allow sufficient exposure of the rib cage laterally. It may be helpful to determine the operative level of the incision with preoperative imaging. Alternatively, one can count the ribs from distal to proximal to isolate the level desired. The head of the rib articulates with the intervertebral cavity formed by adjacent vertebrae. The fifth rib articulates with the T4-5 disc space. Identification of the level of interest is essential before the start of the procedure. The location of the patient's midline is reconfirmed by palpating the spinous processes.

Various locations of incisions have been described in the past. A median or paramedian incision may be made straight or curved centered over the desired vertebral level. Traditionally, a curvilinear incision about 8 cm lateral to the intended spinous process and 10 to 13 cm long has been used (Fig. 18–13).[17] After the skin incision is made with a knife, the incision is deepened through the superficial and deep fascia to the muscle of the trapezius or latissimus dorsi if at lower thoracic levels. The surgeon transects through the fibers of the trapezius close to the transverse processes of the ribs. The remaining muscles are taken down off the rib of interest in a parallel fashion. The exposure can be widened by dissecting the rib just superior to the one of interest. The muscle attachments are carefully detached from the desired rib with a periosteal elevator (Fig. 18–14A). Also, any muscle attachment is dissected from the transverse process and lamina to provide clear exposure of the operative level (Fig. 18–14B).

The rib and its arthrodial junction can now be disarticulated (Fig. 18–14C). The lateral division can be accomplished 6 to 8 cm from midline; this depends on the extent of pathology that needs to be addressed. Care should be taken not to injure the neurovascular bundle during resection. Identification of the nerve to its dural sleeve in the intervertebral foramen may aid in its safe retraction and allow one to locate the spinal cord reliably. After lateral division, the rib is lifted out of its periosteal bed and disarticulated from the costo-transverse process. This bone can be saved for bone graft and used for fusion if appropriate. When cleared of any muscle, the transverse process may also be resected at its junction with the lamina and pedicle.

Next, the lateral pedicle is identified, and the neurovascular bundle is protected with further dissection. The surgeon subperiosteally dissects along the pedicle and upper and lower vertebral body to separate the pleura from the vertebral wall (Fig. 18–14D). By now, the site of the abscess for irrigation, if present, may have been encountered. Further exposure can be obtained by taking down the pedicle or resecting the facets. If the surgeon intends to dissect to the front of the spine to address fractures or perform a biopsy, he or she must take care to elevate the prevertebral fascia.

KEY POINTS

1. The operative level is localized with intraoperative imaging before incision.

2. The transverse process is clearly exposed by removing any soft tissue and muscle.

3. The neurovascular bundle should be protected during rib resection.

4. The exposure is widened by taking down an additional rib cephalad or caudad.

Lateral Extracavitary Approach

In 1976, Larson and colleagues at the Medical College of Wisconsin expanded on the work of Menard and Capener in the treatment of Pott disease.[37] The lateral extracavitary approach

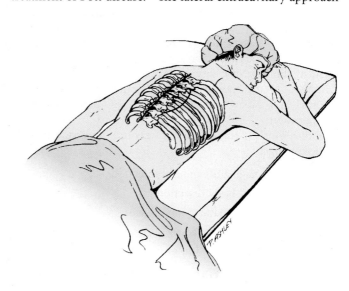

FIGURE 18–13 Median or paramedian incision may be made straight or curved centered over desired vertebral level. Traditionally, curvilinear incision about 8 cm lateral to intended spinous process and 10 to 13 cm long has been used.

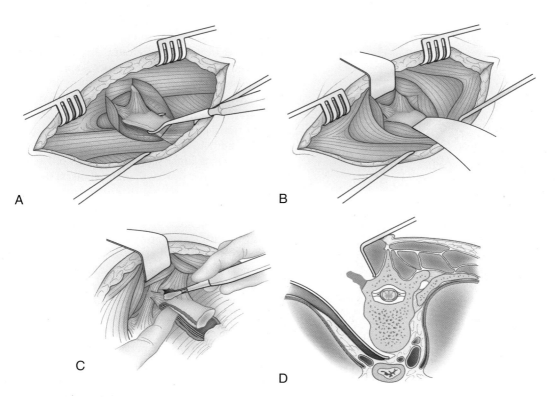

A

B

C

D

FIGURE 18–14 A, Muscle attachments are carefully detached from desired rib with periosteal elevator. **B,** Muscle attachments from transverse process and lamina are detached to give clear exposure of rib and its articulation to spine. **C,** Rib and its arthrodial junction can now be disarticulated. **D,** Subperiosteal dissection is done along pedicle and upper and lower vertebral body to separate pleura from vertebral wall.

allows for simultaneous exposure of posterior elements of the spine and anterior vertebral body and builds on the success of other approaches, such as costotransversectomy, to gain better access to the ventral thecal sac. This approach has evolved since its inception, and its use has expanded beyond treating just vertebral osteomyelitis and Pott disease. Today, the lateral extracavitary approach is used for various applications, including access to vertebral body tumors, treatment of infections, intraspinous decompression of neural lesions, and treatment of thoracic disc disease. Access can be obtained from C7 down to the thoracolumbar junction. It avoids thoracotomy and laparotomy and many of their associated complications.

Indications for the lateral extracavitary approach include the following:

- Abscess drainage and epidural infections
- Partial vertebral body resection
- Treatment of traumatic spine injuries
- Thoracic disc herniations
- Biopsy and decompression of neoplasms

The patient is placed in a prone position on a Jackson frame or other radiolucent table with chest bolsters to allow the abdomen to hang freely. The surgeon should ensure the patient is secured appropriately to the bed. With the patient appropriately secured, the surgeon can safely rotate the bed slightly to the contralateral side and facilitate exposure of the ventral thecal sac across the midline. Care should be taken to ensure

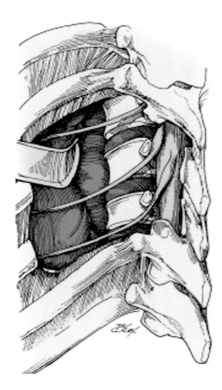

FIGURE 18–15 When posterolateral structures of transverse process and pedicle have been removed, exposure should be adequate for discectomy.

that the head is resting comfortably in the head rest and no pressure is placed on the orbits of the eyes. The anesthesiologist often confirms that the endotracheal tube (if general anesthesia is used) is well secured but also not encroaching on the corners of the mouth. The arms are placed in a position of comfort and are well padded.

Fluoroscopy or intraoperative x-ray may be used to isolate the level to be treated. This area should be widely draped and sufficient space should be allowed in case a thoracotomy becomes necessary during the case. The skin is prepared in the usual sterile manner.

A midline incision over the spinous processes centered over the operative level of interest can be employed. This incision and approach are similar to costotransversectomy. The skin incision is made with a No. 10 blade knife and deepened through the superficial and deep fascia to the muscle of the trapezius and latissimus dorsi if one is at the lower thoracic levels. This incision can also be extended laterally by 8 cm to the operative side if a wider exposure is needed, resulting in a hockey stick–type incision. Next, transection is through the fibers of the trapezius close to the transverse processes of the ribs. A plane is developed to expose the lateral edge of the paraspinal muscles. Self-retaining retractors are useful in maintaining good exposure throughout the approach. The underlying erector spinae muscles are dissected in a subperiosteal fashion off the transverse process and reflected medially. The ribs are identified and stripped of any muscle attachments subperiosteally as well as in a circumferential fashion. This can be done with a Doyen rib dissector.

The exposure can be widened by dissecting the rib just superior to the level of interest. This widening may be necessary if the surgeon intends on performing more extensive work than just a discectomy. Any muscle attachment is dissected from the transverse process and lamina to provide clear exposure of the operative level.

After exposure, the transverse process, rib head, and costotransverse ligaments are identified and divided. Resection of the transverse process is accomplished, and removal of the targeted rib is completed. With the lateral extracavitary approach, a larger section (≤12 cm) of rib is resected, which allows a wider view of the ventral thecal sac. The lateral section of the rib is cut with a rib cutter, and the medial articulation is disarticulated from its vertebral body and costal attachments. Care must be taken not to damage the pleural lining as the ventral vertebral body is approached.

With the rib resected and the transverse process removed, the neurovascular bundle can be followed to the neuroforamen. The pedicle is encountered here and can be removed with a rongeur or a high-speed drill. Care should be taken not to injure the thecal sac while in close proximity with the drill.

When the posterolateral structures of the transverse process and pedicle have been removed, exposure should be adequate enough for discectomy (Fig. 18–15). The posterior vertebral body can be taken down with curets, a drill, or a pituitary rongeur. Further exposure can be developed toward the midline by decompressing the vertebral body. If this decompression is undertaken, a thin layer of cortical bone just ventral to the thecal sac should be maintained to protect the canal contents. This layer can be taken down in a controlled fashion after the remaining anterior cortical and cancellous bone has been decompressed. Corpectomy can proceed from the ipsilateral side of the vertebral body to the extent of the contralateral pedicle. The corpectomy may be facilitated by rotating the secured patient away from the surgeon 20 to 30 degrees.

After exposure of the posterior and ventral surfaces, stabilization can be accomplished with the use of autograft or other interbody device. If may be helpful to verify placement with intraoperative fluoroscopy. Pedicle screw instrumentation of adjacent segments may also be done through a separate fascial incision. With decompression completed, closure should be performed in a sequential fashion. A deep or subcutaneous drain can be placed, and any pleural breaches should be repaired. If the breach is significant, chest tube placement may be necessary.[38] If a chest tube is placed, a postoperative chest x-ray should be obtained to confirm its placement and track its function.

Although this procedure provides excellent exposure of the thecal sac, it can be technically demanding. This approach may have significant operative blood loss, and the surgeon should be prepared for intraoperative transfusion or use of a Cell Saver during the case. The operative time may also be extensive and use of a warmer may be beneficial to the patient.

KEY POINTS

1. The lateral extracavitary approach is similar to costotransversectomy, but provides additional exposure from a wider rib section (12 cm vs. 6 cm).

2. The ventral thecal sac is protected during corpectomy by leaving a thin shell of dorsal cortical bone until this can be depressed into the ventral body.

3. Improved visualization can be achieved during vertebral body resection toward the contralateral pedicle by rotating the patient away from the operative side by 20 to 30 degrees.

4. The surgeon should repair any breach in the pleural lining before complete closure and be prepared to place a chest tube if necessary.

Summary

There are numerous posterior approaches to the thoracic spine. Many of these approaches have been refined and their use expanded on from the original pioneering authors. With each procedure, there are inherent risks and cautions that should be recognized and acknowledged. As medicine advances and new techniques are presented, users of these new techniques should always ensure that they understand the human anatomy and always put patient safety first.

PEARLS

1. During anterior cervical procedures, approaching the cervicothoracic junction from the left is preferred because the recurrent laryngeal nerve has a more reliable course on this side.

2. For thoracic cases, the initial incision is made into the parietal pleura at the disc space, where it is relatively safer.

3. During thoracoabdominal cases, careful attention should be paid to the diaphragm and abdominal muscle during closure to help minimize the risk of a hernia formation.

4. During a transpedicular approach, intraoperative imaging is helpful for localizing a given level and determining depth of resection.

5. During a corpectomy, the ventral thecal sac is protected by leaving a thin shell of dorsal cortical bone until this can be depressed into the ventral body.

PITFALLS

1. During anterior cervical approaches, if the carotid artery is not identified, dissection into the vascular plane can occur and injure the artery and other adjacent neurologic structures.

2. An improper rib count may lead to wrong level surgery, so the count should be double-checked when identifying the rib level; one may also count proximally from the 12th rib up.

3. During a thoracolumbar approach, if one does not elevate the psoas muscle subperiosteally, the lumbar roots may be injured.

4. Retracting the spinal cord during any procedure may cause irreversible damage and permanent neurologic deficits.

5. A breach in the pleural lining that is left unrepaired before wound closure may cause serious postoperative complications.

KEY REFERENCES

1. Kothe R, O'Holleran JD, Liu W, et al: Internal architecture of the thoracic pedicle: An anatomic study. Spine 21:264-270, 1996.
    In this study, data are presented that provide the surgeon with additional information about the internal structure of the thoracic pedicle, which is especially useful for pedicle screw fixation in the thoracic spine. The authors quantify the internal structure of the pedicle in the thoracic spine.

2. McCormack BM, Benzel EC, Adams MS, et al: Anatomy of the thoracic pedicle. Neurosurgery 37:303-308, 1995.
    The authors describe the thoracic pedicle anatomy (interpedicular distance, transverse and sagittal pedicle widths, transverse and sagittal pedicle angles, and distance from the axis of the pedicle to the axis of the transverse process) by assessing 11 cadavers of elderly people. This article presents a previously unreported morphometric finding: the rostral-caudal distance from the thoracic pedicle to the midpoint of the base of the transverse process.

REFERENCES

1. Tew JM Jr, Mayfield FH: Complications of surgery of the anterior cervical spine. Clin Neurosurg 23:424-434, 1976.

2. Kilburg C, Sullivan HG, Mathiason MA: Effect of approach side during anterior cervical discectomy and fusion on the incidence of recurrent laryngeal nerve injury. J Neurosurg Spine 4:273-277, 2006.

3. Daniels AH, Riew KD, Yoo JU, et al: Adverse events associated with anterior cervical spine surgery. J Am Acad Orthop Surg 16:729-738, 2008.

4. Lu J, Ebraheim NA, Nadim Y, et al: Anterior approach to the cervical spine: Surgical anatomy. Orthopedics 23:841-845, 2000.

5. Miscusi M, Bellitti A, Peschillo S, et al: Does recurrent laryngeal nerve anatomy condition the choice of the side for approaching the anterior cervical spine? J Neurosurg Sci 51:61-64, 2007.

6. Liu YL, Hao YJ, Li T, et al: Trans-upper-sternal approach to the cervicothoracic junction. Clin Orthop Relat Res 467:2018-2024, 2008.

7. Kim DH: Surgical Anatomy and Techniques to the Spine. Philadelphia, WB Saunders, 2006.

8. Campos JH: Lung isolation techniques. Anesthesiol Clin North Am 19:455-474, 2001.

9. Fessler RG, Sekhar LN: Atlas of Neurosurgical Techniques: Spine and Peripheral Nerves. New York, Thieme, 2006.

10. Whang PG, Vaccaro AR: Thoracolumbar fracture: Posterior instrumentation using distraction and ligamentotaxis reduction. J Am Acad Orthop Surg 15:695-701, 2007.

11. Kirkpatrick JS: Thoracolumbar fracture management: Anterior approach. J Am Acad Orthop Surg 11:355-363, 2003.

12. Vaccaro AR, Bono CM: Minimally Invasive Spine Surgery. New York, Informa Healthcare, 2007.

13. Landreneau RJ, Hazelrigg SR, Mack MJ, et al: Postoperative pain-related morbidity: Video-assisted thoracic surgery versus thoracotomy. Ann Thorac Surg 56:1285-1289, 1993.

14. Hazelrigg SR, Landreneau RJ, Boley TM, et al: The effect of muscle-sparing versus standard posterolateral thoracotomy on pulmonary function, muscle strength, and postoperative pain. J Thorac Cardiovasc Surg 101:394-400; discussion 400-391, 1991

15. Mayer HM: Minimally Invasive Spine Surgery: A Surgical Manual, 2nd ed. Berlin; New York, Springer, 2006.

16. Magee DJ. Orthopedic Physical Assessment, 4th ed. Philadelphia, Saunders, 2002.

17. Hoppenfeld S, DeBoer P, Hutton R: Surgical Exposures in Orthopaedics: The Anatomic Approach, 2nd ed. Philadelphia, JB Lippincott, 1994.

18. Kothe R, O'Holleran JD, Liu W, et al: Internal architecture of the thoracic pedicle: An anatomic study. Spine 21:264-270, 1996.

19. Banta CJ 2nd, King AG, Dabezies EJ, et al: Measurement of effective pedicle diameter in the human spine. Orthopedics 12:939-942, 1989.

20. Berry JL, Moran JM, Berg WS, et al: A morphometric study of human lumbar and selected thoracic vertebrae. Spine 12:362-367, 1987.

21. Krag MH, Weaver DL, Beynnon BD, et al: Morphometry of the thoracic and lumbar spine related to transpedicular screw placement for surgical spinal fixation. Spine 13:27-32, 1988.

22. Panjabi MM, Takata K, Goel V, et al: Thoracic human vertebrae: Quantitative three-dimensional anatomy. Spine 16:888-901, 1991.

23. Zindrick MR, Wiltse LL, Doornik A, et al: Analysis of the morphometric characteristics of the thoracic and lumbar pedicles. Spine 12:160-166, 1987.

24. Moran JM, Berg WS, Berry JL, et al: Transpedicular screw fixation. J Orthop Res 7:107-114, 1989.

25. Roy-Camille R, Saillant G, Mazel C: Plating of thoracic, thoracolumbar, and lumbar injuries with pedicle screw plates. Orthop Clin North Am 17:147-159, 1986.

26. Kim YW, Lenke LG, Kim YJ, et al: Free-hand pedicle screw placement during revision spinal surgery: Analysis of 552 screws. Spine 33:1141-1148, 2008.

27. McCormack BM, Benzel EC, Adams MS, et al: Anatomy of the thoracic pedicle. Neurosurgery 37:303-308, 1995.

28. Vaccaro AR, Albert TJ: Spine Surgery: Tricks of the Trade, 2nd ed. New York, Thieme, 2009.

29. Yasuoka SPH, MacCarty C: Incidence of spinal column deformity after multilevel laminectomy in children and adults. J Neurosurg 57:441-445, 1982.

30. Hoppenfeld S, DeBoer P, Hutton R, et al: Surgical Exposures in Orthopaedics: The Anatomic Approach. Philadelphia, JB Lippincott, 1984.

31. Shikata J, Yamamuro T, Shimizu K, et al: Combined laminoplasty and posterolateral fusion for spinal canal surgery in children and adolescents. Clin Orthop Relat Res (259):92-99, 1990.

32. Wood KB, Blair JM, Aepple DM, et al: The natural history of asymptomatic thoracic disc herniations. Spine 22:525-529; discussion 529-530, 1997.

33. Patterson RH Jr, Arbit E: A surgical approach through the pedicle to protruded thoracic discs. J Neurosurg 48:768-772, 1978.

34. Perot PL Jr, Munro DD: Transthoracic removal of midline thoracic disc protrusions causing spinal cord compression. J Neurosurg 31:452-458, 1969.

35. Logue V: Thoracic intervertebral disc prolapse with spinal cord compression. J Neurol Neurosurg Psychiatry 15:227-241, 1952.

36. Campbell WC, Edmonson AS, Crenshaw AH: Campbell's Operative Orthopaedics, 6th ed. St. Louis, CV Mosby, 1980.

37. Lifshutz J, Lidar Z, Maiman D: Evolution of the lateral extracavitary approach to the spine. Neurosurg Focus 16:E12, 2004.

38. Vaccaro AR: Fractures of the Cervical, Thoracic, and Lumbar Spine. New York, Marcel Dekker, 2003.

19 CHAPTER

Anterior Exposure to Lumbosacral Spine: Anatomy and Techniques

David S. Wernsing, MD
Richard Balderston, MD

There has been an increasing need for access surgery to the lumbosacral spine. In the past, the need for access was due to the prevalence of Pott disease from tuberculosis with associated spinal osteomyelitis, severe fractures of the spine, or malignant involvement and destruction of the spine. With evolution of the understanding of the pain mechanism in spine disease, there has been a significant increase in the number of spinal fusion procedures. With progress continuing in the development of artificial disc constructs, the need for complete anterior access to the lumbar spine continues to increase. The surgeon who performs anterior spine access procedures must be intimately familiar with the anatomy of the lumbar spine region and adept at recognizing potential hazards to minimize the risk of complications during approach surgery.

Anatomy

Detailed knowledge of the anatomy surrounding the lumbar spine is mandatory to approach the spine with a minimum of risk. By taking advantage of the avascular tissue planes of the abdominal wall and with a thorough knowledge of the anatomic structures to be encountered, the surgeon can gain access to the retroperitoneal space with only a small amount of tissue division.

Abdominal Wall

The superficial layers of the abdominal wall include the skin, subcutaneous fascia, and fatty layers separating them. The muscular wall of the abdomen is composed of differing layers depending on the medial or lateral location of examination. The abdominal wall is composed of three muscle layers lateral to the abdominal rectus muscle—the external and internal oblique muscles and the transversus abdominis muscle. Each layer has associated fascial extensions that come together to make up the anterior and posterior rectus sheath surrounding the rectus muscle medially. Deep to these layers is the transversalis fascia and the peritoneum with a variable amount of preperitoneal fat interspersed between these two

layers. As this layer progresses laterally, the peritoneum thickens and becomes less densely adherent to its adjacent tissue layer.

The posterior musculature includes the psoas major muscle immediately lateral to the lumbar spine. Lateral to the psoas muscle is the quadratus lumborum muscle superiorly and the iliacus muscle inferiorly transitioning at approximately the L4 level. At the more superior disc levels (approximately L2-3 and cephalad), the tendinous and muscular slips of the diaphragm start to form anteriorly on the spine itself. The right crus of the diaphragm inserts into L3, and the left crus inserts into L2. They are tendinous at this point and need to be taken down to expose L2-3. For L3-4, the right crus needs to be taken down for exposure all the way to the right side. These do not need to be repaired.

Retroperitoneal Structures

The primary nonvascular system of concern for the access surgeon is the genitourinary tract. On the left side, the ureter courses with its blood supply and the gonadal vessels until the ureter tracks medially over the iliac vessels at approximately the level of the common iliac artery bifurcation. More superiorly, the left kidney and its surrounding perirenal fat and fascia are encountered. Care must be taken when mobilizing the ureter to avoid devascularizing it with excessive dissection; this can be accomplished by maintaining the ureteral packet with the peritoneum, to which it is adherent.

Vascular Anatomy: Variability, Bifurcations, Iliolumbar Vein, Segmental Vessels, and Middle Sacral Vessels

The distal aorta and the distal vena cava with their respective bifurcations provide the primary structures of consequence to the immediate anterior surface of the lumbosacral region. The aorta sits to the left of the vena cava, in approximation with the midline of the spine, with its major branches typically crossing anterior to the venous branches of the cava. The vena cava sits to the right side of the spine, which is why right-sided approaches are more hazardous.

The vascular anatomy is reviewed in a caudad-to-cephalad order because this is the order of most common to least common levels of approach. The vasculature at the L5-S1 level generally consists of the middle sacral vessels, which can be divided between ligatures or cauterized, depending on their size. The vena cava bifurcation is generally superior to the L5-S1 disc and overlies the L5 vertebral body on the right side, although in a small percentage of individuals this is seated as low as the inferior edge of the L5-S1 disc itself. It bifurcates to the left and right common iliac veins.

Rarely, anomalous venous drainage may be present across the sacral spine. This may include a single vessel as a bridging iliac vein to a confluent venous plexus across the region. The iliolumbar vein typically branches off posterior to the common iliac vein at the L5 vertebral level and is an important consideration for exposure for the L4-5 disc space above. Most of the time, it may be identified within 2 cm of the L4-5 disc space. In a small percentage of patients, it may not be present. The common iliac artery can be easily visualized lateral to the vein and is usually bifurcating into the internal and external iliac arteries at the L5-S1 level.

The vascular anatomy at the L4-5 level is the most variable of all the levels and can provide either a boon or a bane to the access surgeon depending on its layout. Much has been described in scoring systems for the degree of difficulty this variability presents; however, it does not alter the general approach strategy. The aortic bifurcation and the cava bifurcation make up the variable vascular distribution for L4-5. This consideration is only for the amount of relative length that would be obtained when mobilizing the left common iliac artery, not for dissecting out the aortic bifurcation itself.

Generally, the caval bifurcation is at the L5 vertebral body. The aortic bifurcation sits between L4 and L5, although it is usually located superior to the L4-5 disc space. The left common iliac artery courses laterally from this and has a variable degree of length and tortuosity to it. Cephalad to the L4-5 level are the segmental vessels that cross over the vertebral bodies to enter the aorta. The dissection is to elevate the left common iliac artery to decrease the amount of tension on the vessel. In some instances of a high-riding aortic bifurcation, the common iliac artery is able to be maintained in a lateral position. Otherwise, complete mobilization is generally needed to maintain this vessel in a right-sided location relative to the face of the L4-5 disc during a left-sided approach.

Lymphatics

The lymphatics run in parallel to the vasculature surrounding the lumbar spine. The fatty tissue encompassing them may be increased in obese individuals or may be increased secondary to inflammatory processes. Disruption of the lymphatics occurs when exposing the L4-5 level and higher, although clinically significant lymphoceles or mild lymphedema is rare. Generally, the lymphatics track to the lateral aspect of the spine region between the vasculature and the psoas muscle.

Nerves

There are several nerves of importance that run in proximity to the field of dissection for a lumbosacral spine approach. In descending order, the somatic nerves lateral to the psoas muscle include the iliohypogastric nerve, ilioinguinal nerve, and lateral femoral cutaneous nerve. The genitofemoral nerve runs along the anterior surface of the psoas muscle before branching into the laterally located femoral branch and the medially located genital branch.

The sympathetic chain runs in parallel to the spine, along the lateralmost aspect of the anterior face of the vertebral body. Small bridging fibers can be seen coursing medially. The superior hypogastric plexus takes its form around the L5 level. These fibers are variable in their substance and can be viewed in forms ranging from a discrete nerve to a diffuse plexus as it courses inferiorly. They form upward to become the left and right hypogastric nerves, which are an important supply of sympathetic function in the pelvis. Injury to this nerve can cause retrograde ejaculation in men. These fibers are relatively adherent to the peritoneum and generally are mobilized as one structure, along with the ureter.

Surgical Approach

Preoperative Considerations

Communication is the mainstay to a successful partnership between the spine surgeon and access surgeon and the supporting surgical team. Before the day of surgery, relevant radiologic imaging will have been obtained and reviewed to determine the surgical plan. Any additional imaging should be pursued at that time to take into account disease processes that the patient may have. Examining plain films for signs of arterial calcifications, which may provide indirect evidence of vascular disease (Fig. 19–1), is particularly useful for the access surgeon. Additionally, the plain film should be evaluated for osteophytes and spondylolisthesis, which can exaggerate misleading anatomic bony features or be an indicator of potential inflammatory changes. A thorough vascular examination should be repeated at the time of surgery. Pulse oximetry on the patient's left lower extremity is a useful adjunct for monitoring arterial flow distal to the area of dissection. Positioning of the patient is important to facilitate intraoperative placement of personnel, fixed retraction, and fluoroscopy machines.

General Considerations

There are two general anatomic routes for anterior exposure to the lumbar spine—transperitoneal and retroperitoneal. Several techniques have been described for both anatomic routes. Generally, these can be distinguished as open techniques and laparoscopic or robotic assisted techniques. These techniques may vary from institution to institution based on access and preference of the spine surgeon, anatomic considerations, and type of spine operation being considered (type of fusion vs. disc replacement vs. oncologic intervention). There are advantages and disadvantages to both techniques, although there is generally a lower complication profile with an anterior retroperitoneal approach versus a transperitoneal approach.

With a higher associated complication rate, the open transperitoneal approach should be used only when extenuating circumstances exist (e.g., revision surgery or prior extensive retroperitoneal surgery) and not for primary open exposures. There are otherwise no advantages to performing a primary case transperitoneally from L2 to S1 because all these levels can be reached via a retroperitoneal route almost all the time. For access surgeons who use robotic or laparoscopic techniques in their transperitoneal approach, this may offset some of the risk.

Open Approaches

Retroperitoneal

The retroperitoneal approach can proceed from various incisions, including vertical midline, paramedian, oblique, and transverse. Extensive lateral incisions should be avoided because this may denervate medially situated rectus muscle. The incision needs to take into account the spinal level and the number of lumbar levels to be exposed. An infraumbilical transverse incision can accommodate most approaches to the L4-5 and L5-S1 disc levels, whereas a more obliquely oriented incision is favored for access to disc levels above L4 (Figs. 19–2 and 19–3). This incision allows for access to the L2-3 disc level and possibly L1-2 disc level in patients with a favorable body habitus.

The operative procedure should begin after an appropriate review of the films and after surgical goals have been established between the access surgeon and the spine surgeon. Communication with all members of the team is important to establish the surgical plan of the case and to decrease the risk of complications. Review of relevant radiographic material by the access surgeon can show potential deviations from normal anatomy and is the first step toward risk reduction. At that time, the relative position of the L4-5 disc level to the superior iliac crest can be identified.

Lateral fluoroscopy can be used to assess the level of the incision (Fig. 19–4). This imaging is done in conjunction with a radiopaque probe or rod to determine the angle of the approach and level, which can be marked on the patient's abdomen. Fluoroscopy can be especially important in obese patients because there may be no other anatomic landmarks palpable to guide the placement of the abdominal incision (Fig. 19–5). In most nonobese patients, palpation by an experienced access surgeon can be used to locate the sacral prominence to identify the L5-S1 disc space. A transverse approach to the L4-5 level should be directed at approximately the level of the superior anterior iliac spine, although fluoroscopic confirmation should be used if there is any question. All of the landmarks can be confirmed by fluoroscopic guidance, and fluoroscopy is especially important in patients who have distorted spine anatomy, had prior spine surgery, or are obese.

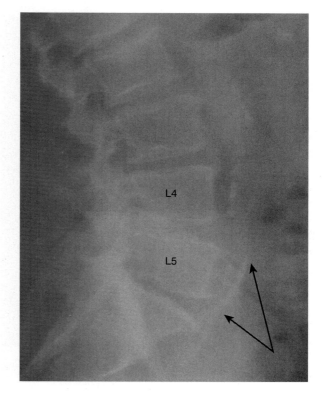

FIGURE 19–1 Calcification of aorta and common iliac artery (*arrow*).

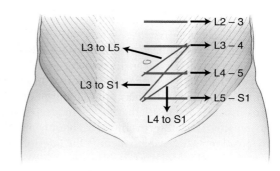

FIGURE 19–2 Approximate level of incision for approach of disc levels.

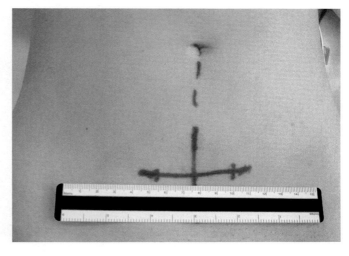

FIGURE 19–3 Skin marking for L5-S1 approach.

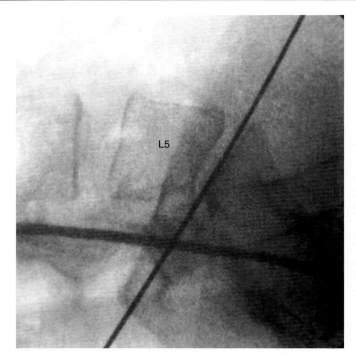

FIGURE 19–4 Radiologic determination of angle of approach for L5-S1 disc level.

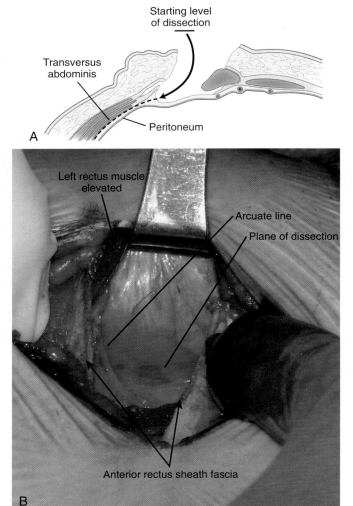

FIGURE 19–6 A, Initial approach to the retroperitoneum. **B,** Initial approach with the peritoneum separating away from the posterior rectus fascia.

When the level has been determined, the incision is made and cautery is used to deepen this to the level of the anterior rectus sheath fascia. The fascia is transversely or obliquely incised, and superior and inferior fascial flaps are raised at the linea alba. Care should be taken in patients who have had previous Pfannenstiel incisions because they may have unrecognized midline incisional hernias. The mobilization of the fascial flaps provides for less tethering of the deeper tissues and rectus muscle. The left rectus muscle is bluntly mobilized to a lateral position, taking care to identify the inferior epigastric vessels and small perforators. By dissecting deep to these vessels, they can be preserved; however, they can be clipped and divided if necessary.

Inspection and gentle finger dissection can be used to identify the inferior edge of the posterior rectus sheath.

This provides the landmark to begin blunt separation of the peritoneal cavity laterally to start the exposure into the retroperitoneal space (Fig. 19–6). Standing on the patient's right side allows the access surgeon to take advantage of the natural

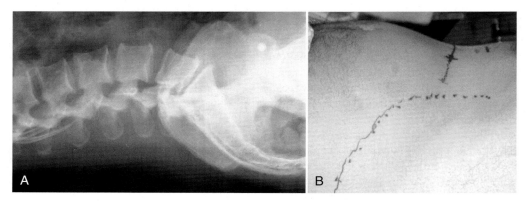

FIGURE 19–5 A, Lateral view of lumbar spine. **B,** Lateral view of patient.

motion of his or her hand to roll the peritoneum in a medial direction, although many surgeons proceed with the approach from the left side to maintain direct visualization of the vasculature (Fig. 19–7). The left ureter easily rolls up as part of this maneuver. The landmark to feel for is the bulge of the psoas muscle and the pulse of the common iliac artery. A common mistake is to persist in aggressive dissection lateral to the psoas muscle thinking that the planes may be adhesed. In almost all virgin retroperitoneal spaces, the blunt dissection should be able to be accomplished easily and without use of force (Fig. 19–8).

When the peritoneum has started to roll medially, and the iliac artery has been palpated, the next landmark to be palpated should be the L5-S1 disc level. Feeling for this

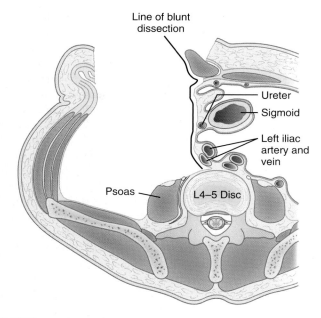

FIGURE 19–8 Approach to retroperitoneum with the peritoneal packet mobilized medially.

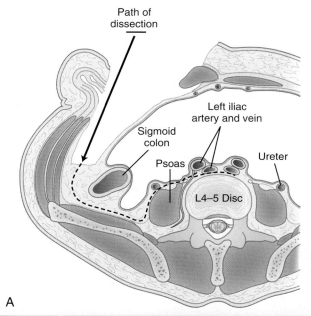

A

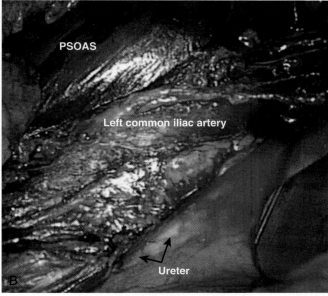

B

FIGURE 19–7 A, Initial line of approach once past the deep lateral margin of the posterior rectus sheath. **B,** View of the retroperitoneal structures with the peritoneal packet partially medialized.

prominence (comparing anatomic structures with the expected findings of the preoperative radiographs) lets the access surgeon confirm that the appropriate plane has been mobilized. In patients who have significantly abnormal anterior spine anatomy, plain films should be used to confirm location. Fixed or table-mounted retraction can be set to hold back the peritoneum and abdominal wall structures with secondary retractors (either table-mounted or hand-held) used for vascular structures. The ureter should be identified in its retroperitoneal course, and care should be taken to protect it. The arterial structures should be gently palpated at this point to evaluate their baseline and to feel for any evidence of plaque disease or thrills. When the initial peritoneal mobilization has been performed, the access surgeon may shift to the patient's left side; this provides for a more direct view of the lateral aspects of the vascular structures.

The L5-S1 disc space can be mobilized with the use of Kittner dissectors. The middle sacral vessels can be mobilized and divided between ligatures or small clips. The surgeon should be judicious in the use of clips because they may become dislodged or caught during dissection of the spine. Blunt dissection generally can be used to expose the entire face of the L5-S1 disc level without significant need for major vascular mobilization (Fig. 19–9). Care should be taken during the mobilization to elevate the superior hypogastric plexus with the peritoneum. This plexus typically feels like a fibrous band within the peritoneal fat and typically elevates with the peritoneal packet.

The L4-5 disc level is generally the most difficult level to provide full access to for the spine surgeon. The degree of difficulty can be established preoperatively with computed tomography (CT) angiography or magnetic resonance angiography, although angiography is generally unnecessary for most routine cases using open techniques. It is also important to look for vascular calcifications because calcification increases the potential risk for complications with an exposure at the L4-5 level. The transverse incision can be lengthened or obliqued based on the body mass and build of the patient.

The exposure can proceed as described earlier. After the retroperitoneum has been exposed, vascular mobilization is needed to access the L4-5 disc. A plain film can be obtained to confirm the disc level. Gentle blunt dissection can be used to mobilize the left common iliac artery. This dissection should be continued distally well onto the external iliac artery to minimize potential trauma to the artery. Generally, the vascular structures should be mobilized as paired structures, to minimize the "hazard" areas. Separating the vein and artery provides a 360-degree perimeter of vascular structures and is not recommended under routine circumstances. If it is a high bifurcation, a thorough mobilization of the left common iliac artery and vein may allow them to be retracted laterally. Gentle Kittner dissection shows the iliolumbar vein as it branches off the posterolateral aspect of the common iliac vein, inferior to the L4-5 disc. If it is not identified within approximately 15 to 20 mm of the disc space, it may not impede the exposure and may be left intact. Aggressive attempts at identifying the iliolumbar vein beyond this range may increase the risk of injury to the nerve roots in the region.

It is important to divide the vessel securely when there appears to be tethering because excessive traction on this structure can cause tearing with associated significant blood loss. Additional mobilization of the segmental vessels immediately adjacent and superior to the L4-5 region is sometimes necessary (Fig. 19–10). Pulse oximetry is important when mobilizing the L4-5 disc space or higher. Before retraction or mobilization, the oxygen saturation and waveform of a left lower extremity pulse oximeter should be evaluated. When retraction has been applied, if the saturation diminishes to zero, the surgeon has approximately 45 to 50 minutes before the retraction should be released to allow for resumption of unimpeded blood flow. The waveform should normalize over a brief period before replacement of the retractors. This can be repeated with periodic release of the retractors every 30 minutes or so after that. If there is not a return to baseline over a few minutes, vascular examination with ultrasound should be performed to minimize the risk of a missed injury or thrombosis.

Approaches to the lumbar spine above L4 can be through a transverse or more obliquely oriented incision. The abdominal wall is divided in layers to expose the peritoneum directly. Care must be taken in using blunt dissection to gain access to the retroperitoneal space. When completed, fixed retraction can be especially useful to maintain the level of exposure without lengthening the incision. Kittner dissection is used to mobilize the disc level, which can be confirmed with plain film evaluation.

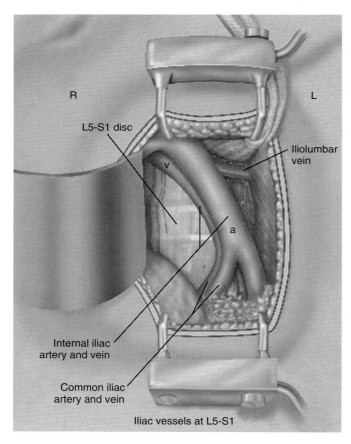

FIGURE 19–9 Exposure of L5-S1 disc.

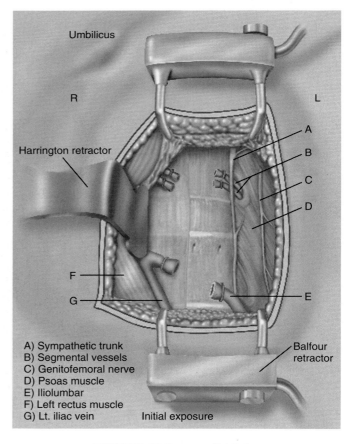

A) Sympathetic trunk
B) Segmental vessels
C) Genitofemoral nerve
D) Psoas muscle
E) Iliolumbar
F) Left rectus muscle
G) Lt. iliac vein

FIGURE 19–10 Exposure of L4-5 disc.

Transperitoneal

The transperitoneal approach is not generally used except in extenuating circumstances (e.g., prior extensive retroperitoneal surgery or revision spine access surgery). This approach starts with an incision in the midline to provide direct visualization of the abdominal cavity. Fixed retraction is generally used to facilitate controlling the small and large bowel to keep it out of the field of dissection. The Trendelenburg position can also be used to assist with maintaining exposure. For the L5-S1 level, the peritoneum superficial to the sacral prominence is incised. Care is taken to identify the vascular structures, and blunt dissection can be used to tease open the area of the face of the disc. Excessive cautery dissection should be minimized to decrease potential injury to the sympathetic nerves and hypogastric plexus. The middle sacral vessels generally need to be divided to complete the exposure.

Additional levels generally can be approached by mobilizing the left colon medially, taking care to identify the left ureter and the left gonadal vessels. This mobilization provides access to the L3-4 and L4-5 disc levels. More cephalad levels would need additional complete mobilization of the left kidney, and these levels are generally best attained via a true retroperitoneal approach.

Laparoscopic or Robotic Approach

Laparoscopic or robotic minimally invasive approaches have been used over the last 10 years as more attention has been given to overall patient recovery and length of stay. The immediacy of improvement with minimally invasive spine approaches has not followed the same pathway as for other general surgical procedures. The improvements in length of stay and cosmesis are sometimes seen but usually at a tradeoff of prolonged operative times and increased complication rates. These approaches are technically more complicated and are not in uniform or widespread use and have generally been superseded by the mini-open approach.[1-3]

As with open approaches, there are two general routes by which access surgeons perform laparoscopic approaches—transperitoneal and retroperitoneal. There are additional permutations to these types of approaches based on the type of spine intervention being performed and on whether the approach is fully laparoscopic or laparoscopic-assisted.

The transperitoneal approach involves the same maneuvers on the inside as described for the open approach. Fluoroscopy is used to site appropriately the level of the approach device being used. Two to four trocars are inserted to provide retraction for the bowel while mobilizing the peritoneum over the L5-S1 disc space. After the exposure has been completed laparoscopically, one of two steps can be taken. If the anterior fusion is being performed through guide tubes, a small incision can be made just large enough to accommodate the guide. It is positioned with lap guidance, and then the spine surgeon performs the fusion. Alternatively, the surgeon may place a small assist device, such as a hand port or wound protector device, to splint open a small incision to allow the spine surgeon to work directly.

Adapting minimally invasive surgery to the retroperitoneal approach has been slightly more challenging. Multiple techniques have been developed, but are based on laparoscopic or laparoscopic-assisted principles. With fluoroscopic guidance, the level of the disc is marked on the patient's abdomen. Using a lateral or oblique approach, an open trocar technique is used to access the retroperitoneal space. A balloon dissector or finger dissection can be used for the initial development of the space. Under direct vision, the balloon is insufflated to develop the retroperitoneal space mechanically. The balloon is then exchanged for a regular 10-mm trocar, and an additional two to three ports are placed as needed; this is usually done in a stepwise fashion as the space is developed further. Soft-tipped retractors and Kittners are used to mobilize the field at the indicated levels, using fluoroscopy as needed for guidance.

After the exposure has been completed in this fashion, the spine surgeon can be set up in a similar fashion as for the laparoscopic transperitoneal approach. This approach may be especially useful in obese patients who need a single-level exposure above L5. This approach would allow for the direct mobilization of the tissue surrounding the level that would otherwise be unable to be obtained without making a larger incision. There may also be an increasing role for this approach for spine surgeons who perform lateral lumbar interbody fusion.

Additional Exposure Considerations

There has been an evolution of the treatment algorithm of back pain with the continued development of motion-preserving disc replacement products. As greater numbers of patients undergo disc replacement, there is likely to be an accompanying need for revision surgery. Although the need for anterior revisions for acute problems has been uncommon, this is likely to increase with time as the parts typically sustain wear and tear as observed for other joint prostheses. For patients who are undergoing surgery at the L5-S1 level, the surgeon may use a right-sided approach to preserve the tissues planes in case it becomes necessary to return to the retroperitoneum.

For all levels, vascular protection "patches" are being used for twofold effect. The first is as a barrier interface to prevent vascular ingrowth and scarring into the discectomy space. Preservation of separate layers helps revision surgeons reaccess the space with less potential morbidity to the vasculature. Second, the inert barrier may provide a guide path through the surrounding scar tissue planes to reach the area of the disc. Although review of strategies for revision access is beyond the scope of this chapter, consideration for possible future revision at the time of the primary procedure would help to reduce the considerable morbidity associated with these procedures.

Complications

Complications secondary to anterior lumbar exposure can be minimized with a thorough knowledge of the anatomy and of

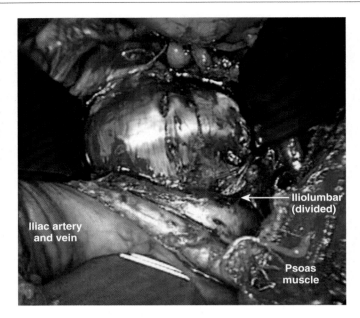

FIGURE 19–11 Anterior view of L4-5 disc.

the spine surgeon's operative technique. There is the potential for complications during the access phase of the operation and during the instrumentation phase, both of which need to be anticipated to minimize the risk.

During the initial exposure, appropriate precautions must be taken in any patient who has had prior lower abdominal surgery or disease states, ranging from procedures such as inguinal hernia repairs to cesarean sections to pathologic gynecologic disease or diverticulitis. Pediatric urologic procedures can be especially dangerous because the details may not be known by the patient. Male patients with prior hernia repairs with mesh may experience same-side testicular pain postoperatively, and this should be discussed ahead of time. Each can contribute to making the tissue planes more difficult to navigate. The access surgeon must always be suspicious for the potential of ventral or incisional hernias in any patient with lower abdominal scars.

Sharp dissection can be used to minimize cautery trauma while dissecting tissue planes around potential hernia sites. As dissection proceeds into the retroperitoneal planes, care must be taken not to apply undue force to mobilize them. Filmy avascular planes should be able to be manipulated with only a small amount of effort. Additional effort or need for cautery may be suggestive of veering into the wrong plane. Care should be taken to include the gonadal vessels and the left ureter en bloc with the medialized peritoneum because this provides the safest first step toward protecting the ureter. If there is doubt about any tubular structure, the surgeon should delay dividing it until it has been completely examined and identified.

Tears in the peritoneum usually can be primarily repaired at this time to help maintain the integrity of the cavity. This repair facilitates retraction and helps minimize potential injury to intra-abdominal organs, especially the intestines. If injury does occur with exposure of luminal contents to the

working field, consideration should be given to deferring further surgical intervention until the bowel injury has had time to heal (minimum of 3 to 5 days, ideally 2 to 3 months). Excessive use of cautery in proximity to the bowel or by metal retractors should also be avoided because of the risk of indirect burn injury. This injury can manifest as a delayed bowel injury several days to weeks later. Also at higher levels of exposure, consideration must be given to protecting the spleen, to minimize potential retractor trauma to this fragile organ.

When the primary retractors are set to hold the peritoneum, the vascular dissection can begin (either under direct vision or with laparoscopic visualization). In noninflamed tissue, gentle vascular mobilization can be accomplished with the use of peanut dissectors and a vein retractor. Clearly identified venous branches should be divided between ligatures to minimize avulsion injuries. The left iliolumbar vein can be easily avulsed during the exposure of the L4-5 disc space if this is not controlled during vascular mobilization (Fig. 19–11). The variable location of this vein may account for part of the significantly higher rate of vascular injury at this level.[4] This vascular injury can lead to significant bleeding, which may be difficult to control if the distal end retracts. Small (<1 mm) venous branches can be cauterized to decrease the risk of larger venous avulsion injury. Most small venous tears can be controlled with mild direct pressure with or without topical thrombotic agents. Venous injuries that are on an exposed surface or in the angle of retraction should be controlled with a small monofilament suture on a taper needle if necessary. This suture decreases the risk of propagation into a large venous injury; however, it may increase the risk of postoperative thrombosis at the site of repair.

Arterial injuries can occur at the time of dissection but are more likely to occur during instrumentation or secondary to retractor compression. Small segmental arteries should be controlled while mobilizing levels greater than L5, and the middle sacral artery can be divided between ligatures along with the vein. Direct major arterial injury is rare but can be catastrophic if it occurs.

The arterial and venous structures are at risk during the period of instrumentation. Vessels that are under tension are more susceptible to extensive sharp injury than when in situ. Both structures can be traumatized by instrumentation against fixed field retraction to cause a scissoring or pinching effect. The ureter is also at risk for this type of injury. Arterial bruising can propagate a small vascular wall hematoma into a thrombotic event secondary to direct or indirect trauma. Thrombosis of the left common iliac artery is the most common arterial complication.[5-7] "Snap" injuries can also occur where the artery is quickly moved from one position to another. In patients who have palpable atherosclerotic plaque disease, there may be an increased risk of thromboembolic events. It is important to perform a full vascular mobilization of the left common and external iliac arteries to decrease the potential risk of injury secondary to stretch or angulation. This injury can give rise to the formation of a plaque lip, which could give rise to a mural thrombosis, which could then propagate. It is important to check frequently the pulse examination of the distal extent of the exposed left external and internal iliac arteries and to use continuous pulse oximetry to minimize potential rare arterial injuries.

Few nerve structures are directly at risk during lumbosacral exposure. The hypogastric nerve is a potential source of injury, however, with significant clinical consequences, especially in men. The expected rate of retrograde ejaculation should be less than 1%, but the reported rate is 0 to 5.9%.[8] The incidence of retrograde ejaculation is increased 10-fold with a transperitoneal approach versus a retroperitoneal approach.[9] Expectant management shows resolution of the problem in 50% to 80% of patients over 6 to 12 months; however, it is best avoided by a retroperitoneal approach and careful dissection. Sympathetic injury can lead to a hyperthermic response in the corresponding left lower extremity with subsequent feeling of increased warmth and mild edema. This condition also resolves over 6 to 12 months, but permanent autoregulatory dysfunction can occur in rare cases. Additional nerve injuries are rare and are usually related to compression injuries of the lateral abdominal wall somatic nerves causing temporary dermal hypoesthesias.

Lymphatic injury is rarely clinically significant, although there are case reports of lymphoceles developing after approach procedures. Generally, if there is a need for aggressive lymphatic dissection, small clips can be applied, especially if lymph is noted to be draining into the surgical field. If a lymphocele develops, percutaneous drainage can be performed with radiologic guidance. Drains should not be left in anticipation of leakage because this may increase the risk of infection.

Infectious complications, although rare, can be devastating and educational. Superficial wound infections can be treated with local drainage and antibiotic therapy and rarely lead to deep infection. Deep space infection is rare and occurs in less than 1% of patients.[10] Presentation of deep infection would lead to concern over a possible missed injury with subsequent field contamination, although this can be supported further by culture results. Late presentation may occur years after the initial operation.

Conclusion

With various techniques evolving over the years, the mini-open retroperitoneal approach is becoming the standard, with decreased complication rate, better cosmesis, and less abdominal wall disruption to provide exposure to the lumbar spine. Access to the lumbar spine can be very successful when performed by a surgeon thoroughly knowledgeable about the anatomy and the potential risks involved. The safest approach is where all the potential risks are identified ahead of time, so that minimal problems occur.

Acknowledgments

The authors extend special thanks to Sal Brau.

PEARLS

1. Plain film or fluoroscopy should be used liberally to identify the appropriate angle of exposure. "Off target" exposures make it difficult for the spine surgeon and increase the risk of the case.

2. Small rents in the peritoneum can be simply repaired to help maintain the field clear of bowel. Larger defects can be left open; care must be taken to retract abdominal contents out of the way.

3. Venous bleeding can almost always be controlled with specific directed pressure, and this may be all that is necessary.

PITFALLS

1. The surgeon should be aware of the pinching effect of retractor blades. These may "scissor" against the instruments used for discectomy and increase the risk of a missed injury.

2. Before closure of the abdomen, the retroperitoneal space should be inspected. The arteries distal to the point of manipulation should be palpated. The pulse should be of similar quality to the beginning. Vascular thrills should be evaluated further and not dismissed.

3. Do not overdissect in the retroperitoneum. This will increase the regional scarring and make it more difficult to perform any future procedures.

4. If a segmental vessel or the iliolumbar vein appears under tension, divide it to minimize the chance of an uncontrolled tear.

KEY POINTS

1. Review exposure needs and plan preoperatively with the team.

2. Provide an adequate exposure safely and efficiently to the appropriate level. Do not overdissect.

3. Provide a safe retraction setup.

4. Monitor the vascular examination preoperatively and postoperatively.

5. Inspect the region completely before removing retractors. Retractor blades should be taken down in a stepwise fashion.

KEY REFERENCES

1. Kaiser MG, Haid RW Jr, Subach BR, et al: Comparison of the mini-open versus laparoscopic approach for anterior lumbar interbody fusion: A retrospective review. Neurosurgery 51:97-103, 2002.
This single-institution retrospective review compares the results of the mini-open anterior lumbar interbody fusion technique with the laparoscopic approach.

2. Brau SA, Delamarter RB, Schiffman ML, et al: Vascular injury during anterior lumbar surgery. Spine J 4:409-412, 2004.

This retrospective review of a prospectively compiled database on 1310 patients undergoing anterior lumbar exposure highlights the safety of the procedure, while showing what vascular injuries can occur.

3. Sasso RC, Kenneth Burkus J, LeHuec JC: Retrograde ejaculation after anterior lumbar interbody fusion: Transperitoneal versus retroperitoneal exposure. Spine 28:1023-1026, 2003.

This prospective study involving 146 men to assess the development of retrograde ejaculation showed a 10-fold increase in this complication in patients undergoing transperitoneal approaches to the lumbar spine.

4. Faciszewski T, Winter RB, Lonstein JE, et al: The surgical and medical perioperative complications of anterior spinal fusion surgery in the thoracic and lumbar spine in adults: A review of 1223 procedures. Spine 20:1592-1599, 1995.

This large, single-institution retrospective review reports the complications of 1223 spine approach procedures.

REFERENCES

1. Chung SK, Lee SH, Lim SR, et al: Comparative study of laparoscopic L5-S1 fusion versus open mini-ALIF, with a minimum 2-year follow up. Eur Spine J 12:613-617, 2003.

2. Kaiser MG, Haid RW Jr, Subach BR, et al: Comparison of the mini-open versus laparoscopic approach for anterior lumbar interbody fusion: A retrospective review. Neurosurgery 51:97-103, 2002.

3. Zdeblick TA, David SM: A prospective comparison of surgical approach for anterior L4-L5 fusion: Laparoscopic versus mini anterior lumbar interbody fusion. Spine 25:2682-2687, 2000.

4. Hamdan AD, Malek JY, Schermerhorn ML, et al: Vascular injury during anterior exposure of the spine. J Vasc Surg 48:650-654, 2008.

5. Oskouian RJ Jr, Johnson JP: Vascular complications in anterior thoracolumbar spinal reconstruction. J Neurosurg 96:1-5, 2002.

6. Kulkarni SS, Lowery GL, Ross RE, et al: Arterial complications following anterior lumbar interbody fusion: Report of eight cases. Eur Spine J 12:55-56, 2003.

7. Brau SA, Delamarter RB, Schiffman ML, et al: Vascular injury during anterior lumbar surgery. Spine J 4:409-412, 2004.

8. Tiusanen H, Seitsalo S, Osterman K, et al: Retrograde ejaculation after anterior interbody fusion. Eur Spine J 4:339-342, 1995.

9. Sasso RC, Kenneth Burkus J, LeHuec JC: Retrograde ejaculation after anterior lumbar interbody fusion: Transperitoneal versus retroperitoneal exposure. Spine 28:1023-1026, 2003.

10. Faciszewski T, Winter RB, Lonstein JE, et al: The surgical and medical perioperative complications of anterior spinal fusion surgery in the thoracic and lumbar spine in adults: A review of 1223 procedures. Spine 20:1592-1599, 1995.

20 CHAPTER

Lateral and Posterior Approaches to Lumbosacral Spine

Yu-Po Lee, MD
Arvind Ravinutala, BS
Steven R. Garfin, MD

Selection of Approach to Lumbar Spine

When the decision to operate has been made, the surgeon must choose the best procedure and approach. When considering the options in the lumbar spine, many factors must be taken into account. First is the location of the pathology. Disease or deformity that primarily involves the vertebral bodies may be most easily approached through the abdomen or flank. The posterior elements are most easily approached through a posterior midline incision. Second, the morbidity of each approach must fit the risk tolerance of each individual patient. It would be advisable to avoid an anterior approach in a young man who has pathology at L5-S1 to avoid the small chance of retrograde ejaculation. With the advent of minimally invasive techniques, such as minimally invasive transforaminal lumbar interbody fusions and minimally invasive lateral interbody fusions, decreasing overall morbidity from blood loss and tissue dissection must be weighed against more complete visualization and disc removal provided by the anterior approach. These are some of the factors that should be considered when deciding on a surgical approach to maximize results and minimize patient morbidity.

Minimally Invasive Lateral Approach to Spine

The concept of minimally invasive spine surgery is attractive to patients and surgeons. Decreased postoperative pain, shorter hospital stay, and quicker return to activities support the use of minimally invasive techniques when achievable. One technique is the lateral access to the spine.[1,2] This technique can be used for multilevel interbody fusions to correct kyphoscoliosis, for interbody support when treating adjacent segment degeneration or multilevel fusions, or to drain a psoas abscess (Fig. 20–1). With this approach, access to the spine from T7 down to L4-5 is possible. L4-5 is often difficult to reach, however, because of a high-riding iliac crest, and the means to access L5-S1 laterally has not been developed.

Technique

After the patient has been intubated and prophylactic antibiotics have been given, the patient is placed in the lateral decubitus position. When correcting a kyphoscoliosis, it is easier to perform the lateral approach on the side of the concavity. The table should be flexed to increase the distance between the iliac crest and the rib cage, and the patient should be secured with tape over the greater trochanter and chest wall (Fig. 20–2). The leg on top should also be flexed to relax the psoas. A cross-table anteroposterior radiograph should be taken, and the table should be rotated to place the patient in a true anteroposterior position. A corresponding lateral fluoroscopic image should also be taken to verify that access to the disc space is possible. Minor adjustments should be made to the table to obtain a true lateral image.

After the patient has been prepared and draped, the lateral image is obtained first. A radiopaque marker is placed over the center of the affected disc space (Fig. 20–3). When this point has been identified, a mark is made. Through this mark, a small incision is made for insertion of the dilators and an expandable retractor, which provides access to the lateral spine. A second mark is made posterior to this first mark at the border between the erector spinae muscles and the abdominal oblique muscles. At this second mark, a transverse incision about 2 cm long is made to accommodate the surgeon's index finger (Fig. 20–4). Finger dissection is used down to the lumbodorsal fascia. A clamp, or scissors, can be used to spread the fascia and muscle fibers and provide entry into the retroperitoneal space.

When an opening is created, the index finger is used to sweep the peritoneum anteriorly and to palpate the psoas muscle (Fig. 20–5A and B). The surgeon uses the index finger to sweep inferiorly to feel the inner table of the iliac crest (if in the lower lumbar spine) to verify that he or she is in the abdominal cavity. When the psoas is identified, the index finger is swept up to the previously made direct lateral mark. A 2-cm incision is made; the external and internal oblique muscles and the transverses abdominis muscles are split, and dilators are placed through this opening. The index finger, which is already in the retroperitoneal space, guides the initial

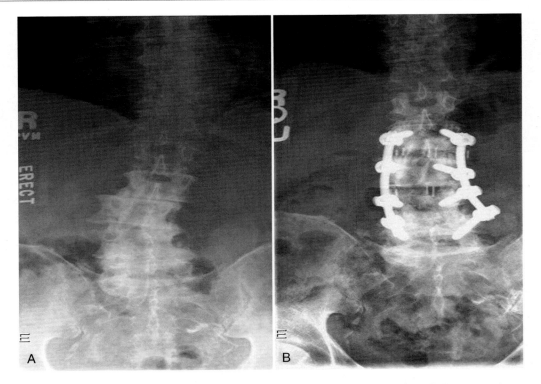

FIGURE 20–1 A, Anteroposterior radiograph of a 69-year-old man with degenerative scoliosis. **B,** Anteroposterior radiograph after L2-3 and L3-4 lateral interbody fusions.

dilator onto the psoas (Fig. 20–5C). The fibers of the psoas are split with the dilator using neurologic monitoring as a safety measure, if desired. A lateral radiograph should be obtained to verify the central position of the dilator at the desired disc space. After the position of the initial dilator is secured by placing a Kirschner wire through the dilator and into the disc space, larger dilators are used to spread the psoas under neurologic monitoring, and then an expandable retractor is placed over the dilators (Fig. 20–5D).

After the retractor is secured to the table, the dilators are removed to provide lateral access to the disc (Fig. 20–6). A

neurologic monitoring probe can be used to check for any nerves that may be crossing the working window of the retractor. If a nerve is detected, the Kirschner wire should be repositioned away from the nerve, and the psoas should be redilated. If this fails, conversion to another means of interbody fusion should be considered because repeated

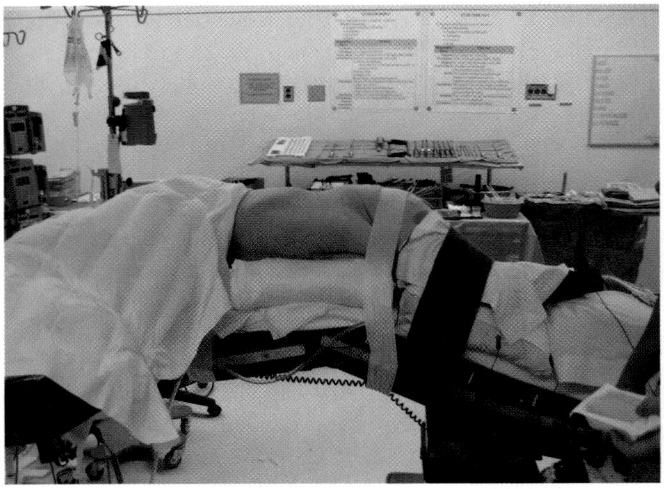

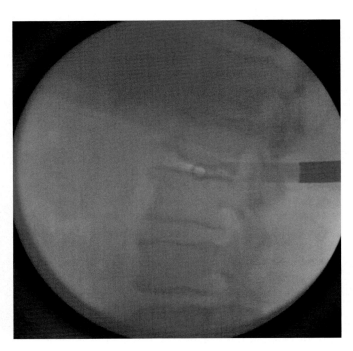

FIGURE 20–2 Patient placed in right lateral decubitus position with table flexed to increase distance between the patient's ribs and iliac crest.

FIGURE 20–3 Fluoroscopic image showing center positioning over disc space. A mark is made on skin corresponding to this mark.

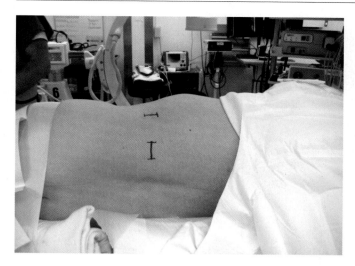

FIGURE 20–4 Two-incision technique shown with lateral and posterolateral marks. Posterolateral incision is made about the length of the surgeon's index finger away from lateral incision. From this mark, the surgeon should also measure the distance to spine to ensure that he or she can reach the psoas from this incision.

positioning of the retractor, or pressure on the nerve, could result in postoperative paresthesias or palsies.

Anteroposterior and lateral radiographs should be taken at this point to verify that the retractor is docked on the disc space and that the retractor is positioned over the center of the disc. When appropriate positioning has been confirmed, the retractor should be secured in place. A lateral discectomy is performed in standard fashion with shavers, curets, and rasps. A Cobb elevator should be used to release the contralateral anulus (Fig. 20–7). Releasing the contralateral anulus loosens the spine in the coronal plane and aids in the correction of coronal plane deformities. Sizers and trials are used to determine the optimal implant size. The implant is filled with the surgeon's graft or fusion enhancer of choice and impacted across. The wound is closed in layers. No drains are typically necessary.

Complications

Because minimally invasive lateral access to the spine is a newer procedure, publications regarding the efficacy and complication rates are sparse. Numbness in the lateral thigh and psoas weakness have been noted by some physicians; however, the rate still remains unknown. To minimize this risk, the retractor is opened just enough to perform the lateral discectomy. Exuberant deployment of the retractor may place undue pressure on the nerve roots or the psoas itself, or both. Also, neurologic monitoring is advised to decrease the possibility of nerve injury.

Injuries to the bowel and vessels have not been reported, but these may occur. It is recommended that this procedure be done at a facility where a general or vascular surgeon is available. One method to decrease the rate of bowel or vascular injury is to place the initial dilator under direct visualization. After the lateral incision has been made, the retractor can

be passed down to the psoas. The initial dilator is then placed through the psoas under direct visualization.

Posterior Approach to Lumbar Spine

The posterior approach through a midline longitudinal incision is the most common approach to the lumbar spine.[3] It provides direct access to the spinous processes, laminae, facets, and even pedicles and lateral aspects of the vertebral bodies at all levels of the lumbar spine. The pedicle starting holes and transverse processes can be reached by dissecting and retracting the paraspinal muscles laterally. Through this approach, it is possible to perform most of the spine procedures currently practiced today, including microdiscectomies, laminectomies, and most fusion procedures. The posterior

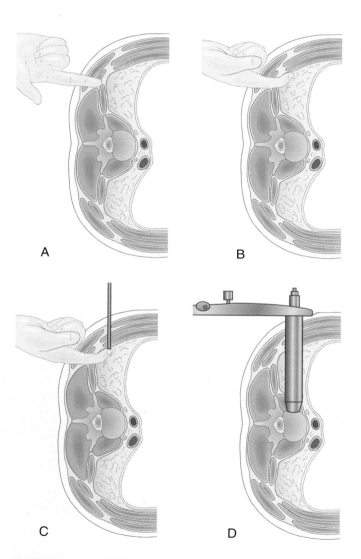

FIGURE 20–5 A and **B,** The surgeon uses digital palpation to sweep abdominal contents anteriorly and create a cavity in retroperitoneal space. **C,** Index finger guides initial dilator down to psoas. **D,** When initial dilator is secured in place with Kirschner wire, larger dilators are used to spread psoas under neurologic monitoring, and retractor is placed over dilators.

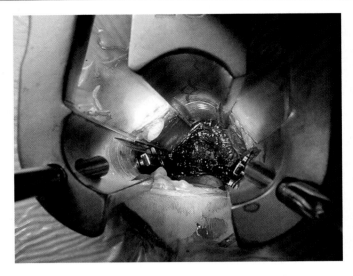

FIGURE 20-6 When retractor is deployed, soft tissue over disc space must be cleared away. Probe is used to detect any nerves that may cross the field.

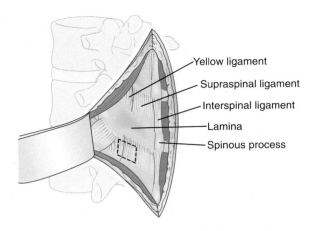

FIGURE 20-8 Dorsal subperiosteal exposure of lumbar spine. (From Benzel E: Spine Surgery: Techniques, Complication Avoidance, and Management. Philadelphia, Churchill Livingstone, 2004.)

Yellow ligament
Supraspinal ligament
Interspinal ligament
Lamina
Spinous process

aspect of the vertebral body and disc space over the lower lumbar levels can be reached after laminectomy by retracting the dura, but the exposure is limited.

Anatomic variations exist among individuals, and this must be taken into account when planning surgery. The intercrestal line typically crosses at L3-4, but this is not a rigid anatomic finding. A lateral radiograph shows where the intercrestal line is. Also, lumbarization or sacralization of the last vertebral segment can confuse the surgeon when localizing the level of pathology. Additionally, a spina bifida occulta or an unusually wide interlaminar space may exist. To avoid inadvertent injury to the dura or nerve roots with a bovie or periosteal elevator during the exposure, the surgeon should study radiographs before surgery to look for these abnormalities.

Technique

The patient is positioned prone to allow the abdomen to hang free of pressure. This position reduces venous plexus filling around the cauda equina by permitting the venous plexus to drain directly into the inferior vena cava. The anesthesiologist should check the eyes, and the surgeon and nurses should assess the bony prominences to ensure that they are well padded. If a microdiscectomy or decompression is to be performed, flexing the lumbar spine on a Wilson frame, or similar table, is recommended to open up the interspinous spaces. If a fusion also is to be performed, placing the patient on a Jackson table is recommended to maintain the lumbar lordosis. A solution containing epinephrine in a 1 : 500,000 concentration may be injected into the subcuticular tissues and muscles to decrease blood loss.

A midline incision is made between the spinous processes of the levels to be exposed, and the erector spinae and multifidus muscles are dissected from the bony elements (spinous processes, interspinous ligaments, laminae, facet joints, and transverse processes) as needed for the levels that must be visualized, using electrocautery or sharp dissection (Fig. 20-8). The paraspinal muscles should be elevated subperiosteally

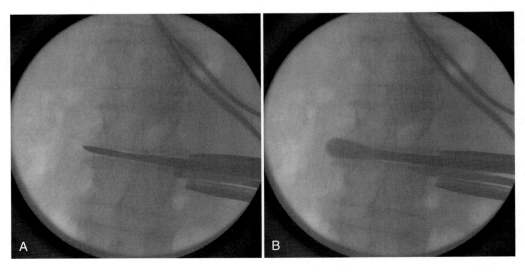

FIGURE 20-7 A and B, Cobb elevator is used to release contralateral anulus. This aids in coronal correction of deformity.

to minimize blood loss. Care should be taken not to injure the facet joint capsules and interspinous ligaments in areas where motion would be expected after the operation. If the transverse processes must be reached, dissection is continued down the lateral side of the facet joints and onto the transverse process itself. The vessels supplying the paraspinal muscles segmentally are close to the facet joints and the pars interarticularis. If these vessels are cut, they can bleed vigorously. Cauterization is necessary to stop these bleeders. The posterior primary rami of the lumbar nerves run with these vessels.

To perform a decompression or a discectomy, it may be necessary to remove the ligamentum flavum. The superficial ligamentum flavum blends laterally into the facet joint capsule. A forward angled or small straight curet is used to detach the superficial and deep layers of the ligamentum flavum from the caudal edge of the cephalad lamina. The surgeon sweeps the curet medial to lateral and advances the curet with each successive sweep to detach the ligamentum flavum from the lamina. The ligamentum flavum typically inserts over the caudal 50% of the undersurface of the lamina. A small, angled elevator is placed under the ligamentum flavum to lift it off the dura and protect the latter. A Kerrison rongeur, pituitary rongeur, or knife can be used to remove the ligamentum flavum. The epidural fat, dura, nerve root, and epidural veins can be seen after the ligamentum flavum has been removed (Fig. 20–9).

If a discectomy or exploration of the disc space is required, it can typically be performed through this opening. A portion of the lamina (laminotomy) may need to be removed to access the disc space adequately. A Penfield No. 4 dissector can be used to help mobilize the traversing nerve root, and a nerve root retractor can be used to retract the nerve roots gently medially. Care must be used not to retract too vigorously to avoid too much tension on the exiting nerve root. Bleeding from the epidural veins commonly occurs. Hemostasis can be obtained with bipolar cautery or the use of cottonoids, absorbable knitted fabric (Surgicel), or thrombin-soaked absorbable gelatin sponge (Gelfoam). Cottonoids can be placed in the cephalad and caudad extremes of the exposure to collapse the vessels and provide a working window.

The key to intracanal anatomy is the pedicle. The disc space is just cephalad to the pedicle, and the intervertebral foramen above the pedicle accommodates the exiting nerve root. The traversing nerve root lies just medial to the pedicle and exits the intervertebral foramen caudally. The disc space can be found by retracting the traversing nerve root medially and exploring the space above the pedicle (Fig. 20–10). The surgeon can use a Penfield No. 4 dissector to feel for the disc space. It should be a raised, white, soft structure.

If a total laminectomy is needed to decompress or expose the dura and nerve roots, the fascia is removed entirely from the tip of the spinous process bilaterally. The muscles are dissected off of the spinous processes and lamina subperiosteally, taking care to protect the facet joints. The pars interarticularis must be exposed fully to avoid transecting it during the decompression. A rongeur can be used to remove the spinous processes.

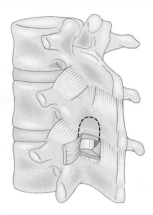

FIGURE 20–9 Removal of ligamentum flavum. (From Benzel E: Spine Surgery: Techniques, Complication Avoidance, and Management. Philadelphia, Churchill Livingstone, 2004.)

The laminectomy may be performed many ways. A high-speed bur may be used to thin the lamina down to a thin cortical shell over the dura, then a Kerrison rongeur is used to remove the lamina. Alternatively, the tip of a rongeur may be inserted under the caudal edge of the cephalad lamina to remove the lamina. The rongeur is used to cut from the underside in an upward direction; this lessens the chance of catching dura. A Kerrison rongeur can be used to complete the laminectomy near the pars and the cephalad edge. To decompress the nerve roots adequately, the lateral recesses and intervertebral foramen must also be explored. A Woodson elevator or dural guide may be used to compress the dura gently and expose the lateral recesses; this exposes the ligamentum flavum in the lateral recess and intervertebral foramen. The ligamentum flavum should be removed to perform an adequate decompression. The medial aspect of the caudal pedicle marks the medial border of the intervertebral foramen.

Osteophytes from the facet joints often compress the exiting nerve root. Care must be taken when removing these osteophytes to avoid injury to the exiting nerve root and to avoid iatrogenic instability caused by too much removal of the facet joint. Typically, removal of less than 50% of the facet joint

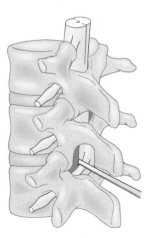

FIGURE 20–10 Exposure of lumbar disc by retracting thecal sac medially. (From Benzel E: Spine Surgery: Techniques, Complication Avoidance, and Management. Philadelphia, Churchill Livingstone, 2004.)

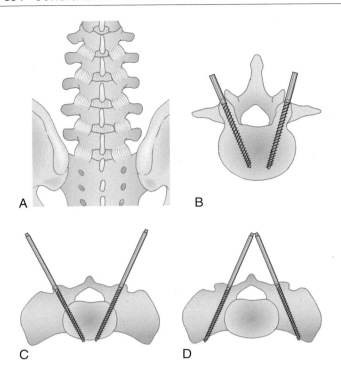

FIGURE 20–11 Illustration of lumbar pedicle entry sites. In lumbar region, the center of pedicles is usually at inferolateral edge of facet joint. (From Herkowitz H, Eismont FJ, Garfin SR, et al [eds]: Rothman-Simeone The Spine, 4th ed. Philadelphia, WB Saunders, 1999.)

preserves its stability. This may necessitate the use of a 1- or 2-mm Kerrison rongeur. The use of a curved Kerrison rongeur can be helpful here. Bearing in mind that the facet joints are oriented sagittally in the lumbar spine, cutting the undersurface of the facet joint provides a greater means of decompressing the nerve roots, while preserving the overall stability of the joint.

With the advent of pedicle screw fixation for the lumbar vertebrae, there are now several additional anatomic relationships that are important at the level of the posterior bony

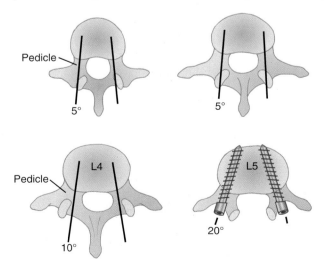

FIGURE 20–12 Transaxial position of pedicle screws. (From Herkowitz H, Eismont FJ, Garfin SR, et al [eds]: Rothman-Simeone The Spine, 4th ed. Philadelphia, WB Saunders, 1999.)

elements.[4] The location of the pedicles is identified by anatomic landmarks and by radiography or image intensification fluoroscopy in the operating room.

In the lumbar region, the center of the pedicles is usually at the inferolateral edge of the facet joint, on an imaginary transverse line bisecting the transverse processes (Fig. 20–11). If there is severe facet arthrosis, the lateral edge of the facet joint may be lateral to the true pedicle entry site, however. In these cases, the surgeon should also refer to the pars interarticularis. The lateral border of the pars typically corresponds to the medial border of the pedicle. In the lumbar region from this point, one may use a pedicle finder, with a 20-degree medial inclination at L5, 10-degree inclination at L4, 5-degree inclination at L3 and L2, and no inclination at L1 (Fig. 20–12). One may follow the progress of the pedicle finder by feeling inside the pedicle with a pedicle feeler and by checking with the image intensifier or by radiographs. In the lateral view, the probe or marker should be parallel to the disc space.

Posterolateral Approach to Lumbar Vertebral Bodies

The posterolateral approach provides direct access to the transverse processes and the mammillary processes of the facets through a longitudinal paraspinal incision, retracting the erector spinae muscles medially.[5,6] This area provides an excellent bed for posterolateral lumbosacral fusion even in the face of preexisting pseudarthrosis, laminar defects, or spondylolisthesis. This approach is the basis for minimally invasive transforaminal lumbar interbody fusions.

Technique

General endotracheal anesthesia is recommended for this procedure. The patient is placed on the operating table in the prone position with chest rolls on either side of the thorax to protect ventilation or on a radiolucent table with chest and hip pads.

A longitudinal paramedian incision is made at the lateral border of the erector spinae muscles (approximately two fingerbreadths from midline) centered over the level of interest. The incision is extended to the lumbar fascia, and the erector spinae muscles are identified. The interval between the erector spinae muscles and the multifidus is found after opening the fascia, and dissection proceeds between these muscles down to the facet joints and the transverse processes of the vertebrae (Fig. 20–13). The paraspinal muscles are retracted medially, the transverse process at the desired level is tagged with a radiopaque marker, and radiographs are obtained to confirm the vertebral level. For a minimally invasive transforaminal interbody fusion, this exposure is adequate to perform a decompression and fusion.

If access to the vertebral body is desired, the dissection can be carried further anteriorly. The transverse process is divided with an osteotome and is retracted laterally with its musculotendinous attachments. The vertebral pedicle is

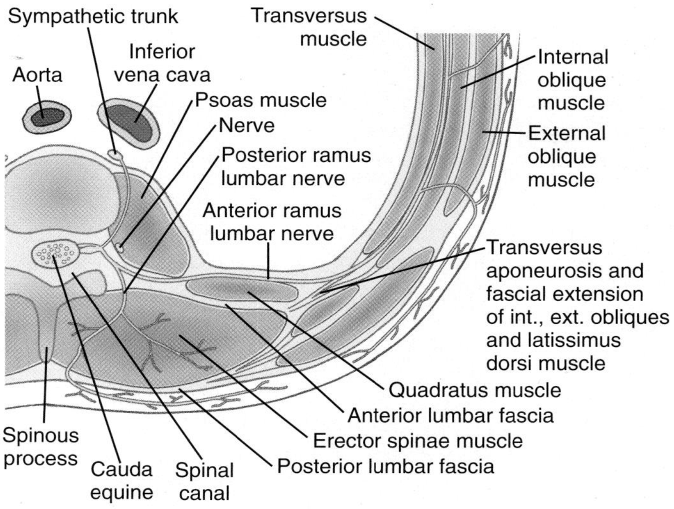

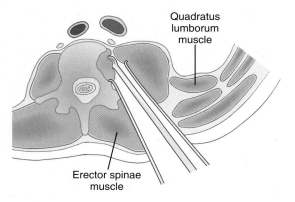

FIGURE 20–13 Cross section of lumbar spine and paraspinal structures at level of L3. (From Herkowitz H, Eismont FJ, Garfin SR, et al [eds]: Rothman-Simeone The Spine, 4th ed. Philadelphia, WB Saunders, 1999.)

palpated, and the lumbar nerves are identified and protected as they leave the foramina above and below the pedicle (Fig. 20–14). The psoas muscle is carefully separated from the vertebra using a periosteal elevator. The lumbar vessels lie on the waist or mid-portion of the vertebral body posterior to the psoas muscle and should be separated from the body during this portion of the dissection. The vessels may be clamped and cauterized if necessary. An opening may be made in the lateral aspect of the vertebral body anterior to the pedicle, using a curet or drill (Fig. 20–15).

The lesion may be identified grossly at this time but should be verified radiographically with a curet placed within the lesion. Through this approach, specimens may be obtained

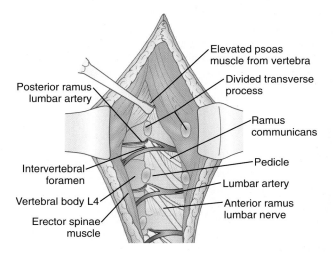

FIGURE 20–14 Lumbar vertebrae as viewed from posterolateral approach. Dissection proceeds directly anterior to stump of transverse process, along pedicle to vertebral body in front. Note lumbar segmental vessels draped over waist or mid-portion of vertebral bodies. By dissecting directly anterior to pedicles, one can avoid these vessels and lumbar nerves leaving neural foramina below pedicles. (From Herkowitz H, Eismont FJ, Garfin SR, et al [eds]: Rothman-Simeone The Spine, 4th ed. Philadelphia, WB Saunders, 1999.)

FIGURE 20–15 Posterolateral approach to lumbar vertebrae, lateral to erector spinae muscle mass and behind psoas. Transverse process is divided and retracted laterally with musculotendinous insertions to gain access to lateral aspect of vertebral body. (From Herkowitz H, Eismont FJ, Garfin SR, et al [eds]: Rothman-Simeone The Spine, 4th ed. Philadelphia, WB Saunders, 1999.)

from the lateral, central, or anterior aspect of the vertebral body or pedicle. The lesion may be curetted, and small chips of cancellous bone graft may be installed to stimulate osteogenesis within a sterile defect. The wound is copiously irrigated with saline and inspected for hemorrhage. The margins are allowed to fall together, and the lumbar fascia is closed with interrupted sutures. The skin is repaired, and the patient is nursed with some form of external spinal support, depending on the postoperative stability of the spine.

PEARLS

1. For lateral interbody fusions, it is often easier to adjust the table to get the perfect anteroposterior and lateral images and have the C-arm rotate between 0 and 90 degrees.

2. For lateral interbody fusions, frequent images should be obtained to ensure good position. Because the surgeon is using a smaller incision and sees less, the surgeon must rely on imaging more to ensure he or she is in the right position.

3. For lateral interbody fusions, MRI should be studied preoperatively to get an idea of where the nerves are. If neurologic monitoring shows the nerve is in the field, the surgeon should be prepared to convert to another form of interbody fusion.

4. To decompress the nerve roots adequately, the lateral recesses and intervertebral foramen must also be explored.

PITFALLS

1. For lateral interbody fusions, aggressive deployment of the retractor or repeated passes with the initial dilator may injure the nerve.

2. For lumbar decompressions, care must be taken to avoid removing too much of the pars or facet joints to avoid iatrogenic instability.

3. When placing pedicle screws, if there is severe facet arthrosis, the lateral edge of the facet joint may be lateral to the true pedicle entry site.

KEY REFERENCES

1. Ozgur BM, Aryan HE, Pimenta L, Taylor WR: Extreme Lateral Interbody Fusion (XLIF): a novel surgical technique for anterior lumbar interbody fusion. Spine J 6:435-443, 2006.
   A good technique paper on the lateral approach to the spine.

2. Regan JJ, Yuan H, McCullen G: Minimally invasive approaches to the spine. Instr Course Lect 46:127-141, 1997.
   A good review on the evolution of minimally invasive approaches to the spine.

3. Birch BD, Desai RD, McCormick PC: Surgical approaches to the thoracolumbar spine. Neurosurg Clin N Am ;8:471-485, 1997.
   A good general review of posterior approaches to the lumbar spine.

4. Stambough JL: Posterior instrumentation for thoracolumbar trauma. Clin Orthop Relat Res (35):73-88, 1997.
   A good review on the placement of pedicle screws in the lumbar spine.

5. Schmidt MH, Larson SJ, Maiman DJ: The lateral extracavitary approach to the thoracic and lumbar spine. Neurosurg Clin N Am 15:437-441, 2004.
   A good technique paper on the extracavitary approach to the thoracic and lumbar spine.

6. Shen FH, Marks I, Shaffrey C, et al: The use of an expandable cage for corpectomy reconstruction of vertebral body tumors through a posterior extracavitary approach: a multicenter consecutive case series of prospectively followed patients. Spine J 8:329-339, 2008.
   A good review on reconstruction of the vertebral body using cages.

REFERENCES

1. Ozgur BM, Aryan HE, Pimenta L, et al: Extreme lateral interbody fusion (XLIF): A novel surgical technique for anterior lumbar interbody fusion. Spine J 6:435-443, 2006.

2. Regan JJ, Yuan H, McCullen G: Minimally invasive approaches to the spine. Instr Course Lect 46:127-141, 1997.

3. Birch BD, Desai RD, McCormick PC: Surgical approaches to the thoracolumbar spine. Neurosurg Clin N Am 8:471-485, 1997.

4. Stambough JL: Posterior instrumentation for thoracolumbar trauma. Clin Orthop Relat Res (335):73-88, 1997.

5. Schmidt MH, Larson SJ, Maiman DJ: The lateral extracavitary approach to the thoracic and lumbar spine. Neurosurg Clin N Am 15:437-441, 2004.

6. Shen FH, Marks I, Shaffrey C, et al: The use of an expandable cage for corpectomy reconstruction of vertebral body tumors through a posterior extracavitary approach: A multicenter consecutive case series of prospectively followed patients. Spine J 8:329-339, 2008.

Lori A. Karol, MD

The prevalence of back pain in children and adolescents is increasing. Although it is assumed that pediatric back pain is rare, more recent studies have shown that more than 50% of children note episodes of back pain by 15 years of age.[1-4] A survey of teenagers revealed that 39% complained of low back pain, but few presented for medical evaluation.[5] Although the number of children and teens complaining of pain is increasing, children and adolescents who have a distinct diagnosis are decreasing in number. A study by Hensinger[6] in 1985 found a specific diagnosis in 84% of children presenting for treatment of back pain. In a study 10 years later, a cause for back pain was identified in only 22% of 217 children evaluated with single photon emission computed tomography (SPECT).[7] The task of the evaluating surgeon is to identify which children are most likely to have an underlying musculoskeletal condition and require a comprehensive evaluation to identify the etiology of their pain.

Studies concur that back pain in young children is worrisome and that a pathologic abnormality can nearly always be identified as the cause of the symptoms. As children reach adolescence, their pain begins to resemble that seen in adults. As the radiologic armamentarium grows, the physician has more choices in the evaluation of these patients, but every child who presents to the physician does not need to undergo every scan available. A complete understanding of the potential causes of back pain enables the physician to evaluate the pediatric patient properly.

History

The initial step in distinguishing which children require symptomatic treatment from children who warrant a complete radiographic evaluation is obtaining a detailed history. The characteristics of the pain are most helpful. Acute pain after trauma is seen with fractures, disc herniations, and apophyseal ring separations. Insidious pain without a clear-cut antecedent event is characteristic of developmental conditions, such as Scheuermann kyphosis, and benign neoplasms. Recurrent pain associated with athletics and relieved by rest leads to suspicion of overuse injuries such as spondylolysis.

Unremitting pain, especially if it is worse at night or wakes the child from sleep, is most worrisome because it is seen in malignancies and infection.[7,8]

The location of pain is very helpful in narrowing down the differential diagnosis. Localized pain may indicate either benign or malignant neoplasms. Lumbar pain may be produced by spondylolysis or spondylolisthesis, whereas pain in the thoracic area may be due to Scheuermann kyphosis. Radiation of pain into the buttocks or legs is seen in herniated discs, apophyseal fractures, and spinal cord or vertebral tumors.

The presence or absence of constitutional symptoms is useful in deciding the potential severity of the underlying condition. Fever in a child with acute back pain points to an infectious or neoplastic etiology. It is important to question the parents about malaise, anorexia, the presence of a rash, or abnormal bruising because back pain can be the presenting complaint in children with leukemia.

Next, a detailed neurologic history must be obtained. Numbness, weakness, decreased ability to walk, and changes in coordination require prompt imaging of the spinal cord. The physician should ask specifically about changes in bowel or bladder function because adolescents are hesitant to admit to these symptoms.

The patient's age is very helpful in directing the evaluation of back pain. Back pain in children younger than 4 years is usually due to either infection or malignancy. A history of fever, limp, and malaise should be sought, and an immediate diagnostic evaluation should be performed. Children in the 1st decade of life commonly present with discitis and osteomyelitis, and malignant neoplasms, but they also may present with benign conditions such as eosinophilic granuloma.[8] Patients older than 10 years are most likely to have back pain secondary to trauma or overuse, resulting in spondylolysis, disc herniations, or apophyseal fractures.[9] Scheuermann kyphosis manifests in adolescence. Teens also rarely present with malignancies, so the physician should always remain cautious while weighing the relative frequency of conditions based on age.

A family history should be taken regarding back pain. Adolescents with ill-defined pain, no constitutional symptoms, no history of excessive athletic activity, no anatomically consistent neurologic complaints, and a positive family history often do not have a musculoskeletal etiology for their pain.[2,8] Psychosomatic pain does occur in this age group, but remains a diagnosis of exclusion.

A complete review of systems should be obtained. Back pain associated with menses is rarely orthopaedic in nature. Flank pain may be renal in origin. A more recent study showed that 5% of children presenting to an emergency department for evaluation of back pain had urinary tract infections.[10]

Physical Examination

The general appearance of the child should be noted. If the child appears systemically ill, immediate evaluation for infection or malignancy is warranted. Whether or not the child can walk and the characteristics of the child's gait are important because the inability to walk can be due to infection or spinal cord compromise. Examination of the skin for dysraphic lesions such as hairy patches or deep sinuses and for café au lait spots is required.

Palpation of the spine can identify the location of the pathologic abnormality. The spine should be inspected for sagittal and coronal alignment. The Adams forward bend test identifies patients with scoliosis, but the presence of scoliosis is usually a symptom of underlying pathology, rather than the cause of the pain. Trunk lean and decompensation may indicate benign or malignant neoplasms or irritating lesions such as herniated discs. Stiffness of the spine should be noted. Usually, thoracic kyphosis increases and lumbar lordosis reverses as a child bends forward. In the presence of significant pain, the child does not allow the spine to move and bends the knees to touch the floor rather than flex the spine. Pain with hyperextension of the spine is often seen in patients with spondylolysis. This pain can be exacerbated further by twisting during hyperextension. Lasègue sign is nearly always positive in patients with herniated discs or fractured apophyses. Straight-leg raise is also diminished in patients with tight hamstrings secondary to spondylolisthesis.

A thorough neurologic examination is crucial in the evaluation of a child with back pain. Motor and sensory function and deep tendon reflexes should be tested. Long tract signs such as clonus and the Babinski reflex must be evaluated to rule out spinal cord compression or abnormality. The abdominal reflex is tested by lightly stroking the four quadrants around the umbilicus in the supine child. Although an absent abdominal reflex is not abnormal, an asymmetrical response may indicate spinal cord abnormalities.

Diagnostic Studies

With the information obtained from the history and physical examination, a focused approach to diagnostic studies can be taken (Table 21–1). If the patient is 10 years of age or younger, if the duration of pain is 2 months or longer, if there is night pain, or if there are constitutional symptoms, standard

TABLE 21–1 Use of Diagnostic Tests

X-ray	History of significant trauma; night pain, fever, or inability to walk; age ≤8 yr; duration of pain >2 mo
Bone scan	Negative plain x-rays with normal neurologic examination; persistent pain; history of athletic overuse
Computed tomography	Positive plain x-ray or bone scan
Magnetic resonance imaging	Abnormal neurologic examination; painful scoliosis in patient <8 yr old; painful left thoracic scoliosis
Laboratory tests	Night pain; fever; age <8 yr; constant pain

radiographs of the spine should be obtained immediately. If the patient is older, the pain is of short duration, and the physical examination is completely normal, the patient may be observed for a short time. Most patients fall between these two groups, and the extent of the radiographic evaluation should be decided on an individual basis.

Radiographs

Plain radiographs are the best screening examination for a child with back pain.[7,11] Anteroposterior and lateral views of the spine should be obtained without pelvic shielding because the shield hides the sacrum, the sacroiliac joints, and the pelvis. The physician should carefully examine the films for alignment, disc space narrowing, endplate irregularities, and lytic or blastic lesions. Each pedicle should be identified on the anteroposterior view. If a question of a lesion arises, a focused coned-down view taken with the patient supine provides better bony detail.

The lateral film should be reviewed for the presence of spondylolysis or spondylolisthesis. As on the anteroposterior view, if there is a question of lysis on the lateral view, a spot lateral view of the lumbosacral junction better visualizes the pars interarticularis. Oblique views of the lumbosacral spine can also show the lysis.

The identification of scoliosis on screening films of a child with back pain should not lead to the conclusion that the curve is the cause of the pain. Although 33% of adolescents with the diagnosis of scoliosis complain of some back pain, it is usually located over the rib prominence and is rarely a presenting complaint.[11] The apex of the curve should be carefully inspected for bony lesions in a child with painful scoliosis.

Bone Scan

If plain radiographs and the neurologic examination are normal, but the patient's symptoms suggest bony pathology, a triphasic technetium bone scan is recommended. Scintigraphy is a highly sensitive but nonspecific tool to localize bony processes. Infections, most benign and malignant bony lesions, and stress fractures have increased bone turnover, which is visualized as increased tracer uptake on scintigraphic images. Pinhole collimation is helpful in localizing the increased

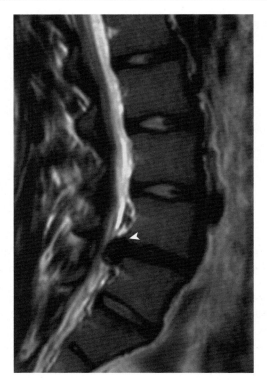

FIGURE 21–1 MRI of a 16-year-old girl with back and right leg pain shows herniated L4-5 disc.

uptake. The study should include the sacroiliac joints and pelvis because pathology in these areas often manifests as back pain.

SPECT combines the physiology of a bone scan with the ability to localize lesions precisely within the vertebra similar to a computed tomography (CT) scan. Increased uptake can be seen in the posterior elements in stress fractures, so SPECT is particularly helpful in diagnosing spondylolysis.[12-15] A study of 100 patients 2 to 18 years old presenting with low back pain found that a negative SPECT scan was most helpful in ruling out an organic cause for back pain of less than 6 weeks' duration.[16]

Computed Tomography

CT provides the best imaging of the vertebral anatomy. It is not used as a screening tool but is useful when a lesion is seen on plain radiography or when bone scintigraphy shows increased uptake. CT can be used to assess the status of the pars interarticularis in patients with spondylolysis. Although bone lesions can be seen on magnetic resonance imaging (MRI), surrounding edema may overestimate the extent of skeletal involvement.

TABLE 21–2 Likely Diagnoses Based on Age

Age <5 yr	Tumor, discitis
Age 5-10 yr	Langerhans cell histiocytosis, discitis, tumor or leukemia
Age 10-18 yr	Scheuermann kyphosis, herniated disc or apophysis, spondylolysis, osteoid osteoma, tumor or leukemia

Magnetic Resonance Imaging

MRI is used to image the neural axis in all children who have an abnormal neurologic examination. MRI can identify spinal neoplasms, cord abnormalities such as syringomyelia and tethers, discitis, and herniated discs. Auerbach and colleagues[16] recommended MRI as the best imaging modality for patients with low back pain of greater than 6 weeks' duration.

Laboratory Tests

Laboratory tests should be obtained at presentation in all young children with back pain and children with night pain, fever, malaise, or easy bruising. A complete blood count with differential should be obtained. Peripheral smear should be ordered looking for abnormal cell lines consistent with leukemia. The erythrocyte sedimentation rate and C-reactive protein should also routinely be studied because they are elevated in infection and malignancy. Urinalysis should be used to screen for renal conditions.

Differential Diagnosis

Table 21–2 summarizes differential diagnoses based on the child's age.

Disc Herniation

Intervertebral disc herniation occasionally occurs in older children and teens. The onset of symptoms is usually related to acute or repetitive trauma.[17] Back pain with radiation into the legs is a complaint in 82% of affected patients.[18] Pain is exacerbated by activity and relieved by rest. As in adults, pain is worsened by sneezing, coughing, or straining.

Physical examination reveals decreased spinal flexibility, with inability to touch the toes. On bending toward the floor, the patient often lists to one side. The straight-leg raise test (Lasègue sign) is positive in 85% of children with herniated discs; objective neurologic findings, such as absent reflexes, motor weakness, and decreased sensation, are less common in children than in adults.[19]

Radiographs are generally normal, although if the child is sufficiently symptomatic, films may show an olisthetic scoliosis or trunk lean. There is an increased incidence of concomitant spinal abnormalities in patients with herniated discs. In particular, congenital spinal stenosis is frequently seen. Other findings include transitional vertebrae or spondylolisthesis.[20]

Disc herniation is seen best on MRI (Fig. 21–1). The involved disc is readily appreciated, and other processes that might produce sciatica, such as epidural abscess and spinal cord tumor, can be ruled out.[8] Herniation of the disc can be differentiated from an avulsed vertebral apophysis on either MRI or CT scan. Correlation of MRI findings with the history and clinical examination is necessary because mild disc bulging can exist as a normal variant.

Treatment is initially conservative, consisting of anti-inflammatory medication and bed rest. Prolonged nonoperative management may lead to persistent pain, however, so if the patient does not respond to symptomatic treatment, disc excision should be performed.[19] Short-term results are very encouraging, with 95% good and excellent results and nearly universal resolution of back and leg pain.[19] Although long-term follow-up shows deterioration in results, with 24% reoperation after 30 years,[21] outcome studies show that patients treated by discectomy as adolescents function better than adults after similar surgery.[22] Surgical technique for adult and pediatric patients is similar. Some early reports indicate pediatric patients can safely undergo endoscopic percutaneous discectomy.[23]

Apophyseal Ring Fracture (Slipped Vertebral Apophysis)

The apophyseal ring fracture, also known as a slipped vertebral apophysis, occurs in adolescents and young adults. The etiology is either acute trauma resulting in rapid flexion and axial compression or cumulative microtrauma. The fracture typically develops at the junction of the posteroinferior vertebral body and the cartilaginous ring apophysis, with posterior displacement of the fragment into the spinal canal.[24] CT scan can show the size and location of the bony fragment, with large central fragments being most common and most likely to result in significant pain if left untreated.[25]

Symptoms mimic a herniated disc, with the sudden onset of severe back pain radiating into the leg. Physical examination shows a positive straight-leg raise test, but as is the case with disc herniations, neurologic signs are infrequently present.

The diagnosis is made radiographically. High-quality lateral radiographs may show an arc-shaped rim of cartilage, cartilage with attached underlying bone, or a small triangular bony fragment lying posterior to the vertebral body. The fragment is best visualized on CT scan.[24] The levels most frequently injured are L4 or S1. Treatment is surgical removal of the avulsed fragment.

Vertebral Fractures

Pediatric patients with spinal fractures present with back pain. If the energy of injury is sufficient that fracture is possible, radiographs should be obtained at once. When compression fractures are seen in children without high-energy trauma, an immediate evaluation should be performed for underlying malignancy.

Developmental Disorders

Spondylolysis and Spondylolisthesis

Spondylolysis refers to a stress fracture of the pars interarticularis, occurring predominantly in the lower lumbar spine. The most frequent level is L5, followed by L4. It is extremely rare to have more than one vertebral level involved. Spondylolysis is bilateral in 80% of cases and unilateral in 20%. More recent

studies show that 50% of young athletes presenting for evaluation of back pain have injuries to the pars interarticularis.[26] The mechanism of injury is repetitive microtrauma in hyperextension, overloading the pars interarticularis, over time leading to stress fracture. Sports linked to a high incidence of spondylolysis are gymnastics, diving, ballet, and football. Gymnasts and football linemen have a fourfold increase in incidence of spondylolysis compared with the general pediatric population.[27]

Symptoms consist of low back pain that is exacerbated by athletic activity and at least partly relieved by rest. The pain is present in the lower back, but can radiate into the legs.

Physical examination may reveal hamstring tightness and loss of normal lumbar mobility. The ability to bend forward to the floor may be diminished. In hyperflexible patients (i.e., gymnasts and ballerinas), motion may seem normal. The patient is usually tender to palpation of the lumbar spine. Hyperextension usually reproduces the back pain, and axial rotation in hyperextension exacerbates the pain.

Lateral radiographs may show lysis across the pars interarticularis, and oblique radiographs can be helpful in less obvious cases (Fig. 21–2). The appearance of a collar on the "Scottie dog" suggests stress fracture. Often, plain radiographs are nondiagnostic. In these cases, scintigraphy can reveal increased tracer uptake at the involved level. The use of SPECT is particularly helpful in localizing increased uptake in the pars interarticularis (Fig. 21–3).[13,14,28] A specific scintigraphic pattern, seen as a triangle of increased signal with increased uptake in the pedicles, has been described.[29] Positive bone scans and SPECT imaging are generally seen in the prefracture

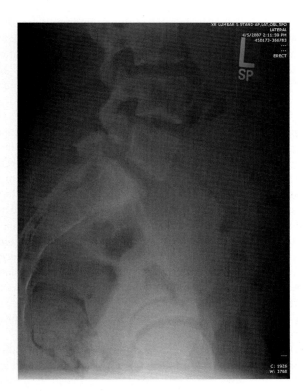

FIGURE 21–2 Lateral radiograph of lumbar spine shows spondylolysis of L5 in a 16-year-old volleyball player.

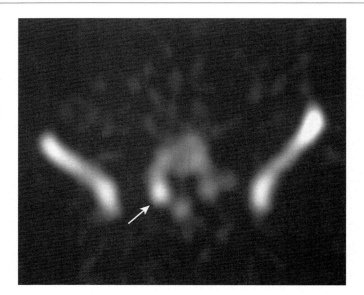

FIGURE 21–3 Increased uptake in pars interarticularis of an adolescent ballerina with spondylolysis.

state and in relatively acute injuries.[30] The bone scan may not be "hot" in chronic spondylolysis.[14]

MRI has also been used to diagnose spondylolysis, but false-positive scans can occur.[31] Better bony definition of the fracture is obtained using CT scans. Additionally, CT is superior to MRI in the assessment of incomplete fractures and in establishing healing in patients with spondylolysis.[32] The pars is imaged by using a reverse gantry angle and obtaining thin slices on the CT scan.[33]

Spondylolysis and spondylolisthesis can produce scoliosis. Curves resulting from these conditions are usually described as olisthetic, are associated with oblique takeoff of the spine from the pelvis, are small in degree, and have little rotation. Spondylolysis and spondylolisthesis occur in patients with idiopathic scoliosis more frequently than in the general population but are usually asymptomatic.

Treatment of spondylolysis is initially nonoperative and primarily involves modifying the patient's level of athletic activity.[34] Cessation of sport until the resolution of symptoms is combined with a concomitant exercise program to stretch the hamstrings and strengthen the paraspinal and abdominal musculature. Resumption of activities is gradual. The patient's technique or training should be modified to minimize recurrent fractures. Use of a antilordotic lumbar orthosis increases the success of nonoperative treatment, particularly in patients with acute injuries and "hot" bone scans.[35,36] A more recent study found resolution of symptoms after bracing correlated with initial increased activity on SPECT scans and with decreased uptake on follow-up scans, whereas SPECT scans for patients whose pain did not improve showed no significant decrease in activity after bracing.[37]

The overall success rate of nonoperative treatment ranges from 73% to 100%.[36] A multicenter study of 436 children and adolescents with CT-proven spondylolysis found 95% excellent results and 100% return to sport without surgery after 3 months of cessation of activity with use of a thoracolumbar

orthosis.[38] Patients who have normal radiographs but are found to have a stress reaction without fracture on further imaging are highly likely to improve (and not progress to radiographic fracture) with conservative treatment.[39,40] Surgery is typically reserved for the few patients whose symptoms are refractory to 6 months of conservative measures and whose pain recurs with activity after initial nonoperative success.[41]

Spondylolisthesis is a related condition in which anterior slippage of a vertebral body occurs on the more distal vertebra. Most often, it is due to bilateral spondylolysis, with the portion of the vertebra anterior to the pars fracture slipping anteriorly. Dysplastic spondylolisthesis occurs in teens who have an elongated but intact pars interarticularis, which allows for the anterior translation without pars fracture.[42]

Patients with spondylolisthesis often present with complaints of low back pain. The pain may radiate into the legs. Physical findings mimic findings of spondylolysis, with the addition of a possible palpable step-off at the area of listhesis. In severe spondylolisthesis, the buttocks may appear "heart-shaped." If there is significant hamstring tightness, gait alterations are seen: The teen appears to be shuffling with posterior pelvic tilt. Patients may have a painful, or olisthetic, scoliosis (Fig. 21–4).

Plain radiographs establish the diagnosis. The slip is easily seen on a spot lateral radiograph of the lumbosacral junction, and the severity of the spondylolisthesis can be classified as the percentage of forward translation of L5 on the sacrum. Abnormal kyphosis is also seen as the cephalad vertebra tips forward on the caudal segment. A characteristic finding on the anteroposterior radiograph, the appearance of "Napoleon's hat," can be seen as L5 moves forward on the sacrum.

Treatment is initially conservative in mild spondylolisthesis and surgical as the magnitude of the slip increases. Surgical treatment of high-grade spondylolisthesis is recommended, but preferred techniques vary among surgeons, and reduction remains controversial.[43] The surgical treatment of spondylolisthesis and spondylolysis is discussed in further detail in Chapter 27.

Scheuermann Kyphosis

Scheuermann kyphosis is a developmental condition that occurs in adolescents and is characterized by increased thoracic kyphosis accompanied by lumbar hyperlordosis. Boys are affected slightly more frequently than girls.

Back pain, which is usually located at the apex of the thoracic kyphosis and may be present in the lower lumbar spine as well, is the presenting symptom. The pain is usually described as aching in nature, does not wake the patient from sleep, and does not radiate. It is exacerbated by vigorous activity and prolonged sitting. The severity of the back pain is variable, with some patients denying significant symptoms and instead presenting for evaluation of poor posture. Neurologic symptoms are highly unusual.

Physical examination of a patient with Scheuermann disease shows increased thoracic kyphosis that is most notable on forward bending, where the apex appears to protrude

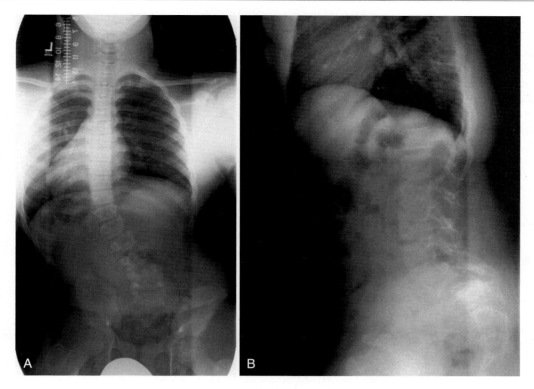

FIGURE 21–4 A, Scoliosis in a 13-year-old boy with low back and leg pain of 6 months' duration. **B,** Lateral radiograph shows spondylolisthesis at L5-S1.

posteriorly. The deformity is usually fairly rigid and does not disappear with hyperextension. There may be concomitant hamstring tightness, with inability to touch the floor with the fingertips.

The diagnosis is made radiographically (Fig. 21–5). Criteria for the diagnosis of Scheuermann disease have been outlined by Sorenson as (1) three contiguous vertebral bodies with greater than 5 degrees of anterior wedging; (2) abnormal disc narrowing; (3) endplate irregularities; and (4) Schmorl nodes, defined as disc herniations into the vertebral bodies.

Most patients with Scheuermann disease can be managed nonoperatively.[44] Physical therapy exercises and nonsteroidal medication can be helpful in relieving symptoms. The role of bracing is controversial. Patients with significant remaining spinal growth may benefit from orthotic treatment; it has been proposed that correction of deformity may be achieved in compliant patients.[45] The Milwaukee brace is the orthosis of choice for the treatment of Scheuermann disease.[46] Surgical correction of deformity and fusion is reserved for patients with severe kyphosis measuring greater than 75 degrees, patients whose symptoms are refractory to conservative measures, and patients who have significant cosmetic concerns.[47] The management of Scheuermann kyphosis is discussed in Chapter 26.

Lumbar Scheuermann Disease

Lumbar Scheuermann disease is a less common variant in which increased kyphosis and endplate changes are seen in the

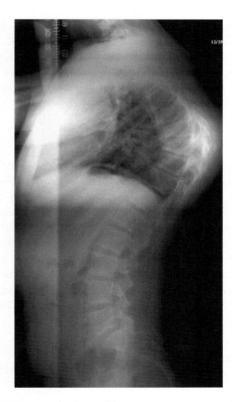

FIGURE 21–5 Anterior wedging of thoracic spine in a 15-year-old boy with Scheuermann kyphosis.

lumbar spine.[48] It also occurs most frequently in adolescence, and its cause is believed to be overuse. Microfractures occur in the vertebral endplates resulting in low back pain. Radiographs reveal endplate irregularities and disc space narrowing, anterior Schmorl nodes, and possible anterior wedging of the affected vertebrae leading to loss of lumbar lordosis. Radiographs may also show associated spondylolysis or scoliosis.[15,49] The radiographic appearance of vertebral changes and disc space narrowing may resemble infection or tumor. Scintigraphy may reveal mildly increased uptake at one or two vertebral levels.[15] MRI shows signal change and dehydration in the lumbar discs, with further disc deterioration occurring over time.[50] Treatment is symptomatic, and pain is usually ameliorated with modification of activity or use of an orthosis.

Idiopathic Scoliosis

Most patients who have idiopathic scoliosis do not complain of back pain, but symptoms are not as uncommon as previously thought. In a study by Ramirez and colleagues,[11] 32% of 2442 children who were thought to have idiopathic curves complained of some degree of back pain. Left-sided thoracic curves, which were associated with spinal cord abnormalities, were the most common factor associated with a positive diagnosis on further evaluation. Plain radiographs were found to be sufficient in the evaluation of typical curves if the neurologic examination was normal. Careful inspection of the apex of the deformity and at the lumbosacral junction (for spondylolysis and spondylolisthesis) occasionally yields a cause for the pain and the scoliosis (see Fig. 21–4). In the absence of neurologic findings on physical examination, MRI was not helpful. A more recent study showed that MRI was useful in identifying neural axis abnormalities in 6% of 104 patients. Back pain and early age of onset of scoliosis were present in patients with MRI abnormalities.[51]

Syringomyelia

Syringomyelia is defined as cystic dilation of the central canal of the spinal cord. The dilation of the cord leads to abnormalities in the neurologic pathways that transmit pain and temperature. Although not always symptomatic, patients may complain of pain. There is a predisposition toward left thoracic scoliosis in patients with syringomyelia.[52] Physical findings include scoliosis, foot deformities such as cavus, decreased sensation, and asymmetrical abdominal reflexes. The syrinx is clearly imaged on MRI. Treatment is neurosurgical decompression, although controversy exists regarding the size of syrinx that requires surgery.

Tethered Spinal Cord

Low back pain may be the presenting complaint in children with tethered spinal cords. The cord normally terminates at the L1-2 level. Persistence of the cord more distally implies tethering. Physical findings include foot deformity, spasticity, or weakness. Radiographs often show coexistent congenital vertebral abnormalities. The diagnosis is made on MRI, where the filum may appear thickened or the conus may be visualized at L3 or distal. Treatment of the symptomatic tethered cord is surgical release.

Idiopathic Juvenile Osteoporosis

Idiopathic juvenile osteoporosis is a rare disease that usually affects children in the first 2 decades of life. Presenting symptoms include back and leg pain owing to compression fractures and pain during weight bearing.[53,54] Radiographic findings include vertebral wedging owing to compression fractures with mildly increased kyphosis. Bone mineral density is decreased, but metabolic laboratory values are normal. The differential diagnosis includes leukemia. Orthotic management of back pain is usually sufficient. Medical management should be under the supervision of a pediatric rheumatologist. The disease is self-limiting, and symptoms resolve during puberty.[55]

Infectious and Inflammatory Etiologies

Discitis

Discitis is defined as a presumed bacterial infection of the intervertebral disc space. It is the most common cause of back pain in young children. The incidence of discitis is greatest in children 5 years old and younger, although it can occur in older children.[56] The etiology is believed to be infectious. In an immature child, blood vessels traverse the vertebral endplates and terminate in the nucleus pulposus. In young children, the disc is vascular, and this allows for seeding of bacteria into the disc space.[57-59] Presenting complaints vary but include back pain, refusal to walk, limping, and abdominal pain. The child usually is systemically ill, and patients often present to the emergency department. Approximately half have fever on presentation.

Physical examination reveals spinal stiffness, and often the spine is held in a flexed position. If asked to retrieve a toy from the floor, a child with discitis squats by bending the knees rather than bend the spine. Young children may exhibit Gowers sign when rising from the floor, using their upper extremities to push up on the legs as a strategy to minimize lumbar motion.[60] Tenderness to palpation of the affected area may be present.

Radiographic findings are usually minimal at the time of presentation. Subtle disc space narrowing and paraspinal soft tissue swelling on the lateral view are the first radiographic changes (Fig. 21–6). Over time, endplate irregularities are seen. Because plain radiographs are usually normal at the time of presentation, further imaging is required. Technetium bone scans show increased uptake on both sides of the affected disc space (Fig. 21–7A). Bone scans are positive in 74% to 100% of children with discitis[61,62]; they lead to earlier diagnosis and treatment. MRI also localizes the infection and delineates the extent of soft tissue involvement (Fig. 21–7B). In patients who are refractory to treatment, MRI is useful in assessing whether or not a soft tissue abscess is present.[63] MRI shows decreased signal on T1-weighted images and increased signal on T2-weighted images. If an abscess is present, there is peripheral enhancement with the administration of gadolinium.[64]

The evaluation of a child with possible discitis also includes obtaining laboratory studies. Elevations of erythrocyte sedimentation rate and C-reactive protein are seen in greater than 90% of children with discitis.[8] The white blood cell count may be elevated, but is less reliable.[57] Blood cultures should be obtained and are positive in greater than 50% of children with discitis.[62]

In the past, the treatment of discitis was controversial, but now there is more agreement that discitis represents a bacterial infection and should be treated with antibiotics.[57,63,65] Cultures of the intervertebral disc are positive in 60% of children, with *Staphylococcus aureus* the most common organism. A more recent study of disc space cultures showed *S. aureus* was cultured in 55% and *Kingella kingae* was cultured in 27% of children with discitis.[66] Because of the preponderance of *S. aureus* and the fact that 40% of cultures from the disc space remain negative, routine aspiration of the affected disc is not recommended.[65] If the patient fails to improve quickly with antistaphylococcal antibiotics, fine-needle aspiration under CT guidance can be useful.[67] Although administration of a second-generation cephalosporin for 3 weeks has been recommended,[65] epidemiologic trends in antibiotic resistance may alter which antibiotic should be chosen. Surgical biopsy and débridement are reserved for patients who fail medical management, have a neurologic deficit, have an abscess on MRI, or whose diagnosis is in question.

The outcome of pediatric discitis is favorable. Ten-year radiographic follow-up has shown narrowed disc space (60% of children) or bony ankylosis (40%), but kyphosis is rare and generally mild, and patients are pain-free.[68]

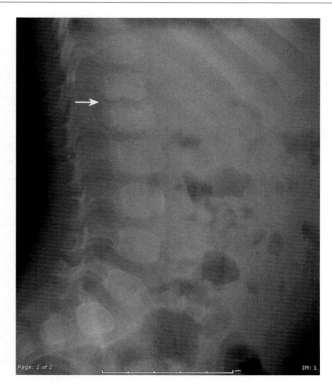

FIGURE 21–6 Disc space narrowing and endplate irregularities in a child with T11-12 discitis.

Disc space infection in infants younger than 1 year of age is usually very aggressive and requires immediate diagnosis and treatment. Infants are often septic at presentation. Residual kyphosis after eradication of the infection has been described.[69]

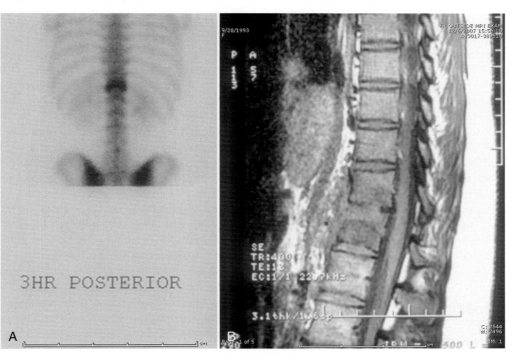

FIGURE 21–7 A, Bone scan in a child with discitis shows increased uptake. **B,** MRI reveals destruction of disc space, erosion of endplates, and vertebral involvement.

Vertebral Osteomyelitis

The distinction between discitis and osteomyelitis in children is blurred. It is believed that osteomyelitis is a continuation of discitis,[58] with the two entities representing a condition termed *infectious spondylitis*. Osteomyelitis produces more notable vertebral body radiographic changes. *S. aureus* is the most common organism.[59]

Opportunistic infections may also affect the vertebral column, especially in immunocompromised patients, such as patients with malignancies or who have had organ transplants. Fungal infections such as coccidioidomycosis are rare, but must be kept in mind in endemic regions.[70]

Tuberculosis is increasing in frequency and is seen most commonly in children from endemic regions. Symptoms include fever, malaise, weight loss, and night sweats. Neurologic findings occur more frequently in tuberculosis than in discitis.[71] Radiographic changes are more advanced in children with tuberculous spondylitis and consist of bony destruction of the vertebral body, kyphosis, soft tissue abscesses, and soft tissue calcifications. CT findings include erosions with calcification and intraspinous, paravertebral, and epidural abscesses.[72,73] Chest radiograph shows evidence of tuberculosis in 67% of children with tuberculous infection of the spine.[72] The purified protein derivative test is usually positive except in children with immunologic challenge, in whom it remains nonreactive. Pathologic examination of tissue from fine-needle aspiration of the affected bone yields a positive diagnosis in 83% of children and teens[74] and shows epithelioid giant cells and caseous necrosis or tubercle bacilli. Polymerase chain reaction has been used for faster identification of the organism.

Ankylosing Spondylitis and Rheumatologic Conditions

Ankylosing spondylitis is a rheumatologic condition characterized by loss of spinal mobility. It may manifest in adolescents as back pain. It occurs more frequently in boys than in girls. Physical findings include loss of lumbar flexibility so that lordosis does not reverse on forward flexion, increased kyphosis, and limited chest expansion with inspiration. Plain radiographs may reveal sclerosis, narrowing, or fusion of the sacroiliac joints. MRI has been shown to be superior to bone scan in identifying inflammation of the sacroiliac joint.[75,76] Laboratory evaluation of patients with ankylosing spondylitis shows a high incidence of HLA-B27. Onset of ankylosing spondylitis before the age of 16 years has been linked to worse functional outcomes than in patients with onset in adulthood.[77] Other rheumatologic conditions linked with back pain include polymyositis, dermatomyositis, and inflammatory bowel disease.

Hematologic Conditions

Sickle Cell Anemia and β-Thalassemia

In a study of pediatric patients presenting to a Canadian emergency department for the evaluation of back pain, 13% were found to have sickle cell anemia.[10] The spine has been reported as the second most common site for pain crisis in these patients, second only to the knee. Anemia is present in 86%.[78] Physical examination reveals tenderness to palpation. Treatment is pain management and admission to the hematology service.

β-thalassemia may also produce pain crises that affect the spine. In a more recent study, 25% of patients with thalassemia complained of low back pain.[79]

Neoplasms

Aneurysmal Bone Cysts

Aneurysmal bone cysts are nonmalignant expansile lytic lesions of bone that are characterized by their vascularity. Although not malignant tumors, they can be locally aggressive. Their etiology is unclear; a few familial cases have been identified.[80] Approximately 15% of aneurysmal bone cysts affect the spinal column, with a predilection for the posterior elements. If of sufficient size, the lesion may extend into the anterior column.[81,82] A large multicenter series of spinal aneurysmal bone cysts documented 30% were located in the cervical spine, 30% were in the thoracic spine, and 40% were in the lumbar spine.[83]

Back pain, which can result from the lesion itself or from an associated pathologic fracture, is the primary symptom. Neurologic compromise is unusual.

Radiographs show an expansile lytic lesion with a "bubbly" appearance. There is expansion of the cortex. CT scans best define the extent of the lesion and reveal the thin rim of surrounding bone (Fig. 21–8). Sacral lesions have been occasionally shown to affect more than one vertebral level.[84]

Treatment of aneurysmal bone cysts is surgical curettage with bone grafting.[85] Because of the vascularity of the cysts, preoperative embolization is very helpful in reducing intraoperative blood loss and improving visualization.[86-88] Spinal cord monitoring during embolization has been advocated to avoid vascular injury to the spinal cord.[89] Scheduling the surgical resection shortly after embolization is necessary to prevent revascularization of the lesion before curettage. When resection of the lesion leads to mechanical instability, simultaneous fusion is recommended.[90] There is a 10% to 14% recurrence rate after curettage and grafting for spinal aneurysmal bone cysts. A four-step surgical program, consisting of curettage, use of a high-speed bur, electrocautery, and bone grafting, with stabilization via short posterior fusion with instrumentation as needed, has been proposed more recently, with all patients disease-free at follow-up.[91]

In limited cases, repeat embolizations and radionuclide ablation have been used to treat spinal aneurysmal bone cysts definitively.[88] Repeat embolization has been advocated in patients who do not have neurologic findings or pathologic fracture, in patients in whom the diagnosis is certain, and in patients whose lesions have recurred.[92]

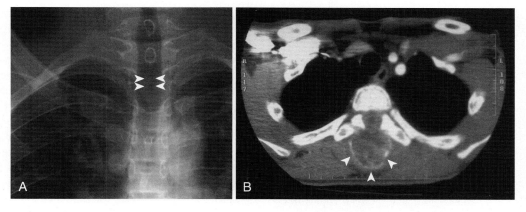

FIGURE 21–8 A, Anteroposterior radiograph of thoracic spine of a 16-year-old boy with lower extremity weakness and loss of bladder function shows absence of the spinous process at T2. **B,** CT scan delineates extent of aneurysmal bone cyst of posterior elements of T2.

Osteoid Osteoma

Osteoid osteoma is the most common benign spinal tumor occurring in children, with presentation occurring in the 2nd decade of life. The tumors typically are located in the posterior elements of the spine. Osteoid osteomas produce back pain that is worse at night and ameliorated by aspirin or nonsteroidal medication.

Physical examination reveals decreased spinal flexibility. Often patient stands with a list. The neurologic examination is generally normal. Plain radiographs are usually insufficient to make the diagnosis, but an olisthetic scoliosis might be apparent. When scoliosis is present, the lesion is usually located in the concavity of the apex of the curve.[93] Bone scan is positive, with distinct increased uptake seen (Fig. 21–9). CT scans provide the best imaging of osteoid osteomas, with a small radiolucent nidus and surrounding sclerosis and new bone apparent (Fig. 21–10). MRI shows increased signal intensity in the muscles and surrounding bone.[94] The MRI appearance and the tendency for enhancement in the soft tissues near the lesion may lead the physician to suspect a malignant tumor.[95]

Long-term administration of nonsteroidal anti-inflammatory medication can provide pain relief in a small group of patients with spinal osteoid osteomas, so a trial of nonsurgical treatment is warranted. Usually, symptoms are sufficient to warrant surgical removal of the nidus, which typically results in immediate pain relief. Intraoperative CT has been used to target the nidus better and minimize bony resection.[96] Newer treatments are under investigation, including percutaneous CT-guided drilling of the nidus with a bur and thermocoagulation.[97,98] When scoliosis has been

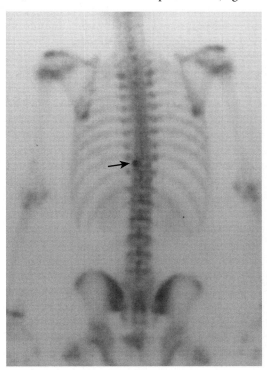

FIGURE 21–9 Bone scan of a 15-year-old boy with a 2-year history of back pain shows increased uptake at T10.

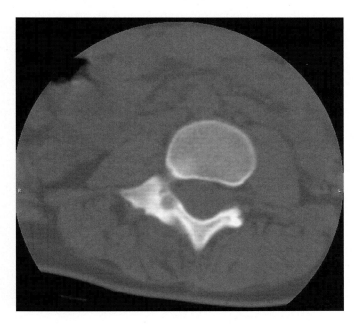

FIGURE 21–10 CT scan shows radiolucent nidus with surrounding bony sclerosis in an 11-year-old child with back pain resulting from an osteoid osteoma.

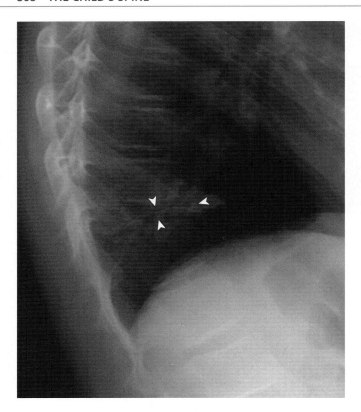

FIGURE 21–11 Lateral radiograph of a 12-year-old boy with vertebra plana of T11 consistent with eosinophilic granuloma. Back pain resolved with conservative treatment.

long-standing, persistence of the deformity is possible after successful removal of the osteoid osteoma.

Osteoblastoma

Although osteoblastoma is a less common benign lesion of the spine, 40% of osteoblastomas are located in the vertebrae. They also are located in the posterior elements of the spine, but because they are by definition larger than osteoid osteomas, they often extend anteriorly into the vertebral bodies.[99] The primary symptom of osteoblastoma is back pain, which is usually less severe than in osteoid osteoma. Neurologic abnormalities may result from the size of the lesion and its encroachment on the spinal canal or neural foramina.[94]

The lesion can be usually seen on plain radiographs, but CT scans are invaluable in assessing the size and extent of osteoblastoma. As in osteoid osteoma, MRI in osteoblastoma can overestimate the extent and aggressiveness of the lesion.[100] Plain radiographs also reveal scoliosis in approximately 40% of affected patients.[93]

Treatment is surgical removal of the lesion, with fusion as needed to address instability based on the size of resection. Recurrence occurs in 10% of osteoblastomas.

Eosinophilic Granuloma (Langerhans Cell Histiocytosis)

Eosinophilic granuloma, also known as Langerhans cell histiocytosis or histiocytosis X, is a peculiar condition of childhood typified by the development of lytic lesions of bone. The lesions may occur singly or affect multiple areas of the skeleton, including the spine. When the condition is associated with systemic involvement, it is known as *Hand-Schüller-Christian disease* or the more severe *Letterer-Siwe disease.* Eosinophilic granuloma has a higher incidence in boys. The average age at diagnosis is 6 years, with most patients in the 1st decade of life.[101]

Vertebral lesions in eosinophilic granuloma occur in 10% to 17% of affected children. Patients may present with back pain or a limp. Occasionally, neurologic signs can be present.

Radiographs show lytic lesions within the vertebral body or, more rarely, the posterior elements. Larger lesions lead to collapse of the vertebral body, which can be symmetrical or asymmetrical (Fig. 21–11). Although vertebra plana (also known as "coin-on-end" appearance) is the classically described spinal lesion in eosinophilic granuloma, only 40% of children with eosinophilic granuloma and vertebral lesions have been reported to have vertebra plana.[102] Skeletal surveys often identify other sites of involvement, which supports the diagnosis. Typical sites of involvement include the skull, the pelvis, and the diaphyses of the long bones. Bone scan is positive in 90% of children with eosinophilic granuloma.[103]

The differential diagnosis includes leukemia, infection, and other malignant tumors such as Ewing sarcoma.[104] If the radiographic appearance is atypical and other peripheral skeletal lesions are not identified, a surgical biopsy of the spinal lesion is warranted. Pathologic specimens show clonal proliferation of Langerhans-type histiocytes, eosinophils, and giant cells.[105]

Most patients with eosinophilic granuloma experience spontaneous resolution of disease. Because the condition seems to be self-limiting, the indications for treatment are few. Back pain resulting from a unifocal spinal lesion can usually be relieved by rest and the use of orthoses.[101,105] Patients with neurologic compromise may be treated with low-dose radiation therapy or with surgical débridement of the lesion and stabilization.[103,106] Radiation therapy has fallen out of favor as treatment for eosinophilic granuloma of the spine because of the potential for secondary malignancies. Multifocal disease, particularly when associated with systemic involvement, is treated with chemotherapy.[107]

The long-term outcome of eosinophilic granuloma in the absence of systemic disease is very good. Recurrence of disease is not seen in children.[107,108] Over time, improvement in vertebral body height is seen, although complete restoration to normal is unusual.[109,110]

Malignant Tumors

Leukemia

Leukemia is the most common pediatric malignancy that produces back pain. Many children first present to the orthopaedic surgeon; 6% to 25% of children with acute leukemia have been reported to present initially with back pain.[111,112] Most of these children are initially misdiagnosed, so the orthopaedic surgeon must have a high level of suspicion to evaluate these patients properly.[113] The history may reveal symptoms of pallor, fatigue, loss of appetite, or fever. The parent should be questioned about a history of bruising or abnormal bleeding.

Radiographic findings are not always initially present but include generalized osteopenia, vertebral compression fractures, and metaphyseal leukemic lines. Vertebral compression fractures occur in 7% of children with acute lymphocytic leukemia (Fig. 21–12).[112,114]

The diagnosis can usually be made on laboratory examination, with abnormalities seen in any or all of the three cell lines—anemia, thrombocytopenia, and leukopenia. The erythrocyte sedimentation rate is usually elevated. Of children with leukemia, 10% or more initially have normal automated counts.[114,115] Inspection of the peripheral smear reveals the diagnosis in some of these children.

Chemotherapy under the direction of a pediatric oncologist is the treatment of choice. Spinal bracing can be prescribed to relieve back pain and prevent further compression fractures.

Vertebral Malignant Tumors

Malignant tumors of the spine cause significant back pain in more than 50% of children at the time of diagnosis.[116] Although rare, these tumors must remain in the differential diagnosis of pediatric back pain. Pain may radiate into the legs, resembling the symptoms of a herniated disc. Patients with disc herniation are in the 2nd decade of life, whereas children with spinal or spinal cord tumors may be younger. Neurologic deficits and reflex changes are uncommon in disc herniation but frequent in tumors.[117]

Vertebral tumors include Ewing sarcoma and osteosarcoma.[118] Osteosarcoma rarely affects the spine.[119] Radiographs are variable, with osteolytic, osteoblastic, and mixed appearances possible. CT and MRI are used to stage the tumor. Treatment is difficult.

Of Ewing sarcomas, 10% occur in the spine, with the sacrum the most frequent site.[120] The average age at presentation is 13.3 years.[121] Relentless back pain is the primary symptom. Neurologic deficits are present in 58% of patients with spinal Ewing tumors.[122] Radiographs may show an expansile lytic lesion with variable vertebral collapse. Cases of Ewing sarcoma that radiographically resemble vertebra plana have been reported, leading to the misdiagnosis of eosinophilic granuloma.[122] MRI delineates the extent of the lesion and its accompanying soft tissue mass.

Spinal Metastasis

Neuroblastoma is the most frequent tumor to metastasize to the spine in children.[123] In a more recent study of 29 malignant spine tumors, neuroblastoma represented one third of all cases.[116] Radiographs usually show diffuse vertebral involvement. The thoracic spine is most frequently involved. An elevation of urinary normetanephrine may help in establishing the diagnosis.[120] Other tumors that involve the spine

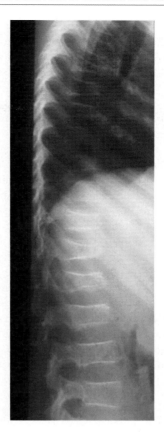

FIGURE 21–12 Osteopenia and multiple compression fractures in a child presenting with back pain owing to leukemia.

include rhabdomyosarcoma, Wilms tumor, and primary neuroectodermal tumors.[124]

Spinal Cord Tumors

Common spinal cord tumors in children are astrocytomas and ependymomas. The onset of symptoms is indolent. Neurologic signs, such as deterioration of gait, delay in motor skills, and loss of bladder control, raise suspicion.[125-127] Back pain is usually present, leading to initial referral to the orthopaedic surgeon in 31% to 58% of patients who are eventually diagnosed with spinal cord tumors.[125,126] Physical examination reveals motor deficits, clonus, and possibly scoliosis. There may be limitation of spinal flexibility. Radiographs can show changes secondary to pressure or expansion of the tumor, including absence or thinning of the pedicle or widening of the intervertebral foramina. Spinal cord tumors are best seen on MRI.

Although uncommon, neurofibromas in children and adolescents with neurofibromatosis can undergo malignant degeneration into neurofibrosarcoma. Back pain in a patient with neurofibromatosis should be evaluated.

Nonorthopaedic Causes of Pain

Intra-abdominal processes, such as inflammatory bowel disease, hydronephrosis, ovarian cysts, endometriosis, and urinary tract infections, can produce back pain. Pain resulting from these conditions is not exacerbated by activity and tends to be more intense at night. Pediatric referral should be made when nonmusculoskeletal causes are suspected.

Psychosomatic Pain (Conversion Reaction)

As discussed in the beginning of this chapter, there are children in whom an organic etiology for back pain cannot be found despite thorough evaluation. Back pain can be influenced by psychosocial factors that alter the patient's perception of pain and the effect of pain on everyday life. Psychosomatic pain remains a diagnosis of exclusion. It is more prevalent in adolescents, particularly in teens whose family members have a history of similar back pain. A detailed social history often reveals problems at home or school, often resulting in anxiety and depression. Treatment is difficult but includes intervention by psychologists and physical therapists. More recent studies show that 71% of children and adolescents who have negative diagnostic evaluations for back pain continue to have pain at an average follow-up of 4.4 years.[7] Even 8 years after initial evaluation, 62% of 58 patients were still symptomatic.[128]

KEY REFERENCES

1. Feldman DS, Hedden DM, Wright JG: The use of bone scan to investigate back pain in children and adolescents. J Pediatr Orthop 20:790-795, 2000.
   SPECT in 170 children with back pain led to no diagnosis in 78%, whereas constant pain, night pain, male gender, and acute symptoms were associated with positive diagnoses such as tumor (4.6%).

2. Selbst SM, Lavelle JM, Soyupak SK, et al: Back pain in children who present to the emergency department. Clin Pediatr 38:401-406, 1999.
   Of 225 children seen in an emergency department over 1 year for back pain, 25% received diagnoses of "trauma," 24% received diagnoses of muscle strains, and 13% received diagnoses of sickle cell crises.

3. Anderson K, Sarwark JF, Conway JJ, et al: Quantitative assessment with SPECT imaging of stress injuries of the pars interarticularis and response to bracing. J Pediatr Orthop 20:28-33, 2000.
   Patients with back pain owing to spondylolysis and positive SPECT responded favorably to orthotic treatment, with decreased uptake seen on repeat scans.

4. Early SD, Kay RM, Tolo VT: Childhood diskitis. J Am Acad Orthop Surg 11:413-420, 2003.
   This is an excellent current review of the spectrum of spinal infections, including pediatric discitis and osteomyelitis, with treatment recommendations.

5. Kayser R, Mahlfeld K, Nebelung W, et al: Vertebral collapse and normal peripheral blood cell count at the onset of acute lymphatic leukemia in childhood. J Pediatr Orthop B 9:55-57, 2000.
   This important article raises awareness of the possibility of leukemia manifesting with back pain and normal laboratory test results.

6. Dormans JP, Moroz L: Infection and tumors of the spine in children. J Bone Joint Surg Am 89(Suppl):79-97, 2007.
   This is a thorough review of the evaluation and treatment of benign and malignant tumors of the spine manifesting in pediatric patients.

REFERENCES

1. Burton AK, Clarke RD, McClune TD, et al: The natural history of low back pain in adolescents. Spine 21:2323-2328, 1996.

2. Balague F, Skovron ML, Nordin M, et al: Low back pain in schoolchildren: A study of familial and psychological factors. Spine 20:1265-1270, 1995.

3. Harreby M, Nygaard B, Jessen T, et al: Risk factors for low back pain in a cohort of 1389 Danish school children: An epidemiologic study. Eur Spine J 8:444-450, 1999.

4. Olsen TL, Anderson RL, Dearwater SR, et al: The epidemiology of low back pain in an adolescent population. Am J Public Health 82:606-608, 1992.

5. Wedderkopp N, Leboeuf-Yde C, Andersen LB, et al: Back pain reporting pattern in a Danish population-based sample of children and adolescents. Spine 26:1879-1883, 2001.

6. Hensinger RN: Back pain in children. In Bradford DS, Hensinger RN (eds): The Pediatric Spine. New York, Thieme, 1985, p 41.

7. Feldman DS, Hedden DM, Wright JG: The use of bone scan to investigate back pain in children and adolescents. J Pediatr Orthop 20:790-795, 2000.

8. Ginsburg GM, Bassett GS: Back pain in children and adolescents: Evaluation and differential diagnosis. J Am Acad Orthop Surg 5:67, 1997.

9. Micheli LJ, Wood R: Back pain in young athletes: Significant differences from adults in causes and patterns. Arch Pediatr Adolesc Med 149:15-18, 1995.

10. Selbst SM, Lavelle JM, Soyupak SK, et al: Back pain in children who present to the emergency department. Clin Pediatr 38:401-406, 1999.

11. Ramirez N, Johnston CE II, Browne RH: The prevalence of back pain in children who have idiopathic scoliosis. J Bone Joint Surg Am 79:364-368, 1997.

12. Bellah RD, Summerville DA, Treves ST, et al: Low back pain in adolescent athletes: Detection of stress injury to the pars interarticularis with SPECT. Radiology 180:509-512, 1991.

13. Bodner RJ, Heyman S, Drummond DS, et al: The use of single photon emission computed tomography (SPECT) in the diagnosis of low-back pain in young patients. Spine 13:1155-1160, 1988.

14. Lusins JO, Elting JJ, Cicoria AD, et al: SPECT evaluation of lumbar spondylolysis and spondylolisthesis. Spine 19:608-612, 1994.

15. Mandell GA, Morales RW, Harcke HT, et al: Bone scintigraphy in patients with atypical lumbar Scheuermann disease. J Pediatr Orthop 13:622-627, 1993.

16. Auerbach JD, Ahn J, Zgonis MH, et al: Streamlining the evaluation of low back pain in children. Clin Orthop 466:1971-1977, 2008.

17. Grobler LJ, Simmons EH, Barrington TW: Intervertebral disc herniation in the adolescent. Spine 4:267-278, 1979.

18. Parisini P, DiSilvestre M, Greggi T, et al: Lumbar disc excision in children and adolescents. Spine 26:1997-2000, 2001.

19. DeLuca PF, Mason DE, Weiand R, et al: Excision of herniated nucleus pulposus in children and adolescents. J Pediatr Orthop 14:318-322, 1994.

20. Epstein JA, Epstein NE, Marc J, et al: Lumbar intervertebral disc herniation in teenage children: Recognition and management of associated anomalies. Spine 9:427-432, 1984.

21. Luukkonen M, Partanen K, Vapalahti M: Lumbar disc herniations in children: A long-term clinical and magnetic resonance imaging follow-up study. Br J Neurosurg 11:280-285, 1997.

22. Durham SR, Sun PP, Sutton LN: Surgically treated lumbar disc disease in the pediatric population: An outcome study. J Neurosurg 92:1-6, 2000.

23. Mayer HM, Mellerowicz H, Dihlmann SW: Endoscopic discectomy in pediatric and juvenile lumbar disc herniations. J Pediatr Orthop B 5:39-43, 1996.

24. Takata K, Inoue S, Takahashi K, et al: Fracture of the posterior margin of a lumbar vertebral body. J Bone Joint Surg Am 70:589-594, 1988.

25. Chang CH, Lee ZL, Chen WJ, et al: Clinical significance of ring apophysis fracture in adolescent lumbar disc herniation. Spine 33:1750-1754, 2008.

26. Sassmannhausen G, Smith BG: Back pain in the young athlete. Clin Sports Med 21:121-132, 2002.

27. Jackson DW, Wiltse LL, Cirinciane RJ: Spondylolysis in the female gymnast. Clin Orthop 117:68-73, 1976.

28. Lawrence JP, Greene HS, Grauer JN: Back pain in athletes. J Am Acad Orthop Surg 14:726-735, 2006.

29. Van der Wall H, Storey G, Magnussen J, et al: Distinguishing scintigraphic features of spondylolysis. J Pediatr Orthop 22:308-311, 2002.

30. Dutton JA, Hughes SP, Peters AM: SPECT in the management of patients with back pain and spondylolysis. Clin Nucl Med 25:93-96, 2000.

31. Yamane T, Yoshida T, Mimatsu K: Early diagnosis of lumbar spondylolysis by MRI. J Bone Joint Surg Br 75:764-768, 1993.

32. Campbell RS, Grainger AJ, Hide IG, et al: Juvenile spondylolysis: A comparative analysis of CT, SPECT, and MRI. Skeletal Radiol 34:63-67, 2005.

33. Harvey CJ, Richenberg JL, Saifuddin A, et al: The radiological investigation of lumbar spondylolysis. Clin Radiol 53:723-728, 1998.

34. Smith JA, Hu SS: Management of spondylolysis and spondylolisthesis in the pediatric and adolescent population. Orthop Clin North Am 30:487-499, 1999.

35. D'Hemecourt PA, Zurakowski D, Driemler S, et al: Spondylolysis: Returning the athlete to sport participation with brace treatment. Orthopedics 25:653-657, 2002.

36. Morita T, Ikata T, Katoh S, et al: Lumbar spondylolysis in children and adolescents. J Bone Joint Surg Br 77:620-625, 1995.

37. Anderson K, Sarwark JF, Conway JJ, et al: Quantitative assessment with SPECT imaging of stress injuries of the pars interarticularis and response to bracing. J Pediatr Orthop 20:28-33, 2000.

38. Kurd MF, Patel D, Norton R, et al: Nonoperative treatment of symptomatic spondylolysis. J Spinal Disord Tech 20:560-564, 2007.

39. Sys J, Michielsen J, Bracke P, et al: Nonoperative treatment of active spondylolysis in elite athletes with normal x-ray findings: Literature review and results of conservative treatment. Eur Spine J 10:498-504, 2001.

40. Takemitsu M, El Rassi G, Woratanarat P, et al: Low back pain in pediatric athletes with unilateral tracer uptake at the pars interarticularis on single photon emission computed tomography. Spine 31:909-914, 2006.

41. Cavalier M, Herman MJ, Cheung EV, et al: Spondylolysis and spondylolisthesis in children and adolescents: I. Diagnosis, natural history, and nonsurgical management. J Am Acad Orthop Surg 14:417-424, 2006.

42. Lonstein JE: Spondylolisthesis in children: Cause, natural history, and management. Spine 24:2640-2648, 1999.

43. Cheung EV, Herman MJ, Cavalier R, et al: Spondylolysis and spondylolisthesis in children and adolescents: II. Surgical management. J Am Acad Orthop Surg 14:488-498, 2006.

44. Tribus CB: Scheuermann's kyphosis in adolescents and adults: Diagnosis and management. J Am Acad Orthop Surg 6:36-43, 1998.

45. Pizzutillo PD: Nonsurgical treatment of kyphosis. Instr Course Lect 53:485-491, 2004.

46. Sachs B, Bradford D, Winter R, et al: Scheuermann kyphosis: Follow-up of Milwaukee brace treatment. J Bone Joint Surg Am 69:50-57, 1987.

47. Lowe JG: Scheuermann's disease. Orthop Clin North Am 30:475-487, 1999.

48. Blumenthal SL, Roach J, Herring JA: Lumbar Scheuermann's: A clinical series and classification. Spine 12:929-932, 1986.

49. Ogilvie JW, Sherman J: Spondylolysis in Scheuermann's disease. Spine 12:251-253, 1987.

50. Heithoff KB, Gundry CR, Burton CV, et al: Juvenile discogenic disease. Spine 19:335-340, 1994.

51. Benli IT, Uzumcujil O, Aydin E, et al: Magnetic resonance imaging abnormalities of neural axis in Lenke-type 1 idiopathic scoliosis. Spine 31:1828-1833, 2006.

52. Akhtar OH, Rowe DE: Syringomyelia-associated scoliosis with and without the Chiari-I malformation. J Am Acad Orthop Surg 16:407-417, 2008.

53. Dimar JR II, Campbell M, Glassman SD, et al: Idiopathic juvenile osteoporosis: An unusual cause of back pain in an adolescent. Am J Orthop 24:865-869, 1995.

54. Smith R: Idiopathic juvenile osteoporosis: Experience of twenty-one patients. Br J Rheumatol 34:68-77, 1995.

55. Tortolani PJ, McCarthy EF, Sponseller PD: Bone mineral density deficiency in children. J Am Acad Orthop Surg 10:57-66, 2002.

56. Early SD, Kay RM, Tolo VT: Childhood diskitis. J Am Acad Orthop Surg 11:413-420, 2003.

57. Ring D, Johnston CE II, Wenger DR: Pyogenic infectious spondylitis in children: The convergence of discitis and vertebral osteomyelitis. J Pediatr Orthop 15:652-660, 1995.

58. Song KS, Ogden JA, Ganey T, et al: Contiguous discitis and osteomyelitis in children. J Pediatr Orthop 17:470-477, 1997.

59. Tay BKB, Deckey J, Hu S: Spinal infections. J Am Acad Orthop Surg 10:188-197, 2002.

60. Mirovsky Y, Copeliovich L, Halperin N: Gowers' sign in children with discitis of the lumbar spine. J Pediatr Orthop B 14:68-70, 2005.

61. Crawford AH, Kucharzyk DW, Ruda R, et al: Discitis in children. Clin Orthop 266:70-79, 1991.

62. Wenger DR, Bobechko WP, Gilday DL: The spectrum of intervertebral disc-space infection in children. J Bone Joint Surg Am 60:100-108, 1978.

63. Ring D, Wenger DR: Magnetic resonance imaging scans in discitis: Sequential studies in a child who needed operative drainage. J Bone Joint Surg Am 76:596-601, 1994.

64. DuLac P, Panuel M, Devred P, et al: MRI of disc-space infection in infants and children: Report of 12 cases. Pediatr Radiol 20:175-178, 1990.

65. Glazer PA, Hu SS: Pediatric spinal infections. Orthop Clin North Am 27:111-123, 1996.

66. Garron E, Viehweger E, Launay F, et al: Nontuberculous spondylodiscitis in children. J Pediatr Orthop 22:321-328, 2002.

67. Hoffer FA, Strand RD, Gebhardt MC: Percutaneous biopsy of pyogenic infection of the spine in children. J Pediatr Orthop 8:442-444, 1988.

68. Kayser R, Mahlfeld K, Greulich M, et al: Spondylodiscitis in childhood: Results of a long-term study. Spine 30:318-323, 2005.

69. Eismont FJ, Bohlman HH, Soni PL, et al: Vertebral osteomyelitis in infants. J Bone Joint Surg Br 64:32-35, 1982.

70. Wrobel CJ, Chappell ET, Taylor W: Clinical presentation, radiological findings, and treatment results of coccidiomycosis involving the spine: Report on 23 cases. J Neurosurg 95:33-39, 2001.

71. Mushkin AY, Kovalenko KN: Neurological complications of spinal tuberculosis in children. Int Orthop 23:210-212, 1999.

72. Magnus KG, Hoffman EB: Pyogenic spondylitis and early tuberculous spondylitis in children: Differential diagnosis with standard radiographs and CT. J Pediatr Orthop 20:539-543, 2000.

73. Morris BS, Varma R, Barg A, et al: Multifocal musculoskeletal tuberculosis in children: Appearances on CT. Skeletal Radiol 31:1-8, 2002.

74. Francis IM, Das DK, Luthra UK, et al: Value of radiologically guided fine needle aspiration cytology (FNAC) in the diagnosis of spinal tuberculosis. Cytopathology 10:390-401, 1999.

75. Blum U, Buitrago-Tellez C, Mundinger A, et al: Magnetic resonance imaging (MRI) for detection of active sacroiliitis: A prospective study comparing conventional radiography, scintigraphy, and contrast enhanced MRI. J Rheumatol 23:2107-2115, 1996.

76. Kurugoglu S, Kanberoglu K, Kanberoglu A, et al: MRI appearances of inflammatory vertebral osteitis in early ankylosing spondylitis. Pediatr Radiol 32:191-194, 2002.

77. Stone M, Warren RW, Bruckel J, et al: Juvenile-onset ankylosing spondylitis is associated with worse functional outcomes than adult-onset ankylosing spondylitis. Arthritis Rheum 53:445-451, 2005.

78. Roger E, Letts M: Sickle cell disease of the spine in children. Can J Surg 42:289-292, 1999.

79. Onur O, Sitti A, Gumruk R, et al: Beta thalassaemia: A report of 20 children. Clin Rheumatol 18:42-44, 1999.

80. DiCaprio MR, Murphy MJ, Camp RL: Aneurysmal bone cyst of the spine with familial incidence. Spine 25:1589-1592, 2000.

81. Hay MC, Paterson D, Taylor TKF: Aneurysmal bone cysts of the spine. J Bone Joint Surg Br 60:406-411, 1978.

82. Vergel De Dios AM, Bond JR, Shives TC, et al: Aneurysmal bone cysts: A clinicopathologic study of 238 cases. Cancer 69:2921-2931, 1992.

83. Cottalorda J, Kohler R, Sales de Gauzy G, et al: Epidemiology of aneurysmal bone cyst in children: A multicenter study and literature review. J Pediatr Orthop B 13:389-394, 2004.

84. Papagelopoulos PJ, Choudhoury SN, Frassica FJ, et al: Treatment of aneurysmal bone cysts of the pelvis and sacrum. J Bone Joint Surg Am 83:1674-1681, 2001.

85. Papagelopoulos PJ, Currier BL, Shaughnessy WJ, et al: Aneurysmal bone cyst of the spine: Management and outcome. Spine 23:621-628, 1998.

86. DeCristofaro R, Biagini R, Boriani S, et al: Selective arterial embolization in the treatment of aneurysmal bone cyst and angioma of bone. Skeletal Radiol 21:523-527, 1992.

87. DeKleuver M, Van der Heul RO, Veraart BB: Aneurysmal bone cyst of the spine: 31 cases and the importance of the surgical approach. J Pediatr Orthop B 7:286-292, 1998.

88. DeRosa GP, Graziano GP, Scott J: Arterial embolization of aneurysmal bone cyst of the lumbar spine: A report of two cases. J Bone Joint Surg Am 72:777-780, 1990.

89. Berenstein A, Young W, Ransohoff J, et al: Somatosensory evoked potentials during spinal angiography and therapeutic transvascular embolization. J Neurosurg 60:777-785, 1984.

90. Ozaki T, Halm H, Hillmann A, et al: Aneurysmal bone cysts of the spine. Arch Orthop Trauma Surg 119:159-162, 1999.

91. Garg SM, Mehta S, Dormans JP: Modern surgical treatment of primary aneurysmal bone cyst of the spine in children and adolescents. J Pediatr Orthop 25:387-392, 2005.

92. Boriani S, DeLure F, Campanacci L, et al: Aneurysmal bone cyst of the mobile spine: Report on 41 cases. Spine 26:27-35, 2001.

93. Saifuddin A, White J, Sherazi Z, et al: Osteoid osteoma and osteoblastoma of the spine: Factors associated with the presence of scoliosis. Spine 23:47-53, 1998.

94. Ozaki T, Liljenqvist U, Hillmann A, et al: Osteoid osteoma and osteoblastoma of the spine: Experiences with 22 patients. Clin Orthop 397:394-402, 2002.

95. Lefton DR, Torrisi JM, Haller JO: Vertebral osteoid osteoma masquerading as a malignant bone or soft-tissue tumor on MRI. Pediatr Radiol 31:72-75, 2001.

96. Rajasekaran S, Kamath V, Shetty AP: Intraoperative Iso-C three-dimensional navigation in excision of spinal osteoid osteomas. Spine 33:E25-E29, 2008.

97. Baunin C, Puget C, Assoun J, et al: Percutaneous resection of osteoid osteoma under CT guidance in eight children. Pediatr Radiol 24:185-188, 1994.

98. Cove JA, Taminiau AH, Obermann WR, et al: Osteoid osteoma of the spine treated with percutaneous computed tomography-guided thermocoagulation. Spine 25:1283-1286, 2000.

99. Boriani S, Capanna R, Donati D, et al: Osteoblastoma of the spine. Clin Orthop 278:37-45, 1992.

100. Shaikh MI, Saifuddin A, Pringle J, et al: Spinal osteoblastoma: CT and MR imaging with pathological correlation. Skeletal Radiol 28:33-40, 1999.

101. Levine SE, Dormans JP, Meyer JS, et al: Langerhans' cell histiocytosis of the spine in children. Clin Orthop 323:288-293, 1996.

102. Floman Y, Bar-On E, Mosheiff R, et al: Eosinophilic granuloma of the spine. J Pediatr Orthop B 6:260-265, 1997.

103. Ghanem I, Tolo VT, D'Ambra P, et al: Langerhans cell histiocytosis of bone in children and adolescents. J Pediatr Orthop 23:124-130, 2003.

104. Papagelopoulos PJ, Currier BL, Galanis E, et al: Vertebra plana caused by primary Ewing sarcoma: Case report and review of the literature. J Spinal Disord Tech 15:252-257, 2002.

105. Willman CL, Busque L, Griffith BB, et al: Langerhans histiocytosis (histiocytosis X): A clonal proliferative disease. N Engl J Med 331:154-160, 1994.

106. Yeom JS, Lee CK, Shin HY, et al: Langerhans' cell histiocytosis of the spine: Analysis of 23 cases. Spine 24:1740-1749, 1999.

107. Garg S, Mehta S, Dormans JP: Langerhans' cell histiocytosis of the spine in children: Long-term followup. J Bone Joint Surg Br 86:1740-1750, 2004.

108. Plasschaert F, Craig C, Bell R, et al: Eosinophilic granuloma: A different behaviour in children than in adults. J Bone Joint Surg Br 84:870-872, 2002.

109. Mammano S, Candiotto S, Balsana M: Cast and brace treatment of eosinophilic granuloma of the spine: Long-term follow-up. J Pediatr Orthop 17:821-827, 1997.

110. Raab P, Hohmann F, Kuhl J, et al: Vertebral remodeling in eosinophilic granuloma of the spine: A long-term follow-up. Spine 23:1351-1354, 1998.

111. Rogalsky RJ, Black GB, Reed MH: Orthopaedic manifestations of leukemia in children. J Bone Joint Surg Am 68:494-501, 1986.

112. Kobayashi D, Satsuma S, Kamegaya M, et al: Musculoskeletal conditions of acute leukemia and malignant lymphoma in children. J Pediatr Orthop B 14:156-161, 2005.

113. Santangelo JR, Thomson JD: Childhood leukemia presenting with back pain and vertebral compression fractures. Am J Orthop 28:257-260, 1999.

114. Meehan PL, Viroslav S, Schmitt EW: Vertebral collapse in childhood leukemia. J Pediatr Orthop 15:592-595, 1995.

115. Kayser R, Mahlfeld K, Nebelung W, et al: Vertebral collapse and normal peripheral blood cell count at the onset of acute lymphatic leukemia in childhood. J Pediatr Orthop B 9:55-57, 2000.

116. Conrad EU III, Olszewski AD, Berger M, et al: Pediatric spine tumors with spinal cord compromise. J Pediatr Orthop 12:454-460, 1992.

117. Martinez-Lage JF, Martinez Robledo A, Lopez F, et al: Disc protrusion in the child: Particular features and comparison with neoplasms. Childs Nerv Syst 13:201-207, 1997.

118. Garg S, Dormans JP: Tumors and tumor-like conditions of the spine in children. J Am Acad Orthop Surg 13:372-381, 2005.

119. Shives TC, Dahlin DC, Sim FH, et al: Osteosarcoma of the spine. J Bone Joint Surg Am 68:660-668, 1986.

120. Dormans JP, Moroz L: Infection and tumors of the spine in children. J Bone Joint Surg Am 89(Suppl):79-97, 2007.

121. Venkateswaran L, Rodriguez-Galindo C, Merchant TE, et al: Primary Ewing tumor of the vertebrae: Clinical characteristics, prognostic factors, and outcome. Med Pediatr Oncol 37:30-35, 2001.

122. Grubb MR, Currier BL, Pritchard DJ: Primary Ewing's sarcoma of the spine. Spine 19:309-313, 1994.

123. Leeson MC, Makely JT, Carter JR: Metastatic skeletal disease in the pediatric population. J Pediatr Orthop 5:261-267, 1985.

124. Lam CH, Nagib MG: Nonteratomatous tumors in the pediatric sacral region. Spine 27:E284-E287, 2002.

125. Parker AP, Robinson RO, Bullock P: Difficulties in diagnosing intrinsic spinal cord tumours. Arch Dis Child 75:204-207, 1996.

126. Pena M, Galasko CS, Barrie JL: Delay in diagnosis of intradural spinal tumors. Spine 17:1110-1116, 1992.

127. Newton HB, Newton CL, Gatens C, et al: Spinal cord tumors: Review of etiology, diagnosis, and multidisciplinary approach to treatment. Cancer Pract 3:207-218, 1995.

128. Mirovsky Y, Yakim I, Halperin N, et al: Non-specific back pain in children and adolescents: A prospective study until maturity. J Pediatr Orthop B 11:275-278, 2002.

Paul D. Sponseller, MD
Beverlie L. Ting, MD

Congenital scoliosis is a progressive three-dimensional deformity of the spine caused by congenital anomalies of the vertebrae that result in an imbalance of the longitudinal growth of the spine. To understand their natural history and their treatment, it is important to understand the embryologic development of vertebrae.

Embryology

Paraxial mesoderm on either side of the notochord condenses to form somites, in a process known as *somitogenesis*. Each somite subdivides further into ventral sclerotome and dorsolateral dermomyotome. During the 4th week of development, cells from the sclerotome region of the somite on each side of the body migrate ventrally and surround the notochord and the neural tube. Each vertebra is formed by sclerotome cells from two somite levels (Fig. 22–1). The cranial and caudal parts of adjacent sclerotomes, which are not ossified yet, fuse with each other.[1] The ventral part of each vertebra forms the body around the notochord, and the dorsal part forms costal processes laterally and the vertebra arch dorsally.

Ossification begins during the 6th week from three primary ossification centers: one in the body (or centrum, formed by early fusion of two centers) and one in each half of the vertebral arch. During the 6th week of development, mesenchymal cells between cranial and caudal parts of the original sclerotome fill the space between two vertebral bodies to contribute to formation of the intervertebral structures.[2] This stage is called the *segmentation stage*.

Somitogenesis relies on the Notch signaling pathway and its interactions with FGF and Wnt signaling; however the precise mechanisms remain unclear.[3-5] Mutations in downstream components and targets of the Notch signaling pathway, such as *Dll3, Mesp2,* and *Lfng,* result in abnormal vertebral development in mouse models and are associated with characteristic vertebral defects seen in patients with spondylocostal dysostosis.[3-7] More recent experimental evidence in vertebrate animal models and human stem cells has revealed the oscillatory nature of gene expression in paraxial mesoderm during somitogenesis.[3,8,9] These findings support the concept that a putative segmentation clock triggers the cyclic expression of genes in the Notch, FGF, and Wnt signaling pathways and is essential for normal vertebral development.

Classification

Two types of basic vertebral anomalies can occur: failures of formation and failures of segmentation.[10]

Failures of Formation

Failure of vertebral formation (type I deformity) can be partial, causing a wedged vertebra with intact pedicles (Fig. 22–2), or complete, causing a hemivertebra with a unilateral pedicle (Fig. 22–3). Hemivertebrae are classified according to their longitudinal growth potential, which in normal vertebrae is provided by growth apophyses on both vertebral ends.

- *Segmented hemivertebra*: Both the superior and the inferior ends of the hemivertebra have growth potential. The shape of adjacent vertebrae is normal.

- *Semisegmented hemivertebra*: Either the superior or the inferior end of the hemivertebra has growth potential. The other end is fused with the adjacent vertebra.

- *Incarcerated hemivertebra*: Both the superior and the inferior ends of the hemivertebra have growth potential, but the adjacent vertebrae compensate for it. The hemivertebra is "carved into" the adjacent levels.

- *Nonsegmented hemivertebra*: There is no growth potential. The hemivertebra is completely fused with vertebrae above and below.

Failures of Segmentation

Failure of segmentation (type II deformity) can be partial, causing a bar (Fig. 22–4), or complete, causing a block vertebra. A congenital bar can be anterior, posterior, lateral, or mixed. In many cases, vertebral anomalies owing to failures of formation and failures of segmentation coexist,[11] occasionally

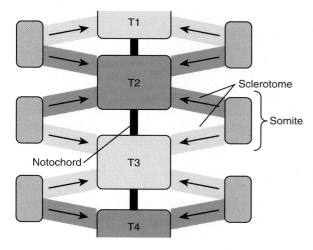

FIGURE 22–1 Each vertebra is formed by a part of four somites.

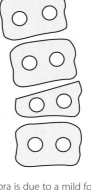

FIGURE 22–2 Wedge vertebra is due to a mild form of unilateral vertebral failure. The vertebra height is asymmetrical on the right and left side.

on several levels, and form a mixed deformity (type III deformity).

Associated Anomalies

Embryologic development of the spine coincides with the development of many other organ systems. It is not rare to have associated anomalies with vertebral deficiencies. These anomalies occur in 30% to 60% of children with congenital spinal anomalies.[11-13] The most common coexistent anomalies involve the spinal cord and the genitourinary tract. Intraspinal anomalies include problems such as tethered cord, diastematomyelia, and syringomyelia. The most common genitourinary defects are renal agenesis, ectopic kidney, duplication, and reflux.

Many of these anomalies are part of the VATER association. The acronym *VATER*[14] includes the following deficiencies: vertebral defects (*V*), anal atresia (*A*), tracheoesophageal fistula (*TE*), radial limb reduction, and renal defects (*R*). The acronym VATER was modified in 1975[15] to *VACTERL* by adding cardiac defect (*C*) and limb defect (*L*) (Fig. 22–5).

Congenital vertebral anomalies are also found with a high incidence in Klippel-Feil syndrome,[16,17] which is characterized by the combination of cervical fusion, limited neck range of motion, short neck, and low hairline. More recently,

congenital scoliosis has been associated with Sprengel deformity, Mayer-Rokitansky-Küster-Hauser syndrome, Jarcho-Levin syndrome, Goldenhar syndrome, and Genoa syndrome.[18-21]

Etiology

Congenital scoliosis is uncommon in the general population. Its true incidence is unknown, but the familial incidence in the congenital scoliosis population is typically 1% to 5%.[13,22-24] It is slightly more common in girls than in boys, with a ratio of 3:2.

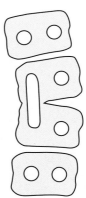

FIGURE 22–4 Congenital unilateral bar. Partial fusion between two vertebrae prevents longitudinal growth on its side.

FIGURE 22–3 Hemivertebrae are classified according to their growth potential. **A,** Segmented hemivertebra. **B,** Semisegmented hemivertebra. **C,** Incarcerated hemivertebra. **D,** Nonsegmented hemivertebra.

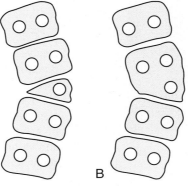
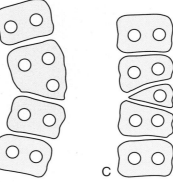
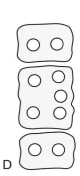

A   B   C   D

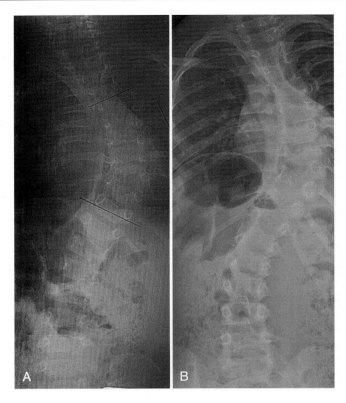

FIGURE 22–5 Congenital scoliosis with VACTERL association managed by observation since birth. **A** and **B,** Right thoracic curve and compensatory lumbar curve remain relatively unchanged from birth at 1 year of age (**A**) and at 8 years of age (**B**).

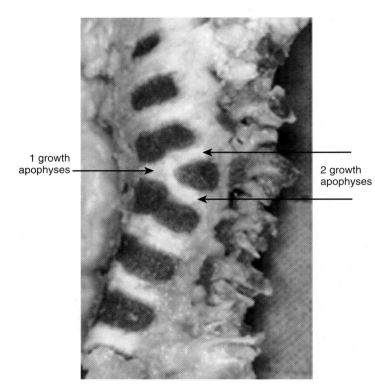

1 growth apophyses

2 growth apophyses

FIGURE 22–6 Hemivertebra forces spine into a curve. There are two growth apophyses on the hemivertebra side and only one on the other side, leading to worsening during growth.

The precise etiology of congenital scoliosis is unclear. Although most cases seem to be sporadic, in contrast to idiopathic scoliosis,[25] the role of genetic and environmental factors is often reported.[6,26,27] The genetic role has been reported in cases of congenital scoliosis in twins,[28-30] but, more recently, several studies have isolated gene mutations.[25,27,31]

Environmental factors have also been implicated in the genesis of congenital scoliosis. Maternal acute carbon monoxide exposure during somite formation induces vertebral anomalies in the offspring of mouse and rabbit models.[26,32] The mechanism of carbon monoxide action remains vague, however. Carbon monoxide could act directly on the cartilaginous spine via resulting hypoxia or a gene mutation.[26] The etiologic theories are clouded further by the finding of an increased incidence of idiopathic scoliosis in families with congenital scoliosis.

Natural History

As with scoliosis of any etiology, congenital scoliosis progresses in 70% of patients during growth. The potential for increase in curvature is related to imbalances in the number of growth apophyses and the location of vertebral anomalies.[33] Without any treatment, about 85% of patients with congenital scoliosis have a curve greater than 41 degrees by maturity.[33] Curves with segmented hemivertebrae are at risk for progression during growth because segmented hemivertebrae act as enlarging wedges (Fig. 22–6). The most progressive anomaly is a convex segmented hemivertebra associated with a concave unilateral bar because there is absolutely no growth potential on the side of the bar. Conversely, a wedge vertebra has only a slight risk of worsening, whereas a complete block or an incarcerated hemivertebra does not cause any progressive scoliosis.

The location of the anomaly also plays a part in the evolution of scoliosis. The most severe anomalies are those located at the thoracolumbar region, whereas the least severe are located at the upper thoracic spine.

The natural history of congenital scoliosis has to take several factors into account:

- Type of anomaly
- Location
- Number of anomalies
- Initial severity of the scoliosis
- Global growth potential balance between each side of the spine

Analysis of these factors allows one to determine the potential for progressive curvature and the most appropriate treatment.

More recent work has focused on the role of the spine and chest wall in lung development, which predominantly occurs by age 5. Congenital defects in the development of the ribs and vertebrae often occur together. Concurrent scoliosis and rib fusions may constrict the thorax and compromise pulmonary development. The inability of the thorax to support normal respiration is termed *thoracic insufficiency syndrome*.[34] Thoracic insufficiency syndrome can be assessed clinically by respiratory rate and the thumb excursion test and radiographically by plain radiographs and computed tomography (CT) volumetric studies. Early fusion of scoliotic deformity before age 9, especially in patients requiring more than four levels of fusion and patients with proximal fusions, also puts these patients at risk for the development of restrictive pulmonary disease.[35] The increasing awareness of the need to preserve pulmonary function has led to a surge in growth-preserving surgical techniques for complex multilevel congenital scoliosis.

Assessment

Physical Examination

The physical examination of a patient with congenital scoliosis is guided by the knowledge of a heightened incidence of other structural and neural anomalies. The examination should begin with an assessment of a patient's existing balance: sagittal plane balance and coronal balance, shoulder malalignment, and any deviation of head and trunk from the center of the pelvis. In addition, it is crucial to assess and document the neurologic status, including strength, reflexes, and presence of any atrophy. Flexibility of the deformity, gait, and limb-length inequality should be checked. Pain, if present, should be localized and quantified. The presence of a dimple or any cutaneous mark on the back should be noted. The examiner should search for other anomalies of the extremities (particularly radial malformation) and range of neck motion.

Imaging

Radiographs

For patients with congenital scoliosis, early plain radiographs are helpful to determine the type of vertebral abnormality. The best period to categorize the deformity is before 4 years of age. If a patient is seen by the orthopaedic surgeon after this age, valuable information may sometimes be gained by examining prior chest radiographs and abdominal or renal films. The spine surgeon learns to check for subtle clues, such as the presence and spacing of pedicles and fused or absent ribs. Later films make it difficult to assess the type of anomaly present because the vertebrae are too ossified, especially in the area of a fusion or bar (Fig. 22–7).

Anteroposterior and lateral films allow one to check the type and the location of deficiency, to measure the spine curvature, and to assess the pedicle width. Measurement of curvature according to the Cobb method[36] can be a challenge,

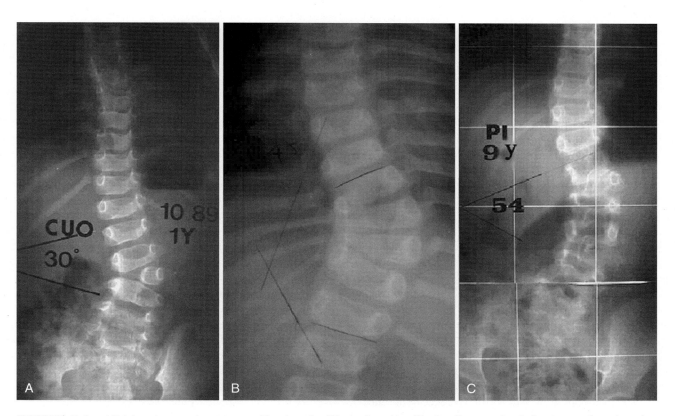

FIGURE 22–7 A and **B,** It is easier to analyze segmented hemivertebra (**A**) or unilateral bar (**B**) when films are taken before 4 years of age than after. **C,** Lumbar segmented hemivertebra in a 9-year-old child.

however.[37] It has been shown that there is an increase in measurement error[38] in congenital scoliosis owing to irregular vertebral landmarks and difficulty in numbering them. It is important always to compare current films against original ones rather than rely on curvature measurement itself. Assessment of curve evolution and compensatory curve development helps to confirm or to refute scoliosis progression. Because compensatory curves involve normally formed vertebrae, they can be more reproducibly measured. If a compensatory curve has not progressed, it is less likely that significant progression has occurred in a congenital curve.

Computed Tomography

CT with three-dimensional reconstruction can be used to identify spinal abnormalities in complex cases in which radiographs are often difficult to interpret.[39] CT scans can also help visualize spinal deformities that are obscured by overlying structures on plain radiographs.

Magnetic Resonance Imaging

Intraspinal anomalies are often associated with congenital scoliosis, but their incidence is variable. Before the introduction of magnetic resonance imaging (MRI), myelography and CT were the procedures of choice, and the incidence of intraspinal anomalies in this context varied widely from 5% to 58%.[17,40] The advent of MRI has led to more accurate discovery of intraspinal anomalies in 30% to 41% of cases.[41-43] The most common anomalies reported are tethered cord, syringomyelia, and diastematomyelia.

Although MRI is typically ordered in cases of unusual curve or of abnormal neurologic examination in idiopathic scoliosis, it seems reasonable to order MRI systematically in congenital scoliosis because of two factors:

1. Intraspinal anomalies are encountered in one third of cases of congenital scoliosis, and some of them may require neurosurgical procedures. Some of these anomalies may require treatment for their own sake (e.g., a large syrinx), whereas others need to be addressed if corrective orthopaedic surgery is planned (e.g., diastematomyelia).
2. There is no clear correlation between detectable neurologic manifestations and MRI findings.[43]

In practice, there is no urgency to order MRI when congenital scoliosis is diagnosed, especially given the need for general anesthesia in young children. It seems more appropriate to order MRI for patients with an abnormal neurologic examination, patients with worsening scoliosis despite a normal physical examination, or patients for whom a surgical procedure is considered.

Finally, a genitourinary assessment is useful at the time of initial diagnosis of congenital vertebral anomaly. This assessment can be performed accurately with renal ultrasonography. Often, MRI of the spine also shows the presence or absence of renal anomalies.[44] Further consultation may be indicated based on the results of this study.

Treatment

Nonoperative Treatment

Congenital vertebral anomalies require close clinical monitoring at periodic intervals during growth. Consistent observation allows for assessment of the evolution of spinal curves. In complex malformations, early treatment is often more straightforward and safer.

In contrast to idiopathic scoliosis, nonoperative treatment has little value in congenital scoliosis. The only potentially useful treatment is bracing of the noncongenital components of a flexible curve. For a few cases with long and flexible curves, progression of scoliosis can be slowed by bracing. Spinal curves in congenital scoliosis are often short and rigid, however. Given the significant time period remaining before skeletal maturity, bracing is rarely, if ever, more than a temporizing solution. Treatment of congenital scoliosis consists of two options: (1) clinical monitoring of static vertebral anomaly and (2) operative treatment of worsening scoliosis.

Operative Treatment

Congenital scoliosis develops because one side of the spine is growing faster than the other. The main principle of operative treatment is to balance growth, with or without deformity reduction. Five major operations have been described: posterior spine fusion, combined anterior and posterior spine fusion, convex hemiepiphysiodesis, hemivertebra excision, and guided growth by vertical expandable prosthetic titanium rib (VEPTR) or growing rods.

Posterior Spine Fusion

Posterior in situ fusion is the simplest and the safest technique (Fig. 22–8). This seemingly simple surgical exposure must be performed with caution, however, because failure to recognize potential posterior laminar defects can lead to neurologic damage. Imaging is useful before the exposure is made because the anomalous area is difficult to localize. After exposure of the posterior elements, the target region should be reconfirmed with radiographs because the hemivertebra or bar seen anteriorly may not have corresponding posterior elements. Fusion must include all vertebrae involved in the congenital curve and should extend laterally to the transverse processes. A postoperative cast or a rigid brace is required for 4 to 6 months to achieve fusion and curve correction.

With this technique, problems may occur, as follows:

- Because the anterior spine remains intact, anterior spinal growth is still active. This active growth can lead to increased rotational deformity with bending of the fusion mass, known as the "crankshaft phenomenon." Risk factors include young age at surgery and large curves at time of arthrodesis. A review of 54 patients with congenital scoliosis reported a 15% crankshaft incidence in patients undergoing posterior spinal fusion before the age of 10 years and

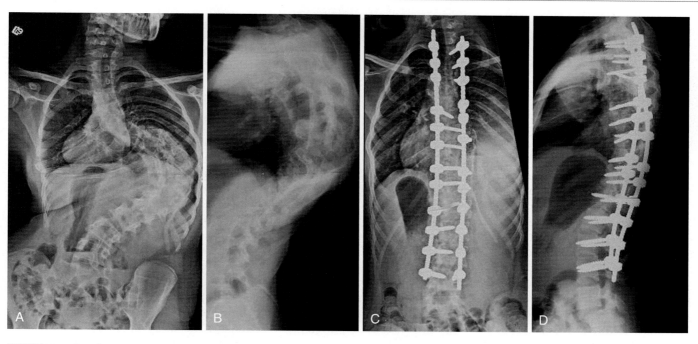

FIGURE 22–8 A and **B,** Severe congenital scoliosis measuring 120 degrees in a 15-year-old girl. **C** and **D,** The patient underwent posterior spinal fusion with instrumentation, right vertebral column resection, and multiple discectomies.

found a positive correlation with earlier surgery and curves greater than 50 degrees.[45]

- There is a risk of unwanted extension of the fusion (owing to difficult localization and short anomalies).

To avoid pseudarthrosis and to obtain greater intraoperative correction, posterior instrumentation can be used. The development of pediatric-sized instrumentation has limited the problem of implant prominence in young children; however, concern for potential neurologic injury persists. Although a more recent review reported no significant increase in neurologic injury,[46] careful intraoperative spinal cord monitoring and possibly an intraoperative wake-up test is recommended to avoid such complications. The surgeon also must carefully consider anatomy because anomalous pedicles and laminae do not always lend themselves well to fixation. Instrumentation becomes more feasible with increasing age, especially after 2 years of age.

Combined Anterior and Posterior Spine Fusion

Performing an anterior approach allows a surgeon to perform discectomy and remove vertebral endplates.[47] Better spine flexibility can be obtained, allowing for better deformity correction. Anterior bone graft is placed for fusion. This bone graft is most appropriate when the anomalous segment is lordotic.

Compared with posterior fusion only, combined anterior and posterior fusion decreases the risk of pseudarthrosis and crankshaft phenomenon and can be performed with posterior instrumentation. In some cases, anterior fusion may be performed by a posterior approach. This approach is most feasible at the thoracolumbar junction, where retropleural dissection may yield substantial exposure of the vertebral anomaly. An element of kyphosis accompanying the scoliosis also facilitates a posterior approach. An endoscopic approach to discectomy and epiphysiodesis has been shown to be an effective alternative. With an anterior approach, vascular anomalies to the cord in congenital scoliosis may confer a higher risk of ischemia after vessel ligation.

Convex Hemiepiphysiodesis

The principle of convex hemiepiphysiodesis is the same as that commonly employed for deformity of growing long bones. Convex hemiepiphysiodesis slows convex side growth while the concave curve still grows, allowing for safe progressive deformity correction. Prerequisites for this procedure include a patient young enough for significant corrective growth (<6 years old), the presence of less than seven involved vertebrae, and significant concave growth potential.[48] This technique requires a combined anterior and posterior exposure, followed by corrective rigid spinal immobilization for 6 months until fusion is complete. The anterior procedure consists of removal of the convex portion of discs and vertebral endplates and fusion of the convex portion with bone graft. A longitudinal rib inlay functions as an effective peripheral tether. The posterior exposure consists of unilateral removal of the facet joints and fusion. The correction is usually modest, on the order of 0 to 20 degrees by maturity. A single posterior approach with transpedicular convex anterior hemiepiphysiodesis has been reported; however, it seems less long-term correction is maintained.[49]

Instrumentation can be used to achieve concave posterior distraction[50] and convex posterior compression.[50,51] This technique allows a surgeon to obtain better intraoperative correction. Because this technique relies on remaining growth to achieve correction, it is most useful in children with intact spinal growth potential in whom involved vertebrae are limited.

Hemivertebra Excision

The operation for hemivertebra excision consists of combined anterior and posterior excision of the hemivertebra, followed by anterior and posterior fusion (Fig. 22–9). Anterior structural graft is useful on the concave side to maintain a normal sagittal contour. If the patient is old enough, instrumentation may be useful anteriorly and posteriorly to maintain good correction and to apply compression. Unless the construct is rigid, postoperative immobilization is usually necessary. Instrumentation may allow the patient to use a brace, however, instead of a cast.

Similar to convex hemiepiphysiodesis, hemivertebra excision can be performed via a single posterior approach.[52-57] This is becoming the most common approach for hemivertebra excision because of improved imaging and monitoring.

Osteotomies

In complex curves with multiple fusions, or previously fused curves, significant trunk imbalance may justify another corrective approach. In these situations, multiple anterior and posterior osteotomies or vertebral column resection allows spinal mobilization. A prerequisite is imaging of the entire spine to rule out anomalies in the canal. After performance of osteotomies, correction may be achieved at the same stage or after a period of corrective halo-gravity traction to correct the curve slowly.

Guided Growth Procedures

More recent concern regarding thoracic insufficiency syndrome in patients with congenital scoliosis, especially after early fusion with traditional growth-arresting surgical techniques, has led to the development of guided growth procedures using growing rods and VEPTR devices.[58] Growing rods allow for continued growth in spinal height before definitive fusion; this presumably optimizes the thoracic volume available for pulmonary development and function. Although complications associated with growing rod procedures are manageable, it is important to inform patients of the risks inherent to undergoing multiple surgical spinal procedures. In a study of early-onset scoliosis patients, dual growing rods lengthened at 6-month intervals were shown to achieve greater curve correction and allow for greater spinal growth compared with single growing rods lengthened after 15 to 20 degrees of curve progression.[59]

Expansion thoracoplasty using VEPTR aims to relieve a constricted concave hemithorax in patients with congenital scoliosis associated with fused ribs (Fig. 22–10).[60] When surgery is performed before 2 years of age, which coincides with the period of rapid lung growth, pulmonary function at 5-year follow-up is significantly better compared with children who undergo surgery at a later age.[61] Significant curve

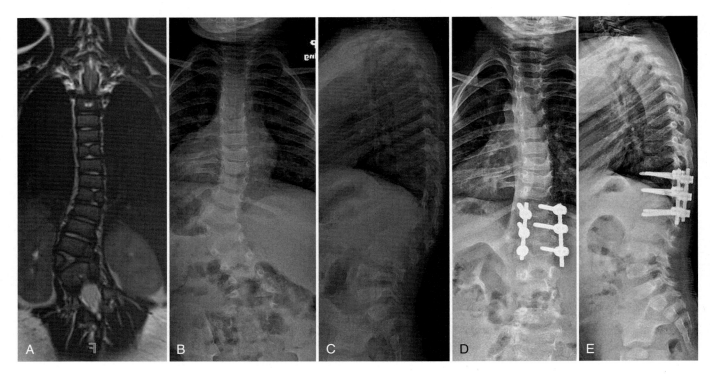

FIGURE 22–9 A-C, A 2-year-old boy with progressive kyphoscoliosis at level of L1 hemivertebra. **D** and **E,** The patient underwent hemivertebra resection and anterior and posterior spinal fusion with posterior spinal instrumentation. He was placed in a cast and maintained good correction postoperatively.

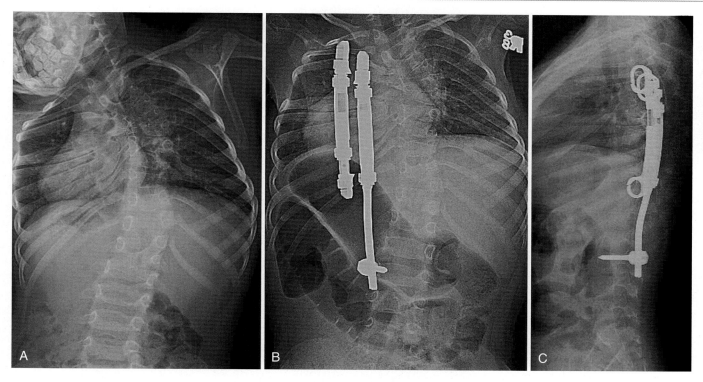

FIGURE 22–10 A, Severe chest deformity associated with congenital scoliosis and multiple rib fusions in a symptomatic 4-year-old child. **B** and **C,** The patient underwent multiple rib osteotomies with the use of VEPTR anchored from rib to rib and from rib to spine.

correction can also be indirectly achieved.[61] The use of VEPTR continues to evolve.

Indications

The problem in congenital scoliosis is usually not whether surgery is needed, but rather when and what kind of surgery is needed. In contrast to idiopathic scoliosis, for which a definitive fusion is delayed until near skeletal maturity, early deformity correction is generally desired to avoid structural spine decompensation[52] and to fuse the fewest vertebrae possible in congenital scoliosis. Patient height at maturity is not significantly diminished by early surgical intervention because in allowing a progressive curve to grow, the only growth that occurs is deformed growth (with increasing rotation and development of compensatory curves) and not vertical growth. Performing early corrective surgery, even with traditional growth-arresting procedures, ultimately allows the child to be taller and straighter.

Surgical means to achieve correction are varied, and their indications depend on many factors, such as the nature of the vertebral anomaly and its location, the curve size and its flexibility, and the child's age. Posterior fusion in situ is reserved for small curves with limited growth potential of the unfused anterior spine to avoid the crankshaft phenomenon. Lordosis in a region with congenital scoliosis is a contraindication to this approach because anterior growth would worsen lordosis. The main indication for a combined anterior and posterior fusion is a deformity with significant growth potential, such as a unilateral bar with a contralateral hemivertebra. This technique prevents bending of the posterior fusion mass.

Convex hemiepiphysiodesis is an appealing procedure to balance spinal growth. Prerequisites include the following:

- Six or fewer involved vertebrae
- Curve less than 70 degrees
- Age younger than 6 years because spinal growth is two thirds complete by this age
- Absence of pathologic congenital kyphosis or lordosis

Hemivertebra excision should be reserved for children with an unacceptable deformity, a fixed lateral translation of the trunk, and a hemivertebra located at the apex of the curve. The safest locations for this operation are the lumbar and lumbosacral spine.

Use of instrumentation depends on surgeon preference, but it is usually reserved for large curves in children older than 5 years, in whom obtaining and maintaining deformity correction with a plaster cast only would be difficult. Intraspinal anomalies should be considered contraindications because of the high risk of neurologic damage.

In a young patient with progressive deformity, growing rods should be considered as an alternative to long spinal fusion because the latter may adversely affect pulmonary function. VEPTR may play a role in deformity correction in patients with congenital scoliosis and concurrent rib fusions. Long-term outcome studies are needed for more informed surgical decision making regarding the use of guided growth procedures.

The treatment of congenital scoliosis is quite different from the treatment of idiopathic scoliosis. The surgeon must adapt to the great variations in every case because the type and time of surgery depend on various factors. Treatment must be based on the complete evaluation of the spine anomaly and knowledge of its potential for progression. Surgery is often indicated to avoid the development of permanent large curves at maturity.

KEY POINTS

1. Assessment of vertebral anomalies is best in early childhood.

2. Progressive deformation is due to imbalance in spine growth. Some vertebral anomalies do not lead to imbalance and are not likely to produce deformity.

3. Bracing has almost no effect on congenital spine curves.

4. Surgery should be performed as early as practical to prevent secondary structural changes.

5. All patients with congenital scoliosis should be evaluated for genitourinary anomalies. They should also undergo panspinal MRI if significant progression occurs or if surgery is indicated.

6. The first available film should be analyzed and used for subsequent comparisons.

7. The measurement error for congenital scoliosis is greater than idiopathic (approximately 10 degrees).

8. Neurologic risk of spine surgery is higher for congenital scoliosis than other types.

9. Congenital anomalies of the posterior elements do not often correlate with anomalies of the bodies and may require three-dimensional CT to previsualize.

10. The surgeon should be aware of midline laminar defects when using a posterior exposure.

KEY REFERENCES

1. Loder RT, Urquhart A, Steen H, et al: Variability in Cobb angle measurements in children with congenital scoliosis. J Bone Joint Surg Br 77:768-770, 1995.
   The measurement variation in congenital scoliosis was found to be 19 degrees in this study.

2. McMaster MJ, Ohtsuka K: The natural history of congenital scoliosis: A study of two hundred and fifty-one patients. J Bone Joint Surg Am 64:1128-1147, 1982.
   This article defined the progression risk and the differences between patterns of anomalies and levels of the spine.

3. Ruf M, Harms J: Hemivertebra resection by a posterior approach: Innovative operative technique and first results. Spine 27:1116-1123, 2002.
   This article revolutionized the treatment of hemivertebrae by showing the safety of a posterior approach.

4. Giampietro PF, Dunwoodie SL, Kusumi K, et al: Progress in the understanding of the genetic etiology of vertebral segmentation disorders in humans. Ann N Y Acad Sci 1151:38-67, 2009.
   This is an excellent review of advances in the understanding of the genetic and environmental factors that contribute to vertebral development.

5. Campbell RM Jr, Smith MD, Mayes TC, et al: The characteristics of thoracic insufficiency syndrome associated with fused ribs and congenital scoliosis. J Bone Joint Surg Am 85:399-408, 2003.
   This article characterizes thoracic insufficiency syndrome, which has led to the development of guided-growth procedures in the treatment of congenital scoliosis.

REFERENCES

1. Larsen WJ, Sherman LS, Potter SS, et al: The fourth week. In: Human Embryology, 3rd ed. New York, Churchill Livingstone, 2001, pp 79-112.

2. Sadler TW, Langman J: Skeletal system. In: Langman's Medical Embryology, 8th ed. Philadelphia, Lippincott Williams & Wilkins, 2000.

3. Dunwoodie SL: Mutation of the fucose-specific beta1,3 N-acetyl-glucosaminyltransferase LFNG results in abnormal formation of the spine. Biochim Biophys Acta 1792:100-111, 2009.

4. Dequeant ML, Pourquie O: Segmental patterning of the vertebrate embryonic axis. Nat Rev Genet 9:370-382, 2008.

5. Giampietro PF, Dunwoodie SL, Kusumi K, et al: Progress in the understanding of the genetic etiology of vertebral segmentation disorders in humans. Ann N Y Acad Sci 1151:38-67, 2009.

6. Bulman MP, Kusumi K, Frayling TM, et al: Mutations in the human delta homologue, DLL3, cause axial skeletal defects in spondylocostal dysostosis. Nat Genet 24:438-441, 2000.

7. Turnpenny PD, Alman B, Cornier AS, et al: Abnormal vertebral segmentation and the notch signaling pathway in man. Dev Dyn 236:1456-1474, 2007.

8. William DA, Saitta B, Gibson JD, et al: Identification of oscillatory genes in somitogenesis from functional genomic analysis of a human mesenchymal stem cell model. Dev Biol 305:172-186, 2007.

9. Aulehla A, Wehrle C, Brand-Saberi B, et al: Wnt3a plays a major role in the segmentation clock controlling somitogenesis. Dev Cell 4:395-406, 2003.

10. Winter RB, Moe JH, Eilers VE: Congenital scoliosis: A study of 234 patients treated and untreated. J Bone Joint Surg Am 50:1-47, 1968.

11. Jaskwich D, Ali RM, Patel TC, et al: Congenital scoliosis. Curr Opin Pediatr 12:61-66, 2000.

12. Jog S, Patole S, Whitehall J: Congenital scoliosis in a neonate: Can a neonatologist ignore it? Postgrad Med J 78:469-472, 2002.

13. Shahcheraghi GH, Hobbi MH: Patterns and progression in congenital scoliosis. J Pediatr Orthop 19:766-775, 1999.

14. Quan L, Smith DW: The VATER association: Vertebral defects, Anal atresia, T-E fistula with esophageal atresia, Radial and

Renal dysplasia. A spectrum of associated defects. J Pediatr 82:104-107, 1973.

15. Nora AH, Nora JJ: A syndrome of multiple congenital anomalies associated with teratogenic exposure. Arch Environ Health 30:17-21, 1975.

16. Chaumien JP, Rigault P, Maroteaux P, et al: [The so-called Klippel-Feil syndrome and its orthopaedic incidences]. Rev Chir Orthop Reparatrice Appar Mot 76:30-38, 1990.

17. Winter RB, Moe JH, Lonstein JE: The incidence of Klippel-Feil syndrome in patients with congenital scoliosis and kyphosis. Spine 9:363-366, 1984.

18. Fisher K, Esham RH, Thorneycroft I: Scoliosis associated with typical Mayer-Rokitansky-Küster-Hauser syndrome. South Med J 93:243-246, 2000.

19. Lapunzina P, Musante G, Pedraza A, et al: Semilobar holoprosencephaly, coronal craniosynostosis, and multiple congenital anomalies: A severe expression of the Genoa syndrome or a newly recognized syndrome? Am J Med Genet 102:258-260, 2001.

20. Larson AR, Josephson KD, Pauli RM, et al: Klippel-Feil anomaly with Sprengel anomaly, omovertebral bone, thumb abnormalities, and flexion-crease changes: Novel association or syndrome? Am J Med Genet 101:158-162, 2001.

21. Mooney JF 3rd, Emans JB: Progressive kyphosis and neurologic compromise complicating spondylothoracic dysplasia in infancy (Jarcho-Levin syndrome). Spine 20:1938-1942, 1995.

22. Purkiss SB, Driscoll B, Cole WG, et al: Idiopathic scoliosis in families of children with congenital scoliosis. Clin Orthop Relat Res (401):27-31, 2002.

23. Winter RB: Congenital scoliosis. Orthop Clin North Am 19:395-408, 1988.

24. Wynne-Davies R: Congenital vertebral anomalies: Aetiology and relationship to spina bifida cystica. J Med Genet 12:280-288, 1975.

25. Giampietro PF, Raggio CL, Blank RD: Synteny-defined candidate genes for congenital and idiopathic scoliosis. Am J Med Genet 83:164-177, 1999.

26. Farley FA, Loder RT, Nolan BT, et al: Mouse model for thoracic congenital scoliosis. J Pediatr Orthop 21:537-540, 2001.

27. Imaizumi K, Masuno M, Ishii T, et al: Congenital scoliosis (hemivertebra) associated with de novo balanced reciprocal translocation, 46,XX,t(13;17)(q34;p11.2). Am J Med Genet 73:244-246, 1997.

28. McKinley LM, Leatherman KD: Idiopathic and congenital scoliosis in twins. Spine 3:227-229, 1978.

29. Ogden JA, Southwick WO: Congenital and infantile scoliosis in triplets. Clin Orthop Relat Res (136):176-178, 1978.

30. Pool RD: Congenital scoliosis in monozygotic twins: Genetically determined or acquired in utero? J Bone Joint Surg Br 68:194-196, 1986.

31. Goshu E, Jin H, Fasnacht R, et al: Sim2 mutants have developmental defects not overlapping with those of Sim1 mutants. Mol Cell Biol 22:4147-4157, 2002.

32. Schwetz BA, Smith FA, Leong BK, et al: Teratogenic potential of inhaled carbon monoxide in mice and rabbits. Teratology 19:385-392, 1979.

33. McMaster MJ, Ohtsuka K: The natural history of congenital scoliosis: A study of two hundred and fifty-one patients. J Bone Joint Surg Am 64:1128-1147, 1982.

34. Campbell RM Jr, Smith MD, Mayes TC, et al: The characteristics of thoracic insufficiency syndrome associated with fused ribs and congenital scoliosis. J Bone Joint Surg Am 85:399-408, 2003.

35. Karol LA, Johnston C, Mladenov K, et al: Pulmonary function following early thoracic fusion in non-neuromuscular scoliosis. J Bone Joint Surg Am 90:1272-1281, 2008.

36. Cobb JR: Outline for the study of scoliosis. Edwards JW, trans. Instructional Course Lecture Vol 5. Ann Arbor, MI, American Academy of Orthopaedic Surgeons, 1948, pp 261-275.

37. Facanha-Filho FA, Winter RB, Lonstein JE, et al: Measurement accuracy in congenital scoliosis. J Bone Joint Surg Am 83:42-45, 2001.

38. Loder RT, Urquhart A, Steen H, et al: Variability in Cobb angle measurements in children with congenital scoliosis. J Bone Joint Surg Br 77:768-770, 1995.

39. Newton PO, Hahn GW, Fricka KB, et al: Utility of three-dimensional and multiplanar reformatted computed tomography for evaluation of pediatric congenital spine abnormalities. Spine 27:844-850, 2002.

40. Blake NS, Lynch AS, Dowling FE: Spinal cord abnormalities in congenital scoliosis. Ann Radiol (Paris) 29(3-4):377-379, 1986.

41. Bradford DS, Heithoff KB, Cohen M: Intraspinal abnormalities and congenital spine deformities: A radiographic and MRI study. J Pediatr Orthop 11:36-41, 1991.

42. Prahinski JR, Polly DW Jr, McHale KA, et al: Occult intraspinal anomalies in congenital scoliosis. J Pediatr Orthop 20:59-63, 2000.

43. Suh SW, Sarwark JF, Vora A, et al: Evaluating congenital spine deformities for intraspinal anomalies with magnetic resonance imaging. J Pediatr Orthop 21:525-531, 2001.

44. Riccio AI, Guille JT, Grissom L, et al: Magnetic resonance imaging of renal abnormalities in patients with congenital osseous anomalies of the spine. J Bone Joint Surg Am 89:2456-2459, 2007.

45. Kesling KL, Lonstein JE, Denis F, et al: The crankshaft phenomenon after posterior spinal arthrodesis for congenital scoliosis: A review of 54 patients. Spine 28:267-271, 2003.

46. Hedequist DJ, Hall JE, Emans JB: The safety and efficacy of spinal instrumentation in children with congenital spine deformities. Spine 29:2081-2086; discussion 2087, 2004.

47. McMaster MJ, Singh H: The surgical management of congenital kyphosis and kyphoscoliosis. Spine 26:2146-2154; discussion 2155, 2001.

48. Winter RB, Lonstein JE, Denis F, et al: Convex growth arrest for progressive congenital scoliosis due to hemivertebrae. J Pediatr Orthop 8:633-638, 1988.

49. Keller PM, Lindseth RE, DeRosa GP: Progressive congenital scoliosis treatment using a transpedicular anterior and posterior convex hemiepiphysiodesis and hemiarthrodesis: A preliminary report. Spine 19:1933-1939, 1994.

50. Shono Y, Abumi K, Kaneda K: One-stage posterior hemivertebra resection and correction using segmental posterior instrumentation. Spine 26:752-757, 2001.

51. Cheung KM, Zhang JG, Lu DS, et al: Ten-year follow-up study of lower thoracic hemivertebrae treated by convex fusion and concave distraction. Spine 27:748-753, 2002.

52. Klemme WR, Polly DW Jr, Orchowski JR: Hemivertebral excision for congenital scoliosis in very young children. J Pediatr Orthop 21:761-764, 2001.

53. Lazar RD, Hall JE: Simultaneous anterior and posterior hemivertebra excision. Clin Orthop Relat Res (364):76-84, 1999.

54. Nakamura H, Matsuda H, Konishi S, et al: Single-stage excision of hemivertebrae via the posterior approach alone for congenital spine deformity: Follow-up period longer than ten years. Spine 27:110-115, 2002.

55. Ruf M, Harms J: Hemivertebra resection by a posterior approach: Innovative operative technique and first results. Spine 27:1116-1123, 2002.

56. Ruf M, Harms J: Posterior hemivertebra resection with transpedicular instrumentation: Early correction in children aged 1 to 6 years. Spine 28:2132-2138, 2003.

57. Suk SI, Chung ER, Kim JH, et al: Posterior vertebral column resection for severe rigid scoliosis. Spine 30:1682-1687, 2005.

58. Vitale MG, Matsumoto H, Bye MR, et al: A retrospective cohort study of pulmonary function, radiographic measures, and quality of life in children with congenital scoliosis: An evaluation of patient outcomes after early spinal fusion. Spine 33:1242-1249, 2008.

59. Thompson GH, Akbarnia BA, Campbell RM Jr: Growing rod techniques in early-onset scoliosis. J Pediatr Orthop 27:354-361, 2007.

60. Campbell RM Jr, Smith MD, Hell-Vocke AK: Expansion thoracoplasty: The surgical technique of opening-wedge thoracostomy. Surgical technique. J Bone Joint Surg Am 86(Suppl 1):51-64, 2004.

61. Campbell RM Jr, Smith MD, Mayes TC, et al: The effect of opening wedge thoracostomy on thoracic insufficiency syndrome associated with fused ribs and congenital scoliosis. J Bone Joint Surg Am 86:1659-1674, 2004.

23
CHAPTER

Idiopathic Scoliosis

Fernando E. Silva, MD
Ronald A. Lehman Jr., MD
Lawrence G. Lenke, MD

Idiopathic scoliosis is the most common cause of spinal deformity; 80% of all scoliosis cases are due to idiopathic scoliosis. Before arriving at the diagnosis of idiopathic scoliosis in a patient, other causes, such as congenital, neuromuscular (developmental or acquired), functional, inflammatory or infectious, pathologic, and intraspinal, have to be discounted. Ponseti and Friedman[1] first described early-onset scoliosis in 1950. Dickson[2] expounded further on that concept and proposed that idiopathic scoliosis be divided into early (0 to 5 years old) and late onset (>5 years old), based on spinal growth velocity noted in these two age groups. Presently, idiopathic scoliosis is divided into three categories based on chronologic age: infantile (birth to 2 years + 11 months), juvenile (3 years to 9 years + 11 months), and adolescent (10 years to 17 years + 11 months).[3] The radiographic diagnosis necessitates measuring the coronal plane angle, using the Cobb method, as equal to or greater than 10 degrees. Patients with curves less than 10 degrees are considered to have spinal asymmetry.[4,5]

Epidemiology

Infantile and juvenile scoliosis are less prevalent than adolescent idiopathic scoliosis. Infantile idiopathic scoliosis is more common in Europe, constituting less than 1% of idiopathic scoliosis cases in the United States, and tends to comprise left-sided thoracic curves, typically occurring in boys. More recent reviews suggest that there might be a decline in its incidence.[6] Juvenile cases are typically diagnosed at age 7 years in girls and 5 years in boys and account for about 10% to 20% of idiopathic scoliosis cases.[3] In contrast to infantile idiopathic scoliosis, juvenile cases tend to occur predominantly in girls and tend to comprise right-sided curves. Between the ages of 3 and 6 years, there seems to be a similar distribution between boys and girls, however, again becoming predominant in girls after age 6 years.

Adolescent idiopathic scoliosis is more prevalent than other types of idiopathic scoliosis. Among adolescents, the prevalence of 10-degree curves is less than 3%, with about 5% of curves showing progression of greater than 30 degrees.[4]

This prevalence decreases as a function of curve magnitude, however, to about 0.3% to 0.5% and 0.1% in curves measuring 20 degrees and 40 degrees.[7] The prevalence of curves greater than 10 degrees is higher among girls, with a 4:1 ratio of girls to boys.[8]

Etiology

Infantile scoliosis occurs roughly in 1 of 10,000 births. Possible causes are thought to occur from intrauterine molding or postnatal pressure on the spinal column from supine positioning while sleeping. Other etiologic factors that have been considered in idiopathic scoliosis include dysfunction in proprioception to maldevelopment in central pattern generators in the spinal cord[9-11] and connective tissue, hormonal, and muscle structural changes.[12] More recent reports in the literature strongly suggest a genetic link. The growth spurt noted among adolescents seems to play a role in progression, as a critical buckling load is reached on the existing curve as the spine grows. In a review of the literature, Kouwenhoven and Castelein[13] concluded many factors may play a role in the initiation and progression of adolescent idiopathic scoliosis at a certain age. The literature suggests, however, that in the observed deformation of the spine, genetics and the unique mechanics of the fully erect posture, which is exclusive to humans, play an important role.

Genetics

The genetics of idiopathic scoliosis seem to be similar in all idiopathic groups. The incidence rate is 11% among first-degree relatives, 2.4% among second-degree relatives, and 1.4% among third-degree relatives.[14] Concordance among monozygotic and dizygotic twins has been reported to range from 73% to 92% and 36% to 63%.[15,16] In 2007, Anderson and colleagues[17] published a population-based study taken from the Danish Twin Registry in which 46,418 twins were registered. From the 34,944 respondents, the concordance rate for monozygotic twins was 13% versus 0% for dizygotic twins. In 2007, Gao and colleagues[18] published a report providing evidence of linkage and association with 8q12 loci. Through further investigation, they discovered the first gene (*CHD7*) associated with a susceptibility to idiopathic scoliosis. In 2008, Kulkarni and colleagues[19] mapped a developmentally critical *CHD* gene to 15q26.1 and when taken together with *CHD7*, this suggested a possible role for *CHD2* in the embryonic development of the spine. More recently in 2009, Gurnett and colleagues[20] published a report of a single multi-generational family in which adolescent idiopathic scoliosis and pectus excavatum segregated as an autosomal dominant condition. Through linkage analysis, the investigators identified a genetic locus for the two conditions on chromosome 18q. Although genetic mapping for idiopathic scoliosis is still in its infancy, great strides are being made to help clinicians better understand the etiology and prevalence of this condition.

Natural History

About 90% of infantile curves show spontaneous resolution, especially among infants who are younger than 1 year when idiopathic scoliosis is diagnosed.[6,21] The curves that typically progress are double curves with a thoracic component. Insight into the curves that can progress can be obtained from the rib-vertebral angle difference (RVAD) and "phase of the rib head."[22] In terms of phase of the rib head, if the head and neck of the convex rib of the vertebral body at the apex of the curve does not overlap the vertebral body, it is termed *phase I*; if it does overlap, it is termed *phase II*. In terms of the latter, curves with RVAD greater than 20 degrees or phase II angles are very likely to progress. Phase II angles are almost certain to progress; RVAD calculation is unnecessary when a curve is noted to be phase II type. Juvenile curves less than 25 degrees also can spontaneously resolve. These curves tend to progress, however, if they are discovered before age 6 years and idiopathic scoliosis is diagnosed or if they are greater than 30 degrees. About 70% of juvenile curve types tend to progress. The RVAD has not proved to be useful as a predictor of curve progression.

Many factors are considered in the natural history of adolescent idiopathic scoliosis. Growth potential, skeletal maturity, curve magnitude, and curve location are important considerations when assessing progression of adolescent idiopathic scoliosis. Although family history, gender, and rotation do not seem to have an effect on progression, growth potential seems to have a significant effect. Peak height growth seems to correlate best with, and is a better predictor of, progression than skeletal maturity. In terms of biomechanics, this likely is secondary to attaining vertebral column height, which leads to a critical buckling load and greater bending moments with eventual curve progression. In girls, peak height growth seems to occur 6 to 12 months before the onset of menarche. In boys, peak height growth seems to correlate with the closure of triradiate cartilages. Larger or double curves tend to progress more than single curves. Additionally, curves can progress after skeletal maturity; thoracic curves greater than 50 degrees and thoracolumbar/lumbar curves greater than 30 degrees can progress on average 1 degree per year.[23,24]

Evaluation

History and Physical Examination

A complete history and physical examination is completed, and any family history of scoliosis is noted. With infantile and juvenile cases in particular, a thorough prenatal and birth and developmental history is obtained. In adolescent cases, growth spurt history, if any at the time of presentation, is noted. This information is imperative in determining peak growth velocity and its implications on curve progression. Symptoms of pain or weakness and how the patient perceives his or her appearance relative to the deformity are especially important with adolescent idiopathic scoliosis.[25] Age at onset of menarche and voice changes in boys are noted as well because they are likely predictors of growth potential and possible curve progression.

During the examination, height, weight, and age (years plus months since last birthday) are recorded. The head is examined with special attention to torticollis and plagiocephaly because the latter has been associated with higher incidence in infantile scoliosis. Possible conditions and anomalies that might be present are buccal and palatal anomalies; café au lait spots; and midline dimples or hair patches or both over the lumbodorsal spine, which can be important clinical clues that an intraspinal pathologic process might be present. Limb laxity is also checked, and genetic counseling and testing is requested when laxity is present.

Trunk shift is evaluated with the patient standing and the hips and knees fully extended. The relationship of the patient's head to the pelvis is also noted in evaluating the overall coronal and sagittal balance. Any shoulder, breast, or pelvic asymmetry is noted.[26] Curve rotation is assessed by performing an Adams forward-bend test and is quantified with a scoliometer. This assessment is modified in infants by laying the patient on the examiner's knee. This test also helps assess the rigidity of the curve, which is an important factor in terms of prognostication. Leg-length discrepancy and pelvic obliquity are evaluated. Alternatively, a sitting forward test can be performed. The latter maneuver can also help rule out plagiocephaly and developmental hip dysplasia, especially in infants. When leg-length discrepancy is the likely cause of the deformity, a shoe lift is used to reevaluate the patient to determine if the curve corrects.

A thorough neurologic examination is performed. The neurologic examination includes all cranial nerves; motor strength; reflexes (including abdominal reflexes), often associated with Chiari malformations; sensory modalities; and gait.[27] Finally, other possible causes of scoliosis, such as congenital, neuromuscular, and syndromic types, must be ruled out. Infection, neoplasms, and spondylolisthesis also must be discounted.

Radiographic Evaluation

Posteroanterior and lateral 36- × 14-inch long cassette views including bending films—with appropriately placed bolsters—for further curve classification and planning bracing or surgical intervention are obtained, and the Cobb angles are measured.[5] Curves greater than 20 degrees in infants and children, neurologic symptoms in all patients with idiopathic scoliosis, and left-sided, sharp angular or irregular curve patterns require further investigation, including screening total spine magnetic resonance imaging (MRI).[28,29] When anomalies of the nervous system are present on MRI, a neurosurgical consultation is indicated.

Classification Systems

There is no formal curve classification system for infantile or juvenile scoliosis. The first treatment-based adolescent idiopathic scoliosis classification was developed in 1983 by King and colleagues.[30] They reported on a series of 405 patients with adolescent idiopathic scoliosis, developing a uniplanar system based on thoracic curves and analyzing only the coronal plane. This system allowed for surgical planning and helped in assessing whether or not a King II curve could be selectively fused.[31] Interobserver and intraobserver reliability of this

traditional thoracic classification system is fair at best, however.[32,33] Additionally, coronal decompensation has been reported after selective fusions.

Lenke and colleagues[34] developed a comprehensive, practical two-dimensional classification system in 2001, which included the sagittal plane as well (Fig. 23–1). The Lenke curve classification includes not only thoracic curves, but also thoracolumbar/lumbar curve patterns. Additionally, this classification allows the surgeon to assess curves in coronal and sagittal planes, and it has been proven reliable in terms of interobserver and intraobserver reliability.[32,33] Its definition of the structural characteristics of a proximal thoracic curve has been deemed reliable, leading to shorter proximal fusions when this curve pattern is nonstructural.[35] The Lenke classification allows a stricter structural curve evaluation, permitting a more objective analysis of when a given curve would tolerate a selective fusion leading to a balanced outcome.[36,37] The latter is clinically significant because one of the most important principles in preventing postoperative decompensation is proper identification of curve patterns, including curves that tolerate selective fusion.[31,38] This three-tiered classification

THE LENKE CLASSIFICATION SYSTEM FOR AIS

Curve type	Proximal thoracic	Main thoracic	Thoracolumbar/lumbar	Description
1	Nonstructural	Structural*	Nonstructural	Main thoracic (MT)
2	Structural†	Structural*	Nonstructural	Double thoracic (DT)
3	Nonstructural	Structural*	Structural†	Double major (DM)
4	Structural†	Structural§	Structural§	Triple major (TM)
5	Nonstructural	Nonstructural	Structural*	Thoracolumbar/lumbar (TL/L)
6	Nonstructural	Structural†	Structural*	Thoracolumbar/lumbar-main thoracic (TL/L-MT)

*Major curve: largest Cobb measurment, always structural; †Minor curve: remaining structural curves; §Type 4 - MT or TL/L can be the major curve

STRUCTURAL CRITERIA (Minor curves)		LOCATION OF APEX (SRS definition)	
Proximal thoracic	– Side bending Cobb ≥25° – T2–T5 Kyphosis ≥+20°	CURVE	APEX
Main thoracic	– Side bending Cobb ≥25° – T10–L2 Kyphosis ≥+20°	Thoracic	T2 to T11/12 disc
Thoracolumbar/lumbar	– Side bending Cobb ≥25° – T10–L2 Kyphosis ≥+20°	Thoracolumbar Lumbar	T12/L1 L1/2 disc to L4

MODIFIERS

Lumbar coronal modifier	Center sacral vertical line to lumbar apex
A	Between pedicles
B	Touches apical body(ies)
C	Completely medial

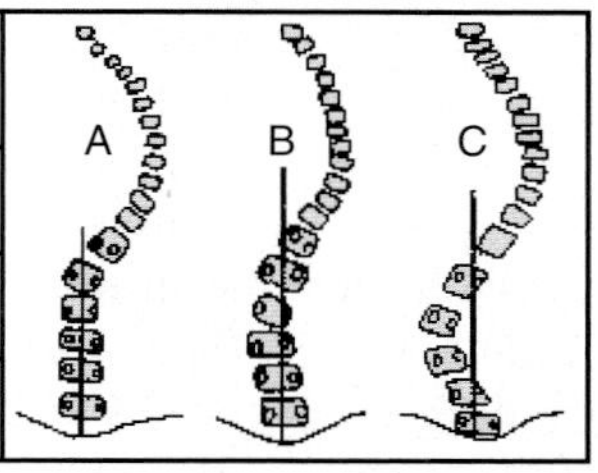

Thoracic sagittal profile T5-T12	
Modifier	Cobb angle
– (Hypo)	<10°
N (Normal)	10°–40°
+ (Hyper)	>40°

Curve type (1–6) + Lumbar coronal modifier (A. B, C) + Thoracic sagittal modifier (–, N, +) = Curve classification (e.g. 1B+): _____

FIGURE 23–1 Lenke adolescent idiopathic scoliosis (AIS) classification system.

combines a curve type (1 through 6) and coronal lumbar and sagittal thoracic modifiers to produce a triad comprehensive curve classification (e.g., 1A−).

More recently, the addition of a lower end vertebra (LEV) modifier has been proposed for the Lenke classification. The LEV of the lowest structural curve was found to be a highly reliable vertebral landmark, and comparison of the LEV with a selected lowest instrumented vertebra (LIV) is an important consideration in the overall evaluation of the surgical treatment of adolescent idiopathic scoliosis.[39] A more detailed postoperative assessment of the distal fusion length is theoretically allowed by comparing the LIV with the LEV. Such a modifier aids in a more thorough evaluation of the Lenke curve classification (e.g., 5CN-L3 when L3 is the LEV of the curve being classified).

Three-Dimensional Classification

Although the Lenke classification system has criteria in the coronal and the sagittal planes that have an impact classification, it still has shortcomings because scoliosis is a known three-dimensional deformity, and the axial or transverse plane is not a component of this system. A task force of the Scoliosis Research Society has been charged with developing a clinically useful three-dimensional analysis and ultimate classification of scoliosis.[40] The key factor in this assessment would be the plane and maximal curvature, which is the three-dimensional deformity that occurs as the spine translates and rotates out of the normal sagittal profile in scoliosis deformities. It is expected that in the next decade much more information will be provided so that three-dimensional analysis and classification will become a standard for all practitioners.

Nonoperative Treatment Options and Indications

Three fundamental treatment options exist for idiopathic scoliosis: observation, bracing and casting, and surgery. These treatment modalities are based on the natural history of idiopathic scoliosis or the potential or probability of curve progression.[4,41] Many modalities have been proposed to slow or halt curve progression, such as electrical stimulation and physical therapy; however, none of these modalities have been scientifically proven to be a viable alternative in the treatment of scoliosis.[42,43]

Observation

Most infantile curves are left-sided; these curves have been known to resolve spontaneously up to 90% of the time, but they can progress.[41] Deciphering which curves will progress can be guided by the RVAD and the relationship of the apical rib head to the vertebral body (i.e., phase I or II).[22] Typically, curves less than 20 degrees are expectantly followed every 6 to 8 months. Infants with curves less than 25 degrees and RVAD less than 20 degrees and children with curves less than 25 degrees should be followed clinically and radiographically

every 6 months. Treatment is instituted for curves greater than 25 degrees. Treatment is also started for a progression of 5 degrees or greater in two consecutive visits or 10 degrees or greater in one follow-up visit. Juvenile curves more often require operative intervention, however.

Bracing and Casting

Bracing[44] is the nonoperative treatment of choice in small but progressive scoliosis in growing children and teens. In about 75% of cases, bracing can control the curve and avoid progression, rendering the curve small enough so that the risk of progression after growth is unlikely.[42] In a younger child, whose growth potential remains a significant issue, bracing allows for continued growth until the patient requires eventual operative treatment because of curve progression. With infantile cases, molded casting followed by bracing used to be the mainstay in nonoperative management. Bracing and casting of these patients comes with potential consequences, however, that include pulmonary restriction, which can have future ramifications.[45,46] Sanders and colleagues[47] found serial casting to be beneficial in the treatment of infantile scoliosis. They reported that curves less than 60 degrees often fully corrected in infants if casting was started before age 20 months.

Adolescents with curves less than 20 degrees at presentation are observed and followed at 4-month and 6-month intervals. For curves between 20 degrees and 30 degrees, bracing is started if a curve progresses 5 degrees or more in two consecutive visits or 10 degrees or more in one visit.

Bracing is usually started the first office visit when the patient is skeletally immature (Risser ≤2) and presents with a 25- to 40-degree curve. Several brace options exist, and deciding which brace to use depends on the apex of the curve and physician preference. Curves with an apex above T6 would likely require the use of a Milwaukee (cervicothoracolumbosacral orthosis) brace.[48] Conversely, curves with apices at T7 or below and above L2 do well in a Boston underarm thoracolumbosacral orthosis brace, and these braces are more socially acceptable because of the lack of a cervical extension. The Charleston bending brace is an option if the child is noncompliant to brace-wear. This brace is typically worn at night, and some studies have shown its efficacy.[49,50] The efficacy of a brace seems to depend on the length of time the brace is worn.[51] When bracing is initiated and pad placement is deemed appropriate, patient follow-up occurs every 4 to 6 months, with in-brace radiographic evaluation and appropriate fitting adjustments made when necessary.

Modifications to the standard thoracolumbosacral orthosis include variations of the Chêneau brace (Jacques Chêneau, Münster, Germany) and the SpineCor dynamic brace (SpineCorporation, Chesterfield, UK). The Chêneau 2000 orthosis allows for a greater amount of initial correction by using a hypercorrected mold and pads, which provide derotational forces.[52] This brace is the first that uses the theory of expansion to allow for active correction by respiratory movements.[53] The SpineCor[54] and TriAC (Boston Brace International, Avon, MA) are nonrigid braces. They work by using straps, which correspond to a specific correcting movement depending on the curve pattern, producing a progressive positional change, dynamic curve correction, and appropriate muscle balance.

Operative Intervention

Operative intervention is usually recommended for patients whose curves progress despite nonoperative management.[54] In infants, operative intervention is controversial; it is occasionally performed in infants with curves greater than 45 degrees or thoracolumbar/lumbar curves greater than 40 degrees. Children are typically more prone to curve progression and are more likely to require operative intervention. Other patients who are likely to benefit from operative intervention are skeletally immature patients with adolescent idiopathic scoliosis with a greater than 40- to 45-degree curve and mature patients with curves greater than 50 degrees.[23,55]

Surgical Techniques

Currently, anterior-only, posterior-only, and circumferential procedures are the mainstay of surgical treatment options.[57] The prevalence of anterior-only and circumferential procedures has declined with a concomitant increase in posterior-only procedures. Surgeons have become aware more recently that early intervention with a definitive anteroposterior fusion for progressive infantile and juvenile curves leads to loss of trunk height development, which can lead to chest wall and lung underdevelopment.[58,59] This problem has promoted innovative techniques to try to control progressive curves surgically without definitive fusion, which include epiphysiodesis,[60,61] growing rod placement (Figs. 23–2 and 23–3),[62] intervertebral stapling (Fig. 23–4),[86] spinal tethering (Fig. 23–5),[66] and the vertical expandable prosthetic titanium rib[67]; the last-mentioned is used more in progressive early-onset scoliosis in which rib and chest wall deformities can be quite severe.[64]

Many surgeons today still prefer to perform an anterior approach in younger patients when there is risk of crankshaft development and especially for thoracolumbar and lumbar major curves (Lenke type 5). With the introduction of pedicle screws, a posterior approach has shown numerous benefits over an anterior procedure, such as better maintenance of the obtained correction, providing more powerful corrective forces, three-column control, and obviating the need for anterior releases and thoracoplasties.[68-74] In addition, a posterior approach avoids the negative consequences of chest cage disruption and pulmonary compromise that can result from an open anterior approach (Fig. 23–6).[75-77] In addition, the thoracic aorta is at risk if an anteriorly placed screw penetrates the vertebral cortex on the opposite side.[78,79]

According to Tis and colleagues,[80] with advances in anterior instrumentation, surgeons theoretically should see a reduction in the rate of rod breakage, pseudarthrosis, and sagittal decompensation and improved correction rates. These authors concluded that open anterior spinal fusion surgery is a safe method for the treatment of thoracic adolescent idiopathic scoliosis. At 5-year follow-up, they reported good coronal and sagittal correction of the main thoracic and compensatory thoracolumbar/lumbar curves, but they also reported that pulmonary function was mildly decreased as with any procedure in which a thoracotomy is performed. Tis and colleagues[80] also concluded that in skeletally immature patients, an open anterior spinal fusion can increase kyphosis; however, newer techniques used in their series seemed to limit progressive kyphosis, which has been noted in previously published reports.

Adolescent curves can typically be surgically treated via an anterior or posterior approach (or both) with instrumentation and fusion.[77] Anterior fusion levels typically extend from end-to-end vertebrae, as measured with the Cobb technique. Short fusions above and below the apex, depending on whether the apex is a disc or a vertebra, have been advocated for flexible thoracolumbar curves.[81] In this technique, if the apex is a

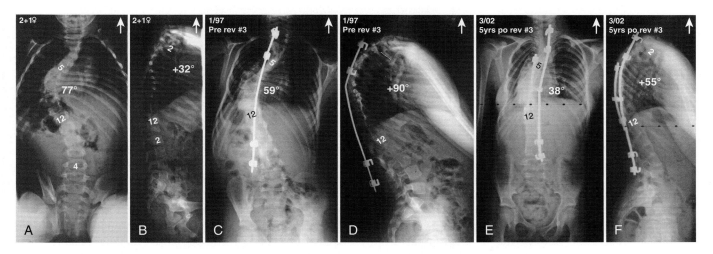

FIGURE 23–2 A and **B,** A girl age 2 years + 1 month who presented with 77-degree left thoracic infantile idiopathic scoliosis. **C** and **D,** She was treated with a posterior single hook growing rod with only partial correction of her deformity and increasing sagittal kyphosis. **E** and **F,** Ultimately, she underwent posterior spinal fusion ending up with overall acceptable coronal and sagittal balance 5 years after fusion.

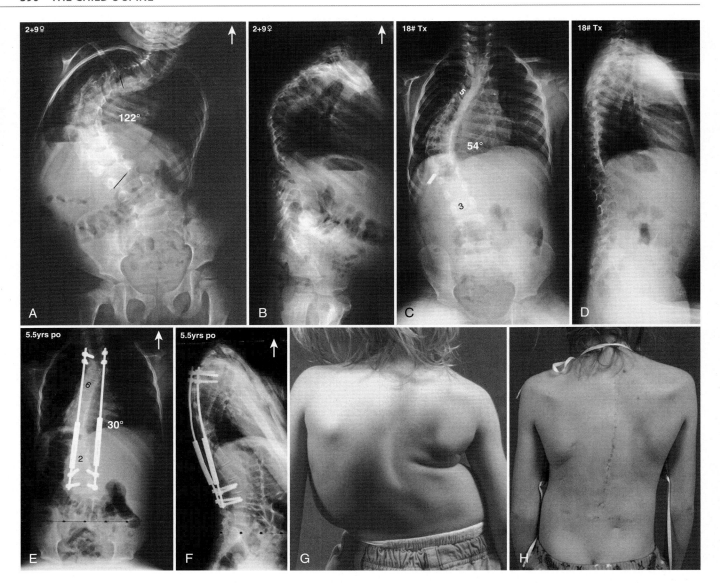

FIGURE 23–3 A and **B,** A girl age 2 years + 9 months who presented with severe infantile-onset idiopathic scoliosis. Her left thoracic curve measured 122 degrees. **C** and **D,** She was placed in halo-gravity traction, and underwent a short apical anterior release and fusion and was prepared for a growing rod construct. **E** and **F,** She had a dual rod, pedicle screw growing rod construct placed, and at 5 years + 6 months after initiation of growing rod construct, she continues to be lengthened with overall good coronal and sagittal balance and acceptable lung fields produced via this treatment. **G** and **H,** Clinical photographs of preoperative and latest lengthening show maintenance of trunk alignment and growth.

vertebral body, the discs above and below the apex are included in the fusion. If the apex is a disc, the two discs above and below the apex are included in the fusion. Brodner[82] predicted fusion levels based on the supine-pull ("stretch") films, ensuring a thorough release is performed to obtain a "bone-on-bone" fusion. Anterior structural grafts have been used to counter the kyphogenesis associated with anterior instrumentation.[77]

Thoracoscopic procedures have been shown to provide advantages over open anterior thoracotomy procedures.[81] Kishan and colleagues[85] showed that anterior thoracoscopy had fewer adverse affects on pulmonary function. Sucato and colleagues[86] found that adding a thoracoscopic release performed in the prone position to a posterior instrumentation

and fusion offered the advantages of minimally invasive surgery and did not require repositioning to perform the posterior procedure. In addition, when double-lung ventilation is used, acute pulmonary complications are significantly reduced. A steep learning curve is required, however, and these techniques have diminished in popularity owing to the proliferation of pedicle screw constructs.

Determining proximal and distal fusion levels is paramount in preventing decompensation because choosing the incorrect levels is the main reason for postoperative decompensation.[26,87] *Adding-on* is another phenomenon that can result if a fusion is stopped "short." Suk and colleagues[88] reported 5-year results of 203 patients in which they found that adding-on occurred in 17 patients who

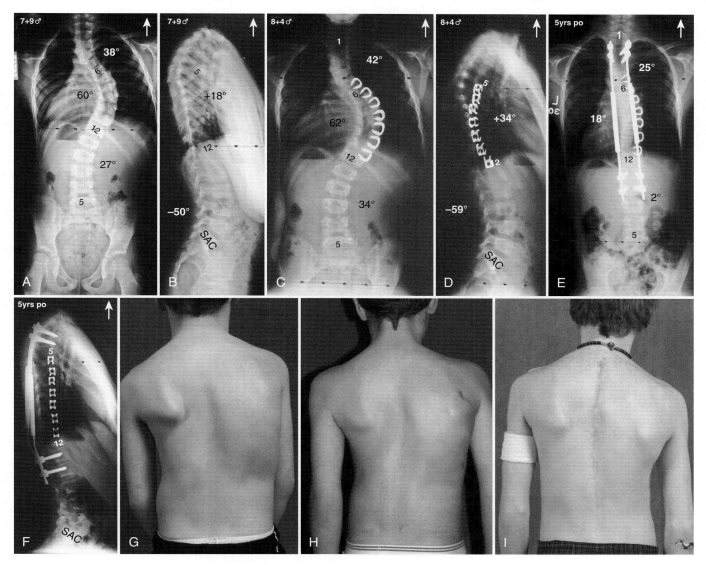

FIGURE 23–4 A and **B,** A boy age 7 years + 9 months who presented with progressive juvenile-onset right thoracic idiopathic scoliosis. His main thoracic curve measured 60 degrees and was progressive despite bracing. **C** and **D,** He had anterior thoracic stapling performed with slow progression of deformity with growth. **E** and **F,** A posterior dual screw-rod growing construct was placed, and 5 years after insertion, his deformity correction has been maintained to 18 degrees of the main thoracic curve with good sagittal profile. **G-I,** Clinical photographs before surgery, status post stapling, and 5 years status post growing rod construct show improvement of truncal deformation.

were fused on average two levels short of the neutral vertebra.

Distal fusion levels are based on the understanding and determination of the end, neutral, and stable vertebrae of the distal structural curve that is to be included in the fusion.[89] Current correction techniques employing pedicular fixation and derotation maneuvers allow for preservation of distal fusion levels, however. When fusing to a vertebra cephalad to the stable vertebra, the intended LIV must touch the central sacral vertical line (CSVL), not have a significant rotation (Nash-Moe grade ≤1.5), and the disc below this proximal vertebra must be parallel or closed on the convexity. In placing thoracic screws, it is essential to follow sequential steps at every screw placement.[68,69] With small pedicles, time should be taken to expand the pedicle to accommodate a screw.[90] Although the authors advocate the use of pedicle screws

whenever possible, when employing hook and rod segmental instrumentation, it is imperative to reverse hook orientation where the discs are reversed in orientation to maintain coronal and sagittal balance.[91] Based on the lumbar modifier, attention must also be paid to the degree of tilt left on the LIV when carrying out selective fusions.

A rough estimate of the degree of tilt to be left on the LIV is equal to the remaining tilt on a preoperative supine film, with judicious use of intraoperative radiographs. This tilt can be assessed on intraoperative full-length radiographs[92]; this is imperative in allowing accommodation of the structural component of the lumbar curves, especially with selective fusions.[37] The lower endplate of the LIV should be horizontal for type A lumbar modifier curves, a mild tilt should be left on type B curves, and an appropriate degree of tilt should be left on the LIV for type C curves. Clinical assessment of the deformity

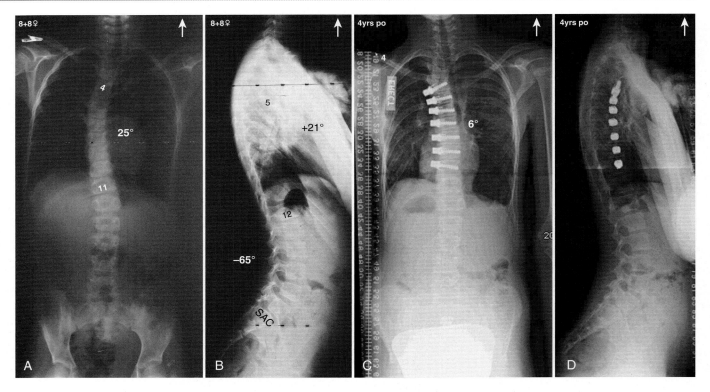

FIGURE 23–5 A and **B,** A girl age 8 years + 8 months who presented with progressive left thoracic scoliosis. She had a positive family history of scoliosis with her mother requiring scoliosis fusion as a child. Her left thoracic curve progressed to 25 degrees with normal sagittal profile. **C** and **D,** She was treated with a single left thoracic mobile tether, with slow progressive correction of her deformity to 6 degrees with a normal sagittal profile 4 years after treatment. She had only one surgery and did not wear a brace postoperatively.

cannot be overemphasized because it plays as important a role as the radiographic findings when deciding whether to perform a selective fusion.

Selective Fusions

A selective fusion is performed when one or more curves present are not included in the fusion. Strictly speaking, the term *selective fusion* is reserved for untreated minor thoracic or lumbar curves that cross the midline. Situations arise when one considers fusing nonstructural, secondary curves for the sake of cosmesis or spinal balance or both.

The Lenke classification system allows a more objective way to decide when to perform selective fusions in patients with adolescent idiopathic scoliosis, especially with type C curve patterns.[37,88] The Lenke system has stricter criteria that define the structural characteristics of individual curves, leading to an objective analysis when choosing which curves can be selectively fused without ensuing clinical imbalance.[33] Radiographic parameters aid in objective analysis of the structural nature of each curve *relative* to the other, such that if parameters match, both curves usually require surgical attention.[54,93] Relative Cobb angle measurements and apical vertebral rotation and apical vertebral translation ratios of the thoracic and thoracolumbar/lumbar curves are important in such analysis and decision processes.[38,39]

Skeletal immaturity and clinical appearance are additional important factors.[31,33,87] The magnitude of the rib and lumbar prominences is important during the clinical analysis and decision making for selective fusion (e.g., is the patient willing to accept a moderate lumbar hump when contemplating a selective thoracic fusion and vice versa). *One cannot overlook the thoracolumbar sagittal profile* because this can lead to curve misclassification and incorrect operative management. As previously noted, based on the lumbar modifier, attention must be paid to the degree of tilt left on the LIV when carrying out selective thoracic fusions, allowing accommodation of the structural lumbar curve (Fig. 23–7).

Selective anterior fusions of major thoracolumbar/lumbar curves associated with minor and partially structural thoracic curves in Lenke 5C and 6C curves can occasionally be considered, provided that the thoracic curve is less than 50 degrees, the thoracic curve bends out to 20 degrees or less, the thoracolumbar/lumbar-to-thoracic Cobb ratio is 1.25 or greater, and the triradiate cartilages are closed.[36] Additionally, such selective fusions should not be undertaken when shoulder depression ipsilateral to the thoracolumbar/lumbar curve exists, the patient is highly skeletally immature, or a clinically unacceptable rib hump is present. To prevent decompensation, if the lumbar curve bends out less than the thoracic curve, the lumbar curve should not be overcorrected because the thoracic curve likely would not compensate to achieve postoperative balance.[87] One study showed an average spon-

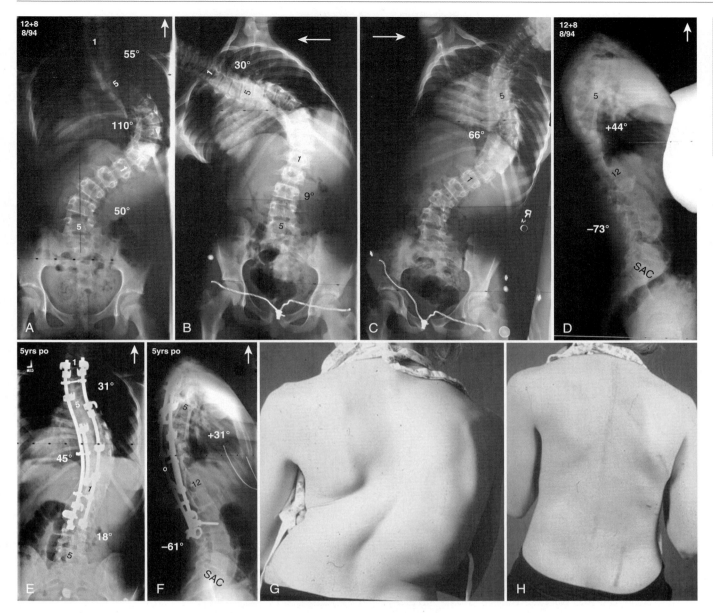

FIGURE 23–6 A-D, A girl age 12 years + 8 months with severe right thoracic adolescent idiopathic scoliosis deformity. Her curve progressed to 110 degrees bending to 66 degrees with overall 44 degrees of thoracic kyphosis—a 4A+ classification. **E** and **F,** She underwent open anterior release and primary posterior hook construct from T2-L3. At 6 years postoperatively, adequate coronal and sagittal alignment and balance is shown. **G** and **H,** Preoperative and postoperative clinical photographs show improved truncal correction with right thoracotomy, posterior midline and iliac crest scars visible.

taneous correction of 14 degrees or 36% improvement of the thoracic curve when selective thoracic fusion was performed.[37]

Adjuncts to Correction

Direct Vertebral Rotation

In the past, curves greater than 75 degrees, curves with less than 50 degrees of correction, and curves needing a thoracoplasty have required anterior releases. With the use of modern techniques of multisegmental pedicle screw fixation and the

addition of DVR techniques, safe and effective procedures demonstrating greater coronal and sagittal realignment along with acceptable cosmesis without the need for an anterior procedure have been reported.[94-96] In the thoracic region, the DVR helps derotate the spine and significantly decreases the rib prominence (Fig. 23–8). Care must be taken to use stiffer rods, prebent in the sagittal profile to prevent inducing hypokyphosis in the thoracic spine. It also helps to obtain better three-dimensional correction in the thoracolumbar/lumbar component of Lenke double major curves and to minimize the LIV tilt/horizontal angle.[94]

A DVR is performed if screw placement is adequate, if the thoracic spine is not overly lordotic or kyphotic, and when

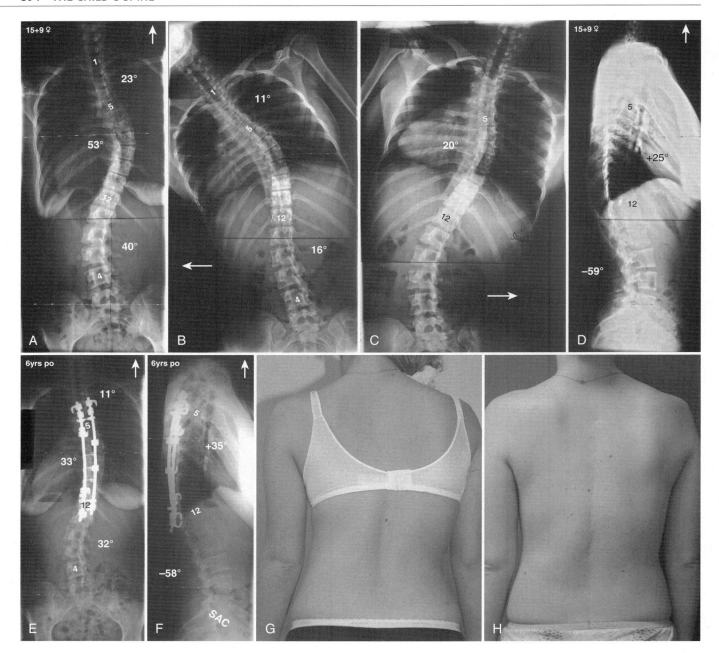

FIGURE 23–7 A-D, A girl age 15 years + 9 months with progressive right thoracic decompensatory left lumbar scoliosis. Her main thoracic curve progressed to 53 degrees, and her nonstructural lumbar curve of 40 degrees side bended to 16 degrees. She had a normal sagittal profile—a 1CN classification. **E** and **F,** She underwent posterior selective thoracic fusion with a hook-rod, Wisconsin wire construct. At 6 years postoperatively, she has near-perfect spinal balance with matched 33-degree thoracic, 32-degree lumbar coronal plane deformities and normal sagittal profile. **G** and **H,** Preoperative and postoperative clinical photographs show improved coronal truncal alignment and balance.

there is a clinically significant thoracic or lumbar prominence. The DVR technique necessitates accurate placement of pedicle screws at the apex of the deformity and the two levels at the proximal and distal extent of the fusion. When the thoracic spine has a (+) sagittal modifier, according to the Lenke classification, a DVR maneuver is not performed because such degrees of kyphosis place considerable strain on the proximal screws. In these patients, the coronal and sagittal deformity is addressed simultaneously by "convex rod" instrumentation first.

Osteotomies

Several osteotomy choices are available to correct sagittal, coronal, and multiplanar deformities associated with previously fused or more severe idiopathic scoliosis curves, including Ponté osteotomy (or Smith-Petersen osteotomy), pedicle subtraction osteotomy, and vertebral column resection. A Smith-Petersen osteotomy is classically described when performing an osteotomy through a fusion mass, whereas the authors describe here an osteotomy of this type in an unfused

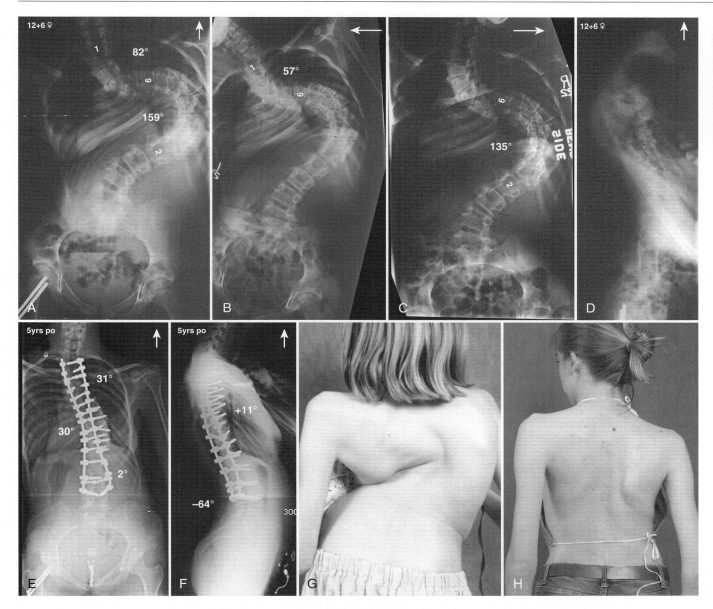

FIGURE 23–8 A-D, A girl age 12 years + 6 months with a severe progressive right thoracic scoliosis. Her curve progressed to 159 degrees bending to only 135 degrees. **E-G,** She underwent posterior single-level vertebrectomy and pedicle screw construct with marked correction of her coronal plane deformity at 5 years postoperatively. **H** and **I,** Preoperative and postoperative clinical photographs show her posterior midline scar.

spine as a Ponté osteotomy, which was the original description of a posteriorly based chevron osteotomy through previously unfused anatomy.

Sagittal imbalance can generally be divided into two types.[97] In type I, the patient is in global positive balance owing to compensating for loss of segmental lordosis or kyphosis. In type II, loss of segmental lordosis or kyphosis is not compensated, leading to global imbalance. When scoliosis is associated with type I, multiple Ponté osteotomies can be performed at the site of maximal loss of segmental kyphosis. Mobility of the anterior column is required. In revision cases, these can be done asymmetrically with the widest portion of the osteotomy at the convexity or at the site of a previous fusion mass. The surgeon must pay attention when performing these osteotomies because the patient can be pitched into the concavity, possibly creating global coronal imbalance.[98] Type II sagittal

imbalance is best managed by the use of pedicle subtraction osteotomy because longer lever arms and greater degrees of correction are often warranted, especially with sharp angular deformities. Anterior column mobility is not required, however, because one pivots the correction anterior to the osteotomy site.

Similar to sagittal imbalance, coronal imbalance can be classified as type A or B. In type A, the shoulders and pelvis are tilted in the opposite direction, whereas in type B, they tilt in the same direction.[97] Typically, single-plane deformities—type A—can be addressed with a single pedicle subtraction osteotomy; additionally, multiple or asymmetrical pedicle subtraction osteotomies can be used when dealing with stiff or kyphoscoliotic cases. Simple trigonometric calculations at the vertebral body where the osteotomy is going to be performed permit precise determination of the angle of bony resection required for global balance.[99] Type B deformities likely require vertebral column resections.

Vertebral column resections can be performed via a combined anterior and posterior approach (i.e., circumferentially) or from a posterior-only approach (Fig. 23–9).[100] Compromised pulmonary function lends consideration, however, to performing a posterior-only approach. The surgeon must balance the potential pulmonary compromise of the patient with the understanding that the extracavitary approach (i.e., posterior-only) requires a higher level of surgical understanding and is technically more demanding.[101,102] As with all things, adherence to safety is the most important principle, and if the surgeon is uncomfortable with a particular approach or technique, a referral should be made. This correction modality is appropriate in the setting of congenital cases, multiplanar or kyphoscoliotic stiff curves, curves previously fused circumferentially, and cases of global imbalance. In the last-mentioned situation, attention must be paid to the shoulders and pelvic tilt direction.

Minimally Invasive Techniques

Minimally invasive spine surgery is a popular concept that uses imaging, retraction, and implant technologies to help surgeons locate the exact area on which they are to operate. This type of procedure is done through incisions of less than 1 inch long; damage to surrounding muscles and other tissues is avoided,

which rapidly increases the healing and reduces recovery time. It also uses technology to perform the surgery more efficiently. One example is a video-assisted thoracoscopic procedure. According to Newton and colleagues,[81] this procedure can be used for an anterior thoracic release or to achieve deformity correction via rod-screw constructs. Because of the small incisions made and the muscle-splitting technique used, a reduction in chest wall disruption and subsequent lung volume decrease, as is the case with an open thoracotomy approach, was noted. This procedure offers comparable curve correction and a faster return to presurgical function.[84-86]

With advances in instrumentation as mentioned previously and the enhanced ability to perform a direct vertebral derotation with posterior pedicle screw constructs, the use of video-assisted thoracoscopic instrumentation procedures has declined substantially. The decision between an anterior and a posterior approach is based purely on surgeon preference at this point.

Postoperative Care

Patients are observed in the intensive care unit overnight. Sitting and standing with assistance is permitted, and physical therapy is started on the 1st postoperative day for patients undergoing a posterior-only procedure. When stable, patients are transferred to the regular floor. As bowel function returns

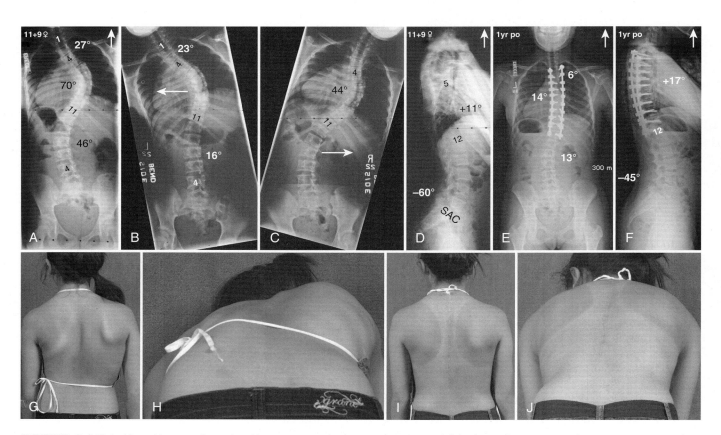

FIGURE 23–9 A-D, A girl age 11 years + 9 months with progressive right thoracic compensatory left lumbar scoliosis. Her main thoracic curve progressed to 70 degrees, and her compensatory 46-degree curve side bended to 16 degrees—a 1CN classification. **E** and **F,** She underwent selective thoracic fusion with a pedicle screw construct with nicely matched 14-degree thoracic and 13-degree lumbar scoliotic curves at 1 year postoperatively with adequate sagittal balance. **G-J,** Preoperative and postoperative clinical photographs show improved truncal correction.

and patients are able to tolerate clear fluids, routine intravenous narcotics are replaced with oral narcotics as needed. Typically, no postoperative bracing is used. When patients are ambulatory, the urinary catheter is removed. On postoperative day 3, the drains are discontinued along with prophylactic antibiotics. After discharge, usually postoperative day 4 or 5, patients resume showering at approximately 2 weeks postoperatively.

Complications

Complications can occur during any of the treatment stages—preoperative, intraoperative, or postoperative.[103] During the preoperative period, inappropriate curve classification and inadequate surgical planning can lead to inappropriate surgical decisions. It is essential to ensure that when performing a selective fusion, appropriate structural curve criteria are met.[87] Choosing inappropriate fusion levels can also be included in the category of preoperative complications, which is discussed later.

Intraoperative complications most commonly result from technical errors, including instrumentation misplacement. Hooks that do not hug the lamina or misplaced pedicle screws can lead to devastating complications including spinal cord deficit. Overcorrection of curves and, conversely, inadequate releases, leading to an unbalanced spine, account for other types of intraoperative complications. Inappropriate decortication, inadequate bone graft material, and the use of bulky crosslinks can result in a higher rate of pseudarthrosis.

Intraoperative neurophysiologic monitoring with somatosensory evoked potentials and motor evoked potentials helps alert the surgeon to any impending intraoperative spinal cord neurologic deficit.[104] These deficits typically occur from spinal cord distraction, from overcorrection, from vascular compromise, or, rarely, directly from instrumentation. If the somatosensory evoked potentials and motor evoked potentials decline past warning criteria, the surgeon should implement a course of action that includes ensuring that the irrigation being used is of adequate temperature, keeping adequate mean arterial blood pressure elevated at a minimum greater than 80 to 90 mm Hg, and reversing instrumentation or spinal correction to the prewarning criteria state. Appropriate-dosed steroid boluses are also considered in accordance with the National Acute Spinal Cord Injury Study (NASCIS) III protocol if motor evoked potentials do not return to baseline within a reasonable time. A wake-up test should also be performed to assess true upper and lower neurologic function. In addition to adhering to the proven sequential technique of free hand screw placement, pedicle screw stimulation provides an added safety measure.[68,69] Judicious use of intraoperative imaging can also be employed, especially with significant deformities.

Postoperative complications can arise from delayed consequences of technical errors, neurovascular compromise, medical comorbidities, and wound infections. Although perioperative antibiotics are commonly used, when wound infections do occur, they generally are treated aggressively with wound irrigation and débridement. Instrumentation well seated on the spine is always left in place; however, the decision to remove or maintain the bone graft is defined by the individual case and surgeon preference. In addition, removal of instrumentation can lead to loss of curve correction and decompensation.[105] Additionally, at final closure, heat-stable, powder antibiotics can be placed inside the wound (deep and superficial to the fascia), and long-term parenteral antibiotics are provided based on the results of intraoperative wound cultures and sensitivities. With delayed or late infections, the instrumentation is initially removed and later replaced because the deformity can progress as the fusion mass is subject to repeated bending forces.[105,106] Also, the fusion mass is inspected further, and any pseudarthrosis noted is repaired at the reinstrumentation stage.

Summary

Understanding and treatment of spinal deformities have broadened; however, idiopathic scoliosis remains a diagnosis of exclusion. With advances in genetic mapping of idiopathic scoliosis, better understanding of the etiology and incidence of the disease is likely in the near future. It is hoped that this better understanding will bring earlier identification, an improved understanding of curve progression risk, and treatment of the condition without the need for major surgery of severe curves. Technologic advances, including the advent of pedicle screw instrumentation and osteotomy techniques, have significantly improved spinal surgeons' ability to treat more rigid curves, while obtaining better correction and maintaining safety.

Possible treatment modalities include close observation, bracing, and surgical intervention. The Lenke classification of adolescent idiopathic scoliosis allows for the identification of appropriate fusion levels and choice of selective fusions, which are imperative for optimal surgical management. Although all curves can be approached posteriorly, one can employ an anterior approach in selected Lenke 1 curve patterns, Lenke 6CN curves, and most Lenke 5CN curves. Selective fusions should be performed whenever possible, and critical curve analysis should be performed preoperatively with all available objective modalities. Direct vertebral rotation offers improved thoracic correction and a decreased need for thoracoplasty. Complex decompensated, large, rigid curves and curves previously fused may require osteotomies to achieve the desired correction. Some pitfalls of scoliosis surgery, such as decompensation and adding-on of a fused curve, can be avoided when these principles are applied.

One must be mindful of the lessons of the past in understanding the assessment and management of spinal deformity. Spinal surgeons constantly must strive for improvements in surgical technique. These improvements can include less invasive approaches, while not forgetting the basic principles of curve selection and fusion techniques. The ultimate goal should be correction of the curve without fusion allowing for continued spinal motion. Safety for patients must be key. This is achieved by appropriate training, careful patient selection, and adherence to the principles of deformity surgery.

The authors would like to acknowledge Jennifer Roth for her assistance in the preparation of this chapter.

PEARLS AND PITFALLS

1. Bracing of the juvenile idiopathic or skeletally immature adolescent idiopathic patient is still a viable option for those with curves between 25° and 45°. Brace compliance, the fit of the orthosis, and the number of hours of brace-wear per day are critical components to success, along with the genetic predisposition towards curve progression.

2. It is important to determine the flexibility of the spinal deformity. Therefore preoperative radiographic assessment should include not only upright radiographs, but also side-bending, supine, push-prone, traction (if applicable), and hyperextension (for hyperkyphosis) radiographs, alone or in combination.

3. Proper classification of AIS curves preoperatively will aid in the regions of the spine to be fused. One must remember to include the thoracolumbar sagittal profile in preoperative planning to prevent misclassification and incorrect surgical management.

4. It is critical to examine shoulder symmetry clinically and radiographically when selecting proximal fusion levels in idiopathic scoliosis patients to obtain optimal shoulder balance after surgery.

5. Distal fusion levels are determined by the relationship among the end, neutral, and stable vertebrae of the distal structural curve to be fused, along with the position of those vertebrae to the CVSL (center sacral vertical line). Most commonly, the distal fusion level will be one level above stable, as long as that level is fairly neutral and the vertebra is at least "touched" by the CSVL on the upright coronal film.

6. Anterior approaches for spinal deformity have diminished in popularity over the last decade. Disadvantages such as chest cage disruption including suboptimal pulmonary function, risk of implants abutting against the major vessels, and the ability to treat only a single curve at a time have limited these approaches over time.

7. The use of posterior instrumentation and fusion with or without various forms of spinal osteotomies has become the mainstay for the surgical management of pediatric and adult idiopathic scoliosis deformities. With the posterior approach, all curve patterns can be managed by surgeons who are familiar with this classic midline posterior approach.

8. Surgical outcomes are based on radiographic parameters and clinical assessment such as scoliometer measurements and shoulder height, as well as questionnaires reported by patients, such as the SRS-30.

9. The use of segmental pedicle screw fixation for the posterior treatment of pediatric and adult idiopathic scoliosis curves has become the primary instrumentation construct. In addition, thorough bone grafting with a combination of autogenous bone, allograft bone, and/or the use of osteobiologics, especially in the adult population, has become routine at many centers throughout North America.

10. Optimal surgical outcomes in the treatment of adult idiopathic scoliosis deformities include proper patient selection, exacting surgical technique, and a well balanced spinal alignment with minimal to no complications.

KEY POINTS

1. Patient evaluation skills and highly specialized technical skills are essential for the scoliosis surgeon.

2. Anterior approaches are possible, but all curves can be addressed posteriorly.

3. Selective fusions should always be considered when appropriate.

4. Adjuncts to posterior correction possibly can help obviate more extensive approaches.

5. Avoidance and treatment of complications in the preoperative, intraoperative, and postoperative periods is important.

6. Some form of spinal cord monitoring is mandatory for all scoliosis corrective procedures.

KEY REFERENCES

1. Lenke LG, Betz RR, Bridwell KH, et al: Intraobserver and interobserver reliability of the classification of thoracic adolescent idiopathic scoliosis. J Bone Joint Surg Am 80:1097-1106, 1998.
   This study showed poor to fair reliability of the King classification of adolescent idiopathic scoliosis, questioning its usefulness as an accurate system.

2. Lenke LG, Betz RR, Harms J, et al: Adolescent idiopathic scoliosis: A new classification to determine extent of spinal arthrodesis. J Bone Joint Surg Am 83:1169-1181, 2001.
   This new two-dimensional treatment-based adolescent idiopathic scoliosis classification system was found to have good to excellent reliability and allows classification of all adolescent idiopathic scoliosis curves.

3. Lenke LG, Betz RR, Clements D, et al: Curve prevalence of a new classification of operative adolescent idiopathic scoliosis: Does classification correlate with treatment? Spine (Phila Pa 1976) 27:604-611, 2002.
   Of 606 consecutive adolescent idiopathic scoliosis cases classified by the Lenke et al system, type 1 main thoracic curves were the most common type (51%), and 90% of curves were fused as predicted by the system.

4. Sanders AE, Baumann R, Brown H, et al: Selective anterior fusion of thoracolumbar/lumbar curves in adolescents: When can the associated thoracic curve be left unfused? Spine (Phila Pa 1976) 28:706-713, 2003.
   Of 49 patients with adolescent idiopathic scoliosis who underwent an anterior selective thoracic fusion, 43 had satisfactory results based on the preoperative thoracolumbar/lumbar-to-thoracic ratio of 1.25 or greater.

5. Edwards CC 2nd, Lenke LG, Peelle M, et al: Selective thoracic fusion for adolescent idiopathic scoliosis with C modifier lumbar curves: 2- to 16- year radiographic and clinical results. Spine (Phila Pa 1976) 29:536-546, 2004.
   Satisfactory results were achieved with selective thoracic fusion of properly selected C modifier lumbar curves with undercorrection of the instrumented thoracic curve (36%) to match the spontaneous correction of the lumbar curve (34%).

REFERENCES

1. Ponseti IV, Friedman B: Prognosis in idiopathic scoliosis. J Bone Joint Surg Am 32:381-395, 1950.

2. Dickson RA: Conservative treatment for idiopathic scoliosis. J Bone Joint Surg Br 67:176-181, 1985.

3. James JI: Idiopathic scoliosis: The prognosis, diagnosis, and operative indications related to curve patterns and the age at onset. J Bone Joint Surg Br 36:36-49, 1954.

4. Bunnell WP: The natural history of idiopathic scoliosis before skeletal maturity. Spine (Phila Pa 1976) 11:773-776, 1986.

5. Cobb JR: Outline for the study of scoliosis. Instr Course Lect 5:261-275, 1948.

6. Fernandes P, Weinstein SL: Natural history of early onset scoliosis. J Bone Joint Surg Am 89(suppl 1):21-33, 2007.

7. Kane WJ, Moe JH: A scoliosis-prevalence survey in Minnesota. Clin Orthop Relat Res 69:216-218, 1970.

8. Pring ME, Wenger DR: Adolescent deformity. In Bono CM, Garfin SR (eds): Spine Orthopedic Surgery Essentials. Philadelphia, Lippincott Williams & Wilkins, 2004, pp 163-164.

9. Moreau A, Wang DS, Forget S, et al: Melatonin signaling dysfunction in adolescent idiopathic scoliosis. Spine (Phila Pa 1976) 29:1772-1781, 2004.

10. Azeddine B, Letellier K, Wang da S, et al: Molecular determinants of melatonin signaling dysfunction in adolescent idiopathic scoliosis. Clin Orthop Relat Res 462:45-52, 2007.

11. Yamamoto H: A postural dysequilibrium as an etiological factor in idiopathic scoliosis [abstract O]. In Programs and Abstracts of the 17th Annual Meeting of the Scoliosis Research Society, Denver, 1982, p 52.

12. Machida M, Dubousset J, Imamura Y, et al: An experimental study in chickens for the pathogenesis of idiopathic scoliosis. Spine (Phila Pa 1976) 18:1609-1615, 1993.

13. Kouwenhoven JW, Castelein RM: The pathogenesis of adolescent idiopathic scoliosis: Review of the literature. Spine (Phila Pa 1976) 33:2989-2998, 2008.

14. Risser JC, Norquist DM, Cockrell BR Jr, et al: The effect of posterior spine fusion on the growing spine. Clin Orthop Relat Res 46:127-139, 1966.

15. Carr AJ: Adolescent idiopathic scoliosis in identical twins. J Bone Join Surg Br 72:1077, 1990.

16. Kesling LK, Reinker KA: Scoliosis in twins: A meta-analysis of the literature and report of six cases. Spine (Phila Pa 1976) 22:2009-2014, 1997.

17. Anderson MO, Thomsen K, Kyvik KO: Adolescent idiopathic scoliosis in twins: A population-based survey. Spine (Phila Pa 1976) 32:927-930, 2007.

18. Gao X, Gordon D, Zhang D, et al: CHD7 gene polymorphisms are associated with susceptibility to idiopathic scoliosis. Am J Hum Genet 80:957-965, 2007.

19. Kulkarni S, Nagarajan P, Wall J, et al: Disruption of chromodomain helicase DNA binding protein 2 (CHD2) causes scoliosis. Am J Med Genet 146A:1117-1127, 2008.

20. Gurnett CA, Alaee F, Bowcock A, et al: Genetic linkage localizes an adolescent idiopathic scoliosis and pectus excavatum gene to 18q. Spine (Phila Pa 1976) 34:E94-E100, 2009.

21. Diedrich O, von Strempel A, Scholz M, et al: Long-term observation and management of resolving infantile idiopathic scoliosis: A 25-year follow-up. J Bone Joint Surg Br 84:1030-1035, 2002.

22. Mehta MH: The rib-vertebra angle in the early diagnosis between resolving and progressive infantile scoliosis. J Bone Joint Surg Br 54:230-243, 1972.

23. Weinstein SL, Ponseti IV: Curve progression in idiopathic scoliosis. J Bone Joint Surg Am 65:447-455, 1983.

24. Weinstein SL, Zavala DC, Ponseti IV: Idiopathic scoliosis: Long-term follow-up and prognosis in untreated patients. J Bone Joint Surg Am 63:702-712, 1981.

25. Lonstein JE: Patient evaluation. In Bradford DS, Lonstein JE, Moe JH, et al (eds): Moe's Textbook of Scoliosis and Other Spinal Deformities, 2nd ed. Philadelphia, WB Saunders, 1987, pp 47-88.

26. Li M, Gu S, Ni J, et al: Shoulder balance after surgery in patients with Lenke Type 2 scoliosis corrected with the segmental pedicle screw technique. J Neurosurg Spine 10:214-219, 2009.

27. Muhonen MG, Menezes AH, Sawin PD, et al: Scoliosis in pediatric Chiari malformations without myelodysplasia. J Neurosurg 77: 69-77, 1992.

28. Dobbs MB, Lenke LG, Szymanski DA, et al: Prevalence of neural axis abnormalities in patients with infantile scoliosis. J Bone Joint Surg Am 84:2230-2234, 2002.

29. Gupta P, Lenke LG, Bridwell KH: Incidence of neural axis abnormalities in infantile and juvenile patients with spinal deformity: Is a magnetic resonance image screening necessary? Spine (Phila Pa 1976) 23:206-210, 1998.

30. King HA, Moe JH, Bradford DS, et al: The selection of fusion levels in thoracic idiopathic scoliosis. J Bone Joint Surg Am 65:1302-1313, 1983.

31. Lenke LG, Bridwell KH, Baldus C, et al: Preventing decompensation in King Type II curves treated with Cotrel-Dubousset instrumentation: Strict guidelines for selective thoracic fusion. Spine (Phila Pa 1976) 17:274S-281S, 1992.

32. Schroeder TM, Blanke KM, Vaughan V, et al: Validation of radiographic software to determine Lenke classification [abstract 54]. In Programs and Abstracts of the 40th Annual Meeting of the Scoliosis Research Society, Miami, 2005, p 93.

33. Lenke LG, Betz RR, Bridwell KH, et al: Intraobserver and interobserver reliability of the classification of thoracic adolescent idiopathic scoliosis. J Bone Joint Surg Am 80:1097-1106, 1998.

34. Lenke LG, Betz RR, Harms J, et al: Adolescent idiopathic scoliosis: A new classification to determine extent of spinal arthrodesis. J Bone Joint Surg Am 83:1169-1181, 2001.

35. Cil A, Pekmezci M, Yazici M, et al: The validity of Lenke's criteria for defining structural proximal thoracic curves in patients with adolescent idiopathic scoliosis [abstract 74]. In Programs and Abstracts of the 40th Annual Meeting of the Scoliosis Research Society, Miami, 2005, p 120.

36. Sanders AE, Baumann R, Brown H, et al: Selective anterior fusion of thoracolumbar/lumbar curves in adolescents: When can the associated thoracic curve be left unfused? Spine (Phila Pa 1976) 28:706-713, 2003.

37. Edwards CC 2nd, Lenke LG, Peelle M, et al: Selective thoracic fusion for adolescent idiopathic scoliosis with C modifier lumbar curves: 2- to 16- year radiographic and clinical results. Spine (Phila Pa 1976) 29:536-546, 2004.

38. Lenke LG, Bridwell KH: Achieving coronal balance using Cotrel-Dubousset instrumentation (C-D.I.). In 8th Proceeding

of the International Congress on Cotrel-Dubousset Instrumentation. Montpellier, Sauramps Medical, 1991, pp 27-32.

39. Lenke LG, Kuklo TR, Sucato DJ, et al: Comparison of the lower-end vertebra (LEV) to the lowest instrumented vertebra (LIV) in adolescent idiopathic scoliosis: A role for the addition of an LEV modifier to the Lenke Classification System [abstract 131]. In Programs and Abstracts of the 13th International Meeting on Advanced Spine Techniques (IMAST), Athens, 2006, p 121.

40. Sangole A, Aubin CE, Labelle H, et al: The central hip vertical axis (CHVA): A reference axis for the Scoliosis Research Society three-dimensional classification of idiopathic scoliosis. Spine (Phila Pa 1976) 35:E530-E534, 2010.

41. Weinstein SL: Idiopathic scoliosis: Natural history. Spine (Phila Pa 1976) 11:780-783, 1986.

42. Nachemson AL, Peterson LE: Effectiveness of treatment with a brace in girls who have adolescent idiopathic scoliosis: A prospective, controlled study based on data from the Brace Study of the Scoliosis Research Society. J Bone Joint Surg Am 77:815-822, 1995.

43. Stone B, Beekman C, Hall V, et al: The effect of an exercise program on change in curve in adolescents with minimal idiopathic scoliosis: A preliminary study. Phys Ther 59:759-763, 1979.

44. Fayssoux RS, Cho RH, Herman MJ: A history of bracing for idiopathic scoliosis in North America. Clin Orthop Relat Res 468:654-664, 2010.

45. Kennedy JD, Robertson CF, Olinsky A, et al: Pulmonary restrictive effect of bracing in mild idiopathic scoliosis. Thorax 42:959-961, 1987.

46. Katsaris G, Loukos A, Valavanis J, et al: The immediate effect of a Boston brace on lung volumes and pulmonary compliance in mild adolescent idiopathic scoliosis. Eur Spine J 8:2-7, 1999.

47. Sanders JO, D'Astous J, Fitzgerald M, et al: Derotational casting for progressive infantile scoliosis. J Pediatr Orthop 29:581-587, 2009.

48. Blount WP, Schmidt AC, Keever ED, et al: The Milwaukee brace in the operative treatment of scoliosis. J Bone Joint Surg Am 40:511-525, 1958.

49. Trivedi JM, Thomson JD: Results of Charleston bracing in skeletally immature patients with idiopathic scoliosis. J Pediatr Orthop 21:277-280, 2001.

50. Clin J, Aubin CE, Parent S, et al: A biomechanical study of the Charleston brace for the treatment of scoliosis. Spine (Phila Pa 1976) 35:E940-E947, 2010.

51. Price CT, Scott DS, Reed FR Jr, et al: Nighttime bracing for adolescent idiopathic scoliosis with the Charleston bending brace: Long-term follow-up. J Pediatr Orthop 17:703-707, 1997.

52. Kotwicki T, Chêneau J: Biomechanical action of a correction brace of thoracic idiopathic scoliosis: Chêneau 2000 orthosis. Disabil Rehabil Assist Technol 3:146-153, 2008.

53. Rigo M, Negrini S, Weiss H, et al: SOSORT consensus paper on brace action: TLSO biomechanics of correction (investigating the rationale for force vector selection). Scoliosis 1:11, 2006.

54. Szwed A, Kolban M, Jaloszewski M: Results of SpineCor dynamic bracing for idiopathic scoliosis. Ortop Traumatol Rehabil 11:427-432, 2009.

55. Reference deleted in proofs.

56. Weinstein SL, Dolan LA, Spratt KF, et al: Health and function of patients with untreated idiopathic scoliosis: A 50-year natural history study. JAMA 289:559-667, 2003.

57. Maruyama T, Takeshita K: Surgical treatment of scoliosis: A review of techniques currently applied. Scoliosis 18:6, 2008.

58. Dobbs MB, Weinstein SL: Infantile and juvenile scoliosis. Orthop Clin North Am 30:331-341, 1999.

59. Lenke LG, Dobbs MB: Management of juvenile idiopathic scoliosis. J Bone Joint Surg Am 89(suppl 1):55-63, 2007.

60. Marks DS, Iqbal MJ, Thompson AG, et al: Convex spinal epiphysiodesis in the management of progressive infantile idiopathic scoliosis. Spine (Phila Pa 1976) 21:1884-1888, 1996.

61. Bylski-Austrow DI, Wall EJ, Glos DL, et al: Spinal hemiepiphysiodesis decreased the sizes of vertebral growth plate hypertrophic zone and cells. J Bone Joint Surg Am 91:854-893, 2009.

62. Akbarnia BA, Marks DS, Boachie-Adjei O, et al: Dual growing rod technique for the treatment of progressive early-onset scoliosis: A multicenter study. Spine (Phila Pa 1976) 30(17 Suppl):S46-S57, 2005.

63. Betz RR, Kim J, D'Andrea LP, et al: An innovative technique of vertebral body stapling for the treatment of patients with adolescent idiopathic scoliosis: a feasibility, safety, and utility study. Spine 28:S255-S265, 2003.

64. Betz RR, Ranade A, Samdani AF, et al: Vertebral body stapling: a fusionless treatment option for a growing child with moderate idiopathic scoliosis. Spine 35:169-176. 2010.

65. Newton PO, Upasani VV, Farnsworth CL, et al: Spinal growth modulation with use of a tether in an immature porcine model. J Bone Joint Surg 90:2695-2706, 2008.

66. Crawford CH III, Lenke LG: Growth modulation by means of anterior tethering resulting in progressive correction of juvenile idiopathic scoliosis: A case report. J Bone Joint Surg Am 92:202-209, 2010.

67. Thompson GH, Akbarnia BA, Campbell RM Jr: Growing rod techniques in early-onset scoliosis. J Pediatr Orthop 27:354-361, 2007.

68. Lenke LG, Rinella A, Kim Y: Freehand thoracic pedicle screw placement. Semin Spine Surg 14:48-57, 2002.

69. Kim YJ, Lenke LG, Bridwell KH, et al: Free hand pedicle screw placement in the thoracic spine: Is it safe? Spine (Phila Pa 1976) 29:333-341, 2004.

70. Good CR, Lenke LG, O'Leary PT, et al: Can posterior-only surgery provide similar radiographic and clinical results as combined anterior (thoracotomy/thoracoabdominal)/posterior approaches for adult scoliosis? Spine (Phila Pa 1976) 35:210-218, 2010.

71. Kioschos HC, Asher MA, Lark RG, et al: Overpowering the crankshaft mechanism: The effect of posterior spinal fusion with and without stiff transpedicular fixation on anterior spinal column growth in immature canines. Spine (Phila Pa 1976) 21:1168-1173, 1996.

72. Burton DC, Asher MA, Lai SM: Scoliosis correction maintenance in skeletally immature patients with idiopathic scoliosis: Is anterior fusion really necessary? Spine (Phila Pa 1976) 25:61-68, 2000.

73. Suk SI, Kim JH, Cho KJ, et al: Is anterior release necessary in severe scoliosis treated by posterior segmental pedicle screw fixation? Eur Spine J 16:1359-1365, 2007.

74. Dobbs MB, Lenke LG, Kim YJ, et al: Anterior/posterior spinal instrumentation *versus* posterior instrumentation alone for the treatment of adolescent idiopathic scoliotic curves more than 90°. Spine (Phila Pa 1976) 31:2386-2391, 2006.

75. Kim YJ, Lenke LG, Bridwell KH, et al: Pulmonary function in adolescent idiopathic scoliosis relative to the surgical procedure. J Bone Joint Surg Am 87:1534-1541, 2005.

76. Lonner BS, Auerbach JD, Estreicher MB, et al: Pulmonary function changes after various anterior approaches in the treatment of adolescent idiopathic scoliosis. J Spinal Disord Tech 22:551-558, 2009.

77. Tis JE, O'Brien MF, Newton PO, et al: Adolescent idiopathic scoliosis treated with open instrumented anterior spinal fusion: Five-year follow-up. Spine (Phila Pa 1976) 35:64-70, 2010.

78. Sucato DJ, Kassab F, Dempsey M: Analysis of screw placement relative to the aorta and spinal canal following anterior instrumentation for thoracic idiopathic scoliosis. Spine (Phila Pa 1976) 29:554-559, 2004.

79. Maruyama T, Takeshita K, Nakamura K, et al: Spatial relations between the vertebral body and the thoracic aorta in adolescent idiopathic scoliosis. Spine (Phila Pa 1976) 29:2067-2069, 2004.

80. Reference deleted in proofs.

81. Hall JE, Millis MB, Snyder BD: Short segment anterior instrumentation for thoracolumbar scoliosis. In Bridwell KH, DeWald RL (eds): The Textbook of Spinal Surgery, 2nd ed. Philadelphia, Lippincott-Raven, 1997, pp 665-674.

82. Brodner W, Mun Yue W, Möller HB, et al: Short segment bone-on-bone instrumentation for single curve idiopathic scoliosis. Spine (Phila Pa 1976) 28:S224-S233, 2003.

83. Geck MJ, Rinella A, Hawthorne D, et al: Comparison of surgical treatment in Lenke 5C adolescent idiopathic scoliosis: Anterior dual rod versus posterior pedicle fixation surgery: A comparison of two practices. Spine (Phila Pa 1976) 34:1942-1951, 2009.

84. Newton PO, Marks M, Faro F, et al: Use of video-assisted thoracoscopic surgery to reduce perioperative morbidity in scoliosis surgery. Spine (Phila Pa 1976) 28:S249-S254, 2003.

85. Kishan S, Bastrom T, Betz RR, et al: Thoracoscopic scoliosis surgery affects pulmonary function less than thoracotomy at 2 years postsurgery. Spine (Phila Pa 1976) 32:453-458, 2007.

86. Sucato DJ, Erken YH, Davis S, et al: Prone thoracoscopic release does not adversely affect pulmonary function when added to a posterior spinal fusion for severe deformity. Spine (Phila Pa 1976) 34:771-778, 2009.

87. Bridwell KH, Lenke LG: Prevention and treatment of decompensation: When can levels be saved and selective fusion be performed in idiopathic scoliosis? Spine State Art Rev 8:643-658, 1994.

88. Suk SI, Lee SM, Chung ER, et al: Selective thoracic fusion with segmental pedicle screw fixation in the treatment of thoracic idiopathic scoliosis: More than 5-year follow-up. Spine (Phila Pa 1976) 30:1602-1609, 2005.

89. O'Brien MF, Kuklo TR, Blanke KM, et al (eds): Radiographic Measurement Manual. Memphis, Medtronic Sofamor Danek, USA, Inc, 2004.

90. Rinella A, Cahill P, Ghanayem A, et al: Thoracic pedicle expansion after pedicle screw placement in a pediatric cadaveric spine: A biomechanical analysis [abstract 35]. In Programs and Abstracts of the 39th Annual Meeting of the Scoliosis Research Society, Argentina, 2004, p 70.

91. Bridwell KH, McAllister JW, Betz RR, et al: Coronal decompensation produced by Cotrel-Dubousset "derotation" maneuver for idiopathic right thoracic scoliosis. Spine (Phila Pa 1976) 16:769-777, 1991.

92. Lehman RA Jr, Lenke LG, Helgeson MD, et al: Do intraoperative radiographs in scoliosis surgery reflect radiographic result? Clin Orthop Relat Res 468:679-686, 2010.

93. Donaldson S, Stephens D, Howard A, et al: Surgical decision making in adolescent idiopathic scoliosis. Spine (Phila Pa 1976) 32:1526-1532, 2007.

94. Keeler KA, Lehman RA, Lenke LG, et al: Direct vertebral rotation (DVR) in the treatment of thoracolumbar/lumbar adolescent idiopathic scoliosis (AIS): Can it optimize correction when fusing to L3? [abstract 137]. In Programs and Abstracts of the 15th International Meeting on Advanced Spine Techniques, Hong Kong, 2008, p 215.

95. Lee SM, Suk SI, Chung ER: Direct vertebral rotation: A new technique of three-dimensional deformity correction with segmental pedicle screw fixation in adolescent idiopathic scoliosis. Spine (Phila Pa 1976) 29:343-349, 2004.

96. Kadoury S, Cheriet F, Beauséjour M, et al: A three-dimensional retrospective analysis of the evolution of spinal instrumentation for the correction of adolescent idiopathic scoliosis. Eur Spine J 18:23-37, 2009.

97. Bridwell KH: Adult spinal deformity revision surgery. In Heary RF, Albert TJ (eds): Spinal Deformity: The Essentials. New York, Thieme Medical Publishers, 2007, pp 240-248.

98. Booth KC, Bridwell KH, Lenke LG, et al: Complications and predictive factors for the successful treatment of flatback deformity (fixed sagittal balance). Spine (Phila Pa 1976) 24:1712-1720, 1999.

99. Ondra SL, Marzouk S, Koski T, et al: Mathematical calculation of pedicle subtraction osteotomy size to allow precision correction of fixed sagittal deformity. Spine (Phila Pa 1976) 31:E973-E979, 2006.

100. Bradford DS, Tribus CB: Vertebral column resection for the treatment of rigid coronal decompensation. Spine (Phila Pa 1976) 22:1590-1599, 1997.

101. Lenke LG, O'Leary PT, Bridwell KH, et al: Posterior vertebral column resection for severe pediatric deformity: Minimum two-year follow-up of thirty-five consecutive patients. Spine (Phila Pa 1976) 34:2213-2221, 2009.

102. Lenke LG, Sides BA, Koester LA, et al: Vertebral column resection for the treatment of severe spinal deformity. Clin Orthop Relat Res 468:687-699, 2010.

103. Lenke LG, Bridwell KH, Erickson MA, et al: Prospective radiographic and clinical outcomes and complications of 756 consecutive operative adolescent idiopathic scoliosis patients [abstract 3]. In Programs and Abstracts of the 44th Annual Meeting of the Scoliosis Research Society, San Antonio, 2009, p 39.

104. Padberg AM, Wilson-Holden TJ, Lenke LG, et al: Somatosensory- and motor-evoked potential monitoring without a wake-up test during idiopathic scoliosis surgery: An accepted standard of care. Spine (Phila Pa 1976) 23:1392-1400, 1998.

105. Potter BK, Kirk KL, Shah SA, et al: Loss of coronal correction following instrumentation removal in adolescent idiopathic scoliosis. Spine (Phila Pa 1976) 31:67-72, 2006.

106. Luhmann SJ, Lenke LG, Bridwell KH, et al: Revision surgery after primary spine fusion for idiopathic scoliosis. Spine (Phila Pa 1976) 34:2191-2197, 2009.

Neuromuscular Scoliosis

Peter O. Newton, MD
Eric S. Varley, DO
Burt Yaszay, MD
Dennis R. Wenger, MD
Scott J. Mubarak, MD

General Principles

Neuromuscular disorders commonly lead to spinal deformities that are some of the most challenging treatment dilemmas addressed by spine surgeons. Despite the various conditions that fall in this category, neuromuscular disorders involve neurologic or muscular deficiencies that produce progressive multiplanar skeletal deformities. Common features of neuromuscular scoliosis include the following:

- *Large curves early in life*: Early neuromuscular insult predisposes patients to rapidly progressive scoliosis.
- *Stiff curves*: These patients are more likely to develop stiff curves because of the early onset of neuromuscular deficiency resulting in limited mobility and secondary contractures.
- *Progressive curves*: As in idiopathic scoliosis, the potential for curve progression is greatest during rapid growth and with loss of ambulation. Increasing weakness or persistent muscle imbalance around the spine in patients with neuromuscular disorders can cause progression of scoliosis independent of growth, however.
- *Long curves*: Less severely affected individuals may have an S-shaped curve with well-balanced double curves. Long C-shaped curves are more likely in severely affected patients with resultant sitting imbalance.
- *Pelvic obliquity*: Lower extremity contractures and imbalanced spinal deformity cause pelvic obliquity, which may impair comfortable sitting for these patients.
- *Sagittal plane deformity*: Gravity and muscular deficiency can also lead to sagittal plane deformity, including thoracic or lumbar hyperkyphosis or lumbar hyperlordosis.

Patients with neuromuscular disorders are challenging because of the complexity of their deformity and fragility of their overall health and are best treated by an experienced surgeon with support from a multidisciplinary team.

Classification

The classification of neuromuscular scoliosis can be based on the underlying disorder: neurologic (e.g., cerebral palsy) or muscular (e.g., muscular dystrophy). Neurologic deficiencies can be broken down further into upper motor neuron dysfunction, as seen in myelomeningocele, or lower motor neuron dysfunction, as seen in spinal muscular atrophy (SMA).

Natural History and Associated Complications

Neuromuscular scoliosis generally begins early in life, is rapidly progressive, and causes significant morbidity. Some patients are capable of ambulation, although many lose their ability to walk early in life or never achieve ambulatory status at all. The use of a wheelchair affords these patients educational and social opportunities that enrich their lives. Spinal deformity can impair comfortable sitting and dramatically reduce the individual's quality of life. Unbalanced curves and significant pelvic obliquity make wheelchair positioning difficult and may cause uneven distribution of weight that may lead to pressure sores (Fig. 24–1). Prominences created by the convexity of a curve may result in skin breakdown; creases within the concavity of the trunk deformity are susceptible to skin maceration and infection (Fig. 24–2). Majd and colleagues[1] showed a correlation between deformity size, functional decline, and decubitus. Large rigid curves restrict lung volume and impair respiration in patients who often already have limited pulmonary capacity. Treatment of neuromuscular scoliosis can also help the caretakers of these patients, improving the ease of transfers, positioning, feeding, and hygiene. The ultimate goal of treatment of patients with neuromuscular scoliosis is the maintenance of as much independence and function as possible. When patients with neuromuscular scoliosis lose the ability to sit comfortably, their quality of life is dramatically decreased. The natural history for a given patient is largely determined by the specific underlying neuromuscular condition and the degree of involvement.

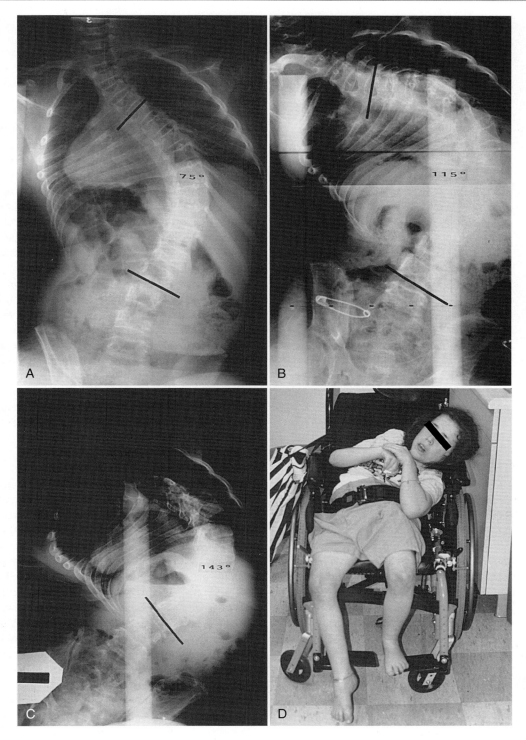

FIGURE 24–1 Progression of scoliosis after skeletal maturity in a patient with cerebral palsy. **A,** At age 15, curve measures 75 degrees. **B,** At age 18, curve measures 115 degrees. **C,** Age 23, curve measures 143 degrees. **D,** The patient is unable to be comfortably positioned in her wheelchair.

Treatment Principles

The basic principles of observing or bracing smaller, flexible curves and surgically fusing larger, more rigid curves in adolescent idiopathic scoliosis apply to the treatment of neuromuscular scoliosis, although with less aggressive parameters.

Observation alone is employed until curves begin to cause functional impairment. Bracing can be a temporizing measure, used primarily to provide sitting support while the patient grows. Eventually, many of these patients require surgical stabilization with a spinal instrumentation and fusion procedure.

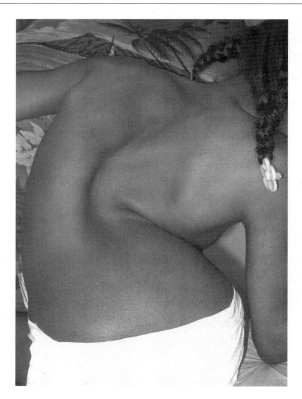

FIGURE 24–2 Severe spinal deformity can lead to skin maceration on concave side of curvature and pressure sores on convex side.

Nonoperative Treatment

Medical Treatment

Spinal Muscle Atrophy

Various medications have been tested to improve the musculoskeletal function of patients with neuromuscular disorders. Randomized placebo-controlled trials have been conducted investigating the efficacy of several medical treatments for SMA, including creatine, phenylbutyrate, gabapentin, and thyrotropin-releasing hormone.[2-5] None of these compounds has proven to be an efficacious drug treatment for SMA.[2]

Cerebral Palsy

Several medical therapies have been investigated for the treatment of spasticity in patients with cerebral palsy. Botulinum toxin has gained a growing acceptance as a treatment of upper and lower limb spasticity. Initial reviews of the literature by the Cochrane Collaboration and others yielded inconclusive evidence that could neither confirm nor deny the efficacy of botulinum toxin in the treatment of spasticity.[6] Inclusion of more recent randomized controlled trials into the analysis has provided evidence that supports the use of botulinum toxin to provide a time-limited benefit to decrease muscle tone in children with upper and lower limb spasticity associated with cerebral palsy.[7] Although evidence for the use of botulinum toxin is not yet conclusive, the evidence trend is in favor of using this therapy to reduce spasticity associated with cerebral palsy.

Intrathecal baclofen is a well-established treatment that has been shown to provide significant benefits in controlling spasticity in patients with cerebral palsy. Intrathecal baclofen has been shown to reduce the need for orthopaedic lower extremity procedures and the rate of postoperative complications associated with these procedures.[8] Concerns have been raised, however, regarding its impact on the progression of scoliosis in patients with spastic quadriplegia. In a retrospective review, Ginsburg and Lauder[9] found a sixfold increase in the rate of scoliosis curve progression at 2-year follow-up in a group of 19 spastic quadriplegic cerebral palsy patients. Caird and colleagues[10] showed a significantly higher rate of complications associated with posterior spinal fusion and instrumentation in a group of 20 spastic cerebral palsy patients with intrathecal baclofen pumps compared with a matched control group. This study was limited by its relatively small sample size and lack of a control group. Shilt and colleagues[11] found no difference in curve progression at 3-year follow-up between 50 cerebral palsy patients treated with intrathecal baclofen and 50 matched control cerebral palsy patients. Based on the current evidence, no significant conclusions can be drawn about the impact of intrathecal baclofen pumps on the progression or treatment of spinal deformity in patients with cerebral palsy. Baclofen can provide significant relief of spasticity, and this evidence must be considered in the context of any potential side effects.

Duchenne Muscular Dystrophy

Advances in general care, glucocorticoid treatment, noninvasive ventilatory support, cardiomyopathy management, and scoliosis management have significantly changed the course of Duchenne muscular dystrophy (DMD). Survival into adulthood is now a realistic possibility for many patients who received optimal treatment.[12] Although gene-based and cellular-based therapies are currently under development for the treatment of DMD, the efficacy of glucocorticoid steroids has been evaluated by several randomized controlled trials. In their Cochrane review and meta-analysis, Manzur and colleagues[13] concluded there is evidence that muscle function and strength are improved in the short-term (6 months to 2 years) with corticosteroid therapy. The authors based their conclusion on six randomized controlled trials and observed that the most effective prednisolone dose seemed to be 0.75 mg/kg/day, given daily.[13] Markham and colleagues[14] showed that glucocorticoid therapy provides the added benefit of retarding the anticipated development of ventricular dysfunction if begun before ventricular dysfunction in their series of 14 DMD patients treated with steroids compared with 23 DMD patients treated without steroids.

Genetic and Family Counseling

Because of the complexity of the medical and psychosocial issues associated with neuromuscular disorders and spinal deformity, care needs to be coordinated with a multidisciplinary team. The primary care physician should be well informed of all orthopaedic issues and play a central role in managing care. Psychosocial support for patients and parents is also vital. Patient advocacy groups have proved to be very useful in helping families cope with the illness and associated surgical care. Physicians may wish to provide information regarding clinical trials or refer families to clinical trial websites (www.clinicaltrials.gov provides a current listing of open clinical trials). Patients and parents may need to be referred for genetic counseling to confirm the patient's diagnosis and aid in family planning.

Bracing

Bracing is a controversial treatment method in idiopathic and neuromuscular scoliosis. Bracing in neuromuscular scoliosis may be used for postural support, although there is incomplete evidence of its efficacy in limiting curve progression (Fig. 24–3). The etiology of the patient's scoliosis and the patient's muscle tone have an impact on the practicality of brace treatment. Patients with spastic disorders generally do not tolerate rigid brace treatment, whereas patients with flaccid paresis are more apt to be compliant with brace treatment. The type of orthoses may play a role in the outcome of the treatment.

Kotwicki and colleagues[15] followed 45 nonambulatory patients with neuromuscular scoliosis treated with a suspension trunk orthosis (STO) and found that the STO slowed curve progression in 23 patients. The STO construction functions contrary to the classic thoracolumbosacral orthosis (TLSO), with the STO not resting against the patient's pelvis but rather directly against the seat. The evidence supporting STO use to prevent curve progression is limited, however, and skin intolerance found in 36 patients complicates its clinical practicality. Although there is limited research on the results of the STO brace, there are numerous studies investigating the TLSO brace. In a study of 15 patients, Shoham and colleagues[16] found that a TLSO reduced scoliotic deformity and pelvic obliquity leading to reduced sitting pressure. These results are contrary to other studies reported in the literature. In a study of 23 patients, Miller and colleagues[17] followed 23 patients with cerebral palsy who wore a rigid Wilmington TLSO for an average of 67 months and concluded that the bracing did not slow progression of their deformity. Olafsson and colleagues[18] followed 90 patients with various neuromuscular conditions treated with a soft Boston orthosis for an average of 3 years after brace treatment. They concluded that brace wear was indicated only in a limited subset of patients—ambulatory patients with hypotonia and short thoracolumbar curves (<40 degrees). In all other patients, brace wear was ineffectual in altering progression but did provide assistance in sitting.

Patients with neuromuscular scoliosis may lack sensate skin to feel pressure from the brace or the muscular control to pull away from the sides of the brace. These patients rarely tolerate the rigid braces often used in idiopathic scoliosis. Patients tend to tolerate soft TLSOs designed to provide improved sitting stability and head and trunk control, while limiting discomfort and skin breakdown (Fig. 24–4).[19]

The impact of the orthosis on pulmonary function is another important factor to consider when contemplating a TLSO for patients with neuromuscular scoliosis. The effect of bracing on pulmonary dysfunction seems to depend on the

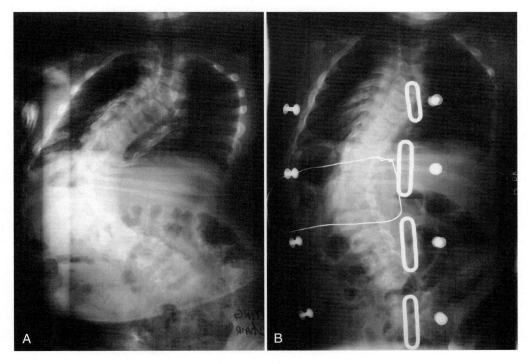

FIGURE 24–3 A and **B,** Bracing in neuromuscular scoliosis is often poorly tolerated. Although it provides modest correction as shown in these radiographs, rigid bracing may lead to excessive skin pressure in patients, who cannot actively pull away from brace.

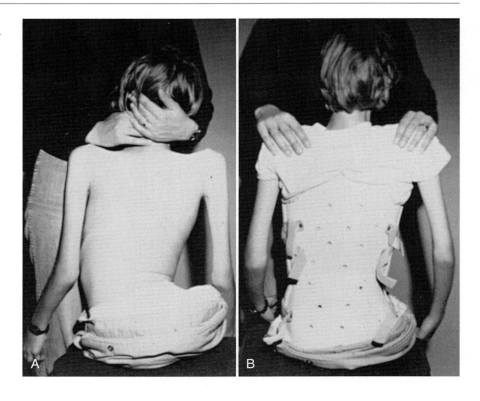

FIGURE 24–4 A and **B,** Soft total-contact TLSO in an older child. Less rigid forms of bracing are better tolerated but do not seem to alter the natural history of curve progression.

level of muscle spasticity. Flaccid patients are more amenable to rigid bracing, although this bracing may significantly decrease chest expansion leading to compromised pulmonary function.[20] Spastic patients seem to be more amenable to soft bracing, which does not seem to compromise pulmonary function,[21] although this bracing has been shown only to enhance seating comfort.[17] Olafsson and colleagues[18] and Bunnell and MacEwen[22] suggested that a subset of patients with minimum deformity and muscle hypotonia or mild spasticity may experience slowing of curve progression by bracing without a negative impact on pulmonary function.

Other factors to evaluate when choosing orthotic treatment for neuromuscular scoliosis include ease of application and obstructions. A bivalved brace may be easier for a caregiver to place, although it cannot provide as much corrective strength as a single opening brace. Winter and Carlson[23] found the two-piece bivalved brace to be a useful support in children with myelomeningocele and SMA. Patients with a stoma or gastrostomy tube require modification of the brace to accommodate these features.

If a patient is not a candidate for bracing or surgery, wheelchair modifications can aid in providing a more comfortable seating position. Modular seating systems can be configured for optimal support of an individual patient (Fig. 24–5). A biomechanical evaluation of seating insert configurations by Holmes and colleagues[24] concluded that three-point force application provides significant sitting support and static correction of scoliosis. Patients with more severe deformity may benefit from custom-molded seatbacks, although these items are expensive, and younger patients may outgrow them quickly.

Operative Treatment

The timing for operative treatment is influenced by curve severity, underlying neuromuscular pathology, and other factors. The curve severity guidelines are loosely based on, but less aggressive than, the guidelines used in idiopathic scoliosis. Fusion should be considered as coronal deformity approaches 40 to 60 degrees. DMD may be an important exception to this concept: Surgery has been advocated when the deformity reaches 20 degrees because of pulmonary considerations.[25] Patients with severely limited respiratory function have been shown to have good outcomes in spinal surgery, however. The sagittal profile is another important consideration because lordotic and kyphotic deformities can also impair sitting balance and pulmonary capacity (Fig. 24–6). Other factors that play a role in the decision to operate include patient age, nutritional status, cardiac function, curve progression, patient comorbidities, and family and caretaker support.

The benefit of scoliosis surgery in this population is a topic of much debate. Many of these patients are poor operative candidates and risk much undergoing involved corrective surgery. Preoperatively, patients may have compromised pulmonary function, limited cardiac capacity, poor bone stock, and high risk for aspiration, which put them in danger of intraoperative or postoperative complications. Correction of large deformities requires extensive exposures and long procedures that can lead to blood loss greater than one to two patient blood volumes. Although many patients already have neurologic compromise, they are still at risk for further compromise because of intraoperative spinal column manipulation. More powerful instrumentation systems have led to less

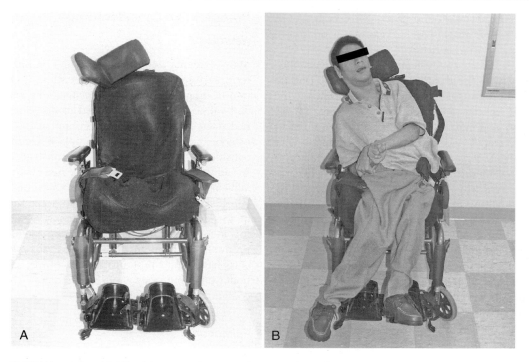

FIGURE 24–5 A and **B,** Wheelchair systems can provide sitting support for patients who are not good candidates for bracing. Custom-molded seatbacks can be made to accommodate substantial spinal deformities.

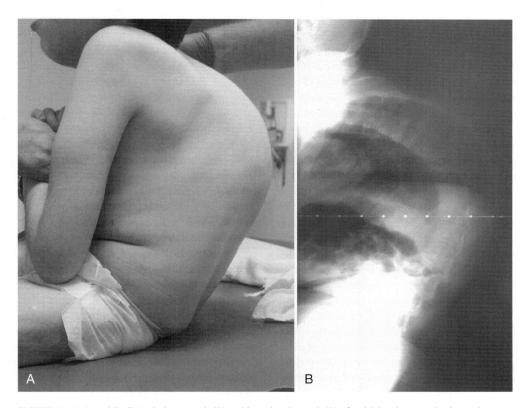

FIGURE 24–6 A and **B,** Clinical photograph (**A**) and lateral radiograph (**B**) of a child with severe kyphosis that impedes balanced sitting.

postoperative decompensation and pseudarthrosis; however, there remains a considerable risk of curve progression, sometimes necessitating revision surgery.[26-28]

Despite the risk of surgery, the benefits of corrective scoliosis surgery for many of these patients are substantial. Halting or slowing curve progression has a positive impact on the functional ability, comfort, and overall quality of life of these patients. Lonstein and Akbarnia[29] reported that more than 50% of patients treated had functional improvement after surgery. In a study of 79 patients with total body spastic cerebral palsy, Comstock and colleagues[27] found that 85% of caretakers surveyed were satisfied with the surgery, reporting improved comfort, sitting ability, and cosmesis for the patients. Bridwell and colleagues[26] found similar trends in a study of 54 patients with neuromuscular disorders with all caretakers reporting benefit from the surgery, specifically in the areas of ease of patient care, skin breakdown, patient comfort, pulmonary complications, and quality of life. Askin and colleagues[30] evaluated 20 patients with neuromuscular scoliosis preoperatively and 6, 12, and 24 months after corrective spinal surgery. The authors noted decreased physical ability at the 6-month time point followed by a return to preoperative function by 12 months and concluded that scoliosis surgery in these patients can stabilize, but not improve, function; however, 75% of patients or caregivers were extremely pleased with the cosmetic results of the surgery. Although most of these patients have deteriorating courses, the correction of spinal deformity seems to improve their function and quality of life.

Although these positive results make a strong case for spine surgery in patients with neuromuscular scoliosis, several review studies have been unable to show a clear benefit of surgical intervention for the patient. Mercado and colleagues[31] evaluated 198 publications and graded their results on the concept of Grades of Recommendation introduced in the *Journal of Bone and Joint Surgery*.[32] These authors concluded that the current literature shows there is poor-quality evidence that spinal fusion improves the quality of life in patients with cerebral palsy or DMD.[31] In a Cochrane Collaboration review, Cheuk and colleagues[33] found that there were no randomized controlled clinical trials available to evaluate the effectiveness of scoliosis surgery in patients with DMD, and so no evidence-based recommendations could be made. Although the practicality of conducting a randomized controlled trial of this nature is questionable, the literature does not provide sufficient evidence to support the role of spinal surgical treatment in patients with neuromuscular scoliosis. It is recommended that the decision for surgical intervention be made based on the needs of the individual patient in consultation with the multidisciplinary neuromuscular care team.

The goal of treatment is preservation of function, which may entail maintaining ambulatory status, maintaining sitting without upper extremity support, or simply allowing assisted comfortable sitting. The decision to operate on a patient with neuromuscular scoliosis is a highly individualized process that should involve a frank and open discussion with the family and patient about the risks and expectations of such a procedure.

Preoperative Considerations

Neurologic

Many patients with neuromuscular scoliosis are on long-term seizure therapy, which has some important operative ramifications. Antiepileptic medications such as phenytoin and valproate have been linked to decreased bone turnover and decreased intestinal absorption of calcium resulting in osteopenia, which may affect implant fixation and should be considered in the selection of construct components.[34,35] In addition, valproate is associated with decreased von Willebrand factor and an increased bleeding time. If possible, consideration should be given to weaning the patient off of this medication, or at least the surgeon should prepare for increased blood loss by having supplementary blood products available during surgery. Preoperative screening of complete blood count, prothrombin time, and partial thromboplastin time may not be predictive of intraoperative coagulopathy.[36]

Pulmonary

Patients with neuromuscular disorders are prone to pulmonary complications, necessitating a thorough preoperative pulmonary assessment. Poor upper airway tone and anatomic deviations can lead to increased risk of airway obstruction during and after surgery. These patients are at high risk for aspiration because of poor oropharyngeal tone and coordination; not only can chronic aspiration lead to pulmonary fibrosis, but also acute aspiration can result in perioperative aspiration pneumonia. Patients may require a dietary change, placement of a gastrostomy tube, or a Nissen fundoplication with gastrostomy tube placement to control this aspiration tendency before undergoing spinal surgery. Reactive airway disease is common in these patients and may necessitate the use of preoperative bronchodilators and inhaled steroids. In addition, these patients may have chronic hypoventilation with carbon dioxide retention and poor oxygenation.

Full pulmonary assessment should be conducted by a pulmonologist and include a chest radiograph, arterial blood gases, and pulmonary function tests if the patient's developmental age is at least 4 years old. Vital capacity that exceeds 500 mL and peak expiratory flow greater than 180 mL/min are associated with decreased perioperative pulmonary complications. Although surgery may be considered in appropriately selected patients with preexisting respiratory failure, Gill and colleagues[37] showed that patients with a forced vital capacity (FVC) of 20% of predicted value can safely be operated on for deformity correction. This prospective observational study followed eight patients on noninvasive night ventilation for respiratory failure with 48 months after surgery and found that all patients recovered well with no major complications. If a patient cannot be assessed with formal pulmonary function tests, other signs of ventilatory capacity must be used, including crying, laughing, and other vocalizations.[38-40]

Nutritional

Proper nutritional balance is crucial for successful surgical outcomes in patients with neuromuscular scoliosis. Many patients are malnourished secondary to a combination of reflux, low calorie intake, and high metabolic demand from frequent illness. Malnourished patients are more prone to perioperative complications such as wound dehiscence, wound infection, and pulmonary complications. Conversely, older patients may be obese, presenting further operative complications associated with their body habitus. Nutritional status should be assessed preoperatively with albumin and total blood lymphocyte levels. Albumin should be greater than 3.5 g/L, and total lymphocyte count should be greater than 1.5 g/L[40]; in a study of 44 patients, Jevsevar and Karlin[41] found that patients had a lower incidence of postoperative infections if they met these criteria.

Gastrointestinal

Because patients with neuromuscular scoliosis are prone to gastrointestinal dysmotility, they are at risk for a postoperative ileus, requiring aggressive hydration, maximized nutritional status, and a rigid daily toilet regimen. In addition, some patients are very thin, and supine positioning and the acute straightening of their deformity put them at risk for superior mesenteric artery syndrome with obstruction of the duodenum. Although less common since the advent of segmental instrumentation and decreased use of casting, this prolonged obstruction carries significant morbidity; identifying at-risk patients and maintaining a high index of suspicion when encountering protracted vomiting is essential.

Cardiovascular

Patients may have cardiac problems secondary to their deformity and other cardiac issues that are comorbidities of the primary disorder. Thoracic cage deformity resulting from scoliosis can cause hypoventilation and subsequent increased pulmonary vascular resistance; this increased vascular resistance can cause right ventricular hypertrophy and eventually cor pulmonale. Patients with DMD may have cardiomyopathy and arrhythmias. The complications associated with arrhythmias may be alleviated with glucocorticoid steroid treatment.[14] Patients with myotonic dystrophy may also have cardiac arrhythmias. Left ventricular hypertrophy can be associated with Friedreich ataxia.

Hematologic

Studies have shown that patients with neuromuscular scoliosis have greater blood loss than patients with idiopathic scoliosis undergoing similar procedures. In this neuromuscular group, the underlying disorder plays a major role in determining the extent of blood loss. In a review article, Shapiro and Sethna[42] found that patients with DMD had the greatest mean levels of blood loss. Much of this difference is due to the requirement

for larger fusions in patients with neuromuscular scoliosis, although osteopenia in these patients may also play a role.[43,44] Preparation for major blood loss—sometimes exceeding 200% of a patient's blood volume—is essential.[38] Often, these patients have already had major surgery, and previous blood loss experience can be used as a guideline for preoperative preparation. Patients should have partial thromboplastin time, prothrombin time, and platelet function evaluated as a part of their preoperative blood work; a more aggressive coagulopathy workup should be conducted if the patient has previously shown a tendency toward excessive blood loss.

Preoperative autologous blood donation should be arranged for patients healthy enough to tolerate this. For a posterior procedure, 4 U of packed red blood cells is generally sufficient; however, the addition of a kyphectomy or an anterior procedure may increase this requirement. Intraoperative blood work may confirm a dilutional coagulopathy necessitating the use of fresh frozen plasma, platelets, or cryoprecipitate to correct this imbalance.

Several pharmacologic agents have been under investigation for their efficacy in reducing blood loss during surgery. Aprotinin, tranexamic acid, and aminocaproic acid have also been investigated to determine their effect on blood loss in spinal surgery. Aprotinin, a serine protease inhibitor, was shown to reduce blood loss in adults, but its production was halted in 2007 by the U.S. Food and Drug Administration (FDA) because of concerns of higher mortality rate after its use in cardiac surgery.

In a prospective, double-blinded, placebo control study of 40 pediatric patients, Neilipovitz and colleagues[45] found that tranexamic acid administration significantly reduced perioperative blood transfusions. These results have been supported by a meta-analysis by Gill and colleagues,[46] which found that tranexamic acid and aminocaproic acid are effective in minimizing blood loss and transfusion in patients undergoing spine surgery. The side effects for tranexamic acid and aminocaproic acid are minor but should be discussed with the patient before using these agents. The surgeon and the anesthesiologist should familiarize themselves with these agents and make a collaborative decision on their use based on the needs and concerns of the individual patient.

Radiographic Assessment

Patients should have a preoperative anteroposterior and lateral film taken of the entire spine preferably in an upright (sitting or standing) position. For assessment of skeletal maturity, a separate anteroposterior radiograph of the pelvis should be considered because scoliosis films often truncate the anatomy necessary to determine skeletal maturity. To assess spinal flexibility, supine bending films or traction films are used. Accurate measurements of the coronal Cobb angle, sagittal Cobb angle, and pelvic obliquity are crucial for complete preoperative planning and postoperative evaluations. In a more recent analysis of the interobserver and intraobserver variability of radiographic measurements of patients with neuromuscular scoliosis, Gupta and colleagues[53] found that neuromuscular

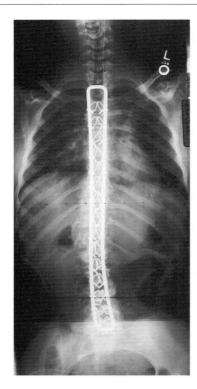

FIGURE 24–7 This one-piece Luque "box" is a modification of the original double Luque rod technique and is a more rigid construct.

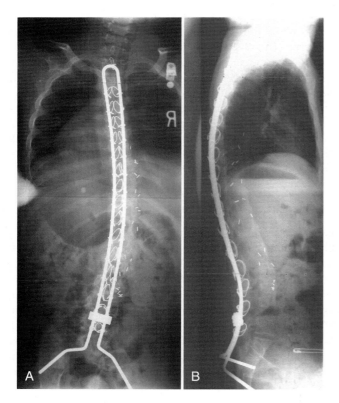

FIGURE 24–8 A and B, Unit rod, as shown here in a patient with cerebral palsy, provides a method for obtaining fixation to pelvis and correction of pelvic obliquity.

radiographs can be reliably analyzed with the use of coronal Cobb angle. Patients who may have congenital spinal anomalies or spinal tethering, such as patients with myelomeningocele, should undergo magnetic resonance imaging (MRI) to evaluate the neural elements fully before surgery. Computed tomography (CT) may also be useful in some patients with severe deformity or in patients with a congenital malformation of the vertebrae.

History of Instrumentation in Neuromuscular Scoliosis

In 1942, Haas[47] published one of the first references to surgical intervention in neuromuscular scoliosis: a case report describing muscle and fascial transfers to obtain complete and permanent correction in one patient. With the introduction of the Harrington rod in 1962, use of this instrumentation with fusion of the spine in patients with neuromuscular scoliosis became the standard. Series using only Harrington rods and posterior spinal fusion have been associated with high incidences of pseudarthrosis (19% to 40%), moderate initial correction (20% to 57%), and loss of correction ranging from 14% to 28%.[29,48] After Harrington rod instrumentation, most patients required bed rest and bracing or casting for up to 1 year.

The introduction of segmental spinal instrumentation by Luque[49] in 1976 led to major advances in the biomechanical stability and correction of these very deformed spines (Fig. 24–7). Several studies revealed that Luque segmental sublaminar wire fixation had fewer complications than Harrington instrumentation and was stable enough so that most patients required no brace or cast postoperatively.[48,50,51] Using the Luque method, the only patients with cerebral palsy requiring postoperative bracing may be patients with athetosis or poor fixation because of severe osteopenia. This is a tremendous advantage because postoperative casting carries the potential for skin and pulmonary complications. Because of these attributes, the Luque technique became the standard method for posterior spinal instrumentation in patients with neuromuscular spinal deformities.

Contouring Luque spinal rods after the technique introduced by Allen and Ferguson[52] (Galveston technique) allowed the rods to be fixed to the pelvis, providing surgeons with a more effective method of controlling pelvic obliquity. Bell, Moseley, and Koreska developed the unit rod, a precontoured U-shaped rod that includes the Galveston portion for pelvic fixation (Fig. 24–8). Studies of patient outcomes with unit rod fixation have revealed excellent correction and maintenance of correction.[54-56] Bulman and colleagues[57] compared the unit rod with double Luque rods and reported superior correction of sagittal and coronal alignment and pelvic obliquity with the unit rod constructs. Tsirikos and colleagues[56] evaluated 287 children treated with unit rod instrumentation to the pelvis with 2-year follow-up and concluded that it offers the advantages of good correction of deformity and pelvic obliquity, a low complication rate, and a 96% caretakers' survey satisfaction rate. Unit rod instrumentation has also been shown to have good results in ambulatory patients, with excellent deformity correction and preservation of ambulatory function at 2.9-year follow-up in 24 patients.[58] Additionally, biomechanical studies have shown that the addition of an L5 pedicle screw increases the construct stiffness and the strength-reducing complications associated with the loss of fixation.[59]

Through a desire to achieve similar correction as the unit rod construct, without the need for pelvic fixation, the U-rod was investigated by McCall and Hayes.[60] This rod is an outgrowth of the unit rod concept except the rod terminates in pedicle screws at the L5 level relying on the iliolumbar ligaments to achieve correction of the pelvic obliquity. In their comparison study of 30 patients with unit rod instrumentation and sacral fusion and 25 patients with U-rod instrumentation and L5 fusion, McCall and Hayes[60] found that the U-rod provided comparable correction of scoliosis and pelvic obliquity in curves with less than 15 degrees L5 tilt at 4 years of follow-up. Regardless of whether the precontoured unit rod or double Luque rods are used, segmental sublaminar wire instrumentation provides simple, inexpensive, and fairly powerful correction of coronal plane deformity. Segmental sublaminar wire instrumentation has limitations in the maintenance of sagittal plane alignment, however, because the sublaminar wiring fails to fix spinal length, and the vertebrae can slide along the smooth rod construct, particularly during trunk flexion (Fig. 24–9A).

Multihook segmental systems such as Cotrel-Dubousset (CD) and Isola have also been shown to be efficacious in patients with neuromuscular scoliosis.[61-63] The comparative efficacy of these two different constructs is inconclusive. In a study of 47 patients with neuromuscular scoliosis, Yazici and colleagues[64] concluded that the Isola instrumentation combined with Galveston pelvic fixation provided correction and maintenance of pelvic obliquity superior to Luque Galveston, unit rod, or CD instrumentation. The results of this study are in contrast to the work of Wimmer and colleagues,[63] who found that there was no difference between Luque Galveston and Isola instrumentation in radiographic outcomes, patient satisfaction, or complication rate. The selection of either of these two instrumentation systems is a choice that relies on surgeon experience and the needs of the individual patient.

In some circumstances, a hybrid system with a combination of hooks, pedicle screws, and sublaminar wires may provide optimal fixation with maximal correction. A biomechanical study conducted at the authors' institution showed that the addition of bilateral L1 pedicle screws to a Luque-Galveston construct on a cadaveric axial skeleton increased construct stiffness by greater than 60%. The addition of selective hooks or screws or both to an otherwise sublaminar wire construct allows use of compressive and distractive force to address the coronal and the sagittal deformities. Additionally, proximal fixation with sublaminar wires compromises the ligaments above, making junctional kyphosis more likely. Hooks (transverse process) or pedicle screws or both may limit this complication in kyphotic patients at greatest risk.

Pelvic and Sacral Fixation

Severe pelvic obliquity secondary to unbalanced scoliotic curves and lower extremity contractures is common and

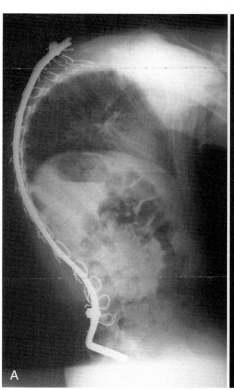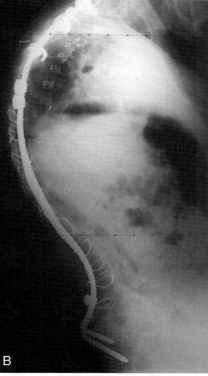

FIGURE 24–9 A, Failure of proximal sublaminar wiring in this construct resulted in increased kyphosis and prominent hardware necessitating revision surgery 3 years after primary procedure. **B,** After proximal revision, the patient developed pullout of the Galveston portion of his construct. This clinical course emphasizes that fixation challenges are present in patients with neuromuscular deformity, particular hyperkyphosis.

A

B

progressive in patients with neuromuscular scoliosis. A solid spinal fusion to the pelvis aids in sitting comfort and balance[1,65]; however, achieving this goal can be troublesome (Fig. 24–9B). Controlling the motion across the lumbosacral joint requires secure fixation to the pelvis to prevent a pseudarthrosis.

Various systems have been proposed to provide fixation to the pelvis. The Galveston technique was the first advancement to improve fusion rates and clinical success in long fusions to the sacrum.[52,53] When paired with either contoured Luque rods or unit rods, it provides powerful coronal correction of pelvic obliquity. This technique places greater forces, however, on the lumbosacral junction, and proper contouring of the rods may be difficult. The initial concern regarding the association between radiolucency around the screw tips ("windshield wiper" sign) and an increased incidence of complications is of little clinical significance (Fig. 24–10).[66,67] Although a biomechanical evaluation of the Galveston technique by Sink and colleagues[28] showed that this construct creates a long lever arm that places considerable cantilever forces at the lumbosacral junction, these forces lead to a high incidence of proximal fixation pullout and distal migration of Galveston rods. The rods also require three-dimensional bending that makes it difficult to contour the rod properly.[68]

Other systems of sacropelvic fixation use an "S" bend (Dunn-McCarthy), which hooks distally over the sacral alae, while the more proximal portion is secured to the lumbar spine at L4 or above with a pedicle screw or infralaminar hook. Reviewing the results of 67 patients, McCarthy and

colleagues[69] found that this technique had decreased operative time compared with Galveston fixation and excellent clinical results, although in 2 of the 67 constructs there was migration of the rods into the pelvis. Other techniques of rod contouring to fix to the pelvis include the Warner-Fackler and McCall techniques, both commonly used in the treatment of myelomeningocele-associated kyphosis in which posterior elements of the lumbar or sacral spine may be absent. In the Warner-Fackler technique,[70] Luque rods are bent to 90 degrees in two places at the distal end, allowing the rods to pass through the S1 foramina and lever against the front of the sacrum to provide sagittal correction (Fig. 24–11). In a slight variation of this technique, McCall[71] described bending Luque rods to 20 to 40 degrees, passing them through the S1 foramina and bending the protruding portion according to the contour of the anterior sacrum. In 16 myelomeningocele patients with hyperkyphosis, McCall[71] found satisfactory correction and maintenance of correction after 5 years of follow-up.

Improvement on the Galveston concept has been the focus of many clinical studies.[69,72-74] The use of S1 screws alone was investigated, but bone quality is generally not substantial enough for successful use in patients with neuromuscular scoliosis. Early and colleagues[72] compared the biomechanical properties of Galveston sacropelvic fixation versus Colorado II sacropelvic plates using S1 screws, S2 alar screws, and iliac screws and found that both methods provided similar construct stiffness with the Colorado II plate limiting L5-S1 motion in flexion-extension. These authors found that addition of a pair of L1 screws increased the construct stiffness by approximately 50% in both fixation techniques.

The use of iliac screw fixation has become a subject of several more recent articles because of its ease of implantation, avoiding the complex lumbosacral three-dimensional Galveston rod contouring. Clinical and biomechanical studies have shown an improved fusion rate and high pullout strengths after the use of iliac screws for caudad lumbosacral fixation.[73,74] In a review of 50 patients treated with one or two bilateral iliac screws, Phillips and colleagues[75] concluded that iliac screws provide a safe and effective means to treat neuromuscular scoliosis at 21 months of follow-up. These authors also noted that two screws in each iliac wing provided a more stable fixation with fewer implant-related complications than using a single screw. In a direct comparison of 20 patients with Galveston rod fixation versus 20 patients with iliac screw fixation, Peelle and colleagues[76] found that both techniques offer similar pelvic fixation with the iliac screw construct allowing additional screw fixation points to the sacrum and lower lumbar vertebrae. The long-term impact of these screws on the sacroiliac joint was investigated in 67 adult patients by Tsuchiya and colleagues,[74] and no evidence of degeneration was observed at 5- to 10-year follow-up.

Although iliac screws provide a promising alternative to Galveston fixation, several studies have shown difficulty with implant prominence causing skin irritation.[77] Peelle and colleagues[76] did not observe this complication in their patient series, however, because they countersunk the screws below the superficial portion of the posterior iliac crest. The patient's

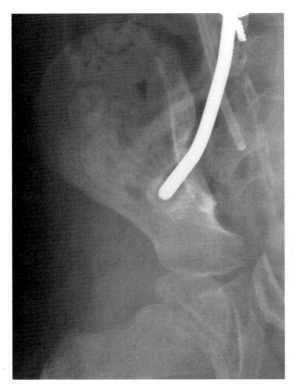

FIGURE 24–10 Radiolucency around rod tip in ilium (windshield wiper effect) suggests lumbosacral pseudarthrosis, which may remain asymptomatic and resolve spontaneously.

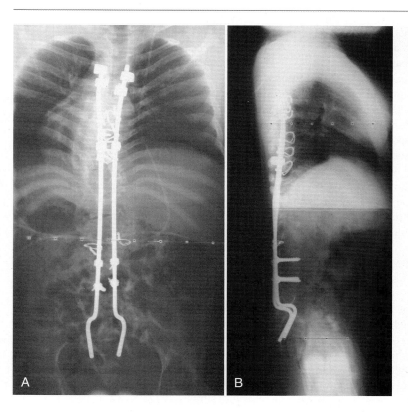

FIGURE 24–11 A and **B,** Warner-Fackler method of pelvic fixation was used after kyphectomy in this patient with myelodysplasia.

body habitus must be considered when selecting the means of sacropelvic fixation. In very small or thin patients, the authors continue to prefer a Galveston rod construct for pelvic fixation. Screw fixation is used when possible, especially in cases with a kyphotic deformity, where the Galveston rod may not optimally resist pelvic flexion (Fig. 24–12).

When patients with neuromuscular scoliosis are instrumented because of the severe obliquity of the pelvis, intraoperative halo-femoral traction may also be beneficial. Previous studies on this traction technique have been described for patients with idiopathic and congenital scoliosis. In nonambulatory patients with neuromuscular scoliosis, surgeons have

FIGURE 24–12 A and **B,** Fixation to pelvis in this patient with cerebral palsy was provided by iliac screws connected to 5.5-mm posterior rod system.

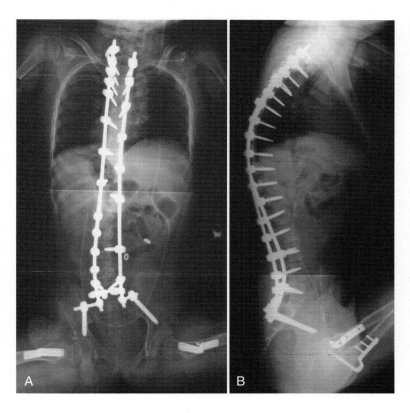

relied on rods or screws inserted into the iliac wings by a cantilever method to level the pelvis. This method has the potential to weaken the bone-construct connection in patients with poor bone stock. In a study of 20 nonambulatory patients with neuromuscular scoliosis with halo-femoral traction and 20 matched patients without halo-femoral traction, Takeshita and colleagues[78] found that halo-femoral traction provided significantly improved lumbar curve and pelvic obliquity correction at 2-year follow-up. These authors had no associated perioperative complications with this technique and found that unilateral femoral traction with corresponding halo traction was able to level the pelvis to an acceptable position before the surgery was begun. When a significant hip flexion contracture exists, traction results in an increase in lumbar lordosis, however, that may be undesirable.

Some authors have argued that the pelvis can be left unfused in patients with slight pelvic obliquity, mild contractures, and little pelvic deformity in the sagittal plane, whereas others have argued that an ambulatory patient should never be fused to the pelvis.[69,79] McCall and colleagues[60] advocated that patients with less than 15 degrees of L5 tilt should be considered for a fusion to L5. These authors believed that this fusion allows greater mobility and improves the patients' ability to carry out activities of daily living. Other studies promote fusion to the pelvis in all patients regardless of ambulatory status. A study by Tsirikos and colleagues[58] of ambulatory cerebral palsy patients with severe pelvic obliquity who were treated with fusion to the pelvis by Luque-Galveston instrumentation found that 23 of 24 patients maintained their ambulatory status. Given the progressive nature of this deformity and the fragility of these patients as operative candidates, the authors generally recommend including the pelvis in the fusion mass for most neuromuscular deformities.

Anterior Spinal Release and Fusion

Indications

The addition of an anterior procedure can assist in the correction of neuromuscular spinal deformity and may be justified in several situations (Fig. 24–13). Anterior release and fusion has generally been indicated in patients with rigid scoliosis, patients with rigid kyphosis, immature patients at risk for the development of crankshaft growth, and patients at risk for pseudarthrosis owing to incompetent posterior elements (myelomeningocele or severe osteopenia).[80] In assessing the rigidity of the deformity, traction and supine bending films are useful but may underrepresent the available flexibility. An anterior release of a large rigid curve increases the overall spine mobility and makes the posterior correction easier with a relatively high fusion rate. In a study by Newton and colleagues,[80] the fusion rate achieved with anterior release combined with posterior corrective instrumentation and fusion was found to be comparable between adolescent patients with neuromuscular scoliosis and idiopathic scoliosis at 3-year follow-up.

Anterior instrumentation and spinal fusion alone and in combination with posterior instrumentation have also been shown to be successful techniques in a subset of patients with neuromuscular scoliosis. The authors' current algorithm indicates an anterior procedure for "severe" curves (most often thoracolumbar). If a near-complete correction of the major curve can be predicted with anterior instrumentation after an aggressive multilevel discectomy, a single rod anterior system is included. If the curve remains rigid after an anterior release, the anterior instrumentation is skipped, and either an apical vertebrectomy is performed, or the correction is achieved after posterior osteotomies (Fig. 24–14). It is important to avoid

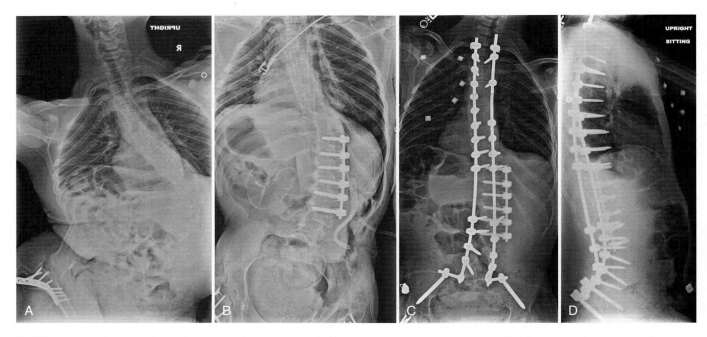

FIGURE 24–13 A, This severe thoracolumbar curve has preoperative Cobb angle of 136 degrees. **B,** Owing to inflexibility, anterior disc excision and anterior instrumentation was used as the first stage of this procedure. **C** and **D,** Posterior instrumentation T2 to pelvis was used in this spastic quadriplegic patient.

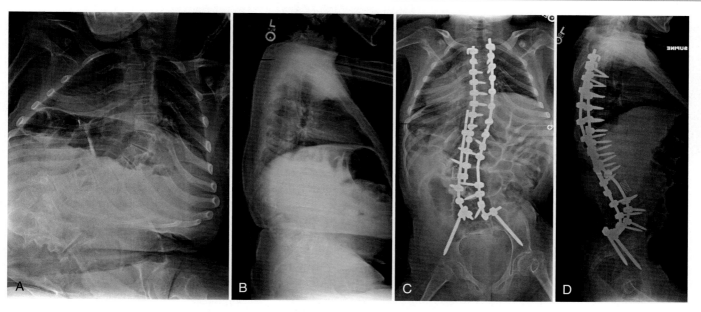

Figure 24-14 A and **B,** This severe 140-degree lumbar curve was upsetting wheelchair sitting balance in this spastic quadriplegic patient. **C** and **D,** This curve was treated with a staged procedure. Anterior release did not provide sufficient flexibility, and anterior L1 and L2 corpectomy was performed. This procedure was followed by T2 to pelvis posterior instrumentation with completion of L1 and L2 corpectomy posteriorly.

"locking in" a poor correction with anterior instrumentation in rigid curves. The goals of achieving a level pelvis and balanced spine must be weighed against the added morbidity of an anterior release or instrumentation procedures or both.

In skeletally immature patients with idiopathic scoliosis, anterior release and fusion reduces anterior overgrowth that results in crankshaft deformity; however, whether this principle can be applied in neuromuscular scoliosis is controversial. In a study of 50 skeletally immature patients with neuromuscular scoliosis treated with posterior instrumentation only, Smucker and Miller[81] noted no significant curve progression at an average of 4 years of follow-up. In contrast, Comstock and colleagues,[27] after review of 60 skeletally immature patients with cerebral palsy who underwent surgical scoliosis correction, concluded that skeletally immature patients have the best correction and long-term outcomes when treated with anterior and posterior procedures.

Instrumentation

The indications for anterior instrumentation have been a subject of investigation more recently. Several studies have shown that anterior instrumentation alone provides acceptable correction without the need for posterior instrumentation in selected short flexible curves that do not include the pelvis or have less than 15 degrees of pelvic obliquity.[82,83] Some studies advocate anterior release followed by posterior instrumentation, whereas others find indications for anterior disc excision and anterior instrumentation before proceeding posteriorly. Anterior instrumentation provides a very powerful means of addressing coronal plane deformities and in many cases simplifies the posterior instrumentation across the levels instrumented anteriorly.

The present options for maximal deformity correction include anterior instrumentation followed by relatively simple posterior fixation versus anterior release and posterior fixation with greater use of posterior osteotomies. The first option also has the advantage of allowing an indefinite time between stages if required. Ultimately, the decision to include an anterior procedure (release or instrumentation) is multifactorial and depends on the experience of the surgeon, the overall health of the patient, and the characteristics of the deformity.

Intraoperative Considerations

Patient Positioning

The patient is positioned for anterior surgery with the apex of the deformity centered over the table break in a nearly lateral position. Flexing the table improves exposure, as does leaning the patient back toward the surgeon. If anterior instrumentation is planned, a direct lateral position is preferred. Posterior surgery is generally performed on a spinal frame; this allows the abdomen to hang free, decreasing the pressure on the vena cava and epidural venous system. This position limits problematic epidural blood loss, particularly when a laminotomy for posterior release and sublaminar wire passage are required at several levels. In a smaller patient, chest rolls may suffice for prone positioning.

Spinal Cord Monitoring

Multimodality monitoring is a useful tool in children with neuromuscular scoliosis. Although patients with true paralysis and myelomeningocele do not benefit from this observation, the use of spinal cord monitoring is helpful for other patients to protect existing extremity function. Current evidence supports the use of transcranial motor evoked potentials (TcMEPs), somatosensory spinal evoked potentials, and 1+ reflex potentials in spinal cord monitoring.[84,85] TcMEPs provide useful data on the motor function and vascular status of the spinal cord, whereas somatosensory spinal evoked potentials provide information on the integrity of the sensory pathways of the dorsal columns. TcMEP monitoring has become a vital component of spinal cord monitoring. In a study of 1121 consecutive patients with adolescent idiopathic scoliosis undergoing spine surgery, Schwartz and colleagues[85] concluded that TcMEP monitoring is the most effective means to detect evolving spinal cord injury. TcMEPs monitor the anterior horn motor neurons, whose high metabolic rate is especially vulnerable to ischemic injury.[86] Because of the complexity and associated hematologic issues of patients with neuromuscular scoliosis, multimodal spinal cord monitoring is highly recommended.

Blood Conservation

Antifibrinolytic agents, hypotensive anesthesia, Cell Saver, subperiosteal dissection, and electrocautery all can reduce blood loss. If an anterior approach is selected, unilateral ligation of the segmental vessels can be performed without significant risk of ischemia of the neural elements. Several studies have concluded that unilateral ligation carries no risk of causing neurologic compromise. Some authors recommend spinal cord monitoring during temporary (10 to 15 minutes) clamping of the segmental vessels before division.[87-89] Periodic intraoperative coagulation panels should also be used to detect a dilutional coagulopathy, which ideally can be treated with early use of fresh frozen plasma, cryoprecipitate, and platelets before disseminated intravascular coagulopathy (DIC) develops. The hematologic status of cerebral palsy patients should be monitored very closely because they typically have increased bleeding that starts earlier in a procedure despite a normal coagulation profile.[90]

Bone Graft

In patients with neuromuscular scoliosis, the autologous iliac crest bone graft is often of poor quality and limited quantity. Also, harvesting may interfere with the placement of pelvic instrumentation. Because these patients need a significant volume of graft given the extent of fusion, supplemental graft in the form of freeze-dried or frozen cancellous allogeneic bone is almost always necessary to supplement local bone graft (facets, spinous process). Although allograft is generally regarded as safe and reliable for fusion augmentation in these patients,[64] evaluation by Sponseller and colleagues[91] of 210 patients with neuromuscular scoliosis revealed an increased risk of infection with the use of allograft. In a study by Yanci and Asher,[92] the rate of pseudarthrosis in patients with neuromuscular scoliosis undergoing surgery with allograft was 2.5%.

Timing of Combined Procedures

The evidence for performing staged versus same-day anterior and posterior procedures is unclear. In a study of 45 patients who underwent combined anterior and posterior surgery, Tsirikos and colleagues[93] found that same-day procedures were associated with longer operative time, greater blood loss, and a higher incidence of medical and technical complications. These results were in contrast, however, to a study by Mohamad and colleagues,[94] who found no difference between single-stage and staged surgical procedures in their review of 175 patients with neuromuscular scoliosis. Further studies on staging combined procedures have focused on the use of traction and defining the curve characteristics that would be most appropriate for a staged procedure. For large, rigid curves, the use of staged surgery with anterior release and halo-pelvic traction as the first stage and posterior instrumentation and fusion as the second stage was investigated by Yamin and colleagues.[95] These authors concluded that patients whose Cobb angle was greater than 80 degrees and flexibility was less than 20% should be treated with this method. Yamin and colleagues[95] also recommended that patients whose spine flexibility was less than 10% with a Cobb angle that remained greater than 70 degrees after the first-stage anterior release and halo-pelvic traction should undergo pedicle subtraction osteotomies in the second-stage surgery.

It is important to anticipate the need for a staged procedure because unplanned staged procedures have a higher complication rate than planned staged procedures.[94] Given the evidence, the authors recommend planning a staged procedure in larger patients with severe deformity or a history of large-volume blood loss in previous surgeries or both. Despite careful planning, hemodynamic instability may force unplanned staging. Blood loss in the posterior procedure tends to be two to three times the blood loss during the anterior procedure; if the surgeon encounters anterior blood loss greater than half the patient's blood volume, a staged procedure should be considered.

Anterior Surgical Approaches

Transthoracic Approach

The standard approach to the thoracic spine is via an open thoracotomy performed on the convexity of the scoliosis. The rib one to two levels above the most cephalad vertebral body to be approached should be removed. The spine can be exposed over approximately six levels between T4 and L1 with this approach. The superficial dissection is in line with the rib, dividing the serratus anterior and latissimus dorsi muscles. The rib is stripped subperiosteally and removed as far posteriorly as possible. With a rib-spreading retractor in place, the parietal pleura is opened longitudinally along the spine. The segmental vessels may be clamped and ligated or maintained, based on the required exposure.

Thoracoscopic Approach

In the thoracic spine, thoracoscopy is an option instead of open thoracotomy. Video-assisted thoracic surgery allows exposure of the entire thoracic spine through three to five intercostal portals. The thoracoscopic approach is less invasive, sparing the chest wall musculature. Investigation has shown that there is less perioperative pulmonary dysfunction associated with this approach in adolescent patients with idiopathic scoliosis. This assertion is supported by Newton and colleagues,[96] who found that comparable correction rates and pulmonary function are present at 5-year follow-up in adolescent patients with idiopathic scoliosis. Although the benefits in adolescent patients with idiopathic scoliosis have been well described, the potential benefits in respiratory function remain unclear in patients with neuromuscular scoliosis.

In a study of perioperative complications after surgical correction in 175 patients with neuromuscular scoliosis, Mohamad and colleagues[94] discussed no positive or negative correlations associated with video-assisted thoracic surgery and pulmonary function. Given this lack of evidence and the technical demands of this technique, the benefits of this procedure must be weighed in the context of the experience of the surgeon and possible complications. Mastery of this less invasive approach may prove to be a valuable tool in treating these fragile patients, however.

Thoracoabdominal Approach

When exposure of the thoracolumbar junction is required, the thoracoabdominal approach extends a thoracotomy incision distally. This extended incision allows exposure from the lower thoracic spine to the sacrum. The diaphragm is detached from the chest wall, which may have pulmonary consequences in patients with limited pulmonary reserve. The thoracotomy approach is combined with a retroperitoneal exposure of the lumbar spine. The diaphragm is divided near the chest wall circumferentially to its origin on the spine at L1.

Retroperitoneal Lumbar Approach

The retroperitoneal approach to the lumbar spine provides exposure from L1 to the sacrum, but placement of instrumentation above L2 often requires a thoracoabdominal exposure. The incision is in line with the 12th rib, curving to parallel the rectus abdominis inferiorly. The three abdominal muscle layers are divided, taking care to identify the translucent layer of peritoneum. The plane between the transversus abdominis and the peritoneum is developed posteriorly. The psoas muscle is reflected posteriorly, exposing the spine. Inferiorly, the iliac vessels and commonly a large iliolumbar vein require careful dissection. The L5-S1 disc can be exposed either by elevating the iliac vessels or by working between the bifurcation anteriorly.

Vertical Expandable Prosthetic Titanium Rib

The vertical expandable prosthetic titanium rib (VEPTR) has gained attention more recently for its role in the correction of early-onset scoliosis and congenital spinal deformities. Hell and colleagues[97] investigated the efficacy of VEPTR in 15 children, 6 of whom were diagnosed with neuromuscular scoliosis. These authors concluded that this technique was safe, effective, and improved sitting ability and cosmesis. These results were supported by a preliminary investigation by Latalski and colleagues, who found that VEPTR considerably improved respiratory capacity in two patients with congenital spinal deformity and one patient with neuromuscular scoliosis.[98] Although these initial results show promise, the clinical application of VEPTR in neuromuscular scoliosis remains a subject that requires further study.

Postoperative Care

Intensive Care Unit

Patients with neuromuscular scoliosis who have undergone extensive spinal surgery are best managed immediately postoperatively in an intensive care unit setting. Ventilatory support is often needed for 24 to 48 hours or more. An intensivist accustomed to caring for these children is invaluable in the early postoperative course.

Bracing

Postoperative bracing is usually not required if the bone quality is sufficient to provide secure implant fixation. In difficult cases, a molded orthosis may be needed; it should be molded after the surgery if significant deformity correction is anticipated. After kyphosis correction, an orthosis may be helpful for reducing the stress on the proximal posterior fixation points.

Complications

The surgical treatment of neuromuscular scoliosis has been shown to have a higher complication rate compared with surgical treatment of idiopathic scoliosis. In the largest study to date of perioperative complications associated with neuromuscular scoliosis surgery, Mohamad and colleagues[94] reported their complication rate to be 33% in 175 patients. These results are consistent with previous studies that found the complication rate to range from 24% to 75%.[66,67,99,100] The factors that are associated with perioperative complications include a history of seizures, unplanned staged surgical procedures, and increased blood loss.[94] Pulmonary issues have been found to be the most prevalent complication of spinal surgery in these patients and should be closely monitored by the multidisciplinary care team.

Wound Infections

The rate of wound infections in this type of surgery is higher than in surgery for adolescent idiopathic scoliosis, ranging from 8% to 15% in the literature. Superficial wound infections are more common than deep wound infections and require close monitoring because they can quickly progress in patients with neuromuscular disorders. Wound infection is also more common in nonambulatory patients with severe involvement and tends to involve multiple gram-negative organisms. A higher rate of wound infection has also been found in patients with sacropelvic fixation with a trend toward a higher rate of deep wound infection.[94] The incidence of deep wound infection may be reduced in patients with neuromuscular disease undergoing spine surgery with an antibiotic-loaded bone graft. In a study of 220 children with cerebral palsy treated with unit rod instrumentation, Borkhuu and colleagues[101] found that the use of gentamicin-impregnated bone graft decreased the incidence of deep wound infection by 11% compared with patients who received bone graft without antibiotics.

In patients with neuromuscular disease, a high index of suspicion must still be maintained, and any suspected infection must be aspirated from deep and superficial layers. A wound infection requires débridement and closure over drains with broad-spectrum antibiotics. Vacuum-assisted closure for deep infections has shown good results with an ease of use and a marked reduction in the need for hardware removal.[102,103] When a wound has been infected, the risk for pseudarthrosis increases.[91,104]

Respiratory Complications

Given the baseline susceptibility of patients with neuromuscular disorders to respiratory complications and the chest wall insult and immobilization associated with scoliosis correction, respiratory complications are common in the postoperative period; the reported incidence ranges from 9% to 22%. These complications include pneumonia, pleural effusion, and atelectasis that may require prolonged intubation.[66,67,100] A preoperative consultation with a pulmonologist to maximize the patient's pulmonary health and aggressive care in the intensive care unit help to reduce the incidence of problems; however, caregivers and patients should be warned that permanent ventilator dependence is a possible sequela of surgery for some patients.

Urinary Tract Infections

The incidence reported in the literature of urinary tract infections in patients with neuromuscular scoliosis is 9% to 22%. Expeditious removal of a urinary catheter inserted for the procedure and adequate hydration may reduce the risk of urinary tract infection. Patients with myelomeningocele often have chronic colonization of bacteria in their bladder. Perioperative prophylactic antibiotics should address these organisms.[66,67,99,100]

Cerebral Palsy

An estimated 25,000 children are diagnosed with cerebral palsy each year. With this huge volume of patients, cerebral palsy has replaced polio as the prototypic neuromuscular disorder. Cerebral palsy is caused by a static upper motor neuron lesion that interferes with the developing motor system. This lesion is usually caused by an anoxic insult in the perinatal period; however, child abuse in young infants is another common cause of brain injury that can lead to cerebral palsy.

Scoliosis in Cerebral Palsy

Scoliosis is common in cerebral palsy with a 25% incidence of spinal deformity in all cerebral palsy patients. The incidence and degree of deformity correlate with the amount of neurologic deficit and ambulatory status. In a study of 272 institutionalized patients, the highest prevalence of scoliosis was found in the most severely affected patients with 75% of spastic quadriplegic and 68% of spastic diplegic patients having at least 10 degrees of spinal deformity. In the above-mentioned study, 44% of patients who could ambulate independently, 54% of patients who could ambulate with assistance, 61% of patients who could sit independently, 75% of patients who could sit with assistance, and 76% of bedridden patients had significant deformity. Although these numbers may be inflated by the fact that the study population was composed entirely of institutionalized patients, they still reveal a trend of increased deformity with increased spasticity and decreased independent mobility.[105,106]

The development of scoliosis in cerebral palsy patients is thought to result partly from persistent primitive reflex patterns and asymmetrical tone in the paraspinous and intercostal muscles. Pelvic obliquity from contractures around the hip plays a role in scoliosis development; however, it is often difficult to isolate this as a contributing factor because pelvic obliquity, hip contractures, and scoliosis often develop simultaneously. Placing patients with a weak trunk and total body involvement into artificial upright sitting positions without appropriate spinal support may encourage gravity-related kyphosis and scoliosis. This suspicion was raised by Madigan and Wallace[106] when they found a 75% incidence of scoliosis in a predominantly institutionalized population comprising "prop sitters" but only a 25% incidence in a population of spastic quadriplegics in which prop sitting was not pursued.

Scoliosis in cerebral palsy has been classified into four categories based on curve pattern (single vs. double) and the presence or absence of pelvic obliquity. Long C curves with pelvic obliquity generally occur in more severely involved nonambulatory patients with spasticity. S curves occur more frequently in sitting or walking patients with little spasticity. S curves seem to be more idiopathic in nature, often without associated pelvic obliquity.[29] Patients with severe involvement and a developmental level less than 6 months seldom attain independent sitting balance. Lack of neuromuscular control prevents proper alignment of the head, and these patients do not develop compensatory curves to bring the shoulders and head over the pelvis.

Curve progression is related to the above-mentioned risk factors and quadriplegia, poor functional status, and a single thoracolumbar curve.[1,107,108] As in idiopathic scoliosis, risk of progression is also related to curve magnitude and to the amount of remaining spinal growth. Because progression of spinal deformity begins at the onset of the neuromuscular condition, patients with cerebral palsy have a much longer time to progress and have the potential for developing larger curves than patients with adolescent idiopathic scoliosis. This period of potential curve progression is prolonged further because these patients often maintain open growth plates into their late teens or early 20s. In adults, Thometz and Simon[108] found that larger curves progress faster than smaller curves; they noted curve progression of 0.8 degree per year in curves less than 50 degrees and 1.4 degrees per year in curves greater than 50 degrees. Even patients who have completed growth are at risk for scoliosis progression.

Treatment Options

Bracing

The natural history of scoliosis in children with cerebral palsy is early onset with a flexible spine deformity between 3 and 10 years of age with a relatively fast progression to a rigid structural curve.[107] Most of the articles in the literature do not support the use of bracing. Bracing can function as a temporizing measure, however, in patients with early-onset, flexible scoliosis or in patients with contraindications for surgery.[15] Spastic cerebral palsy patients have poor tolerance for bracing because of the spasticity of their limbs inhibiting brace application, the incidence of skin pressure irritation, and sometimes increasing respiratory problems.[15,17] A soft brace may be used owing to the lack of practicality of dynamic bracing, although it becomes mainly a sitting support rather than a treatment modality. For patients who cannot tolerate bracing, wheelchair seating systems can facilitate upright posture and allow patients to participate in more activities with greater social interaction.

Surgical Management

Various techniques and instrumentation exist for surgical scoliosis correction in cerebral palsy patients. In patients with hypotonia, a thoracolumbar or lumbar curve that does not extend to the pelvis, and a pelvic obliquity less than 15 degrees, fusion to L5 without sacropelvic fixation may occasionally be appropriate.[60] For most cerebral palsy patients with spinal deformity, an extensive posterior fusion with instrumentation from the upper thoracic level (T1 or T2) to the pelvis is indicated. The most common instrumentation systems used have been the combination of Luque wires and a unit rod or two Galveston rods. Luque-Galveston constructs maybe modified with iliac screw fixation to aid in the ease of insertion and to provide safe, reliable correction.[74,75] Several studies have shown the efficacy of these methods in cerebral palsy patients. Boachie-Adjei and colleagues[100] retrospectively reviewed 45 patients treated with Luque-Galveston constructs and found 53% correction of scoliosis and 50% correction of pelvic obliquity. The correction was maintained at an average of 3 years of follow-up despite a 6.5% pseudarthrosis rate. Benson and colleagues[99] reported on a cohort of 50 patients also treated with Luque-Galveston instrumentation who showed a 65% scoliosis correction rate with maintenance of correction at 40

months of follow-up. Only one patient in this series had a pseudarthrosis (2%).

Other studies have reported successful correction using the unit rod system in cerebral palsy patients. Bulman and colleagues[57] compared 15 patients instrumented with Luque-Galveston constructs to 15 patients with unit rod instrumentation and concluded that the unit rod provided significantly improved correction and maintenance of correction of both scoliosis and pelvic obliquity at 2 years after surgery. Although the power of this study is limited by its small size and short follow-up, the findings are echoed in the results of other studies. Westerlund and colleagues[109] reported 66% scoliosis correction and 75% pelvic obliquity correction that was maintained at an average of 5 years' follow-up. Tsirikos and colleagues[56] retrospectively reviewed 287 cerebral palsy patients treated with unit rod instrumentation and found a 68% correction of scoliosis and 71% correction in pelvic obliquity at 2-year follow-up.

More recently, there has been a trend toward using more hooks and screws in neuromuscular constructs. Segmental screw fixation common in idiopathic scoliosis may result in improved fixation with a reduced complication rate.[110] Although this instrumentation shows great promise, follow-up studies are insufficient to clarify this issue.

Surgical correction of scoliosis and pelvic obliquity may also be improved with the use of intraoperative traction. In a comparison study of patients with and without asymmetrical intraoperative halo-pelvic traction, Vialle and colleagues[111] concluded that intraoperative traction resulted in reduced anesthetic duration and improved correction of scoliosis and pelvic obliquity. These results are supported by Takeshita and colleagues,[78] who found that halo-femoral traction improved scoliosis and pelvic obliquity surgical correction in nonambulatory patients with neuromuscular disorders.

Sagittal plane deformities are also common problems in cerebral palsy patients with scoliosis and require a different approach than that required for coronal plane deformities. Lumbar hyperlordosis and thoracic hyperkyphosis can impair sitting balance and comfort. Hyperkyphosis can be exacerbated by pelvic obliquity and gravity in a patient who sits unsupported propped up and is associated with an increased incidence of instrumentation pullout and failure.[28] Sagittal plane kyphotic deformities require treatment similar to treatment of the deformity in Scheuermann disease with or without an anterior release and a hybrid system of hooks and pedicle screws to apply segmental compression across the kyphotic segments.

Authors' Recommendations

For gravity-dependent mild scoliosis or hypotonic kyphosis in children younger than 10 years, the authors recommend a Plastizote body jacket. This body jacket supports the spine, assists head control, and is well tolerated by the patient. The orthosis usually lasts more than 2 years before it is outgrown. For more rigid curves between 30 degrees and 50 degrees or in less rapidly growing patients older than 12 years, a rigid total-contact orthosis may be tried. Although less well

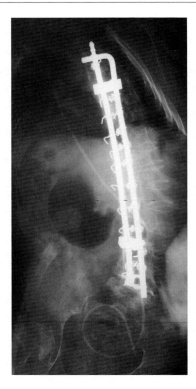

FIGURE 24–15 This patient with cerebral palsy presented at age 17 with Harrington-Luque instrumentation from T4 to L4 done 5 years previously. At presentation, the patient had 85-degree C-shaped scoliosis with marked pelvic obliquity, rotational deformity, and resultant sitting difficulties. In most nonambulatory patients who have adequate spinal length, fusion to pelvis is recommended to avoid this dilemma.

tolerated, a total-contact orthosis provides better correction and may delay the need for surgery by providing greater sitting support.

As discussed earlier, defining the precise indications for surgical intervention in patients with scoliosis and cerebral palsy is difficult. The authors recommend that surgery be considered when scoliosis greater than 50 to 70 degrees exists, taking into consideration the patient's functional, mental, and general health status. The decision to proceed with surgery of this magnitude requires a thoughtful analysis and discussion with the family and caregivers. If Luque instrumentation is used posteriorly, when possible, 5.5- to 6.35-mm rods and a combination of infralaminar hooks, pedicle screws, and double 16- to 18-gauge wires should be used to maximize correction and rigidity. Smaller diameter rods (4.5 to 4.75 mm) should be used only in very small patients for fear of rod breakage. Anterior fusion should be considered in patients with rigid curves greater than 60 to 80 degrees, in skeletally immature patients, or in patients with fixed pelvic obliquity. In severe curves with marked pelvic obliquity, the correction of the pelvic obliquity and the certainty of permanent correction are often enhanced by the addition of anterior lumbar instrumentation.

The use of pedicle screws and aggressive posterior osteotomies has reduced the use of anterior surgery for some patients. For the most flexible cases, an all-posterior hybrid construct is appropriated; the authors prefer pelvic fixation with iliac bolts over Galveston rods. If the curve is more rigid, Ponte-type osteotomies are added, and the density of pedicle screws is increased. Patients with curves that do not correct to less than 70 degrees on side bending are considered for an anterior procedure, most often at the thoracolumbar junction. If, after complete disc excision (including the posterior longitudinal ligament), the spine is now flexible enough for near-complete correction, the correction is achieved with an anterior rod system. If the spine remains rigid after discectomy, performing an apical vertebral excision is considered. In either case, an anterior rod is avoided when residual rigidity remains, and the correction is achieved with the posterior instrumentation.

All cerebral palsy patients with limited ambulatory capacity should be fused inferiorly to include the pelvis, even if their pelvic obliquity is correctable, because of the potential for increased obliquity owing to persistent muscle imbalances (Fig. 24–15). Most patients do not require postoperative immobilization. In patients with poor bone stock or a motion disorder undergoing fusion to the pelvis, a brace is considered for 3 to 6 months after surgery.

Myelodysplasia

Myelodysplasia is characterized by a persistent open neural arch owing to failed proliferation of neuroectodermal cells in early embryonic development and has been associated with maternal hyperthermia and folate deficiency. The spinal deformity comes from a congenital malformation of levels at the defect, often resulting in a regional hyperkyphosis, and from the muscle imbalance around the spine distal to the lesion (Fig. 24–16).

Scoliosis in Myelodysplasia

The incidence of scoliosis in patients with myelodysplasia (spina bifida) varies in the literature from 52% to 90%.[112,113] In a more recent study of 141 patients by Trivedi and colleagues,[113] the authors defined scoliosis in myelodysplasia as curvature greater than 20 degrees and concluded that new curvature could develop as late as 15 years of age.[112] In this cohort of patients, 89% of patients with the last intact laminar arch located in the thoracic region had scoliosis, whereas 44% and 12% had scoliosis if their last intact laminar arch was in the upper and lower lumbar regions. From this trend, Trivedi and colleagues[113] concluded that the last intact laminar arch was the most useful early predictor of scoliosis risk, although ambulatory status and clinical motor levels were also useful predictors.

Myelodysplastic spine is one of the most difficult treatment dilemmas in scoliosis management. These patients present with congenital malformations (Fig. 24–17), often in the form of severe kyphosis preventing comfortable sitting and causing skin breakdown that may necessitate separate and early intervention. The risk of deformity from weak, spastic paraspinal musculature and asymmetrical hip contractures remains, often requiring more definitive surgical correction in the

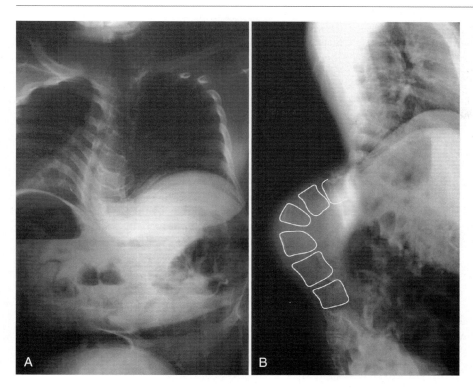

FIGURE 24–16 A and B, Severe progressive kyphosis in this patient with thoracic level myelomeningocele caused skin breakdown problems and difficulty with self-catheterization before she underwent kyphectomy and instrumentation as shown in Figure 24–11.

preteen or teen years. Surgical correction for myelodysplasia presents unique problems because of the absent posterior elements, increasing the dependence on anterior fusion and fixation. In addition, the posterior approach for surgical correction traverses the poor-quality skin and scar tissue that results from the defect and the early neurosurgical repair (Fig. 24–18).

There may be an association between myelodysplasia patients with a tethered spinal cord and rapidly progressive scoliosis.[114] Most of these patients have some variation of cord tethering as a residuum of the defect and its neurosurgical closure. In patients with unexpected rapid curve progression or increased trunk spasticity (hypertonicity), a tethered

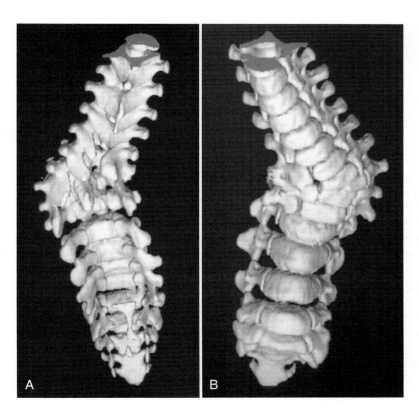

FIGURE 24–17 A and B, Three-dimensional CT scan shows absence of posterior elements and congenital vertebral anomalies that make myelomeningocele spinal deformities challenging treatment dilemmas.

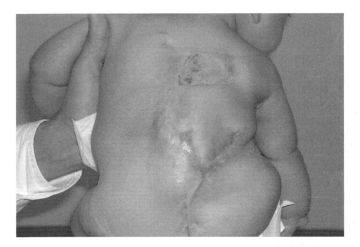

FIGURE 24–18 An infant with severe scarring from original neurosurgical closure of spinal defect.

cord with or without hydromyelia should be considered. Studies such as MRI or myelography may help define the anatomy; however, the literature does not support a causal relationship between scoliosis and Chiari malformation or syringomyelia.[114] Thoughtful teamwork with a neuroradiologist, neurologist, and neurosurgeon helps clarify these issues. Surgical release of a tethered cord can result in scoliosis stabilization, maintenance of motor function, and decreased back pain.[115] Pierz and colleagues[116] evaluated 21 cases of de-tethering, however, and concluded that improvement or stabilization of scoliosis after de-tethering is less likely in patients with curves greater than 40 degrees or thoracic level defects or both. Given the high incidence of scoliosis and the tendency for rapid progression in these patients, annual follow-up evaluations with posteroanterior and lateral radiographs should closely track coronal and sagittal spinal deformity and hip contractures and trunk spasticity.

Treatment Options

Bracing

Bracing in myelodysplasia is even more difficult and less successful than in other neuromuscular disorders. Studies show that braces offered as a temporizing measure rarely yield effective curve control. Although Muller and Nordwall,[117] after evaluating 21 myelodysplasia patients treated with bracing, concluded that deformity progression can be halted in patients with curves less than 45 degrees, a more recent study by Olafsson and colleagues[18] reviewed outcomes in 20 patients and reported a successful outcome in only 20% of patients. Bracing is difficult in these patients because of pressure sores, especially prevalent over kyphotic deformities at the level of the neurologic defect. Obesity, poor-quality and insensate skin, decreased vital capacity, and obstructing stomal bags also contribute to the difficulty of brace wear in these patients. In the study by Olafsson and colleagues,[18] half of the patients stopped wearing their braces because of discomfort. Custom-molded

or modular wheelchair inserts offer another temporizing measure for comfortable upright posture until surgery is conducted.

Surgical Management

Definitive surgical management need only be delayed until patients reach 10 to 12 years of age because growth hormone deficiency limits their growth, and truncal height has reached its maximum around this time. Indications for operative management are similar to the indications for other neuromuscular disorders, although a curve that is rapidly progressive in a patient with myelodysplasia may be treated earlier at 40 to 50 degrees. Because a significant hip flexion-abduction contracture can produce lumbar lordosis and scoliosis, the hip contracture should be surgically released before any attempt at surgical correction of the spine.

Anterior Fusion

As previously discussed, anterior fusion is very important in myelodysplasia because the anterior spine provides a large surface for bony fusion in the lumbar spine, in contrast to the deficient posterior elements at these levels. A thoracoabdominal retroperitoneal approach from the convex side of the curve and division of the diaphragm allows anterior disc excision and bone grafting; this may be combined with posterior instrumentation to provide curve correction in select patients (Fig. 24–19). Use of anterior instrumentation alone has a specific role in the treatment of myelodysplasia scoliosis. In a study of 14 myelodysplasia patients treated with a Texas Scottish Rite Hospital anterior construct alone, Sponseller and colleagues[118] concluded that anterior instrumentation was successful in a select group of patients with thoracolumbar curves less than 75 degrees, compensatory curves less than 40 degrees, no hyperkyphosis, and no syrinx in the spinal cord. Basobas and colleagues[82] found excellent surgical correction and maintenance with an anterior instrumentation and fusion procedure in their study of 11 myelodysplasia patients at 5-year follow-up. In patients with a lumbar curve and fixed pelvic obliquity, anterior instrumentation provides a powerful means of correcting the deformity (Fig. 24–20).

Posterior Fusion

Although essential to a solid fusion in most myelodysplasia patients, the posterior procedure is difficult because of the poor quality of overlying tissue, decreased paraspinal muscle vascularity, and missing posterior elements. Posterior fusion in combination with anterior fusion is recommended by several authors. In a study of 50 patients, Banit and colleagues[119] concluded that posterior fusion alone yielded a much higher pseudarthrosis rate of 16% than rates reported for anterior and posterior fusion combined. Parsch and colleagues[120] reviewed results of 54 myelomeningocele patients treated surgically and also concluded that anterior and posterior instrumented fusion resulted in the best correction and lowest complication rate.

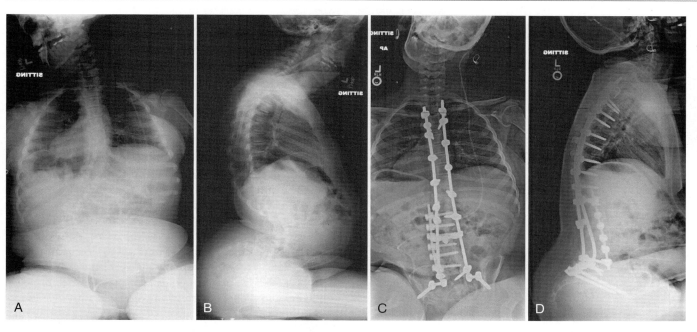

FIGURE 24–19 **A** and **B,** This young patient with myelodysplasia presented with 80 degrees of scoliosis and severe lordosis. **C** and **D,** Severe lordosis was treated with anterior instrumentation from T12 to L5 followed by posterior instrumentation from T3 to pelvis.

Luque or unit rods with sublaminar wiring can be used in segments of the spine in which the posterior elements are intact, although supplementation with screws and hooks increases construct stability. In regions in which the posterior elements are missing, pedicle screws are stronger, although the atypical anatomy makes accurate screw placement difficult. In addition, pedicle screws may be prominent particularly in a kyphotic region because the lateral bony columns are often subcutaneous.

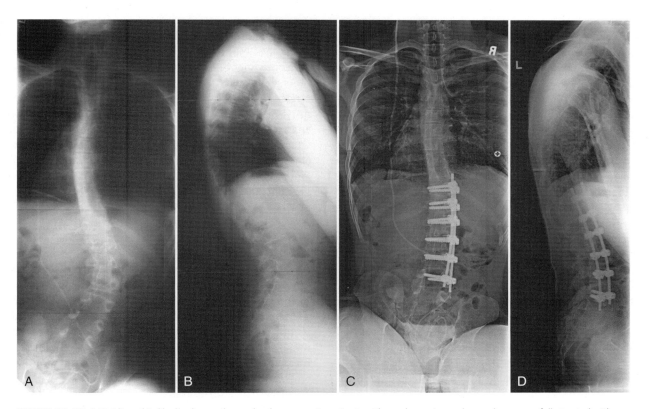

FIGURE 24–20 **A-D,** Idiopathic-like lumbar or thoracolumbar curves in patients with myelomeningocele may be successfully treated with anterior instrumentation only.

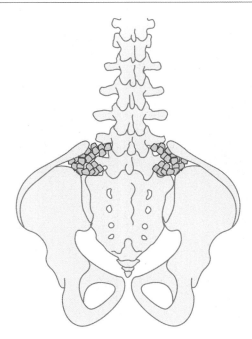

FIGURE 24–21 This bone grafting technique increases the chance of stable fusion by including the wing of the ilium and the sacrum.

Fusion to the Pelvis

There is considerable controversy over whether the pelvis should be included in the fusion mass. Lindseth and colleagues[121] contended that this is necessary only if there is a component of kyphosis in the lumbar spine or if pelvic obliquity is greater than 15 degrees. They noted an increased incidence of ischial ulcers in patients left with residual pelvic obliquity and fusion to the pelvis probably because the rigid, long, curved segment prevents easy shifting of weight between ischial tuberosities. A prospective evaluation of 11 myelomeningocele patients treated with anterior and posterior instrumented fusion to the lumbar spine revealed good correction of coronal and sagittal plane deformities with fair maintenance of correction. From this experience, the authors of the study concluded that, with the advent of more stable segmental instrumentation, the pelvis could be spared to allow more lumbosacral mobility and to avoid the morbidities associated with pelvic fusion.[122] Similar results have been found in a select group of myelodysplasia patients with anterior-only instrumentation and fusion where pelvic obliquity can be corrected without pelvic fixation.[82]

The most predictable approach from the standpoint of the spinal deformity is fusion to the pelvis. In patients with limited activity, the authors recommend fusion to the pelvis to ensure a straight spine over a level pelvis. In ambulatory or very active patients who play recreational activities, such as wheelchair basketball, the pelvis may be spared with the knowledge that a later revision may be required.

Various options are available for instrumentation to the pelvis. The Galveston modification of Luque rods is a commonly used system, although it may not provide as much stability as the Warner-Fackler modification in correcting kyphosis. As previously described, the Warner-Fackler method involves two 90-degree bends in the distal end of a Luque rod allowing the rod to pass through the S1 foramina and lever against the anterior aspect of the sacrum (see Fig. 24–11).[70] In a small series of nine patients treated with kyphectomy and this method of pelvic fixation, Thomsen and colleagues[123] reported excellent correction and maintenance of kyphosis correction at an average of 28 months of follow-up. The authors described two instances of complications (loss of rod connection and migration) both at about 32 months after surgery and concluded that this technique, although effective, should be limited to patients weighing less than 30 kg. McCall described a similar technique with Luque rods passed through the S1 foramina and bent once to 20 to 40 degrees depending on sacral inclination. In his series of 16 patients, McCall[71] reported good correction of kyphosis and excellent maintenance after 57 months of follow-up. Iliac screw fixation has also been shown to afford equivalent maintenance of pelvic obliquity and scoliosis correction compared with the Galveston technique.[75,76]

True fusion to the pelvis (to the wing of the ilium rather than just to the sacrum) can be achieved by suturing the detached iliac crest apophysis to the transverse process of the spine at L3 or L4 and filling the created triangle with bone graft (Fig. 24–21). Pseudarthrosis is common in fusions to the pelvis, and the authors still advise a conservative immobilization protocol.

Major and minor complications are more common in myelomeningocele patients than in other patients with neuromuscular scoliosis. Reports of the incidence of wound infections range from 19% to 43%.[124] Many patients have minor complications, such as urinary tract infections or minor wound dehiscence. Major complications, including massive blood loss and instrumentation failure, are more common in myelomeningocele scoliosis than in idiopathic scoliosis or other neuromuscular conditions.[119,124] Pseudarthrosis rates range from 16% to 50% in the literature.[119,125] In addition, the proximity of procedures to the dural sac and the abnormal anatomy increase the risk of shunt compromise and failure. By attending to detail and applying all that is currently known about myelomeningocele scoliosis surgery (careful anterior and posterior fusion, segmental attachment, cautious remobilization), the major complication rate can be reduced to 15% or less.

Kyphosis Treatment

As already noted, bracing is extremely difficult in the severe kyphosis associated with myelomeningocele. Kyphosis is relentlessly progressive (3 to 8 degrees per year) and can become pathologic in 20% of patients. Because surgical correction is complex and difficult, many children are left untreated and seem to function reasonably well, although skin breakdown over the kyphosis, pressure on abdominal contents, and loss of trunk height remain problems. Indications for surgery include progressive kyphosis, skin breakdown over the kyphosis, respiratory compromise, and concern regarding the effect of severe trunk shortening (Fig. 24–22).[71,126]

Kyphosis in myelomeningocele can be corrected, but intra-operative or perioperative death is frequent enough to give pause to all who treat this disorder. Death can occur from uncontrolled bleeding or problems with cerebrospinal fluid dynamics. The advent of segmental spinal instrumentation has made kyphectomy with fusion at least moderately predictable. The segmental attachment must extend well into the thoracic spine to control the large sagittal plane bending moments.

Basic principles include a long midline posterior approach with exposure of five or six levels of normal closed laminae proximally and distal exposure down to the mid-sacral level. The sac and cord are retracted or resected, with care being taken to repair the dura slightly distal to and separate from the cord transection to avoid tying off the central canal and disturbing cerebrospinal fluid dynamics.[127] In most cases, retracting the scarred thecal sac allows sufficient exposure.[126] The spine is prepared for segmental attachment by passing laminar wires or hooks through all normal laminae proximally. The distal segments can be attached by pedicle screw fixation or by screws placed directly into the vertebral bodies. Because the bleeding encountered with osteotomy may force a rapid finish, complete preparation is essential for a successful instrumentation.

The vertebral bodies making up the cranial two thirds of the kyphosis are excised, allowing one to "fold in" the remaining proximal and distal spinal segments (Fig. 24–23). Care

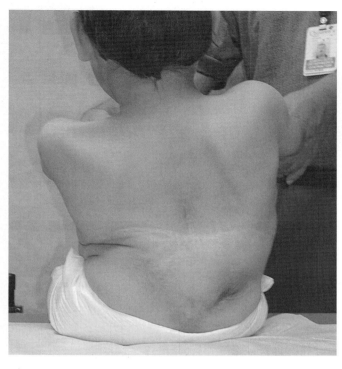

FIGURE 24–22 Lumbar gibbus on this patient with thoracic level myelomeningocele was causing sitting difficulties and loss of trunk height before he underwent kyphectomy and spinal fusion.

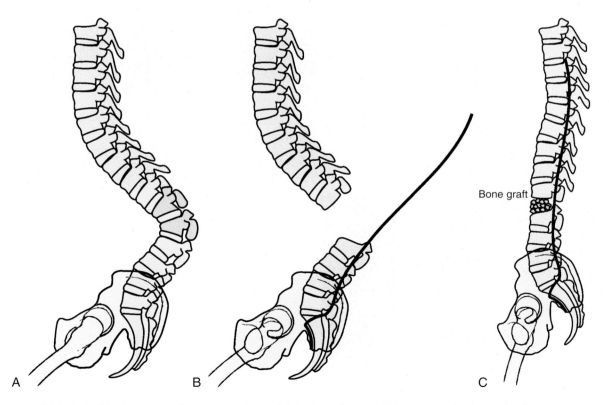

Bone graft

A   B   C

FIGURE 24–23 Sagittal diagram describing sequence for performing kyphectomy. **A,** Spine is exposed, dural sac is tied off or retracted, and kyphotic segment of spine is excised. **B,** To improve mobility of remaining segments, discs can be excised, and lower two or three pairs of ribs can be sectioned from their origins. **C,** Two segments of spine are "folded inward," bone grafted (from the excised segments), and wired to previously contoured rods.

must be taken when the vertebrectomy is performed because the kidneys may be present in the concavity of the deformity and may sustain inadvertent injury. Often ribs 10 to 12 must be transected bilaterally to free the proximal segment enough so that the spine folds inward. The rods are positioned posterior to the infolded segments and secured in place. Posterolaterally placed polyaxial screws may be used to augment wiring and provide greater construct rigidity (Fig. 24–24). In a study of seven myelomeningocele patients, Kocaoglu and colleagues[128] found that the addition of polyaxial screws provided greater correction capacity and a low instrumentation profile in patients with a kyphectomy and Luque instrumentation. The excised vertebrae provide adequate bone graft, applied anteriorly and posteriorly.

Spinal Muscular Atrophy

Affecting 1 in 10,000 newborns, SMA is a fairly common autosomal recessive disorder that is characterized by varying degrees of degeneration of the anterior horn cells that results in a symmetrical muscle paralysis of the trunk and proximal musculature. The etiology of SMA has been linked to mutations in the *SMN1* gene, whose exact cellular function is unknown. Absence or deficiency of this inhibitory protein allows increased motor neuron death that leads to progressive muscle paralysis, eventually causing respiratory insufficiency and scoliosis (Fig. 24–25).[129] Although there are more severe forms, 80% of patients live to adulthood and achieve sitting balance.[130]

Spinal Muscular Atrophy Types

SMA is broken down into three types. First described in the 1890s, type I is also known as *Werdnig-Hoffman disease* or *acute infantile SMA*. In this form, children are born with a normal appearance but by 6 months begin to show signs of muscle weakness with poor head control, absent reflexes, and respiratory insufficiency, which is the cause of death by 2 to 3 years of age.[131] Children with type II SMA—the *chronic infantile* or *Dubowitz* form—experience the onset of muscle weakness between 6 and 19 months of age but do not have the same severity of symptoms. They attain sitting balance but rarely are able to walk independently. Although respiratory impairment

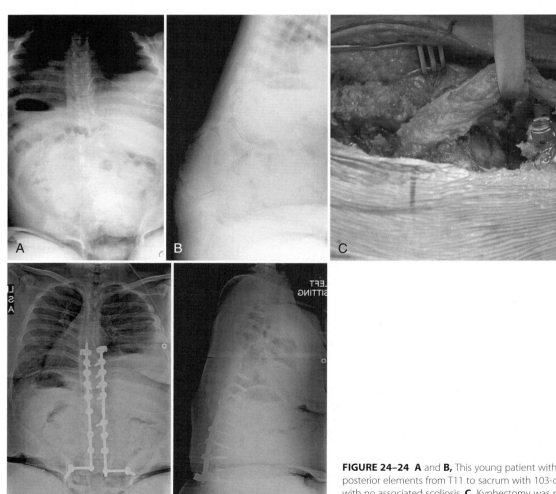

FIGURE 24–24 A and **B,** This young patient with spina bifida was missing posterior elements from T11 to sacrum with 103-degree focal lumbar kyphosis with no associated scoliosis. **C,** Kyphectomy was performed with excision of L2 and L3 vertebrae. **D** and **E,** Posterior instrumentation and fusion was used from T7 to pelvis.

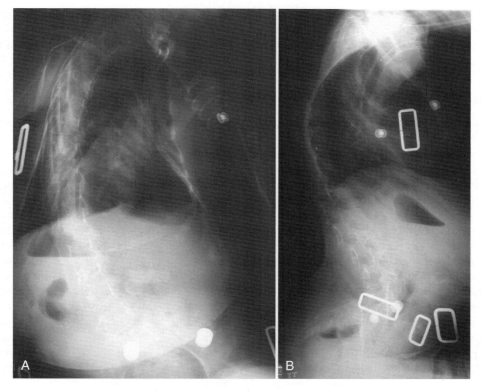

FIGURE 24–25 A and **B,** This patient's bell-shaped thoracic cage, characteristic of spinal muscular atrophy, has been compromised further by severe scoliosis.

is not as severe as in type I, respiratory complications are common. Type III SMA is also termed the *chronic juvenile form* of the disease or *Kugelberg-Welander syndrome* and is characterized by onset after 2 years with milder impairment; most children develop the ability to walk at some time, although many lose this ability around puberty.[132]

Scoliosis in Spinal Muscular Atrophy

The natural history of scoliosis in SMA depends on whether the patient has type I, II, or III; however, these types represent a spectrum of disease, and the distinctions between types may not be absolute. One should be guarded in making unqualified predictions of prognosis based on type.

All patients with type I SMA develop curves greater than 15 degrees. Surgical intervention is not warranted in these patients because of their short life span; a body jacket provides good support for balanced and comfortable sitting. Patients with type II also develop curves greater than 15 degrees, although the onset of spinal deformity occurs later, between 2 and 4 years of age. Most of these patients do not ambulate and are likely to experience rapidly progressive scoliosis. The prevalence of spinal deformity in type III patients is varied, but it typically develops in about half of patients.[133] Some of these patients are independent walkers and more likely to escape spinal deformity.[131,134,135]

Scoliosis in SMA tends to progress. In 52 cases of SMA, Granata and colleagues found an increase in curve magnitude of 8 degrees per year, despite brace use. They likewise showed a significant increase in curve progression when a patient with mild involvement stopped walking. In 13 nonwalking SMA patients, these investigators found a 3-degree per year curve progression. Walking patients with mild involvement showed only a 0.6-degree per year progression.[136] The curve most often seen with SMA is a C-shaped thoracolumbar curve. Kyphosis can also be seen with these spinal deformities but is typically not severe.

Treatment Options

Bracing

As with other neuromuscular diseases, bracing is mainly a temporizing measure to aid in sitting while patients attain more trunk height and vertebral size before surgical intervention. The effectiveness of bracing depends on the type of SMA, the severity of the deformity, and the remaining growth of the patient. Early studies reported delay of progression in a limited subset of patients with milder forms of SMA.[131,135] No studies have documented correction of deformity with dynamic bracing, however, because many patients do not have the muscular control to pull away from the sides of the brace. The evidence for brace application is still inconclusive because no current studies stratify their results based on age and SMA type. When bracing is elected to provide support for comfortable, balanced sitting before or in lieu of surgery, pulmonary function must also be considered. SMA patients are abdominal breathers because the disease affects intercostal muscle and diaphragmatic function. Because bracing significantly restricts abdominal movement and tidal volume, pretreatment pulmonary function should be a consideration in choosing this treatment modality.[132]

Surgical Management

Several studies have supported the use of segmental instrumentation to the pelvis for the definitive management of scoliosis in SMA. Brown and colleagues[137] evaluated 40 patients with SMA who were treated with posterior fusions and concluded that there were fewer complications and better maintenance of correction with Luque instrumentation compared with Harrington instrumentation. A study by Bentley and colleagues[138] reported a 51% surgical correction rate of coronal deformity in 33 SMA patients with good maintenance of correction. Fusion should be performed before the patient's curve becomes too stiff; periodic bending films and examinations are important for the timing of fusion.

Spinal fusion almost always results in a loss of function. Evaluating 40 patients with preoperative and postoperative functional and strength testing, Furumasu and colleagues[139] found that the straight but rigid spine was not always an immediate advantage to patients. The increased length of the spine creates a longer lever arm against which weakened proximal muscles have to work. These investigators reported an increased use of assistive devices, such as mobile arm supports, reachers, and lapboards. In this study, stronger patients were still able to maintain function, but weaker patients lacked the strength and flexibility to move their trunk in daily activities. Other studies have also noted a postoperative loss of function[137,140]; Aprin and colleagues[141] noted increased preservation of preoperative function in 22 patients who underwent preoperative and postoperative physical therapy. Spinal fusion does not stabilize pulmonary function. In a study of eight patients—4 with SMA type II and 4 with SMA type III—Chng and colleagues[142] reported a continued decline in pulmonary function at 44 months after spinal fusion and instrumentation. These authors noted that this decline was less marked than the natural history of SMA and that it was most likely secondary to the progressive neuromuscular weakness of the disease.

Ultimately, spinal fusion limits the progressive decline in spinal deformity and pulmonary function that characterizes SMA. A straight spine over a level pelvis allows comfortable sitting and the use of upper extremities in daily functions and is undoubtedly a great benefit to these patients. The timing of fusion should be an individual decision that takes into account the patient's comfort, functional status, and overall health. As with DMD, fusion needs to be performed before pulmonary function has declined to a level at which pulmonary complications are prohibitive.

Authors' Recommendations

The authors' use bracing in early flexible curves as soon as progression is documented. The goal in bracing is to temporize, allowing the child to achieve as much sitting height as possible. Spinal fusion may be delayed until approximately 10

to 12 years of age, unless the curve is uncontrollable by bracing and is greater than 40 degrees. Surgical intervention with hybrid spinal instrumentation and fusion to the pelvis is the method of choice. In very young Risser 0 patients, anterior fusion without division of the diaphragm rarely may be considered to prevent the crankshaft phenomenon but must be weighed against the pulmonary risk. Most patients are treated by posterior-only methods, particularly if pedicle screws can be inserted.

Duchenne Muscular Dystrophy

The most common hereditary neuromuscular condition, DMD is a sex-linked recessive disorder that affects 1 in 3500 boys. A deficiency of the muscle cell membrane stabilization protein dystrophin results in cell membrane leakage and gradual deterioration with fatty infiltration.[143] These patients typically present with progressive muscle weakness at 3 to 5 years of age. DMD patients are young boys with delayed onset of walking, a wide-based gait, a wide-based stance with pronounced lordosis and pseudohypertrophy of the calves. Gower sign of DMD is a characteristic way in which these patients rise up from the floor using all four limbs to get into a "bear position" and then pushing off of their thighs with their upper extremities to force hip extension and right the trunk. In this manner, these children overcome their proximal muscle weakness. Elevated creatine kinase level (5000 to 15,000 U/L) is a good screening test. Definitive diagnosis is established by either a genetic analysis or a muscle biopsy specimen revealing decreased levels or absence of dystrophin.[144-146]

The clinical course of these patients is fairly predictable. Patients usually use a wheelchair full-time by 10 to 12 years of age. The incidence of spinal deformity and rate of scoliosis progression in these patients are controversial. Several studies have found that DMD scoliosis increases at a rate of 15 to 30 degrees yearly and may exceed 100 degrees if untreated (Fig. 24–26).[147-150] In contrast, a 10-year retrospective study of 123 DMD patients by Kinali and colleagues[151] found a highly variable rate of the presence and the progression of scoliosis in children with DMD. Despite this inconsistency, skeletally immature patients with a Cobb angle progression to greater than 20 degrees generally continue to progress. The association of the severity of spinal deformity and decline in pulmonary function has been well described. Respiratory failure generally leads to death in the late teens or early 20s, although advances in treatment have improved prognosis.[152]

Scoliosis in Muscular Dystrophy

More than any other form of neuromuscular disorder, pulmonary function and life expectancy are directly correlated with spinal deformity. FVC begins to decline at the age patients stop standing. From that time, the restrictive effects of thoracic cage deformity and loss of respiratory muscle function cause pulmonary function to decline 4% for each 10 degrees of deformity and each year of age (Fig. 24–27).[153] Smith and colleagues[150] reviewed the natural history of DMD in 51 boys and

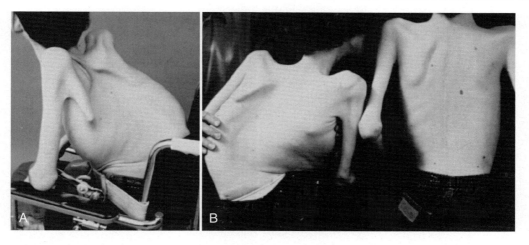

FIGURE 24–26 A and **B,** Clinical photograph of two brothers with severe scoliosis secondary to muscular dystrophy. The boy on the right underwent a successful posterior spinal instrumentation and fusion, achieving good sitting balance. His older brother had already lost too much pulmonary function to tolerate surgery. He is unable to sit well, even with support.

found that the rate of progression of scoliosis was inversely related to the age of death. Although most studies have failed to identify a protective role of spinal surgery on pulmonary function,[151,152,154] Galasko and colleagues[155] reported a stabilization of pulmonary function at 3-year follow-up. The study by Galasko and colleagues[155] compared 32 patients who underwent spinal fusion and 23 patients who refused surgery; the FVC remained stable for 3 years postoperatively in the fused group compared with an 8% per year average decline in patients not operated on.[155] Although the impact of spinal surgery on pulmonary function is unknown, the relationship between pulmonary decline and progression of scoliosis has been shown by Kennedy and colleagues[154] to be 3% to 5% per year. When scoliosis progression has reached 20 to 30 degrees, many authors recommend surgery (Fig. 24–28).[25,156,157] Glucocorticoid treatment seems to be affecting the natural history of this condition, but it is unclear how the surgical indications for spinal fusion should be modified.

Treatment Options

The preoperative evaluation of DMD patients must take into account other comorbidities of their disease. Pulmonary function testing should be done before surgery to assess the severity of preoperative respiratory compromise. Although more recent studies have reported successful spinal surgery at FVC of less than 35%,[158] previous work associated this lowered FVC value with increased postoperative morbidity.[157] Similar to the progressive decline in pulmonary function over time, the severity of cardiac dysfunction also increases with age. DMD patients are likely to develop cardiomyopathy and arrhythmias in the 2nd decade of life, and an electrocardiogram, a chest radiograph, and an echocardiogram should be done to screen for cardiac problems. Despite the fact that many of these patients are obese, they should be evaluated for malnutrition because wound healing complications and increased infections rates have been reported.[159] DMD is also associated with a tendency for increased blood loss caused by

poor vasoconstrictive function owing to a lack of dystrophin in vessel smooth muscle; preparation for major operative blood loss should be made.[160] Additionally, patients with dystrophic myopathies have an increased risk of malignant hyperthermia.[161]

Surgical Management

Long fusions from T2 to either L5 or the pelvis are recommended. The distal extent of the fusion has been an area of much research and remains a controversial subject. Mubarak and colleagues[157] determined that instrumentation and fusion to L5 was effective in mild deformities with pelvic obliquity less than 15 degrees at 34-month follow-up. Sengupta and colleagues[162] found similar results in their review of posterior fusions in 50 patients and concluded that fusion to L5 with pedicle screw instrumentation is adequate if done soon after patients lose walking ability. These results were supported further by McCall and Hayes,[60] who found that fusion to L5

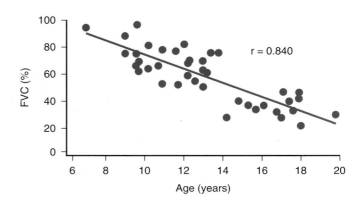

FIGURE 24–27 Percentage of forced vital capacity (FVC) versus age in patients with Duchenne muscular dystrophy. FVC percentage was found to be the parameter of pulmonary function that most strongly correlated with age and thoracic Cobb angle measurement. (From Kurz LT, Mubarak SJ, Schultz P, et al: Correlation of scoliosis and pulmonary function in Duchenne muscular dystrophy. J Pediatr Orthop 3:347, 1983.)

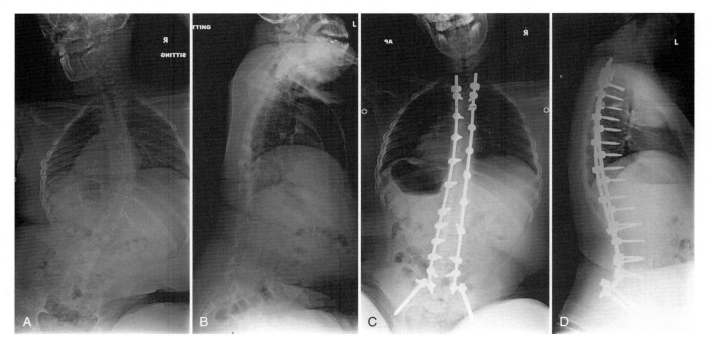

FIGURE 24–28 A-D, Preoperatively, this boy with Duchenne muscular dystrophy had 20 degrees of scoliosis and 30 degrees of thoracolumbar region kyphosis. He underwent posterior instrumentation and fusion from T3 to L5 at age 13 to retard further progression of spinal deformity. Treating the patient early allowed stopping short of pelvis.

was a viable alternative to fusion to the pelvis in patients with less than 15 degrees of L5 tilt.

Given the limitations of a minimal curve size and pelvic obliquity, fusion to the pelvis is the most common method of spinal fixation in DMD patients. Luque rods with the Galveston technique of pelvic fixation are a well-studied technique that offers acceptable results. Brook and colleagues[163] reviewed results of Luque and Luque-Galveston instrumentation in 17 patients and found an average of 63% correction and good maintenance of correction. Bentley and colleagues[138] reviewed 64 patients treated with posterior fusion and reported a 47% correction rate with good maintenance of correction. The authors recommended fusion to T4 stating that the lower level of fusion allows more freedom of movement for feeding and upper extremity use. Unit rods have also been evaluated in DMD patients and provide acceptable results; however, placement of the rods into the iliac wings makes this technique challenging.[163] The Dunn-McCarthy technique with S-shaped rods looped over the sacral alae has been shown to provide good results in DMD patients. This technique has gained popularity because of its dependable fixation in patients with osteopenia and ease of placement in the kyphotic lumbar spine that is often seen in DMD patients.[69,156]

More recent advances in segmental pedicle screw fixation have resulted in their promotion as an alternative to more traditional hook-wire and Galveston pelvic fixation techniques. Hahn and colleagues[164] reported results of 20 DMD patients treated with pedicle screw–alone fixation and concluded that pedicle screws combined with iliac screws provided a stable construct that eliminated the need for a combined anterior procedure at minimum 2-year follow-up. These authors found that this technique limited blood loss

compared with sublaminar wiring, had no implant loosening, and allowed early mobilization leading to no pulmonary complications. Pedicle screw fixation with a free-hand technique has been shown to be as safe and accurate as in other conditions.[165]

Authors' Recommendations

In patients with DMD, spinal fusion is performed when curves reach 20 degrees and FVC is greater than 40%. Preoperative FVC of less than 30% to 35% is correlated with a high incidence of major respiratory complications. The surgical technique recommended by the authors is segmental instrumentation (mainly with pedicle screws) and posterior fusion from the high thoracic level (T2 or T3 down to L5). Usually, the intensive care unit stay is 2 days, and the average hospital stay is 8 days. If the pelvic obliquity is greater than 10 degrees or the scoliosis curve is greater than 40 degrees, the authors consider instrumentation to the pelvis to correct this obliquity and ensure a level pelvis. The ultimate goal in the treatment of deformity in DMD is the maintenance of upright sitting balance and maximal pain-free function. Many of the authors' patients are now older than 20 years with an upright posture, minimal wheelchair difficulties, and improved quality of life.

Rett Syndrome

Rett syndrome is a developmental disorder of unknown etiology that occurs in 1 in 20,000 females. The syndrome is linked to a mutation in the *MeCP2* gene located on the X

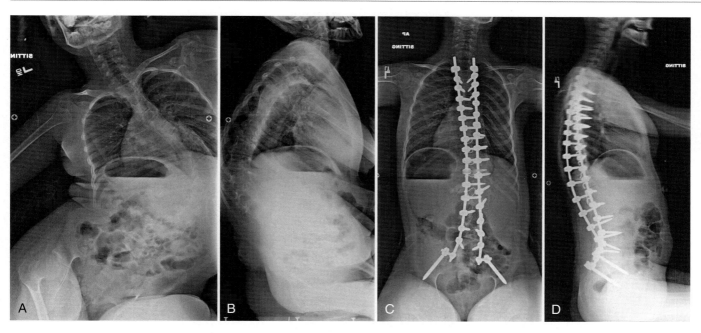

FIGURE 24–29 A-D, This 9-year-old girl with Rett syndrome has 80 degrees of spinal deformity, despite bracing. Because her triradiate cartilage remained open, she underwent anterior thoracoscopic release and posterior instrumentation from T2 to pelvis.

chromosome, which encodes a deacetylator that regulates the transcription of certain genes. Patients appear normal at birth but begin the stepwise deterioration characteristic of Rett syndrome. The syndrome has four stages. In the first stage, generally occurring when patients are 6 to 18 months of age, signs of the syndrome include developmental stagnation, slowed head and brain growth, and generalized hypotonia. From approximately age 1 to 3 years, patients begin to regress developmentally and exhibit autisticlike symptoms. In the third stage, between age 2 and 10 years, patients have seizures, exhibit ataxia, exhibit mental retardation, and perform stereotypic gestures such as repetitive hand wringing. During this phase, scoliosis and spasticity can be seen. In the fourth stage, patients exhibit upper and lower motor neuron signs with increased rigidity and muscle wasting. Scoliosis is most likely to develop in this final stage (Fig. 24–29).[166]

Scoliosis in Rett Syndrome

The incidence of scoliosis increases as patients get older: 8% of girls with Rett syndrome have scoliosis at age 5, 40% have it by age 11, and 80% have it by age 20. The deformity can be rapidly progressive; Lidstrom and colleagues[167] reported on 78 patients with Rett syndrome and reported progression rates of 20 to 41 degrees per year in the 10 most severe cases. Because scoliosis in Rett syndrome has this potential for progression, yearly evaluation of the spine should be conducted after the age of 5 years.[168]

The treatment for Rett syndrome is similar to treatment for cerebral palsy. Bracing has a limited role in treatment, although it may provide support for comfortable sitting until surgery is performed.[169] As with cerebral palsy, the authors recommend that if sitting comfort and balance become compromised,

treatment with segmental instrumentation is indicated. Spinal surgery is indicated when the curve exceeds 40 degrees. Long-term outcome of surgery in patients with Rett syndrome has shown good results. In a prospective study of 23 girls with Rett syndrome and neuromuscular scoliosis, Larsson and colleagues[170] found improved seating position and patient satisfaction at 6-year follow-up. These authors reported that all patients who could walk preoperatively maintained ambulation postoperatively. They also noted that patients and parents reported an overall improvement in well-being with better sitting posture and improved breathing. As with all patients with neuromuscular disorders who undergo scoliosis surgery, spinal cord monitoring is advocated.[171]

PEARLS

1. Neuromuscular spinal deformities are often complex, multiplanar, and rigid.

2. Segmental instrumentation reduces the risk of progression. Hooks and screws add to construct rigidity compared with sublaminar wires alone.

3. Hyperkyphosis increases the risk of implant failure or junctional kyphosis or both. Segmental posterior compression instrumentation reduces this risk.

PITFALLS

1. Blood loss should be anticipated. The surgeon should minimize blood loss during exposure and consider use of a pharmacologic agent to reduce blood loss during surgery. Transfusion should be done early, and clotting factors should be replaced (fresh frozen plasma) before coagulopathy develops.

2. The surgeon needs to be aware of infrapelvic causes of obliquity, such as hip contracture.

3. Preoperative nutritional supplementation, often via a gastrostomy tube with fundoplication, should be considered.

4. Postoperative intensive care unit support is crucial to negotiating major spinal surgery safely in these medically compromised patients.

KEY REFERENCES

1. Karol LA: Scoliosis in patients with Duchenne muscular dystrophy. J Bone Joint Surg Am 89:155-162, 2007.
   This review article provides a comprehensive review of nonoperative and operative management of scoliosis in patients with Duchenne muscular dystrophy.

2. Luque ER: Segmental spinal instrumentation for correction of scoliosis. Clin Orthop Relat Res (163):192-198, 1982.
   This article provides the classic description of the technique that became the standard method of segmental fixation in neuromuscular scoliosis.

3. Tokala DP, Lam KS, Freeman BJ, et al: Is there a role for selective anterior instrumentation in neuromuscular scoliosis? Eur Spine J 16:91-96, 2007.
   This report of good short-term clinical and radiographic outcomes presents selection criteria for selective anterior instrumentation in patients with neuromuscular scoliosis.

4. Trivedi J, Thomson JD, Slakey JB, et al: Clinical and radiographic predictors of scoliosis in patients with myelomeningocele. J Bone Joint Surg Am 84:1389-1394, 2002.
   The risk of scoliosis in patients with myelodysplasia is substantial. This article presents the correlation with the level of paralysis.

REFERENCES

1. Majd ME, Muldowny DS, Holt RT: Natural history of scoliosis in the institutionalized adult cerebral palsy population. Spine 22:1461-1466, 1997.

2. Bosboom WM, Vrancken AF, van den Berg LH, et al: Drug treatment for spinal muscular atrophy types II and III. Cochrane Database Syst Rev CD006282, 2009.

3. Mercuri E, Bertini E, Messina S, et al: Randomized, double-blind, placebo-controlled trial of phenylbutyrate in spinal muscular atrophy. Neurology 68:51-55, 2007.

4. Miller RG, Moore DH, Dronsky V, et al: A placebo-controlled trial of gabapentin in spinal muscular atrophy. J Neurol Sci 191:127-131, 2001.

5. Tzeng AC, Cheng J, Fryczynski H, et al: A study of thyrotropin-releasing hormone for the treatment of spinal muscular atrophy: A preliminary report. Am J Phys Med Rehabil 79:435-440, 2000.

6. Ade-Hall RA, Moore AP: Botulinum toxin type A in the treatment of lower limb spasticity in cerebral palsy. Cochrane Database Syst Rev CD001408, 2000.

7. Lukban MB, Rosales RL, Dressler D: Effectiveness of botulinum toxin A for upper and lower limb spasticity in children with cerebral palsy: A summary of evidence. J Neural Transm 116:319-331, 2009.

8. Gerszten PC, Albright AL, Johnstone GF: Intrathecal baclofen infusion and subsequent orthopedic surgery in patients with spastic cerebral palsy. J Neurosurg 88:1009-1013, 1998.

9. Ginsburg GM, Lauder AJ: Progression of scoliosis in patients with spastic quadriplegia after the insertion of an intrathecal baclofen pump. Spine 32:2745-2750, 2007.

10. Caird MS, Palanca AA, Garton H, et al: Outcomes of posterior spinal fusion and instrumentation in patients with continuous intrathecal baclofen infusion pumps. Spine 33:E94-E99, 2008.

11. Shilt JS, Lai LP, Cabrera MN, et al: The impact of intrathecal baclofen on the natural history of scoliosis in cerebral palsy. J Pediatr Orthop 28:684-687, 2008.

12. Manzur AY, Kinali M, Muntoni F: Update on the management of Duchenne muscular dystrophy. Arch Dis Child 93:986-990, 2008.

13. Manzur AY, Kuntzer T, Pike M, et al: Glucocorticoid corticosteroids for Duchenne muscular dystrophy. Cochrane Database Syst Rev CD003725, 2008.

14. Markham LW, Kinnett K, Wong BL, et al: Corticosteroid treatment retards development of ventricular dysfunction in Duchenne muscular dystrophy. Neuromuscul Disord 18:365-370, 2008.

15. Kotwicki T, Durmala J, Czubak J: Bracing for neuromuscular scoliosis: Orthosis construction to improve the patient's function. Disabil Rehabil Assist Technol 3:161-169, 2008.

16. Shoham Y, Meyer S, Katz-Leurer M, et al: The influence of seat adjustment and a thoraco-lumbar-sacral orthosis on the distribution of body-seat pressure in children with scoliosis and pelvic obliquity. Disabil Rehabil 26:21-26, 2004.

17. Miller A, Temple T, Miller F: Impact of orthoses on the rate of scoliosis progression in children with cerebral palsy. J Pediatr Orthop 16:332-335, 1996.

18. Olafsson Y, Saraste H, Al-Dabbagh Z: Brace treatment in neuromuscular spine deformity. J Pediatr Orthop 19:376-379, 1999.

19. Letts M, Rathbone D, Yamashita T, et al: Soft Boston orthosis in management of neuromuscular scoliosis: A preliminary report. J Pediatr Orthop 12:470-474, 1992.

20. Berven S, Bradford DS: Neuromuscular scoliosis: Causes of deformity and principles for evaluation and management. Semin Neurol 22:167-178, 2002.

21. Leopando MT, Moussavi Z, Holbrow J, et al: Effect of a Soft Boston Orthosis on pulmonary mechanics in severe cerebral palsy. Pediatr Pulmonol 28:53-58, 1999.

22. Bunnell WP, MacEwen GD: Non-operative treatment of scoliosis in cerebral palsy: Preliminary report on the use of a plastic jacket. Dev Med Child Neurol 19:45-49, 1977.

23. Winter RB, Carlson JM: Modern orthotics for spinal deformities. Clin Orthop Relat Res 74-86, 1977.

24. Holmes KJ, Michael SM, Thorpe SL, et al: Management of scoliosis with special seating for the non-ambulant spastic cerebral palsy population—a biomechanical study. Clin Biomech (Bristol, Avon) 18:480-487, 2003.

25. Sussman M: Duchenne muscular dystrophy. J Am Acad Orthop Surg 10:138-151, 2002.

26. Bridwell KH, Baldus C, Iffrig TM, et al: Process measures and patient/parent evaluation of surgical management of spinal deformities in patients with progressive flaccid neuromuscular scoliosis (Duchenne's muscular dystrophy and spinal muscular atrophy). Spine 24:1300-1309, 1999.

27. Comstock CP, Leach J, Wenger DR: Scoliosis in total-body-involvement cerebral palsy: Analysis of surgical treatment and patient and caregiver satisfaction. Spine 1998;23:1412-1424; discussion 1424-1425, 1998.

28. Sink EL, Newton PO, Mubarak SJ, et al: Maintenance of sagittal plane alignment after surgical correction of spinal deformity in patients with cerebral palsy. Spine 28:1396-1403, 2003.

29. Lonstein JE, Akbarnia A: Operative treatment of spinal deformities in patients with cerebral palsy or mental retardation: An analysis of one hundred and seven cases. J Bone Joint Surg Am 65:43-55, 1983.

30. Askin GN, Hallett R, Hare N, et al: The outcome of scoliosis surgery in the severely physically handicapped child: An objective and subjective assessment. Spine 22:44-50, 1997.

31. Mercado E, Alman B, Wright JG: Does spinal fusion influence quality of life in neuromuscular scoliosis? Spine 32:S120-S125, 2007.

32. Wright JG, Einhorn TA, Heckman JD: Grades of recommendation. J Bone Joint Surg Am 87:1909-1910, 2005.

33. Cheuk DK, Wong V, Wraige E, et al: Surgery for scoliosis in Duchenne muscular dystrophy. Cochrane Database Syst Rev CD005375, 2007.

34. Farhat G, Yamout B, Mikati MA, et al: Effect of antiepileptic drugs on bone density in ambulatory patients. Neurology 58:1348-1353, 2002.

35. Sheth RD, Wesolowski CA, Jacob JC, et al: Effect of carbamazepine and valproate on bone mineral density. J Pediatr 127:256-262, 1995.

36. Chambers HG, Weinstein CH, Mubarak SJ, et al: The effect of valproic acid on blood loss in patients with cerebral palsy. J Pediatr Orthop 19:792-795, 1999.

37. Gill I, Eagle M, Mehta JS, et al: Correction of neuromuscular scoliosis in patients with preexisting respiratory failure. Spine 31:2478-2483, 2006.

38. Pruijs JE, van Tol MJ, van Kesteren RG, et al: Neuromuscular scoliosis: Clinical evaluation pre- and postoperative. J Pediatr Orthop B 9:217-220, 2000.

39. Soudon P, Hody JL, Bellen P: Preoperative cardiopulmonary assessment in the child with neuromuscular scoliosis. J Pediatr Orthop B 9:229-233, 2000.

40. Winter S: Preoperative assessment of the child with neuromuscular scoliosis. Orthop Clin North Am 25:239-245, 1994.

41. Jevsevar DS, Karlin LI: The relationship between preoperative nutritional status and complications after an operation for scoliosis in patients who have cerebral palsy. J Bone Joint Surg Am 75:880-884, 1993.

42. Shapiro F, Sethna N: Blood loss in pediatric spine surgery. Eur Spine J 13(Suppl 1):S6-S17, 2004.

43. Kannan S, Meert KL, Mooney JF, et al: Bleeding and coagulation changes during spinal fusion surgery: A comparison of neuromuscular and idiopathic scoliosis patients. Pediatr Crit Care Med 3:364-369, 2002.

44. Meert KL, Kannan S, Mooney JF: Predictors of red cell transfusion in children and adolescents undergoing spinal fusion surgery. Spine 27:2137-2142, 2002.

45. Neilipovitz DT, Murto K, Hall L, et al: A randomized trial of tranexamic acid to reduce blood transfusion for scoliosis surgery. Anesth Analg 93:82-87, 2001.

46. Gill JB, Chin Y, Levin A, et al: The use of antifibrinolytic agents in spine surgery: A meta-analysis. J Bone Joint Surg Am 90:2399-2407, 2008.

47. Haas S: Spastic scoliosis and obliquity of the pelvis. J. Bone Joint Surg 24:774-780, 1942.

48. Sullivan JA, Conner SB: Comparison of Harrington instrumentation and segmental spinal instrumentation in the management of neuromuscular spinal deformity. Spine 7:299-304, 1982.

49. Luque ER: Segmental spinal instrumentation for correction of scoliosis. Clin Orthop Relat Res (163):192-198, 1982.

50. Herring JA, Wenger DR: Segmental spinal instrumentation: A preliminary report of 40 consecutive cases. Spine 7:285-298, 1982.

51. Taddonio RF: Segmental spinal instrumentation in the management of neuromuscular spinal deformity. Spine 7:305-311, 1982.

52. Allen BL Jr, Ferguson RL: The Galveston technique for L rod instrumentation of the scoliotic spine. Spine 7:276-284, 1982.

53. Gupta MC, Wijesekera S, Sossan A, et al: Reliability of radiographic parameters in neuromuscular scoliosis. Spine 32:691-695, 2007.

54. Bell DF, Moseley CF, Koreska J: Unit rod segmental spinal instrumentation in the management of patients with progressive neuromuscular spinal deformity. Spine 14:1301-1307, 1989.

55. Dias RC, Miller F, Dabney K, et al: Surgical correction of spinal deformity using a unit rod in children with cerebral palsy. J Pediatr Orthop 16:734-740, 1996.

56. Tsirikos AI, Lipton G, Chang WN, et al: Surgical correction of scoliosis in pediatric patients with cerebral palsy using the unit rod instrumentation. Spine 33:1133-1140, 2008.

57. Bulman WA, Dormans JP, Ecker ML, et al: Posterior spinal fusion for scoliosis in patients with cerebral palsy: A comparison of Luque rod and Unit Rod instrumentation. J Pediatr Orthop 16:314-323, 1996.

58. Tsirikos AI, Chang WN, Shah SA, et al: Preserving ambulatory potential in pediatric patients with cerebral palsy who undergo spinal fusion using unit rod instrumentation. Spine 28:480-483, 2003.

59. Erickson MA, Oliver T, Baldini T, et al: Biomechanical assessment of conventional unit rod fixation versus a unit rod pedicle screw construct: a human cadaver study. Spine 29:1314-1319, 2004.

60. McCall RE, Hayes B: Long-term outcome in neuromuscular scoliosis fused only to lumbar 5. Spine 30:2056-2060, 2005.

61. Guidera KJ, Hooten J, Weatherly W, et al: Cotrel-Dubousset instrumentation: Results in 52 patients. Spine 18:427-431, 1993.

62. Neustadt JB, Shufflebarger HL, Cammisa FP: Spinal fusions to the pelvis augmented by Cotrel-Dubousset instrumentation for neuromuscular scoliosis. J Pediatr Orthop 12:465-469, 1992.

63. Wimmer C, Wallnofer P, Walochnik N, et al: Comparative evaluation of Luque and Isola instrumentation for treatment of

neuromuscular scoliosis. Clin Orthop Relat Res 439:181-192, 2005.

64. Yazici M, Asher MA, Hardacker JW: The safety and efficacy of Isola-Galveston instrumentation and arthrodesis in the treatment of neuromuscular spinal deformities. J Bone Joint Surg Am 82:524-543, 2000.

65. Pritchett JW: The untreated unstable hip in severe cerebral palsy. Clin Orthop Relat Res (173):169-172, 1983.

66. Broom MJ, Banta JV, Renshaw TS: Spinal fusion augmented by Luque-rod segmental instrumentation for neuromuscular scoliosis. J Bone Joint Surg Am 71:32-44, 1989.

67. Gau YL, Lonstein JE, Winter RB, et al: Luque-Galveston procedure for correction and stabilization of neuromuscular scoliosis and pelvic obliquity: A review of 68 patients. J Spinal Disord 4:399-410, 1991.

68. Allen BL Jr, Ferguson RL: The Galveston technique of pelvic fixation with L-rod instrumentation of the spine. Spine 9:388-394, 1984.

69. McCarthy RE, Bruffett WL, McCullough FL: S rod fixation to the sacrum in patients with neuromuscular spinal deformities. Clin Orthop Relat Res (364):26-31, 1999.

70. Warner WC Jr, Fackler CD: Comparison of two instrumentation techniques in treatment of lumbar kyphosis in myelodysplasia. J Pediatr Orthop 13:704-708, 1993.

71. McCall RE: Modified Luque instrumentation after myelomeningocele kyphectomy. Spine 23:1406-1411, 1998.

72. Early S, Mahar A, Oka R, et al: Biomechanical comparison of lumbosacral fixation using Luque-Galveston and Colorado II sacropelvic fixation: Advantage of using locked proximal fixation. Spine 30:1396-1401, 2005.

73. Schwend RM, Sluyters R, Najdzionek J: The pylon concept of pelvic anchorage for spinal instrumentation in the human cadaver. Spine 28:542-547, 2003.

74. Tsuchiya K, Bridwell KH, Kuklo TR, et al: Minimum 5-year analysis of L5-S1 fusion using sacropelvic fixation (bilateral S1 and iliac screws) for spinal deformity. Spine 31:303-308, 2006.

75. Phillips JH, Gutheil JP, Knapp DR Jr: Iliac screw fixation in neuromuscular scoliosis. Spine 32:1566-1570, 2007.

76. Peelle MW, Lenke LG, Bridwell KH, et al: Comparison of pelvic fixation techniques in neuromuscular spinal deformity correction: Galveston rod versus iliac and lumbosacral screws. Spine 31:2392-2398; discussion 2399, 2006.

77. Stevens DB, Beard C: Segmental spinal instrumentation for neuromuscular spinal deformity. Clin Orthop Relat Res (242):164-168, 1989.

78. Takeshita K, Lenke LG, Bridwell KH, et al: Analysis of patients with nonambulatory neuromuscular scoliosis surgically treated to the pelvis with intraoperative halo-femoral traction. Spine 31:2381-2385, 2006.

79. Whitaker C, Burton DC, Asher M: Treatment of selected neuromuscular patients with posterior instrumentation and arthrodesis ending with lumbar pedicle screw anchorage. Spine 25:2312-2318, 2000.

80. Newton PO, White KK, Faro F, et al: The success of thoracoscopic anterior fusion in a consecutive series of 112 pediatric spinal deformity cases. Spine 30:392-398, 2005.

81. Smucker JD, Miller F: Crankshaft effect after posterior spinal fusion and unit rod instrumentation in children with cerebral palsy. J Pediatr Orthop 21:108-112, 2001.

82. Basobas L, Mardjetko S, Hammerberg K, et al: Selective anterior fusion and instrumentation for the treatment of neuromuscular scoliosis. Spine 28:S245-S248, 2003.

83. Tokala DP, Lam KS, Freeman BJ, et al: Is there a role for selective anterior instrumentation in neuromuscular scoliosis? Eur Spine J 16:91-96, 2007.

84. Costa P, Bruno A, Bonzanino M, et al: Somatosensory- and motor-evoked potential monitoring during spine and spinal cord surgery. Spinal Cord 45:86-91, 2007.

85. Schwartz DM, Auerbach JD, Dormans JP, et al: Neurophysiological detection of impending spinal cord injury during scoliosis surgery. J Bone Joint Surg Am 89:2440-2449, 2007.

86. de Haan P, Kalkman CJ, de Mol BA, et al: Efficacy of transcranial motor-evoked myogenic potentials to detect spinal cord ischemia during operations for thoracoabdominal aneurysms. J Thorac Cardiovasc Surg 113:87-100; discussion 101, 1997.

87. Leung YL, Grevitt M, Henderson L, et al: Cord monitoring changes and segmental vessel ligation in the "at risk" cord during anterior spinal deformity surgery. Spine 30:1870-1874, 2005.

88. Tsirikos AI, Howitt SP, McMaster MJ: Segmental vessel ligation in patients undergoing surgery for anterior spinal deformity. J Bone Joint Surg Br 90:474-479, 2008.

89. Winter RB, Lonstein JE, Denis F, et al: Paraplegia resulting from vessel ligation. Spine 21:1232-1233; discussion 1233-1234, 1996.

90. Sarwark J, Sarwahi V: New strategies and decision making in the management of neuromuscular scoliosis. Orthop Clin North Am 38:485-96, v, 2007.

91. Sponseller PD, LaPorte DM, Hungerford MW, et al: Deep wound infections after neuromuscular scoliosis surgery: A multicenter study of risk factors and treatment outcomes. Spine 25:2461-2466, 2000.

92. Yazici M, Asher MA: Freeze-dried allograft for posterior spinal fusion in patients with neuromuscular spinal deformities. Spine 22:1467-1471, 1997.

93. Tsirikos AI, Chang WN, Dabney KW, et al: Comparison of one-stage versus two-stage anteroposterior spinal fusion in pediatric patients with cerebral palsy and neuromuscular scoliosis. Spine 28:1300-1305, 2003.

94. Mohamad F, Parent S, Pawelek J, et al: Perioperative complications after surgical correction in neuromuscular scoliosis. J Pediatr Orthop 27:392-397, 2007.

95. Yamin S, Li L, Xing W, et al: Staged surgical treatment for severe and rigid scoliosis. J Orthop Surg 3:26, 2008.

96. Newton PO, Upasani VV, Lhamby J, et al: Surgical treatment of main thoracic scoliosis with thoracoscopic anterior instrumentation: A five-year follow-up study. J Bone Joint Surg Am 90:2077-2089, 2008.

97. Hell AK, Hefti F, Campbell RM Jr: [Treatment of congenital scoliosis with the vertical expandable prosthetic titanium rib implant]. Orthopade 33:911-918, 2004.

98. Latalski M, Fatyga M, Gregosiewicz A: The vertical expandable prosthetic titanium rib (VEPTR) in the treatment of scoliosis

and thoracic deformities: Preliminary report. Orthop Traumatol Rehabil 9:459-466, 2007.

99. Benson ER, Thomson JD, Smith BG, et al: Results and morbidity in a consecutive series of patients undergoing spinal fusion for neuromuscular scoliosis. Spine 23:2308-2317; discussion 2318, 1998.

100. Boachie-Adjei O, Lonstein JE, Winter RB, et al: Management of neuromuscular spinal deformities with Luque segmental instrumentation. J Bone Joint Surg Am 71:548-562, 1989.

101. Borkhuu B, Borowski A, Shah SA, et al: Antibiotic-loaded allograft decreases the rate of acute deep wound infection after spinal fusion in cerebral palsy. Spine 33:2300-2304, 2008.

102. Canavese F, Gupta S, Krajbich JI, et al: Vacuum-assisted closure for deep infection after spinal instrumentation for scoliosis. J Bone Joint Surg Br 90:377-381, 2008.

103. Gabriel A, Heinrich C, Shores J, et al: Outcomes of vacuum-assisted closure for the treatment of wounds in a paediatric population: Case series of 58 patients. J Plast Reconstr Aesthet Surg 62:1428-1436, 2009.

104. Szoke G, Lipton G, Miller F, et al: Wound infection after spinal fusion in children with cerebral palsy. J Pediatr Orthop 18:727-733, 1998.

105. Kalen V, Conklin MM, Sherman FC: Untreated scoliosis in severe cerebral palsy. J Pediatr Orthop 12:337-340, 1992.

106. Madigan RR, Wallace SL: Scoliosis in the institutionalized cerebral palsy population. Spine 6:583-590, 1981.

107. Saito N, Ebara S, Ohotsuka K, et al: Natural history of scoliosis in spastic cerebral palsy. Lancet 351:1687-1692, 1998.

108. Thometz JG, Simon SR: Progression of scoliosis after skeletal maturity in institutionalized adults who have cerebral palsy. J Bone Joint Surg Am 70:1290-1296, 1988.

109. Westerlund LE, Gill SS, Jarosz TS, et al: Posterior-only unit rod instrumentation and fusion for neuromuscular scoliosis. Spine 26:1984-1989, 2001.

110. Teli M, Elsebaie H, Biant L, et al: Neuromuscular scoliosis treated by segmental third-generation instrumented spinal fusion. J Spinal Disord Tech 18:430-438, 2005.

111. Vialle R, Delecourt C, Morin C: Surgical treatment of scoliosis with pelvic obliquity in cerebral palsy: The influence of intra-operative traction. Spine 31:1461-1466, 2006.

112. Dunteman RC, Vankoski SJ, Dias LS: Internal derotation osteotomy of the tibia: Pre- and postoperative gait analysis in persons with high sacral myelomeningocele. J Pediatr Orthop 20:623-628, 2000.

113. Trivedi J, Thomson JD, Slakey JB, et al: Clinical and radiographic predictors of scoliosis in patients with myelomeningocele. J Bone Joint Surg Am 84:1389-1394, 2002.

114. Dias MS: Neurosurgical causes of scoliosis in patients with myelomeningocele: An evidence-based literature review. J Neurosurg 103:24-35, 2005.

115. Sarwark JF, Weber DT, Gabrieli AP, et al: Tethered cord syndrome in low motor level children with myelomeningocele. Pediatr Neurosurg 25:295-301, 1996.

116. Pierz K, Banta J, Thomson J, et al: The effect of tethered cord release on scoliosis in myelomeningocele. J Pediatr Orthop 20:362-365, 2000.

117. Muller EB, Nordwall A: Brace treatment of scoliosis in children with myelomeningocele. Spine 19:151-155, 1994.

118. Sponseller PD, Young AT, Sarwark JF, et al: Anterior only fusion for scoliosis in patients with myelomeningocele. Clin Orthop Relat Res (364):117-124, 1999.

119. Banit DM, Iwinski HJ Jr, Talwalkar V, et al: Posterior spinal fusion in paralytic scoliosis and myelomeningocele. J Pediatr Orthop 21:117-125, 2001.

120. Parsch D, Geiger F, Brocai DR, et al: Surgical management of paralytic scoliosis in myelomeningocele. J Pediatr Orthop B 10:10-17, 2001.

121. Lindseth RE, Dias LS, Drennan JC: Myelomeningocele. Instr Course Lect 40:271-291, 1991.

122. Wild A, Haak H, Kumar M, et al: Is sacral instrumentation mandatory to address pelvic obliquity in neuromuscular thoracolumbar scoliosis due to myelomeningocele? Spine 26:E325-E329, 2001.

123. Thomsen M, Lang RD, Carstens C: Results of kyphectomy with the technique of Warner and Fackler in children with myelodysplasia. J Pediatr Orthop B 9:143-147, 2000.

124. Geiger F, Parsch D, Carstens C: Complications of scoliosis surgery in children with myelomeningocele. Eur Spine J 8:22-26, 1999.

125. Ward WT, Wenger DR, Roach JW: Surgical correction of myelomeningocele scoliosis: A critical appraisal of various spinal instrumentation systems. J Pediatr Orthop 9:262-268, 1989.

126. Nolden MT, Sarwark JF, Vora A, et al: A kyphectomy technique with reduced perioperative morbidity for myelomeningocele kyphosis. Spine 27:1807-1813, 2002.

127. Ko AL, Song K, Ellenbogen RG, et al: Retrospective review of multilevel spinal fusion combined with spinal cord transection for treatment of kyphoscoliosis in pediatric myelomeningocele patients. Spine 32:2493-2501, 2007.

128. Kocaoglu B, Erol B, Akgulle H, et al: Combination of Luque instrumentation with polyaxial screws in the treatment of myelomeningocele kyphosis. J Spinal Disord Tech 21:199-204, 2008.

129. Nicole S, Diaz CC, Frugier T, et al: Spinal muscular atrophy: Recent advances and future prospects. Muscle Nerve 26:4-13, 2002.

130. Dubowitz V: Benign infantile spinal muscular atrophy. Dev Med Child Neurol 16:672-675, 1974.

131. Evans GA, Drennan JC, Russman BS: Functional classification and orthopaedic management of spinal muscular atrophy. J Bone Joint Surg Br 63:516-522, 1981.

132. Tangsrud SE, Carlsen KC, Lund-Petersen I, et al: Lung function measurements in young children with spinal muscle atrophy: A cross sectional survey on the effect of position and bracing. Arch Dis Child 84:521-524, 2001.

133. Sucato DJ: Spine deformity in spinal muscular atrophy. J Bone Joint Surg Am 89(Suppl 1):148-154, 2007.

134. Merlini L, Granata C, Bonfiglioli S, et al: Scoliosis in spinal muscular atrophy: Natural history and management. Dev Med Child Neurol 31:501-508, 1989.

135. Schwentker EP, Gibson DA: The orthopaedic aspects of spinal muscular atrophy. J Bone Joint Surg Am 58:32-38, 1976.

136. Granata C, Merlini L, Magni E, et al: Spinal muscular atrophy: Natural history and orthopaedic treatment of scoliosis. Spine 14:760-762, 1989.

137. Brown JC, Zeller JL, Swank SM, et al: Surgical and functional results of spine fusion in spinal muscular atrophy. Spine 14:763-770, 1989.

138. Bentley G, Haddad F, Bull TM, et al: The treatment of scoliosis in muscular dystrophy using modified Luque and Harrington-Luque instrumentation. J Bone Joint Surg Br 83:22-28, 2001.

139. Furumasu J, Swank SM, Brown JC, et al: Functional activities in spinal muscular atrophy patients after spinal fusion. Spine 14:771-775, 1989.

140. Phillips DP, Roye DP Jr, Farcy JP, et al: Surgical treatment of scoliosis in a spinal muscular atrophy population. Spine 15:942-945, 1990.

141. Aprin H, Bowen JR, MacEwen GD, et al: Spine fusion in patients with spinal muscular atrophy. J Bone Joint Surg Am 64:1179-1187, 1982.

142. Chng SY, Wong YQ, Hui JH, et al: Pulmonary function and scoliosis in children with spinal muscular atrophy types II and III. J Paediatr Child Health 39:673-676, 2003.

143. Pennisi E: Genetics: Hopping to a better protein. Science 322:1454-1455, 2008.

144. Ashton EJ, Yau SC, Deans ZC, et al: Simultaneous mutation scanning for gross deletions, duplications and point mutations in the DMD gene. Eur J Hum Genet 16:53-61, 2008.

145. Biggar WD, Klamut HJ, Demacio PC, et al: Duchenne muscular dystrophy: Current knowledge, treatment, and future prospects. Clin Orthop Relat Res (401):88-106, 2002.

146. McDonald CM, Abresch RT, Carter GT, et al: Profiles of neuromuscular diseases: Duchenne muscular dystrophy. Am J Phys Med Rehabil 74:S70-S92, 1995.

147. Cambridge W, Drennan JC: Scoliosis associated with Duchenne muscular dystrophy. J Pediatr Orthop 7:436-440, 1987.

148. Miller F, Moseley CF, Koreska J: Spinal fusion in Duchenne muscular dystrophy. Dev Med Child Neurol 34:775-786, 1992.

149. Robin GC, Brief LP: Scoliosis in childhood muscular dystrophy. J Bone Joint Surg Am 53:466-476, 1971.

150. Smith AD, Koreska J, Moseley CF: Progression of scoliosis in Duchenne muscular dystrophy. J Bone Joint Surg Am 71:1066-1074, 1989.

151. Kinali M, Messina S, Mercuri E, et al: Management of scoliosis in Duchenne muscular dystrophy: A large 10-year retrospective study. Dev Med Child Neurol 48:513-518, 2006.

152. Miller F, Moseley CF, Koreska J, et al: Pulmonary function and scoliosis in Duchenne dystrophy. J Pediatr Orthop 8:133-137, 1988.

153. Kurz LT, Mubarak SJ, Schultz P, et al: Correlation of scoliosis and pulmonary function in Duchenne muscular dystrophy. J Pediatr Orthop 3:347-353, 1983.

154. Kennedy JD, Staples AJ, Brook PD, et al: Effect of spinal surgery on lung function in Duchenne muscular dystrophy. Thorax 50:1173-1178, 1995.

155. Galasko CS, Delaney C, Morris P: Spinal stabilisation in Duchenne muscular dystrophy. J Bone Joint Surg Br 74:210-214, 1992.

156. Karol LA: Scoliosis in patients with Duchenne muscular dystrophy. J Bone Joint Surg Am 89(Suppl 1):155-162, 2007.

157. Mubarak SJ, Morin WD, Leach J: Spinal fusion in Duchenne muscular dystrophy—fixation and fusion to the sacropelvis? J Pediatr Orthop 13:752-757, 1993.

158. Harper CM, Ambler G, Edge G: The prognostic value of preoperative predicted forced vital capacity in corrective spinal surgery for Duchenne's muscular dystrophy. Anaesthesia 59:1160-1162, 2004.

159. Ramirez N, Richards BS, Warren PD, et al: Complications after posterior spinal fusion in Duchenne's muscular dystrophy. J Pediatr Orthop 17:109-114, 1997.

160. Noordeen MH, Haddad FS, Muntoni F, et al: Blood loss in Duchenne muscular dystrophy: Vascular smooth muscle dysfunction? J Pediatr Orthop B 8:212-215, 1999.

161. Flick RP, Gleich SJ, Herr MM, et al: The risk of malignant hyperthermia in children undergoing muscle biopsy for suspected neuromuscular disorder. Paediatr Anaesth 17:22-27, 2007.

162. Sengupta DK, Mehdian SH, McConnell JR, et al: Pelvic or lumbar fixation for the surgical management of scoliosis in Duchenne muscular dystrophy. Spine 27:2072-2079, 2002.

163. Brook PD, Kennedy JD, Stern LM, et al: Spinal fusion in Duchenne's muscular dystrophy. J Pediatr Orthop 16:324-331, 1996.

164. Hahn F, Hauser D, Espinosa N, et al: Scoliosis correction with pedicle screws in Duchenne muscular dystrophy. Eur Spine J 17:255-261, 2008.

165. Modi HN, Suh SW, Fernandez H, et al: Accuracy and safety of pedicle screw placement in neuromuscular scoliosis with free-hand technique. Eur Spine J 17:1686-1696, 2008.

166. Guidera KJ, Borrelli J Jr, Raney E, et al: Orthopaedic manifestations of Rett syndrome. J Pediatr Orthop 11:204-208, 1991.

167. Lidstrom J, Stokland E, Hagberg B: Scoliosis in Rett syndrome: Clinical and biological aspects. Spine 19:1632-1635, 1994.

168. Bassett GS, Tolo VT: The incidence and natural history of scoliosis in Rett syndrome. Dev Med Child Neurol 32:963-966, 1990.

169. Keret D, Bassett GS, Bunnell WP, et al: Scoliosis in Rett syndrome. J Pediatr Orthop 8:138-142, 1988.

170. Larsson EL, Aaro S, Ahlinder P, et al: Long-term follow-up of functioning after spinal surgery in patients with Rett syndrome. Eur Spine J 18:506-511, 2009.

171. Master DL, Thompson GH, Poe-Kochert C, et al: Spinal cord monitoring for scoliosis surgery in Rett syndrome: Can these patients be accurately monitored? J Pediatr Orthop 28:342-346, 2008.

25 CHAPTER

Thoracoscopic Approach for Spinal Conditions

Peter O. Newton, MD
Eric S. Varley, DO
Burt Yaszay, MD
Dennis Wenger, MD
Scott Mubarak, MD

Thoracoscopic Anterior Release and Fusion

Mack and colleagues[1] first introduced endoscopic spine techniques in 1993. Since that time, thoracoscopy, also known as video-assisted thoracic surgery (VATS), has evolved to become a valuable tool in the treatment of spinal deformity and other spinal conditions. The goals of thoracoscopic anterior spinal surgery are essentially the same as the goals of open surgery, but they are accomplished with less invasive techniques. Specifically, the goal of VATS in the surgical management of idiopathic scoliosis is to perform a safe, reproducible, and effective procedure that results in improvement in spinal alignment and balance in all planes and axial derotation comparable to, or better than, that obtained with an open procedure.[2] In addition to idiopathic scoliosis, thoracoscopy has been used for anterior releases in kyphosis, hemiepiphysiodeses and hemivertebrectomies, excision of spinal tumors, and treatment of spinal trauma.

VATS offers several possible advantages over an open approach, including reduced postoperative pain, reduced trauma to the chest wall, decreased intraoperative blood loss, reduced pulmonary morbidity, access to more vertebral levels, and improved cosmesis. Although posterior procedures remain the "gold standard" for surgical treatment of most spinal disorders, VATS is a beneficial procedure for a subset of spine patients.

Indications

Scoliosis

Thoracic scoliosis has various etiologies (idiopathic, neuromuscular, syndrome related) that are frequently not diagnosed and treated until the curve is relatively large and stiff. Anterior surgery has been most frequently used as a means to achieve a complete discectomy and release of the anterior spine; this results in greater curve flexibility and prevents the "crankshaft" phenomenon in young patients. Although no strict guidelines on the magnitude and flexibility of the

spinal curvature that requires release have been established, generally curves with a Cobb angle greater than 70 to 75 degrees and a bend correction less than 50% are considered appropriate for release. When sufficient segmental mobility of the released vertebra has been achieved, posterior instrumentation is placed to correct the deformity (Fig. 25–1).

Lenke[3] reported on a combined anterior VATS release and fusion followed by posterior instrumentation in the treatment of adolescent idiopathic scoliosis that had an average preoperative curve of 82 degrees (range 41 to 125 degrees) with postoperative correction of 70% to 28 degrees (range 5 to 60 degrees). Similarly, Newton and colleagues[4] reported a series of 112 pediatric spinal deformity cases with an average preoperative curve of 80 degrees that received an anterior release combined with posterior instrumentation and found a 67% correction in idiopathic scoliosis and a 52% correction in neuromuscular scoliosis. More recent studies have called into question the utility of the anterior release, however, in the age of modern segmental pedicle screw instrumentation.[5,6] Suk and colleagues[6] found an average correction of 66% when posterior pedicle screws alone were used in preoperative thoracic curves of 80 degrees with a flexibility of 45%. Although modern pedicle screw constructs offer a similar correction, an anterior release may still be indicated to optimize coronal and axial plane correction, improve sagittal alignment by increasing thoracic kyphosis, and prevent crankshaft growth.

Children and young adolescents (Risser 0, open triradiate cartilage) with progressive scoliosis are known to be at risk for crankshaft deformity when treated with a posterior fusion alone.[7] These results were reported for children using hook and wire fixation, however, and not modern pedicle screw instrumentation. Although there has been concern regarding adequate pedicle size in children to accommodate pedicle screws, Catan and colleagues[8] performed a magnetic resonance imaging (MRI) analysis of thoracic pedicle morphology in preadolescent patients with idiopathic scoliosis and found that the anatomic measurements were compatible with pedicle screw instrumentation. Sarlak and colleagues[9] reported more recently a series of seven children (average age 7.4 years) with

FIGURE 25–1 **A** and **B,** Preoperative posteroanterior (**A**) and lateral (**B**) radiographs of large stiff curve. **C** and **D,** Postoperative posteroanterior (**C**) and lateral (**D**) radiographs. Thoracoscopic anterior spinal release and discectomy and combined posterior spinal instrumentation and fusion provide acceptable correction.

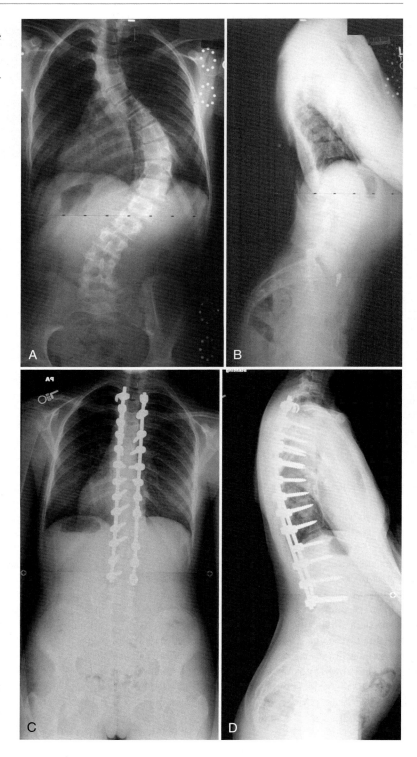

scoliosis with an average preoperative thoracic curve of 56 degrees who were treated with posterior segmental pedicle screw instrumentation and 5 years of follow-up. These authors found a 57% correction rate with no evidence of crankshaft phenomenon in four patients but found a slight increase in Cobb angle and a significant increase in angle of trunk rotation (ATR) suggesting crankshaft phenomenon in two patients.[9] Given the lack of clear evidence on the appropriate treatment of these cases, an anterior fusion may be a viable option to limit anterior growth and prevent this late increasing deformity.[10] Thoracoscopic disc excision and fusion provides a minimally invasive option and minimizes the risk of pulmonary complications in these young patients with progressive deformity.[11-13]

Patients with spinal deformity associated with Marfan syndrome, neurofibromatosis 1, and prior spinal irradiation may have an increased risk of pseudarthrosis after an isolated posterior scoliosis correction. In cases such as these, an anterior fusion procedure may improve the odds of successful arthrodesis, especially when autogenous bone graft is used.[4]

Kyphosis

Controversy exists regarding the need for anterior procedures in cases of thoracic kyphosis.[14-16] In previous studies, Papagelopoulos and colleagues[17] and Sturm and colleagues[18] found that posterior correction with hook or hybrid fixation alone did not provide adequate strength to maintain correction in patients with progressive kyphosis. Because of the lack of satisfactory results with posterior hook or hybrid instrumentation, combined anterior and posterior approaches to treatment of kyphotic deformity have been investigated. In a retrospective analysis of 32 patients with Scheuermann kyphosis treated with a combined anterior release followed by posterior segmental hybrid instrumentation, Lowe and Kasten[19] found that a combined approach resulted in a 51% correction of the deformity with no major postoperative complications. Herrera-Soto and colleagues[20] specifically investigated the use of thoracoscopy in these patients and found similar benefits to scoliosis patients, including decreased blood loss and less morbidity compared with an open thoracotomy.

In a series of 39 patients with Scheuermann kyphosis, Lee and colleagues[15] compared posterior-only thoracic segmental pedicle screw constructs with combined anterior and posterior constructs. These authors found a similar correction rate between both techniques, with an increase in complications in the combined anterior and posterior group. Although posterior segmental pedicle instrumentation seems to offer a similar correction rate to a combined anterior and posterior approach, no recommendations can be made based on the current evidence.[14] The optimal treatment approach to progressive kyphosis must be based on the surgeon's judgment and experience for each individual patient.

Congenital Deformity

Operative management of congenital scoliosis depends on the type of vertebral anomaly, its location, the age of the patient, and the potential continued growth of the child. Although various techniques are available, thoracoscopy also has been applied to the treatment of congenital scoliosis.[4,12,21] Several methods of surgical treatment have been employed in these patients with limited results. In a study with 12 years of follow-up in patients with congenital scoliosis, Kesling and colleagues[22] found that 15% of 54 patients who received a posterior arthrodesis developed crankshaft phenomenon.

Given the lack of satisfactory results with previous posterior-only techniques, anterior surgery may be considered in these patients The anterior portion of circumferential arthrodesis and growth-modifying hemiepiphysiodesis are theoretically possible via the endoscopic approach. First reported by Roaf,[23] hemiepiphysiodesis has been described more recently by Samdani and Storm,[24] who reported that a convex hemiepiphysiodesis is best performed on children 5

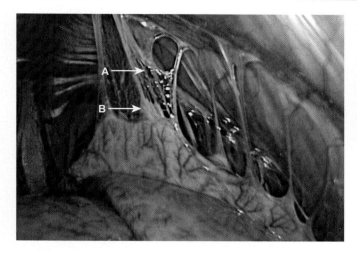

FIGURE 25–2 Endoscopic view of pleural adhesions indicated by *arrows A* and *B*.

years of age with a short curve less than 40 degrees and scoliosis involving five or fewer segments using a combined anterior and posterior approach. In this combined anterior and posterior hemiepiphysiodesis procedure, the convex halves of the discs are removed anteriorly, followed by a posterior arthrodesis and casting.[25] Although a lower thoracic level hemivertebra occasionally may be indicated for excision, doing so thoracoscopically is challenging. Many patients undergoing treatment for congenital scoliosis are younger than 5 years of age and require anterior fusion over very few levels of the spine and may not benefit from a thoracoscopic approach. The use of VATS in these patients must be decided on a case-by-case basis.

Contraindications

As suggested earlier, the small size of the patient is a relative contraindication to thoracoscopy. Lung deflation is more difficult in these cases because standard size double-lumen and bronchial blocking endotracheal tubes are too large. Another contraindication is the presence of a markedly reduced working distance between the chest wall and the spine. In severe cases of scoliosis, the reduced distance limits the field of vision (the endoscope is too close to the spine to obtain any perspective) and the maneuverability of the working instruments. A minimum distance of 2 to 3 cm of working space between the rib cage and the spinal column is required to provide adequate visualization. If the distance is less than 2 cm, thoracoscopy is not advised. Body weight of less than 30 kg is a relative contraindication because the relative benefits of thoracoscopy seem to be reduced in small patients.[26]

Visualization of the surgical field is mandatory in all surgical approaches, and it may be compromised in thoracoscopic surgery by incomplete deflation of the lung or pleural adhesions that prevent collapse away from the chest wall and spine. Pleural adhesions (Fig. 25-2) can be anticipated in patients with a history of prior ipsilateral thoracic surgery or significant pulmonary infection, both of which should discourage the surgeon from using the thoracoscopic approach.

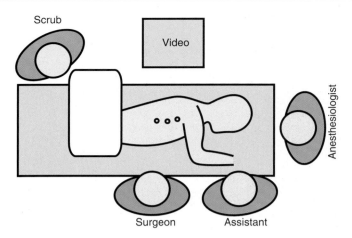

FIGURE 25–3 Diagrammatic setup in operating room shows position of surgeon, assistants, scrub nurse, and monitor for endoscopic surgery.

Surgical Technique

Much of the equipment required for spinal thoracoscopy is common to all endoscopic surgery. An endoscope (10-mm diameter, 0- and 45-degree angle viewing), video camera, light source, and monitor have become standard in nearly all modern operating rooms. Access through the chest wall between the ribs is maintained with plastic tubular "ports." These ports provide a path to place the endoscope and working instruments into the chest cavity.

Patient positioning has traditionally been in the lateral decubitus position (Fig. 25–3). Some studies have suggested that in select cases prone positioning may be possible, avoiding the need to reposition the patient for the posterior procedure or even allowing simultaneous anterior release and posterior instrumentation.[27-29] Although the ability to convert to an open approach may be restricted, it has been shown that the prone position does not adversely affect postoperative pulmonary function.[30] This approach necessitates a more posterior portal placement, however, and may limit the anterior extent of spinal exposure and disc excision.

The role of the anesthesiologist is crucial in the success and safety of thoracoscopic surgery.[31] Spinal cord monitoring is advised using somatosensory and transcranial motor evoked potentials. Complete ipsilateral lung deflation is essential to prevent lung parenchymal injury from passing instruments and to allow visualization of the spine. Double-lumen endotracheal tubes are preferred in patients large enough (>45 kg) to accept these devices. In children (<45 kg), selective intubation of a single lung is often required as an alternative. A small balloon advanced into the main stem bronchus blocks ventilation to the lung on the operative side. In nearly all patients with normal preoperative pulmonary function, single-lung ventilation can be tolerated. The surgeon and anesthesiologist should be aware of the increased risk of developing postoperative mucous plugs as a result of single-lung ventilation.

After lung deflation, portals are established through the chest wall (Fig. 25–4). The orientation of these portals may vary depending on the pathology, although in most cases of deformity release and fusion they are best placed in a linear relationship along the anterior axillary line. Owing to the site of diaphragm insertion, the inferior portals require a slightly more posterior placement to maintain an intrathoracic position. Initial exposure of the spine often requires gentle retraction of the lung, at least until it becomes completely atelectatic (Fig. 25–5). The vasculature including the azygos vein and subclavian artery is identified before the introduction of surgical instruments to prevent inadvertent injury (Fig. 25–6). The vertebral levels are confirmed by identifying the first rib partially hidden beneath the subclavian artery and counting down distally (Fig. 25–7). Division of the pleura overlying the spine may be performed either longitudinally, over the length of the spine to be fused, or transversely, at each disc space.

Treatment of the segmental vessels (Fig. 25–8) may be similarly individualized with either division or preservation, depending on the needs of the case or preference of the surgeon. In most cases, the authors prefer a longitudinal pleural exposure with division of the segmental vessels using Harmonic laparoscopic coagulating sheers (Ethicon Endo-Surgery, Cincinnati, Ohio). Division of the segmental

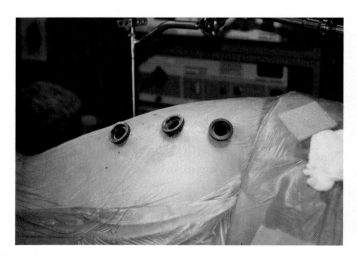

FIGURE 25–4 Proper placement of portals is necessary for multilevel discectomies with the patient in lateral position.

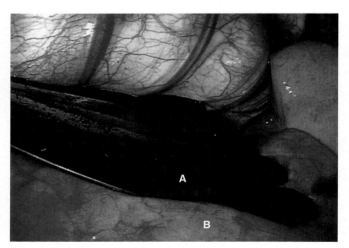

FIGURE 25–5 Intraoperative endoscopic view of fan retractor (A) placed on lung (B) to aid in complete deflation.

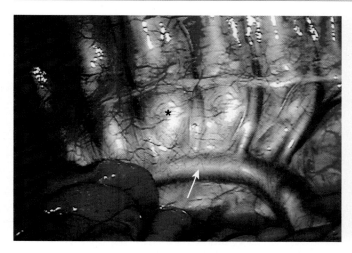

FIGURE 25–6 Endoscopic view of thoracic cavity shows spine (*asterisk*), segmental vessels, azygos vein (*arrow*), and atelectatic lung.

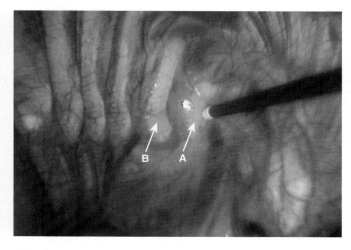

FIGURE 25–7 Peanut dissector is used to palpate first rib (*A*). Second rib (*B*) is most obvious.

vessels allows greater anterior spinal exposure for more complete annular release. Blunt dissection of the pleura to the contralateral side of the spine is performed exposing approximately 270 degrees of the disc perimeter. After division of the pleura, any remaining areolar tissue is divided, and packing sponges are used to create a space between the anterior spine and the pleura.

Possible levels that can be accessed thoracoscopically are T2-L1. Exposure of the T12-L1 disc and L1 vertebral body requires division of a small segment of the diaphragm insertion, which can be accomplished by extending the pleural incision distally into the diaphragm. The proximal thoracic spine in the right chest is often covered by the confluence of the segmental veins, which may appear daunting at the T3 and T4 levels. With slow cautious use of the ultrasonic devices, these vessels can be sealed and divided safely, however, exposing the upper thoracic spine. Disc excision techniques are similar to techniques used in open surgery. An annulotomy is performed with the electrocautery or Harmonic scalpel. A rongeur is an excellent tool for most of the disc excision. Specially designed endoscopic rongeurs are available in extended lengths with various angles (straight, up, right, left) to reach the depths of each disc space (Fig. 25–9).

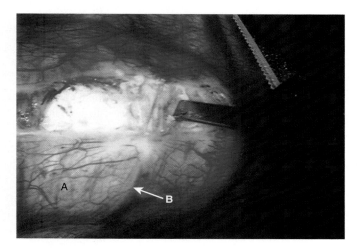

FIGURE 25–8 After division of pleura (*A*), Harmonic laparoscopic coagulating sheers are applied to segmental vessel (*B*).

Awareness of the discectomy path is vital to avoid damage to the neural elements and to prevent excess bone excision, which causes increased bleeding and suboptimal visualization. An angled curet may also be used to remove residual endplate

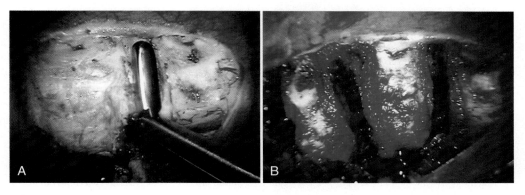

FIGURE 25–9 **A,** Discectomy can be done with rongeur or curet or both with complete removal of anulus fibrosus, nucleus pulposus, and both endplates of cartilage. **B,** Appearance after multilevel discectomies completed. Empty disc space can be temporarily packed with Surgicel for hemostasis control before application of bone graft.

cartilage and expose the cancellous bony surface required for fusion. Bleeding from the bone can be limited by using the avascular plane of dissection between the cartilage endplate and the vertebral body in immature patients. The key to a comprehensive discectomy is optimal visualization deep into the disc space; this not only allows complete removal of all disc tissue, but also prevents injury to the posterior longitudinal ligament and neural elements.

When the discectomy is complete, either allogeneic cancellous or autogenous (rib or iliac crest) bone graft is placed into the disc space with an endoscopic tubular plunger (Fig. 25–10). The method and type of bone grafting also seems to be important to the success of arthrodesis. This may be crucial only in selected cases; however, all patients are at some risk for pseudarthrosis after posterior instrumentation and fusion procedures. In a study of 112 patients treated with an anterior release followed by posterior instrumentation, Newton and colleagues[4] compared the grade of arthrodesis between patients who received autogenous versus allogeneic bone graft. These authors found the disc space was fused in 88% of the autograft group compared with 72% of the allograft group at 2-year follow-up.[4] When autograft is not available, either allograft bone or demineralized bone matrix may be used because they have been shown to result in similar fusion rates.[4,32] Although autogenous bone graft is optimal for patients at greatest risk for pseudarthrosis, the risk-to-benefit ratio must be analyzed on a case-by-case basis.

Outcomes

The thoracoscopic approach has several advantages compared with an open thoracotomy approach. These advantages, including pulmonary function, reduced recovery period, less pain, and improved cosmesis, are realized, however, only if the efficacy of the spinal procedure equals that of open surgery. Experimental animal and clinical studies suggest comparable efficacy in experienced hands. Several studies have been conducted to evaluate the learning curve necessary to be experienced in this technique.[12,33,34] Newton and colleagues[12] found that there was a slight decrease in operative time throughout the course of the first 65 patients treated at their institution and concluded that thoracoscopy had a steep but not prohibitive learning curve. In a more recent study by Son-Hing and colleagues,[33] the learning curve was found to be short with appropriate training and resulted in an excision of a greater amount of disc tissue and a decrease in operative time, while providing similar curve correction to an open thoracotomy.

Several experimental studies have been done to analyze the extent of disc excision possible with thoracoscopic techniques. Biomechanical evaluations of the instability resulting from discectomy were equivalent between open and endoscopic approaches in various animal models.[34-37] The extent of endplate bony exposure has also been shown to be similar with the two approaches experimentally.[34,38] In a histomorphometric study of 32 pigs (160 discs), Zhang and colleagues[34] found that there was not a learning curve associated with the amount of disc material excised (>50% in 94% of the discs in this study), but a learning curve was present for the thoroughness of the endplate excision in thoracoscopic discectomy. Because the purpose of the endplate excision is to remove the growth potential and expose a cancellous bony surface for fusion, added care must be taken during the endplate removal step of this procedure.

The clinical results of thoracoscopic anterior release and fusion in patients with spinal deformity have been generally favorable although poorly controlled.[39] Although there was an increase in the use of this method during the 1990s, it has since declined in popularity with the widespread adoption of posterior segmental pedicle screw instrumentation. Despite more recent studies that have called the necessity of this technique into question for large, stiff curves, there may be a subset of patients who benefit from this procedure.[5,6,40] Studies by Luhmann and colleagues[5] and by Suk and colleagues[6] looked at curves with an average of 80 degrees main thoracic Cobb angle and an average flexibility of 45%. Both groups of investigators concluded that a similar coronal correction can be achieved with posterior segmental pedicle screw fixation as with a combined anterior and posterior procedure. These studies did not examine deformity on the extreme end of curves greater than 100 degrees with less than 25% flexibility, however. In a more recent study of 21 patients with an average preoperative Cobb angle greater than 110.5 degrees and flexibility of 13%, Yamin and colleagues[40] found a staged procedure to provide a safe and effective treatment with a mean correction rate of 65.2%. These authors recommended that patients with a Cobb angle greater than 80 degrees and flexibility less than 20% should be treated with a staged anterior release and posterior pedicle screw instrumentation with the addition of halo-pelvic traction to correct the deformity.[40]

Evaluation of VATS perioperative and postoperative data reveals an increase in operative time compared with open thoracotomy but a decrease in blood loss, chest tube drainage, and pulmonary morbidity and an increase in patient satisfaction. The time to perform thoracoscopic surgery has ranged

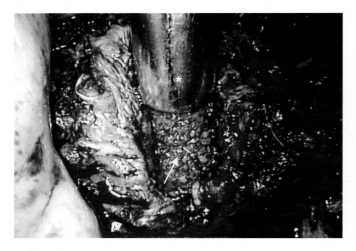

FIGURE 25–10 Morcellized bone graft (*arrow*) is introduced into disc space using tubular plunger (*asterisk*).

from 90 minutes to 4 hours with a decrease in operative time as experience is gained. The total operative time per disc level excised averages 20 to 40 minutes. Studies on the learning curve for VATS have been performed by Newton and colleagues[12] as well as by Son-Hing and colleagues.[33] VATS operative time decreased 26% to 30% and operative time per disc decreased 15% to 24% between the first seven and last seven patients in both series.[12,33] As surgeons gain experience with improved thoracoscopic techniques, instrumentation, and training, the operative time has been shown to be less for VATS compared with an open approach.[33]

The reported blood loss and chest tube drainage have been comparable to open procedures with blood loss generally averaging less than 300 mL.[12,33,41,42] In cases of excessive blood loss, conversion to open thoracotomy may be required. The incidence of major complications for either VATS or open thoracotomy is less than 1%.[12,33,43] The most common complications associated with VATS are pulmonary, such as atelectasis, pleural effusions, pneumothorax, and excessive chest tube drainage.[12,33,42,43] Faro and colleagues[44] compared pulmonary function after an open versus a thoracoscopic anterior procedure and found that pulmonary function recovered more quickly with VATS, and this difference was maintained after 2 years of follow-up. As with all anterior spinal surgery, these risks exist and must be minimized. Although the instrumentation, techniques, and support for VATS continue to improve, this approach is technically demanding, and proper training is essential to the success of this procedure.

Thoracoscopic Anterior Scoliosis Instrumentation

Over the past decade, spinal surgical techniques have evolved to minimize soft tissue disruption in an effort to improve functional outcomes and accelerate the rehabilitation process. Since the first thoracoscopic instrumentation and fusion of idiopathic scoliosis in 1996, this technique has been developed based on the principles of open thoracic anterior scoliosis instrumentation. The rationale for anterior spinal fusion compared with posterior fusion for idiopathic scoliosis is the potential to preserve vertebral motion segments, to reduce intraoperative blood loss, to reduce muscle disruption, to achieve greater coronal plane correction and increased thoracic kyphosis restoration, and to improve spontaneous correction of the unfused lumbar and cephalad thoracic curves.[4,43,45,46] The goal of anterior thoracoscopic instrumentation in the surgical management of idiopathic scoliosis is to perform a safe, reproducible, and effective procedure that results in improvement in spinal alignment and balance in all planes and axial rotation comparable to, or better than, that obtained with an open procedure.[2] Although early studies described high rates of pseudarthrosis, implant failure, and loss of fixation, more recent studies have shown comparable results between thoracoscopic anterior instrumentation and fusion and posterior and open anterior techniques.[45-49]

Indications

Anterior instrumentation and fusion has been used in various spinal conditions and studied extensively in adolescent patients with idiopathic scoliosis. Although the curve patterns amenable to this approach continue to be elucidated, in general, structural adolescent or adult (with normal bone density) thoracic curves may be considered for selective thoracic anterior instrumentation (Fig. 25–11).[50] A review of the pediatric spine literature reveals that anterior instrumentation and fusion has been primarily evaluated in moderate thoracic, thoracolumbar, and lumbar curves between 40 and 70 degrees with flexibility greater than 50%.[51,52] Anterior instrumentation and fusion is kyphogenic and may be a valuable tool in patients with significant hypokyphosis. Eight or fewer vertebrae may be included in the arthrodesis, and the fusion may extend from T4 to L1.[52]

The radiographic parameters are not the sole indications; the decision to perform an anterior procedure must be considered in the context of the overall patient evaluation. The patient's level of maturity and pulmonary status are also important factors to consider. Anterior fusion eliminates growth potential and may be useful in preventing crankshaft phenomenon; however, eliminating this potential in very young children may result in posterior column overgrowth (kyphosis). Specific age parameters have yet to be determined, and the decision must be made based on the needs of the individual patient and the surgeon's experience.

Contraindications

Contraindications for thoracoscopic instrumentation are similar to the contraindications for anterior release and fusion. The procedure is contraindicated if the patient has severe or acute respiratory insufficiency. Previous severe respiratory infections and ipsilateral thoracic surgery are also relative contraindications because pleural adhesions complicate thoracoscopic visualization. In addition to general thoracoscopic contraindications, large stiff curves and hyperkyphosis measuring 40 degrees or greater (from T5 to T12) are relative contraindications. Patients with osteopenia or poor bone stock are also not good candidates for this technique. Additionally, in patients in whom a single rod construct is being considered, a seizure disorder and a suspicion that the patient would be noncompliant with postoperative orders are also contraindications because of concerns of implant loosening. Given that thoracoscopic visualization extends from T4 to L1, thoracoscopic instrumentation should not be attempted for double major curves or curves that extend beyond these end points.[52-54]

Surgical Technique

Before surgery, full-length standing posteroanterior and lateral radiographs, side-bending radiographs, and pulmonary function tests are obtained. The same surgical technique principles apply as with a thoracoscopic release and fusion. Portal placement is the same as with a release procedure. Care is

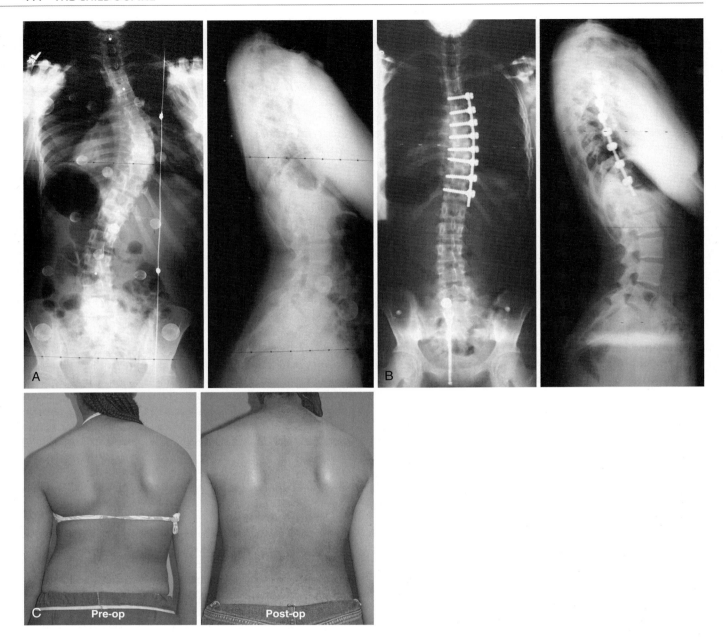

FIGURE 25–11 A, Preoperative posteroanterior and lateral radiographs of a patient with adolescent idiopathic scoliosis. **B,** Postoperative posteroanterior and lateral radiographs after thoracoscopic instrumentation from T5 to T12 with correction of deformity. **C,** Clinical appearance of the patient before and after thoracoscopic anterior instrumentation and fusion with excellent trunk balance and shoulder symmetry.

taken with the posterior portal placement along the posterior axillary line because screw placement in the posterior aspect of the vertebral bodies is accessed through these channels. After the portals are placed, a thorough discectomy and end-plate preparation are performed as described previously for the anterior release and fusion surgical technique. Spinal instrumentation and curve correction is performed under the guidance of fluoroscopy and endoscopy.

Either a single-rod or dual-rod system may be used depending on the size of the vertebrae, the concerns for rod breakage, and the experience of the surgeon. Single-rod systems offer a greater ease of implantation; however, biomechanical studies have suggested that dual-rod constructs are more stable than single-rod constructs.[55,56] Also, in their series of 60 patients with 2 to 5 years of follow-up, Hurford and colleagues[57] reported that dual-rod constructs provided a similar curve correction rate to single-rod constructs but with a significantly improved SRS questionnaire outcome and no reported cases of pseudarthrosis. The length of the cephalad-most screw is templated on the preoperative posteroanterior radiograph (usually 27.5 or 30 mm), and this screw is placed first. The screws are optimally positioned 1 to 2 mm anterior to the rib head in the middle of the vertebral body with approximately 10 degrees of subtle anterior angulation.

The path of each screw is approximately parallel to the endplates (Fig. 25–12). Penetration of the far cortex greatly

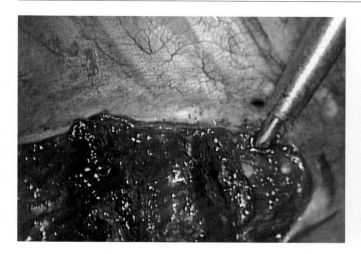

FIGURE 25–12 Screws are placed along path parallel to endplates.

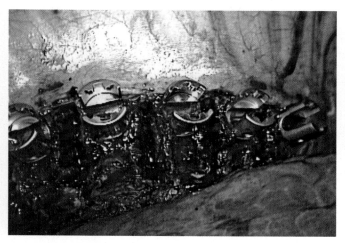

FIGURE 25–13 Care must be taken in screw placement to ensure that screws are aligned to accept rod.

enhances the fixation and is mandatory at the proximal levels to reduce the risk of screw pullout. Care must be taken to avoid placing successive screws increasingly anterior in the vertebral body because this may negatively affect fixation and restoration of kyphosis and potentially place the aorta at increased risk of iatrogenic injury.[58] Although there have been concerns regarding vertebral body screws placed thoracoscopically, Qiu and colleagues[59] showed that there is no statistically significant difference in the accuracy of vertebral body screw placement in thoracoscopic versus mini-open thoracotomy approaches. When the proper screw length has been selected, a pilot hole is created with an awl and the tapped advanced under fluoroscopic guidance. A bicortical screw (5.5 to 7.5 mm in diameter) is placed into the vertebra. Screw position is confirmed again fluoroscopically, and the remaining screws are placed in a similar fashion.

After all the screws are placed (Fig. 25–13), the length of the rod is determined with a calibrated rod-measuring device. A rod of appropriate length is cut and contoured to the desired level of postoperative scoliosis and kyphosis. The rod is sequentially loaded into the screws and secured with locking nuts (Fig. 25–14). Fully seating the rod into the screws may be accomplished with either a rod pusher or the use of a reduction device. Several styles of compressors have been developed to compress between levels. This compression is an important component to the anterior correction of scoliosis but must be performed in a cautious manner, particularly at the upper levels where screw fixation may be tenuous.

Bone grafting is crucial to the success of this procedure. As mentioned previously in the section on thoracoscopic release, autogenous graft provides the optimal base for a solid fusion and is recommended.[4,32] At the lower levels of the thoracic spine, distal to T11, structural anterior support may be required to aid in maintaining proper sagittal alignment.

Outcomes

In 1998, Picetti and colleagues[60] were the first to report a clinical case of multilevel anterior scoliosis correction performed thoracoscopically. Early studies reported high rates of

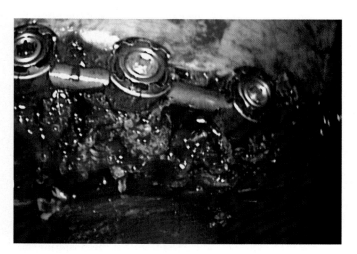

FIGURE 25–14 Endoscopic view of locked single rod anterior screw and rod construct.

pseudarthrosis, implant failure, and loss of fixation.[54,61,62] Since that time, the initial learning curve has been overcome,[12,63] and comparable results have been reported between thoracoscopic anterior procedures and open anterior and posterior techniques.* Early and midterm results of thoracoscopic anterior instrumentation have been favorable. In a series of 45 patients with adolescent idiopathic scoliosis, Norton and colleagues[2] found an overall curve correction 87.3% (51.6 degrees preoperatively to 6.6 degrees postoperatively), an average hospital stay of 2.9 days, and a return to school after 2 to 4 weeks. Newton and colleagues[46] reported that radiographic findings, pulmonary function, and clinical measures remained stable between 2 and 5 years' follow-up in their series of 23 patients treated with VATS instrumentation. In the Norton series,[2] three patients had transient pulmonary complications, and in the Newton series,[46] three patients had an implant failure that necessitated a surgical revision in one patient. Both series found no significant loss of correction after an average 4.6-year (Norton series) and 5.3-year (Newton series) follow-up.

*References 2, 4, 13, 45, 46, 49, 64.

Although operative time is longer in VATS cases compared with an open anterior or posterior procedure, operative time does decrease with experience. Lonner and colleagues[63] reported a significant reduction in operative time from 6 hours in their first 28 cases to 4 hours 30 minutes in the last 15 cases. Studies by Lonner and colleagues[13] and Wong and colleagues[65] compared VATS with standard posterior procedures and found a decrease in intraoperative blood loss and a reduced hospital stay in the Lonner study and a reduced intensive care unit stay in the Wong study. When pulmonary function is evaluated, VATS has been shown to result in better recovery of pulmonary function compared with open techniques and similar return to function as in standard posterior techniques.[13,44] Similarly, in regard to shoulder girdle function, Ritzman and colleagues[66] found that VATS was comparable to posterior instrumentation, which were both better than open anterior surgery. Further comparison by Lonner and colleagues[13] of the impact of VATS versus posterior spinal instrumentation and fusion on the patients' quality of life using the SRS-22 instrument revealed that patients who underwent VATS scored higher in the self-image, mental health, and total domains despite similar curve corrections.

In all of the aforementioned studies, VATS was compared with a mix of posterior spinal fusion instrumentation anchors (wires, hooks, screws). Although many of these past studies focused on the outcomes of thoracoscopic instrumentation compared with open anterior or posterior hybrid instrumentation, more recently VATS has been directly compared with posterior segmental pedicle screw constructs. Lonner and colleagues[45] performed a matched-pair analysis of 34 patients with adolescent idiopathic scoliosis with single thoracic curves of approximately 50 degrees. The patients had equivalent radiographic results, patient-based clinical outcomes, and complication rates with the exception that the posterior thoracic pedicle screw group had a slightly better major curve correction (63.8% vs. 57.3%). These authors concluded that VATS offers the advantages of reduced blood loss (371 mL vs. 1018 mL), fewer total levels fused (5.9 vs. 8.9), and preservation of nearly one caudal fusion level. The disadvantages included increased operative time (325 minutes vs. 246 minutes) and slightly less improved pulmonary function.

The evidence regarding which scoliosis patients would be the best candidates for VATS is unclear. The authors advise that the patient's age, curve properties, and risk factors must be carefully considered in context of surgeon experience when electing to use this approach. Although posterior pedicle screw instrumentation remains the "gold standard," VATS may still play a valuable role in optimally selected patients.

Treatment of Other Thoracic Spine Conditions

The thoracoscopic approach has been applied to thoracic and thoracolumbar reconstruction in cases of metastatic tumors, infection, fractures, and herniated discs. The clinical benefits compared with open thoracotomy include less postoperative pain and a faster recovery. The technical demands of treating these conditions may be greater, but theoretically any lesion situated anteriorly and compressing the spinal cord can be addressed with this technique.

Tumor

Approximately 70% of all spinal tumors are located on the thoracic spine with 85% of these tumors on the ventral surface of the vertebral body and epidural space.[67,68] Current treatment options include surgery, radiation, and chemotherapy. Patchell and colleagues[69] found that significantly more patients treated with direct surgical decompression followed by radiation were able to walk after treatment than patients who were treated with radiotherapy alone. An anterior approach to this decompression offers the advantages of direct cord decompression with tumor resection, immediate interbody reconstruction and stabilization, and a lower wound complication rate than posterior incisions.[68] Although traditional open transthoracic vertebrectomies have been used, they are associated with significant morbidity.[70]

Advances in endoscopic expandable interbody cages have made the excision and stabilization of these tumors possible through a thoracoscopic approach.[68,71] Thoracoscopy has been shown to have substantial clinical benefits in patients with tumors, including reduced postoperative pain, shorter intensive care unit and hospital stays, faster return to activity, and reduced complication rates.[68,71,72] These benefits are especially important because these patients have a mean survival of only 8 to 12 months.[68] Although data on large case series are pending, thoracoscopy is a promising treatment modality for these patients.

Trauma

In principle, the treatment of thoracic spinal injuries (e.g., burst fractures, multiple compression fractures, dislocations) involves correction of malposition, decompression of the spinal canal, and stabilization. To achieve these goals, anterior column reconstruction or decompression or both are often required. Because of the morbidity associated with conventional open thoracotomy, a thoracoscopic procedure has been developed to provide a less invasive solution. Although a thoracoscopic approach requires a longer operative time, it has been shown to have good clinical results in trauma patients with burst fractures. Beisse and colleagues[73] reported 371 patients who underwent thoracoscopic anterior reconstruction and fusion with instrumentation for spinal trauma. The average duration of surgery was 6 hours, and this gradually decreased to an average of 2.5 to 3 hours as the surgeon gained experience and skill. An 85% to 90% fusion rate was observed with the thoracoscopic technique, which Beisse and colleagues[73] believed was comparable with the standard approach.

Thoracic Disc Herniation

Surgical treatment is required for herniated discs that cause neurologic symptoms that are refractory to conservative care. Myelopathy is the strongest indication for surgery to prevent permanent damage to the spinal cord. Approaches for treatment of thoracic disc herniation include the posterior transpedicular approach, posterolateral approach, and anterior transthoracic approach (thoracotomy and thoracoscopy). The endoscope provides a magnified view of the entire ventral surface of the spine and spinal cord. Discectomy and rib head excision provide access to the spinal canal, which must be clearly visualized to ensure the decompression is complete. Anand and Regan[74] reported the outcome of 100 such cases performed endoscopically. These authors reported that thoracoscopic surgery for thoracic disc herniation has an overall long-term satisfaction rate of 84% and a clinical success rate of 70% for refractory thoracic disc disease.

Future of Thoracoscopic Spinal Surgery

The role of thoracoscopy in the treatment of spinal pathology continues to evolve. Midterm reports show favorable outcomes using these techniques, but further work remains to define which patients are the optimal candidates for a thoracoscopic procedure. As thoracoscopy continues to progress, new techniques, new instrumentation, and experienced mentors will make it possible to expand its use. A cautious optimism is prudent for all surgeons participating in the growth of this field. When done well in properly selected patients, the thoracoscopic approach has clear advantages over open thoracotomy; however, substantial experience and sound judgment are required. Although this technique has a role to play in the current surgical management of pediatric deformity, the next generation of anterior growth modulating strategies may be ideally amenable to a thoracoscopic approach.

PEARLS

1. Proper patient selection is essential.
2. Portal placement should be optimized.
3. Visualization can be maintained by maintaining single-lung ventilation and minimizing bleeding.
4. Surgeons should master discectomy and fusion before proceeding to instrumentation.
5. A mini-open approach should be used as needed to augment exposure.

PITFALLS

1. Lung injury can result from incomplete atelectasis.
2. Loss of perspective or orientation within the chest can be avoided by looking through the portal directly.
3. Bleeding needs to be controlled. The surgeon can control bleeding from segmental vessels with a Harmonic scalpel, bone bleeding with wax, and bleeding from epidural veins with bipolar cautery and hemostatic agents.
4. Pseudarthrosis can be avoided by performing a thorough discectomy and endplate excision. Complete autogenous bone grafting (if possible) is recommended. Pseudarthrosis is more difficult to avoid at lower thoracic levels.

KEY POINTS

1. Thoracoscopic spinal procedures are technically demanding.
2. Although performed through relatively small incisions, thoracoscopic surgeons have the potential to perform procedures of similar magnitudes to open procedures in properly selected cases.
3. Visualization is the key to performing surgery safely and effectively. This is critical in thoracoscopic surgery as well.

KEY REFERENCES

1. Lonner BS, Kondrachov D, Siddiqi F, et al: Thoracoscopic spinal fusion compared with posterior spinal fusion for the treatment of thoracic adolescent idiopathic scoliosis: Surgical technique. J Bone Joint Surg Am 89(Suppl 2 Pt 1):142-156, 2007.
   This article provides a thorough description of the thoracoscopic fusion and instrumentation technique and a detailed comparison with posterior fusion and instrumentation. The study concludes that thoracoscopic spinal instrumentation compares favorably with posterior fusion in terms of coronal plane curve correction and balance, sagittal contour, complications, pulmonary function, and patient-based outcomes.
2. Reddi V, Clarke DV Jr, Arlet V: Anterior thoracoscopic instrumentation in adolescent idiopathic scoliosis: A systematic review. Spine 33:1986-1994, 2008.
   The authors present a systematic review of the outcomes of anterior thoracoscopic instrumentation. The authors performed a literature review and analyzed eight articles that met their inclusion criteria. They concluded that the evidence remains unclear and the benefit-to-risk ratio must be weighed carefully when electing to use thoracoscopic instrumentation.
3. Newton PO, Upasani VV, Lhamby J, et al: Surgical treatment of main thoracic scoliosis with thoracoscopic anterior instrumentation: A five-year follow-up study. J Bone Joint Surg Am 90:2077-2089, 2008.
   This article reports a midterm 5-year follow-up study on the outcome of thoracoscopic instrumentation. The radiographic findings, pulmonary function, and clinical measures remain stable between the 2- and 5-year assessment points.
4. Arlet V: Anterior thoracoscopic spine release in deformity surgery: A meta-analysis and review. Eur Spine J 9(Suppl 1):S17-S23, 2000.
   The author presents an update on endoscopic spine release in spinal deformities based on a review of 10 selected articles and analysis of the outcome of 151 procedures.

REFERENCES

1. Mack MJ, Acuff TE, Ryan WH: Implantable cardioverter defibrillator: The role of thoracoscopy. Ann Thorac Surg 56:739-740, 1993.

2. Norton RP, Patel D, Kurd MF, et al: The use of thoracoscopy in the management of adolescent idiopathic scoliosis. Spine 32:2777-2785, 2007.

3. Lenke LG: Anterior endoscopic discectomy and fusion for adolescent idiopathic scoliosis. Spine 28(15 Suppl):S36-S43, 2003.

4. Newton PO, White KK, Faro F, et al: The success of thoracoscopic anterior fusion in a consecutive series of 112 pediatric spinal deformity cases. Spine 30:392-398, 2005.

5. Luhmann SJ, Lenke LG, Kim YJ, et al: Thoracic adolescent idiopathic scoliosis curves between 70 degrees and 100 degrees: Is anterior release necessary? Spine 30:2061-2067, 2005.

6. Suk SI, Kim JH, Cho KJ, et al: Is anterior release necessary in severe scoliosis treated by posterior segmental pedicle screw fixation? Eur Spine J 16:1359-1365, 2007.

7. Dubousset J, Herring JA, Shufflebarger H: The crankshaft phenomenon. J Pediatr Orthop 9:541-550, 1989.

8. Catan H, Buluc L, Anik Y, et al: Pedicle morphology of the thoracic spine in preadolescent idiopathic scoliosis: Magnetic resonance supported analysis. Eur Spine J 16:1203-1208, 2007.

9. Sarlak AY, Atmaca H, Buluc L, et al: Juvenile idiopathic scoliosis treated with posterior arthrodesis and segmental pedicle screw instrumentation before the age of 9 years: A 5-year follow-up. Scoliosis 4:1, 2009.

10. Lapinksy AS, Richards BS: Preventing the crankshaft phenomenon by combining anterior fusion with posterior instrumentation: Does it work? Spine 20:1392-1398, 1995.

11. Gonzalez Barrios I, Fuentes Caparros S, Avila Jurado MM: Anterior thoracoscopic epiphysiodesis in the treatment of a crankshaft phenomenon. Eur Spine J 4:343-346, 1995.

12. Newton PO, Shea KG, Granlund KF: Defining the pediatric spinal thoracoscopy learning curve: Sixty-five consecutive cases. Spine 25:1028-1035, 2000.

13. Lonner BS, Kondrachov D, Siddiqi F, et al: Thoracoscopic spinal fusion compared with posterior spinal fusion for the treatment of thoracic adolescent idiopathic scoliosis. J Bone Joint Surg Am 88:1022-1034, 2006.

14. Lowe TG, Line BG: Evidence based medicine: Analysis of Scheuermann kyphosis. Spine 32(19 Suppl):S115-S119, 2007.

15. Lee SS, Lenke LG, Kuklo TR, et al: Comparison of Scheuermann kyphosis correction by posterior-only thoracic pedicle screw fixation versus combined anterior/posterior fusion. Spine 31:2316-2321, 2006.

16. Bradford DS, Ahmed KB, Moe JH, et al: The surgical management of patients with Scheuermann's disease: A review of twenty-four cases managed by combined anterior and posterior spine fusion. J Bone Joint Surg Am 62:705-712, 1980.

17. Papagelopoulos PJ, Klassen RA, Peterson HA, et al: Surgical treatment of Scheuermann's disease with segmental compression instrumentation. Clin Orthop Relat Res (386):139-149, 2001.

18. Sturm PF, Dobson JC, Armstrong GW: The surgical management of Scheuermann's disease. Spine 18:685-691, 1993.

19. Lowe TG, Kasten MD: An analysis of sagittal curves and balance after Cotrel-Dubousset instrumentation for kyphosis secondary to Scheuermann's disease: A review of 32 patients. Spine 19:1680-1685, 1994.

20. Herrera-Soto JA, Parikh SN, Al-Sayyad MJ, et al: Experience with combined video-assisted thoracoscopic surgery (VATS) anterior spinal release and posterior spinal fusion in Scheuermann's kyphosis. Spine 30:2176-2181, 2005.

21. Vitale MG, Matsumoto H, Bye MR, et al: A retrospective cohort study of pulmonary function, radiographic measures, and quality of life in children with congenital scoliosis: An evaluation of patient outcomes after early spinal fusion. Spine 33:1242-1249, 2008.

22. Kesling KL, Lonstein JE, Denis F, et al: The crankshaft phenomenon after posterior spinal arthrodesis for congenital scoliosis: A review of 54 patients. Spine 28:267-271, 2003.

23. Roaf R: The treatment of progressive scoliosis by unilateral growth-arrest. J Bone Joint Surg Br 45:637-651, 1963.

24. Samdani AF, Storm PB: Other causes of pediatric deformity. Neurosurg Clin N Am 18:317-323, 2007.

25. Winter RB: The surgical treatment of congenital spine deformity: General principles and helpful hints. Iowa Orthop J 15:79-94, 1995.

26. Early SD, Newton PO, White KK, et al: The feasibility of anterior thoracoscopic spine surgery in children under 30 kilograms. Spine 27:2368-2373, 2002.

27. King AG, Mills TE, Loe WA Jr, et al: Video-assisted thoracoscopic surgery in the prone position. Spine 25:2403-2406, 2000.

28. Lieberman IH, Salo PT, Orr RD, et al: Prone position endoscopic transthoracic release with simultaneous posterior instrumentation for spinal deformity: A description of the technique. Spine 25:2251-2257, 2000.

29. Sucato DJ, Elerson E: A comparison between the prone and lateral position for performing a thoracoscopic anterior release and fusion for pediatric spinal deformity. Spine 28:2176-2180, 2003.

30. Sucato DJ, Erken YH, Davis S, et al: Prone thoracoscopic release does not adversely affect pulmonary function when added to a posterior spinal fusion for severe spine deformity. Spine 34:771-778, 2009.

31. Lischke V, Westphal K, Behne M, et al: Thoracoscopic microsurgical technique for vertebral surgery—anesthetic considerations. Acta Anaesthesiol Scand 42:1199-1204, 1998.

32. Weinzapfel B, Son-Hing JP, Armstrong DG, et al: Fusion rates after thoracoscopic release and bone graft substitutes in idiopathic scoliosis. Spine 33:1079-1083, 2008.

33. Son-Hing JP, Blakemore LC, Poe-Kochert C, et al: Video-assisted thoracoscopic surgery in idiopathic scoliosis: Evaluation of the learning curve. Spine 32:703-707, 2007.

34. Zhang H, Sucato DJ, Hedequist DJ, et al: Histomorphometric assessment of thoracoscopically assisted anterior release in a porcine model: Safety and completeness of disc discectomy with surgeon learning curve. Spine 32:188-192, 2007.

35. Connolly PJ, Ordway NR, Sacks T, et al: Video-assisted thoracic diskectomy and anterior release: A biomechanical analysis of an endoscopic technique. Orthopedics 22:923-926, 1999.

36. Wall EJ, Bylski-Austrow DI, Shelton FS, et al: Endoscopic discectomy increases thoracic spine flexibility as effectively as open discectomy: A mechanical study in a porcine model. Spine 23:9-15; discussion 15-16, 1998.

37. Newton PO, Cardelia JM, Farnsworth CL, et al: A biomechanical comparison of open and thoracoscopic anterior spinal release in a goat model. Spine 23:530-535; discussion 536, 1998.

38. Huntington CF, Murrell WD, Betz RR, et al: Comparison of thoracoscopic and open thoracic discectomy in a live ovine model for anterior spinal fusion. Spine 23:1699-1702, 1998.

39. Arlet V: Anterior thoracoscopic spine release in deformity surgery: A meta-analysis and review. Eur Spine J 9(Suppl 1): S17-S23, 2000.

40. Yamin S, Li L, Xing W, et al: Staged surgical treatment for severe and rigid scoliosis. J Orthop Surg 3:26, 2008.

41. Krasna MJ, Jiao X, Eslami A, et al: Thoracoscopic approach for spine deformities. J Am Coll Surg 197:777-779, 2003.

42. Levin R, Matusz D, Hasharoni A, et al: Mini-open thoracoscopically assisted thoracotomy versus video-assisted thoracoscopic surgery for anterior release in thoracic scoliosis and kyphosis: A comparison of operative and radiographic results. Spine J 5:632-638, 2005.

43. Upasani VV, Newton PO: Anterior and thoracoscopic scoliosis surgery for idiopathic scoliosis. Orthop Clin North Am 38:531-540, vi, 2007.

44. Faro FD, Marks MC, Newton PO, et al: Perioperative changes in pulmonary function after anterior scoliosis instrumentation: Thoracoscopic versus open approaches. Spine 30:1058-1063, 2005.

45. Lonner BS, Auerbach JD, Estreicher M, et al: Video-assisted thoracoscopic spinal fusion compared with posterior spinal fusion with thoracic pedicle screws for thoracic adolescent idiopathic scoliosis. J Bone Joint Surg Am 91:398-408, 2009.

46. Newton PO, Upasani VV, Lhamby J, et al: Surgical treatment of main thoracic scoliosis with thoracoscopic anterior instrumentation: A five-year follow-up study. J Bone Joint Surg Am 90: 2077-2089, 2008.

47. Newton PO, Parent S, Marks M, et al: Prospective evaluation of 50 consecutive scoliosis patients surgically treated with thoracoscopic anterior instrumentation. Spine 30(17 Suppl):S100-S109, 2005.

48. Lowe TG, Alongi PR, Smith DA, et al: Anterior single rod instrumentation for thoracolumbar adolescent idiopathic scoliosis with and without the use of structural interbody support. Spine 28:2232-2241; discussion 2241-2242, 2003.

49. Grewal H, Betz RR, D'Andrea LP, et al: A prospective comparison of thoracoscopic vs open anterior instrumentation and spinal fusion for idiopathic thoracic scoliosis in children. J Pediatr Surg 40:153-156; discussion 156-157, 2005.

50. Deviren V, Metz LN: Anterior instrumented arthrodesis for adult idiopathic scoliosis. Neurosurg Clin N Am 18:273-280, 2007.

51. Reddi V, Clarke DV Jr, Arlet V: Anterior thoracoscopic instrumentation in adolescent idiopathic scoliosis: A systematic review. Spine 33:1986-1994, 2008.

52. Lonner BS, Kondrachov D, Siddiqi F, et al: Thoracoscopic spinal fusion compared with posterior spinal fusion for the treatment of thoracic adolescent idiopathic scoliosis: Surgical technique. J Bone Joint Surg Am 89(Suppl 2 Pt 1):142-156, 2007.

53. Picetti GD, Pang D: Thoracoscopic techniques for the treatment of scoliosis. Childs Nerv Syst 20(11-12):802-810, 2004.

54. Picetti GD 3rd, Pang D, Bueff HU: Thoracoscopic techniques for the treatment of scoliosis: early results in procedure development. Neurosurgery 51:978-984; discussion 984, 2002.

55. Fricka KB, Mahar AT, Newton PO: Biomechanical analysis of anterior scoliosis instrumentation: Differences between single and dual rod systems with and without interbody structural support. Spine 27:702-706, 2002.

56. Lowe TG, Enguidanos ST, Smith DA, et al: Single-rod versus dual-rod anterior instrumentation for idiopathic scoliosis: A biomechanical study. Spine 30:311-317, 2005.

57. Hurford RK Jr, Lenke LG, Lee SS, et al: Prospective radiographic and clinical outcomes of dual-rod instrumented anterior spinal fusion in adolescent idiopathic scoliosis: Comparison with single-rod constructs. Spine 31:2322-2328, 2006.

58. Sucato DJ, Kassab F, Dempsey M: Analysis of screw placement relative to the aorta and spinal canal following anterior instrumentation for thoracic idiopathic scoliosis. Spine 29:554-559; discussion 559, 2004.

59. Qiu Y, Wang WJ, Wang B, et al: Accuracy of thoracic vertebral screw insertion in adolescent idiopathic scoliosis: A comparison between thoracoscopic and mini-open thoracotomy approaches. Spine 33:2637-2642, 2008.

60. Picetti G 3rd, Blackman RG, O'Neal K, et al: Anterior endoscopic correction and fusion of scoliosis. Orthopedics 21:1285-1287, 1998.

61. Picetti GD 3rd, Ertl JP, Bueff HU: Endoscopic instrumentation, correction, and fusion of idiopathic scoliosis. Spine J 1:190-197, 2001.

62. Sucato DJ: Thoracoscopic anterior instrumentation and fusion for idiopathic scoliosis. J Am Acad Orthop Surg 11:221-227, 2003.

63. Lonner BS, Scharf C, Antonacci D, et al: The learning curve associated with thoracoscopic spinal instrumentation. Spine 30:2835-2840, 2005.

64. Lonner BS, Auerbach JD, Estreicher M, et al: Video-assisted anterior thoracoscopic spinal fusion versus posterior spinal fusion: A comparative study utilizing the SRS-22 outcome instrument. Spine 34:193-198, 2009.

65. Wong HK, Hee HT, Yu Z, et al: Results of thoracoscopic instrumented fusion versus conventional posterior instrumented fusion in adolescent idiopathic scoliosis undergoing selective thoracic fusion. Spine 29:2031-2038; discussion 2039, 2004.

66. Ritzman TF, Upasani VV, Pawelek JB, et al: Return of shoulder girdle function after anterior versus posterior adolescent idiopathic scoliosis surgery. Spine 33:2228-2235, 2008.

67. Byrne TN, Borges LF, Loeffler JS: Metastatic epidural spinal cord compression: Update on management. Semin Oncol 33:307-311, 2006.

68. Kan P, Schmidt MH: Minimally invasive thoracoscopic approach for anterior decompression and stabilization of metastatic spine disease. Neurosurg Focus 25:E8, 2008.

69. Patchell RA, Tibbs PA, Regine WF, et al: Direct decompressive surgical resection in the treatment of spinal cord compression caused by metastatic cancer: A randomised trial. Lancet 366:643-648, 2005.

70. Walsh GL, Gokaslan ZL, McCutcheon IE, et al: Anterior approaches to the thoracic spine in patients with cancer: Indications and results. Ann Thorac Surg 64:1611-1618, 1997.

71. Dickman CA, Rosenthal D, Karahalios DG, et al: Thoracic vertebrectomy and reconstruction using a microsurgical thoracoscopic approach. Neurosurgery 38:279-293, 1996.

72. Kaiser LR, Shrager JB: Video-assisted thoracic surgery: The current state of the art. AJR Am J Roentgenol 165:1111-1117, 1995.

SECTION

IV

73. Beisse R, Muckley T, Schmidt MH, et al: Surgical technique and results of endoscopic anterior spinal canal decompression. J Neurosurg Spine 2:128-136, 2005.

74. Anand N, Regan JJ: Video-assisted thoracoscopic surgery for thoracic disc disease: Classification and outcome study of 100 consecutive cases with a 2-year minimum follow-up period. Spine 27:871-879, 2002.

26
CHAPTER

Pediatric Kyphosis: Scheuermann Disease and Congenital Deformity

Steven S. Agabegi, MD
Namdar Kazemi, MD
Alvin H. Crawford, MD

The normal adult spine has four curves in the sagittal plane. In utero and at birth, there are two primary kyphotic curves in the thoracic spine and sacrococcygeal region. The lordotic curves in the cervical and lumbar spine are compensatory curves and develop as a child holds his or her head upright and begins to stand and walk.[1] Lordotic curves are considered secondary and compensate for the degree of kyphosis in the primary curves to allow a balanced spine in the sagittal plane.

There is great variability in defining the normal range of thoracic kyphosis. As measured by the Cobb method, the normal range of thoracic kyphosis is 20 to 45 degrees.[2,3] Normal kyphosis increases with age and is slightly greater in women.[3] Thoracic kyphosis is measured on a lateral radiograph using the Cobb method from the superior endplate of T2 to T5 depending on visibility to the inferior endplate of T12. The thoracolumbar junction is normally neutral or slightly lordotic (0 to 10 degrees of lordosis). Any degree of kyphosis at the thoracolumbar junction is considered abnormal. Lumbar lordosis is measured from the superior endplate of L1 to the superior endplate of S1, and normal values are 40 to 65 degrees.

The importance of achieving a neutral sagittal balance has been emphasized in recent years in the evaluation and treatment of various kyphotic deformities. The C7 plumb line should fall through the posterosuperior corner of the L5-S1 disc space. If it falls anterior to this point, there is positive sagittal balance, and if it falls posterior to this point, there is negative sagittal balance. Jackson and McManus[4] reported values in asymptomatic adults with a mean sagittal vertical axis offset of 0.5 cm (± 2.5 cm SD). According to these data, offset greater than 2.5 cm anteriorly or posteriorly is considered beyond the normal range. A positive sagittal balance is poorly tolerated because intradiscal pressures increase in the lumbar spine, and the posterior spinal musculature is placed at a mechanical disadvantage leading to back pain.

Scheuermann Disease

In 1921, the Danish radiologist Scheuermann described a pathologic condition and distinguished it from passively correctable postural humpback when he noted the development of painful fixed kyphosis in 105 children.[5] Scheuermann likened the entity to the femoral head abnormality described by Calvé and Perthes and named it *osteochondritis deformans juvenilis dorsi.* Several terms have been used in the past to describe this entity, including *kyphosis dorsalis juvenilis,* but *Scheuermann disease* and *Scheuermann kyphosis* are the most common.[6]

Scheuermann disease is the most common cause of severe thoracic kyphosis in adolescents with reported prevalence of 1% to 8%.[7-9] The prevalence is approximately equal in boys and girls. Approximately one third of patients have concomitant scoliosis, which is usually mild.[10]

In 1964, Sorensen[11] defined the radiographic criteria that have now become widely accepted for diagnosing Scheuermann disease: anterior vertebral wedging greater than 5 degrees on three or more consecutive vertebrae at the apex of the curve. Associated radiographic findings include endplate irregularities and Schmorl nodes (herniation of disc into vertebral endplates). Schmorl nodes are not specific to Scheuermann disease and can be found in various conditions. Scheuermann disease is typically diagnosed at age 10 to 12 years. Sorenson's criteria are typically not present in patients younger than age 10 because the ring apophysis has not ossified before this age.

There are two curve patterns in Scheuermann disease. The thoracic type is most common, and its apex is located between T7 and T9. The thoracolumbar type has also been referred to as "atypical" Scheuermann disease; its apex is located between T10 and T12, and it is more likely to become symptomatic in adult life.[10] Vertebral endplate changes, Schmorl nodes, and disc space narrowing are much more common in the thoracolumbar form of Scheuermann disease. Sorenson's criteria (three consecutive wedged vertebrae) are unnecessary to diagnose the thoracolumbar form of Scheuermann disease.

Lumbar Scheuermann disease is a distinct entity in which significant degenerative changes are present in the lumbar spine (typically L1-4) without vertebral wedging or significant kyphotic deformity (Fig. 26–1). Schmorl nodes and endplate irregularities are common. Lumbar Scheuermann disease is

FIGURE 26–1 A and **B,** A 16-year-old girl with back pain and lumbar Scheuermann disease, with typical endplate changes at T12-L1 and L1-2.

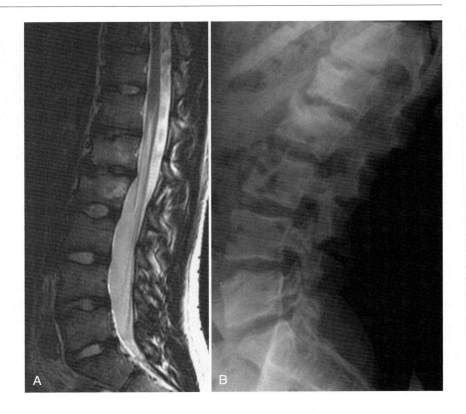

more common in males, especially laborers who engage in heavy lifting activites.

Other causes of kyphosis include congenital kyphosis, postlaminectomy kyphosis, myelomeningocele, posttraumatic kyphosis, neuromuscular kyphosis, infections, tumors, and various metabolic conditions. The main differential diagnosis in patients with Scheuermann disease is postural kyphosis, in which the spine is flexible without structural vertebral wedging.

Etiology

Although the etiology of Scheuermann disease is unknown, several theories exist. Scheuermann's initial description suggested that the condition results from avascular necrosis of the vertebral ring apophyses, which leads to a premature growth arrest with resultant wedging of the anterior portion of the vertebral bodies, and mentioned that it resembled Legg-Calvé-Perthes disease of the hip.[5,6] Schmorl and Junghans[12] hypothesized that herniation of disc material into the vertebral body endplates occurred as a result of inherent weakening of the cartilaginous endplate, with resultant damage to the endplate causing growth disturbance and kyphosis. Schmorl nodes are not specific to kyphotic deformities, however, and are found in normal spines.

Genetic factors have also been proposed. An autosomal dominant inheritance pattern with incomplete penetrance and variable expression in families with Scheuermann disease has been described.[13-15] Three cases of Scheuermann kyphosis in monozygotic twins have been reported in the English literature,[11,16,17] supporting the genetic etiology hypothesis.

Other etiologies of the deformity have been attributed to defective endplates, upright posture, juvenile osteoporosis, increased release of growth hormone, defective formation of collagen fibrils with subsequent weakening of vertebral endplates, strenuous manual labor, trauma, vitamin A deficiency, epiphysitis, poliomyelitis, prolonged sitting, and osteochondrosis.[18-23] Mechanical factors have also been proposed to play a role in pathogenesis, owing to partial reversal of vertebral wedging with brace treatment and thickening of the anterior longitudinal ligament.[10,24]

Clinical Evaluation

The clinical evaluation begins with a complete history and physical examination. The deformity is often attributed to poor posture in an adolescent, delaying diagnosis and treatment.[10] One should inquire about the onset of the deformity and the location of pain. If the patient has pain, it is usually mild and aggravated by prolonged sitting or exercise and typically is near the apex of the kyphotic deformity.[10] Spondylolysis and spondylolisthesis have been noted with an increased incidence in patients with Scheuermann disease and can be a source of low back pain.[25] There is a 50% incidence of spondylolysis in Scheuermann kyphosis,[25] presumably resulting from increased stress on the pars interarticularis in the lower lumbar spine as a result of hyperlordosis. With significant deformity, the erector spinal musculature is placed at a mechanical disadvantage, which may also contribute to pain that is common with this condition.

The Adams forward bending test is used to evaluate any deformity in the coronal plane. On the Adams test, the deformity of Scheuermann disease is sharply angulated compared with the harmonious curve of a postural kyphosis. The flexibility of the deformity should be assessed with a prone hyperextension maneuver. Typically, the kyphosis is fixed and remains visible with spine hyperextension, and patients cannot voluntarily correct the deformity.

Increased lumbar lordosis is often noted in these patients as compensation for the kyphotic deformity to maintain overall sagittal balance. It is important to assess coronal and sagittal balance. Lowe and Kasten[26] studied the sagittal contour of 24 patients with Scheuermann kyphosis and found that most patients with Scheuermann kyphosis have negative balance before surgery and have slightly more negative balance after surgery. Lumbar hyperlordosis was reduced from an average of 75 degrees before surgery to 55 degrees after surgery.

Tightness and contracture of pectoral and hamstring muscles is common.[27] One should look for cutaneous lesions, foot deformities, or muscle contractures. These may signal an underlying neurologic problem. A complete neurologic examination should be performed. Although neurologic findings are rare in Scheuermann disease, spinal cord compression has been reported.[18,28-31] Causes of cord compression include thoracic disc herniation, dural cysts, or severe kyphosis.

Imaging Studies

Routine radiographs include standing posteroanterior and lateral 36-inch films. Sorenson's criteria (three consecutive wedged vertebrae of ≥ 5 degrees) are used as diagnostic criteria. On the lateral view, the fists are placed in the supraclavicular fossa to visualize the upper thoracic spine better. Arm position has a tendency to displace the C7 plumb line. Patients with Scheuermann kyphosis typically have normal or negative sagittal balance, however. It is important to be consistent with the methods used when obtaining x-rays in the preoperative and postoperative periods. A supine hyperextension bolster lateral view is useful in assessing the flexibility of the deformity and can help differentiate it from postural kyphosis.[32] Other radiographic abnormalities that may be present, such as spondylolysis, scoliosis, disc space narrowing, and endplate irregularities, should be noted.

All patients with a rapidly progressive kyphosis, neurologic abnormalities, or any evidence of congenital kyphosis should undergo magnetic resonance imaging (MRI). One report showed transient paraparesis owing to thoracic spinal stenosis and recommended preoperative MRI in patients undergoing surgical correction.[33] Thoracic disc herniations are known to occur with increased frequency in patients with Scheuermann disease.[34,35] The issue of whether all surgical patients should undergo MRI preoperatively is controversial; the authors' practice is to obtain MRI in all patients before surgery to rule out stenosis, disc herniation, or other pathologies.

Natural History

Several early studies suggested an ominous natural history for Scheuermann disease, with significant back pain, embarrassment about physical appearance, interference with social functioning, and cardiopulmonary failure.[11,36-40] Ponte and colleagues[36] showed in their series that all curves greater than 45 degrees progressed during the adolescent growth spurt and continued to increase after age 30. Sorensen[11] reported a 50% incidence of pain during the adolescent growth spurt, and a high rate of pain was noted in patients with kyphosis greater than 60 degrees.[37] Other studies noted the often unremitting and incapacitating nature of the pain, progressive nature of the deformity, risk of cardiopulmonary failure, and unacceptable appearance of the deformity in untreated adults.[38-40] Aggressive surgical treatment was recommended to prevent these problems in the future.[40]

In 1993, Murray and colleagues[18] provided the first long-term follow-up study on the natural history of untreated Scheuermann disease in patients with an average age of 53 years and average kyphosis of 71 degrees. These investigators found that 64% of patients (compared with 15% of controls) reported back pain. The proportion of patients who had pain that interfered with their daily lives was not significantly different, however, from control subjects. Their data suggested that although patients with Scheuermann disease may have some functional limitations, they do not have major interference with their lives. Murray and colleagues[18] found that their patients adapted reasonably well to this condition and recommended that surgical treatment should be carefully reviewed. Other reports have also suggested the generally benign natural history of this condition.[41-43]

The natural history is more favorable when the deformity is in the thoracic spine, rather than the thoracolumbar spine. Back pain is much more common in the latter. It is believed that thoracolumbar kyphosis has a higher incidence of progression because of the lack of support provided by the surrounding rib cage.[44] When a thoracolumbar kyphosis exceeds 50 to 55 degrees, the deformity is readily apparent, especially in thin patients, and pain is common.[44] The thoracolumbar spine is typically neutral to slightly lordotic, and any degree of kyphosis may be clinically apparent. In adults, degenerative disc disease is frequently seen at the apical segments of the kyphosis and may be a source of back pain.[45,46]

Although progression of deformity can be rapid during the adolescent growth spurt, it is unknown whether the deformity would progress after skeletal maturity is reached. Thoracic curves greater than 80 degrees and thoracolumbar curves greater than 55 to 60 degrees may be at risk of progression after skeletal maturity, although the true incidence of progression is unknown.[10,44] If nonsurgical treatment is chosen for curves of this magnitude, periodic follow-up is recommended into adulthood.

Pulmonary failure secondary to severe deformity is very rare. Murray and colleagues[18] found that lung volume, lung mechanics, and diffusing capacity were not significantly affected and were normal in patients with curves less than 100 degrees. They found that as the deformity reaches 100 degrees, restrictive lung disease occurs more often when the curve apex is between T1 and T8.

Nonsurgical Treatment

Nonoperative treatment consists of observation, exercise and physical therapy, or bracing and casting. As is the case with the management of all spinal deformities, diligent observation is the mainstay of nonoperative treatment. In a skeletally immature patient with a mild deformity, periodic observation every 6 months is recommended to document progression. Exercise and physical therapy are useful to treat associated back pain and to improve muscle tone and posture. There is no evidence that exercise improves the kyphotic deformity or reverses endplate changes. Adolescents with kyphosis less than 60 degrees are treated with a physical therapy and exercise program, with periodic radiographs until the patient is skeletally mature. Most adults with untreated Scheuermann disease respond well to a back exercise program if the kyphosis is not severe.

Skeletally immature adolescents with kyphosis greater than 60 degrees are considered for a brace. Applying a brace to a patient with Scheuermann kyphosis tends to be more challenging than applying one to a patient with idiopathic scoliosis. The apex of a typical thoracic Scheuermann kyphosis is usually at or above T8, and a traditional thoracolumbosacral orthosis (TLSO) does not extend high enough to provide substantial corrective forces. The Milwaukee brace or serial hyperextension casts are the most effective in this regard, but are poorly tolerated because of appearance issues. The Milwaukee brace is most effective in a skeletally immature patient with a flexible kyphosis greater than 55 to 60 degrees, who is highly motivated and has the appropriate body habitus. Patients with larger curves, patients with vertebral wedging greater than 10 degrees, and skeletally mature patients do not usually respond to bracing. An underarm TLSO is indicated when the apex of the curve is at or below T11, but in the senior author's experience, relief of symptoms as opposed to correction is the main indication for a TLSO in these patients.

The use of the Milwaukee brace for the treatment of scoliosis was first reported by Blount and colleagues in 1958.[47] In 1959, Moe began treating Scheuermann kyphosis with the Milwaukee brace.[38] In 75 patients who completed treatment, the kyphosis improved by 40%, and the vertebral wedging improved by 42%. Bradford and colleagues[38] reported factors that limited the amount of correction included kyphosis greater than 65 degrees, skeletal maturity, and vertebral wedging averaging more than 10 degrees.

Sachs and colleagues[32] found that curves less than 74 degrees in skeletally immature patients can be successfully treated in a Milwaukee brace. They reported 120 patients with Scheuermann disease who were treated with the Milwaukee brace with more than 5 years of follow-up; 76 patients had improvement in kyphosis, 10 patients had no change in kyphosis, and 24 patients had worsening of deformity compared with initial studies. One third of patients with an initial kyphosis of 75 degrees or greater subsequently underwent surgery. Results showed that treatment with the Milwaukee brace consistently improved kyphosis by approximately 50% during the active phase of treatment, but some loss of correction occurred over time. The final result showed improvement in 69% of patients.

Gutowski and Renshaw[48] reported 75 patients treated with either a Milwaukee or Boston brace. For compliant patients, the average improvement in kyphosis was 27% in the Boston orthosis group and 35% in the Milwaukee orthosis group, despite the fact that patients in the former group were younger and had smaller, more flexible curves. Compliance with orthosis wearing was twice as likely with the Boston orthosis (61% compliance vs. 29% compliance for Milwaukee orthosis). Results in patients who wore their orthoses at least 16 hours per day were equal to results in patients with 23 hours of daily wear. The Boston brace provided satisfactory correction in curves less than 70 degrees and had better compliance. For larger curves, a Milwaukee brace was recommended.

Ponte and colleagues[36] reported on 1043 patients treated with casts for 8 to 16 months, followed by Milwaukee brace and physical therapy until skeletal maturity. Patients had a mean initial curve of 57 degrees and at 3-year follow-up had a mean 62% wedge improvement and 40% curve correction.

Before considering brace treatment, a hyperextension x-ray over bolster (patient supine with bolster at apex of deformity) is helpful to assess the potential efficacy of a brace. If the deformity is flexible, a brace may help. If the deformity is totally rigid, a brace is unlikely to be helpful, and casting may be better in this situation. A lateral radiograph in the brace should show correction of the kyphosis to within the normal range (<45 degrees).

If bracing is chosen, physical therapy should be initiated for trunk stabilization and postural exercises and to stretch the pectoral and hamstring muscles. The brace should be worn for 23 hours a day. To get a meaningful correction with brace treatment in Scheuermann disease, correction of the vertebral wedging deformity by bone remodeling is necessary. In contrast to scoliosis, in which bracing does not correct the curve, bracing in Scheuermann disease may help achieve some curve correction. After 12 to 18 months of bracing, partial reversal of anterior wedging of vertebral bodies is often noted.[10] Loss of correction can occur, however, after discontinuation of the brace. Montgomery and Hall[24] reported an average loss of correction of 15 degrees in 21 patients 18 months or more after they stopped wearing the brace. Brace treatment initially leads to some correction by opening the disc spaces, which close down again unless sufficient time is allowed to reverse the wedging of the vertebral bodies.

The authors consider a brace for curves of 55 to 70 degrees in skeletally immature patients (Risser 0 to 2) with the proper body habitus and motivation to wear a Milwaukee brace. A preliminary hyperextension plaster cast can be used to improve flexibility before application of a Milwaukee brace. The authors generally consider a brace or cast only if the deformity is flexible enough to allow at least 40% correction. In a skeletally immature patient with flexible deformities, the authors have developed the "four 6's" program, consisting of a hyperextension Risser cast for 6 weeks, Milwaukee brace for 6 months, weaning out of the brace for 6 weeks, and sleeping only in the brace for 6 months. This contract with teenage patients has resulted in improved compliance and satisfactory outcomes.

During bracing, follow-up radiographs are taken at 4- to 6-month intervals, and patients are followed to skeletal maturity. Patients and parents should expect a gradual loss of correction after the brace is discontinued.

Indications for Surgery

Surgical indications for patients with Scheuermann kyphosis are controversial because the true natural history of the disease with regard to curve progression has not been defined. Controversial issues are the importance of cosmesis, degree of pain and disability that warrants surgical intervention, and various opinions on the natural history of curves 65 to 80 degrees. These factors must be weighed against the risks of surgical intervention. Treatment decisions should be individualized after a thorough discussion with the patient and parents.

Generally accepted surgical indications include a progressive thoracic kyphosis greater than 75 to 80 degrees in a skeletally immature patient; thoracolumbar kyphosis exceeding 50 to 55 degrees that is associated with pain unresponsive to conservative treatment; progression of deformity despite bracing; and cosmetic deformity that the surgeon, patient, and family consider significant and unacceptable. Other factors to consider are patient age, location of the kyphosis, and extent to which the kyphosis is sharp and angular. If the apex is at the thoracolumbar junction, the deformity typically appears more significant clinically and is more likely to be disabling into adulthood because of the inability of the lumbar spine to compensate for the deformity. If the deformity is very sharp and angular, more consideration should be given to surgical treatment. Generally, pulmonary or neurologic compromise does not occur until the curve is greater than 100 degrees, and these are rarely indications for surgery.

Neurologic compromise is an indication for surgery, but it rarely occurs in Scheuermann disease. Cord compression may be due to disc herniation at the apex, severe kyphosis, and extradural cysts.[34] Similarly, pulmonary compromise is rare and does not occur until the curve is greater than 100 degrees.[7,18,40,43]

Surgical Treatment

The surgical options for Scheuermann disease include posterior-only correction and fusion, combined anterior and posterior fusion, and anterior-only procedures. Historically, the surgical treatment of Scheuermann disease consisted of apical anterior release and fusion followed by posterior fusion. This approach originated from work by Bradford and colleagues[49] in 1975, in which they found an unacceptably high rate of correction loss after posterior-only fusion with Harrington compression instrumentation. These investigators reported a 9% pseudarthrosis rate and 23% risk of instrumentation complications. In 1980, work from the same institution showed solid fusion and good maintenance of correction with anterior release and fusion followed by posterior compression instrumentation in 24 patients.[39]

The efficacy of combined anterior release and posterior fusion is well documented in the literature.[39,50-52] Anterior release traditionally has been recommended for patients with severe, rigid deformities that do not correct to less than 50 degrees on a hyperextension lateral radiograph. With use of modern pedicle screw instrumentation, the indications for performing an anterior release are less common, however, and even severe deformities are being successfully treated with a posterior-only approach.

The anterior release can be performed through an open thoracotomy or thoracoabdominal approach depending on the location of the apex of the deformity or can be performed through a video-assisted thoracoscopic surgery approach.[53,54] The senior author has achieved excellent results with simultaneous video-assisted thoracoscopic surgery release and posterior fusion and instrumentation in the prone position (Fig. 26–2). The levels requiring anterior release typically include six to eight segments centered around the apex of the deformity. The anterior longitudinal ligament and entire disc are removed, and the space is packed with fibular structural allograft bone. In very severe deformities, an intervening period of halo-femoral traction may be considered between the anterior and posterior procedures.

Anterior release and fusion ensures that correction is reliably achieved and solid fusion is obtained. There is, however, the obvious morbidity of the additional operating time and reported complications including hemothorax, pneumothorax, and pulmonary embolism.[7,50,55] There may be potential negative effects on pulmonary function, which may not return to baseline even at 2 years postoperatively.[56-58] Although anterior surgery has benefits in achieving correction of severe deformities, the additional surgery is not without consequence.

Over the last 3 decades, several studies have shown good results with posterior-only fusion and instrumentation with various constructs.[37,55,59-62] Speck and Chopin[37] found posterior-only fusion to be adequate in skeletally immature patients, but that combined anterior and posterior surgery is needed for skeletally mature patients.

In 1984, Ponte and colleagues[63] described shortening of the posterior column by employing multiple osteotomies and posterior compression instrumentation and fusion. The Ponte osteotomy is similar to the Smith-Peterson osteotomy except that it is performed at multiple levels in the thoracic spine (Figs. 26–3 and 26–4). Smith-Peterson's original osteotomy was in the lumbar spine, at one level, in patients with rheumatoid arthritis.[64] After Ponte's description in 1984,[65] this procedure did not gain popularity for many years, especially among North American surgeons, until pedicle screw instrumentation became popular in the thoracic spine. As pedicle screws became more widely used and the ability to obtain strong, three-column fixation in the spine became possible, several studies have documented successful results with posterior-only treatment of more severe deformities.[66,67]

Lee and colleagues[67] compared posterior-only fusion (18 patients) with combined anterior and posterior fusion (21 patients) and found better correction and fewer complications in the posterior-only group at a mean 2-year follow-up. The anterior and posterior group did not have Ponte osteotomies, and hybrid hook and screw constructs were used, whereas the

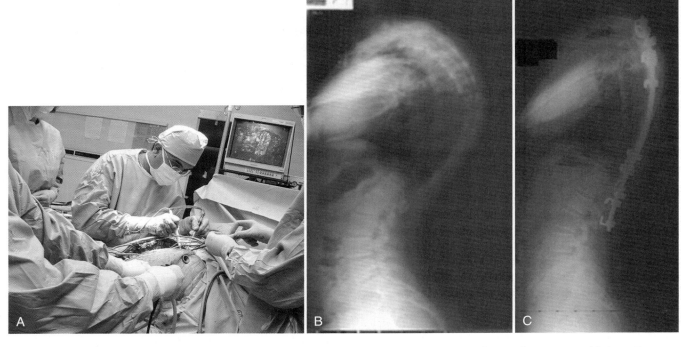

FIGURE 26–2 A-C, A 17-year-old boy underwent simultaneous prone video-assisted thoracoscopic surgery release and posterior spinal fusion with excellent correction of kyphosis.

posterior-only group had Ponte osteotomies (in 67%) and had all pedicle screw constructs.

Geck and colleagues[66] obtained good correction in 17 patients employing multiple osteotomies and pedicle screw fixation, averaging 9.3 degrees of correction per osteotomy

across the apex. There is growing evidence that anterior release may be unnecessary to obtain satisfactory correction of even severe deformities if multilevel segmental osteotomies are performed in conjunction with pedicle screw fixation.[66-68] Hosman and colleagues[68] suggested that posterior-only correction is

FIGURE 26–3 A and **B,** A 15-year-old boy with Scheuermann kyphosis, significant mid-back pain, and progression underwent posterior-only correction with multilevel Ponte osteotomies and pedicle screw instrumentation.

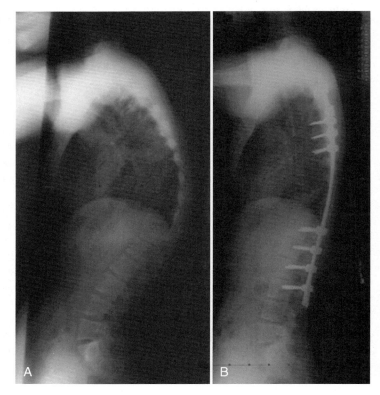

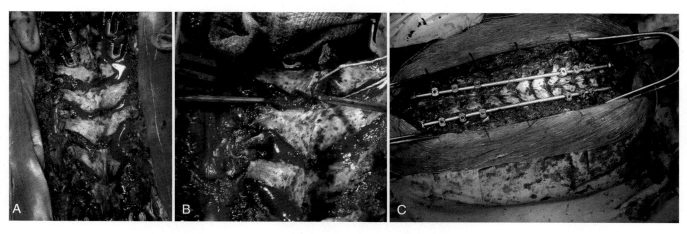

FIGURE 26–4 A-C, Multilevel Ponte osteotomies performed on the patient shown in Figure 26–3. Removal of ligamentum flavum and superior and inferior facets out through neural foramen allows shortening of posterior column and correction of kyphosis.

often adequate for correcting up to a 100-degree kyphosis to a physiologic range of 40 to 50 degrees without an anterior release.

Most patients with Scheuermann kyphosis can be managed by posterior fusion and instrumentation alone. A combined anterior and posterior procedure also has a long-standing successful track record. For very severe deformities (>100 degrees) that are rigid, an anterior release performed through an open or thoracoscopic approach is preferred to obtain some flexibility of the spine.

The posterior-only approach for more rigid deformities consists of performing Ponte or Smith-Peterson osteotomies through the apical kyphotic segments. Instrumentation options include all-pedicle screws or a hybrid construct of hooks and pedicle screws, depending on the preference of the surgeon. Successful results have been obtained regardless of the type of instrumentation. The authors prefer to use pedicle screws placed bilaterally at all levels with correction achieved by cantilever forces and by compression. Shortening the posterior column is an important component of surgical treatment.

Surgical Principle

Degree of Deformity Correction

Surgical treatment of Scheuermann kyphosis should aim to correct the thoracic kyphosis to the high-normal range of thoracic kyphosis (40 to 50 degrees). Overcorrection of a kyphotic deformity can lead to neurologic complications, postoperative sagittal malalignment, and proximal junctional kyphosis. The last condition may occur as a result of forces being transferred to the proximal junction after an aggressive corrective maneuver.[10,51,68] Lowe and Kasten[26] recommended that no more than 50% of the preoperative kyphosis be corrected and that the final kyphosis should never be less than 40 degrees. These authors also found that the negative sagittal balance is worsened postoperatively, and this may predispose patients to junctional kyphosis.[26]

Selection of Fusion Levels

Proper selection of fusion levels is crucial to avoid complications related to junctional decompensation. The proximal extent of the fusion should be the proximal end vertebra in the measured kyphotic deformity.[7,26,55,69] There has been considerable debate regarding the optimal distal extent of the fusion. Traditionally, it has been suggested to extend the distal fusion level to the first lordotic disc beyond the end vertebra to minimize risk of junctional kyphosis.[26,60] Some authors have advocated the inclusion of L1,[20] including the inferior neutral vertebra, whereas others have advocated including L2 in the fusion. Poolman and colleagues[70] advocated the inclusion of the second lordotic disc below the kyphotic deformity. More recently, Cho and colleagues[71] emphasized the importance of the sagittal stable vertebra, defined as the most proximal vertebra touched by the posterior sacral vertical line. The posterior sacral vertical line is a line drawn vertically from the posterior-superior corner of the sacrum on the lateral upright radiograph. Cho and colleagues[71] found that distal junctional problems were more common when the fusion level was to the first lordotic vertebra rather than down to the sagittal stable vertebra. They recommended extending the distal end of the fusion to the vertebra that touches the posterior sacral vertical line.

Complications

The most worrisome complication of surgical treatment of Scheuermann disease is neurologic deficit. The 1999 Morbidity and Mortality Report of the Scoliosis Research Society reported the risk of neurologic injury during surgery for Scheuermann disease to be 1 per 700 cases. Surgical treatment of kyphotic deformities is associated with a higher incidence of neurologic complications than treatment of coronal deformities because the spinal cord is lengthened anteriorly after correction, which may compromise its anterior vascular supply.[72]

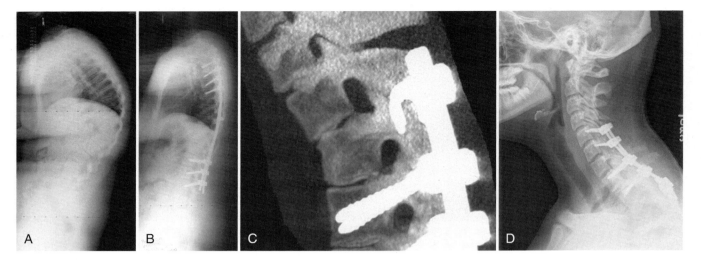

FIGURE 26–5 A-D, An 18-year-old woman noticed prominence of her neck 1 year postoperatively. She had developed proximal junctional kyphosis, which was revised with extension of fusion to cervical spine.

Neurologic complications during deformity surgery can be caused by direct trauma to the neural elements (during instrumentation or osteotomies); stretch injury to the spinal cord during corrective maneuvers; or a vascular insult to the spinal cord, whether secondary to stretch or disruption of vascular supply or secondary to hypotension.[73-75] A preexisting spinal canal stenosis may increase the risk of neurologic injury during correction (Tribus[33]), and although controversial, the authors believe that preoperative MRI should be obtained to rule out any compressive lesions. Overcorrection of a kyphotic deformity is hazardous to the neural elements because the spinal cord is lengthened, and no more than a 50% correction (from preoperative kyphosis) should be attempted.

Distraction has been shown to induce spinal cord injury in feline studies by a reduction in cord perfusion.[76,77] Cantilever forces used during corrective maneuvers increase the length of the anterior column, which may have the same effect as distraction. Caution should be used during correction, which should ideally be a gentle combination of cantilever forces and compressive forces to shorten the posterior column.

Junctional Kyphosis

Proximal junctional kyphosis is defined as kyphosis measured from one segment cephalad to the upper end instrumented vertebra to the proximal instrumented vertebra, with an abnormal value defined as 10 degrees or greater (Fig. 26–5).[78] Similarly, distal junctional kyphosis is defined as kyphosis measured from one segment caudal to the end instrumented vertebra to the distal instrumented vertebra, with abnormal value again being 10 degrees or more of kyphosis (Fig. 26–6).[78]

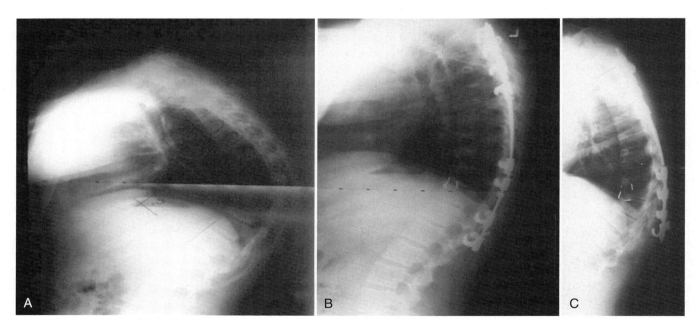

FIGURE 26–6 A-C, A patient underwent surgical treatment of Scheuermann kyphosis and developed distal junctional kyphosis after surgery. This case illustrates the importance of extending fusion below first lordotic disc.

In a retrospective multicenter review of 78 patients with Scheuermann kyphosis treated surgically, there was a 32% incidence of proximal junctional kyphosis and 5% incidence of distal junctional kyphosis.[78] The investigators found that proximal junctional kyphosis was related to stopping the fusion caudal to the proximal end vertebra and is influenced by pelvic incidence. Distal junctional kyphosis was always associated with fusion cephalad to the sagittal stable vertebra. Despite the high rate of proximal junctional kyphosis, the problem was clinically problematic or required reoperation in only 5.1% of cases.

Lowe and Kasten[26] reported a radiographic rate of proximal junctional kyphosis of 30% ranging from 12 to 49 degrees and of distal junctional kyphosis of 28% ranging from 10 to 30 degrees. In their study, proximal junctional kyphosis was related to greater than 50% correction of the curve magnitude in 5 of 10 patients who developed proximal junctional kyphosis. Proximal junctional kyphosis was also related to fusing short of (caudal to) the proximal Cobb end vertebrae by one or two levels. The authors recommended correcting kyphosis to no less than 40 degrees.

To prevent proximal junctional kyphosis, the authors prefer to place transverse process hooks one level above the end instrumented vertebra without disruption of the interspinous ligament at the cephalad level. Placement of pedicle screws at the most cephalad level of the construct risks damage to the interspinous ligament owing to the angle needed to place these screws.

Although earlier studies reported a high incidence of pseudarthrosis with a posterior-only procedure,[39,49] the use of modern instrumentation and techniques has resulted in a low rate of pseudarthrosis in adolescents. The tensile forces applied to a kyphotic deformity likely increase the incidence of pseudarthrosis in patients with Scheuermann disease as opposed to patients with idiopathic scoliosis, but this is unproven. Thorough preparation of the fusion bed with decortication and use of allograft bone is recommended. The authors do not use iliac crest autograft, but it is a viable option if other risk factors for pseudarthrosis exist.

Other reported complications include pulmonary embolus, pleural effusion, persistent back pain, instrumentation failure, and superior mesenteric artery syndrome.[8,26,49,52] Daniels and colleagues[79] reported a case of acute celiac artery occlusion resulting in necrosis of the stomach after combined anterior and posterior fusion, with 50% correction of the curve.

Congenital Kyphosis

The first description of congenital kyphosis in the English language was by Greig[80] in 1916 when he reported a 2-year-old child with a posterior hemivertebra. In 1932, Van Schrick[81] differentiated failure of vertebral body formation versus failure of segmentation as the cause of congenital kyphosis in four patients.

By definition, a vertebral anomaly is present at birth, but the clinical deformity may not manifest until much later. Congenital kyphosis develops prenatally as a result of growth deficits of the centrum occurring during the late stages of chondrification and ossification, leading to hypoplasia or aplasia of the vertebral body.[82,83] The defect is thought to be due to inadequate vascularization of the vertebral body during fetal development. Most vertebral malformations occur between days 20 and 30 of fetal development.[84]

Congenital kyphosis is less common than congenital scoliosis, but it is associated with a higher risk of neurologic compromise and progression of deformity if untreated.[85] Congenital kyphosis and kyphoscoliosis are not separate entities but rather a spectrum of spinal deformities caused by vertebral anomalies. If one side of the vertebra is involved more than the other, concomitant scoliosis may develop. In most cases, the deformity involves the coronal plane to some extent.

Classification

Van Schrick[81] was the first to classify this condition into failure of vertebral body formation and failure of segmentation. Winter and colleagues[86] described three types in 1973 based on their classic review of 130 patients with kyphotic deformity of the spine owing to congenital vertebral anomalies. They classified the deformities as type I, congenital failure of vertebral body formation; type II, congenital failure of vertebral body segmentation; and type III, mixed failure of formation and segmentation. Type I was the most common with most deformities in the thoracolumbar region followed by the upper thoracic region and the least deformities occurring in the lumbar spine. Failure of segmentation was symmetrical and produced pure kyphosis. Failure of vertebral body formation was often asymmetrical producing scoliosis and kyphosis. In the series by McMaster and Singh,[87] 65% of patients had anterior failure of vertebral body formation; 20% had segmentation defects, 10% had mixed anomalies, and 5% could not be classified (Fig. 26–7).

Type I deformity is due to partial failure of vascularization of the cartilaginous centrum of the vertebral body.[87] These deformities are the most common type. The absence of two growth plates anteriorly with continued growth of posterior elements results in a sharp angular kyphosis and can lead to spinal cord compression. The prognosis is considerably worse than the unsegmented type (type II). The natural history involves relentless progression if untreated.

McMaster and Singh[87] further classified type I deformities into four patterns of malformations: posterolateral quadrant vertebra (35%), posterior hemivertebra (7%), butterfly vertebra (13%), and anterior wedged vertebrae (5%). If the failure of formation is purely anterior, a pure kyphosis results. More commonly, the defect is anterolateral with a posterior corner hemivertebra (posterolateral quadrant type), resulting in kyphoscoliosis. McMaster and Singh[87] noted that the posterolateral quadrant vertebra has the worst prognosis, progresses relentlessly, and has a high rate of spinal cord compression. This anomaly is due to a complete failure of formation of the anterolateral portion of the vertebral body, leaving a posterolateral fragment of bone of varying size attached to one pedicle and the neural arch.[87] Defects of formation are treated

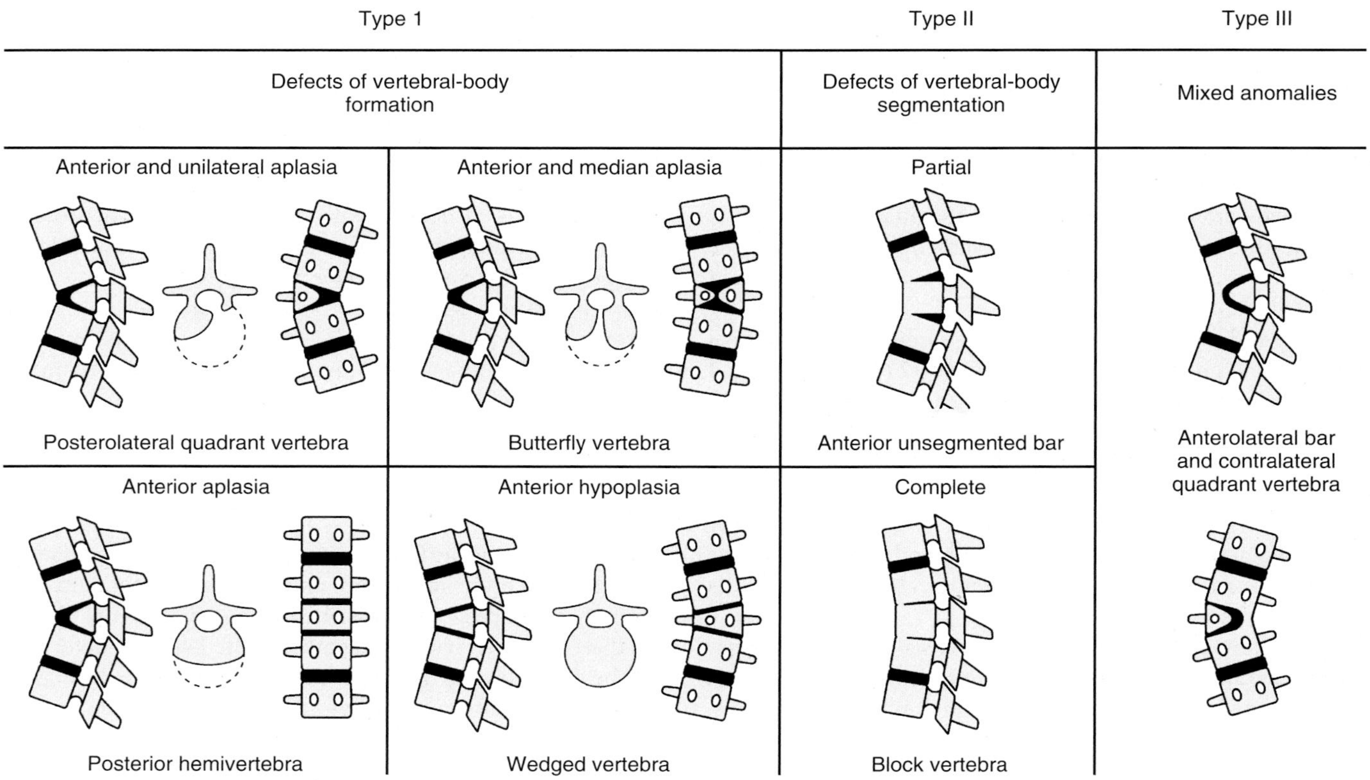

FIGURE 26–7 Congenital kyphosis type I results from defects in vertebral body segmentation, and congenital kyphosis type III results from mixed anomalies. (From McMaster MJ, Singh H: Natural history of congenital kyphosis and kyphoscoliosis. J Bone Joint Surg Am 81:1369, 1999.)

surgically because of the high risk of progression and potential neurologic complications if left untreated.

Dubousset[88] classified type I deformities into two types: a well-aligned spinal canal and a dislocated canal. Shapiro and Herring[89] and Zeller and colleagues[90] used the terms *congenital vertebral displacement* (Shapiro and Herring) and *congenital dislocated spine* (Zeller and colleagues) to describe deformities in which anterior and posterior elements were abnormal and there was posterior displacement of anomalous vertebrae. Zeller and colleagues[90] described the "step-off" sign as the loss of continuity of the posterior cortex of adjacent vertebral bodies as a half of a congenital dislocated spine.

Patients with type II deformity have a better prognosis in terms of rate of progression of deformity and neurologic complications. This deformity is secondary to bony metaplasia in the anterior portion of the anulus fibrosus, resulting in an anterior unsegmented bar.[87] There is no longitudinal growth, but posterior growth continues resulting in a kyphotic deformity. The rate of progression is slow, and spinal cord compression does not occur.[87] McMaster and Singh[87] subdivided defects of vertebral body segmentation into partial (anterior unsegmented bar) or complete (block vertebrae) failure of segmentation.

Imaging Studies

In younger children, vertebral anomalies may be difficult to appreciate on plain films because of incomplete ossification.

Computed tomography (CT) scans with three-dimensional reconstructions are useful for precisely defining the nature of the deformity. Flexion and extension lateral radiographs are useful to assess flexibility of the deformity. MRI is recommended preoperatively in all cases to rule out intraspinal anomalies, which can be present in 5% to 37% of patients with congenital kyphosis and scoliosis.[91,92] MRI is also useful in identifying cord compression or cord signal changes that may result from the angular kyphosis.

Clinical Evaluation

Numerous associated anomalies can accompany congenital spinal deformities, including renal and cardiopulmonary anomalies, chest deformities (pectus carinatum or excavatum), intraspinal anomalies (e.g., diastematomyelia, tethered cord, Arnold-Chiari malformation, syringomyelia). Proper workup of congenital deformities includes renal ultrasound, cardiac echocardiogram, and MRI of the brain and entire spine.

Progression can be insidious, and at each follow-up examination, the initial radiograph, the previous radiograph, and the present radiograph should be reviewed, using the same levels for comparison. Failure to recognize progression can lead to a severe deformity, requiring more extensive surgery with higher risks. During periods of rapid spinal growth (birth to 5 years and during the adolescent growth spurt), more frequent evaluation (every 6 months) is wise. During the "dormant" phase of growth (5 to 10 years), yearly evaluation is adequate. Even if the absolute magnitude of the kyphotic deformity is not increasing, its flexibility may worsen over time, and this may be an indication for earlier surgery.

A complete neurologic examination is crucial. Before surgery, urodynamic testing should be considered in patients with large curves because it may detect subtle preexisting myelopathy in high-risk patients (especially young children).

Natural History

The natural history of congenital kyphosis depends on the type of deformity, age of the patient and amount of growth remaining, and location of the deformity. Winter and colleagues[86] found type I deformities to have the worst prognosis and to progress rapidly, followed by type III and type II. McMaster and Singh[87] found the most rapid progression to occur in type III deformities, followed by type I and II. The posterolateral quadrant vertebra has the worst prognosis.

Kyphosis resulting from defects of formation progresses an average of 7 degrees per year and is most rapid during the adolescent growth spurt.[86] Progression is most likely to occur during rapid periods of growth (birth to 3 years and adolescent growth spurt). Type II deformities progress an average of 5 degrees per year.[93] Progression rate is slower in type II deformities because bony bar formation of the anterior disc occurs later in childhood, and the growth discrepancy between the posterior and anterior elements is not as great as type I deformities.

Neurologic involvement and spinal cord compression occur primarily with anterior failure of vertebral body formation (type I or III) because of the acute angular kyphosis over a short segment. The rate of neurologic involvement has been estimated to be around 18%.[87] This rate is likely to be much higher if all patients were untreated. Neurologic compromise is most common during the adolescent growth spurt when progression is most rapid. The greatest risk of spinal cord compression occurs when the apex is at the mid-thoracic region (T4-9) because this is a vascular watershed area. The onset of cord compression can occur at any age, but is most common during the adolescent growth spurt. All patients who develop neurologic deficit progress to paraplegia if left untreated.[87] Progressive neurologic deficit should be immediately treated surgically.

Type II deformities (failure of segmentation) produce a more rounded kyphosis compared with the angular gibbous deformity that occurs with failure of formation.[86,93] These deformities occur most often in the lower thoracic and thoracolumbar region. They are less likely to progress and rarely cause neurologic compromise because of the more gradual kyphosis that is spread out over several segments (as opposed to the sharp angular kyphosis of type I deformities).

Treatment

Nonoperative treatment in congenital kyphosis primarily consists of diligent observation to document progression of the deformity (Fig. 26–8). Bracing and casting is believed to be ineffective in congenital kyphosis.[86,94] Progression can be insidious, and radiographs may show small degrees of progression over months that may be deemed insignificant. However, over a 2- to 3-year time frame, the progression may be much more significant. At each follow-up evaluation, current radiographs should be compared with the initial radiographs to document progression more precisely. In all cases of congenital kyphoscoliosis, especially with type I deformities, it is crucial to obtain a posteroanterior radiograph and a lateral radiograph at each visit because the scoliosis may appear to be stable but the lateral view may show significant progression of the kyphosis owing to a hemivertebra. The authors refer to such a hemivertebra as a "snake in the grass" (Fig. 26–9).

The importance of observation was highlighted by a more recent report by Campos and colleagues,[95] who described seven patients with early thoracolumbar kyphosis associated with single lumbar vertebral hypoplasia, which appeared similar to a failure of formation (Fig. 26–10). All patients had spontaneous correction of alignment over time. In all seven patients, the anomaly was limited to one lumbar level (L1 or L2), and the defect was limited to the superior portion of the anterior half of the vertebral body without posterior malformations. The investigators recommended a brief period of observation to document progression versus spontaneous correction. If progression was documented or if the deformity persisted at age 3 years, further workup was recommended.

Surgical Treatment

The guiding principle of operative treatment of congenital kyphosis is early fusion to prevent severe deformity and to allow for some correction with growth.[85] If curves with a bad prognosis are recognized at an early age, simple prophylactic surgical treatment can prevent progression and neurologic complications. The surgical treatment of congenital kyphosis can be challenging, and many factors must be considered when deciding on the operative plan, such as type of vertebral anomaly, patient age and amount of growth remaining, severity of deformity, and presence or absence of spinal cord compression or neurologic deficits or both.[85]

All operations should be performed with spinal cord monitoring, including motor evoked potentials, somatosensory evoked potentials, and electromyography monitoring. Traction is contraindicated because of the high incidence of neurologic complications.[86,96] Because of the rigidity of the kyphosis at the apex, traction primarily causes correction of the ends of the curve, which are more flexible. This correction lengthens the spine and pulls the spinal cord against the unforgiving apical bone, which leads to more compression of the cord and resulting neurologic complications.

The treatment of type I deformities is almost always surgical because of the high risk of progression and neurologic sequelae if deformities are left untreated. The presence of a posterolateral quadrant vertebra mandates early prophylactic surgical treatment before the child is 5 years of age and before the kyphosis is 50 degrees.[87] Traditionally, this treatment was

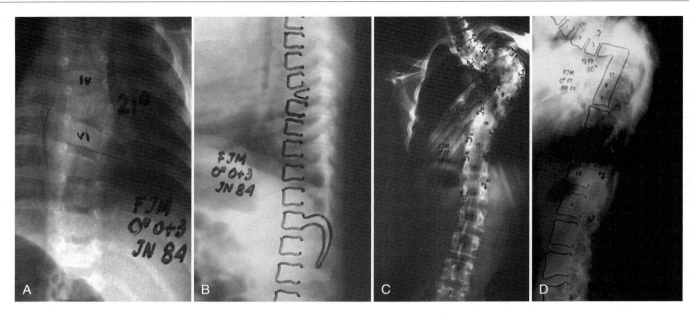

FIGURE 26–8 A-D, T5 hemivertebra initially diagnosed at age 3 months. The patient did not follow up until age 17, when he became paraplegic and wheelchair-dependent with severe spinal deformity. (Courtesy of R. Maenza, MD, Italian hospital, Buenos Aires, Argentina.)

best achieved by a posterior growth arrest procedure, which is essentially a posterior (convex) hemiepiphysiodesis. More recently, hemivertebra excision performed through an all-posterior approach has been used for these deformities, and this is discussed later in the chapter. In situ fusion can be done with or without instrumentation, extending one level above to one level below the abnormal vertebra. If the deformity is less than 50 to 55 degrees, and there is growth potential anteriorly, creating a posterior tether allows some gradual correction in the presence of continuing anterior growth. This also eliminates the risk of spinal cord compression.

Although cases reported earlier did not use instrumentation, pseudarthrosis rates were relatively high, and re-exploration of the fusion mass was routinely recommended for this reason. Earlier reports recommended prolonged bed rest (up to 6 months) after surgery. The use of spinal instrumentation, specifically pedicle screw instrumentation, has been shown to be safe and effective in very young patients with congenital spinal deformities[97,98] and improves the fusion rate, making re-exploration and prolonged bed rest unnecessary. The authors prefer to use allograft bone because fusion rates tend to be high in young patients. The fundamental principles of fusion surgery, including facet excision and thorough decortication, must be adhered to for optimal results. Postoperatively, the authors immobilize very young children in a brace given their inability to restrict their activities.

The surgical treatment of older patients (>5 years old) with more severe deformities (>55 to 60 degrees) has traditionally been a combined anterior and posterior fusion. Several studies have documented the inefficacy of posterior fusion alone for

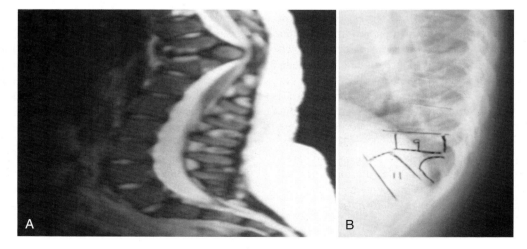

FIGURE 26–9 A and **B,** Hemivertebra causing severe cord compression. This deformity is often not well appreciated on posteroanterior view and can be missed if proper imaging is not performed. The authors refer to such a "hidden" anomaly on posteroanterior view as a "snake in the grass."

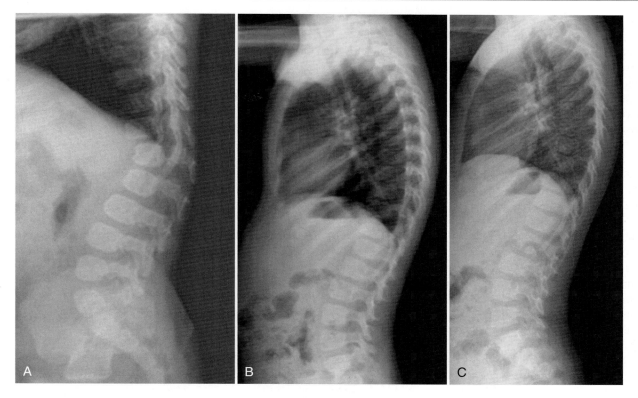

FIGURE 26–10 A-C, A 6-month-old boy with wedging deformity of L1 vertebra, which spontaneously corrected over time. The patient was braced with a TLSO. Lateral x-rays show deformity at 6 months of age (**A**), 3.5 years of age (**B**), and 4.5 years of age (**C**). This case highlights the importance of diligent observation of all congenital deformities and performing surgery only if progression is documented.

these patients,[85,99,100] and a combined anterior and posterior fusion with or without instrumentation has been recommended.[24,86,96] Winter and colleagues[86] made this recommendation in a review of 94 patients in whom progressive congenital kyphosis had been treated after the age of 5 years. Some degree of vertebral resection is necessary to obtain satisfactory correction. McMaster and Singh[85] recommended anterior strut grafting and instrumented posterior fusion because of the substantial rate of pseudarthrosis and deformity progression with posterior fusion alone. Large curves place the posterior fusion at a mechanical disadvantage in the absence of anterior fusion, leading to a high pseudarthrosis rate. Older patients (>5 years old) lack sufficient spinal growth to produce an appreciable correction. Other studies have corroborated these findings that posterior fusion alone, with or without instrumentation, is insufficient for a type I or type III kyphotic deformity greater than 50 degrees.[24,96] McMaster and Singh[85] recommended fusing the entire deformity in older patients with large curves (longer fusion than in younger patients with smaller curves).

The anterior and posterior procedures can be done in 1 day or can be staged, depending on the preference of the surgeon. The anterior procedure is done through a transthoracic, transthoracic-retroperitoneal, or purely retroperitoneal approach depending on the location of the deformity. When exposure is obtained, the segmental vessels are ligated, and periosteal flaps are created. The segmental vessels should be ligated as anteriorly as possible to avoid disruption of the

collateral circulation, which lies closer to the foraminal regions. Complete discectomies are performed. Rib strut grafts are placed from end vertebra to end vertebra, creating slots in the vertebral bodies.

The above-mentioned studies were completed before pedicle screw instrumentation became widely used. The superior three-column fixation that is obtained with pedicle screws may obviate the need for an anterior surgery in many patients, even patients with severe deformities.

An alternative to early in situ posterior fusion for a hemivertebra is complete resection of the hemivertebra. Traditionally, hemivertebra excisions have been done through combined anterior and posterior exposures. More recent reports have shown this procedure to be safe and effective through a posterior-only approach,[101-103] and this is the authors' preference. Shono and colleagues[104] reported on one-stage posterior hemivertebra resection and fusion and instrumentation in 12 patients 8 to 24 years old with kyphoscoliosis. Satisfactory correction of the scoliosis (from 49 degrees to 18 degrees) and the kyphosis (from 40 degrees to 17 degrees) was obtained, without neurologic complications or pseudarthrosis. Ruf and Harms[97,101] described a similar approach in children 15 months old, mostly in congenital scoliosis, with successful outcomes. The location of a hemivertebra in congenital kyphosis or kyphoscoliosis (at the apex of kyphotic deformity) makes it amenable to resection from a posterior approach with visualization of the spinal cord during correction. This approach allows for correction and short segment fusion without concern regarding continued growth of the anterior column that may lead to future progression or crankshaft phenomenon.

Patients with spinal cord compression and neurologic deficits require decompression of the spinal cord. This decompression can be done either from an anterior approach or posteriorly from a costotransversectomy approach. Laminectomies alone are contraindicated because the compression is from the ventral aspect of the cord, and laminectomies create further mechanical instability. If the deformity is severe and spinal cord compression exists, the apex of the deformity may be so far posterior that cord decompression may be more feasible from a posterior approach. In such cases, a vertebral body resection is performed through bilateral costotransversectomies or a transpedicular approach. After the body is resected, the spinal column is shortened in such cases to obtain some bony apposition anteriorly. In severe gibbous deformities, decompression is technically more feasible from a posterior approach. A cage can be inserted anteriorly if the deformity allows it.

With surgical treatment of kyphosis, some lengthening of spine usually results. The kyphotic apex is stiff, so the normal, flexible spine corrects and lengthens around a relatively fixed deformity. This situation can be a significant stress on the vascularity of the spinal cord. Every effort should be made to shorten the spine with correction.

A type II kyphosis does not require immediate surgical treatment, unless the deformity is already sufficiently severe to require correction, or the curve is shown to be progressive under observation.[85] If a type II deformity is detected early and has been noted to be progressive, but the curve is not severe and is within acceptable limits, a posterior fusion alone (one level above to one level below the congenital kyphosis) is sufficient to prevent further progression.[24,86,93,96] These deformities have no potential for anterior growth because of ossification of anterior disc spaces. For more severe curves in which substantial correction is necessary, traditionally an anterior approach has been recommended to perform osteotomies of the unsegmented areas, discectomies and fusion, and posterior fusion and instrumentation.[93] All patients who undergo surgical treatment should be observed to skeletal maturity because adding-on of additional vertebrae above and below the fused segment can occur during the adolescent growth spurt.

Complications

Pseudarthrosis and Progressive Deformity

Techniques to obtain a solid fusion more reliably include combined anterior and posterior fusion, use of instrumentation, proper facet decortication, and use of autogenous bone graft. With use of modern spinal instrumentation and proper technique, pseudarthrosis rates are low in young children even with a posterior-only fusion.[98,105] Pseudarthrosis typically leads to progression of the deformity, and if any progression is noted in the postoperative period, re-exploration of the fusion mass is recommended. For severe curves (>55 to 60 degrees), the most reliable means of avoiding these complications is by performing a combined anterior and posterior fusion.

Neurologic Complications

The rate of neurologic complications is higher in the surgical treatment of congenital kyphosis than other spinal deformities, especially in older patients with large deformities.[96] As mentioned previously, traction is contraindicated in the treatment of congenital kyphosis. Neurologic complications are more likely to occur if attempts are made to obtain maximum correction of the curve with use of instrumentation. Partial correction is preferable, and the goal is to obtain a balanced spine in the coronal and sagittal planes, rather than maximal correction. Spinal cord monitoring is mandatory, and the use of the wake-up test is recommended if the patient can cooperate.

PEARLS

1. Surgical correction of Scheuermann kyphosis can be accomplished in most cases by posterior-only fusion with multilevel Ponte osteotomies. Complete removal of the inferior and superior facets and ligamentum flavum allows the posterior column to be shortened.

2. A combination of cantilever forces and compression is used to obtain correction in Scheuermann kyphosis.

3. MRI is recommended before surgical correction of Scheuermann kyphosis. The presence of stenosis or disc herniation may alter the operative plan.

4. In a very young child with congenital deformity, fusion should be as short as possible. In an adolescent patient, the entire deformity should be addressed.

5. Although bracing and casting are not very effective in congenital deformities, casting may be considered in a very young infant as a temporizing measure to allow further growth before surgery is performed.

PITFALLS

1. Overcorrection of a kyphotic deformity can lead to neurologic injury because the spinal cord is lengthened. No more than 50% correction (from preoperative kyphosis) should be attempted.

2. Selection of proper fusion levels and preservation of the supraspinous ligament at the proximal end of the construct can help prevent a junctional kyphosis. The possibility of a junctional kyphosis should be discussed with the patient and family preoperatively.

3. All patients with congenital kyphosis require diligent observation. Not all patients experience progression, and early surgery in the absence of documented progression should be avoided.

4. In patients with congenital scoliosis, the lateral radiograph should be critically examined. The scoliosis may appear to be stable, but the kyphosis may be progressing.

KEY POINTS

1. The natural history of Scheuermann disease is generally benign, and most patients do not experience significant disability in adulthood.

2. A Milwaukee brace is recommended in skeletally immature patients with curves of 55 to 70 degrees.

3. Surgical indications include a progressive thoracic kyphosis greater than 75 to 80 degrees in a skeletally immature patient; thoracolumbar kyphosis exceeding 50 to 55 degrees that is associated with pain unresponsive to conservative treatment; progression of deformity despite bracing; or cosmetic deformity that the surgeon, patient, and family consider significant and unacceptable.

4. Patients diagnosed with congenital kyphosis should undergo MRI of the entire spine to rule out intraspinal anomalies.

5. Diligent, periodic observation of all patients with congenital kyphosis is crucial; without such observation, severe deformities with neurologic sequelae may develop.

6. The natural history of congenital kyphosis, particularly type I deformities, is unfavorable. Insidious progression of the deformity can occur with growth, and surgery is recommended if progression is noted.

7. Goals of treatment are early fusion to prevent severe deformity, to halt progression, and to achieve head and trunk balance.

8. In a very young child, fusion should be as short as possible; the entire deformity should be addressed in adolescent patients.

9. Postoperatively, patients should be followed to skeletal maturity to ensure that progression of the primary or compensatory curves does not occur.

KEY REFERENCES

1. Winter RB, Moe JH: The results of spinal arthrodesis of congenital spinal deformities in patients younger than five years old. J Bone Joint Surg 64-A:419-432, 1982.
   Authors reviewed the results of spinal fusion for congenital deformity in 49 patients younger than age 5.

2. Winter RB, Moe JH, Lonstein JE: The surgical treatment of congenital kyphosis: A review of 94 patients age 5 years or older with 2 years or more follow-up in 77 patients. Spine 10:224-231, 1985.
   Authors reviewed the results of spinal fusion for congenital kyphosis in 77 patients older than age 5.

3. Murray PM, Weinstein SL, Spratt KF: The natural history and long-term follow-up of Scheuermann's kyphosis. J Bone Joint Surg Am 75:236-248, 1993.
   This was the first long-term follow-up study on the natural history of Scheuermann disease.

4. McMaster MJ, Singh H: Natural history of congenital kyphosis and kyphoscoliosis. A study of one hundred and twelve patients. J Bone Joint Surg Am 81:1367-1383, 1999.

Authors further classified type 1 deformities into four patterns of malformations. They noted that the posterolateral quadrant vertebra has the worst prognosis, progresses relentlessly, and has a high rate of spinal cord compression.

5. Lowe TG: Scheuermann's disease. Orthop Clin North Am 30:475-487, 1999.
   This review article discusses the natural history, diagnosis, and treatment of Scheuermann disease.

6. Campos MA, Fernandes P, Dolan LA, Weinstein SL: Infantile thoracolumbar kyphosis secondary to lumbar hypoplasia. J Bone Joint Surg Am 90:1726-1729, 2008.
   This is a report on seven patients with early thoracolumbar kyphosis with lumbar hypoplasia. All cases resolved without surgical treatment.

REFERENCES

1. Bernhardt M: Normal spinal anatomy: Normal sagittal plane alignment. In Bridwell KH, DeWald RL (eds): The Textbook of Spinal Surgery, vol 1, 2nd ed. Philadelphia, Lippincott-Raven, 1997, pp 185-191.

2. Bernhardt M, Bridwell K: Segmental analysis of the sagittal plane alignment of the normal thoracic and lumbar spine and thoracolumbar junction. Spine 14:717-721, 1989.

3. Fon GT, Pitt MJ, Thies AC Jr: Thoracic kyphosis: Range in normal subjects. AJR Am J Roentgenol 134:979-983, 1980.

4. Jackson RP, McManus AC: Radiographic analysis of sagittal plane alignment and balance in standing volunteers and patients with low back pain matched for age, sex, and size: A prospective controlled clinical study. Spine 19:1611-1618, 1994.

5. Scheuermann HW: Kyphosis douselis juveniles. Orthop Chir 41:305, 1921.

6. Scheuermann HW: Kyphosis juveniles (Scheuermann's kaukheit). Clin Orthop Relat Res 128:5-7, 1977.

7. Wenger DR, Frick SL: Scheuermann kyphosis. Spine 24:2630-2639, 1999.

8. Tribus CB: Scheuermann's kyphosis in adolescents and adults: Diagnosis and management. J Am Acad Orthop Surg 6:36-43, 1998.

9. Scoles PV, Latimer BM, DiGiovanni BF, et al: Vertebral alterations in Scheuermann's kyphosis. Spine 16:509-515, 1991.

10. Lowe TG: Scheuermann's disease. Orthop Clin North Am 30:475-487, 1999.

11. Sorensen KH: Scheuermann's Juvenile Kyphosis: Clinical Appearances, Radiography, Aetiology, and Prognosis. Copenhagen, Enjar Munksgaard Forlag, 1964.

12. Schmorl G, Junghans H: Die Gesunde und Kranle Wirbel-seule in Roentgenbild. Leipzig, Thieme Verlag, 1932.

13. Findlay A, Conner AN, Conner JM: Dominant inheritance of Scheuermann's juvenile kyphosis. J Med Genet 26:400-403, 1989.

14. McKenzie L, Sillence D: Familial Scheuermann disease: A genetic and linkage study. J Med Genet 29:41-45, 1992.

15. Nielsen OG, Pilgaard P: Two hereditary spinal diseases producing kyphosis during adolescence. Acta Paediatr Scand 76:133-136, 1987.

16. Carr AJ: Idiopathic thoracic kyphosis in identical twins. J Bone Joint Surg Br 72:144, 1990.

17. Graat HCA, Van Rhijn LW, Schrander-Stumpel CTRM, et al: Classical Scheuermann disease in male monozygotic twins. Spine 27:E485-E487, 2002.

18. Murray PM, Weinstein SL, Spratt KF: The natural history and long-term follow-up of Scheuermann's kyphosis. J Bone Joint Surg Am 75:236-248, 1993.

19. Ippolito E, Ponseti IV: Juvenile kyphosis: Histological and histochemical studies. J Bone Joint Surg Am 63:175, 1981.

20. Ascani E, La Rosa G: Scheuermann kyphosis. In Weinstein SL (ed): The Pediatric Spine: Principles and Practice. New York, Raven Press, 1994, pp 557-584.

21. Lambrinudi L: Adolescent and senile kyphosis. BMJ 2:800, 1934.

22. Bradford DS, Daher YH: Vascularized rib grafts for stabilization of kyphosis. J Bone Joint Surg Br 68:357, 1986.

23. Lopez RA, Burke SW, Levine DB, et al: Osteoporosis in Scheuermann's disease. Spine 13:1099, 1988.

24. Montgomery SP, Hall JE: Congenital kyphosis. Spine 4:360-364, 1982.

25. Ogilvie JW, Sherman J: Spondylolysis in Scheuermann's disease. Spine 12:251-253, 1987.

26. Lowe TG, Kasten MD: An analysis of sagittal curves and balance after Cotrel-Dubousset instrumentation for kyphosis secondary to Scheuermann disease: A review of 32 patients. Spine 19:1680-1685, 1994.

27. Somhegyi A, Ratko I: Hamstring tightness and Scheuermann's disease (commentary). Am J Phys Med Rehab 72:44, 1993.

28. Bhojraj SY, Dandawate AV: Progressive cord compression secondary to thoracic disc lesions in Scheuermann's kyphosis managed by posterolateral decompression, interbody fusion and pedicular fixation: A new approach to management of a rare clinical entity. Eur Spine J 3:66, 1994.

29. Klein DM, Weiss RL, Allen JE: Scheuermann's dorsal kyphosis and spinal cord compression: Case report. Neurosurgery 18:628, 1986.

30. Lesoin F, Leys D, Rousseaux M, et al: Thoracic disk herniation and Scheuermann's disease. Eur Neurol 26:145, 1987.

31. Yablon JD, Kasdon DL, Levine H: Thoracic cord compression in Scheuermann's disease. Spine 13:896, 1988.

32. Sachs B, Bradford DS, Winter R, et al: Scheuermann kyphosis: Follow-up of Milwaukee brace treatment. J Bone Joint Surg Am 69:50-57, 1987.

33. Tribus CB: Transient paraparesis: A complication of the surgical management of Scheuermann's kyphosis secondary to thoracic stenosis. Spine 26:1086-1089, 2001.

34. Bradford DS, Garcia A: Neurological complications in Scheuermann's disease: A case report and review of the literature. J Bone Joint Surg Am 51:567-572, 1969.

35. Chiu KY, Luk KD: Cord compression caused by multiple disc herniations and intraspinal cyst in Scheuermann's disease. Spine 20:1075-1079, 1995.

36. Ponte A, Gebbia F, Eliseo F: Non-operative treatment of adolescent hyperkyphosis. Orthop Trans 9:108, 1985.

37. Speck GR, Chopin DC: The surgical treatment of Scheuermann's kyphosis. J Bone Joint Surg Br 68:189-193, 1986.

38. Bradford DS, Moe JH, Montalvo FJ, et al: Scheuermann's kyphosis and roundback deformity: Results of Milwaukee brace treatment. J Bone Joint Surg Am 56:740-758, 1974.

39. Bradford DS, Ahmed KB, Moe JH, et al: The surgical management of patients with Scheuermann's disease: A review of twenty-four cases managed by combined anterior and posterior spine fusion. J Bone Joint Surg Am 62:705-712, 1980.

40. Bradford DS: Vertebral osteochondrosis (Scheuermann's kyphosis). Clin Orthop Relat Res 158:83-90, 1981.

41. Travaglini F, Conte M: Cifosi 25 anni. Progress in patologia vertebrate. In Goggia A (ed): Le cifosi, vol 5. Bologna, Goggia, 1982, p 163.

42. Travaglini F, Conte M: Untreated kyphosis: 25 years later. In Gaggi A (ed): Kyphosis. Bologna, Italian Scoliosis Research Group, 1984, p 21.

43. Lowe TG: Scheuermann disease. J Bone Joint Surg Am 72:940-945, 1990.

44. Lowe TG: Kyphosis of the thoracic and thoracolumbar spine in the pediatric patient: Surgical treatment. Instr Course Lect Pediatrics 189-196, 2006.

45. Harreby M, Neergaard K, Hesselsoe G, et al: Are radiologic changes in the thoracic and lumbar spine of adolescence risk factors for low back pain in adults? A 25 year prospective cohort study of 640 school children. Spine 20:2298-2302, 1995.

46. Paajaanen H, Alanen A, Erkintalo M, et al: Disc degeneration in Scheuermann disease. Skeletal Radiol 18:523-526, 1989.

47. Blount WP, Schmidt AC, Bidwell RG: Making the Milwaukee brace. J Bone Joint Surg Am 40:526-528, 1958.

48. Gutowski WT, Renshaw TS: Orthotic results in adolescent kyphosis. Spine 13:485-489, 1988.

49. Bradford DS, Moe JH, Montalvo FJ, et al: Scheuermann's kyphosis: Results of surgical treatment by posterior spine arthrodesis in twenty-two patients. J Bone Joint Surg Am 57:439-448, 1975.

50. Herndon WA, Emans JB, Micheli LJ, et al: Combined anterior and posterior fusion for Scheuermann's kyphosis. Spine 6:125-130, 1981.

51. Lowe TG: Double L-rod instrumentation in the treatment of severe kyphosis secondary to Scheuermann's disease. Spine 12:336-341, 1987.

52. Lim M, Green DW, Billinghurst JE, et al: Scheuermann kyphosis: Safe and effective surgical treatment using multisegmental instrumentation. Spine 29:1789-1794, 2004.

53. Herrera-Soto JA, Parikh SN, Al-Sayyad MJ, et al: Experience with combined video-assisted thoracoscopic surgery (VATS) anterior spinal release and posterior spinal fusion in Scheuermann's kyphosis. Spine 30:2176-2181, 2005.

54. Yang C, Askin G, Yang SH: Combined thoracoscopic anterior spinal release and posterior correction for Scheuermann's kyphosis [in Chinese]. Zhonghua Wai Ke Za Zhi 42:1293-1295, 2004.

55. Papagelopoulos PJ, Klassen RA, Peterson HA, et al: Surgical treatment of Scheuermann disease with segmental compression instrumentation. Clin Orthop Relat Res 139-149, 2001.

56. Vedantam R, Lenke LG, Bridwell KH, et al: A prospective evaluation of pulmonary function in patients with adolescent

idiopathic scoliosis relative to the surgical approach used for spinal arthrodesis. Spine 25:82-90, 2000.

57. Graham EJ, Lenke LG, Lowe TG, et al: Prospective pulmonary function evaluation following open thoracotomy for anterior spinal fusion in adolescent idiopathic scoliosis. Spine 25:2319-2325, 2000.

58. Wong CA, Cole AA, Watson L, et al: Pulmonary function before and after anterior spinal surgery in adult idiopathic scoliosis. Thorax 51:534-536, 1996.

59. Taylor TC, Wenger DR, Stephen J, et al: Surgical management of thoracic kyphosis in adolescents. J Bone Joint Surg Am 61:496-503, 1979.

60. Sturm PF, Dobson JC, Armstrong GW: The surgical management of Scheuermann's disease. Spine 18:685-691, 1993.

61. Otsuka NY, Hall JE, Mah JY: Posterior fusion for Scheuermann kyphosis. Clin Orthop Relat Res 134-139, 1990.

62. Johnston CE, Elerson E, Dagher G: Correction of adolescent hyperkyphosis with posterior-only threaded rod compression instrumentation: Is anterior spinal fusion still necessary? Spine 30:1528-1534, 2005.

63. Ponte A, Vero B, Siccardi GL: Surgical treatment of Scheuermann's hyperkyphosis. In Winter RB (ed): Progress in Spinal Pathology: Kyphosis. Bologna, Aulo Gaggi, 1984, pp 75-80.

64. Smith-Peterson MN, Larson CB, Aufrank OE: Osteotomy of the spine for correction of flexion deformity in rheumatoid arthritis J Bone Joint Surg Am 27:1-11, 1945.

65. Ponte A: Posterior column shortening for Scheuermann's kyphosis. In Haher TR, Merola AA (eds): Surgical Techniques for the Spine. New York, Thieme Verlag, 2003, pp 107-113.

66. Geck MJ, Macagno A, Ponte A, et al: The Ponte procedure: Posterior only treatment of Scheuermann's kyphosis using segmental posterior shortening and pedicle screw instrumentation. J Spinal Disord Tech 20:586-593, 2007.

67. Lee SS, Lenke LG, Kuklo TR, et al: Comparison of Scheuermann kyphosis correction by posterior-only thoracic pedicle screw fixation versus combined anterior/posterior fusion. Spine 31:2316-2321, 2006.

68. Hosman AJ, de Kleuver M, Anderson PG, et al: Analysis of the sagittal plane after surgical management for Scheuermann's disease: A view on overcorrection and the use of an anterior release. Spine 27:167-175, 2002.

69. de Jonge T, Ilés T, Bellyei A: Surgical correction of Scheuermann kyphosis. Int Orthop 25:70-73, 2001.

70. Poolman RW, Been HD, Ubags LH: Clinical outcome and radiographic results after operative treatment of Scheuermann disease. Eur Spine J 11:561-569, 2002.

71. Cho KJ, Lenke LG, Bridwell KH, et al: Selection of the optimal distal fusion level in posterior instrumentation and fusion for thoracic hyperkyphosis: The sagittal stable vertebra concept. Spine 34:765-770, 2009.

72. Cheh G, Lenke LG, Padberg AM, et al. Loss of spinal cord monitoring signals in children during thoracic kyphosis correction with spinal osteotomy: Why does it occur and what should you do? Spine 33:1093-1099, 2008.

73. Wilburg G, Thompson GH, Shaffer JW, et al: Postoperative neurological deficits in segmented spinal instrumentation. J Bone Joint Surg Am 66:1178-1188, 1984.

74. Winter B: Spine update: Neurologic safety in spinal deformity surgery. Spine 22:1527-1533, 1997.

75. Othman Z, Lenke LG, Bolon SM, et al: Hypotension-induced loss of intraoperative monitoring data during surgical correction of Scheuermann kyphosis: A case report. Spine 29:E258-E265, 2004.

76. Dolan EJ, Transfeldt EE, Tator CH, et al. The effect of spinal distraction on regional spinal cord blood flow in cats. J Neurosurg 53:756-764, 1980.

77. Yeoman PM, Gibson MJ, Hutchinson A, et al: Influence of induced hypotension and spinal distraction on feline spinal somatosensory evoked potentials. Br J Anaesth 63:315-320, 1989.

78. Lonner BS, Newton P, Betz R, et al: Operative management of Scheuermann's kyphosis in 78 patients: Radiographic outcomes, complications, and technique. Spine 32:2644-2652, 2007.

79. Daniels AH, Jurgensmeier D, McKee J, et al: Acute celiac artery compression syndrome after surgical correction of Scheuermann kyphosis. Spine 34:E149-E152, 2009.

80. Greig DM: Congenital kyphosis. Edinburgh Medical Journal February 1916.

81. Van Schrick F: Die angeborene Kyphose. Z Orthop Chir 56:238-259, 1932.

82. Tsou PM: Embryology of congenital kyphosis. Clin Orthop 128:18-25, 1977.

83. Tsou PM, Yau A, Hodgson AR: Embryogenesis and prenatal development of congenital vertebral anomalies and their classification. Clin Orthop 152:211-231, 1980.

84. Rivard CH, Narbaitz R, Uhthoff HK: Congenital vertebral malformations: Time of induction in human and mouse embryo. Orthop Rev 8:135, 1979.

85. McMaster MJ, Singh H: Surgical management of congenital kyphosis and kyphoscoliosis. Spine 26:2146-2155, 2001.

86. Winter RB, Moe JH, Wang JF: Congenital kyphosis: Its natural history and treatment as observed in a study of one hundred and thirty patients. J Bone Joint Surg Am 55:223-256, 1973.

87. McMaster MJ, Singh H: Natural history of congenital kyphosis and kyphoscoliosis: A study of one hundred and twelve patients. J Bone Joint Surg Am 81:1367-1383, 1999.

88. Dubousset J: Congenital kyphosis and lordosis. In Weinstein SL (ed): The Pediatric Spine. New York, Raven Press, 1994, pp 245-258.

89. Shapiro J, Herring J: Congenital vertebral displacement. J Bone Joint Surg Am 75:656-662, 1993.

90. Zeller RD, Ghanem I, Dubousset J: The congenital dislocated spine. Spine 21:1235-1240, 1996.

91. Basu PS, Elsebaie H, Noordeen ChM: Congenital spinal deformity: A comprehensive assessment at presentation. Spine 27:2255-2259, 2002.

92. Suh S-W, Sarwark JF, Vora A, et al: Evaluating congenital spine deformities for intraspinal anomalies with magnetic resonance imaging. J Pediatr Orthop 21:5525-5531, 2001.

93. Mayfield JK, Winter RB, Bradford DS, et al: Congenital kyphosis due to defects of anterior segmentation. J Bone Joint Surg Am 62:1291-1301, 1980.

94. James JI: Kyphoscoliosis. J Bone Joint Surg Br 37:414-426, 1955.

95. Campos MA, Fernandes P, Dolan LA, et al: Infantile thoracolumbar kyphosis secondary to lumbar hypoplasia. J Bone Joint Surg Am 90:1726-1729, 2008.

96. Winter RB, Moe JH, Lonstein JE: The surgical treatment of congenital kyphosis: A review of 94 patients age 5 years or older with 2 years or more follow-up in 77 patients. Spine 10:224-231, 1985.

97. Ruf M, Harms J: Pedicle screws in 1- and 2-year-old children: Technique, complications, and effect on further growth. Spine 27:E460-E466, 2002.

98. Hedequist DJ, Hall JE, Mans JB: The safety and efficacy of spinal instrumentation in children with congenital spine deformities. Spine 29:2081-2086, 2004.

99. Kim HW, Weinstein SL: Atypical congenital kyphosis: Report of two cases with long-term follow-up. J Bone Joint Surg Br 80:25-30, 1998.

100. Winter RB, Moe JH: The results of spinal arthrodesis of congenital spinal deformities in patients younger than five years old. J Bone Joint Surg Am 64:419-432, 1982.

101. Ruf M, Harms J: Posterior hemivertebra resection with transpedicular instrumentation: Early correction in children aged 1 to 6 years. Spine 28:2132-2138, 2003.

102. Nakamura H, Matsuda H, Konishi S, et al: Single-stage excision of hemivertebrae via the posterior approach alone for congenital spine deformity: Follow-up period longer than ten years. Spine 27:110-115, 2002.

103. Suk SI, Kim JH, Kim WJ: Posterior vertebral column resection for severe spinal deformities. Spine 27:2374-2382, 2002.

104. Shono Y, Abumi K, Kaneda K: One-stage posterior hemivertebra resection and correction using segmental posterior instrumentation. Spine 26:752-757, 2001.

105. Kim YJ, Otsuka NY, Flynn JM: Surgical treatment of congenital kyphosis. Spine 26:2251-2257, 2001.

27 CHAPTER

Spondylolysis and Spondylolisthesis

Suken A. Shah, MD

Faisal Mahmood, MD

K. Durga Nagraju, MD, DNB

Andrew H. Milby, MD

Spondylolysis is defined as a defect in the pars interarticularis of the posterior vertebral arch and is a common cause of back pain and disability.[1] In addition, spondylolysis may lead to instability of the spinal column and result in anterior translation of the vertebral body relative to the level inferior to the defect. This translation in the setting of spondylolysis is termed *spondylolisthesis,* from the Greek roots, *spondylos,* meaning "vertebrae," and *olisthesis,* meaning "to slip."[2] Even in the absence of symptoms from the pars defects themselves, spondylolisthesis may lead to clinically significant radiculopathy and progressive neurologic deficits secondary to nerve root impingement. Both conditions vary in their presentations and require judicious application of conservative and surgical treatment strategies.

The clinical syndrome of spondylolisthesis was first described in 1782 by the Belgian obstetrician Herbiniaux,[3] before an understanding of its pathophysiology. Herbiniaux reported a bony prominence anterior to the sacrum that created an impediment to vaginal delivery in a cohort of his patients. In 1853, the German physician Robert[4] reported on specific defects in the pars interarticularis; these defects were first labeled spondylolysis by Killian in 1854.[2] Killian[2] proposed that forces imposed by the body's weight caused subluxation of the lumbosacral facets and subsequent vertebral body subluxation. A short time later, in 1855, anatomic studies by Robert and Lambl revealed that a neural arch defect typically preceded the subluxation.[5] Robert freed the fifth lumbar vertebra successfully of surrounding soft tissue and showed that a neural arch defect was required for slippage to occur.[6]

In 1881, Neugebauer[7] detailed the clinical and anatomic manifestations of the deformity and suggested that lysis, elongation, and angulation of the pars interarticularis could lead to spondylolisthesis. In his travels through Europe in 1888, Neugebauer came across 10 specimens in which there was gross displacement of the fifth lumbar vertebra. He aptly termed this phenomenon *spondyloptosis,* from the Greek *ptosis,* meaning "falling off or down," to indicate a vertebra that is completely dislocated. Neugebauer initially attributed the deformity to traumatic injury; however, he later proposed that it was due to a congenital abnormality of neural arch ossification. This theory of abnormal ossification was questioned by Lane, who, in 1893, posited that spondylolisthesis was due to modification of the interarticular part of the fifth lumbar vertebra by pressure from the inferior facet of L4 superiorly and from the superior sacral process inferiorly.

Pathophysiology

As understanding of spondylolisthesis progressed, classifications of common subtypes emerged. The most widely used classification system today was described by Wiltse.[8-11] This system represents a further development of the classification described by Newman and Stone,[12] who, in 1962, reported the long-term outcomes of 319 patients with spondylolisthesis. In their series, spondylolisthesis was classified in terms of radiographic appearance and proposed etiology.

Wiltse separated spondylolisthesis into five main groups (Table 27–1). Type I, also known as *congenital* or *dysplastic spondylolisthesis,* is secondary to a congenital defect of the superior sacral facet or the inferior L5 facet or both with gradual anterior translation of the L5 vertebra. Type II, also known as *lytic* or *isthmic spondylolisthesis,* involves a defect in the isthmus or pars interarticularis. Type II is classified further into three subtypes: Type IIA represents a spondylolysis or a stress fracture of the pars region. Type IIB represents an intact but elongated pars caused by repeated stress and bony remodeling. Type IIC represents an acute traumatic fracture of the pars leading to anterolisthesis; this is the rarest of the subtypes. It is not the pars defect itself but the anterior translation that allows the lesion to be termed *spondylolisthesis.* Type III is degenerative in origin and is a disease of older adults that develops as a result of facet arthritis and remodeling. Such long-standing intersegmental instability can lead to either anterolisthesis or posterolisthesis. As the disease progresses, the articular processes may become more horizontally shaped, creating the potential for rotational deformity as well. Type IV is a post-traumatic disruption of posterior elements other than the pars (as in type IIC). This disruption is a gradual event and not an acute fracture-dislocation as seen in type IIC. Type V involves the destruction of the posterior elements in the setting of a pathologic process, such as malignancy, Paget

TABLE 27-1 Spondylolisthesis Classification by Wiltse[18]

Type	Description
I	Congenital dysplastic
II	Isthmic—defect at pars interarticularis
IIA	Spondylolytic—stress fracture of pars interarticularis
IIB	Elongation of pars interarticularis
IIC	Acute or traumatic fracture of pars interarticularis
III	Degenerative—long-standing intersegmental instability
IV	Post-traumatic—defects of posterior elements (aside from pars interarticularis)
V	Pathologic

disease, tuberculosis, or giant cell tumors. Additionally, an iatrogenic spondylolisthesis may occur after facetectomy.

Wiltse type I and type II constitute most cases, and these are the focus of this chapter. Although the classification schemes described allow for the systematic study of these disparate disease entities, they are of no proven prognostic value in the prediction of deformity progression.

The extent to which spondylosis depends on genetic or developmental factors is controversial. In 1982, Marchetti and Bartolozzi[13] divided spondylolisthesis into developmental and acquired subtypes. Developmental etiologies included elongation of the pars, lytic lesions, and traumatic events, whereas acquired etiologies included iatrogenic, pathologic, and degenerative conditions. In 1994, a revised classification system subclassified the developmental group further into high or low dysplastic. In these two subgroups, the pars interarticularis was described as being either osteolytic or elongated. Traumatic lesions were incorporated into the acquired group, and the iatrogenic etiology was relabeled as postsurgical (Table 27-2). Although developmental abnormalities of the posterior arch are typically insufficient to cause spondylolysis in the absence of other inciting factors, they may play a significant role in the predisposition to spondylolysis and subsequent spondylolisthesis.

A significant genetic predisposition is suggested by the observation that spondylolysis occurs in 15% to 70% of

first-degree relatives of individuals with the disorder.[14-22] Spondylolisthesis also shows a strong familial association, with an incidence in first-degree or second-degree relatives of approximately 25% to 30%.[5,9,11,23] A radiographic study by Wynne-Davies and Scott[15] showed that dysplastic spondylolisthesis has a familial incidence of 33%, whereas the isthmic variant has a familial incidence of 15%. Compared with the incidence in the general population, this represents a fourfold and twofold increased familial risk in patients with dysplastic and isthmic spondylolisthesis. Wynne-Davies and Scott[15] suggested a multifactorial autosomal dominant pattern of inheritance with incomplete penetrance. Wiltse[22] suggested, however, that a cartilaginous defect in the vertebrae may be of autosomal recessive inheritance with varying expressivity. Additionally, the correlation between spina bifida occulta and spondylolisthesis strengthens the suggestion of a hereditary contribution.

In combination with developmental susceptibilities, certain activities are risk factors for spondylolysis because of the nature of the biomechanical stresses imparted on the pars interarticularis. Biomechanical analyses have shown that hyperextension and persistent lordosis increase shear stresses at the neural arch.[24-27] Wiltse and colleagues[28] hypothesized that most cases of isthmic spondylolysis should be considered fatigue fractures caused by repetitive load and stress as opposed to a single traumatic event, although a traumatic event may lead to completion of a fracture already in development. Farfan and colleagues[29] hypothesized that a single event leads to the initial microfracture in the pars, with fractures occurring as a result of repetitive overload. As a result of these biomechanical data, activities that involve hyperextension of the lumbar spine, such as gymnastics, weightlifting, diving, football, and volleyball, have been implicated as causative factors in the development of spondylolysis.[27,30-32]

Persistent lumbar lordosis may also increase susceptibility to spondylosis; Ogilvie and Sherman[14] reported a 50% prevalence of asymptomatic spondylolysis in patients with Scheuermann kyphosis. The tendency toward progression of slippage during adolescence and the observation that girls are several times more likely to have an increase in deformity are also suggestive of a hormonal role in the development of spondylolisthesis.[23]

Epidemiology

The exact prevalence of spondylolysis is uncertain because it is asymptomatic in a large proportion of patients. Reports regarding the prevalence of spondylolysis are based primarily on painful or symptomatic spondylolysis or cases associated with listhesis. The prevalence in whites has been reported as 3% to 6% with a male-to-female ratio of 2:1.[33-35] Roche and Rowe[35] examined 4200 cadaveric specimens and found an overall prevalence of spondylolysis of 4.2%. Considerable ethnic variability exists in the prevalence of spondylolysis, with a lower prevalence in African Americans (1.8% to 2.4%) than in whites (5.6%).[36-39] The highest prevalence has

TABLE 27-2 Spondylolisthesis Classification by Marchetti and Bartolozzi[13]

Developmental	
High dysplastic	Interarticular lysis
	Elongation of pars interarticularis
Low dysplastic	Interarticular lysis
	Elongation of pars interarticularis
Acquired	
Traumatic	Acute or stress fracture
Postsurgical	Direct or indirect effect of surgery
Pathologic	Local or systemic pathology
Degenerative	Primary or secondary

been reported in the Eskimo population, with rates of 13% in adolescent patients and 54% in adults.[40] Although this prevalence may suggest a genetic predisposition, it has also been posited that Eskimos, who carry their infants in a papoose, place undue stress on the pars interarticularis.[36]

The reported incidence of isthmic spondylolisthesis ranges from 2.6% to 4.4%.[5,41-43] In the largest prospective radiographic study, Fredrickson and colleagues[41] evaluated 500 patients at age 6 years with a 20-year follow-up. A pars defect was appreciated in 4.4% of 6-year-old children. By age 12, 5.2% of the cohort were noted to have the defect (85% participation rate). This increased to 6% by age 18; however, most of the nonaffected patients had dropped out of the study (34% participation rate). Back pain had developed in only four of the patients, and one patient required an operative procedure to decompress a herniated disc at a level cephalad to the spondylolisthesis. Pars defects at L5 were noted to be bilateral in 78% of cases, with most of these progressing to spondylolisthesis. As a corollary to this study, Fredrickson and colleagues[41] also evaluated 500 newborns and found no evidence of spondylolysis or spondylolisthesis. The only reported case of a pars lesion in a newborn has been published by Borkow and Kleiger.[44] Isthmic spondylolisthesis is rare in children younger than 5 years old, with only a few reported cases.[43,45,46]

In spondylolysis, the pars interarticularis defect may be unilateral or bilateral. If the defect is bilateral, the chance of progression to listhesis is greater. The most common location of a spondylitic defect is L5 (85%),[47] and the defect may be observed as high as L2; multilevel defects are seen infrequently. Rarely, multiple defects may be seen at the same level. Ariyoshi and colleagues[48] reported a case of spondylolysis at three sites in L5 involving the bilateral pars interarticularis and the center of the right lamina.

The most common site of isthmic spondylolisthesis is at the L5-S1 level secondary to osteolysis at L5. Estimates show that this lesion is located at the L5 pars interarticularis in 90% of type II cases, at L4 in 5%, and in more cephalad vertebrae in the remaining 5% of cases.[11] Additionally, authors reported spina bifida occulta at the same level in 30% of patients with pars lesions. The incidence of spina bifida associated with spondylolisthesis has been reported to range from 24% to 70%.[9,23,49,50] Age at presentation with isthmic spondylolisthesis follows a bimodal distribution. One peak occurs between the ages of 5 and 7 years, and the second occurs in the teenage years.[9,19,49,51] The incidence in athletes who subject themselves to excessive lumbar posturing, such as gymnasts, soccer players, pitchers, cricket bowlers, and divers, is higher than in the general population.[53-60]

In pediatric patients, dysplastic and isthmic are the most commonly encountered subtypes, with the latter representing 85% of the cases. As with spondylolysis, isthmic (type II) spondylolisthesis is two times more frequent in boys than girls.[35] Dysplastic spondylolisthesis, similar to its isthmic counterpart, is also most commonly found at the L5-S1 junction. The incidence is two times higher in girls,[61,62] and based on more recent published reports, it accounts for 14% to 21% of total cases.[62,63]

History and Physical Examination

Spondylolysis may be discovered incidentally or may manifest with low back pain typically in the teenage years.[64] In approximately half of cases, the onset of low back pain is associated with a history of trauma or an inciting event.[23,65,66] Usually these patients complain of focal low back pain, only rarely radiating to the buttocks or posterior thigh, which becomes worse with activity or on hyperextension of the spine.[31,67-70] Lifting and weight bearing can exacerbate the pain, and a forced lumbar extension often intensifies the symptoms. Neurologic involvement is rare in isolated spondylolysis. Medical professionals who have little experience with spondylolysis often assume the defect to be a sequela of trauma requiring immediate immobilization and surgical intervention. In these cases, it is the responsibility of the spine surgeon to offer reassurance that imminent neurologic compromise is highly unlikely.[71,72]

Physical examination of the lumbar spine reveals focal tenderness in acute cases and mild discomfort in chronic cases. Patients maintain a full range of forward flexion (unless the hamstrings are tight) that is usually painless, but hyperextension movement leads to an exacerbation of symptoms as does lateral bending or rotation. Other associated physical signs are an antalgic gait, increased lumbar lordosis, and hamstring tightness. A single-leg hyperextension test is used for the diagnosis and differentiation of unilateral spondylolysis from bilateral lysis. This test is performed by the patient bearing weight on one leg with the hip and knee of the other leg flexed, while hyperextending the lumbar spine. This maneuver is performed on both sides; asymmetrical low back pain indicates unilateral spondylolysis. Bilateral lesions show symmetrical or asymmetrical pain with this maneuver.[73,74] The neurologic examination in isolated spondylolysis is generally normal, with radicular findings suggestive of foraminal stenosis owing to inflammation or instability.

Spondylolisthesis may manifest in a similar fashion but is also typically associated with hamstring tightness. This tightness manifests as a muscle spasm of the posterior thighs associated with a fixed flexion at the hip and knees. An increased popliteal angle is present on straight-leg raise. Increased popliteal angle is almost always observed universally, even in low-grade spondylolisthesis. Electromyographic and neurologic abnormalities are typically absent; this suggests that there is not a neurologic basis for the hamstring tightness, but that it likely results from the patient's attempts to maintain global sagittal balance.[63,75] Other authors hypothesize that tightness results as a sequela of chronic nerve root irritation from the instability and micromotion of the involved segment.[75-78] Patients often ambulate and stand with increased flexion at the hips and knees, also known as the Phalen-Dickson sign.[76] This flexed posturing increases as the amount of slippage increases. The patient may also exhibit a shuffled or short-stepped gait.[78]

Patients with spondylolisthesis may initially present with focal neurologic deficits or radiculopathy, although this is uncommon. Bilateral radicular symptoms are more commonly observed than unilateral radiculopathy. Typically, the

L5 root is involved with pain radiating to the buttocks and posterior thigh or weakness of the extensor hallucis longus. Constant loading of the pars defects may hinder bony healing, resulting in a fibrous union that may be a persistent source of pain. Local expansion of fibrocartilaginous scar tissue within the area of the pars defect may cause nerve root compression. Tension on the nerve root also increases with progression of olisthesis, increasing further the likelihood of radicular symptoms with disease progression.[72] In higher grade subluxations, traction of the cauda equina over the sacrum may exist. This traction may lead to signs and symptoms of cauda equina compression, such as perineal paresthesia, decreased sphincter tone, and urinary retention. Additionally, traction of the cauda is thought to create a reflex spasm of the hamstrings.[79,80]

Higher grade spondylolisthesis results in a palpable step-off over the spinous processes. In isthmic spondylolisthesis, the step-off is typically found at the L4-5 junction, as the neural arch of the L5 vertebrae does not translate anteriorly with the body but remains within its geographic location in relation to the sacrum. In dysplastic spondylolisthesis, the neural arch is still attached to the vertebral body and slides anteriorly with the body, producing a palpable step-off that is typically appreciated at the lumbosacral junction. Lumbosacral kyphosis with a retroverted sacrum results in heart-shaped, flattened buttocks. In severe cases, the trunk appears grossly shortened, and the rib cage lies within close proximity to the iliac crests.

Scoliosis also may be associated with spondylolisthesis.[12,25,81-85] The incidence has been reported to be 60%. Scoliosis may result because of a combination of hamstring and paraspinal muscle spasm, rotational deformity, or truncal asymmetry. If scoliosis is secondary to spondylolisthesis (nonstructural), it usually resolves after treatment of the olisthesis. The patient may also have an adolescent idiopathic curve with a low-grade spondylolisthesis that was detected incidentally on radiographic evaluation.

Radiographic Evaluation

Many imaging modalities may be useful in the diagnosis and evaluation of spondylolisthesis. Radiographic evaluation of spondylolisthesis begins with plain radiographs, including lateral, anteroposterior, and oblique views.[86] The anteroposterior view should be angled 15 degrees to the inclination of the L5-S1 disc (Ferguson view). This view not only allows for visualization of the presence of sacral spinal bifida, but also evaluates the size of the lumbar transverse processes and height of the disc.

The defect in isthmic spondylolysis is visualized as lucency in the region of the pars interarticularis. The lucency is commonly described as having the appearance of a collar or a "broken neck on the Scotty dog" seen in lateral oblique radiographs. A spot lateral view is able to identify only 19% of pars defects,[33,87] whereas oblique lateral views can detect the pars defect in 84% of cases.[88] It is important to take right and left oblique views because pars defects may be unilateral in some cases, and the collar may be visible in only one projection.

Although oblique views are most sensitive in diagnosing spondylolysis, the lateral view is optimal for appreciating the degree of olisthesis in spondylolisthesis. The lateral view should be performed with the patient standing. Flexion-extension views may assess for the presence of associated instability. This subtle movement may be an important pain generator and is essential for further treatment planning. Additionally, these views show the extent of postural reduction of the lumbosacral angulation and translation that may be obtained without formal release.

Because the sensitivity of plain radiographs is limited, radionuclide (technetium 99mm) bone imaging may be a good option in cases of suspected spondylolysis with negative plain radiographs. A bone scan identifies pars interarticularis stress fractures that can be missed in oblique radiographs because a stress reaction may be present without a bony defect. Patients who have had a recent trauma or performed strenuous activity and are symptomatic have a bone scan showing increased uptake in the spondylolytic area; however, patients with chronic low backache can have normal bone scans if the defect is chronic, is sclerotic, and has lost its blood supply. Single photon emission computed tomography (SPECT) is more sensitive and provides more details than plain x-rays and technetium bone scan.[89,90] A "hot" scan insinuates increased activity, and the patient may benefit from orthotic immobilization, whereas a "cold" scan suggests a chronic lesion that is not metabolically active and is unlikely to respond to immobilization alone.[72]

Thin-cut axial computed tomography (CT) is highly accurate at visualizing osseous anatomy and is superior to plain radiography in its ability to show dysplastic facets and pars defects. CT may also be used after plain radiographs or bone scan to assess the healing potential of an identified pars defect.[91] In addition to showing spondylolysis accurately, CT may identify changes in the apophyseal joints associated with degenerative and reverse spondylolisthesis and can show minimal degrees of spondylolisthesis by the presence of a pseudobulging disk.[92]

Magnetic resonance imaging (MRI) is a highly sensitive imaging technique that allows for additional visualization of soft tissue and neural structures and is recommended in all cases associated with neurologic findings. MRI offers the distinct advantage of being able to image the spine in any plane without exposure to ionizing radiation. Sagittal thin slices (3-mm slice thickness for T1-weighted images and 4-mm slice thickness for T2-weighted images) are able to identify 95% of pars defects, with T1-weighted images being more sensitive than T2-weighted images.[93] In the early course of the disease, MRI helps in identifying the stress reaction at the pars interarticularis before the end-stage bony defect.[94,95] In more acute presentations in which plain radiographs may be negative, a fat saturation technique can be applied to minimize signal from fat and to bring out signal from fluid structures such as bone edema. MRI also allows for evaluation the spinal cord and its associated elements with greater anatomic detail and without the procedural risks associated with CT myelography. MRI may show the degree of impingement of neural elements by fibrous scar tissue at the spondylolytic defect. Additionally, involvement of adjacent discs should be evaluated because abnormal biomechanics can lead to early degenerative changes at adjacent levels.

The most commonly used radiographic grading system for spondylolisthesis is the one proposed by Meyerding in 1932.[95a] The degree of slippage is measured as the percentage of distance the anteriorly translated vertebral body has moved forward. On the lateral radiograph, a line is drawn along the posterior sacral border. A line perpendicular to this is drawn at the superior part of the sacrum. The anterior translation or displacement of the inferior border of L5 as a proportion of the width of S1 is expressed as a percentage. The Meyerding classification grades increasing olistheses from I to IV (Table 27–3). Spondyloptosis, in which the fifth lumbar vertebra has slipped forward over 100% of the gliding plane past the sacral promontory, is referred to as grade V. Spondylolysis without olisthesis is referred to as grade 0.

Although the Meyerding classification system quantifies translational subluxation in the anteroposterior plane, it does not quantify the sagittal rotation of a vertebral body that may coexist in spondylolisthesis. This angular displacement is referred to as the *slip angle,* and as with the Meyerding grading system, the erect lateral radiograph is the basis for measurement. The slip angle is calculated by measuring the angle formed by the intersection of two lines: (1) a line perpendicular to the posterior cortex of the sacrum and (2) a line paralleling the inferior endplate of L5. In the normal spine, slip angle values should be close to zero. The slip angle quantifies the lumbosacral kyphosis and was shown by Boxall and colleagues[63] to be the most useful tool in determining the risk of the progression in a skeletally immature patient. A slip angle greater than 55 degrees is associated with a high probability and increased rate of progression.

Sacral inclination or pelvic tilt refers to the vertical position of the sacrum. It is the angle formed by the intersection of two lines: (1) a line perpendicular to the floor and (2) a line parallel to the posterior cortex of the sacrum. Normal values are greater than 30 degrees. With an increasing slip, lumbosacral kyphosis is increased, and the sacrum is forced into a more vertical orientation decreasing the pelvic tilt.

In 1983, Wiltse and Winter[96] proposed a classification that separated the tangential movement seen in low-grade slips (grade I and II) from the angular and tangential movement that was appreciated in high-grade slips (grade III or higher). The three measurements that were factored were degree of slip, vertebral wedging, and sacral rounding. These authors recommended the forward displacement of the fifth lumbar vertebra in relationship to the sacrum be measured as an actual percentage as first described by Taillard[42] and later recommended by Laurent and Osterman.[97] It was stressed that even a small degree of progression should be measured, and this was not quantifiable on the Meyerding scale. Sacral tilt as described previously and sagittal rotation or slip angle were also used. The method for measuring slip angle, which Wiltse and Winter[96] termed *sagittal rotation,* was modified by measuring the angle formed by the intersection of two lines: (1) a line extending off the anterior cortex of the L5 vertebral body and (2) a line off the posterior border of the first sacral

TABLE 27–3 Meyerding Classification*

Grade	Percentage of Slippage (A/B)
0	0 (spondylolysis)
I	0-25%
II	25%-50%
III	50%-75%
IV	75%-100%
V	Vertebral body completely displaced (spondyloptosis)

*Grades 0 and V were added later on.

vertebrae. Wiltse and Winter[96] believed the endplates of the L5 and S1 bodies to be unreliable osseous structures secondary to osseous hyperplasia.

Conservative Management

Treatment of spondylolysis mainly focuses on pain relief, core muscle strengthening, and restoration of full lumbar range of motion. Achieving these goals enables the patient to return to normal activity without any restrictions. Management of spondylolysis depends on the severity of the symptoms and level of activity. Initial conservative management in the form of activity restriction and bracing (for pain relief) relieves symptoms in patients with spondylolysis. It is likely that most lesions do not heal with bone but become a stable fibrous union that remains relatively asymptomatic.

Conservative management of spondylolysis includes complete cessation of activity, rehabilitation with strengthening of the abdominal and paraspinal musculature, minimization of pelvic tilt, and perhaps antilordotic bracing.[98] Conservative management protocols also depend on several factors such as disease involvement (spondylolysis vs. spondylolisthesis), level and laterality of the defect (unilateral vs. bilateral pars defects), duration since injury (acute vs. chronic), and age of the patient.[99] Many authors prefer to use a total-contact, low-profile polyethylene orthosis, which is designed to maintain an antilordotic posture and extends from just below the nipples to 1 inch above the greater trochanter. The brace is worn for 23 hours/day for minimum of 3 to 6 months.[100] If clinical symptoms improve, the brace can be gradually weaned through a period of part-time wear.

Excellent clinical outcomes have been reported with a course of activity restriction and bracing that prevents repetitive hyperextension movements at the lumbar spine.[100-103] Good to excellent results with brace therapy have been shown in 80% of patients with grade 0 or I spondylolisthesis.[100,104,105] Bell and colleagues[104] showed prevention of increased slip angle and 100% reduction of pain in 28 patients with grade I or II spondylolisthesis after a mean brace treatment of 25 months. In a series of 82 symptomatic patients with various degrees of spondylolisthesis, Pizzutillo and Hummer[105] reported that nonoperative treatment of grade II or less was shown to relieve pain reliably in two thirds of patients. A study by Steiner and Micheli[100] showed radiographic evidence of healing pars defects in 12 of 67 patients with spondylolysis or grade I spondylolisthesis after treatment in a modified Boston brace. Excellent or good results were achieved in 78% with return to full activities. Patients with spondylolysis and grade I spondylolisthesis may return to full activity and sports with resolution of symptoms and documented lack of slip progression. Controversy exists regarding postbrace activity level for patients with grade II spondylolisthesis. The general consensus is that after successful brace treatment a child with grade II spondylolisthesis may return to sports that do not involve hyperlordotic posturing.[18,26,27]

Patients with acute pars interarticularis fractures are best treated with immediate initiation of bracing for pain relief and restriction from athletic activity with continued mobilization for activities of daily living. Anderson and colleagues[107] used clinical evaluation and SPECT imaging to compare the rate of response to early versus late initiation of bracing. In this study, patients with early bracing showed rapid relief of symptoms, a short bracing time, and rapid reduction of SPECT ratio. Patients showing a spondylolytic defect on plain radiography but whose bone scans were negative were determined to have inactive (terminal) spondylolytic defects, pseudarthrosis, or old unhealed fractures.[73,108] Athletes with low back pain and increased uptake on SPECT scan at the pars interarticularis but no defect on radiographs typically respond to a period of rest and active rehabilitation; very few athletes develop defects or persistent back pain.[109]

As the understanding of spinal biomechanics has progressed, Panjabi[110] posited the concept of specific training of lumbar muscles in chronic low back pain. According to his concept, specific training of muscles around the lumbar spine improves the dynamic stability and controls segmental spinal motion. The local muscular system that controls the lumbar spine consists of lumbar multifidus, internal oblique, and transverse abdominis.[110] A randomized trial by O'Sullivan of 44 patients who were treated with two different protocols showed that a specific strengthening program was more effective than generalized back strengthening exercises.[98] Along with exercises that target specific core muscle groups with the spine in neutral position, strengthening of hip flexors and hamstring stretching are important and recommended.[100,101,111]

Patients with low-grade dysplastic spondylolisthesis are less likely than patients with isthmic spondylolisthesis to respond to conservative measures,[5] but conservative therapy is still recommended as the initial modality. The importance of radiographic and neurologic follow-up should be stressed to these patients because they are at a higher risk for slip progression owing to facet hypoplasia. Radiographic follow-up is recommended at least annually until skeletal maturity and more frequently during peak height velocity before puberty. Documentation of slip percentage, angle, sacral inclination, wedging, and pelvic tilt is recommended as part of proper documentation of progression of the deformity.

Surgical Treatment

Surgical intervention is indicated for patients with persistent pain, progressive spondylolisthesis, or neurologic symptoms who fail conservative management. Treatment approach is influenced by the level of spinal maturity, degree of slippage, symptoms, the patient's activity level, and expected progression. In contrast to a comparable adult, an asymptomatic adolescent may be a candidate for surgical intervention because of expected progression of deformity in a high-grade slip, which may lead further to mechanical and neurologic dysfunction. In a skeletally immature patient with slippage greater than 50% or a mature adolescent with a slip greater than 75%, operative intervention is recommended even if the patient is asymptomatic.[106,112,113] Surgical decompression is also indicated when a patient has neural compromise, with a radiculopathy or bowel or bladder dysfunction.[114-116]

Surgical treatment options may be broadly divided into two categories: direct repair of the pars defects versus arthrodesis of the involved segments to prevent slip progression with or without decompression of affected neural structures. Procedures for direct fixation of pars defects include Buck technique,[117] Scott wiring,[118] and repair with an ipsilateral pedicle screw and hook.[119,120]

Fusion of the involved level has been widely advocated as treatment of symptomatic spondylolysis.[106,121] The long-term effects of fusion in a young patient must be considered, however, owing to the potential for adjacent segment degeneration.[122,123] Based on their simulated lumbar fusion studies in cadavers, Weinhoffer and colleagues[124] concluded that increased intradiscal pressure at the level of fusion could lead to accelerated degeneration at the adjacent discs. Kinematic studies of adjacent vertebra after fusion have shown disc degeneration, increased stress at the facet joints, hypertrophy of the facets, and hypermobility at the adjacent level.[123,125,126] Based on these kinematic studies and the goal of preserving motion when possible, isolated repair of the pars interarticularis defect is the preferred treatment for symptomatic pars defects in patients with no slip or disc degeneration at that level and relief from the diagnostic injection. Fusion is an option if an attempt at pars repair is unsuccessful, the lamina is dysplastic, the defect is very large, or disc degeneration or listhesis is present. Some authors maintain that results for fusion are better at L5 because of the narrow lamina at L5 and the steep lordotic angle that may be present.[127]

To increase the probability of response to surgical treatment, Wu and colleagues[128] reported on the use of preoperative diagnostic pars injection at the site of the defect. In their series of 100 patients who had failed conservative management, the pain generator was confirmed by injecting 1.5 mL of bupivacaine (Marcaine) into the lytic area. Reproduction of similar pain and pain relief of at least 70% of the usual pain quality for more than 6 hours were considered as a positive response, and these patients subsequently showed an excellent outcome after repair of the defect.[128]

Buck fusion is an open technique in which the fibrous tissue at the pars defect is identified, thoroughly débrided, and stabilized with a 4.5-mm stainless steel cortical screw in compression.[117] Buck[117] concluded that this technique was indicated only in cases in which the gap was smaller than 3 to 4 mm. Various studies showed 88% to 100% defect healing and satisfactory results with his technique.[129-131] Direct repair using a screw is a demanding procedure, however; owing to the narrowness of the lamina, a minimal displacement or malposition of the screw can lead to implant failure or complications such as nerve root irritation, injury to the posterior arch or dura, or pseudarthrosis.[132,133]

In the Scott technique, a stainless steel wire is looped from the transverse processes to the spinous process of the level involved and tightened, in conjunction with local iliac crest bone graft.[118] This wire creates a tension band construct, placing the pars defect under compression, and holds the bone graft in place. Bradford and Iza[134] reported 80% good to excellent results and 90% radiographic healing of the defects. This technique requires greater surgical exposure, with extensive stripping of the muscles to expose the transverse process. Complications such as wire breakage are common with this technique. Salib and Pettine[135] modified this technique by passing a wire around the cortical screws introduced into both pedicles and tightening it beneath the spinous process. Biomechanical tests show that fixation of the wire to the pedicle screw does not increase the stiffness of the system.[136] Both cerclage techniques have good defect healing rates of 86% to 100%.[118,135,137,138] Songer and Rovin[139] modified this construct by replacing the wire with a cable tied up to a pedicle screw and then passed and wrapped around the contralateral lamina. This system provides solid fixation, and the authors reported excellent outcome in five of seven patients and 100% solid union in all patients.

Morscher and colleagues[140] introduced a new technique to repair the pars defect with a laminar hook, which is loaded with compression by a spring placed against a screw threaded in the articular process. Healing rates with this technique range from 56% to 82%.[140-144] The major drawback of this procedure is screw penetration to the inferior articular process of the cephalad vertebra, which can lead to screw loosening or breakage.[145] Gillet and Petit[146] introduced the concept of the rod screw construct, in which the rod is firmly fixed to the spinous process, and published excellent outcomes in 6 of 10 patients.

Taddonio, using the Cotrel-Dubousset system, first introduced a repair using pedicle screw fixation.[221] Tokuhashi and Matsuzaki[127] reported excellent outcomes with the Isola pediculolaminar system. Kakiuchi[147] reported similar results using Texas Scottish Rite Hospital instrumentation system; with this technique, hooks are fixed at the lamina and connected with a rod to an ipsilateral pedicle screw after compression. Roca and colleagues[148] reported 92% excellent results with their new pedicle screw hook construct system in adolescents, but they have not recommended this technique for patients older than 20 years. Pellise and colleagues[149] advised 1-mm thin cuts to assess the pars anatomy, but 2.5-mm cuts help in assessing bone healing after direct repair in spondylolysis.

The authors' preferred technique for pars repair is to use minimal access tubes or retractors to obtain exposure of the pars defect and débride the fibrous tissue and hypertrophic nonunion with a bur and curets to bleeding bone, but care must be taken not to enlarge the defect further and destabilize the segment. Iliac crest bone graft is placed into the defect, and a cannulated laminar screw is placed percutaneously over a predrilled guidewire from the ipsilateral inferior lamina across the defect to engage the cortical bone of the pedicle or superior endplate for compression, avoiding the facet joint. Additional graft (or bone graft replacement) is placed over the defect, extending from the lamina to the junction of the transverse process. The patient is immobilized in a low-profile thoracolumbosacral orthosis for 12 weeks (hip joint locked with a leg extension for the first 6 weeks) and then progressed to rehabilitation. Healing is checked at 6 months, and the patient is allowed to resume all sports.

For a pediatric patient with grade I or II spondylolisthesis, dysplastic spondylolisthesis at the lumbosacral junction, or a slip secondary to a defect of the L5 pars who has failed conservative treatment, posterior in situ fusion is recommended from L5 to S1. With the widespread use of pedicle screws and the myriad screw options that are available, numerous studies have been performed supporting the use of transpedicular fixation. Transpedicular fixation has been shown to increase the rate of fusion, and a positive correlation has been reported between successful fusion and clinical outcome.[150-156] Other series have not shown a statistically significant difference between instrumented and noninstrumented posterior fusions.[157,158] In one study of 10 patients in a cohort who had the working diagnosis of spondylolisthesis, 5 underwent instrumented fusion, 4 of whom achieved an excellent or good outcome, compared with 2 of 5 who underwent a noninstrumented fusion.[159]

Lenke and colleagues[160] performed noninstrumented in situ fusions in 56 pediatric patients with isthmic spondylolisthesis. Based on radiographic evidence, only 50% showed a solid fusion mass, whereas 33% showed radiographic changes highly unlikely or with no evidence of a fusion mass. Despite poor fusion rates, overall clinical improvement was noted in greater than 80% of the cohort with preoperative symptoms of back or leg pain or hamstring tightness. A trend for improved clinical outcome with increased rigidity of fixation has been noted.[151] Pedicle screw fixation systems have been shown to be mechanically superior to other fixation while allowing for the selective segmental force without extension to adjacent levels.[161] Additionally, the use of instrumentation obviates the need for postoperative casting in a compliant patient. If exposure of midline structures and decompression is not warranted, the paraspinal approach described by Wiltse and colleagues[11,162] is recommended because it avoids neural arch defects, minimizes soft tissue trauma, and improves visualization of posterolateral structures. Additionally it helps maintain position of the bone graft and may promote fusion. During surgical dissection, care must be taken to protect facets at levels cephalad to the proposed fusion because this may create instability or degeneration later on. Minimally invasive techniques are available.

The method of immobilization after an in situ posterior fusion ranges from bed rest to bilateral pantaloon spica casts for 6 months. Literature can be found to support either end of the spectrum.[112,163-169] Boxall and colleagues[63] and Sherman and colleagues[170] compared in situ patients who were immobilized in a cast or orthosis with patients who were treated with bed rest.[63,170] Each study showed no statistical difference in the fusion rate based on immobilization methods.

Decompression is warranted in patients with neurologic findings. Patients with low-grade spondylolisthesis generally do not have significant neurologic symptoms. In an adult patient with radiculopathy, it may be acceptable to perform only a decompressive procedure as described in 1955 by Gill and colleagues.[114] The removal of loose posterior elements and cartilaginous tissue can increase vertebral column instability and further progression of deformity, however—an unacceptable risk in the pediatric spine.[171,172] Although a wide decompression may be warranted, it should be augmented with spinal fusion in a growing child.[114] Studies have also shown an increased risk of progression of deformity in patients with L5 laminectomy and posterior fusion versus patients with posterior fusion alone.[172-174]

Treatment of high-grade spondylolisthesis is a topic of great debate. Symptomatic patients with high-grade spondylolisthesis tend to fare poorer with nonoperative treatment compared with their counterparts with low-grade spondylolisthesis.[175] In high-grade spondylolisthesis, correction of the slip angle rather than the degree of anterior listhesis should be addressed. Although studies show that patients with greater than 50% of slippage may not have a poor nonoperative outcome,[176] fusion is the general treatment of choice among spinal surgeons. In determining the most appropriate procedure, one must take into account all presenting symptoms, neurologic function, radiographic findings, clinical deformity, patient's age, and the surgeon's experience.

As with low-grade spondylolisthesis, in situ fusion was a described treatment for pediatric patients with high-grade spondylolisthesis; however, cranial extension including L4 is recommended.[165] A Wiltse approach is suggested unless decompression is warranted. As reported by Pizzutillo and colleagues,[177] bone graft placement at the level of or anterior to the transverse processes extending to the sacral ala helps to ensure a large posterolateral fusion mass, which can effectively counteract shear forces at the lumbosacral junction. Allograft or autograft or both may be used, balancing the rate of successful fusion versus the potential for donor site pain and morbidity.[173,178-181]

Postoperative progression of deformity has been appreciated in patients and has been attributed to pseudarthrosis, lack of postoperative immobilization, lack of graft consolidation or maturation, or deterioration of the solid fusion mass. Progression has been appreciated in patients with a solid fusion mass as evidenced by radiography. Patients with a greater preoperative deformity are at higher risk.[165,168,172,182,183] The advance of slippage is usually minor in these cases, and studies have shown that radiographic evidence of pseudarthrosis does not always lead to pain.[63,160,184] Studies with long-term follow-up of patients with high-grade spondylolisthesis show in situ fusion to be a viable solution in maintenance of symptom relief and prevention of degenerative arthrosis of mobile cephalad spinal segments.[163,185-187]

Grzegorzewski and Kumar[168] found no radiographic pseudarthrosis in 21 patients with high-grade spondylolisthesis treated with in situ fusion, postoperative immobilization in a pantaloon spica cast, and 4 months of bed rest. Although five patients showed evidence of slip progression, two of whom showed an increased slip angle within the 1st year, only four patients had symptoms of back pain after postoperative follow-up of almost 13 years. Overall reports show radiographic evidence of successful fusion to range from 71% to 100% and relief of back pain and neurologic symptoms to range from 74% to 100% in patients after in situ fusion.[1,165,170,175] Patients with high-grade spondylolisthesis who are at risk of developing pseudarthrosis are patients who require a wide decompression secondary to L5 radiculopathy or sacral root symptoms and patients with excessive mobility at the L5-S1 junction. Patients with hypoplastic transverse processes, spina bifida, and sacral malformation are also at risk of pseudarthrosis.

Transsacral fusion using either fibular graft or mesh case has been shown more recently to be a viable treatment option. By providing an anterior column support and fusion bed, increased structural stability can be achieved. Smith and Bohlman[187] suggested a modification to posterolateral fusion to decrease the incidence of pseudarthrosis and progression of deformity. Eleven patients with high-grade spondylolisthesis were treated in a single-stage procedure involving spinal decompression, in situ posterolateral arthrodesis with autologous iliac crest graft, and anterior arthrodesis with a fibular graft inserted from the posterior approach. A cannulated drill was used to develop a transsacral osseous tunnel extending into the L5 vertebral body. A mid-diaphyseal fibular graft was harvested, trimmed, and inserted into this tunnel, acting as a dowel in the lumbosacral junction. Preoperative neurologic findings were sensory deficits in all but one patient and cauda equina syndrome in five patients. Six patients had prior spinal operations that had failed. The average duration of follow-up was 64 months showing a solid fusion mass with complete or major neurologic recovery in all patients. Average time to solid fusion was 12 weeks.

In a patient with sagittal balance and high-grade spondylolisthesis, an in situ procedure or partial reduction can be performed, and a cage or fibular dowel can be inserted anteriorly from L5 into S1 or posteriorly with a retrograde direction from S1 into L5. Posterior insertion of the transvertebral cage or fibular graft is advantageous because it obviates the need for an anterior approach to the lumbosacral region, which has its own drawbacks. There is less blood loss and less risk of injury to great vessels. Because the entire procedure can be done with the patient in one position and with one incision, operative time is also greatly reduced. A partial reduction can be performed by use of concave rods, and fusion should be augmented with posterior instrumentation.

Mahmood and colleagues[188] presented a case series in which a transsacral mesh cage was used in lieu of a fibular strut graft. Partial reduction was accomplished with a pedicle screw curved rod construct after which an osseous tunnel was established and a transsacral cage impregnated with bone graft was inserted from a posterior approach. A distinct benefit of using a cage is increased biomechanical stability, as studies have shown fibular strut resorption, deformation, and even fracture.[189-191] Additionally, the use of a cage avoids potential donor site morbidity.[192,193] Average radiographic and clinical follow-up of these patients was 38 months showing evidence of fusion and relief of symptoms.

There is no clear indication for when reduction of a high-grade spondylolisthesis is necessary, as opposed to performing a fusion with mild correction of the slip angle. Many authors suggest an in situ fusion or mild correction is indicated for patients who exhibit sagittal balance and acceptable slip angle. When considering reduction, improvement of slip angle should be the primary objective rather than improvement of grade of listhesis. In patients with a high-grade slip, a larger slip angle correlates with increased risk of progression of deformity.[75,77] Reduction of spondylolisthesis results in improved sagittal balance, improvement in cosmesis, and a biomechanically stable fusion mass. In addition, by reducing the deformity, canal stenosis is improved, and tension on nerve roots and the cauda equina is reduced. Improvement of overall sagittal alignment leads to improved posture, improved gait, and increased function. Reduction of spondylolisthesis in skeletally immature patients is recommended for patients with a high slip angle (>45 degrees), patients with severe sagittal imbalance, and patients who are at high risk of developing a pseudarthrosis with in situ fusion.[63,163,194]

Numerous methods of reduction have been described. The earliest reported reduction was published in 1936 by Jenkins,[194a] who used longitudinal traction followed by anterior fusion; however, the reduction could not be maintained. Since his initial report, variations of Jenkins' described technique have been published.[163,185,195-205] Reduction techniques may be as minimally invasive as external casting after bone graft placement or as complex as staged procedures involving multiple posterior and anterior approaches.

Reduction with external casting is particularly beneficial in young patients, in whom pedicle screw fixation is not feasible. After an open procedure in which posterior elements are decorticated and bone graft is placed around the proposed fusion site, the surgical wound is closed. The patient is placed on an antilordotic frame or spica table with extension of the spine to reduce the lumbosacral kyphosis. The patient should be awake for this part of the procedure to report any changes in neurologic function. If this is impossible, the use of neuro-monitoring may help in the neurologic assessment during the reduction. To hold the reduction, the spica cast should be extended to the trunk and incorporate at least one thigh. Burkus and colleagues[166] showed that the use of pantaloon spica cast immobilization led to a decrease in sagittal translation of more than 5% in three quarters of patients treated with cast immobilization and a decrease in the slip angle of more than 5% in 58% of patients treated with cast immobilization. Of the patients who did not undergo cast immobilization, 45% had an increase in sagittal translation of more than 5%, and 56% had an increase in slip angle of more than 5 degrees.

In patients in whom instrumentation can be placed, reduction followed by instrumentation for stability is recommended. Published procedures include halo-femoral or halo-pelvic traction and anteroposterior fusion followed by application of a pantaloon spica cast to apply anteriorly directed pressure.[163,199] Other authors have described anterior release with partial reduction and anterior interbody fusion,[206] intraoperative closed reduction followed by instrumented posterior fusion,[207] and a two-stage procedure with a posterior decompression and halo-skeletal traction followed by interbody fusion.[208] Drawbacks to these procedures included lengthy preoperative hospitalization for traction and lengthy postoperative immobilization in a cast. The study by Burkus and colleagues[166] compared patients treated with a pure in situ fusion with patients who underwent posterior fusion and were reduced postoperatively in a pantaloon spica cast. Reduction was found to be safe, and fusion rates were noted to higher, in addition to less chance of late slip and slip angle progression in patients who were treated with a reduction.

Mehdian and Arun[209] published a three-stage procedure using a combined anterior and posterior approach performed in one operative sitting. In the first stage, a laminectomy of L5 is performed with wide decompression of the L4-S1 nerve roots. L5-S1 discectomy was performed next followed by an osteotomy of the posterosuperior aspect of S1. The second stage consisted of a transperitoneal approach to the L5-S1 level, allowing removal of the anterior disc protrusion and associated thickened anulus fibrosus, effectively allowing posterior translation of the superior body. In the final stage, the patient is repositioned prone and instrumented from L4-S1. Bilateral pedicle screws are initially placed at L4 and S1, and a reduction can be performed with the assistance of curved rods, after which bilateral L5 pedicle fixation points can be established. Cages may be inserted in the L5-S1 interspace to promote a solid arthrodesis.

The authors' preferred method for treating high-grade slips with significant lumbosacral kyphosis is postural reduction with positioning under anesthesia and a wide decompression of the L5 and S1 nerve roots bilaterally. The dysplastic L5-S1 disc is removed with a transforaminal approach, and the dome of the sacrum is osteotomized (sacroplasty) to facilitate gentle reduction. Reduction pedicle screws are used to reduce the slip gently, an interbody graft is placed, and the construct is compressed posteriorly to obtain lordosis.

Treatment of severe deformity, including spondyloptosis, can be challenging to the most experienced spine surgeon. The natural history of spondyloptosis is unclear because of its rarity and because it is frequently not reported separately from high-grade spondylolisthesis (grade III and IV). Most authors agree that in a symptomatic patient, benign neglect is not a viable option. The surgical management of spondyloptosis in children is variably documented in the literature. Some authors propose that posterior fusion in situ with or without decompression is a safe and reliable procedure,[168] whereas others suggest that reduction of the slipped vertebra may prevent some of the adverse sequelae of in situ fusion, which include nonunion, bending of the fusion mass, and persistent or increasing lumbosacral deformity.[191,210-212] Many investigators advocate a combined anterior and posterior fusion using instrumentation. An in situ circumferential fusion as described by Smith and Bohlman[187] has the lowest risk for iatrogenic nerve injury.

Resection of the L5 vertebra with reduction of L4 onto S1 was initially described by Gaines and Nichols in 1985.[213] The initial stage of the procedure involves an anterior L5 vertebrectomy in which the L5 body is removed to the base of the pedicles. The second stage is performed through a midline posterior approach involving resection of the now loose L5 posterior elements, decompression, and instrumented reduction through transpedicular instrumentation of L4 onto S1.[213,214] Lehmer and colleagues[214] performed a retrospective review evaluating indications, techniques, results, and patient satisfaction. Of patients, 25% were found to require reoperation secondary to delayed union or instrumentation failure. Three quarters were noted to have early postoperative neurologic deficits, more than half of which were present preoperatively, and most resolved. All three patients with preoperative cauda equina syndrome recovered postoperatively, and patient questionnaires revealed a high patient satisfaction rate.

As with other lumbar fusion surgery, the most common complication from an operative intervention is pseudarthrosis. Reported rates vary from 0% to 39%,[83,164,166,169,215] and pseudarthrosis occurs more frequently in fusions performed for lytic (type IIA) spondylolisthesis.[216] X-rays often show lucency around pedicle screws, instrumentation failure, progression of slip angle, or increased vertebral displacement.

Reports exist of increase in spondylolisthesis even with an uninstrumented solid arthrodesis as shown radiographically.* In most of these reports, x-rays and not CT was used to assess fusion mass, and many of these cases may have been pseudarthroses. Increased slip was reported in noninstrumented fusions, providing a sound argument for instrumented fusion.

As per the 2003 Mortality and Morbidity report of the Scoliosis Research Society, the incidence of neurologic complications with lytic spondylolisthesis surgery is 3.1%.[217] Radiculopathy is the most common surgical complication after reduction. Intraoperative manipulation can cause direct dural trauma injuring multiple sacral and lumbar nerve roots and resulting in postoperative deficits. The L5 nerve roots are most commonly involved, and reports show variable rates of resolution, with the highest risk associated with aggressive reductions of high-grade listhesis.[218-220]

Cauda equina syndrome is a potentially disastrous complication that can occur as a result of intraoperative technique, as a result of postoperative conditions, or with no apparent antecedent cause.[208,219,221-223] Schoenecker and colleagues[116] described 12 cases after in situ arthrodesis for grade III or IV L5-S1 spondylolisthesis. During the procedures, there was no evidence of compromise of the cauda equina. Of 12 patients, 5 showed complete recovery, and 7 had permanent residual deficits manifested by bowel and bladder dysfunction. Although the exact etiology is unknown, it may be related to vascular phenomena, transient anterior displacement of L5 during the surgical exposure causing laminar impingement on the sacral dome, or a period of hyperextension during patient positioning.[224] With reduction of the deformity, the risk is far greater. If cauda equina syndrome is suspected, surgical decompression is imperative. Sacroplasty and resection of the adjacent disc or

lamina of L5 or both is recommended because it is thought to facilitate neurologic recovery.[116]

With surgical advancements in technique and instrumentation, new biologic and mechanical fusion adjutants, neuromonitoring, and advanced imaging, it is hoped that further reductions in complication rates may be achieved despite the risks inherent to these highly invasive procedures.

Summary

The treatment of patients with spondylolisthesis can be a challenge for the most experienced spinal specialists. With an increasing number of pediatric athletes and improvements in diagnostic imaging techniques, more patients with spondylolisthesis are presenting to the clinician's office. To address the patient's needs best, one first must establish a proper diagnosis, quantify the deformity, and understand properly the etiology of the disease and its risk of progression.

Most pediatric patients with low-grade slips can be treated effectively with nonoperative modalities such as immobilization, activity and sports restriction or modification, analgesia, and physical therapy. Severe spondylolisthesis in adolescents can be cosmetically and functionally debilitating and poses a challenge to the treating spinal surgeon. Management of high-grade spondylolisthesis often requires larger procedures with increased associated risks. In addition to fusion with or without instrumentation, reduction of the listhesis may be beneficial in certain high-grade lesions. With the increased risks and complexity of the reduction procedure, strict selection criteria must be applied to select proper surgical candidates. Improvement of the slip angle should be the primary objective in considering a patient for deformity reduction. Additionally, sagittal alignment and overall balance should be considered during the decision-making process. All risks must be thoroughly communicated to the patient and family before the decision is made to proceed with surgical intervention.

PEARLS

1. Spondylolysis is often discovered incidentally. In asymptomatic cases, patients may need no treatment other than monitoring for progression to spondylolisthesis.

2. Various surgical options have been described for direct fixation of the pars interarticularis in spondylosis and for decompression and fusion for spondylolisthesis. The risks and benefits of each of these options must be carefully considered before recommending surgical treatment.

PITFALL

1. Spondylolisthesis may be associated with neurologic findings attributable to canal stenosis or nerve root impingement. MRI is recommended in cases with neurologic findings. Surgical intervention may be required even in asymptomatic cases if progressive translation is observed.

---

*References 8, 63, 106, 168, 169, 177.

KEY POINTS

1. Spondylolysis is defined as a defect in the pars interarticularis and is likely multifactorial in etiology with activity-related, degenerative, and genetic components.

2. Spondylolysis is a common cause of back pain, particularly in young adults and athletes engaging in repetitive hyperextension activities.

3. Most cases of symptomatic spondylolysis respond to conservative management, including bracing, activity modification, and analgesia.

4. Spondylolisthesis is defined as the anterior translation of a superior vertebral body relative to an inferior vertebral body and may occur as a result of insufficiency of the pars interarticularis (isthmic spondylolisthesis), following spondylolysis, or in the absence of spondylolysis (degenerative spondylolisthesis).

KEY REFERENCES

1. Meyerding HW: Spondylolisthesis. Surg Gynecol Obstet 54: 371-377, 1932.
   The first description of a systematic approach to the radiographic staging of spondylolisthesis.

2. Wiltse LL: The etiology of spondylolisthesis. J Bone Joint Surg Am 44-A:539-560, 1962.
   An early example from a series of works characterizing the disparate etiologies of spondylolisthesis.

3. Buck JE: Direct repair of the defect in spondylolisthesis: Preliminary report. J Bone Joint Surg Br 52:432-437, 1970.
   Description of operative technique for direct repair of defects in the pars interarticularis.

4. Fredrickson BE, Baker D, McHolick WJ, et al: The natural history of spondylolysis and spondylolisthesis. J Bone Joint Surg Am 66:699-707, 1984.
   An epidemiologic overview of spondylolysis and rates of radiographic progression to spondylolisthesis.

5. Bell DF, Ehrlich MG, Zaleske DJ: Brace treatment for symptomatic spondylolisthesis. Clin Orthop Relat Res (236):192-198, 1988.
   Clinical series showing good response to conservative treatment of symptomatic low-grade spondylolisthesis with antilordotic orthoses.

6. Panjabi MM: The stabilizing system of the spine: Part I. Function, dysfunction, adaptation, and enhancement. J Spinal Disord 5:383-389, 1992.
   A description of spinal biomechanics and the ramifications of spondylolisthesis.

7. Osterman K, Schlenzka D, Poussa M, et al: Isthmic spondylolisthesis in symptomatic and asymptomatic subjects, epidemiology, and natural history with special reference to disk abnormality and mode of treatment. Clin Orthop Relat Res (297):65-70, 1993.
   Retrospective analysis of 35 years of data on rates of slip progression, response to treatment, and indications for operative intervention in isthmic spondylolisthesis.

8. Lenke LG, Bridwell KH, Bullis D, et al: Results of in situ fusion for isthmic spondylolisthesis. J Spinal Disord 5:433-442, 1992.
   Series of noninstrumented fusions suggesting an incomplete correlation between fusion rates and symptomatic improvement.

REFERENCES

1. Bradford DS, Hu SS: Spondylolysis and spondylolisthesis. In Weinstein SL (ed): The Pediatric Spine: The Principles and Practice. New York, Raven Press, 1994, pp 585-601.

2. Killian HF: Schilderungen neuer beckenformen and ihres verhaltens im leben. Mannheim, Verlag von Bassermann & Mathy, 1854.

3. Herbiniaux G: Traite sur divers accouchemens labprieux, et sur polypes de la matrice. Bruxelles, JL, DeBoubers, 1782.

4. Robert C: Eine cigenthumliche Angeborene lodose, Wahrscheinlich Bedingt durch eine Verschiebung des Korpers des letzen Lendenwirbels auf die Vordere fiache des ersten Kreuzbeinwirbels (spondylolisthesis killian) nebst Bemerkungen uber die Mechanic diser Bekenformation. Monatsschr Beburtskund Frauenkrankheiten, 2nd ed. 1853, pp 429-432.

5. Ganju A: Isthmic spondylolisthesis. Neurosurg Focus 13:E1, 2002.

6. Newell RL: Spondylolysis: An historical review. Spine (Phila Pa 1976) 20:1950-1956, 1995.

7. Neugebauer FL: Aetiologie der sogenannten Spondylolisthesis. Arch Gynäkol (20):133, 1882.

8. Wiltse L, Newman PH, Macnab I: Classification of spondylolysis and spondylolisthesis. Clin Orthop Relat Res 117:23-29, 1976.

9. Wiltse L, Rothman S: Spondylolithesis: Classification, diagnosis, and natural history. Semin Spine Surg 1:78-94, 1989.

10. Wiltse L, Rothman S: Spondylolisthesis: Classification, diagnosis, and natural history. Semin Spine Surg 5:264-280, 1993.

11. Wiltse L, Winter RB: Terminology and measurement of spondylolisthesis. J Bone Joint Surg Am 65:768-772, 1983.

12. Newman PH, Stone K: The etiology of spondylolisthesis: With a special investigation. J Bone Joint Surg Br 45:39-59, 1963.

13. Marchetti PG, Bartolozzi P: Classification of spondylolisthesis as a guidance for treatment. In DeWald RL, Bridwell KH, (eds): The Textbook of Spinal Surgery, Vol 2. Philadelphia, Lippincott Wilkins & Williams, 1997, pp 1211-1254.

14. Ogilvie JW, Sherman J: Spondylolysis in Scheuermann's disease. Spine (Phila Pa 1976) 12:251-253, 1987.

15. Wynne-Davies R, Scott JH: Inheritance and spondylolisthesis: A radiographic family survey. J Bone Joint Surg Br 61:301-305, 1979.

16. Friberg S: Studies on spondylolisthesis. Acta Chir Scand Suppl 55, 1939.

17. Albanese M, Pizzutillo PD: Family study of spondylolysis and spondylolisthesis. J Pediatr Orthop 2:496-499, 1982.

18. Wiltse LL: Spondylolisthesis in children. Clin Orthop Relat Res 21:156-163, 1961.

19. Wiltse LL, Widell EH, Jackson DW: Fatigue fracture: The basic lesion in isthmic spondylolisthesis. J Bone Joint Surg Am 57:17-22, 1975.

20. Laurent LE: Spondylolisthesis. Acta Orthop Scand 35(Suppl):1-45, 1958.

21. Shahriaree H, Sajadi K, Rooholamini SA: A family with spondylolisthesis. J Bone Joint Surg Am 61:1256-1258, 1979.

22. Wiltse LL: The etiology of spondylolisthesis. J Bone Joint Surg Am 44-A:539-560, 1962.

23. Newman PH: Degenerative spondylolisthesis. Orthop Clin North Am 6:197-199, 1975.

24. Dietrich M, Kurowski P: The importance of mechanical factors in the etiology of spondylolysis: A model analysis of loads and stresses in human lumbar spine. Spine (Phila Pa 1976) 10:532-542, 1985.

25. Krenz J, Troup JD: The structure of the pars interarticularis of the lower lumbar vertebrae and its relation to the etiology of spondylolysis, with a report of a healing fracture in the neural arch of a fourth lumbar vertebra. J Bone Joint Surg Br 55:735-741, 1973.

26. Letts M, Smallman T, Afanasiev R, et al: Fracture of the pars interarticularis in adolescent athletes: A clinical-biomechanical analysis. J Pediatr Orthop 6:40-46, 1986.

27. Schulitz KP, Niethard FU: Strain on the interarticular stress distribution: Measurements regarding the development of spondylolysis. Arch Orthop Trauma Surg 96:197-202, 1980.

28. Wiltse LL, Widell EH Jr, Jackson DW: Fatigue fracture: The basic lesion is isthmic spondylolisthesis. J Bone Joint Surg Am 57:17-22, 1975.

29. Farfan HF, Osteria V, Lamy C: The mechanical etiology of spondylolysis and spondylolisthesis. Clin Orthop Relat Res (117):40-55, 1976.

30. Jackson DW, Wiltse LL, Cirincoine RJ: Spondylolysis in the female gymnast. Clin Orthop Relat Res (117):68-73, 1976.

31. Ciullo JV, Jackson DW: Pars interarticularis stress reaction, spondylolysis, and spondylolisthesis in gymnasts. Clin Sports Med 4:95-110, 1985.

32. Semon RL, Spengler D: Significance of lumbar spondylolysis in college football players. Spine (Phila Pa 1976) 6:172-174, 1981.

33. Amato M, Totty WG, Gilula LA: Spondylolysis of the lumbar spine: Demonstration of defects and laminal fragmentation. Radiology 153:627-629, 1984.

34. Fredrickson BE, Baker D, McHolick WJ, et al: The natural history of spondylolysis and spondylolisthesis. J Bone Joint Surg Am 66:699-707, 1984.

35. Roche MB, Rowe GG: The incidence of separate neural arch and coincident bone variations: A summary. J Bone Joint Surg Am 34:491-494, 1952.

36. Yochum TR, et al: Natural history of spondylolysis and spondylolisthesis. In Yochum TR, Rowe LJ (eds): Essentials of Skeletal Radiology. Baltimore, Williams & Wilkins, 1987, pp 243-272.

37. Osterman K, Schlenzka D, Poussa M, et al: Isthmic spondylolisthesis in symptomatic and asymptomatic subjects, epidemiology, and natural history with special reference to disk abnormality and mode of treatment. Clin Orthop Relat Res 297:65-70, 1993.

38. Stewart T: The age incidence of neural arch defects in Alaskan natives, considered from the standpoint of etiology. J Bone Joint Surg Am 35:937, 1953.

39. Wong LC: Rehabilitation of a patient with a rare multi-level isthmic spondylolisthesis: A case report. JCCA J Can Chiropr Assoc 48:142-151, 2004.

40. Simper LB: Spondylolysis in Eskimo skeletons. Acta Orthop Scand 57:78-80, 1986.

41. Fredrickson B, Baker D, McHolick WJ, Yuan HA, et al: The natural history of spondylolysis and spondylolisthesis. J Bone Joint Surg Am 66:699-707, 1984.

42. Taillard WF: Etiology of spondylolisthesis. Clin Orthop Relat Res (117):30-39, 1976.

43. Beguiristain JL, Díaz-de-Rada P. Spondylolisthesis in preschool children. J Pediatr Orthop 225-230, 2004.

44. Borkow SE, Kleiger B: Spondylolisthesis in the newborn: A case report. Clin Orthop Relat Res 81:73-76, 1971.

45. Taillard WF: Etiology of spondylolisthesis. Clin Orthop Relat Res 117:30-39, 1976.

46. Turner RD, Bianco AJ Jr: Spondylolisthesis and spondylolysis in children and teen-agers. J Bone Joint Surg Am 53:1298-1306, 1971.

47. Patel DR, Nelson TL: Sports injuries in adolescents. Med Clin North Am 84:983-1007, 2000.

48. Ariyoshi M, Nagata K, Sonoda K, et al: Spondylolysis at three sites in the same lumbar vertebra. Int J Sports Med 20:56-57, 1999.

49. Grobler LJ, Wiltse LL: Classification, non-operative, and operative treatment of spondylolisthesis. In The Adult Spine: Principles and Practice, Vol 2. New York, Raven Press, 1991, pp 1655-1704.

50. Saraste H: The etiology of spondylolysis: A retrospective radiographic study. Acta Orthop Scand 56:253-255, 1985.

51. Baker DR, McHollick W: Spondyloschisis and spondylolisthesis in children. J Bone Joint Surg Am 38:933-934, 1956

52. Reference deleted in proofs.

53. Soler T, Calderon C: The prevalence of spondylolysis in the Spanish elite athlete. Am J Sports Med 28:57-62, 2000.

54. Wimberly RL, Lauerman WC: Spondylolisthesis in the athlete. Clin Sports Med 21:133-145, 2002.

55. Stinson JT: Spondylolysis and spondylolisthesis in the athlete. Clin Sports Med 12:517-528, 1993.

56. Standaert CJ: Spondylolysis in the adolescent athlete. Clin J Sport Med 12:119-122, 2002.

57. Lundin DA, Wiseman DB, Shaffrey CI: Spondylolysis and spondylolisthesis in the athlete. Clin Neurosurg 49:528-547, 2002.

58. Jackson DW, Wiltse LL, Cirincoine RJ: Spondylolysis in the female gymnast. Clin Orthop Relat Res (117):68-73, 1976.

59. Herman MJ, Pizzutillo PD, Cavalier R: Spondylolysis and spondylolisthesis in the child and adolescent athlete. Orthop Clin North Am 34:461-467, 2003.

60. MacDonald J, D'Hemecourt P: Back pain in the adolescent athlete. Pediatr Ann 36:703-712, 2007.

61. Wiltse L, Jackson DW: Treatment of spondylolisthesis and spondylolysis in children. Clin Orthop Relat Res 117:92-100, 1976.

62. Newman PH: Surgical treatment of spondylolisthesis in the adult. Clin Orthop Relat Res 117:106-111, 1976.

63. Boxall D, Bradford DS, Winter RB, et al: Management of severe spondylolisthesis in children. J Bone Joint Surg Am 61:479-495, 1979.

64. Arriaza BT: Spondylolysis in prehistoric human remains from Guam and its possible etiology. Am J Phys Anthropol 104:393-397, 1997.

65. El Rassi G, Takemitsu M, Woratanarat P, et al: Lumbar spondylolysis in pediatric and adolescent soccer players. Am J Sports Med 33:1688-1693, 2005.

66. Harvell JC Jr, Hanley EN Jr: Spondylolysis and spondylolisthesis. In Pang D (ed): Disorders of the Pediatric Spine. New York, Raven Press, 1995, pp 561-574.

67. Hambly MF, Wiltse LL, Peek RD: Spondylolisthesis. In Watkins RG, Williams L, Lin P, et al (eds): The Spine in Sports. St Louis, Mosby, 1996, pp 157-163.

68. Micheli LJ, Wood R: Back pain in young athletes: Significant differences from adults in causes and patterns. Arch Pediatr Adolesc Med 149:15-18, 1995.

69. Comstock CP, Carragee EJ, O'Sullivan GS: Spondylolisthesis in the young athlete. Physician Sports Med 22:39-46, 1994

70. Anderson S: Assessment and management of pediatric and adolescent patients with low back pain. Phys Med Rehabil Clin North Am 2:157-185, 1991.

71. Loman Y, Margulies JY, Nyska M, et al: Effect of major axial skeleton trauma on preexisting lumbosacral spondylolisthesis. J Spinal Disord 4:353-358, 1991.

72. Luhmann S, O'Brien MF, Lenke L: Spondylolysis and spondylolisthesis. In Morrissy RT, Weinstein SL (ed): Lovell and Winter's Pediatric Orthopaedics, Vol 2, 6th ed. Philadelphia, Lippincott Williams & Wilkins, 2006, pp 839-870.

73. Weiker GG: Evaluation and treatment of common spine and trunk problems. Clin Sports Med 8:399-417, 1989.

74. Ralston S, Weir M: Suspecting lumbar spondylolysis in adolescent low back pain. Clin Pediatr (Phila) 37:287-293, 1998.

75. Barash HL, Galante JO, Lanthert CL, et al: Spondylolisthesis and tight hamstrings. J Bone Joint Surg Am 52:1319-1328, 1970.

76. Phalen GS, Dickson JA: Spondylolisthesis and tight hamstrings. J Bone Joint Surg Am 43:505-512, 1961.

77. Deyerle WM: Lumbar nerve-root irritation in children. Clin Orthop Relat Res 21:125, 1961.

78. Meyers LL, Dobson SR, Wiegand D, et al: Mechanical instability as a cause of gait disturbance in high-grade spondylolisthesis: A pre- and postoperative three-dimensional gait analysis. J Pediatr Orthop 19:672-676, 1999.

79. Guntz E, Schluter K: Dysplasia of the neural arch and its clinical manifestations (spondylolisthesis). Clin Orthop Relat Res 8:71-90, 1956.

80. Jones PH, Love JG: Tight filum terminae. AMA Arch Surg 73:556-566, 1956.

81. Libson E, Bloom RA, Shapiro Y: Scoliosis in young men with spondylolysis or spondylolisthesis: A comparative study in symptomatic and asymptomatic subjects. Spine (Phila Pa 1976) 9:445-447, 1984.

82. Papagelopoulos PJ, Peterson HA, Ebersold MJ, et al: Spinal column deformity and instability after lumbar or thoracolumbar laminectomy for intraspinal tumors in children and young adults. Spine (Phila Pa 1976) 22:442-451, 1997.

83. Seitsalo S, Osterman K, Poussa M: Scoliosis associated with lumbar spondylolisthesis: A clinical survey of 190 young patients. Spine (Phila Pa 1976) 13:899-904, 1988.

84. Lindholm TS, Ragni P, Ylikoski M, et al: Lumbar isthmic spondylolisthesis in children and adolescents. Spine (Phila Pa 1976) 15:1350-1355, 1990.

85. McCarroll JR, Miller JM, Bitter MA: Lumbar spondylolysis and spondylolisthesis in college football players. A prospective study. Am J Sports Med 14:404-406, 1986.

86. Lowe RW, Hayes TD, Kaye J, et al: Standing roentgenograms in spondylolisthesis. Clin Orthop Relat Res 117:80-84, 1976.

87. Libson E, Bloom RA, Dinari G: Symptomatic and asymptomatic spondylolysis and spondylolisthesis in young adults. Int Orthop 6:259-261, 1982.

88. Standaert CJ, Herring SA: Spondylolysis: A critical review. Br J Sports Med 34:415-422, 2000.

89. Bodner RJ, Heyman S, Drummond DS, et al: The use of single photon emission computed tomography (SPECT) in the diagnosis of low-back pain in young patients. Spine (Phila Pa 1976) 13:1155-1160, 1988.

90. Bellah RD, Summerville DA, Treves ST, et al: Low-back pain in adolescent athletes: Detection of stress injury to the pars interarticularis with SPECT. Radiology 180:509-512, 1991.

91. Congeni J, McCulloch J, Swanson K: Lumbar spondylolysis: A study of natural progression in athletes. Am J Sports Med 25:248-253, 1997.

92. Teplick JG, Laffey PA, Berman A, et al: Diagnosis and evaluation of spondylolisthesis and/or spondylolysis on axial CT. AJNR Am J Neuroradiol 7:479-491, 1986.

93. Udeshi UL, Reeves D: Routine thin slice MRI effectively demonstrates the lumbar pars interarticularis. Clin Radiol 54:615-619, 1999.

94. Harvey CJ, Richenberg JL, Saifuddin A, et al: The radiological investigation of lumbar spondylolysis. Clin Radiol 53:723-728, 1998.

95. Yamane T, Yoshida T, Mimatsu K: Early diagnosis of lumbar spondylolysis by MRI. J Bone Joint Surg Br 75:764-768, 1993.

95a. Meyerding HW: Spondylolisthesis. Surg Gynecol Obstet 54:371-377, 1932.

96. Wiltse LL, Winter RB: Terminology and measurement of spondylolisthesis. J Bone Joint Surg Am 65:768-772, 1983.

97. Laurent LE, Osterman K: Operative treatment of spondylolisthesis in young patients. Clin Orthop Relat Res (117):85-91, 1976.

98. O'Sullivan PB, Phyty GD, Twomey LT, et al: Evaluation of specific stabilizing exercise in the treatment of chronic low back pain with radiologic diagnosis of spondylolysis or spondylolisthesis. Spine (Phila Pa 1976) 22:2959-2967, 1997.

99. Fujii K, Katoh S, Sairyo K, et al: Union of defects in the pars interarticularis of the lumbar spine in children and adolescents: The radiological outcome after conservative treatment. J Bone Joint Surg Br 86:225-231, 2004.

100. Steiner ME, Micheli LJ: Treatment of symptomatic spondylolysis and spondylolisthesis with the modified Boston brace. Spine (Phila Pa 1976) 10:937-943, 1985.

101. Blanda J, Bethem D, Moats W, et al: Defects of pars interarticularis in athletes: A protocol for nonoperative treatment. J Spinal Disord 6:406-411, 1993.

102. Daniel JN, Polly DW Jr, Van Dam BE: A study of the efficacy of nonoperative treatment of presumed traumatic spondylolysis in a young patient population. Mil Med 160:553-555, 1995.

103. Morita T, Ikata T, Katoh S, et al: Lumbar spondylolysis in children and adolescents. J Bone Joint Surg Br 77:620-625, 1995.

104. Bell DF, Ehrlich MG, Zaleske DJ: Brace treatment for symptomatic spondylolisthesis. Clin Orthop Relat Res (236):192-198, 1988.

105. Pizzutillo PD, Hummer CD III: Nonoperative treatment of pain adolescent spondylosis and spondylolisthesis. J Pediatr Orthop 9:538-540, 1989.

106. Hensinger RN: Spondylolysis and spondylolisthesis in children and adolescents. J Bone Joint Surg Am 71:1098-1107, 1989.

107. Anderson K, Sarwark JF, Conway JJ, et al: Quantitative assessment with SPECT imaging of stress injuries of the pars interarticularis and response to bracing. J Pediatr Orthop 20:28-33, 2000.

108. Dutton JA, Hughes SP, Peters AM: SPECT in the management of patients with back pain and spondylolysis. Clin Nucl Med 25:93-96, 2000.

109. Takemitsu M, El Rassi G, Woratanarat P, et al: Low back pain in pediatric athletes with unilateral tracer uptake at the pars interarticularis on single photon emission computed tomography. Spine (Phila Pa 1976) 31:909-914, 2006.

110. Panjabi MM: The stabilizing system of the spine: Part I. Function, dysfunction, adaptation, and enhancement. J Spinal Disord 5:383-389, 1992.

111. Kurd MF, Patel D, Norton R, et al: Nonoperative treatment of symptomatic spondylolysis. J Spinal Disord Tech 20:560-564, 2007.

112. Harris IE, Weinstein SL: Long-term follow-up of patients with grade-III and IV spondylolisthesis: Treatment with and without posterior fusion. J Bone Joint Surg Am 69:960-969, 1987.

113. Bell DL, Ehrlich MG, Zaleske DJ: Brace treatment for symptomatic spondylolisthesis. Clin Orthop Relat Res 236:192-198, 1988.

114. Gill GG, Manning JG, White HL: Surgical treatment of spondylolisthesis without spine fusion: Excision of the loose lamina with decompression of the nerve roots. J Bone Joint Surg Am 37:493-520, 1955.

115. Gill GG: Long-term follow-up evaluation of a few patients with spondylolisthesis treated by excision of the loose lamina with decompression of the nerve roots without spinal fusion. Clin Orthop Relat Res (182):215-219, 1984.

116. Schoenecker P, Cole HO, Herring J, et al: Cauda equina syndrome after in situ arthrodesis for severe spondylolisthesis at the lumbosacral junction. J Bone Joint Surg Am 72:369-377, 1990.

117. Buck JE: Direct repair of the defect in spondylolisthesis: Preliminary report. J Bone Joint Surg Br 52:432-437, 1970.

118. Nicol RO, Scott JH: Lytic spondylolysis: Repair by wiring. Spine (Phila Pa 1976) 11:1027-1030, 1986.

119. Ivanic GM, Pink TP, Achatz W, et al: Direct stabilization of lumbar spondylolysis with a hook screw: Mean 11-year follow-up period for 113 patients. Spine (Phila Pa 1976) 28:255-259, 2003.

120. Lundin DA, Wiseman D, Ellenbogen RG, et al: Direct repair of the pars interarticularis for spondylolysis and spondylolisthesis. Pediatr Neurosurg 39:195-200, 2003.

121. Nachemson A: Repair of the spondylolisthetic defect and intertransverse fusion for young patients. Clin Orthop Relat Res (117):101-105, 1976.

122. Lehmann TR, Spratt KF, Tozzi JE, et al: Long-term follow-up of lower lumbar fusion patients. Spine (Phila Pa 1976) 12:97-104, 1987.

123. Lee CK: Accelerated degeneration of the segment adjacent to a lumbar fusion. Spine (Phila Pa 1976) 13:375-377, 1988.

124. Weinhoffer SL, Guyer RD, Herbert M, et al: Intradiscal pressure measurements above an instrumented fusion: A cadaveric study. Spine (Phila Pa 1976) 20:526-531, 1995.

125. Axelsson P, Johnsson R, Stromqvist B: The spondylolytic vertebra and its adjacent segment: Mobility measured before and after posterolateral fusion. Spine (Phila Pa 1976) 22:414-417, 1997.

126. Mihara H, Onari K, Cheng BC, et al: The biomechanical effects of spondylolysis and its treatment. Spine (Phila Pa 1976) 28:235-238, 2003.

127. Tokuhashi Y, Matsuzaki H: Repair of defects in spondylolysis by segmental pedicular screw hook fixation: A preliminary report. Spine (Phila Pa 1976) 21:2041-2045, 1996.

128. Wu SS, Lee CH, Chen PQ: Operative repair of symptomatic spondylolysis following a positive response to diagnostic pars injection. J Spinal Disord 12:10-16, 1999.

129. Buck J: Further thoughts on direct repair of the defect in spondylolysis. J Bone Joint Surg Br 61:123, 1979.

130. Beckers L: Buck's operation for treatment of spondylolysis and spondylolisthesis. Acta Orthop Belg 52:819-823, 1986.

131. Buring K, Fredensborg N: Osteosynthesis of spondylolysis. Acta Orthop Scand 44:91-92, 1973.

132. Ebraheim NA, Xu R, Darwich M, et al: Anatomic relations between the lumbar pedicle and the adjacent neural structures. Spine (Phila Pa 1976) 22:2338-2341, 1997.

133. Lu J, Ebraheim NA, Biyani A, et al: Screw placement in the lumbar vertebral isthmus. Clin Orthop Relat Res (338):227-230, 1997.

134. Bradford DS, Iza J: Repair of the defect in spondylolysis or minimal degrees of spondylolisthesis by segmental wire fixation and bone grafting. Spine (Phila Pa 1976) 10:673-679, 1985.

135. Salib RM, Pettine KA: Modified repair of a defect in spondylolysis or minimal spondylolisthesis by pedicle screw, segmental wire fixation, and bone grafting. Spine (Phila Pa 1976) 18:440-443, 1993.

136. Deguchi M, Rapoff AJ, Zdeblick TA: Biomechanical comparison of spondylolysis fixation techniques. Spine (Phila Pa 1976) 24:328-333, 1999.

137. Johnson GV, Thompson AG: The Scott wiring technique for direct repair of lumbar spondylolysis. J Bone Joint Surg Br 74:426-430, 1992.

138. Hambly MF, Wiltse LL: A modification of the Scott wiring technique. Spine (Phila Pa 1976) 19:354-356, 1994.

139. Songer MN, Rovin R: Repair of the pars interarticularis defect with a cable-screw construct: A preliminary report. Spine (Phila Pa 1976) 23:263-269, 1998.

140. Morscher E, Gerber B, Fasel J: Surgical treatment of spondylolisthesis by bone grafting and direct stabilization of spondylolysis by means of a hook screw. Arch Orthop Trauma Surg 103:175-178, 1984.

141. Albassir A, Samson I, Hendricks L: [Treatment of painful spondylolysis using Morscher's hook]. Acta Orthop Belg 56:489-495, 1990.

142. Hefti F, Seelig W, Morscher E: Repair of lumbar spondylolysis with a hook-screw. Int Orthop 16:81-85, 1992.

143. Pavlovcic V: Surgical treatment of spondylolysis and spondylolisthesis with a hook screw. Int Orthop 18:6-9, 1994.

144. Winter M, Jani L: Results of screw osteosynthesis in spondylolysis and low-grade spondylolisthesis. Arch Orthop Trauma Surg 108:96-99, 1989.

145. Sales de Gauzy J, Vadier F, Cahuzac JP: Repair of lumbar spondylolysis using Morscher material: 14 children followed for 1-5 years. Acta Orthop Scand 71:292-296, 2000.

146. Gillet P, Petit M: Direct repair of spondylolysis without spondylolisthesis, using a rod-screw construct and bone grafting of the pars defect. Spine (Phila Pa 1976) 24:1252-1256, 1999.

147. Kakiuchi M: Repair of the defect in spondylolysis: Durable fixation with pedicle screws and laminar hooks. J Bone Joint Surg Am 79:818-825, 1997.

148. Roca J, Iborra M, Cavanilles-Walker JM, et al: Direct repair of spondylolysis using a new pedicle screw hook fixation: Clinical and CT-assessed study: an analysis of 19 patients. J Spinal Disord Tech 18(Suppl):S82-S89, 2005.

149. Pellise F, Toribio J, Rivas A, et al: Clinical and CT scan evaluation after direct defect repair in spondylolysis using segmental pedicular screw hook fixation. J Spinal Disord 12:363-367, 1999.

150. Yuan HA, Garfin SR, Dickman CA, et al: A historical cohort study of pedicle screw fixation in thoracic, lumbar, and sacral spinal fusions. Spine (Phila Pa 1976) 19(20 Suppl):2279S-2296S, 1994.

151. Zdeblick TA: A prospective, randomized study of lumbar fusion: Preliminary results. Spine (Phila Pa 1976) 18:983-991, 1993.

152. Bjarke Christensen F, Stender Hansen E, Laursen M, et al: Long-term functional outcome of pedicle screw instrumentation as a support for posterolateral spinal fusion: Randomized clinical study with a 5-year follow-up. Spine (Phila Pa 1976) 27:1269-1277, 2002.

153. Deguchi M, Rapoff AJ, Zdeblick TA: Posterolateral fusion for isthmic spondylolisthesis in adults: Analysis of fusion rate and clinical results. J Spinal Disord 11:459-464, 1998.

154. Bono CM, Lee CK: Critical analysis of trends in fusion for degenerative disc disease over the past 20 years: Influence of technique on fusion rate and clinical outcome. Spine (Phila Pa 1976) 29:455-463; discussion Z5, 2004.

155. Chang P, Seow KH, Tan SK: Comparison of the results of spinal fusion for spondylolisthesis in patients who are instrumented with patients who are not. Singapore Med J 34:511-514, 1993.

156. Ricciardi JE, Pflueger PC, Isaza JE, et al: Transpedicular fixation for the treatment of isthmic spondylolisthesis in adults. Spine (Phila Pa 1976) 20:1917-1922, 1995.

157. Moller H, Hedlund R: Surgery versus conservative management in adult isthmic spondylolisthesis—a prospective randomized study: Part 1. Spine (Phila Pa 1976) 25:1711-1715, 2000.

158. Moller H, Hedlund R: Instrumented and noninstrumented posterolateral fusion in adult spondylolisthesis—a prospective randomized study: Part 2. Spine (Phila Pa 1976) 25:1716-1721, 2000.

159. de Loubresse CG, Bon T, Deburge A, et al: Posterolateral fusion for radicular pain in isthmic spondylolisthesis. Clin Orthop Relat Res (323):194-201, 1996.

160. Lenke LG, Bridwell KH, Bullis D, et al: Results of in situ fusion for isthmic spondylolisthesis. J Spinal Disord 5:433-442, 1992.

161. Shirado O, Zdeblick TA, McAfee PC, et al: Biomechanical evaluation of methods of posterior stabilization of the spine and posterior lumbar interbody arthrodesis for lumbosacral isthmic spondylolisthesis: A calf-spine model. J Bone Joint Surg Am 73:518-526, 1991.

162. Wiltse LL, Bateman JG, Hutchinson RH, et al: The paraspinal sacrospinalis-splitting approach to the lumbar spine. J Bone Joint Surg Am 50:919-926, 1968.

163. Cheung EV, Herman MJ, Cavalier R, et al: Spondylolysis and spondylolisthesis in children and adolescents: II. Surgical management. J Am Acad Orthop Surg 14:488-498, 2006.

164. Hensinger RN, Lang JR, MacEwen GD: Surgical management of spondylolisthesis in children and adolescents. Spine (Phila Pa 1976) 1:207-216, 1976.

165. Poussa M, Schlenzka D, Seitsalo S, et al: Surgical treatment of severe isthmic spondylolisthesis in adolescents: Reduction or fusion in situ. Spine (Phila Pa 1976) 18:894-901, 1993.

166. Burkus JK, Lonstein JE, Winter RB, et al: Long-term evaluation of adolescents treated operatively for spondylolisthesis: A comparison of in situ arthrodesis only with in situ arthrodesis and reduction followed by immobilization in a cast. J Bone Joint Surg Am 74:693-704, 1992.

167. Bosworth DM, Fielding JW, Demarest L, et al: Spondylolisthesis: A critical review of a consecutive series of cases treated by arthrodesis. J Bone Joint Surg Am 37:767-786, 1955.

168. Grzegorzewski A, Kumar SJ: In situ posterolateral spine arthrodesis for grades III, IV, and V spondylolisthesis in children and adolescents. J Pediatr Orthop 20:506-511, 2000.

169. Newton PO, Johnston CE 2nd: Analysis and treatment of poor outcomes following in situ arthrodesis in adolescent spondylolisthesis. J Pediatr Orthop 17:754-761, 1997.

170. Sherman FC, Rosenthal RK, Hall JE: Spine fusion for spondylolysis and spondylolisthesis in children. Spine (Phila Pa 1976) 4:59-66, 1979.

171. Wiltse LL, Jackson DW: Treatment of spondylolisthesis and spondylolysis in children. Clin Orthop Relat Res (117):92-100, 1976.

172. Seitsalo S, Osterman K, Hyvärinen H, et al: Severe spondylolisthesis in children and adolescents: A long-term review of fusion in situ. J Bone Joint Surg Br 72:259-265, 1990.

173. Al-Sayyad MJ, Abdulmajeed TM: Fracture of the anterior iliac crest following autogenous bone grafting. Saudi Med J 27:254-258, 2006.

174. Davis IS, Bailey RW: Spondylolisthesis: Long-term follow-up study of treatment with total laminectomy. Clin Orthop Relat Res 88:46-49, 1972.

175. Frennered AK, et al: Midterm follow-up of young patients fused in situ for spondylolisthesis. Spine (Phila Pa 1976) 16:409-416, 1991.

176. Beutler WJ, Fredrickson BE, Murtland A, et al: The natural history of spondylolysis and spondylolisthesis: 45-year follow-up evaluation. Spine (Phila Pa 1976) 28:1027-1035; discussion 1035, 2003.

177. Pizzutillo PD, Mirenda W, MacEwen GD: Posterolateral fusion for spondylolisthesis in adolescence. J Pediatr Orthop 6:311-316, 1986.

178. Cricchio G, Lundgren S: Donor site morbidity in two different approaches to anterior iliac crest bone harvesting. Clin Implant Dent Relat Res 5:161-169, 2003.

179. Jenis LG, Banco RJ, Kwon B: A prospective study of autologous growth factors (AGF) in lumbar interbody fusion. Spine (Phila Pa 1976) 6:14-20, 2006.

180. Seiler JG 3rd, Johnson J: Iliac crest autogenous bone grafting: Donor site complications. J South Orthop Assoc 9:91-97, 2000.

181. Silber JS, Anderson DG, Daffner SD, et al: Donor site morbidity after anterior iliac crest bone harvest for single-level anterior cervical discectomy and fusion. Spine (Phila Pa 1976) 28:134-139, 2003.

182. Krenz J, Troup JD: The structure of the pars interarticularis of the lower lumbar vertebrae and its relation to the etiology of spondylolysis, with a report of a healing fracture in the neural arch of a fourth lumbar vertebra. J Bone Joint Surg Br 55:735-741, 1973.

183. Stanton RP, Meehan P, Lovell WW: Surgical fusion in childhood spondylolisthesis. J Pediatr Orthop 5:411-415, 1985.

184. Johnson JR, Kirwan EO: The long-term results of fusion in situ for severe spondylolisthesis. J Bone Joint Surg Br 65:43-46, 1983.

185. Ploumis A, Hantzidis P, Dimitriou C: High-grade dysplastic spondylolisthesis and spondyloptosis: Report of three cases with surgical treatment and review of the literature. Acta Orthop Belg 71:750-757, 2005.

186. Smith JA, Hu SS: Management of spondylolysis and spondylolisthesis in the pediatric and adolescent population. Orthop Clin North Am 30:487-499, 1999.

187. Smith MD, Bohlman HH: Spondylolisthesis treated by a single-stage operation combining decompression with in situ posterolateral and anterior fusion: An analysis of eleven patients who had long-term follow-up. J Bone Joint Surg Am 72:415-421, 1990.

188. Mahmood F, Emami A, Hwang K, et al: Trans-sacral mesh cage with partial reduction for treatment of high-grade spondylolisthesis. Presented at the 13th International Meeting on Advanced Spinal Techniques, Hong Kong, 2008.

189. Roca J, Ubierna MT, Cáceres E, et al: One-stage decompression and posterolateral and interbody fusion for severe spondylolisthesis: An analysis of 14 patients. Spine (Phila Pa 1976) 24:709-714, 1999.

190. Smith JA, Deviren V, Berven S, et al: Clinical outcome of trans-sacral interbody fusion after partial reduction for high-grade l5-s1 spondylolisthesis. Spine (Phila Pa 1976) 26:2227-2234, 2001.

191. Bohlman HH, Cook SS: One-stage decompression and posterolateral and interbody fusion for lumbosacral spondyloptosis through a posterior approach: Report of two cases. J Bone Joint Surg Am 64:415-418, 1982.

192. Lee EH, Goh JC, Helm R,et al: Donor site morbidity following resection of the fibula. J Bone Joint Surg Br 72:129-131, 1990.

193. Youdas JW, Wood MB, Cahalan TD, et al: A quantitative analysis of donor site morbidity after vascularized fibula transfer. J Orthop Res 6:621-629, 1988.

194. Lenke LG, Bridwell KH: Evaluation and surgical treatment of high-grade isthmic dysplastic spondylolisthesis. Instr Course Lect 52:525-532, 2003.

194a. Jenkins JA: Spondylolisthesis. Br J Surg 24: 80-86, 1936.

195. Aota Y, Kumano K, Hirabayashi S, et al: Reduction of lumbar spondylolisthesis using a CDI pedicle screw system. Arch Orthop Trauma Surg 114:188-193, 1995.

196. Bell GR, Gurd AR, Orlowski JP, et al: The syndrome of inappropriate antidiuretic-hormone secretion following spinal fusion. J Bone Joint Surg Am 68:720-724, 1986.

197. Boachie-Adjei O, Do T, Rawlins BA: Partial lumbosacral kyphosis reduction, decompression, and posterior lumbosacral transfixation in high-grade isthmic spondylolisthesis: Clinical and radiographic results in six patients. Spine (Phila Pa 1976) 27:E161-E168, 2002.

198. Bridwell KH: Surgical treatment of high-grade spondylolisthesis. Neurosurg Clin N Am 17:331-338, 2006.

199. Dubousset J: Treatment of spondylolysis and spondylolisthesis in children and adolescents. Clin Orthop Relat Res (337):77-85, 1997.

200. Hu SS, Bradford DS, Transfeldt EE, et al: Reduction of high-grade spondylolisthesis using Edwards instrumentation. Spine (Phila Pa 1976) 21:367-371, 1996.

201. Poussa M, Remes V, Lamberg T, et al: Treatment of severe spondylolisthesis in adolescence with reduction or fusion in situ: Long-term clinical, radiologic, and functional outcome. Spine (Phila Pa 1976) 31:583-590; discussion 591-592, 2006.

202. Rengachary SS, Balabhandra R: Reduction of spondylolisthesis. Neurosurg Focus 13:E2, 2002.

203. Schwend RM, Waters PM, Hey LA, et al: Treatment of severe spondylolisthesis in children by reduction and L4-S4 posterior segmental hyperextension fixation. J Pediatr Orthop 12:703-711, 1992.

204. Weisskopf M, Ohnsorge JA, Wirtz DC, et al: [Reduction of spondylolisthesis by temporary adjacent segment distraction]. Z Orthop Ihre Grenzgeb 144:511-515, 2006.

205. Yan DL, Pei FX, Li J, et al: Comparative study of PILF and TLIF treatment in adult degenerative spondylolisthesis. Eur Spine J 17:1311-1316, 2008.

206. Muschik M, Zippel H, Perka C: Surgical management of severe spondylolisthesis in children and adolescents: Anterior fusion in situ versus anterior spondylodesis with posterior transpedicular instrumentation and reduction. Spine (Phila Pa 1976) 22:2036-2042; discussion 2043, 1997.

207. Matthiass HH, Heine J: The surgical reduction of spondylolisthesis. Clin Orthop Relat Res (203):34-44, 1986.

208. Schoenecker PL, Cole HO, Herring JA, et al: Cauda equina syndrome after in situ arthrodesis for severe spondylolisthesis

at the lumbosacral junction. J Bone Joint Surg Am 72:369-377, 1990.

209. Mehdian S, Arun R: Reduction of severe adolescent isthmic spondylolisthesis: A new technique. Spine (Phila Pa 1976) 30:E579-E584, 2005.

210. Al-Sebai MW, Al-Khawashki H: Spondyloptosis and multiple-level spondylolysis. Eur Spine J 8:75-77, 1999.

211. Ferris LR, Ho E, Leong JC: Lumbar spondyloptosis: A long term follow up of three cases. Int Orthop 14:139-143, 1990.

212. Hilibrand AS, Urquhart AG, Graziano GP, et al: Acute spondylolytic spondylolisthesis: Risk of progression and neurological complications. J Bone Joint Surg Am 77:190-196, 1995.

213. Gaines RW, Nichols WK: Treatment of spondyloptosis by two stage L5 vertebrectomy and reduction of L4 onto S1. Spine (Phila Pa 1976) 10:680-686, 1985.

214. Lehmer SM, Steffee AD, Gaines RW Jr: Treatment of L5-S1 spondyloptosis by staged L5 resection with reduction and fusion of L4 onto S1 (Gaines procedure). Spine (Phila Pa 1976) 19:1916-1925, 1994.

215. Lamberg T, Remes V, Helenius I, et al: Uninstrumented in situ fusion for high-grade childhood and adolescent isthmic spondylolisthesis: Long-term outcome. J Bone Joint Surg Am 89:512-518, 2007.

216. Lee C, Dorcil J, Radomisli TE: Nonunion of the spine: A review. Clin Orthop Relat Res (419):71-75, 2004.

217. Montgomery D, SRS Morbidity and Mortality Committee: Report of changing surgical treatment trends for spondylolisthesis. Presented at Scoliosis Research Society Pre-Meeting Course, Quebec City, Quebec, 2003.

218. Albrecht S, Kleihues H, Gill C, et al: [Repositioning injuries of nerve root L5 after surgical treatment of high degree spondylolistheses and spondyloptosis—in vitro studies]. Z Orthop Ihre Grenzgeb 136:182-191, 1998.

219. Ogilvie JW: Complications in spondylolisthesis surgery. Spine (Phila Pa 1976) 30(6 Suppl):S97-S101, 2005.

220. Petraco DM, Spivak JM, Cappadona JG, et al: An anatomic evaluation of L5 nerve stretch in spondylolisthesis reduction. Spine (Phila Pa 1976) 21:1133-1138; discussion 1139, 1996.

221. DeWald RL, Faut MM, Taddonio RF, et al: Severe lumbosacral spondylolisthesis in adolescents and children: Reduction and staged circumferential fusion. J Bone Joint Surg Am 63:619-626, 1981.

222. Maurice HD, Morley TR: Cauda equina lesions following fusion in situ and decompressive laminectomy for severe spondylolisthesis: Four case reports. Spine (Phila Pa 1976) 14:214-216, 1989.

223. O'Brien JP, Mehdian H, Jaffray D: Reduction of severe lumbosacral spondylolisthesis: A report of 22 cases with a ten-year follow-up period. Clin Orthop Relat Res (300):64-69, 1994.

224. Ogilvie J: Complications in spondylolisthesis surgery. Spine (Phila Pa 1976) 30:S97-S101, 2005.

SECTION

IV

Cervical, Thoracic, and Lumbar Spinal Trauma of the Immature Spine

Justin B. Hohl, MD
Clinton J. Devin, MD
Catherine J. Fedorka, MD
Joon Yung Lee, MD

Epidemiology

Spine injuries involve 1% to 5% of children admitted to trauma centers, making these injuries relatively uncommon in pediatric patients.[1,2] The true incidence may be higher given the challenges of obtaining a reliable examination and necessary images in children compared with adults.[1-3] A high index of suspicion is warranted in children with polytrauma and children who have sustained a head injury; 40% to 50% of children with a head injury also have a cervical spine injury.[3,4]

The level of spine involvement and mechanism vary with age. The cervical spine is most commonly involved in all pediatric patients; children younger than 8 years of age are more susceptible to upper cervical spine injuries, and children older than 8 more commonly sustain subaxial cervical spine injuries.[5] Thoracic and lumbar spine injuries also increase in incidence as children age and the spine takes on the biomechanical characteristics of an adult.[5]

Traffic-related incidents account for nearly one third of all pediatric spine injuries; however, other mechanisms of injury are unique to particular age groups.[5] In neonates, birth trauma is the most common cause of spine trauma with an incidence of 1 in 60,000 live births.[6] Excessive distraction or hyperextension of the cervical spine is thought to be the mechanism, occurring in breach deliveries and large neonates.[7] Spinal cord injury should always be suspected in neonates with hypotonia or cardiopulmonary instability. Injuries in infants and young children should raise suspicion for nonaccidental trauma. Imaging studies show avulsion fractures of the spinous processes or multilevel compression fractures in conjunction with rib fractures, long bone fractures, cutaneous lesions, and other characteristic injuries of abuse.[8,9] In older children and adolescents, sports-related injuries and diving accidents occur more frequently.[5] Recognizing these unique mechanisms of injury helps to raise the suspicion of a spine injury for the treating clinician.

Developmental Anatomy and Biomechanics

Understanding the developmental anatomy allows identification of normal radiographic variants and synchondroses versus true pathology. The atlas and axis undergo unique development, whereas the subaxial cervical spine, thoracic spine, and lumbar spine follow a similar pattern of maturation. The atlas develops from three primary centers of ossification: the anterior arch and two neural arches.[10] The two neural arches are visible at birth and develop into the lateral masses. The anterior arch is radiographically visible at birth in only 20% of infants, and in the remaining infants it ossifies over the subsequent year. Measuring the atlanto-dens interval (ADI) is unreliable in infants younger than 1 year old. The synchondrosis between the two neural arches located posteriorly closes by age 3. Ossification between the anterior arch and the two neural arches occurs by age 7.[11]

The axis (C2) is formed by five primary centers of ossification. The odontoid process is formed by two parallel ossification centers that fuse in utero during the 7th fetal month. A secondary ossification center occurs at the tip of the odontoid, termed the *os terminale,* arising between ages 3 and 6 years and fusing by age 12 years. The remaining primary centers of ossification are the body and two neural arches. The body typically fuses with the odontoid by age 6 years, but this synchondrosis can persist until age 11. The neural arches fuse anterior to the body by age 6 and posterior by age 3, similar to the atlas. Fractures can occur through the synchondrosis of the odontoid peg, recognized by soft tissue swelling and asymmetrical gapping of this synchondrosis with associated tilting of the dens.[12]

The subaxial cervical spine (C3-7), thoracic spine, and lumbar spine all develop in a similar fashion. There are three primary ossification centers: the two neural arches and the body. The neural arches fuse to the body anteriorly by age 6 and posteriorly by age 3. Secondary centers of ossification can exist at the tips of the transverse processes, spinous process, and superior and inferior aspects of the vertebral body. These areas ossify in early adulthood and can be mistaken for fracture.[10,11] The vertebral bodies of the subaxial cervical spine first ossify posteriorly with progression anteriorly as the child ages. This process replaces a cartilage scaffold with bone, and the vertebral body takes on its characteristic rectangular shape by age 7. Until age 7, it is acceptable to have anterior wedging of the subaxial cervical vertebrae, and this should not be confused with anterior compression fractures. This normal wedging can be profound at C3.

Children with a spine injury are typically divided by age: younger than or older than 8 years old. The biomechanics and injury patterns seen in children younger than 8 years differ from the patterns seen in children older than 8. The spine typically assumes adult characteristics and size by age 8 to 10 years. From birth until age 8, children are usually more susceptible to upper cervical spine injuries. In addition, it is more common for children in this younger age group to have a neurologic injury and subluxation or complete dislocation rather than a fracture.[2,13-16] Proposed reasons for the increased incidence of upper cervical spine injuries in this younger age group are listed in Table 28–1. These unique characteristics are important to keep in mind when transporting and evaluating a young child.

Transport and Evaluation

Proper care of pediatric spine injuries begins at the scene of the accident. In a child with polytrauma, a spine injury must be assumed to exist until proved otherwise with appropriate precautions and immobilization undertaken. Children should be initially placed in a well-fitting cervical collar and immobilized on a spine board. Commercial collars often do not fit appropriately, preventing adequate immobilization. In this case, sandbags can be placed on each side of the head to prevent motion.

Herzenberg and colleagues[17] were the first to note that the transport of young children (<8 years old) on a standard adult spine board tended to cause excessive flexion of the cervical spine. It was noted in all cases that the cervical spine was forced into relative kyphosis because of the disproportionately large head relative to the chest. This flexed position could potentially jeopardize the cervical cord if the mechanism of injury was a flexion force, which is often the case in motor vehicle accidents. To obtain a neutral position, Herzenberg and colleagues[17] recommended pediatric spine boards with a cutout for the occiput. Alternatively, a standard spine board can be used with a towel roll placed under the shoulders allowing the head to drop into mild extension, as shown in Figure 28–1.

In a subsequent study, Curran and colleagues[18] prospectively evaluated these modified transportation methods for achieving neutral alignment of the cervical spine. They obtained supine lateral radiographs of the cervical spine in 118 pediatric trauma patients and measured the sagittal alignment using the Cobb method. They determined that only 60% of the patients were within 5 degrees of neutral alignment using

TABLE 28–1 Risk Factors in Children Younger than 8 Years Old for Developing Upper Cervical Spine Injuries
Disproportionately large head and weak neck muscles
Fulcrum of movement centered at C2-3
Ligamentous and joint capsule laxity
Horizontal orientation facet joints
Increased cartilage-to-bone ratio with relative anterior wedging of vertebrae and incomplete ossification of odontoid process

this method. This study highlights the point that very young children may need even more relative chest elevation and as the child approaches age 8 this decreases. This point was confirmed by Nypaver and Treloar,[19] who evaluated the height of back elevation needed in children younger than 4 years versus children older than 4 to achieve neutral cervical spine alignment. Children younger than four required 5 mm additional elevation.

Although it is unknown how alignment during transport affects outcome, the authors follow the recommendations of Herzenberg and colleagues[17] regarding spine board immobilization, keeping in mind that very young children may need additional elevation to achieve neutral alignment. A clinical guideline is to evaluate the child from the side after immobilization, aligning the external auditory meatus with the shoulder. A well-fitting cervical collar should be placed, transport should occur on a spine board with a cutout for the occiput or alternatively elevating the shoulders, sand bags should be placed on either side of the head to prevent rotation, and the head should be taped to the spine board.

Clinical evaluation of a child thought to have an injury to the spine is often hampered by an inability to obtain an accurate history and a thorough physical examination. The clinician should have a heightened suspicion of spine injury in nonverbal children, owing to a 23-fold increased likelihood of missing a cervical spine injury.[20] The mechanism of injury should be taken into account when considering the likelihood of an occult spine injury. Additionally, the presence of associated injuries, including facial trauma, head injuries, thoracic

Emergency transport and positioning of young children

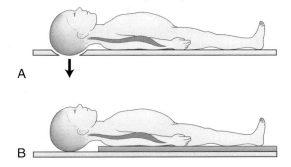

FIGURE 28–1 Emergency transport and positioning of young children. (From Herzenberg JE, Hensinger RN, Dedrick DK, et al: Emergency transport and position of young children who have an injury of the cervical spine: The standard backboard may be hazardous. J Bone Joint Surg Am 71:15-22, 1989.)

wall injuries, and abdominal injuries, increases the likelihood of spine trauma. Abdominal injuries, particularly injuries of the small bowel, are associated with flexion distraction injuries of the thoracolumbar spine.[21] Spinal injuries can occur at multiple levels with noncontiguous fractures occurring in 16%.[22]

The cervical collar is carefully removed, with an assistant stabilizing the head so that the patient or examiner does not inadvertently move the head during the examination. The cervical spine is visually inspected and palpated for malalignment, asymmetry, interspinous widening, and tenderness. Cervical spine injuries often manifest with torticollis, whereby the child's head is fixed in a rotated and tilted position. Attention is turned to the thoracolumbar spine. The log-roll maneuver should be done with someone keeping the head and neck in alignment with the rest of the spine and trunk. Cervical in-line traction should be avoided in young children because of the increased risk of ligamentous and atlanto-occipital injuries. The thoracolumbar spine is inspected and palpated.

A thorough neurologic examination, as performed in adults, should be carefully documented. If a neurologic deficit is identified, frequent examinations should be performed to detect a change in the deficit. Throughout the sensory, motor, and reflex examination, the contralateral extremity should always be used as a comparison to detect subtle injuries.

Plain Radiography of Cervical Spine

Imaging of the spine should be done if a child meets any of the following criteria: The child is nonverbal secondary to age or altered mental status, intoxication is present, a neurologic deficit exists or there is a history of a transient deficit, neck pain is present, there is a history of a high-risk mechanism of injury, physical signs of neck trauma or lap belt trauma are present, or painful distracting injuries are present.[23] Additionally, unexplained cardiorespiratory instability can be an indication of a high cervical spine injury and should be evaluated appropriately.

The three-view cervical spine series may not be as applicable in pediatric patients with polytrauma, but likely still has a role in patients without polytrauma. The supine lateral cervical radiograph has a reported sensitivity of 79% to 85% in pediatric patients.[24] This sensitivity is dependent on seeing all seven cervical vertebrae, including the occipitocervical and cervicothoracic junction. Lally and colleagues[25] found that all seven cervical vertebrae were seen in only 57% of children on the initial cervical spine series. The addition of the anteroposterior and open-mouth odontoid views increases the sensitivity to approximately 94% if ideal images can be obtained, which can be extremely challenging in an uncooperative child.[26] Buhs and colleagues[27] showed that the open-mouth odontoid view did not provide additional information in children younger than 9 that was not already appreciated on the anteroposterior and lateral views. In its place, these authors recommended use of computed tomography (CT) from the occiput to C2.

The use of flexion and extension radiographs during the initial evaluation has come into question. Ralston and colleagues[28] disputed the need for these dynamic studies in the acute setting. These investigators had blinded radiologists retrospectively review static and flexion-extension radiographs on 129 children. They found that if the static x-rays were normal, the flexion-extension views would reveal no abnormality. Dwek and Chung[29] confirmed these findings, retrospectively evaluating 247 children in whom static and flexion-extension radiographs had been obtained in the trauma setting. They found the flexion-extension view helpful in ruling out an injury in only four patients who were originally thought to have abnormal static films. These dynamic studies are helpful in evaluating for instability after an appropriate time of closed treatment. In the delayed setting, flexion-extension radiographs can confirm either healing and resultant stability or the need for operative treatment.

Interpretation of the cervical spine series requires an understanding of the normal anatomy and the anatomic variants of the immature spine that can mimic trauma. Special attention should be given to the upper cervical spine including the atlantoaxial and atlanto-occipital region given the propensity of injuries to this area in children and the subtle radiographic findings.[30] Several methods for evaluating the craniocervical junction using the lateral x-ray have been described. The "rule of 12's" is thought to be the most sensitive method, whereby the distance between the basion and tip of the odontoid process should be 12 mm or less, and a line drawn parallel along the posterior aspect of the body of C2 including the odontoid should come within 12 mm of the basion. The distance from the tip of the odontoid to the basion is unreliable in children younger than 13 because of incomplete ossification of the odontoid; however, the line drawn parallel to the back of the C2 body and odontoid peg should be less than 12 mm from the basion.[22] A gap of more than 5 mm from the occipital condyle to the C1 facet also represents a disruption of the occipitocervical junction.[31]

The atlantoaxial articulation is best evaluated with the ADI. In children, the normal ADI can be up to 5 mm. If the ADI exceeds 5 mm on lateral flexion and 4 mm on lateral extension, the transverse atlantal ligament is likely disrupted.[32] When the ADI exceeds 10 to 12 mm, the alar and apical ligaments have failed with a high risk of cord compression.[33] The extent of cord compression at the atlantoaxial joint can be determined using Steel's rule of thirds,[34] which is based on dividing the inner diameter of the C1 ring into thirds. One third of the space should be occupied by the odontoid; one third, by the spinal cord; and one third, by the space available for the cord. When the dens migrates posteriorly by greater than one third of this space, the transverse ligament has been disrupted, and the spinal cord is likely being compressed.

Swischuk[35] described the posterior cervical line (spinolaminar line) to help diagnose pathologic angulation and translation in the upper cervical spine. The posterior cervical line is formed by drawing a line from the anterior aspect of the spinous process of C1 to the anterior aspect of the spinous process of C3. The line should pass within 1.5 mm of the anterior aspect of the spinous process of C2 on flexion-extension radiographs; otherwise, a true injury should be suspected.

Many normal anatomic variants should be recognized so as to not be confused with a "true" traumatic injury. A normal finding on extension radiographs in 20% of children is overriding of the anterior arch of the atlas on the odontoid. This finding is incomplete ossification of the dens.[36] Another common variant noted on cervical spine x-rays in an immature spine is pseudosubluxation of C2 on C3 and less commonly C3 on C4. Cattell and Filtzer[36] were the first to appreciate this normal finding in a study involving 160 pediatric patients with no history of cervical spine trauma. On dynamic radiographs, 46% of children younger than 8 years showed 3 mm of anteroposterior motion of C2 on C3; 14% of children had radiographic pseudosubluxation of C3 on C4.[36,37] Based on this study and others, 4 mm of translation is considered normal.[6,28,36,38]

The absence of cervical lordosis on static lateral x-rays can be a normal finding in 14% of children up to age 16.[22] This normal variant can be differentiated from a more ominous sign of posterior ligamentous injury by assessing the posterior intraspinous distance. Each intraspinous distance should not be more than 1.5 times greater than the intraspinous distance directly above and below a given level. The only exception to this rule is the C1-2 intraspinous distance, which can be greater than 1.5 times the distance of the level below. This normal increased mobility is thought to be secondary to the stout posterior ligaments linking C1 to the occiput.[39,40]

Another challenge unique to the developing spine is differentiating a synchondrosis that has not yet ossified from a true fracture. A synchondrosis typically shows well-corticated sclerotic margins. Another helpful aid in differentiating a subtle fracture from a synchondrosis is evaluation of the prevertebral soft tissues. The retropharyngeal space (at C2) should be less than 7 mm and the retrotracheal space (at C6) should be less than 14 mm in children. In simplistic terms, the retropharyngeal space should be one half the anteroposterior distance of a cervical vertebral body, and the retrotracheal space can be up to a full cervical vertebral body. The retropharyngeal soft tissue can be falsely increased with expiration, such as in a crying child.[41] The lateral cervical spine x-ray should be repeated, attempting to obtain the radiograph during inspiration, to determine if a true abnormality exists.

Plain Radiography of Thoracic Spine

Currently, conventional radiography is being used for screening of the thoracolumbar spine, but there are shortcomings of this modality. It is often difficult to obtain satisfactory views of the upper two or three thoracic vertebrae, and the swimmer's view can be used to counter obstruction by the shoulders. These screening radiographs should be obtained when the patient arrives and is on the spine board, to help expedite the process of thoracolumbar spine clearance. The same four lines that were evaluated in the cervical spine should have a smooth contour in the thoracolumbar spine. In addition, the facet joints should be symmetrical, and there should not be widening between the spinous process.

Burst fractures are best seen on a CT scan; subtle findings on conventional radiography include interpedicular widening on the anteroposterior projection and small cortical defects at the posterosuperior corner of the vertebral body on the lateral projection. Improper radiographs are the leading cause of missed injury and subsequent neurologic deterioration in large series of trauma patients, supporting the argument for increased use of CT.[42,43]

Computed Tomography and Magnetic Resonance Imaging of Spine

The use of helical CT has replaced conventional radiography as the screening tool of choice for the adult cervical spine in the setting of blunt trauma.[44,45] One concern in children is the exposure to radiation and potential risk of developing thyroid cancer. Some estimates have been four times the radiation dose in the helical CT group compared with conventional radiographs.[46,47] CT scan with reconstructions should be used for the correct indications.

There is growing evidence that CT is superior to plain radiography for evaluating the thoracolumbar spine in adults. This evidence has relevance in patients with polytrauma who are being evaluated with a traumagram. These studies, originally targeted for evaluation of the thoracic and abdominal contents, have been shown to be very sensitive at screening for thoracolumbar spine injury. Multiple prospective studies have shown a higher sensitivity for CT (93% to 100%) compared with plain radiography (33% to 74%) with improved interobserver variability.[37,48-50] This information can likely be extrapolated to pediatric patients, but further studies need to be performed before CT scans with sagittal and coronal reconstructions replace conventional radiography for thoracolumbar spine clearance.

Magnetic resonance imaging (MRI) is useful for evaluating a neurologic deficit and soft tissue involvement, to help with preoperative planning, and to assist with cervical spine clearance in an obtunded patient. MRI in this age group can be difficult because these young patients often need sedation to prevent movement during data acquisition. MRI should be obtained in patients with evidence of a neurologic deficit, and some investigators would argue that it should be obtained in patients with a transient deficit. A transient deficit can be an indication of a more serious ligamentous and neurologic injury and subsequent need for immobilization.[51]

In a study of 74 children suspected to have a cervical spine injury based on plain radiography, MRI confirmed the plain radiography diagnosis in 66% and altered the diagnosis in 34%.[52] Keiper and colleagues[53] obtained MRI in children who had clinical symptoms consistent with a cervical spine injury despite having negative plain x-rays and CT studies. There were 16 abnormal results in 52 children, with posterior soft tissue injury being the most common injury. Four of these patients eventually underwent surgical stabilization, and MRI assisted with preoperative planning. MRI can be especially helpful in clearing the cervical spine in obtunded patients. Frank and colleagues[54] showed the effectiveness of MRI at decreasing time to cervical spine clearance, length of time in the pediatric intensive care unit, and length of time in the hospital.

Spine Clearance

Early cervical spine clearance has multiple benefits and helps avoid complications. Cervical collars have known complications, including skin breakdown around the neck, dysphagia, pulmonary complications, increased intracranial pressure, and decubitus ulcers.[38,55,56] After a cervical collar has been placed on a child, formal clearance must be obtained before it can be removed. Clinical clearance of the cervical spine has been evaluated using the National Emergency X-Radiography Utilization Study (NEXUS), which was originally developed for adults. NEXUS has been used as a decision-making instrument to determine the need for radiography. The criteria in adults for clinical clearance are absence of neck pain, neurologic symptoms, distracting injuries, or altered mental status (owing to injury, age, or intoxication). If any one of these four criteria is present, the patient is considered to be high risk and must be radiographically cleared. If none of these criteria are present, the collar can be cleared without further imaging.

Application of NEXUS criteria in pediatric patients was studied in a prospective multicenter study. All 30 cervical spine injuries were placed correctly into the high-risk group, and, more importantly, no cervical spine injuries were noted in the low-risk group. Additionally, use of NEXUS criteria decreased pediatric cervical spine imaging by 20%.[57] These rules cannot be safely applied in children too young to cooperate with an examination, in children in the presence of a high-energy mechanism, or in children with associated injuries that heighten the suspicion of a spine injury. The Canadian C-Spine Rule has gained popularity in the adult literature, showing a higher sensitivity than NEXUS (99.4% vs. 90.7%) and a higher specificity (45.1% vs. 36.8%), but to the authors' knowledge it has not been studied in children.[58]

It has been shown that an efficient, multidisciplinary approach can facilitate rapid clearance of the cervical spine, decreasing average time to 7.5 hours in nonintubated patients and 19.4 hours in intubated patients.[23] This rapid clearance is dependent on a system that is safe and user-friendly enough to allow the primary team to perform the clearance. Anderson and colleagues[59] evaluated the percent of cervical spines cleared by spine specialists before versus after initiation of a clearance protocol, noting a 60% increase in spines cleared by nonspine physicians without any late injuries detected.

A spine clearance protocol should incorporate a thorough history and physical examination with judicious use of imaging modalities. Imaging should begin with plain anteroposterior and lateral radiographs. An open-mouth odontoid view should be obtained in children older than 8 who have the ability to cooperate; otherwise, a CT scan from occiput to C2 should be performed. Children undergoing a CT scan to evaluate for head injury should have the cervical spine with reconstructions included, and this scan can be used for clearance.

Children with no evidence of injury on plain radiography or CT scan who have persistent pain should remain in the cervical collar with later clearance in the clinic with dynamic radiographs. In the presence of a neurologic deficit or a history of a transient deficit before arrival, MRI of the entire spine should be obtained. If spinal cord injury without radiographic abnormality (SCIWORA) is suspected, the cervical collar should remain in place, spine precautions should be continued, and the patient should be admitted for observation because there can be delayed deterioration.[60,61]

Clearing the cervical spine in an unconscious patient can be facilitated by a standard protocol. If the patient returns to a normal mental status, the protocol for a conscious patient can be used. There have been reports of delayed neurologic deterioration in patients with altered mental status and unrecognized ligamentous injury that subluxated on mobilization.[62] The two modalities available for evaluating ligamentous injury in an obtunded patient include fluoroscopic flexion-extension and MRI. Fluoroscopic flexion-extension examination can be labor-intensive, and in an adult series, it was difficult to visualize the cervicothoracic junction.[63] Because of these problems, many investigators believe that MRI is superior for evaluating ligamentous injury.

MRI has been found to be most sensitive for detecting a ligamentous injury at postinjury day 2 or 3.[64] Stassen and colleagues[65] used MRI within their protocol at a Level I adult trauma center for assisting in cervical spine clearance. All obtunded patients with a negative CT scan of the cervical spine underwent MRI on postinjury day 3 if they could not be clinically cleared. MRI allowed clearance of the cervical collar in 60% of subjects, and there was no delayed neurologic sequela. The remaining patients were treated in a cervical collar for 6 weeks without complication.

The best available evidence indicates that MRI is the most sensitive study for detecting posterior ligamentous disruption and should be the primary study in obtunded patients.[66] Equivocal MRI findings can be evaluated further with flexion-extension radiographs, or the physician can forgo further study and treat the patient with a collar for 6 weeks. At the termination of the 6-week period, the patient should undergo a flexion-extension series to ensure adequate healing. Expedient clearance of the thoracolumbar spine in a child with polytrauma is also very important to prevent skin breakdown, respiratory complications, and ileus. At the authors' institution, the CT traumagram, with sagittal and coronal reconstructions, is used to augment the clinical examination and clear the thoracolumbar spine.

Spinal Cord Injury in Children

The mechanism of spinal cord injury differs depending on age.[22] Children younger than 8 years old more often sustain spinal cord insult involving the upper cervical spine, secondary to ligamentous injury often with no discernible bony changes. Children older than 8 have spinal cord injuries with associated fractures owing to biomechanics of the spine that more closely mirror the biomechanics of the adult spine. A thorough neurologic examination should be obtained to determine the level involved and whether the lesion is complete or incomplete. It is important to note whether there is sacral sparing as indicated by sensation at the anal muco-cutaneous junction (S4-5 dermatome) on the left and the right side, ability to contract the anal sphincter voluntarily, and deep anal sensation. This sacral sparing indicates continuity of long tracts with improved likelihood for return of neurologic function.[67] The Frankel classification and American Spinal Injury Association (ASIA) Impairment Scale have been used in pediatric patients to provide a standardized description of injury.

Damage to the spinal cord has been categorized into primary and secondary injury. Primary injury occurs at the time of the accident leading to structural damage of the neural elements and supporting blood supply. Secondary injury occurs within minutes of the trauma setting off a cascade of events that result in ischemia, increased cell membrane permeability, pathologic electrolyte shift, edema, and production of free radicals.[68] This process continues to evolve over the subsequent days, and medical and surgical strategies are directed at mitigating secondary injury. Current treatments of interest include support of spinal cord perfusion, steroids, and early versus delayed decompression.

During transport and initial evaluation, it is crucial to prevent hypotension and to keep oxygen saturations high in patients suspected to have a spinal cord injury so as to help protect the spinal cord blood perfusion.[69] Animal and adult studies have shown improved outcome in subjects aggressively managed to prevent spinal cord ischemia.[70-72] This practice has been accepted by many pediatric trauma centers and includes admitting patients to the intensive care unit and accurately monitoring volume status and blood pressure. The mean arterial pressure should be maintained at greater than 80 mm Hg for 7 days.

Steroids are stabilizing agents; they act as a powerful anti-inflammatory decreasing edema and scavenging oxygen free radicals. High-dose methylprednisolone is administered to children based on data collected in adults. The recommendations on timing and dose are based on studies performed in patients as reported in the National Acute Spinal Cord Injury Study III.[73,74] Methylprednisolone is administered intravenously at a loading dose of 30 mg/kg over 15 minutes followed by 5.4 mg/kg/hr continuous infusion. If administration of the steroid is initiated within 3 hours of injury, the infusion should be continued for 23 hours. If steroid administration is started at 3 to 8 hours after injury, it should be continued for the subsequent 48 hours.

Steroids should not be given if a child presents after 8 hours or if the spinal cord injury is secondary to penetrating trauma. In this setting, there are significant risks with little to no benefit.[75] The National Acute Spinal Cord Injury Study III[73,74] excluded all children younger than 13 years of age. There are no equivalent data in young children, and in this age group the use of steroids is not evidence based.

The indications for early operative intervention for pediatric patients with spinal cord injury include radiographic confirmation of spinal cord compression in the setting of an incomplete injury or progressive deficit, an open spinal injury, and a grossly unstable spine in patients who are neurologically intact. To the authors' knowledge, there have been no well-designed prospective studies in pediatric patients evaluating the effect and timing of decompression.[76]

Functional outcomes depend on the level of injury and whether it is complete or incomplete. Patients with injuries above C4 may be dependent on a respirator, and phrenic nerve pacemakers can be implanted. Patients with C3 lesions can shrug their shoulders and often have neck motion, permitting operation of equipment with sip/puff controls, voice activation, eyebrow or eye blink, and head or chin controls. Patients with C6 lesions are often able to propel a manual wheelchair with the assistance of fusions and tendon transfers. At least partial recovery after a complete spinal cord injury has been reported in 10% to 25% of patients.[22,69,75,77] In a series reported by Wang and colleagues,[78] 64% of patients showed at least partial recovery after spinal cord injury. Of patients with complete injuries, 25% eventually became ambulatory. Recovery was seen up to 1 year after injury.

Children are also better able to adapt to an injury. Anderson and colleagues[79] interviewed 161 adults who had sustained a spinal cord injury as a child and found that 64% lived independently, and approximately 50% of patients reported being satisfied with their quality of life. Concerning outcomes from operative versus nonoperative treatment of spine fractures associated with spinal cord injuries, one study showed that patients in the operative group were able to use their wheelchair 5.2 weeks earlier.[80] Early activity is crucial in paralyzed patients to avoid pulmonary complications, disuse osteopenia, and complications from insensate skin.[67]

Complications unique to pediatric patients with a spinal cord injury are susceptibility to development of post-traumatic deformity and growth arrest.[81] Causes can be divided into intrinsic, extrinsic, and iatrogenic factors. Intrinsic factors include injury to the vertebral apophyses resulting in abnormal growth and change in biomechanics from altered shape of the vertebral body and loss of posterior ligamentous support. This change in biomechanics can alter the forces on the vertebral apophyses, exacerbating the deformity further.[82] Extrinsic factors include weak trunk muscles in the setting of gravity and spasticity with a contracture. Iatrogenic factors include improperly instrumented segments and use of a laminectomy without fusion. The risk of developing a deformity, in the setting of a laminectomy without fusion, is approximately 50%, with a much higher incidence in the cervical and thoracic spine.[83] Nonoperative treatment with a brace can help slow the progression of deformity, temporizing the situation and allowing the child maximum time to grow before performing a fusion.[84] Performing surgical correction and fusion needs to take into account remaining growth. An estimate of remaining growth can be determined by multiplying 0.7 mm times the number of segments fused times the number of years of remaining growth.[85]

Posterior fusion in young children has the added drawback of crankshaft phenomenon. This phenomenon occurs with continued growth of the anterior column in the setting of a fused posterior column. With continued anterior growth, the apical vertebral body rotates producing a scoliotic curvature.[86] Delaying surgery must be balanced with addressing curves while they are still supple. The goals of surgery include halting progression, obtaining correction, and balancing the spine and pelvis to equalize sitting skin pressure. Indications include a scoliotic curve of greater than 40 degrees and kyphotic curves of greater than 60 degrees. Anterior release may be needed if the deformity is rigid as shown on bending films. Including the sacrum in the fusion construct is recommended if pelvic obliquity exists.

Spinal Cord Injury Without Radiographic Abnormality

The biomechanical differences in the spine of children younger than 8 years place them at risk of SCIWORA.[22] This entity was first described by Pang and Wilberger[87] in 1982 before the use of MRI. The term *SCIWORA* was developed to describe spinal cord injuries without overt vertebral column disruption as displayed by conventional x-rays, CT scans, myelograms, and dynamic flexion-extension radiographs. SCIWORA excludes injuries secondary to penetrating trauma, secondary to electrical shock, secondary to obstetric complication, and in association with congenital anomalies. The incidence of SCIWORA in patients with spinal cord injury for ages birth to 17 was reported to be 35% in earlier literature.[61] As MRI has become more widely used, the incidence in children with spinal cord injuries is reported to be 3%.[5] This change likely reflects an improvement in imaging quality and the ability to detect subtle injuries previously missed, rather than a change in actual injury type. More recently, Bosch and colleagues[88] found that recurrent SCIWORA was an uncommon entity, which occurred only in low-energy sports-related injuries, resulting in transient neurologic symptoms, with full recovery in all cases.

MRI is the study of choice for evaluation of patients suspected to have SCIWORA. There are extraneural soft tissue changes and intraneural changes. The changes seen on MRI are secondary to edema and methemoglobin, a processed form of hemoglobin. Edema is seen as isointense on T1 and hyperintense on T2; extracellular methemoglobin is seen as hyperintense on T1 and hyperintense on T2. MRI changes in the extraneural tissues can be detected within hours of injury because the blood is quickly metabolized into a form easily seen on MRI. Intraneural changes can take days to be detectable because of the delayed metabolism of a hemorrhage into a form visible on MRI.[89,90] It is recommended that MRI be obtained at the time of presentation to rule out a compressive lesion that needs to be surgically addressed and at 6 to 9 days after injury to improve detection of intraneural injuries related to SCIWORA.[61]

The recommended duration of immobilization in a brace has been controversial, with the concern for delayed neurologic deterioration or reinjury motivating the recommendation for a brace. Bosch and colleagues[88] found that immobilization did not prevent recurrent SCIWORA, and it did not improve the outcomes of primary SCIWORA after instability was properly ruled out. A meta-analysis by Launay and colleagues[60] showed that patients immobilized for 8 weeks had a 17% chance of developing recurrent SCIWORA, whereas no patients immobilized for 12 weeks had recurrent SCIWORA develop. Based on this information, it is recommended that children be immobilized for 12 weeks with flexion and extension views of the injured region at 12 weeks to detect instability.

Atlanto-occipital Dislocation

Atlanto-occipital dislocations were previously thought to be rare injuries that were fatal and usually found on autopsy.[91,92] More recently, this injury has been identified more frequently with a higher survival rate, particularly among children. Increased survival is possibly due to faster response by emergency personnel, improved cervical immobilization, and faster diagnosis by emergency department physicians.[92-97]

The atlanto-occipital joint is a condylar joint with minimal bony stability and is stabilized primarily by ligaments. In children, the occipital condyles are less cup-shaped, and the articulation is more horizontal, potentially explaining the higher incidence of dislocation among children compared with adults.[30,31,95] Ligamentous stability is provided primarily by the tectorial membrane, the anterior longitudinal ligament, the nuchal ligament, and the paired alar ligaments.

Dislocation of the atlanto-occipital joint is usually due to a deceleration mechanism, such as a motor vehicle accident or pedestrian-vehicle accident in which the head violently moves forward, causing separation of the condyles and the atlas. Diagnosing dislocation based on physical examination findings can be difficult because of varied presentation and concomitant traumatic brain injury. Neurologic function can range from a normal examination to flaccidity (early), absent deep tendon and sacral reflexes (early), poikilothermy, spasticity (late), urinary retention (late), priapism (late), and autonomic dysreflexia (late).

On lateral plain films, the distance between the tip of the basion and dens is known as the *dens-basion distance,* which is normally less than or equal to 10 mm.[98] Additionally, the Powers ratio is the distance from the basion to the posterior aspect of the arch of the atlas divided by the distance from the anterior tubercle of the atlas to the rim of the foramen magnum, which is normally between 0.7 and 1, with a value greater than 1 indicating anterior atlanto-occipital dislocation.[99] These traditional radiographic criteria have been called into question because of accuracy, leading some to advocate using CT and MRI for diagnosis.[93,94,100] More recently, it has been suggested that a condyle-C1 interval of greater than 4 mm, as measured on a reformatted CT scan, is valuable in identifying atlanto-occipital dislocation.[100]

Although initial treatment of atlanto-occipital dislocation is immobilization in a halo or Minerva cast, most unstable injuries should be managed by posterior occipitoatlantal fusion with internal fixation. Wire fixation or fixation with a contoured rod and wires can be used from occiput to C1 to preserve C1-2 motion. If the stability of the C1-2 junction is questionable, fusion from occiput to C2 may be considered.

Fractures of the Atlas

A fracture of the ring of C1 is a rare injury in children that can occur when an axial load forces the occipital condyles into the lateral masses, resulting in fractures that involve the anterior and posterior rings (Jefferson fracture).[101-105] Children differ from adults because they can have plastic deformation of the ring and a single fracture and hinging on a synchondrosis. Instability exists when there is disruption of the transverse ligament. This disruption is determined on the anteroposterior cervical spine film by adding the overhang of the C1 lateral mass relative to the C2 lateral mass on the left and right sides. If the sum is greater than or equal to 7 mm, instability exists and should be treated with traction and a halo or Minerva cast. Cases with sums less than 7 mm can be treated with a well-fitting cervical orthosis.[105] Surgical stabilization of C1 fractures is rarely required.

Atlantoaxial Instability

Instability at the level of C1-2 can be secondary to traumatic ligamentous injury or chronic disease processes, including inflammatory diseases, malignancy, bone dysplasias, and congenital craniofacial malformations. Down syndrome is well reported in the literature, and there are other reports of atlantoaxial subluxation associated with Reiter syndrome, Larsen syndrome, juvenile rheumatoid arthritis, Morquio syndrome, and Kniest syndrome.[106-112]

In traumatic atlantoaxial injury, the transverse ligament is disrupted, resulting in an increased ADI. The ADI is the distance as measured on a lateral cervical x-ray between the posterior aspect of the anterior ring of C1 and the anterior cortex of the dens. Active flexion views may be required to observe subluxation, and CT scans can show avulsions of the transverse ligament. In children, the normal distance is 4.5 mm, whereas in adults it is 3 mm. Acute rupture of the transverse ligament is rare in children, accounting for 10% of cervical spine injuries.[113,114] Alternatively, the ligament itself may be intact but can be avulsed from its attachment to C1. Surgical stabilization of C1-2 after reduction in extension is generally recommended, followed by immobilization for 8 to 12 weeks in a halo brace, Minerva cast, or cervical orthosis. To document stability after fixation, flexion and extension views are recommended.

In Down syndrome, the frequency of atlantoaxial instability has been reported to approach 10% to 30% by adolescence.[107,115-118] Instability in patients with Down syndrome is attributed to laxity of the transverse ligament and C1-2 joint capsules. Nearly 98% to 99% of patients are asymptomatic but should be followed closely,[119-121] with some authors recommending yearly neurologic and radiographic examination.[122] Surgery is indicated in symptomatic patients and asymptomatic patients with an ADI greater than 10 mm or with less than 14 mm of space available for the spinal cord on lateral films.[123] There is a high reported surgical complication rate for these patients, including the risk of pseudarthrosis, wound infection and dehiscence, adjacent level disease, and neurologic injury.[117,124]

Surgical fixation for atlantoaxial arthrodesis originated with posterior wire stabilization and structural bone grafting, as popularized by Gallie in 1939[125] and Brooks and Jenkins in 1978.[126] This technique requires the passage of wires into the spinal canal, with the potential risk of spinal cord injury.[127,128] Additionally, a wire construct often lacks sufficient stability[129,130] resulting in nonunion rates of 30% even with a halo vest postoperatively.[43,50,51,131-133]

The C1-2 posterior transarticular screw, or Magerl screw (1986), has a decreased rate of nonunion[127,134-138] but carries the risk of injuring the vertebral artery.[139] Segmental C1-2 fixation was introduced by Goel and Laheria in 1994[140] using a plate and lateral mass screws and then by Harms and Melcher in 2001[141] using polyaxial C1 lateral mass screws and C2 pedicle screws with a rod. This approach offers the distinct advantage of being able to insert the screws and then achieve the reduction compared with the Magerl screw technique, in which an anatomic reduction must be achieved before screw insertion. Figure 28–2 shows a 6-year-old boy who had atlantoaxial subluxation.

Atlantoaxial Rotatory Subluxation

Atlantoaxial rotatory subluxation, also known as *rotatory fixation* if it has persisted for more than 3 months, is a frequent cause of torticollis in children. The most common etiologies are trauma and infection, although congenital and iatrogenic causes also exist. Patients present with neck pain; headaches; and a cock-robin position, in which the head is rotated to one side with some lateral flexion. In acute subluxations, movement is painful and accompanied by sternocleidomastoid spasms. The child often has the ability to make the deformity worse but cannot correct it. In fixed deformities, the pain subsides, but the lack of motion persists; neurologic deficits are rare.[142]

The mechanism of injury is often trivial trauma, whereby the neck is rotated and tilted, resulting in subluxation of C1 on C2.[143,144] The infectious etiology is known as *Grisel syndrome* and most commonly occurs after an upper respiratory tract infection but can also occur after tonsillectomy, pharyngoplasty, or retropharyngeal abscess.[145] Because of the anastomoses between the veins and lymphatics draining the pharynx and periodontoid plexus, inflammation in the pharynx can lead to attenuation of the transverse ligament or synovium or both surrounding C1-2, resulting in subluxation.

X-ray examination can be challenging because of the difficulty in positioning a patient with torticollis, but anteroposterior and open-mouth odontoid images should be obtained in as close to a neutral position as possible.[146] The lateral masses appear different in size because one is rotated anteriorly and one posteriorly, and the distances from the lateral masses to the dens are asymmetrical. Two-dimensional and three-dimensional CT scans have largely replaced cineradiography and can show superimposition of the atlas on the axis in a rotated position.[147,148]

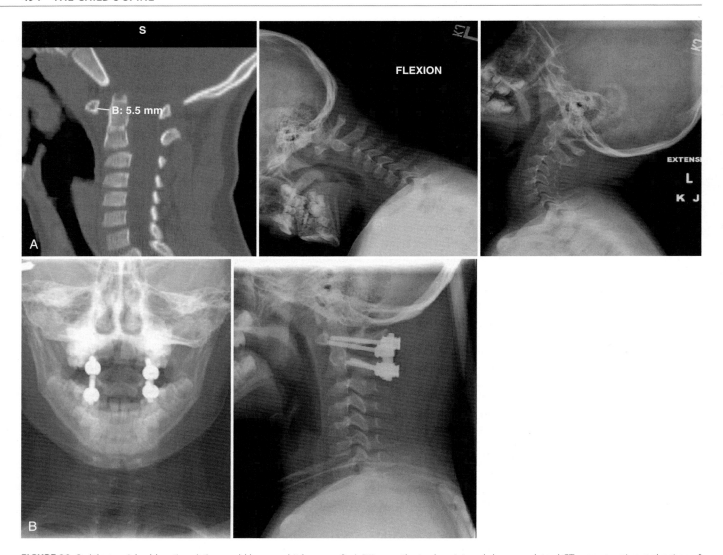

FIGURE 28–2 Atlantoaxial subluxation. A 6-year-old boy was hit by a car. **A,** A 5.5-mm atlanto-dens interval shown on lateral CT reconstruction at the time of injury. **B,** After 3 months of conservative treatment in cervical collar, instability is shown on flexion and extension lateral cervical x-rays. **C,** Postoperative x-rays after C1-2 fusion.

Treatment options depend on the timing of injury and duration of symptoms,[149] with some children likely never receiving medical attention because of spontaneous reduction. In patients whose symptoms have persisted less than 1 week, they can be treated with a soft collar, anti-inflammatories, and home exercises. If spontaneous reduction does not occur after a week, the patients should be put in head halter traction and bed rest, which usually relieves the symptoms if they have persisted less than 1 month. In cases of atlantoaxial rotatory subluxation that have endured more than 1 month, reduction with head halter traction is unlikely,[150] but halo traction can be used to attempt reduction. More weight can be used with the halo, while applying a rotation to the right and left to assist the reduction. Documentation of the reduction should be performed by CT scan, and then the patient must remain in the halo vest for 6 weeks. If reduction is unable to be maintained, posterior fusion of C1-2 is recommended. Additionally, fusion is recommended if the halo immobilization fails after 6 weeks, if the subluxation has been present for more than 3 months, or if the patient has instability or neurologic compromise.[151]

Odontoid Fractures

Odontoid fractures are one of the most common cervical spine fractures in children, reported to represent up to 75% of all cervical spine fractures owing to the large head-to-body size ratio.[152] In children, the most common mechanism is falling, whereas in young adults the mechanism is typically high-velocity trauma such as motor vehicle accidents.

Fractures of the odontoid in children typically occur through the synchondrosis, which is a cartilage line at the base of the odontoid. Fractures that reduce spontaneously can look like a Salter I injury or appear to be normal on plain films. CT scans with three-dimensional reconstructions can assist in identifying minimally displaced odontoid fractures,[153] and MRI can show bone and soft tissue edema around a minimally displaced fracture.

Most odontoid fractures are displaced anteriorly with an intact anterior periosteal sleeve that can help stabilize the fracture when immobilized in extension and help encourage healing.[148,154-156] Treatment of displaced fractures is by closed reduction via an extension or hyperextension maneuver with immobilization in a halo cast or Minerva jacket for children younger than 3 years. Most fractures heal uneventfully after 6 to 8 weeks, at which time documentation of stability with flexion-extension views is recommended. In cases that are difficult to reduce, head halter or halo traction, and rarely manipulation under general anesthesia, is necessary. The need for surgical fixation is unusual because of the excellent results from closed treatment.[157-159]

Os Odontoideum

Os odontoideum is an unsupported round ossicle that is separated from the body of the axis by a transverse gap. Some authors propose that os odontoideum is due to an unrecognized fracture that is distracted by the alar ligaments and results in nonunion,[33,142,160-168] whereas other authors suggest that it is congenital because of its association with congenital syndromes.[169-171] Presentation ranges from asymptomatic to frank myelopathy. Diagnosis can usually be made on routine x-rays, with lateral flexion-extension views showing the degree of displacement of C1 on C2. Measuring the distance between C1 and the ossicle is not helpful, however, because they move together. Instead, one should evaluate the space available for the cord or the relationship of the body of the axis to the posterior aspect of the anterior arch of C1. More recently, investigators have suggested using dynamic (real-time) MRI to aid in diagnosis of instability.[172]

There is debate in the literature regarding management of patients with os odontoideum. Some authors advocate conservative management with yearly clinical and radiographic evaluation of patients with a stable os odontoideum.[161,173-175] There are reports, however, of decompensation and death in asymptomatic patients who have been followed conservatively.[161,176,177] Many surgeons favor surgical stabilization of patients with an os odontoideum.[175,177-180] Options include methods for C1-2 arthrodesis as already discussed.[180,181]

Hangman's Fracture

A hangman's fracture, or traumatic spondylolisthesis, is a fracture of the bilateral pars interarticularis of C2. This name derives from the fact that the fracture resembles the injury associated with a judicial hanging. Because the fracture fragments separate and decompress the cord, neurologic injury is unusual. Most of these injuries occur in children younger than 2 years, likely because of the large head size and poor muscle control. X-rays often show anterior subluxation of C2 on C3 with lucencies anterior to the pedicles of the axis. Persistent synchondroses of the axis have been reported that can be confused with hangman's fractures.[133,182-184] Treatment consists of immobilization for 8 to 12 weeks in a Minerva jacket, halo, or cervical orthosis. Pizzutillo and colleagues[185] reported healing in four of five children treated in a Minerva jacket or

halo cast. If nonunion occurs, anterior or posterior arthrodesis can stabilize the fracture.[151]

Lower Cervical (Subaxial) Spine Injuries

Traumatic injuries to the lower cervical spine (C3-7) are rare in young children and infants but are more common in adolescents and older children. Children younger than age 9 account for only 22% to 31% of pediatric lower cervical spine injuries, whereas children older than age 10 account for 70% to 73%.[186] One should suspect a cervical spine injury if the patient is unconscious, has cervical rigidity, has muscle guarding, has neck pain, has radicular pain, has numbness, or has neurologic deficits.[186] In infants, motor weakness and hypotonia should raise suspicion of a cervical spine injury.

Compression Fractures

Compression fractures are the most common fracture in the pediatric lower cervical spine. Trauma causing flexion and axial loading leads to a loss of vertebral height. When evaluating a child, one must be careful not to mistake normal cervical wedging for a compression fracture. Ossification is incomplete until age 7 years, and normal anterior wedging of the lower cervical spine until this age is considered normal. This wedging is usually most notable at the C3 vertebra.[187] Compression fractures are usually considered stable injuries and can be treated nonoperatively. With immobilization, these fractures normally heal in 3 to 6 weeks. Flexion and extension films should be obtained at 2 to 4 weeks to confirm stability and alignment of the fracture.

Facet Fractures and Dislocations

Facet fractures and dislocations are the second most common lower cervical spine injuries in children and most commonly occur in adolescents.[151] Unilateral dislocations often affect the nerve root, whereas bilateral dislocations affect the spinal cord.[188] The cartilaginous components are overlapped and locked causing a "perched facet" on x-ray, which indicates a true dislocation. Treatment for a unilateral dislocation is initially traction and reduction if the patient is awake and able to cooperate with an examination. If the dislocation cannot be reduced, open reduction and arthrodesis is warranted. Bilateral facet fractures and dislocations are considered unstable, and reduction and stabilization is required.[151] Figure 28-3 shows a 6-year-old girl with bilateral lumbar facet dislocations.

Burst Fractures

Burst fractures in the subaxial spine are rare in pediatric patients. These injuries occur secondary to axial loading. Retropulsed fragments and occult laminar fractures can compromise the spinal canal. CT is a useful modality in determining canal compromise and bony involvement. A burst fracture

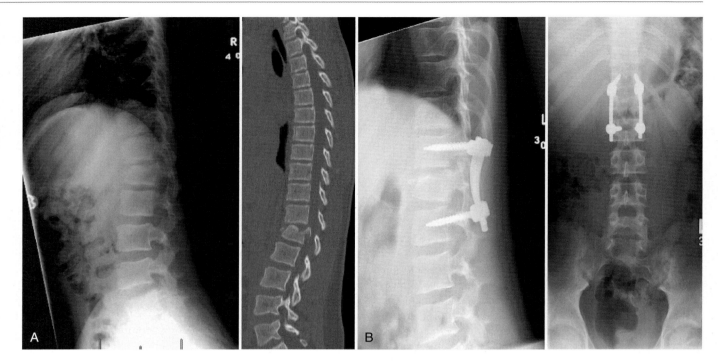

FIGURE 28–3 Lumbar burst fracture. A 14-year-old boy was in a motor vehicle accident and had 50% retropulsion of L1 vertebral body. **A,** Lateral x-ray and sagittal CT reconstruction. **B,** Postoperative result after decompression and fusion.

with no neurologic deficit and minimal spinal canal compromise can be treated with traction followed by halo immobilization. If imaging shows significant canal compromise or the patient has neurologic deficits, surgical decompression and fixation is recommended typically via anterior arthrodesis. This is one of the few instances where anterior fusion is recommended in children because the need for stability outweighs the risk of developing a deformity secondary to destruction of the anterior growth plate. In older children and adolescents, anterior instrumentation can be used without as much risk of kyphotic deformity.[151]

Vertebral Growth Plate Fractures

In contrast to adults, lower cervical spine injuries in children can occur through the synchondrosis at the cartilaginous endplate. The primary ossification centers fuse by 7 to 8 years of age, but the secondary ossification centers can remain open until 25 years of age.[189] MRI can be used to assess the growth plate because it may be difficult to differentiate normal lucency of a synchondrosis from a traumatic lesion on x-ray. Fracture of the synchondrosis can lead to anterior or posterior displacement of the endplate. Anterior displacement can be treated conservatively with a cervical orthosis until the fracture has healed. Posterior displacement of the endplate is treated with an anterior surgical approach to reduce the bony nucleus resulting in spinal decompression and alignment. The patient should remain in a cervical orthosis for 4 to 5 months.[190]

Pediatric Halo

Halo immobilization is often used in the treatment of pediatric cervical spine injuries, even in infants. Presized halos and vests are used in adults, and these often work for adolescents. Prefabricated halos and vests are also available for children and infants, but because of the wide variability in size in children, custom vests and rings may be necessary. CT is recommended before pin placement to help determine bone structure. The pediatric skull is thickest anterolaterally and posterolaterally, and pins should be placed accordingly, with attention to the supraorbital and supratrochlear nerves.[191] The number of pins required varies with age. Children younger than 2 years require 8 to 10 pins, but by age 5 years only 4 pins may be necessary.[188] Pins should be inserted perpendicular to the skull to improve pin-bone interface.[192] The amount of torque required during pin insertion decreases with age, with 2 to 4 inch-pounds required for younger children and standard torque of 6 to 8 inch-pounds in adolescents. There can be great variation in pressures with different torque wrenches, however, and they should be calibrated before halo placement on a child.[193] Pins should not be retightened at 48 hours in children. In adolescents, retightening can be done at 48 hours, however.[151]

Complications are common with halo immobilizers in children. Dormans and colleagues[194] reported a complication rate of 68% but noted that most complications were minor, and all patients were able to wear the halo until fracture healing occurred. The most common complications include superficial pin tract infection and pin loosening. Serious but less common complications include dural penetration, supra-orbital and supratrochlear nerve injury, pin scars, and deep pin infections.

Thoracolumbar Classification Systems

Thoracolumbar fractures in children are uncommon but can cause significant morbidity and mortality, requiring a high index of suspicion for these injuries. Two classification systems for thoracolumbar spine injuries are discussed here: the Denis classification and the Thoracolumbar Injury Classification and Severity (TLICS) scale.

Denis[195] described a three-column classification system. The anterior column consists of the anterior ligament, the anterior anulus fibrosus, and the anterior part of the vertebral body. The middle column contains the posterior longitudinal ligament, the posterior anulus fibrosus, and the posterior wall of the vertebral body. The posterior column comprises the supraspinous and infraspinous ligaments, the posterior capsule, and the ligamentum flavum. Denis[195] used this system to classify thoracolumbar injuries as compression fractures, burst fractures, flexion-distraction injuries, or fracture-dislocation injuries. He also classified the stability of these fractures based on the number of columns affected. If two or more columns fail, the fracture is considered unstable accord-ing to Denis.[195]

The Spine Trauma Study Group developed the TLICS scale. Three primary axes were identified to help analyze and manage fracture patterns: (1) injury morphology, (2) integrity of the posterior ligamentous complex, and (3) neurologic status. The three primary axes are divided further into subgroups. Mor-phology is determined from radiographs, MRI, and CT scan using one of three morphologic categories: (1) compression, which can be classified further with a burst component, (2) translation and rotation, and (3) distraction. The integrity of the posterior ligamentous complex is categorized as (1) intact, (2) disrupted, or (3) indeterminate. The neurologic status is categorized as intact, nerve root injury, complete spinal cord injury, or incomplete spinal cord injury. The TLICS score is based on these principles, and specific values are assigned to each subgroup with lesser point values for less severe injuries. These scores can help guide surgical treatment. Patients with a score of 3 or less are generally treated nonoperatively depend-ing on the type of injury. Patients with a score of 5 or greater generally require surgical fixation. Patients with a score of 4 fall in the intermediate zone where treatment is up to the discretion of the surgeon.[187]

Compression Fractures

Compression fractures are the most common thoracolumbar fracture pattern.[196] The severity of the fracture is based on the percentage of height lost, but regardless of severity, these frac-tures are rarely associated with neurologic deficit. It is impor-tant to determine if the injury is acute or chronic because these

injuries can commonly occur as a result of falls. MRI or a bone scan can be used to determine acuity. Compression fractures are nearly always stable injuries, but one must be sure to examine the posterior soft tissues to rule out a flexion-distraction injury. Additionally, a CT scan should be obtained to rule out a burst fracture. Treatment options depend on whether the fracture is isolated or if contiguous fractures are present. Isolated compression fractures are best treated with an extension orthosis. These fractures usually heal in 4 to 6 weeks, but x-rays should be obtained to monitor alignment. Contiguous compression fractures can result in kyphosis. If kyphosis greater than 40 degrees is present, surgical treatment should be considered. The preferred surgical treatment is gen-erally posterior instrumentation spanning one to two levels above and below the injured vertebra, with decompression if a neurologic deficit exists.[196]

Burst Fractures

Burst fractures involve, at a minimum, the anterior and middle columns.[195] These injuries are most common in the lower tho-racic and upper lumbar regions. Cord injury can occur with retropulsion of bony fragments at the thoracolumbar junction resulting in conus medullaris or cauda equina syndromes. There have been few studies of burst fractures in immature patients. Most investigators believe that conservative treat-ment is warranted if the posterior ligament column is intact and there are no neurologic deficits. Treatment should include an extension molded cast or a thoracic, lumbar, or sacral orthosis. The goal is to allow the patient to maintain an upright position allowing ambulation.

If there is injury to the posterior ligamentous complex, surgical treatment may be used to protect the integrity of the spine. Anterior and posterior approaches can be used.[197] The posterior approach allows for decompression and direct frac-ture reduction. The anterior approach allows direct canal decompression through corpectomy of the fractured verte-brae.[196] Figure 28–4 shows a 13-year-old boy with a lumbar burst fracture.

Chance Fractures

Chance fractures, or flexion-distraction injuries, are most often caused by lap belt injuries in motor vehicle accidents. With frontal impact, the lap belt causes the axis of rotation to be the anterior spine, causing distractive forces on the poste-rior spine and anterior vertebral compression. According to the Denis classification, this is a three-column injury and is unstable.[195] The classic finding on x-ray is an "empty facet" sign. The inferior articular process of the superior vertebrae is no longer in contact with the superior articular process of the inferior vertebrae, and the facet appears empty.[196] Treatment of Chance fractures is based on severity of the injury. If only bony fractures are present with no injury to the ligamentous complexes, a hyperextension cast can be used. If ligamentous disruption is present, surgical treatment is necessary. Young children can be treated surgically with posterior wiring com-bined with a cast, whereas older children and adolescents can

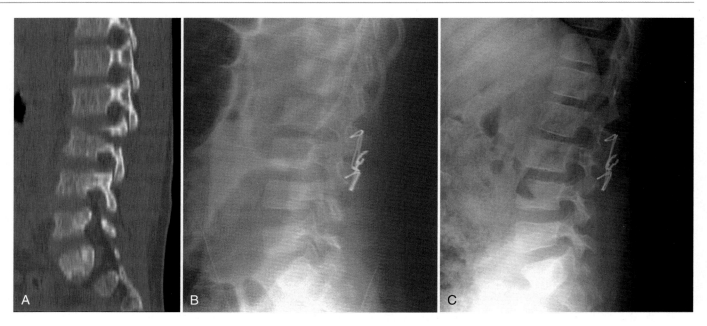

FIGURE 28–4 Lumbar Chance fracture. A 5-year-old boy was restrained by a lap belt in a motor vehicle accident. **A,** Sagittal CT reconstruction shows L2 Chance fracture. **B,** Postoperative image after spinous process wiring. **C,** Image 3 years postoperatively.

undergo segmental fixation.[196,198] Figure 28–5 shows a Chance fracture in a 5-year-old boy.

Fracture-Dislocations

Fracture-dislocations in the thoracolumbar spine are three-column injuries and are very unstable.[195] These injuries nearly always require surgical stabilization. If complete spinal cord injury is present, internal fixation is warranted because it may aid the rehabilitation process. Children younger than 10 years should undergo longer fusions to reduce the occurrence of paralytic scoliosis later on.

Limbus Fractures

Limbus fractures occur at the posterior vertebral endplate when disc material herniates between the unfused peripheral ring apophysis of the epiphyseal endplates and central cartilage. These fractures often manifest as low back pain in adolescents and young adults, although they can be identified in older patients as well.[199] These lesions are usually located in the lower lumbar spine and appear on x-rays as a corner defect in the endplate and a wedge-shaped piece of bone posterior to the body or disc space. CT and MRI can more fully delineate the bony defect and disc injury. These injuries are less likely to resorb on their own and often require surgical decompression in symptomatic patients.

Depending on the size of the lesion, the disc (calcified or noncalcified) and bony fracture can be removed via an extended laminotomy, hemilaminectomy, or laminectomy. In the absence of routine disc herniation, the discectomy can be performed in standard fashion, thus identifying the fracture as the endplate is exposed.[199]

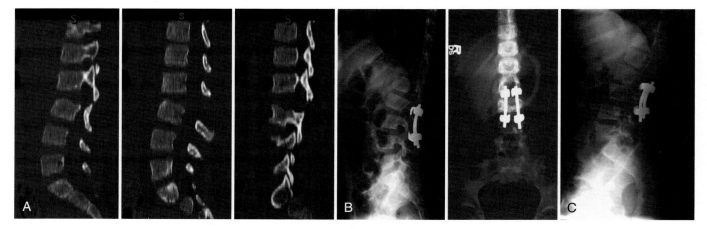

FIGURE 28–5 Bilateral lumbar facet dislocation. A 6-year-old girl was in a motor vehicle accident. **A,** Sagittal CT reconstructions show bilateral L2-3 facet dislocations. **B,** Postoperative image after L2-3 fusion with pedicle hook instrumentation. **C,** Image 3 years postoperatively.

KEY POINTS

1. Traumatic injury to the pediatric spine is relatively rare; injuries in children younger than 8 years old typically affect the upper cervical spine because of the large head size, whereas older children are more likely to sustain subaxial cervical spine injuries and thoracolumbar injuries as the spine takes on the biomechanical characteristics of an adult.

2. During transport, children younger than 4 years often require a cutout region for the occiput or elevation of the shoulders to accommodate the disproportionately large head and to keep the cervical spine in neutral alignment.

3. Spine imaging in an injured child should begin with a trauma x-ray series. Young children who cannot cooperate may require a CT scan from the occiput to C2. A CT traumagram including sagittal and coronal reconstructions of the cervical, thoracic, and lumbar spine is acceptable, and x-rays are not needed. MRI can be used to evaluate a neurologic deficit and determine if a ligamentous injury exists.

4. In spinal cord injury in pediatric patients, there is a susceptibility to development of post-traumatic deformity and growth arrest, and surgical correction and fusion needs to take into account remaining growth.

5. Evaluation of cervical and lumbar trauma in children requires an understanding of developmental anatomy to differentiate trauma from age-appropriate findings. Evidence of soft tissue swelling and sharp edges at the suspected fracture are more indicative of trauma. Injuries that are unique to children include atlantoaxial rotatory instability, birth injuries, and limbus fractures. Generally, young children more often have ligamentous injuries, whereas older children and adolescents have bony injuries as the spine takes on adult characteristics.

KEY REFERENCES

1. Herzenberg JE, Hensinger RN, Dedrick DK, et al: Emergency transport and positioning of young children who have an injury of the cervical spine: The standard backboard may be hazardous. J Bone Joint Surg Am 71:15-22, 1989.
   This article addresses the importance of accounting for the disproportionately large head in children during transport by using a backboard with an occipital cutout or elevating the shoulders.

2. Brown RL, Brunn MA, Garcia VF: Cervical spine injuries in children: A review of 103 patients treated consecutively at a level one pediatric trauma center. J Pediatr Surg 36:1107-1114, 2001.
   This article reports the increased prevalence of upper cervical spine injuries and SCIWORA in young children.

3. Bilston LE, Brown J: Pediatric spinal injury type and severity are age and mechanism dependent. Spine 32:2339-2347, 2007.

This article shows that injury is age and mechanism dependent. Falls are the most common mechanism in children younger than 8 years old, minor neck injuries are more common in children older than 8 years, and sporting injuries are most common in older boys. Motor vehicle accidents cause the most serious spinal trauma in children.

4. Vaccaro AR, Lehman RA Jr, Hurlbert RJ, et al: A new classification of thoracolumbar injuries: The importance of injury morphology, the integrity of the posterior ligamentous complex, and neurologic status. Spine 30:2325-2333, 2005.
   The composite injury severity score derived from this classification system assigns 1 to 4 points to three critical components of an injury: integrity of the posterior ligamentous complex, injury morphology, and neurologic status. Fractures with scores of 3 points or less are considered nonoperative cases. Fractures with scores of 4 points can be considered for nonoperative or operative intervention. Fractures with scores of 5 or more points are considered surgical cases.

5. Mayfield JK, Erkkila, JC, Winter RB: Spine deformity subsequent to acquired childhood spinal cord injury. J Bone Joint Surg Am 63:1401-1411, 1981.
   This article found that children who had spinal cord injury before the adolescent growth spurt were much more likely to have progressive spinal deformity than children who were injured after the growth spurt.

REFERENCES

1. Cirak B, Ziegfeld S, Knight V, et al: Spinal injuries in children. J Pediatr Surg 39:607-612, 2004.

2. Kokoska ER, Keller M, Rallo MC, et al: Characteristics of pediatric cervical spine injuries. J Pediatr Surg 36:100-105, 2001.

3. d'Amato C: Pediatric spinal trauma. Clin Orthop Relat Res (432):34-40, 2005.

4. Givens TG, Polley K, Smith GF, et al: Pediatric cervical spine injury: A three-year experience. J Trauma 41:2310-2314, 1996.

5. Bilston LE, Brown J: Pediatric spinal injury type and severity are age and mechanism dependent. Spine 32:2339-2347, 2007.

6. Vogel LC: Unique management needs of pediatric spinal cord injury in patients: Etiology and pathophysiology. J Spinal Cord Med 20:10-13, 1997.

7. Leventhal HR: Birth injuries of the spinal cord. J Pediatr 56:447-453, 1960.

8. Ranjith RK, Mullet J, Burke TE: Hangman's fracture caused by suspected child abuse. J Pediatr Orthop 11:329-332, 2002.

9. Rooks VJ, Sisler C, Burton B: Cervical spine injury in child abuse: Report of two cases. Pediatr Radiol 28:193-195, 1998.

10. Bailey DK: The normal cervical spine in infants and children. Radiology 59:712-719, 1952.

11. Herman MJ, Pizzutillo P: Cervical spine disorders in children. Clin Orthop Relat Res 30:457-466, 1999.

12. Bohn D, Armstrong D, Becker L, et al: Cervical spine injuries in children. J Trauma 30:463-469, 1990.

SECTION IV

13. Eleraky M, Theodore N, Adams M, et al: Pediatric cervical spine injuries: Report of 102 cases and review of literature. J Neurosurg Spine 92:12-17, 2000.

14. Finch G, Barnes M: Major cervical spine injuries in children and adolescents. J Pediatr Orthop 186:811-814, 1998.

15. Nuckley D, Hersted S, Eck M, et al: Developmental biomechanics of the cervical spine: Tension and compression. J Biomech 38:2266-2275, 2005.

16. Ouyang J, Zhu Q, Zhao W, et al: Biomechanical assessment of the pediatric cervical spine under bending and tensile loading. Spine 30:716-723, 2005.

17. Herzenberg JE, Hensinger R, Dedrick DK, et al: Emergency transport and position of young children who have an injury of the cervical spine: The standard backboard may be hazardous. J Bone Joint Surg Am 71:15-22, 1989.

18. Curran C, Dietrich A, Bowman MJ, et al: Pediatric cervical spine immobilization: Achieving neutral position. J Trauma 39:729-732, 1995.

19. Nypaver M, Treloar D: Neutral cervical spine positioning in children. Ann Emerg Med 23:208-211, 1994.

20. Laham JL, Cotcamp D, Gibbons PA, et al: Isolated head injuries versus multiple trauma in pediatric patients: Do the same indications for cervical spine evaluation apply? Pediatr Neurosurg 21:221-226, 1994.

21. Slotkin JR, Lu Y, Wood KB: Thoracolumbar spinal trauma in children. Neurosurg Clin N Am 18:621-630, 2007.

22. Hadley MN, Zabramski JM, Browner CM, et al: Pediatric spinal trauma: Review of 122 cases of spinal cord and vertebral column injuries. J Neurosurg 68:18-24, 1988.

23. Lee SL, Sena M, Greenholz SK, et al: A multidisciplinary approach to the development of a cervical spine clearance protocol: Process, rationale, and initial results. J Pediatr Surg 38:358-362, 2003.

24. Bonadio WA: Cervical spine trauma in children: General concepts, normal anatomy, radiographic evaluation. Am J Emerg Med 11:158-165, 1993.

25. Lally KP, Senac M, Hardin WD, et al: Utility of the cervical spine radiograph in pediatric trauma. Am J Surg 158:540-542, 1989.

26. Baker C, Kadish H, Schunk JE: Evaluation of pediatric cervical spine injury. Am J Emerg Med 17:230-234, 1999.

27. Buhs C, Cullen M, Klein M, et al: The pediatric trauma C-spine: Is the "odontoid" view necessary? J Pediatr Surg 35:994-997, 2000.

28. Ralston ME, Chung K, Barnes PD, et al: Role of flexion-extension radiographs in blunt pediatric cervical spine injury. Acad Emerg Med 8:237-245, 2001.

29. Dwek JR, Chung C: Radiography of cervical spine injury in children: Are flexion-extension radiographs useful for acute trauma? AJR Am J Roentgenol 174:1617-1619, 2000.

30. Bucholz RW, Burkhead WZ: The pathological anatomy of fatal atlanto-occipital dislocations. J Bone Joint Surg Am 61:148-250, 1979.

31. Kaufman RA, Carroll CD, Buncher CR: Atlantooccipital junction: Standards for measurement in normal children. AJNR Am J Neuroradiol 8:995-999, 1987.

32. Roche C, Carty H: Spinal trauma in children. Pediatr Radiol 31:677-700, 2001.

33. Fielding JW, Cochran JB, Lawsing JF, et al: Tears of the transverse ligament of the atlas: A clinical and biomechanical study. J Bone Joint Surg Am 56:1683-1691, 1974.

34. Steel HH: Anatomical and mechanical considerations of the atlanto-axial articulation. J Bone Joint Surg Am 50:1481-1482, 1968.

35. Swischuk LE: Anterior displacement of C2 in children. Radiology 122:759-763, 1977.

36. Cattell HS, Filtzer D: Pseudosubluxation and other normal variations in the cervical spine in children. J Bone Joint Surg Am 47:1295-1309, 1965.

37. Sheridan R, Peralta R, Rhea J, et al: Reformatted visceral protocol helical computed tomographic scanning allows conventional radiographs of the thoracic and lumbar spine to be eliminated in the evaluation of blunt trauma patients. J Trauma 55:665-669, 2003.

38. Stambolis V, Brady S, Klos D, et al: The effects of cervical bracing upon swallowing in young, normal, healthy volunteers. Dysphagia 18:39-45, 2003.

39. Naidich JB, Naidich TP, Garfein C, et al: The widened interspinous distance: A useful sign of anterior cervical dislocation in the supine frontal projection. Radiology 123:113-116, 1977.

40. Bonadio W: Cervical spine trauma in children, II: Mechanisms and manifestations of injury, therapeutic considerations. Am J Emerg Med 11:256-278, 1993.

41. Ardran GM, Kemp F: The mechanism of changes of the cervical airway in infancy. Med Radiogr Photogr 44:26-38, 1968.

42. Davis JW, Phreaner DL, Hoyt DB, et al: The etiology of missed cervical spine injuries. J Trauma 34:342-346, 1993.

43. Gerrelts BD, Petersen EU, Mabry J, et al: Delayed diagnosis of cervical spine injuries. J Trauma 31:1622-1626, 1991.

44. Grogan EL, Morris JAJ, Dittus RS, et al: Cervical spine evaluation in urban trauma centers: Lowering institutional costs and complications through helical CT scan. J Am Coll Surg 200:160-165, 2005.

45. Nunez DBJ, Zuluaga A, Fuentes-Bernardo DA, et al: Cervical spine trauma: How much more do we learn by routinely using helical CT? RadioGraphics 16:1307-1318, 1996.

46. Fearon T, Vucih J: Normalized pediatric organ-absorbed doses from CT examinations. AJR Am J Roentgenol 148:171-174, 1987.

47. Huda W, Bissessur K: Effective dose equivalents, HE, in diagnostic radiology. Med Physics 17:998-1003, 1990.

48. Gestring ML, Gracias VH, Feliciano MA, et al: Evaluation of the lower spine after blunt trauma using abdominal computed tomographic scanning supplemented with lateral scanograms. J Trauma 53:9-14, 2002.

49. Hauser CJ, Visvikis G, Hinrichs C, et al: Prospective validation of computed tomographic screening of the thoracolumbar spine in trauma. J Trauma 55:228-234, 2003.

50. Wintermark M, Mouhsine E, Theumann N, et al: Thoracolumbar spine fractures in patients who have sustained severe trauma: Depiction with multi-detector row CT. Radiology 277:681-689, 2003.

51. Brown RL, Brunn MA, Garcia VF: Cervical spine injuries in children: A review of 103 patients treated consecutively at a level 1 pediatric trauma center. J Pediatr Surg 36:1107-1114, 2001.

52. Flynn JM, Closkey RF, Mahboubi S, et al: Role of magnetic resonance imaging in the assessment of pediatric cervical spine injuries. J Pediatr Orthop 22:573-577, 2002.

53. Keiper MD, Zimmerman RA, Bilaniuk LT: MRI in the assessment of the supportive soft tissues of the cervical spine in acute trauma in children. Neuroradiology 40:359-363, 1998.

54. Frank JB, Lim CK, Flynn JM, et al: The efficacy of magnetic resonance imaging in pediatric cervical spine clearance. Spine 27:1176-1179, 2002.

55. Davis JW, Parks SN, Detlefs CL, et al: Clearing the cervical spine in obtunded patients: The use of dynamic fluoroscopy. J Trauma 39:435-438, 1995.

56. Kolb JC, Summers RL, Galli RL: Cervical collar-induced changes in intracranial pressure. Am J Emerg Med 17:135-137, 1999.

57. Viccellio P, Simon H, Pressman BD, et al: A prospective multicenter study of cervical spine injury in children. Pediatrics 108:E20, 2001.

58. Stiell IG, Clement CM, McKnight RD, et al: The Canadian C-spine rule versus the NEXUS low-risk criteria in patients with trauma. N Engl J Med 349:2510-2518, 2003.

59. Anderson RC, Kan P, Hansen KW, et al: Cervical spine clearance after trauma in children. Neurosurg Focus 20:E3, 2006.

60. Launay F, Leet AI, Sponseller PD: Pediatric spinal cord injury without radiographic abnormality: A meta-analysis. Clin Orthop Relat Res 433:166-170, 2005.

61. Pang D: Spinal cord injury without radiographic abnormality in children, 2 decades later. Neurosurgery 55:1325-1342, 2004.

62. Levi AD, Hurlbert J, Anderson P, et al: Neurologic deterioration secondary to unrecognized spinal instability following trauma: A multicenter study. Spine 31:451-458, 2006.

63. Bolinger B, Shartz M, Marion D: Bedside fluoroscopic flexion and extension cervical spine radiographs for clearance of the cervical spine in comatose trauma patients. J Trauma 56:132-136, 2005.

64. Ajani AE, Cooper DJ, Scheinkestel CD, et al: Optimal assessment of cervical spine trauma in critically ill patients: A prospective evaluation. Anaesth Intensive Care 26:487-491, 1998.

65. Stassen NA, Williams VA, Grestring ML, et al: Magnetic resonance imaging in combination with helical computed tomography provides safe and efficient method of cervical spine clearance in the obtunded patient. J Trauma 60:171-177, 2006.

66. Diaz JJ, Aulino JM, Collier B, et al: The early work-up for isolated ligamentous injury of the cervical spine: Does computed tomography scan have a role? J Trauma 59:897-904, 2005.

67. Marino RJ, Ditunno JFJ, Donovan WH, et al: Neurologic recovery after traumatic spinal cord injury: Data from the Model Spinal Cord Injury Systems. Arch Physical Med Rehabil 80:1391-1396, 1999.

68. Amar AP, Levy ML: Pathogenesis and pharmacological strategies for mitigating secondary damage in acute spinal cord injury. Neurosurgery 44:1027-1039, 1999.

69. Zivin JA, DeGirolami U: Spinal cord infarction: A highly reproducible stroke model. Stroke 11:200-202, 1980.

70. Zach GA, Seiler W, Dollfus P: Treatment results of spinal cord injuries in the Swiss Paraplegic Centre of Basel. Paraplegia 14:58-65, 1976.

71. Vale FL, Burns J, Jackson AB, et al: Combined medical and surgical treatment after acute spinal cord injury: Results of a prospective pilot study to assess the merits of aggressive medical resuscitation and blood pressure management. J Neurosurg 87:239-246, 1997.

72. Levi L, Wolf A, Belzerg H: Hemodynamic parameters in patients with acute cervical cord trauma: Description, intervention, and prediction of outcome. Neurosurgery 33:1007-1017, 1993.

73. Bracken MB, Shepard MJ, Holford TR, et al: Administration of methylprednisolone for 24 or 48 hours or tirilazad mesylate for 48 hours in the treatment of acute spinal cord injury. JAMA 277:1597-1604, 1997.

74. Bracken MB, Shepard MJ, Holford TR, et al: Methylprednisolone or tirilazad mesylate administration after acute spinal cord injury: 1-year follow-up. J Neurosurg 89:699-706, 1998.

75. Heary RF, Vaccaro AR, Mesa JJ, et al: Steroids and gunshot wounds to the spine. Neurosurgery 41:576-583, 1997.

76. Fehlings MG, Perrin RG: The timing of surgical intervention in the treatment of spinal cord injury: A systematic review of recent clinical evidence. Spine 31:S28-S35, 2006.

77. Pang D, Pollack IF: Spinal cord injury without radiographic abnormality in children—the SCIWORA syndrome. J Trauma 29:654-664, 1989.

78. Wang MY, Hoh DJ, Leary SP, et al: High rates of neurological improvement following severe traumatic pediatric spinal cord injury. Spine 29:1493-1497, 2004.

79. Anderson CJ, Vogel LC, Willis KM, et al: Stability of transition to adulthood among individuals with pediatric-onset spinal cord injuries. J Spinal Cord Med 29:46-56, 2006.

80. Jacobs RR, Asher MA, Snider RK: Thoracolumbar spinal injuries: A comparative study of recumbent and operative treatment in 100 patients. Spine 5:463-477, 1980.

81. Pouliquen JC, Kassis B, Glorion C, et al: Vertebral growth after thoracic or lumbar fracture of the spine in children. J Pediatr Orthop 17:115-120, 1997.

82. Vaccaro AR, Silber JS: Post-traumatic spinal deformity. Spine 26:S111-S118, 2001.

83. Yasuoka S, Peterson HA, MacCarty CS: Incidence of spinal column deformity after multilevel laminectomy in children and adults. J Neurosurg 57:441-445, 1982.

84. Mayfield JK, Erkkila JC, Winter RB: Spine deformity subsequent to acquired childhood spinal cord injury. J Bone Joint Surg Am 63:1401-1411, 1981.

85. Moe JH, Kharrat K, Winter RB, et al: Harrington instrumentation without fusion plus external orthotic support for the treatment of difficult curvature problems in young children. Clin Orthop Relat Res 185:35-45, 1984.

86. Dubousset J, Herring JA, Shufflebarger H: The crankshaft phenomenon. J Pediatr Orthop 9:541-550, 1989.

87. Pang D, Wilberger JEJ: Spinal cord injury without radiographic abnormalities in children. J Neurosurg 57:114-129, 1982.

88. Bosch MD, Vogt MT, Ward WT: Pediatric spinal cord injury without radiographic abnormality. Spine 27:2788-2800, 2002.

89. Grabb PA, Pang D: Magnetic resonance imaging in the evaluation of spinal cord injury without radiographic abnormality in children. Neurosurgery 35:406-414, 1994.

90. Flanders AE, Schaefer DM, Doan HT, et al: Acute cervical spine trauma: Correlation of MR imaging findings with degree of neurologic deficit. Radiology 177:25-33, 1990.

91. Davis D, Bohlman H, Walker AE, et al: The pathological findings in fatal craniospinal injuries. J Neurosurg 34:603-613, 1971.

92. Montane I, Eismont FJ, Green BA: Traumatic occipitoatlantal dislocation. Spine 15:112-116, 1991.

93. Farley FA, Graziano GP, Hensinger RN: Traumatic atlanto-occipital dislocation in a child. Spine 17:1539-1541, 1992.

94. Matava MJ, Whitesides TE, Davis PC: Traumatic atlanto-occipital dislocation with survival. Spine 18:1897-1903, 1993.

95. Papadopoulos SM, Dickman CA, Sonntag VKH, et al: Traumatic atlanto-occipital dislocation with survival. Neurosurgery 28:574-579, 1991.

96. Rockswold GL, Sljeskog EL: Traumatic atlantooccipital dislocation with survival. Minn Med 62:151-154, 1979.

97. Woodring JH, Selke ACJ, Duff DE: Traumatic atlantooccipital dislocation with survival. AJR Am J Roentgenol 137:21-24, 1981.

98. Wholey MH, Bruwer AJ, Baker HLJ: The lateral roentgenogram of the neck (with comments on the atlanto-odontoid-basion relationship). Radiology 71:350-356, 1958.

99. Powers B, Miller MD, Kramer RS, et al: Traumatic anterior atlanto-occipital dislocations. Neurosurgery 4:12-17, 1979.

100. Gerlock AJJ, Mirfahkraee M, Benzel EC: Computed tomography of traumatic atlanto-occipital dislocation. Neurosurgery 12:316-319, 1983.

101. Judd DB, Liem LK, Petermann G: Pediatric atlas fracture: A case of fracture through a synchondrosis and review of the literature. Neurosurgery 46:991-995, 2000.

102. Jefferson G: Fracture of the atlas vertebra: Report of four cases and a review of those previously recorded. Br J Surg 7:407-422, 1919-1920.

103. Marlin AE, Gayle RW, Lee JF: Jefferson fractures in children. J Neurosurg 58:277-279, 1983.

104. Mikawa Y, Watanabe R, Yamano Y, et al: Fractures through a synchondrosis of the anterior arch of the atlas. J Bone Joint Surg Br 69:483, 1987.

105. Richards PG: Stable fractures of the atlas and axis in children. J Neurol Neurosurg Psychiatry 47:781-783, 1984.

106. Hensinger RN, DeVito PD, Tagsdale CG: Stable fractures of the atlas and axis in children. J Bone Joint Surg Am 68:189-198, 1986.

107. Burke SW, French HG, Roberts JM, et al: Chronic atlantoaxial instability in Down syndrome. J Bone Joint Surg Am 67:1356-1360, 1985.

108. Dawson EG, Smith L: Atlanto-axial subluxation in children due to vertebral anomalies. J Bone Joint Surg Am 61:582-587, 1979.

109. Hammerschlag W, Ziv I, Wald U, et al: Cervical instability in an achondroplastic infant. J Pediatr Orthop 8:481-484, 1988.

110. Kobori M, Takahashi H, Mikawa Y: Atlanto-axial dislocation in Down's syndrome: A report of two cases requiring surgical correction. Spine 11:195-200, 1986.

111. Kransdorf MJ, Wherle PA, Moser RPJ: Atlantoaxial subluxation in Reiter's syndrome. Spine 13:13-14, 1988.

112. Miz GS, Engler GL: Atlanto-axial subluxation in Larsen's syndrome: A case report. Spine 12:411-412, 1987.

113. McGrory BJ, Klassen RA, Chao EY, et al: Acute fracture and dislocations of the cervical spine in children and adolescents. J Bone Joint Surg Am 75:988-995, 1993.

114. Lui TN, Lee ST, Wong CW, et al: C1-C2 fracture-dislocations in children and adolescents. J Trauma 40:408-411, 1996.

115. American Academy of Pediatrics. Atlanto-axial instability in Down syndrome: Subject review. Pediatrics 96:151-154, 1995.

116. Pueschel SM, Scolia FH: Atlantoaxial instability in individuals with Down syndrome: Epidemiologic, radiographic, and clinical studies. Pediatrics 4:555-560, 1987.

117. Segal LS, Drummond DS, Zanotti RM, et al: Complications of posterior arthrodesis of the cervical spine in patients who have Down syndrome. J Bone Joint Surg Am 73:1547-1560, 1991.

118. Windell J, Burke SW: Sports participation of children with Down syndrome. Orthop Clin North Am 34:439-443, 2003.

119. Pueschel SM, Scolia FH, Tupper TB, et al: Skeletal anomalies of the upper cervical spine in children with Down syndrome. J Pediatr Orthop 10:607-611, 1990.

120. Cohen WI: Atlantoaxial instability: What's next? Arch Pediatr Adolesc Med 152:119-122, 1998.

121. Merrick I, Ezra E, Josef B, et al: Musculoskeletal problems in Down syndrome. European Paediatric Orthopaedic Society Survey: The Israeli sample. J Pediatr Orthop B 9:610-619, 2000.

122. Caird MS, Wills BPD, Dormans JP: Down syndrome in children: The role of the orthopaedic surgeon. J Am Acad Orthop Surg 14:610-619, 2006.

123. Ferguson RI, Putney ME, Allen BLJ: Comparison of neurologic deficits with atlanto-dens intervals in patients with Down syndrome. J Spinal Disord 10:246-252, 1997.

124. Sherk HH, Whitaker LA, Pasquariello PS: Fascial malformations and spinal anomalies: A predictable relationship. Spine 7:526-531, 1982.

125. Gallie W: Fractures and dislocation of the cervical spine. Am J Surg 46:495-499, 1939.

126. Brooks AL, Jenkins EB: Atlanto-axial arthrodesis by the wedge compression method. J Bone Joint Surg Am 60:279-284, 1978.

127. Coyne TJ, Fehlings MG, Wallace MC, et al: C1-C2 posterior cervical fusion: Long-term evaluation of results and efficacy. Neurosurgery 37:688-692, 1995.

128. Smith MD, Phillips WA, Hensinger RN: Complications of fusion to the upper cervical spine. Spine 16:702-705, 1991.

129. Crisco JJI, Panjabi MM, Oda T, et al: Bone graft translation of four upper cervical spine fixation techniques in a cadaveric model. J Orthop Res 9:835-836, 1991.

130. Grob D, Crisco JJD, Panjabi MM, et al: Biomechanical evaluation of four different posterior atlantoaxial fixation techniques. Spine 17:480-490, 1992.

131. Hajek PD, Lipka J, Hartline P, et al: Biomechanical study of C1-C2 posterior arthrodesis techniques. Spine 18:173-177, 1993.

132. Naderi S, Crawford NR, Song GS, et al: Biomechanical comparison of C1-C2 posterior fixations: Cable, graft, and screw combinations. Spine 23:1946-1955, 1998.

133. Smith T, Skinner SR, Shonnard NH: Persistent synchondrosis of the second cervical vertebra simulating a hangman's fracture in a child. J Bone Joint Surg Am 75:1228-1230, 1993.

134. Dickman CA, Sonntag VK: Surgical management of atlanto-axial nonunions. J Neurosurg 83:248-253, 1995.

135. Grob D, Magerl F: Surgical stabilization of C1 and C2 fractures. Orthopade 16:46-54, 1987.

136. Grob D, Jeanneret B, Aebi M, et al: Atlanto-axial fusion with transarticular screw fixation. J Bone Joint Surg Br 73:972-976, 1991.

137. Jeanneret B, Magerl F: Primary posterior fusion C1/C2 in odontoid fractures: Indications, technique, and results of transparticular screw fixation. J Spinal Disord 5:464-475, 1992.

138. Stillerman CB, Wilson JA: Atlanto-axial stabilization with posterior transarticular screw fixation: Technical description and report of 22 cases. Neurosurgery 32:948-954, 1993.

139. Madawi AA, Casey AT, Solanki GA, et al: Radiological and anatomical evaluation of the atlantoaxial transarticular screw fixation technique. J Neurosurg 86:961-968, 1997.

140. Goel A, Laheria V: Plate and screw fixation for atlanto-axial subluxation. Acta Neurochir 129:47-53, 1994.

141. Harms J, Melcher RP: Posterior C1-C2 fusion with polyaxial screw and rod fixation. Spine 26:2467-2471, 2001.

142. Fielding JW, Hawkins RJ: Atlanto-axial rotary fixation (fixed rotary subluxation of the atlanto-axial joint). J Bone Joint Surg Am 59:37-44, 1977.

143. Coutts MB: Atlanto-epistropheal subluxations. Arch Surg 29:297-311, 1934.

144. Crook TB, Enyon CA: Traumatic atlantoaxial rotatory subluxation. Emerg Med J 22:671-672, 2005.

145. Wetzel FT, Larocca H: Grisel's syndrome: A review. Clin Orthop Relat Res 240:141-152, 1989.

146. Maheshwaran S, Sgouros S, Jeyapalan K, et al: Imaging of childhood torticollis due to atlanto-axial rotatory fixation. Childs Nerv Syst 11:667-671, 1995.

147. Geehr RB, Rothman SLG, Kier EL: The role of computed tomography in the evaluation of upper cervical spine pathology. Comput Tomogr 2:79-97, 1978.

148. Scapinelli R: Three dimensional computed tomography in infantile atlantoaxial rotatory fixation. J Bone Joint Surg Br 76:367-370, 1994.

149. Phillips WA, Hensinger RN: The management of the rotatory atlanto-axial subluxation in children. J Bone Joint Surg Am 71:664-668, 1989.

150. Burkus JK, Deponte RJ: Chronic atlantoaxial rotatory fixation: Correction by cervical traction, manipulation, and branching. J Pediatr Orthop 6:631-635, 1986.

151. Warner WC, Hedequist DJ: Cervical spine injuries in children. In Beaty JH, Kasser JR (eds): Rockwood and Wilkins' Fractures in Children, 6th ed. Philadelphia, Lippincott Williams & Wilkins, 2006, pp 776-816.

152. Sherk HH: Fractures of the atlas and odontoid process. Orthop Clin North Am 9:973-984, 1978.

153. Sherburn EW, Day RA, Kaufman BA, et al: Subdental synchondrosis fracture in children: The value of a 3-dimensional computerized tomography. Pediatr Neurosurg 25:256-259, 1996.

154. Apple JS, Kirks DR, Merten DF, et al: Cervical spine fractures and dislocations in children. Pediatr Radiol 17:45-49, 1987.

155. Ries MD, Ray S: Posterior displacement of an odontoid fracture in a child. Spine 11:1043-1044, 1986.

156. Shaw BA, Murphy KM: Displaced odontoid fracture in a 9-month-old child. Am J Emerg Med 1:73-75, 1999.

157. Godard J, Hadji M, Raul JS: Odontoid fractures in the child with neurologic injury: Direct osteosynthesis with a corticospongious screw and literature review. Childs Nerv Syst 13:105-107, 1997.

158. Price E: Fractured odontoid process with anterior dislocation. J Bone Joint Surg Br 42:410-413, 1960.

159. Schippers N, Konings D, Hassler W, et al: Typical and atypical fractures of the odontoid process in young children: Report of two cases and a review of the literature. Acta Neurochir 138:524-530, 1996.

160. Fielding JW: Cineroentgenography of the normal cervical spine. J Bone Joint Surg Am 39:187-190, 1957.

161. Fielding JW, Hensinger RN, Hawkins RJ: Os odontoideum. J Bone Joint Surg Am 62:376-383, 1980.

162. Fielding JW, Stillwell WT, Chynn KY, et al: Use of computed tomography for the diagnosis of atlanto-axial rotatory fixation. J Bone Joint Surg Am 60:1102-1104, 1978.

163. Hawkins RJ, Fielding JW, Thompson WJ: Os odontoideum: Congenital or acquired. J Bone Joint Surg Am 58:413-414, 1976.

164. Hukda S, Ora H, Okabe N, et al: Traumatic atlantoaxial dislocation causing os odontoideum in infants. Spine 5:207-210, 1980.

165. Kuhns LR, Loder RT, Farley FA, et al: Nuchal cord changes in children with os odontoideum: Evidence for associated trauma. J Pediatr Orthop 18:815-819, 1998.

166. Ricciardi JE, Kaufer H, Louis DS: Acquired os odontoideum following acute ligament injury. J Bone Joint Surg Am 58:410-412, 1976.

167. Stillwell WT, Fielding JW: Acquired os odontoideum. Clin Orthop Relat Res 135:71-73, 1978.

168. Verska JM, Anderson PA: Os odontoideum: A case report of one identical twin. Spine 22:706-709, 1997.

169. Giannestras NJ, Mayfield FH, Maurer J: Congenital absence of the odontoid process. J Bone Joint Surg Am 46:839-843, 1964.

170. Sherk HH, Dawoud S: Congenital os odontoideum with Klippel-Feil anomaly and fatal atlanto-axial instability. Spine 6:42-45, 1981.

171. Wollin DG: The os odontoideum. J Bone Joint Surg Am 45:1459-1471, 1971.

172. Hughes TBJ, Richman JB, Rothfus WE: Diagnosis of os odontoideum using kinematic magnetic resonance imaging: A case report. Spine 24:715-718, 1999.

173. Clements WD, Mezue W, Matthew B: Os odontoideum: Congential or acquired? That's not the question. Injury 26:640-642, 1995.

174. Spierings EL, Braakman R: The management of os odontoideum: Analysis of 137 cases. J Bone Joint Surg Br 64:422-428, 1982.

175. Dai L, Yuan W, Ni B, et al: Os odontoideum: Etiology, diagnosis, and management. Surg Neurol 53:106-108, 2000.

176. Michaels L, Prevost MJ, Crang DF: Pathologic changes in a case of os odontoideum (separate odontoid process). J Bone Joint Surg Am 51:956-972, 1996.

177. Klimo PJ, Kan P, Rao G, et al: Os odontoideum: Presentation, diagnosis, and treatment in a series of 78 patients. J Neurosurg Spine 9:332-342, 2008.

178. Lowry DW, Pollack IF, Clyde B, et al: Upper cervical spine fusion in the pediatric population. J Neurosurg 87:671-676, 1997.

179. Taggard DA, Menezes AH, Ryken TC: Treatment of Down syndrome-associated craniovertebral junction abnormalities. J Neurosurg 93:205-213, 2000.

180. Wang J, Vokshoor A, Kim S, et al: Pediatric atlantoaxial instability: Management with screw fixation. Pediatr Neurosurg 30:70-78, 1999.

181. Brockmeyer DL, York JE, Apfelbaum RI: Anatomic suitability of C1-C2 transarticular screw placement in pediatric patients. J Neurosurg 92:7-11, 2000.

182. Matthews LS, Vetter LW, Tolo VT: Cervical anomaly stimulating hangman's fracture in a child. J Bone Joint Surg Am 64:299-300, 1982.

183. Nordstrom REA, Lahdenrants TV, Kaitila II, et al: Familial spondylolisthesis of the axis vertebra. J Bone Joint Surg Br 68:704-706, 1986.

184. Williams JPI, Baker DH, Miller WA: CT appearance of congential defect resembling the hangman's fracture. Pediatr Radiol 29:549-550, 1990.

185. Pizzutillo PD, Rocha EF, D'Astous J, et al: Bilateral fractures of the pedicle of the second cervical vertebra in the young child. J Bone Joint Surg Am 68:892-896, 1986.

186. Dogan S, Safavi-Abbasi S, Theodore N, et al: Pediatric subaxial cervical spine injuries: Origins, management, and outcome in 51 patients. Neurosurg Focus 20:E1, 2006.

187. Rihn JA, Anderson DT, Harris E, et al: A review of the TCLIS system: A novel, user-friendly thoracolumbar trauma classification system. Acta Orthop 79:461-466, 2008.

188. McCall T, Fasset D, Brockmeyer D: Cervical spine trauma in children: A review. Neurosurg Focus 20:E5, 2006.

189. Lawson JP, Ogden JA, Bucholz RW, et al: Physeal injuries of the cervical spine. J Pediatr Orthop 7:428-435, 1987.

190. Vaille R, Mary P, Schmider L, et al: Spinal fracture through the neurocentral synchondrosis in battered children: A case report. Spine 31:E345-E349, 2006.

191. Garfin SR, Roux R, Botte MJ, et al: Skull osteology as it affects halo pin placement in children. J Pediatr Orthop 6:434-435, 1986.

192. Copley LA, Pepe MD, Tan V, et al: A comparison of various angles of halo pin insertion in an immature skull model. Spine 24:1777-1780, 1999.

193. Copley LA, Dormans JP, Pepe MD, et al: Accuracy and reliability of torque wrenches used for halo application in children. J Bone Joint Surg Am 85:2199-2204, 2003.

194. Dormans JP, Criscitiello AA, Drummond DS, et al: Complications in children managed with immobilization in a halo vest. J Bone Joint Surg Am 77:1370-1373, 1995.

195. Denis F: The three column spine and its significance in the classification of acute thoracolumbar spinal injuries. Spine 6:817-831, 1983.

196. Newton PO: Thoracolumbar spine fractures. In Beatty JH, Kasser JR (eds) Rockwood and Wilkins' Fractures in Children, 6th ed. Philadelphia, Lippincott Williams & Wilkins, 2006, pp 816-830.

197. Wood K, Butterman G, Mehbod A, et al: Operative compared with nonoperative treatment of a thoracolumbar burst fracture without neurological deficit. J Bone Joint Surg Br 85:773-781, 2003.

198. Rumball K, Jarvis J: Seat belt injuries of the spine in young children. J Bone Joint Surg Br 74:571-575, 1992.

199. Epstein NE: Lumbar surgery for 56 limbus fractures emphasizing noncalcified type III lesions. Spine 17:1489-1496, 1992.

29 CHAPTER

The Immature Spine and Athletic Injuries

Robert Eilert, MD

Most spine injuries in athletically active children and adolescents are chronic, resulting from repetitive demand on the immature spine during participation in sports. The most serious injuries are acute as a result of direct trauma. The age at which a child can be considered an athlete varies and may be 3 years old when a child puts on skis or 10 years old when he or she begins to ride bulls (Fig. 29–1). Several sports, such as skiing, football, and horseback riding, involve increased risk of acute traumatic events, making spine fracture a significant concern when considering an adolescent athlete. This chapter discusses the initial evaluation and on-field management of spine fractures; the complete treatment of spine fractures is covered elsewhere.

According to surveys of patients seen in sports medicine specialty clinics, the most common cause of back pain in adolescent athletes is stress fracture, or *spondylolysis*. Spine hyperextension and repeated twisting contribute to the high rate of spondylolysis seen in sports such as gymnastics, football, and weightlifting. The rate of spondylolysis in gymnasts is 20% compared with 5% to 6% in the general population.[1]

Less aggressive sports such as golf can also cause adolescent back pain and spine injury. The golf swing places significant torque on the spine and surrounding muscles and can produce strains and sprains, which are minor injuries that interfere with performance. In all sports, appropriate strength training, routine stretching, and good technique are imperative for young athletes to avoid injury and to continue participation in sports throughout their lifetime.

The most effective technique in screening for serious disease is a good patient history, and diagnosing spine injury is no exception. Although helpful, a radiograph is seldom definitive in diagnosing the cause of back pain. Radiography is imperative for diagnosis of an acute fracture, but back pain without a specific injury is usually treated on the basis of a careful history and a thorough physical examination.

Understanding the requirements of the particular sport and gaining knowledge of the training schedule of the athlete are important when performing the patient history. For example, a gymnast with no history of sudden trauma who practices 3 hours daily has a chronic stress that may account for her back pain. A young gymnast's developing spine, given

insufficient recovery time, is highly susceptible to repetitive trauma.

Return to sport is a major goal for an athlete, and the physician needs to be aware of the demands of the specific sport to determine when return to participation is reasonable. The physician should take heed of a young athlete who is reluctant to return to sport after an injury. Family dynamics often influence when a child is willing to resume activity.

Physical activity is the normal function of the musculoskeletal system. The American Academy of Orthopaedic Surgeons (AAOS) has encouraged physical activity as health promoting for all ages in its "Get Up, Get Out, Get Moving" program. The keys to maintaining a healthy spine are good nutrition and proper exercise. Good nutrition includes avoiding obesity and not smoking. Exercise programs should include strengthening for power and endurance and stretching to improve joint range of motion and muscle length.

Principles of Diagnosis

The initial treatment of low back pain usually begins without a specific diagnosis. A nonspecific diagnosis is satisfactory as long as the patient's condition improves. In contrast, the narrow area in which surgery offers reliable benefit to the patient requires a carefully determined, specific diagnosis.

History

A good patient history depends on effective patient-physician communication. When a patient presents with low back pain, the history is important to rule out serious diagnoses rather than leading to a definitive diagnosis. The physician brings knowledge of possible causes and treatments to the interview and assembles a differential diagnosis. The patient wants to tell his or her story and brings knowledge of timelines and anecdotal details.

The term *interview* implies an interaction with the patient as opposed to the traditional notion of extracting information from the patient. When allowed to tell his or her story, an adult patient takes an average of 90 seconds.[2] Adolescents tend to

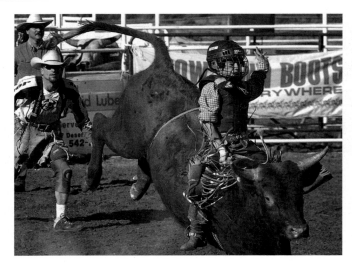

FIGURE 29–1 This 10-year-old boy is following the traditions of ranch life in Colorado where rodeo is a part of life. He won his first big belt buckle in competition at 8 years old.

be more taciturn and talk less than the average adult. The average physician cuts off the patient with a question after 18 seconds because he or she has formed a differential diagnosis. Such interruption stops the flow of information, and often the patient is never permitted to relate pertinent facts.

The use of a visual pain scale facilitates consistent documentation. The patient's assessment of the intensity of the pain using a visual scale (Fig. 29–2) often stimulates a description of the circumstances that exacerbate or alleviate that pain. When making the differential diagnosis, the physician can classify the clinical syndrome into one of three categories: (1) nonmechanical back or leg pain (or both), (2) mechanical back or leg pain (or both), and (3) sciatica.

Warning signs for possible cancer include a history of cancer or constitutional symptoms such as fever or weight loss. Risk factors for infection include a history of recent bacterial infection, intravenous drug use, or an immunocompromised state. Patients with a spine cancer or spine infection often have pain that is not diminished by rest. Warning signs of possible spine fracture are major trauma (e.g., motor vehicle accident, blunt trauma, fall from a height), prolonged corticosteroid use, and osteoporosis. Symptoms suggestive of *cauda equina syndrome,* which requires urgent surgical consultation, include saddle anesthesia (found in 75% of patients); recent onset of bladder or bowel dysfunction (with urinary retention the most common symptom); and severe or progressive

weakness of the lower extremities,[3] especially involving both lower extremities.

There are several findings to note when ascertaining psychosocial contributions to nonorganic back pain, as follows[4]:

1. *Superficial nonanatomic tenderness.* Lightly pinching or rolling the skin should not affect the deep structures, which might cause true pain.

2. *Patient's response to positive stimulation such as axial loading.* Lightly placing one's hand on top of the head should not significantly increase pressure in the low back.

3. *Distraction.* One should look for a significant difference in straight-leg raising ability in the seated versus the supine position.

4. *Overreaction.* An overly loquacious patient or behavior disproportionate to the stimulus should be noted.

5. *Disturbances in sensation or distribution of pain or weakness that do not follow anatomic patterns.*

Symptoms and signs that suggest back pain from nonmechanical causes, such as subclinical pyelonephritis, kidney stones, or dissecting aneurysm, should also be considered.

Genetics

The "wild card" in the etiology of sciatic pain is genetics. Ala-Kokko[5] noted that scientific studies have identified specific versions of the genes encoding collagen, aggrecan, vitamin D receptor, and matrix metalloproteinase-3 that have significant associations with lumbar disc disease. Many other genes may also play a role in disc disease.[6-8]

Physical Examination

The physical examination should take into consideration the three reasons for orthopaedic consultation: pain, deformity, and dysfunction. Although there is poor correlation between physical findings, symptoms, and treatment outcome, an examination of the patient's back is necessary. The purpose of physical examination is to confirm the impression gained from the history, if possible, and to look for surprises. Many obvious anatomic abnormalities can be visualized only when the patient's back is bare. The physical examination usually helps to exclude a serious disease rather than identify one. The "three S's" of an abnormal spine examination are apparent to observation: *spasm, scoliosis,* and *spondylolisthesis.*

0	2	4	6	8	10

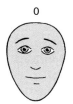 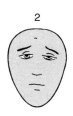 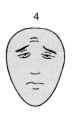 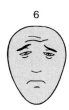 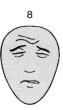 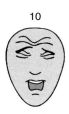

FIGURE 29–2 Bieri faces. Drawings are neutral in terms of gender and ethnicity. The patient indicates a number that corresponds to his or her pain between 0 and 10.

Watching the patient move in flexion, extension, and rotation gives a visible assessment of pain. How a patient moves is as important to note as the range of motion. Whether the patient can bend to the knees, below the knees, or to the toes provides a rough measure of flexibility. Observing spinal rotation allows one to evaluate the facet joints.

After checking range of motion and palpating for tenderness and muscle spasm, the physician should observe the rotational symmetry of the spine using the Adams forward-bend test and noting whether the pelvis is level. It is worthwhile to observe the effect of compression of the pelvis while the patient is lying on his or her back because this is a nonspecific test for sacroiliac joint disorders.

Observing standing posture in the coronal and sagittal planes is important to document evidence of deformity. Special tests such as one-leg standing (the stork test) and compression tests for the neck (Spurling test) are indicated when one suspects spondylolysis or compression neuropathy. Anisomelia can be diagnosed by measuring limb lengths from the anterior superior iliac spine to the medial malleolus.

The neurologic examination requires close attention to detail and begins by having the patient heel walk and toe walk. Both functions demand strength, coordination, and cooperation one would expect from an athletic child. Testing deep tendon reflexes is important, especially if they are asymmetrical; testing the abdominal reflexes is essential to detecting hydromyelia.

The straight-leg raise test or Lasègue sign is a test for nerve root irritation or inflammation. A positive response is the reproduction of radicular pain. Pain on the opposite side or a positive "cross straight-leg raise test" is significant for diagnosis of a herniated disc. The straight-leg raise test can simultaneously provide evidence of sciatica and hamstring contracture.

Imaging

Modern imaging techniques such as computed tomography (CT) and magnetic resonance imaging (MRI) permit accurate visualization of anatomic defects in the spine. Although both techniques are powerful diagnostic tools, the defects revealed by CT or MRI are not always causative with regard to the patient's pain. The literature is replete with cases in which anatomic defects are present on MRI or CT in completely asymptomatic patients.

The Cochrane group performed a meta-analysis of the literature and concluded that there is no correlation between radiographic changes and back pain.[9] Contrary to that opinion, researchers in Tokyo reported a study in which they correlated preparticipation spinal radiographs with the incidence of back pain and disability among young football players.[10] They followed 171 high school and 742 college football players over a 1-year period. High school players with spondylolysis had a higher incidence of low back pain (79.8%) than players with no radiographic abnormality (37.1%). College players with spondylolysis, disc space narrowing, and spinal instability had a higher incidence of low back pain (80.5%, 59.8%, and 53.5%) than players with normal radiographs (32.1%).

College players with spondylolysis had a higher incidence of low back pain than players with disc space narrowing and spinal instability.

How can this incongruence of findings be explained? It is believed that asymptomatic abnormalities in the general population, particularly abnormalities seen with aging, may become symptomatic with vigorous physical activity. Abnormal spine radiographs in a young athlete should be considered a risk factor for injury.

Magnetic Resonance Imaging of the Spine

MRI technology takes advantage of the high hydrogen content of the molecules that make up biologic tissues. Hydrogen atoms have a specific "spin" property associated with them, and the "spin" state can be altered in the presence of a strong magnetic field. Alterations in the "spin" properties of hydrogen atoms in biologic tissues can be detected by MRI technology, and highly sensitive visual images are produced.

Although MRI is a very sensitive and accurate assessment of spinal anatomy, it cannot distinguish between painful and painless structures in the spine. A patient may have severe back pain and MRI may reveal no abnormalities, or the converse may be true. It can be difficult for the physician to correlate MRI findings with the patient's signs and symptoms to make a clinical diagnosis. Typically, it is unnecessary to obtain MRI at the onset of spine-related pain because most cases of back and neck pain resolve within 2 to 12 weeks with proper conservative treatment. MRI is indicated when more aggressive treatments (e.g., injections or surgery) are contemplated.

Bone Scan or Bone Scintigraphy

Bone scan or bone scintigraphy is not as specific as MRI or CT but is very sensitive to changes in metabolic activity of bone. Increased metabolic activity is seen with inflammation, infection, and tissue proliferation owing to tumors such as osteoid osteoma. Bone scintigraphy uses a short-lived radioactive pharmaceutical agent to label specific tissues or structures and ultimately to visualize them via scintillation-mediated imaging. Gamma emissions from the radiopharmaceutical are detected by a gamma camera, converted to light photons, amplified with photomultiplier tubes, and digitized via computer to present a high-resolution (4 to 6 mm) two-dimensional image.

Single Photon Emission Computed Tomography

With single photon emission computed tomography (SPECT), gamma camera detectors rotate around the patient in small increments (usually 3- or 6-degree steps), and emission data are obtained from different plane angles. Computer algorithms break the image into pixels, each of which represents an approximately 6-mm area of the planar image. Pixel data are used to render clinically useful volumetric images. SPECT is arguably the best screening examination for significant spinal abnormality versus nonspecific back pain in children and the first examination that should be ordered. Auerbach[11] showed that SPECT exceeded MRI or plain radiography in accurately defining spondylolysis in a series of 100 children with significant back pain.

Principles of Treatment and Rehabilitation

Acute Treatment

When pain onset is acute and severe, bed rest may be necessary for 2 or 3 days for initial pain control. A longer period of bed rest quickly becomes counterproductive. The key to recovery is modified activity within a minimal range to start, followed by gentle progression of activity. The sooner the athlete begins a level of tolerated activity, the quicker and more effective is the recovery. Research and experience have dispelled the notion that prolonged absolute rest is beneficial for treatment of back pain.[12]

Nonsteroidal anti-inflammatory drugs can be potent when given with muscle relaxants, but the duration of medication should be no longer than 10 days. Opioid administration is rarely necessary for more than a few days. Local anesthetic injections into the facet joints or into trigger points can be useful treatments and may help to diagnose disease related to the facet joint or fibromyalgia.

Passive physical therapy modalities such as ice, massage, or heat can be helpful in initial treatment, but the athlete needs to begin active rehabilitation and assume responsibility for his or her recovery. Strengthening should begin as soon as possible, and bracing should be minimized.

Bracing

Bracing is effective in some cases, if used intermittently and primarily as a tool for returning to activity. If used as a "crutch," extended time in a brace produces atrophy and loss of motion. The Cochrane Collaboration reported a meta-analysis on the use of braces for low back pain in 2004.[13] There was moderate evidence that lumbar supports are no more effective for primary prevention than other types of treatment or no intervention. The authors found no data promoting the effectiveness of lumbar supports for secondary prevention. This opinion is consistent with the generally held concept that passive treatment such as bracing should be limited to acute pain relief and that active rehabilitation is an early goal for return to participation in sports and prevention of future injury. Spinal manipulation can provide short-term improvement, but the evidence for longer term relief is inconclusive.[14]

Traction

Traction has historically been used to treat low back pain. Current thought remains disparate, however, regarding the therapeutic value of traction.[15] Multiple reviewers have concluded that traction as a treatment for back pain is an outmoded technology that has fallen out of favor.

Rehabilitation

The rehabilitation program consists of stages—building a foundation of fundamentals and moving through increasingly difficult levels of activity. Physical rehabilitation should be designed to be sport specific and diagnosis specific. A gymnast with spondylolysis needs a program avoiding hyperextension while the bone is allowed to heal. As rehabilitation goals, he or she needs to stay active in the maneuvers that do not stress the back and to maintain general fitness.

Generally, rehabilitation begins with flexion and extension cycles to reduce joint stiffness and relax elastic structures. There should be minimal loading of the spine during this stage. Hip and knee range of motion exercises are added next to offload the spine, followed by specific muscle training. Focus is first placed on the anterior abdominal muscles and maintaining the spine in neutral position, followed by lateral muscle exercises for side support of quadratus lumborum and abdominal wall muscles; finally, an extensor muscle program is added. Repetitions and movement duration should be closely monitored by the therapist.

Core Stabilization

A core stabilization program is based on the principle of coordinated muscle contraction. This contraction is done from a neutral, pain-free position. Finding and maintaining a pain-free position is fundamental to reestablishing isometric muscle control. Flexibility training should not be approached until strength has been regained.

Flexibility

Exercise programs that load the spine throughout the range of motion have poorer outcomes. Greater mobility is associated with poorer outcomes as well. The range of motion of the spine has little predictability for future low back pain. Programs emphasizing trunk stabilization with a neutral spine have had the most success.[16-18] These programs emphasize increasing the range of motion of the hips and knees.

Muscle Performance (Strength versus Endurance)

The term *strength* is defined as the maximum force a muscle can produce during a single exertion to create joint torque. The term *endurance* refers to the ability to maintain a force for a period of time. Muscle performance includes strength and endurance. The few studies available suggest that endurance has a much greater prophylactic value than strength.[19] The emphasis should be placed on endurance and should precede strengthening exercises in a gradual, progressive exercise program (i.e., longer duration, lower effort exercises).

Sport-Specific Exercise

The physical therapist, trainer, physician, and coach must collaborate in designing a sport-specific rehabilitation program.

New exercises should closely simulate the sport. Progress should be slow enough to develop an awareness of muscle function. The buildup to maximum performance requires time and patience.

Deep Water Running and Swimming

Walking in a swimming pool is a gentle strengthening exercise for the back. Deep water running is excellent for treating athletes with back pain. The buoyancy of the water helps to unload the spine. Athletes run in the deep end of a swimming pool, normally with the aid of a flotation vest. Water is about 800 times denser than air, so resistance met during water running is greater than when running on land. Deep water running can help to maintain aerobic performance for 6 weeks in trained endurance athletes; sedentary individuals can appreciate significantly increased maximal oxygen uptake. During spine rehabilitation programs, deep water running can be used for maintenance training, but deep water running is not a substitute for conventional training.[20-22] Swimming is an excellent exercise for the back, but caution is advised for the novice. The swimming strokes can produce or exacerbate back injury if proper technique is not practiced.

Cycling

Although bicycling is generally considered a healthy form of non–weight-bearing, low-impact exercise, it is important to avoid prolonged flexion in a seated position. A more upright posture is easier on the intervertebral disc, so the upright mountain bike posture is preferred to the flexed racing bike posture. Avoiding the vibration of rough terrain is also logical, making stationary cycling a more reasonable option in the early stages of rehabilitation.

Program Guidelines

The following caveats should be considered when prescribing and monitoring any "return to sport" rehabilitation program[23]:

1. Low back exercises are most beneficial when performed daily.[24]

2. The "no pain—no gain" approach when exercising the spine may cause tissue damage associated with certain specific repeated movements.[25]

3. General exercise programs that include cardiovascular training (e.g., walking) have been shown to be effective for rehabilitation of individuals with low back pain and for injury prevention.[26]

4. Intervertebral discs are more hydrated early in the morning after rising from bed; it is unwise to perform full-range spinal motions (bending) shortly after rising.[27]

5. More repetitions of less demanding exercises assist in the enhancement of endurance and strength. Evidence indicates that endurance has more protective value than strength, and strength gains should not be overemphasized at the expense of endurance.[19]

6. There is no such thing as an ideal set of exercises for all individuals. Although science at present cannot evaluate the optimal exercises for each situation, the combination of science and clinical experience should be used to select an exercise program.

7. Individuals need to be patient and stick with the program. Increased function and pain reduction may not occur for 3 months in some individuals.[28]

Education

Several studies have documented the value of patient education in the treatment of spine problems.[29] Education has been shown to be as valuable to the patient's recovery as physical therapy. In 2004, Frost and colleagues[29] measured the effectiveness of routine physical therapy compared with a single assessment session and advice from a physical therapist for patients with low back pain. They used a multicenter, randomized controlled trial in seven British National Health Service physiotherapy departments. These authors concluded that routine physical therapy was no more effective than a single assessment and advice session from a physiotherapist in treating low back pain.

In the physician's office, handouts are an excellent source of education and can be reference guides for the patient during rehabilitation activities (Table 29–1). Good preprinted handouts are available from multiple sources, such as the

TABLE 29–1 Ways to Avoid Overuse Injuries

1. *Use good technique*	An overhand pitch produces less strain than a side-arm pitch
2. *If it hurts, don't do it*	"No pain—no gain" is a poor concept. You feel the fatigue of a good workout, but you must recognize the pain of going beyond fatigue to injury
3. *Stop when fatigued*	Avoid the temptation of an extra repetition. Sprints are best done after a rest
4. *Increase duration gradually*	It takes time for the body to respond to increased demand and to strengthen
5. *Rest for a time after major increases*	It is better to alternate 3 hard days with an easy day and then rest for 2 days
6. *Quit when you are tired*	When you have exhausted the glycogen stored in your muscles, your technique falters, and you are prone to injury
7. *Do preventive exercises*	Keep your body in balance by stretching to gain full range of motion and loosening contractures
8. *Remember your old injuries*	When you recall your old injuries, you can work to avoid repeating them
9. *Warm up slowly*	Use gentle stretching and gradually increasing effort to limber up muscles and deep breathing to stimulate the heart and lungs

Krames (http://www.krames.com/) or the AAOS (http://www.aaos.org/) websites. Personalizing the handouts gives the athlete assurance in his or her provider's interest and commitment to the rehabilitation plan and confidence in the treatment plan on leaving the office. With the availability of digital radiography, it is inexpensive to give the patient a copy of his or her radiograph to take home. Being educated regarding the nature of the injury and being part of the rehabilitation team, and not merely the subject, motivates the athlete and can bring about speedier and more complete recovery.

Return to Play

For the athlete, returning to play is a central issue and may be measured in terms of games missed as opposed to return of fitness. Generally, the athlete can return to play when there is no pain with sport-specific activities and when full range of motion and strength have been recovered. There is no definitive test to measure when that point is reached. Gradual improvement in pain and progression in performing functional activities are predictive of a good prognosis.

Disorders and Treatment

Low Back Pain in Adolescent Athletes

When a physician sees a child with back pain, he or she needs to rule out serious disorders, begin acute care, and anticipate a rehabilitation program that allows the child to return to normal physical activity. Careful evaluation is important; treatment is usually nonspecific. An open-ended interview to hear the patient's story and expectations is the most valuable assessment instrument. Obtaining a detailed description of the pain is paramount.

The description of pain needs to include its location, duration, onset, and characteristic. If pain is associated with a particular activity or position, that information is helpful for diagnosis. Even with the most aggressive diagnostic workups and follow-ups, however, an organic cause for back pain in adolescents is found only about half of the time.

Lumbar spine pain or low back pain accounts for 5% to 8% of athletic injuries.[30] Injuries are often due to poor conditioning of the spine, poor biomechanics, or repetitive stresses placed on the spine by the nature of the sport. Overuse injuries from repeated lumbar hyperextension may be common in children participating in sports such as gymnastics, volleyball, and rowing.

Historical studies show that the correct diagnosis of acute low back pain is established on the first visit only 2% of the time. After 6 weeks, the diagnostic accuracy increases to 15%, and it increases to 30% at 3 months.[31] The physician's initial visit is best used to rule out serious disorders, such as disc herniation or malignant disease. Although less than 1% of back pain complaints are related to serious spine pathology or require emergent treatment, such as neoplasm or cauda equina syndrome, it is important to exclude these conditions and reassure the patient accordingly.

Aggressive diagnostic workup may be deferred and implemented only for patients who do not improve within 3 or 4 weeks. Often, pain resolves without much treatment, and the athlete continues participation. With severe or prolonged pain that prompts medical consultation, a diagnostic workup is appropriate for guiding the treatment.

Back pain that follows an acute injury is usually attributed to muscle strain. There is little scientific evidence showing muscle strain as a back pain generator, however, probably because pain produced by an injury cannot be differentiated to the various soft tissues of the back.[32] The pain may be localized or diffuse. The patient frequently relates that more stiffness occurred after a night's sleep. This type of back pain attributed to muscle strain tends to improve with time.

Growth is not linear, and as growth spurts occur, an imbalance between new length of bone and old length of muscles occurs. These contractures, whether of the hamstrings or other muscles adjacent to the spine, can produce limited motion and pain with athletic activities.

An adolescent with normal musculoskeletal structure may have back pain from poor standing and sitting posture. The typical profile is of lumbar hyperlordosis, thoracic hyperkyphosis, and contracted hamstrings. Radiographs are unnecessary to make the diagnosis or to institute a program of stretching and postural correction.

Mechanical backache secondary to poor posture is more common in sedentary children. Athletic children are less likely to report nonspecific back pain than their nonathletic counterparts. Children who do not walk to school and have a poor self-image of their health in general report more back pain. Multivariate analysis showed that the incidence of low back pain in adolescents is inversely related to time spent doing physical activity (e.g., regular walking or bicycling) and directly related to television or computer time.[33]

Posture and inactivity contribute to low back pain. The intervertebral discs have the highest fluid content in the morning, which influences the pressure generated on spinal tissues during flexion.[34] Avoidance of flexion after arising in the morning significantly reduces nonspecific back pain.[35]

Plain radiographs are indicated at the time of the first visit if there is a history of severe trauma, loss of neurologic function, or history of malignancy. For an adolescent athlete with a high-risk factor because of a repetitive hyperextension maneuver, oblique views are appropriate for evaluation of the pars interarticularis.

Spondylolysis

Spondylolysis is a stress fracture of the pars interarticularis. It is generally considered to be a low-risk fracture that heals on its own. The fracture occurs most frequently at L5, followed by L4 and L3. Spondylolysis occurs in 5% to 6% of the general population.[1] The lesion is usually asymptomatic and appreciated only incidentally on a radiograph. Generally, no single traumatic event causes spondylolysis; rather, repetitive stress produces fatigue defects, and a single event may complete the fracture. These fractures may develop fibrous nonunion or heal in an elongated state.[36]

The incidence of pars defects is greater in adolescent athletes than in the general population and is a particular clinical problem for this population.[37] Sports that require repetitive hyperextension or extension combined with rotation such as gymnastics, wrestling, and weightlifting are more often associated with a stress fracture of the pars interarticularis. White female gymnasts experience a rate of spondylolysis (11%) five times that of the general white female population.[38] Certain participants in sports such as diving, weightlifting, wrestling, and gymnastics have disproportionately high rates of spondylolysis. A study of elite Spanish athletes showed the highest rates of spondylolysis in gymnasts and weightlifters followed by throwing athletes and rowers.[39] Other reports suggest that a wide variety of sports increase the risk of spondylolysis, including soccer, volleyball, and baseball.[40]

A major concern for patients with defects in the pars interarticularis is the progressive development of symptomatic spondylolisthesis. The incidence of progressive spondylolisthesis is low (3% to 10%) and mainly occurs during adolescence.[41,42] There is no known correlation between active sports participation and either the occurrence or the progression of spondylolisthesis.

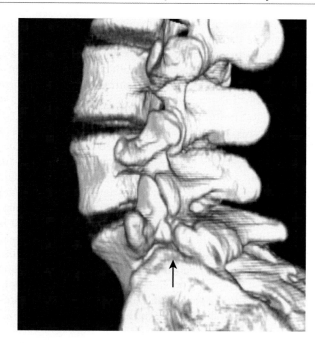

FIGURE 29–3 Spondylolysis. Three-dimensional CT scan shows pars interarticularis defect at end of *arrow*.

Clinical Presentation

Pain may begin after acute injury, or there may be acute exacerbation of mild symptoms present for weeks or months. Lumbar spinal extension or rotation activities are particularly associated with the generation of symptomatic low back pain. Commonly, affected patients have a hyperlordotic posture and hamstring contractures. The classic test during physical examination is to have the patient stand on one leg and lean backward. If the lesion is unilateral, the pain is most often produced by standing on the ipsilateral leg. This test is not definitive but contributes to the diagnosis.

Spondylolysis is a bone lesion and in most patients does not produce a neurologic deficit. Any nerve root signs would suggest an alternative pathology, such as a herniated nucleus pulposus (HNP).

Diagnostic Imaging

Spondylolysis cannot be diagnosed by history and physical examination alone. The key to establishing the diagnosis of spondylolysis is visual confirmation of the pars lesion. The determination of a symptomatic spondylolytic lesion has become more sophisticated with the use of nuclear imaging, CT, and MRI.

A defect in the pars interarticularis is apparent in Figure 29–3, which shows a three-dimensional CT scan. The classic description of this appearance on the oblique view radiograph is that of a collar on the "Scottie dog." Approximately 20% of the pars interarticularis lesions are seen only on the lateral oblique views, and CT may be necessary to show it.

Magnetic resonance imaging should be used as the primary investigation for adolescents with back pain and suspected stress reactions of the pars interarticularis. Single-photon emission computed tomography (SPECT) use is limited by the high rate of false-positive and false-negative results and by considerable ionizing radiation exposure.[42a]

For an adolescent with low back pain, normal radiographs, and a negative bone scan, spondylolysis is ruled out. Other causes should be investigated. MRI may be ordered under these circumstances to rule out disc pathology or other causes for pain in nonosseous tissues. Similarly, adolescents with back pain, positive radiographs, and negative bone scan warrant MRI to investigate further the basis for pain.

Treatment

Most patients with symptomatic spondylolysis do well with conservative treatment.[43] The main goals of treatment are amelioration of pain, return to activity, and prevention of recurrence. Treatment modalities include rest, medication, and bracing, alone or in combination. Many pars interarticularis lesions heal with early care, particularly early-stage unilateral defects. Osseous healing is unnecessary to achieve an excellent clinical outcome with full return to activities, although this healing is desirable when possible.

Activity restriction is important to limit pain. Running, jumping, and sport-specific activities that produced the pain should be eliminated for 4 to 6 weeks. Contact and collision sports are not allowed, and hyperextension activities should specifically be eliminated.

Physical therapy has been proved quite effective in the treatment of spondylolysis. Patients with a specific and carefully managed exercise program show significant reduction in pain intensity and functional disability levels.[44,45] Therapy should include exercises to increase hamstring flexibility and to strengthen deep core muscles in the abdomen and the lumbar region.[46]

The role of bracing is difficult to define. A rigid brace is not mandatory for the treatment of symptomatic spondylolysis. Many surgeons begin bracing immediately for spondylolysis, whereas others reserve bracing for patients who do not progress with their conservative program or who experience increasing pain. The main advantage of a brace may be that it promotes better posture.

Various studies have determined that only 9% to 15% of cases of symptomatic spondylolysis or grade 1 spondylolisthesis require surgery.[42,47-49] The indications for surgery are progressive slip, intractable pain, development of neurologic defects, and segmental instability associated with pain. Pain alone can be controlled by activity modification and medication and is not an indication for surgery. Surgical treatment is directed at repairing the fracture in the pars interarticularis using bone grafting and internal fixation. Various techniques using wires and screws have been advocated. The technique by Chen and Lee,[50] using a pedicle screw and laminar hook, has the advantage of not violating the facet joints, while providing excellent stabilization for healing.

Return to Activity

When follow-up examination reveals no discomfort and pain is well controlled with ordinary daily activities, a low level of sports participation is appropriate. Return to sport can be achieved after 4 to 6 weeks of modified activity. Activity intensity can increase as tolerated. Continued therapy should focus on core strengthening, improvement in posture, and avoidance of hyperextension.

Preventing recurrence is a major goal of treatment. A maintenance fitness program should be included in any workout regimen that is prescribed. Any low back pain that is worsened by extension or twisting should prompt a reduction in activity and increased periods of rest. If these precautions are instituted at the first sign of symptoms, a long course of rest and rehabilitation may be avoided.

Spondylolisthesis

Spondylolisthesis occurs when there is a bilateral defect in the pars interarticularis and one vertebra slips forward relative to the vertebra beneath it. The incidence of spondylolisthesis in athletes is the same as in the general population. No substantiated criteria are available for predicting which cases of spondylolysis will progressively slip, resulting in spondylolisthesis. Patients with dysplastic posterior elements have a higher risk of slip progression. Radiographic studies have shown a strong correlation between slip progression and a more vertical inclination of the superior plate of S1.[51,52] Most cases of spondylolisthesis are mild, unlikely to progress, and cease to progress after growth is complete. With mild spondylolisthesis, there is no increased rate of disability and no reason to restrict participation in sports.

Isthmic spondylolisthesis is the type seen in young athletes, excluding the rare cases of congenital absence of facet joints. Bilateral stress fractures of the pars interarticularis are the distinguishing pathology of spondylolisthesis. The stress fractures are unusual in that they occur in young people and rarely heal spontaneously. The only suspected causative factor, other than familial predisposition, is minor or repetitive hyperextension.

Symptoms associated with spondylolisthesis are dull low back pain exacerbated by activity, particularly hyperextension and rotation. Sports requiring repetitive rotation and extension under load, such as gymnastics, football, wrestling, hockey, pole vaulting, diving, and throwing sports, have been incriminated as causative factors in multiple studies.[53,54] Typical of mechanical-type pain, rest tends to alleviate the pain.

During the examination the findings of paravertebral muscle spasm, hamstring contractures, and limited flexibility may be dramatic. Kyphosis associated with severe grades of slip flattens the profile of the buttocks and creates a sagittal postural malalignment (Fig. 29–4). A step-off at the lumbosacral level may be palpable.

Weakness, loss of sensation, and a positive straight-leg raise test are usually absent, differentiating spondylolisthesis from a herniated disc. If radiculopathy is present, the L5 root is usually involved. Cauda equina syndrome has been reported in severe cases owing to nerve root stretch over the dome of the sacrum.[55]

The diagnosis is easily confirmed by a lateral radiograph of the lumbar spine. The severity of the slip is graded either by the quartile classification of Meyerding or, more commonly, as a percentage of displacement relative to the top of the sacrum. There is consensus that kyphosis is a more important measure of the deformity than displacement.[56] The slip angle and sacral inclination are used to describe the sagittal plane deformity.

The treatment of a young athlete with spondylolisthesis is based on the same principles as the population at large, but the desire of the individual to continue sports participation must be considered as well. The age of the patient, the severity and duration of pain, and the degree of deformity all must be considered when formulating a treatment plan. A young, minimally symptomatic patient with a less than 25% slip requires little restriction of activity but should be monitored for progression. Initial flexion-extension lateral radiographs are useful for assessing instability. Serial lateral films at yearly intervals can document any progression of slipping, unless symptoms warrant more frequent follow-up. If the degree of slip is 25% to 50%, the consensus is that the athlete should be restricted from collision sports such as gymnastics and football. If the patient is truly asymptomatic, continued participation may be reasonable as a matter of judgment and cooperation.

Surgical stabilization is recommended for an immature patient with documented progression. Stabilization by spinal fusion is also recommended for slips greater than 50%, even if the patient is asymptomatic.

If the patient still has unremitting, disabling pain after a 6-month program of conservative treatment, certain surgical decisions are made: in situ fusion versus reduction, whether to perform decompression, whether to perform anterior and posterior fusion, and plus or minus bed rest. The debate over

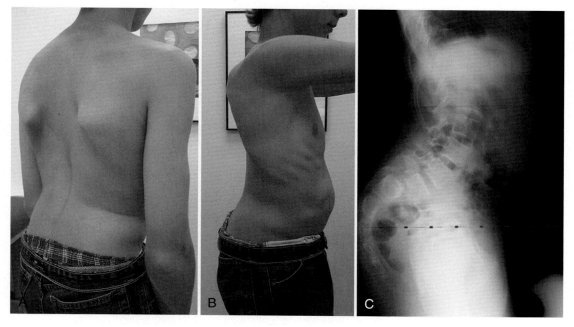

FIGURE 29–4 A-C, Spondylolisthesis. Paravertebral muscle spasm is striking. Sagittal imbalance produced by severe slip made clinical diagnosis evident before radiograph was obtained.

these issues remains. In situ fusion is the "gold standard" with well-documented long-term excellent outcomes.[57] Isolated removal of the laminar fragment, or Gill procedure, is contra-indicated because further progression is common after that procedure.

Absolute indications for decompression are motor deficit and bowel or bladder dysfunction.[56] Some surgeons do not perform decompression even with motor or sensory signs because these signs tend to improve with a solid fusion.[58] Many surgeons perform a decompression at the time of fusion if weakness, sensory loss, or radicular pain is present, particularly in instances of severe slip. With severe degrees of slip, anterior fusion with or without reduction of the kyphotic deformity can be done using pedicle screw fixation and anterior interbody cages.

Although various methods for reduction of spondylolisthesis are advocated, many are associated with a significant rate of temporary or permanent nerve root damage. Reduction should be done only after wide decompression of the nerve roots, and significant nerve damage may still occur. Return to vigorous athletic participation is not guaranteed after surgery even if the fusion is solid. Most surgeons recommend against any but the least demanding of sports after such a major spine procedure. The decision regarding participation should be delayed until the outcome of surgery is clear.

Lumbar Scheuermann Disease (Juvenile Disc Disease)

The classic radiographic criteria for the diagnosis of Scheuermann disease is kyphosis of the thoracic spine with wedging of 15 or more degrees over three vertebrae.[59] Scheuermann disease is associated with endplate changes such as irregularity

of the apophyseal ring and Schmorl nodes. The causes of Scheuermann disease, which has been attributed to juvenile osteoporosis, are controversial. This condition affects 0.4% to 8.3% of the general population and causes irregularities in ossification and endochondral growth in the thoracic spine in adolescents and young adults.[59] The disease leads to various pathologic changes at the junction of the vertebral body and the intervertebral disc, resulting in pronounced wedging of the vertebral bodies and progressive kyphosis in severe cases. According to various studies, it causes back pain in 20% to 60% of cases and occasionally causes severe deformity of the spine.[59]

An increased frequency of radiologic abnormalities of the thoracolumbar spine has been reported among young athletes in various sports, such as soccer, gymnastics, water-ski jumping, or wrestling, compared with nonathletes.[60-70] Although the origins of typical Scheuermann disease[71] have been a matter of controversy,[67,72] atypical Scheuermann disease is considered to be strongly associated with trauma or excessive loading of the spine, especially in the flexed posture and during growth spurts.[60,67,73] Axial compression forces apparently cause vertebral endplate bulging, whereas compression of the immature spine in flexion is considered to cause anterior intravertebral disc herniation (marginal Schmorl nodes).[61,66,67,72-75] Abnormalities of the vertebral ring apophysis are thought to be the result of failure in tension shear, analogous to Osgood-Schlatter avulsion at the knee (Fig. 29–5).[68]

In 1985, Greene and colleagues[72] described back pain and vertebral changes in the lumbar spine similar to changes seen in Scheuermann disease of the thoracic spine. These changes were accompanied by mechanical low back pain. In 1994, Heithoff and colleagues[76] saw similar changes on MRI and coined the term *juvenile discogenic disease.* Their group

FIGURE 29–5 A and **B,** Juvenile disc disease. This 14-year-old baseball player presented with irritative scoliosis and pain localized to upper lumbar level. Note endplate irregularity and erosion anteriorly at L1-2 level on lateral radiograph.

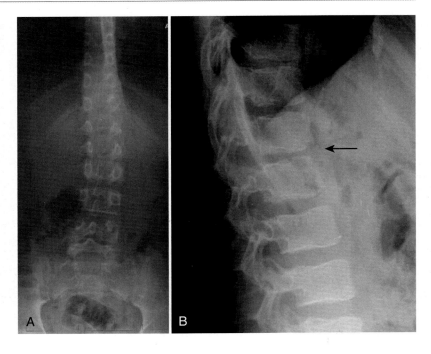

detected evidence of thoracolumbar Scheuermann disease and multilevel disc disease of the lower lumbar spine in 9% of the subjects studied. The patients ranged in age from 7 to 66, but most were young: Slightly less than half of the patients were younger than 30; 9% were younger than 21. Males outnumbered females 3:1. Disc degeneration was found most frequently at the L5-S1 level, followed in order by L4-5 and L3-4. Of patients, 80% showed evidence of substantial degeneration at more than one lumbar level, and 53% had disc herniations involving at least one lower lumbar level.

Heithoff and colleagues[76] suspected that a substantial number of young adults have a combination of painful multilevel disc degeneration and lumbar spine changes typical of Scheuermann disease. In their view, both conditions may be caused by an underlying genetic defect in disc structure. It has been estimated that 80% of young patients requiring disc surgery have a genetic predisposition to disc degeneration.[76] Juvenile discogenic disease has been statistically associated with athletic activity and repetitive trauma. Most patients can be treated nonoperatively, but a subset have concurrent spinal stenosis, which may require decompression.[77]

Herniated Nucleus Pulposus

Acute disc herniation, or HNP, is relatively rare in children and adolescents compared with adults. Reports suggest that only 0.5% to 4% of surgically managed HNP occurs in patients younger than 18.[78-82] Despite the low incidence, approximately 10% of severe back pain in skeletally immature patients is due to disc herniation.[83,84] High-risk activities include weightlifting and collision sports such as football.[84] HNP has also been associated with injuries sustained during gymnastics, basketball, baseball, and wrestling.[85] Nearly 95% of herniations occur

from L4 to S1 and are fairly evenly distributed between L4-5 and L5-S1.[80,85] The L3-4 level is affected in only 5% of patients.[85]

The presenting symptoms of HNP in children differ from the symptoms seen in adults. The profile of an adolescent with HNP includes the presence of tension signs and sciatic scoliosis, without localizing neurologic signs. Most patients present with low back pain, with or without leg pain.[84,85] Associated leg pain is seen far less often than in adults (<20% of the time).[74] In children, the herniation is thought to be more central and the volume of extruded disc material less than in adults.[79,84] Actual rupture of the disc is rare in children.[86]

Physical examination often reveals an abnormal gait or scoliosis owing to paraspinal muscle spasm.[84,85] Nerve tension signs, such as a positive straight-leg raise test, are present in greater than 80% to 90% of patients, and the crossed-leg raise test is positive in more than 50%.[79,84,85,87] Objective motor weakness may be present in 40%, with the extensor hallucis longus most commonly affected, and deep tendon reflexes at the knee and ankle are decreased in approximately 40% of patients.[85]

MRI is a very effective way to image the disc, spinal cord, and nerve roots and because of its noninvasive nature is a commonly used imaging technique. MRI has been shown to detect 100% of symptomatic herniations (Fig. 29–6).[88] Herniation is associated with endplate changes, with marrow signal intensity changes on MRI, and with increased cartilage in the material removed during surgery. There is a correlation of marrow signal intensity changes on MRI and the biology of the removed material. Avulsion-type disc herniation is common.[89]

Conservative treatment is as outlined for nonspecific low back pain. The literature suggests, however, that the overall outcomes of conservative treatment are generally poor.

Recommendations suggest a 2- to 4-week trial of conservative management followed by surgical excision of the disc if symptoms have not resolved.[85]

Indications for surgical excision of the disc include persistent symptoms despite conservative management, cauda equina syndrome, progressive neurologic deficits, and reinjury.[84,85] Many authors have reported greater than 90% good to excellent results after surgical excision.[80,82,85,90] After surgical excision, low back pain and leg pain resolved within 3 weeks, and neurologic findings resolved after 3 months.[80] Long-term follow-up studies show excellent outcomes, including absence of pain and no activity limitations.[80,82,90]

Apophyseal Ring Fracture

Bone fragments at the posterior vertebral endplate have been given numerous names, such as posterior marginal node; limbus fracture; fracture of the vertebral rim, ring, or endplate; epiphyseal dislocation; and apophyseal ring fracture.[91] This condition is unique to adolescents[84] and was first described by Skobowytsh-Okolot in 1962.[81,92] Endplate fracture was discovered in 20% of patients younger than 21 years and in 33% of patients younger than 17 who were undergoing lumbar disc surgery.[93] The overall prevalence is only 0.07% of all patients of all ages undergoing disc surgery. There is a strong male predominance, with 85% of cases occurring in boys; 66% of cases are related to a traumatic event such as weightlifting, heavy work, or sports injury.[81] Associations have also been found with Scheuermann disease.[94]

Hyperextension of the lumbar spine[95] and rapid flexion together with axial compression to the vertebral column such as occurs with weightlifting are two proposed mechanisms of apophyseal ring injury.[81,84,96] The presenting symptoms of an apophyseal ring fracture are similar to the symptoms seen with HNP—back, buttock, and posterior thigh pain. Symptoms are worse with coughing, sneezing, sports, and prolonged sitting.[84] Pain may radiate down one or both legs. The straight-leg raise test is positive, and contralateral straight-leg raise is frequently positive. Paraspinal muscle spasm, lumbar tenderness, scoliosis, intermittent claudication, paraparesis, and cauda equina syndrome have been reported.[81,84]

Plain radiographs can be useful and show the avulsed fragment in approximately 40% of cases.[81,91] This fragment appears as an arcuate or wedge-shaped bone fragment posterior to the vertebral body or disc space. Alternatively, it can appear as a bony ridge on the posterior surface of the vertebral body. MRI may show a defect in the posterior vertebral rim. The fragment may be seen as a low signal area lying posteriorly but can be difficult to distinguish from cortical bone and posterior longitudinal ligament. MRI may be diagnostic in only 22% of cases.[91] CT is an excellent imaging study for these fractures because it can define the bony fragment, any associated disc prolapse, vertebral defect, and severity of any associated stenosis in approximately 75% of cases. CT should be considered if MRI fails to show an expected HNP or ring fracture.[91]

A trial of short-term rest, use of nonsteroidal anti-inflammatory drugs, and physical therapy is indicated. If

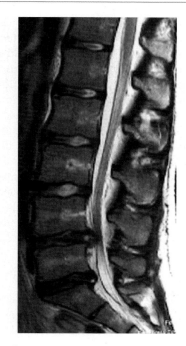

FIGURE 29–6 Herniated nucleus pulposus. This 15-year-old wrestler has black bulging disc at L4-5 highlighted by a white dot on MRI. (Courtesy Charles Burton, MD.)

symptoms fail to resolve after 2 to 4 weeks or if there is progressive neurologic involvement or cauda equina syndrome, surgical excision of the fragment and any associated disc material should be performed.[84] Good to excellent results have been reported after surgical excision in nearly all pediatric cases of avulsed ring fracture.

Cervical Spine Injuries

Traumatic neck injuries in young athletes may be to bone, nerve, or soft tissue. The order of incidence is as follows[97]:

1. Nerve root or brachial plexus neurapraxia (burners)
2. Cervical strains (muscular injury)
3. Disc injury with neck pain only
4. Cervical sprains (ligament injury)
5. Disc herniation with radicular symptoms
6. Transient spinal cord compression secondary to stenosis
7. Fractures

On-Field Examination

If a cervical spine injury is suspected, the physician or trainer should appreciate any spinal pain, altered perception of touch, numbness, and weakness in, or difficulty moving, the extremities. Any player with signs of head trauma, such as disturbed vision, headache, staggering gait, disorientation, or memory loss, should not participate further.

For an ambulatory athlete complaining of pain or spasm in the neck, the physician should localize the tenderness and evaluate for muscle spasm. The physician should evaluate neck range of motion and perform a motor and sensory examination of the extremities. On failing the examination, the athlete should be removed from competition and immobilized in a cervical collar. Alarming signs associated with a cervical fracture are acute torticollis, resistance to any motion, and the patient using the hands to support the head. If the player is unconscious, the presumption is that a cervical spine injury exists, and the neck is immobilized. Any facemask should be removed, but the helmet should be left in place. The player should be immobilized before being moved. Players with persistent or severe pain should be given a prompt radiologic evaluation. Return to participation depends on complete resolution of symptoms and normal radiographs.

Field Treatment of Cervical Fractures

Fractures of the cervical spine are relatively rare. The on-field treatment protocol should be well rehearsed and efficient, however. The minimal equipment includes tools or instruments necessary to remove the facemask, a cervical collar, and a backboard. Such an extensive setup may be impractical, but the medical attendant is well advised to know what emergency medical services are available, such as a well-equipped ambulance. A cell phone or other communication capability should be available on the sideline. The key is advance planning.

Lifting an individual high enough to insert a backboard beneath requires a chief who carefully links the head to the chest and six additional people to lift. If a team has not practiced or there are not six individuals immediately trained and available, the athlete should not be moved until there is adequate assistance to immobilize and transport him or her without incurring additional damage. Instructions for the prehospital care of a spinal cord injury on an athletic field are published online by an interdisciplinary task force.[98]

Prevention of Catastrophic Injuries to the Cervical Spine in Football

According to Cantu and Mueller[99] of the National Center for Catastrophic Sport Injury Research, prevention is related to teaching and enforcing good technique in blocking and tackling and the proper use of well-fitted equipment. Cantu and Mueller[99] noted, "The football helmet is not the cause of cervical spine injuries. Poorly executed tackling and blocking technique are the major problems." The neck should be kept upright, avoiding use of the helmet and facemask as the initial and primary contact point in blocking and tackling. Rules against spearing should be strongly enforced, and athletes should strengthen their necks for further protection in the event of a miss-hit. Cantu and Mueller[99-104] stated that being prepared for the treatment and transport of a player with a major spine injury can mean the difference between life and death. That means having a plan and practicing the teamwork necessary for a successful transport.

Cervical Peripheral Nerve Injuries

Stingers or Burners

"Burners" or "stingers" are common injuries to the neck in collision sports such as football, hockey, or diving. A high percentage of football players, especially defensive players, experience burners during their playing career. Other sports in which burners occur include wrestling, backpacking, sledding, skiing, horseback riding, boxing, weightlifting, and climbing.

Burners are caused by either compression or distraction. An asymmetrical axial load on the neck causing compression in the neuroforamen can injure the peripheral nerve root. If the athlete falls directly on the shoulder and the head is distracted away from the shoulder, traction is applied to the nerve root and the brachial plexus. When the cervical spine is hyperextended, hyperflexed, or laterally flexed to the opposite side, the angle between the shoulder and neck is increased beyond the normal range, stretching the brachial plexus.

Symptoms are a severe burning or searing pain in the shoulder and arm associated with loss of sensation and weakness of the arm. The pain may be decreased by abducting the shoulder; this can be achieved by asking the athlete to place a hand on the top of the head. Spurling maneuver is a diagnostic test that reproduces the compression mechanism of injury. The patient's neck is extended, laterally flexed to the involved side, and rotated to the involved side with axial loading applied while in that position. The burning or searing pain is reproduced. Extension-compression mechanisms are most common, followed by brachial stretch and direct blow mechanisms.[105]

Burners are best prevented by enforcing the rules on spearing, by strengthening and conditioning the neck, and by proper use of good-quality protective equipment. Shoulder pads are protective equipment for the neck in football. An A-frame design to the shoulder pads brings lateral stability to the base of the neck, preventing lateral tilt while allowing rotation of the head, which occurs at C1-2 (50%). The base of the shoulder pad needs to extend down well on the chest anteriorly and posteriorly to link the chest to the base of the neck. It is almost impossible to prevent extension of the head. The player needs to learn to block with the shoulder and keep the head down so that the opposing player is not contacted with a facemask or the helmet.

Initial treatment for this injury is removal from participation and rest, followed by strengthening exercises of the neck and, finally, careful stretching and restoration of range of motion. Because the pain, paresthesias, and weakness typically last only a few seconds or minutes, these injuries fall into the Seddon classification of neurapraxia. Occasionally, athletes with more severe injuries experience a prolonged recovery period that may last hours to several weeks and may lead to a prolonged loss of time from competition.[106-113] Return to play criteria include full range of motion of the neck associated with complete return of arm strength and sensation.

Burners may occur many times during the season, ranging from a transient nerve irritation without residual damage to a complete avulsion of the nerve root from the spinal cord with permanent deficit. Burners are symptoms of injury to either the brachial plexus or a nerve root and must be evaluated systematically.

Quan and Bird[114] proposed a classification of peripheral nerve injuries that correlates well with electrodiagnostic studies and prognoses, based on earlier classifications by Seddon[114a] and Sunderland.[114b] This classification scheme is useful for diagnosis and advice in individual cases (Table 29–2).

Cervical Stenosis

Congenital cervical stenosis is a risk factor for cervical spine injuries.[115] Two studies have analyzed the relationship of burners to cervical stenosis in college football players at the University of Iowa and Tulane University.[105,116] Burners were more common in players with spinal stenosis as defined by the Torg ratio, especially the occurrence of repeated episodes of neurapraxia. The Torg ratio is defined as the ratio of the spinal canal width to the width of the vertebral body at the same level and is most narrow at C7. These studies suggest that a Torg ratio of 0.7 to 0.8 or lower is high risk. For players with cervical stenosis, the risk of burners is three times that of players without stenosis (Fig. 29–7).

Transient Spinal Cord Compression

Torg and colleagues[117] described the syndrome of transient quadriplegia, considered to represent a "neurapraxia of the cervical spinal cord." This syndrome includes bilateral upper extremity and lower extremity neurologic involvement with no associated fracture or dislocation. It usually resolves within 36 hours. The transient quadriplegia was associated with developmental spinal stenosis, either as an isolated entity or associated with congenital abnormalities, cervical instability, or intervertebral disc disease. The authors noted statistically significant spinal stenosis in all patients who incurred episodes of transient quadriparesis.[117,118] They also noted that there was "no evidence that the occurrence of neurapraxia of the cervical spinal cord predisposes an individual to permanent neurological injury."[117]

Fracture

Fracture of the Thoracolumbar Spine

Fracture or dislocation of the thoracolumbar spine is unusual. The typical mechanism is an axial load, as from a fall onto the buttocks from a height or at a relatively rapid speed. The injury is usually a relatively benign compression fracture occurring in the lower thoracic spine or at the thoracolumbar junction. Some compression fractures are not easily seen on plain radiographs (Fig. 29–8). When there is significant pain or tenderness using spot radiographs, CT or MRI can aid in identification and localization of the fracture. Any neurologic findings require special evaluation.

TABLE 29–2 Quan and Bird Classification of Nerve Injury

Type of Injury	Mode of Recovery	Time to Recovery
Conduction block (neurapraxia)	Remyelination of focal segment involved	2-12 wk
Limited axonal loss	Collateral sprouting from surviving motor axons	2-6 mo
Intermediate axonal loss	Collateral sprouting and axonal regeneration from site of injury	2-6 mo
Severe axonal loss	Axonal regeneration	2-18 mo
Complete nerve discontinuity	No recovery without nerve grafting	2-18 mo

Data from Quan D, Bird SJ: Nerve conduction studies and electromyography in the evaluation of peripheral nerve injuries. Univ Pa Orthop J 12:45-51, 1999.

Sacral Stress Fracture

Sacral stress fractures occur almost exclusively in individuals participating in running sports at an elite level. Treatment includes a brief period of limited weight bearing followed by progressive mobilization, physical therapy, and return to sport in 1 to 2 months, after the pain has resolved.

Treatment of spine fractures generally falls into two categories: closed and open. With closed treatment, the fracture is reduced if necessary, and the patient is immobilized in a body cast. Reduction is the primary technique for decompression of the spinal cord. If reduction is not required, the patient is fitted with a brace for comfort.

With open treatment, a surgical procedure is performed to reduce or secure severely displaced or unstable fractures.

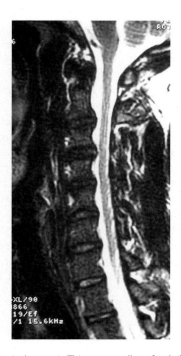

FIGURE 29–7 Cervical stenosis. This young college football lineman has Torg ratio of 0.4 and is at great risk to continue the sport because of congenital spinal stenosis.

FIGURE 29–8 Thoracolumbar fracture in a 16-year-old horsewoman. Fracture was aligned and stabilized by three-level fusion. Anatomic details are clear on three-dimensional CT scan.

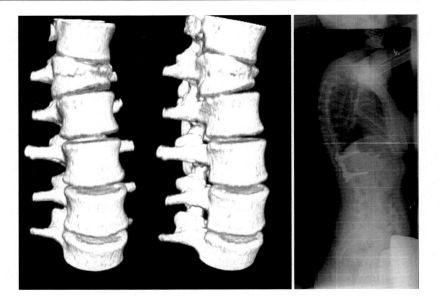

Open procedures are indicated when two or three of the pillars of the vertebral column are disrupted. Internal fixation is usually required. Pedicle screws and rods are the current devices used for posterior fixation. Anterior fixation with plates and screws is less common. Bone grafting to obtain spinal fusion and biologic long-term stabilization are the final parts of the procedure. Factors to consider when deciding when and if an athlete should return to play after spine fracture are healing, rehabilitation, risk of reinjury, and neurologic status.

Iliac Apophysitis

Apophyseal injuries are a unique injury in adolescent athletes and are associated with skeletal immaturity and repetitive microtrauma. With iliac apophysis involvement, the patient usually presents with back pain localized to the iliac crest, which facilitates diagnosis. There is local tenderness, which is exacerbated by resisted lateral bending and extension. Radiographs are normal. The treatment is conservative for 3 to 6 weeks, during which time the pain predictably resolves.

The typical athlete affected is an adolescent runner. Clancy and Foltz[119] described a series of 21 young distance runners, in all of whom pain resolved with alteration of training and rest. As the apophysis closes at the end of growth, even the most recalcitrant cases resolve, similar to Osgood-Schlatter disease of the knee. There are a couple of case reports of avulsion of the apophysis in older teenagers that was surgically repaired, but this is rare.[120,121]

Tumor

Spine cancers in children are rare. Children 7 to 15 years old with spine infection or tumor tend to present with back, pelvic, or abdominal pain.[122] Intradural spinal metastasis pain is a characteristically cramping pain. The physician should take note of back pain that increases with recumbency and keeps the patient awake at night. Progressive pain is characteristic of tumors, not trauma-induced pain. The pain of cancer tends to be constant.

Neoplasia of the spine may originate in either the neural or the osseous elements. Most bony spine tumors of childhood are benign, but they usually cause pain or an irritative scoliosis (Fig. 29–9). Osteoid osteoma is a small, sclerotic, irritative lesion of the posterior spinal elements. The pain is worse at night and is relieved by aspirin or other anti-inflammatory drugs. Although the natural history is for spontaneous resolution of the pain over years, patients do not often tolerate long-term pain well.

Osteoblastoma is a larger version of the same process. Osteoid osteoma and osteoblastoma may manifest as stiffness or scoliosis with or without pain. The lesion may not be apparent on plain radiographs. Bone scan is intensely positive and an excellent first supplemental imaging study in children.

Eosinophilic granuloma in the spine produces a flattening of the vertebra, or *vertebra plana*, rarely with neurologic compromise. Some degree of vertebral regrowth occurs with time in this benign condition. Conservative treatment is indicated if the diagnosis is clear.

Bony malignancies are rare and include leukemia, Ewing sarcoma, and osteosarcoma in bone and neuroblastoma or astrocytoma in the spinal cord. In the absence of actual bone destruction, these tumors may show subtle signs of pressure owing to their growth, such as separation or thinning of the pedicles or scoliosis.

Spinal cord tumors such as astrocytoma or ependymoma are more likely to manifest as extremity weakness, gait disturbance, or scoliosis. Precisely because they are rare, these serious lesions should always be kept in mind. MRI is the study of choice for diagnosis.

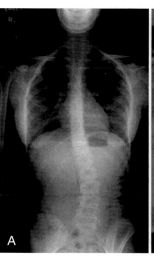
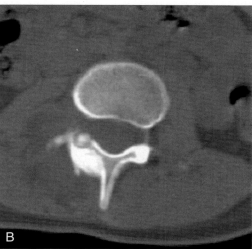

FIGURE 29–9 Osteoid osteoma. Tumor did not show on MRI done for this 14-year-old softball pitcher who presented with back pain and scoliosis. **A,** SPECT scan was hot at L3. **B,** CT scan clearly delineates pathologic lesion. Irritative scoliosis corrected spontaneously after tumor was excised.

PEARLS

1. Back pain in an active adolescent athlete is due to spondylolysis until proven otherwise.

2. An open-ended history taken from the patient is the most cost-effective diagnostic tool and worth the time.

PITFALLS

1. Do not perform a cursory nonfocused history and examination for adolescent back pain.

2. Do not jump to surgery before implementing effective nonoperative treatment for back pain.

KEY POINTS

1. Most spine sports injuries in children are chronic injuries resulting from overuse rather than acute injuries secondary to direct trauma.

2. Encouraging the patient to relate his or her history by attentive listening is helpful in determining a differential diagnosis more quickly and accurately.

3. The most common cause of chronic back pain in adolescent athletes is stress fracture or spondylolysis.

4. Sports employing repeated hyperextension maneuvers, such as gymnastics, provide the mechanism for increased stress on the pars interarticularis, which is the site of spondylolysis.

5. Screening radiographs seldom augment a benign history in making a diagnosis. For patients who do not improve in 3 to 4 weeks, CT and MRI can be helpful for diagnosis.

6. Nonoperative treatment is effective for most back pain in children. Spondylolysis, spondylolisthesis, or the rare condition HNP may require operative treatment. Vigorous postoperative rehabilitation may return the athlete to sport.

7. Flexibility is the first priority in treating back pain, with strengthening exercises employed only after a good range of motion has been obtained. Sport-specific exercises are important to prevent reinjury on return to full activity.

KEY REFERENCES

1. Bono CM: Low back pain in athletes. J Bone Joint Surg Am 86:382-396, 2004.
   This review focuses on spondylolysis and degenerative lumbar disc disease as the major sources of chronic pain in athletes, while pointing out that most low back pain in athletes is due to self-limited sprains or strains. Although these injuries usually respond to nonoperative treatment, the author found direct repair of recalcitrant defects to be the usual course recommended in the literature. Whether the disc changes are worse than changes seen in the general population is debatable. The author advocates anterior interbody fusion for a patient who does not respond to a directed conservative program.

2. Brodke DS, Ritter SM: Nonoperative management of low back pain and lumbar disc degeneration. J Bone Joint Surg Am 86:1810-1818, 2004.
   This review article summarizes the treatment options for nonspecific low back pain, including bed rest, medications, physical therapy, manipulation, braces, and injections. The authors acknowledge that a specific pain generator should be sought and that scientific evidence is lacking to support any particular mode of treatment.

3. Ginsburg GM, Bassett GS: Back pain in children and adolescents: Evaluation and differential diagnosis. J Am Acad Orthop Surg 5:67-78, 1997.
   The authors document the differential diagnosis for back pain in children to include spondylolysis, spondylolisthesis, Scheuermann kyphosis, disc herniations, infections, and tumors. They discuss the appropriate tests for early detection and treatment with a rationale for selecting the most appropriate study.

4. McGill SM: Low back exercises: Evidence for improving exercise regimens. Phys Ther 78:754-765, 1998.
   This review article documents the biomechanical evidence from the laboratory that can be used to guide the scientific choice of an exercise program for back pain. The author

recommends that an exercise program load tissues to strengthen them, while avoiding injury from overexertion. The relative importance of strength, flexibility, and endurance is explored. Specific exercises are described to enhance the stability of the back for rehabilitation and health maintenance.

5. Salminen JJ, Erkintalo MO, Pentti J, et al: Recurrent low back pain and early disc degeneration in the young. Spine 24:1316-1321, 1999.
   The authors studied a group of 14-year-old Finnish boys and girls prospectively who had chronic low back pain and compared them with a similar sample of 40 patients who were asymptomatic. The risk of reporting recurrent low back pain up to age 23 years was 16 times as high in the group with early degenerative disc findings. Significant changes included disc protrusion and Scheuermann-type changes on MRI of the lumbar spine.

6. Standaert CJ, Herring SA: Spondylolysis: A critical review. Br J Sports Med 34:415-422, 2000.
   The authors based their review on more than 125 articles addressing spondylolysis. They found no controlled clinical trials. Their conclusions were that isthmic spondylolysis is a fatigue fracture of the pars interarticularis, which is more often symptomatic in adolescent athletes. Treatment by activity modification and exercise is usually successful, with symptomatic relief occurring with or without healing of the skeletal defect. Multiple imaging studies have been recommended, and bracing was used in some studies. Rarely, surgery is indicated.

REFERENCES

1. Fredrickson B, Baker D, McHolick WJ, et al: The natural history of spondylolysis and spondylolisthesis. J Bone Joint Surg Am 66:699-707, 1984.

2. Langewitz W, Denz M, Keller A, et al: Spontaneous talking time at start of consultation in outpatient clinic: Cohort study. BMJ 325:682-683, 2002.

3. Rydevik B: Neurophysiology of cauda equina compression. Acta Orthop Scand Suppl 251:52-55, 1993.

4. Waddell G, McCulloch JA, Kummel E, et al: Nonorganic physical signs in low-back pain. Spine 5:117-125, 1980.

5. Ala-Kokko L: Genetic risk factors for lumbar disc disease. Ann Med 34:42-47, 2002.

6. Solovieva S, Leino-Arjas P, Saarela J, et al: Possible association of interleukin 1 gene locus polymorphisms with low back pain. Pain 109:8-19, 2004.

7. Tolonen J, Gronblad M, Virri J, et al: Oncoprotein c-Fos and c-Jun immunopositive cells and cell clusters in herniated intervertebral disc tissue. Eur Spine J 11:452-458, 2002.

8. Wang YJ, Lu WJ, Shi Q, et al: Gene expression profile of degenerated cervical intervertebral disc tissues in rats. Chin J Traumatol 7:330-340, 2004.

9. Van Tulder MW, Assendelft WJ, Koes BW, et al: Spinal radiographic findings and nonspecific low back pain: A systematic review of observational studies. Spine 22:427-434, 1997.

10. Iwamoto J, Abe H, Tsukimura Y, et al: Relationship between radiographic abnormalities of lumbar spine and incidence of low back pain in high school and college football players: A prospective study. Am J Sports Med 32:781-786, 2004.

11. Auerbach JA: Towards an evidence-based approach for imaging in evaluation of back pain in children. Ottawa, POSNA, 2005.

12. Brodke D, Ritter S: Nonoperative management of low back pain and lumbar disc degeneration. J Bone Joint Surg Am 86:1810-1818, 2004.

13. van Tulder MW, Jellema P, van Poppel MN, et al: Lumbar supports for prevention and treatment of low back pain. Cochrane Database Syst Rev CD001823, 2000.

14. Meade TW, Dyer S, Browne W, et al: Low back pain of mechanical origin: Randomised comparison of chiropractic and hospital outpatient treatment. BMJ 300:1431-1437, 1990.

15. Ramos G, Martin W: Effects of vertebral axial decompression on intradiscal pressure. J Neurosurg 81:350-353, 1994.

16. Saal JA, Saal JS: Nonoperative treatment of herniated lumbar intervertebral disc with radiculopathy: An outcome study. Spine 14:431-437, 1989.

17. Bridger RS, Orkin D, Henneberg M: A quantitative investigation of lumbar and pelvic postures in standing and sitting: Interrelationships with body position and hip muscle length. Int J Indust Ergonom 9:235-244, 1992.

18. McGill SM, Norman RW: Low back biomechanics in industry in the prevention of injury. In Grabiner M (ed): Current Issues in Biomechanics. Champaign, IL, Human Kinetics Publishers, 1992.

19. Alaranta H, Luoto S, Heliovaara M, et al: Static back endurance and the risk of low-back pain. Clin Biomech (Bristol, Avon) 10:323-324, 1995.

20. Dowzer CN, Reilly T, Cable NT: Effects of deep and shallow water running on spinal shrinkage. Br J Sports Med 32:44-48, 1998.

21. Dowzer CN, Reilly T, Cable NT, et al: Maximal physiological responses to deep and shallow water running. Ergonomics 42:275-281, 1999.

22. Reilly T, Dowzer CN, Cable NT: The physiology of deep-water running. J Sports Sci 21:959-972, 2003.

23. McGill SM: Low back exercises: Evidence for improving exercise regimens. Phys Ther 78:754-765, 1998.

24. McGill S: Low back exercises: Prescription for the healthy back and when recovering from injury. In: Resource Manual for Guidelines for Exercise Testing and Prescription, 7th ed. Indianapolis, American College of Sports Medicine, 2005.

25. McGill SM: The biomechanics of low back injury: Implications on current practice in industry and the clinic. J Biomech 30:465-475, 1997.

26. Nutter P: Aerobic exercise in the treatment and prevention of low back pain. Occup Med 3:137-145, 1988.

27. Adams MA, Dolan P: Recent advances in lumbar spinal mechanics and their clinical significance. Clin Biomech (Bristol, Avon) 10:3-19, 1995.

28. Potvin J, Norman R: Can fatigue compromise lifting safety? In Proceedings of the Second North American Congress on Biomechanics, Chicago, August 24-28, 1992, pp 513-514.

29. Frost H, Lamb SE, Doll HA, et al: Randomised controlled trial of physiotherapy compared with advice for low back pain. BMJ 329:708, 2004.

30. Loud KJ, Micheli LJ: Common athletic injuries in adolescent girls. Curr Opin Pediatr 13:317-322, 2001.

31. Nachemson AL: Advances in low-back pain. Clin Orthop Relat Res 201:266-278, 1985.

32. Andersson G: The epidemiology of spinal disorders. In Frymoyer J, Weinstein J, Ducker T, et al (eds): The Adult Spine: Principles and Practice. Philadelphia, Lippincott-Raven, 1991, pp 107-146.

33. Szpalski M, Gunzburg R, Balague F, et al: A 2-year prospective longitudinal study on low back pain in primary school children. Eur Spine J 11:459-464, 2002.

34. Adams MA, Dolan P, Hutton WC, et al: Diurnal changes in spinal mechanics and their clinical significance. J Bone Joint Surg Br 72:266-270, 1990.

35. Snook SH, Webster BS, McGorry RW, et al: The reduction of chronic nonspecific low back pain through the control of early morning lumbar flexion: A randomized controlled trial. Spine 23:2601-2607, 1998.

36. Cyron BM, Hutton WC: The fatigue strength of the lumbar neural arch in spondylolysis. J Bone Joint Surg Br 60:234-238, 1978.

37. Herman MJ, Pizzutillo PD, Cavalier R: Spondylolysis and spondylolisthesis in the child and adolescent athlete. Orthop Clin North Am 34:461-467, 2003.

38. Jackson DW, Wiltse LL, Cirincoine RJ: Spondylolysis in the female gymnast. Clin Orthop Relat Res (117):68-73, 1976.

39. Soler T, Calderon C: The prevalence of spondylolysis in the Spanish elite athlete. Am J Sports Med 28:57-62, 2000.

40. El-Rassi G, Takemitsu M, Glutting J, et al: Clinical outcome and return to athletics after nonoperative treatment of spondylolysis in children. Poster Exhibit. Scoliosis Research Society, Buenos Aires, 2004.

41. Bono CM: Low-back pain in athletes. J Bone Joint Surg Am 86:382-396, 2004.

42. Logroscino G, Mazza O, Aulisa G, et al: Spondylolysis and spondylolisthesis in the pediatric and adolescent population. Childs Nerv Syst 17:644-655, 2001.

42a. Leono A, Cianfoni A, Cerase A, et al: Lumbar spondylolysis: a review. Skeletal Radiol May 2010 (Epub ahead of print).

43. Cavalier R, Herman MJ, Cheung EV, et al: Spondylolysis and spondylolisthesis in children and adolescents: I. Diagnosis, natural history, and nonsurgical management. J Am Acad Orthop Surg 14:417-424, 2006.

44. McNeely ML, Torrance G, Magee DJ: A systematic review of physiotherapy for spondylolysis and spondylolisthesis. Man Ther 8:80-91, 2003.

45. O'Sullivan PB, Phyty GD, Twomey LT, et al: Evaluation of specific stabilizing exercise in the treatment of chronic low back pain with radiologic diagnosis of spondylolysis or spondylolisthesis. Spine 22:2959-2967, 1997.

46. Salminen JJ, Erkintalo MO, Pentti J, et al: Recurrent low back pain and early disc degeneration in the young. Spine 24:1316-1321, 1999.

47. Standaert CJ, Herring SA: Spondylolysis: A critical review. Br J Sports Med 34:415-422, 2000.

48. Dubousset J: Treatment of spondylolysis and spondylolisthesis in children and adolescents. Clin Orthop Relat Res 337:77-85, 1997.

49. Cheung EV, Herman MJ, Cavalier R, et al: Spondylolysis and spondylolisthesis in children and adolescents: II. Surgical management. J Am Acad Orthop Surg 14:488-498, 2006.

50. Chen JF, Lee ST: A physiological method for the repair of young adult simple isthmic lumbar spondylolysis. Chang Gung Med J 23:92-98, 2000.

51. Labelle H, Roussouly P, Berthonnaud E, et al: Spondylolisthesis, pelvic incidence, and spinopelvic balance: A correlation study. Spine 29:2049-2054, 2004.

52. Curylo LJ, Edwards C, DeWald RW: Radiographic markers in spondyloptosis: Implications for spondylolisthesis progression. Spine 27:2021-2025, 2002.

53. Berk RH: [Lumbar spine injuries in pediatric and adolescent athletes]. Acta Orthop Traumatol Turc 38(Suppl 1):S58-S63, 2004.

54. Wimberly RL, Lauerman WC: Spondylolisthesis in the athlete. Clin Sports Med 21:133-145, 2002.

55. Teitz CC, Cook DM: Rehabilitation of neck and low back injuries. Clin Sports Med 4:455-476, 1985.

56. Burkus JK, Lonstein JE, Winter RB, et al: Long-term evaluation of adolescents treated operatively for spondylolisthesis: A comparison of in situ arthrodesis only with in situ arthrodesis and reduction followed by immobilization in a cast. J Bone Joint Surg Am 74:693-704, 1992.

57. Lonstein JE: Spondylolisthesis in children: Cause, natural history, and management. Spine 24:2640-2648, 1999.

58. Zindrick MR, Wiltse LL, Doornik A, et al: Analysis of the morphometric characteristics of the thoracic and lumbar pedicles. Spine 12:160-166, 1987.

59. Sorensen K: Scheuermann's Juvenile Kyphosis: Clinical Appearances, Radiography, Aetiology and Prognosis. Copenhagen, Mundsgaard, 1964.

60. Commandre F, Gagnerie G, Zakarian M: The child, the spine and sports. J Sports Med Phys Fitness 28:11-19, 1988.

61. Goldstein J, Berger P, Windier G: Spine injuries in gymnasts and swimmers: An epidemiologic investigation. Am J Sports Med 19:463-468, 1991.

62. Hellstrom M, Jacobsson B, Sward L: Radiologic abnormalities of the thoraco-lumbar spine in athletes. Acta Radiol 31:127-132, 1990.

63. Matheson G, Clement D, McKenzie D: Stress fractures in athletes: A study of 320 cases. Am J Sports Med 15:46-58, 1987.

64. Micheli L: Low back pain in the adolescent: Differential diagnosis. Am J Sports Med 7:362-364, 1979.

65. Ohlen G, Wredmark T, Spangfort E: Spinal sagittal configuration and mobility related to low-back pain in the female gymnast. Spine 14:847-850, 1989.

66. Sward L, Hellstrom M, Jacobsson B: Back pain and radiologic changes in the thoraco-lumbar spine of athletes. Spine 15:124-129, 1990.

67. Sward L, Hellstrom M, Jacobsson B: Disc degeneration and associated abnormalities of the spine in elite gymnasts: A magnetic resonance imaging study. Spine 16:437-443, 1991.

68. Sward L, Hellstrom M, Jacobsson B: Vertebral ring apophysis injury in athletes: Is the etiology different in the thoracic and lumbar spine? Am J Sports Med 21:841-845, 1993.

69. Tall R, DeVault W: Spinal injury in sport: Epidemiologic considerations. Clin Orthop Relat Res 12:441-448, 1993.

70. Tsai L, Wredmark T: Spinal posture, sagittal mobility, and subjective rating of back problems in former female elite gymnasts. Spine 18:872-875, 1993.

71. Scheuermann V: Kyphosis juvenilis (Scheuermann's Krankheit). Fortschr Rontgenstr 53:1-16, 1936.

72. Greene T, Hensinger R, Hunter L: Back pain and vertebral changes simulating Scheuermann's disease. J Pediatr Orthop 5:1-7, 1985.

73. Sward L, Eriksson B, Peterson L: Anthropometric characteristics, passive hip flexion, and spinal mobility in relation to back pain in athletes. Spine 15:376-382, 1990.

74. Schmorl G: Zur Kenntnis der Wirbelkorperepiphyse und der an ihr vorkommenden Verletzungen. Arch Klin Chir 153:35-45, 1928.

75. Siffert R: Classification of the osteochondroses. Clin Orthop Relat Res 158:10-18, 1981.

76. Heithoff KB, Gundry CR, Burton CV, et al: Juvenile discogenic disease. Spine 19:335-340, 1994.

77. Dimar JR 2nd, Glassman SD, Carreon LY: Juvenile degenerative disc disease: A report of 76 cases identified by magnetic resonance imaging. Spine J 7:332-337, 2007.

78. Durham SR, Sun PP, Sutton LN: Surgically treated lumbar disc disease in the pediatric population: An outcome study. J Neurosurg 92:1-6, 2000.

79. Epstein JA, Epstein NE, Marc J, et al: Lumbar intervertebral disk herniation in teenage children: Recognition and management of associated anomalies. Spine 9:427-432, 1984.

80. Ishihara H, Matsui H, Hirano N, et al: Lumbar intervertebral disc herniation in children less than 16 years of age: Long-term follow-up study of surgically managed cases. Spine 22:2044-2049, 1997.

81. Martinez-Lage JF, Poza M, Arcas P: Avulsed lumbar vertebral rim plate in an adolescent: Trauma or malformation? Childs Nerv Syst 14:131-134, 1998.

82. Parisini P, Di Silvestre M, Greggi T, et al: Lumbar disc excision in children and adolescents. Spine 26:1997-2000, 2001.

83. Ikata T, Morita T, Katoh S, et al: Lesions of the lumbar posterior end plate in children and adolescents: An MRI study. J Bone Joint Surg Br 77:951-955, 1995.

84. Sassmannshausen G, Smith BG: Back pain in the young athlete. Clin Sports Med 21:121-132, 2002.

85. DeLuca PF, Mason DE, Weiand R, et al: Excision of herniated nucleus pulposus in children and adolescents. J Pediatr Orthop 14:318-322, 1994.

86. Shillito J Jr: Pediatric lumbar disc surgery: 20 patients under 15 years of age. Surg Neurol 46:14-18, 1996.

87. Ginsburg GM, Bassett GS: Back pain in children and adolescents: Evaluation and differential diagnosis. J Am Acad Orthop Surg 5:67-78, 1997.

88. Gibson J, Waddell G: Surgery for degenerative lumbar spondylosis. Cochrane Database Syst Rev CD001352, 2005.

89. Hassard GH, Carmack WL, Dixon J, et al: Rehabilitation: A team approach to total patient care. The rehabilitation team. J Pract Nurs 28:22-25, 1978.

90. Papagelopoulos PJ, Shaughnessy WJ, Ebersold MJ, et al: Long-term outcome of lumbar discectomy in children and adolescents sixteen years of age or younger. J Bone Joint Surg Am 80:689-698, 1998.

91. Beggs I, Addison J: Posterior vertebral rim fractures. Br J Radiol 71:567-572, 1998.

92. Skobowytsh-Okolot B: "Posterior apophysis" in L.IV—the cause of neuroradicular disturbance. Acta Orthop Scand 32:341-351, 1962.

93. Banerian KG, Wang AM, Samberg LC, et al: Association of vertebral end plate fracture with pediatric lumbar intervertebral disk herniation: Value of CT and MR imaging. Radiology 177:763-765, 1990.

94. Dietemann JL, Runge M, Badoz A, et al: Radiology of posterior lumbar apophyseal ring fractures: Report of 13 cases. Neuroradiology 30:337-344, 1988.

95. Keller RH: Traumatic displacement of the cartilaginous vertebral rim: A sign of intervertebral disc prolapse. Radiology 110:21-24, 1974.

96. Lippit A: Fracture of the vertebral body end plate and disk protrusion causing subarachnoid block in an adolescent. Clin Orthop Relat Res 11:112-115, 1974.

97. Proctor MR, Cantu RC: Head and neck injuries in young athletes. Clin Sports Med 19:693-715, 2000.

98. Kleiner D, Almquist J, Bailes J, et al: Prehospital care of the spine-injured athlete: A document from the Inter-Association Task Force for Appropriate Care of the Spine-Injured Athlete. Dallas, National Athletic Trainers Association, 2001.

99. Cantu RC, Mueller FO: Catastrophic spine injuries in football (1977-1989). J Spinal Disord 3:227-231, 1990.

100. Cantu RC, Mueller FO: Catastrophic football injuries: 1977-1998. Neurosurgery 47:673-675; discussion 675-677, 2000.

101. Cantu RC, Mueller FO: Catastrophic spine injuries in American football, 1977-2001. Neurosurgery 53:358-362; discussion 362-363, 2003.

102. Cantu RC, Mueller FO: Brain injury-related fatalities in American football, 1945-1999. Neurosurgery 52:846-852; discussion 852-843, 2003.

103. Mueller FO, Cantu RC: Catastrophic injuries and fatalities in high school and college sports, fall 1982-spring 1988. Med Sci Sports Exerc 22:737-741, 1990.

104. Mueller FO, Cantu RC: The annual survey of catastrophic football injuries: 1977-1988. Exerc Sport Sci Rev 19:261-312, 1991.

105. Meyer SA, Schulte KR, Callaghan JJ, et al: Cervical spinal stenosis and stingers in collegiate football players. Am J Sports Med 22:158-166, 1994.

106. Albright JP, McAuley E, Martin RK, et al: Head and neck injuries in college football: An eight-year analysis. Am J Sports Med 13:147-152, 1985.

107. Albright JP, VanGilder J, el-Khoury GY, et al: Head and neck injuries in sports. In Scott WN, Nisonson B, Nicholas JA (eds): Principles of Sports Medicine. Baltimore, Williams & Wilkins, 1984, pp 40-86.

108. Bergfeld JA, Hershman E, Wilbourn A: Brachial plexus injury in sports: A five year follow-up. Orthop Trans 12:743-744, 1988.

109. Clancy WG Jr, Brand RL, Bergfield JA: Upper trunk brachial plexus injuries in contact sports. Am J Sports Med 5:209-216, 1977.

110. Funk FF, Wells RE: Injuries of the cervical spine in football. Clin Orthop Relat Res 109:50-58, 1975.

111. Rockett FX: Observations on the "burner": Traumatic cervical radiculopathy. Clin Orthop Relat Res 164:18-19, 1982.

112. Speer KP, Bassett FH 3rd: The prolonged burner syndrome. Am J Sports Med 18:591-594, 1990.

113. Watkins RG: Neck injuries in football players. Clin Sports Med 5:215-246, 1986.

114. Quan D, Bird SJ: Nerve conduction studies and electromyography in the evaluation of peripheral nerve injuries. Univ Pa Orthop J 12:45-51, 1999.

114a. Seddon HJ: Three types of nerve injuries. Brain 66:237, 1943.

114b. Sunderland SA: A classification of peripheral nerve injuries producing loss of function. Brain 74:491-516, 1951.

115. Eismont FJ, Clifford S, Goldberg M, et al: Cervical sagittal spinal canal size in spine injury. Spine 9:663-666, 1984.

116. Castro FP Jr, Ricciardi J, Brunet ME, et al: Stingers, the Torg ratio, and the cervical spine. Am J Sports Med 25:603-608, 1997.

117. Torg JS, Pavlov H, Genuario SE, et al: Neurapraxia of the cervical spinal cord with transient quadriplegia. J Bone Joint Surg Am 68:1354-1370, 1986.

118. Pavlov H, Torg JS, Robie B, et al: Cervical spinal stenosis: Determination with vertebral body ratio method. Radiology 164:771-775, 1987.

119. Clancy WG Jr, Foltz AS: Iliac apophysitis and stress fractures in adolescent runners. Am J Sports Med 4:214-218, 1976.

120. Doral MN, Aydog ST, Tetik O, et al: Multiple osteochondroses and avulsion fracture of anterior superior iliac spine in a soccer player. Br J Sports Med 39:e16, 2005.

121. Pointinger H, Munk P, Poeschl GP: Avulsion fracture of the anterior superior iliac spine following apophysitis. Br J Sports Med 37:361-362, 2003.

122. Dormans JP, Moroz L: Infection and tumors of the spine in children. J Bone Joint Surg Am 89(Suppl 1):79-97, 2007.

Asheesh Bedi, MD
Robert N. Hensinger, MD

Congenital anomalies of the cervical spine occur infrequently and receive little attention when pathologic conditions of the spine are considered. These spinal abnormalities have a great impact on affected individuals, however, and physicians who deal with problems of the spine should be familiar with the diagnosis and management of these anomalies. These structural defects originate early in fetal development; when they are discovered in childhood, they appear to be static and unchanging. This appearance is deceptive, however, because with further growth many may prove to be capable of dramatic change and progressive deformity, particularly in the cervical spine, and may be life-threatening. Many anomalies are not discovered until a complication occurs. Anomalies of the occipitocervical junction often remain undetected until late childhood or adolescence, and some remain hidden well into adulthood.

Other anomalies of the spine, although recognized in early life, may not become clinically significant until adulthood. During the growing years, a delicate balance is struck between the congenitally distorted bony elements of the vertebral column and the neurologic elements. Later, in adult life, factors such as aging or intercurrent trauma may alter this relationship. A patient with an os odontoideum may gradually develop laxity of the supporting structures after countless flexion-extension movements of the neck or may develop serious instability of the atlantoaxial joint and spinal cord compression after a seemingly trivial injury. Individuals with Klippel-Feil syndrome may gradually develop symptoms of degenerative arthritis at the hypermobile articulations adjacent to the cervical synostosis.

Diagnosis and assessment of these congenital spinal conditions are hampered by the difficulties encountered during radiographic evaluation. In a normal child, the pattern of vertebral growth and ossification has wide variation and often is incomplete until late in the 2nd decade. Fixed bony deformities often prevent proper positioning for standard views. Nonstandard views and oblique projections add to diagnostic confusion and hinder complete assessment of the patient. Dynamic computed tomography (CT) scans, magnetic resonance imaging (MRI), cineradiography, myelography, and arteriography are sometimes helpful in the evaluation of these conditions and should be available to a physician engaged in treating the more complex problems.

This chapter is especially concerned with the treatment of these spinal anomalies. Too often a policy of observation is adopted, whereas more vigorous management could control, ameliorate, and even occasionally correct the deformity. Sufficient information is available about the natural history of these anomalies, and attention must now be directed to the results of treatment. Operative stabilization of a patient with chronic atlantoaxial instability may prevent a neurologic disaster.

Physicians who treat these children must be concerned with their total care. It is tempting to focus attention on the problems of the spine to the exclusion of all others, but it is imperative to be aware of the high incidence of associated anomalies with vertebral malformations. Recognition of a vertebral abnormality should stimulate a thorough and intensive search for associated anomalies. Poor management of these related problems, particularly urinary complications, may nullify a well-planned and well-executed orthopaedic program. Particular emphasis is placed on related anomalies of the central nervous system, which may be subtle in their manifestation yet have a great impact on the patient's social and educational adjustment to life.

A hearing deficit may be unrecognized until well into the school years. Mirror motions of the upper extremities may limit effective two-handed activity, such as playing a piano or climbing a ladder. These and other learning disabilities can be an important part of the condition yet may not be appreciated by the physician, teacher, or parent. Early recognition and appropriate treatment of these problems can substantially contribute to the general well-being of the child.

Basilar Impression

Basilar impression (or invagination) is a deformity of the bones of the base of the skull at the margin of the foramen magnum. The floor of the skull appears to be indented by the upper cervical spine, and the tip of the odontoid is more cephalad, sometimes protruding into the opening of the foramen magnum, and it may encroach on the brainstem. This deformity increases the risk of neurologic damage from injury, circulatory embarrassment, or impairment of cerebrospinal fluid flow. In 1939, Chamberlain[1] first called attention to the clinical significance of this anomaly with the following vivid description:

> The changes shown by the roentgenogram give the impression of softening of the base of the skull and moulding through the force of gravity. It is as though the weight of the head has caused the ears to approach the shoulders, while the cervical spine, refusing to be shortened, has pushed the floor of the posterior fossa upward into the brain space.

The terms *platybasia* and *basilar impression* are often used as synonyms, but they are not related anatomically or pathologically. Platybasia has no clinical significance; it is merely an anthropologic term used to denote flattening of the angle formed by the intersection of the plane of the anterior fossa with the plane of the clivus. Basilar impression, which is invagination in the region of the foramen magnum, does have clinical significance. Patients with symptomatic basilar impression are seldom found to have an associated platybasia.

There are two types of basilar impression: (1) primary, a congenital abnormality often associated with other vertebral defects, such as atlanto-occipital fusion, hypoplasia of the atlas, bifid posterior arch of the atlas, odontoid abnormalities, Klippel-Feil syndrome, and Goldenhar syndrome,[2] and (2) secondary, a developmental condition usually attributed to softening of the osseous structures at the base of the skull, with the deformity developing later in life. Secondary basilar invagination is a potentially devastating sequelae of osteogenesis imperfecta, Hajdu-Cheney syndrome, and other osteochondrodysplasias.[3] Although the precise etiology remains unclear, it has been suggested that the axial load from the cranium and its contents lead to recurrent microfractures in the region of the foramen magnum and precipitate flattening and infolding of the posterior skull base. This theory has been supported by intraoperative findings of thickened, proliferative callus at the skull base in patients with osteogenesis imperfecta.[4,5] This thickened callus is also seen in conditions such as osteomalacia, rickets, Paget disease, renal osteodystrophy, rheumatoid arthritis, neurofibromatosis, and ankylosing spondylitis.[6]

Radiographic Features

Basilar impression is difficult to assess radiographically. Many measurement schemes have been proposed; those most commonly referred to are the Chamberlain,[1] McGregor,[7] and McRae lines in the lateral radiograph (Fig. 30–1) and the Fischgold-Metzger line in the anteroposterior projection. The Chamberlain line[1] (a line drawn from the dorsal marginal hard palate to the posterior lip of the foramen magnum) is seldom used because the posterior lip of the foramen magnum (opisthion) is difficult to define on a standard radiograph (Fig. 30–2A) and is often itself invaginated in basilar impressions.

The McGregor line (a line drawn from the upper surface of the posterior edge of the hard palate to the most caudal point of the occipital curve of the skull) is easier to identify (see Figs.

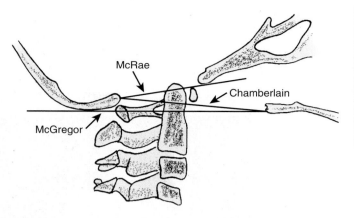

FIGURE 30–1 Lateral craniometry. Drawing indicates three lines used to determine basilar impressions. Chamberlain line (1939) is drawn from posterior lip of foramen magnum (opisthion) to dorsal margin of hard palate. McGregor line (1948) is drawn from upper surface of posterior edge of hard palate to most caudal point of occipital curve of skull. McRae line (1953) defines opening of foramen magnum. McGregor line is best method for screening because bony landmark can be clearly defined at all ages on routine lateral radiograph.

30–1 and 30–2) and is preferable. The position of the tip of the odontoid is measured in relation to this baseline, and a distance of 4.5 mm above McGregor line is considered to be on the extreme edge of normality.[7] The study of normal variations by Hinck and colleagues[8] showed a wide range of normality, however, and difference between males and females.

The McRae line defines the opening of the foramen magnum and is derived from McRae's observation that if the tip of the odontoid lies below the opening of the foramen magnum, the patient is likely to be asymptomatic. The McRae line is an accurate guide in the clinical assessment of patients with basilar impression.

A criticism of the lateral lines (McGregor and Chamberlain) is that the hard palate is not actually a part of the skull and may be distorted by an abnormal facial configuration or a highly arched palate, independent of a craniovertebral anomaly. In addition, the patient may have an abnormally long or short odontoid or an abnormality of the axis or occipital facets, which can diminish the value of the measurements. Upper cervical spine measurements on plain radiographs have an unacceptable interobserver reliability and intraobserver reproducibility. Although there are multiple factors for the wide variation between observers, many authors have suggested that the basion and opisthion are difficult to localize on radiographs and may be altered significantly by small changes in patient position.[9]

Since the advent of CT and MRI, the diagnosis of basilar invagination can be made directly rather than based on craniometric lines.[10] These techniques have largely replaced the older tomography techniques, particularly the anteroposterior measurement of Fischgold and Metzger,[10,11] which was previously the most accurate method. The mean and range of normal distances from the odontoid peg to the most frequently used skull baseline employing MRI was 1.2 mm (median 1.5 mm, SD 3 mm) below Chamberlain line; 0.9 mm

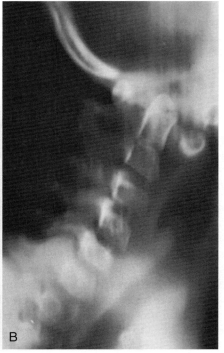

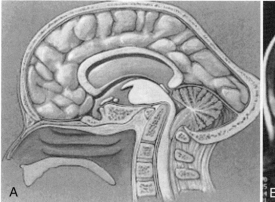

FIGURE 30–2 A 6-year-old girl presented with a history of unusual gait and recent episode of unconsciousness after mild head trauma. **A,** Routine lateral radiograph suggests that odontoid is displaced proximally into opening of foramen magnum. McGregor line has been drawn from most caudal portion of occiput to hard palate. Tip of odontoid is more than 5 mm above this line, indicating basilar impression. **B,** Lateral laminagraph shows subluxation of C1 and C2 and that tip of odontoid is above opening of foramen magnum (McRae line).

(median 1.1, SD 3 mm) below McGregor line; and 4.6 mm (median 4.8, SD 2.6) below McRae line.[10] MRI also allows direct assessment of the degree of neural compression and identifies the presence of associated pathologic processes, such as Chiari malformation, hydrocephalus, syringomyelia, or cerebellar herniation (Fig. 30–3).[4] The lateral reference lines on plain radiographs are still very useful screening tools, however.[12,13]

Clinical Features

Patients with basilar impression frequently have a deformity of the skull or neck (e.g., a short neck in 78%, asymmetry of the face or skull or torticollis in 68%).[14] These physical findings are often noted in patients without basilar impression (Klippel-Feil syndrome, occipitalization) and are not considered pathognomonic.

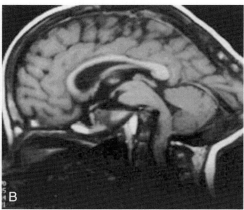

FIGURE 30–3 Secondary basilar invagination with osteochondrodysplasia. **A,** Sagittal drawing shows acute cervicomedullary angle, ventrally compressed brainstem, herniated hindbrain, and invaginated clival-atlantoaxial complex. **B,** Sagittal MRI shows these key findings in an 11-year-old girl with Hajdu-Cheney syndrome. (Images adapted from Sawin PD, Menezes AH: Basilar invagination in OI and related osteochondral dysplasias. J Neurosurg 86:950-960, 1997.)

The symptoms (or lack of them) even in severe basilar impression are difficult to explain.[13,14] The more segments involved in a patient with Klippel-Feil syndrome, the more likely it is that the odontoid will be superior.[13] Basilar impression is frequently associated with anomalous neurologic conditions, such as Arnold-Chiari malformation[14] and syringomyelia,[15,16] which can cloud the clinical picture further. Symptoms are generally due to crowding of the neural structures at the level of the foramen magnum, particularly the medulla oblongata. The neurologic sequelae of basilar invagination are determined by the degree of cephalad migration of the clivus-atlas-dens complex. In addition to the direct compression of the ventral brainstem, the dens creates a fulcrum for traction on the cervical cord. Cerebellar dysfunction may arise from direct compression or reflect secondary herniation from the posterior fossa.

There is an unusually high incidence of basilar impression in northeast Brazil,[17] and the work of De Barros and colleagues[14] has been helpful in delineating the symptoms and signs. Patients who were symptomatic with pure basilar impression had the dominant complaints of motor and sensory disturbances, and 85% had weakness and paresthesia of the limbs. In contrast, patients who were symptomatic with pure Chiari malformation were more likely to have cerebellar and vestibular disturbances (unsteadiness of gait, dizziness, and nystagmus). In both conditions, there may be impingement of the lower cranial nerves as they emerge from the medulla oblongata, particularly the trigeminal (V), glossopharyngeal (IX), vagus (X), and hypoglossal (XII) nerves.[14] Headache and pain in the nape of the neck, in the distribution of the greater occipital nerve, are common findings.[14,18]

Posterior encroachment may cause blockage of the aqueduct of Sylvius, and the presenting symptoms may be from increased intracranial pressure or hydrocephalus.[7,14] Compression of the cerebellum with vestibular involvement or herniation of the cerebellar tonsils (Chiari malformation) is a frequent finding,[14] leading to vertical or lateral nystagmus in 65% of cases. These symptoms may be caused not by direct pressure from the posterior rim of the foramen magnum but rather by a thickened band of dura invisible on plain radiographs; this has prompted several authors to recommend routine MRI evaluation. If this situation is unrecognized, bony decompression alone (without opening the dura) would be unsuccessful in obtaining remission of symptoms or halting progression of the neurologic injury.[14]

There is a high incidence of vertebral artery anomalies in basilar impression, atlanto-occipital fusion, and absence of the C1 facet.[19] In addition, the vertebral arteries may be compressed as they pass through the crowded foramen magnum, causing symptoms suggestive of vertebral artery insufficiency, such as dizziness, seizures, mental deterioration, and syncope.[7,19,20] These symptoms may occur alone or in combination with symptoms of spinal cord compression.[7,14,19,21] Michie and Clark[22] and Bachs and colleagues[23] theorized that one explanation for the frequent association of syringomyelia or syringobulbia and basilar impression is that the vertebral arteries and the anterior spinal artery are compromised in the region of the foramen magnum, with subsequent degeneration of the spinal cord and medulla. Arteriographic studies are unavailable to confirm this thesis. Children with occipitocervical anomalies may be more susceptible to vertebral artery injury and brainstem ischemia, particularly children who undergo skull traction for correction of scoliosis. Moderate amounts of traction (<15 lb) that normally would be well tolerated may compromise these abnormal vessels. Careful radiographic evaluation of the occipitocervical junction should precede any use of skull traction, even if only minimal traction forces are planned.[24]

Although this condition is congenital, many patients do not develop symptoms until the 2nd or 3rd decade of life.[13,14] These delayed symptoms may be due to a gradually increasing instability from ligamentous laxity caused by aging, similar to the delayed myelopathies reported after atlantoaxial dislocations or the increasing instability of C1 and C2 in patients with odontoid agenesis.[25] These individuals often develop premature cervical osteoarthritis, as found in the family studies of Gunderson and colleagues.[21] Chamberlain[1] and others theorized that the young developing brain may be more tolerant of compressive effects, which later prove deleterious to older tissues. Similarly, arteriosclerotic changes in the vertebral arteries may make these vessels more susceptible to minor constrictions. Symptoms frequently occur in older patients in whom a congenital anomaly would not ordinarily be considered. Patients with this malformation have been mistakenly diagnosed as having multiple sclerosis, posterior fossa tumors, amyotrophic lateral sclerosis, or traumatic injury. It is important to survey this area whenever such a diagnosis is considered and whenever this malformation is suspected.

Treatment

Treatment depends on the cause of the symptoms and often requires the teamwork of an orthopaedist, neurosurgeon, neurologist, and radiologist. It is possible to have a severe basilar impression without neurologic symptoms, and a search for associated conditions must be conducted. Hydrocephalus from aqueductal stenosis, if present, must be addressed first with ventricular shunting before any other surgical interventions.[4]

Treatment of symptomatic basilar invagination is dictated by the severity of ventral neural compression and reducibility of the deformity. An initial attempt should be made to realign the cervical spine and decompress the neural elements by head positioning and, in some cases, halo traction. Plain radiographs and MRI may be used to determine the adequacy of reduction and neural decompression. Patients who respond to such closed reduction methods may be treated with suboccipital craniectomy and upper cervical laminectomy, followed by occipitocervical arthrodesis. More recent reports suggest that many of the physical changes can be reversed by atlantoaxial distraction fixation surgery.[26,27] Most authors suggest opening the dura to look for a tight posterior dural band.[14] Brainstem compression not relieved by traction demands anterior decompression and resection of the offending anterior atlas, odontoid, or distal clivus. Posterior decompression and fusion are also necessary and may be performed immediately after or as a staged procedure.[28]

Posterior fossa decompression alone for symptomatic secondary basilar invagination typically provides only transient relief of symptoms, followed by recurrent neurologic deterioration months to years after the index procedure. Studies have shown that secondary basilar invagination in patients with osteochondrodysplasia tends to progress even after occipitocervical fusion with infolding of the skull base around the fusion mass and progressive forward bending.[3] Prolonged bracing with an orthotic device and lifelong surveillance may be prudent to halt further recurrence or symptomatic progression.[4] These recommendations are generalizations regarding treatment, and appropriate references should be consulted in the evaluation of individual patients.

Atlantoaxial Instability

The clinical significance of a bony anomaly in the region of the atlantoaxial joint is primarily related to its influence on the stability of this articulation. The precipitating factor may be an abnormal odontoid, atlanto-occipital fusion, or laxity of the transverse atlantal ligament, but the end result is narrowing of the spinal canal (encroachment) and impingement on the neural elements.[29] It is important not to lose sight of this basic problem, but frequently it becomes obscured in radiographic detail, conflicting reports, and unusual clinical symptoms and signs. It is important to review atlantoaxial instability before a detailed discussion of the individual anomalies that may be contributory.

Pathomechanics

The articulation between C1 and C2 is the most mobile part of the vertebral column and normally has the least stability of any of the vertebral articulations. The normal cervical spine permits about 90 degrees of rotatory motion; 50% of this motion occurs in the atlantoaxial joint. Considerable shifting from side to side (lateral slide) also occurs as a component of this rotatory motion. Flexion and extension are permitted to a limited degree (normally about 10 degrees of extension and 5 degrees of forward flexion); more than 10 degrees of flexion indicates subluxation.[30] The odontoid acts as a bony buttress to prevent hyperextension, but the remaining normal range of motion is maintained and is solely dependent on the integrity of the surrounding ligaments and capsular structures.

The articulation between the condyles of the skull and the atlas (atlanto-occipital joint) normally allows only a few degrees of flexion-extension—a slight nodding motion of the head. In rotation, the atlas and head turn as a unit. The articulation between the axis and C3 permits some flexion-extension but is similarly restricted in rotation. The atlantoaxial joint is extremely mobile but structurally weak and is located between two relatively fixed points, the atlanto-occipital and C2-3 joints.

Motion of the atlantoaxial articulation is usually accentuated in patients with bony anomalies of the occipitocervical junction. An excellent example is a patient with atlanto-occipital fusion, who is frequently found to have compensatory hypermobility of the atlantoaxial joint. If this same patient has an associated synostosis of C2-3, it is reasonable to expect that this additional stress on the atlantoaxial articulation may eventually lead to significant instability.[28,29,31,32] This assumption has clinical support in that 60% of patients with symptomatic atlanto-occipital fusion have associated fusion of C2-3.[29,32,33]

Nonetheless, it is unusual for patients to become symptomatic before the 3rd decade. It must be assumed that at least initially a delicate balance is struck between the hypermobile articulation and the adjacent spinal cord. Motion is maintained without neurologic compromise. This relationship must be altered before symptoms develop. In a symptomatic patient, trauma is immediately suspected, but statistically it is not often associated or is of a minor nature.

More likely, the degenerative changes of aging cause the lower cervical articulations to become more rigid. This gradual restriction of motion below places an increased demand on the ligaments and capsular structures of the atlantoaxial articulation, with the development of instability.[34] With aging, the central nervous system itself becomes less tolerant of intermittent compression, and its ability to recover is diminished. There is evidence to suggest that intermittent compression is more harmful or irritating to the spinal cord than static, constant compression.[35] Arteriosclerosis and loss of elasticity from aging affect the vertebral arteries, making them more sensitive to compression at the foramen magnum.[36]

As a consequence, a symptomatic patient often presents with a puzzling clinical picture. Only a few patients present initially with a history of head or neck trauma, neck pain, torticollis, quadriparesis, or signs of high spinal cord compression, any of which would facilitate the diagnosis. A changing, intermittent pattern of symptoms is more typical than the localized pattern suggested by the radiographs alone. Many patients mistakenly receive the diagnosis of a diffuse demyelinating disease such as multiple sclerosis or amyotrophic lateral sclerosis.

In patients with basilar impression or atlanto-occipital fusion, the clinical findings suggest that the major damage is occurring anteriorly from the odontoid. The symptoms and signs of pyramidal tract irritation, muscle weakness and wasting, ataxia, spasticity, hyperreflexia, and pathologic reflexes are commonly found.[33,37] Autopsy findings consistently show that the brainstem is indented by the abnormal odontoid.[37,38] Other, less common complaints include diplegia, tinnitus, earaches, dysphasia, and poor phonation, all of which are due to cranial nerve or bulbar irritation from direct pressure of the odontoid on the medulla.

If the primary area of impingement is posterior from the rim of the foramen magnum, the dural band, or the posterior ring of the atlas (typical of odontoid anomalies), symptoms are referable to the posterior columns with alterations in deep pain and vibratory responses and proprioception. If there is also an associated cerebellar herniation, nystagmus, ataxia, and incoordination may be observed. Symptoms referable to vertebral artery compression—dizziness, seizures, mental deterioration, and syncope—may occur alone or in combination with symptoms of spinal cord compression.[34]

In children, the presenting symptoms may be quite subtle and nonspecific. Perovic and colleagues[39] reported that in most of their patients the only presenting symptom was generalized weakness, manifested as lack of physical endurance, a history of frequent falling, or the child's asking to be carried. Pyramidal tract signs appeared later, and posterior column signs and sphincter disturbances were less frequently encountered.[39] Similarly, in achondroplasia, retardation of motor skills and increasing hydrocephalus may be the only clinical manifestation of impending quadriparesis secondary to basilar stenosis.

Atlantoaxial instability is commonly associated with other anomalies of the spine, many of which lead to scoliosis. Patients with congenital scoliosis, Down syndrome, spondyloepiphyseal dysplasia, osteogenesis imperfecta, and neurofibromatosis all can have significant atlantoaxial instability, which may be unrecognized. Radiologic surveys, particularly flexion-extension views of the C1-2 articulation, should be obtained before administration of general anesthesia or preliminary spinal traction in the management of the scoliosis.

Atlantoaxial Instability and Down Syndrome

Spitzer and colleagues[40] were the first to describe occipitoatlantal instability and atlantal hypoplasia in Down syndrome. Generalized ligamentous laxity and flat facets predispose to hypermobility and pathologic motion at the craniovertebral and atlantoaxial articulations. Depending on patient age at the time of the study, 10% to 40% of these patients have radiologically detectable atlantoaxial instability.[40,41]

The natural history of atlantoaxial instability in patients with Down syndrome is not well known. Burke and colleagues[42] reported 7 of 32 patients developing atlantoaxial instability over a 13-year period. Morton and colleagues[43] found no evidence of de novo atlantoaxial instability in 67 patients with Down syndrome over a 5-year period. In addition, a direct correlation between neurologic deterioration and atlantoaxial instability has not been established. Ferguson and colleagues[44] identified 17 of 84 patients with atlantoaxial instability on plain radiographs but could not correlate any difference in neurologic symptoms with radiographic findings. Taggard and colleagues[45] did not find such a benign relationship between C1-2 instability and neurologic function, however, reporting acute neurologic deterioration in six patients after a minor fall or intubation for a general anesthetic.

Radiographic Features

The atlas-dens interval (ADI) is the space seen on the lateral radiograph between the anterior aspect of the dens and the posterior aspect of the anterior ring of the atlas (Fig. 30–4). In children, the ADI should be no greater than 4 mm,[30] particularly in flexion, where the greatest distance can be noted. The upper limit of normal in adults is less than 3 mm. Occasionally, the space between the odontoid and the ring of C1 forms

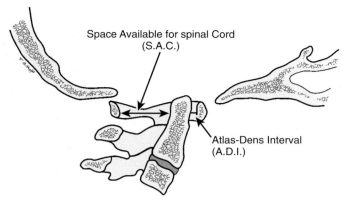

FIGURE 30–4 Atlantoaxial joint showing normal atlas-dens interval (ADI), normal space available for spinal cord (SAC), distance between posterior aspect of odontoid, and nearest posterior structure.

a "V" shape in flexion; in this situation, the ADI is measured at the mid-portion of the odontoid. A subtle increase in the ADI in the neutral position may indicate disruption of the transverse atlantal ligament. The ADI is a valuable aid in the evaluation of acute injury, when standard flexion-extension views would be potentially hazardous.[30,46] Fielding and colleagues[47] noted that the shift of C1-2 does not exceed 3 mm in adults if the transverse ligament is intact. The transverse ligament ruptures within the range of 5 mm.[48] Similar data for children are unavailable.

The ADI is of limited value in evaluating chronic atlantoaxial instability owing to congenital anomalies, rheumatoid arthritis, or Down syndrome. In these conditions, the odontoid is frequently found to be hypermobile with a widened ADI, particularly in flexion (Fig. 30–5), but not all are symptomatic, and all do not require surgical stabilization.[42,48] In this situation, attention should be directed to the amount of space available for the spinal cord (SAC). Determining the SAC is accomplished by measuring the distance from the posterior aspect of the odontoid or axis to the nearest posterior

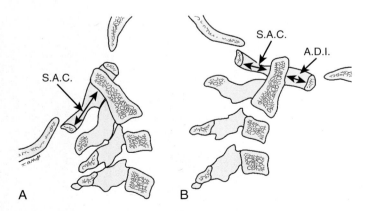

FIGURE 30–5 Atlantoaxial instability with intact odontoid. **A,** Extension—forward sliding of atlas with increased atlas-dens interval (ADI) and decreased space available for spinal cord (SAC). **B,** Flexion—ADI and SAC return to normal as intact odontoid provides bony block to subluxation in hyperextension.

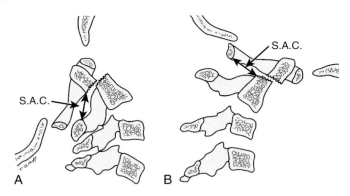

FIGURE 30–6 Atlantoaxial instability with os odontoideum, absent odontoid, or traumatic nonunion. **A,** Extension—forward sliding of atlas with reduction of space available for spinal cord (SAC) but no changes in atlas-dens interval (ADI). **B,** Flexion—posterior subluxation with reduction in SAC and no change in ADI.

structure (foramen magnum or posterior ring of the atlas).[29,32,49] This measurement is particularly helpful in evaluating a patient with nonunion of the odontoid or os odontoideum because in both conditions the ADI may be normal, yet in flexion or extension there may be considerable reduction in the space available for the spinal cord (Fig. 30–6).[50] Lateral flexion-extension views should be conducted voluntarily by the patient, particularly a patient with a neurologic deficit (Fig. 30–7). Most symptomatic patients exhibit significant instability.

Patients with a normal odontoid process and an attenuated or ruptured transverse atlantal ligament are particularly at risk; with anterior shift of the atlas over the axis, the spinal cord is easily damaged by direct impingement against the intact odontoid process,[50,51] such as in atlanto-occipital fusion. The situation is less dangerous if the odontoid process is absent or fractured and is carried forward with the atlas (os odontoideum).[47] In a large series of patients with os odontoideum reported by Fielding and colleagues,[47] the average displacement was 1 cm, mostly either anterior or posterior, but some were unstable in all directions.

In patients with multiple anomalies, the usual radiographic views are not always reliable in confirming the presence or absence of an odontoid.[39] Similarly, in patients with abnormal bone, such as patients with Morquio syndrome or spondyloepiphyseal dysplasia, the odontoid may be present but dysplastic, blending with the surrounding abnormal bone, and cannot be differentiated. In these situations, adequate visualization can be obtained by using lateral laminagraphic techniques (see Fig. 30–2) or with a CT scan with reconstruction views.[52,53] When the exact cut at the level of the odontoid is determined, it is repeated in flexion-extension to ascertain the stability of the atlantoaxial articulation. Extension views should not be ignored. Many patients have been found to have significant posterior subluxation.[29,47,54] Dynamic (flexion-extension) CT scans have been used to show this area, particularly with lateral reconstruction, and have replaced the laminagraphs.[51-53]

Dynamic MRI provides direct vision of the neurologic structures and in many cases the site of bony impingement and cord compression that may not be appreciated on routine views.[52,55-57] CT scans have been extremely helpful in evaluating anomalies of the upper cervical spine. Three-dimensional reconstruction aids in visualizing anatomic relationships. Dynamic CT or MRI flexion and extension views are difficult to perform and time-consuming, but they can provide graphic evidence of looseness.[58] MRI similarly has been helpful in showing the relationship of the neurologic structures to the bony anatomy, such as the Chiari malformation and syringomyelia.[55,58] Also, the transverse atlantal ligament can be visualized with MRI.[55]

Steel[59] called attention to the checkrein effect of the alar ligaments and how they form the second line of defense after disruption of the transverse atlantal ligament (Fig. 30–8). This

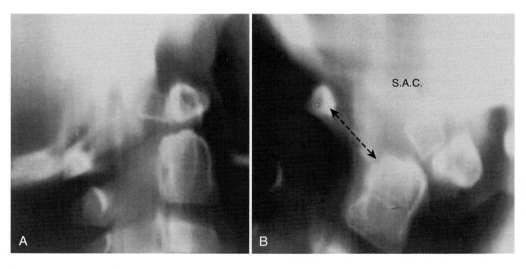

FIGURE 30–7 Lateral flexion-extension radiography of os odontoideum. **A,** Extension. **B,** Flexion. Odontoid ossicle is fixed to anterior ring of atlas and moves with it in flexion and extension and lateral slide. Space available for spinal cord (SAC) decreases with flexion, and ossicle moves into spinal canal with extension.

secondary stability no doubt plays an important role in patients with chronic atlantoaxial instability.[60] Steel's anatomic studies provided a simple rule that is helpful to physicians evaluating this area. He defined the "rule of thirds": The area of the vertebral canal at C1 can be divided into one third odontoid; one third spinal cord; and one third "space," which represents a safe zone in which displacement can occur without neurologic impingement and is roughly equivalent to the transverse diameter of the odontoid (usually 1 cm).[59]

In chronic atlantoaxial instability, it is of prime importance to recognize when the patient has exceeded the "safe zone" of Steel and enters the area of impending spinal cord compression. At this point, the second line of defense, the alar ligaments, has failed, and there is no longer a margin of safety (see Fig. 30–8).[48] Experimentally, Fielding and colleagues[48] found that after rupture of the transverse ligament, the alar ligaments are usually inadequate to prevent further displacement of C1-2 when a force similar to that which ruptured the transverse ligament is applied. Although the alar ligaments appear thick and strong, they stretch with relative ease and permit significant displacement.

McRae[33] was first to call attention to the relationship of neurologic symptoms and the sagittal diameter of the spinal canal (SAC) (see Fig. 30–4). He noted that his patients with atlanto-occipital fusion with less than 10 mm of available space behind the odontoid or atlas were always symptomatic. With the availability of more clinical data, this measurement has been more specifically defined. After an extensive review of the literature, Greenberg[34] determined that in adults spinal cord compression always occurs if the sagittal diameter of the cervical canal behind the dens is 14 mm or less. Cord compression is possible between 15 mm and 17 mm and never occurs if the distance is 18 mm or more. Variations in patient size and the presence or absence of soft tissue elements affect the clinical significance of the measurement, however. Jauregui and colleagues[56] refined these measurements further for children. MRI may be helpful in assessing the integrity of the transverse atlantal ligament.[55] In some patients, myelography has shown a ventral impingement secondary to a thick wad of radiolucent soft tissue posterior to the dysplastic odontoid and the body of the axis.[39]

Data on normal variations in sagittal and transverse diameter of the cervical spine have been collected for infants, children, and young adults.[46,61,62] As might be expected, these measurements generally are smaller than in adults and follow a predictable growth curve. Clinical significance is determined via two parameters: (1) comparison of the absolute diameter with the known norms for that vertebral level and age, and (2) comparison of successive vertebral levels within the same individual. Variations in the latter are more sensitive in determining an abnormality involving a single vertebra because there is good correlation between adjacent levels in the same child. These measurements should be readily available when evaluating the growing spine for pathologic narrowing and expansion.[63] The transparencies developed by Haworth and Keillor[61] are particularly helpful in this regard and provide an efficient screening test for assessing the transverse diameter of the spinal canal in the growing child. The sagittal diameter of

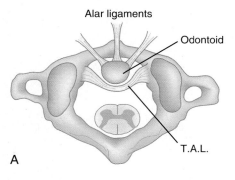

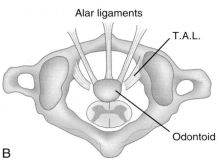

FIGURE 30–8 Atlantoaxial joint as viewed from above. **A,** Normal. **B,** Disruption of transverse atlantal ligament (TAL): Odontoid occupies safe zone of Steel. Intact alar ligaments (second line of defense) prevent spinal cord compression.

the cervical canal is largest at C1 and gradually narrows in size until C5-7. The appearance is similar to a funnel, and enlargement in the outline suggests an intraspinal mass, even if the absolute measurements do not exceed the upper limits of normal.[63]

In children, there are several normal variations in cervical spine mobility that can be alarming to physicians who are unaware of them. Cattell and Filtzer[64] called attention to the frequent (20%) finding of overriding of the anterior arch of the atlas on the odontoid with extension of the neck. This variation is due to normal elasticity of ligaments and diminishes with growth; it is not present after age 7 years. Pseudosubluxation of 3 mm of C2 on C3 can be found in more than one half of children younger than age 8 years (Fig. 30–9).[64-66] Swischuk[66] suggested a posterior cervical line that is useful in differentiating physiologic from pathologic anterior displacement of C2 on C3. Less frequently, hypermobility occurs at the C3-4 interspace. Recognition becomes particularly important when evaluating a young child who has Klippel-Feil syndrome or has undergone recent trauma.

The normal pattern of ossification of the cervical spine in children can pose problems in radiographic interpretation. At birth, the odontoid is separated from the body of the axis by a wide cartilaginous band, which represents the vestigial disc space, referred to as the *neurocentral synchondrosis* (see section on anomalies of odontoid). On the lateral radiograph, this lucent line is similar in appearance to an epiphyseal growth plate. This line may be confused with the jointlike articulation between the odontoid and the body of the atlas found in os odontoideum; this is present in nearly all children at age 3 and

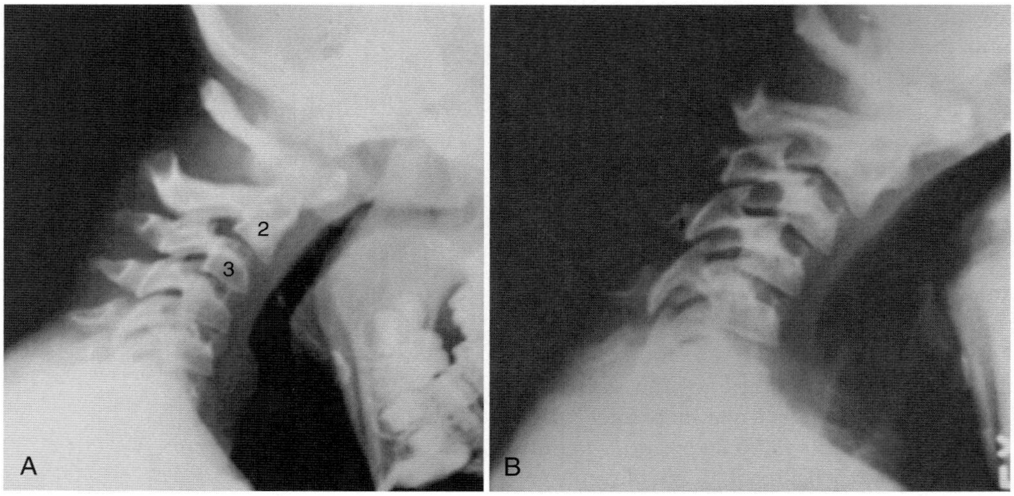

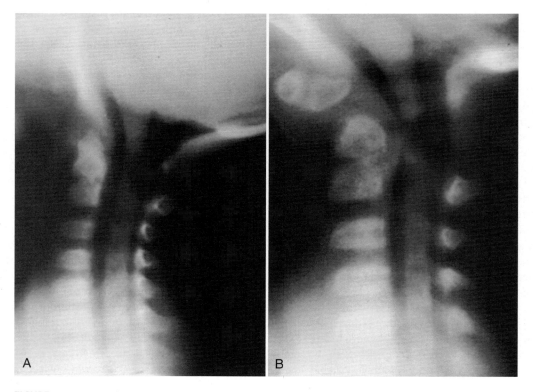

FIGURE 30–9 A, Pseudosubluxation of C2 on C3 in a child at age 5 years. **B,** At age 10, flexion view of cervical spine shows normal motion without pseudosubluxation. This normal variation can be found in more than half of children younger than age 8 years.

absent in most by age 6. Consequently, the diagnosis of os odontoideum in children must be confirmed by showing motion between the odontoid and the body of the axis. Atlantoaxial fusion may be difficult to diagnose in a young child because a significant portion of the ring of C1 is unossified at birth. There is usually a 5- to 9-mm gap posteriorly, which ossifies by age 4.[31] The anterior arch of the atlas is invisible in 80% of infants, and the entire ring may not be completely ossified until age 10 years.[31,53]

Myelography can be helpful in defining an area of constriction. In this regard, gas or water-soluble contrast agent (metrizamide) myelography should be used in preference to myelography with oil contrast media (Fig. 30–10).[33,39,67,68] CT in conjunction with metrizamide myelography is particularly

FIGURE 30–10 Normal gas myelography-polytomography. **A,** A 3-year-old dwarf presented with slightly abnormal odontoid, no atlantoaxial instability, and no neurologic signs or symptoms. **B,** Atlantoaxial instability without cord compression and myelopathy was noted in a 7-year-old dwarf with congenitally detached odontoid that dislocates forward with anterior arch of atlas. Posterior ring of atlas is absent, and posterior impingement of spinal cord against axis is avoided. (Courtesy Steven E. Kopits, MD, and Milos Perovic, MD.)

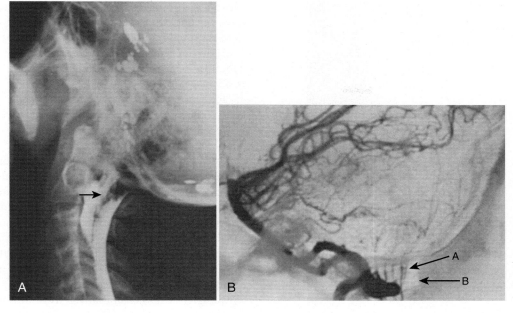

FIGURE 30–11 A 12-year-old child presented with nystagmus and cerebellar ataxia. **A,** Myelography shows Arnold-Chiari malformation with herniation of cerebellar tonsils through foramen magnum. *Arrow* indicates distal migration of tonsils. **B,** Vertebral arteriography in same patient shows inferior cerebellar vessels looping down to spinal canal. *Arrow A* indicates inferior cerebellar vessels; *arrow B* indicates posterior ring of atlas. (Courtesy Frank Lee, MD.)

helpful in evaluating children with rotational deformities or compromise of the neural canal in the upper cervical spine.[51,67,68]

MRI allows a more complete and accurate examination of the soft tissues and brainstem and assists in identifying the area of direct impingement in individuals with occipitocervical anomalies.[57] Dynamic flexion-extension MRI allows for improved selection of patients for cervical arthrodesis and allows direct determination of the need for concurrent anterior or posterior decompression of neural elements.[52,58] Surgical stabilization may be avoided or delayed in individuals with mild radiographic instability without spinal cord compromise.

Excessive motion at the occiput-C1 may lead to compression of the vertebral arteries.[53] Vertebral arteriography is helpful in evaluating patients who exhibit symptoms of transient brainstem ischemia.[24,69,70] If cerebellar herniation (Chiari malformation) is suspected, arteriography combined with myelography can show the anomaly (Fig. 30–11).[68]

Treatment

Effective treatment generally can be provided only if the exact cause of symptoms has been determined by a careful correlation of the clinical and radiologic findings. Before surgical intervention, reduction of the atlantoaxial articulation should be achieved by either positioning or traction.[28,60,65,71] Operative reduction should be avoided, if possible, because it is associated with increased morbidity and mortality rates.[72,73] The patient should be maintained in the reduced position preoperatively until spinal cord edema and local irritation resolve; this is usually accompanied by improvement of the neurologic status and often remission of symptoms. If neurologic symptoms are unchanged with reduction and rest, the physician should carefully seek other causes.

Various techniques for surgical stabilization of atlantoaxial instability have been used in pediatric patients with good results.[60,74] Sublaminar wiring, C1-2 transarticular screws, transoral decompression with posterior plating, and laminectomy with Steinmann pin occipitocervical fusion all have been reported with good results (Fig. 30–12).[28,45] Choice of surgical procedure for stabilization must be individualized based on clinical presentation and surgeon expertise.[28,71]

Too little attention has been paid in the past to occult respiratory dysfunction in patients with atlantoaxial instability.[74,75] Many patients have an unrecognized decrease in vital capacity and chronic alveolar hypoventilation as a result of the neurologic injury to the brainstem.[18,76] Similarly, gag and cough reflexes are often depressed,[74] and the patient may experience a deterioration of pulmonary function in the postoperative period.[76] Periods of apnea and respiratory distress during surgery or in the immediate postoperative period have frequently resulted in death or have required prolonged respiratory support.[76] Preoperative pulmonary evaluation can be helpful in limiting the severity of respiratory complications. If pulmonary function is significantly reduced or if gag and cough reflexes are depressed, consideration should be given to preoperative tracheostomy.[74] Equipment for mechanical respiratory support must be immediately available during the postoperative period.[76]

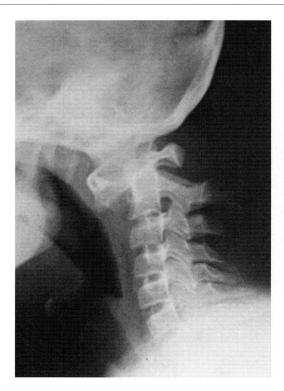

FIGURE 30–12 An 11-year-old child with Down syndrome presented with gross atlantoaxial instability. The patient's gait was clumsy. Physical examination revealed poor coordination of the extremities. There was no other evidence of motor or sensory impairment of pathologic reflexes. The patient had no symptoms referable to the cervical spine 2 years after surgical stabilization.

Laxity of Transverse Atlantal Ligament

Laxity of the transverse atlantal ligament is a diagnosis of exclusion suggested by the clinical occurrence of chronic atlantoaxial dislocation without a predisposing cause.[33] There is no history of trauma, congenital anomaly, infection, or rheumatoid arthritis to account for the radiologic finding. Most patients with this condition have the typical symptoms of atlantoaxial instability and require surgical stabilization.

Laxity of the transverse atlantal ligament is unusually common in patients with Down syndrome, with a reported incidence of 15% (Fig. 30–13).[42,77] The lesion may be found in all age groups, with no age preponderance.[42] These patients seem to have rupture or attenuation of the transverse atlantal ligament with encroachment of the safe zone of Steel (see Fig. 30–8), but at least initially they are protected by the checkrein action of the alar ligaments from spinal cord compression (see Fig. 30–13). In other words, many patients have excessive motion, but relatively few are symptomatic, and most cases are discovered only by radiologic survey.[78] If radiographs of the upper cervical spine indicate an ADI of more than 5 mm, instability is considered to be present. Usually, if symptoms are present, instability of greater than 7 to 10 mm is found. MRI can be helpful in assessing the integrity of the transverse atlantal ligament.[55]

Complete data are unavailable regarding the best way to manage this problem.[42,77,78] Very little is known about the natural history, despite radiographic examination of hundreds of children.[78] Studies have indicated that some children experience progressive looseness with time; others who manifest small degrees of instability can occasionally become stable.[42] Currently, radiographic examination on a routine basis is recommended for children with Down syndrome, particularly children who compete in athletics.[77] Any child with Down syndrome who has a musculoskeletal complaint, such as subluxing patella, dislocating hips, or unsteady gait, should be investigated. In addition, evaluation of the cervical spine should be a part of the preoperative assessment in these cases.

A patient with Down syndrome and no evidence of radiographic instability requires no activity restrictions other than avoidance of collision sports.[42-44] With current knowledge, prophylactic stabilization is not indicated. When a patient

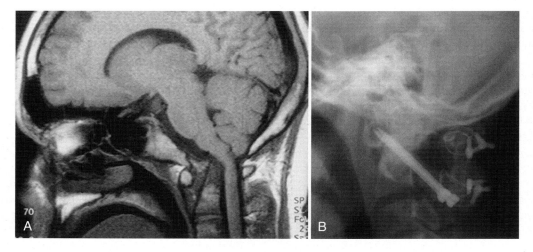

FIGURE 30–13 A 16-year-old developmentally delayed child presented with insidious onset of bilateral upper extremity hyperreflexia and gait ataxia. **A,** Sagittal T1-weighted MRI shows cervicomedullary compression and increased atlantoaxial interval. **B,** Postoperative lateral radiograph shows reduction of deformity and fixation with transarticular screws augmented with sublaminar wires and bone graft. (Adapted from Taggard DA, Menezes AH, Ryken TC: Treatment of Down's syndrome-associated craniovertebral junction anomalies. J Neurosurg Spine 93:205-213, 2000.)

develops atlantoaxial instability and is neurologically intact, any sport with the potential to stress the cervical spine should be avoided. The Special Olympics has identified gymnastics, high jump, diving, butterfly and breast stroke swimming, and pentathlon to be at-risk activities.[42] The use of a cervical collar in these patients is controversial. Progressive instability, neurologic symptoms, or both are indications for surgical stabilization.[34,42]

Occipitoatlantal Instability

Occipitoatlantal instability is a rare condition often caused by trauma or, less commonly, congenital abnormalities.[79,80] Previously, most patients did not survive this injury, but with improved resuscitative measures, the problem has been reported more frequently. Clinical and neurologic manifestations include cardiorespiratory arrest, motor weakness, quadriplegia, torticollis, pain in the neck, vertigo, and projectile vomiting.[79] Surgical stabilization is usually necessary. Anomalies of the upper cervical spine can also lead to this condition, and it has been reported in association with Down syndrome. The curvature of the occipital condyle in healthy children increases by 60% from infancy to adolescence.[80] Patients who have Down syndrome and occipitoatlantal instability fail to develop this curved architecture in the occipital condyle.[80]

Atlanto-occipital Fusion (Occipitalization, Occipitocervical Synostosis, Assimilation of Atlas)

Atlanto-occipital fusion is characterized by a partial or complete congenital union between the atlas and the base of the occiput (Fig. 30–14). It ranges from total incorporation of the atlas into the occipital bone to a bony or fibrous band uniting one small area of the atlas to the occiput.[81] Basilar impression is commonly associated with occipitocervical synostosis; other associated anomalies include Klippel-Feil syndrome, occipital vertebrae, and condylar hypoplasia.[31,32]

Occipitocervical synostosis, basilar impression, and odontoid anomalies are the most common developmental malformations of the occipitocervical junction. Incidence ranges from 1.4 to 2.5 per 1000 children.[31,82] Gholve and colleagues[32] found a predominance in boys of 80%.

Clinical Features

Most patients have an appearance similar to that in Klippel-Feil syndrome, with a short, broad neck; a low hairline; torticollis; a high scapula; and restricted neck movements.[35,37,83] The skull may be deformed and shaped like a "tower." Kyphosis and scoliosis are frequent. Other associated anomalies occasionally seen include dwarfism, funnel chest, pes cavus, syndactylies, jaw anomalies, cleft palate, congenital ear deformities, hypospadias, and sometimes genitourinary tract defects.

Neurologic symptoms do not usually occur until the 3rd or 4th decade but can manifest during childhood.[32,84] Symptoms progress in a slow, unrelenting manner and may be initiated by traumatic or inflammatory processes. Symptoms rarely begin dramatically, but they have been reported as a cause of sudden death.[85] It is difficult to explain why neurologic problems develop so late and progress so slowly in these patients. It may be that the frequently associated atlantoaxial instability progresses with age and the resultant added demands placed on this articulation, producing gradual spinal cord or vertebral artery compromise.

McRae and Barnum[83] suggested that the key to development of neurologic manifestations lies with the odontoid and its position, an indication of the degree of actual or relative

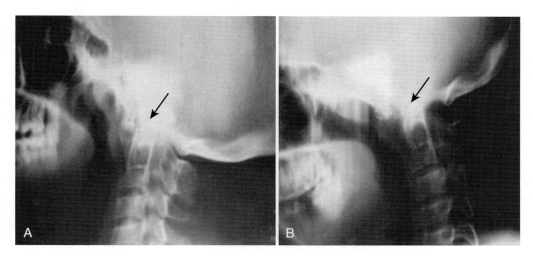

FIGURE 30–14 A 22-year-old patient presented with symptomatic atlanto-occipital fusion and hypermobile odontoid. **A** and **B**, Lateral laminagraphs in extension (**A**) and flexion (**B**) show odontoid extending well into opening of foramen magnum (McRae line); with flexion, odontoid moves posteriorly with impingement of brainstem. (Courtesy Dr. Donald L. McRae, MD.)

basilar impression. If the odontoid lies below the foramen magnum, the patient is usually asymptomatic.[33] With the decrease in vertical height of the atlas, the odontoid may project well into the foramen magnum, producing brainstem pressure, a fact well documented by autopsy.[37,38]

Anterior compression of the brainstem from the backward-projecting odontoid is most common (see Fig. 30–14). This compression produces various findings, depending on the location and the degree of pressure. Pyramidal tract signs and symptoms (spasticity, hyperreflexia, muscle weakness and wasting, and gait disturbances) are most common, but cranial nerve involvement (diplopia, tinnitus, dysphagia, and auditory disturbances) may be seen less often. Compression from the posterior lip of the foramen magnum or the constricting band of dura may disturb the posterior columns, resulting in loss of proprioception, vibration, and tactile discrimination. Nystagmus, a common occurrence, is probably due to posterior cerebellar compression.

Vascular disturbances from vertebral artery involvement may occasionally result in syncope, seizures, vertigo, and unsteady gait, among other signs and symptoms of brainstem ischemia.[15,53] Disturbed mechanics of the cervical spine may result in a dull aching pain in the posterior occiput and neck with episodic neck stiffness and torticollis.[15] Tenderness noted in the area of the posterior scalp may be due to irritation of the greater occipital nerve. The following most common signs and symptoms occur, in decreasing order of frequency: pain in the occiput and neck, vertigo, unsteady gait, paresis of the limbs, paresthesias, speech disturbances, hoarseness, double vision, syncope, auditory noise or disturbance, and interference with swallowing. Acute respiratory failure secondary to hypoventilation and sleep apnea may occur.[15] All these may be manifestations of underlying atlantoaxial instability, which, as an isolated lesion, may produce neck pain, headaches, and neurologic deficits from cord or root irritation and, rarely, sudden death.[34,73]

Radiographic Features

Standard radiographs of this area can be difficult to interpret. Tomography, CT, and MRI may be necessary to clarify the pathologic condition (see Fig. 30–14).[15,52,53,84,85] Most commonly, the anterior arch of the atlas is assimilated into the occiput, usually in association with a hypoplastic posterior arch. The condition may range from total incorporation of the atlas into the occipital bone to a bony or fibrous band uniting one small area of the atlas to the occiput. CT scans are often necessary to show bony continuity of the anterior arch of the atlas with the occiput. Posterior fusion is not usually evident because this portion of the ring may be represented only by a short bony fringe on the edge of the foramen magnum. Despite its innocuous radiologic appearance, this fringe is frequently directed downward and inward, can compromise the spinal canal posteriorly, and has been found to create a groove in the spinal cord. It is usually assumed that the assimilated atlas is fused symmetrically to the occipital opening, but several autopsy specimens have shown a posterior positioning of the atlas.[83] This position, in effect, pushes the odontoid posteriorly, narrowing the spinal canal and the space available for the spinal cord.

Ossification of the atlas proceeds from paired centers—one for each of the lateral masses. These progress posteriorly into the neural arches, which are fully ossified at birth except for a gap of 5 to 9 mm posteriorly that closes by the 4th year.[53] The anterior arch of the atlas is invisible in 80% of neonates. This area most commonly ossifies from a single center, which appears during the 1st year of life and fuses to the remainder of the atlas by the 3rd year.[31,34,53,86,87] A persistent bifid anterior and posterior arch of the atlas beyond age 4 years is observed in skeletal dysplasias, Goldenhar syndrome, Down syndrome, Conradi syndrome, and atlas assimilation.[88] In an extensive review of CT scans from 1104 patients, Senoglu and colleagues[89] found a 3.35% incidence. None had neurologic deficits or needed intervention. Rarely, hyperplasia of the posterior arch occurs and has been associated with myelopathy.[90]

There is varying loss of height of the atlas, allowing the odontoid to project upward into the foramen magnum and creating a "relative" basilar impression (see Fig. 30–14). The position of the odontoid relative to the foramen magnum was described earlier (see section on basilar impression). McRae[38,83] measured the distance from the posterior aspect of the odontoid to either the posterior arch of the atlas or the posterior lip of the foramen magnum (SAC), which was closer. He stated that a neurologic deficit would be present if this distance was less than 19 mm. This distance should be determined in flexion because this position most dramatically reduces the space available for the cord.

Flexion-extension stress films (see Fig. 30–14) often show posterior displacement of the odontoid from the anterior arch of the atlas of 12 mm.[83] Associated atlantoaxial instability has been reported to develop eventually in 50% of patients[29,31]; this is determined by measuring the distance from the anterior border of the odontoid to the posterior aspect of the anterior arch of the atlas. A distance greater than 4 mm in young children who probably have considerable cartilage present and 3 mm in older children and adults is considered pathologic.[86,87,91] The odontoid itself often has an abnormal shape and direction; it frequently is longer, and its angle with the body of the axis is directed more posteriorly.[73,83]

McRae[33] was the first to note the frequent occurrence of congenital fusion of C2-3 (70%) and C1-2 instability in patients with atlanto-occipital fusion (Fig. 30–15). This occurrence suggests that greater demands are placed on the atlantoaxial articulation, particularly in flexion and extension when the joints above and below are fused.[37,83] von Torklus and Gehle[31] noted that approximately 50% of patients develop late onset of atlantoaxial instability and the resultant potential for compromise of the spinal cord.[29]

Gholve and colleagues[32] used a morphologic classification: zone 1, a fused anterior arch; zone 2, fused lateral masses; zone 3, a fused posterior arch; and a combination of fused zones. In their study, 57% had atlantoaxial instability, with almost half of those having an associated C2-3 fusion. Spinal canal encroachment occurred in 37%, with almost half of these patients having clinical findings of myelopathy. The highest prevalence of spinal canal encroachment (63%) was noted in patients with occipitalization in zone 2.

Another commonly associated abnormality is the presence of a constricting band of dura posteriorly. This band has been found to create a groove in the spinal cord and may be the primary cause of symptoms. The band cannot be visualized on routine radiographs, and it does not correlate with the presence or absence of the posterior bony fringe of the atlas. Consequently, CT and MRI should be an integral part of the evaluation. Water-soluble contrast material (metrizamide) alone or in conjunction with CT can visualize the spinal canal and its contents. A properly performed study yields valuable information regarding the presence of a dural band; tonsillar herniation; and the size, shape, and position of the spinal cord in the spinal canal.[35,92]

Treatment

Management of this uncommon problem may be hazardous. In contrast to anomalies of the odontoid, surgical intervention carries a much higher risk of morbidity and mortality.[37,73,93] Nonoperative methods such as cervical collars, braces, plaster, and traction should be attempted initially in some patients. These methods are often helpful in patients with persistent complaints of head and neck pain and are particularly helpful if symptoms follow minor trauma or infection. If neurologic deficits are present, immobilization may achieve only temporary relief. Patients presenting with evidence of a compromised situation in the upper cervical area must take precautions not to expose themselves to undue trauma.

With anterior spinal cord signs and symptoms owing to an unstable atlantoaxial complex, an occiput-to-C2 fusion is suggested, with preliminary traction to attempt reduction, if necessary. If reduction is possible and there are no neurologic signs, surgical intervention carries an improved prognosis.[34,37,73] Operative reduction should be avoided because this has frequently resulted in death.[72,73]

Transoral resection of the odontoid should be considered if there is irreducible ventral compression.[28,94] Resection of the odontoid through an anterior approach may destabilize the upper cervical spine. In a large study, Dickman and colleagues[95] noted that 11 of 19 patients (40%) developed craniovertebral junction instability after transoral removal of the odontoid, 8 of whom did not have clinical or radiographic evidence of instability preoperatively. Instability was more common if there was a congenital bony malformation or if the patient required posterior decompression for an associated condition, such as Chiari malformation or syrinx.[95]

Posterior signs and symptoms and myelographic evidence of bony or dural compression, depending on the degree of neurologic involvement, may be indications for a posterior decompression and stabilization of the occiput to C2.[71,96-99] Satisfactory occipital cervical stabilization and fusion can be obtained by using a halo brace in the postoperative period.[98] Internal fixation can facilitate postoperative management for certain patients, however. Internal fixation of the occipital cervical junction can pose problems, and several fixation techniques have been found helpful.[27,28,71] The addition of a cervical

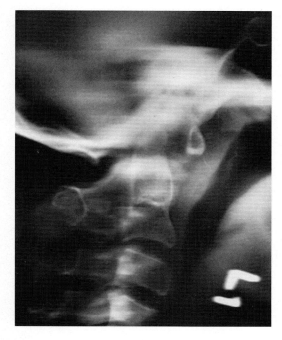

FIGURE 30–15 A 23-year-old man presented with Klippel-Feil syndrome, ataxic gait, hyperreflexia, and a history of several episodes of unconsciousness. Lateral laminagraph of cervical spine and base of skull shows C2-3 fusion and fusion of ring at C1 to opening of foramen magnum (occipitalization). Odontoid is hypermobile. Patients with this pattern of fusion are at great risk. With aging, odontoid may become hypermobile, and space available for spinal cord posteriorly may be compromised.

laminectomy may increase C1-2 instability or lead to the late development of a cervical kyphosis, particularly if the laminectomy involves several levels.[96,100] In these cases, the patient should be managed expectantly with appropriate internal stabilization or a halo vest.[82,96]

Anomalies of Ring of C1

Anomalies of the posterior arch can be characterized as median clefts or hypoplasia. Geipel[101] found defects in the posterior arch, most of which were median clefts, in 4% of 1613 autopsies. Currarino and colleagues[102] developed a classification scheme (types A to E) for congenital defects of the posterior arch of C1 (Fig. 30–16). Greater than 90% are the type A *median cleft* variant. These patients are usually asymptomatic, and their anomaly is incidentally identified on radiographic studies.[89] Types C and D are accompanied by a free-floating posterior tubercle. These patients may experience neck pain and neurologic symptoms before discovery of the anomaly. The free posterior tubercle has been shown to move with neck extension and in some cases may migrate anteriorly and traumatize the spinal cord with neck extension. MRI studies have shown signal abnormality of the posterior spinal cord at the C1-2 level consistent with this mechanism of injury (Fig. 30–17).[102]

Dubousset[103] called attention to a previously unrecognized problem with the ring of C1, the hemiatlas. Although there had been an occasional case report, Dubousset[103] presented

Type

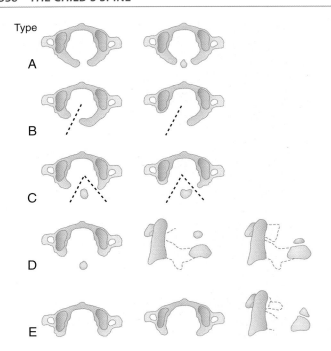

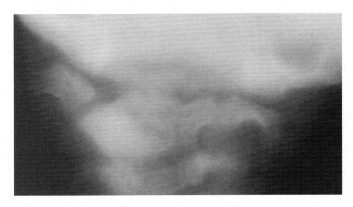

FIGURE 30–18 Absence of C1 facet in a 5-year-old child with severe, progressive torticollis. Laminagraph shows hemiatlas, with complete absence of left portion of C1 ring. (Courtesy Dr. Luther C. Fisher III, MD.)

FIGURE 30–16 Classification system for posterior C1 ring anomalies. *Type A* is small midline failure of fusion. *Type B* defects are unilateral clefts of variable size, ranging from small gap to complete absence of hemiarch. *Type C* indicates bilateral defects with preservation of most of dorsal arch. *Type D* is complete absence of posterior arch with retained, midline tubercle. *Type E* is complete posterior arch and tubercle deficiency. (Adapted from Currarino G, Rollins N, Diehl JT: Congenital defects of the posterior arch of the atlas. Spine 47:267-271, 2000.)

the first large study to review the problem in depth. He reported 17 patients in whom he was able to document absence of the facet of C1, which led to a severe and progressive torticollis in young children (Fig. 30–18). Initially, the deformity is flexible and can be passively corrected. As the child ages,

the torticollis becomes more severe and eventually fixed. Radiographic diagnosis using tomography or CT has been helpful in identifying this deformity. Use of traction to align the head and neck at the time of the study assists in highlighting the problem. If the patient is passively correctable, a single posterior fusion, occiput to C2, is performed. A halo cast is applied postoperatively to maintain the head in a satisfactory alignment until the fusion is complete.

Although the time at which this becomes a fixed deformity was not defined, Dubousset[103] reported good results in teenagers. This deformity can accompany Klippel-Feil syndrome with anomalies of the lower cervical spine as well. Dubousset[103] found an increased incidence of anomalies of the vertebral vessels in these children and suggested arteriographic evaluation before the use of traction or surgical intervention, which could further compromise a precarious blood supply to the midbrain and spinal cord.

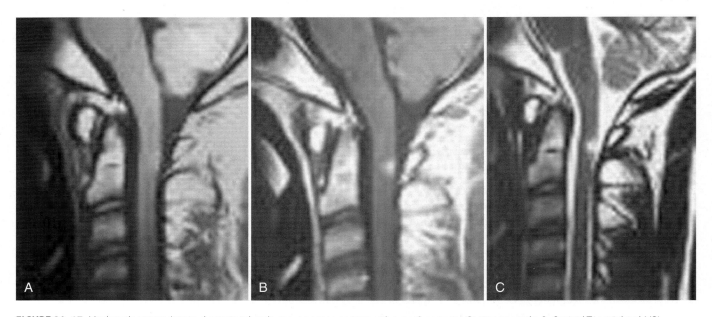

FIGURE 30–17 Myelopathy secondary to dynamic tubercle movement in patient with type C posterior C1 ring anomaly. **A,** Sagittal T1-weighted MRI. **B,** Sagittal T1-weighted MRI with contrast medium enhancement. **C,** Sagittal T2-weighted MRI of cord contusion at C1-2 level. (Adapted from Currarino G, Rollins N, Diehl JT: Congenital defects of the posterior arch of the atlas. Spine 47:267-271, 2000.)

Anomalies of Odontoid (Dens)

Congenital anomalies of the odontoid can lead to an unstable atlantoaxial complex, with potential neurologic sequelae and death owing to spinal cord pressure.[50] Several gradations or variations of anomalies of the odontoid exist, ranging from aplasia (complete absence) to hypoplasia (partial absence) to os odontoideum (Fig. 30–19).

Aplasia or agenesis of the odontoid is a complete absence of development. Hypoplasia is a partially developed odontoid, ranging in size from a short, stubby, peglike projection to an odontoid of almost normal size.[104] Os odontoideum is an anomaly in which the odontoid process is divided by a wide transverse gap, leaving the apical segment without support

from the base.[105] Distinguishing aplasia or hypoplasia from os odontoideum is of limited importance because these anomalies usually lead to atlantoaxial instability and the clinical signs, symptoms, and treatment are identical. The only distinctive features are radiographic.

Incidence

The frequency of these anomalies is unknown; similar to many anomalies that may be asymptomatic, they are probably more common than is recognized. They are often incidental findings or are seen in patients sustaining trauma or with symptoms sufficient to require radiographic investigation.

In the authors' experience, aplasia is extremely rare. Many previous reports have confused aplasia for hypoplasia, and, as

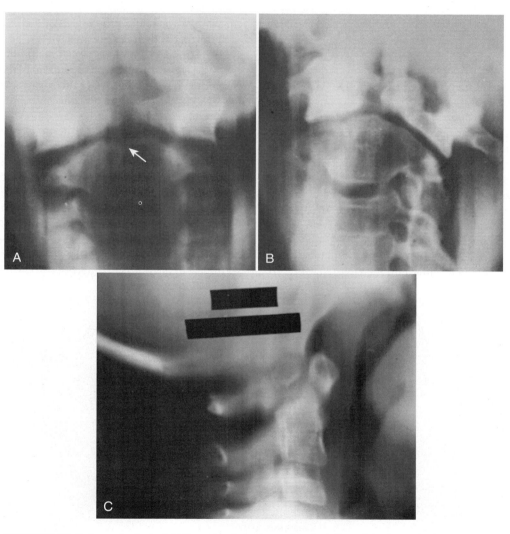

FIGURE 30–19 A, Agenesis of odontoid (open-mouth laminagraphic view). Note slight depression between superior articular facets of axis (*arrow*). A short bony remnant in this position is termed *odontoid hypoplasia*. **B,** Os odontoideum (open-mouth laminagraphic view). Os odontoideum is an oval or round ossicle, usually approximately half the normal size of odontoid, with smooth cortical border of uniform thickness. Jointlike articulation between os odontoideum and body of axis appears radiologically as wide radiolucent gap and usually extends above level of superior facets. **C,** Lateral radiograph of os odontoideum. Odontoid ossicle is fixed to anterior ring of atlas and moves with it in flexion and extension and lateral slide. A short bony remnant usually projects superiorly from body of C2.

previously emphasized, aplasia probably has been a misnomer because it almost never describes an associated absence of the portion below the articular facets that contributes to the body of the axis. Hypoplasia and os odontoideum are infrequently reported and can be considered rare.[54,104,106-109] With more recent awareness, these lesions are being recognized more commonly, however, than previous literature might indicate—especially os odontoideum.[47] In a large series reported by Wollin,[109] the average age of diagnosis was 30 years, but in a later series it was 18.9 years, suggesting earlier recognition.[47] An increasing number of children with these anomalies are being discovered.

In conditions such as Down syndrome, Morquio syndrome, Klippel-Feil syndrome, and some skeletal dysplasias, odontoid anomalies in association with ligamentous laxity producing atlantoaxial instability are much more common than in the general population.[40,42,50,110-115] Associated regional malformations may occur, but in contrast to many congenital cervical anomalies, they are rare.[50,104,108,116]

Development of Odontoid

The body of the odontoid is derived from the mesenchyme of the first cervical sclerotome and is actually the centrum of the first cervical vertebra, which becomes separated from the atlas during development to fuse with the remainder of the axis.[82,114,117] The apex of the odontoid process is derived from the mesenchyme of the most caudal occipital sclerotome or proatlas. Ossification of these two segments of the odontoid proceeds along separate lines.

Between the 1st and 5th prenatal months, the dens begins to ossify from two centers, one on each side of the midline. By the time of birth, they have fused into a single mass.[86,87,91] Occasionally, the right and left halves of the odontoid are not fused at birth, and a longitudinal midline cleft may be seen.

At birth, the tip of the odontoid has not ossified, is V-shaped, and is known as a *dens bicornis* (Fig. 30–20). A separate ossification center within the "V," known as a *summit ossification center* or *ossiculum terminale*, usually appears at age 3 years and fuses with the remainder of the dens by age 12.[86,87,118] Cattell and Filtzer[64] found an ossiculum terminale in 26% of 70 normal children 5 to 11 years old.

An ossiculum terminale may never appear or may occasionally fail to fuse with the dens; it is then called an *ossiculum terminale persistens*. It is occasionally discernible as either a cyst or an area of increased density. These developmental anomalies are of little clinical significance.[50,119] Sherk and Nicholson[114] reported a rare case of quadriplegia and death, however, in a child with Down syndrome that was directly attributable to atlantoaxial instability secondary to an ossiculum terminale. A similar occurrence in an otherwise normal child has been reported.[120] The ossiculum terminale usually is firmly bound to the main body of the dens by cartilage and consequently is seldom the source of instability.

At birth, the dens is separated from the body of the axis by a cartilaginous band (see Fig. 30–20) that represents the epiphyseal growth plate. This plate does not run across the base of the dens at the level of the superior articular facets of the axis but lies well below this level within the body of the axis (see Fig. 30–20B). The part of the odontoid below the articular facets contributes to the body of the axis. On the open-mouth view, the odontoid fits like a "cork in a bottle," lying sandwiched between the neural arches (see Fig. 30–20B). This epiphyseal line is present in almost all children by age 3 years and in 50% of children by age 4, but it is absent in most by age 6.[64,91] It rarely persists into adolescence and adult life. If present, the line is not seen at the base of the dens where a fracture would be anticipated but lies well below the level of the superior articular facets within the body of the axis. In a young child, the unossified portions of the odontoid may give

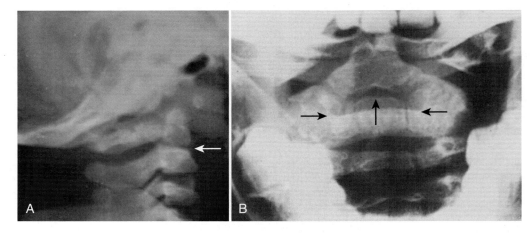

FIGURE 30–20 A, Radiograph of a 6-month-old newborn. Odontoid is normally formed and recognizable on routine radiographs at birth but is separated from the body of the axis by a broad cartilaginous band (*arrow*), similar in appearance to an epiphyseal plate. It represents the vestigial disc space and is referred to as *neurocentral synchondrosis*. **B,** Neurocentral synchondrosis is not at anatomic base of dens, at the level of superior articular facets of axis. This open-mouth view shows that embryologic base of odontoid is below articular facets and contributes a substantial portion to body of axis. This radiolucent line is present in nearly all children at age 3 years and in 50% by age 4; it is absent in most individuals by age 5.

the false impression of odontoid hypoplasia. Similarly, one may erroneously conclude that the child has C1-2 instability because the anterior arch of the atlas commonly may slide upward and may protrude beyond the ossified portion of the odontoid[64] on the lateral extension radiograph (Fig. 30–21).

The blood supply to the odontoid is from two sources. The vertebral arteries provide an anterior ascending artery and a posterior ascending artery that arise at the level of C3 and pass ventral and dorsal to the body of the axis and the odontoid, anastomosing in an apical arcade in the region of the alar ligaments. These arteries supply small penetrating branches to the body of the axis and the odontoid. Lateral to the apex of the odontoid, the anterior ascending arteries and apical arcade receive anastomotic derivatives from the carotids by way of the base of the skull and the alar ligaments. This curious arrangement of the blood supply is necessary because of the embryologic development and anatomic function of the odontoid. The transient neurocentral synchondrosis between the odontoid and the axis prevents the development of any significant vascular channels between the two structures. The body of the odontoid is surrounded entirely by synovial joint cavities, and its fixed position relative to the rotation of the atlas precludes vascularization by direct branches from the vertebral arteries at the C1 segmental level.

Etiology and Pathogenesis

A congenital etiology for os odontoideum has been assumed, and two theories have been advanced:

1. Failure of fusion of the apex or ossiculum terminale to the odontoid—this is unlikely because the fragment is too small and never approximates the size of the os odontoideum.

2. Failure of fusion of the odontoid to the axis—this too is doubtful because one would expect a crater or depression of C2 because a substantial portion of C2 is derived from the odontoid, and this has not been reported.

There is more often an associated short, stubby projection or hypoplastic odontoid remnant in the area of the odontoid base.[105,109] Hypoplasia and os odontoideum can be acquired secondary to trauma or, rarely, infection.[33,47,109,118,121-123] Several cases of "os odontoideum" that developed several years after trauma when a normal odontoid was initially present have been reported (see Fig. 30–21).[41,122-124] Most patients have a significant episode of trauma before the diagnosis of os odontoideum.[47]

Fielding and colleagues[47] suggested that most evidence favors an unrecognized fracture in the region of the base of the odontoid as the most common cause and less often a congenital origin. They postulated that after fracture of the odontoid there may be only slight separation of the fragments, but, with time, contracture of the alar ligaments, which attach to the tip of the odontoid, exerts a distraction force that pulls the fragment away from the base and closer to their origin at the occiput (Fig. 30–22). The blood supply to the odontoid is precarious because it passes up along the sides of the odontoid, is easily traumatized, and contributes to poor fracture healing or callus formation that may retard retraction of the fragment. The position of the odontoid adjacent to the ring of C1 is maintained by the intact transverse atlantal ligament.

The blood supply to the fragment is maintained by the proximal arterial arcade, from the carotid to the alar ligaments, and may be sufficient to maintain only a portion of the odontoid. Similarly, the blood supply to the proximal portion of the odontoid can be interrupted by excessive traction on

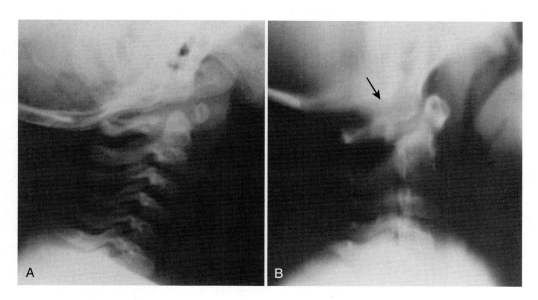

FIGURE 30–21 A, Lateral radiograph of a 5-year-old boy who at age 2 years fell from a sofa shows normal-appearing odontoid and cervical spine. The child complained of pain in neck and occiput and presented with torticollis. Symptoms and signs gradually resolved over 1 month. **B,** The child was asymptomatic until age 5, when over a period of 6 months he developed increasing neck pain and stiffness without neurologic findings. Radiographs showed os odontoideum and 7 mm of motion with flexion-extension. The patient subsequently underwent C1-2 stabilization.

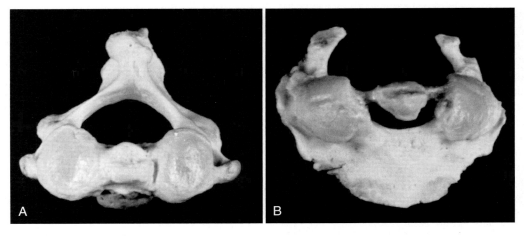

FIGURE 30–22 A, Anatomic specimen of os odontoideum from a 17-year-old boy with multiple congenital anomalies who died of renal disease. Previous bony attachment of odontoid to axis was rough and blunted. Fibrocartilage pseudarthrosis was between os odontoideum and C2. **B,** Occiput and occipital joints, with os odontoideum suspended between facets. Transverse ligament was intact but loosened during preparation of specimen. Alar ligaments remain attached to tip of os odontoideum. Ligaments are shortened and appear to have pulled residual odontoid tip closer to their origin on occiput. Os odontoideum was firmly attached by soft tissue to occiput and ring of C1 and moved freely with these structures on C2. Foramen magnum is incomplete posteriorly. Posterior ring of C1 (not pictured) was intact and otherwise normal in its appearance. Spinal cord was narrowed and attenuated at level of C1.

these ligaments.[47] A familial form[125] and os odontoideum in identical twins with no history of trauma have been reported.[126,127] It is probable that congenital and post-traumatic forms of hypoplasia and os odontoideum exist.[115] Failure of fusion of the apex of the odontoid (derived from the proatlas) to the main body of the atlas (derived from the first cervical sclerotome) is thought to result in the congenital form of os odontoideum.

The free ossicle of the os odontoideum usually appears fixed to the anterior arch of the atlas and moves with it in flexion and extension (see Fig. 30–7).[49,115] Instability can reduce the SAC but not the ADI.[30] The instability may be predominantly anterior or posterior or grossly unstable in all directions.[47,49,60] In a group of patients requiring surgery, the average displacement was 11 mm.

There is controversy regarding the presence of associated bony anomalies in the area of the hypoplastic dens or os odontoideum. In the authors' experience, these changes are occasionally present, but with improved awareness they will undoubtedly be found more often. The posterior arch of C1 may be hypoplastic, whereas the anterior arch is hypertrophied.[34,49,54] Hypertrophy of the C1 anterior arch can be a useful sign of a chronic pathologic condition of C1-2.[53,115,128] If the posterior ring of C1 is narrow and there is abnormal anterior displacement of C1, there is less available space for the cord and an increased danger of neurologic sequelae.

Clinical Features

Patients may present clinically with no symptoms, local neck symptoms, transitory episodes of paresis after trauma, or frank myelopathy secondary to cord compression.[50,73,129] Minor trauma is commonly associated with the onset of symptoms, often of sufficient degree to warrant radiologic evaluation of the cervical spine. Symptoms may be mechanical owing to local irritation of the atlantoaxial articulation, such as neck pain, torticollis, or headache. Neurologic symptoms are due to C1-2 displacement and spinal cord compression. An important factor differentiating os odontoideum from other anomalies of the occipitovertebral junction is that these patients seldom have symptoms referable to cranial nerves[107] because the area of the spinal cord impingement is below the foramen magnum.

If clinical manifestations are limited to neck pain and torticollis (local joint irritation) without neurologic involvement (40% of cases),[49,106] the prognosis is excellent.[47,107,130,131] Similarly, patients who exhibit only transient weakness of the extremities and dysesthesia after trauma usually have complete return of function. Patients in whom there is an insidious onset and slowly progressive neurologic impairment have a greater potential for permanent deficit.[47,116] Sudden death has been reported.[108] Damage may be mixed, with involvement of the anterior and the posterior spinal cord structures. Weakness and ataxia are more common complaints than sensory loss. Spasticity, increased deep tendon reflexes, clonus, loss of proprioception, and sphincter disturbances in various combinations have all been described, however.[49]

A few patients may have symptoms and signs of cerebral and brainstem ischemia, seizures, mental deterioration, syncope, vertigo, and visual disturbances.[60,117,131,132] In these patients, there typically is a paucity of cervical spinal cord signs and symptoms, and it is presumed that the patients are experiencing vertebral artery compression at the foramen magnum or just below it.[133-135] The diagnosis can be confusing, and many patients are misdiagnosed or thought to have progressive neurologic illness. Whenever Friedreich ataxia, multiple sclerosis, or other unexplained neurologic complaint is encountered, survey of the occipitocervical junction is suggested.

Radiographic Features

Recommended radiographic views are open-mouth, anteroposterior, lateral, flexion-extension, and CT reconstructions.[42] Dynamic flexion-extension CT scans are valuable because plain films do not always show the anomaly or the extent of motion (Fig. 30–23; see Fig. 30–7).

Cineradiography has been valuable for understanding odontoid anomalies, particularly anomalies that cause atlantoaxial instability,[129,136] but owing to high radiation exposure it has been largely replaced by dynamic CT scans in flexion and extension and CT reconstruction.[51,57] Most children with these lesions have a predominance of either anterior or posterior instability, but these can exist together.[49]

Normal Variations

At birth, the normal odontoid can be visualized in the lateral view with its epiphyseal plate (see Fig. 30–20). A mistaken impression of hypoplasia may be given by a lateral extension radiograph because the anterior arch of the atlas may slide upward and protrude beyond the ossified tip of the dens, especially in very young patients.[137]

Agenesis or Hypoplasia of Odontoid

Agenesis or hypoplasia of odontoid is an extremely rare anomaly that may be recognized from birth onward and is best seen in the open-mouth view, which is sometimes difficult to obtain in infancy (see Fig. 30–19). The diagnostic feature is the absence of the basilar portion of the odontoid, which normally dips down into and contributes to the body of the axis. This basilar portion is well below the level of the superior articular facets of the axis. The lateral view is of little help in distinguishing this anomaly from hypoplasia.

The most common form of hypoplasia manifests as a short, stubby peg of odontoid projecting just above the lateral facet articulations (see Fig. 30–19). Tomography is necessary to confirm whether an os odontoideum is present in addition to the hypoplasia.

In patients with multiple anomalies, the usual radiographic views are not always reliable in confirming the presence or absence of an odontoid. Similarly, in patients with abnormal bone, such as in Morquio syndrome and spondyloepiphyseal dysplasia,[50] the odontoid may be present but dysplastic, blending with the surrounding abnormal bone, and cannot be differentiated. In these situations, good results have been obtained by using lateral laminagraphic techniques (see Fig. 30–23) or dynamic CT scans in flexion and extension to ascertain the stability of the atlantoaxial articulation. The extension view should not be ignored. Many patients have been found with significant posterior subluxation.[47,54] Giannestras and colleagues[54] reported a youngster who became quadriparetic from prolonged hyperextension while lying prone watching television.

Os Odontoideum

In os odontoideum, there is a jointlike articulation between the odontoid and the body of the axis that appears radiologically as a wide radiolucent gap (see Fig. 30–19B and C). This gap may be confused with the normal neurocentral

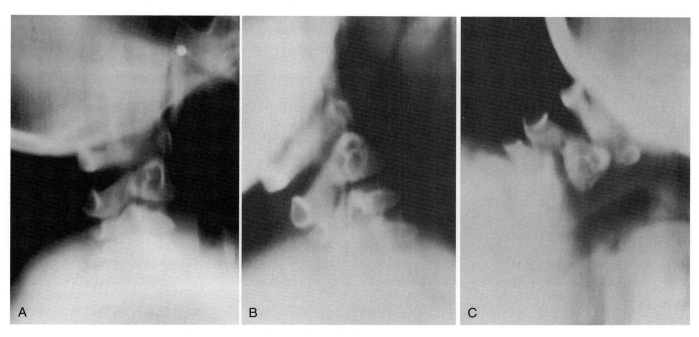

FIGURE 30–23 A 7-year-old child was diagnosed with spondyloepiphyseal dysplasia. **A,** Odontoid was discovered to be absent in this patient. **B** and **C,** Lateral laminagraphs show stable atlantoaxial articulation in extension (**B**) and flexion (**C**). The patient was neurologically normal.

synchondrosis (see Fig. 30–19) before age 5 years. In children, the diagnosis of os odontoideum is confirmed by showing motion between the odontoid and the body of the axis. In adults, the diagnosis of os odontoideum is suggested by observing a radiolucent defect between the dens and the body of the axis.

The radiologic appearance of os odontoideum may be similar to a traumatic nonunion, and often they cannot be differentiated.[33,109] In os odontoideum, the gap between the free ossicle and the axis usually extends above the level of the superior facets and is wide with a smooth edge. The ossicle is usually approximately one half the normal size of the odontoid and is round or oval, and the cortex is of uniform thickness. In traumatic nonunion, the gap between the fragments is characteristically narrow and irregular and frequently extends into the body of the axis below the level of the superior facets of the axis. The bone fragments appear to "match," and there is no marginal cortex at the level of the fracture or the rounded-off appearance found with os odontoideum.[118] The odontoid ossicle is fixed firmly to the anterior ring of the atlas and moves with it in flexion, extension, and lateral slide. The anterior portion of the atlas is usually hypertrophied, and the posterior portion of the ring may be hypoplastic or absent.[47,107,128]

Recommended radiographic views are open-mouth and lateral flexion-extension views. The literature supports that plain radiographs are sufficient to establish the diagnosis of os odontoideum. Spierings and Braakman[138] and Watanabe and colleagues[129] studied flexion-extension radiographs in patients with os odontoideum and attempted to correlate radiographic measurements with myelopathy. The degree of C1-2 instability measured by anteroposterior translation did not correlate with neurologic deficits, but the space available for the cord with neck extension (SAC) was significantly smaller in the myelopathic group. A critical anteroposterior diameter for cervical myelopathy was identified as 13 mm.[129,138]

CT reconstructions are indicated when routine views are unsatisfactory in showing the anomaly. Lateral flexion-extension stress views should be conducted voluntarily by patients, particularly patients with a neurologic deficit. The degree of anteroposterior displacement of the atlas on the axis should be documented (Fig. 30–24). The os odontoideum moves with the ring of C1, and consequently measurements of its relationship to C1 are of little value. Measurements can be made using a line projected superiorly from the posterior border of the body of the axis to a line projected inferiorly from the posterior border of the anterior arch of the atlas. Measurements greater than 3 mm should be considered pathologic. Most symptomatic patients exhibit significant instability.[47] In a large series reported by Fielding and colleagues,[47] the average measurement was 1 cm; most were either anterior or posterior, but some were unstable in all directions.[129]

When instability has been long-standing, it becomes multidirectional, and the C1-2 articulation is very unstable.[129] Watanabe and colleagues[129] noted that patients who have more than 20 degrees of sagittal plane rotation have a higher rate of myelopathy (86%), and patients with myelopathy have a high rate of instability (40%). The greater the sagittal plane rotation and looseness, the more likely is spinal cord compression.

CT scan can help to define the anatomy of the craniocervical junction, including the completeness of the atlas ring and the position of the transverse foramina at C1 and C2. CT scan has also been shown to aid in distinguishing os odontoideum from a post-traumatic odontoid nonunion (Fig. 30–25).[139]

MRI is helpful for evaluating the SAC. MRI studies have shown a direct correlation between cord signal abnormality and the degree of myelopathy measured clinically.[140] Dynamic MRI as described by Hughes and colleagues[141] allows direct visualization of motion of the os odontoideum, atlas, and axis and surrounding motion throughout the full range of motion of the cervical spine (Fig. 30–26). New open MRI

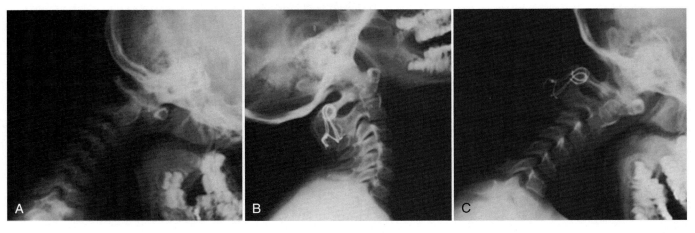

FIGURE 30–24 A 7-year-old child had a 1-year history of peculiar posturing and neck stiffness. **A,** Flexion radiograph showed os odontoideum and subluxation of C1-2. Degree of anteroposterior displacement of atlas on axis should be documented. Os odontoideum moves with ring of C1, and consequently measurements of its relationship to C1 are of little value. Measurements can be made using a line projected inferiorly from posterior border of anterior arch of atlas. **B** and **C,** Extension (**B**) and flexion (**C**) radiographs after posterior stabilization. Reduction must be accomplished before surgery; if wire stabilization is selected, care must be taken to avoid further flexion of neck during surgery.

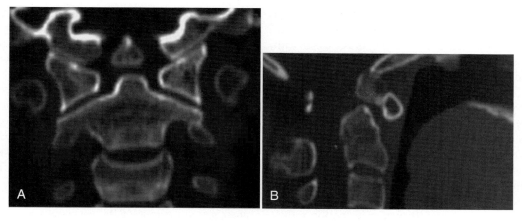

FIGURE 30–25 A and **B,** Coronal (**A**) and sagittal (**B**) CT scans of upper cervical spine clearly show os odontoideum.

configurations allow analysis of the cervical spine in the physiologic upright position, supporting the weight of the head; this may assist in identifying subtle pathology that is not apparent in the nonphysiologic, supine position.

Treatment

Patients with congenital anomalies of the odontoid lead a precarious existence. The concern is that a trivial insult superimposed on an already weakened and compromised structure may be catastrophic. In the authors' experience, patients with these problems either have or develop gross atlantoaxial instability and with it the possibility of progressive myelopathies or even death.[49]

The natural history of os odontoideum is variable, and predictive factors for instability have not been identified.[49] Indications for surgical stabilization include an os odontoideum in association with occipitocervical pain or os odontoideum with myelopathy. Other factors that may assist in surgical decision making are the severity of C1-2 instability and other associated osseous anomalies. Neural decompression must address anterior bony or soft tissue impingement of the spinal cord or compression posteriorly from the dorsal arch of C1.

Patients with local symptoms or transient myelopathies may expect recovery, at least temporarily.[107,130,131] Cervical traction or immobilization may be helpful in such circumstances. Surgical stabilization is indicated if there is neurologic

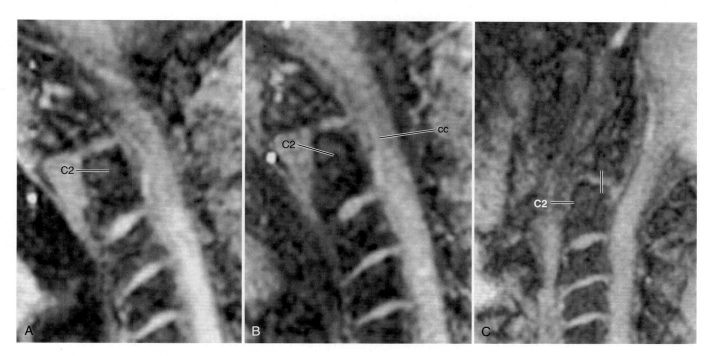

FIGURE 30–26 Dynamic MRI of cervical spine showing cord compression in a patient with os odontoideum. **A,** Sagittal MR in neutral position. **B,** Cervical spine in flexion shows retrolisthesis of os with cord compression. **C,** Cervical spine in extension shows reduction of os to C2 body and relief of cord compression. (Adapted from Hughes TB, Richman JD, Rothfus WE: Diagnosis of os odontoideum using kinematic MRI. Spine 24:715-718, 1999.)

involvement (even if transient), if there is instability of 10 mm or more in flexion and extension, if there is progressive instability, or if there are persistent neck complaints associated with atlantoaxial instability.

Considerable controversy exists over the role of prophylactic stabilization in asymptomatic patients with instability.[49,65,107,130,135] Surgical treatment is not required for every patient in whom an os odontoideum is identified. Patients who have no neurologic symptoms or instability at C1-2 can be managed with periodic observation. The lack of C1-2 instability at initial diagnosis does not guarantee that instability will not develop in these patients, however, or that they are not at higher risk for spinal cord injury with trauma. For this reason, longitudinal follow-up with flexion-extension radiographs of these patients is recommended.

Klimo and colleagues[49] recommended surgical stabilization for all patients with os odontoideum. The safety of stability, and with it the ability to lead a normal active life, must cause one to weigh the possible complications of surgery against the catastrophic dangers of instability with secondary cord pressure. In the pediatric age group, it may be difficult or impossible to curtail activity, even in the presence of marked instability.[47,60,142] If possible, reduction of the atlantoaxial articulation must be accomplished before surgery either by careful positioning of the patient or by skull traction. Manipulative reduction during surgery is discouraged because it has proved extremely hazardous and may result in respiratory distress, apnea, or death.[65] Ideally, the patient should be maintained in the reduced position several days before surgery to allow recovery of neurologic function and to lessen spinal cord irritation. When fusion is undertaken, regardless of the indication, preoperative halo traction is often required to achieve reduction, which may have to be continued during surgery and postoperatively until transfer to a suitable immobilization device.[107,143]

The suggested method of stabilization is posterior cervical fusion of C1-2. Posterior C1-2 arthrodesis in the treatment of os odontoideum provides effective stabilization in most patients. Posterior Gallie and Brook sublaminar wiring techniques with iliac crest bone graft and halo immobilization have been reported with favorable fusion results.[71,144-153] This method is not without risk because slight flexion is often required to pass the wire beneath the posterior ring of the atlas, and it can have tragic results.[107,144] When attempting posterior stabilization using a wire technique in small children, the spinous process of C2 may be small or poorly developed or not yet completely ossified. In this situation, a threaded Kirschner wire through the spinous process, as described by Mah and colleagues,[154] can be very helpful in improving the stability of the wiring technique.

In a patient with a marginally functioning neurologic status, it may be wiser to perform an occiput-to-C2 arthrodesis and plan to maintain immobilization in extension during the postoperative period.[107] In this regard, the halo vest is helpful. Incomplete development of the posterior ring of C1 is uncommon but is reported to occur with increased frequency in patients with os odontoideum.[47] The completeness of the C1 arch should be evaluated preoperatively because a large gap may preclude wire fixation.[148] If wire fixation is employed, excessive tightening of the wire should be avoided. The articulation is frequently unstable in flexion and extension, and posterior dislocations may occur, owing to overcorrection, with disastrous results.

In patients who have a highly mobile but reducible C1-2 articulation, several authors have reported good results using transarticular screws.[41,71,144,149,150,152] Atlantoaxial transarticular screws have been shown to be feasible in pediatric patients, and the superior biomechanical stability may eliminate the need for prolonged postoperative halo vest immobilization (see Fig. 30–12).[149,155] A preoperative CT scan with reconstruction views is essential with this technique to define the C1-2 anatomy and course of the vertebral arteries.[41] An aberrant path of the vertebral vessels that are at risk with screw placement is a contraindication for the procedure.[41] Other techniques have been described. Lateral mass screws and transarticular screws have been used with good success being reported.[152,156-158] Lateral mass screws and fixation to the skull occiput have comparable strength.[156] The carotid artery can be hit with a lateral mass screw.[159]

With transarticular fixation of C1-2, the lamina of C1 can be removed without the necessity of extending the fusion to the occiput. The cervical fusion of C1-2 is generally reliable and safe; however, in patients with spinal cord compression, fixed dislocations, or congenital ligamentous laxity, particularly in patients with Down syndrome, extra caution should be employed.[148,160] Smith and colleagues[160] reported significant problems with C1-2 stabilization, particularly in patients who are very unstable or have a myelopathy. Patients with failed fusions or irreducible dislocations were at high risk for perioperative neurologic complications.

Patients in whom the C1-2 dislocation is unreducible after an adequate trial of traction pose a difficult management problem.[161] In this situation, posterior decompression by laminectomy has been associated with increased morbidity and mortality.[107] In addition, posterior decompression alone may potentiate C1-2 instability, and if performed it must be accompanied by occiput-to-C2 arthrodesis.[47,161] For patients with no neurologic deficit, a simple in situ posterior fusion is the least hazardous procedure. If reduction of the C1-2 dislocation is considered necessary or if the clinical situation precludes posterior stabilization, an anterior approach should be considered.[28,34,162] The lateral retropharyngeal approach described by Whitesides and McDonald[162] provides anterior exposure of the C1-2 articulation adequate to perform decompression, reduction, and stabilization. This route may be used in place of the transoral or mandibular and tongue-splitting approaches, which are associated with an increased incidence of infection.[28,162] Associated myelopathy can be addressed with reduction of the deformity, dorsal or ventral decompression, and occipitocervical fusion.

A common clinical problem is differentiation between a fractured odontoid and os odontoideum. Discovery is usually made after trauma in both conditions, and an accurate diagnosis may be impossible by radiographic techniques alone. In this situation, a period of immobilization (skull traction or cast) is recommended. Overdistraction, particularly in children, should be avoided because it can lead to os odontoideum.[47] If the lesion represents an acute fracture, healing usually occurs. If a congenital or traumatic nonunion is present, surgical stabilization is necessary if atlantoaxial instability is shown.

Summary

Anomalous development of the odontoid is uncommon; the clinical significance lies in its potential to produce serious neurologic sequelae owing to atlantoaxial instability. Although there are several recognized variations (aplasia, hypoplasia, and os odontoideum), clinically they share the same signs and symptoms, and treatment is identical. Symptoms are usually due to instability of the atlantoaxial joint, with compression of the spinal cord anteriorly against the axis or posteriorly from the ring of the atlas. Patients may present with no symptoms, persistent neck complaints, or transient or permanent neurologic deficits or may die suddenly. Symptoms from cranial nerve irritation seldom occur, but symptoms of cerebral and brainstem ischemia are occasionally noted owing to compression of the vertebral arteries in the area of the atlas.

If the condition is suspected, the diagnosis can usually be confirmed on lateral flexion-extension radiographs. CT scans with reconstruction views are often very helpful. Flexion-extension stress radiographs are also necessary to determine the presence and degree of atlantoaxial instability.

The role of prophylactic surgical stabilization is not yet established. If marked instability is shown or if there are clinical findings of neurologic compromise, there is general agreement that surgical fusion should be performed. Operative reduction should be avoided, and preoperative correction by traction or positioning is preferred. Posterior surgical stabilization of the C1 and C2 vertebrae is sufficient if this can be accomplished without flexing the head further. In this situation, occiput-to-C2 stabilization is recommended to avoid all possibility of further neurologic trauma during the procedure.

Klippel-Feil Syndrome (Congenital Synostosis of Cervical Vertebrae, Brevicollis)

In 1912, Klippel and Feil[163] published the first complete description of the clinical aspects and pathology of the syndrome that bears their name. Their attention was attracted to a patient with the unusual clinical findings of marked shortening of the neck, a low posterior hairline, and severe restriction of neck motion. The patient died, and at the postmortem examination Klippel and Feil discovered a complete fusion of the cervical vertebrae. Subsequently, Feil collected 13 additional examples and published a thesis[164] in 1919 that included his findings from this larger group and a review of the literature. The term *Klippel-Feil syndrome* in its present usage refers to all patients with congenital fusion of the cervical vertebrae, whether it involves two segments, congenital block vertebrae (Fig. 30–27), or the entire cervical spine (Fig. 30–28).

Feil originally suggested a system of classification based on the extent and type of the cervical fusion, but except for the area of genetics,[165,166] this classification has not proved

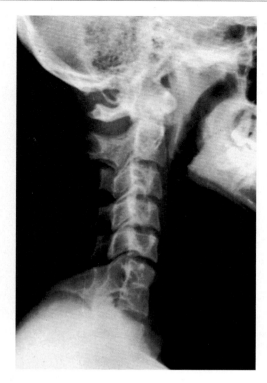

FIGURE 30–27 Congenital block vertebrae at C6-7. Symptoms are directly related to number and level of involved vertebrae; this represents the most benign form of Klippel-Feil syndrome.

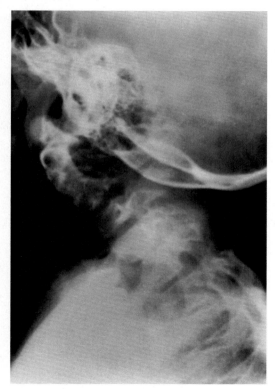

FIGURE 30–28 A 12-year-old girl presented with Klippel-Feil syndrome and iniencephaly—enlarged foramen magnum and absent posterior laminae. Note fixed hyperextension and long segment of cervical fusion (C2-6) and abnormal occipitocervical articulation. This pattern could be viewed as a more elaborate variation of C2-3 pattern of McRae. Flexion-extension and rotational forces are concentrated in area of abnormal occipitocervical junction. These patients may be at risk of developing instability with aging.

TABLE 30–1 Abnormalities Associated with Klippel-Feil Syndrome

	%
Common Abnormalities	
Scoliosis	60
Renal abnormalities	35
Sprengel deformity	30
Deafness	30
Synkinesis	20
Congenital heart disease	14
Less Common Abnormalities	
Ptosis	
Duane contracture	
Lateral rectus palsy	
Facial nerve palsy	
Syndactyly	
Hypoplastic thumb	
Upper extremity hypoplasia	
Neurenteric cyst	

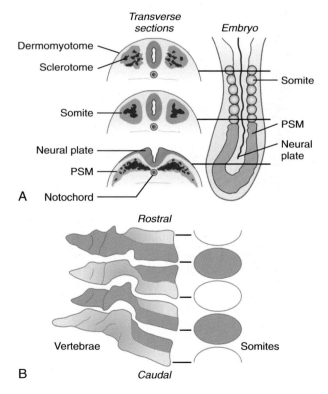

FIGURE 30–29 A, Embryologic differentiation of mesoderm into pairs of somites on either side of spinal cord. Somites divide further to form ventral sclerotome and dorsal dermomyotome. **B,** Cells from rostral and caudal half of adjacent somites fuse to form future vertebral bodies and arches. Defects in this process have been theorized in Klippel-Feil syndrome. PSM, paraspinal muscles. (Adapted from Tracy MR, Dormans JP, Kusumi K: Klippel-Feil syndrome. Clin Orthop 424:183-190, 2004.)

clinically useful. As additional patients were discovered and radiographic techniques improved, it became apparent that certain anomalies of the occipitocervical junction (see sections on basilar impression, atlanto-occipital fusion, and anomalies of odontoid) should be considered separately from the original syndrome. Although these conditions occur commonly in conjunction with fusion of the lower cervical vertebrae, their significance depends on how they influence the atlantoaxial joint. Their prognostic and therapeutic implications are distinctly different, and they occur with sufficient frequency to warrant individual analysis.

Between 20 and 30 days' gestational age, the paraxial mesoderm undergoes cephalad-to-caudal segmentation into spherical, discrete somites. As somites mature, they subdivide into sclerotomes, myotomes, and dermatomes. The sclerotomes, precursors of the adult vertebral bodies, undergo resegmentation such that the caudal section of one somite fuses with the cephalad segment of the adjacent one to form a vertebral body (Fig. 30–29).[167]

Congenital cervical fusion is the result of failure of normal segmentation of the cervical somites during the 3rd to 8th weeks of life. With the exception of a few patients in whom this condition is inherited,[21,166,168,169] the etiology is as yet undetermined. Klippel-Feil syndrome has been theorized to result from disruption of this embryologic segmentation process. Pedigree analysis and molecular studies in animal models are ongoing to define specific genetic abnormalities that may explain these congenital spinal anomalies. Pedigree analysis of a large affected family has identified the first human Klippel-Feil locus (*SGM1*). This gene is disrupted by a heritable paracentric inversion of chromosome 8. The function of this locus remains to be defined, however. *Drosophila* and mouse models have identified genes in the HOX, PAX, and Notch signaling pathways to play a key role in segmentation and somitogenesis. In particular, *Pax1* and *Pax9* are strongly expressed in the vertebral column in mice and play central roles in somite segmentation. Future molecular genetics studies will continue to define the genetic basis for these congenital cervical anomalies.[167] Klippel-Feil anomaly has been associated with fetal alcohol syndrome, but it is unlikely that this is a common mechanism.[170]

The effect of this embryologic abnormality is not limited to the cervical spine—the entire fetus may be adversely affected. Patients with Klippel-Feil syndrome, even patients with minor cervical lesions, may have other, less apparent or even occult defects in the genitourinary,[112,171,172] nervous,[92,173] and cardiopulmonary systems[174-176] and even hearing impairment.[112,177-179] Many of these "hidden" abnormalities may be more detrimental to the patient's general well-being than the obvious deformity of the neck. In the review by Hensinger and colleagues,[112] a high incidence of related congenital anomalies was found (Table 30–1), emphasizing that all patients with Klippel-Feil syndrome should be thoroughly investigated.

Clinical Features

The classic clinical description of Klippel-Feil syndrome is a triad—low posterior hairline, short neck, and limitation of neck motion—but less than half of patients have all three signs (Figs. 30–30 and 30–31).[112,180] The presence of these signs is directly related to the degree of cervical spine involvement. Clinically, the most consistent finding is limitation of neck motion.[166] If fewer than three vertebrae are fused or if only the lower cervical segments are fused, the patient generally has no detectable limitation.[166] In addition, many patients with marked cervical involvement are able to compensate with hypermobility at the unfused joints and to maintain a deceptively good range of motion.[112] Several patients seen by the authors have 90 degrees of flexion-extension, occurring at the only open interspace (Fig. 30–32). Generally, flexion-extension is better preserved than rotation or lateral bending. Rarely, patients have no detectable motion and fixed hyperextension of the neck; this is usually associated with iniencephaly (absence of the posterior cervical laminae and an enlarged foramen magnum) (see Fig. 30–28).[181]

Unless extreme, shortening of the neck is a subtle finding. Similarly, the low posterior hairline is not constant (see Figs. 30–30 and 30–31). Less than 20% of patients with Klippel-Feil syndrome have obvious facial asymmetry, torticollis, or webbing of the neck.[112,166] When extreme, webbing of the neck is called *pterygium colli* and consists of large skin folds extending from the mastoid to the acromion (see Fig. 30–31).[182] The underlying muscles may be involved, but surgical release generally does not result in improved neck motion.

Sprengel deformity occurs in 15% to 35% of cases unilaterally or bilaterally (Fig. 30–33).[112,165,166,171,183,184] At the 3rd week of gestation, the scapula develops from mesodermal tissue high in the neck at the level of C4. It descends into the thoracic position by the 8th week, or approximately at the same time that the Klippel-Feil lesion is thought to occur.[165,166] It is logical to expect a significant relationship between these two anomalies. Occasionally, there is a bony bridge between the cervical spine and scapula, an omovertebral bone, or connection to the clavicle.[185] Its removal may permit an increase in neck and shoulder motion.

Probably for the same embryologic reasons, other clinical findings are occasionally apparent (see Table 30–1), including ptosis of the eye, Duane contracture (contracture of the lateral rectus muscle),[166] lateral rectus palsy, facial nerve palsy, neurenteric cyst,[186] and cleft or high-arched palate.[187,188] Abnormalities of the upper extremities include syndactyly, hypoplastic thumb, supernumerary digits, and hypoplasia of the upper extremity, which may represent an interruption of the embryonic blood supply.[189] Abnormalities of the lower extremities are infrequent.

With the exception of the anomalies that involve the atlantoaxial joint, no symptoms can be directly attributed to the fused cervical vertebrae. All symptoms commonly associated with Klippel-Feil syndrome originate at the open segments where the remaining free articulations may become compensatorily hypermobile.[180,190,191] Owing to the increased demands placed on these joints or in response to trauma, this hypermobility can lead to frank instability or early degenerative arthritis.[180,183,190]

Symptoms may arise from two sources: (1) mechanical symptoms owing to irritation of the joint and (2) neurologic

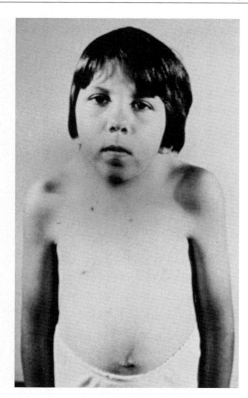

FIGURE 30–30 A 9-year-old child with Klippel-Feil syndrome. Note short neck with tendency toward webbing, mild torticollis, and asymmetry of eye level. The patient clinically has marked restriction of neck motion, impaired hearing, and mirror motions (synkinesia) of upper extremities.

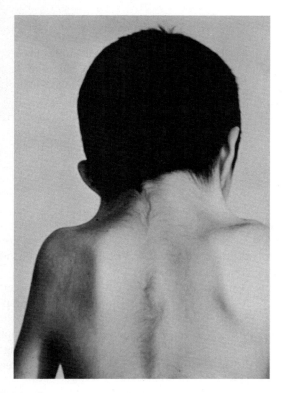

FIGURE 30–31 Extreme form of webbing of neck—pterygium colli. Note low posterior hairline.

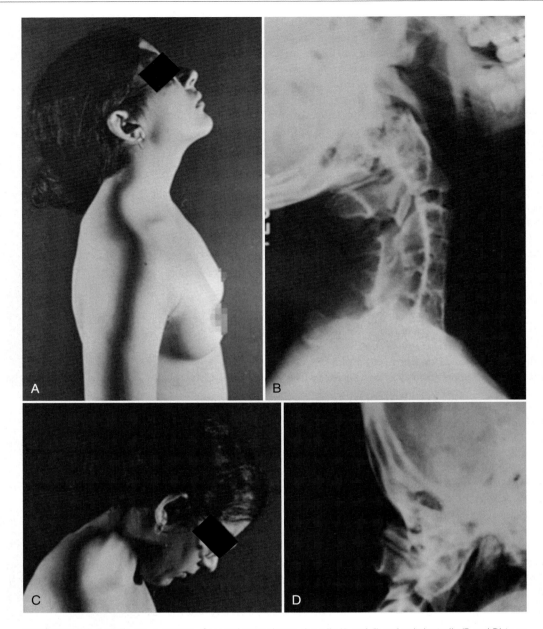

FIGURE 30–32 A-D, Flexion-extension of cervical spine shown clinically (**A** and **C**) and radiologically (**B** and **D**) in an 18-year-old woman with Klippel-Feil syndrome. Most neck motion is occurring at C3-4 disc space. Clinically, the patient is able to maintain adequate 90-degree range of flexion-extension. She is asymptomatic at present, but with aging this hypermobile articulation may become unstable.

symptoms owing to root irritation or spinal cord compression. Patients with a short segment fusion are less likely to develop symptoms[166,192] because the loss of motion is adequately compensated by the remaining free segments. Patients with synostosis of the lower cervical spine are at less risk because the limitation is minimal and can be adequately compensated by the more normally mobile joints above. Most patients who develop symptoms are in the 2nd or 3rd decade of life,[166,180,190] suggesting that the instability is in part a function of time with increasing ligament laxity.

Neurologic symptoms are generally localized to the head, neck, and upper extremities and result from direct irritation or impingement of the cervical nerve roots with radicular symptoms in the upper extremities.[22] The symptoms can usually be localized to the hypermobile joints adjacent to the fused segments.[193] There may be constriction and narrowing of the nerve root at the foramen from osteophytic spurring.[22,180] If joint instability is progressive or if there is appropriate trauma, the spinal cord may be involved to varying degrees, ranging from mild spasticity, hyperreflexia, and muscular weakness to sudden complete quadriplegia after minor trauma.[166,183,194,195] Syncope and neurologic compromise may be associated with mechanical compromise of the vertebral arteries secondary to hypermobility, with ischemic episodes or emboli.[196,197]

FIGURE 30–33 A 6-year-old child with Klippel-Feil syndrome and Sprengel deformity on left. **A,** Frontal view. **B,** Posterior view. **C,** Radiographic appearance shows posterior vertebral anomalies of cervical spine and high left scapula. The patient subsequently had left scapuloplasty.

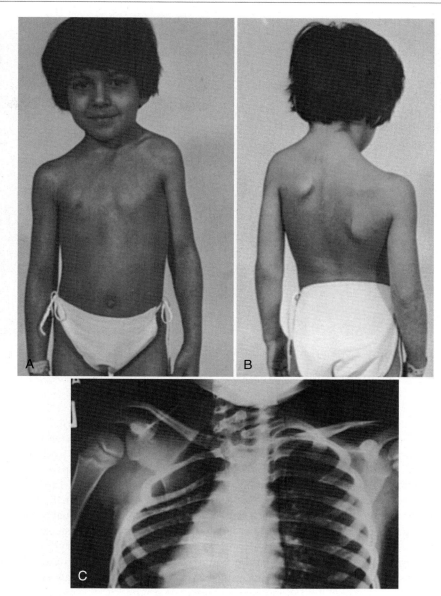

Radiographic Features

In a child with severe involvement, an adequate radiographic evaluation can be difficult. Fixed bony deformities frequently prevent proper positioning, and overlapping shadows from the mandible, occiput, or foramen magnum may obscure the upper vertebrae (Fig. 30–34). In this situation, flexion-extension views may provide the information necessary to assess stability. Another technique that has gained wide acceptance in the diagnosis of cervical instability is CT.[51,180] This technique coupled with flexion-extension of the cervical spine can delineate more precisely the presence or absence of spinal cord compression. CT can be enhanced further by contrast myelography. With MRI, the relationship between the bony elements and neurologic structures can be viewed directly in flexion and extension to show the origin of neural compression.[57,187,198] Use of MRI is particularly helpful for patients who have abnormal bone, such as patients with Morquio disease.[199]

With these techniques, the space available for the spinal cord can be measured directly rather than inferred by use of the ADI.[57] Knowledge of the normal variations in cervical spine mobility, particularly in children, is important in evaluating patients with Klippel-Feil syndrome.[64,200] Pseudosubluxation of C2 on C3 with flexion can be observed in 45% of normal children younger than 8 years of age (see Fig. 30–9).[64] Marked angulation at a single interspace during flexion, rather than a uniform arc of vertebral motion, can be observed in normal children (16%)[201] and may be misinterpreted as vertebral fusion below.

Fusion of cervical vertebrae is the hallmark of Klippel-Feil syndrome. This fusion may be simply synostosis of two bodies (congenital block vertebrae) (Fig. 30–35; see Fig. 30–27) or massive fusion of vertebrae, which was found in Klippel and Feil's first patient (see Fig. 30–28).[163]

Aside from vertebral fusion, flattening (wasp waist) and widening of the involved vertebral bodies, an increase in the

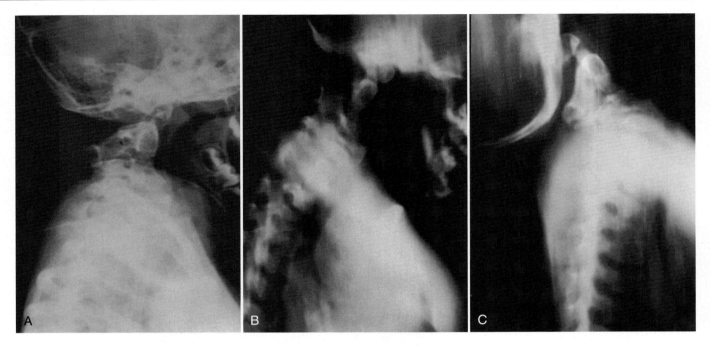

FIGURE 30–34 A 6-year-old boy presented with Klippel-Feil syndrome. **A,** Routine lateral radiograph of cervical spine. Overlapping shadows from shoulder and occiput obscure much of cervical spine. **B,** Lateral laminagraph in flexion shows anterior hemivertebra, probably C4, and congenital fusion of C2-3, C6-7, and T3-4. **C,** Lateral laminagraph in extension shows absence of posterior ring of C1 and unstable C1-2 articulation. Flexion-extension laminagraphs are helpful in providing information necessary to evaluate children with severe deformity, particularly if vertebral instability is suspected.

space available for the spinal cord, and absent disc spaces are the most common findings.[202,203] Hypoplasia of the disc space or remnants of it can often be seen (see Fig. 30–35). In a young child, narrowing of the cervical disc space cannot always be appreciated because the ossification of the vertebral body is incomplete, and the unossified endplates may give the false impression of a normal disc space (Fig. 30–36). With continued growth, the ossification of the vertebral bodies is completed, however, and the fusion becomes obvious.[191] If fusion is suspected in a child, it may be confirmed by flexion-extension views (Fig. 30–37). Juvenile rheumatoid arthritis (Fig. 30–38), rheumatoid spondylitis, and infection can mimic the radiographic findings, but usually the clinical history and physical examination indicate the correct diagnosis.

Hemivertebrae are common (Fig. 30–39); they occurred in 74% of patients in the review of Gray and colleagues,[166] and the incidence increases with the number of segments fused.

Fusion of posterior elements usually parallels fusion of the vertebral bodies. In a young child, particular attention should be paid to the laminae because fusion posteriorly is often more apparent than anteriorly in early life (Fig. 30–40).[112,191]

The sagittal and transverse diameters of the spinal canal are usually normal. Narrowing of the spinal canal, if it occurs, is usually seen in adult life and is due to degenerative changes (osteoarthritic spurs) or hypermobility.* Enlargement of the cervical canal is uncommon; if found, it may indicate conditions such as syringomyelia, hydromyelia, or Arnold-Chiari malformation.[62,206] The intervertebral foramina are usually smooth in contour but are frequently smaller than normal and oval rather than circular (Fig. 30–41). Posterior spina bifida is common (45%), but anterior spina bifida is rare. Rarely, there is complete absence of the posterior elements. This condition

_____

*References 64, 178, 193, 198, 204, 205.

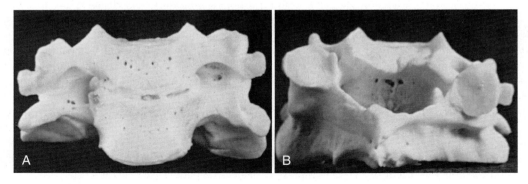

FIGURE 30–35 Postmortem specimen of congenital block of vertebra of C3-4. **A,** Anterior view. **B,** Posterior view. Specimen shows complete fusion, but remnants of cartilaginous vertebral bodies can still be seen.

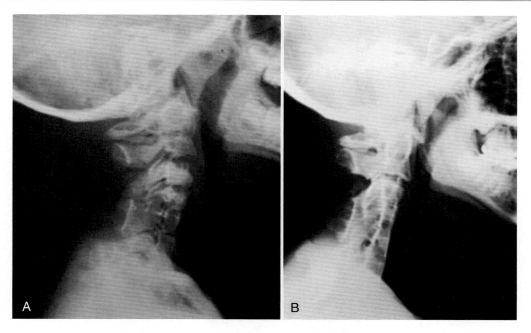

FIGURE 30–36 A, Lateral radiograph of an 8-year-old child shows posterior fusion of laminae and spinous process but incomplete fusion of vertebral bodies anteriorly. **B,** At age 19, there is complete fusion of vertebral bodies at C2-3 and C4-7. Unossified cartilage of vertebral bodies in children can give false appearance of normal disc space.

is usually accompanied by enlargement of the foramen magnum and fixed hyperextension of the neck, referred to as *iniencephaly* (see Fig. 30–28).[181]

All these defects may extend into the upper thoracic spine, particularly in patients with severe involvement. A disturbance of the upper thoracic spine on a routine chest radiograph may be the first clue to an unrecognized cervical synostosis. With a high thoracic congenital scoliosis, the radiographic evaluation should routinely include lateral views of the cervical spine.

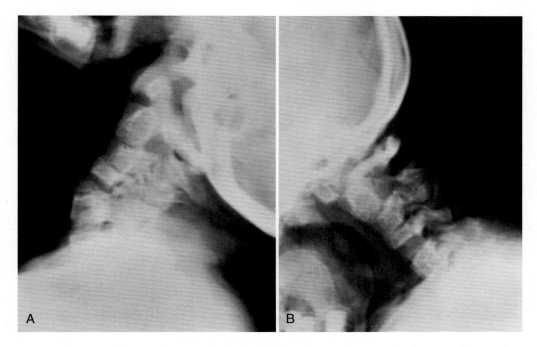

FIGURE 30–37 A 3-year-old child presented with Klippel-Feil syndrome and congenital scoliosis. **A** and **B,** Lateral flexion-extension radiographs of cervical spine show that neck motion occurs predominantly between C4 and C5. Flexion-extension views are helpful in determining type and extent of congenital fusion in young children.

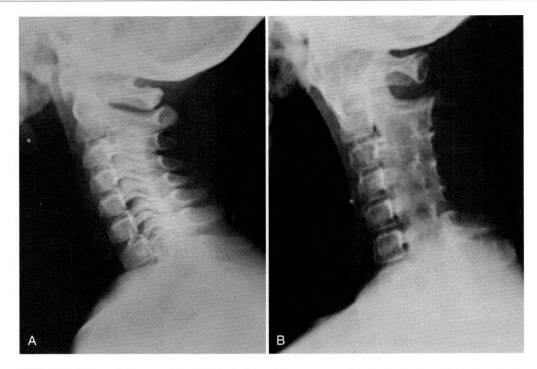

FIGURE 30–38 Juvenile rheumatoid arthritis. **A,** Radiographic appearance of cervical spine in a patient at age 5, at onset of rheumatoid process. **B,** Same patient at age 10 with complete fusion of laminae posteriorly and severely restricted neck motion. With further growth, these vertebral bodies would be expected subsequently to fuse.

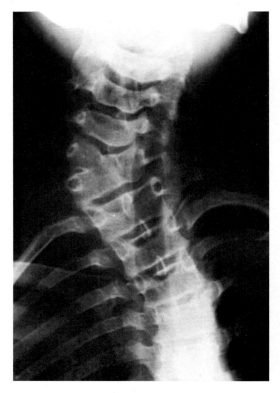

FIGURE 30–39 A 14-year-old patient presented with cervical hemivertebrae. Hemivertebrae are common in Klippel-Feil syndrome but usually are found in dorsal or lumbar vertebral segments.

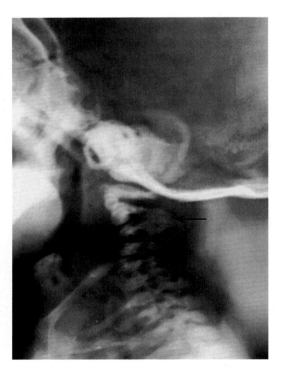

FIGURE 30–40 A 3-month-old infant presented with Klippel-Feil syndrome. Radiograph shows posterior fusion of laminae of C2-3 (*arrow*). In young children, particular attention should be paid to laminae because fusion posteriorly is often more apparent than anteriorly in early life.

Patterns of Cervical Motion

One can gain insight into the problem of instability by reviewing the lateral flexion-extension films of a patient with Klippel-Feil syndrome. The type or pattern of cervical motion depends on the location and extent of the fused cervical vertebrae. Patients with fusion of the lower cervical vertebrae or with more than two disc spaces between fused segments seem to be at low risk for serious problems.

Pizzutillo and colleagues[190] reviewed patients from the Alfred I. DuPont Institute and patients reported in the literature to determine the long-term problems found in Klippel-Feil syndrome. In their classification, these investigators noted that patients who have upper segment instability were more likely to be younger and to have neurologic problems. Conversely, degenerative changes were more common in older patients with low segment hypermobility. This finding emphasizes the importance of screening the upper cervical spine in a young child for instability. There are three high-risk patterns of cervical spinal motion that potentially have a poor prognosis, from either early instability or late degenerative osteoarthritis.[207]

Pattern 1 is fusion of C2 and C3 with occipitalization of the atlas. Complications associated with this pattern were first reported by McRae in 1953,[33] and they received substantial support in the literature.[22,208] Flexion-extension is concentrated in the area of C1 and C2. With aging, an odontoid can become hypermobile, narrowing the spinal canal and compromising the spinal cord and brainstem.

Pattern 2 is a long fusion with an abnormal occipitocervical junction (see Fig. 30–28). This is similar to the C2-3 fusion of McRae and could be reviewed as a more elaborate variation. The force of flexion-extension and rotation is concentrated in the area of the abnormal odontoid or poorly developed ring of C1, which cannot withstand the wear and tear of aging.[204,207,208] It is important to differentiate this pattern from the pattern in a patient with a long fusion and a normal C1-2 articulation (Fig. 30–42), which is usually compatible with a normal life expectancy.

Pattern 3 is a single open interspace between two fused segments (Fig. 30–43). In this situation, cervical spine motion is concentrated at the single open articulation. In some patients, this hypermobility may lead to frank instability or degenerative osteoarthritis (Fig. 30–44).* This pattern can be easily recognized because the cervical spine appears to angle or hinge at the open segment. Samartzis and colleagues[203] studied cervical fusion patterns in patients with Klippel-Feil syndrome. They developed a classification system in which type I described a single fusion; type II described multiple, noncontiguous fusions; and type III described multiple, contiguous fusions. Samartzis and colleagues[203] found that type I was associated with axial neck symptoms, and types II and III were associated with radicular and myelopathic symptoms.

*References 22, 166, 183, 190, 193, 203, 204, 207.

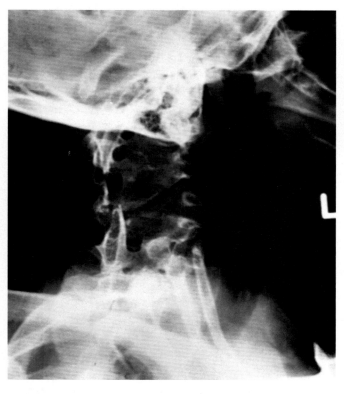

FIGURE 30–41 Oblique view of cervical spine shows smooth contour of intervertebral foramina, which are frequently smaller than normal and oval rather than circular.

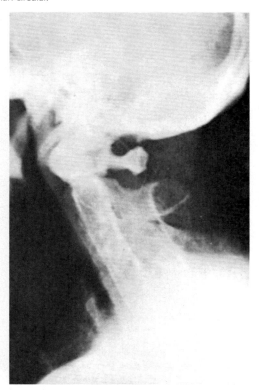

FIGURE 30–42 Radiograph of a 45-year-old man with Klippel-Feil syndrome. The patient has complete fusion of C2-7. Flexion-extension occurs only at atlantoaxial articulation. There are no symptoms referable to neck, despite two previous serious falls. This pattern seems to be relatively safe because normal occipitocervical junction serves as protection from late instability.

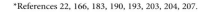

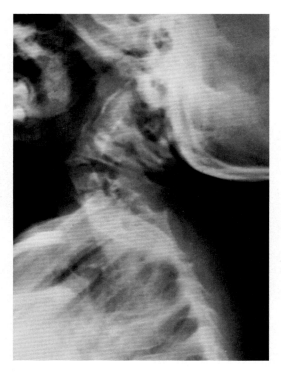

FIGURE 30–43 Open interspace between two fused segments. This 7-year-old child with Klippel-Feil syndrome has flexion-extension motion of neck occurring primarily at one interspace. Cervical spine appears to angle or hinge at this point. This pattern is worrisome because wear and tear of aging may lead to early degenerative change or instability and narrowing of spinal cord.

Associated Conditions

Scoliosis

Scoliosis is the most frequent anomaly found in association with the syndrome.[112,171,209,210] Of these patients, 60% have a significant degree of scoliosis (>15 degrees by the Cobb method).[112,210] Most of these patients require treatment and should be followed through the growth years. Radiographic examinations should include lateral views of the spine because increasing kyphosis may make the need for treatment of the scoliosis more urgent. If the deformity is recognized early, many children can be successfully managed with standard spinal orthoses. At present, most of these patients have required posterior spinal stabilization, partly owing to late recognition.[112,171,173,194]

Two types of scoliosis can be identified: congenital scoliosis, owing to vertebral anomalies and differential growth patterns (Fig. 30–45), and compensatory scoliosis, below the area of vertebral involvement. In the authors' series, congenital scoliosis is more common (55%), and in more than half of the children, the curvature was progressive and required treatment.[112] Progressive curves are more likely associated with children who have extensive fusions.[210] Most children (75%) required posterior spinal fusion to arrest an increasing deformity, and the remainder were controlled with a brace or cast.[112] Progressive scoliosis frequently occurred in the normal-appearing vertebrae below the primary congenital curve. If only the congenitally involved segments are examined in follow-up, an increasing compensatory scoliosis in the lower

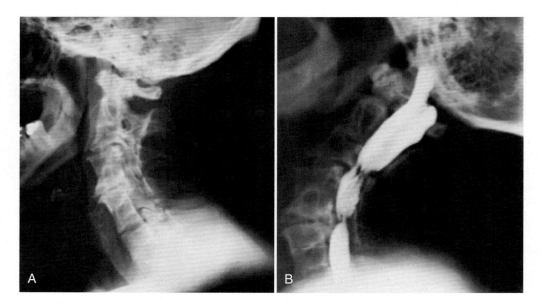

FIGURE 30–44 A 54-year-old man presented with a 4-month history of persistent neck pain with radiation into upper extremities. He had no history of neck complaints but a long history of occipital headaches. He recently noted paresthesias in upper and lower extremities. Neurologic examination and electromyography were normal. **A,** Lateral radiograph of cervical spine shows congenital fusion between C2-3, C4-5, and C6-7. Note marked changes of degenerative osteoarthritis with large osteophyte formation at open interspace of C3-4 and C5-6. **B,** Myelography during extension of cervical spine shows narrowing of spinal canal owing to large osteoarthritic spurs at C3-4 and C5-6. The patient subsequently underwent spine stabilization with relief of neck complaints.

vertebrae may not be recognized, and its significance may not be appreciated until serious deformity results.[207]

When surgical intervention is required, the same principles apply as used in congenital scoliosis. When spinal fusion is performed, the orthopaedist should carefully consider the overall alignment of the patient's spine. The temptation to achieve maximal radiologic correction of the mobile segments must be tempered by careful consideration of the congenitally fixed segments. Failure to observe this principle may result in an unbalanced spine; the patient will have traded one deformity for another that may be even worse than the original.

Documented progression of scoliosis, whether in the congenitally distorted elements or in the compensatory curve below, demands immediate and appropriate treatment to prevent serious additional deformity. Progressive scoliosis in the thoracic spine may seriously compromise pulmonary function.[112,174] More subtle occult abnormalities can lead to respiratory difficulty in some patients with Klippel-Feil syndrome.[211] Abnormal rib spacing, congenital fusion of the ribs, and deformed costovertebral joints may inhibit full expansion of the rib cage during respiration.[212] Although not causing an angular deformity, fusion of the thoracic vertebrae may decrease the size of the thoracic cage. A dwarf with spondylothoracic deformity may represent a severe form of this problem, leading to early respiratory death.[213]

Also, Krieger and colleagues[75] reported on the relationship of occult respiratory dysfunction and craniovertebral anomalies. They noted that in addition to the obvious problems of bony impingement or traction on the brainstem, these patients may have subtle hydrocephalus, which may adversely affect respiratory function. This information has particular application when cervical distraction devices are contemplated in the treatment of scoliosis (halo-femoral or halo-pelvic traction). When considering the use of such devices, the physician should be aware that children with Klippel-Feil syndrome may be more susceptible to neurologic or vascular injury and that the presence of cervical anomalies may preclude the use of cervical distraction.[112]

Renal Abnormalities

More than one third of children with Klippel-Feil syndrome can be expected to have a significant urinary tract anomaly. These anomalies are often asymptomatic in young children. Previously, the authors recommended that such anomalies be evaluated with intravenous pyelography (Fig. 30–46).[112] It has been found, however, that ultrasonography offers a noninvasive way to screen adequately for the anomalies associated with this syndrome.[201] The pronephros, the embryologic tissue destined to become the genitourinary tract, develops between the 7th and 14th somites, in the same region and at the same time as the cervical spine,[212,214] quite similar to the scapulae in Sprengel deformity. The most frequent abnormality is unilateral absence of a kidney. Other abnormalities include a double collecting system, renal ectopia, horseshoe kidney, and hydronephrosis from ureteropelvic obstruction. In the authors'

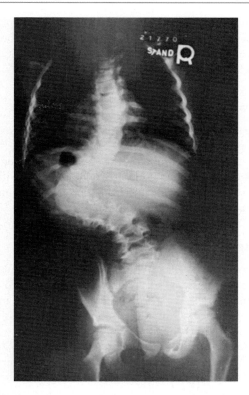

FIGURE 30–45 Radiograph of an 8-year-old child with Klippel-Feil syndrome and deafness. Severe kyphoscoliosis subsequently required spine correction and stabilization.

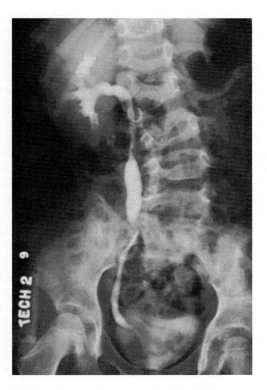

FIGURE 30–46 Radiograph of a 10-year-old child with Klippel-Feil syndrome shows multiple vertebral anomalies, unilateral absence of kidney, and hydroureter. Ureteral reimplantation was required for ureteral reflux and hydronephrosis.

series, 2 of 50 patients developed severe pyelonephritis in the remaining kidney, requiring renal transplantation.[112] In Klippel and Feil's original case report, the patient died of nephritis.[163]

Cardiovascular Abnormalities

The literature notes the association of Klippel-Feil syndrome with congenital heart disease (4.2% to 14%).[112,175,176,194] The most common lesion reported has been an interventricular septal defect occurring alone or in combination with other defects, such as patent ductus arteriosus and abnormal position of the heart and aorta.

Deafness

The association of hearing impairment and deafness in Klippel-Feil syndrome (>30%) has been reported in the otology literature,[177-179,205] but it is seldom mentioned in orthopaedic reports.[112,171] Other defects include absence of the auditory canal and microtia.

Jalladeau[205] published the first report of deafness. Stark and Borton[179] noted that detailed audiologic data were not yet available, and the precise defect is often unknown. There is no characteristic audiologic anomaly, and all types of hearing loss (conductive, sensorineural, and mixed) have been described. These patients should undergo a complete audiometric evaluation when they are discovered. The relationship between hearing loss and speech-language retardation is well documented, and early detection of hearing impairment can lessen the retardation by permitting early initiation of speech and language training.[179]

Mirror Motions (Synkinesis)

Synkinesis consists of involuntary paired movements of the hands and occasionally the arms. The patient is unable to move one hand without similar reciprocal motion of the opposite hand. Mirror motion was first described by Bauman,[173] who found it in four of six patients with Klippel-Feil syndrome. This condition has been noted to occur occasionally in normal preschool children and patients with cerebral palsy or Parkinson disease, but most patients with this condition have Klippel-Feil syndrome.[165] Approximately 20% exhibit mirror motions clinically.[112] Baird and colleagues,[92] using electromyography to examine 13 patients with Klippel-Feil syndrome, found 10 patients with electrically detectable paired motion in the opposite extremity. This finding suggests that many patients may be subclinically affected and may be more clumsy at two-handed activities. Some authors have suggested that synkinesis should be included as part of the syndrome.[92,165]

The etiology of synkinesis is unknown, but it seems to be a separate congenital neurologic defect not caused by bony impingement or irritation of the spinal cord.[212,215] The examination of two autopsy specimens suggests that the clinical findings are due to inadequate or incomplete decussation of the pyramidal tracts in conjunction with a dysraphic cervical

spinal cord. As a consequence, cerebral control over the upper extremities must follow less direct pathways located in the extrapyramidal system, and affected patients require more extensive practice to dissociate the movements of the individual extremities.

Synkinesis is most pronounced in young children, particularly children younger than 5 years. The condition tends to decrease with age. Occupational therapy has been helpful in teaching control over the extremities, or at least in disguising the reciprocal motion to a tolerable cosmetic level. Still, many patients may find discriminating two-handed activity difficult, such as playing the piano, typing, sewing, or ladder climbing.[216]

Treatment

A patient with Klippel-Feil syndrome with minimal involvement can be expected to lead a normal active life with no or only minor restrictions or symptoms. Many patients with severe involvement can have the same good prognosis if early and appropriate treatment is instituted when needed; this is particularly applicable in the area of associated scoliosis and renal abnormalities. Prevention of further deformity or complications can be of great benefit. The actual treatment of Klippel-Feil syndrome is confined mostly to the area of associated conditions and is discussed under the respective headings.

At present, treatment choices for the cervical spine anomalies are quite limited. Patients with major areas of cervical synostosis or high-risk patterns of cervical spinal motion should be strongly advised to avoid activities that place stress on the cervical spine. In these patients, the mobile articulations are under greater mechanical demands and are less capable of protecting them against traumatic insults.

As discussed, sudden neurologic compromise or death after minor trauma has been reported in patients with Klippel-Feil syndrome and is usually due to disruption at the hypermobile articulation.[22,166,183] The role of prophylactic surgical stabilization in asymptomatic patients has not yet been defined. There is no satisfactory definition of when the risk of instability warrants further reduction of neck motion.

For symptomatic patients with mechanical problems, the usual treatment measures for degenerative osteoarthritis are applicable and include traction, a cervical collar, and analgesics. Symptoms that suggest neurologic compromise require careful consideration and evaluation by a neurologist, neurosurgeon, and orthopaedist (see Fig. 30–44). The exact area of irritation must be determined before surgical intervention. Attempts should be made preoperatively to obtain reduction of the bony architecture in advance of surgical stabilization. Also, the anesthesiologist may need to plan for airway management and be prepared for difficult intubation.[217] The physician must be mindful that there are other associated abnormalities in the brainstem and in the spinal cord itself that may be contributing to the symptoms.

Treatment of the cosmetic aspects of this deformity has met with limited success. Occasionally, children with the fixed torticollis posture may be improved with bracing. Bracing requires long-term application, however, and excellent patient cooperation. Correction of the bony deformity by direct means, such as wedge osteotomy or hemivertebrae excision, has been done on a limited basis.[218] Ruf and colleagues[218] reported hemivertebrae resection for correction of head tilt. Occasionally, carefully selected patients who have cervical congenital scoliosis may obtain some correction and improvement of appearance by use of the halo vest combined with posterior cervical fusion. Bonola[219] described a method of rib resection to attain apparent increase in neck length and motion. This procedure is an extensive surgical experience, however, and is a great risk to the patient. No subsequent reports have appeared in the literature. More recently, the vertical expandable prosthetic titanium rib (VEPTR) has been used to correct cervical tilt along with congenital thoracic scoliosis in thoracic insufficiency syndrome.[220] Early results of this treatment have been promising.

Soft tissue procedures, Z-plasty, and muscle resection may achieve cosmetic improvement in properly selected patients.[171] These procedures can restore a more natural contour to the shoulders and neck and an apparent increase in neck length. Neck motion is generally not increased, and the scars may be extensive, particularly in a patient with a large skin web. If an omovertebral bone is present or an abnormal connection to the clavicle,[185] its removal may permit an increase in neck and shoulder motion. The risk of brachial plexus injury from traction is higher in patients with Klippel-Feil syndrome because there are likely to be anomalous origins of the cervical nerve roots in these patients. Iniencephaly and absence of the posterior cervical elements (see Fig. 30–28) may be associated with Sprengel deformity and must be identified if surgical correction is considered.[181]

Summary

Klippel-Feil syndrome is an uncommon condition caused by congenital fusion of two or more cervical vertebrae. Most affected individuals are asymptomatic or have a mild restriction of neck motion. If symptoms referable to the cervical spine occur, it is usually in adult life and is due to degenerative arthritis or instability of the hypermobile articulations adjacent to the area of synostosis. Most patients respond to conservative treatment measures; a small percentage require judicious surgical stabilization. Cosmetic surgery is of limited benefit in treatment of the neck deformity.

The relatively good prognosis of the cervical lesion is overshadowed by the "hidden" or unrecognized associated anomalies. The high incidence of significant scoliosis, renal anomalies, deafness, neurologic malformations, Sprengel deformity, and cardiac anomalies should be of great concern to the physician. Early recognition and treatment of these problems may be of substantial benefit, sparing the patient further deformity or serious illness.

Muscular Torticollis (Wry Neck)

Muscular torticollis is a common condition usually discovered in the first 6 to 8 weeks of life. The deformity is caused by contracture of the sternocleidomastoid muscle, with the head tilted toward the involved side and the chin rotated toward the contralateral shoulder (Fig. 30–47A). If the infant is examined within the first 4 weeks of life, a mass or "tumor" is usually palpable in the neck (Fig. 30–48).[221] It is generally a nontender, soft enlargement that is mobile beneath the skin and attached to or located within the body of the sternocleidomastoid muscle. Ultrasonography may be helpful in confirming the mass.[222] The mass attains maximal size within the 1st month of life and then gradually regresses. If the child is examined after 4 to 6 months of age, the mass is usually absent, and the contracture of the sternocleidomastoid muscle and the torticollis posture are the only clinical findings (Fig. 30–49). The mass is frequently unrecognized and was undetected in 80% of the patients of Coventry and Harris.[223]

If the condition is progressive, deformities of the face and skull can result and are usually apparent within the 1st year.[224]

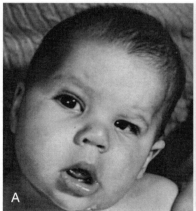
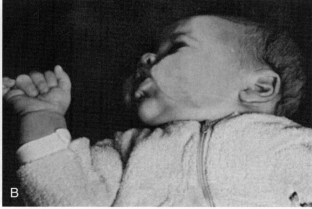

FIGURE 30–47 A 6-month-old infant presented with right-sided congenital muscular torticollis. **A,** Note rotation of skull and asymmetry and flattening of face on side of contracted sternocleidomastoid. **B,** Same patient with head resting on glass and photographed from below. Note how face conforms to surface. When the infant sleeps, usually prone, it is more comfortable to have affected side down, and consequently face remodels to conform to bed.

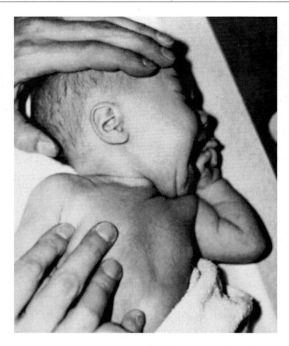

FIGURE 30–48 A 6-week-old infant presented with swelling in region of sternocleidomastoid. Mass is usually soft, nontender, and mobile beneath skin but is attached to muscle.

Flattening of the face on the side of the contracted sternocleidomastoid muscle may be particularly impressive (see Fig. 30–47A). The deformity is probably due to the position the child assumes when sleeping (see Fig. 30–47B). In a study of children in the United States, it was found that they generally sleep prone,[225] and in this position it is more comfortable to have the affected side down. As a consequence, the face remodels to conform to the bed. In children who sleep supine, reverse modeling of the contralateral aspect of the skull is

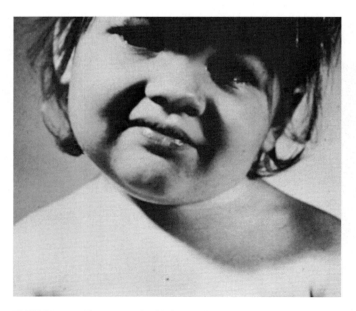

FIGURE 30–49 This 18-month-old child had torticollis that was resistant to stretching exercises and required surgical release.

evident. The Back to Sleep Campaign has altered sleep patterns.[226] If the condition remains untreated during the growth years, the level of the eyes and ears becomes distorted and may result in considerable cosmetic deformity. More recent reports suggest that infants with torticollis are at an increased risk for early gross motor delay, but most normalize in the 1st year of life. The delay seemed more strongly associated with little or no time prone when awake than with congenital muscular torticollis.[227]

Etiology

At present, congenital muscular torticollis is believed to be the result of local compression of the soft tissues of the neck at the time of delivery.[228] It is usually unilateral, but bilateral torticollis has been reported.[224] Birth records of affected children show a preponderance of breech or difficult deliveries or primiparous births.[162,229] The deformity has occurred after otherwise normal deliveries, however, and has been reported in infants born by cesarean section.[221,229] Davids and colleagues[228] found that MRI studies of the sternocleidomastoid muscle in infants with congenital muscular torticollis have signal changes similar to changes observed in the forearm and leg after compartment syndrome. That finding, coupled with cadaveric dissections, shows that there is a fascial covering of the entire sternocleidomastoid muscle; a review of the children treated by Davids and colleagues[228] strongly suggests that congenital muscular torticollis represents a compartment syndrome.

Microscopic examinations of resected surgical specimens and experimental work with dogs[230] suggest that the lesion is due to occlusion of the venous outflow of the sternocleidomastoid muscle. This occlusion results in edema, degeneration of muscle fibers, and eventual fibrosis of the muscle body. Coventry and Harris[223] suggested that the clinical deformity is related to the ratio of fibrosis to remaining functional muscle. If sufficient normal muscle is present, the sternocleidomastoid stretches with growth, and the child is not likely to develop the torticollis posture, whereas if there is a predominance of fibrosis, there is very little elastic potential.

Pathologic studies showed that with time the fibrosis of the sternal head may entrap and compromise the branch of the accessory nerve to the clavicular head of the muscle (progressive denervation), leading to a late increase in the deformity.[231] Some evidence suggests that the problem may be due to uterine crowding or "packaging syndrome" because in three of four children the lesion is on the right side.[221,228,229] Also, 5% to 20% of children with congenital muscular torticollis have congenital dysplasia of the hip, which is believed to be due to restriction of infant movement in the tight maternal space.[232-234] Boys with developmental dysplasia of the hip were nearly five times more likely to have congenital muscular torticollis.[233] Radiographs of the cervical spine should be obtained to rule out congenital anomaly of the cervical spine or C1-2 rotatory subluxation.[235,236]

Ultrasonography is now widely accepted to be one of the most sensitive tests for the diagnosis of congenital muscular torticollis and developmental hip dysplasia. Tien and colleagues[237] found that a homogeneous, hyperechoic mass within the sternocleidomastoid muscle was diagnostic of congenital muscular torticollis. They found the coexistence of developmental hip dysplasia and torticollis to be 17%; 8.5% of children with identifiable hip dysplasia required some treatment.

Treatment

Conservative Measures

Excellent results can be obtained with conservative measures in most patients.[221,223,229,238,239] Of the patients reported by Coventry and Harris,[223] 90% responded to stretching exercises alone. Cheng and colleagues[240] showed that controlled manual stretching was safe and effective in the treatment of greater than 95% of patients with congenital muscular torticollis when seen before the age of 1 year. The most important prognostic factors for success were minimal initial rotational deficit, age younger than 1 year at presentation, and lack of a palpable tight band or tumor in the affected sternocleidomastoid muscle.

Exercises are performed by the patient, with guidance from the physical therapist and physician. Standard maneuvers include positioning of the ear opposite the contracted muscle to the shoulder and touching the chin to the shoulder on the affected side. When adequate stretching has been obtained in the neutral position, these maneuvers should be repeated with the head hyperextended, to achieve maximal stretching and prevent positions of the crib and toys so that the neck is stretched when the infant tries to reach and grasp. Children should be examined for plagiocephaly because the findings may be subtle.[241] The use of a "sleeping helmet" has been suggested to reduce the deformity and hasten face and skull remodeling.[242]

Surgery

If the condition persists beyond 1 year of age, nonoperative measures are rarely successful.[238] Similarly, established facial asymmetry and limitation of normal motion of more than 30 degrees usually preclude a good result and lead to surgical intervention and poor cosmesis (Fig. 30–50).[238] A good (but not perfect) cosmetic result can be obtained, however, in children 5 to 7 years of age (Fig. 30–51).[223,236,239,243,244] Asymmetry of the skull and face improves as long as adequate growth potential remains after the deforming pull of the sternocleidomastoid is removed (Fig. 30–52).[223,236,243] Shim and colleagues[245] showed that patients older than 8 years, including patients who were skeletally mature, benefit from unipolar or bipolar release of the sternocleidomastoid and postoperative physical therapy. These authors preferred to wait until the child was old enough to comply with the postoperative exercise and bracing.[246] All patients had improved functional and cosmetic results postoperatively.

Surgery consists of resection of a portion of the distal sternocleidomastoid muscle (see Fig. 30–50). At least a 1-cm segment of the tendon should be removed to guard against recurrence of the deformity. A transverse incision is made low

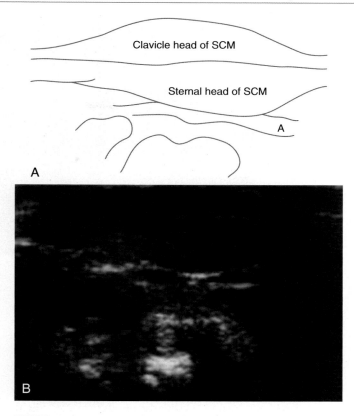

FIGURE 30–50 A, Diagram showing abnormal appearance of sternocleidomastoid (SCM) in congenital muscular torticollis. **B,** Ultrasonography shows homogeneous, hyperechoic mass on SCM. (Adapted from Tien YC, Su JY, Lin GT, et al: Ultrasonographic study of the coexistence of muscular torticollis and dysplasia of the hip. J Pediatr Orthop 21:343-347, 2001.)

in the neck to coincide with a normal skin fold.[247] It is important not to place the incision near or very near the clavicle because scars in this area tend to spread and are cosmetically unacceptable (see Fig. 30–51).[121] Similarly, closure with a subcuticular suture is preferred.[166]

The most common postoperative complaint is disfiguring scarring.[221,229,247] The two heads of the sternocleidomastoid are identified, and both are sectioned (see Fig. 30–50). It is important to release the investing fascia around the sternocleidomastoid because this, too, is frequently contracted.[221] Rotation of the chin and head at this point generally reveals the adequacy of the surgery, and palpitation of the neck shows any extraneous tight bands that could lead to partial recurrence of incomplete correction (see Fig. 30–52).[229] In an older child, an accessory incision (bipolar) is often required to section the muscle at its origin on the mastoid process. The whole muscle should not be excised because this may lead to reverse torticollis[229] or additional deformity from asymmetry in the contour of the neck.[221]

The postoperative regimen includes passive stretching exercises performed in the same manner as those done preoperatively. The exercises should begin as soon as the patient can tolerate manipulation of the neck. Occasionally, head traction at night is helpful, particularly in an older child. Bracing or cast correction may be necessary if the deformity has been

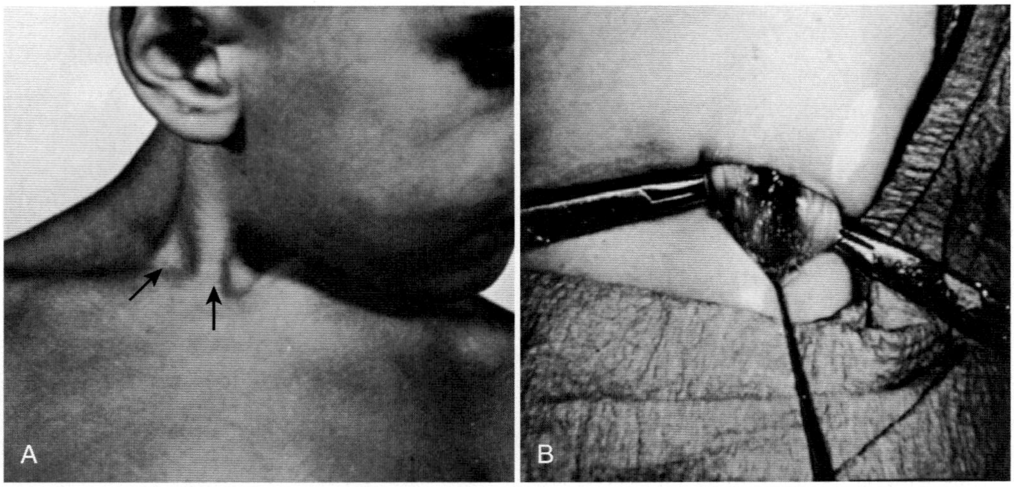

FIGURE 30–51 **A,** Clinical appearance of a 6-year-old child with congenital muscular torticollis. Note appearance of two heads of sternocleidomastoid (*arrows*). **B,** Operative exposure of the same patient shows complete replacement with fibrous tissue of two heads of sternocleidomastoid.

of long duration or if the torticollis posture has become a strong habit.[248] Results of surgery have been uniformly good, with a low incidence of complications or recurrence, and almost all patients are pleased with the results.[221,223,229,238] Slight restriction of the neck motion and anomalous reattachment occur frequently[229,247] but are generally unnoticed by the patient. If the patient is young, the facial asymmetry can be expected to resolve completely, unless there is persistence of the torticollis, particularly from residual fascial bands (Fig. 30–53; see Fig. 30–52).[229]

Differential Diagnosis

Torticollis is a common childhood complaint. The etiology is diverse, and identifying the cause can pose a difficult diagnostic problem (Tables 30–2 and 30–3).

Congenital muscular torticollis is the most common cause of wry neck posture in infants and young children, but there are other problems that lead to this unusual posture. Head tilt and rotatory deformity of the head and neck (torticollis) usually indicate a problem at C1-2, whereas head tilt alone

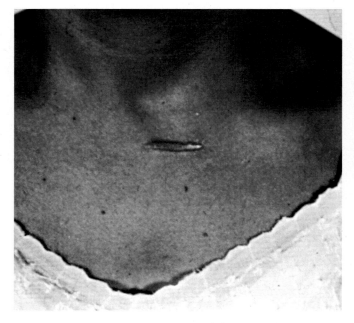

FIGURE 30–52 An 18-year-old patient after resection of portion of sternocleidomastoid. Incision was placed too near clavicle and consequently spread, becoming cosmetically unacceptable.

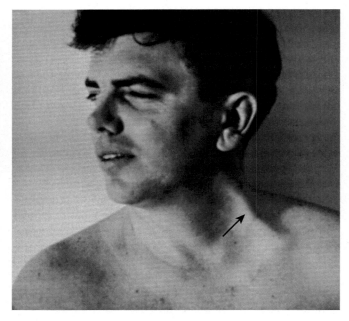

FIGURE 30–53 A 23-year-old man underwent release of sternocleidomastoid. There is residual fascial band (*arrow*) and slight restriction of neck motion.

indicates a more generalized problem in the cervical spine. If the posturing of the head and neck is noted at or shortly after birth, congenital anomalies of the cervical spine should be considered. Bony anomalies of the cervical spine, particularly anomalies that involve C1-2, typically manifest as a rigid deformity, and the sternocleidomastoid muscle is not contracted or in spasm.

Gyorgyi[249] examined 20 cases of congenital torticollis and found the following coexisting anomalies: congenital cervical fusions, asymmetrical facet joints, basilar impression, atlanto-axial dislocation, assimilation of the atlas, and deformities of the odontoid process. Gyorgyi[249] noted that in children with congenital torticollis, 40% had a history of breech presentation. Many occipitocervical malformations manifest as torticollis.[31,33,38,112] De Barros and colleagues[14] noted that 68% had basilar impression, most commonly unilaterally. Approximately 20% of patients with Klippel-Feil syndrome have associated torticollis.[112,250] With asymmetrical development of the occipital condyles or the facets of C1, the head tilt may result in a torticollis unless compensated for by a tilt of the lower cervical spine similar to that which occurs in the milder forms.[14,103,166]

If torticollis is noted in the weeks after delivery, the usual cause is congenital muscular torticollis. If the child is younger than 2 months of age, a palpable lump may be found in the sternocleidomastoid. Congenital muscular torticollis is painless, is associated with a contracted or shortened sternocleidomastoid muscle, and is unaccompanied by any bony abnormalities or neurologic deficit. Soft tissue problems are less common and include abnormal skin webs or folds (pterygium colli), which maintain the torticollis posture. Tumors in the region of the sternocleidomastoid, cystic hygroma, branchial cleft cyst, and thyroid teratoma are rare but should be considered.

Inflammatory conditions include local irritation from cervical lymphadenitis, which may lead to the appearance of a wry neck or tilt of the head. Another less frequent cause is a retropharyngeal abscess after inflammation of the posterior pharynx or tonsillitis.[251] Children with polyarticular juvenile rheumatoid arthritis frequently develop involvement of the cervical joints. Torticollis and limitation of cervical motion may be the only clinical signs. Spontaneous atlantoaxial rotatory subluxation may follow acute pharyngitis.[250,252] Radiographic confirmation is difficult, and the CT methods for evaluation suggested by Phillips and Hensinger[252] should be used. Early diagnosis and reduction of the displacement are important.[252,253] If it becomes fixed, it poses a considerable treatment problem.[252] A rare inflammatory cause is acute calcification of a cervical disc,[254,255] which can be visualized on routine radiographic study of the neck (Fig. 30–54).

Traumatic causes should always be considered and carefully excluded early in the evaluation. If unrecognized, they may have serious neurologic consequences. Generally, torticollis most commonly follows injury to the C1-2 articulation. Minor trauma can lead to spontaneous C1-2 subluxation. Fractures or dislocation of the odontoid may not be apparent in the initial radiographic views (see Fig. 30–18), and consequently a high index of suspicion and careful follow-up are

required. Children with bone dysplasia, Morquio syndrome, spondyloepiphyseal dysplasia, and Down syndrome have a high incidence of C1-2 instability and should be evaluated routinely.

Intermittent torticollis can occur in a young child. A seizurelike disorder termed *benign paroxysmal torticollis of infancy* has many neurologic causes, including drug intoxication. Similarly, Sandifer syndrome, involving gastroesophageal reflux with sudden posturing of the trunk and torticollis,

TABLE 30–2 Differential Diagnosis of Torticollis

Congenital	Acquired
Occipitocervical anomalies	Neurogenic
Basilar impressions	Spinal cord tumors
Atlanto-occipital fusion	Cerebellar tumors (posterior fossa)
Odontoid anomalies	Syringomyelia
Hemiatlas	Ocular dysfunction
Pterygium colli (skin web)	Bulbar palsies
Congenital muscular torticollis	Traumatic (particularly C1-2)
Klippel-Feil syndrome	Subluxations
	Dislocations
	Fractures
	Inflammatory
	Cervical adenitis
	Spontaneous hyperemic atlantoaxial rotatory subluxation
	Tuberculosis
	Typhoid
	Rheumatoid arthritis
	Acute calcification of disc
	Miscellaneous
	Sandifer syndrome (hiatal hernia with esophageal reflux)

TABLE 30–3 Torticollis Caused by Bony Anomalies

Congenital Anomalies of Craniocervical Junction	Acquired Anomalies of Craniocervical Junction
Klippel-Feil syndrome	Traumatic
Atlanto-occipital synostosis (unilateral)	Subluxations
Odontoid anomalies	Dislocations
Aplasia	Fractures
Hypoplasia	Inflammatory
Os odontoideum	Rheumatoid arthritis
Occipital vertebra	Idiopathic
Asymmetry of occipital condyles (hypoplasia)	Atlantoaxial rotatory displacement
	Subluxation
	Fixation

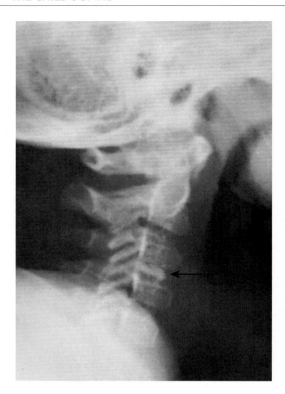

FIGURE 30–54 A 6-year-old girl presented with acute onset of torticollis and neck pain but no history of trauma or recent infection. Lateral radiograph of cervical spine shows acute calcification of disc between C3 and C4 (*arrow*). The child was treated conservatively with a neck collar, and there was spontaneous resolution of torticollis and symptoms over a 2-week period. Disc calcification was still radiologically visible at 6 months after onset of symptoms but not at 12 months.

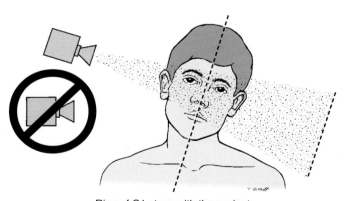

Ring of C1 stays with the occiput

FIGURE 30–55 Obtaining a satisfactory radiograph may be hampered by the patient's limited ability to cooperate; fixed bony deformity; and overlapping shadows from mandible, occiput, and foramen magnum. A helpful guide is that the atlas moves with the occiput; if x-ray beam is directed 90 degrees to lateral of skull, satisfactory view of occipitocervical junction usually results.

is being recognized more often, particularly in neurologically handicapped children, such as children with cerebral palsy.[256]

Neurologic disorders, particularly space-occupying lesions of the central nervous system, such as tumors of the posterior fossa or spinal column, chordoma, and syringomyelia, are often accompanied by torticollis. Generally, there are additional neurologic findings, such as long tract signs and weakness in the upper extremities. Uncommon neurologic causes include dystonia musculorum deformans and problems of hearing and vision that can result in head tilt.[257] Although uncommon, hysterical and psychogenic causes exist, but these should be diagnosed only after other causes are carefully excluded.

Radiographic Features

All children with torticollis should be evaluated with radiography to exclude a bony abnormality or fracture. Radiographic interpretation of congenital torticollis may be difficult because of the fixed abnormal head position and the restricted motion. In children with a painful wry neck, it may be impossible to position them appropriately for a standard view of the occipitocervical junction. A helpful guide is that the atlas moves with the occiput; if the x-ray beam is directed 90 degrees to the lateral skull, a satisfactory view of the occipitocervical junction usually results. Flexion-extension stress films, dynamic CT scan, or cineradiography may be necessary to confirm atlantoaxial instability. The bony anomalies that may be present in congenital torticollis are documented in the sections on anomalies of odontoid, Klippel-Feil syndrome, and basilar impression.

Rotatory subluxation of C1 and C2 presents a unique problem. Plain radiographs seldom differentiate the position of C1 and C2 during subluxation from that in a normal child whose head is rotated because both give the same picture. Open-mouth views have been difficult to obtain and interpret. Lack of cooperation and decreased neck motion on the part of the child can make it impossible to obtain these special views. Fielding and Hawkins[250] recommended cineradiography, but the radiation dosage is relatively high, and patient cooperation may be difficult to obtain because of muscle spasm.

The normal relationship between the occiput and the atlas is thought to be rarely affected in atlantoaxial rotatory subluxation. A lateral radiograph of the skull may show the relative position of the atlas and axis more clearly than a lateral radiograph of the cervical spine, in which tilting of the head also tilts the atlas, and overlapping shadows make interpretation difficult (Fig. 30–55). Similarly, if during CT scans the child is in the torticollis position, the image may be interpreted by the radiologist as showing rotation of C1 and C2. Conversely, in a child with rotatory subluxation, the rotation of C1 and C2 may be within the range of normal, as is usually the case. Early in this condition, the radiologist may attribute the finding to patient positioning.[245] This dilemma can be resolved by paying close attention to proper positioning of the patient, obtaining CT cuts at the level of C1, and rotating the head to the right and left and showing the facets to be locked in that position.[245]

KEY POINTS

1. Patients with osteochondrodysplasias, such as osteogenesis imperfecta, have bone softening and are at increased risk for developing basilar impression.

2. CT and MRI have become the imaging modalities of choice to evaluate basilar invagination and associated compression of neural elements.

3. Separation of the anterior ring of C1 from the odontoid of more than 4.5 mm is suggestive of failure of the transverse atlantal ligament.

4. When there is occipitalization and an accompanying fusion of C2-3, there is a 70% risk of failure of the transverse atlantal ligament.

5. Nonunion of an odontoid fracture and os odontoideum can occur in children and must be differentiated.

6. Klippel-Feil syndrome is often associated with other problems, such as Sprengel deformity, scoliosis, and renal anomalies.

7. Congenital muscular torticollis represents a compartment syndrome of the sternocleidomastoid muscle.

KEY REFERENCES

1. Aronson DD, Kahn RH, Canady A, et al: Instability of the cervical spine after decompression in patients who have Arnold-Chiari malformation. J Bone Joint Surg Am 73:898-906, 1991.
   This article identified the importance of occipitocervical stabilization after posterior decompressive procedures.

2. Chamberlain WE: Basilar impression (platybasia): A bizarre developmental anomaly of the occipital bone and upper cervical spine with striking and misleading neurologic manifestations. Yale J Biol Med 11:487, 1939.
   Chamberlain was the first to identify this clinical problem and the concept that the upper cervical spine seemed to indent the occiput.

3. Currarino G, Rollins N, Diehl JT: Congenital defects of the posterior arch of the atlas: A report of seven cases including an affected mother and son. AJNR Am J Neuroradiol 15:249-254, 1994.
   This article highlights the importance of C1 ring anomalies and their relationship to neurologic symptoms.

4. De Barros MC, Faria W, Ataide L, et al: Basilar impression and Arnold-Chiari malformation: A study of 66 cases. J Neurol Neurosurg Psychiatry 1:596, 1968.
   This study of a large population of Brazilian patients with this deformity helped to define neurologic findings and the natural history of the condition.

5. Fielding JW, Griffin PO: Os odontoideum: An acquired lesion. J Bone Joint Surg Am 56:187, 1974.
   The authors postulated the concept of a traumatic and a congenital origin of os odontoideum.

6. Fielding JW, Hawkins RJ, Ratzan S: Fusion for atlantoaxial instability. J Bone Joint Surg Am 58:400, 1976.
   In this landmark article, the authors discussed fusion for atlantoaxial instability.

7. Hall JE, Simmons ED, Danylchuk K, et al: Instability of the cervical spine and neurological involvement in Klippel-Feil syndrome: A case report. J Bone Joint Surg Am 92:460-462, 1990.
   This important article identifies instability and neurologic compromise at a hypermobile articulation.

8. Hensinger RN, Lang JR, MacEwen GD: The Klippel-Feil syndrome: A constellation of related anomalies. J Bone Joint Surg Am 56:1246, 1974.
   The authors completed a large series that studied Klippel-Feil syndrome in a large population and identified different patterns of cervical motion.

9. Locke GR, Gardner JI, Van Epps EF: Atlas-dens interval (ADI) in children: A survey based on 200 normal cervical spines. AJR Am J Roentgenol 97:135, 1966.
   These authors were the first to define the ADI in children.

10. McAfee PC, Bohlman HH, Han JS, et al: Comparison of nuclear magnetic resonance imaging and computed tomography in the diagnosis of upper cervical spinal cord compression. Spine 11:295, 1986.
    These authors helped to define the new role of CT and MRI in evaluating basilar invagination.

11. McRae DL: Bony abnormalities in the region of the foramen magnum: Correlation of the anatomic and neurologic findings. Acta Radiol 40:335, 1953.
    This was the first study to delineate differences and the significance of abnormalities of the cervical spine.

12. McRae DL, Barnum AS: Occipitalization of the atlas. AJR Am J Roentgenol Radium Ther Nucl Med 70:23, 1953.
    This article was one of the first on the subject of occipitalization and the potential for myelopathy complicating congenital atlantoaxial dislocation.

13. Sawin PD, Menezes AH: Basilar invagination in osteogenesis imperfecta and related osteochondral dysplasias: Medical and surgical management. J Neurosurg 86:950-960, 1997.
    This series addressed treatment and outcomes of basilar invagination in patients with osteochondrodysplasias.

REFERENCES

1. Chamberlain WE: Basilar impression (platybasia): A bizarre developmental anomaly of the occipital bone and upper cervical spine with striking and misleading neurologic manifestations. Yale J Biol Med 11:487, 1939.

2. Gosain AK, McCarthy JG, Pinto RS: Cervicovertebral anomalies and basilar impression in Goldenhar syndrome. Plast Reconstr Surg 93:498-506, 1994.

3. Menezes AH: Specific entities affecting the craniocervical region. Childs Nerv Syst 24:1169-1172, 2008.

4. Sawin PD, Menezes AH: Basilar invagination in osteogenesis imperfecta and related osteochondral dysplasias: Medical and surgical management. J Neurosurg 86:950-960, 1997.

5. Brooks BL, Gall C, Wang AM, et al: Osteogenesis imperfecta associated with basilar impression and cerebral atrophy: A case report. Comput Med Imaging Graph 13:363-367, 1989.

6. Epstein BS, Epstein JA: The association of cerebellar tonsillar herniation with basilar impression incident to Paget's disease. AJR Am J Roentgenol Radium Ther Nucl Med 107:535, 1969.

7. McGregor M: The significance of certain measurements of the skull in the diagnosis of basilar impression. Br J Radiol 21:171, 1948.

8. Hinck VC, Hopkins CE, Savara BS: Diagnostic criteria of basilar impression. Radiology 76:572, 1961.

9. Clay WC, Sturm PF, Hatch RS, et al: Intraobserver reproducibility and interobserver reliability of cervical spine measurements. J Pediatr Orthop 20:66-74, 2000.

10. Cronin CG, Lohan DG, Mhuircheartaigh JN, et al: MRI evaluation and measurement of the normal odontoid ped position. Clin Radiol 62:897-903, 2007.

11. Fischgold H, Metzger J: Étude radiotomographique de l'impression basilaire. Rev Rhum Mal Osteoartic 19:261, 1952.

12. Adam AM: Skull radiographic measurements of normals and patients with basilar impression: Use of Landzert's angle. Surg Radiol Anat 9:225, 1987.

13. Samartzis D, Kalluri P, Herman J, et al: Superior odontoid migration in the Klippel-Feil patient. Eur Spine J 16:1489-1497, 2007.

14. De Barros MC, Faria W, Ataide L, et al: Basilar impression and Arnold-Chiari malformation: A study of 66 cases. J Neurol Neurosurg Psychiatry 1:596, 1968.

15. Bassi P, Corona C, Contri P, et al: Congenital basilar impression: Correlated neurologic syndromes. Eur Neurol 32:238-243, 1992.

16. Kohno K, Sakaki S, Nakamura H, et al: Foramen magnum decompression for syringomyelia associated with basilar impression and Chiari I malformation: Report of three cases. Neurol Med Chir 31:715-719, 1991.

17. da Silva JA: Basilar impression and Arnold-Chiari malformation: Surgical findings in 209 cases. Neurochirurgia 35:189-195, 1992.

18. Ali MM, Russell N, Awada N, et al: A craniocervical malformation presenting as acute respiratory failure. J Emerg Med 14:569-572, 1996.

19. Bernini F, Elefante R, Smaltino F, et al: Angiographic study on the vertebral artery in cases of deformities of the occipitocervical joint. AJR Am J Roentgenol Radium Ther Nucl Med 107:526, 1969.

20. Dickinson LD, Tuite GF, Colon GP, et al: Vertebral artery dissection related to basilar impression: Case report. Neurosurgery 36:835-838, 1995.

21. Gunderson CH, Greenspan RH, Glaser GH, et al: Klippel-Feil syndrome: Genetic and clinical re-evaluation of cervical fusion. Medicine 46:491-511, 1967.

22. Michie I, Clark M: Neurological syndromes associated with cervical and craniocervical anomalies. Arch Neurol 18:241, 1968.

23. Bachs A, Barraquer-Bordas L, Barraquer-Ferre L, et al: Delayed myelopathy following atlantoaxial dislocations by separated odontoid process. Brain 78:537, 1955.

24. Barker R, Fareedi S, Thompson D, et al: The use of CT angiography in the preoperative planning of cervical spine surgery in children. Childs Nerv Syst 25:955-959, 2009.

25. Fromm GH, Pitner SE: Late progressive quadriparesis due to odontoid agenesis. Arch Neurol 9:291, 1963.

26. Goel A, Shah A: Reversal of longstanding musculoskeletal changes in basilar invagination after surgical decompression and stabilization. J Neurosurg Spine 10:220-227, 2009.

27. Goel A, Shah A, Rajan S: Vertical mobile and reducible atlantoaxial dislocation. J Neurosurg Spine 11:9-14, 2009.

28. Kumar R, Kalra SK, Mahapatra AK: A clinical scoring system for neurological assessment of high cervical myelopathy: Measurements in pediatric patients with congenital atlantoaxial dislocations. Neurosurgery 61:987-994, 2007.

29. Hosalkar HS, Sankar WN, Wills BPD, et al: Congenital osseous anomalies of the upper cervical spine. J Bone Joint Surg Am 90:337-348, 2008.

30. Locke GR, Gardner JI, Van Epps EF: Atlas-dens interval (ADI) in children: A survey based on 200 normal cervical spines. AJR Am J Roentgenol 97:135, 1966.

31. von Torklus D, Gehle W: The Upper Cervical Spine. New York, Grune & Stratton, 1972.

32. Gholve PA, Hosalkar HS, Ricchetti ET, et al: Occipitalization of the atlas in children. J Bone Joint Surg Am 89:571-578, 2007.

33. McRae DL: Bony abnormalities in the region of the foramen magnum: Correlation of the anatomic and neurologic findings. Acta Radiol 40:335, 1953.

34. Greenberg AD: Atlantoaxial dislocations. Brain 91:655, 1968.

35. Spillane JD, Pallis C, Jones AM: Developmental abnormalities in the region of the foramen magnum. Brain 80:11, 1957.

36. Nagashima C: Atlanto-axial dislocation due to agenesis of the os odontoideum or odontoid. J Neurosurg 33:270, 1970.

37. Bharucha EP, Dastur HM: Craniovertebral anomalies (a report on 40 cases). Brain 87:469, 1964.

38. McRae DL: The significance of abnormalities of the cervical spine. AJR Am J Roentgenol 84:3, 1960.

39. Perovic NM, Kopits SE, Thompson RC: Radiologic evaluation of the spinal cord in congenital atlanto-axial dislocations. Radiology 109:713, 1973.

40. Spitzer R, Rabinowitch JY, Wybar KC: A study of the abnormalities of the skull, teeth, and lenses in mongolism. Can Med Assoc J 84:567-572, 1961.

41. Reilly CW, Choit RL: Transarticular screws in the management of C1-C2 instability in children. J Pediatr Orthop 26:582-588, 2006.

42. Burke SW, French HG, Roberts JM, et al: Chronic atlanto-axial instability in Down syndrome. J Bone Joint Surg Am 67:1356-1360, 1985.

43. Morton RE, Khan MA, Murray-Leslie C, et al: Atlantoaxial instability in Down syndrome: A five-year follow up study. Arch Dis Child 72:115-119, 1995.

SECTION

IV

44. Ferguson RL, Putney ME, Allen BL: Comparison of neurological deficits with atlanto-dens intervals in patients with Down syndrome. J Spinal Disord 10:246-252, 1997.

45. Taggard DA, Menezes AH, Ryken TC: Treatment of Down syndrome-associated craniovertebral junction anomalies. J Neurosurg Spine 93:205-213, 2000.

46. Hinck VC, Hopkins CE, Savara BS: Sagittal diameter of the cervical spinal canal in children. Radiology 79:97, 1962.

47. Fielding JW, Hensinger RN, Hawkins RJ: Os odontoideum. J Bone Joint Surg Am 62:376, 1980.

48. Fielding JW, Cochran GV, Lawsing JF III, et al: Tears of the transverse ligament of the atlas. J Bone Joint Surg Am 56:1683, 1974.

49. Klimo P Jr, Kan P, Rao G, et al: Os odontoideum: Presentation, diagnosis, and treatment in a series of 78 patients. J Neurosurg Spine 9:332-342, 2008.

50. Hensinger RN: Osseous anomalies of the craniovertebral junction. Spine 111:323, 1986.

51. Roach JW, Duncan D, Wenger DR, et al: Atlanto-axial instability and spinal cord compression in children: Diagnosis by computerized tomography. J Bone Joint Surg Am 66:708, 1984.

52. Gupta V, Khandelwal N, Mathuria SN, et al: Dynamic magnetic resonance imaging evaluation of craniovertebral junction abnormalities. J Comput Assist Tomogr 31:354-359, 2007.

53. Smoker WRK, Khanna G: Imaging the craniocervical junction. Childs Nerv Syst 24:1123-1145, 2008.

54. Giannestras NJ, Mayfield FH, Provencio FP, et al: Congenital absence of the odontoid process: A case report. J Bone Joint Surg Am 46:839, 1964.

55. Dickman CA, Mamourian A, Sonntag VK, et al: Magnetic resonance imaging of the transverse atlantal ligament for the evaluation of atlantoaxial instability. J Neurosurg 75:221-227, 1991.

56. Jauregui N, Lincoln T, Mubarak S, et al: Surgically related upper cervical spine canal anatomy in children. Spine 18:1939-1944, 1993.

57. McAfee PC, Bohlman HH, Han JS, et al: Comparison of nuclear magnetic resonance imaging and computed tomography in the diagnosis of upper cervical spinal cord compression. Spine 11:295, 1986.

58. Weng MS, Haynes RJ: Flexion and extension cervical MRI in pediatric population. J Pediatr Orthop 16:359-363, 1996.

59. Steel HH: Anatomical and mechanical considerations of the atlanto-axial articulations. J Bone Joint Surg Am 50:1481, 1968.

60. Fielding JW, Hawkins RJ, Ratzan SA: Spine fusion for atlanto-axial instability. J Bone Joint Surg Am 58:400, 1976.

61. Haworth JB, Keillor GW: Use of transparencies in evaluating the width of the spinal canal in infants, children and adults. Radiology 79:109, 1962.

62. Naik DR: Cervical spinal canal in normal infants. Clin Radiol 21:323, 1970.

63. Dolan KD: Expanding lesions of the cervical spinal canal. Radiol Clin North Am 15:203, 1977.

64. Cattell HS, Filtzer DL: Pseudosubluxation and other normal variations in the cervical spine in children. J Bone Joint Surg Am 47:1295, 1965.

65. Garber JN: Abnormalities of the atlas and axis vertebrae, congenital and traumatic. J Bone Joint Surg Am 46:1782, 1964.

66. Swischuk LE: Anterior displacement of C2 in children: Physiologic or pathologic? Radiology 12:759-763, 1977.

67. Geehr RB, Rothman SLG, Kier EL: The role of computed tomography in the evaluation of upper cervical spine pathology. Comput Tomogr 2:79, 1978.

68. Resjo M, Harwood-Nash DC, Fitz CR: Normal cord in infants and children examined with computed tomographic metrizamide myelography. Radiology 130:691, 1979.

69. Bhatnagar M, Sponseller PD, Carroll C IV, et al: Pediatric atlantoaxial instability presenting as cerebral and cerebellar infarcts. J Pediatr Orthop 11:103-107, 1991.

70. Miyata I, Imaoka T, Masaoka T, et al: Pediatric cerebellar infarction caused by atlantoaxial subluxation: Case report. Neurol Med Chir 34:241-245, 1994.

71. Ahmed R, Trynelis VC, Menezes AH: Fusions at the craniovertebral junction. Childs Nerv Syst 24:1209-1224, 2008.

72. Sinh G, Pandya SK: Treatment of congenital atlanto-axial dislocations. Proc Aust Assoc Neurol 5:507, 1968.

73. Wadia NH: Myelopathy complicating congenital atlanto-axial dislocation (a study of 28 cases). Brain 90:449, 1967.

74. Grantham SA, Dick HM, Thompson RC Jr, et al: Occipitocervical arthrodesis: Indications, technic and results. Clin Orthop 65:118, 1969.

75. Krieger AJ, Rosomoff HL, Kuperman AS, et al: Occult respiratory dysfunction in a craniovertebral anomaly. J Neurosurg 31:15, 1969.

76. Reddy KR, Rao GS, Devi BI, et al: Pulmonary function after surgery for congenital atlantoaxial dislocation. J Neurosurg Anesthesiol 21:196-201, 2009.

77. Pueschel SM, Scola FH: Atlantoaxial instability in individuals with Down's syndrome: Epidemiologic, radiographic, and clinical studies. Pediatrics 80:555, 1987.

78. Davidson RG: Atlantoaxial instability in individuals with Down's syndrome: A fresh look at the evidence. J Bone Joint Surg Am 47:1295, 1965.

79. Georgopoulos G, Pizzutillo PD, Lee MS: Occipitoatlantal instability in children: A report of five cases and review of the literature. J Bone Joint Surg Am 69:429, 1987.

80. Browd SR, McIntyre JS, Brockmeyer D: Failed age-dependent maturation of the occipital condyle in patients with congenital occipitoatlantal instability and Down syndrome: A preliminary analysis. J Neurosurg Pediatrics 2:359-364, 2008.

81. Chandraraj S, Briggs CA: Failure of somite differentiation at the craniovertebral region as a cause of occipitalization of the atlas. Spine 17:1249-1251, 1992.

82. Macalister A: Notes on the development and variations of the atlas. J Anat Physiol 27:519, 1983.

83. McRae DL, Barnum AS: Occipitalization of the atlas. AJR Am J Roentgenol Radium Ther Nucl Med 70:23, 1953.

84. Malhotra V, Leeds NE: Case report 277. Skeletal Radiol 12:55-58, 1984.

85. Hadley LA: The Spine. Springfield, IL, Charles C Thomas, 1956.

86. Bailey DK: The normal cervical spine in infants and children. Radiology 59:712, 1962.

87. Caffey J: Paediatric X-ray Diagnosis. Chicago, Year Book Medical Publishers, 1967.

88. Menezes AH: Craniocervical developmental anatomy and its implications. Childs Nerv Syst 24:1109-1122, 2008.

89. Senoglu M, Safavi-Abbasi S, Theodore N, et al: The frequency and clinical significance of congenital defects of the posterior and anterior arch of the atlas. J Neurosurg Spine 7:399-402, 2007.

90. Musha Y, Mizutani K: Cervical myelopathy accompanied with hypoplasia of the posterior arch of the atlas. J Spinal Disord Tech 22:228-232, 2009.

91. Fielding JW: The cervical spine in the child. Curr Pract Orthop Surg 5:31, 1973.

92. Baird PA, Robinson GC, Buckler WS: Klippel-Feil syndrome. Am J Dis Child 113:546, 1967.

93. Nicholson JS, Sherk HH: Anomalies of the occipitocervical articulation. J Bone Joint Surg Am 50:295, 1968.

94. DiLorenzo N: Craniocervical junction malformation treated by transoral approach: A survey of 25 cases with emphasis on postoperative instability and outcome. Acta Neurochir 118:112-116, 1992.

95. Dickman CA, Locantro J, Fessler RG: The influence of transoral odontoid resection on stability of the craniovertebral junction. J Neurosurg 77:525-530, 1992.

96. Aronson DD, Kahn RH, Canady A, et al: Instability of the cervical spine after decompression in patients who have Arnold-Chiari malformation. J Bone Joint Surg Am 73:898-906, 1991.

97. Fehlings MG, Errico T, Cooper P, et al: Occipitocervical fusion with a five-millimeter malleable rod and segmental fixation. Neurosurgery 32:198-207, 1993.

98. Letts M, Slutsky D: Occipitocervical arthrodesis in children. J Bone Joint Surg Am 72:1166-1170, 1990.

99. Rea GL, Mullin BB, Mervis LJ, et al: Occipitocervical fixation in nontraumatic upper cervical spine instability. Surg Neurol 40:255-261, 1993.

100. McLaughlin MR, Wahlig JB, Pollack IF: Incidence of postlaminectomy kyphosis after Chiari decompression. Spine 22:613-617, 1997.

101. Geipel P: Zur Kenntnis der Spina bifida das Atlas. Forstschr Rontgenstr 42:583-589, 1930.

102. Currarino G, Rollins N, Diehl JT: Congenital defects of the posterior arch of the atlas: A report of seven cases including an affected mother and son. AJNR Am J Neuroradiol 15:249-254, 1994.

103. Dubousset J: Torticollis in children caused by congenital anomalies of the atlas. J Bone Joint Surg Am 68:178, 1986.

104. Stevens JM, Chong WK, Barber C, et al: A new appraisal of abnormalities of the odontoid process associated with atlanto-axial subluxation and neurological disability. Brain 117:133-148, 1994.

105. Michaels L, Prevost MJ, Crong DF: Pathological changes in a case of os odontoideum (separate odontoid process). J Bone Joint Surg Am 51:965, 1969.

106. Gwinn JL, Smith JL: Acquired and congenital absence of the odontoid process. Am J Roentgenol Radium Ther Nucl Med 88:424, 1962.

107. Minderhoud JM, Braakman R, Penning L: Os odontoideum: Clinical, radiological, and therapeutic aspects. J Neurol Sci 89:521, 1969.

108. Schiller F, Nieda I: Malformations of the odontoid process: Report of a case and clinical survey. Calif Med 86:394, 1957.

109. Wollin DG: The os odontoideum: Separate odontoid process. J Bone Joint Surg Am 45:1459, 1963.

110. Curtis BH, Blank S, Fisher RL: Atlantoaxial dislocation in Down's syndrome. JAMA 205:464, 1968.

111. Dzenitis AJ: Spontaneous atlantoaxial dislocation in a mongoloid child with spinal cord compression: Case report. J Neurosurg 25:458, 1966.

112. Hensinger RN, Lang JR, MacEwen GD: The Klippel-Feil syndrome: A constellation of related anomalies. J Bone Joint Surg Am 56:1246, 1974.

113. Martel W, Fishler JM: Observation of the spine in mongoloidism. Am J Roentgenol Radium Ther Nucl Med 97:630, 1966.

114. Sherk HH, Nicholson JL: Ossiculum terminale and mongolism. J Bone Joint Surg Am 51:957, 1969.

115. Sankar WN, Wills BPD, Dormans JP, et al: Os odontoideum revisited: The case for a multifactorial etiology. Spine 31:979-984, 2006.

116. Basset FH, Goldner JL: Aplasia of the odontoid process. Proc Am Acad Orthop Surg 50:833, 1968.

117. Shapiro R, Youngsberg AS, Rothman SLG: The differential diagnosis of traumatic lesions of the occipito-atlanto-axial segment. Radiol Clin North Am 3:505, 1971.

118. Rothman RH, Simeone FA: The Spine, 2nd ed. Philadelphia, WB Saunders, 1982.

119. Evarts CM, Lonsdale D: Ossiculum terminale: An anomaly of the odontoid process: Report of a case of atlantoaxial dislocation with cord compression. Cleve Clin Q 37:73, 1970.

120. Swoboda B, Hirschfelder H, Hohmann D: Atlantoaxial instability in a 7-year-old boy associated with traumatic disrupture of the ossiculum terminale (apical odontoid epiphysis). Eur Spine J 4:248-251, 1995.

121. Ahlback I, Collert S: Destruction of the odontoid process due to axial pyogenic spondylitis. Acta Radiol [Diagn] (Stockh) 10:394, 1970.

122. Fielding JW: Disappearance of the central portion of the odontoid process. J Bone Joint Surg Am 47:1228, 1965.

123. Fielding JW, Griffin PO: Os odontoideum: An acquired lesion. J Bone Joint Surg Am 56:187, 1974.

124. Freiberger RH, Wilson PD Jr, Nicholas JA: Acquired absence of the odontoid process. J Bone Joint Surg Am 47:1231, 1965.

125. Phillips PC, Lorentsen KJ, Shropshire LC, et al: Congenital odontoid aplasia and posterior circulation stroke in childhood. Ann Neurol 23:410-413, 1988.

126. Kirlew KA, Hathout GM, Reiter SD, et al: Os odontoideum in identical twins: Perspectives on etiology. Skeletal Radiol 22:525-527, 1993.

127. Morgan MK, Onofrio BM, Bender CE: Familial os odontoideum: Case report. J Neurosurg 70:636-639, 1989.

128. Holt RG, Helms CA, Munk PL, et al: Hypertrophy of C-1 anterior arch: Useful sign to distinguish os odontoideum from acute dens fracture. Radiology 173:207-209, 1989.

129. Watanabe M, Toyama Y, Fujimura Y: Atlantoaxial instability in os odontoideum with myelopathy. Spine 21:1435-1439, 1996.

130. McKeever FM: Atlantoaxial instability. Surg Clin North Am 48:1375, 1968.

131. Rowland LP, Shapiro JH, Jacobson HG: Neurological syndromes associated with congenital absence of the odontoid process. Arch Neurol Psychiatry 80:286, 1958.

132. Ford FK: Syncope, vertigo, and disturbances of vision resulting from intermittent obstruction of the vertebral arteries due to a defect in the odontoid process and excessive mobility of the axis. Bull Johns Hopkins Hosp 91:168, 1952.

133. Kikuchi K, Nakagawa H, Watanabe K, et al: Bilateral vertebral artery occlusion secondary to atlantoaxial dislocation with os odontoideum: Implication for prophylactic cervical stabilization by fusion: Case report. Neurol Med Chir 33:769-773, 1993.

134. Takakuwa T, Hiroi S, Hasegawa H, et al: Os odontoideum with vertebral artery occlusion. Spine 19:460-462, 1994.

135. Gillman CL: Congenital absence of the odontoid process of the axis: Report of a case. J Bone Joint Surg Am 41:340, 1959.

136. Hosono N, Yonenobu K, Ebara S, et al: Cineradiographic motion analysis of atlantoaxial instability in os odontoideum. Spine 16(Suppl):S480-S482, 1991.

137. Elliott S: The odontoid process in children: Is it hypoplastic? Clin Radiol 39:391-393, 1988.

138. Spierings EL, Braakman R: The management of os odontoideum: Analysis of 37 cases. J Bone Joint Surg Br 64:422-428, 1982.

139. Fagan AB, Askin GN, Earwaker JW: The jigsaw sign: A reliable indicator of congenital etiology in os odontoideum. Eur Spine J 13:295-300, 2004.

140. Yamashita Y, Takahashi M, Sakamoto Y, et al: Atlantoaxial subluxation: Radiography and magnetic resonance imaging correlated to myelopathy. Acta Radiol 30:135-140, 1989.

141. Hughes TB, Richman JD, Rothfus WE: Diagnosis of os odontoideum using kinematic magnetic resonance imaging. Spine 24:715-718, 1999.

142. Shepard CN: Familial hypoplasia of the odontoid process. J Bone Joint Surg Am 48:1224, 1966.

143. Greenberg AD, Scovillo WB, Davey LM: Transoral decompression of atlantoaxial dislocation due to odontoid hypoplasia: Report of two cases. J Neurosurg 28:266, 1968.

144. Levy ML, McComb JG: C1-C2 fusion in children with atlantoaxial instability and spinal cord compression: Technical note. Neurosurgery 38:211-215, 1996.

145. Huang CI, Chen IH: Atlantoaxial arthrodesis using Halifax interlaminar clamps reinforced by halo vest immobilization: A long-term follow-up experience. Neurosurgery 38:1153-1156, 1996.

146. Moskovich R, Crockard HA: Atlantoaxial arthrodesis using interlaminar clamps: An improved technique. Spine 17:261-267, 1992.

147. Dickman CA, Crawford NR, Paramore CG: Biomechanical characteristics of C1-2 cable fixations. J Neurosurg 85:316-322, 1996.

148. Smith MD, Phillips WA, Hensinger RN: Fusion of the upper cervical spine in children and adolescents: An analysis of 17 patients. Spine 16:695-701, 1991.

149. Brockmeyer D, Apfelbaum R, Tippets R, et al: Pediatric cervical spine instrumentation using screw fixation. Pediatr Neurosurg 22:147-157, 1995.

150. Coyne TJ, Fehlings MG, Wallace MC, et al: C1-C2 posterior cervical fusion: Long-term evaluation of results and efficacy. Neurosurgery 37:688-693, 1995.

151. Stabler CL, Eismont FJ, Brown MD, et al: Failure of posterior cervical fusions using cadaveric bone graft in children. J Bone Joint Surg Am 67:370-375, 1985.

152. Menendez JA: Techniques of posterior C1-C2 stabilization. Neurosurgery 60(Suppl 1):s1-103-s1-s111, 2007.

153. Visocchi M, Fernandez E, Ciampini A, et al: Reducible and irreducible os odontoideum in childhood treated with posterior wiring, instrumentation and fusion. Past or present? Acta Neurochir (Wien) 151:1265-1274, 2009.

154. Mah JY, Thometz J, Emans J, et al: Threaded K-wire spinous process fixation of the axis for modified Gallie fusion in children and adolescents. J Pediatr Orthop 9:675-679, 1989.

155. Grob D, Crisco JJ III, Panjabi MM, et al: Biomechanical evaluation of four different posterior atlantoaxial fixation techniques. Spine 17:480-490, 1992.

156. Bambakidis NC, Feiz-Erfan I, Horn EM, et al: Biomechanical comparison of occipitoatlantal screw fixation techniques. J Neurosurg Spine 8:143-152, 2008.

157. Haque A, Price AV, Sklar FH, et al: Screw fixation of the upper cervical spine in the pediatric population. J Neurosurg Pediatrics 3:529-533, 2009.

158. Chamoun RB, Relyea KM, Johnson KK, et al: Use of axial and subaxial translaminar screw fixation in the management of upper cervical spinal instability in a series of 7 children. Neurosurgery 64:734-739, 2009.

159. Hoh DJ, Maya M, Jung A, et al: Anatomical relationship of the internal carotid artery to C-1: Clinical implications for screw fixation of the atlas. J Neurosurg Spine 8:335-340, 2008.

160. Smith MD, Phillips WA, Hensinger RN: Complications of fusion to the upper cervical spine. Spine 16:702-705, 1991.

161. Dyck P: Os odontoideum in children: Neurological manifestations and surgical management. Neurosurgery 2:93, 1978.

162. Whitesides TE, McDonald AP: Lateral retropharyngeal approach to the upper cervical spine. Orthop Clin North Am 9:1115, 1978.

163. Klippel M, Feil A: Un cas d'absence des vertèbres cervicales avec cage thoracique remontant jusqu'à la base du crane. Nouv Icon Salpet 25:223, 1912.

164. Feil A: L'absence et la diminution des vertèbres cervicales (étude clinique et pathogenique): Le syndrome de réduction numérique cervicale. Thèses de Paris, 1919.

165. Erskine CA: An analysis of the Klippel-Feil syndrome. Arch Pathol 41:269, 1946.

166. Gray SW, Romaine CB, Skandalakis JF: Congenital fusion of the cervical vertebrae. Surg Gynecol Obstet 118:373, 1964.

167. Tracy MR, Dormans JP, Kusumi K: Klippel-Feil syndrome: Clinical features and current understanding of etiology. Clin Orthop 424:183-190, 2004.

168. Clarke RA, Kearsley JH, Walsh DA: Patterned expression in familial Klippel-Feil syndrome. Teratology 53:152-157, 1996.

169. Clarke RA, Singh S, McKenzie H, et al: Familial Klippel-Feil syndrome and paracentric inversion inv(8)(q22.2q.23.3). Am J Hum Genet 57:1364-1370, 1995.

170. Schilgen M, Loeser H: Klippel-Feil anomaly combined with fetal alcohol syndrome. Eur Spine J 3:289-290, 1994.

171. McElfresh E, Winter R: Klippel-Feil syndrome. Minn Med 56:353, 1973.

172. Ramsey J, Bliznak J: Klippel-Feil syndrome with renal agenesis and other anomalies. AJR Am J Roentgenol 113:460, 1971.

173. Bauman GI: Absence of the cervical spine: Klippel-Feil syndrome. JAMA 98:129, 1932.

174. Baga N, Chusid EL, Miller A: Pulmonary disability in the Klippel-Feil syndrome. Clin Orthop 67:105, 1969.

175. Morrison SG, Perry LW, Scott LP: Congenital brevicollis (Klippel-Feil syndrome) and cardiovascular anomalies. Am J Dis Child 115:614, 1968.

176. Nora JJ, Cohen M, Maxwell GM: Klippel-Feil syndrome with congenital heart disease. Am J Dis Child 102:858, 1961.

177. McLay K, Maran AG: Deafness and the Klippel-Feil syndrome. J Laryngol Otol 83:175, 1969.

178. Palant DI, Carter BL: Klippel-Feil syndrome and deafness. Am J Dis Child 123:218, 1972.

179. Stark EW, Borton TE: Hearing loss and the Klippel-Feil syndrome. Am J Dis Child 123:233, 1972.

180. Ulmer JL, Elster AD, Ginsberg LE, et al: Klippel-Feil syndrome: CT and MRI of congenital abnormalities of cervical spine and cord. J Comput Assist Tomogr 17:215-224, 1993.

181. Sherk HH, Shut L, Chung S: Iniencephalic deformity of cervical spine with Klippel-Feil anomalies and congenital elevation of the scapula. J Bone Joint Surg Am 56:1254, 1974.

182. Frawley JM: Congenital webbing. Am J Dis Child 29:799, 1925.

183. Shoul MI, Ritvo M: Clinical and roentgenological manifestations of the Klippel-Feil syndrome (congenital fusion of the cervical vertebrae, brevicollis): Report of eight additional cases and review of the literature. AJR Am J Roentgenol 68:369, 1952.

184. Samartzis D, Herman J, Lubicky JP, Shen FH: Sprengel's deformity in Klippel-Feil syndrome. Spine 32:E512-E516, 2007.

185. Mooney JF III, White DR, Glazier S: Previously unreported structure associated with Sprengel deformity. J Pediatr Orthop 29:26-28, 2009.

186. Gumerlock MK, Spollen LE, Nelson MJ, et al: Cervical neurenteric fistula causing recurrent meningitis in Klippel-Feil sequence: Case report and literature review. Pediatr Infect Dis J 10:532-535, 1991.

187. Guille JT, Miller A, Bowen JR, et al: The natural history of Klippel-Feil syndrome: Clinical, roentgenographic, and magnetic resonance imaging findings at adulthood. J Pediatr Orthop 15:617-626, 1995.

188. Prasad VS, Reddy DR, Murty JM: Cervicothoracic neurenteric cyst: Clinicoradiological correlation with embryogenesis. Childs Nerv Syst 12:48-51, 1996.

189. Bavinck JN, Weaver DD: Subclavian artery supply disruption sequence: Hypothesis of a vascular etiology for Poland, Klippel-Feil, and Mobius anomalies. Am J Med Genet 23:903-918, 1986.

190. Pizzutillo PD, Woods MW, Nicholson L: Risk factors in the Klippel-Feil syndrome. Orthop Trans 11:473, 1987.

191. Samartzis D, Kalluri P, Herman J, et al: The extent of fusion within the congenital Klippel-Feil segment. Spine 33:1637-1642, 2008.

192. Samartzis D, Herman J, Lubicky JP, et al: Classification of congenitally fused cervical patters in Klippel-Feil patients. Spine 31:E798-E804, 2006.

193. Hall JE, Simmons ED, Danylchuk K, et al: Instability of the cervical spine and neurological involvement in Klippel-Feil syndrome: A case report. J Bone Joint Surg Am 92:460-462, 1990.

194. Forney WR, Robinson SJ, Pascoe DJ: Congenital heart disease, deafness, and skeletal malformations: A new syndrome? J Pediatr 68:14, 1966.

195. Illingworth RS: Attacks of unconsciousness in association with fused cervical vertebrae. Arch Dis Child 31:8, 1956.

196. Born CT, Petrik M, Freed M, et al: Cerebrovascular accident complicating Klippel-Feil syndrome: A case report. J Bone Joint Surg Am 79:1412-1415, 1988.

197. Ross CA, Curnes JT, Greenwood RS: Recurrent vertebrobasilar embolism in an infant with Klippel-Feil anomaly. Pediatr Neurol 3:181-183, 1987.

198. Ritterbusch JF, McGinty LD, Spar J, et al: Magnetic resonance imaging for stenosis and subluxation in Klippel-Feil syndrome. Spine 16(Suppl):S539-S541, 1991.

199. Kulkarni MV, Williams JC, Yeakley JW, et al: Magnetic resonance imaging in the diagnosis of the cranio-cervical manifestations of the mucopolysaccharidoses. Magn Res Imaging 5:317, 1987.

200. Sullivan RC, Bruwer AJ, Harris L: Hypermobility of the cervical spine in children: A pitfall in the diagnosis of cervical dislocation. Am J Surg 95:636, 1958.

201. Drvaric DM, Ruderman RJ, Conrad RW, et al: Congenital scoliosis and urinary tract abnormalities: Are intravenous pyelograms necessary? J Pediatr Orthop 7:441, 1987.

202. Nguyen VD, Tyrrel R: Klippel-Feil syndrome: Patterns of bony fusion and a wasp-waist sign. Skeletal Radiol 22:519-523, 1993.

203. Samartzis D, Kalluri P, Herman J, et al: The role of congenitally fused cervical segments upon the space available for the cord and associated symptoms in Klippel-Feil patients. Spine 33:1442-1450, 2008.

204. Baba H, Maezawa Y, Furusawa N, et al: The cervical spine in the Klippel-Feil syndrome: A report of 57 cases. Int Orthop 19:204-208, 1995.

205. Jalladeau J: Malformations congénitales associées syndrome de Klippel-Feil. Thèse de Paris, 1936.

206. Yousefzadeh DK, El-Khoury GY, Smith WL: Normal sagittal diameter and variation in the pediatric cervical spine. Pediatr Radiol 144:319, 1982.

207. Hensinger RG: Congenital anomalies of the cervical spine. Clin Orthop 264:16-38, 1991.

208. Shen FH, Samartzis D, Herman J, et al: Radiographic assessment of segmental motion at the atlantoaxial junction in the Klippel-Feil patient. Spine 31:171-177, 2006.

209. Theiss SM, Smith MD, Winter RB: The long-term follow-up of patients with Klippel-Feil syndrome with congenital scoliosis. Spine 22:1219-1222, 1997.

210. Thomsen MN, Schneider U, Weber M, et al: Scoliosis and congenital anomalies associated with Klippel-Feil syndrome types I-III. Spine 22:396-401, 1997.

211. Rosen CL, Novotny EJ, D'Andrea LA, et al: Klippel-Feil sequence and sleep-disordered breathing in two children. Am Rev Respir Dis 147:202-204, 1993.

212. Avery LW, Rentfro CC: The Klippel-Feil syndrome: A pathologic report. Arch Neurol Psychiatry 36:1068, 1936.

213. Moseley JE, Bonforte RJ: Spondylothoracic dysplasia: A syndrome with congenital heart disease. Am J Dis Child 102:858, 1961.

214. Moore WB, Matthews TJ, Rabinowitz R: Genitourinary anomalies associated with Klippel-Feil syndrome. J Bone Joint Surg Am 57:355, 1975.

215. Gunderson CH, Solitare GB: Mirror movements in patients with the Klippel-Feil syndrome: Neuropathologic observations. Arch Neurol 18:675, 1968.

216. Notermans SLH, Go KG, Boonstra S: EMG studies of associated movements in a patient with Klippel-Feil syndrome. Psychiatr Neurol Neurochir 73:257, 1970.

217. Stallmer ML, Vanaharam V, Mashour GA: Congenital cervical spine fusion and airway management: A case series of Klippel-Feil syndrome. J Clin Anesth 20:447-451, 2008.

218. Ruf M, Jenson R, Harms J: Hemivertebra resection in the cervical spine. Spine 30:380-385, 2005.

219. Bonola A: Surgical treatment of the Klippel-Feil syndrome. J Bone Joint Surg Br 38:440, 1956.

220. Campbell RM, Adcox BM, Smith MD, et al: The effect of midthoracic VEPTR opening wedge thoracostomy on cervical tilt associated with congenital thoracic scoliosis in patients with thoracic insufficiency syndrome. Spine 32:2171-2177, 2007.

221. Ling CM, Low YS: Sternomastoid tumor and muscular torticollis. Clin Orthop 86:144, 1972.

222. Chan YL, Cheng JC, Metreweil LC: Ultrasonography of congenital muscular torticollis. Pediatr Radiol 22:356-360, 1992.

223. Coventry MB, Harris LE: Congenital muscular torticollis in infancy: Some observations regarding treatment. J Bone Joint Surg Am 41:815, 1959.

224. Babu MKV, Lee P, Mahadev A, et al: Congenital bilateral sternocleidomastoid contracture: A case report. J Pediatr Orthop B 18:145-147, 2009.

225. Brackbill Y, Douthitt TC, West H: Psychophysiological effects in the neonate of prone versus supine placement. J Pediatr 82:2, 1973.

226. National Institutes of Health: National Institute of Child Health and Human Development. Back to Sleep Campaign. Available at http://www.nichd.nih.gov/sids/. Accessed July 30, 2009.

227. Ohman A, Nilsson S, Lagerkvist A-L, et al: Are infants with torticollis at risk of a delay in early motor milestones compared with a control group of healthy infants? Dev Med Child Neurol 51:545-550, 2009.

228. Davids JR, Wenger DR, Mubarak SJ: Congenital muscular torticollis: Sequela of intrauterine or perinatal compartment syndrome. J Pediatr Orthop 13:141-147, 1993.

229. MacDonald C: Sternomastoid tumor and muscular torticollis. J Bone Joint Surg Br 51:432, 1969.

230. Brooks B: Pathologic changes in muscle as a result of disturbances of circulation. Arch Surg 5:188, 1922.

231. Sarant JB, Morrissy RT: Idiopathic torticollis: Sternocleidomastoid myopathy and accessory neuropathy. Muscle Nerve 4:374, 1981.

232. Hummer DC Jr, MacEwen GD: The coexistence of torticollis and congenital dysplasia of the hip. J Bone Joint Surg Am 54:1255, 1972.

233. von Heideken J, Green DW, Burke SW, et al: The relationship between developmental dysplasia of the hip and congenital muscular torticollis. J Pediatr Orthop 26:805-808, 2006.

234. Minihane KP, Grayhack JJ, Simmons TD, et al: Developmental dysplasia of the hip in infants with congenital muscular torticollis. Am J Orthop 37:E155-E158, 2008.

235. Brougham DI, Cole WG, Dickens DR, et al: Torticollis due to a combination of sternomastoid contracture and congenital vertebral anomalies. J Bone Joint Surg Br 71:404, 1989.

236. Slate RK, Posnick JC, Armstrong DC, et al: Cervical spine subluxation associated with congenital muscular torticollis and craniofacial asymmetry. Plast Reconstr Surg 91:1187, 1993.

237. Tien YC, Su JY, Lin GT, et al: Ultrasonographic study of the coexistence of muscular torticollis and dysplasia of the hip. J Pediatr Orthop 21:343-347, 2001.

238. Canale ST, Griffin DW, Hubbard CN: Congenital muscular torticollis: Long-term follow-up. J Bone Joint Surg Am 64:810, 1982.

239. de Chalain TM, Katz A: Idiopathic muscular torticollis in children: The Cape Town experience. Br J Plast Surg 45:397, 1992.

240. Cheng JC, Wong MW, Tang SP, et al: Clinical determinants of the outcome of manual stretching in the treatment of congenital muscular torticollis in infants. J Bone Joint Surg Am 83:679-687, 2001.

241. Rogers GF, Oh AK, Mulliken JB: The role of congenital muscular torticollis in the development of deformational plagiocephaly. Plast Reconstr Surg 123:643-652, 2009.

242. Clarren FA: Muscular torticollis. J Bone Joint Surg Am 30:556, 1948.

243. Wirth CJ, Hagena FW, Wuelker N, et al: Biterminal tenotomy for the treatment of congenital muscular torticollis: Long-term results. J Bone Joint Surg Am 74:427, 1992.

244. Lee IJ, Lim SY, Song HS, et al: Complete tight fibrous band release and resection in congenital muscular torticollis. J Plastic Reconstr Aesthet Surg 63:947-953, 2010.

245. Shim JS, Noh KC, Park SJ: Treatment of congenital muscular torticollis in patients older than 8 years. J Pediatr Orthop 24:683-688, 2004.

246. Shim JS, Jang HP: Operative treatment of congenital torticollis. J Bone Joint Surg Br 90:934-939, 2008.

247. Staheli LT: Muscular torticollis: Late results of operative treatment. Surgery 69:469, 1971.

248. Akazawa H, Nakatsuka Y, Miyake Y, et al: Congenital muscular torticollis: Long-term follow-up of thirty-eight partial resections of the sternocleidomastoid muscle. Arch Orthop Trauma Surg 112:205-209, 1993.

249. Gyorgyi G: Les changements morphologiques de la région occipitocervicale associés au torticollis. J Radiol Electrol Med Nucl 45:797, 1965.

250. Fielding JW, Hawkins RJ: Atlanto-axial rotatory fixation (fixed rotatory subluxation of the atlanto-axial joint.) J Bone Joint Surg Am 59:37, 1977.

251. Bredenkamp JR, Maceri DR: Inflammatory torticollis in children. Arch Otolaryngol Head Neck Surg 116:310, 1990.

252. Phillips WA, Hensinger RN: The management of rotatory atlanto-axial subluxation in children. J Bone Joint Surg Am 71:664, 1989.

253. Been HD, Kerkhoffs GM, Maas M: Suspected atlantoaxial rotatory fixation-subluxation. Spine 32:E163-E167, 2007.

254. Melnick JC, Silverman FN: Intervertebral disk calcification in childhood. Radiology 80:399, 1963.

255. Schechter LS, Smith A, Pearl M: Intervertebral disk calcification in childhood. Am J Dis Child 123:608, 1972.

256. Sutcliff J: Torsion spasms and abnormal postures in children with hiatus hernia: Sandifer's syndrome. Prog Pediatr Radiol 2:190, 1969.

257. Williams CR, O'Flynn E, Clarke NM, et al: Torticollis secondary to ocular pathology. J Bone Joint Surg Br 78:620, 1996.

31 CHAPTER Congenital Anomalies of the Spinal Cord

Joel A. Bauman, MD
Daniel M. Schwartz, PhD
William C. Welch, MD
Leslie N. Sutton, MD

Developmental abnormalities of the spinal cord may occur in isolation or in association with abnormalities of the bony spine and visceral structures. The term *spinal dysraphism* refers to a group of congenital anomalies of the spine in which the midline structures fail to fuse. If the lesion is confined to the bony posterior arches at one or more levels, it is termed *spina bifida*. Simple spina bifida of the lower lumbar spine is a common radiographic finding, especially in children, and by itself carries no significance; in contrast, bony spina bifida may accompany any of several complex anomalies involving the spinal cord; nerve roots; dura; and bladder, rectum, and genital organs. In these cases, spinal dysraphism is a major source of disability in children and adults.

Spinal dysraphism is generally divided into two distinct syndromes: (1) *Spina bifida cystica,* which includes myelomeningocele, is characterized by herniation of the spinal cord and nerves through a defect in the skin and is readily apparent at birth and even visible on prenatal imaging studies. (2) *Spina bifida occulta* is less obvious; the nervous structures are covered by full-thickness skin, and the external signs are often subtle. It is important to recognize this condition as early as possible because surgery is usually performed prophylactically to prevent progressive neurologic damage.

Myelomeningocele

Myelomeningocele is the most common significant birth defect involving the spine. The condition is manifest at birth and is characterized by herniation of a malformed spinal cord through a defect in the bony canal and skin. It almost always results in permanent disability regardless of medical intervention and often deprives the victim of "those qualities held in high esteem by our society—independence, physical powers and intelligence."[1] In the past, it was assumed that all of the neurologic dysfunction that occurs with myelomeningocele arose from disordered embryogenesis. More recent work suggests, however, that at least some of the spinal cord damage is acquired in utero,[2] and fetal surgery to close the spinal defect is now being performed at selected centers.

Embryology

Myelomeningocele is one of a group of neural tube defects that also includes anencephaly, encephalocele, and craniorachischisis. The most severe of these are incompatible with life and occur earliest in embryogenesis.

By 18 days of development, the embryo is a flattened oval disc with all three germ layers present. A longitudinal depression, the neural groove, appears in the neural plate, which is destined to become the brain and spinal cord. By 22 days, the neural groove has deepened, and fusion of the adjacent tissue begins the transformation of the flat neural plate into a hollow neural tube. The entire process is called *neurulation,* which begins in the dorsal midline and simultaneously progresses cephalad and caudad. The final portions of the tube to close are the rostral opening (the anterior neuropore, at 24 days) and the caudal opening (the posterior neuropore, at 28 days). By the 1st month of gestation, the entire process has been completed. The development of the meninges begins after closure of the posterior neuropore, as does formation of the bony laminae.[3]

Myelomeningocele presumably occurs when the posterior neuropore fails to close or if it reopens as the result of distention of the central canal of the spinal cord with cerebrospinal fluid (CSF). The spinal abnormality is only one component of a complex of central nervous system abnormalities, which include the Chiari II malformation, hydrocephalus, and brain anomalies such as partial agenesis of the corpus callosum and gyral malformations. McLone and Naidich[4] attempted to explain these associations with their "unified theory." It is hypothesized that the open spinal defect allows excessive drainage of CSF in utero and that this results in collapse of the rhombencephalic vesicle, resulting in a small posterior fossa volume. Growth of the cerebellum and brainstem within a small posterior fossa results in downward herniation and caudal displacement of the cerebellar vermis and brainstem into the cervical spinal canal (the Chiari II malformation). Because the outlet of the fourth ventricle is occluded by impacted brain tissue, obstructive hydrocephalus develops either in the fetal period or in the newborn period after closure of the myelomeningocele eliminates the spinal defect as a drainage pathway.

Epidemiology

The incidence of myelomeningocele ranges from less than 1 case per 1000 live births in the United States to almost 9 cases per 1000 in areas of Ireland. The etiology of myelodysplasia is unknown, and evidence exists for environmental and multi-factorial genetic influences. A role for genetic risk factors is supported by numerous studies documenting familial aggregation of this condition. In addition, several lines of evidence point to the potential importance of maternal nutritional status as a determinant of the risk for having a child with spina bifida. Indirect support is provided by studies that indicate that season of conception, socioeconomic status, and degree of urbanization may be related to the risk of spina bifida. Several micronutrients (vitamins C and B_{12}, zinc, and folic acid) have been implicated as potential risk factors as well.[5]

Folic acid is the most extensively studied micronutrient. In August 1991 after the Medical Research Council Vitamin Study Group report was published, the U.S. Centers for Disease Control and Prevention (CDC) advised that women with a history of an affected pregnancy should take 4 mg of folic acid daily, starting at the time they planned to become pregnant.[6] A dose of 0.4 mg was later recommended for all women of childbearing age capable of becoming pregnant. It was anticipated that these recommendations would have a substantial impact on the risk of neural tube defects in the offspring of such women. Most affected pregnancies (approximately 95%) occur in women with no history of a prior affected fetus or child, however.[7] It has been suggested that fortification of the food supply may be more effective than individual supplementation for the prevention of neural tube defects.

Prenatal Diagnosis

More recent developments in prenatal diagnosis of fetal anomalies have made antenatal recognition of myelomeningocele commonplace. Families at risk are routinely offered amniocentesis for amniotic α-fetoprotein and acetylcholinesterase, which are important in separating open lesions from skin-covered masses such as myelocystocele. Screening ultrasonography performed on mothers when the fetus is at 16 to 20 weeks of gestation has also proved valuable.[8] Other anomalies may be detected, and ultrasonography may detect skin-covered lesions such as lipomyelomeningocele. The cardinal finding is splaying of the posterior elements of the spine in the axial plane in the lumbosacral region. Indirect signs are the lemon sign, which refers to a bilateral concave contour of the frontal bones of the skull, and the banana sign, which describes anterior curvature of the cerebellar hemispheres. Hydrocephalus is also readily detected. In referral centers, diagnostic sensitivity is close to 100% in diagnosing spina bifida.[9]

Prenatal magnetic resonance imaging (MRI), using ultra-fast T2-weighted sequences, may also be used to characterize the Chiari II malformation and other associated anomalies.[10] Fetal MRI may detect spinal cord abnormalities in instances where ultrasonography can detect only bony abnormalities.[11] Studies indicate that such prenatal imaging studies can help to determine prognosis. Specifically, lesion level determined by prenatal imaging studies seems to predict neurologic deficit and ambulatory potential, but the degree of fetal ventriculomegaly and the extent of hindbrain deformity are not predictive.[12] Families can be professionally counseled regarding the expected prognosis and offered conventional treatment, abortion, or the possibility of fetal closure. Patients of low socioeconomic class, who are most at risk for neural tube defects, often do not present for prenatal care until after 24 weeks of gestation, when screening is no longer of value.

The value of prenatal diagnosis of spinal dysraphism is that an opportunity is provided to terminate the pregnancy, to evaluate the fetus for possible fetal surgery, and to determine the best mode of delivery. It has been proposed that children with myelomeningocele sustain traumatic damage to the placode and nerves when they are delivered vaginally and that children electively delivered by cesarean section before the onset of labor have improved motor levels.[13] Other investigators have found little benefit to this strategy,[12] but in the United States cesarean delivery has become routine.

Initial Evaluation

The initial assessment of a newborn infant with a myelomeningocele begins with a detailed examination to evaluate general well-being and to seek associated anomalies. Fatal urologic or cardiac anomalies may be evident that would favor nonoperative treatment. Some infants may have abnormal facies suggesting Down syndrome, and although chromosomal studies should be obtained, these are most often normal, and the facial appearance becomes normal with age. Approximately 85% of infants with myelomeningocele present with hydrocephalus or develop it within the newborn period.[14] A large head circumference or bulging fontanel suggests the need for early head ultrasonography via the fontanel. Stridor, apnea, or bradycardia in the absence of overt intracranial hypertension suggests a symptomatic Chiari II malformation and hindbrain dysfunction, which carries a poor prognosis.

The myelomeningocele is inspected. If the sac is intact, it should not be ruptured. The red granular neural placode is surrounded by the pearly zona epithelioserosa, which interfaces with full-thickness skin. This tissue must be excised at the time of surgery to prevent epidermoid inclusion cysts from developing later in life. Most myelomeningoceles are slightly oval, with the long axis oriented vertically. If the lesion is more horizontally oriented, it may be easier to close it horizontally. If the sac has ruptured, the placode is readily visible. A vertically oriented groove within the placode represents the opened central canal of the spinal cord and may be dripping CSF. The spinal level of the lesion and its size are estimated. Associated kyphosis or scoliosis is noted.

The neurologic examination is difficult in neonates, and it is easy to mistake reflex motion for voluntary movement. Fixed contractures and foot deformity suggest paralysis of the spinal segments innervating the joints. Any movement in response to painful stimulation of the same extremity must be viewed as potentially reflexive. Crying in response to a painful stimulus suggests intact sensation at that level. Table 31–1 lists the segmental innervation of the lower extremities and may be used as a guide in assigning a functional level. It is best, however, to document function of the individual muscle groups rather than simply to record a spinal level.

Virtually all patients with myelomeningocele have abnormal bladder function, but it is difficult to assess this in the newborn period. A patulous anus lacking in sensation and a distended bladder on physical examination or ultrasonography confirm a neurogenic bladder. A renal and bladder ultrasound examination is performed to evaluate the upper tracts and to assess the adequacy of emptying.

Initial Management

The ethics of selecting newborn infants with severe congenital anomalies for aggressive or "conservative" management is controversial, and a thorough discussion is beyond the scope of this chapter. In the United States, most fetuses with myelomeningocele are detected prenatally, and termination is carried out if the family wishes. When the decision is made to continue the pregnancy, most children undergo closure either in the fetal period or postnatally. Ideally, a counseling session is carried out at 18 to 24 weeks of gestation when there is opportunity to consider elective termination of the pregnancy or surgery before birth. This counseling is performed by a multidisciplinary team that is expert in managing the pregnancy and is familiar with the care of children with myelomeningocele of all ages and can offer a realistic discussion regarding long-term prognosis. In some instances, the defect is unexpected, and the parents are informed of the likely outcome as soon as possible after the delivery.

Management of an Unrepaired Newborn

Closure is usually performed 24 to 48 hours after birth to prevent ventriculitis. It is vital to emphasize to the family that surgical closure of the myelomeningocele is a lifesaving measure but does not alter preexisting deficits. A very few infants are so severely affected that no realistic benefit can follow aggressive management. For these infants, antibiotics are not given, and they are discharged home to the care of the parents. It is understood that if the infant survives or if the parents change their minds and opt for aggressive treatment, the infant again becomes a candidate for surgical intervention.

Pending plans for definitive care, the infant is nursed in the prone position with a sterile saline-soaked gauze dressing loosely applied to the sac or placode. Broad-spectrum antibiotics (ampicillin and cefotaxime) are begun intravenously pending discussion with the parents. If there is no sign of overt hydrocephalus, the back is closed initially, and hydrocephalus is treated with a ventriculoperitoneal shunt at a separate procedure if needed. In patients with hydrocephalus and intracranial hypertension at birth, it may be advisable to perform both procedures at the same time because failure to treat the hydrocephalus may allow continued leakage of CSF into the back

TABLE 31–1 Innervation of Leg Muscles

Hip flexion	L1-3
Hip adduction	L2-4
Knee extension	L2-4
Ankle inversion	L4
Toe extension	L5-S1
Hip abduction	L5-S1
Hip extension	L5-S1
Knee flexion	L5-S2
Ankle plantar flexion	S1-2

Data from Sharrard WJW: The segmental innervation of the lower limb muscles in man. Ann R Coll Surg 35:106-122, 1964.

and threaten the closure and because the infant is exposed to a single anesthetic. The goal of back closure is to seal, using multiple tissue layers, the spinal cord and subarachnoid space against entry of bacteria from the skin. At the same time, the surgeon must preserve whatever neurologic function remains and attempt to prevent tethering of the spinal cord. The cross-sectional anatomy of a typical myelomeningocele is shown in Figure 31–1.

The infant is positioned in the prone position under general anesthesia. Rolls are placed under the chest and hips to allow the abdomen to hang freely and minimize epidural bleeding (Fig. 31–2A). If the sac is intact, fluid is aspirated and sent for culture. The surgeon gently attempts to approximate the base of the sac or defect vertically and then horizontally to determine which direction would produce the smallest skin defect. An elliptical incision is made, oriented along that axis, outside the junction of the normal, full-thickness skin and the thin, pearly zona epithelioserosa. Full-thickness skin forming the base of the sac is viable and should not be excised. This incision is carried through the subcutaneous tissue until the

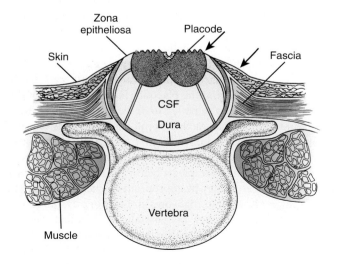

FIGURE 31–1 Cross-sectional anatomy of typical lumbosacral myelomeningocele. CSF, cerebrospinal fluid.

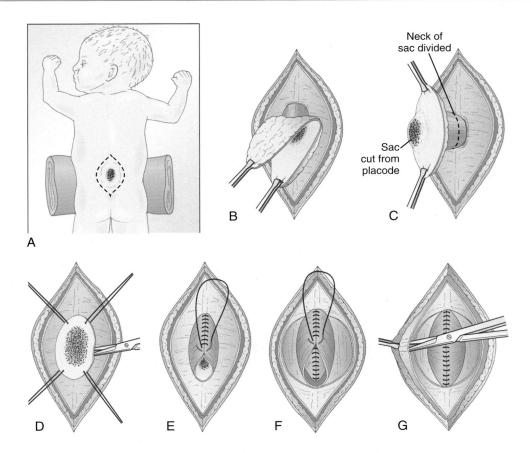

FIGURE 31–2 Technique for closure of myelomeningocele (see text). **A,** The infant is placed in prone position with towel rolls under hips. An elliptic incision is outlined just outside zona epithelioserosa, which may be oriented on vertical or horizontal axis. **B,** Incision is to level of lumbodorsal fascia. The apices of the island of skin within incision are grasped with clamps, and skin is undermined medially until dural sac is seen to funnel through fascial defect. **C,** Dural sac is first incised at its base. Skin is excised from placode and discarded, allowing placode to fall into spinal canal. **D,** Everted dura is undermined and reflected medially to envelop placode. The placode itself may be folded medially and sewn into a tube at this point. **E,** Dural layer is closed with nonabsorbable suture, using a running stitch. **F,** Fascia is incised to muscle, undermined, and reflected medially to create second layer of closure. **G,** Skin is undermined using blunt techniques to permit closure.

glistening layer of everted dura or fascia is encountered. The base of the sac is mobilized medially until it is seen to enter the fascial defect (Fig. 31–2B).

The sac is entered by radially incising the cuff of skin surrounding the placode. This skin is sharply excised circumferentially around the placode and discarded, with care being taken to avoid damaging the placode (Fig. 31–2C). All of the zona epithelioserosa is removed to prevent later development of an epidermoid cyst. At this point, the placode is floating freely inside the everted dura (Fig. 31–2D). In some thoracic myelomeningoceles, the placode is large and "thinned out," and there is complete paraplegia below the level of the defect. In these instances, it may be appropriate to excise the placode to prevent spasticity and high-pressure bladder dysfunction.

In some cases, it may be possible to "reconstruct" the placode so that it fits better within the canal and to reconstruct the tubular form of the spinal cord so that a pial surface is in contact with the dural closure. The purpose of this reconstruction is to prevent retethering. Reconstruction is accomplished by interrupted 6-0 sutures to approximate the pia-arachnoid-neural junction of one side with the other. The central canal is closed along its entire length.

Attention is now directed toward the dura, which is everted and loosely attached to the underlying fascia. It is undermined and reflected medially on each side until enough has been mobilized to effect closure (Fig. 31–2E). The dura is very thin anteriorly where the root sleeves exit and is easily torn. When it is free, the dura is closed in a watertight fashion with 4-0 nonabsorbable suture material.

Particularly if the dural closure is suboptimal, it is desirable also to close the fascia as a separate layer. The fascia is incised laterally in a semicircular fashion on either side, elevated from the underlying muscle, and reflected medially (Fig. 31–2F). It is closed with 4-0 suture over the underlying dural closure. The fascia is poor at the caudal end of a lumbar myelomeningocele or with sacral lesions, and the closure may be incomplete.

Mobilization of the skin is by blunt dissection with scissors or a finger; it may be necessary to free it anteriorly to the abdomen (Fig. 31–2G). In most instances, the closure is easiest in the mid-sagittal (vertical) plane, but occasionally less tension is required for a horizontal closure. A two-layer closure is performed. The epidermis may be closed with absorbable suture material and tissue glue if there is little tension, but interrupted nonabsorbable suture material is preferred for large defects.

Very large lesions require special techniques. There is often an associated gibbous deformity, and it is helpful to use a rongeur to remove the everted lamina, which, if left in place, would produce pressure points on the skin closure. Large circular defects may be closed by an S-shaped skin opening, allowing the use of rotation flaps (Fig. 31–3). Alternatively, a Z-rhomboid flap, tissue expanders, or latissimus dorsi myocutaneous flaps may be employed. Lateral relaxing incisions with split-thickness skin grafting have been described, but should be avoided if possible because the cosmetic result is poor. Alternatively, allogeneic skin grafts such as Alloderm (Lifecell, Branchburg, NJ) can be sewn directly to the edges of an approximated closure and may offer a better cosmetic result.[15] In rare cases where patients are referred late for surgery, significant scarring of the placode can occur. Tissue expansion is particularly useful in such cases.[16]

Large defects occasionally undergo dehiscence, owing to tension on the skin closure or superficial infection. This dehiscence is usually evident by 7 days postoperatively. In most cases, the underlying fascial and dural closures remain intact. The dehiscence may be treated by removing the sutures to the point of good skin closure, débriding the devitalized tissue, and beginning a program of saline wet-to-dry dressings. When a good granulation bed is observed, the wound can simply be allowed to granulate and contract or may be secondarily closed or repaired with a skin graft with or without tissue expansion.[17] For persistent wound breakdown, the pedicled "propeller" flap can be used as a vascularized salvage procedure.[18] CSF leakage is treated by a ventricular diversion procedure, even if the ventricles are small.

Cervical meningoceles and myelomeningoceles are uncommon. Despite the high spinal level, the actual spinal cord involvement is often minor, and the prognosis is good. Many of these lesions are actually meningoceles with a small clump of gliotic tissue at the base of the sac or myelocystoceles that are characterized by a "sac within a sac." The outer cyst is in continuity with the subarachnoid space, and the inner cyst is in continuity with the distended central canal. These lesions should be operatively explored in early infancy for cosmetic regions and to untether the spinal cord.

Closure Before Birth

In a few centers, a fetus with spina bifida may be a candidate for in utero treatment because this condition is routinely detected before 20 weeks of gestation (Fig. 31–4). There is evidence that neurologic deterioration occurs during gestation. Normal lower extremity movement can be seen on ultrasound studies of affected fetuses before 17 and 20 weeks of gestation, whereas most late-gestation fetuses and newborns have some degree of deformity and paralysis. Such deterioration could be the result of exposure of neural tissue to

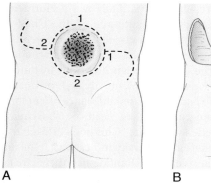 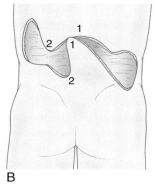

FIGURE 31–3 A, Z-plasty closure for large circular skin defects. Horizontal, S-shaped skin incision is used with defect in the center. **B,** Closure is accomplished by approximating points of the skin edge to troughs of opposing skin edge.

amniotic fluid and meconium or direct trauma as the exposed neural placode impacts against the uterine wall. Theoretically, such deterioration could be reduced or eliminated by in utero closure of the lesion.

Some animal studies (in which a model for spina bifida is created by laminectomy and exposure of the fetal spinal cord to the amniotic fluid) have shown improved leg function if the lesion is closed before birth.[19] Although other animal studies have failed to show behavioral improvement, they have documented the presence of somatosensory evoked potentials (SSEPs) in the treated myelomeningocele group compared with an absence of SSEPs in the untreated group.[20] There is also evidence that the Chiari II malformation, which occurs in most individuals with spina bifida, is acquired and could potentially be prevented by in utero closure.[21]

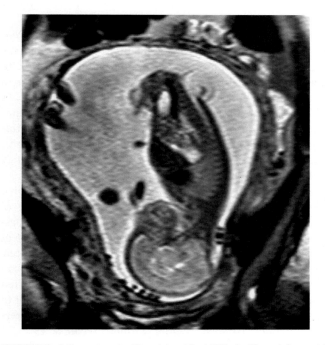

FIGURE 31–4 Fast spin-echo T2-weighted fetal MRI of a 20-week fetus with myelomeningocele. The sac is intact.

In 1997, in utero repair of spina bifida was performed by hysterotomy at Vanderbilt University and at The Children's Hospital of Philadelphia.[22,23] Fetuses treated in utero were subsequently delivered by cesarean section, ideally at around 36 weeks of gestation. The early experience at both institutions suggested that compared with infants treated postnatally, fetuses treated in utero had a decreased incidence of hindbrain herniation and possibly a decreased need for shunting.[24,25] The combined experience at the Children's Hospital of Philadelphia and Vanderbilt University indicates that the incidence of hydrocephalus requiring shunting in patients treated in utero is less than that of historical controls stratified by spinal level who received standard postnatal care.[26,27] It is hypothesized that fetal closure of the spinal lesion reduces the need for shunting by eliminating the leakage of CSF, which puts back-pressure on the hindbrain. The hindbrain hernia can be reduced, and the obstruction of the outflow from the fourth ventricle is relieved.[28]

It is now estimated that more than 330 in utero spina bifida closures have been performed.[29] The procedure seems to be generally well tolerated by the expectant mothers. The fetal death rate is about 5% and is due to uncontrollable labor and premature birth. One analysis of leg function in children treated prenatally revealed no significant difference from a set of historical controls treated with conventional postnatal repair. Many of the children evaluated in this series had lower limb paralysis at the time of the surgery, however, which may have diluted any possible benefit.[30] Data from the Children's Hospital of Philadelphia suggested possibly better leg function in patients who already had intact leg movement shown by ultrasound before fetal sugery.[31] Problems with delayed development of dermoid inclusion cysts and tethered cord may adversely affect long-term outcome.[32] The preliminary experience suggests that children treated in utero have the same urodynamic abnormalities that are seen in conventionally treated children with spina bifida.[33,34]

To date, outcomes for spina bifida infants treated in utero have been assessed relative to outcomes in conventionally treated, historical controls.[14] Such comparisons are prone to substantial bias, however, because fetuses who undergo in utero closure represent a highly selected subset of cases. In addition, the medical management of spina bifida is continuously improving, making comparisons with historical controls particularly problematic. Definitive answers about the benefits of fetal closure can be obtained only by a properly designed and conducted randomized trial.

A consortium of three institutions (Children's Hospital of Philadelphia, Vanderbilt University, and University of California San Francisco) undertook an unblinded, randomized, controlled trial of conventional versus in utero treatment of spina bifida (MOMS: Management of Myelomeningocele Study). Pregnant women who receive a prenatal diagnosis of spina bifida between 16 and 25 weeks of gestation are referred to a central screening center. Eligible subjects who consent to participate in the trial are assigned to one of the three centers and randomly assigned to either in utero repair at 19 to 25 weeks of gestation or cesarean delivery after demonstration of lung maturity followed by conventional postnatal repair at the study center. The primary study end points are the need for a shunt procedure at 1 year, and fetal and infant mortality. Secondary end points are neurologic function, cognitive outcome, and maternal morbidity. The study is expected to enroll 200 subjects and is estimated to close in 2011. It is hoped that the trial will be completed before other institutions begin performing in utero repair of spina bifida, which at this time remains of unproven benefit.

Surgical Complications

Latex Allergy

An increased incidence of allergy to latex, as found in surgical gloves, balloons, and urinary catheters, has been well documented in children with spinal dysraphism.[35] Allergy to latex is a type I, immediate, IgE-mediated reaction that can lead to anaphylaxis and death. Sensitization presumably arises from repeated exposure, at home and in the operating room. In many centers, all children with spina bifida are managed in a latex-free environment, and surgical procedures are preceded by prophylactic medications.

Late Deterioration

Myelomeningocele is a birth defect; although there are often severe neurologic sequelae, they should remain static. Any sign of worsening in a child or adult with spina bifida should provoke an intense search for a cause, which is usually treatable. Possible reasons for neurologic deterioration include uncontrolled hydrocephalus, Chiari malformation, hydromyelia, tethered cord syndrome, epidermoid or dermoid inclusion cyst, basilar impression, cervical instability, kyphoscoliosis, obesity, and reactive depression. Even with modern diagnostic techniques, it may prove difficult to determine which of the above-listed factors is responsible for worsening in a particular patient. This is true partly because the anatomic changes (e.g., Chiari malformation or tethered cord) are present in most children with myelodysplasia, whether or not they are symptomatic.

Tethered Cord

Approximately 20% to 30% of patients with myelomeningocele experience spinal cord tethering, which may result in progressive loss of function similar to that seen with occult spinal dysraphism.[36,37] This phenomenon does not seem to be reduced by fetal repair, in which inclusion cysts have been found in 19% of patients who underwent fetal repair.[38] Signs and symptoms usually appear during the 1st decade of life when growth is rapid and include back and leg pain, decrease in urinary control, gait difficulty and leg weakness, hip dislocation, progressive foot deformity, and possibly scoliosis. Urinary and gait difficulties are complaints confined to patients with low-level lesions, who are already functioning quite well neurologically and have the most to lose. In more severely affected patients who may already be wheelchair bound, pain may be the only manifestation of cord tethering and may be confused with appendicitis, hernia, urinary tract infection, or traumatic arthritis associated with abnormal posture or gait.

Workup consists of MRI of the brain and complete spine, including sagittal and axial views. A "myelo survey" set of images, consisting of a limited brain study and T1-weighted sagittal views through the entire spine, can be obtained, which limits the time needed for the examination. This survey invariably shows a Chiari II malformation, a low-lying dorsally displaced spinal cord, and perhaps an associated diastematomyelia or hydromyelia; however, these same findings are noted in asymptomatic patients, and their presence does not by itself indicate the need for surgery. It is important that all children with myelomeningocele be carefully followed by a specialty team of clinicians, including an orthopaedist, urologist, pediatrician, and physical therapist, so that subtle signs of deterioration can be documented because the decision to operate is made largely on clinical grounds.

The surgical procedure to release a tethered spinal cord in a patient with myelomeningocele is similar to surgery for a lipomyelomeningocele. Patients are operated on in the prone position with rolls under the chest and hips. A vertical midline incision is used, regardless of the type of closure used for the initial myelomeningocele closure. The most caudal normal lamina above the palpable spina bifida defect is identified and removed, and the underlying normal (but low-lying) spinal cord is identified. With the aid of magnification, the dorsally and laterally attached placode is carefully dissected free from adhesions, working in a caudal direction. This is best done with sharp instruments. When the spinal cord has been released, it falls into the patulous sac of the anterior spinal canal. Any associated diastematomyelia or dermoid inclusion cyst is removed. The dura is closed primarily or with a graft.

As with lipomyelomeningocele, the aim of surgery is to prevent further deterioration of function, but occasionally improvement is seen, even in preexisting deficits of long-standing duration. Reigel[39] reported improvement in bladder function in five of nine patients with recent deterioration and in 77% of patients with gait difficulty and motor weakness. Pain almost invariably is relieved. Retethering can occur, and if new symptoms suggest this as an etiology, reoperation is indicated. An evidence-based review of the literature concluded that aggressive tethered cord release should be performed in adults within 5 years of symptom onset.[40] Post–myelomeningocele repair patients tend to fare worse, however, than adult patients with closed dysraphism.

Hydromyelia

The routine availability of MRI has heightened awareness of this entity, which may be found in 68% of myelomeningocele patients.[36] Hydromyelia presumably is the result of hydrodynamic forces arising from persistent fetal or untreated hydrocephalus that forces CSF down the central canal of the spinal cord.[4] This explanation accounts for the frequency of symptomatic hydromyelia in patients with unshunted ventriculomegaly and patients considered to have "compensated" hydrocephalus, whose nonfunctional shunts were not revised because they lacked overt signs or symptoms of intracranial hypertension.[41] An alternative explanation has been proposed by Oldfield and colleagues,[42] who used dynamic MRI to study CSF flow. They suggested that a systolic pressure wave in the cranial compartment is transmitted in a pistonlike manner to the cerebellar tonsils, causing a systolic spinal CSF pressure wave that pushes CSF into the cord through its outer surface.

Symptoms of hydromyelia in spina bifida differ from symptoms in classic syringomyelia. The latter entity typically produces a dissociated sensory loss (relative loss of pain and temperature modalities with preservation of light touch), atrophy, and fasciculations primarily affecting the shoulder girdle and hands. When found in association with myelomeningocele, hydromyelia typically results in progressive bladder dysfunction, spasticity of upper and lower extremities, quadriparesis, and generally preserved sensation. The myelomeningocele repair may become swollen and tender. Symptoms may be due in part to the direct effects of the hydrocephalus stretching the cortical motor fibers. Hydromyelia may also be seen with progressive scoliosis. Spinal cord tethering may be the primary underlying etiology, however, of scoliosis and hydromyelia in these cases.[43]

Workup consists of MRI of the brain, followed by MRI of the entire spine to visualize the extent of the hydromyelia and the associated Chiari malformation and tethered spinal cord (Fig. 31–5). The hydromyelia cavity may be localized to a few spinal segments or extend throughout the length of the spinal cord. There may be multiple cavities and septations.

Treatment of symptomatic hydromyelia begins with a ventriculoperitoneal shunt or shunt revision if the ventricles are enlarged. If the ventricles are small or if the hydromyelia persists without improvement in symptoms after this procedure, a Chiari decompression is performed. MRI of the spine is

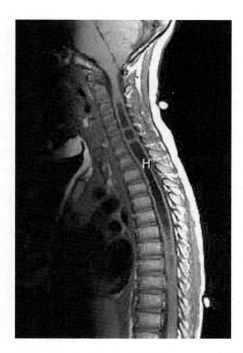

FIGURE 31–5 T1-weighted mid-sagittal MRI of a patient with Chiari malformation and large septated hydromyelia (H).

repeated 3 to 6 months after decompression, and a hydromyelia shunt is considered at that time if the syrinx has not improved. The shunt is usually placed from the hydromyelia to the pleural cavity; this is ideally done in the thoracic area but should be at the spinal level where the cavity is largest. The shunt is made to drain at a very low pressure. Follow-up MRI is done when the patient is stable. Shunt failure is common.

Other procedures have been described. Terminal ventriculostomy was advocated by Gardner and colleagues[44] for classic syringomyelia, but the myelotomy tends to scar closed with time. In addition, the negative pressure provided by the pleural end of a shunt provides more decompression than simply allowing the hydromyelia to communicate with the subarachnoid space. Park and colleagues[45] advocated posterior fossa decompression and plugging of the obex to prevent CSF fluid from the fourth ventricle from entering the central canal in patients in whom ventriculoperitoneal shunt revisions do not alleviate symptoms. This is a formidable procedure, however, and recurrent vomiting may occur from irritation or compression of the brainstem at the obex.

Chiari Malformation

The Chiari malformations are anomalies of craniovertebral function characterized by downward displacement of the cerebellar vermis, tonsils, and cervicomedullary junction into the spinal canal. The following five types are described:

Type I becomes symptomatic primarily in young adults or adolescents without myelomeningocele. The medulla and cerebellar tonsils extend downward into the cervical spinal canal as a tongue of tissue plastered against the dorsal surface of the spinal cord, rarely below C2. There may be associated hydromyelia, but hydrocephalus is uncommon. Symptoms include lower cranial nerve palsies, vertigo, oscillopsia, truncal ataxia, headache, and syncope in association with the Valsalva maneuver. In addition, the classic symptoms of syringomyelia, such as scoliosis, weakness and atrophy of the hands, and dissociated sensory loss, may be seen if there is an associated hydromyelia of the spinal cord.

Type II nearly always occurs in association with myelomeningocele, and symptoms may be apparent in infancy, childhood, or adulthood. Anatomically, the cerebellum is small, as is the posterior fossa, and the foramen magnum is large. The vermis projects as a tongue of tissue into the cervical spinal canal, and the vermis tongue and fourth ventricle may extend as low as the thoracic spine. Commonly, there is a kink in the medulla, and the cervical nerve roots are seen to project in an upward direction. Hydrocephalus is present in 90% of cases. Type II lesions typically manifest in infancy with inspiratory stridor owing to vocal cord paralysis, weakness in feeding, bradycardia, apnea, or "blue spells." Patients are often erroneously diagnosed as having croup or asthma.[46] In older children and adults, symptoms are similar to symptoms seen with type I lesions.

Type III is uncommon and consists of cervical spina bifida with cerebellar hernia. It is usually fatal in the newborn period.

Type IV is occasionally described, consisting of agenesis of the cerebellum. This is not a form of hindbrain herniation.

Type 0 has been reported[47]; this describes patients without spina bifida who have hydromyelia but no tonsillar herniation. It is theorized that a functional obstruction of the outlets of the fourth ventricle occurs, either from an occult web or from ventral distortion.

MRI of the brain and spine is the procedure of choice for initial evaluation because the lesion is readily visualized and associated abnormalities are easily excluded. Mid-sagittal views show the tongue of cerebellum extending below the foramen magnum in type I lesions (see Fig. 31–5) and the "vermian pseudotumor," consisting of the fused brainstem and cerebellum, in type II lesions.

Chiari type II lesions manifesting in an infant with myelomeningocele are particularly difficult to manage. When symptoms are severe, the brainstem nuclei may be irreversibly damaged, and the patient would not improve with surgical decompression.[46] This situation has prompted a trend toward earlier intervention, when improvement may still be possible.[48] If shunt function is shown to be optimal with shunt tap or imaging, Chiari decompression should be undertaken.

Patients are operated on in the prone position. A midline incision is used to expose the suboccipital bone and the cervical spine down to the level of the cerebellar hernia as seen on MRI, and a laminectomy is performed. The tonsillar hernia can usually be seen through the translucent dura, which is opened in the midline, beginning at the lowest point of the laminectomy and progressing cephalad. In this way, MRI-compatible clips or a running suture can be used to control bleeding from the anomalous venous sinuses in the posterior fossa. The dural opening should include the fibrous band usually present at the foramen magnum; however, because the foramen magnum is typically large and the venous sinuses are caudally displaced, the dural incision should rarely be carried above the level of the foramen magnum. It may be possible to open the fourth ventricle and establish CSF flow to the subarachnoid space, but dense adhesions and distorted anatomy often may make this unwise. As in Chiari I repair, the dura is left open, or a dural graft is employed, and the muscles, fascia, and skin are closed as usual.[49]

If the child does not improve, and stridor and apnea persist, a frank discussion with the family is indicated. Options include tracheostomy and feeding gastrostomy and long-term ventilator therapy, if needed. Such treatment seriously reduces the quality of life, and some families may opt to withdraw support. Late complications include cervical instability or deformity from the laminectomy. Rarely, symptoms may recur, and computed tomography (CT) may show bone overgrowth of a previous area of decompression. Reoperation may be beneficial in selected instances.

Older children and adults with Chiari malformations who present with type I symptoms respond to decompression more favorably, presumably because the cranial nerve nuclei are functional and symptoms are due to compression. The surgical procedure is the same as that described earlier.

Shunt Malfunction and Arrested Hydrocephalus

Any neurologic deterioration in a patient with myelomeningocele should prompt a thorough investigation of the shunt. Some patients have nonfunctioning shunts and ventriculomegaly yet have no overt symptoms of intracranial hypertension or may have never received shunts and have baseline ventriculomegaly. These patients have been described as having "compensated" or "arrested" hydrocephalus. It has been suggested that some of these patients might benefit from shunting or shunt revision, which in some instances may result in improved neuropsychological functioning.[50]

Summary

Signs or symptoms of worsening in a patient with myelodysplasia should provoke a thorough evaluation. The importance of careful history taking and physical examination cannot be overemphasized because radiologic studies often reveal a plethora of abnormalities, and only an astute clinician can discern which is responsible for a particular complaint. If symptoms involve only the lower extremities and sphincters, possible causes include decompensated hydrocephalus, hydromyelia, and tethered cord. If the upper extremities or brainstem is involved, possible causes include hydrocephalus, hydromyelia or hydrobulbia, cervical instability, basilar impression, kyphoscoliosis, and Chiari malformation. Sometimes the clinician is forced simply to treat the various lesions serially until symptoms improve.

Outcome

Significant progress has been made in the understanding and management of myelomeningocele over the past 25 years, particularly in the widespread use of multidisciplinary teams of specialists to manage children with this condition. More recent population-based data indicate that 1-year survival of individuals with spina bifida is approximately 92%[51] and that 78% of all individuals with spina bifida survive to age 17 years.[52] Mortality continues into the adult years[53]: 57% of patients die by the 4th decade of life.[54] Death is due to problems associated with the Chiari II malformation, restrictive lung disease secondary to chest deformity, shunt malfunction, and urinary sepsis. Perineal sensation and urinary continence may be predictive of survival.[55]

Approximately 75% of young children with myelomeningocele are ambulatory to some extent, although most require braces and crutches. The likelihood that a child will ambulate is related to the level of the lesion; virtually all patients with sacral and lumbosacral lesions walk, but only half of patients with thoracic or thoracolumbar lesions walk with the use of braces and crutches. Patients with high-level lesions often can walk as young children but become wheelchair users as they get older, gain weight, or simply discover that wheelchair locomotion requires less energy and is faster than ambulation with crutches. A more recent report compared ambulatory potential between patients delivered by cesarean section and patients who underwent a trial of labor. Compared with the elective cesarean group, patients in the trial of labor group were more likely to be ambulatory at 2 years (independently ambulant 7% vs. 28%, ambulant with assistance 63% vs. 65%, or wheelchair bound 30% vs. 7%) and at 10 years (independently ambulant 5% vs. 21%, ambulant with assistance 30% vs. 54%, or wheelchair bound 65% vs. 25%). There was no statistical difference based on mode of delivery.[56]

Overall, approximately 75% of surviving infants have normal intelligence (IQ >80). This percentage decreases slightly to approximately 70% for surviving adults.[57] Numerous factors predict poor intellectual outcome. In one study, the mean IQ of infants who were not shunted was 104; of infants shunted without complications, it was 91; and of infants shunted who had complications such as ventriculitis or anoxia, it was 70.[58] Intelligence is also related to the level of the lesion: Approximately 55% of infants with thoracic lesions have significant developmental delay compared with only 25% of infants with lesions at lower levels.[59]

The cause of mental retardation in children with myelodysplasia remains controversial. McLone and colleagues[60] attributed it to ventriculitis, but this does not account for all cases, and it is likely that in most cases forebrain dysfunction is simply part of the complex of anomalies associated with myelodysplasia. With respect to fetal surgery, preliminary evidence from the Children's Hospital of Philadelphia showed that two thirds of surviving patients are within normal cognitive range at 2 years of age.[27] Because cognitive function seems to be related to shunting, it is hoped that a decrease in overall shunting rate may improve overall intelligence in this population.

Although virtually all children with myelomeningocele have abnormal bladder function, urinary continence with the use of clean intermittent catheterization approaches 90% in children 5 to 9 years old. Ongoing urologic care is essential.[61] Scoliosis is present in 49%, with 43% eventually requiring spinal fusion, for which the procedural complication rate is extremely high.[62] Of children, 23% have at least one seizure. A tethered cord release is performed in 32%, with 97% having improvement or stability of preoperative symptoms.[53]

Occult Spinal Dysraphism and Tethered Cord

In contrast to open spinal dysraphism, the anomalies included in the group of occult spinal dysraphisms may not be obvious at birth. No neural tissue is exposed, although there is often a visible cutaneous sign in the lumbosacral region. Included in this group are such diverse entities as lipomyelomeningocele, hypertrophied filum terminale, congenital dermal sinus, neurenteric cyst, sacral agenesis diastematomyelia (split cord malformations), myelocystocele, and anterior sacral meningocele. These conditions most often become symptomatic because of spinal cord tethering but may also manifest as recurring bouts of meningitis or spinal abscess. They may also be found incidentally in the evaluation of anorectal anomalies. Early

TABLE 31–2 Presenting Symptoms and Signs of Occult Spinal Dysraphism

	%
Leg weakness	48
Cutaneous abnormality	48
Foot deformity	39
Urinary incontinence	36
Fecal incontinence	32
Sensory abnormality	32
Recurrent urinary tract infection	20
Gait abnormality	16
Scoliosis	14

Adapted from James H, Walsh J: Spinal dysraphism. Curr Prob Pediatr 11:1-25, 1981.

recognition of these lesions is important because they result in progressive symptoms, and prophylactic operative treatment is indicated in most cases.

Embryology

After closure of the neural tube, the fetal spine is covered by ectoderm, and the low lumbar and sacrococcygeal segments have not developed.[3] At this point, the caudal end of the neural tube blends with a large aggregate of undifferentiated cells, the *caudal cell mass.* A series of vacuoles in this mass coalesce and achieve continuity with the central canal of the previously formed neural tube (at roughly 29 days' gestation), a process called *canalization.* The third phase involves *retrogressive differentiation,* during which the previously formed tail structures undergo a precise, ordered necrosis, leaving only the filum terminale, the coccygeal ligament, and the terminal ventricle of the conus as remnants by 11 weeks. Cell rests with potential for differentiation may be left within these structures, accounting for the development of lipomas, hamartomas, ectopic renal tissue, and the rare malignancy occasionally found in association with occult spinal dysraphism. Failure of the caudal cell mass to regress presumably gives rise to the hypertrophied filum terminale.

The bony vertebrae develop subsequently. The sacrococcygeal vertebrae also undergo regressive changes to decrease the number of segments originally present. Some vertebral malformations found in conjunction with neural defects arise during this period and may be part of a more generalized complex of anomalies involving other structures, such as the rectum, bladder, and genitalia (see section on caudal regression syndromes).

Pathogenesis

Symptoms may be caused in several ways. First, abnormal formation of the spinal cord and roots during embryogenesis may result in permanent deficits manifest at birth, as seen in myelomeningocele. Second, local masses growing within the rigid bony spinal canal may compress the conus medullaris or cauda equina and cause mechanical distortion or ischemia,

with consequent dysfunction of these neural elements in a progressive fashion.[63] This mechanical distortion may account for the acceleration of symptoms seen in some patients with significant weight gain in whom a lipoma enlarges in proportion to other body fat stores.

Finally, symptoms may be produced by traction on the spinal cord. Early in embryonic development, there is a progressive and rapid ascent of the conus within the bony spinal canal owing to faster growth of the vertebral bodies compared with the spinal cord. This "ascent of the conus" in children is slight, being only one segment, from L3 to L2 in the period from the 26th week of intrauterine life until maturity.[64] Nonetheless, if the conus is tethered to the bony spinal canal, as often occurs in dysraphism, there is loss of mobility of the conus during spinal flexion and extension. Experimentally, spinal cord tethering has been shown to interfere reversibly with spinal cord oxidative metabolism[65] and is probably the major cause of progressive neural damage in older children and adults with dysraphism lesions.

Clinical Manifestations

Bony spina bifida occulta at L5-S1 is a common radiologic finding in children and adults and is usually associated with no symptoms or signs. Unless other findings are present, no further evaluation or treatment is required. Signs of clinically significant spina bifida occulta may be in the form of cutaneous, neurologic, orthopaedic, urologic, or rectal abnormalities (Table 31–2).

Cutaneous Syndrome

Cutaneous abnormalities indicative of an underlying spinal dysraphism are situated on or near the midline, usually in the lumbrosacral region, but occasionally in the thoracic region or the neck.[66] A wide variety of abnormalities are seen.

A striking finding is the hairy patch (hypertrichosis), also known as "faun's tail," which always occurs in the midline. It may be small but more commonly is a wide, diamond-shaped patch in the lumbar or lower thoracic area (Fig. 31–6). Frequently, the patient's mother has trimmed the hair for years before presentation to the physician. If the dysraphism is in the cervical or upper thoracic region, there is usually a smaller patch of silky hair. The underlying abnormality may not be confined to the level of the hairy patch, and it is important to image the entire spine. Hypertrichosis may occur with any of the types of dysraphism but is particularly associated with split cord malformations.[67]

Subcutaneous lipomas at or near the midline of the lumbosacral spine may indicate an underlying intradural lipoma. These are nontender, poorly circumscribed soft masses of fat that are continuous with the normal subcutaneous tissue and with the intraspinal portion of a lipomyelomeningocele. The overlying skin is normal, hairy, or dimpled, and there may be an associated angioma or skin tag (Fig. 31–7). Other conditions may manifest as skin-covered masses overlying the caudal spine (Table 31–3). Often, an older patient gives a history of having had the superficial mass removed for cosmetic reasons.

Pigmented nevi may be red to brown with mottling. Cutaneous port-wine angiomas in the suboccipital area ("stork bites") are usually not significant. Hemangiomas in the lumbosacral area are frequently associated with an underlying dysraphism.

Atretic meningoceles may also be seen, consisting of a central area of thin, pearly skin surrounded by a halo of red, pink, or brown (spinal aplasia cutis). These represent myelomeningoceles or meningoceles that have partially healed spontaneously. Dimples at the tip of the coccyx (coccygeal pits) are frequent findings in normal newborns and usually have no significance.[68] Deep dimplelike depressions higher in the spine may be the external stigma of an epithelialized tract that connects with the filum terminale, spinal cord, or intraspinal dermoid cyst and require further investigation. The meningocele manqué is a skin blemish sometimes referred to as a "cigarette burn" because it resembles a small scar with loss of skin in the midline. When this blemish is obvious at birth, it may cause concern of CSF leakage, but this seldom occurs. Other cutaneous lesions that may be associated with a tethered cord include rudimentary caudal appendages ("tails") and asymmetrical gluteal folds.

Neurologic Syndrome

Muscle weakness and gait disturbance are usually apparent at 2 years of age when a child begins to walk. On examination, there may be striking muscular atrophy and leg-length asymmetry. The deep tendon reflexes may be normal, increased, or

TABLE 31–3 Differential Diagnosis of Skin-Covered Lesions Overlying the Spine

Myelocystocele
Meningocele
Lipomyelomeningocele
Sacrococcygeal teratoma
Duplication of rectum
Abscess
Hemangioma
Bone malformation or tumor
Epidermoid or dermoid
Pilonidal cyst
Chondroma
Neuroblastoma
Glioma
Chordoma
Hamartoma

absent, giving the pattern of a mixed upper and lower motor neuron lesion. Patchy sensory loss is present, particularly in the distal leg and perineum. Pain in the back with a radicular component is frequent in older children or adults.[69]

Orthopaedic Syndrome

The most frequent orthopaedic finding is unilateral or bilateral cavovarus deformity of the foot, with or without leg-length discrepancy (Fig. 31–8). There may also be "claw toes." The

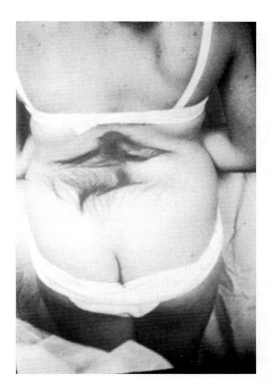

FIGURE 31–6 Hypertrichosis in a young woman, indicating underlying tethered cord.

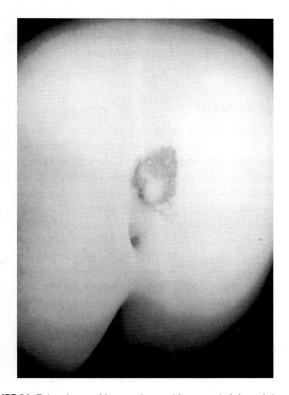

FIGURE 31–7 Lumbosacral hemangioma with congenital dermal sinus tract below.

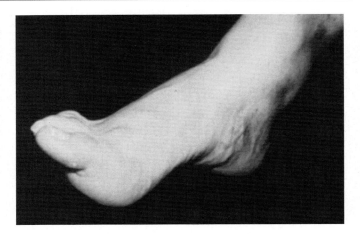

FIGURE 31–8 Foot deformity with tethered cord. The high arch is typical and may be accompanied by hammer toes and leg-length inequality.

abnormal gait is the result of orthopaedic deformity and muscular weakness. It is presumed that the foot deformity is due to lack of, or weak innervation of, antagonistic muscles of the lower extremity.[70] Scoliosis, especially if found in a young child or a boy or if noted to be rapidly progressive or accompanied by pain, also suggests an underlying spinal cause.

Urologic Syndrome

Occult spinal dysraphism should always be considered when one encounters infants with an abnormal voiding pattern, new-onset urinary or fecal incontinence in a previously toilet-trained child, or urinary tract infection in a child of any age. As opposed to older children, most infants with occult spinal dysraphism have normal results on urodynamic testing.[71] This fact underscores the importance of recognizing the syndrome as early as possible so that prophylactic surgery can be performed.

Anorectal Anomalies

Anorectal anomalies, including vesicointestinal fissures, cloacal extrophy, rectovesical fistulas, and imperforate anus, are frequently associated with an underlying tethered cord.[72] The overall incidence of tethered cord with imperforate anus is 35% and may be increased in boys.[73] In many cases, no cutaneous abnormality is seen, and radiographic screening is indicated in these patients.

Radiologic Investigation

Spine MRI is the imaging study of choice to screen for occult spinal dysraphism. Bony anatomy is poorly seen but is of secondary importance in planning an operative approach for most lesions. A fibrous tract extending from a cutaneous coccygeal pit to the bony coccyx represents a persistent coccygeal ligament and is of no clinical significance. The presence of fat in the filum is a frequent incidental finding on MRI. Generally, if the conus is at the normal level (at or above the L2-3 interspace) and if the patient has no clinical signs or symptoms of

a tethered cord, surgery is not warranted. Fat occurring very close to the conus may represent a special case, however, because this finding is associated with clinical tethering.[74] A tethered cord may be suspected when the conus lies at the L2-3 level or below in a child or adult or if the conus is dorsally displaced.

Diffusion-weighted imaging may differentiate epidermoid cysts from arachnoid cysts.[75] Postoperative studies may be difficult to interpret. The conus rarely ascends significantly after successful surgery, and even in asymptomatic patients the conus is shown to be dorsally displaced postoperatively. Although MRI is currently the best screening test for spinal cord tethering, it may not be useful for ruling out postoperative retethering. Some authors have proposed that imaging in the prone position to evaluate cord motion might be useful, but this has not been of value clinically.[76,77]

Ultrasonography through the infant spine or through congenital spina bifida or laminectomy defects has also been used to screen for occult spinal dysraphism.[76,77] Although the level of the conus is readily seen, it is difficult to assign a specific spinal level to its termination. Sometimes one can visualize the tethering element, such as a hypertrophied filum or lipoma. Spinal cord motion has also been used to assess tethering.[78] Ultrasonography may be useful as a screening test when the probability of a tethered cord is low, but MRI is preferable if an occult dysraphic lesion is strongly suspected.

Cases of tethered spinal cord with the conus in normal position on imaging studies have been described.[79] Tethering is suspected on the basis of the typical clinical syndrome and confirmed at surgery. Mechanisms included hypertrophied filum terminale, meningocele manqué, and split cord malformation. This situation is uncommon, but when typical symptoms are present, surgical exploration is justified.

Specific Entities

Lipomyelomeningocele

Lipomyelomeningocele occurs at a rate of 1 in 4000 live births and in contemporary series is the most common cause of tethered cord syndrome.[80] The term *lipomyelomeningocele* is misleading, in that it suggests herniation of neural elements through a spina bifida defect into a meningeal sac. The neural elements remain within the spinal canal, and only the lipoma itself may protrude through the spina bifida defect to manifest as a subcutaneous mass. Some authors have used the term *lipoma of the cauda equina*, but the fatty mass is invariably attached to the conus medullaris or filum terminale rather than to the cauda equina. Chapman[81] classified lipomyelomeningoceles as lesions that attach to the *caudal* end of the conus, lesions that insert *dorsally*, and lesions that are *transitional*.

If the lipoma inserts onto the dorsal surface of the conus, there is usually a substantial subcutaneous mass, which may be asymmetrical. Along the lateral interface of the attachment of the lipoma to the spinal cord, the dura and pia are also fused (Fig. 31–9). Sensory roots emerge just anterior to this *lateral line of fusion*. As a result, neither the sensory roots nor the motor roots are actually within the lipoma. Alternatively, the lipoma may join the conus at its caudal end. The remaining mass may lie entirely within the spinal canal or extend dorsally through the spina bifida defect (Fig. 31–10). The fatty tumor may replace the filum terminale, or there may be a separate filum that lies anteriorly. The nerve roots usually lie ventral to the fatty mass but may lie within the fibrous ventral portion of the mass itself. Transitional forms may occur, which are often the most difficult to manage surgically. Probably the rarest subtype is the *chaotic lipomyelomeningocele,* described by Pang and colleagues,[82] which has a prominent ventral component. MRI often defines the type of lipomyelomeningocele, which is helpful in understanding the anatomy that is encountered at operation.

Lipomyelomeningocele is only one form of occult spinal dysraphism, and elements of other forms may coexist. Some patients may have associated anorectal or urogenital anomalies,[83] and the pathologic anatomy may include elements of myelocystocele, diastematomyelia, or thickened filum.[80] Despite the superficial resemblance of lipomyelomeningocele to open dysraphism (myelomeningocele), it is rare for patients to have associated hydrocephalus, gyral anomalies, or Chiari malformations. The relationship of Chiari type I malformation found in association with lipomyelomeningocele has been controversial, but a more recent study found a 13% incidence of Chiari I malformations in patients with lipomyelomeningocele. There was no difference, however, in hindbrain herniation or posterior fossa volumes of lipomyelomeningocele patients with or without Chiari I malformation.[84] It is unclear that CSF overdrainage occurring during untethering procedures has any relationship to tonsillar herniation.[85] Cadaver experimentation has not shown downward tonsillar descent with conus medullaris traction.[86] As with myelomeningocele, there is an association with hydromyelia, particularly in the terminal spinal segments.[87] The cognitive

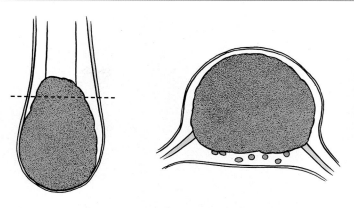

FIGURE 31–10 Caudally inserting lipomyelomeningocele. *Left,* Lipoma inserts on low-lying conus. *Right,* Cross section through lipoma, below level of cord. Nerve roots of cauda equina usually pass ventrally and may be adherent.

impairments characteristic of children with myelomeningocele seem to be absent, however, in children with spinal lipomas.[88]

The specific cause of lipomyelomeningocele is unknown. Familial occurrence has been reported in two siblings but seems to be extraordinarily rare.[89] Other neural tube defects such as myelomeningocele may be found in 2% to 5% of siblings, suggesting a possible genetic predisposition to open and closed neural tube defects.[90] An environmental cause has not been established, although a case of maternal use of valproic acid and a child with lipomyelomeningocele has been reported.[91]

The usual presentation of lipomyelomeningocele varies according to the age of the patient. Newborns and infants up to age 1 year typically present with a skin-covered lumbosacral mass (Fig. 31–11). There may be associated hair, sinuses, tags, or nevi. Children 1 year of age or older present with progressive signs or symptoms of tethered spinal cord, as previously

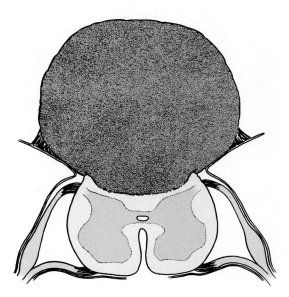

FIGURE 31–9 Cross-sectional anatomy of dorsally inserting lipomyelomeningocele. There is a broad lateral attachment between lipoma and lateral dura. Nerve roots emerge anterior to fatty mass.

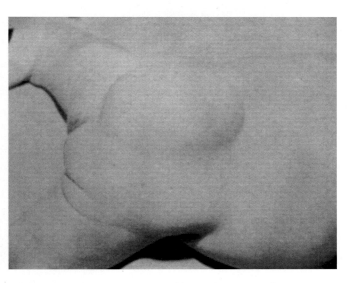

FIGURE 31–11 Typical presentation of lipomyelomeningocele in a newborn as skin-covered mass.

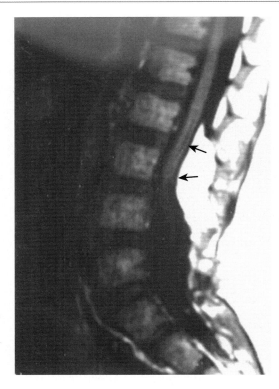

FIGURE 31–12 T1-weighted sagittal MRI of dorsally inserting lipomyelomeningocele. Cord is low lying, and lipoma attaches broadly along its dorsal aspect, tethering conus to spinal canal (*arrows*).

described. Adults may present with back pain and sciatica or acute neurologic deterioration associated with lifting, falls, exercise, or assuming positions of spinal flexion. It has been suggested that the lipoma may enlarge or shrink with overall body fat.[92]

With frequent use of in utero screening, the diagnosis of lipomyelomeningocele is increasingly made prenatally with ultrasonography. The finding of an echogenic mass in the lumbosacral area without accompanying hydrocephalus may suggest the diagnosis, but it may be impossible to exclude myelomeningocele using this technique. High-resolution ultrasonography has also been used as a screening test for newborns with suspected tethered cords, but MRI is the study of choice.

MRI should be performed in sagittal and axial planes. Fatty tumors are readily visualized on T1-weighted images as areas of increased signal intensity because of their short relaxation times. The conus is low, extending to the caudal portion of the thecal sac. The lipoma may insert dorsally (Fig. 31–12) or caudally (Fig. 31–13) and may or may not include the filum. In some instances, the conus may be at the normal level (at or above the L1-2 disc space), but the filum may be thickened and of fatty density. If these patients have other clinical signs or symptoms of tethered cord syndrome, they should be considered to have a tethered cord, and exploration should be carried out.[79] An associated syrinx or hydromyelic cavity frequently may be seen within the terminal spinal cord, corresponding to a dilated terminal ventricle (Fig. 31–14). A large

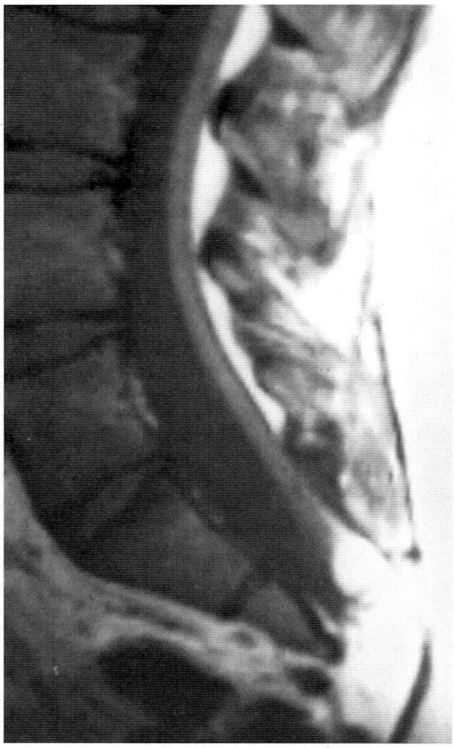

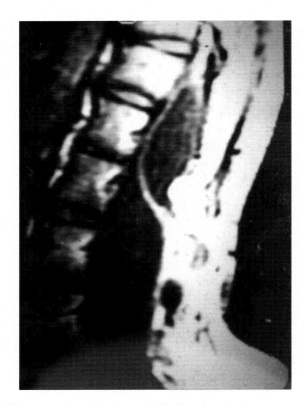

FIGURE 31–14 T1-weighted sagittal MRI of large terminal hydrosyringomyelia. This patient had previously undergone resection of a lipomyelomeningocele and presented with new-onset incontinence. Lesion was successfully treated with syringosubarachnoid shunt.

FIGURE 31–13 T1-weighted sagittal MRI of caudally inserting lipomyelomeningocele. Lipoma tethers conus to caudal end of thecal sac.

neurogenic bladder may also be seen. Lipomyelomeningocele must be distinguished from epidural lipomatosis, which is a rare condition in which fat accumulates in the dorsal epidural space, usually in the thoracic region, as the result of the use of exogenous corticosteroids or from corticosteroid-secreting tumors.

Urologic evaluation is recommended and should include ultrasonography of the bladder and urodynamic studies. More recent work has indicated that the presence of lipomyelo-meningocele is predictive of a worse urologic outcome, in contrast to tethered cord syndrome without dysraphism, in which abnormal urodynamic studies alone are not predictive of poor urologic outcome.[93]

Most neurosurgeons recommend that all children with skin-covered lumbosacral masses, with or without associated neurologic, urologic, or orthopaedic abnormalities, should undergo exploration, preferably in infancy. The surgeon must be prepared to manage a lipomyelomeningocele properly before undertaking the exploration of any midline spinal mass, to avoid damaging neural structures. The first operative procedure stands the best chance of success because scar formation and distorted anatomy found at reoperation compound the difficulties inherent in the procedure.[94] Although some authors have questioned the value of prophylactic surgery,[95] most believe that infants and children with tethered cord syndrome should have prophylactic surgery at the time the lesion is discovered, preferably in the first 6 months of life.[95-98] Early surgery is most likely to untether the cord effectively and, because tethered cord syndrome is progressive, is most likely to maximize functional outcome. An adult patient with a lipomyelomeningocele and nonprogressive symptoms may be followed nonoperatively, although this situation is uncommon. Adult patients who become symptomatic should be offered surgery.[99] The patient should be warned of the possibility that permanent worsening may occur.

Goals of surgery are (1) to untether the spinal cord from the lipoma itself, the filum terminale, or both and (2) to remove the lipomatous mass insofar as this is possible to prevent retethering and to relieve direct compression. It is also desirable to decrease the size of the subcutaneous mass for cosmetic reasons and (3) to reconstruct the dural canal and prevent CSF leakage and to allow sufficient room for the neural elements. This last goal often requires a dural graft. The surgeon must provide sufficient room to allow the conus to float freely within the dural sac and prevent retethering owing to surgical scarring.

General anesthesia is used. Muscle relaxants are avoided for portions of the procedure during which nerve stimulation may be employed. Several authors have described the use of SSEP monitoring, bladder manometry, or rectal sphincter and lower extremity electromyography (EMG) as adjuncts (see section on neurophysiologic monitoring).

The pediatric patient is placed in the prone position with towel rolls underneath the chest and iliac crest to allow the abdomen to hang freely. Adult patients are placed in the kneeling position with a binder to support the buttocks. The operative site is scrubbed with preparation solution, and after this is damp dried, a transparent adhesive plastic drape impregnated with iodine is applied over the skin. A separate plastic "apron" excludes the anus from the operative field.

Magnification with loupes is helpful, and the operative microscope may be required for portions of the dissection. An elliptical skin incision surrounding the subcutaneous mass is made along a vertical axis, with hemostasis being obtained by applying straight mosquito hemostats. The subcutaneous tissue is incised in a circumferential fashion down to the lumbodorsal fascia (Fig. 31–15). The ellipse must be narrow enough to allow skin closure at the end of the procedure but broad enough to resect most of the subcutaneous mass. The subcutaneous fat is incised in a circumferential fashion down to the lumbodorsal fascia using the monopolar cautery. When an anatomic cleavage plane becomes evident, the lipoma is mobilized medially by blunt dissection with the use of a sponge and periosteal elevator so that the stalk can be visualized as it traverses the fascial defect. A self-retaining retractor is inserted, and the lowest intact laminar arch above the bony defect is palpated. The fascia over this spinous process is opened with the cutting cautery, and the laminae are exposed.

A laminectomy of this segment is done, exposing the underlying normal dura. It may be helpful at this point to amputate the large subcutaneous mass with the skin attached at the level of its stalk. Starting at the level of normal dura cephalad to the mass, the epidural fat is melted with the bipolar cautery until the dural defect with fatty tissue extruding through it is encountered. A midline dural opening is made above the defect, exposing the spinal cord (Fig. 31–16). As the dural opening is carried inferiorly toward the defect, a transverse band of thick fibrous tissue is noted at the rostral end of the lipoma stalk, which acts to kink the spinal cord. This is opened widely along with the dura. The dural opening is extended caudad on either side of the exiting lipoma circumferentially.

At this point, the lipoma usually is found to correspond to one of the types described by Chapman.[81] Lipomas that insert into the conus dorsally can be removed from the dorsal aspect of the cord in a plane superficial to the lateral lines of fusion

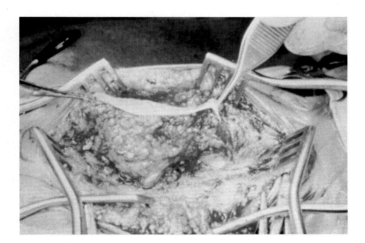

FIGURE 31–15 Initial operative exposure of lipomyelomeningocele. A vertically oriented elliptical skin incision has been made, and subcutaneous lipoma has been followed to fascial defect where it enters spinal canal.

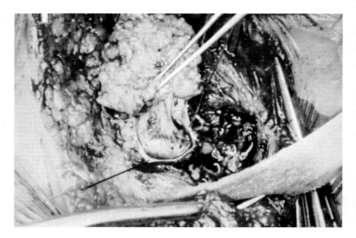

FIGURE 31–16 One-level laminectomy has been performed superior to spina bifida defect (*right*), and dura has been opened. The lipoma can be seen inserting at caudal end of spinal cord and connecting with subcutaneous fat.

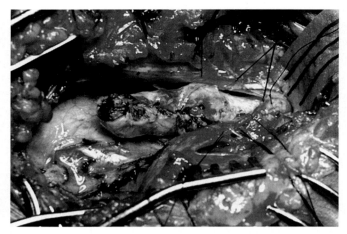

FIGURE 31–18 Lipoma has been largely removed from conus, allowing pial stitches to be placed to reconfigure tubular structure of cord. This may aid in preventing retethering. (From Sutton LN: Lipomyelomeningocele. Neurosurg Clin N Am 6:325-338, 1995.)

of lipoma, conus, and meninges, with the nerve roots emerging anteriorly. Simultaneously, the lines of fusion are divided laterally, first on one side and then on the other, with bipolar cautery and microscissors or a knife blade over a dissector (Fig. 31–17). The CO_2 laser has been helpful in shaving down the mass of the lipoma. The filum is identified and divided.

Lipomas that insert caudally into the conus must be sectioned distal to any functional roots, which may be identified using electrical stimulation and EMG. It is unnecessary to remove all the gross lipoma; to attempt this risks damage to the conus and nerve roots. Simple division of the lipoma releases the point of tethering and fulfills the goal of the operation. Pang and colleagues[100] reported a decreased rate of

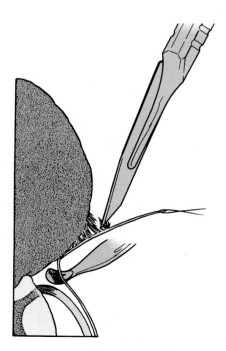

FIGURE 31–17 Lateral attachment between lipoma and dura is sharply divided, while dissector protects underlying nerve roots.

retethering, however, after a very aggressive sharp excision of the lipoma.

After the lipoma has been largely removed from the spinal cord, it is sometimes possible to reapproximate the pial edges of the cord to reconstitute the normal tubular configuration (Fig. 31–18); this does not improve neurologic function but may serve to deter retethering. If the thecal sac is capacious, a fine suture may be used to anchor the conus to the ventral dura to discourage dorsal tethering. If a terminal syrinx is seen on preoperative MRI, a midline myelotomy may be performed to provide communication with the subarachnoid space.

When the cord is free of adhesions, the dura is closed. In some cases, the dura may be approximated and closed with a running locked suture of 4-0 nylon. In many situations, this closure results in stricture of the canal, however, with the likelihood of scar formation and retethering. If there is any doubt, an elliptical graft is sutured to the dural edges. This may be technically very difficult if the dural edge is anteriorly located in the spinal canal. Acellular human dermis (Alloderm) is a convenient graft material. Alternatively, artificial substances such as Gore-Tex (Gore, Newark, DE)[101] may be used to deter scar formation, but it is difficult to obtain a watertight closure with these materials, and tethering often occurs to the pseudodura that forms beneath the graft. Often the superficial subcutaneous tissue layers in the closure are inadequate for a truly watertight closure, and the dural repair becomes of primary importance to avoid a CSF fistula. The patient is placed in steep reverse Trendelenburg position, and a Valsalva maneuver is performed to ensure the closure is adequate. It may be useful to seal the suture line with tissue glue.

The fascia is closed if possible. If a large fascial defect prevents approximation, lateral fascial flaps are elevated and reflected medially, as in the fascial closure in the standard myelomeningocele repair. In closing the skin, it may be advisable to tack the subcutaneous layer to the underlying fascia to obliterate any dead space. The skin itself is closed with absorbable suture and tissue glue.

Patients are kept recumbent for 48 hours. Patients who experience difficulty with voiding in the immediate postoperative period are treated with judicious urinary catheterization to prevent unnecessary straining that might threaten the dural closure. Infants are diapered below the dressing to avoid fecal soiling of the incision.

Patients, particularly those in whom a significant mass has been left, are cautioned to avoid excessive weight gain. These patients often require urologic or orthopaedic referral and close neurosurgical follow-up.

Surgery is relatively safe. The major postoperative complications are CSF leaks and wound breakdown because it is difficult sometimes to obtain good tissue for surgical repair. A persistent subcutaneous collection or frank leak requires re-exploration of the operative site and meticulous closure. An external spinal drainage catheter carefully inserted above the lamina defect through a Tuohy needle for 1 week is useful in protecting the closure after re-exploration. Persistent fever with sterile CSF cultures and a cellular reaction postoperatively may reflect a mild allergic reaction to the graft. This allergic reaction may persist for several months if untreated but usually resolves with a short course of corticosteroids. The incidence of a new permanent neurologic deficit after initial surgery for lipomyelomeningocele is 3% to 6% in experienced hands and is usually confined to a lower root.[80]

Re-exploration of previously operated lipomyelomeningoceles is tedious. Tissue planes are obliterated, and nerve roots often pass within the substance of the lipoma and scar tissue. For this reason, definitive surgery is required at the primary procedure.

Surgical treatment for lipomyelomeningocele is basically prophylactic and is aimed at preventing progression of fixed deficits or development of new deficits in infants and asymptomatic children or adults. Data documenting the progressive nature of untreated lipomyelomeningocele are compelling. Hoffman and colleagues[102] reported 12 patients who initially were neurologically and functionally intact and were untreated or inappropriately treated. Only one of these patients remained intact, whereas the others experienced deterioration over time. After appropriate repair, there was a halt in further deterioration, but few patients improved in function. Patients who are discovered at a younger age (because of cutaneous abnormality) are more likely to remain symptom-free if they undergo appropriate surgery than patients in whom surgery is deferred.[80] Despite these data, other investigators have pointed out that retethering results in late deterioration in 46% of patients with conus lipomas who underwent prophylactic surgery, which is no different from the natural history of the disease.[95]

Lipomas that asymmetrically interface with the cord present a particular challenge because of their lack of "safe space" at the placode-dural interface. Cochrane and colleagues[103,104] reported that an asymmetrically located lipoma inserting laterally or ventrally into dura is more likely associated with earlier neurologic deterioration after surgery compared with symmetrically located placodes.

In symptomatic patients, 20% of patients who undergo an appropriate operation note improvement in stance and gait[105];

in about 39%, there may be improved bowel or bladder function.[98] Deformities of the feet do not improve and may continue to worsen even after successful surgery because abnormal muscular innervation and gait lead to progressive deformity. Continued orthopaedic surveillance and physical therapy are indicated.

The neurologic and urologic status of a patient with a lipomyelomeningocele should remain stable after successful surgery, although orthopaedic deformity may progress because of persistent muscular weakness and imbalance. Any significant deterioration in a patient's status (e.g., new-onset incontinence, pain, or progressive weakness) should provoke a search for a cause. Possible causes include hydromyelia; retethering; infection; and a separate process not addressed by the previous surgery, such as an unrecognized diastematomyelia superior to the operated lipomyelomeningocele.

Hydromyelia is a frequent accompaniment of lipomas and was seen in 6 of 43 patients evaluated at the authors' institution by MRI and in 19% of patients reported by Iskandar and colleagues.[106] If noted on the preoperative scan, hydromyelia may be addressed at the same time as the lipomyelomeningocele procedure by terminal ventriculostomy, which connects the hydromyelia with the subarachnoid space. If a symptomatic hydromyelia recurs, treatment is best accomplished by a syringopleural or syringosubarachnoid shunt.[107]

Assuming that no other pathologic process is found, one must be concerned about the possibility of spinal cord retethering. The incidence of this phenomenon is unknown. Various authors have reported symptomatic retethering to occur in 20% of cases,[108] but the incidence may be much higher. It is likely that virtually all patients experience anatomic retethering within a few weeks of surgery for lipomyelomeningocele but that the dorsal reattachment is at a higher spinal level, and symptoms are relieved because the spinal cord is no longer stretched. Symptomatic retethering can occur at virtually any time after initial surgery, from weeks to more than 10 years.

The onset of new pain or neurologic or urologic signs or symptoms in a previously operated lipomyelomeningocele patient should prompt repeat MRI of the lumbosacral area, despite the fact that postoperative studies are often unrevealing and difficult to interpret. Immediate postoperative MRI in successfully untethered patients would continue to show a low-lying conus and a dorsally displaced spinal cord, and these findings neither confirm nor rule out retethering in a postoperative patient. Because MRI of the spine must be performed with the patient in the supine position to prevent movement artifact from respiration, the spinal cord tends to migrate to the dorsal position, even if no tethering is present. It has been suggested that ultrasound evaluation through the laminectomy defect is helpful in this situation. The finding of prominent pulsation of the spinal cord is reassuring that retethering has not occurred, and its absence is more worrisome, but the value of this remains to be proved.

Developments in MRI technology have allowed assessment of spinal cord pulsations using phase-motion imaging techniques. McCullough and colleagues[109] reported in a small group of patients that cervical spinal cord pulsation peak velocity is decreased in patients with tethering and that it improves after successful surgery. Such techniques would be valuable in diagnosing retethering in patients in whom static images are nondiagnostic. Experience with this technique at the authors' institution has been disappointing, in that the range of cervical and lumbar cord pulsation velocities in normal individuals is so broad that there is considerable overlap with patients with obviously tethered cords. Another technique that is helpful in some instances is prone-supine metrizamide CT-myelography. In contrast to MRI, it is possible to perform an adequate image with the patient in the prone position using this technique, and ventral migration of the conus with contrast material seen dorsal to the cord rules out retethering.

Until more definitive radiographic techniques become available, retethering remains a clinical diagnosis. Most authorities re-explore any patient in whom significant radicular pain develops or in whom unequivocal deterioration occurs, regardless of radiologic studies. Strategies to minimize the likelihood of retethering are important, particularly at reoperation. These include (1) removal of as much of the lipoma as is safe, to reduce the bulk of the conus; (2) creation of a capacious thecal sac, using a graft; (3) closure of the pia in dorsally inserting lipomas; (4) the use of a dural graft "sandwich" of Silastic or Gore-Tex sheeting for the inner layer and a biologic dural substitute for a watertight outer dural closure; and (5) the use of stay sutures to center the conus in the thecal sac. Retethering is usually found to be due to dense scar, usually dorsal and lateral to the conus.

Despite the technical challenges inherent in the procedure, reoperation for recurrent tethering is usually rewarding, at least in the short-term. Successful repeat untethering can be performed in approximately 90% of patients.[94] Pain is relieved in most patients, and gait and motor dysfunction improve in about half of patients. The prognosis for improvement in genitourinary dysfunction and scoliosis is less optimistic.

Sacral Agenesis and Caudal Regression Malformations

Numerous anomalies involving the caudal spine have been described, ranging in severity from simple agenesis of the coccyx to complex malformations of the thoracic and sacral spine, lower extremities, spinal cord, genitourinary system, and gastrointestinal tract. The most common of these include the VACTERL syndrome[110] (*v*ertebral anomalies, *a*nal atresia, *c*ardiac anomalies, *t*racheoesophageal fistula, *e*sophageal atresia, *r*enal and *l*imb anomalies), the OEIS complex (*o*mphalocele, cloacal *e*xstrophy, *i*mperforate anus, and *s*pinal deformities), and sacral agenesis. The most severe form includes fusion of the legs, a condition that has been termed *sirenomelia*, or the mermaid syndrome.[111] A subset of patients with these anomalies are at risk for late deterioration, and detailed imaging should be followed by prophylactic surgery in some cases.[112]

Because imperforate anus and the genitourinary tract are involved in these malformations, embryogenesis must account for these systems and the spine. Primordia of these three organ systems in the embryo originate in a common structure, the *caudal eminence* or *tailbud*. This pluripotential structure arises as a continuation of the primitive streak and ultimately gives rise to all of the structures of the caudal embryo, including the caudal spinal cord. This forms as a solid mass, initially separate from the neural tube, which undergoes programmed necrosis or *retrogressive differentiation* to form the filum terminale, cauda equina, and conus medullaris. During this process, a localized dilation of the central canal, the *ventriculus terminalis,* arises in the conus. Non-neural structures including the hindgut (giving rise to the distal colon, rectum, and anus) and *urogenital sinus* (bladder, urethra, and genitalia) also arise from the caudal eminence. As part of this process, the cloaca is divided longitudinally by the *urorectal membrane* and the *cloacal membrane,* which fuse to partition the cloaca into the urogenital sinus and anorectal canal. The cloacal membrane eventually ruptures to become a perforate anus. Cloacal folds ultimately differentiate into male or female genitalia.

Severe multiorgan cases of caudal agenesis presumably arise from an embryonic insult to the caudal eminence. Failure of somite differentiation causes failure of corresponding spinal cord and notochord segments. Failure of retrogressive differentiation gives rise to lipomas, myelocystoceles, and related conditions. Related hindgut and urogenital anomalies arise from disturbances of the cloaca. Early dehiscence of the cloacal membrane can result in cloacal exstrophy, in which the posterior wall of the cloaca herniates through a pelvic defect, everting the central bowel field between two hemibladder fields. Because the caudal eminence induces some mesodermal structures, including the metanephros, renal anomalies may follow as well.[112,113]

Evidence suggests extrinsic and genetic factors in the causation of caudal regression syndromes. A history of preexisting or gestational maternal diabetes mellitus is obtained in 16% to 49% of cases,[112,114] although caudal spine anomalies occur in only 1% of infants born to diabetic mothers.[115] Most cases are sporadic, although rare familial forms have been reported, and an association with chromosome 7q has been described.[116] Drugs have been implicated in some cases.[117]

The severity of the defect determines the presentation. Newborns may have simple imperforate anus or severe anomalies, including omphalocele, cloacal exstrophy, ambiguous genitalia, and tracheoesophageal fistula. The likelihood of a tethered cord is related to the number of anomalies that are present. Overall, tethering is present in 24% of children with anorectal malformations and in 43% of children with complex malformations.[118] Sacral agenesis is suspected by flattening of the buttocks, shortening of the intergluteal cleft, and prominence of the iliac crests. A soft, skin-covered mass overlying the lumbosacral area suggests a myelocystocele or lipomyelomeningocele with tethered spinal cord. The lower extremities may exhibit abnormalities consistent with the involved vertebral segments. Hammer toes, calcaneovalgus or equinovarus ankle deformities, and contractures of involved joints are similar to findings in myelomeningocele or other forms of tethered cord. Paralysis, atrophy, and incompetent sphincter muscles reflect the myotomes of involvement. Sensation is relatively spared, and the sensory level may be several spinal segments below the motor level.[112] Anomalies higher in the nervous system generally are absent, but a case of Chiari I malformation has been reported.[119]

MRI of the lower spine is the most useful study and should be obtained in suspected cases. Fetal diagnosis of myelocystocele has been described, and it is vital to distinguish this lesion from a myelomeningocele with an intact sac (Fig. 31–19).[120] From the neurosurgical standpoint, the goal is to determine if spinal cord tethering is present and, if so, to delineate the mechanism. Pang[112] classified the appearance of lumbosacral agenesis into five types, based primarily on the appearance of the sacrum. From a practical standpoint, one can divide these anomalies into anomalies with a high conus and anomalies with a low conus. High symmetrical sacral agenesis is correlated with a truncated, club-shaped conus ending around T11 or T12. Tethering is not present, although dural canal stenosis has been reported as the cause of delayed deterioration in a few patients. Paradoxically, the lower, asymmetrical forms of sacral dysgenesis are more likely to have a low-lying tethered cord. Mechanisms of tethering include myelocystocele, typical hypertrophied filum terminale, and lipomyelomeningocele. Myelocystocele is particularly associated with these anomalies and is characterized by a trumpetlike cystic dilation of the caudal central canal, which is extensively tethered to the caudal spinal canal (Fig. 31–20).

Initial management of infants with complex, multisystem anomalies usually does not involve neurosurgery and instead consists of closure of an omphalocele, bowel and possibly urinary diversion, and reconstructive surgery for tracheo-esophageal fistula. MRI of the spine is obtained electively, when the infant is stable. Patients with the conus at a high level do not usually require neurosurgical intervention. Patients with low-lying, tethered cords undergo untethering procedures electively, at about 3 months of age, or when their general condition permits. Even infants with high motor levels should undergo prophylactic untethering. Often the motor level descends over several months, presumably as the infant recovers from spinal cord shock associated with delivery. Untethering is also indicated to preserve sensation. Surgery is similar to surgery for tethered spinal cord without sacral anomalies. Surgery for a myelocystocele consists of defining normal spinal cord anatomy above the lesion, identifying the terminal cyst, resecting the sac and any lipoma, untethering the cord, and reconstructing the dural sac.

Patients who do not have tethered cords and patients who have undergone successful untethering procedures should remain with stable deficits. Patients who experience new neurologic problems later in life should undergo repeat MRI looking for signs of retethering, hydromyelia, or dural stenosis. Patients with complex anomalies require long-term surveillance by a team consisting of a pediatric orthopaedist, urologist, and general surgeon.

Split Cord Anomalies

Split cord malformations are anomalies in which the spinal cord is divided along a portion of its length to form a double tube. Classically, two distinct forms, diastematomyelia and

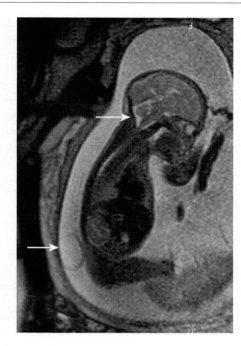

FIGURE 31–19 Fetal MRI shows lumbosacral mass with thick skin (*large arrow*). No Chiari malformation is present (*small arrow*), and α-fetoprotein was normal in amniotic fluid. This was confirmed to be a myelocystocele at birth.

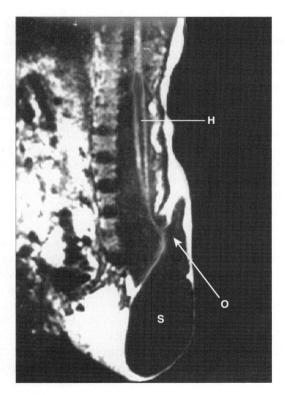

FIGURE 31–20 Sagittal MRI of myelocystocele. S, myelocystocele sac, which is a continuation of central canal, or hydromyelia (H); O, opening through which cerebrospinal fluid communicates to fill sac.

diplomyelia, have been described. The term *diastematomyelia* derives from the Greek words *diastema* ("cleft") and *myelos* ("medulla") and refers to the split in the spinal cord and not, as frequently misapplied, to the intervening bony or cartilaginous spur that often separates the two hemicords. It has been distinguished from *diplomyelia* (from the Greek *diplos*, meaning "double"), which, strictly speaking, refers to a condition in which the spinal cord is completely duplicated (i.e., two complete sets of anterior and posterior horns, with anterior and posterior roots emerging from medial and lateral surfaces of both hemicords). Investigators working more recently maintain that diplomyelia and diastematomyelia are different manifestations of the same pathologic entity and prefer the unifying term *split cord malformation*.[67,121,122] The two hemicords in split cord malformation may exist within a single dural envelope (type II) or, more commonly, are enclosed within separate dural tubes (type I).[67,123] The defect may be at any spinal level, but is most common in the lower thoracic or upper lumbar areas.[124-126]

The embryogenesis of split cord malformation is not fully understood, but the most logical explanation is that suggested by Bremer[127] and amplified by others.[121,128] Any viable theory must explain the frequent association of diastematomyelia with vertebral anomalies, spina bifida, and gut malformations and the equal involvement of the ventral and the dorsal aspects of the neural tube.

In early embryonic development, the neurenteric canal connects the yolk sac (primitive intestinal cavity) with the amniotic cavity through the proliferating primitive knot, which is destined to become the brain and spinal cord. If this canal or an accessory canal persists, the entodermal lining of the yolk sac can herniate through the fistula and split the notochord, neural tube, and migrating mesenchymal elements that are to form the vertebrae. A temporary persistence of this communication results in hemivertebrae: If the herniated entoderm continues to differentiate, it results in a neurenteric cyst; if the tract attaches to the gut, intestinal malrotation or duplications may result. The cuff of pluripotential mesenchymal cells that condense around the entodermal sinus determines the nature of the split cord. The mesenchyme may differentiate into bone, cartilage, or fibrous tissue to form the median septum, which may or may not induce its own investing meninges. A thin membranous septum may be found within the cleft, which may not be seen on imaging studies, suggesting a diagnosis of true diplomyelia.

Whether or not the hemicords possess medial rootlets depends on the location of the neural crest cells within the spinal cord. If they are far lateral and unaffected by the split, only one set of dorsal roots develops on the lateral aspect of the hemicord. If the cell mass is bisected by the split, each hemicord has its own set of paramedian dorsal roots. If the neurenteric tract persists further dorsally to involve the cutaneous ectoderm, a true myelomeningocele occurs. This is also the explanation for the cutaneous signature that often accompanies the malformation. Because normal ascent of the spinal cord continues through this sequence of events, the septum usually lies cephalad to the vertebral defect, and the septum is found at the caudal end of the cleft at surgery.

Clinically, split cord malformation occurs predominantly in girls.[123-125] The largest series reported a female-to-male ratio of 1.5:1.[129] The condition may be asymptomatic, or patients may present with symptoms of spinal cord dysfunction or scoliosis. The clinical findings are no different from findings in other cases of spina bifida occulta. Most patients have a midline thoracic or lumbar cutaneous abnormality. The incidence is 50% to 80%.[63,124,125,130] The level of the skin lesion does not correspond to the level of the split cord malformation. The most common finding is a hairy patch (40%), but other abnormalities include dimples, hemangiomas, lipomas, sinus tracts, or myelomeningocele or meningocele.[125]

Historically, virtually all patients were reported to have significant congenital spinal deformity[124,126] averaging 60 degrees during the growth years. Some modern series report a lower incidence, perhaps because of more widespread imaging.[129,131] The incidence increases with age throughout childhood and is more likely to occur with higher lesions.[123,126] Scoliosis is widely attributed to associated vertebral anomalies such as hemivertebrae, spina bifida, or spinal canal widening rather than to spinal cord dysfunction. In instances of tethering, neural traction may also influence curve development, however.[132] The incidence of split cord malformation among patients with congenital scoliosis is estimated to be 4.9%.[124] The type of scoliosis is nonspecific, apart from the equal incidence of right-sided or left-sided curves, and some authors have recommended obtaining imaging studies of the spinal cord before undertaking surgical treatment of patients with congenital scoliosis.[124,125]

Neurologic symptoms occur as a result of spinal cord tethering and may not arise until adulthood. Symptoms are typical of the tethered cord syndrome and include back pain, gait disturbance, muscular atrophy or deformity of the calf or foot, and spasticity or sensory abnormalities below the level of the lesion with trophic skin changes. Urologic abnormalities occur in 30% to 50% of cases.[129,133] These abnormalities are nonspecific, and other disease entities, such as spinal cord tumor, Friedreich ataxia, and syringomyelia, must be considered. The traction force exerted on the spinal cord may result in brainstem or spinal cord symptoms as the result of an acquired Chiari malformation.[134] Similarly, the spinal traction associated with corrective casts for scoliosis or operative intervention may lead to precipitous paraparesis.[135] Late deterioration in adults has been reported after a blow to the back,[136] after saddle block anesthesia,[133] or simply with associated spondylosis.[133] Adult patients may also show progressive myelopathy without a precipitating event, which may recover after surgery.[70] Pain is present in some children and in virtually all adults. It is usually sharp and localizes to the level of the affected spinal segment.

Split cord malformations are now diagnosed in the fetal period using ultrasonography and fetal MRI.[137] Associated visceral anomalies occur and include horseshoe or ectopic kidney, utero-ovarian malformation, and anorectal malformations. Associated spine anomalies include myelomeningocele and Klippel-Feil syndrome.[138] The classic radiographic appearance of split cord malformation is a fusiform interpedicular widening of the spinal canal on the anteroposterior view with a midline oval bony mass projecting posteriorly from the vertebral body. The spike may be invisible on lateral views. Particularly in early infancy, the spur may be invisible and may not be in continuity with the vertebral body or laminae, supporting the view that the septum is calcified from a separate ossification center.[126] Even in childhood and adult cases, the septum may be cartilaginous and invisible on plain radiographs. In such cases, widening of the neural canal should alert the clinician to the possibility of the diagnosis, and generally the adjacent pedicles should not be widened, as would be seen with an expanding intraspinal tumor.[125] In addition to the widened canal, spina bifida is frequently associated, as are other vertebral anomalies. Scoliosis and kyphosis are common, and their incidence increases with age.[125] This observation reinforces the importance of early detection because the chance of scoliosis developing increases the longer that patients are left without treatment.

MRI is the current procedure of choice for evaluation of split cord malformation (Fig. 31–21). A coronal study shows the split nicely, but sagittal views may not show each hemicord separately, and the study may mistakenly be considered normal. Severe scoliosis may make MRI difficult to interpret because the twisted cord weaves in and out of the imaging plane. In these cases, myelography with axial CT slices after the injection of contrast material is the procedure of choice. The entire spine should be evaluated for the possibility of secondary lesions, such as an associated tight filum terminale, a lipoma, a dermoid cyst or teratoma,[139] or a second spur.

Indications for surgery include progressive neurologic deficit and prophylactically before treatment of scoliosis. Application of a cast or halo pelvic traction for severe kyphoscoliosis may result in paraplegia if the point of tethering is not relieved.[135] Similarly, it is advisable to remove the bony spike as a separate procedure before operative correction of scoliosis. Although it is technically feasible to perform both procedures at a single sitting,[140] removal of the septum may result in early loss of evoked potentials owing to spinal cord manipulation, which reduces the safety of the corrective procedure. In addition, instrumentation of the spine is best avoided with intradural procedures when there is a possibility of a CSF leak.

Management of an asymptomatic patient with split cord malformation is controversial. Most investigators working more recently have urged that asymptomatic children and children who are neurologically stable should undergo prophylactic surgery within the first 2 years of life and cited tethering as the cause of progressive symptoms.[67,122] The older literature states that surgery carries potential risk of neurologic worsening and noted that many patients with split cord malformation remain asymptomatic (or with fixed deficit) throughout growth, favoring a conservative approach.[130,141] A compromise would be to consider the relationship of the septum to the intermedullary cleft in deciding the likelihood of progression owing to tethering. An asymptomatic patient may be followed nonoperatively if the septum is separated from the inferior portion of the cleft, but if the septum is at the caudal end of the cleft or higher, prophylactic surgery is advisable. To stratify risk of neurologic deterioration after

surgery, Mahapatra and Gupta[129] proposed a classification scheme based on the amount of bony septum that straddles the intramedullary cleft. Logically, the highest risk cases are cases in which the bony septum maximally occupies the region of cord split.

The role of surgery in a patient with a cleft but no apparent septum is also unclear. In such patients, there seems to be no reason for tethering, but Pang[67,122] found that at operation these patients essentially always have an unrecognized midline fibrous point of tethering and recommended that these lesions be surgically explored. Finally, the indications for surgery in a patient with myelomeningocele and associated split cord malformation are unclear, although it seems logical to explore such a patient and untether the cord in the face of progressive symptoms referable to the lesion.

The surgical technique described by Matson and colleagues[142] and Meacham[143] is employed. Intraoperative evoked potential recording and rectal manometry have been described,[144] but their value is unproved. In the thoracic spine, the level of the lesion is marked radiographically before the procedure. The patient is positioned as for a standard laminectomy. The paraspinal muscles on each side of the midline are freed and retracted laterally as in any standard laminectomy, but vigorous blunt dissection with a periosteal elevator is avoided because a spina bifida may coexist with the bony septum. The laminectomy is initiated at least one segment above and below the septum and carried out around the bony spike itself, exposing the dural cleft. The cleft usually extends cephalad to the spur but hugs it tightly caudad. A septal elevator is used to free the septum from the surrounding dura, and the superficial portion of the septum is removed by a rongeur or high-speed drill with a diamond bur within the investing

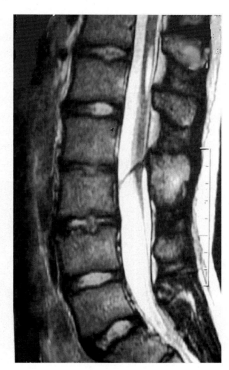

FIGURE 31–21 T2-weighted MRI in sagittal plane shows bony spike penetrating through spinal cord (type I split cord malformation).

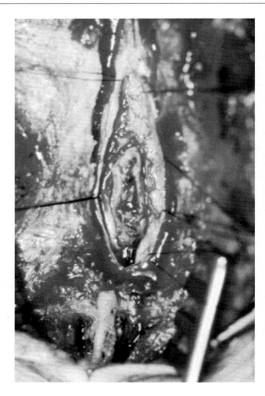

FIGURE 31–22 Operative exposure of split cord malformation (type I). Dura has been opened around bone spur, which has been partially removed.

dural sheath, which serves to protect the spinal cord. The inferior portion of the spur may extend anterior to the spinal cord at the inferior portion of the cleft, and in this case final removal is deferred until the dural compartment has been opened.

The bony spike frequently has large blood vessels within it, and bleeding is managed with bone wax and cautery. The bleeding associated with the epidural venous plexus surrounding the bony spur and deep to the two hemicords may be substantial and should be controlled with bipolar cautery as the spur is removed. When the cleft is decompressed and the cord moves cephalad, bleeding may be difficult to control.

The dura is opened circumferentially around the cleft, and all intradural adhesions at the cleft side are divided (Fig. 31–22). The island of dura and the remainder of the spike are

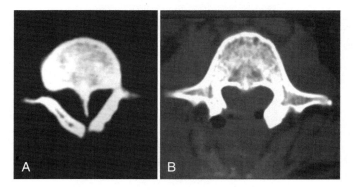

FIGURE 31–23 A and **B,** CT scans before (**A**) and after (**B**) removal of bone spur. The entire spur and its investing dura must be removed to untether cord and prevent regrowth.

removed to the level of the anterior spinal canal (Fig. 31–23). A small midline myelotomy at the caudal portion of the cleft may be required to accomplish this. Type II lesions, in which the two hemicords reside within a common dural sleeve, are managed initially by laminectomy over the region of the abnormality. The dura is opened in a paramedian manner because the hemicords are often tethered dorsally at the midline. Fibrous bands arise from the caudal end of the cleft and are displaced inferiorly as they tether to the dorsal dura. These are sharply divided. Median rootlets are often present and are nonfunctional. They may be sectioned if necessary to release the hemicords.[122] It is neither necessary nor desirable to close the anterior dura. The posterior dura is closed with a graft if necessary. If there is an associated tethering lesion apart from the split cord malformation, this should be addressed at the same time. A separate laminectomy or laminotomy may be required to section a filum terminale.

The procedure should be considered largely prophylactic, although there may be improvement in half of symptomatic patients.[99] Long-standing deficits and scoliosis are unlikely to improve, but pain is almost always alleviated. Bladder and autonomic symptoms are least likely to improve.[129] Complications include CSF leakage and worsening of neurologic status. Cases of type II malformation in which there is an oblique septum and a small, delicate hemicord seem to have a higher risk of cord injury.[67] Failure to improve or late deterioration after operation may be due to failure to remove the tethered spur entirely, failure to address a second lesion such as a hypertrophied filum, or (rarely) regrowth of the septum.[145]

Anterior Sacral Meningocele and Currarino Triad

Anterior meningocele is a rare condition in which there is a herniation of the dural sac through a defect in the anterior surface of the spine, usually in the sacrum. The sac is composed of an outer dural membrane and an inner arachnoid membrane. It contains CSF and occasionally neural elements. If the sac is large, it may manifest as a pelvic mass.

Since its original description in 1837 by "a distinguished surgeon" who preferred to remain anonymous,[146] several hundred cases of anterior sacral meningocele have been reported. In 1981, Currarino and colleagues[147] described the association of anorectal anomalies, sacral bony anomalies, and a presacral mass, which has been termed the *Currarino triad*. The presacral mass in these cases is an anterior sacral meningocele, a teratoma, or both. The triad is a form of split notochord malformation and is inherited as an autosomal dominant trait in 50% of patients.[148] The varied presentations may bring patients to the attention of a wide range of specialists, including urologists, colorectal surgeons, gynecologists, pediatric surgeons, orthopaedic surgeons, and neurosurgeons. When the condition is properly diagnosed and treated, the cure rate is high; if it is improperly managed, meningitis may result in death.

Most anterior sacral meningoceles are congenital, as evidenced by their frequent appearance in infants and young children, the associated anomalies of pelvic organs, and familial incidence.[149] In contrast to the typical posterior myelomeningocele, there is no accompanying hydrocephalus or association with Chiari malformations. In the Currarino triad, there is an abnormal adhesion between endoderm and ectoderm, or there are abnormalities of the notochord that cause a failure of the mesoderm to fuse in the midline. The notochord and somites fuse to form vertebral bodies, separating the endoderm and ectoderm. If the notochord is split, anterior fusion of the vertebral body fails, and a fistula between the gut and the spinal canal is formed. Partial resorption of this connection forms an anterior sacral meningocele or a retrorectal enteric cyst. The combination of mesodermal tissue with these enteric and neuroectodermal elements leads to formation of a presacral teratoma.[150] Genes in the terminal region of chromosome 7q have been linked with sacral dysgenesis[116,151] and may play a role in these malformations.

The lesion is detected far more commonly in women than in men, but in children the sex incidence is approximately equal. Most likely, there is really no sex predilection, and the lesion simply remains undetected in many men.[152] Most clinical manifestations are caused by pressure of the sac on adjacent pelvic structures such as the rectum, bladder, uterus, and sacral nerve roots. Constipation is the most common symptom, particularly in infants and children. Many patients report use of laxatives and enemas. Urinary difficulties may be due to direct pressure of the mass or to pressure on sacral nerve roots. Midline lumbosacral back pain occurs in some patients and may radiate to the perineal area or inner thighs. Some patients report relief after a bowel movement. Headache may be due to either high or low intracranial pressure. Classically, the headache begins in childhood with sudden onset with Valsalva maneuver, as during straining or defecation. In later life, it may accompany coitus.[153] The headache is reproduced when the pelvic mass is compressed on digital examination. When the patient stands, the meningocele fills with fluid, which may cause a secondary low-pressure headache.

Meningitis may be either septic or aseptic and may be recurrent.[154] Bacterial meningitis may be spontaneous owing to microperforations of the rectum allowing passage of bacteria into the sac, or may result from traumatic rupture of the sac during childbirth. Meningitis may also result from attempted needle aspiration of the sac. Aseptic meningitis has been described, presumably from irritation secondary to an associated dermoid.[155] In women of childbearing age, anterior meningocele may result in obstructed labor or rupture of the sac during delivery.[153]

The cardinal sign is a smooth, cystic mass palpable on rectal or pelvic examination. It is usually adherent to the sacrum. The mass is detectable on routine abdominal examination only when it is enormous. The differential diagnosis of masses includes dermoids, chordomas, and osseous or metastatic tumors.[156]

Radiologic evaluation of the sacrum usually shows some abnormality, classically the "scimitar" sacrum. The anteroposterior radiograph shows a well-circumscribed lucent defect on one side of the sacrum corresponding to the sac, and there is no surrounding bony destruction.[153] Urologic contrast studies often show compression of the bladder and uterus and duplication of the ureters or renal pelvis. CT-myelography of the pelvis may be indicated in some cases and is performed with water-soluble contrast medium to show a small communication between the subarachnoid space and the meningocele sac. MRI is often sufficient to show the communication (Fig. 31–24). Heterogeneous signal intensity on T1-weighted and T2-weighted sequences may suggest a teratoma.[157]

Surgical treatment of symptomatic lesions is generally advisable because there is no possibility of spontaneous regression, and in untreated patients there is a 30% mortality rate owing to pelvic obstruction at the time of labor or to erosion into the rectum followed by meningitis.[152,153] An asymptomatic lesion may be followed without the need for surgery if there is no possibility of pregnancy and if the lesion does not enlarge on repeated rectal examination.

Aspiration through the rectum or vagina or percutaneously should not be performed. If a cyst is discovered at laparotomy for other reasons and CSF is obtained on aspiration, the operation should be terminated, and radiologic studies should be performed to define the extent of the lesion and the nature of its communication with the subarachnoid space.

Surgical treatment via laparotomy has been described historically and has been advocated more recently.[152,158] Most modern authors favor sacral laminectomy as the initial approach, however.[159] This approach allows visualization of the intraspinal contents and resection of adhesions or division of an abnormal filum terminale. Nerve roots can be protected, and there is usually good visualization of the opening into the meningocele to allow suturing. The goal of surgery is to untether the spinal cord, decompress the sac, and obliterate the

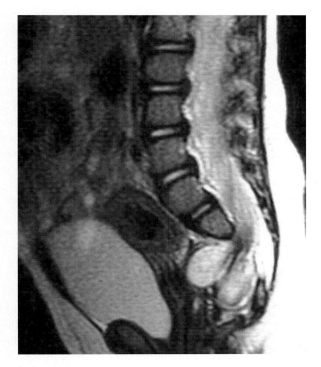

FIGURE 31–24 Mid-sagittal MRI of anterior sacral meningocele in a child. The communication was oversewn by posterior approach.

CSF fistula. It is unnecessary to remove the lining of the pelvic cyst, which may be densely adherent to the rectum. If the dura is fragile or cannot be mobilized sufficiently to allow suture even with a fascial graft, a posterior pelvic operation or laparotomy should be performed with the assistance of an experienced abdominal surgeon.[160]

The technique of sacral laminectomy has been reviewed.[161] Antibiotic coverage and bowel preparation are begun 48 hours before surgery in case the rectum is inadvertently entered during the procedure. Under general anesthesia, the patient is placed in the prone position with the chest and abdomen supported, and the anus is draped out of the field with a plastic sheet. A lumbosacral laminectomy is performed from L5 to S4, and the posterior dura is opened longitudinally.

Nerve roots within the dural canal are carefully retracted laterally, and the filum terminale is divided, exposing the anterior defect in the dura leading to the sac. If no roots enter the sac and the neck is narrow, CSF may be suctioned from the sac, and the anterior dura may be oversewn with 4-0 nonabsorbable suture. If the sac inserts caudad and is merely a terminal extension of the dural canal without nerve roots within it, the terminal sac may be amputated and the caudal sac reconstructed. If the anterior defect is wide and cannot be mobilized into the field sufficiently for primary closure, digital collapse of the sac through the rectum as the sac is ligated may be helpful, or a fascial graft may be sewn to the edges of the defect. If roots exit through the ostium, the dura has to be plicated around them to permit their exit. If it proves impossible to close a widened stalk, a second procedure with an abdominal approach is necessary. The posterior dura is closed in a watertight fashion. Postoperatively, special care must be taken to protect the wound from fecal contamination, and stool softeners may be given to prevent straining.

The lithotomy position is used in case an abdominal procedure is required.[152] After a urethral catheter is placed, a midline incision is extended from the symphysis pubis to above the umbilicus. The procedure is carried out similar to an abdominoperineal resection of the rectum. The wall of the meningocele is exposed by opening the peritoneum on the right side of the rectum and dissected between the wall of the cyst and the fibrous capsule, keeping the sac intact. When the base has been identified, the sac is opened, and nerve roots are identified. The meningocele is resected at its base, leaving enough membrane to effect a watertight closure. The incision is closed without drains.

Surgical results reported in the recent literature have been generally good.[158,162] Complications include meningitis or neurologic deterioration in cases in which nerve roots have been found within the sac.

Congenital Dermal Sinus and Dermoid Cysts

The term *dermal sinus* describes a group of congenital malformations in which a tubular tract lined with squamous epithelium extends from the skin overlying the spine inward to varying depths. Termination of the sinus may be in the subcutaneous tissue, bone, dura, subarachnoid space, or filum terminale; within an intradural dermoid expansion; or within a neuroglial mass inside the spinal cord. These cysts may occur in the occipital region of the head or at any level of the spine above the coccygeal area but are most commonly in the lumbosacral area, where they may be confused with pilonidal sinuses or coccygeal dimples that have no connection with the spinal canal.

In early development, the terminal portion of the neural tube and the coccygeal vertebrae are intimately related and perhaps fused to the overlying epithelium. As the spine begins to elongate, the sacrococcygeal ligament applies traction on the overlying skin, producing a dimple in the skin overlying the sacrococcygeal region. There is no connection with the spinal canal, but MRI may show the fibrous connection to the coccyx. These coccygeal pits are reported to occur in about 4% of children.[163] Some authors have suggested that a "traction test" to determine the rostral or caudal direction of the tract may be useful,[164] but a more useful test is simply to feel the tip of the coccyx directly beneath the dimple. No treatment is necessary except local cleanliness.

The embryonic defect in true congenital dermal sinus is believed to occur early in fetal life at the time the ectoblast differentiates into cutaneous and neural ectoderm. The cleavage between the two layers of ectoderm is incomplete at this point (*incomplete dysjunction*), giving rise to the sinus, and as the neural groove closes to create the neural tube, cutaneous ectodermal elements are invaginated within the neural tube, which may subsequently develop into an intraspinal dermoid growth. As the conus ascends, the sinus tract elongates. When there is an associated defect of mesodermal organization around the tract, spina bifida results.

More superficial sinus tracts that do not penetrate to the spinal canal are explained as failure of fusion of the cutaneous ectoderm after it has separated from the neuroectoderm. Focal enlargement of the tract may occur at any point to form dermoid or epidermal inclusion cysts. The dermal elements are typically intramedullary in the thoracic region and adherent to multiple nerve roots of the cauda equina in the lumbosacral region. Similar dermal inclusions occur in myelomeningoceles[165] and after lumbar puncture. Pilonidal sinuses are acquired lesions in adults and are believed to result from repeated trauma or an inflammatory reaction secondary to penetration of broken strands of hair. It is possible that some pilonidal sinuses in adults represent chronic infection within a superficial congenital dermal sinus, and the distinction between these entities may be blurred. In practice, the term *pilonidal sinus* should be reserved for acquired lesions in adults.

Congenital dermal sinuses may be detected during routine examination of an infant or child or deliberately sought after recurrent bouts of meningitis or local infection at the level of the skin.[166] The sinus occurs in the skin as a deep depression, usually in the lumbar region, which may be accompanied by nevi or hypertrichosis. Sinus tracts may occur in the cervical or thoracic regions.[167] Occasionally, multiple sinuses are encountered. There may be a history of an accompanying purulent or clear discharge. Local infection of the sinus tract with staphylococci or *Escherichia coli* is common. The opening of the sinus tract is invariably in the midline and may be extremely small. Such a sinus opening occurring above the sacrococcygeal region should be explored and excised. Probing and injection of dyes are inadvisable.

Patients may also present with signs of spinal cord or cauda equina compression, from either an expanding dermoid within the spinal canal or an intraspinal abscess. Whether the condition is of gradual or sudden onset, the patient may present with lower extremity weakness, sphincter incontinence, or root irritation and meningismus. Pain in the back and legs is usual with abscess formation or meningitis owing to rupture of the irritating contents of the dermoid cyst. In chronic cases, motor weakness, foot deformity, and reflex changes occur. A young child may refuse to walk.

Dimples below the top of the intergluteal crease require no investigation beyond physical examination. Ultrasound may be a useful screening test,[168] but MRI is indicated in higher lesions to follow the depth of the tract, to determine the level of the conus, and to evaluate the spinal canal for inclusion cysts or abscesses (Fig. 31–25).[169] The tract may be difficult to visualize, and surgical exploration of pores above the sacral region may be indicated even if radiologic studies do not clearly show a communication with the thecal sac. Sinus tracts in the cervical region should be evaluated with cranial MRI because the dermoid tumor and tract may extend into the posterior fossa.

Prophylactic surgery is performed as early as possible to excise the entire tract.[166,167] In asymptomatic patients, the lesions may be explored and the tract followed to its termination. A surgeon undertaking such an operation must be prepared to perform an extensive intradural dissection because the tract may extend for a considerable distance. The operation is begun with an elliptical skin incision surrounding the sinus opening and any abnormal skin surrounding it. The tract is sharply dissected and followed through the fascia. A laminectomy is performed if the tract appears to continue to the dura. If the tract attaches to the dura, the dura is opened lateral to the entrance point, and the intradural contents are inspected. Any intradural tract must be followed to its termination even if this involves an extensive laminectomy to the conus because remaining tissue has the capacity to grow into a large dermoid inclusion. Occasionally, it may be unclear if an intradural tract is a hypertrophied filum or a true sinus tract, and frozen section may be useful.

Intradural cysts are completely removed without violating the capsule if possible. If the cyst has ruptured or is infected, a dense arachnoiditis with scarred nerve roots prevents complete excision.[170] In this event, judicious intracapsular removal of purulent material and dermoid elements is performed, but no attempt is made to remove the scarred capsule wall from the nerve roots. If a cervical or thoracic tract terminates in a neuroglial mass, the tract is amputated at the mass, and no attempt is made to remove it. A watertight dural closure is made except in patients in whom closure would compress residual infected dermoid cyst material, in which case the dura may be left open, and the muscle and fascia are closed.

The outcome is usually favorable when all elements of the tract and associated dermal cysts are excised. Subtotally resected dermoids with root attachment warrant follow-up.

Filum Terminale Syndrome

The hypertrophied filum terminale constitutes a relatively uncommon cause of tethered cord syndrome. In its pure form, the conus is bound into a low position by a thickened filum terminale, but more complex variations include filum lipomas, traction bands, and *meningocele manqué*, a term used to describe aborted or atrophic meningocele sacs that tether the conus.

Patients present with a typical tethered cord syndrome. Cutaneous abnormalities are noted in approximately half of the patients[171] and may consist of a sinus tract, a hairy nevus, a hemangioma, an accessory appendage (tail), or an area of atretic skin. Other symptoms include orthopaedic deformity (scoliosis, leg or foot atrophy), progressive weakness, and urologic dysfunction (urinary incontinence, bladder distention, loss of perineal sensation). Back pain is often prominent in teenage and adult patients. The condition is rarely familial.[171,172] This condition is often suspected in association with imperforate anus, and an incidence of 35% has been reported.[73] The condition is also suspected in children with voiding dysfunction, particularly if there is associated impaired bladder sensation or poor bladder emptying. The value of screening MRI is controversial in these patients.[173,174]

Radiologic investigation usually shows a simple posterior lumbosacral spina bifida but may reveal other vertebral anomalies. Further workup consists of studies to evaluate the level of the conus and may include MRI or supine myelography with CT. Barson[175] measured the level of conus termination in

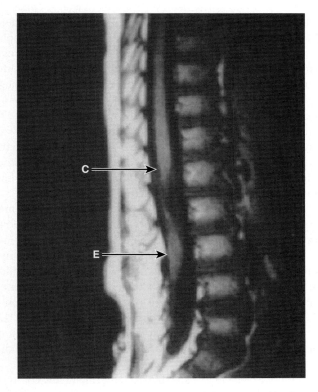

FIGURE 31–25 MRI of spinal congenital dermal sinus tract and lumbar dermoid inclusion cyst. C, conus; E, epidermoid.

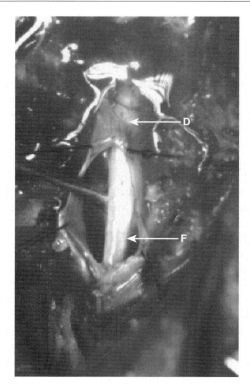

FIGURE 31–26 Intraoperative photograph of hypertrophied filum terminale. After stimulating fatty filum and eliciting no response on electromyography, filum was sectioned. D, dural sac; F, thickened filum terminale.

normal infants and children and reported that on average the adult level (L1-2) is reached by 2 months of age. A conus tip below the L2-3 interspace in a child older than 5 years is definitely abnormal. A filum thicker than 2 mm at myelography is also abnormal. Although MRI may suggest the diagnosis with the finding of a low conus on sagittal and axial views, the filum itself may be poorly seen. If the clinical history is suggestive, myelography in the supine position with a follow-up metrizamide CT scan may be worthwhile even in the face of a normal MRI study. A few patients have been reported who have the typical skin and neurologic manifestations of tethered cord syndrome yet have the conus at the normal spinal level on imaging studies. At operation, these patients had thickened or fatty fila and evidence of tethering.[79,176]

The term *minimal tethered cord syndrome* is sometimes applied to such a scenario,[177] in which the patient exhibits urologic dysfunction but lacks the MRI evidence of tethering. In these cases, division of the filum to relieve urinary symptoms must be guided by strong clinical suspicion. In adults, fat in the filum within 13 mm of the conus has been correlated with neurologic dysfunction, independent of conus position.[74] Conversely, the presence of an asymptomatic fatty filum terminale on MRI is a normal variant, occurring in 0.24% of patients. If the conus is at a normal level, no further workup or treatment is required.[178]

If there is evidence of spinal cord tethering (a low conus or clinical symptoms), prophylactic surgery is recommended at the time the entity is discovered to prevent progression of

symptoms and to relieve chronic back pain. A few children with spinal cord tethering have been reported to show no deterioration over a period of a few years,[179] but most investigators believe that most patients eventually show progression of symptoms and that prophylactic surgery is indicated. A laminectomy is performed above or below the bifid segment, and the dura is opened. The filum is coagulated and sectioned as low as possible (Fig. 31–26). In some reported cases, clips placed at the cut ends of the filum have separated by 2.5 cm on postoperative radiographs.[171] If it proves difficult to identify the filum clearly, it can be electrically stimulated or followed to its termination by performing an extensive sacral laminectomy. Often, small but functional rootlets are intimately attached to the filum and must be identified and dissected away before sectioning.

Terminal syringohydromyelia is reported with meningocele manqué and with tight filum anomalies and may be symptomatic.[180,181] This condition is usually treated by untethering the cord and repeating imaging a few months later. If the terminal syrinx persists and is believed to be the cause of symptoms, shunting the cyst to the subarachnoid space, pleura, or peritoneum may be required.

The results of surgery are favorable in relieving back pain and preventing the progression of existing deficits, and often some long-standing neurologic deficits may improve. In the series by Anderson,[105] urinary incontinence improved in 14 of 33 patients, and weakness and numbness of the legs lessened postoperatively in one third. Back and leg pains were relieved in virtually all children and adults in several series.[69,105,182] Retethering is rare but is reported.[183]

Neurenteric Cyst

Although neurenteric cysts are quite rare, they are well-described entities consisting of cystic structures within the spinal canal or anterior to the vertebral bodies in the mediastinum, abdomen, or neck. Ventral cysts may have connections via a stalk to the meninges and spinal cord through a tunnel-like defect in the vertebral bodies. The cyst wall resembles foregut tissue histologically, and in the literature these lesions are also referred to as *enterogenous cysts*.[184] They may occur in isolation or as part of a more complex group of spinal anomalies, including Klippel-Feil syndrome, spinal lipoma, and syringomyelia.[185,186] They may occur at any spinal level, but most are between C3 and T7.[187]

Early in the development of the human embryo there is a communication between the yolk sac (destined to become the gut) and the dorsal surface of the embryo called the *neurenteric canal*. This fistulous tract transiently connects the future enteric cavity with the neural groove in the region of the coccyx. Bremer[188] pointed out that abnormal accessory neurenteric canals may persist cephalad to the coccygeal tip and can give rise to cysts along the persistent tract. The tract also gives rise to associated vertebral anomalies: a widened vertebral body resulting from bony proliferation in an attempt to fill the gap after disappearance of the tract or a circular defect in the vertebral body produced by the persistent tract that forces bone to form around it. Because the accessory neurenteric tract can be elongated and stretched during growth, the canal may become divided into noncommunicating diverticula that lie at some distance from each other (e.g., in the thoracic cavity and spinal canal). The tendency for the cysts to lie to the right of the vertebral column has been ascribed to the developmental process of gastric and gut rotation.[189] Persistence of only a portion of the tract results in a cyst only within the spinal canal.[190] The cysts are usually anteriorly located within the canal (Fig. 31–27), although dorsally located ones are described.[191]

Neurenteric cysts within the spinal canal or ventral masses are similar pathologically. They may be thick, well-defined capsules or delicate, clear walls that may be confused with spinal arachnoid cysts. They are described as strawberry-colored[192] or whitish[190] and when in the spinal canal may be intradural-extramedullary[193] or intramedullary.[194] The cyst fluid is usually described as clear or milky and quite gelatinous. There may or may not be a ventral dural defect.

Histologically, the cyst wall typically is formed of endodermal ciliated columnar epithelium resting on a basement membrane and may contain gastric parietal and chief cells or mucin-producing goblet cells (Fig. 31–28).[193] The epithelial cells are positive for keratin markers. Some investigators have made a distinction between neurenteric cysts, with well-differentiated gastrointestinal epithelium and a clear connection of the spinal cyst and the chest and abdomen, and "teratomatous cysts," which have less differentiated epithelium and no ventral connection.[195,196]

Neurenteric cysts are usually detected in childhood,[190,193,194,197,198] although adult patients have been reported.[197,199,200] Neurenteric cysts have been detected by prenatal MRI or ultrasound.[201] The diagnosis is suggested by the combination of a thoracic cystic mass with vertebral anomalies. In early childhood, the lesion may manifest as a chest or abdominal mass with cardiorespiratory compromise[202,203] or as a neck mass with tracheal compression or may be detected because of vertebral anomalies seen on a radiograph. Adults and older children tend to present with signs of spinal cord compression in the cervical or thoracic regions,[204] which may be acute or follow trivial trauma.[205] In addition to motor weakness, burning dysesthesias may occur when aggravated by coughing or sneezing or recumbency. Rarely, a neurenteric fistula may lead to meningitis with bowel organisms.[204] Associated malrotation of the gut[206] and diaphragmatic hernia[207] may be found.

Plain radiographs may show widening of the neural canal, cleft vertebrae, or fusion of vertebral segments.[207] An anterior soft tissue mass may be seen in the chest, neck, or abdomen, and the association of such a mass with vertebral anomalies should suggest the diagnosis. The presence of the classic circular defect through the vertebral body, although diagnostic, is not essential.[207] Patients in whom the diagnosis is suspected should undergo MRI[208] and possibly myelography with water-soluble contrast medium and postmyelogram CT to define the bony anatomy and establish the presence or absence of a communication between the spinal canal and a ventral mass. MRI shows a cystic mass and its relationship with the spinal cord.[190]

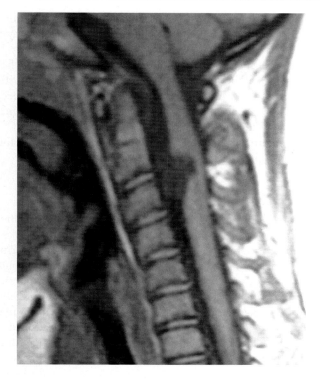

FIGURE 31–27 MRI of cervical spine shows anteriorly placed neurenteric cyst compressing spinal cord and causing myelopathy.

The treatment of neurenteric cysts varies with location and presentation. An intraspinal lesion can be corrected first, at a separate procedure, or as part of a combined procedure, such as thoracotomy, to excise the prevertebral lesion. Because the spinal mass is largely cystic, the traditional treatment has been a wide laminectomy with cyst drainage and conservative resection of cyst wall.[197] Some authors have advocated radical resection of the entire cyst wall, however, which may require a lateral approach[200] or corpectomy[189,199] to approach lesions located ventral to the spinal cord. A cyst-subarachnoid shunt has been described,[206] but the thick nature of the fluid and its possible irritation of the meninges make this unlikely to be useful in most cases. If there is an anterior dural defect,

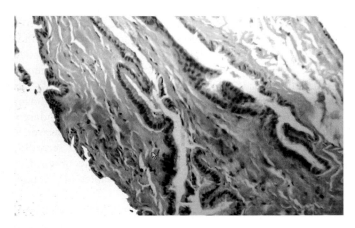

FIGURE 31–28 Light microscopy with hematoxylin and eosin staining of neurenteric cyst. Epithelium resembles gut.

this may be plugged with a muscle or fascial graft from a posterior approach or ligated or sutured if a thoracotomy is performed.

Patients generally recover neurologic function if the deficit is not severe at the time of operation. Good outcomes can still be attained with subtotal resection.[209] Recurrence has been noted after incomplete resection, but the reported recurrence rate in subtotally resected cysts ranges from 11% to 75%.[204,209] In children in particular, delayed kyphosis or swan neck deformity may follow extensive laminectomy.

Intraoperative Neurophysiologic Monitoring

The routine use of intraoperative neurophysiologic monitoring to help guide the surgical management of tethered cord syndrome is controversial, and consequently this monitoring is perhaps underused. Although there have been few published studies on the efficacy of intraoperative neurophysiologic monitoring during release of tethered spinal cord, the authors' clinical experience over 2 decades has been positive, as has been the experience of others.[210,211] Application of a multimodality neuromonitoring protocol has been helpful in (1) identifying functional neural elements that may otherwise have been sacrificed, particularly in the case of a thickened filum terminale; (2) identifying the level of exiting nerve root when faced with ambiguous anatomy; (3) warning of excessive surgical traction on nerve root or spinal cord during manipulation and untethering; (4) assessing the functional properties of each hemicord in patients with diastematomyelia; (5) identifying emerging spinal cord injury; and (6) providing an overall sense of security to the neurosurgeon.

The techniques used in the authors' practice to assess spinal cord and nerve root function and integrity include spontaneous and stimulated EMG, multipulse transcranial motor evoked potentials, and SSEPs. The first two EMG monitoring modalities are used to identify nerve root presence and assess their function in real time. Transcranial motor evoked potentials and SSEPs provide information about the functional integrity of the efferent motor and afferent sensory spinal cord tracts. Transcranial motor evoked potentials are of additional value in verifying nerve root function, serving as a cross-check to spontaneous and stimulated EMG. The details of this technique have been published.[212-215]

Neurophysiologic monitoring of spinal cord and nerve root function is most applicable to operations for spina bifida occulta and least beneficial in cases of spina bifida cystica. Children with myelomeningocele often have severe neurologic deficits that preclude reliable monitoring; SSEPs are invariably absent in high-level dysraphism. Neuromonitoring of myelomeningocele patients with low-level lesions undergoing untethering procedures is potentially helpful, however. A detailed description of the specific stimulus and recording parameters for each of these neurophysiologic monitoring modalities may be found elsewhere (see Chapter 14). EMG is briefly discussed here.

Of all the intraoperative neurophysiologic monitoring modalities, intraoperative EMG plays the greatest role in preserving neural function in patients undergoing spinal cord untethering. Lipomas and fibrous adhesions obscure surgical anatomy, making it difficult to differentiate between neural and non-neural tissue. Likewise, it is often impossible to visualize low sacral nerve root fascicles that may be entwined in a thickened filum terminale, placing the patient at risk for complications of bowel, bladder, and sexual function when the filum is sectioned.

The preferred EMG monitoring technique is 10-channel recording from five bipolar subdermal needle electrode pairs inserted into the left and right adductor, quadriceps, tibialis anterior, gastrocnemius, and external anal sphincter muscles. In infants and young children, limited perianal space may preclude two distinct bipolar electrode pairs for the left and right sides; the left electrode is referenced to the right and vice versa. This electrode montage provides nerve root coverage from L2 to S4 segments. Although manometric monitoring of anal sphincter tone has been described,[144,216] the combination of spontaneous and stimulated EMG is sufficient by itself.[217] Urinary bladder manometry has been advocated as an additional technique to assess urinary sphincter tone because the parasympathetic fibers innervating the detrusor muscle do not travel with the pudendal nerves.[218] This method is cumbersome, however, and not routinely implemented. A sixth EMG channel, rectus abdominis-iliopsoas, is sometimes added when it is necessary to monitor T12-L1 nerve roots.

The EMG monitoring paradigm must consist of continuous, real-time spontaneous muscle activity and intermittent electrically stimulated compound muscle action potential recordings. Spontaneous EMG is used to identify excessive root traction during lipoma resection or untethering, whereas stimulated EMG is imperative for differentiating between neural and non-neural elements and for verifying anatomic level. Reliance on either one of these two EMG modalities alone results in failure to identify root traction, irritation, or the presence of functional nerve root.

To achieve focal stimulation for valid stimulated EMG recordings, a hand-held concentric bipolar stimulating electrode is used. Monopolar stimulators such as those often used for cranial nerve stimulation produce too much current spread, precluding individual nerve root identification. The authors employ a gradual "stair-step" approach to nerve root stimulation beginning at a low constant current and continuing until a compound muscle action potential is recorded. Generally, compound muscle action potentials for sensory nerve roots are elicited between 1 mA and 4 mA, depending on the vertebral level, whereas motor roots have significantly larger compound muscle action potentials and depolarize at much lower current levels (0.1 to 0.2 mA) at short stimulus durations (50 μsec). Nerve root fascicles often require higher current intensity (e.g., 5 to 8 mA) to depolarize and present responses of small amplitude compared with their root trunk counterparts. When attempting to confirm the absence of neural element within the filum, the stimulation intensity should be increased to 10 to 20 mA (depending on stimulus duration) to ensure that no root fascicle is present on the dorsal, ventral, or medial surfaces. If using voltage parameters, the threshold should be up to 100 V for filum sectioning.[219]

KEY POINTS

1. A prospective multicenter trial is now under way to evaluate the efficacy of fetal closure of myelomeningocele at fetal age less than 26 weeks.

2. Reasons for late deterioration in a patient with a myelomeningocele include decompensated hydrocephalus, Chiari malformation, hydromyelia, tethered cord, epidermoid, basilar invagination, spinal deformity, split cord malformation, obesity, and depression.

3. In the setting of a lumbosacral mass detected prenatally, the absence of elevated α-fetoprotein levels in amniotic fluid and absence of a Chiari malformation on ultrasound are more suggestive of a skin-covered dysraphism, such as a myelocystocele, rather than an open neural tube defect.

4. Retethering after prior surgery for tethered cord is a clinical diagnosis and not a radiographic one.

5. Patients with occult dysraphism rarely have associated Chiari malformations, hydrocephalus, or cognitive impairment.

6. When performing surgery for occult dysraphism, the surgeon should always define the normal anatomy above the lesion before entering the lesion itself.

7. Adult patients with tethered cord are at risk for deterioration despite the fact that they have achieved full linear growth.

8. Tethered cord syndrome may occur even when the conus ends at an apparently normal anatomic level (T12-L2).

9. The development of fetal MRI and ultrasound has facilitated increasingly accurate in utero diagnostics of open and closed neural tube defects.

10. Ambulation status, intelligence, and life expectancy in myelomeningocele patients are all largely affected by the initial level of the neural tube defect.

KEY REFERENCES

1. Luthy D, Wardinsky T, Shurtleff D: Cesarean section before the onset of labor and subsequent motor function in infants with myelomeningocele diagnosed antenatally. N Engl J Med 324:662-666, 1991.
   This classic article first suggested that cesarean delivery improves outcome with myelomeningocele. It is now controversial, and other articles have failed to show an improved outcome with cesarean delivery.

2. McLone D, Naidich T: Developmental morphology of the subarachnoid space, brain vasculature, and contiguous structures, and the cause of the Chiari II malformation. AJNR Am J Neuroradiol 13:463-482, 1992.
   This article provides the most convincing explanation for the embryologic association of myelomeningocele, Chiari malformation, hydrocephalus, and hydromyelia and explains reversal of the Chiari malformation with fetal surgery.

3. Sutton L, Adzick N, Bilaniuk L, et al: Improvement in hindbrain herniation demonstrated by serial fetal magnetic resonance imaging following fetal surgery for myelomeningocele. JAMA 282:1826-1831, 1999.

4. Bruner J, Tulipan N, Paschall R, et al: Fetal surgery for myelomeningocele and the incidence of shunt-dependent hydrocephalus. JAMA 282:1819-1825, 1999.
   The articles by Sutton and colleagues and Bruner and colleagues appeared simultaneously and first reported the possible benefit of fetal surgery for myelomeningocele.

5. Tubbs R, Elton S, Grabb P, et al: Analysis of the posterior fossa in children with the Chiari 0 malformation. Neurosurgery 48:1050-1054, 2001.
   This article first described the finding of hydromyelia without visible Chiari malformation and recommended surgical exploration for this condition.

6. Chapman P: Congenital intraspinal lipomas: Anatomic considerations and surgical treatment. Childs Brain 9:37-47, 1982.
   This article describes the surgical anatomy of a lipomyelomeningocele. The classification is still useful to anyone performing this surgery.

7. Kulkarni A, Pierre-Kahn A, Zerah M: Conservative management of asymptomatic spinal lipomas of the conus. Neurosurgery 54:868-875, 2004.
   This is a very controversial article that recommends against prophylactic surgery for asymptomatic patients with lipomyelomeningocele.

8. Pang D, Dias M, Ahab-Barmada M: Split cord malformation: I. A unified theory of embryogenesis for double cord malformations. Neurosurgery 31:451-480, 1992.

9. Pang D: Split cord malformation: II. Clinical syndrome. Neurosurgery 31:481-500, 1992.
   Two articles by Pang and colleagues and Pang together describe the embryogenesis, classification, and management of the various forms of split cord malformations.

10. Warder D, Oakes W: Tethered cord syndrome and the conus in a normal position. Neurosurgery 33:374-378, 1993.
    This article first described the clinical and radiographic syndrome of symptomatic tethering with conus at a normal level.

REFERENCES

1. French B: Midline fusion defects and defects in formation. In Youmans J (ed): Neurological Surgery, 3rd ed. Philadelphia, WB Saunders, 1990, pp 1081-1235.

2. Stiefel D, Meuli M: Scanning electron microscopy of fetal murine myelomeningocele reveals growth and development of the spinal cord in early gestation and neural tissue destruction around birth. J Pediatr Surg 42:1561-1565, 2007.

3. Lemire RJ: Normal and Abnormal Development of the Human Nervous System. Hagerstown, MD, Harper & Row, 1975.

4. McLone D, Naidich T: Developmental morphology of the subarachnoid space, brain vasculature, and contiguous structures,

and the cause of the Chiari II malformation. AJNR Am J Neuroradiol 13:463-482, 1992.

5. Little J, Elwood J: Epidemiology of neural tube defects. In Kiely M (ed): Reproductive and Perinatal Epidemiology. Boca Raton, FL, CRC Press, 1991, pp 251-336.

6. Prevention of neural tube defects: Results of the Medical Research Council Vitamin Study. MRC Vitamin Study Research Group. Lancet 338:131-137, 1991.

7. Botto L, Moore C, Khoury M, et al: Neural tube defects. N Engl J Med 341:1509-1519, 1999.

8. Babcook C: Ultrasound evaluation of prenatal and neonatal spina bifida. Neurosurg Clin N Am 6:203-218, 1995.

9. Nadel A, Green J, Holmes L, et al: Absence of need for amniocentesis in patients with elevated levels of maternal serum alpha-fetoprotein and normal ultrasonographic examinations. N Engl J Med 323:557-561, 1990.

10. Simon E, Goldstein R, Coakley F, et al: Fast MR imaging of fetal CNS anomalies in utero. AJNR Am J Neuroradiol 21:1688-1698, 2000.

11. von Koch CS, Glenn OA, Goldstein RB, et al: Fetal magnetic resonance imaging enhances detection of spinal cord anomalies in patients with sonographically detected bony anomalies of the spine. J Ultrasound Med 24:781-789, 2005.

12. Cochrane D, Aronyk K, Sawatzky B, et al: The effect of labor and delivery on spinal cord function and ambulation in patients with meningomyelocele. Child Nerv Syst 7:312-315, 1991.

13. Luthy D, Wardinsky T, Shurtleff D: Cesarean section before the onset of labor and subsequent motor function in infants with myelomeningocele diagnosed antenatally. N Engl J Med 324:662-666, 1991.

14. Rintoul N, Sutton L, Hubbard A, et al: A new look at myelomeningoceles: Functional level, vertebral level, shunting, and the implications for fetal intervention. Pediatrics 109:409-413, 2002.

15. Danish SF, Samdani AF, Storm PB, et al: Use of allogeneic skin graft for the closure of large meningomyeloceles: Technical case report. Neurosurgery 58(4 Suppl 2):ONS-E376; discussion ONS-E376, 2006.

16. Mowatt DJ, Thomson DN, Dunaway DJ: Tissue expansion for the delayed closure of large myelomeningoceles. J Neurosurg 103(6 Suppl):544-548, 2005.

17. Arnell K: Primary and secondary tissue expansion gives high quality skin and subcutaneous coverage in children with a large myelomeningocele and kyphosis. Acta Neurochir (Wien) 148:293-297; discussion 297, 2006.

18. Murakami M, Hyakusoku H, Ogawa R: The multilobed propeller flap method. Plast Reconstr Surg 116:599-604, 2005.

19. Meuli M, Meuli-Simmen C, Yingling C, et al: In utero surgery rescues neurological function at birth in sheep with spina bifida. Nat Med 1:342-347, 1995.

20. Julia V, Sancho MA, Albert A, et al: Prenatal covering of the spinal cord decreases neurologic sequelae in a myelomeningocele model. J Pediatr Surg 41:1125-1129, 2006.

21. Osaka K, Tanimura T, Hirayama A, et al: Myelomeningocele before birth. J Neurosurg 49:711-724, 1978.

22. Adzick N, Sutton L, Crombleholme T, et al: Successful fetal surgery for spina bifida. Lancet 352:1675-1676, 1998.

23. Tulipan N, Bruner J: Myelomeningocele repair in utero: A report of three cases. Pediatr Neurosurg 28:177-180, 1998.

24. Sutton L, Adzick N, Bilaniuk L, et al: Improvement in hindbrain herniation demonstrated by serial fetal magnetic resonance imaging following fetal surgery for myelomeningocele. JAMA 282:1826-1831, 1999.

25. Bruner J, Tulipan N, Paschall R, et al: Fetal surgery for myelomeningocele and the incidence of shunt-dependent hydrocephalus. JAMA 282:1819-1825, 1999.

26. Tulipan N, Sutton L, Bruner J, et al: The effect of intrauterine myelomeningocele repair on the incidence of shunt-dependent hydrocephalus. Pediatr Neurosurg 38:27-33, 2003.

27. Johnson MP, Gerdes M, Rintoul N, et al: Maternal-fetal surgery for myelomeningocele: Neurodevelopmental outcomes at 2 years of age. Am J Obstet Gynecol 194:1145-1150; discussion 1150-1152, 2006.

28. Sutton L, Sun P, Adzick N: Fetal neurosurgery. Neurosurgery 48:124-142, 2001.

29. Fichter MA, Dornseifer U, Henke J, et al: Fetal spina bifida repair—current trends and prospects of intrauterine neurosurgery. Fetal Diagn Ther 23:271-286, 2008.

30. Tubbs R, Chambers M, Smyth M, et al: Late gestational intrauterine myelomeningocele repair does not improve lower extremity function. Pediatr Neurosurg 38:128-132, 2003.

31. Johnson M, Sutton L, Rintoul N, et al: Fetal myelomeningocele repair: Short term clinical outcomes. Am J Obstet Gynecol 189:482-487, 2003.

32. Mazzola C, Albright A, Sutton L, et al: Dermoid inclusion cysts and early spinal cord tethering after fetal surgery for myelomeningocele. N Engl J Med 347:256-259, 2002.

33. Holzbeierlein J, Pope JI, Adams MC, et al: The urodynamic profile of myelodysplasia in childhood with spinal closure during gestation. J Urol 164:1336-1339, 2000.

34. Holmes NM, Nguyen HT, Harrison MR, et al: Fetal intervention for myelomeningocele: Effect on postnatal bladder function. J Urol 166:2383-2386, 2001.

35. Ellsworth P, Mergueria P, Klein R, et al: Evaluation and risk factors of latex allergy in spina bifida patients: Is it preventable. J Urol 150:691-693, 1993.

36. Talamonti G, D'Aliberti G, Collice M: Myelomeningocele: Long-term neurosurgical treatment and follow-up in 202 patients. J Neurosurg 107(5 Suppl):368-386, 2007.

37. Phuong L, Schoeberl K, Raffel C: Natural history of tethered cord in patients with meningomyelocele. Neurosurgery 50:989-993; discussion 993-995, 2002.

38. Danzer E, Adzick NS, Rintoul NE, et al: Intradural inclusion cysts following in utero closure of myelomeningocele: Clinical implications and follow-up findings. J Neurosurg Pediatr 2:406-413, 2008.

39. Reigel D: Tethered spinal cord. Concepts Pediatr Neurosurg 4:142-150, 1983.

40. George TM, Fagan LH: Adult tethered cord syndrome in patients with postrepair myelomeningocele: An evidence-based outcome study. J Neurosurg 102(2 Suppl):150-156, 2005.

41. Hall P, Campbell R, Kalsbeck J: Meningomyelocele and progressive hydromyelia: Progressive paresis in myelodysplasia. J Neurosurg 43:457-463, 1975.

42. Oldfield E, Murasko K, Shawker T, et al: Pathophysiology of syringomyelia associated with Chiari I malformation of the cerebellar tonsils: Implications for diagnosis and treatment. J Neurosurg 80:3-15, 1994.

43. Dias MS: Neurosurgical causes of scoliosis in patients with myelomeningocele: An evidence-based literature review. J Neurosurg 103(1 Suppl):24-35, 2005.

44. Gardner W, Bell H, Poolos P, et al: Terminal ventriculostomy for syringomyelia. J Neurosurg 46:609-617, 1977.

45. Park T, Cail W, Maggio W, et al: Progressive spasticity and scoliosis in children with myelomeningocele: Radiologic investigation and surgical treatment. J Neurosurg 62:367-375, 1985.

46. Bell W, Charney E, Bruce D, et al: Symptomatic Arnold-Chiari malformation: Review of experience with 22 cases. J Neurosurg 66:812-816, 1987.

47. Tubbs R, Elton S, Grabb P, et al: Analysis of the posterior fossa in children with the Chiari 0 malformation. Neurosurgery 48:1050-1054, 2001.

48. Pollack I, Pang D, Albright A, et al: Outcome following hindbrain decompression of symptomatic Chiari malformations in children previously treated with myelomeningocele closure and shunts. J Neurosurg 77:881-888, 1992.

49. Danish SF, Samdani A, Hanna A, et al: Experience with acellular human dura and bovine collagen matrix for duraplasty after posterior fossa decompression for Chiari malformations. J Neurosurg 104(1 Suppl):16-20, 2006.

50. Mataro M, Poca M, Sahuquillo J, et al: Cognitive changes after cerebrospinal fluid shunting in young adults with spina bifida and assumed arrested hydrocephalus. J Neurol Neurosurg Psychiatry 68:615-621, 2000.

51. Bol KA, Collins JS, Kirby RS: Survival of infants with neural tube defects in the presence of folic acid fortification. Pediatrics 117:803-813, 2006.

52. Hunt G: Open spina bifida: Outcome for a complete cohort treated unselectively and followed into adulthood. Dev Med Child Neurol 32:108-188, 1990.

53. Bowman R, McLone D, Grant J, et al: Spina bifida outcome: A 25 year prospective. Pediatr Neurosurg 34:114-120, 2001.

54. Hunt GM, Oakeshott P: Outcome in people with open spina bifida at age 35: Prospective community based cohort study. BMJ 326:1365-1366, 2003.

55. Oakeshott P, Hunt GM, Whitaker RH, et al: Perineal sensation: An important predictor of long-term outcome in open spina bifida. Arch Dis Child 92:67-70, 2007.

56. Lewis D, Tolosa J, Kaufmann M, et al: Elective cesarean delivery and long-term motor function or ambulation status in infants with meningomyelocele. Obstet Gynecol 103:469-473, 2004.

57. Oakeshott P, Hunt GM: Long-term outcome in open spina bifida. Br J Gen Pract 53:632-636, 2003.

58. Mapstone T, Rekate H, Nulsen F, et al: The mean IQ of infants who were not shunted was 104, of those shunted without complications it was 91, and of those shunted who had complications it was 70. Childs Brain 11:112-118, 1984.

59. Sutton L, Charney E, Bruce D: Myelomeningocele—the question of selection. Clin Neurosurg 33:371-382, 1986.

60. McLone D, Czyzewski D, Raimondi A, et al: Central nervous system infection as a limiting factor in the intelligence of children with myelomeningocele. Pediatrics 70:338-342, 1982.

61. Stone A: Neurourologic evaluation and urologic management of spinal dysraphism. Neurosurg Clin N Am 6:269-277, 1995.

62. Ko AL, Song K, Ellenbogen RG, et al: Retrospective review of multilevel spinal fusion combined with spinal cord transection for treatment of kyphoscoliosis in pediatric myelomeningocele patients. Spine 32:2493-2501, 2007.

63. James C, Lassman L: Spinal dysraphism: Spinal cord lesions associated with spina bifida occulta. Physiotherapy 48:154-157, 1962.

64. Till K: A study of congenital malformations of the lower back. J Bone Joint Surg 51:415-422, 1969.

65. Yamada S, Iacono R, Andrade T, et al: Pathophysiology of tethered cord syndrome. Neurosurg Clin N Am 6:311-324, 1995.

66. Steinbok P, Cochrane D: The nature of congenital posterior cervical or cervicothoracic midline cutaneous mass lesions. J Neurosurg 75:206-212, 1991.

67. Pang D: Split cord malformation: Part II. Clinical syndrome. Neurosurgery 31:481-500, 1992.

68. Gibson P, Britton J, Hall D, et al: Lumbosacral skin markers and identification of occult spinal dysraphism in neonates. Acta Paediatr 84:208-209, 1995.

69. Pang D, Wilberger J: Tethered cord syndrome in adults. J Neurosurg 57:32-47, 1982.

70. Sharrard W: The mechanism of paralytic deformity in spina bifida. Cerebr Palsy Bull 4:310, 1962.

71. Keating M, Rink R, Bauer S, et al: Neurourological implications of the changing approach in management of occult spinal lesions. J Urol 140:1299-1301, 1988.

72. Morimoto K, Takemoto O, Wakayama A: Tethered cord associated with anorectal malformation. Pediatr Neurosurg 38:79-82, 2003.

73. Golonka N, Haga L, Keating R, et al: Routine MRI evaluation of low imperforate anus reveals unexpected high incidence of tethered spinal cord. J Pediatr Surg 37:966-969, 2002.

74. Bulsara K, Zomorodi A, Enterline D, et al: The value of magnetic resonance imaging in the evaluation of fatty filum terminale. Neurosurgery 54:375-379, 2004.

75. Kukreja K, Manzano G, Ragheb J, et al: Differentiation between pediatric spinal arachnoid and epidermoid-dermoid cysts: Is diffusion-weighted MRI useful? Pediatr Radiol 37:556-560, 2007.

76. Vernet O, O'Gorman A, Farmer J, et al: Use of the prone position in the MRI evaluation of spinal cord retethering. Pediatr Neurosurg 25:286-294, 1996.

77. Witkamp T, Vandertop W, Beek F, et al: Medullary cone movement in subjects with a normal spinal cord and in patients with a tethered cord. Radiology 220:208-212, 2001.

78. Lam W, Ai V, Wong V, et al: Ultrasound measurement of lumbosacral spine in children. Pediatr Neurol 30:115-121, 2004.

79. Warder D, Oakes W: Tethered cord syndrome and the conus in a normal position. Neurosurgery 33:374-378, 1993.

80. Kanev P, Bierbrauer K: Reflections on the natural history of lipomyelomeningocele. J Neurosurg 22:137-140, 1995.

81. Chapman P: Congenital intraspinal lipomas: Anatomic considerations and surgical treatment. Childs Brain 9:37-47, 1982.

82. Pang D, Zovickian J, Oviedo A: Long term outcome of total and near total resection of spinal cord lipomas and radical recon-

struction of the neural placode: Part I. Surgical technique. Neurosurgery 65:511-528, 2009.

83. Appignani B, Jaramillo D, Barmes P, et al: Dysraphic myelodysplasias associated with urogenital and anorectal anomalies: Prevalence and types seen with MR imaging. AJR Am J Roentgenol 163:1199-1203, 1994.

84. Tubbs RS, Bui CJ, Rice WC, et al: Critical analysis of the Chiari malformation Type I found in children with lipomyelomeningocele. J Neurosurg 106(3 Suppl):196-200, 2007.

85. Waldau B, Grant G, Fuchs H: Development of an acquired Chiari malformation Type I in the setting of an untreated lipomyelomeningocele: Case report. J Neurosurg Pediatr 1:164-166, 2008.

86. Tubbs RS, Loukas M, Shoja MM, et al: Observations at the craniocervical junction with simultaneous caudal traction of the spinal cord. Childs Nerv Syst 23:367-369, 2007.

87. Brophy J, Sutton L, Zimmerman R, et al: Magnetic resonance imaging of lipomyelomeningocele and tethered cord. Neurosurgery 25:336-340, 1989.

88. Friedrich W, Shurtleff D, Shaffer J: Cognitive abilities and lipomyelomeningocele. Psychol Rep 73:467-470, 1993.

89. Seeds J, Powers S: Early prenatal diagnosis of familial lipoelomeningocele. Obstet Gynecol 72:469-471, 1988.

90. Sebold CD, Melvin EC, Siegel D, et al: Recurrence risks for neural tube defects in siblings of patients with lipomyelomeningocele. Genet Med 7:64-67, 2005.

91. Carter B, Stewart J: Valproic acid prenatal exposure: Association with lipomyelomeningocele. Clin Pediatr 28:81-85, 1989.

92. Endoh M, Iwasaki Y, Koyanagi I, et al: Spontaneous shrinkage of lumbosacral lipoma in conjunction with a general decrease in body fat: Case report. Neurosurgery 43:150-151, 1998.

93. Macejko AM, Cheng EY, Yerkes EB, et al: Clinical urological outcomes following primary tethered cord release in children younger than 3 years. J Urol 178(4 Pt 2):1738-1742; discussion 1742-1743, 2007.

94. Herman J, McLone D, Storrs B, et al: Analysis of 153 patients with myelomeningocele or spinal lipoma reoperated upon for a tethered cord. Pediatr Neurosurg 19:243-249, 1993.

95. Kulkarni A, Pierre-Kahn A, Zerah M. Conservative management of asymptomatic spinal lipomas of the conus. Neurosurgery 54:868-875, 2004.

96. Wu H, Kogan B, Baskin L, et al: Long-term benefits of early neurosurgery for lipomyelomeningocele. J Urol 160:511-514, 1998.

97. Xenos C, Sgouros S, Walsh R, et al: Spinal lipomas in children. Pediatr Neurosurg 32:295-307, 2000.

98. Kang J, Lee K, Jeun S, et al: Role of surgery for maintaining urological function and prevention of retethering in the treatment of lipomeningomyelocele: Experience recorded in 75 lipomeningomyelocele patients. Child Nerv Syst 19:23-29, 2003.

99. Huttmann S, Krauss J, Collmann H, et al: Surgical management of tethered spinal cord in adults: Report of 54 cases. J Neurosurg 95(Suppl):173-178, 2001.

100. Pang D, Zovickian J, Oviedo A: Long term outcome of total and near total resection of spinal cord lipomas and radical reconstruction of the neural placode: Part II: Outcome analysis and preoperative profiling. Neurosurgery 66:253-272, 2010.

101. Aliredjo R, de Vries J, Menovsky T, et al: The use of Gore-Tex membrane for adhesion prevention in tethered spinal cord surgery: Technical case reports. Neurosurgery 44:674-677, 1999.

102. Hoffman H, Taecholarn C, Hendrick E, et al: Lipomyelomeningoceles and their management. Concepts Pediatr Neurosurg 5:107-117, 1985.

103. Cochrane DD, Finley C, Kestle J, et al: The patterns of late deterioration in patients with transitional lipomyelomeningocele. Eur J Pediatr Surg 10(Suppl 1):13-17, 2000.

104. Cochrane DD: Cord untethering for lipomyelomeningocele: Expectation after surgery. Neurosurg Focus 23:1-7, 2007.

105. Anderson R: Occult spinal dysraphism: A series of 73 cases. Pediatrics 55:826-834, 1975.

106. Iskandar B, Oakes W, McLaughlin C, et al: Terminal syringohydromyelia and occult spinal dysraphism. J Neurosurg 81:513-519, 1994.

107. Chapman P, Frim D: Symptomatic syringomyelia following surgery to treat retethering of lipomyelomeningoceles. J Neurosurg 82:752-755, 1995.

108. Colak A, Pollack I, Albright A: Recurrent tethering: A common long-term problem after lipomyelomeningocele repair. Pediatr Neurosurg 29:184-190, 1998.

109. McCullough D, Levy L, DiChiro G, et al: Toward the prediction of neurological injury from tethered spinal cord: Investigation of cord motion with magnetic resonance. Pediatr Neurosurg 16:3-7, 1990-1991.

110. Quinn T, Adzick N: Fetal surgery. Obstet Gynecol Clin North Am 24:143-157, 1997.

111. Valenzano M, Paoletti R, Rossi A, et al: Sirenomelia: Pathological features, antenatal ultrasonographic clues, and a review of current embryogenic theories. Hum Reprod Update 5:82-86, 1999.

112. Pang D: Sacral agenesis and caudal spinal cord malformations. Neurosurgery 32:755-778, 1993.

113. Estin D, Cohen A: Caudal agenesis and associated caudal spinal cord malformations. Neurosurg Clin N Am 6:377-391, 1995.

114. O'Neill O, Piatt J, Pitchell P, et al: Agenesis and dysgenesis of the sacrum: Neurosurgical implications. Pediatr Neurosurg 22:20-28, 1995.

115. Banta J, Nichols O: Sacral agenesis. J Bone Joint Surg Am 51:693-703, 1969.

116. Schrander-Stumpel C, Schrander J, Fryns J, et al: Caudal deficiency sequence in 7q terminal deletion. Am J Med Genet 30:757-761, 1988.

117. Rojansky N, Fasouliotis S, Ariel I, et al: Extreme caudal agenesis: Possible drug-related etiology? J Reprod Med 47:241-245, 2002.

118. Levitt M, Patel M, Rodriguez G, et al: The tethered spinal cord in patients with anorectal malformation. J Pediatr Surg 32:462-468, 1997.

119. Tubbs R, Smyth M, Oakes W: Chiari malformation and caudal regression syndrome: A previously unreported association. Clin Dysmorphol 12:147-148, 2003.

120. Midrio P, Silberstein H, Bilaniuk L, et al: Prenatal diagnosis of terminal myelocystocele in the fetal surgery era: Case report. Neurosurgery 50:1152-1155, 2002.

121. Pang D, Dias M, Ahab-Barmada M: Split cord malformation: Part I: A unified theory of embryogenesis for double cord malformations. Neurosurgery 31:451-480, 1992.

122. Dias M, Pang D: Split cord malformations. Neurosurg Clin N Am 6:339-358, 1995.

123. Ersahin Y, Mutluer S, Kocaman S, et al: Split cord malformations in children. J Neurosurg 88:57-65, 1998.

124. Winter R, Haven J, Moe JH, et al: Diastematomyelia and congenital spinal deformities. J Bone Joint Surg Am 56:27-39, 1974.

125. Keim H: Diastematomyelia and scoliosis. J Bone Joint Surg Am 55:1425-1435, 1973.

126. Hilal S, Marton K, Pollack E: Diastematomyelia in children: Radiographic study of 34 cases. Neuroradiology 112:609-621, 1974.

127. Bremer J: Developmental posterior enteric remnants and spinal malformations: The split notocord syndrome. Arch Dis Child 35:76-86, 1960.

128. Dias M, Walker J: The embryogenesis of complex dysraphic malformations: A disorder of gastrulation? Pediatr Neurosurg 18:229-253, 1992.

129. Mahapatra AK, Gupta DK: Split cord malformations: A clinical study of 254 patients and a proposal for a new clinical-imaging classification. J Neurosurg 103(6 Suppl):531-536, 2005.

130. Eid K, Hochberg J, Saunders D: Skin abnormalities of the back in diastematomyelia. Plast Reconstr Surg 63:534-539, 1979.

131. Akay K, Izci Y, Baysefer A, et al: Split cord malformation in adults. Neurosurg Rev 27:99-105, 2004.

132. Tubbs RS, Oakes WJ, Heimburger RF: The relationship of the spinal cord to scoliosis. J Neurosurg 101(2 Suppl):228-233, 2004.

133. English W, Maltby G: Diastematomyelia in adults. J Neurosurg 27:260-264, 1967.

134. Davis E: Diastematomyelia with early Arnold-Chiari syndrome and congenital dysplastic hip. Clin Orthop 52:179-185, 1967.

135. Shorey W: Diastematomyelia associated with dorsal kyphosis producing paraplegia. J Neurosurg 12:300-305, 1955.

136. Hamby W: Pilonidal cyst, spina bifida occulta and bifid spinal cord: Report of a case with review of the literature. Arch Pathol 21:831-838, 1963.

137. Sonigo-Cohen P, Schmit P, Zerah M, et al: Prenatal diagnosis of diastematomyelia. Child Nerv Syst 19:555-560, 2003.

138. David K, Copp A, Stevens J, et al: Split cervical spinal cord with Klippel-Feil syndrome: Seven cases. Brain 119:1859-1872, 1996.

139. Uzum N, Dursun A, Baykaner K, et al: Split-cord malformation and tethered cord associated with immature teratoma. Child Nerv Syst 21:77-80, 2005.

140. Samdani AF, Asghar J, Pahys J, et al: Concurrent spinal cord untethering and scoliosis correction: Case report. Spine 32:E832-E836, 2007.

141. James C, Lassman L: Diastematomyelia: A critical survey of 24 cases submitted to laminectomy. Arch Dis Child 39:125-130, 1964.

142. Matson D, Woods R, Campbell J, et al: Diastematomyelia (congenital clefts of the spinal cord): Diagnosis and surgical treatment. Pediatrics 6:98-112, 1950.

143. Meacham W: Surgical treatment of diastematomyelia. J Neurosurg 27:78-85, 1967.

144. Pang D, Casey K: Use of an anal sphincter pressure monitor during operations on the sacral spinal cord and nerve roots. Neurosurgery 13:562-568, 1983.

145. Pang D, Parrish R: Regrowth of diastematomyelic bone spur after extradural resection. J Neurosurg 59:887-890, 1983.

146. Bryant T: Case of deficiency of the anterior part of the sacrum with a thecal sac in the pelvis, similar to the tumour of spina bifida. Lancet 1:358, 1837.

147. Currarino G, Coln D, Votteler T: Triad of anorectal, sacral and presacral anomalies. AJR Am J Roentgenol 137:395-398, 1981.

148. Bentley JF, Smith JR: Developmental posterior enteric remnants and spinal malformations: The split notochord syndrome. Arch Dis Child 35:76-86, 1960.

149. Chatkupt S, Speer M, Ding Y, et al: Linkage analysis of a candidate locus (HLA) in autosomal dominant sacral defect with anterior meningocele. Am J Med Genet 52:1-4, 1994.

150. Gegg C, Vollmer D, Tullous M, et al: An unusual case of complete Currarino triad: Case report, discussion of the literature and embryogenic implications. Neurosurgery 44:658-662, 1999.

151. Wang J, Spitz L, Hayward R, et al: Sacral dysgenesis associated with terminal deletion of chromosome 7q: A report of two families. Eur J Pediatr 158:902-905, 1999.

152. Amacher A, Drake C, McLaughlin A: Anterior sacral meningocele. Surg Gynecol Obstet 126:986-994, 1968.

153. Oren M, Lorber B, Lee S, et al: Anterior sacral meningocele: Report of 5 cases and review of the literature. Dis Colon Rectum 20:492-505, 1977.

154. Haga Y, Cho H, Shinoda S, et al: Recurrent meningitis associated with complete Currarino triad in an adult—case report. Neurol Med Chir (Tokyo) 43:505-508, 2003.

155. Quigley M, Schinco F, Brown J: Anterior sacral meningocele with an unusual presentation. J Neurosurg 61:790-792, 1984.

156. Vogel EH: Anterior sacral meningocele as a gynecologic problem: Report of a case. Obstet Gynecol 36:766-768, 1970.

157. Vliegen RF, Beets-Tan RG, van Heurn LW, et al: High resolution MRI of anorectal malformation in the newborn: Case reports of Currarino syndrome and anocutaneous fistula. Abdom Imaging 27:344-346, 2002.

158. Ashley WW Jr, Wright NM: Resection of a giant anterior sacral meningocele via an anterior approach: Case report and review of literature. Surg Neurol 66:89-93; discussion 93, 2006.

159. Lee SC, Chun YS, Jung SE, et al: Currarino triad: Anorectal malformation, sacral bony abnormality, and presacral mass—a review of 11 cases. J Pediatr Surg 32:58-61, 1997.

160. Samuel M, Hosie G, Holmes K: Currarino triad—diagnostic dilemma and a combined surgical approach. J Pediatr Surg 35:1790-1794, 2000.

161. Smith HP, Davis CH Jr: Anterior sacral meningocele: Two case reports and discussion of surgical approach. Neurosurgery 7:61-67, 1980.

162. Sanchez AA, Iglesias CD, Lopez CD, et al: Rectothecal fistula secondary to an anterior sacral meningocele. J Neurosurg Spine 8:487-489, 2008.

163. Haworth JC, Zachary RB: Congenital dermal sinuses in children: Their relation to pilonidal sinuses. Lancet 269:10-14, 1955.

164. Humphreys R: Clinical evaluation of cutaneous lesions of the back: Spinal signatures that do not go away. In Loftus C (ed): Clinical Neurosurgery, vol 43. Baltimore, Williams & Wilkins, 1995, pp 175-187.

165. Martinez-Lage JF, Masegosa J, Sola J, et al: Epidermoid cyst occurring within a lumbosacral myelomeningocele: Case report. J Neurosurg 59:1095-1097, 1983.

166. Ackerman LL, Menezes AH: Spinal congenital dermal sinuses: A 30-year experience. Pediatrics 112(3 Pt 1):641-647, 2003.

167. Ackerman LL, Menezes AH, Follett KA: Cervical and thoracic dermal sinus tracts: A case series and review of the literature. Pediatr Neurosurg 37:137-147, 2002.

168. Lin K, Wang H, Chou M, et al: Sonography for detection of spinal dermal sinus tracts. J Ultrasound Med 21:903-907, 2002.

169. Barkovich AJ, Edwards M, Cogen PH: MR evaluation of spinal dermal sinus tracts in children. AJNR Am J Neuroradiol 12:123-129, 1991.

170. van Aalst J, Beuls EA, Cornips EM, et al: Anatomy and surgery of the infected dermal sinus of the lower spine. Childs Nerv Syst 22:1307-1315, 2006.

171. Fitz CR, Harwood Nash DC: The tethered conus. Am J Roentgenol Radium Ther Nucl Med 125:515-523, 1975.

172. Love JG, Daly DD, Harris LE: Tight filum terminale: Report of condition in three siblings. JAMA 176:31-33, 1961.

173. Wraige E, Borzyskowski M: Investigation of daytime wetting: When is spinal cord imaging indicated? Arch Dis Child 87:151-155, 2002.

174. Pippi Salle JL, Capolicchio G, Houle AM, et al: Magnetic resonance imaging in children with voiding dysfunction: Is it indicated? J Urol 160(3 Pt 2):1080-1083, 1998.

175. Barson AJ: The vertebral level of termination of the spinal cord during normal and abnormal development. J Anat 106(Pt 3):489-497, 1970.

176. Selcuki M, Vatansever S, Inan S, et al: Is a filum terminale with a normal appearance really normal? Childs Nerv Syst 19:3-10, 2003.

177. Selden NR: Minimal tethered cord syndrome: What's necessary to justify a new surgical indication? Neurosurg Focus 23:1-5, 2007.

178. Uchino A, Mori T, Ohno M: Thickened fatty filum terminale: MR imaging. Neuroradiology 33:331-333, 1991.

179. Jamil M, Bannister CM: A report of children with spinal dysraphism managed conservatively. Eur J Pediatr Surg 2(Suppl 1):26-28, 1992.

180. Sade B, Beni-Adani L, Ben-Sira L, et al: Progression of terminal syrinx in occult spina bifida after untethering. Childs Nerv Syst 19:106-108, 2003.

181. Erkan K, Unal F, Kiris T: Terminal syringomyelia in association with the tethered cord syndrome. Neurosurgery 45:1351-1359; discussion 1359-1360, 1999.

182. van Leeuwen R, Notermans NC, Vandertop WP: Surgery in adults with tethered cord syndrome: Outcome study with independent clinical review. J Neurosurg 94(2 Suppl):205-209, 2001.

183. Souweidane MM, Drake JM: Retethering of sectioned fibrolipomatous filum terminales: Report of two cases. Neurosurgery 42:1390-1393, 1998.

184. Lea ME, Sage MR, Bills D, et al: Enterogenous cyst of the cervical spinal canal. Australas Radiol 36:327-329, 1992.

185. Puca A, Cioni B, Colosimo C, et al: Spinal neurenteric cyst in association with syringomyelia: Case report. Surg Neurol 37:202-207, 1992.

186. Whiting DM, Chou SM, Lanzieri CF, et al: Cervical neurenteric cyst associated with Klippel-Feil syndrome: A case report and review of the literature. Clin Neuropathol 10:285-290, 1991.

187. Agnoli AL, Laun A, Schonmayr R: Enterogenous intraspinal cysts. J Neurosurg 61:834-840, 1984.

188. Bremer JL: Dorsal intestinal fistula; accessory neurenteric canal; diastematomyelia. AMA Arch Pathol 54:132-138, 1952.

189. Schmidbauer M, Reinprecht A, Schuster H, et al: Atypical vertebral artery in a patient with an intra- and extraspinal cervical neurenteric cyst. Acta Neurochir (Wien) 109(3-4):150-153, 1991.

190. Devkota UP, Lam JM, Ng H, et al: An anterior intradural neurenteric cyst of the cervical spine: Complete excision through central corpectomy approach—case report. Neurosurgery 35:1150-1153; discussion 1153-1154, 1994.

191. Macdonald RL, Schwartz ML, Lewis AJ: Neurenteric cyst located dorsal to the cervical spine: Case report. Neurosurgery 28:583-587; discussion 587-588, 1991.

192. Levin P, Antin SP: Intraspinal neurenteric cyst in the cervical area. Neurology 14:727-730, 1964.

193. Kumar R, Jain R, Rao KM, et al: Intraspinal neurenteric cysts—report of three paediatric cases. Childs Nerv Syst 17:584-588, 2001.

194. Agrawal D, Suri A, Mahapatra AK, et al: Intramedullary neurenteric cyst presenting as infantile paraplegia: A case and review. Pediatr Neurosurg 37:93-96, 2002.

195. Hes R: Neurenteric cyst or teratomatous cyst. J Neurosurg 80:179-180; author reply 180-181, 1994.

196. Daszkiewicz P, Roszkowski M, Przasnek S, et al: Teratoma or enterogenous cyst? The histopathological and clinical dilemma in co-existing occult neural tube dysraphism. Folia Neuropathol 44:24-33, 2006.

197. Kim CY, Wang KC, Choe G, et al: Neurenteric cyst: Its various presentations. Childs Nerv Syst 15(6-7):333-341, 1999.

198. Rizk T, Lahoud GA, Maarrawi J, et al: Acute paraplegia revealing an intraspinal neurenteric cyst in a child. Childs Nerv Syst 17:754-757, 2001.

199. Takase T, Ishikawa M, Nishi S, et al: A recurrent intradural cervical neurenteric cyst operated on using an anterior approach: A case report. Surg Neurol 59:34-39; discussion 39, 2003.

200. Song JK, Burkey BB, Konrad PE: Lateral approach to a neurenteric cyst of the cervical spine: Case presentation and review of surgical technique. Spine 28:E81-E85, 2003.

201. Fernandes ET, Custer MD, Burton EM, et al: Neurenteric cyst: Surgery and diagnostic imaging. J Pediatr Surg 26:108-110, 1991.

202. Gilchrist BF, Harrison MW, Campbell JR: Neurenteric cyst: Current management. J Pediatr Surg 25:1231-1233, 1990.

203. Superina RA, Ein SH, Humphreys RP: Cystic duplications of the esophagus and neurenteric cysts. J Pediatr Surg 19:527-530, 1984.

204. de Oliveira RS, Cinalli G, Roujeau T, et al: Neurenteric cysts in children: 16 consecutive cases and review of the literature. J Neurosurg 103(6 Suppl):512-523, 2005.

205. Midha R, Gray B, Becker L, et al: Delayed myelopathy after trivial neck injury in a patient with a cervical neurenteric cyst. Can J Neurol Sci 22:168-171, 1995.

206. Silvernail WI Jr, Brown RB: Intramedullary enterogenous cyst: Case report. J Neurosurg 36:235-238, 1972.

207. Neuhauser EB, Harris GB, Berrett A: Roentgenographic features of neurenteric cysts. Am J Roentgenol Radium Ther Nucl Med 79:235-240, 1958.

208. Ellis AM, Taylor TK: Intravertebral spinal neurenteric cysts: A unique radiographic sign—"the hole-in-one vertebra." J Pediatr Orthop 17:766-768, 1997.

209. Garg N, Sampath S, Yasha TC, et al: Is total excision of spinal neurenteric cysts possible? Br J Neurosurg 22:241-251, 2008.

210. Sala F, Krzan MJ, Deletis V: Intraoperative neurophysiological monitoring in pediatric neurosurgery: Why, when, how? Childs Nerv Syst 18(6-7):264-287, 2002.

211. von Koch CS, Quinones-Hinojosa A, Gulati M, et al: Clinical outcome in children undergoing tethered cord release utilizing intraoperative neurophysiological monitoring. Pediatr Neurosurg 37:81-86, 2002.

212. Schwartz D, Wierzbowski L, Fan D, et al: Intraoperative neurophysiological monitoring during spine surgery. In Vaccaro A, Betz R, Zeidman S (eds): Principles and Practices of Spine Surgery. St. Louis, Mosby, 2003, pp 115-126.

213. Schwartz D, Vacarro A: Neurophysiologic monitoring during cervical spine surgery. In Clark C (ed): The Cervical Spine, 4th ed. Philadelphia, Lippincott Williams & Wilkins, 2005, pp 238-244.

214. Hilibrand AS, Schwartz DM, Sethuraman V, et al: Comparison of transcranial electric motor and somatosensory evoked potential monitoring during cervical spine surgery. J Bone Joint Surg Am 86:1248-1253, 2004.

215. Fan D, Schwartz DM, Vaccaro AR, et al: Intraoperative neurophysiologic detection of iatrogenic C5 nerve root injury during laminectomy for cervical compression myelopathy. Spine 27:2499-2502, 2002.

216. Ikeda K, Kubota T, Kashihara K, et al: Anorectal pressure monitoring during surgery on sacral lipomeningocele: Case report. J Neurosurg 64:155-156, 1986.

217. James HE, Mulcahy JJ, Walsh JW, et al: Use of anal sphincter electromyography during operations on the conus medullaris and sacral nerve roots. Neurosurgery 4:521-523, 1979.

218. Krassioukov AV, Sarjeant R, Arkia H, et al: Multimodality intraoperative monitoring during complex lumbosacral procedures: Indications, techniques, and long-term follow-up review of 61 consecutive cases. J Neurosurg Spine 1:243-253, 2004.

219. Khealani B, Husain AM: Neurophysiologic intraoperative monitoring during surgery for tethered cord syndrome. J Clin Neurophysiol 26:76-81, 2009.

Spinal Disorders Associated with Skeletal Dysplasias and Metabolic Diseases

Vernon T. Tolo, MD

Spinal disorders associated with skeletal dysplasias and metabolic diseases may be called orthopaedic trivia by some. None of these conditions are found in a large number of patients, and the numbers of syndromes and subclassifications seem to be almost endless. More than 200 types of short stature syndromes have been described to date, and the mapping of the human genome has led to discovery and clarification of many new metabolic disorders. Despite the relative rarity of these conditions in any spine surgeon's practice, it is important for physicians and surgeons to know enough features of these disorders to allow for their early recognition and diagnosis. Because the natural history of spinal disorders in each of these syndromes is often quite different, it is important initially to establish as accurate a diagnosis as possible, particularly in disorders in which spinal deformity or stenosis may lead to spinal cord compression.[1]

It is often possible to identify and diagnose a skeletal dysplasia at birth by a combination of physical findings, family history, and imaging studies. With many metabolic disorders, the findings at birth may not be easily recognizable, and there often is a delay in diagnosis, which is usually based on serum or urine studies or on biopsy material.

The physical findings most important in identifying the diagnosis relate to body length and to body proportions. If an infant below the 5th percentile for height has average-sized family members, further workup is indicated. If an infant or toddler moves below the 5th percentile in the first few years of life, further evaluation should be done.

Skeletal dysplasias can be divided into two major groups: dysplasias with short limbs and a relatively normal trunk and dysplasias with a short trunk and relatively normal limbs. If an infant has short limbs, it is helpful in establishing possible diagnoses to determine whether the shortening affects the proximal limb (rhizomelia), the forearm or lower leg (mesomelia), or the hand and foot (acromelia). With short limbs, radiographs are very useful to allow distinction between syndromes in which the metaphysis is primarily involved and syndromes in which the epiphysis is primarily involved. If a short trunk dominates the physical findings, it can be assumed that spinal involvement of some type is present. Most often in infants, this short trunk is due to platyspondyly, although

shortness of the trunk at any age may also be related to severe spinal deformity.

Radiographs, particularly the lateral spine radiograph, may often provide specific clues to the correct diagnosis even in a newborn or infant. Additional useful physical findings include facial features, hand and foot abnormalities, and angular deformity of the legs. The physical and imaging findings combined with a consultation with a geneticist should allow for earlier recognition of the correct syndrome or metabolic disorder so that the appropriate spinal problems can be more closely observed, and the family can benefit from early genetic counseling regarding having additional children.

Skeletal Dysplasias

Achondroplasia

Achondroplasia is the most common skeletal dysplasia requiring treatment of spinal disorders. The genetic defect in fibroblast growth factor receptor 3 function is located at chromosome 4p16.3. Hypochondroplasia has a similar genetic defect with lesser expression, and individuals with hypochondroplasia are taller than individuals with achondroplasia. Achondroplasia is recognizable at birth to allow an early diagnosis in nearly all cases. Short limbs with humeral and femoral shortening (rhizomelia) are present together with the characteristic facial features of frontal bossing and nasal bridge depression. Head size is often large compared with other body segments, and hydrocephalus may be present, although most infants with achondroplasia do not require ventriculoperitoneal shunting. The diagnosis can be confirmed by an anteroposterior spinal radiograph, which even at birth shows narrowing of the interpediculate distances in the lumbar spine.

At birth, an infant with achondroplasia has hypotonia in the trunk and in the extremities, and parents should be advised to expect a modest delay in the infant's developmental milestones. Generally, children sit by about 6 months of age and walk at about 12 months of age, but children with achondroplasia usually sit independently between 9 and 12 months of age and walk by about 18 to 24 months of age.

The cause of hypotonia remains unclear regarding whether it is constitutional or the result of a partial neurologic deficit. There was speculation that foramen magnum stenosis might be the cause of the hypotonia, but this has been shown not to be the case.[2] Some hypotonia may result from spinal cord compression at the foramen magnum because there is a relative increased frequency of sleep apnea in infants with achondroplasia, sometimes leading to sudden death.[3] Sleep apnea monitors are often used for the first several months in many of these infants, and if sleep apnea is clinically significant, evaluation of potential spinal cord compression at the foramen magnum is needed.[4,5] This evaluation includes not only careful recording of sleep monitor findings, but also sleep laboratory studies for apnea and oxygen saturation levels and computed tomography (CT) and magnetic resonance imaging (MRI) of the brainstem and upper cervical spine.

Somatosensory evoked potential (SSEP) monitoring has been shown to be helpful in establishing the diagnosis of cervical myelopathy in these patients.[6] If SSEP testing is done, subcortical recording of SSEPs from stimulation of the median nerve is more sensitive and specific in diagnosing high cervical myelopathy than stimulation of the posterior tibial nerve.[7]

There are three major contributing causes that may lead to sleep apnea or respiratory problems in achondroplasia: foramen magnum stenosis, midface hypoplasia, and small chest size. Chest circumference in achondroplasia is generally below the 3rd percentile, but this measurement is the same in infants with or without apneic problems. Midface hypoplasia may lead to snoring and upper airway respiratory compromise and has been implicated as the major reason for repeated otitis media in these children. The most common cause of apnea in infants with achondroplasia is upper cervical spinal cord compression at the foramen magnum, where imaging studies have repeatedly shown a significant decrease in cross-sectional area of the foramen. Although the sagittal plane dimension of the foramen magnum is relatively normal, the loss of area for the spinal cord from the severe side-to-side foramen magnum narrowing, with consequent spinal cord compression, seems to be the underlying cause of apnea in many of these infants.

Previous studies have divided this foramen magnum area compression into two major types—the first involving cervical cord compromise from direct impingement of the posterior rim of the foramen magnum and the second caused by the posterior foramen magnum rim invaginating into the ring of the atlas. In these studies, it is stressed that the neural compression is of the high cervical spinal cord, not of the brainstem itself.[8] Autopsy studies have noted histologic changes in the upper cervical spinal cord similar to changes seen in the central cord syndrome, and some authors believe that if one avoids placing the head of a young child with achondroplasia in hyperextension, the risk of spinal compression is lessened.[9] Persistent foramen magnum compression may play a role in the later finding of a syrinx in the cervical spinal cord.[10]

Some degree of foramen magnum stenosis is present in essentially all children with achondroplasia. By using CT to measure the size of the foramen magnum, it has been shown that 96% have a foramen magnum size smaller than 3 standard deviations below the mean.[8] How and whom to treat remains unclear, however. One study of 32 children with achondroplasia showed 28% with a history of sleep apnea and 22% with abnormal sleep study results, both of which improved in the 6 children who had foramen magnum decompression.[6] Foramen magnum decompression has been reported to be performed more safely and successfully when combined with external ventricular drainage to manage the abnormal cerebrospinal fluid dynamics in this compressive condition.[11] Diverse symptoms and signs such as ataxia, incontinence, and respiratory problems have been reported to be successfully treated by foramen magnum decompression and atlas laminectomy in patients ranging in age from 7 months to 30 years.[12] Some authors recommend that prophylactic cervicomedullary decompression be done, even in asymptomatic children, if T2-weighted MRI signal changes in the spinal cord are present.[13]

Although successful foramen magnum decompression has been reported in infants,[14] other authors maintain that if appropriate sleep apnea monitoring is continued until the child is 2 or 3 years old, there is a natural relative increase in the foramen magnum size with growth, relieving enough of the spinal cord compression to avoid the need for surgical treatment.[15] Reported mortality and morbidity rates from foramen magnum decompression are thought by these authors to be greater than if no treatment except sleep monitoring is done. It is rarely necessary to perform foramen magnum decompression in older children or in adults. If a child has required cervicomedullary decompression, there seems to be an increased risk for symptomatic thoracolumbar stenosis requiring laminectomies before adolescence.[16]

In the cervical spine below the foramen magnum in achondroplasia, the principal spinal disorder is diffuse spinal stenosis. Although a small spinal canal is present from birth, signs or symptoms of neural compression in the lower cervical spine are usually not noted until middle age or later.[17] At those ages, neural compression results from osteophytes that develop with time from degenerative disc changes. The cumulative effect of previous small cervical spine dimensions and osteophyte compression leads to neurologic deficits that require treatment. If pain or sensory changes in the upper extremities are the only findings, conservative care with a cervical orthosis and anti-inflammatory medications is used initially.

If a motor deficit in the upper or lower extremities is present and pain is unrelieved by nonoperative treatment, laminectomy at multiple levels is needed.[18,19] MRI defines the levels of compression, which are usually multiple. As a result, when laminectomy of the cervical spine is needed in achondroplasia, often most of the cervical spine below the axis needs to have the laminae removed to relieve the neural compression. In addition, these patients may need laminectomies in the thoracic and lumbar spine, and some patients with achondroplasia require laminectomy decompression from the skull to the sacrum.[20] Foraminotomies are needed at levels shown on MRI to have neural foraminal stenosis from adjacent osteophytes. After multilevel laminectomy, cervical spine fusion is generally not needed in adults, but in the rare instance that cervical laminectomy in a child with achondroplasia should become needed, there is an increased chance of postlaminectomy kyphosis, and careful follow-up evaluation is needed. Although atlantoaxial instability is commonly seen in some other skeletal dysplasias, this instability is rarely seen in achondroplasia.[21,22]

Of all the spinal segments, the middle and upper thoracic spine is the least involved in spinal deformity or cord compression in achondroplasia. The most common spinal deformities and stenosis, with subsequent neurologic problems, occur in the thoracolumbar and lumbar spine. Thoracolumbar kyphosis is usually present at birth to some degree but is more noticeable when the infant begins to sit (Fig. 32–1A). As sitting begins, the entire spine appears kyphotic, at least partly owing to the generalized hypotonia present at this age. Although some authors have advocated limiting infants to a reclined, rather than a fully upright, sitting position to avoid the development of thoracolumbar kyphosis,[23] this does not seem to be necessary in clinical practice. In more than 90% of children with achondroplasia, thoracolumbar kyphosis improves without treatment as the standing position is assumed and lumbar lordosis develops. Because walking typically is achieved by 18 to 24 months of age, this is the time that the resolution of the thoracolumbar kyphosis begins, followed by the gradual continual improvement over the subsequent 2 to 3 years.

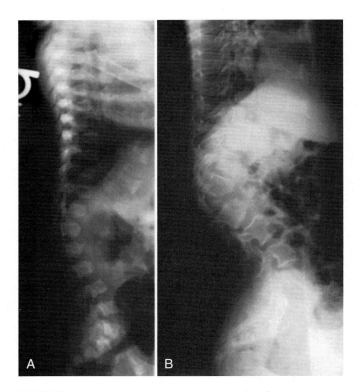

FIGURE 32–1 A, Lateral spinal radiograph at 6 months of age shows early thoracolumbar kyphosis. Most of these deformities resolve by 2 or 3 years of age. If the apical vertebra remains wedged by age 5 or 6 years, surgery is recommended. **B,** Lateral radiograph (same child as **A**) of spine at age 10 years shows persistent wedging of L1 at thoracolumbar junction, which requires anterior and posterior spinal fusion.

A lateral spinal radiograph shows initial relative anterior wedging of the thoracolumbar vertebrae, but this generally resolves as standing and walking occur, with the radiograph showing a gradual filling in of the anterior aspects of the vertebral bodies at the thoracolumbar apex. In the author's experience, bracing to correct this kyphosis has limited value, and the use of a thoracolumbosacral orthosis (TLSO) is poorly tolerated by many children with achondroplasia, partly owing to the difficulty they have with TLSO wear in reaching their feet owing to their short extremities. An orthosis that uses a soft front while supporting the kyphosis has been reported to be successful,[24-27] although proper patient selection for bracing remains problematic. The use of stretching exercises for the hip flexion contractures (always present in this condition), as a means to decrease lumbar lordosis and control the thoracolumbar kyphosis, has been advocated, but documentation of the effectiveness of this passive stretching program is difficult, particularly when most thoracolumbar kyphoses resolve with no treatment.[28]

In a few young patients with achondroplasia, thoracolumbar kyphosis does not improve and becomes progressively worse with time. If there is significant wedging of one or more of the thoracolumbar vertebrae at 5 or 6 years of age, surgical treatment is needed to allow partial correction and prevent continued progression of the deformity (Fig. 32–1B).[29] This approach is based on review of early childhood x-rays of teenagers later requiring treatment for severe thoracolumbar kyphosis and neurologic deficits. It is generally possible by age 5 or 6 years to determine whether or not the thoracolumbar wedging would improve without treatment or progress to a more severe deformity. Using this approach at this earlier age, the kyphotic deformity generally can be corrected better and more safely, leading to the prevention of localized increased kyphosis and early spinal cord compression.

As thoracolumbar kyphosis increases, so does the compensatory lumbar lordosis. Because the lumbar spine capacity decreases as lumbar lordosis increases, control of the thoracolumbar kyphosis seems to delay the onset of lumbar spinal stenosis symptoms. Whether this early kyphosis fusion will eventually lead to less of a need for decompressive lumbar laminectomy has not been determined. Circumferential fusion of the kyphosis thoracolumbar area in children younger than 2 years has been reported to lead to hypoplastic vertebral bodies and iatrogenic spinal stenosis, apparently as a result of inhibition of circumferential vertebral growth after the fusion.[30] In an average-sized individual, it has been shown, however, that the spinal canal achieves its adult dimensions by age 6 years, so circumferential fusion after this age should not lead to iatrogenic stenosis.

In young children with persistent thoracolumbar kyphosis at age 6, the author's favored surgical technique involves a combined anterior and posterior spinal fusion on the same operative day.[29] The child is positioned with a beanbag and tape in a lateral decubitus position with the table tilted about 20 degrees, to allow for simultaneous exposures for the anterior and posterior spinal surgery. Through a thoracoretroperitoneal approach, anterior discectomies are done at three or four levels at the apex of the kyphotic deformity. Because the surgical approach at this level commonly involves an approach through the rib bed of either the 10th or the 11th rib, the portion of the rib removed is saved for an anterior strut graft.

The operating table is then tilted about 20 degrees the other direction to allow exposure of the posterior spine. Through the posterior incision, facetectomies are completed through the levels to be fused, and pedicle screws are placed at the end vertebrae. Because this surgery is usually done on children with no neurologic signs or symptoms, laminectomy is not needed. (If laminectomies are done, there is little bone contact space remaining at the thoracolumbar levels for fusion to occur.) Dual rods are contoured to allow for about 50% correction of the kyphosis and are inserted into the pedicle screws.

Motor evoked potentials and SSEPs must be carefully obtained during and after this correction phase. If there is a change in evoked potentials, the rods are removed. When the evoked potentials have returned to baseline, replacement of the rods, with greater kyphosis bent into these, is done. The final correction is that at which the evoked potentials have remained at baseline and safe correction has been obtained. Decortication of the laminae and transverse processes is done, and bone graft is placed. The table is tilted to its original position, and the rib strut graft is inserted into a channel cut in the apical vertebral bodies to allow the graft to sit into these vertebral bodies as it is anchored in the end vertebrae. Local bone graft is used to graft further the space left by the discectomies. Both wounds are closed in the usual fashion. If the anterior surgery is done first and the strut graft is applied, there is a possibility that this strut graft will displace when the posterior instrumentation and correction occurs. For this reason, the author prefers the simultaneous combined anterior and posterior approaches in the above-described manner.

In the author's surgical series of more than 25 patients with achondroplasia with kyphotic deformity requiring surgical treatment, more than half have temporarily lost SSEPs at the time of the initial correction of the kyphosis. None of these patients have had permanent neurologic deficit postoperatively. If the SSEPs are lost, however, the rod must be removed and bent into more kyphosis before reinsertion of the rods. Postoperatively, a TLSO brace may be used for about 3 months during the day to allow for some protection for the instrumentation and fusion, but the child remains ambulatory at all times. After 3 months postoperatively, sports activity restrictions are stopped, and full activity is resumed (Fig. 32–2). In another series of 12 immature patients with achondroplasia treated with pedicle screw posterior instrumentation and fusion, no loss of evoked potentials was noted, and overall mean kyphosis correction was 50%.[31] The exact cause of this neurologic compromise is unclear but may be related to buckling of the ligamentum flavum with kyphosis correction, leading to further spinal canal compromise.

An alternative approach has been reported to treat persistent thoracolumbar kyphosis in which spinal instrumentation is placed in the anterior spine rather than in the posterior spine.[32] An anterior strut bone graft is placed, and posterior fusion, without instrumentation, is done. This posterior fusion is repeated about 4 months after the initial surgery. A body jacket cast is used for 6 months, and a brace is used for another 3 months. Using this approach in four patients, Ain and Shirley[32] obtained solid fusion, kyphosis correction of 23% to 31%, and no worsening of neurologic function.

Although clinically the principal thoracic and lumbar problem in preadolescent children with achondroplasia is persistent thoracolumbar kyphosis, neurologic compromise from spinal stenosis is the most common spinal disorder in teenagers and adults. Lutter and Langer[33] separated these neurologic manifestations into four types: I, progressive, insidious onset; II, intermittent claudication; III, nerve root compression; and IV, acute onset of paraplegia. Types I and II are the most common. In type I, there is a slow but progressive onset of back pain, associated with lower extremity paresthesias and sensory loss.

Urologic function is often impaired, subclinically at first but later leading to incontinence.[34] If urologic problems are suspected in the initial stages, voiding cystourethrogram can help to diagnose urinary control problems. If voiding cystourethrogram is abnormal, MRI of the thoracic and lumbar spine is indicated. If significant spinal stenosis is present, laminectomy decompression is needed to reverse the urologic problems. In one series of 22 pediatric patients with achondroplasia with symptoms and signs of spinal claudication and requiring laminectomy surgery, 77% had bladder incontinence. These patients requiring laminectomy at this young age had narrower lumbar interpediculate distances and greater thoracolumbar kyphosis than young patients with achondroplasia not requiring laminectomy.[35]

In achondroplasia with type II with neurologic manifestations, there is also a slow, progressive onset of symptoms, with the patient first noting a decreased ability to walk distances. Pain and weakness in the legs result when standing and walking occur, and these symptoms are relieved by the patient squatting, sitting, leaning forward, or lying down. These all are spinal positional changes that flex the lumbar spine to allow more room for the cauda equina and relieve the spinal claudication symptoms. It has been shown in a stillborn infant with achondroplasia that the capacity or space within the lumbar spine is nearly doubled by fully flexing the lumbar spine when compared with the extended or lordotic position.[28]

In this setting, the initial office neurologic examination of the lower extremities may be normal, even if significant spinal stenosis is present. The normal findings may be partly due to the fact that the patient has been sitting in the waiting room with a flexed lumbar spine for a time and has relieved the signs and symptoms of spinal stenosis that are present when standing. It is often helpful to have the patient walk up and down the hall for a few minutes until the symptoms of spinal claudication return, at which time the lower extremity neurologic examination is repeated, often finding weakness, particularly involving the muscles that dorsiflex the ankle. If these physical findings are present and the history suggests spinal claudication, MRI of the thoracic *and* lumbar spine is needed to evaluate the need for surgical treatment with decompressive laminectomy.

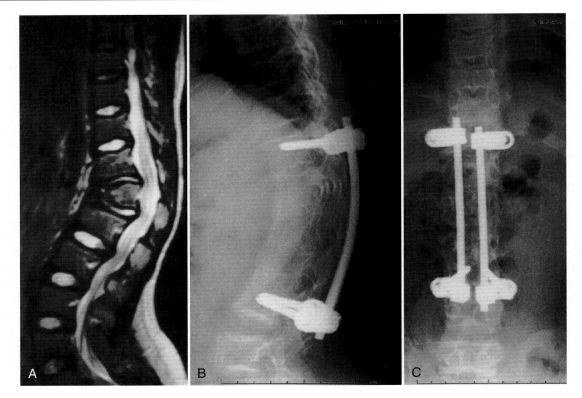

FIGURE 32–2 A 9-year-old boy with achondroplasia had persistent thoracolumbar kyphosis. **A,** MRI showed kyphosis and failure of anterior vertebral body to form. **B** and **C,** Radiographs 2 years after anterior discectomy with strut graft and posterior instrumentation and fusion. Neurologic status remains normal.

Patients with type III neurologic manifestations have more obvious unilateral radicular signs and symptoms to allow an appropriate diagnosis. A positive straight-leg raising test is present in most cases in the lower extremities. Lumbar spine MRI usually allows for identification of the specific point of femoral or sciatic nerve root compression. Acute paraplegia, or type IV manifestation, is uncommon and probably occurs most often after significant trauma. In most instances, before the trauma, there have been signs or symptoms of one of the other types, most often type I or II.

For any of these types, if neurologic deficits are suspected from the history or shown on physical examination, MRI is indicated to localize the site of abnormality. The problem most common in the interpretation of MRI is to determine which level is causing the neurologic signs or symptoms because there is diffuse stenosis usually present in the lower thoracic spine and the entire lumbar spine. Imaging studies show that the primary stenosis is from the narrowing of the interpediculate distances because the anteroposterior dimension of the spinal canal is relatively more normal until osteophytes from disc degeneration protrude into the spinal canal.[36,37] Occasionally, CT myelography may be used to evaluate for levels of spinal stenosis, but if this is done, the myelographic dye should be placed via cisternal puncture in the upper cervical spine and not by lumbar puncture because lumbar puncture, with loss of cerebrospinal fluid, may lead to increased neurologic deficits in achondroplasia.[38]

The selection of the surgical procedures best suited to the individual patient with achondroplasia depends on the physical examination and the imaging findings. In a patient with type III neurologic manifestations, a limited laminectomy, disc excision, and foraminotomy generally suffice to relieve the symptoms. More commonly, in the other types of neurologic manifestations, multilevel decompressive laminectomy is the surgical treatment of choice.[39,40] Laminoplasty was reported to be successful for complete relief of symptoms in 71% of 35 patients with achondroplasia and lumbar stenosis, but the use of this procedure has not been widespread.[41] Even if multilevel laminectomy is done in these patients, fusion may not be needed unless there is a preexisting thoracolumbar kyphosis of about 30 degrees or more. If there is preexisting kyphosis at this level, pedicle screw fixation with dual-rod instrumentation is used with no instrumentation, no matter how small, within the spinal canal at the thoracic levels without laminectomy, although posterior pedicle screws can be used with laminectomy.

In situations with marked thoracolumbar kyphosis and multilevel stenosis on MRI, it is often difficult to determine the exact level of neurologic compromise. Generally, if depressed knee and ankle deep tendon reflexes and leg weakness are present, lumbar laminectomy seems to suffice for treatment. If there is MRI evidence of significant anterior spinal cord compression at the apex of a thoracolumbar kyphosis, and hyperreflexia is present together with leg weakness and sensory changes, anterior partial vertebrectomy or posterior pedicle subtraction osteotomy to decompress the anterior spinal cord at the apex of the kyphosis may be needed, in addition to multilevel lumbar and lower thoracic laminectomies. A report of four patients with achondroplasia and marked kyphosis who had decompression through a pedicle subtraction osteotomy noted that there was a mean kyphosis correction of 44%, but that, despite final improvement in neurologic status, transient postoperative weakness was noted in two of the four patients.[42]

In achondroplastic patients without coincident kyphosis but with neurologic deficits secondary to the diffuse stenosis, multilevel laminectomy is the treatment of choice (Fig. 32–3).[39,40] Before surgery, it is essential to view the entire thoracic and lumbar spine on MRI to assess for *all* levels of stenosis that may be causing lower extremity weakness. It is important to decompress all levels that appear to have neural compression on MRI, and most often the levels for laminectomy extend from around T10 to S1. If only a single-level or double-level laminectomy is done at what appear to be the most involved areas, recurrence of new symptoms within months of the decompressive surgery is common as new levels of compression develop adjacent to the initial sites of decompression.

Because of the severe spinal stenosis present in achondroplasia, with the absence of epidural fat and concurrent loss of most of the subarachnoid space seen at the time of surgery, special precautions and surgical techniques are needed to complete these laminectomies more safely.[34] The use of rongeurs within the spinal canal during laminectomy should be limited, owing to the severe stenosis. A postoperative increase in neurologic deficits is common, even if extreme care is taken during the laminectomy procedure. The use of a high-speed

bur to transect the lamina on each side just medial to the facet or at the facet level is recommended. After the laminae have been transected, the posterior elements are lifted dorsally with a clamp, with the intent to avoid placing instruments within the stenotic spinal canal, which may injure the neural elements.

Foraminotomies can be done as needed after the laminae are removed, but MRI studies showed that although the foramina in achondroplasia lumbar spines were smaller than in control groups, the percentage of foraminal space occupied by the nerve root was similar between the two groups. The conclusion was that spinal stenosis symptoms arose from the central canal stenosis, not from foraminal stenosis. It would seem that foraminotomies in these patients are usually not needed.[43] Unless there is increased kyphosis in the area of laminectomies, the author has noted that fusion may not be needed, even if laminectomies include removal of the facets. It has been reported more recently, however, that 10 skeletally immature patients with achondroplasia required spinal instrumentation and posterior fusion after laminectomies across the thoracolumbar region.[44]

After extensive laminectomy surgery, as described earlier, there may be areas of thinned dura that later form pseudomeningoceles and lead to later neurologic deterioration or pain or both. Using the paraspinal muscles to obliterate the dead space left by removal of the bony laminae seems to be helpful in decreasing the formation of these postlaminectomy pseudomeningoceles.[34] Ain and colleagues[45] reported that 61% of 98 achondroplasia patients undergoing laminectomy

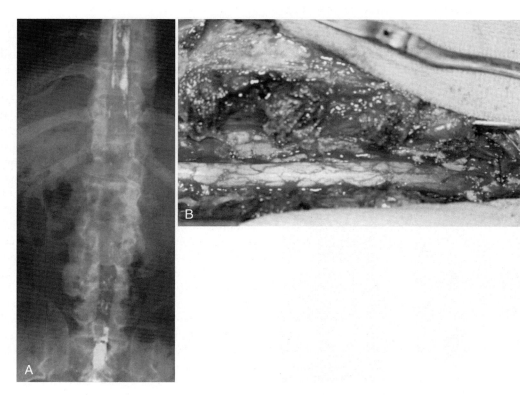

FIGURE 32–3 A and **B,** Radiograph (**A**) and photograph (**B**) of multiple-level laminectomy generally needed for spinal stenosis in achondroplasia. If multiple levels are not included, recurrence of symptoms a few months after limited decompression is common.

surgery had at least one perioperative complication, including 37% with dural tears, 23% with neurologic complications, 9% with infection, and 1 death.

Signs and symptoms of recurrent spinal stenosis may occur years after initial decompressive laminectomies. The most common cause of recurrent stenosis seems to be facet hypertrophy and disc disease, although scar tissue may form over the decompressed dural sac as well. MRI studies with gadolinium enhancement often help to visualize the scar tissue present and where the cauda equina compression has recurred. In one series of eight patients with restenosis, repeat decompression helped improve motor function in some, but three of these patients had significant complications.[46]

In patients with significant thoracolumbar kyphosis and lumbar spine stenosis, both of these conditions can be a possible cause of the underlying neurologic deficit.[47] In this setting, MRI of the entire spine is used to ascertain all levels of compression. To treat lumbar spinal stenosis and anterior spinal cord compression at the apex of the kyphosis, anterior decompression and fusion at the apex of the kyphosis, together with a posterior multilevel laminectomy and instrumented fusion, is needed.[29,47] Anterior decompression and fusion may be done through an anterior approach by vertebrectomy and strut bone graft fusion at the apex of the deformity or by an approach through the pedicles for anterior decompression with cage and bone graft stabilization. After posterior decompression at multiple levels is completed, pedicle screw and rod instrumentation is inserted, and bone graft is placed to complete the fusion. The pedicle anatomy of the thoracic and lumbar spine has been shown by CT to be markedly different from that of the normal spine. In addition to other findings

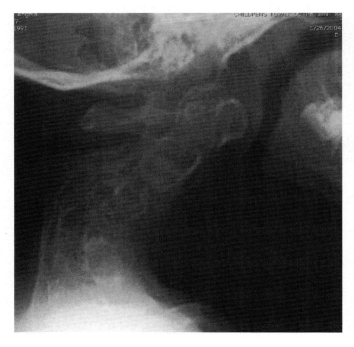

FIGURE 32–4 Lateral cervical spine radiograph of an 8-year-old girl with diastrophic dysplasia 2 years after two-level vertebrectomy with anterior strut graft and posterior fusion for 90-degree kyphosis.

reported, all pedicles are directed cranially, the pedicle starting points diverge from T9 to L5, and the maximal screw path length is at L2.[48,49] Instead of stainless steel implants, titanium spinal implants are used to obtain better images at MRI if there is a subsequent need to evaluate the spinal cord further.

Diastrophic Dysplasia

Diastrophic dysplasia has several typical features that allow this diagnosis to be made at birth. Although in most countries the incidence is about 1 per 1 million, Finland has a much higher number of patients with this disorder and has been the source of much of the current literature on the natural history of patients with diastrophic dysplasia. There is a genetic defect in diastrophic dysplasia sulfate transportase, and the chromosomal location for this defect is at 5q31-q34.

Characteristic diagnostic features include micromelia with markedly short stature; "hitchhiker's thumb"; stiff proximal interphalangeal joints of the fingers; severe equinovarus foot deformity; and, within a few weeks of birth, the formation of external ear cysts, which lead to scarring and the classic "cauliflower ear" appearance.[50] Intelligence is normal. A cleft palate is present in about 25% of these children.

The spine has several areas of involvement in diastrophic dysplasia. All patients have spina bifida of the cervical spine, although symptoms directly related to this anatomic feature do not seem to occur.[51,52] Upper cervical abnormalities seen in some of the other skeletal dysplasias, such as foramen magnum stenosis and atlantoaxial instability, are not present in diastrophic dysplasia.[53] The primary cervical spine abnormality in this condition is mid-cervical kyphosis,[54,55] although a review of 122 patients from Finland found only a 4% incidence of cervical kyphosis.[56] At a young age, many patients with diastrophic dysplasia have mild cervical kyphosis, but most of these cases resolve with time and growth, by an average of 7 years of age.[51,57]

Why cervical kyphosis worsens in a few patients and not in most patients is unclear, but the presence of the bifid cervical spinous processes may play a role. In children in whom kyphosis does not resolve by itself, significant wedging of the apical vertebrae can occur. If progressive kyphosis is noted, cervical fusion is indicated to prevent severe deformity. If cervical kyphosis becomes severe, spinal cord compression occurs, and death may result from this cervical spinal cord compression. At autopsy, neuropathologic examination has shown neurolytic changes in the anterior columns of the spinal cord as a result of anterior cord compression, so treatment of progressive kyphosis at an earlier stage is preferable. In these children, with stiffness of all joints a feature of the condition, it is often difficult to elucidate clearly neurologic functional changes, and liberal use of radiography and MRI is necessary to allow for early detection and ongoing evaluation of cervical kyphosis, together with possible spinal cord compression.

In patients with progressive cervical kyphosis, anterior and posterior fusion is recommended for optimal stabilization (Fig. 32-4). A halo brace is used to allow partial correction and postoperative immobilization until the fusion is solid. The kyphotic neck is usually relatively stiff, and aggressive attempts to correct the kyphosis are more likely to lead to iatrogenic neurologic injury. Laminectomy does not have a role here. If there is spinal cord compression that requires treatment, anterior decompression with vertebrectomies at the apex is the surgical approach of choice.

Kyphoscoliosis is the primary spinal disorder in the thoracic spine. In one study, 40% of children with diastrophic dysplasia developed mild to moderate scoliosis.[58] In these patients, this deformity is not large enough to require treatment except for periodic follow-up, although occasionally a brace is used for a time. About 30% of patients with this condition develop a severe, rigid, progressive thoracic scoliosis associated with a sharply angular mid-thoracic kyphosis. In a more recent study from Finland, of 86 patients with diastrophic dysplasia and scoliosis, 11 cases were severe, 41 cases were "idiopathic-like," and 33 cases were mild and nonprogressive.[59]

In a review of 43 patients with diastrophic dysplasia,[60] if significant kyphoscoliosis was to develop, the onset of the spinal deformity was before age 4 years. In another review of 88 patients, 70 had scoliosis measuring an average of 42 degrees (range 11 to 188 degrees).[61] Lung function generally has been shown to be relatively normal in diastrophic dysplasia, but pulmonary function declines with increasing thoracic kyphoscoliosis.[62]

Imaging studies, such as tomography or three-dimensional CT reconstructions of the spine, often show a wedge-shaped vertebra at the apex of the thoracic kyphoscoliosis, similar to what one would see with a congenital hemivertebra.[60] Although orthotic treatment can be attempted early if there is flexibility proven on lateral bending radiographs, most of these early-onset deformities are very stiff. The treatment goal is to prevent progressive deformity rather than to wait and treat a severe deformity, an approach that is analogous in many ways to the treatment approach used for congenital scoliosis or kyphosis.

Submuscular spinal instrumentation without fusion to allow continued growth can be used in some cases, if there is a large curve in a young child (Fig. 32–5), but significant flexibility of the spine must be shown before this type of instrumentation treatment. If there is no real correction on lateral bending radiographs, anterior and posterior spinal fusion and posterior spinal instrumentation with modest correction is recommended at the stage at which progression has been proven greater than 50 degrees. Spinal growth in diastrophic dysplasia seems to be complete by about age 8 years, so definitive spinal fusion can be done in this condition at an earlier age than with most childhood spinal deformities with less fear of inhibiting later trunk growth.

Some of the most severe cases of kyphoscoliosis the author has seen have been in patients with diastrophic dysplasia (Fig. 32–6). These deformities may be severe enough to cause swallowing difficulties owing to the aberrant path taken by the esophagus. Despite the severity of these deformities, neurologic signs and symptoms related to spinal cord compression in the thoracic and lumbar regions are very rare, in contrast to what is expected from severe kyphotic deformities in general. In patients with diastrophic dysplasia, if neurologic defects or paraplegia is present in conjunction with severe thoracic kyphoscoliosis, the cause is usually iatrogenic, secondary to surgical attempts to instrument and correct the spinal deformity aggressively. There is minimal flexibility in these severe curves, so motor evoked potential and SSEP monitoring is required intraoperatively when spinal instrumentation and fusion is performed to detect early any neurologic changes from overstretching of the spinal cord in the face of a rigid spine. The vertebrae and the spinal canal in this condition are of sufficient size to accept appropriately sized pedicle screws, hooks, and wires or cables as part of spinal instrumentation. A goal in treating patients with scoliosis and diastrophic dysplasia is, however, to detect this deformity early, monitor this closely, and fuse the spinal deformity area before it progresses to a severe degree. Anterior and posterior fusion at an early age for progressive curves seems to be the best approach in treatment to prevent the severe deformity seen in the past in some adults with this condition.[63]

Most patients with diastrophic dysplasia also have a marked lumbosacral lordosis. The sacrum itself also develops a lordotic position with growth. This lordosis is exaggerated further by posterior vertebral body wedging that occurs in L5. In addition, owing to hip flexion contractures that are always present, lumbar lordosis is increased even more when the patient is standing. This standing hip and spine position is also partially compensatory for knee flexion contractures, which are common in these patients. In a study of walking difficulties in patients with diastrophic dysplasia, the walking difficulties were only rarely related to low lumbar spinal stenosis, however.[64] In some patients with diastrophic dysplasia, interpediculate narrowing in the L5 and S1 vertebrae is seen on radiographs and MRI, but decompressive laminectomy is rarely required.[60,61] There is no interpediculate narrowing in the upper lumbar spine.

Spondyloepiphyseal Dysplasia

There are two forms of spondyloepiphyseal dysplasia—the congenita and the tarda types—and they are very distinct from one another.

Spondyloepiphyseal Dysplasia Tarda

Spondyloepiphyseal dysplasia tarda affects only males and is inherited as an X-linked recessive condition. This condition is caused by mutations in the *SEDL* gene in chromosomal location Xp22.2-p22.1.[65] At birth, normal body proportions seem to be present, and the diagnosis is commonly not established until late childhood or early adolescence. The trunk is short but not dramatically so; radiographs show platyspondyly,[66] a characteristic hump-shaped buildup of bone in the central and posterior aspects of the vertebral body, and a delay in ossification of the vertebral ring apophysis. Scoliosis and kyphosis are uncommon; although low back pain may result from a combination of disc degenerative disease and increased lumbar lordosis, the spine is not the most important feature of this condition. Multiple disc herniations have been reported.[67]

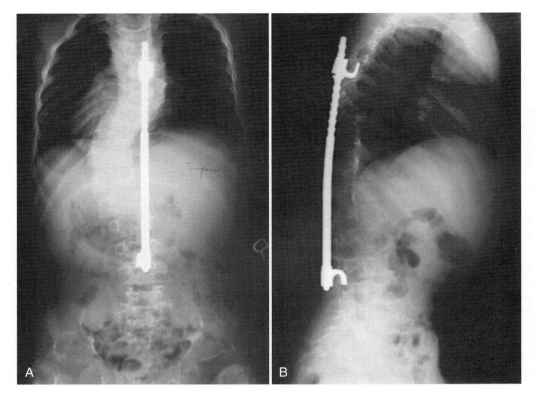

FIGURE 32–5 A, Anteroposterior spinal radiograph of a 5-year-old boy with diastrophic dysplasia. Scoliosis was corrected from 70 degrees to 40 degrees by this submuscular rod without fusion. Although braces must still be worn, these rods are useful in this condition in which young children frequently have severe progressive scoliosis. Definitive instrumentation and fusion can usually be accomplished by age 9 or 10 years. **B,** Radiograph shows progressive kyphosis that often occurs above distraction instrumentation without fusion, if multiple lengthenings are necessary.

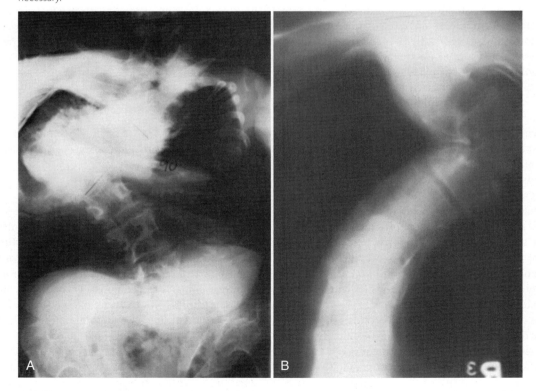

FIGURE 32–6 A, Anteroposterior spinal radiograph of a girl with diastrophic dysplasia; in this condition, some of the most severe cases of scoliosis and kyphosis seen with skeletal dysplasias are present. **B,** Tomogram of thoracic spine in a child with diastrophic dysplasia. This tomogram shows a finding common in this condition when severe scoliosis is present at a young age. The resemblance to congenital kyphoscoliosis may help explain why progression may be so rapid and eventual curve magnitude so severe.

The most common reason that patients with spondyloepiphyseal dysplasia present to an orthopaedist is for treatment of hip pain and stiffness (Fig. 32–7).[65] Premature hip osteoarthritis is a feature of this condition, often starting in the preadolescent years and progressing with age. Increased lumbar lordosis may be exaggerated by hip flexion contractures from hip arthritis. Total hip arthroplasty is commonly needed in early adult life. If this condition is suspected in a child, a family history of the need for hip replacement in early adult life may help make the diagnosis of spondyloepiphyseal dysplasia tarda.

Spondyloepiphyseal Dysplasia Congenita

From the spine point of view, spondyloepiphyseal dysplasia congenita is of much more concern than spondyloepiphyseal dysplasia tarda. Inherited as an autosomal dominant condition, spondyloepiphyseal dysplasia congenita has a defect in type II collagen, on the α_1 chain. The chromosomal location of this defect is 12q13.11-q13.2. Other related skeletal dysplasias with type II collagen abnormalities include Kniest syndrome, Stickler syndrome, and Strudwick spondylometaepiphyseal dysplasia.

Spondyloepiphyseal dysplasia congenita is recognizable at birth with imaging findings in conjunction with short-trunk dwarfism.[68] There is delayed ossification in the vertebral bodies, and coxa vara is present. Hands and feet are of relatively normal size. As the child ages, there continues to be absent or delayed ossification of the femoral heads and irregularities in the epiphyseal and the metaphyseal areas of the long bones. From the medical standpoint, retinal detachment is common in this condition, and the parents need to be aware of this to arrange periodic eye evaluations.

Atlantoaxial instability is the most commonly seen cervical spine problem in children with spondyloepiphyseal dysplasia congenita, with nearly half of children having this finding.[50,69] In infancy, some hypotonia is present, but this should resolve with age. Failure to attain motor milestones progressively in the lower or upper extremities should direct attention to the cervical spine because atlantoaxial instability is often found early in childhood, sometimes at 1 year of age.

Cervical spine radiographs in a young child may be difficult to interpret. In a normal child, there is increased flexibility and motion on flexion and extension compared with an adult, so this has to be taken into consideration. In addition, in spondyloepiphyseal dysplasia congenita, there is a delay in posterior element ossification, so it is even more difficult to delineate clearly instability with flexion and extension radiographs in the upper cervical spine. Because odontoid hypoplasia is the underlying anatomic abnormality, the abnormal motion may be either excessive flexion motion or excessive extension motion (Fig. 32–8).

Although radiographs are the first step in the evaluation of upper cervical stability, flexion-extension sagittal plane MRI is extremely useful not only to view the anatomic abnormalities, but also to see if there is indentation into the spinal cord or narrowing of the spinal canal in either full flexion or full extension positions. If MRI findings are normal except for

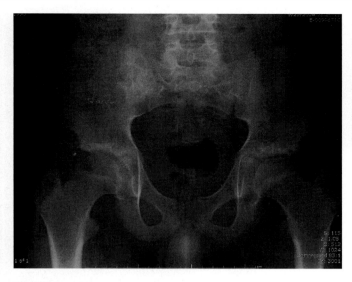

FIGURE 32–7 Anteroposterior radiograph of pelvis shows early abnormalities in hips of a 10-year-old boy with spondyloepiphyseal dysplasia tarda. Note relative flattening of lumbar vertebrae. Hip replacement surgery in early adult life is common in this condition.

odontoid hypoplasia and there is 5 mm or less of motion on flexion and extension lateral cervical spine radiographs, ongoing follow-up is indicated periodically throughout childhood. If there is more than 5 mm of motion with neck extension and flexion or if there is indentation or signal change at the cervical spinal cord, posterior upper cervical spinal fusion is indicated. Laminectomy at the upper cervical spine is generally not needed in patients with spondyloepiphyseal dysplasia congenita and has no role as the only treatment for upper cervical cord compression caused by atlantoaxial instability. If the upper cervical spine sagittal canal diameter is narrowed and myelopathy is present, C1 laminectomy may be indicated in addition to occiput-C2 posterior fusion.[70]

Upper cervical fusion may include only C1 and C2 but commonly extends from the occiput to C2 in these young children; partly owing to the lack of ossification of the posterior elements at this level at this age, this fusion usually is needed. It is more difficult to obtain secure wire fixation of the laminae, and if the instability is excessive, C1 extension movement and overreduction can occur with posterior wiring. To stabilize the upper cervical spine, the author prefers to use a halo brace, applied in the operating room as the first step in the fusion surgery. The number of halo pins used increases in younger children to obtain adequate stability, with six to eight pins usually placed for children younger than 5 years. In these young children, torque screwdrivers are used to tighten the pins to 3 or 4 psi rather than the 6 to 7 psi used in older individuals (Fig. 32–9).

Placement in the halo brace in the operating room is done before prone positioning so that turning the patient under anesthesia is safer for the cervical spine. Obtaining evoked potentials in the upper and lower extremities should be considered before placing the child prone and again after the child is positioned for posterior upper cervical surgery. The back of the halo brace is removed, and radiographs of the atlantoaxial

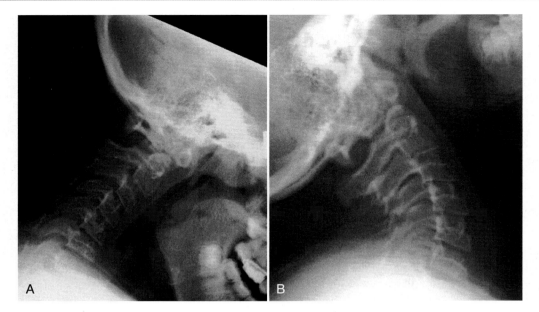

FIGURE 32–8 A 12-year-old girl with spondyloepiphyseal dysplasia congenita has odontoid hypoplasia and 5 mm of motion between C1 and C2 with flexion and extension. In this instance, abnormal motion is mainly in extension, with front of ring of C1 riding over hypoplastic odontoid. MRI in flexion and extension shows no spinal cord signal change and no apparent compression. Periodic monitoring with flexion-extension radiographs and MRI continues.

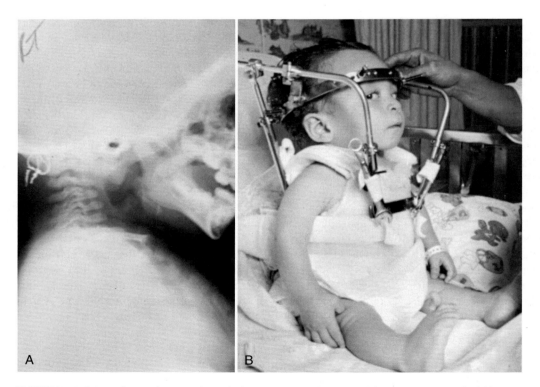

FIGURE 32–9 A, Lateral cervical spine radiograph shows occipitoaxial wiring and fusion in an 18-month-old boy with spondyloepiphyseal dysplasia. Atlantoaxial instability was present on flexion-extension lateral neck radiographs. Flexion MRI showed spinal cord compression. After fusion, motor development of upper and lower extremities improved dramatically. **B,** An 18-month-old boy with spondyloepiphyseal dysplasia had occipitoaxial fusion for atlantoaxial instability. Reduction was obtained preoperatively by this halo brace, which was left on intraoperatively and for 3 months postoperatively. In children of this age, six or eight halo pins are generally necessary for fixation.

area are obtained to confirm that anatomic alignment is present before surgical preparation and draping. The posterior neck and the iliac crest are prepared and draped into the surgical field.

In cervical spine surgery in a young child, care is taken to avoid exposing more of the posterior laminae than is needed because unintended extension of the intended fusion levels can occur just from periosteal stripping of distal laminae. The author prefers to fuse from the occiput to C2, in most cases without any wiring or instrumentation. The occiput is cleared subperiosteally, as are C1 and C2 to just lateral to the facets. A high-speed bur is used to remove the outer layer of cortex on the occiput, and a squared-off "box" is constructed at the base of the occiput for placing the bone graft. A corticocancellous piece of iliac crest bone, long enough to extend from the occiput box to the distal aspect of the C2 lamina and wide enough to cover both sides of the lamina at C1 and C2, is carefully removed from the lateral posterior iliac crest. It is important to ensure this corticocancellous bone graft is long enough to extend from the occiput to C2. Extra strips of cancellous bone graft are also obtained. This bone graft is bent using bone benders and trimmed so that the proximal end fits nicely into the occipital box and the lower end contacts the C1 and C2 laminae on each side.

Decortication of the laminae of C1 and C2 is completed with a high-speed bur, and cancellous bone graft is laid directly on the decorticated laminae. The corticocancellous strips are placed dorsal to the cancellous bone, and a two-layer or three-layer muscle closure is used to hold the corticocancellous bone strips firmly in place. The author has used this technique on many occasions. Employing halo brace immobilization for 3 months, the author has not noted slippage of the graft in children of this age, even without internal fixation. In a series of patients with skeletal dysplasia (including several with spondyloepiphyseal dysplasia congenita) treated for atlantoaxial instability, 92% achieved a solid fusion, and 88% had improvement in neurologic function.[71]

Instability or stenosis is not a problem in the thoracic and lumbar spine in this condition, although some degree of spinal deformity may be seen. Platyspondyly is present throughout but does not seem to cause much of a problem; a mild thoracolumbar kyphosis that does not require treatment may be present. If there is a progressive scoliosis, orthotic treatment with a TLSO is initially tried and often is sufficient treatment. If there is progressive scoliosis, posterior segmental spinal instrumentation and spinal fusion is possible using standard-sized spinal implants because the spine in patients with spondyloepiphyseal dysplasia congenita has a normal spinal canal size. As in all cases of spinal instrumentation for scoliosis, spinal cord monitoring is used intraoperatively.

Pseudoachondroplasia

Pseudoachondroplasia is a short-limbed form of dwarfism that is inherited in an autosomal dominant fashion and has a defect in cartilage oligomeric matrix protein. This defect is located at chromosome 19p13.1. This dysplasia is not usually diagnosed at the time of birth largely because the facial appearance is normal. Although the body proportions are similar to proportions found in achondroplasia, there is a great deal of difference between these two dysplasias.

In pseudoachondroplasia, there is a normal facial appearance; epiphyseal and metaphyseal changes are evident in the long bones on radiographs; and spinal radiographs show flattened vertebral bodies with a central, anterior tonguelike projection and normal interpediculate distances throughout the spine (Fig. 32–10). The primary orthopaedic problems in this dysplasia that require treatment are the angular deformities of the lower extremities requiring corrective osteotomy (often more than once) and premature osteoarthritis of the hips requiring total hip arthroplasty at a relatively early age.

Despite the radiographic appearance of some vertebral flattening, trunk height is relatively normal. Increased lumbar lordosis is common, partly from the spine itself and partly from hip flexion contractures. Proximal femoral extension osteotomies can improve lumbar lordosis if the lordosis remains flexible, but this lordosis becomes more fixed with increasing age. Thoracic kyphosis often initially appears as compensatory to lumbar lordosis, but with time and growth, it may become a fixed and progressive deformity that requires treatment. Orthotic treatment is used initially, but surgery may be needed, particularly if anterior vertebral body wedging is seen on radiographs. This is not the type of kyphosis seen with achondroplasia, in which one or two apical vertebrae are involved, but is caused by multiple levels, each having a lesser amount of wedging. Scoliosis may be seen, but there is nothing characteristic of this in pseudoachondroplasia. If spinal instrumentation and fusion becomes necessary for either kyphosis

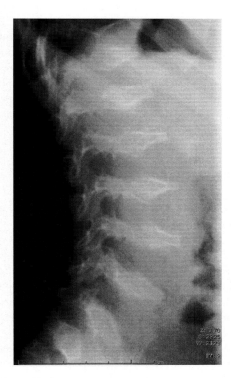

FIGURE 32–10 Lateral radiograph of spine of a 6-year-old boy with pseudoachondroplasia shows characteristic vertebral shape, with anterior mid-vertebral projections, seen in this dysplasia.

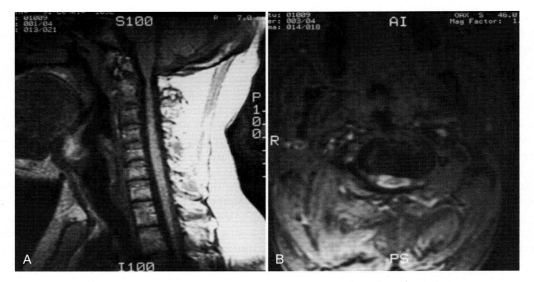

FIGURE 32–11 A and **B,** MRI of cervical spine in a boy with pseudoachondroplasia shows marked narrowing of spinal cord at atlantoaxial level, with flattening of spinal cord seen on transverse cuts. Flexion-extension lateral cervical spine radiographs showed 9 mm of atlantoaxial motion. Posterior atlantoaxial fusion is needed in these cases.

or scoliosis, standard-sized spinal instrumentation can be used. In contrast to achondroplasia, in which no instrumentation should be placed within the spinal canal, patients with pseudoachondroplasia have a normal-sized spinal canal.

Atlantoaxial instability, a condition essentially never seen in achondroplasia, is not unusual in pseudoachondroplasia. This instability may be due partly to the generalized laxity present in all joints in this dysplasia and is not usually a result of odontoid hypoplasia seen in other skeletal dysplasias. Upper cervical instability caused by os odontoideum has been reported in 60% of 15 patients with pseudoachondroplasia, but no surgery was needed in this group.[72] It is recommended that before any orthopaedic procedures that require anesthesia, flexion and extension lateral cervical radiographs should be obtained to evaluate these patients for instability. If atlantoaxial instability is diagnosed, posterior atlantoaxial instrumentation and fusion is needed (Fig. 32–11).

Mucopolysaccharidoses

Several syndromes have been described with abnormal metabolism of mucopolysaccharides. Sanfilippo syndrome (mucopolysaccharidosis [MPS] type III) and Scheie syndrome (MPS type V or type I-S) rarely have spinal manifestations, although Scheie syndrome may have dural thickening that can lead to neurologic deficits.[73] In the remaining types, short-trunk dwarfism is usually seen, and thoracolumbar kyphosis is common. In addition, cervical spine abnormalities are often seen.

MPS is not usually diagnosed at birth but often can be diagnosed in the 1st year of life. Diagnosis is usually made in early childhood, with some syndromes diagnosed earlier than others because some are associated with more dysmorphic changes and with more developmental delay. The specific

diagnosis is established by appropriate serum and urine studies and by culture of either fibroblasts or leukocytes to elucidate the specific MPS syndrome. Molecular studies are also available to classify and type these syndromes further. It is important to establish the exact diagnosis early because the prognosis and natural history of each MPS condition differ widely, varying from expected death in early childhood to survival into late adult life. Similarly, the severity of spinal involvement varies widely from one syndrome to another. Enzyme replacement therapy and bone marrow transplantation therapy have been used in some MPS syndromes, primarily Hurler syndrome, in which survival has been significantly enhanced. The orthopaedic and spinal manifestations still need to be monitored as the child grows.

Significant anesthetic and other perioperative considerations need to be taken into account in this group of patients if surgery of any type is planned.[74,75] At the time of surgery, intubation is often difficult and frequently requires use of fiberoptic intubation techniques. Care must be taken postoperatively to monitor breathing owing to airway compromise. An intensive care unit stay postoperatively is recommended because reintubation, if needed, may be very difficult.[74,76,77]

Hurler Syndrome (Mucopolysaccharidosis Type I)

Although an infant with Hurler syndrome appears normal at birth, short stature becomes apparent early along with delays in motor and mental development. Thoracolumbar kyphosis is present at birth but often is not noted initially, even though anterior beaking of the apical vertebral bodies is seen if radiographs were obtained. By 2 years of age, corneal clouding, coarse facial features with a large tongue and large lips, stiff joints, and hernias are obvious, and further motor and mental deterioration is noted. Many of these physical signs develop in the 1st year of life, and early diagnosis is key to an improved

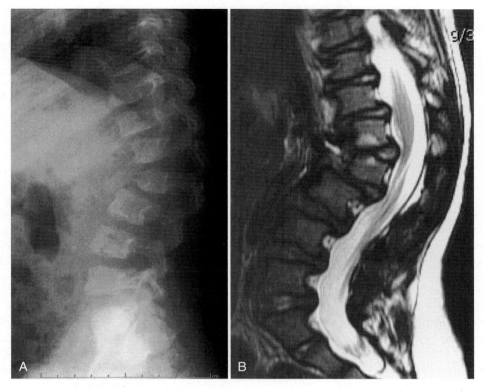

FIGURE 32–12 A and **B,** Lateral spine radiograph (**A**) and MRI (**B**) of a 6-year-old child with Hurler syndrome who has received a bone marrow transplant. Although underlying metabolic condition is treated well with bone marrow transplant, the spine and other orthopaedic problems seen in this condition need to be followed closely as growth progresses.

prognosis. Laboratory studies show excessive dermatan sulfate and heparan sulfate secretion. Atlantoaxial instability may be present.[78,79]

In the past, surgical treatment was not usually indicated for the spine or hip abnormalities seen in Hurler syndrome because death in early childhood was expected. More recently, bone marrow transplantation and enzyme replacement therapy have been used in these patients, however, with significant improvement in quality of life, survival, and life expectancy. Although these therapies can delay or prevent cardiac and neurologic deterioration in Hurler syndrome, numerous orthopaedic manifestations are present that usually require treatment, such as progressive thoracolumbar kyphosis or atlantoaxial instability.[80,81] In one group of 10 patients followed for a mean of 8.7 years after bone marrow transplantation, all showed a decrease, however, in the amount of odontoid dysplasia.[82] In another group of patients with Hurler syndrome who underwent bone marrow transplantation, high lumbar kyphosis was the most common spinal problem seen (Fig. 32–12).[83]

Hunter Syndrome (Mucopolysaccharidosis Type II)

Hunter syndrome is a lysosomal storage disease with a defect in iduronate-2-sulfatase that leads to a buildup of certain glycosaminoglycans and adverse neurologic effects. It is inherited in a X-linked recessive manner, affecting only males, and appearance at birth is normal. These children grow normally for about 2 years, at which time an abnormality is suspected. Life expectancy may extend well into adult life, although death in the 2nd decade of life may occur because of cardiopulmonary problems. Some noncharacteristic vertebral changes are present, but lumbar kyphosis may be marked and require surgical treatment.[84] Evaluation of the upper cervical spine is needed because MRI studies may show anterior spinal cord compression secondary to a thickening of the soft tissue posterior to the odontoid, owing to deposition of the mucopolysaccharide.[85]

Morquio Syndrome (Mucopolysaccharidosis Type IV)

As with the other MPS syndromes, patients with Morquio syndrome appear relatively normal at birth and for the first year or so, at which time parental concern may be raised by a change in physical features and a developmental delay. The thoracolumbar kyphosis characteristic of this condition is present at birth but may not be noted initially. If kyphosis is noted, it may be confused with congenital kyphosis because the child otherwise appears relatively normal. Thoracolumbar kyphosis in Morquio syndrome differs radiographically from congenital kyphosis: The spine in Morquio syndrome has anteroinferior vertebral beaking of the vertebral bodies adjacent to the apical wedged vertebra, whereas congenital kyphosis from a hemivertebra rarely involves more than one level.

As the child becomes older, short stature is more noticeable, together with genu valgum, pectus carinatum, and corneal clouding. Laboratory findings include increased keratan sulfate in the urine and a defect in N-acetyl-hexosamine 6-sulfate sulfatase in fibroblasts. Radiographs of long bones show irregularities in ossification of epiphyses, and hip subluxation is common with growth. Decreased exercise tolerance and decreasing ability to walk longer distances is common with increasing age in childhood and before adolescence. This decreased exercise tolerance may be a result of the hip instability and knee valgus, but evaluation of the cervical and thoracolumbar spine is necessary to rule out spinal cord compression as the cause of progressively decreasing exercise tolerance.

The most common spinal problem requiring treatment is odontoid hypoplasia, which leads to atlantoaxial instability.[55,86-88] Compression at the upper cervical spine is compounded by the frequent presence of an anterior soft tissue mass from the deposition of mucopolysaccharide. Odontoid hypoplasia is present in most children with Morquio syndrome, and evaluation of the cervical spine is needed before orthopaedic surgery for the hips or legs.[89] Instability is most often noted between 6 and 12 years of age. Lateral cervical spine radiographs are obtained in flexion and extension, and if there is more than 5 mm of motion, posterior upper cervical spinal fusion is needed.

In addition to instability, there is extradural soft tissue thickening, which is a contributing cause to the compression here that is often worse than is apparent from the radiographs alone.[90] As with other dysplasias, if the radiographs are unclear regarding what instability may be present, a sagittal view MRI study with the neck in flexion and in extension is useful. When instability is present, posterior cervical fusion has been shown to be beneficial even with long-term follow-up.[71,91] The author prefers occipitoaxial fusion without instrumentation, using iliac crest bone graft for fusion and a halo brace for immobilization for 3 months until fusion is complete (Fig. 32–13). In some children with Morquio syndrome, there may be midcervical or lower cervical spine stenosis or instability below the atlantoaxial level. The more levels of the cervical spine that require decompression and fusion, the harder airway access becomes, owing to a combination of limited neck motion and a progressive pectus carinatum deformity.

Thoracolumbar kyphosis is present at birth, and the degree of kyphotic deformity often does not progress significantly. Most of the time, serial examination and lateral spinal radiographs with the child standing suffice for management. If there is documented kyphosis progression with growth, a TLSO can be used, although in the author's experience this brace is not tolerated well by these children because it is an additional impediment to their limited ability to move about. It may be difficult to differentiate diminished lower extremity function between the lower extremities themselves (hip and knee problems) and thoracolumbar spinal cord and cauda equina compression. MRI of the thoracolumbar kyphosis often shows some degree of intrusion of the protruding discs on the thecal sac, to the extent of causing some spinal cord flattening.

In a young child, use of instrumentation inside the spinal canal has been known to cause neurologic deficits in the lower extremities in some cases (Fig. 32–14). If it is determined that surgery is needed to treat thoracolumbar kyphosis, it may be safer to combine pedicle screw instrumentation and fusion with multilevel laminectomy (Fig. 32–15) or to use anterior spinal instrumentation.[92]

Maroteaux-Lamy Syndrome (Mucopolysaccharidosis Type VI)

Children with Maroteaux-Lamy syndrome appear normal at birth, and short-trunk dwarfism is noted by age 2 or 3 years. Many of the physical features resemble Hurler syndrome, but intelligence is normal. Diagnostic findings include increased urinary excretion of dermatan sulfate and arylsulfatase B deficiency in fibroblasts and white blood cells. This syndrome typically has hip involvement, which on radiographs resembles Legg-Perthes disease. Stenosis at the level of the foramen magnum and upper cervical spine, probably resulting from thickening of the posterior longitudinal ligament, can be improved by laminectomy when neurologic symptoms and signs are present.[93] Thoracolumbar kyphosis is common, and the vertebrae are flattened on spinal radiographs. Laminectomy may be needed if MRI findings correlate with lower extremity loss of function. Spinal fusion should be considered for progressive kyphotic deformity. Spinal cord monitoring is essential, and pedicle screw instrumentation should be attempted because placing implants within the spinal canal has been known to lead to iatrogenic neurologic deficits.

Miscellaneous Syndromes

Kniest Syndrome

The clinical features of Kniest syndrome are closely related to the features found with spondyloepiphyseal dysplasia congenita. Life expectancy and intelligence are normal. Imaging findings outside of the spine include metaphyseal widening of the long bones, coxa vara, delay in epiphyseal ossification, and sometimes angular deformity of the lower extremities.[94,95] These children walk with a marked external foot progression angle because of femoral external rotation. The presence of coronal and sagittal vertebral clefts has been reported in 63% of infants with Kniest syndrome and may be helpful in establishing a diagnosis.[96]

Odontoid hypoplasia with resultant atlantoaxial instability is the most common spinal problem requiring treatment.[97] Use of flexion-extension lateral cervical spine radiographs or flexion-extension sagittal view MRI allows for serial evaluation of this instability to determine any need for posterior occipitoaxial fusion. The criteria for surgery and surgical technique are the same as described earlier for spondyloepiphyseal dysplasia congenita. Scoliosis is common but because of the limited trunk growth does not always require treatment. Periodic thoracolumbar spine radiographs are indicated, however, for evaluation and identification of patients who would benefit from either orthotic or surgical treatment. If

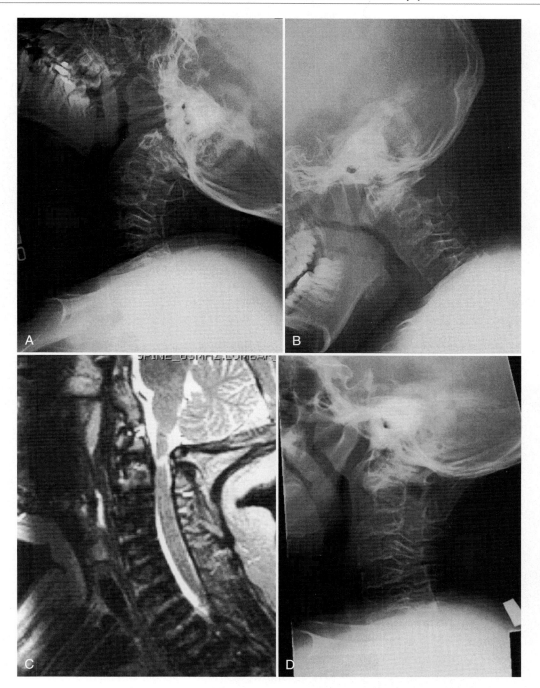

FIGURE 32–13 A and **B,** Lateral extension and flexion cervical spine radiographs show increased and abnormal motion at C1-2 associated with odontoid hypoplasia in a 9-year-old child with Morquio syndrome. **C,** MRI of cervical spine shows signal change within spinal cord at C1-2 indicative of instability at this spinal level with cord compression. **D,** Lateral cervical spine radiograph after occiput-to-C2 posterior fusion.

surgical treatment is needed, small but standard spinal instrumentation can be used. Finally, excessive lumbar lordosis is present, in part from the spine and in part from the expected hip flexion contractures usually present. Because proximal femoral osteotomy is often used to treat coxa vara and external femoral rotation, it is recommended that this femoral osteotomy also include an extension component, which allows some correction of the flexible component of the excessive lumbar lordosis.

Metatropic Dysplasia

Metatropic dysplasia is rare; the name is derived from the apparent change in body proportions with increasing age. This condition seems to be not only a disorder of endochondral ossification, but also seems to be associated with defects in the longitudinal proliferation and maturation of chondrocytes and in the production of normal matrix. The uncoupling of endochondral and perichondral growth seen in this condition

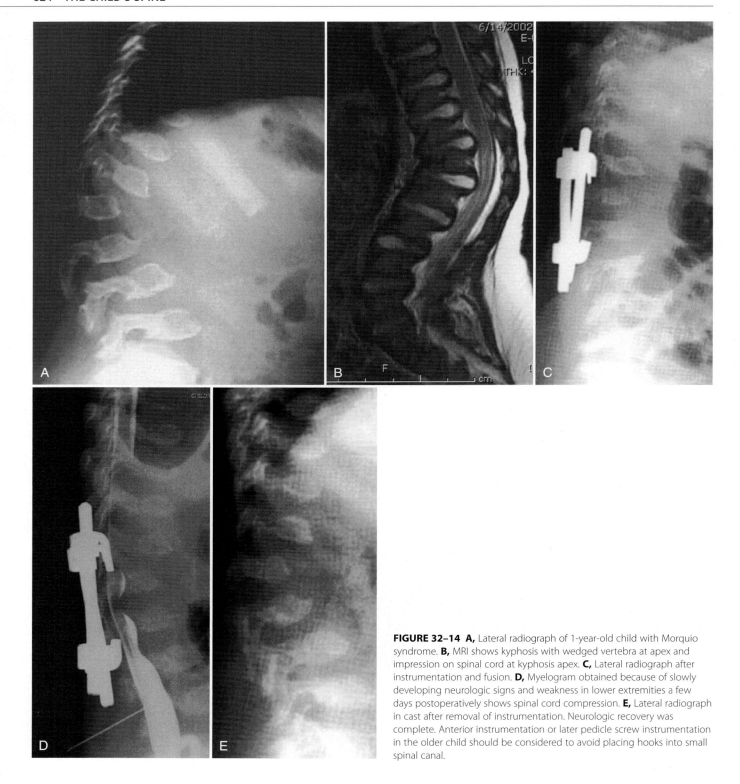

FIGURE 32–14 A, Lateral radiograph of 1-year-old child with Morquio syndrome. **B,** MRI shows kyphosis with wedged vertebra at apex and impression on spinal cord at kyphosis apex. **C,** Lateral radiograph after instrumentation and fusion. **D,** Myelogram obtained because of slowly developing neurologic signs and weakness in lower extremities a few days postoperatively shows spinal cord compression. **E,** Lateral radiograph in cast after removal of instrumentation. Neurologic recovery was complete. Anterior instrumentation or later pedicle screw instrumentation in the older child should be considered to avoid placing hooks into small spinal canal.

may explain why the long bones are dumbbell-shaped, as is seen on radiographs in this dysplasia.[98] As growth occurs, the trunk becomes disproportionately short owing to flattened vertebrae and scoliosis or hyperkyphosis. Life expectancy usually extends into early adulthood. Scoliosis or kyphosis appears early in childhood and is difficult to manage. Orthotic management is attempted early, but growing rod instrumentation without fusion with or without apical fusion should be considered in young children with severe scoliosis. Definitive spinal instrumentation and fusion, commonly involving anterior and posterior fusion, is usually needed by preadolescence if not earlier.

Odontoid hypoplasia has also been reported to be commonly present in this condition and may require upper cervical fusion.[99] More recently, cervical spinal stenosis has been reported to be a common feature of this condition, and decompressive laminectomy may be needed in addition to fusion in the upper cervical spine.[100] An additional feature of metatropic dysplasia that should be considered is the presence of enlarged ventricles on head CT scans.

Mucolipidoses

There are some parallels between MPS syndromes and mucolipidoses (ML) even though the underlying metabolic defect is different, with thoracolumbar kyphosis being present in ML type II and type III. In ML type II, there are physical features similar to the features of Hurler syndrome; children with this type usually die in early or middle childhood. ML type II and type III have a similar biochemical abnormality, but ML type III has milder clinical manifestations, and life expectancy extends well into adult life. Progressive thoracolumbar or upper lumbar kyphosis is treated with posterior spinal instrumentation and fusion, usually anterior and posterior. Carpal tunnel syndrome is common in ML type III and requires median nerve decompression often in adolescence.

Chondrodysplasia Punctata

Also known as Conradi-Hünermann syndrome, chondrodysplasia punctata can be diagnosed at birth by short limbs; ichthyosis; flat facial features; and, in particular, radiographic findings of punctate calcification in the epiphyses at the ends of the long bones. These stippled epiphyses are present even in very young children. Coronal and sagittal vertebral clefts are present in 79% of infants with this dysplasia.[96]

Atlantoaxial instability, in one reported case leading to death from cervical cord compression,[101] and upper cervical stenosis can be seen, so cervical spine imaging is needed in chondrodysplasia punctata (Fig. 32–16).[102-105] Scoliosis is common and often has its onset in early childhood. There are two main types of scoliosis: One slowly progresses with growth, and the other is a dysplastic type that is rapidly progressive. Orthotic treatment may suffice in curves with slower progression, but spinal instrumentation and anterior and posterior fusion is needed in larger dysplastic curves.[106] Growth hormone has been successful in some patients in improving their final height. Life expectancy and intelligence are normal if the child survives the newborn period.

Camptomelic Dysplasia

The most prominent feature in camptomelic dysplasia at birth is bowing of the long bones of the lower extremities. Delayed ossification of the mid-thoracic pedicles is very useful in helping to establish this diagnosis. Cervical kyphosis is reported in 38%,[107] and spinal cord injury as a result of this cervical kyphosis has been reported.[108] Scoliosis and thoracic hyperkyphosis develop very early in childhood and often

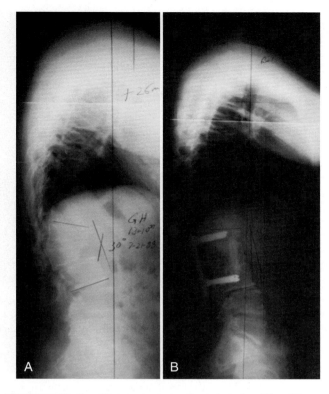

FIGURE 32–15 A and **B,** Lateral spinal radiographs before (**A**) and 7 months after (**B**) laminectomy and spinal fusion in a teenager with thoracolumbar kyphosis associated with Morquio syndrome. Although most kyphotic deformities in Morquio syndrome are minimally progressive or nonprogressive, careful follow-up with growth is needed. Surgical treatment is indicated with progressive kyphosis despite bracing and when abnormal neurologic signs and symptoms are present. If neurologic deficit is present, atlantoaxial region should be evaluated carefully. Instability here is common in Morquio syndrome. (Courtesy of Marc A. Asher, MD, Kansas City, KS.)

develop into severe deformity. Many of these children die in early childhood from pulmonary causes. Orthotic treatment is difficult because of the pulmonary compromise seen in these children. If patients survive past early childhood and have progressive kyphoscoliosis, spinal instrumentation and fusion has been reported to be successful.[107]

Parastremmatic Dysplasia

Parastremmatic dysplasia is an exceedingly rare, short-trunk dwarfism associated with angular deformity of the lower extremities. Radiographs show abnormalities at the epiphyseal and metaphyseal regions of the long bones. Spinal radiographs show flattened vertebral bodies with irregular endplate ossification. Kyphoscoliosis is present in nearly all cases, and either orthotic or surgical treatment, depending on the severity of the deformity, is indicated as these patients survive to adulthood.

Spondyloepimetaphyseal Dysplasia with Joint Laxity

Early development of severe and progressive kyphoscoliosis during infancy is seen in spondyloepimetaphyseal dysplasia with joint laxity. Left untreated, this deformity leads to death

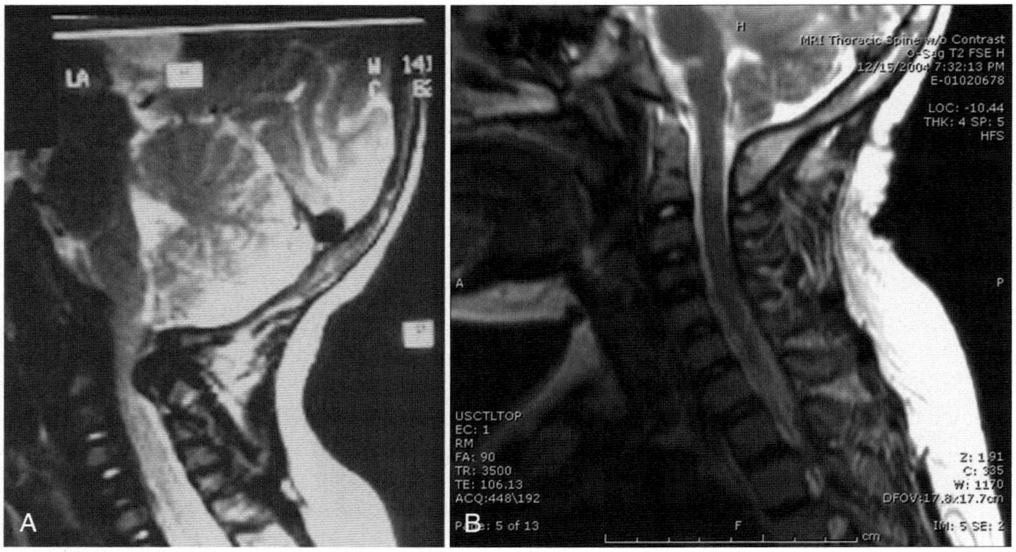

FIGURE 32–16 A, Lateral cervical spine radiograph in a 7-year-old girl with chondrodysplasia punctata shows cervical stenosis with cervical spinal cord compression, leading to weakness when walking. **B,** Lateral cervical spine radiograph 1 year after C1 laminectomy and occipitocervical posterior fusion, with neurologic signs and symptoms resolved.

in early childhood resulting from either spinal cord compression or cardiorespiratory failure in most patients.[109]

Spondylometaphyseal Dysplasia, Kozlowski Type

The Kozlowski type of spondylometaphyseal dysplasia is a short-trunk dwarfism that is usually not diagnosed until preschool age. Platyspondyly causes the short trunk, and kyphosis is common. Life expectancy is normal, and the kyphotic deformity needs to be followed and treated according to how severe it becomes.[110]

Summary

There continues to be finer and more precise molecular and genetic definition of the defects in each of the skeletal dysplasias and metabolic conditions noted in this chapter, and the time may come when the underlying defect causing these short stature syndromes can be treated early enough and effectively enough to prevent many of the clinical manifestations seen in these dysplasias today. That day is not yet here, however. For now, it is important to recognize when a dysplasia is present and to make an accurate diagnosis of which dysplasia the patient has. By knowing the diagnosis, it is possible to monitor these children and later adults for the spinal and other orthopaedic conditions known to be a part of the diagnosed dysplastic condition and to treat these spinal and orthopaedic problems early and more effectively. Although a few metabolic conditions noted here are associated with mental deficiency, patients with skeletal dysplasia are of normal intelligence and enjoy an excellent quality of life. By recognizing the spinal problems most common in each of these skeletal dysplasia conditions, the orthopaedist can

contribute greatly to ensuring that this quality of life is preserved and enhanced.

PEARLS

1. Upper cervical instability and odontoid hypoplasia are very common in SED congenital and Morquio syndrome. MRI evaluation is useful to diagnose, and posterior upper cervical fusion is commonly needed.

2. Diastrophic dysplasia patients with significant scoliosis by age 4 require early fusion to prevent the development of severe thoracic kyphoscoliosis.

3. Before beginning treatment, establish the correct diagnosis with the help of a geneticist.

PITFALLS

1. Avoid placing implants and instruments inside the stenotic spine in achondroplasia patients. You are likely to cause an iatrogenic neurologic deficit.

2. Whenever you see a thoracolumbar kyphosis in an infant, consider the possibility of either Morquio or Hurler syndrome, as well as congenital kyphosis.

KEY POINTS

1. With more than 200 skeletal dysplasia conditions described, it is essential to diagnose the particular dysplasia correctly before treatment of any spinal disorder.

2. The key radiographs to aid diagnosis are an anteroposterior view of both lower extremities from hip to ankle and a lateral view of the spine. Referral to a geneticist should be included in this evaluation.

3. The spine in achondroplasia has stenosis from the foramen magnum to the sacrum. The regions that most commonly require decompression are the thoracolumbar and lumbar areas. Because of the marked stenosis, spinal instrumentation and surgical instruments must be kept out of the spinal canal, or iatrogenic neurologic injury may occur. The surgeon should be aware of the subtle signs and symptoms of early neurologic compromise and evaluate with imaging studies early.

4. If thoracolumbar kyphosis present at birth in achondroplasia does not resolve by age 5 or 6 years, surgical treatment is indicated to prevent progressive worsening.

5. Patients with diastrophic dysplasia require early evaluation for cervical kyphosis and for early-onset thoracic kyphoscoliosis, both of which can progress to severe deformity if not treated at a young age.

6. In spondyloepiphyseal dysplasia congenita, odontoid hypoplasia is common with atlantoaxial instability, occurring frequently at an early age and requiring posterior fusion in most patients.

7. Pseudoachondroplasia has body proportions similar to achondroplasia, but there is no spinal stenosis. Upper cervical instability may occur along with generalized joint laxity present in this condition.

8. If the diagnosis is made in infancy, MPS I or Hurler syndrome can be treated with bone marrow transplantation or enzyme replacement therapy to prevent the cardiac and mental deterioration that previously led to death by age 5 years. The orthopaedic manifestations are still present, however, requiring management similar to that for MPS IV or Morquio syndrome.

9. MPS I and MPS IV have odontoid hypoplasia and frequent atlantoaxial instability, requiring posterior cervical fusion in nearly all these patients.

10. The thoracolumbar kyphosis present at birth with MPS I and MPS IV can be mistakenly diagnosed as a congenital kyphosis and delay early treatment of the MPS condition. If an inferior lip projects out from more than one vertebra at the thoracolumbar kyphosis on a lateral spine radiograph, the infant should be evaluated for possible MPS conditions.

KEY REFERENCES

1. Sciubba DM, Noggle JC, Marupudi NI, et al: Spinal stenosis surgery in pediatric patients with achondroplasia. J Neurosurg 106(5 Suppl):372-378, 2007.
This is a retrospective review of 44 patients younger than 21 years with achondroplasia who had laminectomies for spinal stenosis, with 85% in the thoracolumbar and lumbar regions. Spinal fusion in the decompressed region was used in 72% of cases. If cervicomedullary decompression was needed previously (>60%), decompressive laminectomies were more commonly needed in the pediatric age range.

2. Ain MC, Chang TL, Schkrohowsky JG, et al: Rates of perioperative complications associated with laminectomies in patients with achondroplasia. J Bone Joint Surg Am 90:295-298, 2008.
This is a review of 98 patients with achondroplasia who underwent decompressive laminectomies. Of patients, 61% had at least one perioperative complication: 37% had a dural tear, 23% had neurologic complications, and 3% had pulmonary complications. There was one death. Complications are common in this patient group with spinal surgery.

3. Remes V, Marttinen E, Poussa M, et al: Cervical kyphosis in diastrophic dysplasia. Spine (Phila Pa 1976) 24:1990-1995, 1999.
This study from Finland reviewed cervical spine radiographs of 120 patients with the diagnosis of diastrophic dysplasia. Cervical kyphosis was present at birth in 96% of the patients with a radiograph in infancy, but most resolved without treatment by the mean age of 7 years. Although most cervical kyphoses improve in this condition, it is necessary to monitor these patients because some develop severe kyphosis and myelopathy.

4. Remes V, Tervahartiala P, Poussa M, et al: Thoracic and lumbar spine in diastrophic dysplasia: A clinical and magnetic resonance imaging analysis. Spine (Phila Pa 1976) 26:187-195, 2001.
MRI of the spine was done from T2-S1 in 88 patients 3 to 56 years old with diastrophic dysplasia. Almost 80% had scoliosis with curves ranging from 11 to 188 degrees. Discs were abnormal and narrow, and facet degeneration and muscle atrophy were widespread. The spinal canal is smaller than normal in diastrophic dysplasia, but this usually does not lead to neurologic symptoms.

5. Ain MC, Chaichana KL, Schkrohowsky JG: Retrospective study of cervical arthrodesis in patients with various types of skeletal dysplasia. Spine (Phila Pa 1976) 31:E169-E174, 2006.
The results of cervical fusion for cervical instability in 25 patients with five different types of skeletal dysplasia are reported, with 92% achieving fusion with the initial procedure. Of patients with progressive neurologic findings, 88% improved. There were few complications.

6. Weisstein JS, Delgado E, Steinback LS, et al: Musculoskeletal manifestations of Hurler syndrome: Long term followup after bone marrow transplantation. J Pediatr Orthop 24:97-101, 2004.
Seven patients with Hurler syndrome treated with bone marrow transplant were evaluated at a mean 7.6 years after transplant. Although bone marrow transplant had a very positive effect in slowing or eliminating the cardiac and mental deterioration seen in Hurler syndrome, it did not alter the musculoskeletal disorders seen in MPS such as Hurler syndrome or Morquio syndrome. Thoracolumbar kyphosis and atlantoaxial instability from odontoid hypoplasia require monitoring and often treatment in patients with Hurler syndrome, even after bone marrow transplant.

REFERENCES

1. Lachman RS: Neurologic abnormalities in the skeletal dysplasias: A clinical and radiological perspective. Am J Med Genet 69:33-43, 1997.

2. Reynolds KK, Modaff P, Pauli RM: Absence of correlation between infantile hypotonia and foramen magnum size in achondroplasia. Am J Med Genet 101:40-45, 2001.

3. Pauli RM, Scott CI Jr, Wassman ER Jr, et al: Apnea and sudden unexpected death in infants with achondroplasia. J Pediatr 104:342-348, 1984.

4. Fremion AS, Garg BP, Kalsbeck J: Apnea as the sole manifestation of cord compression in achondroplasia. J Pediatr 104:398-401, 1984.

5. Reid CS, Pyeritz RE, Kopits SE, et al: Cervicomedullary compression in young patients with achondroplasia: Value of comprehensive neurologic and respiratory evaluation. J Pediatr 110:522-530, 1987.

6. Nelson FW, Hecht JT, Horton WA, et al: Neurological basis of respiratory complications in achondroplasia. Ann Neurol 24:89-93, 1988.

7. Li L, Muller-Forell W, Oberman B, et al: Subcortical somatosensory evoked potentials after median nerve and posterior tibial nerve stimulation in high cervical cord compression of achondroplasia. Brain Dev 30:499-503, 2008.

8. Wang H, Rosenbaum AE, Reid CS, et al: Pediatric patients with achondroplasia: CT evaluation of the craniocervical junction. Radiology 164:515-519, 1987.

9. Yang SS, Corbett DP, Brough AJ, et al: Upper cervical myelopathy in achondroplasia. Am J Clin Pathol 68:68-72, 1977.

10. Hecht JT, Butler IJ, Scott CI Jr: Long-term neurological sequelae in achondroplasia. Eur J Pediatr 143:58-60, 1984.

11. Carson B, Winfield J, Wang H, et al: Surgical management of cervicomedullary compression in achondroplastic patients. In Nicoletto B, Kopits SE, Ascani E, et al (eds): Human Achondroplasia: A Multidisciplinary Approach. New York, Plenum Press, 1988, pp 207-214.

12. Ryken TC, Menezes AH: Cervicomedullary compression in achondroplasia. J Neurosurg 81:43-48, 1994.

13. Benglis DM, Sandberg DI: Acute neurological deficit after minor trauma in an infant with achondroplasia and cervicomedullary compression: Case report and review of the literature. J Neurosurg 107(2 Suppl):152-155, 2007.

14. Keiper GL Jr, Koch B, Crone KR: Achondroplasia and cervicomedullary compression: Prospective evaluation and surgical treatment. Pediatr Neurosurg 31:78-83, 1999.

15. Wassman ER Jr, Rimoin DL: Cervicomedullary compression with achondroplasia [letter]. J Pediatr 113:411, 1988.

16. Sciubba DM, Noggle JC, Marupudi NI, et al: Spinal stenosis surgery in pediatric patients with achondroplasia. J Neurosurg 106(5 Suppl):372-378, 2007.

17. Kahonovitz N, Rimoin DL, Sillence DO: The clinical spectrum of lumbar spine disease in achondroplasia. Spine (Phila Pa 1976) 7:137-140, 1982.

18. Morgan DF, Young RF: Spinal neurological complications of achondroplasia: Results of surgical treatment. J Neurosurg 52:463-472, 1980.

19. Pyeritz RE, Sack GH, Udvarhelyi GB: Cervical and lumbar laminectomy for spinal stenosis in achondroplasia. Johns Hopkins Med J 146:203-206, 1980.

20. Uematsu S, Wang H, Kopits SE, et al: Total craniospinal decompression in achondroplastic stenosis. Neurosurgery 35:250-257, 1994.

21. Gulati DR, Rout D: Atlantoaxial dislocation with quadriparesis in achondroplasia: Case report. J Neurosurg 40:394-396, 1974.

22. Hammerschlag W, Ziv I, Wald U, et al: Cervical instability in an achondroplastic infant: Case report. J Pediatr Orthop 8:481-484, 1988.

23. Hall JG: Kyphosis in achondroplasia: Probably preventable. J Pediatr 112:166-167, 1988.

24. Kopits SE: Thoracolumbar kyphosis and lumbosacral hyperlordosis in achondroplastic children. In Nicoletti B, Kopits SE, Ascani E, et al (eds): Human Achondroplasia: A Multidisciplinary Approach. New York, Plenum Press, 1988, pp 241-255.

25. Siebens AA, Hungerford DS, Kirby NA: Achondroplasia: Effectiveness of an orthosis in reducing deformity of the spine. Arch Phys Med Rehabil 68:384-388, 1987.

26. Siebens AA, Kirby N, Hungerford DS: Orthotic correction of sitting abnormality in achondroplastic children. In Nicoletti B, Kopits SE, Ascani E, et al (eds): Human Achondroplasia: A Multidisciplinary Approach. New York, Plenum Press, 1988, pp 313-320.

27. Winter RB, Herring JA: Kyphosis in an achondroplastic dwarf. J Pediatr Orthop 3:250-252, 1983.

28. Siebens AA, Hungerford DS, Kirby NA: Curves of the achondroplastic spine: A new hypothesis. Johns Hopkins Med J 142:205-210, 1978.

29. Tolo VT: Surgical treatment of kyphosis in achondroplasia. In Nicoletti B, Kopits SE, Ascani E, et al (eds.): Human Achondroplasia: A Multidisciplinary Approach. New York, Plenum Press, 1988, pp 257-259.

30. Sensenbrenner JA: Achondroplasia with hypoplastic vertebral bodies secondary to surgical fusion. Birth Defects 10:356-357, 1974.

31. Ain MC, Browne JA: Spinal arthrodesis with instrumentation for thoracolumbar kyphosis in pediatric achondroplasia. Spine (Phila Pa 1976) 29:2075-2080, 2004.

32. Ain MC, Shirley ED: Spinal fusion for kyphosis in achondroplasia. J Pediatr Orthop 24:541-545, 2004.

33. Lutter LD, Langer LO: Neurologic symptoms in achondroplastic dwarfs—surgical treatment. J Bone Joint Surg Am 59:87-92, 1977.

34. Uematsu S, Wang H, Hurko O, et al: The subarachnoid fluid space in achondroplastic spinal stenosis: The surgical implications. In Nicoletti B, Kopits SE, Ascani E, et al (eds): Human Achondroplasia: A Multidisciplinary Approach. New York, Plenum Press, 1988, pp 275-281.

35. Schkrohowsky JG, Hoernschemeyer DG, Carson BS, et al: Early presentation of spinal stenosis in achondroplasia. J Pediatr Orthop 27:119-122, 2007.

36. Lutter LD, Lonstein JE, Winter RE, et al: Anatomy of the achondroplastic lumbar canal. Clin Orthop Relat Res 126:139-142, 1977.

37. Lonstein JE: Anatomy of the lumbar spinal canal. Basic Life Sci 48:219-226, 1988.

38. Suss RA, Udvarhelyi GB, Wang H, et al: Myelography in achondroplasia: Value of a lateral C1-2 puncture and non-ionic, water-soluble contrast medium. Radiology 149:159-163, 1983.

39. Alexander E Jr: Significance of the small lumbar spinal canal: Cauda equina compression syndromes due to spondylosis. Part 5: Achondroplasia. J Neurosurg 31:513-519, 1969.

40. Streeten E, Uematsu S, Hurko O, et al: Extended laminectomy for spinal stenosis in achondroplasia. In Nicoletti B, Kopits SE, Ascani E, et al (eds): Human Achondroplasia: A Multidisciplinary Approach. New York, Plenum Press, 1988, pp 261-273.

41. Thomeer RT, van Dijk JM: Surgical treatment of lumbar stenosis in achondroplasia. J Neurosurg 96(3 Suppl):292-297, 2002.

42. Qi X, Matsumoto M, Ishii K, et al: Posterior osteotomy and instrumentation for thoracolumbar kyphosis in patients with achondroplasia. Spine (Phila Pa 1976) 31:E606-E610, 2006.

43. Modi HN, Suh SW, Song HR, et al: Lumber nerve root occupancy in the foramen in achondroplasia: A morphometric analysis. Clin Orthop Relat Res 466:907-913, 2008.

44. Ain MD, Shirley ED, Pirouzmanesh A, et al: Postlaminectomy kyphosis in the skeletally immature achondroplast. Spine (Phila Pa 1976) 31:197-201, 2006.

45. Ain MC, Chang TL, Schkrohowsky JG, et al: Rates of perioperative complications associated with laminectomies in patients with achondroplasia. J Bone Joint Surg Am 90:295-298, 2008.

46. Ain MC, Elmaci I, Hurko O, et al: Reoperation for spinal restenosis in achondroplasia. J Spinal Disord 13:168-173, 2000.

47. Hancock DO, Phillips DG: Spinal compression in achondroplasia. Paraplegia 3:23-33, 1965.

48. Srikumaran U, Woodard EJ, Leet AI, et al: Pedicle and spinal canal parameters of the lower thoracic and lumbar vertebrae in the achondroplast population. Spine (Phila Pa 1976) 32:2423-2431, 2007.

49. Kumar CP, Song HR, Lee SH, et al: Thoracic and lumbar pedicle morphometry in achondroplasia. Clin Orthop Relat Res 454:180-185, 2007.

50. Walker BA, Scott CI, Hall JG, et al: Diastrophic dwarfism. Medicine (Baltimore) 51:41-59, 1972.

51. Bethem D, Winter RB, Lutter L: Disorders of the spine in diastrophic dwarfism: A discussion of nine patients and review of the literature. J Bone Joint Surg Am 62:529-536, 1980.

52. Herring JA: The spinal disorder in diastrophic dwarfism. J Bone Joint Surg Am 60:177-182, 1978.

53. Remes V, Tervahartiala P, Poussa M, et al: Cervical spine in diastrophic dysplasia: An MRI analysis. J Pediatr Orthop 20:48-53, 2000.

54. Hensinger RN: Kyphosis secondary to skeletal dysplasias and metabolic disease. Clin Orthop Relat Res 128:113-128, 1977.

55. Kopits SE: Orthopaedic complications of dwarfism. Clin Orthop Relat Res 114:153-179, 1976.

56. Remes VM, Marttinen EJ, Poussa MS, et al: Cervical spine in patients with diastrophic dysplasia—radiographic findings in 122 patients. Pediatr Radiol 32:621-628, 2002.

57. Remes V, Marttinen E, Poussa M, et al: Cervical kyphosis in diastrophic dysplasia. Spine (Phila Pa 1976) 24:1990-1995, 1999.

58. Poussa M, Merikanto J, Ryoppy S, et al: The spine in diastrophic dysplasia. Spine (Phila Pa 1976) 16:881-887, 1991.

59. Remes V, Poussa M, Peltonen J: Scoliosis in patients with diastrophic dysplasia: A new classification. Spine (Phila Pa 1976) 26:1689-1697, 2001.

60. Tolo VT, Kopits SE: Spinal deformity in diastrophic dysplasia. Orthop Trans 7:31-32, 1983.

61. Remes V, Tervahartiala P, Poussa M, et al: Thoracic and lumbar spine in diastrophic dysplasia: A clinical and magnetic resonance imaging analysis. Spine (Phila Pa 1976) 26:187-195, 2001.

62. Remes V, Helenius I, Peltonen J, et al: Lung function in diastrophic dysplasia. Pediatr Pulmonol 33:277-282, 2002.

63. Matsuyama Y, Winter RB, Lonstein JE: The spine in diastrophic dysplasia: The surgical arthrodesis of thoracic and lumbar deformities in 21 patients. Spine (Phila Pa 1976) 15:2325-2331, 1999.

64. Reems V, Poussa M, Lonnqvist T, et al: Walking ability in patients with diastrophic dysplasia: A clinical, electroneurophysiological, treadmill and MRI analysis. J Pediatr Orthop 24:546-551, 2004.

65. Fiedler J, Bergmann C, Brenner RE: X-linked spondyloepiphyseal dysplasia tarda: Molecular cause of heritable disorder associated with early degenerative joint disease. Acta Orthop Scand 74:737-741, 2003.

66. Fiedler J, Frances AM, LeMerrer M, et al: X-linked spondyloepiphyseal dysplasia tarda: Molecular cause of heritable platyspondyly. Spine (Phila Pa 1976) 28:478-482, 2003.

67. Nakamura I, Hoshino Y: Multiple disc herniations in spondyloepiphyseal dysplasia tarda: A case report. Int Orthop 22:404-406, 1998.

68. Spranger J, Wiedemann HR: Dysplasia spondyloepiphysaria congenita. Helv Paediatr Acta 21:598-611, 1966.

69. Takeda E, Hashimoto T, Tayama M, et al: Diagnosis of atlantoaxial subluxation in Morquio's syndrome and spondyloepiphyseal dysplasia congenita. Acta Paediatr Jpn 33:633-638, 1991.

70. Miyoshi K, Nakamura K, Haga N, et al: Surgical treatment for atlantoaxial subluxation with myelopathy in spondyloepiphyseal dysplasia congenita. Spine (Phila Pa 1976) 29:E488-E491, 2004.

71. Ain MC, Chaichana KL, Schkrohowsky JG: Retrospective study of cervical arthrodesis in patients with various types of skeletal dysplasia. Spine (Phila Pa 1976) 31:E169-E174, 2006.

72. Shetty GM, Song HR, Unnikrishman R, et al: Upper cervical spine instability in pseudoachondroplasia. J Pediatr Orthop 27:782-787, 2007.

73. Sostrin RD, Hasso AN, Peterson DI, et al: Myelographic features of mucopolysaccharidoses: A new sign. Radiology 125:421-424, 1977.

74. Morgan KA, Rehman MA, Schwartz RE: Morquio's syndrome and its anaesthetic considerations. Paediatr Anaesth 12:641-644, 2002.

75. Dullenkopf A, Holzmann D, Feurer R, et al: Tracheal intubation in children with Morquio syndrome using the angulated video-intubation laryngoscope. Can J Anaesth 49:198-202, 2002.

76. Belani KG, Krivit W, Carpenter BL, et al: Children with mucopolysaccharidosis: Perioperative care, morbidity, mortality, and new findings. J Pediatr Surg 28:403-408, 1993

SECTION

IV

77. Tobias JD: Anesthetic care for the child with Morquio syndrome: General versus regional anesthesia. J Clin Anesth 11:242-246, 1999.

78. Brill CB, Rose JS, Godmilow L, et al: Spastic quadriparesis due to C1-C2 subluxation in Hurler syndrome. J Pediatr 92:441-443, 1978.

79. Thomas SL, Childress MH, Quinton B: Hypoplasia of the odontoid with atlanto-axial subluxation in Hurler's syndrome. Pediatr Radiol 15:353-354, 1985.

80. Weisstein JS, Delgado E, Steinback LS, et al: Musculoskeletal manifestations of Hurler syndrome: Long term followup after bone marrow transplantation. J Pediatr Orthop 24:97-101, 2004.

81. Malm G, Gustafsson B, Berglund G, et al: Outcome in six children with mucopolysaccharidosis type III, Hurler syndrome, after haematopoietic stem cell transplantation (HSCT). Acta Paediatr 97:1108-1112, 2008.

82. Hite SH, Peters C, Krivit W: Correction of odontoid dysplasia following bone-marrow transplantation and engraftment (in Hurler syndrome MPAS 1H). Pediatr Radiol 30:464-470, 2000.

83. Tandon V, Williamson JB, Cowie RA, et al: Spinal problems in mucopolysaccharidosis I (Hurler syndrome). J Bone Joint Surg Br 78:938-944, 1996.

84. Benson PF, Button LR, Fensom AH, et al: Lumbar kyphosis in Hunter's disease (MPS II). Clin Genet 16:317-322, 1979.

85. Parsons VJ, Hughes DG, Wraith JE: Magnetic resonance imaging of the brain, neck and cervical spine in mild Hunter's syndrome (mucopolysaccharidoses type II). Clin Radiol 51:719-723, 1996.

86. Nelson J, Thomas PS: Clinical findings in 12 patients with MPS IV A (Morquio's disease): Further evidence for heterogeneity. Part III: Odontoid dysplasia. Clin Genet 33:126-130, 1988.

87. Blaw MF, Langer LO: Spinal cord compression in Morquio-Brailsford disease. J Pediatr 74:593-600, 1969.

88. Lipson SJ: Dysplasia of the odontoid process in Morquio's syndrome causing quadriparesis. J Bone Joint Surg Am 59:340-344, 1977.

89. Hughes DG, Chadderton RD, Cowie RA, et al: MRI of the brain and craniocervical junction in Morquio's disease. Neuroradiology 39:381-385, 1997.

90. Stevens JM, Kendall BE, Crockard HA, et al: The odontoid process in Morquio-Brailford's disease: The effects of occipito-cervical fusion. J Bone Joint Surg Br 73:851-858, 1991.

91. White KK, Steinman S, Mubarak SJ: Cervical stenosis and spastic quadriplegia in Morquio disease (MPS IV): A case report with twenty-six year followup. J Bone Joint Surg Am 91:438-442, 2009.

92. Dalvie SS, Noordeen MH, Vellodi A: Anterior instrumented fusion for thoracolumbar kyphosis in mucopolysaccharidosis. Spine (Phila Pa 1976) 26:E539-E541, 2001.

93. Thorne JA, Javadpour M, Hughes DG, et al: Craniovertebral abnormalities in type VI mucopolysaccharidosis (Maroteaux-Lamy syndrome). Neurosurgery 48:849-852, 2001.

94. Bethem D, Winter RB, Lutter L, et al: Spinal disorders of dwarfism: Review of the literature and report of eighty cases. J Bone Joint Surg Am 63:1412-1425, 1981.

95. Lachman RS, Rimoin DL, Hollister DW, et al: The Kniest syndrome. Am J Roentgenol Radium Ther Nucl Med 123:805-814, 1975.

96. Westvik J, Lachman RS: Coronal and sagittal clefts in skeletal dysplasias. Pediatr Radiol 28:764-770, 1998.

97. Merrill KD, Schmidt TL: Occipitoatlantal instability in a child with Kniest syndrome. J Pediatr Orthop 9:338-340, 1989.

98. Boden SD, Kaplan FS, Fallon MD, et al: Metatropic dwarfism: Uncoupling of endochondral and perichondral growth. J Bone Joint Surg Am 69:174-184, 1987.

99. Shohat M, Lachman R, Rimoin DL: Odontoid hypoplasia with vertebral cervical subluxation and ventriculomegaly in metatropic dysplasia. J Pediatr 114:239-243, 1989.

100. Leet AL, Sampath JS, Scott CI Jr, et al: Cervical spinal stenosis in metatropic dysplasia. J Pediatr Orthop 26:347-352, 2006.

101. Afshani E, Girdany BR: Atlanto-axial dislocation in chondrodysplasia punctata: Report of the findings in two brothers. Radiology 102:399-401, 1972.

102. Khanna AJ, Braverman ME, Valle D, et al: Cervical stenosis secondary to rhizomelic chondrodysplasia punctata. Am J Med Genet 99:63-66, 2001.

103. Goodman P, Dominguez R: Cervicothoracic myelopathy in Conradi-Hunermann disease: MRI diagnosis. Magn Reson Imaging 8:647-650, 1990.

104. Violas P, Fraisse B, Chapuis M, et al: Cervical spine stenosis in chondrodysplasia punctata. J Pediatr Orthop B 16:443-445, 2007.

105. Garnier A, Dauger S, Eurin D, et al: Brachytelephalangic chondrodysplasia punctata with severe spinal cord compression: Report of four new cases. Eur J Pediatr 166:127-131, 2007.

106. Mason DE, Sanders JO, MacKenzie WG, et al: Spinal deformity in chondrodysplasia punctata. Spine (Phila Pa 1976) 27:1995-2002, 2002.

107. Coscia MF, Bassett GS, Bowen JR, et al: Spinal abnormalities in camptomelic dysplasia. J Pediatr Orthop 9:6-14, 1989.

108. Lekovic GP, Rekate HL, Dickman CA, et al: Congenital cervical instability in a patient with camptomelic dysplasia. Childs Nerv Syst 22:1212-1214, 2006.

109. Kozlowski K, Beighton P: Radiographic features of spondylo-epimetaphyseal dysplasia with joint laxity and progressive kyphoscoliosis: Review of 19 cases. Fortschr Roentgenstr 141:337-341, 1984.

110. Kozlowski KS: Chondrodysplasia spondylometaphysealis. Birth Defects 11:183-185, 1975.

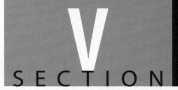

SECTION V

ARTHRITIS AND INFLAMMATORY DISORDERS

David G. Borenstein, MD

Rheumatologic disorders of the axial skeleton are an important cause of spinal pain. These inflammatory disorders affect the bones, joints, ligaments, tendons, and muscles that are anatomic components of the spine. The most important rheumatic disorders that cause inflammation of the joints of the axial skeleton are the seronegative spondyloarthropathies and rheumatoid arthritis (RA). The spondyloarthropathies are characterized by damage of the sacroiliac joints, axial skeleton, and peripheral large joints and the absence of rheumatoid factor. The seronegative spondyloarthropathies include ankylosing spondylitis (AS), reactive arthritis, psoriatic arthritis, and enteropathic arthritis. Genetic factors predispose patients to these illnesses. Environmental factors play a role as triggers of the inflammatory response in genetically predisposed individuals, but these factors have been only partially identified.

RA, a disease that causes chronic inflammation of the synovial lining of the joints, affects the cervical spine at the atlantoaxial junction and the subaxial apophyseal joints. These changes occur most commonly in patients with diffuse disease of long duration. Cervical spine involvement in RA is associated with a wide range of symptoms and signs, from mild neck pain and headaches to severe neurologic dysfunction consisting of radiculopathy, paresthesias, incontinence, quadriplegia, and sudden death.

In the seronegative spondyloarthropathies and RA, joint pain is most severe in the morning and improves with activity. Physical examination reveals localized tenderness with palpation and limitation of motion in all planes of motion of the axial skeleton. Laboratory abnormalities are consistent with systemic inflammatory disease but are nonspecific except for the presence of rheumatoid factor in 80% of patients with RA. Radiographic evaluation identifies characteristic joint space narrowing, sclerosis, and fusion in the sacroiliac joints; vertebral body squaring; and ligamentous calcification that may help in the differential diagnosis of a patient with spinal arthritis.

Although there are no cures for these illnesses, medical therapy consisting of nonsteroidal anti-inflammatory drugs (NSAIDs), cyclooxygenase (COX)-2 inhibitors, and disease-modifying antirheumatic drugs (DMARDs) can be effective in controlling symptoms and improving function. Newer therapies in the form of tumor necrosis factor (TNF)-α and interleukin-1 inhibitors offer the potential to prevent joint inflammation and destruction to a greater degree than with prior therapies.

The prognosis and course of these rheumatic conditions are rarely related to the extent of spine disease alone. Occasionally, atlantoaxial subluxation secondary to RA or the spondyloarthropathies may result in catastrophic neurologic dysfunction. In most circumstances, the status of disease in other areas of the musculoskeletal system and the severity of constitutional symptoms have a greater effect on the patient's daily existence.

Ankylosing Spondylitis

AS is a chronic inflammatory disease characterized by a variable symptomatic course and progressive involvement of the sacroiliac and axial skeletal joints. It is the prototype of the seronegative spondyloarthropathies. This disease complex is characterized by axial skeletal arthritis; the absence of rheumatoid factor in serum (seronegative); the lack of rheumatoid nodules; and the presence of a tissue factor on host cells, human leukocyte antigen (HLA)-B27.

Epidemiology

AS affects 1% to 2% of whites, which is equal to the prevalence for RA. A strikingly high association between HLA-B27 and AS has been shown. HLA-B27 is present in more than 90% of white patients with AS compared with a frequency of 7% to 8% in a normal white population.[1] In North American whites, with a prevalence of HLA-B27 of 7%, the frequency of AS is 0.2%.[2] A positive family history of AS or related spondyloarthropathy increases the risk to 30% among HLA-B27–positive first-degree relatives compared with HLA-B27–positive control subjects (1% to 4%).[3]

The male-to-female ratio is reported in the range of 3:1. Women tend to be less symptomatic, however, and develop less severe disease. Women may also present more often with cervical spine disease with minimal lumbar spine symptoms.

The overall pattern of illness may be similar in men and women.[4]

Pathogenesis

The pathogenesis of AS is unknown. A genetic predisposition to AS and to the seronegative spondyloarthropathies in general exists. A genetically determined host response to an environmental factor in genetically susceptible individuals seems to be the most likely basis for the pathogenesis of the spondyloarthropathies. The presence of HLA-B27 is not sufficient to develop AS; this is supported by the facts that not all individuals with HLA-B27 develop disease, that HLA-B27 even in a homogeneous form does not cause disease, and that a few patients with AS do not have HLA-B27.

Enthesitis is the hallmark that distinguishes the spondyloarthropathies from other forms of arthritis.[5] An enthesis is a dynamic structure undergoing constant modification in response to applied stress. This area is a target for inflammation. Although entheses are primarily affected in the spondyloarthropathies, inflammation of these structures is insufficient to explain the alterations that occur in joints (sacroiliac). Synovitis plays an important role. Synovitis may be a secondary event, however, after initiation with an enthesitis.[6]

AS is a disease of the synovial and cartilaginous joints of the axial skeleton, including sacroiliac joints, spinal apophyseal joints, and symphysis pubis. The large appendicular joints, hips, shoulders, knees, elbows, and ankles are also affected in 30% of patients. The inflammatory process is characterized by chondritis (inflammation of cartilage) or osteitis (inflammation of bone) at the junction of the cartilage and bone in the spine. As opposed to RA, which is associated with osteoporosis as an early manifestation of disease, the inflammation of AS is characterized by ankylosis of joints and ossification of ligaments surrounding the vertebrae (syndesmophytes) and other musculotendinous structures, such as the heels and pelvis.

Clinical History

The classic AS patient is a man 15 to 40 years old with intermittent dull low back pain. The associated stiffness is slowly progressive, measured in months to years. AS rarely occurs in individuals older than 50 years. Patients with spondyloarthropathy initiated after age 50 are more likely to have a non-AS spinal inflammatory disorder, such as psoriatic spondylitis.[7] Back pain, which occurs throughout the disease in 90% to 95% of patients, is greatest in the morning and is increased by periods of inactivity. Patients may have difficulty sleeping because of pain and stiffness; they may awaken at night and find it necessary to leave bed and move about for a few minutes before returning to sleep. Fatigue can be a major symptom and correlates with level of disease activity, functional ability, global well-being, and mental health status.[8]

Back pain improves with exercise. The mode of onset is variable, with most patients developing pain in the lumbosacral region. Peripheral joints (hips, knees, and shoulders) are initially involved in a few patients, and occasionally acute iridocyclitis (eye inflammation) or heel pain may be the first manifestation of disease. Occasionally, individuals older than 50 years may present with mild symptoms despite extensive spinal involvement.[9] Conversely, back pain may be severe, with radiation into the lower extremities, mimicking acute lumbar disc herniation. Patients have symptoms related to the piriformis syndrome. The belly of the piriformis muscle crosses over the sciatic nerve. Inflammation in the sacroiliac joint, where the muscle attaches, results in muscle spasm and nerve compression. There are no abnormal, persistent neurologic signs associated with the sciatic pain. The symptoms are reversible with medical therapy that relieves joint inflammation. This symptom complex of radicular pain is referred to as *pseudosciatica*.

Patients usually have a moderate degree of intermittent aching pain localized to the lumbosacral area. Paraspinal musculoskeletal spasm may also contribute to the discomfort. With progression of the disease, pain develops in the dorsal and cervical spine and rib joints.

Flattening of the lumbar spine and loss of normal lordosis are consistent with spinal involvement. Thoracic spine disease causes decreased motion at the costovertebral joints, reduced chest expansion, and impaired pulmonary function. In 81% of patients, the initial symptoms are back pain; back stiffness; thigh, hip, or groin pain; and sciatica. Pain in peripheral joints is the initial complaint in 13% of patients, pain in the chest is the initial complaint in 2%, and generalized aches are the initial complaint in 1%.

Cervical spine disease occurs less frequently than lumbosacral involvement in AS and at a later time in the course of the illness. Studies of large groups of AS patients report cervical spine involvement to range from 0% to 53.9%. The primary symptom of cervical spine disease is neck stiffness and pain. Patients may develop intermittent episodes of torticollis. Involvement of the cervical spine causes the head to protrude forward, making it difficult to look straight ahead.

Peripheral joint arthritis (hips, knees, ankles, shoulders, and elbows) occurs in 30% of patients within the first 10 years of disease. Hip disease is the most frequent limiting factor in mobility rather than spinal stiffness. Ankylosis may also occur in cartilaginous joints, such as the symphysis pubis, sternomanubrial, and costosternal joints. Erosions of the plantar surface of the calcaneus at the attachment of the plantar fascia result in an enthesitis (inflammation of an enthesis—attachment of tendon to bone). This inflammation causes a fasciitis and periosteal reaction, which causes heel pain and the formation of heel spurs. Achilles tendinitis is another enthesitis associated with heel pain and AS.

Neurologic Complications

Atlantoaxial Subluxation

Neurologic complications of AS are secondary to nerve impingement or trauma to the spinal cord. In a study of 33 patients with AS and neurologic complications, cervical abnormalities were the most common cause of neurologic compromise.[10] Atlantoaxial subluxation occurs in the setting of AS but less often than in RA.[11] In a study of 103 AS patients, 21% had atlantoaxial subluxations. Vertical subluxation is a rare complication. About one third of patients have progression of subluxations. Five of the 22 patients with subluxation required surgical fusion.[12] Rarely, symptoms of atlantoaxial subluxation may be the presenting manifestation of AS.[13] Significant instability may occur without symptoms in RA because of generalized ligamentous laxity and erosion of bone. AS patients have symptoms and signs of nerve impingement more frequently in the setting of instability secondary to the immobilized state of the calcified structures surrounding the spine. Spinal cord compression is associated with myelopathic symptoms, including sensory deficits, spasticity, paresis, and incontinence.

Spinal Fracture

The other change is the loss of normal flexibility because of ankylosis of the spinal joints and ligaments. The spine in this ankylosed state is much more brittle and is prone to fracture, even with minimal trauma. The most common location for fracture is the cervical spine, although dorsal and lumbar spine fractures have also been described.[14,15] The occurrence of traumatic cervical spine injury is 3.5 times greater in AS patients than in the normal population.[16] The frequency of AS as the cause of spinal cord injury is 0.3% to 0.5%.[17] The lower cervical spine (C6-7) is the most frequent location for fracture, which is often associated with a fall. Patients who develop fractures may complain of nothing more than localized pain and decreased or increased spinal motion, but severe sensory and motor functional loss corresponding to the location of the lesion may develop. The onset of neurologic dysfunction may be delayed for weeks after initial trauma.

The diagnosis of fracture may be delayed because of the difficulty of detecting fractures in osteoporotic bone with plain radiographs. Magnetic resonance imaging (MRI) of these patients may identify the location of the fracture.[15] Neurologic deficits may persist despite surgical intervention in 85.7% of patients.[18] A mortality rate of 35% to 50% may be found particularly in AS patients who are elderly, who have complete cord lesions, or who develop pulmonary complications after fracture.[19]

Spondylodiscitis

Another complication of long-standing AS is spondylodiscitis, a destructive lesion of the disc and its surrounding vertebral bodies. This lesion is associated with new onset of localized pain in the spine, which uncharacteristically for a patient with AS is improved with bed rest. The cause of these lesions may be localized inflammation or minor trauma. MRI evaluation reveals increased activity in the central portion of the vertebral endplate confirming this area as an area of enthesitis. In most cases, external immobilization is effective in controlling symptoms, and surgical fusion is reserved for more severely affected patients.

Extra-articular Manifestations

AS is also associated with many nonarticular abnormalities. Constitutional manifestations of disease, such as fever, fatigue, and weight loss, are seen in a few patients with active disease, particularly patients with peripheral joint manifestations. Iritis, inflammation of the anterior uveal tract of the eye, may be the presenting complaint of 25% of patients with AS and is present in 40% of patients over the course of the disease. Cardiac involvement occurs in 10% of patients with disease durations of 30 years or longer. A fibrosing lesion causes the aortic valve and proximal root to thicken. Aortic disease may be more common in patients with peripheral arthritis. Mild features include tachycardia, conduction defects, and pericarditis. AS causes cardiac conduction disturbances, particularly bradyarrhythmias. The most serious cardiac abnormality is proximal aortitis, which results in aortic valve insufficiency, heart failure, and death. Prosthetic valve replacement may forestall cardiac deterioration. Pulmonary involvement is manifested by decreased chest expansion, which limits lung capacity, particularly with severely kyphotic individuals.

Physical Examination

A careful musculoskeletal examination is necessary, particularly of the lumbosacral spine, to discover the early findings of limitation of motion of the axial skeleton, which is especially noticeable with lateral bending or hyperextension. Percussion over the sacroiliac joints elicits pain in most circumstances. Other tests that may be helpful in identifying sacroiliac joint dysfunction place stress on the joint. The tests to be considered include a FABER (flexion abduction and external rotation of the hip) maneuver, Gaenslen test (pressure on a hyperextended thigh with a contralateral flexed hip), Yoeman's test (hyperextension of the thigh with a prone patient), and distraction of the pelvic wings anteriorly and posteriorly.

Measurements of spinal motion, including Schober test (lumbar spine motion), lateral bending of the lumbosacral spine, occiput to wall (cervical spine motion), and chest expansion, are important in ascertaining limitations of motion and following the progression of the disease. Paraspinous muscles may be tender on palpation and in spasm, resulting in limitation of back motion. Finger-to-floor measurements should be done but are more to determine flexibility, which is more closely associated with hip motion than with back mobility. Rotation may be checked with the patient seated. This position fixes the pelvis, limiting pelvic rotation. Chest expansion is measured at the fourth intercostal space in men and below the breasts in women. Patients raise their hands over their head and are asked to take a deep inspiration. Normal expansion is 2.5 cm or greater. Cervical spine evaluation includes measurement of all planes of motion. Peripheral joint examination is also indicated. Careful hip examination is necessary to determine the potential loss of function involved with simultaneous arthritis of the back and hip. Examination of the eyes, heart, lungs, and nervous system may uncover unsuspected extra-articular disease.

Laboratory Data

Laboratory results are nonspecific and add little to the diagnosis of AS. Mild anemia is present in 15% of patients. The erythrocyte sedimentation rate is increased in 80% of patients with active disease. Patients with normal sedimentation rates with active arthritis may have elevated levels of C-reactive protein.[20] Rheumatoid factor and antinuclear antibody are characteristically absent. Histocompatibility testing (for HLA) is positive in 90% of AS patients but is also present in an increased percentage of patients with other spondyloarthropathies (reactive arthritis, psoriatic spondylitis, and spondylitis with inflammatory bowel disease). It is not a diagnostic test for AS. HLA testing may be useful in a young patient with early disease for whom the differential diagnosis may be narrowed by the presence of HLA-B27.

Radiographic Evaluation

Characteristic changes of AS in the sacroiliac joints and lumbosacral spine are helpful in making a diagnosis but may be difficult to determine in the early stages of the disease.[21] The areas of the skeleton most frequently affected include the sacroiliac, apophyseal, discovertebral, and costovertebral joints. The disease affects the sacroiliac joints initially and then appears in the upper lumbar and thoracolumbar areas. Subsequently, in ascending order, the lower lumbar, thoracic, and cervical spine are involved. The radiographic progression of disease may be halted at any stage, although sacroiliitis alone is a rare finding except in some women with spondylitis or in men in the early stage of disease.

Evaluation of the sacroiliac joints is difficult on a conventional anteroposterior supine view of the pelvis because of bony overlap and the oblique orientation of the joint. A Ferguson view of the pelvis (x-ray tube tilted 15 to 30 degrees in a cephalad direction) provides a useful view of the anterior portion of the joint, the initial area of inflammation in sacroiliitis. Radiographic evaluation of the sacroiliac joints is based on five observations: (1) distribution, (2) subchondral mineralization, (3) cystic or erosive bony change, (4) joint width, and (5) osteophyte formation. The symmetry of involvement must be compared with the same areas of the joint (superior-fibrous, inferior-synovial) and with the iliac (thinner cartilage) and sacral (thicker cartilage) sides of the joint.

Sacroiliitis is a bilateral, symmetrical process in AS. During the next stage, the articular space becomes "pseudowidened" secondary to joint surface erosions. With continued inflammation, the area of sclerosis widens and is joined by proliferative bony changes that cross the joint space. In the final stages of sacroiliitis, complete ankylosis with total obliteration of the joint space occurs (Fig. 33–1). Ligamentous structures surrounding the sacroiliac joint may also calcify. The radiographic changes associated with sacroiliitis may be graded from 0 (normal) to 5 (complete ankylosis).

In the lumbar spine, osteitis affecting the anterior corners of vertebral bodies is an early finding. The inflammation associated with osteitis causes loss of the normal concavity of the

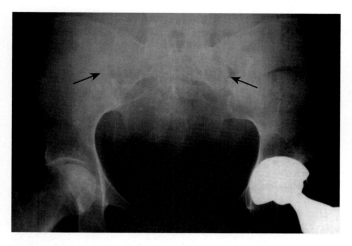

FIGURE 33–1 Ankylosing spondylitis. Anteroposterior view of pelvis of a 38-year-old woman with a 15-year history of ankylosing spondylitis shows bilateral fused sacroiliac joints (*arrows*). She underwent hip replacement because of destructive disease secondary to spondyloarthropathy.

anterior vertebral surface, resulting in a "squared" body (Fig. 33–2).

While osteopenia of the bony structures appears, calcification of disc and ligamentous structures emerges. Thin, vertically oriented calcifications of the anulus fibrosus and anterior and posterior longitudinal ligaments are termed *syndesmophytes*. *Bamboo spine* is the term used to describe the spine of a patient with AS with extensive syndesmophytes encasing the axial skeleton (Fig. 33–3).

The apophyseal joints are also affected in the illness. As the disease progresses, fusion of the apophyseal joints occurs.

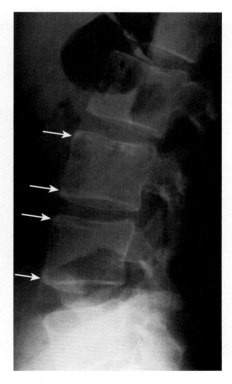

FIGURE 33–2 Ankylosing spondylitis. Lateral view of lumbosacral spine shows "squaring" of all lumbar vertebral bodies (*arrows*).

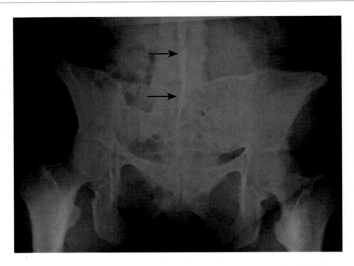

FIGURE 33–3 Ankylosing spondylitis. Anteroposterior view of pelvis of a 64-year-old man with 40 years of ankylosing spondylitis and bamboo spine. Sacroiliac joints are fused, and interspinous ligaments are calcified (*arrows*).

Radiographs of the spine may show the loss of joint space and complete fusion of the joints. Cervical spine ankylosis may be particularly severe (Fig. 33–4). Complete obliteration of articular spaces between the posterior elements of C2-7 results in a column of solid bone. Patients with complete ankylosis of the apophyseal joints and syndesmophytes may develop extensive bony resorption of the anterior surface of the lower cervical vertebrae late in the course of the illness. Bone under the ligaments connecting the spinous processes may also be eroded in the setting of apophyseal joint ankylosis.

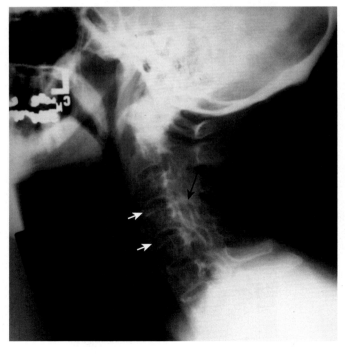

FIGURE 33–4 Ankylosing spondylitis. Lateral view of cervical spine of the patient in Figure 33–3. Radiograph shows anterior syndesmophytes (*white arrows*) and fusion of posterior zygapophyseal joints (*black arrow*).

The C1-2 joints may become eroded and partially dislocated. Synovial tissue around the dens may cause erosion of the odontoid process. Further damage of the surrounding ligaments results in instability that is measured by the movement of the odontoid process from the posterior aspect of the atlas with flexion and extension views of the cervical spine. Widening of the space is indicative of a dynamic subluxation. No movement of the distance between the atlas and axis suggests a fixed subluxation. In addition to atlantoaxial subluxation, migration of the odontoid into the foramen magnum and rotary subluxation may occur. Subaxial subluxation is more characteristic of RA than AS. Computed tomography (CT) detects erosions on both sides of the joint that are frequently missed by plain radiographs.

MRI with fat saturation or contrast medium–enhanced images are able to detect early inflammatory lesions in the sacroiliac joints and the lumbar spine.[22] From a diagnostic and clinical perspective, plain radiographs normally provide adequate information at a reasonable cost. Plain radiographs remain the usual radiographic technique used for the diagnosis of AS. MRI is a good choice for young women with suspected sacroiliitis as a means of decreasing radiographic exposure.

Differential Diagnosis

Two sets of diagnostic criteria exist for AS. The Rome clinical criteria, used in studies of AS, include bilateral sacroiliitis on radiologic examination and low back pain for more than 3 months that is not relieved by rest, pain in the thoracic spine, limited motion in the lumbar spine, and limited chest expansion or iritis. When the Rome criteria proved to lack sensitivity in identifying patients with spondylitis, they were modified at a New York symposium in 1966 (Table 33–1). The modified criteria included a grading system for radiographs of the sacroiliac joints in addition to limited spine motion, chest expansion, and back pain.[23] Although these criteria are used mostly for studies of patient populations, they are helpful in the office setting. The European Spondyloarthropathy Study Group developed a preliminary classification system for spondyloarthropathy in general (Table 33–2).[24]

Although spondyloarthropathies are a common inflammatory musculoskeletal disorder, this group of illnesses is frequently overlooked by nonrheumatologists. A delay in diagnosis from the onset of symptoms and referral to a rheumatologist ranged from 6 to 264 months. Individuals who are misdiagnosed by primary care physicians have mild to moderate disease, with atypical presentations, and are women.[25] The differential diagnosis of spinal pain includes other spondyloarthropathies and herniated intervertebral disc. Characteristics of these specific diseases are listed in Table 33–3. The inflammatory disorders are discussed briefly here.

Psoriatic Arthritis

Patients with psoriasis who develop a characteristic pattern of joint disease have psoriatic arthritis.[26] The prevalence of psoriasis is 1% to 3% of the population. Classic psoriatic arthritis

TABLE 33–1 Diagnostic Criteria for Ankylosing Spondylitis

Rome Criteria

A. Clinical criteria
1. Low back pain and stiffness for >3 mo not relieved by rest
2. Pain and stiffness in thoracic region
3. Limited motion in lumbar spine
4. Limited chest expansion
5. History of evidence of iritis or its sequelae

B. Radiologic criterion
1. Radiograph showing bilateral sacroiliac changes characteristic of ankylosing spondylitis

Diagnosis

Criterion B + 1 clinical criterion or 4 clinical criteria in absence of radiologic sacroiliitis

New York Criteria

A. Clinical criteria
1. Limitation of motion of lumbar spine in anterior flexion, lateral flexion, and extension
2. History of or presence of pain at dorsolumbar junction or in lumbar spine
3. Limitation of chest expansion to ≤1 inch

B. Radiologic criteria (sacroiliitis)

Grade 3: Unequivocal abnormality, moderate or advanced sacroiliitis with one or more erosions, sclerosis, widening, narrowing, or partial ankylosis

Grade 4: Severe abnormality, total ankylosis

Diagnosis

Definite grade 3-4: Bilateral sacroiliitis +1 clinical criterion

Grade 3-4: Unilateral or grade 2 bilateral sacroiliitis with clinical criterion 1 or 2 and 3

Probable grade 3-4: Bilateral sacroiliitis alone

TABLE 33–2 European Spondyloarthropathy Study Group Classification: Criteria for Spondyloarthropathy

Inflammatory spinal pain or synovitis
Asymmetrical
Predominantly in lower extremities

And one of the following:
Positive family history
Psoriasis
Inflammatory bowel disease (sensitivity 77%)
Alternate buttock pain (specificity 89%)
Enthesopathy

Adding:
Sacroiliitis (sensitivity 86%; specificity 87%)

is described as involving distal interphalangeal joints and associated nail disease alone.[27] This pattern occurs in 5% of patients. The most common form of the disease, affecting 70% of patients with psoriatic arthritis, is an asymmetrical oligoarthritis; a few large or small joints are involved. Dactylitis, diffuse swelling of a digit, is most closely associated with this form of the disease. Skin activity and joint symptoms do not correlate, and patients with little skin activity may experience continued joint pain and stiffness.

Psoriatic spondyloarthropathy is found in 5% to 23% of patients with psoriatic arthritis. Patients who develop axial skeletal disease, sacroiliitis, or spondylitis are usually men who have onset of psoriasis later in life. HLA-B27 is more common in individuals with axial disease. Sacroiliac involvement may be unilateral or bilateral. Percussion over the sacroiliac joints can elicit symptoms over the affected side. Patients may

TABLE 33–3 Differential Diagnosis of Ankylosing Spondylitis

	Ankylosing Spondylitis	Reactive Syndrome	Psoriatic Arthritis	Enteropathic Arthritis	Herniated Nucleus Pulposus
Sex	Male	=	=	=	=
Age at onset	15-40	Any age	30-40	15-45	20-40
Presentation	Back pain	GI, GU Infection	Extremity arthritis Psoriasis Back pain	Abdominal pain	Radicular pain
Sacroiliitis	Symmetrical	Symmetrical	Asymmetrical	Symmetrical	–
Axial skeleton	+	±	±	+	–
Peripheral joints	Lower	Lower	Upper	Lower	–
Enthesopathy	+	±	+	–	–
ESR	Elevated	Elevated	Elevated	Elevated	Normal
Rheumatoid factor	–	–	–	–	–
HLA-B27	90%	90%	60%	50%	8%
Course	Continuous	Self-limited	Continuous	Continuous	Episodic or continuous
Therapy	NSAIDs TNF	NSAIDs Antibiotics	NSAIDs Methotrexate	NSAIDs Corticosteroids	NSAIDs Epidural corticosteroids
Disability	Hip	—	Lower extremity	Lower extremity	Neurologic dysfunction

ESR, erythrocyte sedimentation rate; GI, gastrointestinal; GU, genitourinary; NSAIDs, nonsteroidal anti-inflammatory drugs; TNF, tumor necrosis factor.

develop spondylitis in the absence of sacroiliitis, and this has maximal tenderness with percussion over the spine above the sacrum. In the cervical spine, limitation of motion is a primary manifestation of neck involvement.

Spondylitis on radiographs is characterized by asymmetrical involvement of the vertebral bodies and nonmarginal syndesmophytes. Joint ankylosis occurs less commonly than in AS. Of patients, 25% can have sacroiliac involvement manifested by sacroiliitis, which can be unilateral or bilateral. Symmetrical involvement—from side to side and severity of disease—predominates over asymmetrical disease. Sacroiliitis may occur without spondylitis. Spinal disease progression occurs in a random rather than orderly fashion, ascending the spine as commonly noted in AS. Cervical spine disease may occur in the absence of sacroiliitis or lumbar spondylitis. Alterations in the cervical spine include joint space sclerosis and narrowing and anterior ligamentous calcification (Fig. 33–5).

Treatment of psoriatic arthritis is similar to treatment of RA. Immunosuppressive agents and TNF-α inhibitors are indicated for the treatment of peripheral arthritis.[28] The benefits for axial disease are being studied. Patients with psoriatic arthritis develop varying degrees of restriction of spinal motion. There is no consistent correlation between the severity of peripheral joint and axial skeletal disease. Rarely, patients with psoriatic arthritis may develop atlantoaxial subluxation with evidence of cervical myelopathy. Fracture after minor trauma may be overlooked for an extended period.[29] This disease should be treated early and aggressively.[30]

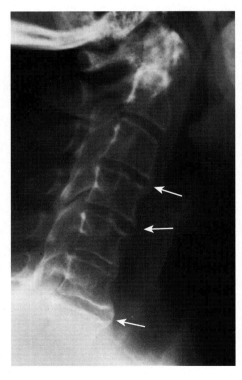

FIGURE 33–5 Psoriatic arthritis. Lateral view of cervical spine of a 45-year-old woman with psoriasis shows anterior syndesmophytes at levels C3-4, C4-5, and C6-7 (*arrows*).

Reactive Arthritis

Reactive arthritis is associated with an infectious agent causing an aseptic inflammation in joints and other organs. This disorder has been associated with the triad of urethritis (inflammation of the lower urinary tract), arthritis, and conjunctivitis formerly referred to as *Reiter syndrome,* a form of reactive arthritis. Reactive arthritis is the most common cause of arthritis in young men and primarily affects the lower extremity joints and the low back. Involvement of the cervical spine is rare. The disease results from the interaction of an environmental factor, usually a specific infection, and a genetically predisposed host. Approximately 1% of patients with the common infection nongonococcal urethritis develop the syndrome. Other authors suggest that 3% of individuals with nonspecific urethritis develop reactive arthritis. The syndrome develops in 0.2% to 15% of all patients with enteric infections secondary to *Shigella, Salmonella, Campylobacter,* and *Yersinia.* The male-to-female ratio in venereal infection is 10:1, and the ratio is 1:1 in large outbreaks secondary to enteric infection.

Reactive arthritis is associated with HLA-B27 in 60% to 80% of individuals. The classic patient with reactive arthritis is a young man about 25 years old who develops urethritis and a mild conjunctivitis, followed by the onset of a predominantly lower extremity oligoarthritis. The conjunctivitis is usually mild and is manifested by an erythema (redness) and crusting of the lids. Arthritis may occur 1 to 3 weeks after the initial infection. In many patients, arthritis is the only manifestation of disease.[31] Back pain is a frequent symptom of patients with reactive arthritis. During the acute course, 31% to 92% of patients may develop pain in the lumbosacral region. Occasionally, the pain radiates into the posterior thighs but rarely below the knees; it may be unilateral. This finding corresponds to the asymmetrical involvement of the sacroiliac joints and is in contrast to the symmetrical involvement of AS.[32] Spondylitis affecting the lumbar, thoracic, and cervical spine occurs less commonly than sacroiliitis, with 23% of patients with severe disease showing such involvement.[33] Neck pain is a rare symptom of patients with reactive arthritis. Constitutional symptoms occur in about one third of patients and include fever, anorexia, weight loss, and fatigue.

On examination, men tend to have involvement in the knees, ankles, and feet, and women have more upper extremity disease. Percussion tenderness over the sacroiliac joints may be unilateral, correlating with asymmetrical involvement in reactive arthritis. The mobility of the lumbosacral and cervical spine should be measured in all planes of motion. Evaluation for enthesopathy, heel pain, or Achilles tendon tenderness is also required.

Sacroiliac involvement may mimic AS (symmetrical disease) or may be asymmetrical in severity of joint changes. Unilateral sacroiliac disease occurs early in the disease process. Variable amounts of sclerosis are associated with erosions. The progression of radiographic changes shows widening of the joint (erosion), then narrowing (fusion). Fusion of the joints occurs less frequently than in AS. Sacroiliitis may be detected in 5% to 10% of individuals early in the illness and in 60% in prolonged illness. Spondylitis is discontinuous in its involvement of the axial skeleton (skip lesions) and is characterized by nonmarginal bony bridging of vertebral bodies. These vertebral hyperostoses are markedly thickened compared with the thin syndesmophytes of AS. Cervical spine disease is associated with hyperostoses at the anteroinferior corners of one or more cervical vertebrae.

The joint and enthesopathic manifestations of reactive arthritis seem to respond better to newer NSAIDs than to aspirin. The drugs are continued as long as the patient remains symptomatic. Oral corticosteroids are less effective in this polyarthritis compared with RA. The role of antibiotic therapy in the acute phase of reactive arthritis is controversial. Antibiotics may be ineffective for *Chlamydia*-associated reactive arthritis.[34] Sulfasalazine has been reported to improve spinal pain and swollen joints in patients with reactive arthritis. The usual dose of sulfasalazine is 2 g/day in divided doses. The immunosuppressive methotrexate is reserved for patients with uncontrolled progression of joint disease and unresponsive, extensive skin involvement. The dose of methotrexate ranges from 7.5 to 25 mg/wk.

The course of the illness is unpredictable. A self-limited illness, lasting 3 months to 1 year, occurs in 30% to 40% of patients. Another 30% to 50% develop a relapsing pattern of illness with periods of complete remission. The final 10% to 25% develop chronic, unremitting disease associated with significant disability.

Enteropathic Arthritis

Ulcerative colitis and Crohn disease are inflammatory bowel diseases. Ulcerative colitis is limited to the colon; Crohn disease, or regional enteritis, may involve any part of the gastrointestinal tract.[35] Inflammation of the gut results in numerous gastrointestinal symptoms, including abdominal pain, fever, and weight loss. These inflammatory diseases are also associated with extraintestinal manifestations, including arthritis. Articular involvement in inflammatory bowel disease includes peripheral and axial skeleton joints. Peripheral arthritis is generally nondeforming and follows the activity of the underlying bowel disease.[36] Axial skeleton disease is similar to AS and follows a course independent of activity of bowel inflammation.

Symptomatic ulcerative colitis usually occurs in adults 25 to 45 years old, and the disease is more common among women than men. Crohn disease occurs in all races and is distributed worldwide. In the United States, the annual incidence of the disease is 4 per 100,000. The disease occurs most often in individuals 15 to 35 years old. Men and women are equally affected. The frequency of peripheral arthritis is 11% in ulcerative colitis and 20% in Crohn disease. Spondylitis occurs in 3% to 4% of both diseases, and radiographic sacroiliitis occurs in 10%. Axial arthritis of inflammatory bowel disease may be a hereditary accompaniment of the disease and not a manifestation of activity of bowel disease itself. Non–HLA-related factors and HLA-B27 may play a role.

Early symptoms of ulcerative colitis are frequent bowel movements with blood or mucus. Mild disease is associated

with some abdominal pain and a few bowel movements per day. Severe disease is characterized by fatigue, weight loss, fever, and extracolonic involvement. Crohn disease is frequently an indolent illness characterized by generalized fatigue, mild nonbloody diarrhea, anorexia, weight loss, and cramping lower abdominal pain. Patients may have symptoms for years before the diagnosis is made.

Articular involvement in inflammatory bowel disease is divided into two forms: peripheral and spondylitic. Axial skeleton involvement in ulcerative colitis and Crohn disease is similar. Spondylitis antedates bowel disease in about one third of patients. This interval may be 10 to 20 years. Of patients, 70% are HLA-B27 positive, 68% have radiographic changes of spondylitis, and 25% have iritis. The spondylitis of inflammatory bowel disease has a course totally independent of the course of the bowel disease. The clinical and radiographic findings are similar to findings of AS, including involvement of shoulders and hips.

Patients with spondyloarthropathy may have decreased motion of the spine in all planes and percussion tenderness over the sacroiliac joints. Rarely, chest expansion is diminished. Patients with more extensive disease have limitation of motion of the cervical spine. Occiput-to-wall measurements document the immobility of the entire axial skeleton, including the cervical spine.

The radiographic changes of spondylitis in inflammatory bowel disease are indistinguishable from classic AS (Fig. 33–6). Findings include squaring of vertebral bodies; erosions; widening and fusion of the sacroiliac joints; symmetrical involvement of sacroiliac joints; and marginal syndesmophytes involving the lumbar, thoracic, or cervical spine.

The factors that help make the diagnosis of enteropathic spondyloarthropathy are the pattern of peripheral arthritis if present (upper extremity disease is uncommon in AS and reactive arthritis; bilateral ankle arthritis is uncommon in psoriatic disease), erythema nodosum, and iritis. Therapy for enteropathic spondylitis is similar to therapy for classic AS. TNF-α inhibitors are effective agents for the bowel and articular disease.[37]

The ultimate course and outcome of these patients depend on the severity of bowel disease. Patients with severe ulcerative colitis have a mortality rate of 10% to 20% over 5 years. Patients with a severe initial attack, continuous clinical activity, involvement of the entire colon, and disease for 10 years or longer have a higher risk of developing cancer of the colon. These patients may require colectomy. Although Crohn disease is associated with frequent recurrences, the overall mortality rate of 5% for the first 5 years of disease is much less than in ulcerative colitis.

Diffuse Idiopathic Skeletal Hyperostosis

Diffuse idiopathic skeletal hyperostosis (DISH) is another disease that may occur in the setting of spondylitis. Patients with AS and DISH should be easily differentiated by careful radiographic evaluation.[38] DISH may cause alterations of the sacroiliac joints.[39] CT of the sacroiliac joints differentiates the hyperostotic joint changes from changes associated with joint

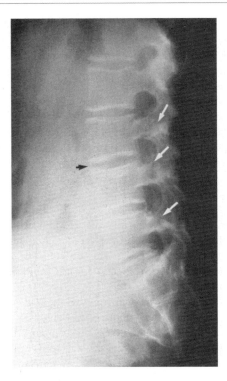

FIGURE 33–6 Enteropathic spondylitis: a lateral view of the lumbar spine demonstrates loss of lumbar lordosis, fusion of the facet joints (*white arrows*), and early syndesmophyte formation (*black arrow*) in the 25-year-old woman with a 9-year history of Crohn's disease. (From Borenstein DG, Weisel SW, Boden SD: Low Back and Neck Pain: Comprehensive Diagnosis and Management, ed 3. Philadelphia, Saunders, 2004.

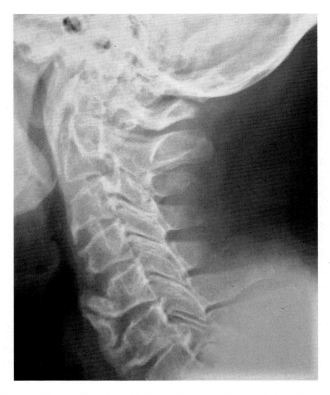

FIGURE 33–7 Diffuse idiopathic skeletal hyperostosis. Lateral view of cervical spine shows large anterior, horizontally oriented osteophytes characteristic of this illness.

erosion and fusion (Fig. 33–7). Also of note is the occurrence of fracture in patients with DISH and patients with AS. The convergence of two common diseases in the same host, a middle-aged man, is likely. The occurrence of AS and DISH of the cervical spine has been reported.[40]

Treatment

The goals of therapy for AS, as with other forms of inflammatory arthritis, are to control pain and stiffness, reduce inflammation, maintain function, and prevent deformity with avoidance of undue toxicity. Patients require a comprehensive program of education, physiotherapy, medications, and other measures. Patients are taught proper posture and mobilizing and breathing exercises to prevent the tendency to stoop forward and lose chest motion. The importance of a firm upright chair for sitting and a hard mattress with no pillows for sleeping is stressed. Physical therapy with range of motion exercises may improve neck movement. Use of braces, splints, and corsets should be avoided.

Nonsteroidal Anti-inflammatory Drugs

Medications to control pain and inflammation are useful to patients with AS. NSAIDs possess antipyretic, analgesic, and anti-inflammatory characteristics. They are anti-inflammatory and analgesic when given long-term in larger doses. Table 33–4 lists NSAIDs currently available for the treatment of spinal disorders. NSAIDs are effective at decreasing pain and improving movement but have not been proven to slow the progression of disease. The benefits of NSAIDs must be balanced against potential toxicities.[41]

Cyclooxygenase Inhibitors

COX-2 inhibitors are a class of NSAIDs that have efficacy equal to COX-1 inhibitors (aspirin, naproxen) with less gastrointestinal toxicity (see Table 33–4). The cardiovascular risk associated with these agents is an active area of research. COX-2 inhibitors should be considered for individuals with increased risks of gastrointestinal bleeding, exclusively. COX-2 inhibitors are effective in osteoarthritis and RA. AS patients were reported to be responsive to celecoxib, a COX-2 inhibitor, in a 6-week controlled study.[42]

Muscle Relaxants

Patients with acute AS may develop severe muscle spasm with associated limited motion that may hinder their return to normal daily activities. In these patients, the addition of muscle relaxant to NSAID helps decrease muscle pain and muscle spasm and improve back motion. Muscle relaxants, such as cyclobenzaprine, at low dosages (5 to 10 mg/day) are helpful while limiting possible drug toxicity. The sleepiness associated with muscle relaxants with long half-lives can be limited by giving the medication 2 hours before bedtime.

TABLE 33–4 Nonsteroidal Anti-inflammatory Drugs*

Drug (Chemical Class)	Trade Name	Size (mg)	Maximum Dose (mg/day)	Frequency (×/day)
Salicylates				
Aspirin	Bayer	81, 325	5200	4-6
Enteric-coated	Ecotrin	325	5200	4-6
Time-release	ZORprin	800	3200	2
Substituted Salicylates				
Diflunisal	Dolobid	250/500	1500	2-3
Salsalate	Disalcid	500/750	3000	2
Choline magnesium trisalicylate	Trilisate	500/750	3000	2
Propionic Acid				
Ibuprofen	Motrin	200, 400, 600, 800	4800	4-6
Naproxen	Naprelan	375, 500	1500	2-3
Ketoprofen	Orudis	50, 75	300	3-4
Extended-release	Oruvail	200		1
Flurbiprofen	Ansaid	50, 100	300	2-3
Oxaprozin	Daypro	600	1800	1-2
Pyrole Acetic Acid				
Sulindac	Clinoril	150, 200	450	2-3
Tolmetin	Tolectin	200, 400, 600	1600	4
Indomethacin	Indocin	25, 50, 75	225	1-3
Benzeneacetic Acid				
Diclofenac sodium	Voltaren	25, 50, 75, 100SR	225	2-3
Diclofenac/misoprostol	Arthrotec	50/75	225	2-3
Oxicam				
Piroxicam	Feldene	10, 20	20	1
Meloxicam	Mobic	7.5, 15	15	1
Pyranocarboxylic Acid				
Etodolac	Lodine	200, 300, 400XL, 500XL	1600	2-4
Meclofenamate	Meclomen	50, 100	400	4
Pyrrolopyrrole				
Ketorolac	Toradol	10	40	4
Naphthylalkanone				
Nabumetone	Relafen	500, 750	2000	2
Cyclooxygenase-2 Inhibitors				
Celecoxib	Celebrex	100, 200, 400	800	2

*Partial list.

Corticosteroids

Systemic corticosteroids are rarely needed and are ineffective for the spinal articular disease of AS. For the occasional patient with continued joint symptoms, adding small doses of corticosteroids (prednisone, 5 mg/day) to maximum doses of NSAIDs may prove to be useful. Larger doses of corticosteroids cause appreciably more toxicity without an increased benefit.

Anti–Tumor Necrosis Factor-α Inhibitors

TNF-α, an inflammatory cytokine, is associated with the inflammatory process that results in the phenotypic expression of AS. Anti–TNF-α therapies are available in the form of infliximab, etanercept, and adalimumab, which inhibit the inflammatory effects of TNF-α. Infusion of intravenous infliximab, 5 mg/kg at 0, 2, and 6 weeks, in a placebo-controlled trial resulted in improvement in axial symptoms and signs, enthesitis, and peripheral arthritis.[43] Open-label extensions of studies for 54 weeks have documented persistent improvement with infliximab infusions at 6-week intervals.[44] In a placebo-controlled, 4-month study of 40 AS patients taking 25 mg of etanercept, 80% of patients receiving the active drug experienced an improvement in morning stiffness, enthesitis, quality of life, erythrocyte sedimentation rate, or C-reactive protein.[45]

The U.S. Food and Drug Administration (FDA) has approved etanercept, 25 mg twice a week, for the treatment of AS. Repeated infusions of infliximab remain effective in AS over a 12-month period.[46] The full benefits of anti–TNF-α therapy in AS remain to be determined. The efficacy of these agents in disease of long duration is less certain. These agents are expensive, and their availability is limited. Toxicities are associated with their use, including the activation of latent tuberculosis.

Prognosis

The general course of AS is benign and is characterized by exacerbations and remissions. Many patients with AS may have sacroiliitis with mild involvement of the lumbosacral spine. Limitation of lumbosacral motion may be mild. The disease can become quiescent at any time. Patients who go on to develop total fusion of the spine may feel better because ankylosis of the spinal joints is associated with decreased pain. In a study of 1492 patients for 2 years, the frequency of patients with a total remission of disease was less than 2%.[47]

Rheumatoid Arthritis

RA is a chronic, systemic, inflammatory disease that causes pain, heat, swelling, and destruction in synovial joints. The joints characteristically affected by RA are small joints of the hands and feet, wrists, elbows, hips, knees, ankles, and cervical spine. Most patients with RA have cervical spine disease manifested as neck pain, headaches, or arm numbness. Signs of cervical spine disease include decreased neck motion with stiffness; undue prominence of the spinous process of the axis (C2); and neurologic dysfunction, including paresthesias, spasticity, incontinence, and quadriplegia. The diagnosis of RA is made in the setting of a history of persistent joint inflammation in the appropriate joints and the presence of specific serum antibodies (rheumatoid factor). The degree of cervical spine destruction in RA does not always correlate with patient complaints and is detected by radiographic evaluation. RA of the cervical spine responds to the same therapy that is effective for the peripheral joints. Surgical intervention with stabilization of the cervical spine is required for persistent neurologic abnormalities.

Epidemiology

The prevalence of RA is 1% to 3% of the U.S. population.[1] RA is found in all racial and ethnic groups. The condition occurs in all age groups but is most common in adults 40 to 70 years old.[48] The male-to-female ratio is approximately 1:3. Symptoms of cervical spine disease occur in 40% to 80% of RA patients. Radiographic evidence of cervical spine involvement is found in 86% of RA patients, whereas neurologic symptoms from cervical spine disease occur less frequently in 10% of patients with radiographic changes. Cervical spine disease usually occurs in the setting of active peripheral disease; however, occasionally neck symptoms may be the initial or predominant symptom without clinical signs of RA in other locations. The lumbar spine is rarely involved in the rheumatoid process. One study suggested that 5% of men and 3% of women with RA have lumbar spine involvement.[49]

Pathogenesis

RA is a chronic immune-mediated disease whose initiation and perpetuation are dependent on T lymphocyte response to unknown antigens.[50] Increased numbers of CD4$^+$ lymphocytes that activate B lymphocytes to produce immunoglobulin are frequently found in synovium from RA patients. The activation of macrophages results in the production of monokines, including TNF-α, and interleukin-1. These factors attract additional lymphocytes and neutrophils. Angiogenesis factors result in the growth of new capillaries. Synovial cells cause tissue destruction by release of activated metalloproteinases, including procollagenase and progelatinase. The inflammatory response is also enhanced by the production of arachidonic acid metabolites.

Cervical Subluxation

In the cervical spine, the structures lined with synovial membrane may be involved in RA. These structures include the atlantoaxial joint. This joint connects the atlas (C1) with the axis (C2) and is responsible for rotation of the skull on the cervical spine. Synovial tissue is located between the atlas and axis and between the ligaments and atlas. Other synovial joints include the zygapophyseal and uncovertebral joints.

RA causes disease in the cervical spine by causing chronic inflammatory changes to occur in the atlanto-occipital, atlantoaxial, zygapophyseal, and uncovertebral joints along with the discs and ligamentous and bursal structures. At the level of the atlantoaxial joint, synovial inflammation of the bursae and ligaments results in laxity of the transverse ligament that holds the atlas and axis together. Normally, the distance between the bones does not exceed 2.5 to 3 mm in adults. The relaxation of supporting ligaments results in excess motion of the axis in relation to the atlas-atlantoaxial subluxation.

Luxation of the atlantoaxial joint may occur anteriorly, posteriorly, superiorly or vertically, or laterally. Anterior subluxation is the most common form and results from insufficiency of the transverse ligament or fracture of the odontoid and occurs in 49% of patients.[51] Posterior subluxation occurs when C1 moves posteriorly on C2 and results from erosion or fracture of the odontoid and occurs in 7% of patients. Vertical or superior subluxation results from destruction of the lateral atlantoaxial joints around the foramen magnum and is found in 38% of patients. Lateral subluxation occurs in 20% with erosion of the lateral mass and odontoid. Abnormal motion of this joint in any direction may result in compression of the cervical spinal cord or medulla oblongata, resulting in the development of neurologic symptoms and signs of myelopathy, including paresthesias, muscle weakness, reflex changes, spasticity, and incontinence. Subluxation of the atlantoaxial joint by the odontoid process of the axis and the posterior arch of the atlas may compress the vertebral arteries. The vertebral arteries are compressed as they travel through the foramina in the transverse processes of C1 and C2. Vertebral artery compression may cause tetraplegia, coma, or sudden death.[52]

Subluxation may occur between cervical vertebrae below the atlantoaxial joint. Common levels include C3-4 and C4-5. Inflammation in the zygapophyseal joints and surrounding bursae undermines the stability of these joints, resulting in excessive motion and angulation of the cervical spine.[53] Intervertebral discs may be invaded by growing synovial tissue, resulting in disc space narrowing. The reported frequency of subaxial subluxation ranges from 7% to 29% of RA patients.[54]

Myelopathy may also occur in patients without atlantoaxial or cervical spine subluxation. In these patients, synovitis from the zygapophyseal joints along with intervertebral disc lesions may compromise the blood supply to the spinal cord through stenosis of vertebral vessels that feed the anterior spinal artery. Ischemic myelopathy is the result. Sudden death may also be a consequence of thrombosis of vertebral vessels.[55]

Clinical History

Patients with RA develop joint pain, heat, swelling, and tenderness. The joint involvement is additive and symmetrical. The joints at greatest risk of being affected by the disease process include the proximal interphalangeal, metacarpocarpal, wrist, elbow, hip, knee, ankle, and metatarsophalangeal joints. In the axial skeleton, the cervical spine is most frequently affected. Patients have joint pain and stiffness, which are most severe in the morning. Activity improves symptoms. The phenomenon of stiffness of a joint with rest occurs frequently with active disease. As a component of systemic inflammation, afternoon fatigue, anorexia, and weight loss are common complaints.

Neck movement frequently precipitates or aggravates neck pain that is aching and deep in quality. Atlantoaxial disease is experienced in the upper part of the cervical spine, and pain radiates over the occiput into the temporal and frontal regions with increasing disease of the C1-2 joint. Occipital headaches are frequently associated with active rheumatoid involvement of the cervical spine. Other symptoms of C1-2 subluxation include a sensation of the head falling forward with flexion of the neck, loss of consciousness or syncope, incontinence, dysphagia, vertigo, convulsions, hemiplegia, dysarthria, nystagmus, or peripheral paresthesias.[56] Peripheral joint erosion is a harbinger of C1-2 subluxation. Development of cervical subluxation occurs in patients who have joint erosions of hands and feet, serum rheumatoid factor, and subcutaneous nodules.

Pain associated with RA in the subaxial segments of the cervical spine is located in the lateral aspects of the neck and clavicles (C3-4) and over the shoulders (C5-6). Neurologic symptoms include paresthesias and numbness. Paresthesias have a burning quality that may be attributed to an entrapment neuropathy (carpal tunnel syndrome) but is sufficiently different not to be confused with joint pain. Patients with sensory symptoms alone may have their symptoms ascribed to arthritis, delaying the diagnosis of cervical myelopathy.[52]

The appearance of spasticity, gait disturbance, muscular weakness, and incontinence (urinary or rectal) indicates significant compression of the spinal cord. Symptoms suggesting vertebrobasilar artery insufficiency include visual disturbances, dizziness, paresthesias of the face, ataxia, and dysarthria.

Physical Examination

Physical examination of a patient with RA with cervical spine disease reveals diffuse peripheral joint involvement characterized by heat, swelling, bogginess, tenderness, and loss of motion. Nodules over the extensor surfaces are noted in 20% of RA patients. Examination of the cervical spine may show tenderness with palpation over the bony skeleton and limitation of all spinal movements. Inspection may show fixation of the head tilted down and to one side. This lateral tilt is caused by the asymmetrical destruction of the lateral atlantoaxial joints. Normal cervical lordosis may also be absent. With the neck flexed, the spinous process of the axis may be prominent in the midline of the neck of a patient with atlantoaxial subluxation. Patients with subaxial subluxation may show abnormalities in the upper extremities. Compression of C6-8 segments causes distinctive numb, clumsy hands and tactile agnosia.[57] Neurologic abnormalities are seen in approximately 7% of RA patients.

Laboratory Data

Abnormal laboratory findings include anemia, elevated erythrocyte sedimentation rate, and increases in serum globulin levels. Thrombocytosis is found in patients with active RA. Rheumatoid factors (antibodies directed against host antibodies) are present in 80% of patients with RA. Antinuclear antibodies are present in 30% of RA patients. C-reactive protein, an acute-phase reactant, may be helpful when obtained in a serial manner to predict individuals who are at increased risk for joint deterioration and as a measure of response to therapy. Individuals with persistent elevations in C-reactive protein are at risk of progressive cervical spine subluxations.[58] Synovial fluid analysis shows inflammatory fluid characterized by poor viscosity, increased numbers of white blood cells, decreased glucose level, and increased protein level.

Radiographic Evaluation

Characteristic radiographic changes of RA in peripheral joints include soft tissue swelling, bony erosion without reactive sclerotic bone, joint space narrowing, and periarticular osteopenia. Radiographic evaluation of the cervical spine includes anteroposterior, lateral with flexion and extension, oblique, and open-mouth frontal projections.

The radiographic criteria for the diagnosis of RA cervical spine disease as proposed by Bland and colleagues[59] are (1) atlantoaxial subluxation of 2.5 mm or more; (2) multiple subluxation of C2-3, C3-4, C4-5, and C5-6; (3) narrow disc spaces with little or no osteophytosis; (4) erosion of vertebrae, especially vertebral plates; (5) odontoid, small, pointed, eroded loss of cortex; (6) basilar impression; (7) apophyseal joint erosion and blurred facets; (8) cervical spine osteoporosis; (9) wide space (>5 mm) between posterior arch of the atlas and spinous process of the axis (flexion to extension); and (10) secondary osteosclerosis, atlantoaxial occipital complex, which may indicate local degenerative change. The normal distance between the odontoid and atlas is 2.5 mm in women and 3 mm in men as measured from the posteroinferior aspect of the tubercle of C1 to the nearest point on the odontoid (Fig. 33–8).[60] The posterior atlanto-odontoid interval is the remaining distance between the posterior surface of the odontoid process and the anterior edge of the posterior ring of the atlas. RA patients with a posterior interval of more than 14 mm did not have neurologic deficits. Posterior subluxation may also occur if the atlas "jumps" over the axis, resting in a dorsal position resulting in posterior subluxation. Vertebrobasilar

artery insufficiency associated with neurologic dysfunction is a manifestation of this form of subluxation.

Upward translocation occurs when the bony and ligamentous integrity of the atlanto-occipital articulations is disrupted. Disease of the occipital condyles, lateral masses of the atlas, and lateral articulations of the axis results in bony erosions or collapse. Erosion of the lateral apophyseal joints allows for a rotational head tilt. The open-mouth view may show narrowing of the atlanto-occipital and atlantoaxial joints and erosion of the odontoid. Subluxation occurs when the lateral masses of the atlas are displaced more than 2 mm with respect to masses of the axis. Bony erosion is the most important factor in the development of severe lateral subluxation.

In addition to changes in the upper cervical spine, radiographic abnormalities, including subaxial subluxation, apophyseal joint narrowing, and disc space narrowing, occur in the lower cervical spine. Subaxial subluxation is present in instances of malalignment of more than 3.5 mm. The stability of flexion and extension of the lower cervical spine depends on the integrity of the anterior and posterior longitudinal ligaments. Greater than 3.5 mm of malalignment is indicative of a mechanically unstable spine. Multiple subluxations may occur, producing a "staircase" appearance on lateral radiographs. Anterior subluxation is more frequent than posterior subluxation. Subaxial subluxation is most notable on a lateral flexion view of the cervical spine (Fig. 33–9). Apophyseal joint disease includes narrowing, erosions, and sclerosis. Disc destruction in the cervical spine is associated with disc space narrowing and is caused by extension of erosive disease from

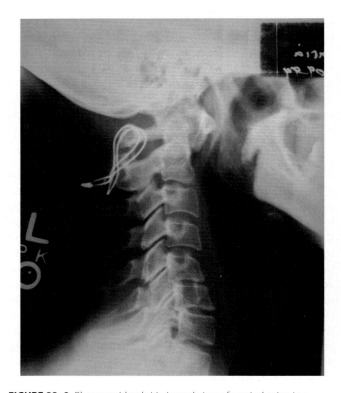

FIGURE 33–8 Rheumatoid arthritis. Lateral view of cervical spine in a 56-year-old woman with more than 20 years of disease. She developed increasing neck pain and dysesthesias in the arms. She had significant dynamic subluxations. C1-2 spinous processes were wired together, and she has had resolution of her symptoms for the subsequent 5 years. (From Borenstein DG, Wiesel SW, Boden SD: Low Back and Neck Pain: Comprehensive Diagnosis and Management, 3rd ed. Philadelphia, Elsevier, 2004.)

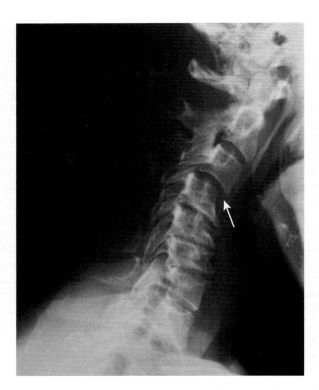

FIGURE 33–9 Rheumatoid arthritis. Lateral view of flexed cervical spine of a 45-year-old woman with 15 years of disease. She has neck and shoulder pain. The neck has anterior subluxation at C3-4 (*arrow*). Cervical lordosis is reversed.

uncovertebral joints or by ongoing trauma to vertebral end-plates secondary to instability. The final stage of apophyseal disease is fibrous ankylosis of one or more levels, which may rarely simulate the appearance of AS.

CT is a useful imaging technique for detecting the extent of bony destruction of structures that may not be easily visualized with plain radiographs. CT detects the position of an eroded odontoid process that may not be seen on open-mouth view radiographs.

MRI is a noninvasive method that is useful in detecting soft tissue abnormalities in the cervical spine of RA patients. It is able to detect pannus around the odontoid and alterations in the substance of the spinal cord. MRI may also be useful in documenting the response of pannus to therapy or the status of the spinal cord in the postoperative state. Compared with CT and plain radiographs, MRI with plain radiographs shows lytic lesions and odontoid erosions and vertical atlantoaxial subluxations more often, shows anterior subluxations as often, and shows lateral subluxations less often.[61]

Differential Diagnosis

RA is a clinical diagnosis based on history of joint pain, distribution of joint involvement, and characteristic laboratory abnormalities (rheumatoid factor). Criteria for the classification of RA were published by the American College of Rheumatology (Table 33–5).[62] In the setting of generalized, active disease, the finding of neck pain associated with multiple abnormalities, including atlantoaxial subluxation, apophyseal joint erosion without sclerosis, disc space narrowing without osteophytes, and multiple subluxations, is most appropriately attributed to RA. The cervical spine abnormalities of AS, psoriatic arthritis, reactive arthritis, enteropathic arthritis, osteoarthritis, and DISH are associated with new bone formation or ligamentous calcification that differentiate them from RA. Occasionally, atlantoaxial subluxation may occur alone in the setting of little peripheral disease. In those circumstances, other disease processes that may cause subluxation include AS, psoriatic arthritis, reactive arthritis, trauma, or local infection.

Treatment

The treatment of RA has undergone a paradigm shift with the advent of new drug therapies directed at control of the factors that mediate the immunologic destruction of joints.[48,63] The previous approach involved an initial conservative approach with few medications prescribed until definite erosions were documented. The treatment for control of generalized RA included a regimen of patient education, physical therapy, NSAIDs, remittive agents (gold, salts, penicillamine, or hydroxychloroquine), corticosteroids, and immunosuppressive agents (methotrexate). The therapy has been organized into a therapeutic pyramid based on the use of less toxic therapies for all patients. Drugs of greater toxicity were added with increasing clinical activity of disease.

A reassessment of the treatment regimen was proposed when additional therapies became available.[64] This regimen

TABLE 33–5 American Rheumatism Association 1987 Revised Criteria for Classification of Rheumatoid Arthritis*

1. Morning stiffness	Morning stiffness in and around joints, lasting at least 1 hr before maximal improvement
2. Arthritis of three or more joint areas	At least 3 joint areas simultaneously have soft tissue swelling or fluid (not bony overgrowth)
3. Arthritis of hand	At least 1 area swollen (as defined above) in a wrist, metacarpophalangeal, or proximal interphalangeal joint
4. Symmetrical arthritis	Simultaneous involvement of proximal interphalangeal, metacarpophalangeal, or metatarsophalangeal joints is acceptable without absolute symmetry
5. Rheumatoid nodules	Subcutaneous nodules, over bony prominences, extensor surfaces, or juxta-articular regions, observed by a physician
6. Serum rheumatoid factor	Demonstration of abnormal amounts of serum rheumatoid factor by any method for which result has been positive in <5% of normal control subjects
7. Radiographic changes	Radiographic change typical of rheumatoid arthritis on posteroanterior hand and wrist radiographs, which must include erosions or unequivocal bony decalcification localized in or most marked adjacent to involved joints (osteoarthritis changes alone do not qualify)

*For classification purposes, a patient is said to have rheumatoid arthritis if the patient has satisfied at least 4 of 7 criteria. Criteria 1 through 4 must have been present for at least 6 wk. Patients with 2 clinical diagnoses are not excluded. Designation as classic, definite, or probable rheumatoid arthritis is not made.
From Arnett FC, Edworthy SM, Block DA, et al: The American Rheumatism Association 1987 revised criteria for the classification of rheumatoid arthritis. Arthritis Rheum 31:315, 1988.

initiated therapy with a multitude of drugs of increased toxicity compared with NSAIDs, with the proposition that the increased morbidity and mortality rates of RA require aggressive initial therapy. The difficulty was the absence of new medicines to control the disorder better. The advent of new agents has offered the opportunity to be more aggressive in preventing lesions before disability occurs.

The American College of Rheumatology has reviewed the available therapies and has proposed new options for the treatment of RA.[65] These new guidelines include data supporting the use of biologic agents in the therapy for RA.

Nonsteroidal Anti-inflammatory Drugs

Medications to control pain and inflammation are useful in patients with RA (see Table 33–4). The choice of agent depends on numerous factors, including drug half-life, formulation, dose range, and tolerability. COX-2 inhibitors are a class of NSAIDs that have efficacy equal to COX-1 inhibitors (aspirin, naproxen) with less gastrointestinal toxicity. COX-2 inhibitors are effective in RA and are associated with fewer gastrointestinal toxicities.[66,67] These agents should be limited to RA

TABLE 33-6 Disease-Modifying Antirheumatic Drugs

Drug	Size (mg)	Dose (mg)	Toxicities	Comment
Hydroxychloroquine	200	200-400	Retinopathy	Requires 6 mo to work
Sulfasalazine	500	1000-2000	Gastrointestinal, anemia	Sulfa allergy
Methotrexate	2.5, 5, 7.5	5-25	Hepatitis, anemia	Requires 6 wk to work
Azathioprine	50	50-300	Hepatitis, leukopenia	Requires 3 mo to work
Leflunomide	10, 20, 100	20	Diarrhea, alopecia	100 × 3 initially; onset at 4 wk
Etanercept (IM) 25	25, 50	50	Injection pain, infections	Requires 6 wk to work
Infliximab (IV)	100	3-5 mg/kg	Nausea, infections	Best with methotrexate
Adalimumab (IM)	40	40 q 2 wk	Nausea, infections	Requires 6 wk to work
Anakinra (IM)	100	100	Injection pain, infections	Best with methotrexate

IM, intramuscular; IV, intravascular.

patients with increased risk of gastrointestinal bleeding until the degree of cardiovascular risk is quantified.

Disease-Modifying Antirheumatic Drugs

Patients who continue to have joint inflammation or who exhibit joint damage (joint space narrowing, bony erosions, or cysts) despite adequate NSAID therapy are candidates for remittive therapy. Remittive agents have a delayed onset of action compared with NSAIDs. Table 33–6 lists DMARDs used for the treatment of RA. Methotrexate at doses of 7.5 to 25 mg/wk is effective in decreasing the inflammation of RA and may slow disease progression. Methotrexate may be given all at once during the week. It is effective over a long duration of therapy.

Leflunomide is an oral pyrimidine inhibitor used to treat RA.[68] The dose is 100 mg for 3 days, than 20 mg or 10 mg daily as tolerated. Toxicities include abnormal liver function tests and diarrhea. Leflunomide and methotrexate can be used together. These patients need to be monitored closely for potential hepatotoxicity.[48]

Systemic corticosteroids are effective in controlling the inflammatory components of RA. Corticosteroids are the most powerful and predictable remedy inducing immediate relief of joint inflammation in RA. Corticosteroids at low doses (5 to 10 mg) have a modest effect on reducing the rate of radiologically detected joint destruction. A prospective trial showed disease-modifying properties of 10 mg of prednisone over a 2-year period.[69] Corticosteroids are also associated with a wide range of toxicities, from hypertension and diabetes to cataracts and obesity.

Anti–Tumor Necrosis Factor-α Inhibitors

Infliximab, etanercept, and adalimumab inhibit the inflammatory effects of TNF-α and are efficacious in the treatment of RA. Infliximab is partly humanized mouse monoclonal antibody directed against TNF-α. It is administered intravenously. Infliximab is added to methotrexate to limit the production of neutralizing antibodies to the mouse component of the agent. In a 30-week trial, combined infliximab and methotrexate was more effective than methotrexate alone in patients with active RA.[70] In a 54-week study, infliximab, 3 mg or 10 mg/kg, and a stable dose of methotrexate prevented radiographic progression to a greater degree than methotrexate alone.[71]

Etanercept is a recombinant form of the p75 TNF receptor fusion protein. Etanercept, 25 mg, is administered by subcutaneous injection twice weekly or 50 mg once a week. Etanercept is more effective than placebo in limiting joint activity in RA.[72] It is also effective and safe when added to methotrexate.[73] This drug is also effective over a 12-month period.[74]

Adalimumab is a fully human monoclonal TNF-α antibody given by subcutaneous injection every 2 weeks at a dose of 40 mg. This anti–TNF-α factor is effective with methotrexate in decreasing joint activity.[75] The concern with anti–TNF-α therapies are the toxicities. Blocking TNF-α increases the risk for serious infection. TNF-α helps to maintain containment of organisms in granulomas. Inhibition of TNF-α has been associated with the reactivation of tuberculosis.[76,77]

Anakinra is a recombinant, nonglycosylated form of human interleukin-1 receptor antagonist. This agent works by competitively inhibiting IL-1 from binding to its receptor site. Anakinra, 100 mg, is given as a daily subcutaneous injection. It has been shown to be an effective agent in combination with methotrexate in the improvement of RA.[78,79]

Immunosuppressive Agents

Immunosuppressive agents are associated with severe toxicities (aplastic anemia and cancer), which limits their benefit to severely affected patients. Only a few patients with RA require this therapy. Immunosuppressive agents used in RA include azathioprine, chlorambucil, cyclophosphamide, and cyclosporine. A combination of cyclosporine and methotrexate may be effective for therapy of patients with severe disease.

Cervical Spine Therapy

Conservative treatment of RA of the cervical spine is supportive. Early aggressive medical management is important to prevent joint destruction. Early DMARD therapy results in better outcomes. Combination therapy used early in the course of RA can limit the development of atlantoaxial and vertical subluxations. Sulfasalazine, methotrexate, hydroxychloroquine, and prednisolone were more effective than a single DMARD with prednisolone in preventing cervical subluxation.[80] Soft cervical collars offer comfort but do not protect against progressive subluxations. Rigid collars can limit anterior subluxations but do not allow reduction of the subluxations in extension. They are poorly tolerated by RA patients with temporomandibular disease.[81]

Prognosis

The course of RA cannot be predicted at time of onset. Some patients develop sustained disease that is associated with joint destruction and resistance to therapy. Patients who are older with seropositive generalized disease with nodules are at greater risk of developing cervical spine disease. Not all patients develop subluxation. In a 5- to 14-year follow-up study, 25% of patients had an increase in subluxation, 50% had no change, and 25% had improvement. In a 5-year study of 106 RA patients, the prevalence of cervical spine subluxation increased from 43% to 70%. In subaxial disease, myelopathy was associated with narrowing of the canal, destruction of spinous processes, axial shortening, younger age of patient, longer duration of disease, higher dose of corticosteroids, and higher stage of disease. Sudden death remains a complication of RA cervical spine disease, particularly in patients with vertical subluxation. Individuals with subluxations had eight times the mortality as RA patients without subluxations.[82]

PEARLS

1. Most HLA-B27–positive individuals (98%) do not have an inflammatory arthropathy of the spine.

2. Enthesopathy is a frequent mechanism of axial and peripheral arthritis in spondyloarthropathies.

3. Plain radiographs are the preferred imaging technique for identification of sacroiliitis.

4. New biologic therapies for treatment of RA and spondyloarthropathies may offer a better opportunity to control inflammation before skeletal damage occurs.

5. AS and enteropathic arthritis share common clinical findings that differ from findings associated with reactive arthritis and psoriatic arthritis.

PITFALLS

1. Patients with spondyloarthropathy may have significant axial disease without pain.

2. A minimal amount of trauma can cause devastating fracture in a patient with a fused spine.

3. Atlantoaxial subluxation may occur without significant degrees of peripheral disease in RA.

4. Inflammatory arthropathies of the axial skeleton are chronic illnesses that do not have a cure.

5. A patient with stable AS of long duration may develop spondylodiscitis with spinal instability that is difficult to treat.

KEY POINTS

1. Inflammatory spinal arthritis is an important, relatively common form of specific low back and neck pain.

2. Most patients with inflammatory spinal arthritis may be identified based on historical and physical examination findings along with plain radiographs

3. New biologic therapies directed at specific cytokines can control the signs and symptoms of inflammatory arthritis and may slow progression of the disease.

KEY REFERENCES

1. Al-Khonizy W, Reveille JD: The immunogenetics of the seronegative spondyloarthropathies. Ballieres Clin Rheumatol 12:567-588, 1998.
   This article provides a lucid discussion of the role of genetics in the predisposition and pathogenesis of inflammatory arthropathies of the spine.

2. American College of Rheumatology Subcommittee on Rheumatoid Arthritis Guidelines: Guidelines for the management of rheumatoid arthritis: 2002 update. Arthritis Rheum 46:328-346, 2002.
   This current listing of new therapies for RA highlights the importance of early aggressive therapy.

3. Braun J, Bollow M, Sieper J: Radiologic diagnosis and pathology of the spondyloarthropathies. Rheum Dis Clin North Am 24:697-735, 1998.
   This is an excellent review of the radiologic methods needed to discover inflammatory alterations of the axial skeleton and the pathologic mechanisms that cause them.

4. Khan MA: Update on spondyloarthropathies. Ann Intern Med 136:896-907, 2002.
   This is an excellent synopsis of current studies reviewing clinical, etiologic, and therapeutic data for the most common spondyloarthropathies.

5. Reiter MF, Boden SD: Inflammatory disorders of the cervical spine. Spine (Phila Pa 1976) 23:2755-2766, 1998.
   The epidemiology, pathogenesis, and surgical considerations of inflammatory arthropathies that damage the cervical spine are reviewed.

REFERENCES

1. Schlosstein L, Terasaki PI, Bluestone R, et al: High association of an HL antigen, W27, with ankylosing spondylitis. N Engl J Med 288:704-706, 1973.

2. Lawrence RC, Helmick CG, Arnett FC, et al: Estimates of the prevalence of arthritis and selected musculoskeletal disorders in the United States. Arthritis Rheum 41:58-67, 1998.

3. Reveille JD, Ball EJ, Khan MA: HLA-B27 and genetic predisposing factors in spondyloarthropathies. Curr Opin Rheumatol 13:265-272, 2001.

4. Gran JT, Ostensen M: Spondyloarthritides in females. Ballieres Clin Rheumatol 12:695-715, 1998.

SECTION V

5. Braun J, Khan MA, Siepper J: Enthesitis and ankylosis in spondyloarthropathy: What is the target of the immune response? Ann Rheum Dis 59:985-994, 2000.

6. McGonagle D, Gibbon W, Emery P: Classification of inflammatory arthritis by enthesitis. Lancet 352:1137-1140, 1998.

7. Caplanne D, Tubach F, Le Parc JM: Late onset spondyloarthropathy: Clinical and biological comparison with early onset patients. Ann Rheum Dis 56:176-179, 1997.

8. Van Tubergen A, Coenen J, Landewe R, et al: Assessment of fatigue in patients with ankylosing spondylitis: A psychometric analysis. Arthritis Rheum 47:8-16, 2002.

9. Mader R: Atypical clinical presentations of ankylosing spondylitis. Semin Arthritis Rheum 29:191-196, 1999.

10. Fox MW, Onofrio BM, Kilgore JE: Neurological complications of ankylosing spondylitis. J Neurosurg 78:871-878, 1993.

11. Sorin S, Askari A, Moskowitz RW: Atlantoaxial subluxation as a complication of early ankylosing spondylitis. Arthritis Rheum 22:273-276, 1979.

12. Ramos-Remus C, Gomez-Vargas A, Hernandez-Chavez A, et al: Two-year follow-up of anterior and vertical atlantoaxial subluxations in ankylosing spondylitis. J Rheumatol 24:507-510, 1997.

13. Hamilton MG, MacRae ME: Atlantoaxial dislocation as the presenting symptom of ankylosing spondylitis. Spine (Phila Pa 1976) 18:2344-2346, 1993.

14. Broom MJ, Raycroft JF: Complications of fractures of the cervical spine in ankylosing spondylitis. Spine (Phila Pa 1976) 13:763-766, 1988.

15. Iplikcioglu AC, Bayar MA, Kokes F, et al: Magnetic resonance imaging in cervical trauma associated with ankylosing spondylitis: Report of two cases. J Trauma 36:412-413, 1994.

16. Detwiler KN, Loftus CM, Godersky JC, et al: Management of cervical spine injuries in patients with ankylosing spondylitis. J Neurosurg 72:210-215, 1990.

17. Bohlman HH: Acute fractures and dislocations of the cervical spine: An analysis of three hundred hospitalized patients and review of the literature. J Bone Joint Surg Am 61:1119-1142, 1979.

18. Rowed DW: Management of cervical spinal cord injury in ankylosing spondylitis: The intervertebral disc as a cause of cord compression. J Neurosurg 77:241-246, 1992.

19. Foo D, Sarkarati M, Marcelino V: Cervical spinal cord injury complicating ankylosing spondylitis. Paraplegia 23:358-365, 1985.

20. Spoorenberg A, van der Heijde D, de Klerk E, et al: Relative value of erythrocyte sedimentation rate and C-reactive protein in assessment of disease activity in ankylosing spondylitis. J Rheumatol 26:980-984, 1999.

21. McEwen C, DiTata D, Ling GC, et al: Ankylosing spondylitis and spondylitis accompanying ulcerative colitis, regional enteritis, psoriasis, and Reiter's disease: A comparative study. Arthritis Rheum 14:291-318, 1971.

22. Bollow M, Enzweiler C, Taupitz M, et al: Use of contrast enhanced magnetic resonance imaging to detect spinal inflammation in patients with spondyloarthritides. Clin Exp Rheumatol 20(Suppl 28):S167-S174, 2002.

23. Bennett PH, Wood PHN: Population studies of the rheumatic diseases. In: Proceedings of the 3rd International Symposium, New York, 1966. Amsterdam, Excerpta Medica, 1968, p 456.

24. Khan MA, van der Linden SM: A wider spectrum of spondyloarthropathies. Semin Arthritis Rheum 20:107-113, 1990.

25. Boyer GS, Templin DW, Bowler A, et al: A comparison of patients with spondyloarthropathy seen in specialty clinics with those identified in a communitywide epidemiologic study. Arch Intern Med 157:2111-2117, 1997.

26. Cohen MR, Reda DJ, Clegg DO: Baseline relationships between psoriasis and psoriatic arthritis: Analysis of 221 patients with active psoriatic arthritis. J Rheumatol 26:1752-1756, 1999.

27. Gladman DD: Psoriatic arthritis. Rheum Dis Clin North Am 24:829-844, 1998.

28. Mease P: Psoriatic arthritis: The role of TNF inhibition and the effect of its inhibition with etanercept. Clin Exp Rheumatol 20(Suppl 28):S116-S121, 2002.

29. Sosner J, Fast A, Kahan BS: Odontoid fracture and C1-C2 subluxation in psoriatic cervical spondyloarthropathy. Spine (Phila Pa 1976) 21:519-521, 1996.

30. Gladman DD: Natural history of psoriatic arthritis. Baillieres Clin Rheumatol 8:379-394, 1994.

31. Arnett FC, McClusky E, Schacter BZ, et al: Incomplete Reiter's syndrome: Discriminating features and HLA-W27 in diagnosis. Ann Intern Med 84:8-12, 1976.

32. Russell AS, Davis P, Percy JS, et al: The sacroiliitis of acute Reiter's syndrome. J Rheumatol 4:293-296, 1977.

33. Good AE: Reiter's syndrome: Long-term follow-up in relation to development of ankylosing spondylitis. Ann Rheum Dis 38:39-45, 1979.

34. Beutler AM, Hudson AP, Whittum-Hudson JA, et al: *Chlamydia trachomatis* can persist in joint tissue after antibiotic treatment in chronic Reiter's syndrome/reactive arthritis. J Clin Rheumatol 3:125-130, 1997.

35. Podolsky DK: Inflammatory bowel disease. N Engl J Med 347:417-429, 2002.

36. Orchard TR, Wordsworth BP, Jewell DP: Peripheral arthropathies in inflammatory bowel disease: Their articular distribution and natural history. Gut 42:387-391, 1998.

37. Van den Bosch F, Kruithof E, De Vos M, et al: Crohn's disease associated with spondyloarthropathy: Effect of TNF-α blockade with infliximab on the articular symptoms. Lancet 356:1821-1822, 2000.

38. Yagan R, Khan MA: Confusion of roentgenographic differential diagnosis of ankylosing hyperostosis (Forestier's disease) and ankylosing spondylitis. Spine State Art Rev 4:561-572, 1990.

39. Durback MA, Edelstein G, Schumacher HR Jr: Abnormalities of the sacroiliac joints in diffuse idiopathic skeletal hyperostosis: Demonstration by computed tomography. J Rheumatol 15:1506-1511, 1988.

40. Williamson PK, Reginato AJ: Diffuse idiopathic skeletal hyperostosis of the cervical spine in a patient with ankylosing spondylitis. Arthritis Rheum 27:570-573, 1984.

41. Miceli-Richard C, Dougados M: NSAIDs in ankylosing spondylitis. Clin Exp Rheumatol 20(Suppl 28):S65-S66, 2002.

42. Dougados M, Behier JM, Jolchine I, et al: Efficacy of celecoxib, a cyclooxygenase-2-specific inhibitor, in the treatment of ankylosing spondylitis: A six-week controlled study with comparison against placebo and against a conventional nonsteroidal anti-inflammatory drug. Arthritis Rheum 44:180-185, 2001.

43. Van den Bosch F, Kruithof E, Baeten D, et al: Randomized double-blind comparison of chimeric monoclonal antibody to tumor necrosis factor alpha (infliximab) versus placebo in active spondyloarthropathy. Arthritis Rheum 46:755-765, 2002.

44. Brandt J, Sieper J, Braun J: Infliximab in the treatment of active and severe ankylosing spondylitis. Clin Exp Rheumatol 20(Suppl 28): S106-S110, 2002.

45. Gorman JD, Sack KE, David JC Jr: Treatment of ankylosing spondylitis by inhibition of tumor necrosis factor alpha. N Engl J Med 346:1349-1356, 2002.

46. Kruithof E, vanden Bosch F, Baeten D, et al: Repeated infusions of infliximab, a chimeric anti-TNF-α monoclonal antibody, in patients with active spondyloarthropathy: One year followup. Ann Rheum Dis 61:207-212, 2002.

47. Kennedy LG, Edmunds L, Calin A: The natural history of ankylosing spondylitis: Does it burn out? J Rheumatol 20:688-692, 1993.

48. Lee DM, Weinblatt ME: Rheumatoid arthritis. Lancet 358:903-911, 2001.

49. Lawrence JS, Sharp J, Ball J, et al: Rheumatoid arthritis of the lumbar spine. Ann Rheum Dis 23:205-217, 1964.

50. Panayi GS: The immunopathogenesis of rheumatoid arthritis. Br J Rheumatol 32(Suppl 1):4-14, 1993.

51. Reiter MF, Boden SD: Inflammatory disorders of the cervical spine. Spine (Phila Pa 1976) 23:2755-2766, 1998.

52. Zeidman SM, Ducker TB: Rheumatoid arthritis: Neuroanatomy, compression, and grading of deficits. Spine (Phila Pa 1976) 19:2259-2266, 1994.

53. Yonezawa T, Tsuji H, Matsui H, Hirano N: Subaxial lesions in rheumatoid arthritis: Radiographic factors suggestive of lower cervical myelopathy. Spine (Phila Pa 1976) 20:208-215, 1995.

54. Halla JT, Hardin JG, Vitek J, et al: Involvement of the cervical spine in rheumatoid arthritis. Arthritis Rheum 32:652-659, 1989.

55. Webb F, Hickman J, Brew D: Death from vertebral artery thrombosis in rheumatoid arthritis. BMJ 2:537-538, 1968.

56. Gordon DA, Hastings DE: Clinical features of rheumatoid arthritis. In Hochberg MC, Silman AJ, Smolen JS, et al (eds): Rheumatology, 3rd ed. Edinburgh, Mosby, 2003, pp 765-780.

57. Chang MH, Liao KK, Cheung SC, et al: "Numb, clumsy hands" and tactile agnosia secondary to high cervical spondylotic myelopathy: A clinical and electrophysiological correlation. Acta Neurol Scand 86:622-625, 1992.

58. Fujiwara K, Fujimoto M, Owaki H, et al: Cervical lesions related to the systemic progression in rheumatoid arthritis. Spine 23:2052-2056, 1998.

59. Bland JH, Van Buskirk FW, Tampas JP, et al: A study of roentgenographic criteria for rheumatoid arthritis of the cervical spine. AJR Am J Roentgenol 95:949-954, 1965.

60. Komusi T, Munro T, Harth M: Radiologic review: The rheumatoid cervical spine. Semin Arthritis Rheum 14:187-195, 1985.

61. Oostveen JCM, van de Laar MAFJ: Magnetic resonance imaging in rheumatic disorders of the spine and sacroiliac joints. Semin Arthritis Rheum 30:52-69, 2000.

62. Arnett FC, Edworthy SM, Block DA, et al: The American Rheumatism Association 1987 revised criteria for the classification of rheumatoid arthritis. Arthritis Rheum 31:315, 1988.

63. Choy EHS, Panayi GS: Cytokine pathways and joint inflammation in rheumatoid arthritis. N Engl J Med 344:907-916, 2001.

64. Wilske KR, Healey LA: Remodeling the pyramid, a concept whose time has come. J Rheumatol 16:565-566, 1989.

65. American College of Rheumatology Subcommittee on Rheumatoid: Arthritis guidelines: Guidelines for the management of rheumatoid arthritis: 2002 update. Arthritis Rheum 46:328-346, 2002.

66. Bombardier C, Laine L, Reicin A, et al: Comparison of upper gastrointestinal toxicity of rofecoxib and naproxen in patients with rheumatoid arthritis. N Engl J Med 343:1520-1528, 2000.

67. Silverstein FE, Faich G, Goldstein JL, et al: Gastrointestinal toxicity with celecoxib vs nonsteroidal anti-inflammatory drugs for osteoarthritis and rheumatoid arthritis: The CLASS study: A randomized controlled trial. JAMA 284:1247-1255, 2000.

68. Kremer JM: Rational use of new and existing disease-modifying agents in rheumatoid arthritis. Ann Intern Med 134:695-706, 2001.

69. Van Everdingen AA, Jacobs JWG, van Reesema DRS, et al: Low-dose prednisone therapy for patients with early active rheumatoid arthritis: Clinical efficacy, disease-modifying properties, and side effects. Ann Intern Med 136:1-12, 2002.

70. Maini R, St. Clair EW, Breedveld F, et al: Infliximab (chimeric anti-tumor necrosis factor α monoclonal antibody) versus placebo in rheumatoid arthritis patients receiving concomitant methotrexate: A randomized phase III trial. Lancet 354:1932-1939, 1999.

71. Lipsky PE, van der Heijde DMFM, St. Clair EW, et al: Infliximab and methotrexate in the treatment of rheumatoid arthritis. N Engl J Med 343:1594-1602, 2000.

72. Moreland LW, Schiff MH, Baumgartner SW, et al: Etanercept therapy in rheumatoid arthritis: A randomized controlled trial. Ann Intern Med 130:478-486, 1999.

73. Weinblatt ME, Kremer JM, Bankhurst AD, et al: A trial of etanercept, a recombinant tumor necrosis factor: Fc fusion protein in patients with rheumatoid arthritis receiving methotrexate. N Engl J Med 340:253-259, 1999.

74. Bathon JM, Martin RW, Fleischmann RM, et al: A comparison of etanercept and methotrexate in patients with early rheumatoid arthritis. N Engl J Med 343:1586-1593, 2000.

75. Weinblatt ME, Keystone EC, Furst DE, et al: Adalimumab, a fully human anti-tumor necrosis factor alpha monoclonal antibody, for the treatment of rheumatoid arthritis in patients taking concomitant methotrexate: The ARMADA trial. Arthritis Rheum 48:35-45, 2003.

76. Keane J, Gershon S, Wise RP, et al: Tuberculosis associated with infliximab, a tumor necrosis factor α-neutralizing agent. N Engl J Med 345:1098-1104, 2001.

77. Baghai M, Osmon DR, Wolk DM, et al: Fatal sepsis in a patient with rheumatoid arthritis treated with etanercept. Mayo Clin Proc 76:653-656, 2001.

78. Cohen S, Hurd E, Cush J, et al: Treatment of rheumatoid arthritis with anakinra: A recombinant human interleukin-1 receptor antagonist, in combination with methotrexate: Results of a twenty-four-week, multicenter, randomized, double-blind, placebo-controlled trial. Arthritis Rheum 46:614-624, 2002.

79. Bresnihan B, Alvaro-Gracia JM, Cobby M, et al: Treatment of rheumatoid arthritis with recombinant human interleukin-1 receptor antagonist. Arthritis Rheum 41:2196-2204, 1998.

80. Neva MH, Kauppi MJ, Kautiainen H, et al: Combination drug therapy retards the development of rheumatoid atlantoaxial subluxations. Arthritis Rheum 43:2397-2401, 2000.

81. Kauppi M, Anttila P: A stiff collar can restrict atlantoaxial instability in rheumatoid atlantoaxial subluxations. Br J Rheumatol 35:771-774, 1996.

82. Riise T, Jacobsen BK, Gran JT: High mortality in patients with rheumatoid arthritis and atlantoaxial subluxations. J Rheumatol 28:2425-2429, 2001.

34
CHAPTER

Surgical Management of Rheumatoid Arthritis

Scott D. Daffner, MD
Sanford E. Emery, MD, MBA

Rheumatoid arthritis is a chronic, progressive, systemic disease with widespread involvement of connective tissues and primarily synovial joints. Women are affected two to three times more often than men with most cases manifesting in the 4th or 5th decades, although patients may be affected at any age. More recent improvements in medical management have correlated with a decrease in hospitalizations for severe rheumatoid disease; however, one study found that although admission for treatment of several medical complications of rheumatoid arthritis decreased significantly from 1983-2001, the rate of admission for cervical spine surgery in this population remained unchanged.[1] The cervical spine is involved in 25% to 90% of patients with rheumatoid arthritis, making it the most commonly affected site after the metatarsophalangeal and metacarpophalangeal joints.[2] In contrast to rheumatoid arthritis of the thoracic and lumbar spine, cervical spine involvement carries significant risks of spinal cord and medullary and vertebral artery compromise and sudden death.[3,4]

Numerous patients with cervical instability may be asymptomatic or may have symptoms indistinguishable from symptoms in patients without instability. Neva and colleagues[5] reviewed 154 patients with rheumatoid arthritis who were on a waiting list for various orthopaedic procedures at a Finnish hospital. Overall, 44% of patients had radiographic evidence of cervical subluxation or prior cervical fusion. When excluding patients with previous fusions, these investigators noted that 69% of patients with radiographic evidence of subluxations reported neck pain compared with 65% of patients without subluxation. Similarly, rates of occipital, temporal, retro-orbital, and upper extremity radicular pain were not significantly different in patients with or without cervical instability. Many patients with significant cervical involvement may be overlooked by the treating physician because of the lack of clear neurologic deficits on physical examination. The physician must be cognizant of the natural history, pathophysiology, clinical presentation, radiologic findings, and treatment options to avoid the grave consequences of rheumatoid disease of the cervical spine.

Historical Perspective

There is some evidence that rheumatoid arthritis was described in the 17th and 18th centuries.[6,7] More concrete evidence points to a period around 1800, according to a description by Landré-Beauvais, a French medical student, in his doctoral thesis.[8] The description of rheumatoid arthritis of the cervical spine occurred much later, with a report in 1890 by Garrod.[9]

Interest increased in the 1950s and 1960s with reports describing cervical instability.[10-13] Articles on the surgical treatment of cervical instability in patients with rheumatoid arthritis followed in the 1960s and 1970s.[14-18] For the most part, C1-2 fusion with Gallie-type[19] wiring and graft techniques were used early on. Brooks and Jenkins,[20] Wertheim and Bohlman,[21] and Clark and colleagues[22] subsequently described modified wiring techniques. Other types of C1-2 fixation emerged later with the use of the Halifax interlaminar clamp,[23] the Magerl transarticular screw technique,[24-28] and posterior C1 lateral mass–C2 pedicle screw fixation.[29]

Foerster[30] originally described occipitocervical procedures in 1927. Kahn and Yglesias[31] were the first to add iliac crest bone graft to occipitocervical fusion in 1935. Hamblen[16] later described the combined use of wires and iliac crest graft for occipitocervical fusion in four patients with rheumatoid arthritis and cervical instability in 1967. In a 1976 report, Brattström and Granholm[14] modified the wiring technique for occipitocervical fusion by adding methyl methacrylate. Modifications of occipitocervical fusion techniques continued in the 1980s with the emergence of the looped rod with iliac crest bone graft, as described by Ransford[32] and Flint[33] and their colleagues and later occipitocervical plating, as described by Grob[34,35] and Smith[36] and their colleagues. Current use of plate or rod fixation extends to the subaxial spine, especially with fixation of the lateral masses described by Magerl and Roy-Camille.[25-27]

Pathophysiology

The inflammatory process in the cervical spine mirrors the inflammatory process in other sites of the body and consists predominantly of T lymphocytes, macrophages, and plasma cells in a hypervascular synoviocyte pannus.[37,38] The inflammatory reaction has a predilection for synovial joints, and the multiple synovial joints[39] of the cervical spine (facets, uncovertebral, atlanto-occipital, atlantodens) are particularly affected. In contrast to the thoracic and lumbar spine, the cervical spine relies heavily on ligaments and joint congruency for stability and so is at greater risk for instability. With significant inflammation, pannus formation and erosion of the joint and capsular structures can occur. Progressive instability can result, manifesting as atlantoaxial (C1-2) instability, subaxial subluxation, cranial settling (also known as *basilar invagination* or *atlantoaxial impaction*), or a combination thereof. Rheumatoid discitis may also occur at the discovertebral junctions with noninfectious erosion of the endplates.[3]

Atlantoaxial instability is the most common instability pattern in the rheumatoid cervical spine and may be the result of the development of periodontoid pannus and progressive inflammatory destruction of the upper cervical spine.[39-41] Pannus formation localizes around the synovial joint formed between the transverse ligament, the posterior arch of the atlas, and the base of the odontoid. The soft tissue may compress the spinal cord and often distends and erodes the surrounding periodontoid-ligamentous structures (alar, apical, and transverse ligaments), the odontoid process (dens), and the lateral articular masses between C1 and C2.[42] Erosion of the dens may lead to the development of occult, atraumatic odontoid fractures.[43] Subsequent static or dynamic instability or subluxation occurs in 50% to 70% of patients.[18,44] Most often, the subluxation is anterior (70%), but lateral, posterior, and rotational subluxations can also occur.[45,46] Anterior subluxation of 0 to 3 mm is normal in adults, subluxation of 3 to 6 mm suggests instability with disruption of the transverse ligament, and subluxation of 9 mm or more suggests disruption of the entire periodontoid-ligamentous and capsular structures with gross instability and is a clear indication for surgery.[18,47,48]

The combination of periodontoid pannus buildup and instability may cause spinal cord and root impingement leading to myeloradiculopathy and sudden death. Delamarter and Bohlman[49] conducted postmortem studies suggesting that paralysis can be due to mechanical neural compression, vascular impairment of the neural structures, or both. Henderson and colleagues[50] reported that diffuse axonal injury with or without frank necrosis may irreversibly affect the spinal cord owing to mechanical damage. These findings may partly explain the smaller diameter and cross-sectional area of the spinal cord found in patients with severe disease.[51] Some evidence suggests that instability promotes worsening periodontoid pannus formation and that stabilization reverses the buildup.[40]

Posterior atlantoaxial subluxation is rare and should raise the possibility of an anterior arch defect of the atlas or erosion or fracture of the odontoid.[48] Patients usually present with myelopathy and posterior kinking of the cord without radiographic compression.[52] Lateral subluxation is defined as more than 2 mm of lateral displacement of the C1-2 lateral masses and occurs in 21% of atlantoaxial subluxations.[48] Lateral subluxations occur more commonly in patients with spinal cord compression than patients without compression and are often accompanied by rotational subluxation.[53]

Subaxial subluxation is the second most common instability pattern and results from destruction of the facet joints, interspinous ligaments, and discovertebral joints.[44,54] These pathologic changes can lead to longitudinal collapse, bony erosion, soft tissue hypertrophy, and sagittal plane instability along multiple spinal segments, causing a "stepladder"-type pattern of deformity. Concurrent spondylodiscitis may occur with pain, neural compression, and instability.

Cranial settling occurs primarily because of bone and cartilage destruction of the atlantoaxial and occipitoatlantal joints in contrast to ligamentous laxity. Although the least common of the three instability patterns, it is the most ominous form. Caudad settling of the cranium and apparent cranial migration of the odontoid are characteristic. As a result, there is an increased risk of sudden death from either static or dynamic stenosis of the foramen magnum and compression of the medulla oblongata (brainstem). Other sequelae include obstructive hydrocephalus or syringomyelia presumably from direct mechanical blockage of normal cerebrospinal fluid flow. In some cases, fixed rotation of the head may occur because of unilateral involvement of the atlantoaxial and occipitoatlantal joints.

Natural History

It is difficult to study the natural history of rheumatoid arthritis because patients are usually treated at some stage of the disease and it would be unethical to do otherwise. From studies on rheumatoid arthritis, it seems consistent that the inflammatory processes in the cervical spine begin early after the onset of rheumatoid arthritis and progress along with peripheral involvement. Atlantoaxial instability may be detected within 2 to 10 years of disease onset in most patients,[55] and there is a strong correlation between cervical spine subluxation and peripheral erosions of the hands and feet.[56] Approximately 10% of patients with cervical spine involvement eventually require surgery.[57]

The natural history of rheumatoid arthritis of the spine without surgical intervention, especially in patients with myelopathy, seems to be progressive disability and risk of sudden death. In one study of 21 patients treated medically, 76% showed deterioration at an average of 6 years of follow-up. All patients in the study became bedridden within 3 years of developing myelopathy, and all died within 7 years with one third dying suddenly for unknown reasons.[58] Risk factors for progression include mutilating articular disease, history of high-dose corticosteroid use, high seropositivity, rheumatoid subcutaneous nodules, vasculitis, and male gender. Other potential but unproven risk factors for cervical involvement include high C-reactive protein level and HLA-Dw2 or HLA-B27 positivity.[59,60] As the disease progresses, pain, neurologic deficits, and sudden death are the primary risks.

Clinical Presentation

Neck pain is the most common symptom in patients with cervical spine involvement. Peripheral erosive changes similarly occur along the apophyseal joints and surrounding soft tissues and may be a source of pain. Cervical instability may cause secondary impingement of the posterior rami of the lesser and greater occipital nerves, which may lead to occipital headaches. Pain in the suboccipital region generally suggests atlantoaxial pathology or cranial settling. Middle or lower cervical pain should suggest subaxial subluxation. These are not hard and fast rules because pain localization in rheumatoid cervical disease may be poor. Subaxial involvement may also lead to painful neck deformity with loss of sagittal plane supporting structures, which may later become fixed deformities owing to postinflammatory ankylosis. Patients may complain of a "clunking" sensation in the neck with neck motion. This sensation is most common in patients with C1-2 instability, owing to spontaneous reduction of the subluxation with neck extension (known as the Sharp-Purser test).[61]

Progressive instability leads to decreased effective canal diameter and brainstem compression. Myelopathy and vertebrobasilar dysfunction may result because of mechanical and ischemic damage to the white and gray matter evidenced on histologic specimens by long tract demyelinization, lateral column necrosis, and focal gliosis.[49] According to Bell,[62] C1-2 instability may lead to a phenomenon termed *cruciate paralysis,* characterized by upper motor neuron dysfunction of the upper extremities with paresis and paralysis and normal lower extremities similar to a mild central cord syndrome after trauma. Pathologically, there is selective injury to the decussating corticospinal tracts of the upper extremities at the level of the cervicomedullary junction with sparing of the uncrossed lower extremity pyramidal and extrapyramidal tracts.

Additional neurovascular changes may occur because of vertebral artery occlusion with decreased flow into the posterior inferior cerebellar artery and cephalad brainstem circulation. Without adequate collateral blood flow, these patients may develop Wallenberg syndrome or lateral medullary infarction. These clinical syndromes are characterized by ipsilateral cranial nerve palsies (cranial nerves V, IX, X, and XI), cerebellar ataxia, Horner syndrome (ptosis, miosis, anhidrosis, and enophthalmos), facial pain, and contralateral loss of pain and temperature sensation.[63] Rarely, patients may develop quadriplegia, quadriplegia with facial muscle paralysis (locked-in syndrome),[64] and sudden death.[38,58]

In contrast to pain symptoms, neurologic signs are less straightforward. Myelopathy is progressive but may not be evident by loss of fine motor control, gait imbalance, or global numbness of the hands, but rather by the slow onset of deteriorating independence and becoming wheelchair bound. In many instances, hand deformities mask motor deficits in the upper extremities, and the patients' deteriorating ambulatory

TABLE 34–1 Ranawat Criteria for Pain and Neural Assessment

Pain Assessment	
Grade 0	None
Grade 1	Mild, intermittent, requiring only aspirin analgesia
Grade 2	Moderate; cervical collar needed
Grade 3	Severe; pain not relieved by either aspirin or collar
Neural Assessment	
Class I	No neural deficit
Class II	Subjective weakness with hyperreflexia and dysesthesias
Class IIIA	Objective findings of paresis and long tract signs, but walking possible
Class IIIB	Quadriparesis with resultant inability to walk or feed oneself

Adapted from Ranawat CS, O'Leary P, Pellici P, et al: Cervical spine fusion in rheumatoid arthritis. J Bone Joint Surg Am 61:1003-1010, 1979.

status may be attributed to large joint involvement rather than myelopathy. Patients must be assessed keeping their global disease in mind. Progression of myelopathy, especially early disease, may be misinterpreted as progression of peripheral disease. A high index of suspicion is necessary in these patients to detect early myelopathy because patients do poorly without early surgical intervention.[38,58]

The Ranawat grading system may provide some useful clinical information in assessing patients with neurologic deficits (Table 34–1).[65] This system classifies pain as none (grade 0), mild (1), moderate (2), or severe (3). Neurologic function falls into three classes: Class I has no neurologic deficit; class II has subjective weakness, dysesthesia, and hyperreflexia; and class III has objective weakness and long tract signs. This last class is subdivided further into class IIIA, in which patients are ambulatory, and class IIIB, in which patients have quadriparesis and are unable to walk. Casey and colleagues[66] reported that only 25% of 55 Ranawat class IIIB patients who underwent surgical decompression and stabilization had a favorable outcome. The mortality rate was 13% after 30 days and 60% by 4 years.

Radiologic Evaluation

Plain radiographs are an effective screening tool for identifying patients with atlantoaxial instability, cranial settling, or subaxial subluxations. Standard anteroposterior, open-mouth (odontoid view), lateral, and controlled flexion-extension plain views should suffice. The flexion-extension views are the most important in detecting whether there is dynamic or static instability in the upper or lower cervical spine and allow for measurement of the anterior atlantodental interval (AADI) and posterior atlantodental interval (PADI). AADI is measured from the anterior surface of the dens to the posterior margin of the anterior ring of the atlas along a transverse axis

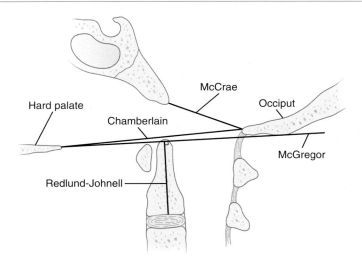

FIGURE 34–1 Drawing of lines for measurements of basilar invagination. *Chamberlain line*: Odontoid tip greater than 6 mm above line. *McCrae line*: Odontoid tip above this line. *McGregor line*: Men, odontoid tip greater than 8 mm above line; women, odontoid tip greater than 9.7 mm above line. *Redlund-Johnell distance*: Men, less than 34 mm; women, less than 29 mm.

of the atlas, whereas PADI is the distance between the posterior surface of the dens and the anterior margin of the posterior ring of the atlas.

Historically, the AADI was used to screen patients who required surgical stabilization for atlantoaxial instability based on an AADI greater than 9 mm, with AADI 0 to 6 mm suggesting instability and AADI 0 to 3 mm being normal.[48] AADI is limited by the occasional difficulty of obtaining accurate measurements in some patients because of erosive changes that distort the normal anatomic landmarks and because it has not been correlated clinically with the mass effect of retrodental pannus that may compress the spinal cord. Boden and colleagues[67] showed that PADI may be more reliable in predicting neurologic outcome because it is a more accurate indicator of the space available for the cord. Patients with a PADI of at least 14 mm were more likely to have neurologic recovery after surgical stabilization, whereas patients with a PADI less than 10 mm had no neurologic recovery. These observations

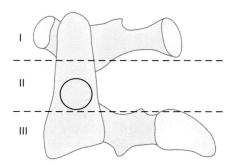

FIGURE 34–2 Station of atlas is determined by dividing odontoid process into thirds in sagittal plane. Normally, anterior ring of atlas should be adjacent to cephalad third of axis (*station I*). If ring of atlas is adjacent to middle third of axis, mild cranial settling is indicated (*station II*). If anterior ring of atlas is adjacent to base of axis, it is considered evidence of severe cranial settling (*station III*). (From Clark CR, Goetz DD, Menezes AH: Arthrodesis of the cervical spine in rheumatoid arthritis. J Bone Joint Surg Am 71:381-392, 1989.)

can also be explained by the anatomy of the spinal cord at the C1 level because the dura requires an average space of 1 mm on the anterior and posterior sides, the cerebrospinal fluid requires 2 mm, and the cord requires 10 mm for a total space of 14 mm.[68]

The open-mouth view is useful to identify lateral subluxation, defined as more than 2 mm of lateral displacement of C1-2 lateral masses, which occurs more commonly in patients with spinal cord compression than in patients without compression.[48,53] Erosive changes of the dens and C1-2 articulations may also be visualized. Taniguchi and colleagues[69] defined the atlantodental lateral shift (ADLS) as a means of assessing lateral atlantoaxial instability. Using dynamic open-mouth odontoid views (taken in maximal left and right lateral bending), ADLS is calculated by dividing the distance from the center of the dens to the medial edge of the C1 lateral mass (in the direction of lateral bending) by the distance between the medial borders of the bilateral C1 lateral masses and is expressed as a percentage. With this method, these investigators noted that in patients with rheumatoid arthritis, the ADLS averaged 14.8% compared with 6.1% in control patients. Among the subgroup of patients with rheumatoid arthritis and increased AADI, the ADLS averaged 20.6% versus 12.7% in patients without anterior atlantoaxial instability.

Posterior subluxation, although rare, may be seen on lateral radiographs of the cervical spine and should be suspected in patients with an absent or fractured odontoid process.[52] The AADI decreases with worsening cranial settling as the arch of the atlas approaches the wider base of the odontoid process and is a potential source of mistaken radiographic improvement.

Cranial settling carries the greatest risk of neurologic deficits and sudden death, especially when superimposed on atlantoaxial instability. As a consequence, several measurement techniques have been used with varying sensitivity and specificity, based on lateral plain radiographs of the upper cervical spine (Fig. 34–1).[70] Most of these techniques assess the relationship between the tip of the odontoid, the hard palate, and the base of the skull. Traditionally, McGregor line (drawn from the posterosuperior tip of the hard palate to the caudad base of the occiput) has been widely used for its simplicity. Cranial settling occurs when the tip of the dens is more than 4.5 mm above this line.

Erosive changes in the odontoid anatomy may make it difficult to analyze many of the measurement techniques, so Redlund-Johnell and Pettersson[71] described a technique that measured the vertical line from the midpoint of the caudad margin of C2 to McGregor line. Cranial settling occurs when the distance is less than 34 mm in men or less than 29 mm in women. Ranawat and colleagues[65] described a similar technique in which the distance along the odontoid was measured from the C2 pedicle to the transverse axis of the ring of C1. This technique avoided problems with changes in odontoid anatomy and identifying the bony landmarks at the base of the skull and hard palate. Cranial settling was positive if the distance was less than 15 mm in men or less than 13 mm in women. Clark and colleagues[22] defined the "station of the atlas" (Fig. 34–2), which indicates the position of the anterior ring of C1 to parts of the body of the axis divided into thirds. Normally, the atlas is adjacent to the upper third (station I) of the axis. Riew and colleagues[70] noted that none of the current radiographic measurements alone had a sensitivity, specificity, or negative or positive predictive value greater than 90% and recommended the combination of the Clark station, Redlund-Johnell criteria, and Ranawat criteria with sensitivity and negative predictive values of 94% and 91%.

Subaxial subluxation is the second most common instability pattern and occurs secondary to inflammatory destruction of the apophyseal and discovertebral joints and supporting soft tissues. White and Panjabi[72] defined radiographic cervical instability as 3.5 mm or more of vertebral translation and greater than 11 degrees of angular changes between adjacent motion segments, although their study is more representative of acute conditions. The space available for the cord should also be considered in these patients because critical stenosis may be present with or without instability. Boden and colleagues[67] correlated anatomic measurements with neurologic findings and reported that a sagittal diameter of less than 14 mm was considered critically stenotic in the rheumatoid subaxial spine. This is in contrast to 13 mm in cervical spondylotic patients who do not have pannus in the canal.

Computed tomography (CT), especially with intrathecal contrast medium, is a valuable addition to plain radiographs in delineating the bony anatomy and identifying cord compression and cranial settling. The degree of medullary compression on CT scans has been shown to correlate with myelopathy.[40] Static or dynamic magnetic resonance imaging (MRI) is the best option, however, to assess the soft tissues and to look for the presence of periodontoid pannus (Fig. 34–3) and spinal cord or brainstem compression.[73-75] MRI is also useful for postoperative evaluation of the periodontoid pannus, which has been shown to decrease after stabilization.[40] Myelopathic signs correlate with MRI findings[75] of a cervicomedullary angle of less than 135 degrees (normal 135 to 175 degrees). This angle measures the intersection of vertical lines drawn along the anterior surface of the brainstem and the cord on sagittal MRI.

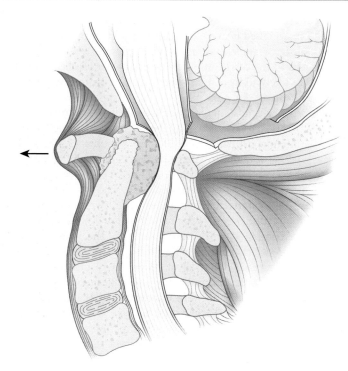

FIGURE 34–3 Illustration showing forward subluxation of atlas on axis, pannus formation around odontoid process, and osseous erosions. There is severe compression of spinal cord between pannus anteriorly and arch of atlas posteriorly. (From Boden SD, Dodge LD, Bohlman HH, et al: Rheumatoid arthritis of the cervical spine: A long term analysis with predictors of paralysis and recovery. J Bone Joint Surg Am 75:1282-1297, 1993.)

Nonsurgical Treatment

Although life expectancy is lower in patients with rheumatoid arthritis, many are living longer with their disease because of more aggressive medical therapy that has slowed disease progression with fewer side effects.[59] Only a few of these patients eventually need surgical stabilization. Patients with early cervical disease and intermittent pain without radiographic instability or myelopathy can be managed with a soft cervical orthosis or trials of physical therapy. Medication options include nonsteroidal anti-inflammatory drugs (NSAIDs); oral steroids (prednisone); and disease-modifying antirheumatic drugs (DMARDs) such as methotrexate, gold, sulfasalazine, hydroxychloroquine, penicillamine, and azathioprine.

In recent years, biologic agents such as tumor necrosis factor (TNF)-α and interleukin-1 antagonists have become increasingly available. The addition of antiresorptive osteopo-

rosis therapy may improve vertebral bone strength in patients with rheumatoid arthritis.[76] Patients should be followed closely for neurologic or radiographic changes. Cervical collars provide support, warmth, some pain relief, and a feeling of stability; however, rigid collars are often poorly tolerated, especially in patients with temporomandibular disease, dental problems, and skin sensitivity, and may have further detrimental effects by blocking spontaneous reduction of anterior atlantoaxial subluxation in extension.

Surgical Management

Indications

Patients with any one or more of the instability patterns described earlier (atlantoaxial instability, cranial settling, subaxial subluxation) associated with or without pain, myelopathy, or neurologic deficits should be considered for early surgery. As noted previously, radiographic indicators for surgery include AADI of 9 mm or more; PADI of less than 14 mm; mobile subaxial subluxation greater than 3.5 mm; cord compression or space available for the cord of less than 14 mm; and cranial settling measured most accurately by the combination of Clark station, Redlund-Johnell criteria, and Ranawat criteria.[70] CT myelography and MRI showing cord compression or a cervicomedullary angle of less than 135 degrees are suggestive of impending neurologic deficits and should be weighed heavily as an indication for surgery within the context of the remaining clinical picture. Patients with headaches in the distribution of the greater or lesser occipital nerve are likely to have atlantoaxial instability and may need C1-2 arthrodesis for pain relief.

Timing of surgical intervention is crucial. In a retrospective review of 110 patients who underwent cervical spine fusion for rheumatoid arthritis, only 3 of 55 patients (5.5%) with early C1-2 fusion for isolated atlantoaxial instability developed subaxial subluxation requiring surgery an average of 9 years later. This review contrasted with a 36% incidence of recurrent cervical instability at a mean of 2.6 years in patients who initially underwent occiput-C3 fusion for atlantoaxial instability combined with cranial settling. The investigators recommended early surgery before the development of cranial settling to decrease the risks of recurrent instability.[39] In a series of 28 patients, Schmitt-Sody and colleagues[77] reported that 7 of 10 patients who were Ranawat class II improved to class I after surgery, whereas only 1 of 11 class III patients improved (class IIIA to class II), and 2 patients deteriorated (class IIIA to class IIIB) postoperatively. Similarly, these authors recommended early surgical stabilization before the development of neurologic symptoms.

Preoperative Assessment

The goals of surgery should be relief of pain, spinal alignment, decompression to relieve neurologic deficits where necessary, and stabilization of the involved motion segments. Thorough preoperative assessment is a prerequisite to good outcome in these often fragile patients. The quality of the bone stock, the presence of irreducible subluxations, and the medical condition of the patients should guide the preoperative decision-making process, including the potential need for awake fiberoptic nasal or endotracheal intubation.[78]

Patients with severe basilar invagination should be considered for preoperative skeletal traction using a halo ring. The ring can be incorporated into a halo vest after surgery. Constant preoperative traction can improve alignment, neurologic symptoms, and pain. Traction may be required for 3 to 7 days or longer,[52,79,80] and some authors have used a halo wheelchair to allow the patient to be more mobile and avoid secondary problems such as decubitus ulcers and infection from prolonged bed rest.[52,79,80] Gentle traction along the midline longitudinal axis with approximately 7 to 12 lb while avoiding hyperflexion or hyperextension is recommended. Patients are monitored with frequent neurologic examinations, and plain radiographs should be obtained to avoid overdistraction during the process. The authors do not routinely use preoperative traction in atlantoaxial instability or subaxial subluxation. Many of these instabilities that moved little on preoperative flexion-extension views are better reduced when the patient is under general anesthesia positioned with the head holder.

When in the operating room, obtaining baseline neurophysiologic data including somatosensory evoked potentials and motor evoked potentials before positioning a myelopathic patient may help prevent cord injury during or after positioning of the head and neck. Finally, the surgical approach should be determined by the underlying pathology and its location, in part analogous to the approach for compressive lesions in patients with cervical spondylosis.[81,82]

Perioperative Management of Rheumatoid Medication

Perioperative management of rheumatoid medications is of utmost importance. Several commonly used agents may act as immune modulators or anti-inflammatories and may place patients at risk for perioperative complications such as wound infections, delayed healing, or delayed fusion. Other medications may potentially have systemic effects if discontinued. The management of medications in the perioperative period frequently requires walking a fine line between patient comfort and reduction of complications. A lack of prospective studies of perioperative medication use among patients with rheumatoid arthritis undergoing orthopaedic procedures makes true evidence-based recommendations difficult. No studies have specifically addressed this issue for patients undergoing spinal procedures.

Because of the risk of increased bleeding time and potentially increased intraoperative blood loss, NSAIDs should be discontinued 3 to 5 half-lives before surgery.[83] In addition, NSAIDs have been previously shown to inhibit bone healing and so should be held as long as possible postoperatively so as not to impair formation of a spinal fusion.

Corticosteroids may produce immunosuppression, which can adversely affect wound and bone healing. Sudden stoppage of long-term corticosteroid therapy may lead to adrenal insufficiency, necessitating the continued use of corticosteroids perioperatively and potentially requiring the use of stress dosing. Generally, perioperative management of corticosteroids depends on the long-term dosage and the potential degree of surgical stress. Most spinal procedures for these patients would be considered highly stressful, and patients on long-term moderate-dose to high-dose regimens (>20 mg/day of prednisone) should receive stress dose steroids on the day of surgery with rapid tapering over 1 to 2 days to their usual long-term dosage.[83,84]

Continued use of methotrexate in the perioperative period has not been shown to increase infection rates.[85] It may affect bone healing, however[86]; this has not been studied in a spinal fusion model. Although withholding methotrexate may increase the likelihood of a flare of rheumatoid symptoms, the authors routinely discontinue its use postoperatively and recommend that patients remain off of methotrexate for 6 to 8 weeks if possible.

Few studies exist to direct perioperative management of the newer biologic agents such as TNF-α and interleukin-1 antagonists. Because of their strong immunoregulatory effects, these agents may predispose patients for opportunistic infections.[83,84] In a retrospective review, Giles and colleagues[87] reported that 10 of 91 (11%) patients with rheumatoid arthritis who underwent an orthopaedic surgical procedure developed early, major postoperative infection (septic arthritis, osteomyelitis, deep wound infection). Of the 10 patients with infection, 7 (70%) were receiving TNF-α inhibitor therapy during the perioperative period. There are no data on the effects of these agents on bone fusion. Current recommendations are to discontinue biologic agents preoperatively (at the end of the dosing cycle), and restart 10 to 14 days postoperatively.

Operative Procedures

Atlantoaxial (C1-2) Instability

Posterior fusion is considered the standard procedure using sublaminar or interspinous wires, hook-claw constructs, or transarticular screws. Gallie[19] and Brooks[20] wiring techniques require the presence of the posterior arch of C1, supplemental bone graft, and external immobilization. Claw-type constructs such as the Halifax clamp are rarely used today because of biomechanical limitations and better options. Transarticular screw fixation is popular because of its multidirectional rigidity, but it requires intraoperative fluoroscopy and preoperative axial imaging to visualize the vertebral artery anatomy. Direct screw fixation of the C1 lateral masses and C2 pedicles, pars, or lamina has been described more recently.[29,88,89]

Wire Techniques

Stand-alone wiring techniques have largely been replaced by transarticular screw or direct screw-rod fixation techniques. Wiring techniques are frequently used as adjuncts to other fixation, particularly for securing bone graft material to help facilitate fusion. In addition, a thorough knowledge of these methods is necessary because their use may be required as a "bailout" in patients with anatomy unfavorable to other techniques.

The Gallie wiring technique plus bone graft was described in 1939 for fracture fixation in the cervical spine.[19] Sublaminar wire fixation is obtained on the C1 ring and around the C2 spinous process (Fig. 34–4). The authors recommend a modification of the Gallie technique. The patient's head is placed in a tong-type holder for rigid positioning. Intraoperative imaging should be used to determine the final position of the head and neck and to confirm adequate reduction of C1. The chin should be tucked to open the space between the occiput and C1 to facilitate passage of sublaminar wire.

An occiput-to-C2 fusion may be safer with or without a C1 laminectomy in cases of an inadequate posterior space available for safe wire passage of an unreducible C1 ring.

A posterior exposure is used, remaining close to the midline with no more than 1.5 cm lateral dissection on the C1 ring to avoid the vertebral artery and the venous plexus between C1 and C2. Cobb elevators are used to expose subperiosteally the base of the occiput to the caudad aspect of the C2 lamina at a minimum. Small curets can be used to develop the plane under the C1 ring for wire passage. A loop is created with a 20-gauge wire with the tip contoured for safe passage under the C1 ring. A nerve hook is used to engage the loop and pull it through approximately 2 cm. The free ends of the 20-gauge wire are fed through the loop, and the wire is cinched down tightly onto the C1 ring at the midline. Alternatively, sutures may be passed underneath C1 with a Mayo needle placed in a reverse manner with the blunt end from caudad to cephalad.

Wires are placed within the suture loops and passed underneath the lamina as the sutures are withdrawn caudally. A bur hole is made at the base of the C2 spinous process, and a second 20-gauge wire is passed through the hole and looped beneath the spinous process and through the hole again to provide stress distribution. Two rectangular blocks of corticocancellous iliac crest bone graft can be harvested and placed over the laminae of C1 and C2 on either side of the midline. The grafts should be near full–thickness to allow for tightening of the wires with less risk of breaking through the fragile bone. The wires are tightened over the graft while watching closely to prevent wire breakthrough. Cancellous chips can be placed around the bone blocks and especially on the ring of C1, where nonunions tend to occur. A drain is typically used, and the wound is closed in layers. If no supplemental internal fixation is used, a halo vest may be needed postoperatively to help maintain reduction. Care must be taken when tightening the wires in the unusual case of a C1 ring that is posteriorly partially dislocated because this tends to subluxate the C1 ring posteriorly. The authors suggest a Brooks technique in this situation.

A Brooks-type modification of the Gallie technique uses bilateral sublaminar wires beneath C1 and C2 (Fig. 34–5). Positioning and exposure are as described for the Gallie technique. A laminotomy may be done between C2 and C3 to facilitate wire passage, a 20-gauge wire is looped, and the

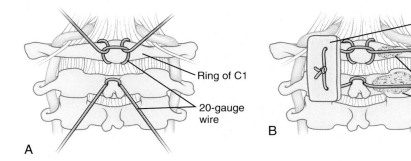

FIGURE 34–4 A and **B,** Modified Gallie-type wiring for posterior C1-2 arthrodesis.

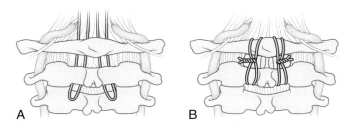

FIGURE 34–5 A and **B,** Brooks-type wiring for posterior C1-2 arthrodesis. Sublaminar wires are passed under C1 and C2 and are tightened down over wedge-shaped, sculpted corticocancellous grafts. Shaping of grafts minimizes chance of graft displacement into canal.

looped end is threaded beneath the lamina of C2 and C1 on either side of the midline. Near full–thickness corticocancellous iliac crest bone grafts are harvested and placed on the lamina of C1 and C2. The grafts should be contoured to fit snugly to reduce the risk of graft slippage. Alternatively, a full bone block may be used with a space in the caudad end to fit around the C2 spinous process. Decortication is unnecessary and risks weakening the lamina. The wires are tightened down in a longitudinal fashion over the bone block on either side. This fixation may provide more rotational stability over the Gallie technique because of fixation on both sides of the midline. A halo vest may be used at the discretion of the surgeon based on the need for maintaining reduction and the adequacy of intraoperative fixation.

Transarticular Screw Fixation

The technique of transarticular screw fixation provides the most rigid fixation for atlantoaxial fusion and can be used in conjunction with wire techniques to provide three-point fixation (Figs. 34–6 and 34–7).[25] It rigidly fixes the C1 and C2 facets, minimizing the need for postoperative external immobilization, which is desired in these patients with fragile skin. Careful preoperative assessment with a CT scan is necessary to define the vertebral artery anatomy adequately. It also ensures that the C2 isthmus is wide enough to accept at least a 3.5-mm screw and that the lateral mass of C1 is reduced and aligned with the superior facet of C2. Other considerations that may preclude the use of this technique include significant cranial settling with collapsed lateral

masses, irreducible subluxations, substantial osteoporosis and osteopenia, comminuted fractures of the atlas and axis vertebrae, and an anomalous vertebral artery.

Patient positioning is the same as with the wire techniques described earlier, but the arm attachment from the tongs to the operating table should be radiolucent to aid visualization with intraoperative fluoroscopy. A longer incision may facilitate angling of the drill guide and screw placement. It is common to use percutaneous stab wounds around the level at the T2-6 spinous process to achieve the correct angle for screw placement. The starting point for drill placement is 3 mm above the C2-3 facet articulation and 2 to 3 mm lateral to the medial border of the C2 facet. The drill guide should be aimed 0 to 10 degrees medially and toward the dorsal cortex of the anterior arch of C1.

Palpation of the medial wall of the pedicle through a laminotomy between C1 and C2 should be considered. Biplanar fluoroscopic images should be obtained before inserting the starting Kirschner wire and during drilling to ensure that the wire hugs the superior cortex of the isthmus to avoid the vertebral artery inferiorly. The vertebral artery is inferior on lateral views and parallel or slightly lateral to the cord on anteroposterior views. The tip of the wire should end about 3 mm short of the anterior cortex of C1 to avoid passing the drill into the oropharynx. Current instrumentations are cannulated and make it easier to place screws. Usually a 3.5-mm or 4.5-mm cannulated screw measuring 40 to 44 mm is adequate. Ideally, wires are drilled on both sides before placing the screws bilaterally. A Gallie-type posterior fixation technique with autologous iliac crest bone graft is used to supplement the fixation. External immobilization devices should be prescribed based on the strength of the construct and bone quality. In many cases, a soft collar is all that is required.

Posterior C1-2 Intra-articular Screw Fixation

A variation is the use of a C1-2 intra-articular interference screw, as described by Tokuhashi and colleagues.[90] In this technique, posterior dissection exposes the C1-2 joints bilaterally. The joint capsule is dissected off the bone and retracted superiorly with the greater occipital nerve. When placing a screw on one side, atlantoaxial subluxation is reduced and maintained by application of a Halifax interlaminar clamp to the contralateral side. A 1-mm Kirschner wire is inserted

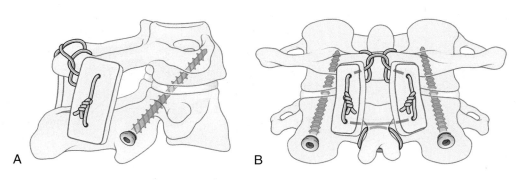

FIGURE 34–6 A and **B,** Transarticular screw technique for C1-2 arthrodesis.

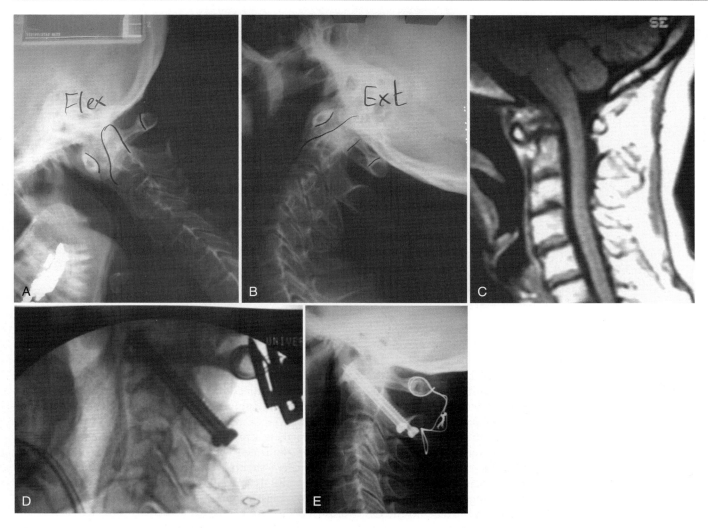

FIGURE 34–7 A 52-year-old woman with long-standing rheumatoid arthritis has neck pain without evidence of frank myelopathy. **A** and **B,** Flexion and extension lateral cervical spine radiograph shows C1-2 instability. There is incomplete reduction in extension. **C,** Sagittal MRI shows pannus around dens. This is likely blocking complete reduction in extension. There is still enough space available for the spinal cord, however, as can be seen on this image. **D** and **E,** Lateral intraoperative fluoroscopic view of C1-2 (**D**) and postoperative lateral radiographic view (**E**) after transarticular screw placement and modified Gallie-type wiring with bone grafting for posterior C1-2 arthrodesis.

directly into the C1-2 joint, and a cannulated tap is used to prepare the site for insertion of the cannulated 5.6-mm or 6.5-mm titanium interference screw. These screws are typically 8 mm or 10 mm long. The procedure is performed on the opposite side. Finally, corticocancellous bone graft is fashioned to fit the intralaminar space and is secured beneath bilateral Halifax clamps. Patients are placed in a cervical collar postoperatively.

In a more recent study, Tokuhashi and colleagues[91] used this technique in 22 patients with rheumatoid arthritis. All patients reported significant improvement in pain, and all patients who were Ranawat class IIIA or above improved neurologically by 2-year follow-up. Atlantoaxial reduction was maintained, and bony fusion was noted in all patients, although four patients eventually had changes in alignment of the subaxial cervical spine (none of which required surgical intervention).

Posterior C1-2 Screw-Rod Constructs

Several methods of posterior C1-2 rigid instrumentation have been described more recently. Harms and Melcher[29] reported a technique involving placement of 3.5-mm polyaxial screws directly into the lateral mass of C1 and into the pars interarticularis or pedicle of C2 bilaterally (Fig. 34–8). Vertical rods are attached to these screws followed by bone grafting to obtain arthrodesis. This method allows for direct manipulation and reduction of C1 on C2 as needed. The advantages of this technique include the theoretical decreased risk to the vertebral artery compared with C1-2 transarticular screws. Bleeding from the venous lakes covering the C1 lateral masses can easily be encountered and is a disadvantage of this technique. This bleeding is usually minimized by meticulous subperiosteal dissection and can typically be controlled by absorbable gelatin sponge (Gelfoam). Either technique

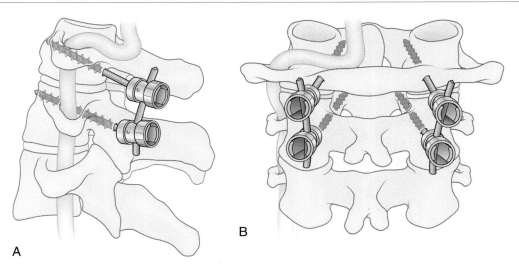

FIGURE 34–8 A and **B,** Posterior C1-2 fixation technique with polyaxial screws and rods. Screws are placed into the lateral masses of C1 and into the pedicles of C2.

requires an intimate knowledge of the anatomy by the operating surgeon aided by good fluoroscopic technique.

For posterior C1-2 screw-rod constructs, first the C1-2 joint is identified because this serves as the anatomic landmark for accurate placement of the C1 lateral mass screw. Removing a small amount of the caudal part of the C1 posterior arch with a bur aids in visualizing the C1 screw starting point. The C2 nerve root can be gently retracted caudally for visualization. The screw is placed in the center of the lateral mass, first using a high-speed bur to create a dimple so that the drill bit does not skid while drilling. The pilot hole is drilled straight or slightly convergent and parallel to the C1 posterior arch in the sagittal direction. The drill hole is typically 18 to 22 mm, which should be confirmed with fluoroscopy. A longer screw than this is needed because the polyaxial screw head needs to be elevated off of the cortex of the lateral mass to accommodate rod fixation.

The entry point for the C2 pedicle screw is in the upper and medial quadrants of the isthmus surface. The direction of the pilot hole is approximately 20 to 30 degrees in a convergent and cephalad direction. The medial border of the C2 pars interarticularis can initially be palpated with a small elevator to help with accurate placement of C2 screws. A typical length for C2 pedicle screws would be 22 to 28 mm, which would again be confirmed with fluoroscopy. In their study, Harms and Melcher[29] did not wire in grafts for their fusion technique; however, this is an option to augment the stability of the screw-rod construct and to help insure a successful arthrodesis (see Fig. 34–7).

An alternative to the C2 pedicle or pars screw is placement of an intralaminar C2 screw (Fig. 34–9). As described by Wright,[88] this technique provides excellent fixation of C2 with virtually no risk of injury to neurovascular structures. Exposure is as described earlier for the placement of C1 lateral mass

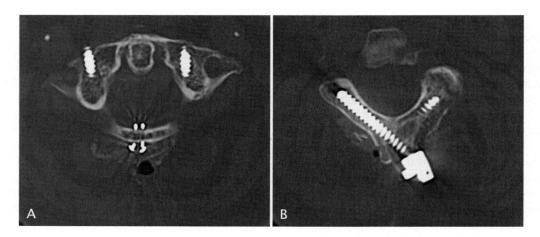

FIGURE 34–9 A and **B,** Posterior C1-2 fixation with placement of C1 lateral mass screws and C2 intralaminar screws. **A,** Axial CT scan through C1 showing location of lateral mass screws. **B,** Axial CT scan through C2 lamina showing bilateral intralaminar screws. Because of the technique required for insertion, the screws are not in exactly the same axial plane.

and C2 pedicle screws. Placement of the C1 lateral mass screws is done by the previously described technique. For placement of the C2 intralaminar screws, a high-speed bur is used to open a small cortical window at the cranial end of the junction of the C2 spinous process and lamina. A hand drill is used to drill the intercortical space of the contralateral lamina to a depth of approximately 30 mm, while maintaining alignment of the drill with the exposed dorsal aspect of the lamina.

After palpation of the drill tract with a ball tip probe, a 4 × 30 mm polyaxial screw is inserted. A starting hole is drilled in the contralateral side at the caudal junction of the spinous process and lamina, and using the same technique, an intralaminar screw is inserted. Care must be taken when inserting the screws to maintain the angle of insertion slightly more shallow than the angle of the lamina, to ensure that any cortical breach occurs dorsally, rather than ventrally into the spinal canal. The polyaxial screw heads from C1 and C2 are connected with a rod. In some instances, because of the angle of the screws relative to one another, offset connectors may need to be used to facilitate rod insertion. The laminae of C1 and C2 may be decorticated, and cortico-cancellous bone graft may be applied (and wired into place if desired).

A more recent biomechanical study examined the relative stability of several C1-2 screw-rod constructs in an odontoid fracture model.[92] Using cadaveric specimens, C1 lateral mass screws were placed and connected to C2 intralaminar screws, C2 pars screws, or C2 pedicle screws. Insertional torque for C2 pedicle screws and intralaminar screws was similar, and both of these were significantly higher than pars screws. Pullout strength was greatest for pedicle screws. In intact models, intralaminar screws provided superior resistance to axial rotation compared with pars screws and similar resistance to pedicle screws. After experimentally induced odontoid fracture, pars and pedicle screws were superior in resisting lateral bending. Although similar to the intralaminar technique, pedicle screws overall provided the greatest stability of C1-2 in all planes, particularly after experimental odontoid fracture. Lapiswala and colleagues[93] noted similar results with C2 intralaminar screws providing less resistance to lateral bending than either C2 pedicle screws or C2-C1 transarticular screws. In their study, all posterior constructs, when supplemented with posterior cable fixation, provided similar stiffness in flexion-extension and axial rotation.

Occipitocervical Fusion

The technique of choice to treat patients with cranial settling or fixed atlantoaxial subluxations causing posterior cord impingement from the ring of C1 is occipitocervical fusion.[52,80,94] In the latter case, an occiput-to-C2 fusion with a C1 laminectomy is preferred. Patient positioning is the same as with the wire techniques described earlier. The base of the occiput from the external occipital protuberance is exposed with caudad extension to the level of the subaxial spine to be fused.

Wiring and Graft Technique

The wiring and graft technique uses corticocancellous bone blocks wired to the occiput and laminae (Fig. 34–10).[52,80,94] The prominent bony protuberance (inion) that is present approximately 2 cm below the external occipital protuberance is the site of wire fixation (approximately 5 to 7 cm from the base of the skull). A 2-mm diamond bur is used to make unicortical holes to form a tunnel with a bridge of superficial cortical bone on each side of the midline. The holes are connected with a towel clamp between the inner and outer tables of the skull. A 20-gauge wire is passed through the tunnel and looped back under and out again to wrap around the bony bridge. A second wire is passed beneath the C1 lamina (if it has not been removed) and looped onto itself to cinch down on the lamina. A wire is passed transversely through the base of the C2 spinous process and looped around and passed back through to distribute stress. Other interspinous or sublaminar wires can be used in more caudad segments as needed. Long, thick corticocancellous iliac crest grafts are harvested, typically 9 to 10 cm in length and 1.5 cm wide.

For occiput-to-C2 fusions, a single block of graft may be used with the caudad end fashioned to fit around the C2 spinous process. A 1.5-mm drill bit is used to place holes through the graft. The wires are threaded through the graft with the cancellous side facing the exposed skull and laminae. The concavity of the central part of the iliac crest facilitates excellent contact between the occiput and the laminae. In severely osteopenic patients, a wire mesh may be placed over the cortical side of the graft to prevent the wires from cutting through the graft.[52] The wires are tightened down cautiously to prevent breakage or cutting through the graft. Cancellous bone chips may be added to the construct. A drain is typically used, and the wound is closed in layers. Without adjuvant fixation, most patients are managed in a halo vest postoperatively, but a two-poster brace or other cervical orthosis may be used based on the stability of the construct.

Occipitocervical Plating

Occipitocervical plating provides more rigid fixation compared with wiring techniques,[34,36,95,96] even in patients with significant osteoporosis. Early instrumentation consisted of acetabular reconstruction plates,[36] but current improvements are more versatile and incorporate plate-rod hybrid constructs (Fig. 34–11). It may be technically challenging to produce the correct amount of contour required at the base of the skull. In longer fusions, it is recommended that fixation is achieved in C2 and in the lower vertebrae before fixation into the skull because the more distal fixation points require more precise anatomic locations. C2 fixation can be done with pedicle screws, transarticular screws, or intralaminar screws (described earlier). Because of their inferior pullout strength, C2 pars screws should not be used unless the fusion is to be carried down into the subaxial cervical spine.

Fixation to the skull requires knowledge of the venous sinus anatomy to avoid bleeding complications. Screws should be placed distal to the transverse sinus, which lies at the level

FIGURE 34–10 Technique of posterior occipitocervical fusion. **A,** Bur hole is made in nuchal bony ridge, staying between cortical table. **B,** 20-gauge wires are passed down; looping the wire through a second time improves the grip and distributes the stress. **C,** Near full–thickness corticocancellous grafts are harvested from ilium. **D,** Grafts are wired in place as shown. Cancellous bone is also packed in crevices. (Modified from Werthein SB, Bohlman HH: Occipitocervical fusion: Indications, technique, and long-term results in thirteen patients. J Bone Joint Surg Am 69:833-836, 1987.)

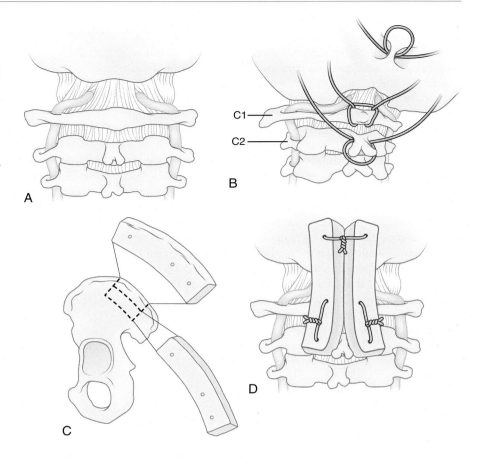

of the external occipital protuberance. The thickness of the skull decreases laterally away from the midline and closer to the foramen magnum.[97] Unicortical fixation is adequate in the thicker areas of the skull, but bicortical fixation can be performed safely. Two to three screws should be used on each side of the midline. A 2-mm diamond bur is used to minimize the chance of a spinal fluid leak, which is common when using more aggressive carbide burs. The holes are tapped, and 3.5- to 4.5-mm screws 6 to 12 mm in length are placed. In case of a spinal fluid leak, bone wax may be sufficient to stop the leak; otherwise, placing the screw usually tamponades the leak. There does not seem to be any adverse effect from breaching the inner table. The head and neck are immobilized in a two-poster brace or a halo vest in patients with osteoporotic bone and questionable fixation. Patients are typically changed to a soft collar for comfort after 8 weeks.

Contoured Loop and Rod Technique

The contoured loop and rod technique was first proposed by Ransford and colleagues in 1986[32] and is used with segmental wiring to provide occipitocervical fixation.[32,98-100] The exposure is similar to that described earlier for plate fixation. Wires are placed in the occiput and beneath the lamina of C1 and the subaxial vertebrae. Earlier constructs relied on a horseshoe-shaped loop of 5⁄32 threaded stainless steel rods. The horizontal limb should be approximately 3.5 to 4 cm wide, and the length

of the occipital portion of the loop should be 2.5 to 3 cm. More recent constructs use a custom-contoured threaded titanium loop with titanium-threaded cables, which allows for postoperative MRI.

Resection of the Odontoid

Mild to moderate cervicomedullary compression can be treated with posterior C1 laminectomy and occipitocervical fusion as described earlier. The pannus resorbs with stabilization.[40] Anterior decompression may be needed, however, to treat an irreducible anterior extradural compression of the cervicomedullary junction by pannus or a severely migrated odontoid.[101,102] The transoral approach is associated with an increased risk of infection with mouth flora; the high retropharyngeal approach is a good alternative in many patients.[103] Supplemental posterior fusion is required unless there is a solid prior posterior fusion mass. In case of a prior posterior fusion, resection of the odontoid without grafting suffices. In cases without prior posterior fusion, anterior strut grafting with iliac crest or fibula is required between C2 or C3 and the clivus, followed by posterior occipitocervical fusion. Posterior stabilization may be staged depending on the medical status of the patient. Thorough preoperative assessment is necessary and includes swallowing and respiratory function considerations, dental assessment, and the presence of a mobile temporomandibular joint to allow about 2.5 to 3 cm of opening.

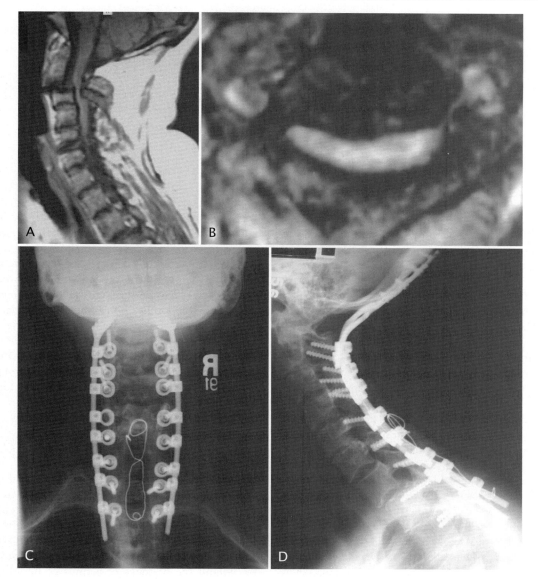

FIGURE 34–11 A 46-year-old woman had a long history of rheumatoid arthritis diagnosed when she was a young girl. She has had chronic neck pain but developed worsening neck pain over the past 6 weeks with increasing numbness of her arms and some truncal numbness. Some weakness of the upper extremities was evident on physical examination. **A** and **B,** MRI shows severe cord compression primarily at C2-3 level. She has multiple levels of subluxation in subaxial spine including C7-T1. **C** and **D,** Anteroposterior and lateral postoperative plain films after posterior decompression at C2-3 followed by long occipitocervical fusion with bone grafting and posterior instrumentation. Screws were placed in pedicles of C7 and T1 for maximum fixation and osteoporotic bone.

Subaxial Fusion

Subaxial subluxations may be fixed or mobile. The fixed types may be best treated with anterior decompression and fusion. Strong consideration should be given to supplemental posterior fixation because anterior column instability may occur from graft resorption or settling into the osteoporotic verte-bral bodies. Mobile subluxations are best treated with traction to realign the spine and posterior instrumented fusion. As noted earlier, a better reduction may be obtained when positioning of the head is done gently with the patient under anesthesia.

Wiring Techniques

Posterior wiring and autogenous bone grafting may provide stable fixation at a high fusion rate. The authors use the triple wire technique described by McAfee and Bohlman (Fig. 34–12).[103] The first 20-gauge wire is woven in a figure-of-eight fashion through holes drilled into the base of the spinous processes of the involved vertebrae. This is the midline tether-ing wire. The wire is typically looped onto itself after passing through the spinous process to help distribute stress; 22-gauge wires can then pass individually through the same holes to loop around the spinous processes at the ends of the segments to be fused. The ends of these wires pass through drill holes

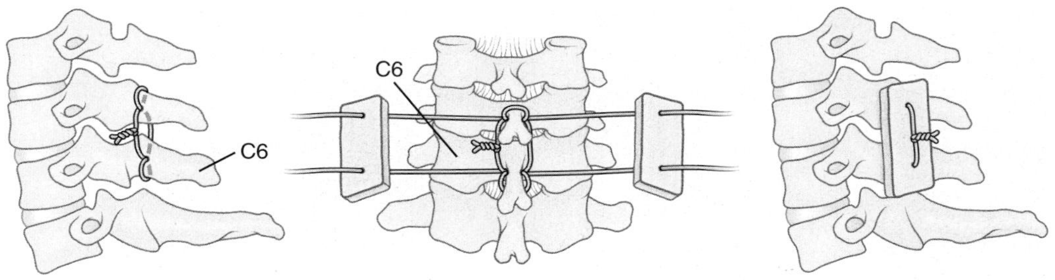

FIGURE 34–12 A-C, Bohlman triple-wire technique for posterior cervical arthrodesis.

in the rectangular corticocancellous iliac crest autografts. The wires are tightened down on the graft to force the graft against the laminae. Decortication is unnecessary. The wound is closed in layers over a drain. A two-poster cervical brace is used for 6 to 8 weeks to allow solid fusion.

Lateral Mass Plating and Screw and Rod Constructs

Lateral mass plating and screw and rod constructs typically provide excellent fixation of the subaxial spine. Several modifications exist in the way the screws are angled in the lateral mass.[25-28] According to An and colleagues,[26] 15 degrees of superior angulation and 30 degrees of lateral angulation best avoids violating the facet joints and the nerve roots. All the techniques avoid the vertebral artery, which lies anterior to the lateral mass. The starting point is 1 mm medial to the center of the lateral mass. Current instrumentations come with standard drill kits. The screws average 14 to 18 mm, depending on the size of the patient. The C7 lateral mass is thin and may require pedicle screw placement or supplemental posterior wiring between the C6 and C7 spinous processes as described earlier. Fluoroscopy is helpful in placing C7 pedicle screws if the shoulders are not in the way, but a C7 laminotomy provides direct palpation of the medial wall of the pedicle for safer screw placement. A 25- to 30-degree medial angulation is recommended.[26] Pedicle screw fixation of all involved levels of the cervical vertebrae has been described frequently in other patient populations but has limitations of pedicle size and risks to the vertebral artery.[104]

Complications

Complications after cervical spine surgery in patients with rheumatoid arthritis include quadriplegia, infection, wound dehiscence, skin problems from external immobilization devices, nonunion, and subaxial subluxation above or below a fused segment. Anterior fusion procedures have risks of graft resorption and anterior column collapse because of the inflammatory process and secondary osteoporosis of the vertebral bodies. Patients undergoing anterior procedures may benefit from adjunctive posterior stabilization.

The progressive nature of rheumatoid disease of the spine demands long-term follow-up to assess for the development of new symptoms in previously asymptomatic segments (see Fig. 34–12). In a study of 51 patients undergoing cervical fusion for instability secondary to rheumatoid arthritis, Clarke

and colleagues[105] reported that at average 8.3-year follow-up, 39% of patients undergoing C1-2 fixation developed subaxial subluxation. Slightly more than half of these patients required extension of fusion for symptomatic or unstable subaxial subluxation. This subluxation occurred most commonly at C3-4 (62% of patients). Of the patients who underwent long posterior fusions (C1 to C6 through T1) for combined atlantoaxial and subaxial instability, none required secondary procedures. Including all involved unstable levels in the initial fusion procedure may reduce the risk of subsequent adjacent level subluxation. Age, presence of atlantoaxial instability, and perioperative complications have been shown to be independent predictors of long-term mortality after cervical surgery in this population.[106]

Thoracolumbar Disease

In contrast to the cervical spine, rheumatoid disease of the thoracic and lumbar spine leads to severe neurologic symptoms less frequently and has received less attention. Cases of thoracic myelopathy, lumbar radiculopathy, and cauda equina syndrome have been reported, however, and seem to be due to bony destruction leading to instability and subluxation with or without the presence of pannus or nodules.[107-109] Radiographic findings include poorly defined margins of the vertebral endplates and a relative lack of osteophytes.[110,111] Involvement of the facet joints may lead to spondylolisthesis and instability on flexion-extension films. Heywood and Meyers[110] postulated that the pathologic process in the lumbar spine begins with synovitis of the facet joints causing functional incompetence, allowing anteroposterior and lateral translation. This synovitis is followed by discitis, which may start as an enthesopathy at the junction of the endplate and disc, resulting in loss of disc height and contributing further to instability. In the thoracic spine, the disease may also spread directly into the spine via the costovertebral joints. Nerve root impingement may be due to spinal instability and direct impingement from rheumatoid pannus.[110]

To correlate radiographic findings with clinical symptoms, Kawaguchi and colleagues[111] studied 106 patients with rheumatoid arthritis and found that 40% of patients complained of back pain, 18% had leg pain and 12% exhibited symptoms of neurogenic claudication. They reported abnormal radiographic findings in 57% of patients, with disc space narrowing the most frequent finding, in 37% of patients; coronal plane deformity in 28%; spondylolisthesis in 23%; and endplate or facet erosion in 20%. Finally, Kawaguchi and colleagues[111] noted a high percentage of osteoporosis, particularly in patients on steroid therapy. Using MRI, Sakai and colleagues[112] reported a 45.2% incidence of lumbar involvement in rheumatoid arthritis and described two distinct patterns of disc destruction: narrowing, in which the disc space progressively collapsed, and ballooning, in which changes in the endplates give the illusion of increasing disc height. Additionally, they found that the degree of lumbar involvement related to the severity of peripheral joint involvement.

The literature regarding surgical treatment of lumbar involvement is sparse. One more recent study retrospectively compared outcomes of 19 patients with rheumatoid arthritis who underwent posterior lumbar decompression and fusion with a matched control group of patients without rheumatoid arthritis.[113] Given the small number of patients in the study, there were no significant differences in complications, fusion, or patient satisfaction between the two groups. Two patients with rheumatoid arthritis showed evidence of loosening of pedicle screws on postoperative radiographs, however, and one patient underwent noninstrumented fusion owing to severe osteoporosis noted intraoperatively. None of the control patients had any hardware complications. In addition, there was a trend toward more wound complications in the rheumatoid arthritis group.

Summary

Most patients with rheumatoid arthritis of the cervical spine can be managed nonoperatively. These patients should be monitored closely, however, because the progression of disease may be silent, and the clinical findings are nonspecific. Screening flexion and extension lateral radiographs should be obtained periodically before neurologic symptoms develop and before any planned surgical procedure that may require general anesthesia, intubation, or manipulation of the cervical spine. The benefits of early detection and surgical intervention in patients with progressive cervical instability cannot be overemphasized, and the current trend is to perform prophylactic fusion before the development of cranial settling or frank neurologic symptoms.[39,51,80] Otherwise, mortality and morbidity significantly increase as patients become less functional and develop Ranawat class III criteria.[51,58,65,79,103] Although surgery in patients with quadriparesis may provide some neurologic and functional recovery, the results are not as predictable as with early surgery.

PEARLS

1. The periodontoid pannus begins to resorb 6 weeks after atlantoaxial fusion.

2. A radiographic AADI of 9 mm or more confirms atlantoaxial instability and is a relative indication for cervical fusion.

3. A PADI of less than 14 mm has a high sensitivity of predicting paralysis and is a more reliable radiographic criterion for

cervical fusion than AADI. A PADI of less than 10 mm is associated with poor motor recovery after fusion, whereas a PADI greater than 14 mm has a higher likelihood of recovery.

4. A cervicomedullary angle of less than 135 degrees (normal 135 to 175 degrees) correlates with myelopathic signs and suggests atlantoaxial instability as the source of myelopathy.

5. Patients with atlantoaxial instability have better outcomes with early surgery before neurologic impairment develops.

PITFALLS

1. Anterior fusion procedures are associated with risk of graft resorption and anterior column collapse owing to the inflammatory process and secondary osteoporosis of the vertebral bodies. Patients undergoing anterior procedures may benefit from adjunctive posterior stabilization.

2. Radiologic improvement of atlantoaxial instability is a "radiographic illusion" and is in reality due to worsening cranial settling as the anterior arch of the atlas approaches the wider base of the odontoid process.

3. Patients with rheumatoid arthritis are at risk for late segmental instability below a previous fusion, and they should be followed long-term.

4. Patients with myelopathy are at significantly increased risk for progression and sudden death if treated nonoperatively.

5. Perioperative upper airway complications are 14 times greater if surgery is done without fiberoptic assistance in patients with rheumatoid arthritis undergoing posterior cervical fusion.

6. Attempts should not be made to pass sublaminar wires beneath a severely stenotic or unreduced C1 arch. A safer option is to fuse from the occiput to the subaxial spine with or without C1 laminectomy.

7. Commonly used rheumatic medications place patients at potential risk for postoperative wound infections, and their effects on spinal fusion are unknown. Most rheumatic medications should be stopped preoperatively and held for as long as possible postoperatively.

8. Patients taking long-term steroids may require perioperative stress dosing.

KEY POINTS

1. Despite improvements in medical management of rheumatoid arthritis, rates of cervical spine surgery have remained constant. The cervical spine is involved in 25% to 90% of patients. Because cervical instability may be asymptomatic in many patients, the clinician must be vigilant to evaluate the cervical spine, particularly in preparation for any proposed surgical management of other structures (e.g., extremities).

2. The inflammatory reaction in rheumatoid arthritis has a predilection for synovial joints, including the facet, occipitoatlantal, and atlantoaxial joints. The resulting joint erosion can lead to instability. The most common instability pattern is atlantoaxial, followed by subaxial instability and

occipitoatlantal instability. Basilar invagination results from cranial settling and can result in sudden death from pressure on the brainstem. Patients frequently present with pain secondary to instability but may also present with neurologic symptoms including myelopathy.

3. Surgical indications include the presence of myelopathy. Radiographic indicators include an AADI 9 mm or greater, PADI less than 14 mm, mobile subaxial subluxation greater than 3.5 mm, space available for the cord less than 14 mm, and cranial settling. Cervicomedullary angle (measured on MRI or CT) less than 135 degrees suggests impending neurologic deficit. Surgical intervention performed early, before the development of cranial settling or ambulatory difficulty, has the best functional outcome.

4. Rheumatoid medications should be managed carefully in the perioperative period. Most drugs act as anti-inflammatories or immune modulators and may increase the risk of perioperative infection and delayed wound healing or bone fusion. There is a paucity of literature relating to perioperative use of rheumatoid medications, particularly with respect to spinal surgery.

5. Modern rigid internal fixation should be used for surgical stabilization whenever possible. Because of variation in patient anatomy, the surgeon must be aware of different fixation options, such as the use of either C2 pedicle screws or C2 interlaminar screws. Similarly, familiarity with classic fixation techniques (e.g., wiring) is necessary because these may sometimes be the only available options. A clear understanding of the anatomy and pathology of the individual patient is necessary to perform safe, effective surgery.

KEY REFERENCES

1. Boden SD, Dodge LD, Bohlman HH, et al: Rheumatoid arthritis of the cervical spine. J Bone Joint Surg Am 75:1282-1297, 1993.

   The authors showed that PADI may be more reliable in predicting neurologic outcome because it is a more accurate indicator of the space available for the cord. Patients with a PADI of at least 14 mm were more likely to have neurologic recovery after surgical stabilization, whereas patients with a PADI less than 10 mm had no neurologic recovery. The critical space available for the cord in the subaxial spine was also shown to be 14 mm.

2. Bundschuh C, Modic MT, Kearney F, et al: Rheumatoid arthritis of the cervical spine: Surface-coil MR imaging. AJNR Am J Neuroradiol 9:565-571, 1988.

   The authors determined that patients with a cervicomedullary angle less than 135 degrees (normal 135 to 175 degrees) were likely to have evidence of brainstem compression, cervical myelopathy, or C2 root pain.

3. Larsson E-M, Holtås S, Zygmunt S: Pre- and postoperative MR imaging of the craniocervical junction in rheumatoid arthritis. AJNR Am J Neuroradiol 152:561-566, 1989.

The authors noted reduction of the periodontoid pannus 6 weeks after surgical stabilization of the atlantoaxial instability.

4. Ranawat CS, O'Leary P, Pellici P, et al: Cervical spine fusion in rheumatoid arthritis. J Bone Joint Surg Am 61:1003-1010, 1979.

   The authors studied 33 patients with cervical instability and devised a classification of pain and neurologic dysfunction that is widely used to assess the functional capacity of patients with rheumatoid arthritis and cervical disease. They also presented an improved method to measure the amount of cranial settling.

5. Riew KD, Hilibrand A, Palumbo MA, et al: Diagnosing basilar invagination in the rheumatoid patient. J Bone Joint Surg Am 83:194-200, 2001.

   The authors noted that none of the traditional radiographic measurements alone had a sensitivity, specificity, or negative or positive predictive value greater than 90% but that the combination of Clark station and Redlund-Johnell, and Ranawat criteria had a sensitivity and negative predictive value of 94% and 91%.

6. Harms J, Melcher R: Posterior C1-C2 fusion with polyaxial screw and rod fixation. Spine (Phila Pa 1976) 26:2467-2471, 2001.

   The authors described the surgical technique for posterior C1 lateral mass and C2 pedicle screw fixation, which has become the preferred method of atlantoaxial fixation.

REFERENCES

1. Ward MW: Decreases in rates of hospitalization for manifestations of severe rheumatoid arthritis, 1983-2001. Arthritis Rheum 50:1122-1131, 2004.

2. Bland JH: Rheumatoid arthritis of the cervical spine. J Rheumatol 3:319-341, 1974.

3. Heywood AWB, Meyers OL: Rheumatoid arthritis of the thoracic and lumbar spine. J Bone Joint Surg Br 68:362-368, 1986.

4. Kawaguchi Y, Matsuno H, Kanamori M, et al: Radiologic findings of the lumbar spine in patients with rheumatoid arthritis, and a review of pathologic mechanisms. J Spinal Disord Tech 16:38-43, 2003.

5. Neva MH, Hakkinen A, Makinen H, et al: High prevalence of asymptomatic cervical spine subluxation in patients with rheumatoid arthritis waiting for orthopaedic surgery. Ann Rheum Dis 65:884-888, 2006.

6. Hansen SE: The recognition of rheumatoid arthritis in the eighteenth century: The contribution of Linné and Bosissier de la Croix de Sauvages. Scand J Rheumatol 22:178-182, 1993.

7. Short CL: The antiquity of rheumatoid arthritis. Arthritis Rheum 17:193-205, 1974.

8. Snorrason E: Landré-Beauvais and his Goutte Asthénique Primitive. Acta Med Scand 142(Suppl 266):115-118, 1952.

9. Garrod AE: A Treatise on Rheumatism and Rheumatoid Arthritis. London, Griffin, 1890.

10. Lourie H, Stewart WA: Spontaneous atlantoaxial dislocation: A complication of rheumatoid disease. N Engl J Med 265:677-681, 1961.

11. Pratt TLC: Spontaneous dislocation of the atlanto-axial articulation occurring in ankylosing spondylitis and rheumatoid arthritis. J Fac Radiol 10:40-43, 1959.

12. Werne S: Spontaneous dislocation of the atlas (as a complication of rheumatoid arthritis). Acta Rheumatol Scand 3:101-107, 1957.

13. Wilson PD Jr, Dangelmajer RC: The problem of atlanto-axial dislocation in rheumatoid arthritis. In Proceedings of the American Orthopaedic Association. J Bone Joint Surg Am 45:1780, 1963.

14. Brattström H, Granholm L: Atlanto-axial fusion in rheumatoid arthritis: A new method of fixation with wire and bone cement. Acta Orthop Scand 47:619-628, 1976.

15. Ferlic DC, Clayton ML, Leidholt JD, et al: Surgical treatment of the symptomatic unstable cervical spine in rheumatoid arthritis. J Bone Joint Surg Am 57:349-354, 1975.

16. Hamblen DL: Occipito-cervical fusion: Indications, technique and results. J Bone Joint Surg Br 49:33-45, 1967.

17. McGraw RW, Rusch RM: Atlanto-axial arthrodesis. J Bone Joint Surg Br 55:482-489, 1973.

18. Rana NA, Hancock DO, Taylor AR, et al: Atlanto-axial subluxation in rheumatoid arthritis. J Bone Joint Surg Br 55:458-470, 1973.

19. Gallie WE: Fractures and dislocations of the cervical spine. Am J Surg 46:495-499, 1939.

20. Brooks AL, Jenkins EB: Atlanto-axial arthrodesis by the wedge compression method. J Bone Joint Surg Am 60:279-284, 1978.

21. Wertheim SB, Bohlman HH: Occipitocervical fusion: Indications, technique, and long-term results in thirteen patients. J Bone Joint Surg Am 69:833-836, 1987.

22. Clark CR, Goetz DD, Menezes AH: Arthrodesis of the cervical spine in rheumatoid arthritis. J Bone Joint Surg Am 71:381-392, 1989.

23. Cybulski GR, Stone JL, Crowell RM, et al: Use of Halifax interlaminar clamps for posterior C1-C2 arthrodesis. Neurosurgery 22:429-431, 1988.

24. Grob D, Jeanneret B, Aebi M, et al: Atlanto-axial fusion with transarticular screw fixation. J Bone Joint Surg Br 73:972-976, 1991.

25. Magerl F, Seeman PS: Stable posterior fusion of the atlas and axis by transarticular screw fixation. In Kehr P, Weidner A (eds): Cervical Spine. Berlin, Springer-Verlag, 1986, pp 322-327.

26. An HS, Gordin R, Renner K: Anatomic considerations for plate-screw fixation of the cervical spine. Spine (Phila Pa 1976) 16(10 Suppl):S548-S551, 1991.

27. Heller JG, Carlson GD, Abitbol JJ, et al: Anatomic comparison of the Roy-Camille and Magerl techniques for screw placement in the lower cervical spine. Spine (Phila Pa 1976) 16(10 Suppl):S552-S557, 1991.

28. Anderson PA, Henley MB, Grady MS, et al: Posterior cervical arthrodesis with AO reconstruction plates and bone graft. Spine (Phila Pa 1976) 16(3 Suppl):S72-S79, 1991.

29. Harms J, Melcher R: Posterior C1-C2 fusion with polyaxial screw and rod fixation. Spine (Phila Pa 1976) 26:2467-2471, 2001.

30. Foerster O: Die Leitungsbahnen des Schmerzgefühls. Berlin, Urban und Schwarzenburg, 1927, p 266.

31. Kahn EA, Yglesias L: Progressive atlanto-axial dislocation. JAMA 105:348-352, 1935.

32. Ransford AO, Crockard HA, Pozo JL, et al: Craniocervical instability treated by contoured loop fixation. J Bone Joint Surg Br 68:173-177, 1986.

33. Flint GA, Hockley AD, McMillan JJ, et al: A new method of occipitocervical fusion using internal fixation. Neurosurgery 21:947-950, 1987.

34. Grob D, Dvorak J, Panjabi M, et al: The role of plate and screw fixation in occipitocervical fusion in rheumatoid arthritis. Spine (Phila Pa 1976) 19:2545-2551, 1994.

35. Grob D, Dvorak J, Panjabi M, et al: Posterior occipitocervical fusion: A preliminary report of a new technique. Spine (Phila Pa 1976) 16(Suppl 3):S17-S24, 1991.

36. Smith MD, Anderson P, Grady MS: Occipitocervical arthrodesis using contoured plate fixation: An early report on a versatile fixation technique. Spine (Phila Pa 1976) 18:1984-1990, 1993.

37. Kontinnen Y, Santavirta S, Bergroth V, et al: Inflammatory involvement of cervical spine ligaments in rheumatoid arthritis. Acta Orthop Scand 57:587, 1986.

38. Mikulowski P, Wollheim FA, Rotmil P, et al: Sudden death in rheumatoid arthritis with atlanto-axial dislocation. Acta Med Scand 198:445-451, 1975.

39. Agarwal AK, Peppelman WC, Kraus DR, et al: Recurrence of cervical spine instability in rheumatoid arthritis following previous fusion: Can disease progression be prevented by early surgery? J Rheumatol 19:1364-1370, 1992.

40. Larsson E-M, Holtås S, Zygmunt S: Pre- and postoperative MR imaging of the craniocervical junction in rheumatoid arthritis. AJR Am J Roentgenol 152:561-566, 1989.

41. Toolanen G, Larsson SE, Fagerlund M: Medullary compression in rheumatoid atlanto-axial subluxation evaluated by computerized tomography. Spine (Phila Pa 1976) 11:191-194, 1986.

42. Chen TY, Lin KL, Ho HH: Morphologic characteristics of atlantoaxial complex in rheumatoid arthritis and surgical consideration among Chinese. Spine (Phila Pa 1976) 29:1000-1004, 2004.

43. Lewandrowski KU, Park PP, Baron JM, et al: Atraumatic odontoid fractures in patients with rheumatoid arthritis. Spine J 6:529-533, 2008.

44. Smith PH, Benn RT, Sharp J: Natural history of rheumatoid cervical luxations. Ann Rheum Dis 31:431-439, 1972.

45. Bogduk N, Major GA, Carter J: Lateral subluxation of the atlas in rheumatoid arthritis: A case report and postmortem study. Ann Rheum Dis 43:341-346, 1984.

46. Rana NA: Natural history of atlanto-axial subluxation in rheumatoid arthritis. Spine (Phila Pa 1976) 14:1054-1056, 1989.

47. Papadopoulos SM, Dickman CA, Sonntag VK: Atlantoaxial stabilization in rheumatoid arthritis. J Neurosurg 74:1-7, 1991.

48. Weissman BN, Aliabadi P, Weinfeld MS, et al: Prognostic features of atlantoaxial subluxation in rheumatoid arthritis patients. Radiology 144:745-751, 1982.

49. Delamarter RB, Bohlman HH: Postmortem osseous and neuropathologic analysis of the rheumatoid cervical spine. Spine (Phila Pa 1976) 19:2267-2274, 1994.

50. Henderson FC, Geddes JF, Crockard HA: Neuropathology of the brainstem and spinal cord in end-stage rheumatoid

arthritis: Implications for treatment. Ann Rheum Dis 52:629-637, 1993.

51. Casey ATH, Crockard HA, Bland JM, et al: Surgery on the rheumatoid cervical spine for the non-ambulant myelopathic patient—too much, too late? Lancet 347:1004-1007, 1996.

52. Lipson SJ: Cervical myelopathy and posterior atlanto-axial subluxation in patients with rheumatoid arthritis. J Bone Joint Surg Am 67:593-597, 1985.

53. Burry HC, Tweed JM, Robinson RG, et al: Lateral subluxation of the atlanto-axial joint in rheumatoid arthritis. Ann Rheum Dis 37:525-528, 1978.

54. Kudo H, Iwano K: Surgical treatment of subaxial cervical myelopathy in rheumatoid arthritis. J Bone Joint Surg Br 73:474-480, 1991.

55. Winfield J, Cooke D, Brook AS, et al: A prospective study of the radiological changes in the cervical spine in early rheumatoid disease. Ann Rheum Dis 40:109-114, 1981.

56. Winfield J, Young A, Williams P, et al: Prospective study of the radiological changes in hands, feet, and cervical spine in adult rheumatoid disease. Ann Rheum Dis 42:613-618, 1983.

57. Pellicci PM, Ranawat CS, Tsairis P, et al: A prospective study of the progression of rheumatoid arthritis of the cervical spine. J Bone Joint Surg Am 63:342-350, 1981.

58. Sunahara N, Matsunaga S, Mori T, et al: Clinical course of conservatively managed rheumatoid arthritis patients with myelopathy. Spine (Phila Pa 1976) 22:2603-2608, 1997.

59. Paimela L, Laasonen L, Kankaanpää E, et al: Progression of cervical spine changes with early rheumatoid arthritis. J Rheumatol 24:1280-1284, 1997.

60. Young A, Corbett M, Winfield J, et al: A prognostic index for erosive changes in the hands, feet, and cervical spines in early rheumatoid arthritis. Br J Rheumatol 27:94-101, 1988.

61. Sharp J, Purser DW: Spontaneous atlantoaxial dislocation in ankylosing spondylitis and rheumatoid arthritis. Ann Rheum Dis 20:47-50, 1961.

62. Bell HS: Paralysis of both arms from injury of the upper portion of the pyramidal decussation: "Cruciate paralysis." J Neurosurg 33:376-380, 1970.

63. Gurley JP, Bell GR: The surgical management of patients with rheumatoid cervical spine disease. Rheum Dis Clin North Am 23:317-332, 1997.

64. Rana NA, Hancock DO, Taylor AR, et al: Upward translocation of the dens in rheumatoid arthritis. J Bone Joint Surg Br 55:471-477, 1973.

65. Ranawat CS, O'Leary P, Pellicci P, et al: Cervical spine fusion in rheumatoid arthritis. J Bone Joint Surg Am 61:1003-1010, 1979.

66. Casey AT, Crockard HA, Bland JM, et al: Predictors of outcome in the quadriparetic nonambulatory myelopathic patient with rheumatoid arthritis: A prospective study of 55 surgically treated Ranawat class IIIb patients. J Neurosurg 85:574-581, 1996.

67. Boden SD, Dodge LD, Bohlman HH, et al: Rheumatoid arthritis of the cervical spine: A long term analysis with predictors of paralysis and recovery. J Bone Joint Surg Am 75:1282-1297, 1993.

68. Koehler PR, Haughton VM, Daniels DL, et al: MR measurement of the normal and pathologic brainstem diameters. AJNR Am J Neuroradiol 6:425-427, 1985.

69. Taniguchi D, Tokunaga D, Hase H, et al: Evaluation of lateral instability of the atlanto-axial joint in rheumatoid arthritis using dynamic open-mouth view radiographs. Clin Rheumatol 27:851-857, 2008.

70. Riew KD, Hilibrand AS, Palumbo MA, et al: Diagnosing basilar invagination in the rheumatoid patient: The reliability of radiographic criteria. J Bone Joint Surg Am 83:194-200, 2001.

71. Redlund-Johnell I, Pettersson H: Radiographic measurements of the craniovertebral region: Designed for evaluation of abnormalities in rheumatoid arthritis. Acta Radiol Diagn 25:23-28, 1984.

72. White AA, Panjabi MM: Clinical Biomechanics of the Spine, ed 2. Philadelphia: JB Lippincott, 1990.

73. Dvorak J, Grob D, Baumgartner H, et al: Functional evaluation of the spinal cord by magnetic resonance imaging in patients with rheumatoid arthritis and instability of upper cervical spine. Spine (Phila Pa 1976) 14:1057-1064, 1989.

74. Bell GR, Stearns KL: Flexion-extension MRI of the upper rheumatoid cervical spine. Orthopedics 14:969-974, 1991.

75. Bundschuh C, Modic MT, Kearney F, et al: Rheumatoid arthritis of the cervical spine: Surface-coil MR imaging. AJR Am J Roentgenol 151:181-187, 1988.

76. Mawatari T, Miura H, Hamai S, et al: Vertebral strength changes in rheumatoid arthritis patients treated with alendronate, as assessed by finite element analysis of clinical computed tomography scans: A prospective randomized clinical trial. Arthritis Rheum 58:3340-3349, 2008.

77. Schmitt-Sody M, Kirchhoff C, Buhmann S, et al: Timing of cervical spine stabilisation and outcome in patients with rheumatoid arthritis. Int Orthop 32:511-516, 2008.

78. Wattenmaker I, Concepcion M, Hibberd P, et al: Upper-airway obstruction and perioperative management of the airway in patients managed with posterior operations on the cervical spine for rheumatoid arthritis. J Bone Joint Surg Am 76:360-365, 1994.

79. van Asselt KM, Lems WF, Bongartz EB, et al: Outcome of cervical spine surgery in patients with rheumatoid arthritis. Ann Rheum Dis 60:448-452, 2001.

80. Peppelman WC, Krauss DR, Donaldson WF III, et al: Cervical spine surgery in rheumatoid arthritis: Improvement of neurologic deficit after cervical spine fusion. Spine (Phila Pa 1976) 18:2375-2379, 1993.

81. Emery SE, Bohlman HH, Bolesta MJ, et al: Anterior cervical decompression and arthrodesis for the treatment of cervical spondylotic myelopathy: Two to seventeen-year follow-up. J Bone Joint Surg Am 80:941-951, 1998.

82. Chin KR, Ozuna R: Options in the surgical treatment of cervical spondylotic myelopathy. Curr Opin Orthop 11:151-157, 2000.

83. Howe CR, Gardner GC, Kadel NJ: Perioperative medication management for the patient with rheumatoid arthritis. J Am Acad Orthop Surg 14:544-551, 2006.

84. Scanzello CR, Figgie MP, Nestor BJ, et al: Perioperative management of medications used in the treatment of rheumatoid arthritis. HSS J 2:141-147, 2006.

85. Grennan DM, Gray J, Loudon J, et al: Methotrexate and early postoperative complications in patients with rheumatoid arthritis undergoing elective orthopaedic surgery. Ann Rheum Dis 60:214-217, 2001.

86. Gerster JC, Bossy R, Dudler J: Bone non-union after osteotomy in patients treated with methotrexate. J Rheumatol 26:2695-2697, 1999.

87. Giles JT, Bartlett SJ, Gelber AC, et al: Tumor necrosis factor inhibitor therapy and risk of serious postoperative orthopedic infection in rheumatoid arthritis. Arthritis Rheum 55:333-337, 2006.

88. Wright NM: Posterior C2 fixation using bilateral, crossing C2 laminar screws: Case series and technical note. J Spinal Disord Tech 17:158-162, 2004.

89. Payer M, Luzi M, Tessitore E: Posterior atlanto-axial fixation with polyaxial C1 lateral mass screws and C2 pars screws. Acta Neurochir 151:223-229, 2009.

90. Tokuhashi Y, Matsuzaki H, Shirasaki Y, et al: C1-C2 intra-articular screw fixation for atlantoaxial posterior stabilization. Spine (Phila Pa 1976) 25:337-341, 2000.

91. Tokuhashi Y, Ajiro Y, Oshima M, et al: C1-C2 Intra-articular screw fixation for atlantoaxial subluxation due to rheumatoid arthritis. Orthopedics 32:1, 2009.

92. Dmitriev AE, Lehman RA, Helgeson MD, et al: Acute and long term stability of atlantoaxial fixation methods: A biomechanical comparison of pars, pedicle, and intralaminar fixation in an intact and odontoid fracture model. Spine (Phila Pa 1976) 34:365-370, 2009.

93. Lapiswala SB, Anderson PA, Oza A, et al: Biomechanical comparison of four C1 to C2 rigid fixative techniques: Anterior transarticular, posterior transarticular, C1 to C2 pedicle, and C1 to C2 intralaminar screws. Neurosurgery 58:516-521, 2006.

94. McAfee PC, Cassidy JR, Davis RF, et al: Fusion of the occiput to the upper cervical spine: A review of 37 cases. Spine (Phila Pa 1976) 16(Suppl 10):S490-S494, 1991.

95. Huckell CB, Buchowski JM, Richardson WJ, et al: Functional outcome of plate fusions for disorders of the occipitocervical junction. Clin Orthop 359:136-145, 1999.

96. Sasso RC, Jeanneret B, Fischer K, et al: Occipitocervical fusion with posterior plate and screw instrumentation: A long-term follow-up study. Spine (Phila Pa 1976) 19:2364-2368, 1994.

97. Roberts DA, Doherty BJ, Heggeness MH: Quantitative anatomy of the occiput and the biomechanics of occipital screw fixation. Spine (Phila Pa 1976) 23:1100-1107, 1998.

98. Fehlings MG, Errico T, Cooper P, et al: Occipitocervical fusion with a five-millimeter malleable rod and segmental fixation. Neurosurgery 32:198-207, 1993.

99. Matsunaga S, Ijiri K, Koga H: Results of a longer than 10-year follow-up of patients with rheumatoid arthritis treated by occipitocervical fusion. Spine (Phila Pa 1976) 25:1749-1753, 2000.

100. Moskovich R, Crockard HA, Shott S, et al: Occipitocervical stabilization for myelopathy in patients with rheumatoid arthritis: Implications of not bone-grafting. J Bone Joint Surg Am 82:349-365, 2000.

101. Kerschbaumer F, Kandziora F, Klein C, et al: Transoral decompression, anterior plate fixation, and posterior wire fusion for irreducible atlantoaxial kyphosis in rheumatoid arthritis. Spine (Phila Pa 1976) 25:2708-2715, 2000.

102. Crockard HA, Calder I, Ransford AO: One-stage transoral decompression and posterior fixation in rheumatoid atlanto-axial subluxation. J Bone Joint Surg Br 72:682-685, 1990.

103. McAfee PC, Bohlman HH: One-stage anterior cervical decompression and posterior stabilization with circumferential arthrodesis: A study of twenty-four patients who had a traumatic or a neoplastic lesion. J Bone Joint Surg Am 71:78-88, 1989.

104. Kast E, Mohr K, Richter HP, et al: Complications of transpedicular screw fixation in the cervical spine. Eur Spine J 15:327-334, 2006.

105. Clarke MJ, Cohen-Gadol AA, Ebersold MJ, et al: Long term incidence of subaxial cervical spine instability following cervical arthrodesis surgery in patients with rheumatoid arthritis. Surg Neurol 66:136-140, 2006.

106. Ronkainen A, Niskanen M, Auvinen A, et al: Cervical spine surgery in patients with rheumatoid arthritis: Longterm mortality and its determinants. J Rheumatol 33:517-522, 2006.

107. Nakamura C, Kawaguchi Y, Ishihara H, et al: Upper thoracic myelopathy caused by vertebral collapse and subluxation in rheumatoid arthritis: Report of two cases. J Orthop Sci 9:629-634, 2004.

108. Hirohashi N, Sakai T, Sairyo K, et al: Lumbar radiculopathy caused by extradural rheumatoid nodules: Case report. J Neurosurg Spine 7:352-356, 2007.

109. Kawaji H, Miyamoto M, Gembun Y, et al: A case report of rapidly progressing cauda equine symptoms due to rheumatoid arthritis. J Nippon Med Sch 72:290-294, 2005.

110. Heywood AWB, Meyers OL: Rheumatoid arthritis of the thoracic and lumbar spine. J Bone Joint Surg Br 68:362-368, 1986.

111. Kawaguchi Y, Matsuno H, Masahiko K, et al: Radiologic findings of the lumbar spine in patients with rheumatoid arthritis, and a review of pathologic mechanisms. J Spinal Disord Tech 16:38-43, 2003.

112. Sakai T, Sairyo K, Hamada D, et al: Radiological features of lumbar spinal lesions in patients with rheumatoid arthritis with special reference to the changes around intervertebral discs. Spine J 8:605-611, 2008.

113. Crawford CH 3rd, Carreon LY, Djurasovic M, et al: Lumbar fusion outcomes in patients with rheumatoid arthritis. Eur Spine J 17:822-825, 2008.

35

CHAPTER

Ankylosing Spondylitis

Serena S. Hu, MD
Dheera Ananthakrishnan, MD, MSE

Ankylosing spondylitis (AS) was first described in the late 1800s by a group of French neurologists. The hallmark of the disease is pain and stiffness of joints, mainly in the axial skeleton. The disease usually affects men in their 2nd and 3rd decades of life. There is some debate about the true male-to-female ratio. It was previously thought that the ratio was almost 10:1; however, it is now accepted that the ratio is much lower, probably about 4:1. The disease in women is usually less severe, possibly leading to what may be perceived as a decreased incidence. AS is an autoimmune condition that often results in chronic pain, disability, deformity, and fractures, much of which is of a spinal etiology. In addition, large joints, most notably the hips, knees, and shoulders, develop early arthritic changes.

The association between the major histocompatibility complex antigen HLA-B27 and AS has been well established.[1-6] Approximately 90% of AS patients are positive for the HLA-B27 antigen, although less than 10% of patients who are HLA-B27 positive manifest the signs and symptoms of AS. First-degree relatives of AS patients who are HLA-B27 positive who are also positive for the antigen have a 30% risk of having AS, in contrast to the prevalence in the general population, which is 1% to 2%. The exact mechanism of the AS and HLA-B27 connection is unknown, although a bacterial association has been proposed.

AS is an inflammatory disease in which joints become arthritic and eroded, followed by autofusion (ankylosis). Microscopic evaluation of early lesions shows lymphocytic infiltrates, plasma cells, and macrophages. The first joints to be affected are usually the sacroiliac joints, followed by the vertebral apophyses, followed by the costovertebral joints. When the costovertebral joints have been fused, chest expansion is much reduced, leading to a decrease in pulmonary function. Enthesopathies are also common, leading to inflammation and erosions of the junction of the anulus and the vertebral endplate. Subchondral marrow edema is a classic finding in enthesopathies associated with AS. Erosions lead to ossification of the endplates, which is manifested by the bridging syndesmophytes seen on plain radiographs. Ankylosis of the facet joints leads to bamboo spine seen on plain radiographs. During the progression of facet ankylosis, patients tend to assume a kyphotic posture to unload the joints and relieve the pain. With time, this compensatory mechanism leads to the fixed deformities of cervicothoracic, thoracic, and lumbar kyphosis commonly seen in AS patients who present to spinal surgeons. These deformities lead to difficulty with horizontal gaze, ambulation, and activities of daily living.

When the spine has become completely ankylosed, it functions as a rigid, brittle beam, leading to an increased incidence of fracture with even minor trauma. These fractures represent the second pressing issue that spine surgeons must deal with when treating patients with AS. Osteoporosis also plays an important role in AS. The greatest decrease in bone mass occurs early in the course of the disease, although the reason for this is unknown.

AS affects peripheral joints as well. The most common joint involved is the hip joint, where protrusio acetabuli can be seen. Hip involvement is often bilateral and often occurs early in the course of the disease. In addition, the presence of thoracic and lumbar kyphosis compounds the problems seen with hip flexion contractures because these conditions contribute to an inability to stand upright. The shoulders, knees, wrists, and hands are also affected but to a much lesser degree.

Nonorthopaedic Manifestations

Although the musculoskeletal system is mainly affected by AS, there are other serious effects of the disease. The most common extraskeletal abnormality is anterior uveitis (approximately 25% of patients), which is usually treated with topical agents and rarely leads to vision loss. Ankylosis in the thoracic spine and at the costovertebral joints leads to markedly diminished chest wall expansion, resulting in restrictive lung disease with decreased lung volumes (vital capacity and total lung volume) and increased dependence on diaphragmatic excursion. Preoperative pulmonary function tests are recommended, as is smoking cessation and aggressive postoperative pulmonary toilet. Some AS patients (25% to 30%) also have a component of ileitis or colitis or both; regardless, all patients for whom surgery is being contemplated should have a preoperative nutritional assessment and be considered for perioperative nutritional supplementation. The incidence of aortic stenosis and aortic valve insufficiency is increased in these patients as well; a preoperative echocardiogram is recommended routinely.

Physical Examination and Diagnosis

A patient with AS is most often a young man who gives a history of vague nonlocalizing back pain, morning stiffness, and possibly increasing difficulty with activities of daily living. Although women are affected with AS, men often present earlier or with more advanced disease. Physical examination and diminished spinal mobility especially in the sagittal plane are usually present. The Schober test is used to evaluate lumbar spinal motion: Points 10 cm above and 5 cm below the lumbosacral junction in the midline are marked on the patient in the fully upright position. With full forward flexion, there should be at least 5 cm of excursion between these two points. Chest expansion is commonly limited to less than 2.5 cm of excursion and is typically measured at the fourth intercostal space. The modified New York diagnostic criteria for AS were outlined in 1984 and are as follows:

1. Sacroiliitis confirmed by radiographs
2. Persistent low back pain greater than 3 months in duration
3. Diminished chest expansion (as just described)
4. Limited range of motion of the lumbar spine in the sagittal and coronal planes

The presence of sacroiliac inflammation and one of the other three criteria is generally considered enough to establish the diagnosis of AS.

Sacroiliitis is usually identified on an anteroposterior pelvis film (with or without a Ferguson view). It is widely accepted that the presence of sacroiliitis is crucial for the diagnosis of AS. Sacroiliac joint destruction is the earliest manifestation of AS. The earliest stages of sacroiliitis show some blurring of the cortical margins; this progresses to subcortical erosions (more commonly on the iliac side because it is less robust than the sacral side). In advanced stages, the sacroiliac joints become completely fused, and the cortical erosions disappear. Sacroiliac joint involvement usually is symmetrical and bilateral. Studies have suggested that the use of bony pelvis computed tomography (CT) or magnetic resonance imaging (MRI) in conjunction with plain radiographs may lead to earlier diagnosis of AS.[7] It has yet to be determined whether this early diagnosis favorably affects clinical outcomes.

Management of Acute Injury

The spinal surgeon is usually not the physician making the initial diagnosis of AS but rather is called on to address spinal deformity caused by AS in the clinic and spinal trauma in an AS patient in an emergency setting. A trauma patient with AS also presents a challenge to the spinal surgeon. The spine in

AS functions as a long rigid beam, acting much like a long bone. This altered biomechanical state, plus the presence of osteoporosis and the lack of ligamentous constraints, significantly decreases the fracture threshold of the ankylosed spine. The key to detecting fractures in these patients is having a high index of suspicion, especially after minor trauma. The cervical and cervicothoracic regions are the most commonly affected. Plain radiography is neither sensitive nor specific in these instances, although it should be used as an initial screen, and the standard radiographic modality used for the diagnosis of fracture in all patients is CT. Epidural hematoma, spinal cord injury, and disc injury can be visualized with MRI techniques.

A patient with AS may present with a progressive neurologic deficit without obvious bony injury or with progression of the deformity and increased pain. Many patients with missed spinal column injuries present at a later time to the clinic or the emergency department with progressive neurologic deficit or worsening of deformity or both. The evaluating clinician must also be aware of possible hyperextension through a fracture at a kyphotic segment, which may result in relatively normal sagittal alignment; attempts to determine the patient's preexisting deformity from history and prior radiographs should always be made. There have been reports of neurologic injury in patients strapped to spine boards in a position of hyperextension when compared with their preinjury alignment.[8-10] Because of the stiff and osteoporotic spine, minor trauma may result in acute angulation or moderately rapid deformity progression. One should refrain from attempting acute correction through such a fracture. The patient should be initially immobilized in a halo vest in the preinjury alignment.

For a patient with a neurologic deficit, MRI is imperative. MRI may reveal an epidural hematoma. Hematomas can occur in these patients owing to bleeding from minor trauma from the osteoporotic bone or from scarred epidural vessels adjacent to a fracture. Evacuation of a hematoma is essential in the presence of progressive neurologic deficit. The decompression required may significantly destabilize the AS patient, and so the surgeon should be prepared to stabilize the spine at the same setting. Usually rigid instrumentation is required, although rarely halo immobilization may be sufficient for some cervical cases. As with instrumentation for elective cases, the screw-bone interface is compromised because of osteoporosis; these constructs should generally be supplemented by external support such as with a halo vest. Laminar hooks may be more rigid in many patients, but external bracing should still be considered.

It is generally accepted that AS patients sustain more spinal fractures and dislocations than individuals without AS.[11-15] Cooper and colleagues[16] retrospectively looked at 158 patients in Rochester, Minnesota, with AS and found a sevenfold increase in the incidence of spinal fractures over that of a cohort of patients without AS. They found no such increase in extremity fractures. The patients with spinal fractures tended to be older and had a greater preinjury involvement of the spine than patients without fractures. Cooper and colleagues[16] also noted that this higher incidence was mainly during the first 5 years after diagnosis and suggested that this was due to a greater percentage of bone density loss during this period, resulting in a decreased fracture threshold. In addition, the dampening structures present in a normal spine have lost their load-absorbing qualities in the ankylosed spine. The intervertebral discs are stiff, as are the ligamentous structures, and the facet joints are ankylosed.

The incidence of neurologic injuries in these patients is quite high, owing to excessive bleeding at the fracture site leaking into the confined epidural space and translation (displacement) at the fracture site. This translation causes direct injury to the spinal cord and persistent bleeding owing to motion, resulting in an enlarging compressive hematoma. Most spinal injuries in AS patients are three-column injuries (owing to stiffening of the load-absorbing structures). These injuries are highly unstable because there are two long lever arms hinging at the fracture site. In addition, the presence of preinjury kyphosis increases the likelihood of translation at the level of the injury, which subsequently increases the likelihood of neurologic injury. Lastly, poor bone stock and difficult radiographic evaluation can lead to a delay in diagnosis. Most of these injuries (60% to 75%) are at the cervicothoracic junction, which is notoriously difficult to evaluate with plain radiographs.

Whang and colleagues[17] compared a cohort of 12 patients with AS who sustained spinal injuries with 18 patients with diffuse idiopathic skeletal hyperostosis (DISH) who sustained spinal injuries. The DISH group represents a group of patients of similar age whose spinal condition results in stiff segments above and below any spinal fracture. Falls from a standing position were the most common mechanism of injury. There was a greater likelihood that the DISH patients did not incur any neurologic deficit (44.4%) compared with AS patients (25% of whom did not have a neurologic deficit). Complication rates were higher in the AS group (42% vs. 33% in the DISH group). There were two deaths in each group related to the injury or its treatment, all of which were considered to be related to the use of the halo vest (aspiration [two deaths], respiratory failure, and multisystem organ failure). Several patients died of unrelated causes during the follow-up period; however, all surviving patients were contacted and were classified as having excellent or good outcomes.

Finkelstein and colleagues[18] looked retrospectively at 21 AS patients with a diagnosis of spinal trauma. One third of these patients had a delay in diagnosis; three had complete spinal cord injuries on presentation, and three experienced neurologic deterioration to complete spinal cord injuries after admission. Finkelstein and colleagues[18] recommended quick screening cervical and thoracic MRI (one film) and screening lumbosacral spine MRI (one film) for diagnosis, in addition to minimal transfers and immediate stabilization. They did not comment on their definitive protocol for treatment of these patients (operative vs. nonoperative).

Hitchon and colleagues[19] retrospectively reviewed 11 patients with AS and thoracic and lumbar fractures. They found 10 of these patients had sustained three-column injuries; 9 patients had extension-type injuries. More than half of these patients had a neurologic deficit (the specifics of which the study authors did not mention); half of these neurologically injured patients had some improvement in function. Hitchon and colleagues[19] recommended surgical intervention for stabilization of thoracic and lumbar three-column injuries because of their inherent instability.

Graham and van Peteghem[20] looked retrospectively at 15 patients over 6 years (1978-1984) comparing types of injuries and treatments. Of patients, 12 had cervical spine injuries; 9 of these had spinal cord injuries. The two patients with thoracic injuries had anterior cord syndromes. There were no compression-type injuries; most injuries resulted from a flexion-extension type of mechanism. The only patient treated with operative intervention was the patient with the lumbar injury, who had hardware failure and had to undergo revision. Two patients died, and three patients had pulmonary complications.

Apple and Anson[21] looked at AS patients with spinal fracture and spinal cord injury, comparing operative versus nonoperative treatments. This study was a retrospective, multicenter study of 59 patients. In the operative group, 37 patients were treated with a variety of procedures. Patients in the nonoperative group were placed in halo traction and then halo vests and placed on bed rest. There were no significant differences between the two groups with regard to motor recovery, fusion complications, or mortality rate (22% in both groups). The nonoperative group did have significantly shorter hospital stays. No analysis of the patients according to type of injury or treatment was done, and no discussion of the deaths was presented.

Hunter and Dubo[12] reviewed the cases of 19 AS patients who had sustained cervical spine fractures. Five of these patients had a complete spinal cord injury, and all of these patients died after their injury. All of these patients were treated nonoperatively. No patient developed neurologic deterioration, and all of the patients with incomplete cord injury regained some function. Hunter and Dubo[12] concluded that nonoperative treatment worked well in these patients, although they suggested that surgery be considered in patients with grossly unstable injuries.

Bohlman retrospectively reviewed 300 patients with cervical spine injuries.[21a] He found only eight patients who carried a preinjury diagnosis of AS. Five of these patients died of pulmonary or gastrointestinal causes. Clinically significant epidural hematomas were found only in the AS patients. Bohlman recommended decompression for patients with progressive neurologic deficit. There was a delay in diagnosis in four patients, all of whom developed spinal cord injuries.

The generally accepted protocol with respect to the management of spine trauma in AS patients is as follows: If the clinician has even the slightest suspicion of spinal injury, the patient should be immobilized in the preinjury position. Plain radiography and fine-cut CT with reconstructions should be obtained. If the patient has a neurologic injury, MRI should be considered, looking for an epidural hematoma. If a fracture is detected and displacement or gross instability is noted, low-weight in-line traction should be used in an attempt to facilitate a reduction. If a reduction is obtained, the patient should be placed in a halo vest for definitive treatment. If a reduction cannot be obtained, internal fixation is recommended, with or without decompression as indicated by the patient's neurologic status. Postoperative immobilization in the form of a halo vest is then recommended. In a patient with a progressive neurologic deficit, MRI is likely to reveal the presence of a hematoma. In a patient with a stable deficit and no hematoma, the cord injury likely occurred at the time of injury; as long as the spine is stable, management of the neurologic injury should be expectant. If the spine is unstable, reduction and stabilization either with traction and a halo vest or with surgery is recommended.

Complications can arise at the time of injury and from treatment of the injury. Deformity and neurologic injury can occur as a result of the injury; treatment with decompression and internal fixation carries risks of nonunion, hardware failure, failure of the bone-screw interface resulting in loss of fixation, and infection. Even halo management has complications. Skull fractures, pin tract infections, intracerebral hemorrhage, and intracranial air all have been reported with halo immobilization in these patients.[9,22] Taggard and Traynelis[24] described a posterior cervical fusion (lateral mass plating) they used in seven AS patients who had sustained fractures. The fusions were supplemented with autologous rib grafts. Postoperatively, the patients were immobilized in collars only, with the exception of one, who was placed in a sternal-occipital-mandibular immobilizer. Fusion occurred in all patients; there were two deaths in quadriplegic patients. Taggard and Traynelis[24] recommended operative intervention as a means of avoiding postoperative halo immobilization.

Deformity

The deformities seen in AS are a result of excessive kyphosis throughout the spine and excessive flexion at the hip joints. All areas of the spine can be affected, with the lumbar spine affected most often, followed by the thoracic and cervical spine. If the physical examination and radiographic examinations indicate that the hip flexion contracture plays a significant role in the overall deformity, hip arthroplasty should be performed before spinal surgical intervention. In this manner, the less morbid operation is performed first; in addition, the spine surgeon can better assess the actual amount of sagittal imbalance attributable to the spine.

The spine surgeon must carefully examine the patient in the standing, seated, and supine positions to determine the major component of the deformity. If a major portion of the deformity corrects on moving from a standing to a seated position, the deformity is mostly from the hip joints, and arthroplasty should be performed first. If the deformity persists on sitting but corrects in the supine position, the deformity is arising from the thoracic, thoracolumbar, or lumbar spine, and a lumbar osteotomy is usually indicated. If the deformity persists even in the supine position, the deformity is in the cervicothoracic area, and an osteotomy in this area is indicated.

From a radiographic standpoint, a full spine lateral radiograph with the neck in a neutral position and the hips in a fully extended position is crucial for surgical planning. This radiograph allows measurement of the chin-brow angle, which is formed by a line from the chin-brow to the floor vertical angle. This measurement is helpful when planning any osteotomy. Ideally, the chin-brow angle should be zero. Suk and colleagues[23] looked at the significance of the chin-brow measurement in assessing the success of surgical intervention. These investigators evaluated 34 AS patients undergoing lumbar or thoracolumbar osteotomies for correction of sagittal imbalance. Preoperative and postoperative chin-brow angles were measured. Clinical outcome assessment involved the Modified Arthritis Impairment Scales (AIMS). This questionnaire consists of three simple questions plus numerous subscales: function, indoor activity, outdoor activity, psychosocial activity, pain, and overall subjectivity. Suk and colleagues[23] found improved postoperative AIMS scores for questions involving looking forward, going up stairs, and going down stairs. There was a negative correlation between chin-brow angles and correction obtained but no correlation between chin-brow angle and clinical outcome. The patients who were overcorrected (to an angle <−10 degrees) had worse scores with regard to looking forward and going down stairs; these results were found to be statistically significant.

When the location of the primary spine deformity is determined, the surgeon must decide what type of osteotomy would be most appropriate. It is preferable to place the osteotomy at the apex of the deformity, but this is not always possible. Thoracic and thoracolumbar osteotomies are limited by the rib cage, the spinal cord, and the conus medullaris. Deformities in these areas are almost always treated with a lumbar osteotomy. By moving the osteotomy inferiorly, one can obtain more sagittal plane alignment owing to a longer lever arm. By overcorrecting at the lumbar level, one can address the thoracic kyphosis and the lumbar kyphosis. If overcorrection is to be performed, the surgeon should take into account if a portion of the deformity is cervicothoracic because the patient's horizontal gaze would be affected and may not be restored.

Preoperative Assessment

A careful history should yield information about the patient's lifestyle, habits, and medications. Smoking cessation is imperative; many surgeons do not undertake the operation while a patient is actively smoking. Nonsteroidal anti-inflammatory drugs should be discontinued at least 2 weeks before surgery. Preoperative pulmonary function tests are indicated because many of these patients have restrictive lung disease. Preoperative echocardiography may also be indicated, as previously mentioned, although cardiac intervention is not often needed. Results of renal function tests should be obtained before surgery; an awareness of tenuous renal function would benefit intraoperative and postoperative fluid management. Many AS patients have a component of renal dysfunction because of long-term use of nonsteroidal anti-inflammatory drugs. Cervical spine flexibility should be assessed by the orthopaedist and the anesthesia service before the procedure; fiberoptic intubation is usually needed because of concomitant ankylosis of the cervical spine.

Historically, most osteotomies in AS patients were performed with the patient awake or using a Stagnara wake-up test for evaluation of spinal cord function before, during, and after a correction. Somatosensory evoked potentials and motor evoked potentials (epidural or transcranial) have become more reliable so that the wake-up test is less frequently needed. The anterior tracts are better monitored by motor evoked potentials. These tracts can be preferentially affected during an extension maneuver when addressing kyphotic deformities, either by direct compression or by impairing the vascular supply to the spinal cord.

A preoperative nutritional assessment (albumin, prealbumin, total protein) should be performed; perioperative nutritional supplementation (tube feedings or parenteral nutritional assessment) may be indicated. Klein and colleagues[25] noted a significant increase in complications such as deep wound infection in patients undergoing lumbar spinal fusion who were malnourished by nutritional parameters preoperatively. Hu and colleagues[26] and Lapp and colleagues[27] showed that supplementation in the form of parenteral nutrition is beneficial in reducing complication rates after reconstructive spine surgery.

Lumbar Osteotomies

The first lumbar osteotomy was described in 1945 by Smith-Petersen.[33] This osteotomy is an opening osteotomy, meaning that the apex of the wedge lies posteriorly, opening up the anterior column during correction (osteoclasis through ossified disc space and anterior longitudinal ligament). Smith-Petersen and colleagues performed multilevel osteotomies in six patients. These osteotomies were V-shaped in the coronal plane, with the point of the "V" at the midline in the interlaminar space. The osteotomies are carried out through the articular processes bilaterally at two or three levels. It is imperative that adequate amounts of lamina and flavum are resected before correction so that compression of the neural elements on closure does not occur.

Cauda equina syndrome has been reported by Simmons[28] as a result of a decrease in canal dimensions. The posteriorly based closing wedge type of osteotomy results in anterior opening at the level of the disc space. This anterior opening can be better achieved in an AS patient than a patient without AS because of the stiffness of the disc space. Complications of an opening wedge osteotomy include superior mesentery artery syndrome and aortic rupture owing to stretching of the abdominal vasculature.[29,30] Vascular complications are rare and tend to occur in older patients with calcific, adherent abdominal vessels.

Lichtblau and Wilson[29] described a patient who underwent closed osteoclasis followed by cast placement. This patient died in the immediate postoperative period of an aortic rupture. His history was significant for a large dose of radiation that was used to treat the ankylosed spine. Fazl and colleagues[30] described an AS patient who sustained a fracture

through the T12-L1 disc space. He was treated with Harrington rod instrumentation and fusion but died 2 days postoperatively from an aortic rupture at the level of the injury. Aortic necrosis was present at autopsy, as were adhesions of the vessels to the spine. More common complications reported include ileus, pneumonia, and root traction injury. Cauda equina syndrome with flaccid paralysis below the level of the injury, although rare, was reported in these studies as well.

Patients originally were immobilized in plaster; segmental instrumentation currently is indicated for these patients. Many investigators have reported their results after multilevel Smith-Petersen osteotomies.[31-33] Nonunion rates resulting in recurrence and progression of deformity were significant. Soon after the original description of this technique, reports of "plugging up" the open disc spaces with interbody fusions showed increased fusion rates and decreased complications.[34] The complications associated with opening wedge osteotomies led to modifications of Smith-Petersen's techniques. In 1949, Wilson and Turkell[34a] described a procedure similar to the Smith-Petersen procedure in which less bone is removed but more osteotomies are created. The anterior longitudinal ligament is not ruptured; the anterior column length is not changed. In 1962, McMaster[32] described the addition of Harrington compression instrumentation to Smith-Petersen osteotomies in 14 patients. This instrumentation was used to close the wedges produced after osteotomy. Postoperatively, the patients were placed in casts for 9 months. Mean correction was 33 degrees at final follow-up. Subjective improvement was found in horizontal gaze and height and posture. McMaster[32] suggested that a slow controlled osteotomy closure was beneficial in terms of overall stability and protection of neural elements. Püschel and Zielke[34b] also performed multiple wedge-shaped Smith-Petersen type osteotomies and used Zielke instrumentation to close the osteotomies. They also recommended a slow correction with a gradual lordosis.

After reports of nonunions and concerns about stretching of the abdominal vasculature and viscera,[35,36,39] Thomasen[37] described a closing wedge osteotomy. He reported on 11 patients in whom he preformed a complete laminectomy at L2, transected the transverse processes, and resected the ankylosed facets at L2-3. The pedicles of L2 were removed in their entirety down to the posterior aspect of the vertebral body. The entire vertebral body was decancellated, followed by removal of the posterior cortex and osteotomies of both lateral cortices. After careful mobilization of the dura above and below L2, Thomasen[37] closed the wedge by gradual flexion of the table. Internal fixation (plates and wiring) was used in six patients; all patients were placed in casts. One patient had a fracture-dislocation above the level of the osteotomy resulting in a cauda equina syndrome; this patient had almost complete return of neurologic function after revision decompression and internal fixation. Correction ranged from 12 to 50 degrees. All patients had subjective improvement of posture and horizontal gaze.

Heinig's eggshell procedure was described in 1984 as a monosegmental osteotomy to be used in the same situations in which one would use Thomasen's procedure.[37] Thomasen leaves the anterior vertebral body cortex intact, whereas Heinig actually describes fracturing this cortex, which decreases the length of the anterior column and the posterior column. As long as more bone is removed posteriorly, restoration of lordosis occurs.

Bradford and colleagues[38] reported in 1987 on a series of 21 patients with AS who underwent single-level or multilevel lumbar or thoracic osteotomies with or without anterior discectomies. All patients had internal fixation posteriorly with a thoracolumbosacral orthosis. Average corrections ranged from 9 to 36 degrees. Complications were noted more frequently in the closing wedge–type osteotomies (neurapraxias and fracture during hook placement). Wake-up tests were used in all patients. In addition, Bradford and colleagues[38] recommended closing-type osteotomies to avoid traction on the spinal cord, wide decompression, and internal fixation to avoid neurologic complications.

In 1990, Hehne and colleagues[39] reported on 177 patients with AS in whom multisegmental opening wedge lumbar and thoracolumbar osteotomies were performed. Hehne and colleagues[39] were the first to report on the use of pedicle screw fixation. Casting and bracing were used postoperatively. Average correction at follow-up (18 to 42 months) was 43 degrees, with horizontal gaze subjectively restored in all cases. Complications included deaths, transient paresis, transient and permanent nerve root injuries, implant failures, and infections. These authors suggested that pedicle screw fixation with multisegmental osteotomies can produce a smoother lordosis than that produced by a monosegmental osteotomy.

In 1992, Jaffray and colleagues[39a] presented three patients in whom a decancellation closing wedge osteotomy was performed. They did not remove the entire pedicle; rather, the inferior aspect of the pedicle was preserved to ensure protection for the exiting nerve root. Pedicle screw fixation plus a postoperative cast was used. Jaffray and colleagues recommended two-level osteotomies (L2 and L4) for patients who needed more correction. Horizontal gaze was corrected in two patients; one patient required a cervicothoracic osteotomy for complete gaze correction. Complications were not discussed.

More recently, Van Royen and De Gast[40] mathematically analyzed the sagittal plane corrections of two patients and determined that the amount of correction needed depends on three parameters: sacral endplate angle, C7 plumb line, and chin-brow angle. The sacral endplate angle reflects the amount of sagittal plane deformity that can be attributed to the hip joints: As the flexion contracture at the hip increases, the pelvis must rotate posteriorly to keep the body center of mass over the pelvis, decreasing the sacral endplate angle. The chin-brow angle has been shown to be a quantifiable parameter that reflects the restoration of horizontal gaze.[40] A mathematical formula was found that determines the ideal location and angle for each particular patient for a closing wedge–type osteotomy centered on the anterior longitudinal ligament.

There have been many retrospective reviews of AS patients treated with various osteotomies for sagittal imbalance. Van Royen and De Gast[40] performed a meta-analysis of 856 AS patients. They found three different techniques described: multisegment (two to three levels) opening wedge osteotomies with rupture of the anterior longitudinal ligament (i.e., Smith-Petersen), multisegment closing wedge osteotomies (Wilson-Turkell), and closing wedge–type osteotomy with pedicle resection and an anterior hinge (Thomasen). After a thorough and careful review, Van Royen and De Gast[40] concluded that although no single technique was clearly superior to the others, the complications associated with closing wedge osteotomies were less serious than the complications associated with the other two groups. In addition, loss of correction was more prevalent in patients treated with opening wedge and polysegmental wedge osteotomies and the closing wedge types.

A handful of studies have attempted to quantify results in terms of patient outcomes using a standardized grading system. In 1995, Halm and colleagues[41] used the modified AIMS questionnaire to evaluate 175 patients retrospectively after lumbar osteotomy. Treatment groups were multisegment Smith-Petersen with Harrington compression instrumentation ($n = 34$), multisegment Smith-Petersen with transpedicular fixation ($n = 136$), and monosegmental Thomasen with segmental fixation ($n = 4$). The investigators found statistically significant improvement in 47 of 60 items. Kim and colleagues[42] used the AIMS questionnaire prospectively in 45 patients with AS who were treated with Thomasen osteotomies at one or two levels. Osteotomies were mainly performed in the lumbar spine (usually L3). Average increase in lumbar lordosis was 34 degrees, with no significant increase in thoracic kyphosis. All parameters measured were significantly improved. Clinical outcome scores were significantly improved in all five categories; no correlation was found between the amount of radiographic correction obtained and clinical outcome as measured by the questionnaire.

Berven and colleagues[43] looked at 13 patients undergoing transpedicular wedge resection. Three of these patients had AS and were having spine surgery for the first time. These investigators also used outcome measures (modified Scoliosis Research Society questionnaire) in a retrospective manner (Figs. 35–1 to 35–4). After 2 years, most of these patients was satisfied and would have the surgery again. The changes in C7 plumb line and lumbar lordosis were statistically significant. Complications included dural tear, transient nerve root injury, pulmonary embolus, and loss of sagittal balance. None of the AS patients showed a loss of sagittal balance at follow-up.

Bridwell and colleagues[44] looked at 27 patients undergoing pedicle subtraction osteotomy, also in a retrospective fashion. Two of these patients had AS. Outcome data (Oswestry and SRS-24) were also obtained retrospectively. Bridwell and colleagues[44] found a significant improvement in sagittal balance and lumbar lordosis and a high level of patient satisfaction. Complications included deep vein thrombosis, myocardial infarction, compartment syndrome, visual field loss, pseudarthrosis, loss of correction, urinary retention, and neurologic deficits (root lesions). The patients with the latter two complications all responded to a central canal decompression.

FIGURE 35–1 A and **B,** Clinical photographs of a patient with ankylosing spondylitis with typical loss of lumbar lordosis, forward sagittal balance, and flexed hips and knees to maintain stance.

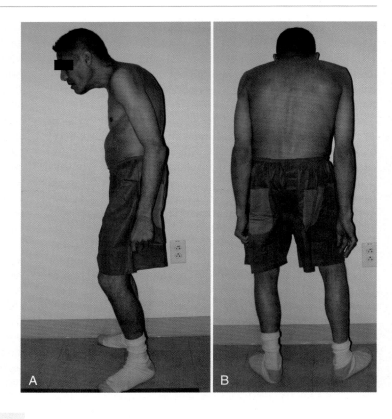

Thoracic Osteotomies

Even when the deformity has been localized to the thoracic spine primarily, lumbar osteotomies are usually recommended. These can be performed below cord and conus level, and they have the advantage of large degrees of correction owing to a long lever arm. Osteotomies performed in the thoracic spine are usually Smith-Petersen, although there have been a handful of studies describing closing wedge osteotomies in the thoracic and thoracolumbar spine.

FIGURE 35–2 Lateral (**A**) and posteroanterior (**B**) radiographs. Note ankylosis of sacroiliac joints, bamboo spine with syndesmophyte formation, and forward sagittal balance. The patient had hip replacement previously for severe hip disease.

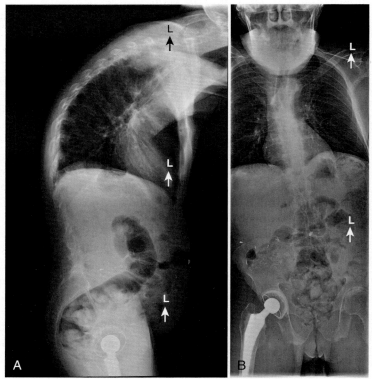

Kawahara and colleagues[45] described a closing-opening wedge osteotomy in the thoracic and thoracolumbar spine. They used this procedure on seven patients with sagittal imbalance. The osteotomy consisted of a partial vertebrectomy with a large posterior wedge that is performed in a manner similar to a costotransversectomy. After bony resection, pedicle screw instrumentation plus temporary correction rods are used to facilitate a closing wedge correction of about 30 degrees. An opening wedge–type maneuver is facilitated, again through the instrumentation, and a spacer or allograft is inserted. Kawahara and colleagues[45] noted good improvement in kyphosis, lordosis, and plumb line. They had no neurologic complications, no nonunions, and no loss of correction (follow-up of 2.2 to 7.5 years).

Cervicothoracic Osteotomy

If the primary deformity has been determined to be in the cervical spine, an osteotomy at the cervicothoracic junction can be done. Patients with these deformities, in addition to the problems with horizontal gaze, also can experience dysphagia and problems related to poor oral intake. The chin-brow angle is of paramount importance when planning a corrective osteotomy in the cervicothoracic region. A key point is not to overcorrect the horizontal gaze because this can lead to inability of patients to see the floor ahead of them. These patients may function better when corrected to a chin-brow angle of about 10 degrees. In 1958, Urist[46] described an osteotomy in

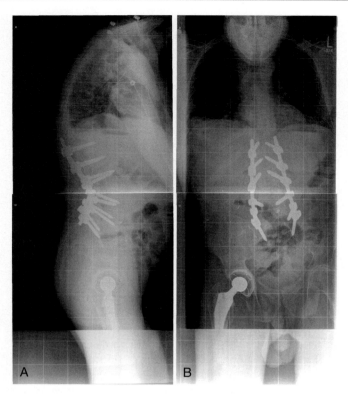

FIGURE 35–3 Lateral (**A**) and posteroanterior (**B**) radiographs after pedicle subtraction osteotomy. Note improved sagittal balance. Closing wedge of L3 is seen on lateral radiograph and can be appreciated by widely divergent screws in L2 compared with L4.

FIGURE 35–4 Patient back (**A**) and side (**B**) views showing clinical correction.

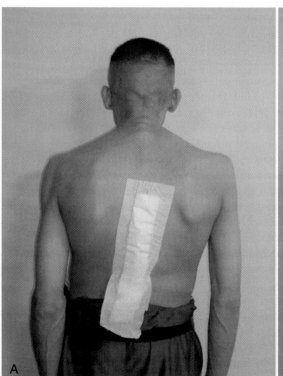

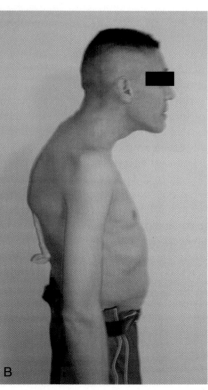

the cervicothoracic region, noting that the canal at this level is quite large and that the C8 nerve root is quite mobile compared with the upper cervical roots. In addition, potential loss of the lower cervical roots is less morbid than loss of the upper cervical roots. Lastly, the vertebral arteries are typically extraosseous at these levels, making resection of the lateral masses less risky.

Careful preoperative planning with radiographic studies is of paramount importance when performing a cervicothoracic osteotomy. Full-length standing lateral spine radiographs are needed to measure the chin-brow angle. Lateral tomography or fine-cut CT with sagittal and coronal reconstructions is performed to delineate the anatomy.[28,46] Axial CT scans can be very helpful in characterizing the distorted anatomy often seen in patients with AS, especially with regard to placement of instrumentation. MRI can help to rule out occult fractures, which should be suspected if there is recent onset of pain or rapid progression of deformity; MRI should be obtained if there is any neurologic deficit. In addition, flexion and extension lateral cervical spine radiographs should be obtained to look for any instability occurring at the occipitocervical and atlantoaxial levels. A subset of AS patients develop instability in these areas as a result of excessive stiffness of the entire spinal column because the stress placed on these upper cervical areas can be quite high. Although the number of AS patients who have occipitocervical or atlantoaxial instability is not as high as the number of AS patients with rheumatoid arthritis, missing this instability can be catastrophic.

The surgeon must carefully examine the preoperative radiographs and CT scans to determine the amount of correction needed. As described by Simmons,[28] the measured chin-brow angle should be transposed onto a neutral cervicothoracic film, with the apex of the angle centered on the posterior longitudinal ligament at the C7-T1 level. By extrapolation, the extent of posterior elements to be resected can be determined.

As originally described by Urist[46] and popularized by Simmons, the procedure was performed under local anesthesia only, with the patient awake in a seated position, in seated halo traction. The seated position carries with it the risk of air embolus in a patient with a patent foramen ovale so that continuous cardiac monitoring is indicated during the procedure.[28,46] With the widespread use of neurophysiologic monitoring, the awake seated position is almost never used for these procedures at the present time except in the case where the severe spinal deformity precludes prone positioning. A baseline set of somatosensory evoked potentials and motor evoked potentials is obtained, and the patient's head is placed in a rigid head holder (three-pin Mayfield). After the flip, a repeat run of neurophysiologic monitoring is obtained.

After a wide and lengthy exposure, a wide cervical decompression at C7 and T1 is performed, including a dorsal unroofing of bilateral C8 nerve roots. The lateral masses at C7 are also resected; in addition, the pedicles at C7 are partially removed to ensure that the C8 nerve roots are not compressed after the correction. Sometimes a portion of the superior aspect of the T1 pedicles must be removed as well. Before the widespread use of instrumentation, postoperative

immobilization consisted of a halo vest or cast that was custom measured or fitted to the patient's torso preoperatively. Currently, sublaminar hooks or lateral mass and pedicle screw instrumentation can be used for rigid stabilization, which greatly reduces the likelihood of translation at the osteoclasis level and subsequent neurologic injury. Lateral mass screws generally do not hold well in these patients with their osteoporotic spines and should be supplemented by halo vest immobilization if the surgeon prefers to use them. Instrumentation is placed three levels above and three levels below C7-T1 after the decompression but before osteoclasis.

After the instrumentation has been placed, a temporary rod is prepared. One surgeon breaks scrub and manipulates the head and neck via the halo ring, facilitating the osteoclasis. The neck is slowly extended about the C7-T1 level, while the scrubbed surgeon watches the decompression site for excessive dural compression. Neurophysiologic signals are carefully monitored during the correction. An audible crack is often heard; the manipulating surgeon should appreciate a decrease in resistance when the osteoclasis has been completed. If the decompression has been planned and executed properly, any residual lateral mass of C7 should be opposed to T1, the C8 nerve roots should be free, and the dura should not be excessively compressed. The halo or Mayfield is resecured to the operative table in the corrected position. The rods are secured into position.

Even with neurophysiologic monitoring, a wake-up test is often performed after correction. Adjustments can be made intraoperatively after the main correction has been obtained. After the instrumentation has been secured, the local bone resected during the osteotomy is used for grafting, supplemented by allograft if the surgeon believes this is indicated, and the wound is closed. The anterior soft tissues are usually tight after being in a shortened position for a long time. The patient is usually kept intubated until the soft tissue edema and the postoperative anterior hematoma lessen. Even with rigid segmental instrumentation, the patient's osteopenia may necessitate placement in a rigid halo vest for the duration of the healing period. Dysphagia is common and usually resolves with time. If the patient's caloric intake is borderline, as is common, it is imperative that these patients receive nutritional supplementation during the healing period, in the form of either tube feedings or parenteral supplementation.

The literature concerning cervicothoracic osteotomies in AS patients is sparse. Simmons[46a] in his original article in 1972 reported on 42 patients who underwent cervicothoracic osteotomy as described by Urist. The operations were performed in the seated position under local anesthesia, and postoperative immobilization consisted of a halo vest. Simmons reported two nonunions successfully treated with anterior fusion, one pulmonary embolus, two myocardial infarctions (one fatal), and one root injury treated with repeat decompression. The patients who did not experience complications all were quite satisfied with their outcomes and had their horizontal gaze restored.

McMaster[32] reported retrospectively on 15 patients with abnormal horizontal gaze who were treated with an extension osteotomy at the cervicothoracic junction. These surgeries were performed in the prone position with a halo jacket in place before the osteotomy. Only three patients had internal fixation. All patients had their horizontal gaze restored. Complications included one patient with delayed postoperative quadriparesis, two nonunions, a C8 nerve root lesion, and subluxation at the osteotomy site. McMaster[32] also treated their nonunions with anterior fusion with subsequent good results.

The remainder of the literature dealing with cervicothoracic osteotomies in AS patients is in the form of case reports. Sengupta and colleagues[46b] addressed the complication of overcorrection resulting in the inability of the patient to look down. They performed a same-day four-stage procedure in the lateral decubitus position with transparent drapes and reported restoration of horizontal gaze in one patient. They recommended this procedure only in extreme cases.

Summary

Spinal reconstructive surgery in a patient with AS is a complex and high-risk procedure. These patients have significant disability from their spinal deformities, however, and can experience significant benefit from correction of their alignment and sagittal imbalance. Careful preoperative planning, a clear understanding of the characteristics of the spines of AS patients, and meticulous intraoperative and postoperative care can lead to measurable improvement in quality of life for these patients.

PEARLS

1. The progression of facet spondylosis causes compensatory kyphosis, which can lead to the fixed deformities of cervicothoracic, thoracic, and lumbar kyphosis commonly seen in AS. These deformities lead to difficulty with horizontal gaze, ambulation, and activities of daily living.

2. Initial immobilization of a patient with AS who has a spinal column fracture should be in the preinjury position because of the potential for injury to the spinal cord if hyperextension from the prior position is performed.

3. Determining the major component of the deformity requires examining the patient in the standing, seated, and supine positions. A truncal forward flexed deformity that corrects when changing from a standing to a seated position is usually due to hip flexion contracture. If the deformity persists on sitting but corrects in the supine position, the deformity is arising from the thoracic, thoracolumbar, or lumbar spine, and a lumbar osteotomy is usually indicated. If the deformity persists in the supine position, the deformity is in the cervicothoracic area.

PITFALLS

1. When the spine has become completely ankylosed, it functions as a rigid, brittle beam, leading to an increased incidence of fracture with even minor trauma.

2. The incidence of neurologic injuries in these patients is quite high, owing to the potential for translation (displacement) at the fracture site. This translation causes direct injury to the spinal cord and persistent bleeding secondary to motion, resulting in an enlarging compressive hematoma.

3. Balancing the achievement of horizontal gaze with the improvement of sagittal balance requires proper planning and staging of lumbar osteotomies relative to cervicothoracic osteotomies, when both are needed.

KEY POINTS

1. Recommended corrective lumbar osteotomies in AS patients are Smith-Petersen osteotomies if disc spaces are still mobile and pedicle subtraction osteotomies if disc spaces are fully autofused.

2. Correction at the time of lumbar osteotomy can be facilitated by positioning the patient so that when the osteotomy is completed, the table can be extended, resulting in the controlled extension of the patient's spine. The use of a supporting frame where the trunk and shoulders are supported separately from the pelvis may be required.

3. For cervicothoracic osteotomy, the patient's head must be held rigidly in a halo or tongs, which can be manipulated to a corrected positive after the osteotomy is completed. Osteotomy is best performed at C7 for maximum canal size, mobility of the nerve roots at this level, and the advantageous vertebral artery position.

KEY REFERENCES

1. Graham B, Van Peteghem PK: Fractures of the spine in ankylosing spondylitis. Spine (Phila Pa 1976) 14:803-807, 1989.
   This is a retrospective review of spinal injuries in AS patients from 1978-1984. The authors reviewed 15 patients and noted a preponderance of cervical injuries and a high rate of neurologic injury.

2. Halm H, Metz-Stavenhagen P, Zielke K: Results of surgical correction of kyphotic deformities of the spine in ankylosing spondylitis on the basis of the modified Arthritis Impact Measurement Scales. Spine (Phila Pa 1976) 20:1612-1619, 1995.
   This is a retrospective review of 175 AS patients who underwent surgical correction of flexion deformities from 1979-1988. The modified AIMS was used as an outcome measure; 47 of 60 items showed significant increases; pain, mobility, depression, and anxiety items were particularly improved.

3. Hehne H, Zielke K, Bohm H: Polysegmental lumbar osteotomies and transpedicled fixation for correction of long-curved kyphotic deformities in ankylosing spondylitis. Clin Orthop Relat Res (258):49-55, 1990.

This is a review of 177 patients with AS in whom segmental pedicle screw fixation and Smith-Petersen osteotomies were performed in the lumbar spine for correction of kyphotic deformities. Harmonious lordosis was obtained, and all patients had restoration of horizontal gaze.

4. Simmons EH: Kyphotic deformity of the spine in ankylosing spondylitis. Clin Orthop Relat Res 128:65-77, 1977.
   This was the first report in the literature of the use of fixation for correction of kyphosis in AS. The technique of cervicothoracic osteotomy at the C7-T1 level was described; 48 patients who underwent this osteotomy were presented.

5. Thomasen E: Vertebral osteotomy for correction of kyphosis in ankylosing spondylitis. Clin Orthop Relat Res 194:142-153, 1985.
   This classic article introduced the technique of Thomasen closing wedge pedicle subtraction osteotomy. The author reviewed 11 patients who underwent the osteotomy, 6 of whom had internal fixation as supplementation.

REFERENCES

1. Brewerton DA, Hart FD, Nicholls A, et al: Ankylosing spondylitis and HL-A27. Lancet 1:904-907, 1973.

2. Calin A: Ankylosing spondylitis. Clin Rheum Dis 11:41-60, 1985.

3. Carbone LD, Cooper C, Michet CJ, et al: Ankylosing spondylitis in Rochester, Minnesota, 1935-1989. Is the epidemiology changing? Arthritis Rheum 35:1476-1482, 1992.

4. Kahn MF, Chamot AM: SAPHO syndrome. Rheum Dis Clin North Am 18:225-246, 1992.

5. Reveille JD: HLA-B27 and the seronegative spondyloarthropathies. Am J Med Sci 316:239-249, 1998.

6. Schlosstein L, Terasaki PI, Bluestone R, et al: High association of an HL-A antigen, W27, with ankylosing spondylitis. N Engl J Med 288:704-706, 1973.

7. Devogelaer JP, Maldague B, Malghem J, et al: Appendicular and vertebral bone mass in ankylosing spondylitis: A comparison of plain radiographs with single- and dual-photon absorptiometry and with quantitative computed tomography. Arthritis Rheum 35:1062-1067, 1992.

8. Broom MJ, Raycroft JF: Complications of fractures of the cervical spine in ankylosing spondylitis. Spine (Phila Pa 1976) 13:763-766, 1988.

9. Moreau W, Wilcox N, Brown MF: Immobilization of spinal fractures in patients with ankylosing spondylitis. Injury 34:372-373, 2003.

10. Podolsky SM, Hoffman JR, Pietrafesa CA: Neurologic complications following immobilization of cervical spine fractures in patients with ankylosing spondylitis. Ann Emerg Med 12:578-580, 1983.

11. Hanson JA, Mirza S: Predisposition for spinal fracture in ankylosing spondylitis. AJR Am J Roentgenol 174:150, 2000.

12. Hunter T, Dubo HI: Spinal fractures complicating ankylosing spondylitis: A long-term followup study. Arthritis Rheum 26:751-759, 1983.

13. Surin VV: Fractures of the cervical spine in patients with ankylosing spondylitis. Acta Orthop Scand 51:79-84, 1980.

14. Verlaan JJ, Diekerhof CH, Buskens E, et al: Surgical treatment of traumatic fractures of the thoracic and lumbar spine: A systematic review of the literature on techniques, complications, and outcome. Spine (Phila Pa 1976) 29:803-814, 2004.

15. Wade W, Saltzstein R, Maiman D: Spinal fractures complicating ankylosing spondylitis. Arch Phys Med Rehabil 70:398-401, 1989.

16. Cooper C, Carbone L, Michet CJ, et al: Fracture risk in patients with ankylosing spondylitis: A population based study. J Rheumatol 21:1877-1882, 1994.

17. Whang PG, Golberg G, Lawrence JP, et al: The management of spinal injuries in patients with ankylosing spondylitis or diffuse idiopathic skeletal hyperostosis: A comparison of treatment methods and clinical outcomes. J Spine Disord Tech 22:77-85, 2009.

18. Finkelstein JA, Chapman JR, Mirza S: Occult vertebral fractures in ankylosing spondylitis. Spinal Cord 37:444-447, 1999.

19. Hitchon PW, From AM, Brenton MD, et al: Fractures of the thoracolumbar spine complicating ankylosing spondylitis. J Neurosurg Spine 97:218-222, 2002.

20. Graham B, van Peteghem PK: Fractures of the spine in ankylosing spondylitis: Diagnosis, treatment, and complications. Spine (Phila Pa 1976) 14:803-807, 1989.

21. Apple DF Jr, Anson C: Spinal cord injury occurring in patients with ankylosing spondylitis: A multicenter study. Orthopedics 18:1005-1011, 1995.

21a. Bohlman HH: Acute fractures and dislocations of the cervical spine. An analysis of three hundred hospitalized patients and review of the literature. J Bone Joint Surg Am 61:1119-1142, 1979.

22. Schroder L, Liljenqvist U, Greiner C, et al: Complications of halo fixation for cervical spine injuries in patients with ankylosing spondylitis—report of three cases. Arch Orthop Trauma Surg 123:112-114, 2003.

23. Suk S, Kim KT, Lee SH, et al: Significance of chin-brow vertical angle in correction of kyphotic deformity of ankylosing spondylitis patients. Spine (Phila Pa 1976) 28:2001-2005, 2003.

24. Taggard DA, Traynelis VC: Management of cervical spinal fractures in ankylosing spondylitis with posterior fixation. Spine (Phila Pa 1976) 25:2035-2039, 2000.

25. Klein JD, Hey LA, Yu CS, et al: Perioperative nutrition and postoperative complications in patients undergoing spinal surgery. Spine (Phila Pa 1976) 21:2676-2682, 1996.

26. Hu SS, Fontaine F, Kelly B, et al: Nutritional depletion in staged spinal reconstructive surgery: The effect of total parenteral nutrition. Spine (Phila Pa 1976) 23:1401-1405, 1998.

27. Lapp MA, Bridwell KH, Lenke LG, et al: Prospective randomization of parenteral hyperalimentation for long fusions with spinal deformity: Its effect on complications and recovery from postoperative malnutrition. Spine (Phila Pa 1976) 26:809-817; discussion 817, 2001.

28. Simmons EH: Kyphotic deformity of the spine in ankylosing spondylitis. Clin Orthop Relat Res (128):65-77, 1977.

29. Lichtblau PO, Wilson PD: Possible mechanism of aortic rupture in orthopaedic correction of rheumatoid spondylitis. J Bone Joint Surg Am 38:123-127, 1956.

30. Fazl M, Bilbao JM, Hudson AR: Laceration of the aorta complicating spinal fracture in ankylosing spondylitis. Neurosurgery 8:732-734, 1981.

31. Law WA: Osteotomy of the spine. Clin Orthop Relat Res (66):70-76, 1969.

32. McMaster MJ: A technique for lumbar spinal osteotomy in ankylosing spondylitis. J Bone Joint Surg Br 67:204-210, 1985.

33. Smith-Petersen MN, Larson CB, Aufranc OE: Osteotomy of the spine for correction of flexion deformity in rheumatoid arthritis. Clin Orthop Relat Res (66):6-9, 1969.

34. Herbert JJ: Technique and results of vertebral osteotomy in 26 cases. Acta Orthop Scand 22:36-58, 1952.

34a. Wilson MJ, Turkel JH: Multiple spinal wedge osteotomy; its use in a case of Marie-Strumpell spondylitis. Am J Surg 77:777-782, 1949.

34b. Püschel J, Zielke K: [Corrective surgery for kyphosis in bekhterev's disease—indication, technique, results (author's transl)]. [Article in German]. Z Orthop Ihre Grenzgeb 120:338-342, 1982.

35. Adams JC: Technique, dangers and safeguards in osteotomy of the spine. J Bone Joint Surg Br 34:226-232, 1952.

36. Camargo FP, Cordeiro EN, Napoli MM: Corrective osteotomy of the spine in ankylosing spondylitis: Experience with 66 cases. Clin Orthop Relat Res (208):157-167, 1986.

37. Thomasen E: Vertebral osteotomy for correction of kyphosis in ankylosing spondylitis. Clin Orthop Relat Res (194):142-152, 1985.

38. Bradford DS, Schumacher WL, Lonstein JE, et al: Ankylosing spondylitis: Experience in surgical management of 21 patients. Spine (Phila Pa 1976) 12:238-243, 1987.

39. Hehne HJ, Zielke K, Bohm H: Polysegmental lumbar osteotomies and transpedicled fixation for correction of long-curved kyphotic deformities in ankylosing spondylitis: Report on 177 cases. Clin Orthop Relat Res (258):49-55, 1990.

39a. Jaffray D, Becker V, Eisenstein S: Closing wedge osteotomy with transpedicular fixation in ankylosing spondylitis. Clin Orthop Relat Res (279):122-126, 1992.

40. Van Royen BJ, De Gast A: Lumbar osteotomy for correction of thoracolumbar kyphotic deformity in ankylosing spondylitis: A structured review of three methods of treatment. Ann Rheum Dis 58:399-406, 1999.

41. Halm H, Metz-Stavenhagen P, Zielke K: Results of surgical correction of kyphotic deformities of the spine in ankylosing spondylitis on the basis of the modified Arthritis Impact Measurement Scales. Spine (Phila Pa 1976) 20:1612-1619, 1995.

42. Kim KT, Suk KS, Cho YJ, et al: Clinical outcome results of pedicle subtraction osteotomy in ankylosing spondylitis with kyphotic deformity. Spine (Phila Pa 1976) 27:612-618, 2002.

43. Berven SH, Deviren V, Smith JA, et al: Management of fixed sagittal plane deformity: Results of the transpedicular wedge resection osteotomy. Spine (Phila Pa 1976) 26:2036-2043, 2001.

44. Bridwell KH, Lewis SJ, Lenke LG, et al: Pedicle subtraction osteotomy for the treatment of fixed sagittal imbalance. J Bone Joint Surg Am 85:454-463, 2003.

45. Kawahara N, Tomita K, Baba H, et al: Closing-opening wedge osteotomy to correct angular kyphotic deformity by a single posterior approach. Spine (Phila Pa 1976) 26:391-402, 2001.

46. Urist MR: Osteotomy of the cervical spine; report of a case of ankylosing rheumatoid spondylitis. J Bone Joint Surg Am 40:833-843, 1958.

46a. Simmons EH: The surgical correction of flexion deformity of the cervical spine in ankylosing spondylitis. Clin Orthop Relat Res 86:132-143, 1972.

46b. Sengupta DK, Khazim R, Grevitt MP, Webb JK: Flexion osteotomy of the cervical spine: a new technique for correction of iatrogenic extension deformity in ankylosing spondylitis. Spine (Phila Pa 1976) 26:1068-1072, 2001.

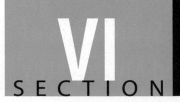

VI
SECTION

CERVICAL DEGENERATIVE DISORDERS

Cervical Spondylosis: Pathophysiology, Natural History, and Clinical Syndromes of Neck Pain, Radiculopathy, and Myelopathy

Sara Jurek, MD
Raj D. Rao, MD

Degenerative changes at the cervical discs and facet joints are ubiquitous in the adult population; these changes are a natural consequence of aging and are asymptomatic in most of the population. *Spondylosis* refers to these age-related degenerative changes within the spinal column.[1] Most patients who present with cervical spondylosis are older than 40 years.[2] Although most of these age-related degenerative changes remain asymptomatic, they can manifest as three main symptom complexes—axial neck pain, upper extremity radiculopathy, or myelopathy—or some combination thereof.[1]

Categorizing the findings at clinical presentation into these distinct divisions simplifies the clinical approach to cervical spondylosis. *Axial neck pain* refers to pain along the spinal column and its related paraspinal musculature. *Cervical radiculopathy* denotes pain radiating into the arm, which may be accompanied by sensory or motor changes in a radicular distribution. *Cervical spondylotic myelopathy* is the development of long tract signs as a result of degenerative changes at the cervical spinal motion segment. This chapter reviews the anatomy, pathogenesis, natural history, and relevant clinical features of patients with axial neck pain, radiculopathy, and myelopathy.

Pathoanatomy

Degenerative changes within the cervical disc lead to loss of disc height, arthrosis in the uncovertebral and facet joints, and motion aberrations between two vertebral bodies.[3] In most patients, desiccation of the disc initiates a cascade of degenerative changes.[4] An alteration in proteoglycan content beginning in the 3rd decade diminishes the ability of the disc to maintain its hydration.[1] The amount of keratin sulfate increases, and the amount of chondroitin sulfate decreases.[4] With these changes in viscoelasticity, the periphery of the disc begins to bear an increasingly greater proportion of the load borne by the disc, with resultant loss of disc height and bulging of the anulus into the spinal canal.

As the disc loses height, the vertebral bodies approach each other, causing infolding of the ligamentum flavum and facet joint capsule and reducing the dimensions of the canal and the foramen.[5] The anterior height of the disc is greater than the posterior height of the disc in a normally configured disc; with degeneration, the ventral portion of the disc loses height to a greater degree than the dorsal portion, and loss of cervical lordosis can occur.[6] A positive feedback cycle ensues with greater force placed on the ventral aspect of the vertebral bodies leading to kyphosis.[4] The uncovertebral and facet joints bear greater loads, accelerating the formation of osteophytes at these joints and at the peripheral vertebral endplate margins. Osteophytes, the posteriorly protruded disc material, and the infolded soft tissue within the canal and neuroforamina all diminish the space available for the spinal cord or nerve root. Radiographically, the C5-6 interspace is the most frequently affected level, followed closely by C6-7.[7]

Pathophysiology

Pathophysiology of Axial Neck Pain

Axial neck pain results from a multitude of potential causes and can be divided geographically into anterior neck pain, which usually stems from sprains and strains of the sternocleidomastoid and other strap muscles and their attachments, and posterior neck pain, which can be subdivided further into subaxial and suboccipital locations.[8] In many patients, subaxial neck pain results from muscular or ligamentous imbalances related to poor posture, faulty ergonomics, or muscle fatigue or stress or both. Muscular pain often occurs as a result of postural adaptations to a primary pain source located in the shoulder, the craniovertebral junction, or the temporomandibular joint.[5]

The physiology of this pain process is not yet fully delineated. Patients with chronic myofascial pain have significantly lower levels of high-energy phosphates in the involved muscle tissue.[9] It is unknown whether the diminished level of high-energy phosphates causes the pain or if it is a result of the pain. Unencapsulated free nerve endings in the neck musculature function as chemonociceptive units. Fatigued muscle

36 Cervical Spondylosis: Pathophysiology, Natural History, and Clinical Syndromes of Neck Pain, Radiculopathy, and Myelopathy   685

SECTION

VI

generates anaerobic metabolites, which accumulate and can stimulate these chemonociceptive nerve endings. These free nerve endings also respond to non-neurogenic pain mediators released as a result of ischemia or injury, such as bradykinin, histamine, serotonin, and potassium ions. Primary muscle pain may result from sensitization of these nerve endings.

Axial neck pain should be attributed to degenerative changes in the cervical discs or facet joints only after careful consideration, owing to the ubiquitous nature of these changes in the spine. Nevertheless, multiple studies suggest that cervical discs and facet joints can generate pain.[10-14] Nerve fibers and nerve endings, containing somatic afferent fibers, innervate the peripheral portion of the intervertebral disc (the outer third of the anulus) and offer a potential mechanism by which degenerative cervical discs generate pain directly. The sinuvertebral nerve, formed by branches of the ventral nerve root and by the sympathetic plexus, innervates the intervertebral disc (Fig. 36–1). When formed, the sinuvertebral nerve turns back into the intervertebral foramen along the posterior aspect of the disc, supplying portions of the anulus, posterior longitudinal ligament, periosteum of the vertebral body and pedicle, adjacent epidural veins, and dura mater.[10] A review of a 12-year cervical discography experience suggests that stimulation of each disc results in consistent and predictable patterns of neck pain (Fig. 36–2).[14]

Degenerative changes at a cervical facet joint can be a source of axial neck pain. Provocative injections into the facet joints of asymptomatic volunteers result in a reproducible pattern of axial neck pain and shoulder girdle pain (Fig. 36–3).[12] Controlled injection of anesthetic into the symptomatic facet joint or into the dorsal primary rami blocks these patterns of facet pain, suggesting that the facet joint plays a role in the development of axial neck pain. C3-4 to C8-T1 facet joints receive their innervation from the medial branches of the cervical dorsal rami above and below each joint, whereas the third occipital nerve innervates the C2-3 facet joint.[11] The presence of mechanoreceptors and nociceptive nerve endings in cervical facet joint capsules further supports a possible role for these structures in the pathogenesis of cervical spine pain.[15] Immunohistochemical studies show the presence of free nerve endings reactive for pain-related peptides located in the synovial folds of the human cervical facet joint.

Suboccipital pain radiating down into the neck or to the back of the ear may be a manifestation of degenerative arthritis in the upper cervical spine. Injection of the atlanto-occipital and atlantoaxial joints results in a reproducible pain pattern in this region, with the atlanto-occipital joints showing the capacity to generate intense and diffuse pain.[16] Wächli and colleagues[17] reported unilateral headaches and atypical facial pain as a result of degenerative changes at the C2-3 level. Some patients with suboccipital headaches presumably have irritation of the greater occipital nerve, which originates from the posterior rami of C2, C3, and C4.[18] The sinuvertebral nerves from C2 and C3 exist as another potential source of suboccipital pain, ascending proximally to innervate the atlantoaxial ligaments, tectorial membrane, and dura mater of the upper cervical cord and posterior cranial fossa.[10]

Pathophysiology of Radiculopathy

Radicular findings in the arm originate from the cervical nerve roots at some point between their origins as nerve rootlets from the spinal cord and their transition into peripheral nerves as they emerge from the neural foramen. Degenerative changes at the cervical motion segment, soft disc herniations, stenosis, intrinsic nerve root pathology, and trauma all can result in these symptoms. Loss of disc height leads to impingement on the nerve root origins from disc bulging, infolding of the facet joint capsule and ligamentum flavum, and osteophyte formation at the disc margins (hard disc formation) and at the uncovertebral and facet joints, all of which result in foraminal stenosis and radiculopathy (Fig. 36–4). Osteophytic spur formation may also compromise the blood supply to the nerve roots. Osteophytes may compress radicular arteries within the dural root sleeves leading to spasm and reduced vascular perfusion. Additionally, blockage of venous outflow may occur, resulting in edema and further compromise of the blood supply of the nerve roots.[19]

Mechanical deformation of the nerve root may lead to motor weakness or sensory deficits. The exact pathogenesis of radicular pain is unclear, but the general belief exists that in addition to the compression, an inflammatory response must occur for pain to develop. Within the compressed nerve root, intrinsic vessels show increased permeability, secondarily resulting in edema of the nerve root. Chronic edema and fibrosis (scar) within the nerve root play a role in altering the response threshold and heighten the sensitivity of the nerve root to pain.[20] Neurogenic chemical pain mediators released from the sensory neuron cell bodies and non-neurogenic mediators released from disc tissue may initiate and perpetuate this inflammatory response (Table 36–1).[21,22]

Dynamic factors in the cervical spinal column affect the amount of nerve root compression. Flexion of the cervical spine lengthens the cervical neural foramina 18% to 31%, whereas extension shortens the foramina 16% to 22%.[23] Rotation to the ipsilateral side narrows the foramen, whereas rotation to the contralateral side widens the foramen. The facet

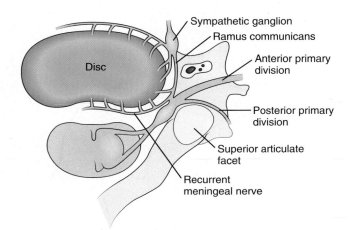

FIGURE 36–1 Cross-sectional anatomy showing dorsal and ventral primary branches of cervical nerve root, origin of sinuvertebral nerve (also known as recurrent meningeal nerve) from the nerve root, and sympathetic plexus. Note proximity of disc, uncovertebral and facet joints, and vertebral artery.

(Figure labels: Sympathetic ganglion; Ramus communicans; Anterior primary division; Disc; Posterior primary division; Superior articulate facet; Recurrent meningeal nerve)

FIGURE 36–2 Axial pain patterns provoked during discography at each cervical level. **A,** C2-3. **B,** C3-4. **C,** C4-5. **D,** C5-6. **E,** C6-7. (From Grubb SA, Kelly CK, Bogduk N: Cervical discography: Clinical implications from 12 years of experience. Spine [Phila Pa 1976] 25:1382-1389, 2000.)

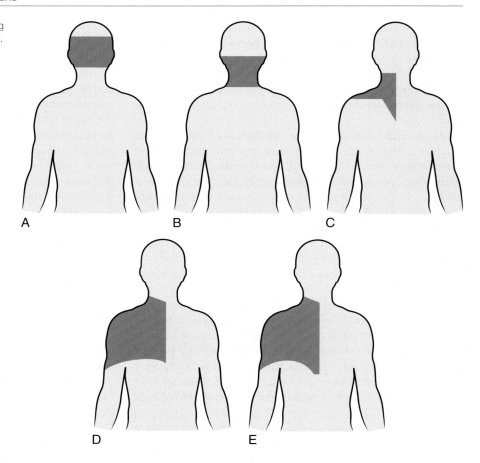

joint capsule and ligamentum flavum buckle with extension, narrowing the foraminal dimensions further. Translation or angulation between vertebral bodies in flexion or extension may result in increased stretch on the nerve root and predispose the individual to radicular symptoms. Patients who do not have nerve root compression with their necks in a static, neutral position may dynamically compress the nerve root during normal activities, resulting in radicular symptoms.

Changes in intrinsic tension within the nerve root have the ability to alter radicular pain. Davidson and colleagues[24] postulated that the decrease in tension within the nerve root caused by a patient resting the hand atop the head—the shoulder abduction sign—relieves radicular pain. These

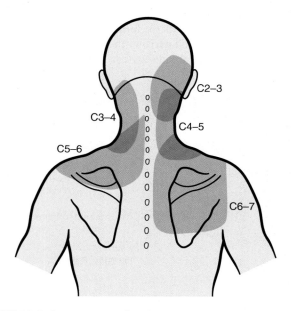

FIGURE 36–3 Composite map of axial pain patterns from facet joints at C2-3 to C6-7. (From Dwyer A, Aprill C, Bogduk N: Cervical zygapophyseal joint pain patterns. I. A study in normal volunteers. Spine [Phila Pa 1976] 15:453-457, 1990.)

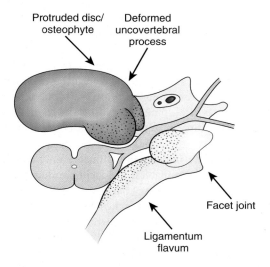

FIGURE 36–4 Nerve root compression in lateral spinal canal from disc, uncovertebral joint, or facet joint pathology can lead to cervical radiculopathy.

investigators also postulated that this change in arm position lifts the sensory root, or dorsal root ganglion, directly cephalad or lateral to the source of compression and that this position decompresses the epidural veins, augmenting pain relief. Another study suggested that the abducted arm position allows relative laxity in the dural ligaments (of Hoffman), resulting in decreased tension on the nerve root.[25]

Often, patients present with radicular pain in an atypical distribution.[26] An anatomic human cadaveric study confirmed the high incidence of intradural connections among C5, C6, and C7 dorsal rootlets (noted to be anatomic variants because of their high incidence rather than anatomic anomalies) and postulated that these variant intradural connections potentially explain the clinical variation and overlapping sensory symptoms frequently observed with cervical spine nerve root compression.[27]

Pathophysiology of Myelopathy

Although it is generally agreed that mechanical compression of the spinal cord is the primary pathophysiologic mechanism resulting in myelopathy, in many patients a combination of this static compression with dynamic factors secondary to motion between the vertebral bodies, a congenitally stenotic canal, changes in the intrinsic morphology of the spinal cord, and vascular factors contributes to the development of myelopathy. A developmentally narrow spinal canal in the anteroposterior plane can contribute to the development of cervical myelopathy. The normal anteroposterior diameter of the cervical spine measures 17 to 18 mm in adults, and the anteroposterior diameter of the spinal cord in the cervical region measures approximately 10 mm. An anteroposterior diameter of the spinal canal less than 13 mm defines congenital cervical stenosis, whereas a diameter greater than 16 mm suggests a relatively low risk of myelopathy (Fig. 36–5A).[28,29] A congenitally narrow spinal canal lowers the threshold at which the cumulative effects of various degenerative structures encroaching on the spinal cord cause signs and symptoms of myelopathy.[30]

A strong association exists between flattening of the cord within the narrowed spinal canal and the development of cervical myelopathy. Penning and colleagues[31] believed that symptoms of cord compression occurred when cross-sectional area of the cord had been reduced by a critical amount (30%) and the remaining transverse area of the cord was less than 60 mm². Houser and colleagues[32] contended that the extent and shape of flattening of the spinal cord serve as an indicator of neurologic deficit: 98% of their patients with severe stenosis manifested by a banana-shaped spinal cord had clinical evidence of myelopathy. Ono and colleagues[33] described an anteroposterior cord compression ratio calculated by dividing the anteroposterior diameter of the cord by the transverse diameter of the cord. A lower anteroposterior compression ratio (<0.40) correlated well with the areas of most severe injury of the cord histologically. The Pavlov ratio, which is the anteroposterior diameter of the spinal canal divided by the anteroposterior diameter of the vertebral body at the same

level, as measured on a lateral radiograph, also indicates static compression; a value of 0.8 or less indicates a developmentally narrow cervical canal and stenosis of the canal.[30,34]

Segmental motion of the cervical spinal column affects the development of cervical myelopathy. Hyperextension of the

TABLE 36–1 Chemical Mediators of Spinal Pain

Neurogenic	Non-neurogenic
Substance P	Bradykinin
Somatostatin	Serotonin
Cholecystokininlike substance	Histamine
Vasoactive intestinal peptide	Acetylcholine
Calcitonin gene-related peptide	Prostaglandin E₁
Gastrin-releasing peptide	Prostaglandin E₂
Dynorphin	Leukotrienes
Enkephalin	diHETE
Gelanin	
Neurotensin	
Angiotensin II	

diHETE, dihydroxyeicosatetraenoic acid
From Chabot MC, Montgomery DM: The pathophysiology of axial and radicular neck pain. Semin Spine Surg 7:2-8, 1995.

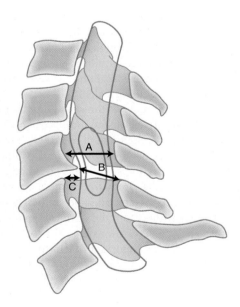

FIGURE 36–5 Radiographic criteria important in pathogenesis of cervical spondylotic myelopathy. **A,** Mid-sagittal diameter of spinal canal is measured as distance from middle of dorsal surface of vertebral body to nearest point on spinolaminar line. Patients in whom osseous canal measures less than 13 mm are considered developmentally stenotic. **B,** Distance of less than 12 mm from posteroinferior corner of vertebral body to anterosuperior edge of lamina of immediately caudal vertebra with neck in extension is suggestive of dynamic stenosis. **C,** Olisthesis (retrolisthesis or anterolisthesis) of greater than 3.5 mm is measure of excessive translation between vertebral bodies. Signal changes within substance of spinal cord, noted on T1-weighted and T2-weighted MRI in some patients, are represented diagrammatically with gray lines. (From Rao RD, Gourab K, David KS: Operative treatment of cervical spondylotic myelopathy. J Bone Joint Surg Am 88:1619-1640, 2006.)

neck narrows the spinal canal by shingling the laminae and buckling the ligamentum flavum ventrally into the canal. Extension and flexion of the neck may alter the diameter of the canal by 2 mm.[35] Angulation or translation between vertebral bodies in flexion or extension may result in narrowing of the space available for the cord (Fig. 36–5B). Particularly during extension, retrolisthesis of a vertebral body can pinch the spinal cord between the inferoposterior margin of a vertebral body and the superior edge of the lamina caudad to it. Forward slippage of a vertebral body may compress the spinal cord between the superoposterior margin of the vertebral body below and the lamina above.[30] Flexion of the spinal column aggravates this forward slippage. Retrolisthesis and anterolisthesis often cause myelopathy in elderly (≥70 years old) patients (Fig. 36–5C).[28,36] Additionally, hypermobility at the third and fourth cervical levels cephalad to a degenerated and stiffened C4-5 segment commonly exists in elderly individuals, potentially resulting in myelopathy at the hypermobile C3-4 level.[37] Research using a spinal cord model showed that the cord is more vulnerable to dynamic, repeated minor loading compared with severe static loading.[38]

Cervical spine flexion and extension cause morphologic changes within the spinal cord itself. Breig and colleagues[39] showed that the spinal cord thickens and shortens with extension, which renders it more susceptible to pressure from the infolded ligamentum flavum or lamina. The spinal cord stretches with flexion, which may subject the cord to higher intrinsic pressure if it presses against a disc or a vertebral body anteriorly. Flexion of the cervical spine may cause stretch (strain) injury to the axons through tensile loading, resulting in increased permeability and myelin injury, rendering these already injured axons more susceptible to secondary injury from other processes, including ischemia.[40]

Barre[41] first proposed in 1924 the possibility that vascular factors play a significant role in the development of cervical myelopathy. The acute development or progression of findings suggests vascular involvement. In two separate canine experiments, cervical cord ischemia superimposed on compression of the cord resulted in a dramatic increase in neurologic findings.[42,43] The effects of compression and ischemia were additive and responsible for the clinical manifestations of myelopathy. These investigations also led to the proposal that ischemia may play an important role in the irreversibility of spinal compression.[42] In a separate dog study, obstruction of the peripheral arterial plexus caused structural changes within the spinal cord.[44]

The classic study by Breig and colleagues[39] established that blood flow through the anterior spinal artery and anterior radicular arteries diminishes when those vessels are tented over a disc or a vertebral body, but that this position does not have a substantial impact on flow through the tortuous posterior spinal arteries. Vessels considered most vulnerable to reduced blood flow include the transverse intramedullary arterioles, arising from the anterior sulcal arteries. These vessels perfuse the gray matter and adjacent lateral columns.[45] Ischemia may also occur from venous congestion.[46] One cell type known to be particularly sensitive to ischemic injury, the oligodendrocyte, plays a principal role in insulating axons

with a myelin sheath. Oligodendrocyte death caused by ischemic insult, likely through the mechanism of oligodendrocyte apoptosis, may explain the demyelination and subsequent irreversible neurologic deficit associated with chronic cervical myelopathy.[40,47]

Severe compression results in pathologic changes within the spinal cord. The central gray matter and the lateral columns show the most changes, with cystic cavitation, gliosis, and demyelination most pronounced caudad to the compression site. The posterior columns and posterolateral tracts show wallerian degeneration cephalad to the site of compression. The irreversibility of these changes may explain why some patients fail to recover after decompressive surgery. The anterior white columns are relatively resistant to infarction, even in cases of severe compression.[48]

Natural History and Epidemiology of Neck Pain, Radiculopathy, and Myelopathy

Axial Neck Pain

Neck pain commonly affects adults of all ages and both sexes almost equally. Few population-based studies exist on the prevalence of neck pain. A study of the Saskatchewan adult population showed that neck pain is more prevalent than commonly thought, with 66% of adults experiencing neck pain during their lifetime and 5% highly disabled by it.[49] Another study showed a 9% point prevalence of neck and shoulder pain.[50] The prevalence of neck pain increases in highly educated individuals and in individuals with a history of injury, headaches, low back pain, or medical comorbidities such as cardiovascular and digestive disorders.[51]

No true natural history studies of axial neck pain exist; all published studies involve some form of treatment in most patients. DePalma and Subin[52] found that most patients with axial symptoms from cervical spondylosis respond favorably to nonoperative treatment. After 3 months of nonoperative treatment, 29% of their patients had total relief of symptoms, 49% improved, and 22% did not improve. Rothman and Rashbaum[53] reported on the 5-year outcome of patients with "predominantly" axial neck pain treated conservatively. They found that 23% of these patients remained partially or totally disabled from their symptoms. At the 5-year follow-up, Rothman and Rashbaum[53] found no significant difference between this group and another similar group of patients who underwent surgery and recommended nonoperative management for "non-neurogenic" axial neck pain symptoms.

Generally, most patients who present early with a single episode of axial neck pain may be reassured that their symptoms will resolve spontaneously. Patients who have persistent or recurrent symptoms that require continued treatment likely fall into a separate group, with approximately one quarter of these patients going on to residual moderate to severe pain. This group should be evaluated more carefully to rule out underlying discogenic or other pathology that may be responsible for their continued symptoms.

Cervical Radiculopathy

In a study of a Midwestern U.S. population, the annual incidence of cervical radiculopathy was found to be 83 per 100,000 population, with a peak incidence in the 6th decade of life.[54] The point prevalence of cervical radiculopathy was found to be 3.5 per 1000 population.[55] As with the natural history of neck pain, no studies on the true natural history of radiculopathy exist, with some form of treatment being provided in most patients. With varying degrees of nonoperative management, 45% of patients with cervical radiculopathy have good resolution of symptoms within 6 weeks of onset; the remaining 55% continue to have a minor to moderate degree of long-term morbidity.

The reported outcomes of cervical radiculopathy vary depending on the study population. Population-based and primary care–based studies suggest a benign natural or nonoperative history of cervical radiculopathy. Good outcomes occur in 71% to 92% of patients after nonoperative measures such as medications, exercise or physical therapy, and traction.[56-59] A population-based study in Rochester, Minnesota, reported that 90% of patients initially diagnosed with cervical radiculopathy were asymptomatic or minimally affected by their condition at 5.9 years of follow-up. Surgery was performed in 26% of this group, but the effects of intervention were not independently analyzed.[54] Studies originating from tertiary referral centers or surgical practices show persistent symptoms and disability in a significant percentage of patients with cervical radiculopathy.

The 1963 study by Lees and Turner[60] on the "natural history" of cervical spondylosis showed the natural history and prognosis to be generally favorable. At long-term follow-up (2 to 19 years) of 51 patients with radiculopathy, 45% had only a single episode of pain without recurrence, 30% had mild continuing symptoms, and 25% had persistent or worsening symptoms. Lees and Turner[60] found that nonoperative treatment helped improve initial symptoms but did not affect end results. Of the patients followed for cervical radiculopathy, none had evidence of myelopathy on follow-up.

Cervical Myelopathy

The true incidence of cervical myelopathy is difficult to ascertain because of the subtle findings in its early stages and the fact that many of the clinical findings of myelopathy are attributed to old age. Similarly, no modern studies on the true natural history of spondylotic myelopathy exist because surgical intervention is so commonly part of the treatment.[61] In 1963, Lees and Turner[60] reported on 44 patients with radiologic and myelographic evidence of myelopathy followed for 3 to 40 years (22 patients for >10 years and 22 additional patients for <10 years). The authors concluded that cervical spondylotic myelopathy follows a protracted clinical course consisting of long periods of relatively stable symptoms punctuated by exacerbations of variable duration. Clark and Robinson[62] showed in a study of 120 patients that the natural history of cervical spondylotic myelopathy consists of progressive deterioration of motor symptoms, with 75% of patients deteriorating stepwise with intervening variable periods of stable disease, 20% deteriorating gradually and steadily, and 5% experiencing a rapid onset of symptoms followed by a lengthy period of quiescence. None of the 120 patients had a return to a normal neurologic state or reversal of symptoms. Nurick[63] retrospectively assessed 37 patients, noting that the neurologic disability manifests early in the course of the disease and subsequently consists of static periods lasting many years. He noted that the prognosis improved for patients presenting with mild disease and that the disability tended to progress in patients older than 60 years. Nurick[63] concluded that spondylotic myelopathy is a benign condition with minimal risk of future neurologic deterioration. Finally, Symon and Lavender[64] argued against the idea that spondylotic myelopathy constitutes a benign disease process and showed in their review that 67% of patients underwent relentless neurologic deterioration without periods of clinical stability. Their analysis of Lees and Turner's data showed that when disability was used as a criterion, only 18% of patients showed improvement.

Clinical Syndromes of Axial Neck Pain, Cervical Radiculopathy, and Myelopathy

Axial Neck Pain

Pain along the posterior neck and trapezius muscles without radiation into the upper extremity is an extremely common, but nonspecific presenting symptom. Patients usually localize the pain to the posterior paraspinal musculature of the neck, with radiation toward the occiput or into the shoulder and periscapular regions. Patients may report stiffness in one or more directions and commonly complain of headaches.[65] Radiating "referred" pain without a dermatomal distribution in the shoulder or arm may accompany the neck pain. Referred pain may be associated with a sensation of warmth or tingling and autonomic phenomena such as piloerection and sweating. Areas of localized pain and tenderness in the posterior muscles of the neck suggest a muscle sprain or a soft tissue injury. Deep palpation of these trigger points produces referred patterns of pain along the course of the myofascial structures.

Determining a position of maximal discomfort may also provide a clue to the underlying pathologic etiology. Anterior neck pain along the sternocleidomastoid muscle belly exacerbated by rotation of the head to the contralateral side most often results from muscular strain. Pain in the posterior neck muscles that worsens with flexion of the head suggests a myofascial etiology. Pain in the posterior aspect of the neck aggravated by extension and especially by rotation of the head to one side may suggest a discogenic component. Suboccipital pain radiating to the back of the ear, occiput, or neck raises the question of pathologic involvement of the upper cervical spine. Limited rotation of the head to one side suggests involvement of the ipsilateral atlantoaxial articulation.

Postural adaptations to pain initiated elsewhere in the body may generate secondary pain in the neck and shoulder girdle. The adaptations and compensatory overuse of normal tissues

TABLE 36-2 Differential Diagnoses of Radiculopathy

Peripheral entrapment syndromes
Rotator cuff or shoulder pathology
Brachial plexitis
Herpes zoster
Thoracic outlet syndrome
Sympathetic mediated pain syndrome
Intraspinal or extraspinal tumors
Epidural abscess
Cardiac ischemia

From Rao R: Neck pain, cervical radiculopathy, and cervical myelopathy: Pathophysiology, natural history and clinical evaluation. J Bone Joint Surg Am 84:1872-1881, 2002.

in the neck and shoulder girdle generate new pain patterns that may remain even after the initial source of pain has resolved. This situation underscores the need to obtain an accurate history on how the neck pain initially presented and how it has evolved over time.

Pathologic processes in the shoulder may manifest with localized pain or referred pain to the neck, which may radiate down the anterior or lateral aspect of the arm. A thorough shoulder examination helps differentiate shoulder pathology from neck pathology. Pain in the neck and shoulder girdle can also be referred from pathologic processes in the heart, lungs, viscera, and temporomandibular joint. Fever, unintended weight loss, and nonmechanical neck pain, especially when worse at night, point to an infectious or neoplastic etiology. Morning stiffness, polyarticular involvement, rigidity, and cutaneous manifestations suggest an inflammatory arthritic element.

Cervical Radiculopathy

Cervical radiculopathy refers to symptoms in a specific dermatomal distribution in the upper extremity. Patients describe sharp pain, tingling, or burning sensations in the involved area. There may be sensory or motor loss corresponding to the nerve root involved, and reflex activity may be diminished.

Patients typically have severe neck and arm pain (frequently unilateral) that precludes them from finding a comfortable position. They may present with the head cocked to the side opposite to their arm pain and sometimes hold the arm over the head, typically resting the wrist or forearm on top of the head—the shoulder abduction sign.[24] The Valsalva maneuver typically exacerbates patients' pain complaints.[66] Extension and lateral rotation of the head to the side of the pain usually aggravate the symptoms—the Spurling maneuver. Aggravation of the symptoms by neck extension often helps differentiate a radicular etiology from muscular neck pain or a shoulder pathologic process with secondary muscle pain in the neck. The Spurling maneuver is particularly useful in differentiating cervical radiculopathy from other upper extremity neck pain etiologies, such as peripheral nerve entrapment,

because it stresses only structures located within the cervical spine by decreasing the size of the intervertebral foramen and impinging further on the involved nerve root.[66,67]

Multiple sources of pain in the neck and upper extremity commonly coexist, and the structures may be compressed at more than one site.[68] Patients with metabolic disorders such as diabetes who have accompanying neuropathy may be more susceptible to radiculopathy and compressive neuropathy. Adaptations to an initial presentation of radiculopathy may result in secondary shoulder pathology, carpal tunnel syndrome, or ulnar nerve irritation persisting long after the initial radicular pain resolves (Table 36-2).

Henderson and colleagues[29] reviewed clinical presentations in 736 patients with cervical radiculopathy: 99.4% had arm pain, 85.2% had sensory deficits, 79.7% had neck pain, 71.2% had reflex deficits, 68% had motor deficits, 52.5% had scapular pain, 17.8% had anterior chest pain, 9.7% had headaches, 5.9% had anterior chest and arm pain, and 1.3% had left-sided chest and arm pain, known as cervical angina. Neurologic deficits corresponded with the offending disc level in approximately 80% of patients with radiculopathy. Another study of 275 patients with cervical radiculopathy noted that 59% of these patients reported headache, frequently occurring ipsilateral to the radicular symptoms.[18]

Occasionally, patients with nerve root compression present with "referred" upper trapezial or interscapular pain without radiating arm pain. The absence of radiating symptoms in a dermatomal fashion does not rule out symptomatic nerve root compression. The clinician should perform a careful physical examination to identify any involved nerve roots, keeping in mind that crossover between myotomes and dermatomes may be present.[67]

C3 radiculopathy results from disc pathology at C2-3 and is unusual. The posterior ramus of C3 innervates the suboccipital region, and involvement of this nerve manifests with pain in this region, often extending to the occiput and back of the ear. No specific neurologic deficits help identify radicular involvement of the C3 nerve root. These patients are difficult to distinguish from patients with other sources of axial neck pain. Unilateral pain, worsening of pain with extension and rotation, and concordant imaging findings may indicate radicular involvement.

C4 radiculopathy may also be a source of unexplained neck and shoulder pain. Patients occasionally have paresthesias or numbness in the lower neck extending laterally to the superior aspect of the shoulder. Diaphragmatic involvement may result from involvement of C3-5 nerve roots.[69,70] Motor deficits in the diaphragm manifest as paradoxical respiration and can be confirmed by fluoroscopic evaluation of the diaphragm during respiration. With paradoxical respiration, the unaffected hemidiaphragm contracts and descends during inspiration; this downward excursion transmits pressure to the abdominal cavity, resulting in upward passive movement of the paralyzed side. A "sniff test," done under fluoroscopy, detects paradoxical movement: Rapidly repeated inspirations through the nostrils normally result in the descent of both hemidiaphragms, but with unilateral diaphragmatic paralysis, there is paradoxical upward motion of the paralyzed side.[71]

C5 radiculopathy classically manifests with pain or paresthesias in an "epaulet" distribution, from the superior aspect of the shoulder extending laterally to the mid-arm. The C5 nerve solely innervates the deltoid muscle, and involvement of C5 can result in profound deltoid weakness. Subtle weakness may also exist in external rotation of the shoulder (supraspinatus and infraspinatus) and elbow flexion (biceps brachialis). The biceps reflex primarily indicates neurologic integrity of C6 but also has a C5 component. Rotator cuff injury and other shoulder pathology manifest in a similar fashion and may coexist with cervical radiculopathy; the shoulder joint must be thoroughly examined in all patients with suspected cervical radiculopathy. Painless shoulder range of motion with good strength in the rotator cuff muscles helps rule out shoulder pathology.

C6 radiculopathy manifests as pain radiating from the base of the neck to the lateral aspect of the elbow, into the radial forearm and radial digits, more commonly involving the thumb. Numbness or paresthesias may exist in the same distribution. Motor deficits may be elicited in the wrist extensors, elbow flexion, and forearm supination. C6 compression most directly affects the brachioradialis reflex; however, subtle changes in the biceps reflex may exist as well.[66] The sensory symptoms may mimic symptoms of carpal tunnel syndrome, which typically involves the radial three and a half digits and causes weakness in the thenar musculature.

C7 is the most frequently involved nerve root in cervical radiculopathy and results from C6-7 disc space pathology. Patients report pain radiating from the neck to the shoulder, down along the triceps, then along the dorsum of the forearm onto the dorsum of the middle finger. Patients usually pronate the forearm while trying to describe the radiation of their symptoms into the dorsum of the hand or long finger, a useful observation when attempting to differentiate the hand symptoms from carpal tunnel syndrome or C6 radiculopathy.[5] Chronic breast pain also has been associated with C7 radiculopathy.[72] Motor weakness exists in the triceps, wrist flexors, and finger extensors with C7 radiculopathy. The triceps reflex may be absent or diminished.

C8 radiculopathy occasionally results from disc herniation or spondylosis at the C7-T1 level. Patients present with paresthesias or pain in a dermatomal distribution along the ulnar border of the arm and forearm, radiating into the ulnar aspect of the hand to the small finger and the ring finger. Numbness usually involves the dorsal and volar aspects of the ulnar two digits and hand. The small muscles of the hand exhibit profound weakness, and patients report difficulty using their hands for routine daily activities. The clinician must differentiate between C8 radiculopathy and ulnar nerve entrapment. C8 radiculopathy may affect function of the flexor digitorum profundus in the index and long fingers and function of the flexor pollicis longus in the thumb, but ulnar nerve entrapment has no effect on these muscles. Ulnar nerve involvement spares all of the short thenar muscles except the adductor pollicis, whereas C8 radiculopathy affects these muscles (Fig. 36–6).

These pain distribution patterns represent classic descriptions and should be used as generalized guidelines for evaluation and diagnosis of compressive radicular pathology.

Because of anatomic variations, chronic conditions, and involvement of multiple levels, the clinical presentation may be less precise.

Cervical Myelopathy

The subtle nature of the clinical findings of early cervical spondylotic myelopathy makes diagnosis a challenge. The physical findings in cervical spondylotic myelopathy can vary significantly depending on the anatomic portion of the cord primarily involved. Sensory symptoms arise from compression at three discrete anatomic locations: (1) the spinothalamic tract, affecting contralateral pain and temperature sensation with light touch often preserved; (2) posterior columns, affecting ipsilateral position and vibration sense, possibly leading to gait disturbances; and (3) dorsal root compression, leading to decreased dermatomal sensation. The motor and reflex examination typically reveals lower motor neuron signs at the levels of the cervical lesions (hyporeflexia and weakness in the upper extremities) and upper motor neuron signs below the lesions (hyperreflexia and spasticity in the lower extremities).[30]

Crandall and Batzdorf[73] described five general categories of cervical spondylotic myelopathy: (1) In transverse lesion syndrome, the corticospinal, spinothalamic, and posterior cord tracts are essentially equally involved. This myelopathy is associated with the longest duration of symptoms, suggesting this category may represent an end stage of the disease. (2) In motor system syndrome, corticospinal tracts and anterior horn cells are involved, resulting in spasticity. (3) In central cord syndrome, motor and sensory deficits affect the upper extremities more severely than the lower extremities. (4) Brown-Séquard syndrome consists of ipsilateral motor deficits with contralateral sensory deficits and seems to be the least advanced form of the disease. (5) Brachialgia and cord syndrome consists of radicular pain in the upper extremity along with motor or sensory long tract signs.

Ferguson and Caplan[74] divided cervical spondylotic myelopathy into four syndromes: (1) medial syndrome, consisting primarily of long tract signs; (2) lateral syndrome, consisting primarily of radicular symptoms; (3) combined medial and lateral syndrome, which constitutes the most common presentation and includes aspects of cord and root involvement; and (4) vascular syndrome, which manifests with rapidly progressive myelopathy and likely represents vascular insufficiency of the cervical spinal cord. A clear-cut sensory or motor pattern may not be present with this syndrome because of the variable injury to the cord resulting from vascular ischemia. A fifth clinical presentation, anterior syndrome, has also been described, consisting of painless weakness in the upper extremities without accompanying symptoms in the lower extremities and without radicular or long tract signs.[30]

The findings in cervical spondylotic myelopathy vary with each patient. Patients may report an insidious onset of clumsiness in the hands or diffuse numbness in the hands resulting in worsening of handwriting or other fine motor skills over the past few months or weeks and difficulty with grasping or holding objects (i.e., trouble with manipulating buttons or

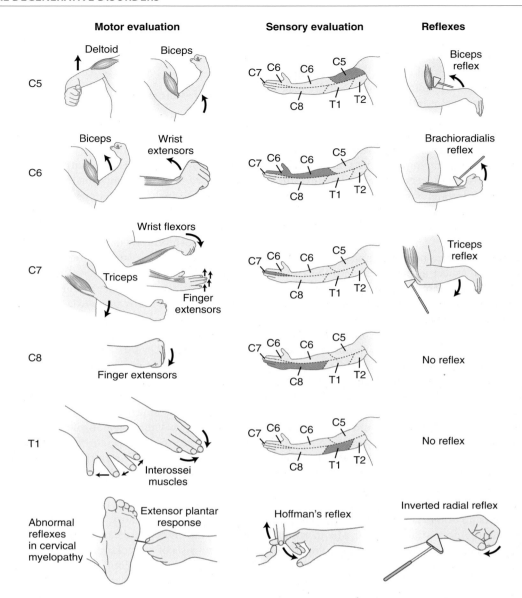

Motor evaluation   **Sensory evaluation**   **Reflexes**

FIGURE 36–6 Neurologic evaluation of a patient with cervical radiculopathy and myelopathy. (From Rao RD, Currier BL, Albert TJ, et al: Degenerative cervical spondylosis: Clinical syndromes, pathogenesis, and management. J Bone Joint Surg Am 89:1360-1378, 2007.)

zippers).[75] Patients frequently experience increasing difficulty with balance that they attribute to age or arthritic hips; relatives may note that the patient's gait has become increasingly clumsy, that the patient holds onto objects to help with balance, and that he or she sustains occasional falls. Nurick[76] developed a system for grading the disability in cervical spondylotic myelopathy on the basis of gait abnormality. Spasticity, muscle weakness, and wasting in the lower extremities with superimposed loss of proprioception result in an unsteady, broad-based gait. Severely affected individuals can be quadriparetic or quadriplegic when first seen.

Physical examination shows exaggerated deep tendon reflexes, sustained clonus, absent or diminished superficial reflexes, and the presence of pathologic reflexes confirming an upper motor neuron lesion. Myelopathy caused by pathology

in the region of the cord cephalad to C3 may result in a hyperactive scapulohumeral reflex (tapping of the spine of the scapula or acromion with a caudally directed force with the seated patient's arm resting at the side results in brisk scapular elevation or humerus abduction or both). This response represents a stretch reflex of the trapezius muscle.[77] Superficial reflexes, such as the abdominal or cremasteric reflex, are often diminished or absent in the presence of upper motor neuron lesions. The pathologic reflexes represent abnormal long tract signs and indicate cord compression.

Patients with moderate to severe spondylotic myelopathy typically exhibit the following pathologic reflexes to varying degrees: (1) the inverted radial reflex—indicative of cord compression at C6 and present when, during elicitation of a brachioradialis reflex, the brachioradialis is hyporesponsive and

36 Cervical Spondylosis: Pathophysiology, Natural History, and Clinical Syndromes of Neck Pain, Radiculopathy, and Myelopathy   693

SECTION

VI

the ipsilateral fingers flex briskly at each hammer tap; (2) the Hoffman reflex—present if the ipsilateral interphalangeal joints of the thumb and index finger flex when the volar surface of the distal phalanx of the long finger is flicked into extension and strongly indicative of cord impingement when asymmetric; and (3) the extensor plantar reflex (also called the Babinski sign)—present when rubbing of the lateral sole of the foot from the heel along a curve to the metatarsal pads with a blunt object causes the hallux to dorsiflex and the lesser toes to fan out (see Fig. 36–6).[30,66] Combined cervical and lumbar involvement is present in 13% of patients with spondylosis, resulting in a potentially confusing clinical picture of lower extremity lower motor neuron findings.[78]

Sensory findings in cervical spondylotic myelopathy also vary. Depending on the exact area of compromise of the cord or nerve root, pain, temperature, proprioception, vibratory, and dermatomal sensations all may be diminished. Presenting findings usually do not include sphincter disturbances. Patients may present with urinary complaints: hesitation, frequency, and, rarely, incontinence or retention. In the study by Crandall and Batzdorf[73] of 62 patients with cervical spondylotic myelopathy, neck pain was present in less than 50% of the patients, and associated radicular pain was present in 38%. Generalized shocklike sensations in the trunk and upper and lower extremities resulting from quick flexion or extension of the neck—the Lhermitte sign—was present in 27% of patients, and sphincter disturbances were present in 44%.

In the past, hand disturbances were primarily attributed to radicular pathology. Several reports have shown findings specific to "myelopathy hand," indicating a high cervical myelopathy above the C5 level.[79,80] Diffuse numbness in the hands is extremely common and is often misdiagnosed as carpal tunnel syndrome or peripheral neuropathy. Clumsiness of the hands results in an inability to perform fine motor tasks. Marked wasting of the intrinsic hand muscles is usually present and progresses insidiously with weakness of finger extension and adduction.[81] Ono and colleagues[80] described two specific signs of myelopathy hand signifying pyramidal tract involvement: (1) the finger-escape sign—when the patient attempts to extend the digits fully with the palm facing down, the ulnar two or three digits tend to drift into abduction and flexion after 30 seconds' duration; and (2) the grip-and-release test—a decreased ability to open and close the fist rapidly because of weakness and spasticity. Normal is greater than 20 grip-and-release movements in 10 seconds. To distinguish between upper motor neuron signs arising from brain pathology versus signs arising from cervical cord pathology, a jaw jerk test may be performed. Closing of the mouth (upward jerking of the mandible) caused by tapping of the lower jaw at a downward angle with the mouth held slightly open constitutes a positive jaw jerk test. This response signifies that the origin of the upper motor neuron findings may be higher up in the brain rather than in the spinal canal and specifically tests cranial nerve V.[82]

Many neurologic conditions resemble cervical spondylotic myelopathy. Multiple sclerosis has distinctive plaques that can be seen on magnetic resonance imaging (MRI) of the brain and spinal cord. The disease is a demyelinating disorder of the central nervous system and causes motor and sensory symptoms but typically has remissions and exacerbations and involvement of the cranial nerves. Amyotrophic lateral sclerosis results in upper and lower motor neuron symptoms, without alteration in sensation. Subacute combined degeneration seen with vitamin B_{12} deficiency causes corticospinal tract and posterior tract symptoms, with greater sensory involvement in the lower extremities. Patients with metabolic or idiopathic peripheral neuropathy have sensory symptoms that may mirror symptoms of myelopathy (Table 36–3).

TABLE 36–3 Differential Diagnoses of Cervical Spondylotic Myelopathy

Peripheral polyneuropathy
Motor neuron disease
Multiple sclerosis
Cerebrovascular disease
Syringomyelia

From Rao R: Neck pain, cervical radiculopathy, and cervical myelopathy: Pathophysiology, natural history and clinical evaluation. J Bone Joint Surg Am 84:1872-1881, 2002.

Summary

Degenerative changes of the cervical spine represent a natural consequence of aging, are ubiquitous in the adult population, and remain asymptomatic in most of the population. When symptoms do arise, clinical syndromes are best grouped into axial neck pain, radiculopathy, and myelopathy, or some combination of these groups. An understanding of the pathophysiology and natural history of these conditions allows the clinician to determine whether cervical spinal pathology is the source of the patient's symptoms and, in many cases, allows localization of the pathology to a specific level within the neck. The natural history suggests that the best treatment, in general, for patients with axial symptoms consists of nonsurgical interventions, whereas some patients with radiculopathy continue to experience disabling pain and may be candidates for surgery. Surgical decompression and stabilization should be considered in patients who continue to have symptoms despite appropriate treatment. Patients with clinically evident myelopathy may be candidates for operative intervention.

PEARLS

1. Axial neck pain is of muscular origin in most patients. In some patients with intractable axial pain, the disc and facet joints may play a role.

2. Radiculopathy is the end result of an inflammatory process within or around the nerve root as a result of mechanical pressure on or chemical irritation of the nerve root.

3. Cervical spondylotic myelopathy occurs as the result of mechanical compression of the spinal cord and is likely augmented by dynamic, congenital, and vascular factors.

PITFALLS

1. Axial neck pain may occasionally be a manifestation of upper cervical radiculopathy.

2. Peripheral nerve entrapment or shoulder pathology may mimic cervical radiculopathy.

3. The presentation of patients with myelopathy may be subtle, with findings in many patients assumed to be the result of old age. Reflexes may be diminished or absent in patients with myelopathy and concomitant peripheral nerve disease or lumbar spinal stenosis.

KEY POINTS

1. Degenerative changes of the cervical spine are generally asymptomatic but can manifest as three main symptom complexes—axial neck pain, upper extremity radiculopathy, or myelopathy—or some combination thereof.

2. Most patients who present early with a single episode of axial neck pain may be reassured that their symptoms will resolve spontaneously; the prognosis in patients who present with a longer duration of symptoms to a tertiary care facility is more guarded.

3. Shoulder joint pathology can mimic or coexist with cervical radiculopathy; the shoulder joint must be carefully evaluated in all patients with suspected cervical radiculopathy.

4. Severe spinal cord compression results in pathologic changes within the spinal cord. Irreversibility of these changes may explain why some patients fail to recover after decompressive surgery.

5. Long tract neurologic findings in cervical spondylotic myelopathy may be masked by concurrent conditions, such as peripheral neuropathy or lumbar spinal stenosis.

KEY REFERENCES

1. Bogduk N, Windsor M, Inglis A: The innervation of the cervical intervertebral discs. Spine (Phila Pa 1976) 13:2-8, 1988.
   This article addresses microdissection and histologic study of cervical intervertebral disc innervation.

2. Cornefjord M, Olmarker K, Farley DB, et al: Neuropeptide changes in compressed spinal nerve roots. Spine (Phila Pa 1976) 20:670-673, 1995.
   This article presents experimental evidence of pain peptide production in nerve root and dorsal root ganglion after compression of the nerve root.

3. Gore DR, Sepic SB, Gardner GM, et al: Neck pain: A long-term follow-up of 205 patients. Spine (Phila Pa 1976) 12:1-5, 1987.
   A 10-year follow-up of patients with neck pain and radiculopathy showed that two thirds of the patients had a favorable result; one third had pain that interfered with their lifestyle.

4. Lees F, Turner JW: Natural history and prognosis of cervical spondylosis. BMJ 2:1607-1610, 1963.
   This article discusses long-term prognosis of cervical spondylosis in two groups of patients: myelopathic and nonmyelopathic.

5. Rao R: Neck pain, cervical radiculopathy, and cervical myelopathy: Pathophysiology, natural history, and clinical evaluation. J Bone Joint Surg Am 84:1872-1881, 2002.
   This is a review of the pathophysiology, natural history, and clinical features of axial neck pain, cervical radiculopathy, and cervical myelopathy.

REFERENCES

1. Roh JS, Teng AL, Yoo JU, et al: Degenerative disorders of the lumbar and cervical spine. Orthop Clin North Am 36:255-262, 2005.

2. Truumees E, Herkowitz HN: Cervical spondylotic myelopathy and radiculopathy. Instr Course Lect 49:339-360, 2000.

3. Geck MJ, Eismont FJ: Surgical options for the treatment of cervical spondylotic myelopathy. Orthop Clin North Am 33:329-348, 2002.

4. Shedid D, Benzel EC: Cervical spondylosis anatomy: Pathophysiology and biomechanics. Neurosurgery 60:S7-S13, 2007.

5. Rao R: Neck pain, cervical radiculopathy, and cervical myelopathy: Pathophysiology, natural history, and clinical evaluation. J Bone Joint Surg Am 84:1872-1881, 2002.

6. Lestini WF, Wiesel SW: The pathogenesis of cervical spondylosis. Clin Orthop Relat Res 69-93, 1989.

7. Gore DR, Sepic SB, Gardner GM, et al: Neck pain: A long-term follow-up of 205 patients. Spine (Phila Pa 1976) 12:1-5, 1987.

8. Wieser ES, Wang JC: Surgery for neck pain. Neurosurgery 60:S51-S56, 2007.

9. Bengtsson A, Henriksson KG, Larsson J: Reduced high-energy phosphate levels in the painful muscles of patients with primary fibromyalgia. Arthritis Rheum 29:817-821, 1986.

10. Bogduk N, Windsor M, Inglis A: The innervation of the cervical intervertebral discs. Spine (Phila Pa 1976) 13:2-8, 1988.

11. Bogduk N, Marsland A: The cervical zygapophysial joints as a source of neck pain. Spine (Phila Pa 1976) 13:610-617, 1988.

12. Dwyer A, Aprill C, Bogduk N: Cervical zygapophyseal joint pain patterns. I: A study in normal volunteers. Spine (Phila Pa 1976) 15:453-457, 1990.

13. Aprill C, Dwyer A, Bogduk N: Cervical zygapophyseal joint pain patterns. II: A clinical evaluation. Spine (Phila Pa 1976) 15:458-461, 1990.

14. Grubb SA, Kelly CK: Cervical discography: Clinical implications from 12 years of experience. Spine (Phila Pa 1976) 25:1382-1389, 2000.

15. McLain RF: Mechanoreceptor endings in human cervical facet joints. Spine (Phila Pa 1976) 19:495-501, 1994.

16. Dreyfuss P, Michaelsen M, Fletcher D: Atlanto-occipital and lateral atlanto-axial joint pain patterns. Spine (Phila Pa 1976) 19:1125-1131, 1994.

36 Cervical Spondylosis: Pathophysiology, Natural History, and Clinical Syndromes of Neck Pain, Radiculopathy, and Myelopathy   695

SECTION

VI

17. Wächli B, Dvorak J, Grob D: Cervical spine disorders and headaches. Twenty-First Annual Meeting of the Cervical Spine Research Society, New York, December 1, 1993.

18. Persson LC, Carlsson JY, Anderberg L: Headache in patients with cervical radiculopathy: A prospective study with selective nerve root blocks in 275 patients. Eur Spine J 16:953-959, 2007.

19. Manifold SG, McCann PD: Cervical radiculitis and shoulder disorders. Clin Orthop Relat Res (368):105-113, 1999.

20. Cooper RG, Freemont AJ, Hoyland JA, et al: Herniated intervertebral disc-associated periradicular fibrosis and vascular abnormalities occur without inflammatory cell infiltration. Spine (Phila Pa 1976) 20:591-598, 1995.

21. Chabot RG, Montgomery DM: The pathophysiology of axial and radicular neck pain. Semin Spine Surg 2-8, 1995.

22. Cornefjord M, Olmarker K, Farley DB, et al: Neuropeptide changes in compressed spinal nerve roots. Spine (Phila Pa 1976) 20:670-673, 1995.

23. Muhle C, Resnick D, Ahn JM, et al: In vivo changes in the neuroforaminal size at flexion-extension and axial rotation of the cervical spine in healthy persons examined using kinematic magnetic resonance imaging. Spine (Phila Pa 1976) 26:E287-E293, 2001.

24. Davidson RI, Dunn EJ, Metzmaker JN: The shoulder abduction test in the diagnosis of radicular pain in cervical extradural compressive monoradiculopathies. Spine (Phila Pa 1976) 6:441-446, 1981.

25. Farmer JC, Wisneski RJ: Cervical spine nerve root compression: An analysis of neuroforaminal pressures with varying head and arm positions. Spine (Phila Pa 1976) 19:1850-1855, 1994.

26. Anderberg L, Annertz M, Rydholm U, et al: Selective diagnostic nerve root block for the evaluation of radicular pain in the multilevel degenerated cervical spine. Eur Spine J 15:794-801, 2006.

27. Tanaka N, Fujimoto Y, An HS, et al: The anatomic relation among the nerve roots, intervertebral foramina, and intervertebral discs of the cervical spine. Spine (Phila Pa 1976) 25:286-291, 2000.

28. Rao RD, Gourab K, David KS: Operative treatment of cervical spondylotic myelopathy. J Bone Joint Surg Am 88:1619-1640, 2006.

29. Henderson CM, Hennessy RG, Shuey HM Jr, et al: Posterior-lateral foraminotomy as an exclusive operative technique for cervical radiculopathy: A review of 846 consecutively operated cases. Neurosurgery 13:504-512, 1983.

30. Bernhardt M, Hynes RA, Blume HW, et al: Cervical spondylotic myelopathy. J Bone Joint Surg Am 75:119-128, 1993.

31. Penning L, Wilmink JT, van Woerden HH, et al: CT myelographic findings in degenerative disorders of the cervical spine: Clinical significance. AJR Am J Roentgenol 146:793-801, 1986.

32. Houser OW, Onofrio BM, Miller GM, et al: Cervical spondylotic stenosis and myelopathy: Evaluation with computed tomographic myelography. Mayo Clin Proc 69:557-563, 1994.

33. Ono K, Ota H, Tada K, et al: Cervical myelopathy secondary to multiple spondylotic protrusions: A clinicopathologic study. Spine (Phila Pa 1976) 2:109-125, 1977.

34. Pavlov H, Torg JS, Robie B, et al: Cervical spinal stenosis: Determination with vertebral body ratio method. Radiology 164:771-775, 1987.

35. Murone I: The importance of the sagittal diameters of the cervical spinal canal in relation to spondylosis and myelopathy. J Bone Joint Surg Br 56:30-36, 1974.

36. Kawaguchi Y, Kanamori M, Ishihara H, et al: Pathomechanism of myelopathy and surgical results of laminoplasty in elderly patients with cervical spondylosis. Spine (Phila Pa 1976) 28:2209-2214, 2003.

37. Mihara H, Ohnari K, Hachiya M, et al: Cervical myelopathy caused by C3-C4 spondylosis in elderly patients: A radiographic analysis of pathogenesis. Spine (Phila Pa 1976) 25:796-800, 2000.

38. Kadanka Z, Kerkovsky M, Bednarik J, et al: Cross-sectional transverse area and hyperintensities on magnetic resonance imaging in relation to the clinical picture in cervical spondylotic myelopathy. Spine (Phila Pa 1976) 32:2573-2577, 2007.

39. Breig A, Turnbull I, Hassler O: Effects of mechanical stresses on the spinal cord in cervical spondylosis: A study on fresh cadaver material. J Neurosurg 25:45-56, 1966.

40. Henderson FC, Geddes JF, Vaccaro AR, et al: Stretch-associated injury in cervical spondylotic myelopathy: New concept and review. Neurosurgery 56:1101-1113, 2005.

41. Barre JA: Troubles pyramidaux et arthrite vertebrale chronique. Medecine 3:58-60, 1924.

42. Hukuda S, Wilson CB: Experimental cervical myelopathy: Effects of compression and ischemia on the canine cervical cord. J Neurosurg 37:631-652, 1972.

43. Gooding MR, Wilson CB, Hoff JT: Experimental cervical myelopathy: Effects of ischemia and compression of the canine cervical spinal cord. J Neurosurg 43:9-17, 1975.

44. Shimomura Y, Hukuda S, Mizuno S: Experimental study of ischemic damage to the cervical spinal cord. J Neurosurg 28:565-581, 1968.

45. Doppman JL: The mechanism of ischemia in anteroposterior compression of the spinal cord. Invest Radiol 10:543-551, 1975.

46. Baron EM, Young WF: Cervical spondylotic myelopathy: A brief review of its pathophysiology, clinical course, and diagnosis. Neurosurgery 60:S35-S41, 2007.

47. Baptiste DC, Fehlings MG: Pathophysiology of cervical myelopathy. Spine J 6:190S-197S, 2006.

48. Ogino H, Tada K, Okada K, et al: Canal diameter, anteroposterior compression ratio, and spondylotic myelopathy of the cervical spine. Spine (Phila Pa 1976) 8:1-15, 1983.

49. Cote P, Cassidy JD, Carroll L: The Saskatchewan health and back pain survey: The prevalence of neck pain and related disability in Saskatchewan adults. Spine (Phila Pa 1976) 23:1689-1698, 1998.

50. Lawrence JS: Disc degeneration: Its frequency and relationship to symptoms. Ann Rheum Dis 28:121-138, 1969.

51. Cote P, Cassidy JD, Carroll L: The factors associated with neck pain and its related disability in the Saskatchewan population. Spine (Phila Pa 1976) 25:1109-1117, 2000.

52. DePalma AF, Subin DK: Study of the cervical syndrome. Clin Orthop Relat Res 38:135-142, 1965.

53. Rothman RH, Rashbaum RF: Pathogenesis of signs and symptoms of cervical disc degeneration. Instr Course Lect 27:203-215, 1978.

54. Radhakrishnan K, Litchy WJ, O'Fallon WM, et al: Epidemiology of cervical radiculopathy: A population-based study from Rochester, Minnesota, 1976 through 1990. Brain 117:325-335, 1994.

55. Salemi G, Savettieri G, Meneghini F, et al: Prevalence of cervical spondylotic radiculopathy: A door-to-door survey in a Sicilian municipality. Acta Neurol Scand 93:184-188, 1996.

56. Honet JC, Puri K: Cervical radiculitis: Treatment and results in 82 patients. Arch Phys Med Rehabil 57:12-16, 1976.

57. Pain in the neck and arm: A multicentre trial of the effects of physiotherapy, arranged by the British Association of Physical Medicine. BMJ 1:253-258, 1966.

58. Martin GM, Corbin KB: An evaluation of conservative treatment for patients with cervical disk syndrome. Arch Phys Med Rehabil 87-92, 1954.

59. Rubin D: Cervical radiculitis: Diagnosis and treatment. Arch Phys Med Rehabil 41:580-586, 1960.

60. Lees F, Turner JW: Natural history and prognosis of cervical spondylosis. BMJ 2:1607-1610, 1963.

61. Rowland LP: Surgical treatment of cervical spondylotic myelopathy: Time for a controlled trial. Neurology 42:5-13, 1992.

62. Clarke E, Robinson PK: Cervical myelopathy: A complication of cervical spondylosis. Brain 79:483-510, 1956.

63. Nurick S: The natural history and the results of surgical treatment of the spinal cord disorder associated with cervical spondylosis. Brain 95:101-108, 1972.

64. Symon L, Lavender P: The surgical treatment of cervical spondylotic myelopathy. Neurology 17:117-127, 1967.

65. Travell JG, Simons DG: Myofascial Pain and Dysfunction: The Trigger Point Manual, vol 2. Baltimore, Williams & Wilkins, 1983.

66. An HS: Cervical root entrapment. Hand Clin 12:719-730, 1996.

67. Rhee JM, Yoon T, Riew KD: Cervical radiculopathy. J Am Acad Orthop Surg 15:486-494, 2007.

68. Massey EW, Riley TL, Pleet AB: Coexistent carpal tunnel syndrome and cervical radiculopathy (double crush syndrome). South Med J 74:957-959, 1981.

69. Cloward RB: Diaphragm paralysis from cervical disc lesions. Br J Neurosurg 2:395-399, 1988.

70. Buszek MC, Szymke TE, Honet JC, et al: Hemidiaphragmatic paralysis: An unusual complication of cervical spondylosis. Arch Phys Med Rehabil 64:601-603, 1983.

71. Malagori K, Fraser RG: The Thorax: Disease. 2nd ed. New York, Marcel Dekker, 1995.

72. LaBan MM, Meerschaert JR, Taylor RS: Breast pain: A symptom of cervical radiculopathy. Arch Phys Med Rehabil 60:315-317, 1979.

73. Crandall PH, Batzdorf U: Cervical spondylotic myelopathy. J Neurosurg 25:57-66, 1966.

74. Ferguson RJ, Caplan LR: Cervical spondylotic myelopathy. Neurol Clin 3:373-382, 1985.

75. Emery SE: Cervical spondylotic myelopathy: Diagnosis and treatment. J Am Acad Orthop Surg 9:376-388, 2001.

76. Nurick S: The pathogenesis of the spinal cord disorder associated with cervical spondylosis. Brain 95:87-100, 1972.

77. Shimizu T, Shimada H, Shirakura K: Scapulohumeral reflex (Shimizu): Its clinical significance and testing maneuver. Spine (Phila Pa 1976) 18:2182-2190, 1993.

78. Edwards WC, LaRocca SH: The developmental segmental sagittal diameter in combined cervical and lumbar spondylosis. Spine (Phila Pa 1976) 10:42-49, 1985.

79. Good DC, Couch JR, Wacaser L: "Numb, clumsy hands" and high cervical spondylosis. Surg Neurol 22:285-291, 1984.

80. Ono K, Ebara S, Fuji T, et al: Myelopathy hand: New clinical signs of cervical cord damage. J Bone Joint Surg Br 69:215-219, 1987.

81. Ebara S, Yonenobu K, Fujiwara K, et al: Myelopathy hand characterized by muscle wasting: A different type of myelopathy hand in patients with cervical spondylosis. Spine (Phila Pa 1976) 13:785-791, 1988.

82. Rhee JM, Riew KD: Cervical spondylotic myelopathy: Including ossification of the posterior longitudinal ligament. In Spivak J (ed): Orthopaedic Knowledge Update Spine, 3rd ed. Rosemont, IL, American Academy of Orthopaedic Surgeons, 2006, pp 235-249.

37 CHAPTER

Medical Myelopathies

Joseph R. Berger, MD

Spinal cord disease may result from a variety of insults. A general classification of these various etiologies is provided in Table 37–1. This chapter addresses the "medical" causes of spinal cord dysfunction.

The nature of the history and the physical findings resulting from these myelopathies is very dependent on the rapidity of onset of the lesion and its specific location in the spinal cord, particularly with respect to the spinal tracts involved. Typically, the chief complaints of patients presenting with these forms of myelopathy are lower extremity weakness and gait disturbance. A sense of stiffness of the legs is common. If the cervical spinal cord is involved, upper extremity weakness is to be expected. Loss of dexterity in the fingers and hands is often perceived by the patient. Frequently, patients may complain of numbness and other sensory abnormalities.

If the illness involves the posterior columns in the cervical region, the patient may exhibit Lhermitte phenomenon, characterized by a sense of lightninglike, electric shocks that generally radiate down the spine and into the extremities on neck flexion. Variants of this phenomenon may occur, and other forms of head and neck movement may precipitate this fleeting discomfort. Spinal cord disease involving the posterior columns in the thoracic region may result in a disquieting bandlike or girdlelike sensation across the chest or abdomen. This phenomenon is a helpful localizing clue. Paresthesias of the distal extremities may also result from these lesions. Urinary urgency and frequency, incontinence of bladder and bowel, and sexual impotence are common.

Generally, but not invariably, a thorough neurologic examination allows the physician to distinguish spinal cord from other causes of these neurologic complaints. The presence of concomitant neurologic illness attributable to disease of the cerebral hemispheres or brainstem, such as hemianopsia, ophthalmoplegia, and dysarthria, does not rule out the possibility of concomitant spinal cord disease, but should suggest that the findings on neurologic examination may be ascribed to a single or multiple lesions higher in the neuraxis than the spinal cord. The physical examination of patients with spinal cord lesions that have developed gradually or who have acute lesions that have been present for several weeks typically reveals a spastic weakness of the involved extremities with associated hyperreflexia and pathologic reflexes. The latter include Hoffman sign (palmar flexion of the thumb when the distal phalanx of the middle finger of the same hand is rapidly tapped) in the upper extremities and Babinski sign (plantar extension of the hallux when the sole of the foot is stroked) in the lower extremities. Several variants of these signs have been described.[1] Superficial reflexes, such as abdominal and cremasteric reflexes, are absent.

In the early period of an acutely developing spinal cord lesion, "spinal shock" is typical, in which a flaccid weakness of the extremities predominates. Although this entity is more common with traumatic lesions of the spinal cord, it may result from infectious, vascular, or other insults to the spinal cord. The presence of a flaccid weakness with areflexia may lead to a false diagnosis of an acute peripheral neuropathy as may be observed with Guillain-Barré syndrome. A careful sensory examination is crucial to distinguish appropriately between these possibilities. A sensory level is to be expected with a spinal cord lesion, but is hardly an invariable finding. Guillain-Barré syndrome is predominantly a motor neuropathy, and when it results in sensory loss, a mild decrease in vibratory sensation in distal extremities is usually observed. Although more severe forms of sensory loss may be seen with this and other causes of peripheral neuropathy, a sensory level is not present.

The appearance of Brown-Séquard syndrome is pathognomonic of spinal cord disease. This syndrome results from an injury to one half of the spinal cord and is characterized by the presence of weakness and loss of position and vibratory sensory perception ipsilateral to the side of the lesion and loss of pinprick and temperature sensory perception on the side of the body contralateral to the lesion. Incomplete forms of Brown-Séquard syndrome are commonly observed.

Acute Idiopathic Transverse Myelitis and Multiple Sclerosis

Patients with acute idiopathic transverse myelitis most often present with paresthesias of the feet, toes, or fingertips.[2] Gradually developing numbness and coincident weakness of the

TABLE 37–1 Etiologies of Myelopathy

Congenital and developmental defects

Trauma

Compromise of spinal canal by degenerative spinal disease and disk herniation

Idiopathic acute or subacute transverse myelitis

Postinfectious and postvaccination myelitis

Multiple sclerosis

Adrenomyeloneuropathy

Infectious myelitis: Viral, bacterial, fungal, parasitic

Epidural abscesses

Arachnoiditis

Vascular disease of the spinal cord: Atherosclerotic, arteriovenous malformation, epidural hematoma

Connective tissue diseases

    Rheumatoid arthritis

    Sjögren syndrome

    Systemic lupus erythematosus

    Wegener disease

Ulcerative colitis

Sarcoid myelopathy

Paraneoplastic myelopathy

Metabolic and nutritional disease of the spinal cord: Vitamin B_{12} deficiency, chronic liver disease, hyperparathyroidism, hyperthyroidism

Toxins

Decompression illness

Electrical injury

Radiation therapy

Necrotic myelopathy of unknown etiology

Heredofamilial degenerations: Hereditary spastic paraplegia, Friedreich ataxia, others

legs follows with subsequent paralysis of the legs. The features of this illness usually evolve over 1 to 3 weeks, but they may develop abruptly. The initial symptoms may be predominantly unilateral, and asymmetrical findings are common. As the illness progresses, upper extremity numbness and weakness and bowel and bladder incontinence may ensue. In some patients, posterior column involvement (decreased vibration and position senses) is spared early but affected later. Occasionally, back (interscapular) pain and, more rarely, calf, arm, or radicular pain may accompany the progressive myelopathy suggesting other pathologic processes, such as an intraspinal neoplasm or epidural abscess. To be considered idiopathic, acute transverse myelitis should be unassociated with a known preceding or concomitant viral infection. The dominant pathologic feature of the spinal cord is demyelination.

Treatment with adrenocorticotropic hormone (ACTH) or corticosteroids has been advocated; the response to therapy may be highly variable, and some studies indicate no benefit.[3] A pilot study of high-dose methylprednisolone in children with acute transverse myelitis showed a significant shortening

of motor recovery compared with historical controls.[4] Approximately one third of patients have a return of a normal gait and bladder function.[2] When recovery to a normal or near-normal level of function occurs, it does so within 1 year of the onset of the illness. Of affected patients, 25% become wheelchair-bound or bedridden, and the remainder have varying degrees of lesser disability.[2]

In some instances, myelopathy develops abruptly. Frequently, a flaccid, areflexic paralysis of the affected limbs accompanies spinal shock. Loss of vision resulting from optic nerve inflammation may accompany this myelopathy. Devic disease (neuromyelitis optica [NMO]) refers to the combination of acute optic neuritis and transverse myelitis. Similar to the more slowly evolving idiopathic transverse myelitis, demyelination is a characteristic neuropathologic hallmark. The pathology has been described as a necrotizing hemorrhagic leukomyelitis. The prognosis of patients with this rapidly evolving myelopathy, particularly when it is accompanied by spinal shock, is worse than the prognosis for the more gradually developing transverse myelitis.[5]

The differential diagnosis of idiopathic transverse myelitis includes multiple sclerosis; infectious myelitis; postinfectious or postvaccination myelitis; and myelopathy associated with vasculitis and connective tissue diseases, such as Behçet disease, systemic lupus erythematosus (SLE), and Sjögren syndrome. Multiple sclerosis may initially manifest as a transverse myelitis; the likelihood of transverse myelitis being the presenting manifestation of multiple sclerosis was previously reported to be 5% to 15%.[2,5-7] Since the advent of more sensitive testing (magnetic resonance imaging [MRI]), this likelihood has been estimated at 42%.[8] If cranial MRI is highly suggestive of multiple sclerosis at the time of onset of myelitis, the risk of progression to clinically definite multiple sclerosis is 50% at 2 years, whereas if cranial MRI is negative, the risk is 5%.[9] A temporal association with a viral illness (Table 37–2), signs and symptoms that develop over a few days, and a monophasic course should suggest the possibility of a viral myelitis.[10]

Spinal cord disease is extremely common in the setting of multiple sclerosis and frequently is responsible for the associated extremity weakness, spasticity, gait abnormalities, and sphincter disturbances. Within 10 to 15 years of the onset of multiple sclerosis, more than 80% of patients exhibit extremity spasticity and weakness, and more than 50% have sphincter disturbances.[11,12] Lhermitte sign has been reported in 38% of patients with clinically definite multiple sclerosis.[13] Approximately 10% of patients with multiple sclerosis have a primary progressive form of the disease. This disorder often affects the spinal cord predominantly and most commonly develops in women older than 40 years.

NMO has been regarded as a variant of multiple sclerosis; however, the occurrence of a unique IgG antibody to the aquaporin-4 channel (NMO-IgG)[14] suggests it is a distinct disorder. NMO may occur as an isolated condition or, more commonly, as recurrent spells of optic neuritis and myelitis. In contrast to the myelitis of multiple sclerosis, which seldom extends beyond two or three segments, the myelitis of NMO is often longitudinally extensive. Optic neuritis or myelitis in isolation may occur with NMO. Treatment recommendations[15] include high-dose intravenous methylprednisolone; plasma exchange; intravenous immunoglobulin; and rituximab, an anti-CD20 antibody directed against B cells.

The diagnostic approach to a patient suspected to have an acute transverse myelitis should begin with a thorough history and physical examination. Evidence of a recent viral illness should be sought. A history of syphilis, connective tissue diseases, or prior neurologic illness may prove essential in arriving at the correct diagnosis. Serologic studies should always include a serum Venereal Disease Research Laboratory (VDRL) test and fluorescent treponemal antibody absorption for syphilis.

MRI of the involved area of the spinal cord is the best radiographic study. MRI may be normal or reveal cord swelling or hyperintense lesions or both on T2-weighted imaging intrinsic to the spinal cord. Miller and colleagues[16] found MRI lesions at the clinically expected level in 64% of patients with a clinical syndrome suggestive of cervical involvement but in only 28% with a suspected thoracic or lumbar lesion. In patients with multiple sclerosis, most lesions are observed in the cervical spinal cord at autopsy and by MRI.[17,18] Lesions on MRI are characteristically T2-weighted hyperintense signal abnormalities, generally less than 10 to 15 mm in length,[18] and multiple, gapped lesions may be observed. Gadolinium enhancement with active disease is often observed.[19] Generally, MRI, if available, negates the need of myelography. If MRI is unavailable, myelography should be performed with water-soluble contrast medium and computed tomography (CT) scan of the affected area. If pain is a significant component of the patient's illness, a CT scan of the appropriate area and a bone scan may be desirable in eliminating the possibility of an epidural abscess or neoplasm.

Cerebrospinal fluid (CSF) examination typically reveals mononuclear pleocytosis, often with 100 to 200 cells, and increased protein. With necrotizing myelopathy, the spinal cord may swell sufficiently to result in a spinal block with an abnormal Queckenstedt test and an extremely high CSF protein (Froin reaction). CSF VDRL, immunoglobulins, basic myelin protein, and viral cultures should be performed.

Somatosensory evoked potentials can be very helpful in ruling in suspected cord lesions. The presence of abnormalities on brainstem auditory evoked potential and visual evoked potential testing would raise the suspicion of multifocal disease (i.e. multiple sclerosis). Absent F waves on nerve conduction testing can also support evidence of a cord lesion.[20]

Adrenomyeloneuropathy

Adrenomyeloneuropathy is a phenotypic variant of the genetic disorder adrenoleukodystrophy, in which myelin sheath abnormalities of the white matter are associated with adrenal insufficiency. Although adrenoleukodystrophy is a sex-linked disorder, it has variable expressions, including mild disease in heterozygous women. Pathologically, the white matter abnormality appears to be a diffuse myelinoclastic sclerosis, but it may occasionally appear as a dysmyelinating condition. The

TABLE 37–2 Viral Etiologies of Myelitis

RNA Viruses	DNA Viruses
Nonenveloped	
Picornaviruses	Hepatitis B
Coxsackieviruses	
Echoviruses	
Polioviruses	
Other enteroviruses	
Hepatitis A	
Encephalomyocarditis virus	
Enveloped	
Togaviruses	Herpesviruses
Arbovirus	Herpes simplex
Rubella	Varicella-zoster
Tick-borne encephalitis virus	Epstein-Barr virus
Retroviruses	Cytomegalovirus
Human immunodeficiency virus type 1	Herpes simiae
Human T-cell lymphotropic virus type I	Poxviruses
Orthomyxoviruses	Vaccinia
Influenza	Variola
Paramyxoviruses	
Measles	
Mumps	
Bunyaviruses	
California encephalitis virus	
Arenavirus	
Lymphocytic choriomeningitis	
Rhabdovirus	
Rabies	

Adapted from Tyler KL, Gross RA, Cascino GD: Unusual viral causes of transverse myelitis: Hepatitis A virus and cytomegalovirus. Neurology 36:855-858, 1986.

neurologic variants are explained by the degree of involvement of brain, spinal cord, and peripheral nerve. Biorefringent material in the adrenal glands and brain observed histopathologically have been shown by sequential extraction methods to be cholesterol esters with high quantities of very long chain fatty acids. Measuring fatty acids in cultured skin fibroblasts from affected individuals, Moser and colleagues[21] showed abnormally large amounts of very long chain fatty acids (C_{24}-C_{30}) and a high ratio of C_{26} to C_{22} fatty acids. The latter has become the preferred method of diagnosing the disorder.

In patients with the spinal-neuropathic form of this disorder, adrenal insufficiency is usually present since early childhood, and a progressive spastic paraparesis and relatively mild peripheral neuropathy develop in the 3rd decade.[22] Other variants affecting the spinal cord have been observed, including a progressive myelopathy in men, a mild spastic paraparesis in women, and combined cerebral and spinal involvement in children and young men. A positive family history is present in approximately 50% of affected individuals. The presence of Addison disease also provides a strong clue to the diagnosis.

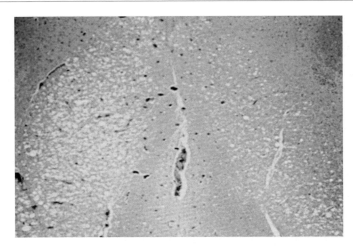

FIGURE 37–1 Microvacuolization of posterior columns of thoracic spinal cord in a patient with HIV-1–related myelopathy.

Addison disease, which is caused by primary adrenal failure, is often accompanied by bronzing of the skin because of excessive secretion of melanocyte-stimulating hormone in association with ACTH.

Infectious Myelopathies

Viral Myelitis

Human Immunodeficiency Virus Infection

Neurologic complications develop in 40% to 60%[23-25] of all patients with acquired immunodeficiency syndrome (AIDS), and neurologic disease heralds human immunodeficiency virus (HIV) infection in 10%[26] to 20%[25] of HIV-infected patients. In retrospective clinical series, spinal cord disease occurring in association with AIDS has been infrequently observed. Levy and colleagues[24] found viral myelitis in 3 of 128 AIDS patients with neurologic symptoms, and the collective incidence of viral myelitis in AIDS was 1% when data were pooled from three different hospital series of neurologic complications of AIDS.[27] The most common form of myelopathy observed with HIV infection has been a unique degeneration of the spinal cord first described by Petito and colleagues.[28] In pathologic series, spinal cord degeneration has been observed in 11%[29] to 22%[28] of unselected cases. These pathologic series suggest that spinal cord disease occurring in association with HIV infection is common but clinically underrecognized.

The prototypic myelopathy observed with HIV infection is a unique degeneration of the spinal cord.[28,30] Petito and colleagues[28] observed this myelopathy in 20 of 89 consecutive autopsies of AIDS patients. Although the clinical presentation of this myelopathy may overlap with the presentation of other myelopathies associated with HIV-1 infection, the pathologic appearance is quite distinct. Clinically, patients complain of leg weakness, unsteadiness, and gait impairment. Incontinence of bladder and bowel often supervenes. In one study, incontinence was observed in 60% of patients.[28] Patients with this disorder often complain of paresthesias and vague discomfort in their legs. Frequently, these complaints are attributed to the general debilitation of the patient, and the true nature of the illness remains undiagnosed until pathologic examination of the spinal cord at the time of autopsy.

On physical examination, a spastic paraparesis is detected with the degree of weakness exceeding the degree of spasticity. Rarely, marked asymmetry of the leg weakness, a monoparesis, or quadriparesis may be found. Gait ataxia is seen, and the heel-to-knee-to-toe test may reveal dysmetria and dyssynergy. Occasionally, weakness is slight or absent on confrontation testing, but hyperreflexia of the lower extremities and extensor plantar responses are noted. Muscle stretch reflexes may also be diminished or absent in this disorder, however, as a result of concomitant peripheral neuropathy. Sensory examination reveals that vibratory and position sense are disproportionately affected compared with pinprick, temperature, or light touch. A significant impairment of the latter modalities suggests the presence of a concomitant peripheral neuropathy. Electrophysiologic studies may reveal a prolonged latency of cortical evoked responses after tibial nerve stimulation. Typically, this myelopathy is seen late in the course of HIV-1 infection; however, it has been described as the presenting manifestation of infection.[31]

Gross examination of the spinal cord and dura is generally normal in HIV-associated myelopathy except when the myelopathy is particularly severe.[28] The striking finding on histologic examination is the loss of myelin and spongy degeneration. The lateral and posterior columns are more severely affected than the anterior columns. Microvacuolization of the white matter of the spinal cord (Fig. 37–1) associated with lipid-laden macrophages bears an uncanny resemblance to the pathology of subacute combined degeneration of the spinal cord. The vacuolization seems to result from intramyelin swelling. Axons are preserved except in areas of marked vacuolization. Microglial nodules may be detected in the spinal cord gray matter, and 20% of the patients in one series also exhibited central chromatolysis of the anterior horn motor cells.[28] Inflammation and intranuclear viral inclusions are generally not seen.

Although HIV has been cultured from the spinal cord, the specific role of HIV in the causation of this illness is uncertain. A similar clinicopathologic condition has been observed in patients with cancer or other immunosuppressive conditions in the absence of HIV infection.[32] The spinal cord pathology is most prominent in the middle and lower thoracic regions. The cord involvement may be asymmetrical and does not seem to be confined to particular tracts.[28] Goldstick and colleagues[30] described involvement of the posterior columns increasing in intensity with rostral progression, whereas pyramidal tract involvement increased caudally. Petito and colleagues[28] were able to correlate the frequency and severity of symptoms to the degree of spinal cord pathology in their series. A potential role of nutritional deficiency as the cause of spinal cord pathology has been suggested.[33] Vacuolar myelopathy is not observed in young children with AIDS; however, pathologic abnormalities of the spinal cord are frequently seen at autopsy.[34] A loss of myelin and axons in the corticospinal tracts seems to be the most common abnormality.

The diagnosis of this illness is one of exclusion. Numerous other myelopathies have been observed in association with HIV infection. An acute myelopathy of uncertain pathogenesis has been noted at the time of seroconversion.[35] Table 37–3 lists other etiologies of spinal cord disease occurring in association with HIV.

The most useful study is MRI of the spinal cord. The author's practice has been generally to forego myelography if MRI of the spinal cord reveals no evidence of mass lesion. The presence of unusual features, such as back pain or radicular findings may dictate a more aggressive diagnostic approach. If MRI is negative, the CSF is examined for the presence of HIV and other pathogens. CSF examination includes viral cultures with specific emphasis on cytomegalovirus and herpes simplex virus (HSV) type 1 and HSV-2. Additionally, routine bacterial and fungal cultures and cryptococcal antigen are obtained. No treatment is known to be effective for this condition, although an aggressive antiretroviral therapy regimen should be tried.

Human T-Cell Lymphotropic Virus Type I

Although thought to be rare in the United States, human T-cell lymphotropic virus type I (HTLV-I) has been observed with increasing frequency in certain subpopulations. A study of volunteer blood donors by the American Red Cross revealed a seropositivity rate of 0.025% among volunteer blood donors.[36] Intravenous drug abusers seem to be at particularly high risk for infection with HTLV-I. Seroprevalence rates in this population range from 7% to 49%.[37,38] In a study of the seroprevalence among female prostitutes in eight areas of the United States, 6.7% were seropositive for HTLV-I and HTLV-II with prevalence rates ranging from 0% in southern Nevada to 25.4% in Newark, New Jersey.[39] A case of transmission of HTLV-I by blood transfusion associated with myelopathy has been confirmed.[40] In 10 native-born cases in the United States, 5 had received blood transfusions, and 6 had multiple sex partners (including one who frequented prostitution and had a history of drug abuse).[41]

In addition to being associated with adult T-cell leukemia/lymphoma, HTLV-I is associated with a chronic progressive myelopathy.[42,43] An association between the presence of seropositivity for HTLV-I and multiple sclerosis has also been suggested,[44] but this remains controversial.

The myelopathy that occurs with HTLV-I has been referred to as *tropical spastic paraparesis* (TSP) or *HTLV-I associated myelopathy* (HAM). This myelopathy is characterized on neuropathologic studies by chronic involvement of the pyramidal tracts chiefly at the thoracic level resulting in spastic lower extremity weakness and a spastic bladder. Paresthesias, pain, and sensory disturbances may also be observed. It is estimated that 1 in 250 individuals infected with HTLV-I develop this progressive myelopathy.[45] The major pathologic features of HTLV-I myelopathy are long tract degeneration and demyelination affecting the pyramidal, spinocerebellar, and spinothalamic tracts associated with hyalinoid thickening of the media and adventitia of blood vessels in the brain, spinal cord, and subarachnoid space with perivascular cuffing with leukocytes, astrocytic gliosis, and foamy macrophages.[46] These lesions may extend from the upper cervical cord to the lumbar regions. Vacuolization may be observed at the periphery of the lesions.

HTLV-II, a related type C retrovirus in the Oncoviridae subfamily also rarely may result in a myelopathy similar to HAM or TSP.[47-53] The epidemiology of this virus is different from HTLV-I because the populations principally affected are American Indians and intravenous drug abusers.[54] The mode of transmission parallels that of HTLV-I and HIV. The rarity of these neurologic disorders accompanying HTLV-II has precluded meaningful analysis of treatment options. The same therapies employed in HAM or TSP have been generally recommended, however.

Enteroviruses

Enteroviruses, particularly poliovirus, can affect the spinal cord. Effective vaccination has made this illness very rare in the Western world. In the United States in the recent past, there were approximately 10 to 15 cases of polio reported yearly; most of these were vaccine associated, although several were imported by immigrants. Paralytic poliomyelitis is a rare complication of poliovirus infection (1% to 2%); most infections

TABLE 37–3 Potential Etiologies of the Myelopathies Associated with Human Immunodeficiency Virus (HIV) Infection

Infectious

Viral

HIV

Acute transient myelopathy occurring at the time of seroconversion[35]

Chronic progressive myelopathy (vacuolar)[28]

Human T-cell lymphotropic virus type I[220,221]

Cytomegalovirus[222]

Herpes simplex[223]

Herpes zoster[224]

Bacterial

Epidural abscess

Mycobacterium tuberculosis[225,226]

Treponema pallidum[227]

Fungal

Cryptococcus neoformans

Others

Parasites

*Toxoplasma gondii*228

Noninfectious Etiologies

Multiple sclerosis–like illness[229]

Tumors[230]

   Plasmacytoma

   Spinal cord astrocytomas

   Others

Epidural hemorrhage secondary to thrombocytopenia

Vascular injury secondary to vasculitis

result in inapparent infection (90% to 95%) or a minor illness with mild systemic symptoms (5% to 10%). The poliovirus has a unique predilection to affect the anterior horn cells of the spinal cord and results in a lower motor neuron type of weakness; this is characterized by a flaccid weakness with wasting, fasciculations, and areflexia. Sensory and sphincter functions are spared. After infection, weakness may arise rapidly over 48 hours or occur in a delayed fashion over weeks. The risk of paralysis increases with age: Infants are rarely paralyzed, adults are paralyzed much more frequently, and risks for children are in between. Other enteroviruses, including coxsackieviruses and echoviruses, may also result in myelitis.

Herpesviruses

Varicella-zoster virus (VZV) is responsible for varicella (chickenpox) and causes shingles in adults. The virus remains latent within the dorsal root ganglia and spreads centrifugally along the corresponding nerves after reactivation resulting in a severely painful, blistering dermatomal eruption. Rarely, when the thoracic dermatomes are involved, the virus may spread centripetally and result in a necrotizing myelopathy.[55] The myelitis complicating VZV infection in immunocompetent individuals typically occurs 1 to 2 weeks after the appearance of the dermatomal rash, although VZV myelitis may develop in the absence of a rash. The myelitis occurs at the level of the affected dermatome and results in paraparesis. In immunosuppressed hosts, such as AIDS patients, VZV myelopathy occurs insidiously and progresses. The disease is suspected by the close temporal relationship to the rash and is confirmed by showing the presence of VZV DNA by polymerase chain reaction in the CSF or VZV antibody in the CSF. Treatment with intravenous acyclovir (10 mg/kg every 8 hours) should be initiated.

Rarely, and usually with primary infection, HSV-2, the etiology of genital herpes, may cause a sacral radiculitis[56] or an ascending myelitis.[57] These neurologic complications are rarely observed with recurrent HSV-2. Epstein-Barr virus,[58,59]

TABLE 37–4 Syphilis of the Spinal Cord

A. Syphilitic meningomyelitis

B. Syphilitic spinal pachymeningitis

   1. Spinal cord gumma

   2. Syphilitic hypertrophic pachymeningitis

C. Spinal vascular syphilis

D. Syphilitic poliomyelitis

E. Tabes dorsalis

F. Miscellaneous

   1. Syringomyelia

   2. Syphilitic aortic aneurysm

   3. Syphilitic vertebral osteitis

   4. Charcot vertebrae

Adapted from Adams R, Merritt H: Meningeal and vascular diseases of the spinal cord. Medicine 23:181, 1944.

the etiologic agent of infectious mononucleosis, and cytomegalovirus[60] may also result in a transverse myelitis at the time of primary infection. In an immunocompromised host, HSV-1, HSV-2, and cytomegalovirus may result in myelitis.

Other Viruses

Many other viruses have been associated with transverse myelitis (see Table 37–2). Of patients with transverse myelitis, 20% to 40% have evidence of preceding or concurrent viral infection.[2,5,7,61,62] Prompted by the increasing availability and efficacy of antiviral therapy and improved diagnostic techniques, in particular, polymerase chain reaction, these percentages are likely to increase.

Myelopathies Resulting from Bacterial Disease

Syphilis

Invasion of the central nervous system (CNS) by *Treponema pallidum* generally occurs within 1 year of syphilitic infection. Abnormal CSF results have been found with an incidence ranging from 13.9% to 70% in untreated patients with primary or secondary syphilis. Although CNS symptoms are infrequent at this stage of the infection, headache and meningismus can be observed during secondary syphilis, and acute meningitis complicates 1% to 2% of secondary syphilis. If left untreated, about 5% of patients with syphilis develop clinical neurosyphilis.

The spinal cord is not immune to the ravages of syphilis. Before the development of effective antibiotics, it was believed that syphilis was the most frequent cause of spinal cord disease. Historically, tabes dorsalis has been the most frequent type with a frequency that was estimated to be 10 times that of other forms of spinal syphilis. Syphilitic meningomyelitis and spinal vascular syphilis were the second and third most common forms of spinal syphilis. Spinal syphilis rarely occurs in the absence of syphilitic involvement at other sites of the neuraxis. It has been estimated that the incidence of pure spinal syphilis is approximately one fifth the incidence of cerebrospinal syphilis.

Syphilis may affect the spinal cord in various ways.[25] The pathology may be predominantly meningovascular or parenchymatous in nature. Gummas may grow within the substance of the cord or compress the cord by growth from the surrounding meninges. The clinical picture of spinal cord compression in syphilis may also arise as a result of hypertrophic pachymeningitis or vertebral lesions secondary to syphilitic osteitis. Table 37–4 presents a classification based on pathology and modified after the one proposed by Adams and Merritt.[63]

Tabes Dorsalis

Tabes dorsalis is the prototypic spinal cord disorder associated with syphilis. It is characterized by incoordination, pains, anesthesia, and various visceral trophic abnormalities.[64] The earliest recognized descriptions of this disorder date to the mid-18th century. By the turn of the 20th century, tabes dorsalis was recognized with increased frequency and, according to Erb, was unequaled in frequency or importance by any other chronic disease of the spinal cord.

Currently, tabes dorsalis probably accounts for no more than 5% of neurosyphilis. Approximately 65% of patients recall a prior history of venereal disease. The latency from infection to the development of tabes dorsalis averages 10 to 15 years, but it ranges from 2 to 38 years. The average age of onset is 40 years with most cases arising in the 4th and 5th decades. Tabes dorsalis is a rare complication of congenital syphilis. It exhibits an equal sex frequency, in contrast to tabes dorsalis occurring in adult syphilis, in which the incidence in men exceeds that in women by 10 : 1.

The clinical course of tabes dorsalis is typically divided into three separate phases. The initial phase is known as the *preataxic phase* or the "period of lightning pain." This phase is insidious in onset and may last months to decades, although it generally averages 3 years in duration. It is characterized by various subjective complaints, the most classic being the "crisis"—a severe lancinating pain. These lightning pains are absolutely characteristic of tabes dorsalis. They occur in 90% of individuals and are the presenting manifestation in 70%. Impotence and sphincter disturbances may also be early features. Physical examination reveals loss of muscle stretch reflexes, sensory loss, a positive Romberg sign, and Argyll Robertson pupils. Argyll Robertson pupils are characterized by intact visual acuity, decreased pupillary light reaction, intact near response, miosis, and irregular pupils. It occurs in classic form in 50% of patients with tabes dorsalis.

In early tabes dorsalis, the tactile sense may be well preserved, but the pain sense is invariably disturbed. Hypalgesia, hyperalgesia, allochiria, pallesthesia, delay in pain perception of 15 seconds after the application of the stimulus, and an aftersensation lasting 30 seconds all may be detected. Loss of deep pain sensation as evidenced by diminished sensation to the application of pressure to the ulnar nerve (Biernacki sign), the Achilles tendon (Abadie sign), and the testicle (Pitres sign) may occur in the absence of significant loss of superficial sensation.

The second phase of tabes is known as the *ataxic phase*. It has a variable duration from 2 to 10 years and is characterized by severe ataxia, affecting the legs chiefly. Generally, the tabetic pains worsen during this period. Arthropathy develops in 5% to 10% as a result of recurrent traumatic injury resulting from loss of deep pain sensation. Proprioceptive loss that results in a slapping gait predisposes the knee joint to this injury. The tarsal joints and hip, ankle, spine, and other joints can be similarly involved.

The third phase is known as the *terminal* or *paralytic phase*. This phase also has an average duration of 2 to 10 years. In this phase of the illness, cachexia, leg stiffness and paralysis, and autonomic dysfunction typified by obstinate constipation and bladder incontinence are prominent. Sepsis from decubitus ulcers and pyelonephritis is frequently the terminal event.

The classic signs of tabes dorsalis are absent in approximately 50% of patients in the early stages of the disease. The most frequently observed findings in these patients are absent ankle jerks and impaired vibratory sensation. In 10% of cases,

tabes dorsalis remains atypical throughout the course of the illness. Tabes dorsalis may also be associated with other complications of neurosyphilis, such as general paresis, syphilitic meningomyelitis, and spinal cord gummas.

The pathology of tabes dorsalis is characterized by changes in the posterior spinal roots and posterior spinal columns (Fig. 37–2). Shrinkage of the spinal cord may be apparent by gross inspection. Leptomeningitis is evidenced by round cell infiltration. The dorsal columns are demyelinated, particularly in the regions of the fasciculus gracilis, root entry zone, and Lissauer tract. Astrocytic proliferation in the posterior columns is accompanied by an increase in connective tissue and thickening of the blood vessel walls. The lower spinal cord bears the brunt of the damage. Nerve fibers in the posterior root are destroyed and replaced by fibrosis. Frequently, lesions

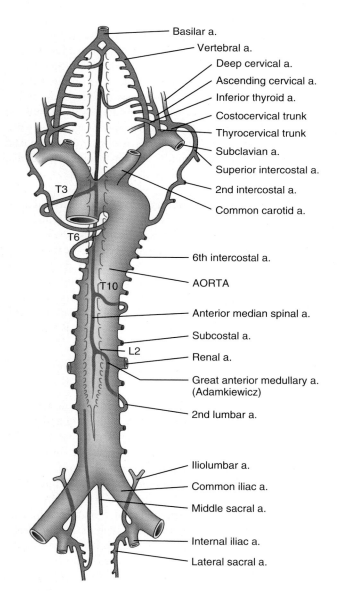

FIGURE 37–2 Representative cross section of lumbar vertebrae and spinal cord with its blood supply. (From Herrick M, Mills PE Jr: Infarction of spinal cord. Arch Neurol 24:228, 1971. Copyright 1971, American Medical Association.)

are observed in the anterior horns, cranial nerves, and brainstem.

Syphilitic Meningomyelitis

Syphilitic meningomyelitis occurs most commonly in individuals 25 to 40 years old, although it may arise in younger and older age groups. In most series, men predominate. The latency from the onset of the infection to the onset of symptoms with syphilitic meningomyelitis varies from 1 to 30 years with most arising within 6 years of infection.[65]

Typically, the patient initially notices a heavy sensation or weakness in the legs. Rarely, symptoms are confined to a single leg. Paresthesias and fleeting pain may accompany the motor disturbance. The onset is slow and gradual, and the symptoms are indistinguishable from symptoms of myelopathy associated with cervical spondylosis. Various subjective complaints have been recorded, including sensations of lower extremity numbness, cold, and tingling and girdle tightness, but objective sensory disturbances are slight. Autonomic dysfunction is also observed. It is generally characterized by precipitate frequency, hesitancy, and impotence. The predominant finding on neurologic examination is a spastic weakness in the extremities, especially the lower extremities. Muscle bulk is preserved, and the muscle stretch reflexes are exaggerated with positive Babinski signs. Sensory loss is slight. Occasionally, Brown-Séquard syndrome, significant amyotrophy, or a clinical picture of transverse myelitis may complicate syphilitic meningomyelitis.

Pathologic examination reveals thickened, inflamed meninges. The cervical region is believed to be the site at which the lesions predominate. The pathologic changes prevail in the periphery of the spinal cord, often with a symmetrical involvement of the lateral columns. The spinal cord dysfunction results from granulomatous invasion, inflammation, and vascular changes. The vascular changes are caused by Heubner and Nissl-Alzheimer endarteritis, lesions of medium and small vessels that are characterized by plasma cell and lymphocytic perivascular cuffing.

Other Forms of Spinal Syphilis

Hypertrophic pachymeningitis[66] is an insidious, slowly progressive syphilitic process that results in spinal root and spinal cord dysfunction. A rare but well-recognized complication of tertiary syphilis is a gumma of the spinal cord. The clinical features of a spinal gumma are indistinguishable from an intramedullary glioma if it arises within the cord or may simulate the appearance of an extramedullary tumor if it arises from the meninges and compresses the spinal cord. Spinal cord infarction is a well-recognized complication of syphilis. Another vascular complication of syphilis is aortitis, which may eventuate in an aortic aneurysm resulting rarely in myelopathy by erosion of the vertebrae and ultimately compression of the spinal cord. Progressive spinal muscular atrophy has been observed in association with neurosyphilis, although the relationship may be coincidental. Occasionally, syphilitic caries may affect the vertebrae, particularly vertebrae of the cervical spine, resulting in

pain, tenderness to palpation, and loss of mobility, and an abnormal spinal curvature in the involved area is noted. Radicular pains are observed in one third of patients. Compression of the spinal cord, although rare, has been reported.

As with other forms of neurosyphilis, the recommended treatment is 12 to 24 million U of aqueous penicillin daily in divided doses administered every 4 hours for 10 to 14 days.[67] Other treatment regimens[68] using doxycycline, ceftriaxone, or erythromycin may be considered if the patient cannot tolerate penicillin. These treatment regimens are not well established in treating symptomatic neurosyphilis, however.

Tuberculosis

Neurologic complications of *Mycobacterium tuberculosis* remain common in some parts of the world but are rare in the developed countries of the Western world. Myelopathy occurring in association with tuberculosis is usually the consequence of tuberculous spondylitis (Pott disease), which accounts for half of all skeletal tuberculosis. Typically, the anterior portion of the vertebral body is affected, with the mycobacterial spread to the vertebrae being hematogenous, lymphatic, or by direct contiguity from the lung.[69] The characteristic radiographic defect is anterior wedging of two adjacent vertebrae with loss of the intervening disk space. The spine is enveloped by pus extruding anteriorly from the affected vertebrae. Myelopathy typically results from pressure on the anterior spinal cord by caseous or granulating tissue, inflammatory thrombosis of the anterior spinal artery, or injury to the cord from spinal instability. The last-mentioned may lead to complete spinal cord transection.

Myelopathy occurring in association with tuberculous infection may also occur as a consequence of intraspinal granulomatous tissue unassociated with a bony lesion and intramedullary tuberculomas. In one study of spinal tuberculosis,[70] 54% of patients had neurologic deficit with bony tuberculous lesions, 39% had neurologic deficit with intraspinal granulomatous tissue occurring in the absence of bony lesions, and 7% had neurologic deficit from intraspinal tuberculomas.

Therapy of patients with spinal tuberculosis requires at least 12 months of antibiotic treatment and surgical decompression in the presence of neurologic abnormalities.[70] In the setting of intraspinal granulomatous disease without significant bony destruction, laminectomy and débridement is adequate[70]; however, more aggressive therapy is warranted when vertebral bodies are involved. A two-stage procedure comprising posterior instrumental stabilization followed by anterior radical decompression permitted earlier mobilization after neurologic recovery.[71] Reports of the frequency of neurologic recovery with spinal tuberculosis vary, but functional recovery rates of 90% have been reported.[71] Thoracic lesions with severe neurologic deficit show the least improvement, whereas lumbar disease has the best outcome.[72]

Other Forms of Bacterial Myelopathy

Numerous other bacterial infections have been associated with myelitis. Rarely, the spinal cord may be seeded by bacteria leading to a suppurative myelitis with abscess formation. In a review by Dutton and Alexander,[73] direct spread for adjacent infections was most commonly observed; however, hematogenous dissemination from endocarditis, pulmonary infections, and other sites was also frequently observed. Organisms isolated in these cases have included staphylococci, streptococci, *Escherichia coli,* and *Nocardia.* Rarely, Whipple disease can manifest as a myelopathy.[74,75]

More often, myelopathies associated with bacterial infection are parainfectious in nature, similar clinicopathologically to myelopathies occurring after viral infection or vaccination. Potential causes[76,77] include scarlet fever, pertussis, whooping cough, mycoplasmal pneumonia, and pneumococcal pneumonia. Myelitis resulting in Brown-Séquard syndrome has also been described with cat-scratch disease.[78] Lyme disease, the result of infection with *Borrelia burgdorferi,* a treponeme, may also result in myelopathy.[79]

Fungal Myelopathies

Fungal disease of the spinal cord is rare. Certain fungi (*Blastomyces, Coccidioides, Aspergillus*) may invade the spinal epidural space. Generally, the spinal cord is compromised by lesions arising from a vertebral osteomyelitic focus or by lesions extending through the intervertebral foramina. Certain fungi that result in granulomatous meningitis (e.g., *Cryptococcus neoformans*) may result in intraspinal or extradural granuloma. Alternatively, these organisms can lead to spinal cord infarction as a result of the associated meningovascular inflammation. Aspergillosis is generally observed only in immunosuppressed patients, with leukemia and lymphoma being common predisposing illnesses. Aspergillosis has been reported to affect the spinal cord in several different ways, including by compromise of the blood supply occurring in association with fungal endarteritis, by direct parenchymal infiltration of the spinal cord, or by cord compression from osteomyelitis and paravertebral mass.[80]

Parasitic Myelopathies

Among the most common parasites that result in spinal cord disease is *Schistosoma,*[81,82] in particular, *Schistosoma haematobium* and *Schistosoma mansoni.* These organisms are seen only in certain geographic regions—the Far East, South America, and Africa. A history of travel to these regions and swimming or bathing in water contaminated with the cercariae that are released from certain aquatic snails may suggest the diagnosis.

Hydatid disease resulting from the larval form of the canine tapeworm, *Echinococcus granulosa,* may result in spinal intramedullary cysts or compress the spinal cord and roots as a consequence of bone invasion. The bone invasion by hydatid disease generally occurs in the lower thoracic region.

Cysticercosis, a particularly common disease in Mexico and Central and South American countries, is the result of infection with the larval form of pork tapeworm, *Taenia solium.* Spinal cord involvement may complicate 5% of cases, although the brain is the preferred site in the CNS.

Cysticercosis most frequently infiltrates the subarachnoid space, but intramedullary fluid-filled cysts are also observed. A slowly progressive myelopathy implicating a lesion in the cervical or thoracic spinal cord is the typical mode of presentation for these lesions. Therapy with albendazole may be effective in eradicating the live parasite.

Paragonimiases, infection with a lung fluke acquired by eating undercooked freshwater crabs, occurs chiefly in China but may be seen in other parts of the world. Spinal cord disease results from extradural or, more rarely, intradural granuloma formation. *Angiostrongylus cantonensis,* the most common cause of eosinophilic meningitis and meningoencephalitis in the world, has also been reported to cause spinal cord disease.[83] In patients with AIDS, toxoplasmosis has been reported in rare instances to cause an abscess of the spinal cord.

Epidural Abscesses

Spinal epidural abscess may manifest as a surgical emergency evolving rapidly over several days or may arise more indolently. *Staphylococcus aureus* is the etiologic agent in greater than 50% of acute spinal epidural abscesses, although a broad spectrum of other organisms may be implicated.[84] The spread of infection may be directly from a focus of osteomyelitis or hematogenously from a distant site, such as skin furuncles or pulmonary infections. Trauma to the back, typically very minor in nature, has been reported by one third of individuals developing spinal epidural abscess.[85] A high degree of suspicion for spinal epidural abscess should be maintained when intravenous drug abusers present with fever and back pain.

Arachnoiditis

Invasion or irritation of the spinal subarachnoid space, as with cases of subarachnoid hemorrhage, meningitis, myelography, spinal or epidural anesthesia, or spinal surgery, can result in arachnoiditis. Arachnoidal inflammation leads to connective tissue proliferation and ultimately to arachnoid thickening, opacification, and adhesion and obliteration of the subarachnoid space. Generally, neurologic complications are the consequence of nerve root involvement; however, in the most severe cases, the nerve roots and the spinal cord may be compressed by bands of connective tissue or cystic loculations of CSF, resulting in myeloradiculopathy. Patients present most frequently with slowly progressive paraparesis, sensory loss, and sphincter dysfunction. Radicular pain of a severe, burning nature may also be present. The pain may not always follow a dermatomal distribution.[86] On examination, weakness, hyporeflexia and sensory deficits can be seen. Diagnosis is made by myelography or MRI. Although some patients, particularly patients with mass lesions resulting in cord compression and myelopathic symptoms, may respond to decompression, surgical exploration with resection of adhesions has not been proven to be beneficial in most patients.

Vascular Disease of the Spinal Cord

Paired segmental arteries arising from the aorta and branches of the subclavian and internal iliac arteries supply blood to the spinal cord (Fig. 37–3).[87] The most important vascular supply to the cervical spinal cord arises from the vertebral artery, which provides the cephalad origin of the anterior median and posterior lateral spinal arteries. The blood supply to the thoracic and lumbar spinal cord arises from the aorta and internal iliac arteries, and segmental branches of the lateral sacral arteries nourish the sacral spinal cord. The segmental branches that arise from the aorta divide into anterior and posterior rami. A branch of the posterior ramus (see Fig. 37–2), the spinal artery, enters the vertebral foramen and branches at irregular intervals into anterior and posterior medullary arteries, which feed the anterior median spinal artery and the posterior spinal arteries. At regular intervals, the spinal artery also branches into the anterior and posterior radicular arteries, which supply the spinal ganglia and roots.

The chief blood supply to the spinal cord comes from the 6 to 8 anterior and 10 or more posterior medullary arteries that arise from the spinal arteries. The most important anterior medullary artery is the artery of Adamkiewicz, which usually approaches the cord on the left side between the T10 and L3 cord segments. Because of the variability of the vascular anatomy of the spinal cord, however, it is impossible to predict the deficits that will occur after occlusion of a specific artery.

Although an anastomosing vascular network can be found over the surface of the spinal cord, the anterior median spinal artery is responsible for nourishing the anterior two thirds of the spinal cord. The territory in its distribution includes the anterior and lateral corticospinal tracts and the lateral spinothalamic tracts, whereas the posterior columns (fasciculus gracilis and cuneatus) are supplied by the posterior spinal arteries.

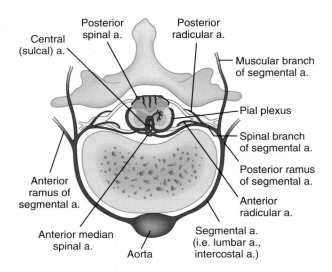

FIGURE 37–3 Anterior view of spinal cord with its segmental blood supply from aorta. (From Herrick M, Mills PE Jr: Infarction of spinal cord. Arch Neurol 24:228, 1971. Copyright 1971, American Medical Association.)

An occlusion of a dominant medullary artery or, more rarely, the anterior median spinal artery results in an ischemic softening of a variable portion of the anterior two thirds of the spinal cord. This entity is referred to as an *anterior spinal artery syndrome* and may arise as the consequence of thrombotic atherosclerotic disease, aortic dissection, embolization, or vasculitis (particularly polyarteritis nodosa) or as a complication of aortic angiography.[88] Cross clamping of the aorta during cardiac surgery for more than 30 minutes may also result in an infarction in this territory. A clinical hallmark of this entity is a dissociated sensory loss in which position and vibratory sensory perception are maintained, but a sensory level to pinprick is present. The latter is accompanied by paralysis below the level of the lesion, which typically manifests in association with spinal shock. Rarely, anastomotic blood flow allows for the preservation of the white matter of the spinal cord, and the gray matter alone is infarcted. Painful segmental spasm and spinal myoclonus may be observed with this condition.[10]

An unusual and seldom clinically diagnosed etiology of vascular injury to the spinal cord results from fibrocartilaginous embolization. The embolization typically follows minor trauma to the vertebrae.[89] Among the reported precipitants have been lifting heavy weights, prolonged coughing, stooping, or falling.[90] Valsalva maneuver has been suggested as a possible contributing factor resulting in the retrograde flow of fibrocartilaginous emboli to the spinal cord. Some investigators have suggested that the fibrocartilaginous debris is forced into the vessels of the spinal leptomeninges and spinal cord through the valveless Batson venous plexus.[91] Minor trauma to the vertebrae before onset was noted in most cases with the time to maximum neurologic deficit ranging from minutes to 24 to 48 hours.[89] Death typically supervenes within 11 months of onset (median 2.5 to 4 months).[89] Multiple emboli have been postulated to occur in some of these instances.[92] Involvement of the anterior spinal artery has also been observed.[93] Spinal MRI reveals characteristics indicative of vascular lesions.[92]

Hemorrhage may occur within the epidural or subdural space or directly into the spinal cord. Trauma, hemorrhagic disorders (particularly administration of anticoagulant therapy), and bleeding from vascular malformations may lead to these complications. These events are usually apoplectic in nature with rapidly developing paralysis and sensory loss. Immediate radiographic demonstration of the region of the hemorrhage and surgical evacuation are indicated.

Vascular malformations are another etiology of hemorrhage into or around the spinal cord. One type of spinal cord vascular malformation is venous angioma, which is found most often on the dorsal portion of the spinal cord. Middle-aged and elderly men are chiefly affected. The slow and temporally irregular development of symptoms resulting from this lesion is believed to be secondary to ischemic compromise and compression of the spinal cord. Another type of spinal cord vascular malformation is arteriovenous malformation, which predominately affects younger patients. It is most often located on the dorsal thoracic or upper lumbar spinal cord. With this lesion, symptoms may be slowly progressive or may appear suddenly. Rapidly developing symptoms may result from occlusion of a key nutrient vessel or hemorrhage. The association of a cutaneous vascular nevus with a vascular malformation of the spinal cord has been referred to as *Klippel-Trenaunay-Weber syndrome*. The syndrome of Alajouanine[94] or angiodyskinetic myelomalacia is a necrotic myelopathy resulting in a slowly evolving amyotrophic paraplegia in men that has been attributed to spinal venous thrombosis. In the absence of a spinal dural arteriovenous fistula, it is likely to be impossible to distinguish this entity from tumor on radiographic imaging.[95] Although its exact nature remains controversial, some investigators have proposed that the lesions are probably acquired rather than congenital.[96]

Venous infarction of the spinal cord can also occur in the absence of an arteriovenous malformation. This spinal cord disorder may be extremely difficult to identify in light of the absence of specific clinical, laboratory, or radiographic findings short of spinal angiography. For this reason, it is likely seldom recognized and underreported. Kim and colleagues[97] classified venous spino-occlusive disease into three types: nonhemorrhagic infarction, hemorrhagic infarction, and embolic infarction. Any region of the spinal cord may be affected, but involvement of the thoracic cord seems to predominate.

Nonhemorrhagic infarction is protracted, seldom accompanied by back pain, evolves slowly, and has survivals averaging approximately 4 years.[97] Hemorrhagic infarction is generally sudden in onset and rapidly progressive. Back pain is observed. The full extent of the spinal cord may be affected.[98] Survival averages approximately 1 month.[97] Hemorrhagic infarction has been reported in association with hypercoagulable syndromes (e.g., Trousseau phenomenon) complicating pancreatic adenocarcinoma.[99] Embolic venous infarction was initially reported by Feigin and colleagues[91] in 1965. This disorder begins precipitously often with pain in the back and extremities. Asymmetrical and dissociated loss of function occurs more commonly in this form of venous spino-occlusive disease.[97]

Myelopathy Secondary to Connective Tissue Diseases

Rheumatoid Arthritis

Rheumatoid arthritis may result in myriad complications involving the spinal cord. Among the major abnormalities of the spine and spinal cord in rheumatoid arthritis are vertebral body erosion,[100] discitis,[101] and spinal cord compression[102] that may be secondary to pannus formation. The most dramatic and frequent abnormality occurs at the atlantoaxial region.[103] Cervical subluxation may assume many forms in this disorder,[103,104] including anterior subluxation, posterior subluxation, vertical subluxation with protrusion of the odontoid, and rotational atlantoaxial subluxation. Other abnormalities include ligamentous calcification, erosion, cystic changes, and spinous process erosion.[104] Cervical subluxation may be asymptomatic, although neck pain is common. Lower

extremity weakness and spasticity, sensory loss, and sphincter disturbances are seen with lesser degrees of frequency. Hyperextension of the cervical spine, such as may occur with endotracheal intubation, in the face of cervical instability secondary to rheumatoid arthritis may cause severe displacement with rapidly evolving myelopathy.

Unusual causes of myelopathy in a patient with rheumatoid arthritis include "epidural lipomatosis" in patients on high-dose corticosteroid therapy[105] and progressive cervical osteomyelitis.[106] Rarely, these patients may develop pseudoaneurysm of the vertebral artery or anterior spinal artery occlusion secondary to compression. Marked C1-2 abnormalities seem to be more frequent in young women with severe, long-standing, seropositive rheumatoid arthritis.[107] MRI may be useful in identifying pannus formation and craniovertebral involvement in rheumatoid arthritis.[108] Many patients stabilize with conservative therapy,[109] and the presence of cervical subluxation does not correlate with decreased survival from rheumatoid arthritis. Surgical craniocervical decompression can be helpful in early cases in which the patients remain ambulatory and are medically stable[110] but is probably not helpful in advanced nonambulatory cases.[111]

Sjögren Disease

Sjögren disease is typically a disease of women 30 to 50 years old characterized by dry eyes (xerophthalmia), dry mouth (xerostomia), and noninflammatory arthritis. Neurologic manifestations are diverse and may reflect peripheral nervous system and CNS involvement. Spinal cord involvement includes progressive myelopathy, acute transverse myelitis, and intraspinal hemorrhage.[112] Recurrent transverse myelitis may be observed. Pathologic examination revealed angiitis and necrotizing myelitis in one instance.[113] Myelopathy related to Sjögren disease can be associated with optic neuropathy or cutaneous vasculopathy.[114,115] The evaluation of Sjögren disease includes Schirmer test, serologic testing for anti-Ro (SSa) and anti-La (SSb) antibodies, and labial biopsy. Anecdotal reports have suggested improvement with corticosteroids and plasma exchange.[116]

Systemic Lupus Erythematosus and Antiphospholipid Antibody Syndrome

Myelopathy is an uncommon manifestation of SLE.[117] In one series of 315 patients with SLE, acute transverse myelopathy was observed in 10 (3.2%).[118] Most patients have evidence of other systemic disease at the time of diagnosis; however, this and other features of CNS lupus may lead to confusion with multiple sclerosis.[119] In a large series of lupus myelopathy, optic neuritis was observed in 48% of patients.[120] The association of optic neuritis and myelopathy may be particularly difficult to distinguish from multiple sclerosis. Typically, patients complain of numbness and weakness of the lower extremities manifesting in a subacute fashion, although in one series the cervical cord was involved in 50%.[118]

SLE-related myelopathy disables two thirds of affected individuals, but the other one third may recover significantly.[121] Sedimentation rate and complement levels seem to be insensitive as markers of disease activity for this condition,[122] and myelopathy is not associated with anti–ribosomal P, anti-ENA, or antiphospholipid antibodies.[118] CSF abnormalities are seen in more than 60% of cases,[118] including increased protein, pleocytosis, and even mildly decreased glucose. MRI may reveal prolongation of T1 or T2 signal in the affected cord, spinal cord enlargement, and contrast enhancement.[123] The presence of a "longitudinal myelitis," characterized by increased signal on T2-weighted imaging over many continuous segments has been suggested as a diagnostic clue, particularly for SLE-related myelopathy associated with antiphospholipid antibody.[124]

Aggressive treatment with intravenous high-dose steroids within 1 week of onset of symptoms has been associated with better outcomes.[125] Other treatment modalities have included cyclophosphamide[120] and plasmapheresis; however, the relative rarity of the syndrome has precluded rational clinical trials, and the effects of these and other therapeutic options remain uncertain. Subarachnoid spinal hemorrhage may occur in association with SLE.[112] Because some cases of SLE-related myelopathy are associated with antiphospholipid antibodies, hypercoagulability or vasculopathy may be partly responsible for the pathogenesis of the disorder.[126]

Isolated myelopathy[127-130] and optic neuropathy associated with myelopathy[131] have been reported to accompany antiphospholipid antibody syndrome. Recurrent transverse myelitis has also been reported.[132,133] Antiphospholipid antibody syndrome is a disorder in which hypercoagulability is associated with antiphospholipid antibodies (lupus anticoagulant, anticardiolipin, and antibodies directed against β_2-glycoprotein I).[134] A wide variety of neurologic disorders may be associated with this disorder.[135] The myelopathy of antiphospholipid antibody syndrome may be recurrent in nature[136] making it difficult to distinguish from multiple sclerosis, particularly when associated with optic neuritis. The disorder may be a variant of SLE. Response to treatment seems to be inconsistent. Recommended therapies have included methylprednisolone, intravenous immunoglobulin, and measures to reduce the antibodies.

Other Autoimmune Myelitides

Transverse myelitis occurring at any level of the spinal cord may complicate polyarteritis nodosa, a disease of small and medium-sized arteries. Cervical spine disease may also be seen with psoriatic arthritis. In 35% of these cases, anklyosing spondylosis occurs with syndesmophytes and ligamentous ossifications. Ankylosing spondylosis may also result in atlantoaxial subluxation in a manner similar to that of rheumatoid arthritis.[137]

Acute transverse myelitis is also known to occur in mixed connective tissue disorder and ulcerative colitis.[138,139] Granulomatous compressive thoracic myelopathy has also been reported as the initial manifestation of Wegener granulomatosis.[140] Immunosuppressive therapy seemed to be partially effective in improving the myelopathic features.

Sarcoid Myelopathy

Sarcoidosis is a chronic idiopathic granulomatous disease that may involve multiple organ systems. Bilateral hilar adenopathy and pulmonary infiltrates are the most common manifestations of the disease. Skin, eyes, heart, bone, and kidney may also be involved. Sarcoid involves the nervous system in only 5% of patients. This involvement may take the form of CNS mass lesions, hydrocephalus, recurrent aseptic meningitis, cranial neuropathies, myopathy, neuropathy, or mononeuropathy multiplex. Granulomatous infiltrates may appear in nearly any structure of the spine and cause arachnoiditis, cauda equina syndrome, intradural and extradural extramedullary granulomas, and intramedullary spinal sarcoidosis.

In the study by Junger and colleagues,[141] the patients were noted to have paraparesis, urinary bladder dysfunction, radiculopathies, chest wall numbness, gait problems, Brown-Séquard syndrome, or limb numbness or pain. The mean age of onset of neurologic symptoms was 35. Evaluation of the CSF revealed mild or moderate pleocytosis (1 to 200 cells/mm^3 [mean 36 cells/mm^3]) and elevated protein (52 to 568 mg/dL [mean 162 mg/dL]).

Definitive diagnostic testing requires biopsy showing noncaseating epithelioid granulomas. As intramedullary biopsy is rarely desirable; biopsy material may be obtained from safer sites (e.g., the lungs) if available. MRI can be normal in some suspected cases of spinal sarcoidosis.[142] Observed changes in spinal sarcoidosis include gadolinium-enhancing nerve roots, enhancing parenchymal spinal cord masses,[143] diffuse spinal cord enlargement, spinal cord atrophy, or focal or diffuse areas of increased T2-weighted signals.[141] Gallium scanning may show uptake in the lungs or parotid, salivary, or lacrimal glands. Systemic disease can be detected by increased serum angiotensin-converting enzyme levels. It is unclear at present whether measurements of CSF angiotensin-converting enzyme levels are helpful in diagnosing nervous system involvement. Serum angiotensin-converting enzyme levels are not informative with respect to CNS involvement.

Spontaneous recovery over months or years can occur in 60% to 80% of patients with isolated pulmonary disease, but very little is known about the natural history of CNS disease. Most authorities proceed aggressively with steroids if neurologic involvement becomes symptomatic. If sarcoidosis is refractory to corticosteroids, cyclosporine, cyclophosphamide, chlorambucil, methotrexate, and radiation therapy have been applied in combinations with steroid with some success.[144,145]

Nutritional Myelopathies

Vitamin B$_{12}$ Deficiency

Vitamin B$_{12}$ deficiency may result from an inadequate dietary intake or from an inability to absorb vitamin B$_{12}$ from the small intestine because of a lack of intrinsic factor. The latter condition is referred to as *pernicious anemia,* although the effects of vitamin B_{12} deficiency on the CNS may occur in the absence of the characteristic megaloblastic anemia. The neurologic disease may occur even in the absence of pathologically abnormal serum levels of vitamin B_{12}. A Schilling test or measurements of methylmalonic acid are warranted when the illness is clinically suspected.

The brain, spinal cord, optic nerve, and peripheral nerves may be adversely affected by the absence of vitamin B_{12}. Typically, the patient comments on a sense of weakness and easy fatigability of the lower extremities that is accompanied by paresthesias. Occasionally, Lhermitte phenomenon is noted. With progression of the disease, a spastic-ataxic gait and loss of vibratory and position sense ensue. The limbs are symmetrically affected. Cognitive and behavioral abnormalities, decreasing visual acuity, and a peripheral neuropathy may be superimposed on the spinal cord symptoms. Physical examination may reveal areas of vitiligo. Hyperpigmentation of the palms and soles is observed in blacks.

The myelopathy that results from vitamin B_{12} deficiency (subacute combined degeneration) is chiefly characterized neuropathologically by foci of demyelination in the posterior and lateral columns of the cervical and upper thoracic spinal cord. The earliest changes of demyelination are fusiform expansions of the myelin sheaths. Subsequently, the myelin degenerates, and if the process is uninterrupted, gliosis and involvement of the axons eventually ensue. Clinical remissions are anticipated when this myelopathy is treated expeditiously with hydroxycobalamin or cyanocobalamin. The mechanism by which vitamin B_{12} deficiency results in demyelination is unknown. It is a cofactor in choline synthesis and important in the conversion of methylmalonyl-CoA to succinyl CoA, both important to the myelin sheath.[146] Fusiform expansion of the myelin sheaths is followed by myelin degeneration.[146,147] If the process is uninterrupted, gliosis and involvement of the axons eventually ensue.[146] After effective therapy, the myelopathy of vitamin B_{12} deficiency not only may resolve clinically, but also radiographically.

Pernicious anemia is treated by intramuscular injection of cyanocobalamin. For the first week, 1000 µg daily is administered, followed by one injection weekly for the next 1 to 3 months and one injection monthly thereafter.

Myelopathy Complicating Copper Deficiency

Copper deficiency may result in spinal cord disease that can be clinically reminiscent of the neurologic manifestations of vitamin B_{12} deficiency.[148] Sensory ataxia with a spastic gait and marked ataxia coupled with a distal axonal sensorimotor neuropathy can be observed.[149] Causes of copper deficiency include prior gastric surgery, excessive zinc ingestion, and malabsorption; however, an underlying cause is not always uncovered.[150] Anemia and neutropenia are often present. Spinal cord disease and peripheral neuropathy developing after gastric bypass surgery should always raise concern about the presence of either vitamin B_{12} deficiency or copper deficiency.[151,152]

Metabolic Myelopathies

Myelopathy Resulting from Portosystemic Shunts

A progressive myelopathy has been observed in association with portosystemic shunting.[153] Although the illness generally accompanies alcoholic cirrhosis, it may arise secondary to other causes of portosystemic shunting. A selective demyelination predominates in the posterior and lateral funiculi of the spinal cord. Hepatic encephalopathy often accompanies the myelopathy. Myelopathy is manifested by an insidiously developing spastic paraparesis and gait with relative preservation of sensory and sphincter function. Hyperparathyroidism and hyperthyroidism have been rarely associated with cervical myelopathies that remit when the endocrinologic derangement is removed.[154-156]

Epidural Lipomatosis or Epidural Hibernomas

The prolonged use of large doses of corticosteroids may result in epidural lipomatosis. Epidural lipomatosis, a deposition of epidural fat, causes a compressive myelopathy. Additionally, it has been reported as an etiology of radiculopathy, cauda equina syndrome, and neurogenic claudication.[105] Spinal MRI should be highly suggestive of the diagnosis.

Paraneoplastic Myelopathies

Paraneoplastic syndromes are syndromes associated with underlying malignancies not caused by direct tumoral invasion or macroscopic metastatic disease. These remote effects of cancer are usually without an identifiable etiology, although some syndromes are associated with circulating antibodies to nervous system tissue or are the result of a presumptive concomitant viral infection. These syndromes generally are uncommon. Approximately 50% of all paraneoplastic syndromes are associated with small cell carcinoma of the lung.[157] The prototypic paraneoplastic syndrome is subacute cerebellar degeneration, which is associated with loss of Purkinje cells in the cerebellar cortex and various circulating antibodies directed against these cells. Paraneoplastic myelopathy is rare[158]—much less common than myelopathy resulting from metastatic epidural spinal cord compression. Myelopathy occurring in association with malignancy can also be secondary to radiation therapy or the result of the combined effects of radiation therapy and intrathecal chemotherapy, especially methotrexate chemotherapy,[159,160] herpes zoster,[161] abscess, or hematoma. These myelopathies may occur in isolation or as part of a syndrome in which encephalomyelitis,[162] cerebellar degeneration, or peripheral radiculoneuropathies are also observed.

The most typical myelopathy is a necrotizing myelopathy. It is a rare entity associated with lymphoma, leukemia, and small cell lung cancer. Myelopathy may manifest before, concomitant with, or after the initial tumor presentation. Clinically, it is characterized by a rapidly ascending spinal cord dysfunction leading to a flaccid areflexic paraplegia.

Myelopathy may manifest asymmetrically and often results in Brown-Séquard syndrome[163]; however, eventually it becomes bilateral and symmetrical. The brainstem may also be involved. There is no effective treatment. One patient with Hodgkin disease and a paraneoplastic myelopathy was believed to respond favorably to intrathecal corticosteroids.[164] CSF usually shows an elevated protein and a mild pleocytosis. Pathologically, there is widespread necrosis of the cord, mostly in the thoracic region.[165] Gray and white matter are involved, and lesions may be identified elsewhere in the CNS. In two cases of "paraneoplastic" necrotizing myelopathy, immunohistochemical studies and electron microscopy revealed convincing evidence of infection with HSV-2.[166]

Other, less common syndromes include a subacute motor neuropathy associated with Hodgkin disease and other malignant lymphomas.[167] It is typically diagnosed at a later stage and sometimes after radiation therapy. The motor weakness is clinically of the lower motor neuron type and involves the legs more than the arms. Sensory loss is mild. The course is benign and may stabilize or improve with specific therapy. Pathologically, neuropathy shows degeneration of the anterior horn cells and resembles an indolent poliomyelitis.[167]

A syndrome of paraneoplastic myelopathy with limbic encephalitis is associated with the antineuronal autoantibody anti-Hu.[168] This syndrome is almost always related to small cell lung cancer, and the presence of anti-Hu should lead to aggressive workup for neoplasms. This antibody is also associated with a subacute generalized sensory neuronopathy.

Although not truly a paraneoplastic disorder, intravascular lymphomatosis should be considered in the differential diagnosis of a patient presenting with an unexplained myelopathy. Spinal cord involvement occurs in approximately one third of patients. Although myelopathy, including conus involvement,[169] may be the heralding feature of the disorder, it seldom remains the only neurologic manifestation.[170] The spinal cord disorder may be indolent or rapidly progressive and may mimic multiple sclerosis or idiopathic transverse myelitis. An initially favorable but incomplete response to corticosteroids may be observed. Damage to the nervous system results from ischemia secondary to occlusion of small-caliber vessels. This disorder is most often the consequence of a clonal expansion of CD20+ B lymphocytes, although T cells and natural killer cells have also been reported. In most cases, the diagnosis remains a conundrum and is established at autopsy.[171] Aggressive therapy with CHOP (cyclophosphamide, hydroxydaunomycin, vincristine [Oncovin], and prednisone) has been associated with long-term survival, but the disease is generally fatal.

Myelopathy Secondary to Radiation Therapy

Myelopathy secondary to radiation therapy is an iatrogenic illness. The incidence is affected by the total dose of radiation delivered, the dose per fraction, and the total volume of tissue irradiated.[172] In a large study by Kagen and colleagues,[173] it was determined that spinal cord injury could be avoided if the total dose delivered was kept to 6000 rads and given over a 30- to 70-day period at a rate not exceeding 200 rads/day or 900 rads/wk.

Two pathophysiologic mechanisms are proposed for this myelopathy: direct damage to the nervous tissue of the spinal cord by irradiation and damage to the vascular supply of the spinal cord. The effects of radiation take the form of an early delayed and late delayed myelopathy. There are no acute effects of radiation on the spinal cord.[172] The incidence of this complication is 2% to 3%[174] but is substantially higher when radiation therapy is combined with hyperthermia.[175]

The early delayed radiation myelopathy usually manifests several weeks after radiation therapy as sensory symptoms and paresthesias. These symptoms may be exacerbated by neck flexion, and a typical Lhermitte phenomenon may be detected. These symptoms are believed to be secondary to demyelination and depletion of oligodendrocytes.[10] The presence of this early delayed myelopathy does not predict the development of a late delayed radiation injury.[176]

Late delayed radiation myelopathy may evolve in two distinct forms: (1) a progressive myelopathy that usually occurs 12 to 15 months after radiation therapy and never before 6 months and (2) a progressive lower motor neuron weakness that occurs 3 to 14 months after radiation. The former is characterized by sensory symptoms similar to early delayed myelopathy, but it is accompanied by an asymmetrical weakness. Frequently, the initial picture is that of Brown-Séquard syndrome, which often progresses to complete transverse myelopathy with spastic paraplegia; truncal sensory level; and bowel, bladder, and sexual dysfunction. The CSF profile is unremarkable except for the frequent presence of a slightly elevated protein. Pathologic changes include areas of necrosis that affect gray and white matter, but white matter seems to be preferentially affected. The posterior columns and posterolateral columns may be especially involved.[172]

There is no specific therapy, although steroids may slow the tempo of the illness. The differential diagnosis includes recurrent tumor or epidural spinal cord compression. The painless nature of the radiation damage is a useful diagnostic clue, particularly when MRI is indeterminate.

Not unexpectedly, the progressive lower motor neuron weakness after radiation therapy is accompanied by pathologic alterations in the anterior horn cells. There is an asymmetrical atrophy with fasciculations and areflexia.[177,178] No sensory or sphincter disturbances are noted. This peculiar myelopathy resembles a paraneoplastic subacute motor neuropathy described in patients with lymphoma.[167]

Toxins

Several agents with industrial, pharmaceutical, and medical applications have been identified as toxins capable of producing myelopathy. Toxic iatrogenic causes of myelopathy include spinal anesthesia and exposure to contrast agents used with myelography and angiography. Spinal anesthesia, with the epidural or intrathecal administration of local anesthetics, has been reported to produce myelopathy.[179,180] Although an extremely rare occurrence, myelopathy following spinal anesthesia may be permanent and includes frank paraplegia, sensory loss, and loss of sphincter function.[181,182]

Some investigators contend that the true incidence of these complications is underreported for medicolegal reasons.[183] In a review of 32,718 cases of epidural or spinal anesthesia,[184] transient paralysis was observed in 48 (0.1%), and permanent paralysis was observed in 7 (0.02%). Similarly, only 3 of 50,000 patients were reported to have permanent lower extremity weakness in a combined series.[185] The first case report of paraplegia after epidural anesthesia was by Davies and colleagues in 1958.[186] The mechanisms of spinal anesthesia–induced myelopathy, particularly myelopathy induced by epidural anesthesia, remain elusive. Possible etiologies[187] include direct neurotoxicity of these agents, toxicity of drug diluents or contaminants, hypotension leading to spinal cord infarction (typically from anterior spinal artery syndrome), epidural hematoma, epidural abscess, trauma from the epidural needle, and exacerbation of an underlying process. In some instances, a surgical procedure, such as renal transplantation, may be contributory or causative. In the latter example, the artery of Adamkiewicz may be inadvertently traumatized. Cases of myelopathy after spinal anesthesia in the setting of spinal cord tumors or herniated discs have been reported.[188]

Although oil-soluble and water-soluble myelographic contrast agents may induce arachnoiditis, which may lead to spinal cord dysfunction, these agents may themselves produce a toxic myelopathy. Although the use of modern contrast agents has essentially eliminated this complication, nearly 6% of patients had permanent myelopathic findings after myelography in early reports.[189] Transient myelopathic symptoms lasting 24 hours have also been reported after administration of water-soluble contrast agents.[77]

Myelopathy as a complication of spinal angiography has been well recognized.[190] Although this complication is most often ascribed to the induction of vasospasm or embolic thrombosis of spinal vessels resulting in ischemic infarction, a direct neurotoxic effect of the angiographic agents has been implicated in some instances.[191,192] Patients may develop pain and spasms immediately on contrast agent injection, or this may be delayed by several hours. Subsequently, patients progress to flaccid paraplegia with frequent sensory and sphincter dysfunction. Partial recovery occurs in about half of the patients, and complete recovery occurs in about 20% within weeks.[77] Many patients are left with a spastic paraplegia.

Although an extremely safe agent when used according to recommendations, nitrous oxide can manifest neurotoxicity when abused or under conditions of chronic exposure.[193,194] Usually long delayed after nitrous oxide exposure, the resulting myeloneuropathy syndrome may include sensory dysesthesias, leg weakness, spasticity, sphincter dysfunction, and ataxia. Thought to result from a nitrous oxide–induced inhibition of vitamin B_{12} use, the symptoms tend to resolve after exposure is discontinued.

Intrathecal administration of antineoplastic agents, such as methotrexate or cytosine arabinoside, has been reported to produce transient and permanent myelopathy.[195-197] Intrathecal steroid administration may initiate an acute meningeal reaction, probably secondary to polyethylene glycol detergent included in the preparation.[198,199] Distinct from problems that are due to a secondary arachnoiditis, this acute syndrome may result in back and leg pain, paresthesias, and sphincter dysfunction. Intravenous heroin administration may also cause an acute transverse myelitis. This syndrome may result from direct drug toxicity, a systemic reaction to the drug itself or to quinine or another drug diluent, a hypersensitivity reaction, or transient spinal cord ischemia.[200]

Iodochlorohydroxyquinolone, a drug used in the treatment of infectious diarrheas, has been reported to cause a syndrome of myeloneuropathy sometimes accompanied by optic atrophy.[201] Seen most frequently in Japan, this syndrome usually follows an episode of abdominal pain or diarrhea and therapy with iodochlorhydroxyquinoline. Although apparently related to the total accumulated dose of the drug, this syndrome might also be related to an enteric virus associated with the patients' initial abdominal symptoms. Patients initially complain of ascending numbness and paresthesias, which develop into a profound sensory loss. Gait ataxia, leg weakness, and sphincter dysfunction are frequent concomitants; optic atrophy and visual loss are seen in about 25% of patients. After discontinuing the drug, complete or near-complete recovery is the rule.

Triorthocresyl phosphates, used as industrial lubricating oils and solvents, are highly neurotoxic. Although accidental occupational exposure is rare, patients are often exposed by ingesting triorthocresyl phosphates in lieu of ethanol or by ingesting cooking oils contaminated with these compounds. Although the most profound neurologic complication of triorthocresyl phosphate ingestion is an acute peripheral neuritis, clinical signs of spinal cord degeneration can be seen in patients with persistent symptoms. Wallerian degeneration of the pyramidal tract and chromatolytic changes in dorsal and ventral horn cells has been identified.[202,203] In patients developing findings of myelopathy, the clinical syndrome is usually permanent.

A peculiar myelopathy seen in India and certain parts of Africa is believed to be the result of a neurotoxin (β-N-oxalylaminoalanine) found in chickpeas, *Lathyrus sativus*. It is most often observed with prolonged consumption of flour made from chickpeas in times of famine when sources of other grains are scarce. Patients complain of the gradual onset of leg weakness, stiffness, and cramping. Paresthesias, formication, and numbness of the legs are frequent. Sphincter disturbances, impotence, and variable involvement of the arms and hands are observed. The prognosis for recovery is poor.

Electrical Injury

Electrical injury of the nervous system results most frequently from accidental exposure to high-tension currents, although lightning and complication of electroshock therapy have also been reported to cause neurologic injury. Although current sufficient to cause damage to the nervous system is usually fatal, individuals who survive such injuries are subject to damage throughout the neuraxis.[77,204] Acutely, patients may have neurologic symptoms referable to cerebral anoxia secondary to cardiac arrhythmias or respiratory arrest. Neural tissue examined shortly after electrical injury shows petechial and perivascular hemorrhages and severe ganglion cell changes. The most abnormal areas of the spinal cord are in the path of the electrical current. Short-term survivors of this acute phase may show focal myelomalacia and mild gliosis on autopsy. Although the pathophysiology is not fully understood, the injury most probably reflects a direct vascular injury to spinal cord vessels, an indirect vascular injury to spinal vasomotor nerves, or a direct effect of current on spinal cord tissue. Pathologic changes noted in long-term survivors postmortem have included demyelination with preservation axons, anterior horn cell loss, and necrosis.

Permanent neurologic manifestations of electrical injury are uncommon. The most characteristic neurologic effect of electrical injury is delayed myelopathy, occurring in 1% to 6% of victims.[205,206] Immediately after electrical injury, patients may complain of paresthesias, pain, urinary dysfunction, or impotence. These symptoms tend to improve rapidly. Occasionally, delays in the onset of neurologic symptoms of up to 6 weeks (averaging 1 week) may be observed. Neurologic signs may worsen over 2 to 14 days.[207] According to Winkelman,[207] one third of patients recover fully, one third have partial recovery, and one third experience no recovery. The last-mentioned is the rule in patients with a complete spinal cord lesion or progression of spinal symptoms over a prolonged period. Rarely, delayed neurologic deficits can appear after a latency of several months.[208,209] The symptoms of delayed myelopathy after electrical injury are typically permanent, but rapid recovery has also been reported.[210]

A cervical myelopathy with atrophic quadriparesis is the most frequent complication; this myelopathy results from current passing from hand to hand.[211,212] With low-voltage injuries (<1000 volts), muscular atrophy from anterior horn cell damage is most common.[77] With higher voltages, more profound injuries occur to the lateral and posterior columns.[77] Pyramidal signs, including spastic weakness, hyperreflexia, and Babinski signs, predominate regardless of the location of the lesion. Sensory findings are less prominent with posterior column dysfunction predominating. Lhermitte phenomenon has been reported rarely.[213] Other forms of electrical injury to the spinal cord result in spinal atrophic paralysis, a syndrome of focal muscular atrophy that typically follows low-tension electrical injury that has a predilection to involve gray rather than white matter and, questionably, amyotrophic lateral sclerosis.

Barotrauma

Spinal cord injury following rapid changes in atmospheric pressure, such as can occur in caisson work, scuba diving, and flying, has been well documented.[214-216] Spinal cord damage results from too-rapid decompression after exposure to significant increases in atmospheric pressure. At higher atmospheric pressures, increasing amounts of gas are dissolved into tissue. The higher tissue concentration of oxygen is used in oxidative metabolism, whereas nitrogen gas, which is inert, remains dissolved only by virtue of the hyperbaric condition. With decompression, the nitrogen is released; when decompression is too rapid, nitrogen bubbles may form and occlude the spinal cord vasculature.

Symptoms tend to develop during or immediately after decompression. Patients frequently complain of interscapular pain followed by lower extremity paresthesias, frank leg weakness, and sphincter disturbances within hours. Examination usually reveals a flaccid paraplegia with loss of pain and temperature sensation and frequent sparing of proprioceptive sensation. In most cases, the thoracic spinal cord is the major site of involvement, whereas combined lesions in the lower cervical and lumbar cord may occur less commonly. Pathologic examination of the cord shows early white matter hemorrhages followed by perivascular demyelination. These changes tend to be most extensive in the posterior and lateral columns, and secondary ascending and descending tract degeneration may be seen over time.

Therapy for decompression myelopathy is recompression followed by controlled slow decompression. If treatment is instituted rapidly, complete recovery is possible. If it is delayed more than a few hours, the chances of recovery are remote.[215,217]

Heredofamilial Degenerations

Numerous genetic neurodegenerative diseases can include spasticity attributable in part or total to spinal cord involvement in their complex of multiple signs and symptoms, but two disorders have quite prominent spastic paraparesis. Hereditary spastic paraplegia appears in autosomal recessive, autosomal dominant, and X-linked forms. A locus for the autosomal recessive form has been found on chromosome 8q; loci for the dominant form have been found at 2p, 14q, and 15q; and a locus for the X-linked form has been found at Xq22. In one family with the X-linked form, this has been shown to be due to a mutation in a proteolipoprotein.[218] There is spastic weakness in the legs, gait difficulties, hyperactive reflexes, and extensor plantar signs. The course is one of slow but relentless progression. There are rare variants with other associated degenerations, such as optic neuropathy. The diagnosis is made by family history and excluding any other causes.[10]

Patients with Friedreich ataxia begin having problems in childhood. There is spastic quadriparesis owing to upper motor neuron degeneration, ataxia from cerebellar degeneration, numbness and foot deformity from neuropathy, nystagmus, tremor, and other problems. There is degeneration of the posterior columns, corticospinal tracts, spinocerebellar tracts, dentate nuclei, cranial nerve nuclei, and myocardial muscle fibers. There is no treatment, and death occurs in young adulthood. It has been found more recently that most cases of the illness are due to trinucleotide repeat expansion in the gene *X25,* which codes for a protein frataxin, on chromosome 9q13. A few cases are due to point mutations in the same gene.[219]

PEARLS

1. The most common form of medical myelopathy is idiopathic transverse myelitis.

2. Idiopathic transverse myelitis may herald multiple sclerosis.

PITFALLS

1. The concurrence of optic neuritis and transverse myelitis may be the consequence of NMO (Devic disease). Assessment of anti-NMO antibody is helpful in diagnosing this disorder because its response to treatment differs from multiple sclerosis.

2. A variety of disorders ranging from viral infections to paraneoplastic syndromes may manifest in a clinically indistinguishable fashion to idiopathic transverse myelitis.

3. Spinal cord swelling and contrast enhancement mimicking an intramedullary spinal cord tumor may occur with these disorders; watchful waiting with repeat clinical assessment and neuroimaging may obviate the need for a spinal cord biopsy.

KEY POINTS

1. Multiple sclerosis is the most common neurologic disorder resulting in myelopathy. Transverse myelitis may be the heralding manifestation of the disorder. At the other end of the clinical spectrum is a slowly evolving myelopathy accompanying primary progressive or secondarily progressive multiple sclerosis.

2. The association of an acute transverse myelitis with optic neuritis may indicate NMO (Devic disease). This disorder is associated with an antibody to the aquaporin-4 channel, and treatment directed against this abnormal immunoglobulin seems to be more effective than other forms of therapy.

3. A broad array of microorganisms is associated with spinal cord disease. Historically, the most common infections were tuberculosis and syphilis. Currently, HIV/AIDS is the most common recognized infectious cause of spinal cord disease. The form of HIV-associated myelopathy most often observed is a vacuolar myelopathy with clinical features similar to subacute combined degeneration occurring with vitamin B_{12} deficiency. This myelopathy typically develops insidiously and is often unrecognized.

4. Clinicians should have a high degree of suspicion for the presence of a spinal epidural abscess in patients presenting with fever and back pain. One third of patients with spinal epidural abscess have a history of preceding back trauma.

5. The nature of the neurologic deficits is often very helpful in recognizing vascular disease of the spinal cord. Paralysis and a dissociated sensory loss characterized by preserved position and vibration perception accompanying a sensory level to pinprick are suggestive of an anterior spinal artery occlusion.

6. The most dramatic and frequent abnormality associated with rheumatoid arthritis occurs in the atlantoaxial region. Hyperextension of the cervical spine may result in a rapidly evolving myelopathy owing to cervical subluxation.

KEY REFERENCES

1. Adams RD, Merritt HH: Meningeal and vascular diseases of the spinal cord. Medicine 23:181, 1944.
   Although published in the middle of the past century, this is the classic work on the spectrum of vascular diseases of the spinal cord. The authors describe in detail the vascular network that supplies the cord and ganglia and address the numerous fashions by which the circulation can be impaired.

2. Kovacs B, Lafferty TL, Brent LH, et al: Transverse myelopathy in systemic lupus erythematosus: An analysis of 14 cases and review of the literature. Ann Rheum Dis 59:120-124, 2000.
   Distinguishing the myelopathy accompanying SLE from idiopathic transverse myelitis is occasionally difficult. A high index of suspicion is necessary. The authors present 14 cases and provide an excellent review of the literature on this important topic.

3. McLean JM, Palagallo GL, Henderson JP, et al: Myelopathy associated with fibrocartilaginous emboli (FE): Review and two suspected cases. Surg Neurol 44:228-235, 1995.
   Fibrocartilaginous embolization with infarction of the spinal cord is often overlooked as a diagnostic entity. The authors present two cases of their own and provide an excellent review of the literature on this topic.

4. Petito CK, Navia BA, Cho ES, et al: Vacuolar myelopathy pathologically resembling subacute combined degeneration in patients with the acquired immunodeficiency syndrome. N Engl J Med 312:874, 1985.
   This is the initial description of the entity referred to as HIV-associated vacuolar myelopathy. The authors address the clinical presentation and the pathologic findings. They show the similarities to subacute combined degeneration of the spinal cord from vitamin B^{12} deficiency and, in a subsequent publication, suggest that this myelopathy is not unique to HIV infection.

5. Vernant JC, Maurs L, Gessain A, et al: Endemic tropical spastic paraparesis associated with human T-lymphotropic virus type I: A clinical and seroepidemiological study of 25 cases. Ann Neurol 21:123, 1987.
   Building on their earlier observations on the association of a unique myelopathy in the setting of HTLV-I seropositivity in a Caribbean population, the authors expand their series and describe in detail the clinical presentation of HAM or TSP.

6. Weinshenker BG, Wingerchuk DM: Neuromyelitis optica: Clinical syndrome and the NMO-IgG autoantibody marker. Curr Top Microbiol Immunol 318:343-356, 2008.
   This is a review of the latest understanding of NMO, or Devic syndrome, with an emphasis on the role of the newly discovered aquaporin-4 antibody in pathogenesis and diagnosis of the disorder.

REFERENCES

1. DeJong RN: Neurological Examination. New York, Harper & Row, 1979.

2. Ropper AH, Poskanzer DC: The prognosis of acute and sub-acute transverse myelopathy based on early signs and symptoms. Ann Neurol 4:51-59, 1978.

3. Kalita J, Misra UK: Is methyl prednisolone useful in acute transverse myelitis? Spinal Cord 39:471-476, 2001.

4. Lahat E, Pillar G, Ravid S, et al: Rapid recovery from transverse myelopathy in children treated with methylprednisolone. Pediatr Neurol 19:279-282, 1998.

5. Lipton HL, Teasdall RD: Acute transverse myelopathy in adults: A follow-up study. Arch Neurol 28:252-257, 1973.

6. Altrocchi PH: Acute transverse myelopathy. Arch Neurol 9:111, 1963.

7. Berman M, Feldman S, Alter M, et al: Acute transverse myelitis: Incidence and etiologic considerations. Neurology 31:966, 1981.

8. Miller DH, Ormerod IE, Rudge P, et al: The early risk of multiple sclerosis following isolated acute syndromes of the brainstem and spinal cord. Ann Neurol 26:635-639, 1989.

9. Lee KH, Hashimoto SA, Hooge JP, et al: Magnetic resonance imaging of the head in the diagnosis of multiple sclerosis: A prospective 2-year follow-up with comparison of clinical evaluation, evoked potentials, oligoclonal banding, and CT. Neurology 41:657-660, 1991.

10. Adams R, Victor M: Diseases of the Spinal Cord. Principles of Neurology, 4th ed. New York, McGraw Hill, 1989.

11. Poser S, Wikstrom J, Bauer HJ: Clinical data and the identification of special forms of multiple sclerosis in 1271 cases studied with a standardized documentation system. J Neurol Sci 40:159-168, 1979.

12. Shepherd DI: Clinical features of multiple sclerosis in northeast Scotland. Acta Neurol Scand 60:218-230, 1979.

13. Kanchandani R, Howe JG: Lhermitte's sign in multiple sclerosis: A clinical survey and review of the literature. J Neurol Neurosurg Psychiatry 45:308-312, 1982.

14. Weinshenker BG, Wingerchuk DM: Neuromyelitis optica: Clinical syndrome and the NMO-IgG autoantibody marker. Curr Top Microbiol Immunol 318:343-356, 2008.

15. Cree B: Neuromyelitis optica: Diagnosis, pathogenesis, and treatment. Curr Neurol Neurosci Rep 8:427-433, 2008.

16. Miller DH, McDonald WI, Blumhardt LD, et al: Magnetic resonance imaging in isolated noncompressive spinal cord syndromes. Ann Neurol 22:714-723, 1987.

17. Oppenheimer DR: The cervical cord in multiple sclerosis. Neuropathol Appl Neurobiol 4:151-162, 1978.

18. Thielen KR, Miller GM: Multiple sclerosis of the spinal cord: Magnetic resonance appearance. J Comput Assist Tomogr 20:434-438, 1996.

19. Thorpe JW, Kidd D, Moseley IF, et al: Serial gadolinium-enhanced MRI of the brain and spinal cord in early relapsing-remitting multiple sclerosis. Neurology 46:373-378, 1996.

20. Syme JA Jr, Kelly JJ Jr: Absent F-waves early in a case of transverse myelitis. Muscle Nerve 17:462-465, 1994.

21. Moser HW, Moser AB, Kawamura N, t al: Adrenoleukodystrophy: Elevated C26 fatty acid in cultured skin fibroblasts. Ann Neurol 7:542-549, 1980.

22. Griffin JW, Goren E, Schaumburg H, et al: Adrenomyeloneuropathy: A probable variant of adrenoleukodystrophy. I. Clinical and endocrinologic aspects. Neurology 27:1107-1113, 1977.

23. Snider WD, Simpson DM, Nielsen S, et al: Neurological complications of acquired immune deficiency syndrome: Analysis of 50 patients. Ann Neurol 14:403-418, 1983.

24. Levy RM, Bredesen DE, Rosenblum ML: Neurological manifestations of the acquired immunodeficiency syndrome (AIDS): Experience at UCSF and review of the literature. J Neurosurg 62:475-495, 1985.

25. Berger JR, Moskowitz L, Fischl M, et al: Neurologic disease as the presenting manifestation of acquired-immunodeficiency-syndrome. South Med J 80:683-686, 1987.

26. Bredesen DE, Messing R: Neurological syndromes heralding the acquired immune-deficiency syndrome. Ann Neurol 14: 141, 1983.

27. Helweg-Larsen S, Jakobsen J, Boesen F, et al: Neurological complications and concomitants of AIDS. Acta Neurol Scand 74:467, 1986.

28. Petito CK, Navia BA, Cho ES, et al: Vacuolar myelopathy pathologically resembling subacute combined degeneration in patients with the acquired immunodeficiency syndrome. N Engl J Med 312:874-879, 1985.

29. de la Monte SM, Ho DD, Schooley RT, et al: Subacute encephalomyelitis of AIDS and its relation to HTLV-III infection. Neurology 37:562-569, 1987.

30. Goldstick L, Mandybur TI, Bode R: Spinal cord degeneration in AIDS. Neurology 35:103-106, 1985.

31. Honig LS, Horoupian DS: Chronic myelopathy as a presenting symptom in HIV infection. Neurology 39(Suppl 1):419, 1989.

32. Kamin SS, Petito CK: Idiopathic myelopathies with white matter vacuolation in non-acquired immunodeficiency syndrome patients. Hum Pathol 22:816-824, 1991.

33. Singh BM, Levine S, Yarrish RL, et al: Spinal cord syndromes in the acquired immune deficiency syndrome. Acta Neurol Scand 73:590-598, 1986.

34. Dickson DW, Belman AL, Kim TS, et al: Spinal cord pathology in pediatric acquired immunodeficiency syndrome. Neurology 39(2 Pt 1):227-235, 1989.

35. Denning DW, Anderson J, Rudge P, et al: Acute myelopathy associated with primary infection with human immunodeficiency virus. BMJ (Clin Res Ed) 294:143-144, 1987.

36. Williams AE, Fang CT, Slamon DJ, et al: Seroprevalence and epidemiological correlates of HTLV-I infection in U.S. blood donors. Science 240:643-646, 1988.

37. Robert-Guroff M, Weiss SH, Giron JA, et al: Prevalence of antibodies to HTLV-I, -II, and -III in intravenous drug abusers from an AIDS endemic region. JAMA 255:3133-3137, 1986.

38. Weiss SH, Ginzburg HM, Saxinger WC, et al: Emerging high rates of human T cell lymphotropic virus type 1 (HTLV-I) and HIV infections among US drug abusers. III International Conference on AIDS, Washington, DC, 1987.

39. Khabbaz RF, Darrow WW, Hartley TM, et al: Seroprevalence and risk factors for HTLV-I/II infection among female prostitutes in the United States. JAMA 263:60-64, 1990.

40. Kaplan JE, Litchfield B, Rouault C,et al: HTLV-I-associated myelopathy associated with blood transfusion in the United States: Epidemiologic and molecular evidence linking donor and recipient. Neurology 41:192-197, 1991.

41. Sheremata WA, Berger JR, Harrington WJ Jr, et al: Human T lymphotropic virus type I-associated myelopathy: A report of

10 patients born in the United States. Arch Neurol 49:1113-1118, 1992.

42. Gessain A, Barin F, Vernant JC, et al: Antibodies to human T-lymphotropic virus type-I in patients with tropical spastic paraparesis. Lancet 2:407-410, 1985.

43. Osame M, Usuku K, , Izumo S, et al: HTLV-I associated myelopathy, a new clinical entity. Lancet 1:1031-1032, 1986.

44. Koprowski H, DeFreitas EC, Harper ME, et al: Multiple sclerosis and human T-cell lymphotropic retroviruses. Nature 318:154-160, 1985.

45. Vernant JC, Maurs L, Gessain A, et al: Endemic tropical spastic paraparesis associated with human T-lymphotropic virus type I: A clinical and seroepidemiological study of 25 cases. Ann Neurol 21:123-130, 1987.

46. Akizuki S, Nakazato O, Higuchi Y, et al: Necropsy findings in HTLV-I associated myelopathy. Lancet 1:156-157, 1987.

47. Berger JR, Svenningsson A, Raffanti S, et al: Tropical spastic paraparesis-like illness occurring in a patient dually infected with HIV-1 and HTLV-II. Neurology 41:85-87, 1991.

48. Harrington WJ Jr, Sheremata W, Hjelle B, et al: Spastic ataxia associated with human T-cell lymphotropic virus type II infection. Ann Neurol 33:411-414, 1993.

49. Jacobson S, Lehky T, Nishimura M, et al: Isolation of HTLV-II from a patient with chronic, progressive neurological disease clinically indistinguishable from HTLV-I-associated myelopathy/tropical spastic paraparesis. Ann Neurol 33:392-396, 1993.

50. Sheremata WA, Harrington WJ Jr, Bradshaw PA, et al: Association of '(tropical) ataxic neuropathy' with HTLV-II. Virus Res 29:71-77, 1993.

51. Lehky TJ, Flerlage N, Katz D, Houff S, et al: Human T-cell lymphotropic virus type II-associated myelopathy: Clinical and immunologic profiles. Ann Neurol 40:714-723, 1996.

52. Peters AA, Oger JJ, Coulthart MB, et al: An apparent case of human T-cell lymphotropic virus type II (HTLV-II)-associated neurological disease: A clinical, molecular, and phylogenetic characterisation. J Clin Virol 14:37-50, 1999.

53. Silva EA, Otsuki K, Leite AC, et al: HTLV-II infection associated with a chronic neurodegenerative disease: Clinical and molecular analysis. J Med Virol 66:253-257, 2002.

54. Lowis GW, Sheremata WA, Minagar A: Epidemiologic features of HTLV-II: Serologic and molecular evidence. Ann Epidemiol 12:46-66, 2002.

55. Rose FC, Brett EM, Burston Jl: Zoster encephalomyelitis. Arch Neurol 11:155-172, 1964.

56. Caplan LR, Kleeman FJ, Berg S: Urinary retention probably secondary to herpes genitalis. N Engl J Med 297:920-921, 1977.

57. Klatersky J, Cappel R, Snoeck JM, et al: Ascending myelitis in association with herpes simplex virus. N Engl J Med 287:182-184 1982.

58. Grose C, Feorino PM: Epstein-Barr virus and transverse myelitis. Lancet 1:892, 1973.

59. Silverstein A : Epstein Barr virus infections of the nervous system. In Vinken P, Bruyn G (eds): Infections of the Nervous System. Amsterdam, North Holland Publishing, 1978.

60. Tyler KL, Gross RA, Cascino GDl: Unusual viral causes of transverse myelitis: Hepatitis A virus and cytomegalovirus. Neurology 36:855-858, 1986.

61. Paine RS, Byers RK: Transverse myelopathy in childhood. AMA Am J Dis Child 85:151-163, 1953.

62. Altrocchi P: Acute transverse myelopathy. Arch Neurol 9:111, 1963.

63. Adams R, Merritt HH: Meningeal and vascular diseases of the spinal cord. Medicine 23:181, 1944.

64. Berger J: Syphilis of the spinal cord. In Davidoff RA (ed): Handbook of the Spinal Cord. New York, Marcel Dekker, 1987.

65. Fisher M, Poser CM: Syphilitic meningomyelitis: A case report. Arch Neurol 34:785, 1977.

66. Gribble LD: Syphilitic spinal pachymeningitis. S Afr Med J 46:1326-1328, 1972.

67. Syphilis: Recommended treatment schedules, 1976. Recommendations established by the Venereal Disease Control Advisory Committee. Ann Intern Med 85:94, 1976.

68. Berger J: Neurosyphilis. In Johnson R (ed): Current Therapies in Neurology. Philadelphia, BC Decker, 1990.

69. Griffiths DL: Tuberculosis of the spine: A review. Adv Tuberc Res 20:92-110, 1980.

70. Nussbaum ES, Rockswold GL, Bergman TA, et al: Spinal tuberculosis: A diagnostic and management challenge. J Neurosurg 83:243-247, 1995.

71. Moon MS, Ha KY, Sun DH, et al: Pott's paraplegia—67 cases. Clin Orthop Relat Res (323):122-128, 1996.

72. Vidyasagar C, Murthy HK: Spinal tuberculosis with neurological deficits. Natl Med J India 9:25-27, 1996.

73. Dutton JE, Alexander GL: Intramedullary spinal abscess. J Neurol Neurosurg Psychiatry 17:303-307, 1954.

74. Clarke CE, Falope ZF, Abdelhadi HA, et al: Cervical myelopathy caused by Whipple's disease. Neurology 50:1505-1506, 1998.

75. Schroter A, Brinkhoff J, Günthner-Lengsfeld T, et al: Whipple's disease presenting as an isolated lesion of the cervical spinal cord. Eur J Neurol 12:276-279, 2005.

76. Miller HG, Gibbons JL, Stanton JB: Para-infectious encephalomyelitis and related syndromes: A critical review of the neurological complications of certain specific fevers. QJM 25:427-505, 1956.

77. Kincaid JC: Myelitis and myelopathy. In: Joynt RJ (ed): Clinical Neurology. New York, Harper & Row, 1982.

78. Pickerill RG, Milder JE: Transverse myelitis associated with cat-scratch disease in an adult. JAMA 246:2840-2841, 1981.

79. Reik L, Steere AC, Bartenhagen NH, et al: Neurologic abnormalities of Lyme disease. Medicine (Baltimore) 58:281-294, 1979.

80. Koh S, Ross LA, Gilles FH, et al: Myelopathy resulting from invasive aspergillosis. Pediatr Neurol 19:135-138, 1998.

81. Suchet I, Klein C, Horwitz T, et al: Spinal cord schistosomiasis: A case report and review of the literature. Paraplegia 25:491-496, 1987.

82. Ferrari TC: Spinal cord schistosomiasis: A report of 2 cases and review emphasizing clinical aspects. Medicine (Baltimore) 78:176-190, 1999.

83. Petjom S, Chaiwun B, Settakorn J, et al: *Angiostrongylus cantonensis* infection mimicking a spinal cord tumor. Ann Neurol 52:99-101, 2002.

84. Kaufman DM, Kaplan JG, Litman N: Infectious agents in spinal epidural abscesses. Neurology 30:844-850, 1980.

85. Baker AS, Ojemann RG, Swartz MN, et al: Spinal epidural abscess. N Engl J Med 293:463-468, 1975.

86. Aldrete JA: Neurologic deficits and arachnoiditis following neuroaxial anesthesia. Acta Anaesthesiol Scand 47:3-12, 2003.

87. Herrick MK, Mills PE Jr: Infarction of spinal cord: Two cases of selective gray matter involvement secondary to asymptomatic aortic disease. Arch Neurol 24:228-241, 1971.

88. Killen DA, Foster JH: Spinal cord injury as a complication of contrast angiography. Surgery 59:969-981, 1966.

89. Bockenek WL, Bach JR: Fibrocartilaginous emboli to the spinal cord: A review of the literature. J Am Paraplegia Soc 13:18-23, 1990.

90. Bots GT, Wattendorff AR, Buruma OJ, et al: Acute myelopathy caused by fibrocartilaginous emboli. Neurology 31:1250-1256, 1981.

91. Feigin I, Popoff N, Adachi M: Fibrocartilaginous venous emboli to the spinal cord with necrotic myelopathy. J Neuropathol Exp Neurol 24:63-74, 1965.

92. McLean JM, Palagallo GL, Henderson JP, et al: Myelopathy associated with fibrocartilaginous emboli (FE): Review and two suspected cases. Surg Neurol 44:228-234; discussion 234-235, 1995.

93. Moorhouse DF, Burke M, Keohane C, et al: Spinal-cord infarction caused by cartilage embolus to the anterior spinal artery. Surg Neurol 37:448-452, 1992.

94. Foix C, Alajouanine T: La myelite necrotique subaigue. Rev Neurol 11:1-42, 1926.

95. Mirich DR, Kucharczyk W, Keller MA, et al: Subacute necrotizing myelopathy: MR imaging in four pathologically proved cases. AJNR Am J Neuroradiol 12:1077-1083, 1991.

96. Koeppen AH, Barron KD, Cox JF: Foix-Alajouanine syndrome. Acta Neuropathol (Berl) 29:187-197, 1974.

97. Kim RC, Smith HR, Henbest ML, et al: Nonhemorrhagic venous infarction of the spinal cord. Ann Neurol 15:379-385, 1984.

98. Roa KR, Donnenfeld H, Chusid JG, et al: Acute myelopathy secondary to spinal venous thrombosis. J Neurol Sci 56:107-113, 1982.

99. Hughes JT: Venous infarction of the spinal cord. Neurology 21:794-800, 1971.

100. Lorber A, Pearson CM, Rene RMl: Osteolytic vertebral lesions as a manifestation of rheumatoid arthritis and related disorders. Arthritis Rheum 4:514, 1961.

101. Blass J: Rheumatoid arthritis of the cervical spine. Bull Rheum Dis 18:471, 1967.

102. Hopkins JS: Lower cervical rheumatoid subluxation with tetraplegia. J Bone Joint Surg Br 49:46-51, 1967.

103. Shannon KM: Connective tissue diseases and the nervous system. In Aminoff MJ (ed): Neurology and General Medicine. New York, Churchill Livingstone, 1989.

104. Bundschuk C, Modic MT, Kearney F, et al: Rheumatoid arthritis of the cervical spine: Surface-coil MR imaging. AJR Am J Roentgenol 151:181, 1988.

105. Perling LH, Laurent JP, Cheek WR: Epidural hibernoma as a complication of corticosteroid treatment: Case report. J Neurosurg 69:613-616, 1988.

106. McGrath H Jr, McCormick C, Carey ME: Pyogenic cervical osteomyelitis presenting as a massive prevertebral abscess in a patient with rheumatoid arthritis. Am J Med 84:363-365, 1988.

107. Halla JT, Hardin JG Jr: The spectrum of atlantoaxial facet joint involvement in rheumatoid arthritis. Arthritis Rheum 33:325-329, 1990.

108. Semble EL, Elster AD, et al: Magnetic-resonance imaging of the craniovertebral junction in rheumatoid-arthritis. J Rheumatol 15:1367-1375, 1988.

109. Smith PH, Sharp J, et al: Natural history of rheumatoid cervical subluxations. Ann Rheum Dis 31: 222-223, 1972.

110. Falope ZF, Griffiths ID, Platt PN, Todd NV: Cervical myelopathy and rheumatoid arthritis: a retrospective analysis of management. Clin Rehabil 16:625-629, 2002.

111. Casey AT, et al: Surgery on the rheumatoid cervical spine for the non-ambulant myelopathic patient—too much, too late? Lancet 347:1004-1007, 1996.

112. Fody EP, Netsky MG, et al: Subarachnoid spinal hemorrhage in a case of systemic lupus erythematosus. Arch Neurol 37:173-174, 1980.

113. Rutan G, Martinez AJ, et al: Primary biliary cirrhosis, Sjogren's syndrome, and transverse myelitis. Gastroenterology 90:206-210, 1986.

114. Harada T, Ohashi T, et al: Optic neuropathy and acute transverse myelopathy in primary Sjogren's syndrome. Jpn J Ophthalmol 39:162-165, 1995.

115. Lyu RK, Chen ST, et al: Acute transverse myelopathy and cutaneous vasculopathy in primary Sjogren's syndrome. Eur Neurol 35:359-362, 1995.

116. Konttinen YT, Kinnunen E, et al: Acute transverse myelopathy successfully treated with plasmapheresis and prednisone in a patient with primary Sjogren's syndrome. Arthritis Rheum 30:339-344, 1987.

117. Ellis SG, Verity MA: Central nervous system involvement in systemic lupus erythematosus: A review of neuropathologic findings in 57 cases, 1955-1977. Semin Arthritis Rheum 8:212-221, 1979.

118. Mok CC, Lau CS, et al: Acute transverse myelopathy in systemic lupus erythematosus: Clinical presentation, treatment, and outcome. J Rheumatol 25:467-473, 1998.

119. Inslicht DV, Stein AB, et al: Three women with lupus transverse myelitis: Case reports and differential diagnosis. Arch Phys Med Rehabil 79:456-459, 1998.

120. Kovacs B, Lafferty TL, et al: Transverse myelopathy in systemic lupus erythematosus: An analysis of 14 cases and review of the literature. Ann Rheum Dis 59:120-124, 2000.

121. Andrianakos AA, Duffy J, et al: Transverse myelopathy in systemic lupus erythematosus: Report of three cases and review of the literature. Ann Intern Med 83:616-624, 1975.

122. Chan KF, Boey ML: Transverse myelopathy in SLE: Clinical features and functional outcomes. Lupus 5:294-299, 1996.

123. Provenzale JM, Barboriak DP, et al: Lupus-related myelitis—serial MR findings. AJNR Am J Neuroradiol 15:1911-1917, 1994.

124. Tellez-Zenteno JF, Remes-Troche JM, Negrete-Pulido RO, et al: Longitudinal myelitis associated with systemic lupus

erythematosus: Clinical features and magnetic resonance imaging of six cases. Lupus 10:851-856, 2001.

125. Harisdangkul V, Doorenbos D, et al: Lupus transverse myelopathy: Better outcome with early recognition and aggressive high-dose intravenous corticosteroid pulse treatment. J Neurol 242:326-331, 1995.

126. Cordeiro MF, Lloyd ME, et al: Ischaemic optic neuropathy, transverse myelitis, and epilepsy in an anti-phospholipid positive patient with systemic lupus erythematosus. J Neurol Neurosurg Psychiatry 57:1142-1143, 1994.

127. Hasegawa M, Yamashita J, et al: Spinal cord infarction associated with primary antiphospholipid syndrome in a young child: Case report. J Neurosurg 79:446-450, 1993.

128. Levine SR, Welch KM: The spectrum of neurologic disease associated with antiphospholipid antibodies: Lupus anticoagulants and anticardiolipin antibodies. Arch Neurol 44:876-883, 1987.

129. Quencer RM: Anticardiolipin antibodies and transverse myelopathy: Expanding our understanding of an elusive clinical problem. AJNR Am J Neuroradiol 19:798-799, 1998.

130. Cuadrado MJ, Khamashta MA, et al: Can neurologic manifestations of Hughes (antiphospholipid) syndrome be distinguished from multiple sclerosis? Analysis of 27 patients and review of the literature. Medicine (Baltimore) 79:57-68, 2000.

131. Aziz A, Conway MD, et al: Acute optic neuropathy and transverse myelopathy in patients with antiphospholipid antibody syndrome: Favorable outcome after treatment with anticoagulants and glucocorticoids. Lupus 9:307-310, 2000.

132. Kim JH, Lee SI, Park SI, Yoo WH: Recurrent transverse myelitis in primary antiphospholipid antibody syndrome—case report and literature review. Rheumatol Int 24:244-246, 2004.

133. Shaharao V, Bartakke S, Muranjan MN, et al: Recurrent acute transverse myelopathy: association with antiphospholipid antibody syndrome. Indian J Pediatr 71:559-561, 2004.

134. Levine JS, Branch DW, Rauch J: The antiphospholipid syndrome. N Engl J Med 346:752-763, 2002.

135. Brey RL, Escalante A: Neurological manifestations of antiphospholipid antibody syndrome. Lupus 7(Suppl 2):S67-S74, 1998.

136. Campi A, Filippi M, et al: Recurrent acute transverse myelopathy associated with anticardiolipin antibodies. AJNR Am J Neuroradiol 19:781-786, 1998.

137. Blau RH, Kaufman RL: Erosive and subluxing cervical spine disease in patients with psoriatic arthritis. J Rheumatol 14:111-117, 1987.

138. Mok CC, Lau CS: Transverse myelopathy complicating mixed connective tissue disease. Clin Neurol Neurosurg 97:259-260, 1995.

139. Ray DW, Bridger J, et al: Transverse myelitis as the presentation of Jo-1 antibody syndrome (myositis and fibrosing alveolitis) in long-standing ulcerative colitis. Br J Rheumatol 32:1105-1108, 1993.

140. Kelley PJ, Toker DE, Boyer P, et al: Granulomatous compressive thoracic myelopathy as the initial manifestation of Wegener's granulomatosis. Neurology 51:1769-1770, 1998.

141. Junger SS, Stern BJ, et al: Intramedullary spinal sarcoidosis: Clinical and magnetic resonance imaging characteristics. Neurology 43:333-337, 1993.

142. Endo T, Koike J, et al: Spinal cord sarcoidosis. Neurology 43:1059-1060, 1993.

143. Lexa FJ, Grossman RI: MR of sarcoidosis in the head and spine: Spectrum of manifestations and radiographic response to steroid therapy. AJNR Am J Neuroradiol 15:973-982, 1994.

144. Agbobu B, et al: Therapeutic considerations in patients with refractory neurosarcoidosis. Arch Neurol 52:875, 1995.

145. Chapelon C, Ziza JM, et al: Neurosarcoidosis: Signs, course and treatment in 35 confirmed cases. Medicine (Baltimore) 69:261-276, 1990.

146. Kunze K, Leitenmaier K: Vitamin B12 deficiency and subacute combined degeneration of the spinal cord. In Vinken PJ, Bruyn GW (eds): Handbook of Clinical Neurology (volume 28) 1976, pp 141-198.

147. Smith W: Nutritional deficiencies and disorders. In Blackwood W, Corsellis J (eds): Greenfield's Neuropathy. London, Edward Arnold, 1977.

148. Kumar N, Gross JB Jr, Ahlskog JE: Copper deficiency myelopathy produces a clinical picture like subacute combined degeneration. Neurology 63:33-39, 2004.

149. Goodman BP, Mistry DH, Pasha SF, Bosch PE: Copper deficiency myeloneuropathy due to occult celiac disease. Neurologist 15:355-356, 2009.

150. Kumar N: Copper deficiency myelopathy (human swayback). Mayo Clin Proc 81:1371-1384, 2006.

151. Berger JR: The neurological complications of bariatric surgery. Arch Neurol 61:1185-1189, 2004.

152. Juhasz-Pocsine K, Rudnicki SA, Archer RL, Harik SI: Neurologic complications of gastric bypass surgery for morbid obesity. Neurology 68:1843-1850, 2007.

153. Plum F, Hindfeldt B: (1976). The neurological complication of liver disease. In Vinken P, Bruyn G (eds): Handbook of Clinical Neurology. Amsterdam, North Holland Publishing, 1976.

154. Heyman SN, Michaeli J, et al: Primary hyperparathyroidism presenting as cervical myelopathy. Am J Med Sci 291:112-114, 1986.

155. Juchet H, Ollier S, et al: Neurologic and psychiatric manifestations of primary hyperparathyroidism: Study of 5 cases. Rev Med Int 14:123-125, 1993.

156. Melamed E, Berman M, et al: Posterolateral myelopathy associated with thyrotoxicosis [Letter]. N Engl J Med 293:778-779, 1975.

157. Swash M, Schwartz MS: Paraneoplastic syndromes. In Johnson RT: Current Therapies in Neurological Diseases—3. Philadelphia, BC Decker, 1990.

158. Norris F: Remote effects of cancer on the spinal cord. In Vinken P, Bruyn G (eds): Handbook of Clinical Neurology. Amsterdam, North Holland, 1979.

159. Cohen ME, Duffner PK, et al: Myelopathy with severe structural derangement associated with combined modality therapy. Cancer 52:1590-1596, 1983.

160. Gagliano RG, Costanzi JJ: Paraplegia following intrathecal methotrexate: Report of a case and review of the literature. Cancer 37:1663-1668, 1976.

161. Muder RR, Lumish RM, et al: Myelopathy after herpes zoster. Arch Neurol 40:445-446, 1983.

162. Henson RA, Urich H: Cancer and the Nervous System. Oxford, Blackwell Scientific, 1982.

163. Handforth A, Nag S, et al: Paraneoplastic subacute necrotic myelopathy. Can J Neurol Sci 10:204-207, 1983.

164. Dansey RD, Hammond-Tooke GD, et al: Subacute myelopathy: An unusual paraneoplastic complication of Hodgkin's disease. Med Pediatr Oncol 16:284-286, 1988.

165. Posner JB: Paraneoplastic syndromes involving the nervous system. In: Aminoff MJ (ed): Neurology and General Medicine. New York, Churchill Livingstone, 1989.

166. Iwamasa T, Utsumi Y, et al: Two cases of necrotizing myelopathy associated with malignancy caused by herpes simplex virus type 2. Acta Neuropathol 78:252-257, 1989.

167. Schold SC, Cho ES, et al: Subacute motor neuronopathy: A remote effect of lymphoma. Ann Neurol 5:271-287, 1979.

168. Dalmau J, Graus F, Rosenblum MK, et al: Anti-Hu-associated paraneoplastic encephalomyelitis/sensory neuronopathy: A clinical study of 71 patients. Medicine (Baltimore) 71:59-72, 1992.

169. Schwarz S, Zoubaa S, et al: Intravascular lymphomatosis presenting with a conus medullaris syndrome mimicking disseminated encephalomyelitis. Neuro-oncol 4:187-191, 2002.

170. Nakahara T, Saito T, et al: (1999). Intravascular lymphomatosis presenting as an ascending cauda equina conus medullaris syndrome: Remission after biweekly CHOP therapy. J Neurol Neurosurg Psychiatry 67:403-406, 1999.

171. Baumann TP, Hurwitz N, et al: Diagnosis and treatment of intravascular lymphomatosis. Arch Neurol 57:374-377, 2000.

172. Delattre J-Y, Posner J: Paraneoplastic syndromes involving the nervous system. In Aminoff M (ed): Neurology and General Medicine. New York, Churchill Livingstone, 1989.

173. Kagen AR, Wollin M, Gilbert HA, et al: Comparison of the tolerance of the brain and spinal cord to injury by radiation. In: Gilbert HA, Kagen AR (eds): Radiation Damage to the Nervous System. New York, Raven Press, 1980.

174. Palmer JJ: Radiation myelopathy. Brain 95:109-122, 1972.

175. Douglas MA, Parks LC, et al: Sudden myelopathy secondary to therapeutic total-body hyperthermia after spinal-cord irradiation. N Engl J Med 304:583-585, 1981.

176. Jones A: Transient radiation myelopathy (with reference to Lhermitte's sign of electrical paraesthesia). Br J Radiol 37:727-744, 1964.

177. Laqueny A, et al: Syndrome de la corne anterieure postradiotherpique. Rev Neurol (Paris) 141:222, 1985.

178. Sadowsky CH, Sachs E Jr, et al: Postradiation motor neuron syndrome. Arch Neurol 33:786-787, 1976.

179. Steen PA, Michenfelder JD: Neurotoxicity of anesthetics. Anesthesiology 50:437-453, 1979.

180. Usubiaga JE: Neurological complications following epidural anesthesia. Int Anesthesiol Clin 13:1-153, 1975.

181. Dripps RD: Anesthesia. Annu Rev Med 5:305-322, 1954.

182. Phillips OC, Ebner H, et al: Neurologic complications following spinal anesthesia with lidocaine: A prospective review of 10,440 cases. Anesthesiology 30:284-289, 1969.

183. Pujol S, Torrielli R: Neurological accidents after epidural anesthesia in obstetrics. Cah Anesthesiol 44:341-345, 1996.

184. Dawkins CJ: An analysis of the complications of extradural and caudal block. Anaesthesia 24:554-563, 1969.

185. Kane RE: Neurologic deficits following epidural or spinal anesthesia. Anesth Analg 60:150-161, 1981.

186. Davies A, Solomon B, et al: Paraplegia following epidural anaesthesia. BMJ 2:654-657, 1958.

187. Ackerman WE, Juneja MM, et al: Maternal paraparesis after epidural anesthesia and cesarean section. South Med J 83:695-697, 1990.

188. Vandam LD, Dripps RD: Exacerbation of pre-existing neurologic disease after spinal anesthesia. N Engl J Med 255:843-849, 1956.

189. Munro D: Fluorescent screen amplification. Radiography 22:102-103, 1956.

190. Hessel SJ, et al: Complications of angiography. Radiology 138:273-281, 1981.

191. Feigelson HH, Ravin HA: Transverse myelitis following selective bronchial arteriography. Radiology 85:663-665, 1965.

192. Killen DA, Foster JH: Spinal cord injury as a complication of aortography. Ann Surg 152:211-230, 1960.

193. Layzer RB: Myeloneuropathy after prolonged exposure to nitrous oxide. Lancet 2:1227-1230, 1978.

194. Blanco G, Peters HA: Myeloneuropathy and macrocytosis associated with nitrous oxide abuse. Arch Neurol 40:416-418, 1983.

195. Shapiro WR, Young DF: Neurological complications of antineoplastic therapy. Acta Neurol Scand Suppl 100:125-132, 1984.

196. Clark AW, Cohen SR, et al: Paraplegia following intrathecal chemotherapy: Neuropathologic findings and elevation of myelin basic protein. Cancer 50:42-47, 1982.

197. Hahn AF, Feasby TE, et al: Paraparesis following intrathecal chemotherapy. Neurology 33:1032-1038, 1983.

198. Mastaglia FL: Neurology and General Medicine. New York, Churchill Livingstone, 1989.

199. Bernat JL: Intraspinal steroid therapy. Neurology 31:168-171, 1981.

200. Richter R: Drug abuse. In Rowland L (ed): Merritt's Textbook of Neurology. Philadelphia, Lea & Febiger, 1984.

201. Sobue I, Ando K, et al: Myeloneuropathy with abdominal disorders in Japan: A clinical study of 752 cases. Neurology 21:168-173, 1971.

202. Chaduri R: Paralytic disease caused by contamination with tricresyl phosphate. Trop Med Hyg 59:98, 1965.

203. Smith HV, Spalding JM: Outbreak of paralysis in Morocco due to ortho-cresyl phosphate poisoning. Lancet 2:1019-1021, 1959.

204. Sprofkin BE: Electrical injuries. In Rowland L (ed): Merritt's Textbook of Neurology. Philadelphia, Lea & Febiger, 1984.

205. Varghese G, Mani MM, et al: Spinal cord injuries following electrical accidents. Paraplegia 24:159-166, 1986.

206. Levine NS, Atkins A, et al: Spinal cord injury following electrical accidents: Case reports. J Trauma 15:459-463, 1975.

207. Winkleman M: Complications of thermal and electrical burns. In Aminoff M (ed): Neurology and General Medicine. New York, Churchill Livingstone, 1995, pp 915-930.

208. Davidson GS, Deck JH: Delayed myelopathy following lightning strike: A demyelinating process. Acta Neuropathol 77:104-108, 1988.

209. Holbrook LA, Beach FX, et al: Delayed myelopathy: A rare complication of severe electrical burns. BMJ 4:659-660, 1970.

210. Clouston PD, Sharpe D: Rapid recovery after delayed myelopathy from electrical burns. J Neurol Neurosurg Psychiatry 52:1308, 1989.

211. Jackson FE, Martin R, et al: Delayed quadriplegia following electrical burn. Milit Med 130:601-605, 1965.

212. Farrell DF, Starr A: Delayed neurological sequelae of electrical injuries. Neurology 18:601-606, 1968.

213. Critchley M: Industrial electrical accidents in their neurological aspect. J State Med 40:459, 1932.

214. Gwozdziewicz J: Changes in the spinal cord of divers connected with chronic forms of caisson disease. Biul Inst Med Morsk Gdansk 16:171-185, 1965.

215. Mastaglia FL, McCallum RI, et al: Myelopathy associated with decompression sickness: A report of six cases. Clin Exp Neurol 19:54-59, 1983.

216. Kim SW, Kim RC, et al: Non-traumatic ischaemic myelopathy: A review of 25 cases. Paraplegia 26:262-272, 1988.

217. Bokeriia LA, Kobaneva RA: Hyperbaric oxygenation in caisson disease. Kilin Med (Mosk) 51:50, 1973.

218. Fink JK, Heiman-Patterson T, et al: Hereditary spastic paraplegia: Advances in genetic research. Hereditary Spastic Paraplegia Working group. Neurology 46:1507-1514, 1996.

219. Campuzano V, Montermini L, et al: Friedreich's ataxia: Autosomal recessive disease caused by an intronic GAA triplet repeat expansion. Science 271:1423-1427, 1996.

220. Aboulafia DM, Saxton EH, et al: A patient with progressive myelopathy and antibodies to human T-cell leukemia virus type I and human immunodeficiency virus type 1 in serum and cerebrospinal fluid. Arch Neurol 47:477-479, 1990.

221. McArthur JC, Griffin JW, et al: Steroid-responsive myeloneuropathy in a man dually infected with HIV-1 and HTLV-I. Neurology 40:938-944, 1990.

222. Tucker T, Dix RD, et al: Cytomegalovirus and herpes simplex virus ascending myelitis in a patient with acquired immune deficiency syndrome. Ann Neurol 18:74-79, 1985.

223. Britton CB, Mesa-Tejada R, et al: A new complication of AIDS: Thoracic myelitis caused by herpes simplex virus. Neurology 35:1071-1074, 1985.

224. McArthur JC: Neurologic manifestations of AIDS. Medicine (Baltimore) 66:407-437, 1987.

225. Doll DC, Yarbro JW, et al: Mycobacterial spinal cord abscess with an ascending polyneuropathy. Ann Intern Med 106:333-334, 1987.

226. Woolsey RM, Chambers TJ, et al: Mycobacterial meningomyelitis associated with human immunodeficiency virus infection. Arch Neurol 45:691-693, 1988.

227. Berger JR: Spinal-cord syphilis associated with human-immunodeficiency-virus infection—a treatable myelopathy. Am J Med 92:101-103, 1992.

228. Herskovitz S, Siegel SE, et al: Spinal cord toxoplasmosis in AIDS. Neurology 39:1552-1553, 1989.

229. Berger JR, Sheremata WA, et al: Multiple sclerosis-like illness occurring with human immunodeficiency virus infection. Neurology 39:324-329, 1989.

230. Weill O, Finaud M, et al: Malignant spinal cord glioma: A new complication of HIV virus infection? Presse Med 16:1977, 1987.

38
CHAPTER

Nonoperative Management of Cervical Disc and Degenerative Disorders

Clayton L. Dean, MD
John M. Rhee, MD

Degenerative, or spondylotic, cervical conditions comprise a spectrum of disorders including degenerative disc disease with axial neck pain, cervical radiculopathy from root compression, and cervical myelopathy from compression of the spinal cord. In most cases, the underlying pathoanatomy begins with degeneration of the cervical disc. Subsequently, the disc can herniate or bulge, causing spinal cord or nerve root compression. Significant loss of disc height may lead to segmental kyphosis. Abnormal kinematics in the motion segment can lead to instability or to the formation of compensatory osteophytes at the level of the disc space and in the uncovertebral joints, which can also cause neural compression. Facet joints may hypertrophy, causing foraminal stenosis, and the ligamentum flavum can hypertrophy or buckle, leading to spinal canal stenosis.

Patients with cervical disc and degenerative disorders often seek medical attention for relief of neck pain, arm pain, weakness, or numbness. Except for individuals with myelopathy or severe, progressive weakness, most patients are initially treated nonoperatively because many have a self-limited course that resolves without surgery. This chapter examines the role of nonoperative management in the treatment of degenerative cervical disorders.

Epidemiology

Population-based cross-sectional surveys have shown that acute and chronic neck pain is widely extant in the general population.[1-3] From the Norwegian registry, Bovim and colleagues[1] showed an overall prevalence of neck pain of 34.4%, with 13.8% of these individuals reporting chronic neck pain of greater than 6 months' duration. Similar numbers were reported for chronic neck pain in Finland.[3] In 2000, Cote and colleagues[2] found that 54% of 1131 subjects had experienced significant neck pain in the previous 6 months, with nearly 5% reporting being highly disabled from neck pain. Many cases of acute neck pain may arise from soft tissue sprains and muscle strains, but ongoing neck pain is more suggestive of a spondylotic source.

Natural History

The natural histories of most nonmyelopathic spondylotic cervical disorders are statistically favorable. In a study of 205 patients with axial neck pain[4] and an average follow-up of 15.5 years, 79% noted improvement with nonoperative care, 43% reported a pain-free state, and 32% continued to complain of moderate to severe persistent pain. The severity of the symptoms at initial presentation and a history of a specific injury were suggestive of long-term persistent symptoms.

In the classic study by Lees and Turner,[5] the natural history of cervical radiculopathy was also shown to be generally favorable. Of 51 patients with radiculopathy and long-term follow-up (2 to 19 years), 45% had only a single episode of pain without recurrence, 30% had mild symptoms, and only 25% had persistent or worsening symptoms. No patients with radiculopathy progressed to myelopathy in their series. On the basis of this study and clinical experience and because it is impossible to identify at the onset of symptoms patients who will or will not improve, nonoperative treatment is generally the initial approach for most patients with cervical radiculopathy. Surgery is reserved for patients with neurologic deficits, progressive dysfunction, or failure to improve after an appropriate course of nonoperative treatment. The definition of what constitutes an appropriate course of nonoperative treatment (in terms of duration and actual regimen) has not been standardized, however.

Although nonoperative treatment is the initial "default" pathway for most patients with nonmyelopathic cervical disorders, it is unclear whether commonly used nonoperative regimens improve on natural history. No controlled trials have compared the various nonoperative regimens (e.g., physical therapy, modalities, traction, medications, manipulation, and immobilization) versus the natural history (i.e., no treatment at all). It is also unclear whether nonoperative treatment outcomes can equal outcomes of surgery.

One series of cervical radiculopathy reported that 20 of 26 (77%) patients had good to excellent results with a progressive program of nonoperative treatment consisting of immobilization, ice, rest, nonsteroidal anti-inflammatory drugs [NSAIDs], traction, postural education and strengthening, oral steroid tapers, acupuncture, and transcutaneous electrical nerve stimulation.[6] Based on comparisons with previously published surgical series, the authors suggested that their nonoperative outcomes were comparable to surgical outcomes and superior to the natural history of cervical radiculopathy. This interpretation of the study is limited, however, by the absence of true controls in the surgical or natural history categories.

Another study retrospectively compared outcomes of surgical versus nonsurgical treatment and found favorable outcomes with the latter[7]; however, meaningful comparisons could not be made between the groups in this study because the surgical patients initially presented with more severe disease. In contrast, the real issue is not whether surgery "works" under the appropriate circumstances: Any surgeon who has treated a patient with cervical radiculopathy who has suffered for months despite conservative treatment who wakes up immediately after surgery with complete resolution of symptoms can attest to that fact. The unresolved question remains, however: Given that many patients improve without surgery, when and in whom should surgery be recommended— and is there a way to predict who needs surgery at the outset to avoid delays in delivering the ultimately needed treatment?

Other factors may affect the natural history of cervical spondylosis. Smoking has been well documented as a risk factor for neck pain[8-10] and has been shown to advance degeneration of the intervertebral disc and connective tissues. Smoking also may contribute to accelerated deterioration of an individual's aerobic fitness. Occupations requiring excessive cervical motion and overhead work may accelerate the process of disc degeneration, as can vibration caused by heavy equipment.[8,10-12] For these individuals, a change in occupation may be necessary to alleviate symptoms. Active litigations claims (e.g., motor vehicle accidents) may provide the patient with incentive to have continued complaints. Likewise, active workers' compensation claims have long been recognized to have an adverse effect on the outcomes of injuries sustained on the job.

Cervical myelopathy, by contrast, is generally considered to be a surgical disorder because myelopathy has been shown to be progressive over time.[13] Surgery has also been shown to have better functional and neurologic outcomes than nonoperative care in myelopathy.[14] It is commonly held that early surgery may improve prognosis in myelopathy by limiting the extent of irreversible spinal cord damage. Nonoperative management of myelopathy is reserved for patients with mild cases, in whom careful follow-up is necessary, or patients with prohibitive surgical risk factors.

Goals of Treatment

The immediate goals of treatment are to control the patient's pain and to minimize the disruption of the patient's everyday life. In addition to treatment, education is important in helping the patient to understand the problem and what to expect in the future.

For patients presenting with an acute problem, pain control is generally the first concern. Although medication is commonly the first line of defense, it needs to be viewed as a temporary measure. Because a painful, immobile cervical spine can limit nearly any activity, return of function may be a slow process in cervical degenerative disease. The longer the patient's activity level is limited, the greater the impact on deconditioning. Activity levels may decline even further as the patient becomes fearful that any motion may cause recurrence or exacerbation of the symptoms. This combination of pain and inactivity may result in a patient with chronic pain if left untreated. Table 38–1 summarizes available nonoperative treatments for cervical degenerative disorders.

Bracing, Immobilization, and Rest

A short course of bed rest is used to treat patients with lumbar disorders; cervical collars are analogously used to manage patients with cervical pathology. Immobilization of the neck is thought to diminish inflammation around an irritated nerve root. Immobilization may also diminish muscle spasm. Alternatively, the warmth provided by wearing the collar may be therapeutic.[15] The efficacy of collars in limiting the duration or severity of problems such as radiculopathy has not been shown, however.[16] In one study of patients with whiplash injury, soft collars did not have an effect on the duration or degree of neck pain.[17]

Although short-term use of collars may be beneficial, prolonged immobilization should be avoided to prevent atrophy of the cervical musculature. Most authors recommend weaning off of the collar over no more than 2 weeks. Because extension can often be more painful than flexion for many patients with acute neck spasm, patients may be more comfortable wearing a traditional soft collar "backwards." Wearing the collar this way promotes relative flexion of the neck and enlargement of the neuroforamina. Similarly, use of an inverted-V–shaped pillow during sleep may be beneficial by promoting neck flexion. Nighttime collar wear may be helpful by maintaining proper cervical alignment during the entire night and protecting the discs from abnormal loads associated with poor sleeping posture. After a few days, the collar may be discontinued from wear in the daytime but may be maintained for longer term at night if the patient desires. Hard collars are typically not used because they can be uncomfortable and too rigid.

Ice, Heat, and Passive Modalities

Cold therapy such as ice often provides quick relief of discomfort for patients with acute pain and spasm. Heat may exacerbate the pain during this immediate period. When motion has started to return, heat is more likely to be beneficial. These measures can generally be tried by the patient at home and do not require the attention of a physician unless they are used

TABLE 38-1 Nonoperative Modalities for Treatment of Cervical Disc and Degenerative Disorders

Modality	Pros	Cons
Cervical collars	Immobilization may decrease inflammation and muscle spasm	Muscle atrophy from prolonged use
Ice or heat	Ice may relieve acute pain and spasm; heat beneficial when regaining motion	Heat may exacerbate pain in acute period
Traction	With neck in flexion may relieve foraminal compression	Avoid in myelopathic patients; if neck extended, may worsen compression of narrowed foramen
NSAIDs	Safe, cost-effective method to decrease inflammation	Gastrointestinal side effects, cardiovascular risks with COX-2 inhibitors
Narcotics	Rapid pain relief in acute period	Constipation, sedation, depression, and potential for abuse
Corticosteroids	May decrease radicular pain acutely	Avascular necrosis, increased blood glucose, unproven long-term benefits
Muscle relaxant	Acute relief of muscle spasms	Sedation, fatigue, abuse potential, limits participation in rehabilitation
Exercise and physical therapy	Well tolerated, aerobic conditioning	No long-term pain benefits shown, forceful passive range of motion may lead to further injury and increased pain
Cervical manipulation	Some anecdotal reports of relief	No objective evidence of improvement in pain; rare potential complications including myelopathy, spinal cord injury, vertebrobasilar artery injury
Cervical steroid injections	Anti-inflammatory effect, interruption of nociceptive input/sympathetic blockade, mechanical disruption of adhesions	Rare complications include dural puncture, meningitis, epidural abscess, intraocular hemorrhage, epidural hematoma, adrenocortical suppression, paralysis

COX-2, cyclooxygenase-2; NSAIDs, nonsteroidal anti-inflammatory drugs.

directly to facilitate an active rehabilitation program. Massage, ultrasound, and iontophoresis all have failed to be of proven long-term efficacy.[18] Other passive modalities that require no effort on the part of the patient may also be of limited value because the patient is not an active participant in his or her own recovery.

Traction

Anecdotally, intermittent home traction is said to help relieve symptoms temporarily in patients with axial neck pain or radiculopathy. Traction has failed to show long-term benefit, however, for patients with axial neck pain or cervical radiculopathy.[19-22] Traction should be avoided in myelopathic patients to prevent stretching of a compromised spinal cord. Some instruction sheets for commonly used home traction units still show the patient with his or her back to the door, leading to an extension traction vector; this may worsen arm pain in patients with radiculopathy if the compromised foramen is narrowed further as a result. Instead, traction with the neck in relative flexion is more likely to lead to symptom relief in the patient with radiculopathy. If there is no response during the first few applications, use of traction should be discontinued.

Medications

The most commonly used medications in the treatment of cervical disc disease are anti-inflammatory agents (including corticosteroids), narcotics, muscle relaxants, and antidepressants.[23]

Nonsteroidal Anti-inflammatory Drugs

NSAIDs are commonly used to treat various musculoskeletal conditions including cervical disc disease. The mechanism of action is related to their anti-inflammatory and analgesic effects. Although these medications are generally very safe, patients who are on long-term NSAID therapy should be monitored for potential liver, kidney, and gastrointestinal problems. Aspirin and ibuprofen are readily available over-the-counter and have good effectiveness at low cost. Selective cyclooxygenase-2 inhibitors are now widely accessible and may diminish the incidence of side effects such as stomach upset, but in controlled trials of osteoarthritis, they do not seem to be any more efficacious than nonselective NSAIDs.[24-26] Cyclooxygenase-2 inhibitors also work without inhibiting platelet function. Although many of these agents seem to be well tolerated by most patients even with a history of gastrointestinal problems, potential cardiovascular risks have tempered their routine use.[27]

Narcotics

Narcotic analgesics may be necessary for symptom relief in the early, severe stages of cervical disc disease. Although mild narcotics are a reasonable choice for a patient with acute pain, they are contraindicated for the long-term management of most patients because of their addictive potential and development of tolerance. Narcotics generally should be used in the acute setting as breakthrough treatment to supplement NSAIDs or in patients who cannot tolerate NSAIDs. They should be weaned off as soon as possible. The side-effect profile of narcotics is well established and includes constipation, sedation, and the possibility of abuse. In addition, little attention is paid to the depressant qualities of narcotics, particularly for patients with chronic pain. This depressant quality may be a particular problem for a patient with a preexisting diagnosis of depression.

As patients develop more tolerance to their current narcotic level, the dosage may need to be increased in a continuous cycle. Newer, extended-release narcotics are attractive because they provide a more even blood level for longer periods. More recent trends have been toward formal pain management programs run by various medical specialists, most commonly anesthesiologists, for the treatment of patients in chronic pain, particularly nonspecific axial neck pain, which generally does poorly with surgery. True multidisciplinary pain programs should include a psychological evaluation and emotional support, while seeking to decrease the patient's pain level and teaching the patient to deal with unresolved pain.

Antidepressants and Anticonvulsants

Antidepressants and anticonvulsants are used in the treatment of chronic neuropathic pain syndromes. Amitriptyline is the antidepressant most commonly used for patients with cervical disc disease.[23] It has an effect on depression and may help to improve sleep patterns, a common problem for patients with pain disorders. It has also shown a modest analgesic benefit in a placebo-controlled trial of lower back pain and lumbar radiculopathy.[28] To the authors' knowledge, no such studies exist for the treatment of cervical radiculopathy, however. There is commonly a time lag of several weeks between the onset of administration of these medications (e.g., gabapentin or amitriptyline) and clinical symptom relief. The role of these agents in acute cervical radiculopathy is unclear.

Oral Corticosteroids

Systemic corticosteroids are often administered to patients with acute neck or arm pain.[23] Oral corticosteroid tapers are most commonly used with good anecdotal results but little clinical data. They may diminish radicular pain acutely, but no long-term benefit in altering the natural history has been shown. Corticosteroids are believed to be more effective, however, in patients with radicular arm pain than in patients with axial pain. Because rare but significant complications such as avascular necrosis of the femoral or humeral head can occur, corticosteroids should be used judiciously. They may be contraindicated in patients with severe diabetes because of effects on blood glucose, and patients being administered steroids need to be counseled appropriately.

Muscle Relaxants

Muscle relaxants are also commonly prescribed for patients with cervical disc disease. As a group, muscle relaxants tend to cause significant sedation and fatigue, and they are increasingly being recognized for their abuse potential. Their depressive effect may be more pronounced when administered simultaneously with narcotics. Muscle relaxants should be used as short-term treatment because they may impair the patient's ability to participate in rehabilitation.

Exercise and Physical Therapy

Physical therapy has not been shown to alter the natural history of cervical radiculopathy.[29,30] A graduated program of physical therapy is commonly prescribed for patients after an initial period of short-term rest or immobilization. Passive modalities have not been proven to be beneficial in the long-term,[31] but they are well tolerated by patients and may reduce pain in the short-term when patients are too symptomatic to participate in an active therapy regimen. As the acute pain resolves, isometric exercises to strengthen the cervical musculature are instituted. The concept of isometric exercises is appealing because the muscles may be strengthened without painful motion of the cervical spine. The concern with isometrics is that contraction of the local musculature, most often the trapezius, results in increased loading of the intervertebral discs, which could exacerbate local pain.

Passive motion is to be avoided in general because patients may be unable to protect themselves from injury at the end point of comfortable motion. Forcible passive motion may result in worsening of pain and further motion loss. Aerobic conditioning may also be helpful in relieving symptoms. Aerobic exercise for individuals with spine pain is generally best limited to low-impact activities. Stationary bicycling, walking, use of a Stairmaster machine, and other nonimpact aerobic exercises are preferred to avoid jarring the cervical spine. Active range of motion and resistive exercises may be added as tolerated. This is the phase of rehabilitation when the patient often notices the most gains. It requires the subject to be an active participant in the treatment of his or her own problem, yet education and assurance from the therapist may be needed to keep the patient participating in the program. It is best for the patient to be involved in a whole-body exercise program with special attention to the shoulder girdle and neck musculature.[30] For a patient with cervical disc disease, special attention should be given to the scapular stabilization muscles, including the trapezius, deltoids, latissimus dorsi, and rhomboids.

The final step in the rehabilitation protocol is a home exercise program. This can be thought of as preventive maintenance for the neck. The home program should include a simple exercise program that does not require fancy equipment but rather inexpensive, accessible items. Postural education, ergonomics, and lifestyle modifications may also be beneficial in preventing recurrences.

Cervical Manipulation

No solid evidence exists of clinical effectiveness of manipulative therapy on the cervical spine.[32] Its efficacy for the treatment of cervical radiculopathy has also not been established.[33-35] The possible mechanisms of action for manipulation are poorly understood, although there are numerous theories.[36]

Although very rare, the potential for catastrophic vascular or spinal cord injury exists. For neck pain and cervicogenic headaches, manipulation probably provides short-term benefits, with a complication rate of 5 to 10 per 10 million manipulations.[33] Reported complications of cervical manipulation include radiculopathy, myelopathy, spinal cord injury, and vertebrobasilar artery injury.[7] The actual incidence of these complications is unknown but probably low. Nevertheless, in the absence of objective evidence showing any proven benefit and given the known (albeit low probability) risks, cervical manipulation is not routinely recommended for patients with cervical radiculopathy and should be avoided in patients with known myelopathy.

Cervical manipulation probably should not be undertaken without an adequate radiographic examination to screen for potential instability. Absolute contraindications for spinal manipulation include vertebral fracture or dislocation, infection, malignancy, spondylolisthesis, myelopathy, vertebral hypermobility, Marfan and Ehlers-Danlos syndromes, osteoporosis, spondyloarthropathies, severe diabetes mellitus, anticoagulation therapy, and objective signs of spinal nerve root compromise.[32]

Cervical Steroid Injections

Although epidural steroid and nerve root injections are commonly described in the nonoperative treatment of lumbar disorders including radiculopathy, they are less commonly reported in the treatment of cervical radiculopathy. One potential reason for the disparity may be the intrinsically greater risks of performing steroid injections into the cervical spine. Because the pathophysiology of disc disease and radiculopathy in the cervical spine is presumably similar to that in the lumbar spine, local steroid injections in the cervical spine should work by the same mechanisms postulated for the lumbar spine. These potential mechanisms include (1) an anti-inflammatory effect, with inhibition of prostaglandin synthesis; (2) interruption of nociceptive input from somatic nerves; (3) a direct membrane-stabilizing effect; (4) blockade of neuropeptide synthesis; (5) sympathetic blockade; (6) the mechanical effect of the injectant breaking up epidural adhesions; and (7) blockade of C fiber activity in the dorsal root ganglion.

The clinical use of cervical epidural and nerve root injections is based largely on these theoretical and other anecdotal considerations because well-designed, placebo-controlled studies are lacking. Few randomized studies have been performed. Stav and colleagues[37] performed a randomized, prospective study in 42 patients with complaints of neck pain with or without radiculopathy. Of patients, 25 received methylprednisolone and lidocaine cervical epidural steroid injections at the C5-6 or C6-7 level, and 17 received the same injectant into the posterior cervical musculature. At 1 week after injection, patients receiving epidural steroids had 76% good to excellent outcomes as assessed by a visual analog scale compared with 36% good to excellent outcomes in patients receiving muscle injections. The results were comparable at 1 year (68% good to excellent results for epidural injections vs. 12%

for muscle injections). This study was not blinded, however, and fluoroscopy was not used to localize the injection. The results were not stratified further according to whether the patient presented with neck pain, arm pain, or both.

There are several retrospective studies on the efficacy of cervical epidural injections, but none are conclusive. Cicala and colleagues[38] found 56% to 80% good to excellent results at 6 months after C7-T1 epidural steroid injections. Most of the patients in the study had neck pain rather than radiculopathy arising from a wide variety of diagnoses. Because the natural history of neck pain is a tendency toward resolution in most patients with time, the lack of a control group in this study makes the results difficult to interpret. In a group of 25 patients with a clinical diagnosis of radiculopathy, Rowlingson and Kirschenbaum[39] showed 64% good to excellent results at 15 months after C6-7 or C7-T1 epidural steroid injections. The interpretation of this study was also impaired by the lack of a control group because the natural history of radicular pain is also one of resolution in most cases. Ferrante and colleagues[40] performed a retrospective analysis of 100 patients to determine which characteristics predicted a favorable outcome with cervical epidural steroid injection. They found that patients older than 50 years and patients with radicular rather than axial neck pain had significantly better outcomes at an average of 13.5 months. Patients with radiculopathy arising from cervical disc herniation did statistically worse.

Selective nerve root blocks are a variant of epidural steroid injections. Instead of coating the epidural space with steroids, the selected root or roots are injected. Proposed advantages over epidural injections include (1) specific targeting of problematic roots, resulting in a greater local concentration of steroid at the desired location; (2) diagnostic information obtained by blocking the pain associated with a symptomatic root, which can be used in surgical planning; and (3) avoidance of the spinal canal and of potential complications associated with entry into the epidural space. Slipman and colleagues[41] reported 60% good to excellent results at 21 months in a retrospective study of selective root blocks. In a prospective study, Vallee and colleagues[42] found 50% good to excellent results at 12 months.

Complications of cervical steroid injections are very rare but can occur. Potential complications include dural puncture, meningitis, epidural abscess, intraocular hemorrhage, adrenocortical suppression, and epidural hematoma. A particularly devastating complication is intrinsic spinal cord injury as a result of improper needle placement. Reports exist of patients who sustained cord injury as proven by magnetic resonance imaging (MRI) after cervical epidural injections, presumably because of oversedation and inability to inform the injectionist of pain related to cord irritation during injection.

Several strategies exist for minimizing the incidence of complications. Interlaminar epidural injections are most safely done at C6-7 or C7-T1 because the epidural space is typically larger there. Epidural injections should also be avoided at the level of a large herniated disc, where the cord may be displaced more posteriorly into the epidural space and preclude safe needle entry. Finally, if a dural puncture inadvertently occurs during attempted epidural steroid injection, the procedure should be aborted rather than repeating it at another level because of the potential for neurotoxicity with introduction of certain medications (e.g., Depo-Medrol formulation of methylprednisolone acetate, which contains ethylene glycol, a substance associated with arachnoiditis) into the cerebrospinal fluid. Reports of complications associated with cervical selective nerve root blocks are rare.

Based on the available data, cervical epidural injections or selective root blocks can be expected to yield 50% to 80% good to excellent results in patients with cervical radiculopathy. It is unclear, however, how these results compare with either the natural history of radiculopathy or surgical management. Selective root blocks are theoretically safer than epidural injections, although both have relatively few reported complications.

Some surgeons use selective root blocks to provide confirmatory diagnostic information for preoperative planning, but evidence showing the validity of doing so has been limited. In their analysis of 101 patients, Sasso and colleagues[43] found that a diagnostic selective nerve root injection could safely and accurately discern the presence or absence of cervical radiculopathy. They noted that in cases in which MRI findings are equivocal, multilevel, or do not agree with the patient's symptoms, the result of a negative diagnostic injection becomes superior in predicting the absence of an offending lesion.

Summary

Because the natural history of cervical disc and degenerative disorders favors resolution, nonoperative treatment is initially recommended for patients who do not have a significant neurologic deficit. Many forms of nonoperative treatment are thought to have at least some short-term benefit in reducing pain. None of the commonly used nonoperative therapies have been proven, however, to alter the natural history of the disease in a controlled, prospective manner. Until such studies are available, empirical and anecdotal evidence must be used.

Generally, physicians should adhere to the dictum of *primum non nocere* when prescribing nonoperative regimens. In the absence of proven benefit, treatments should be used only if they are associated with a reasonably low level of risk. A program of gradual, progressive nonoperative treatment seems most reasonable, adding therapies in a stepwise fashion as failure of symptoms to resolve dictates. Short-term bracing and rest, NSAIDs, oral corticosteroid taper, short-term narcotics, physical therapy, and corticosteroid injections can be used judiciously by the treating physician. In patients with myelopathy, progressive or severe neurologic dysfunction, or failure to improve despite time and nonoperative treatment, surgical management should be considered. In properly selected patients, surgical management generally yields excellent outcomes. Patients with nonspecific chronic axial neck pain tend to do poorly with nonoperative and surgical treatment.

PEARLS

1. Population based cross-sectional surveys have shown that acute and chronic neck pain is widely extant in the general population.

2. The natural histories of most nonmyelopathic spondylotic cervical disorders are statistically favorable, with most cases responding to a course of nonoperative treatment. Surgery is reserved for patients with neurologic deficits, progressive dysfunction, or failure to improve after an appropriate course of nonoperative treatment.

3. A short-term course of cervical immobilization is thought to diminish inflammation around an irritated nerve root and diminish muscle spasm.

4. Oral medications, including NSAIDs, narcotic analgesics, antidepressants and anticonvulsants, systemic corticosteroids, and muscle relaxants, have been shown to provide symptom control for patients with cervical disc disease.

5. Based on available data, cervical epidural injections or selective nerve root blocks can be expected to yield 50% to 80% good to excellent results in patients with cervical disc disease and radiculopathy.

PITFALLS

1. The definition of what constitutes an appropriate course of nonoperative treatment in terms of duration and actual regimen has not been standardized.

2. Cervical manipulation should not be undertaken without an adequate radiographic examination to screen for potential instability. Reported complications include radiculopathy, myelopathy, spinal cord injury, and vertebrobasilar artery injury.

3. Although short-term use of collars may be beneficial, prolonged immobilization should be avoided to prevent atrophy of the cervical musculature.

4. Traction should be avoided in myelopathic patients to prevent stretching of a compromised spinal cord. If there is no response to traction during the first few applications, use of traction should be discontinued.

5. Complications of cervical steroid injections are rare but devastating when they occur. These include dural puncture, meningitis, epidural abscess, intraocular hemorrhage, adrenocortical suppression, and epidural hematoma.

KEY POINTS

1. Most cases of cervical disc and degenerative disorders are self-limited and may be treated nonoperatively. An organized, multidisciplinary approach is often required to achieve a successful outcome.

2. Several modifiable factors have been identified, including smoking, obesity, occupational hazards, and psychological factors. These factors should be identified, and patients should be encouraged to alter these behaviors accordingly.

3. Initial treatment of acute pain can include a brief trial of rest and immobilization with a soft cervical collar. Medications including narcotics, NSAIDs, oral steroids, and antidepressants can be beneficial under the correct circumstances and with proper supervision.

4. Participation in an active rehabilitation protocol seems much more likely to be successful than use of passive modalities. A home exercise program that uses inexpensive, accessible equipment may help to prevent future episodes of pain and increase the chances of long-term success.

5. Cervical epidural injections, or selective root blocks, may help in treating radicular arm pain. It is unclear, however, whether injections alter the overall natural history of radiculopathy or surgical management. Patients with radiculopathy seem to have better outcomes with injection than patients with neck pain alone. Selective root blocks are theoretically safer than epidural injections, although both have relatively few reported complications.

6. Patients with myelopathy, severe or progressive neurologic symptoms, or failure to improve with time are good candidates for surgery. Generally, myelopathy and refractory radiculopathy are good indications for surgery, whereas axial neck pain from disc degeneration is not.

KEY REFERENCES

1. Lees F, Turner JWA: Natural history and prognosis of cervical spondylosis. BMJ 2:1607-1610, 1963.
   In this classic study, the natural history of cervical radiculopathy was shown to be generally favorable.

2. Gore D, Sepic S, Gardner G, et al: Neck pain: A long term follow-up of 205 patients. Spine (Phila Pa 1976) 12:1-5, 1987.
   In this study of 205 patients with axial neck pain and an average follow-up of 15.5 years, 79% noted improvement with nonoperative care, 43% reported a pain-free state, and 32% continued to complain of moderate to severe persistent pain. The severity of the symptoms at initial presentation and a history of a specific injury were suggestive of long-term persistent symptoms.

3. Dillin W, Uppal GS: Analysis of medications used in the treatment of cervical disc degeneration. Orthop Clin North Am 23:421-433, 1992.
   This article presents an analysis of commonly used medications for the treatment of cervical disc disease.

4. Tan JC, Nordin M: Role of physical therapy in the treatment of cervical disk disease. Orthop Clin North Am 23:435-449, 1992.
   This study highlights the role of physical therapy and suggests that it is best for patients to be involved in a whole-body exercise program with special attention to the shoulder girdle and neck musculature.

5. Sasso RC, Macadaeg K, Nordmann D, et al: Selective nerve root injections can predict surgical outcome for lumbar and cervical radiculopathy: Comparison to magnetic resonance imaging. J Spinal Disord Tech 18:471-478, 2005.

This analysis of 101 patients found that a diagnostic selective nerve root injection could safely and accurately discern the presence or absence of cervical radiculopathy. The investigators noted that in cases in which MRI findings are equivocal, multilevel, or do not agree with the patient's symptoms, the result of a negative diagnostic injection becomes superior in predicting the absence of an offending lesion.

REFERENCES

1. Bovim G, Schrader H, Sand T: Neck pain in the general population. Spine (Phila Pa 1976) 19:1307-1309, 1994.

2. Cote P, Cassidy J, Carroll L: The factors associated with neck pain and its related disability in the Saskatchewan population. Spine (Phila Pa 1976) 25:1109-1117, 2000.

3. Makela M, Heliovara M, Sievers K, et al: Prevalence, determinants and consequences of chronic neck pain in Finland. Am J Epidemiol 134:1356-1367, 1991.

4. Gore D, Sepic S, Gardner G, et al: Neck pain: A long term follow-up of 205 patients. Spine (Phila Pa 1976) 12:1-5, 1987.

5. Lees F, Turner JWA: Natural history and prognosis of cervical spondylosis. BMJ 2:1607-1610, 1963.

6. Saal JS, Saal JA, Yurth EF: Nonoperative management of herniated cervical intervertebral disc with radiculopathy. Spine (Phila Pa 1976) 21:1877-1883, 1996.

7. Heckmann JG, Lang CJ, Zobelein I, et al: Herniated cervical intervertebral discs with radiculopathy: An outcome study of conservatively or surgically treated patients. J Spinal Disord 12:396-401, 1999.

8. Frymoyer JL, Pope M, Constanza ML, et al: Epidemiologic studies of low back pain. Spine (Phila Pa 1976) 5:419-423, 1980.

9. Holmes S, Nachemson A: Nutrition of the intervertebral disc: Acute effects of cigarette smoking: An experimental animal study. Int J Microcirc Clin Exp 3:406, 1985.

10. Kelsey J, Githens P, O'Connor T, et al: Acute prolapsed lumbar intervertebral disc: An epidemiologic study with special reference to driving automobiles and cigarette smoking. Spine (Phila Pa 1976) 9:608-613, 1984.

11. Anderson G: Epidemiologic aspects of low back pain in industry. Spine (Phila Pa 1976) 6:53-60, 1981.

12. Kelsey J, Githens P, White A, et al: An epidemiologic study of lifting and twisting on the job and risk for acute prolapsed lumbar intervertebral disc. J Orthop Res 2:61-66, 1984.

13. Nurick S: The natural history and the results of surgical treatment of the spinal cord disorder associated with cervical spondylosis. Brain 95:101-108, 1972.

14. Sampath P, Bendebba M, Davis JD, et al: Outcome of patients treated for cervical myelopathy: A prospective, multi-center study with independent clinical review. Spine (Phila Pa 1976) 25:670-676, 2000.

15. Kurz LT: Cervical disc disease: Nonoperative treatment. In Herkowitz HN, Rothman RH, Simeone FA (eds): Rothman-Simeone, The Spine, 4th ed. Philadelphia, WB Saunders, 1999, p 496.

16. Naylor JR, Mulley GP: Surgical collars: A survey of their prescription and use. Br J Rheumatol 30:282-284, 1991.

17. Gennis P, Miller L, Gallagher EJ, et al: The effect of soft cervical collars on persistent neck pain in patients with whiplash injury. Acad Emerg Med 3:568-573, 1996.

18. Philadelphia Panel Evidence-Based Clinical Practice Guidelines on Selected Rehabilitation Interventions for Neck Pain. Phys Ther 18:1701-1717, 2001.

19. Pain in the neck and arm: A multicentre trial of the effects of physiotherapy, arranged by the British Association of Physical Medicine. BMJ 5482:253-258, 1966.

20. Moeti P, Marchetti G: Clinical outcome from mechanical intermittent cervical traction for the treatment of cervical radiculopathy: A case series. J Orthop Sports Phys Ther 31:207-213, 2001.

21. Moeti P, Marchetti G: Erratum: Clinical outcome from mechanical intermittent cervical traction for the treatment of cervical radiculopathy: A case series. J Orthop Sports Phys Ther 31:538, 2001.

22. Swezey RL, Swezey AM, Warner K: Efficacy of home cervical traction therapy. Am J Phys Med Rehabil 78:30-32, 1999.

23. Dillin W, Uppal GS: Analysis of medications used in the treatment of cervical disc degeneration. Orthop Clin North Am 23:421-433, 1992.

24. Bensen WG: Antiinflammatory and analgesic efficacy of COX-2 specific inhibition: From investigational trials to clinical experience. J Rheumatol Suppl 60:17-24, 2000.

25. Bensen WG, Zhao SZ, Burke TA, et al: Upper gastrointestinal tolerability of celecoxib, a COX-2 specific inhibitor, compared to naproxen and placebo. J Rheumatol 27:1876-1883, 2000.

26. Day R, Morrison B, Luza A, et al: A randomized trial of the efficacy and tolerability of the COX-2 inhibitor rofecoxib vs ibuprofen in patients with osteoarthritis. Rofecoxib/Ibuprofen Comparator Study Group. Arch Intern Med 160:1781-1787, 2000.

27. Graham DJ, Campen D, Hui R, et al: Risk of acute myocardial infarction and sudden cardiac death in patients treated with cyclo-oxygenase 2 selective and non-selective non-steroidal anti-inflammatory drugs: Nested case-control study. Lancet 365:475-481, 2005.

28. Atkinson JH, Slater MA, Williams RA, et al: A placebo-controlled randomized clinical trial of nortriptyline for chronic low back pain. Pain 76:287-296, 1998.

29. Levine MJ, Albert TJ, Smith MD: Cervical radiculopathy: Diagnosis and nonoperative management. J Am Acad Orthop Surg 4:305-316, 1996.

30. Tan JC, Nordin M: Role of physical therapy in the treatment of cervical disk disease. Orthop Clin North Am 23:435-449, 1992.

31. Santiesteban AJ: The role of physical agents in the treatment of spine pain. Clin Orthop Relat Res 24-30, 1983.

32. LaBan MM, Taylor RS: Manipulation: An objective analysis of the literature. Orthop Clin North Am 23:451-459, 1992.

33. Haldeman S, Kohlbeck FJ, McGregor M: Unpredictability of cerebrovascular ischemia associated with cervical spine manipulation therapy: A review of sixty-four cases after cervical spine manipulation. Spine (Phila Pa 1976) 27:49-55, 2002.

34. Stevinson C, Honan W, Cooke B, et al: Neurological complications of cervical spine manipulation. J R Soc Med 94:107-110, 2001.

35. Schellhas KP, Latchaw RE, Wendling LR, et al: Vertebrobasilar injuries following cervical manipulation. JAMA 244:1450-1453, 1980.

36. Pickar JG: Neurophysiological effects of spinal manipulation. Spine J 2:357-371, 2002.

37. Stav A, Ovadia L, Sternberg A, et al: Cervical epidural steroid injection for cervicobrachialgia. Acta Anaesthesiol Scand 37:562-566, 1993.

38. Cicala RS, Thoni K, Angel JJ: Long-term results of cervical epidural steroid injections. Clin J Pain 5:143-145, 1989.

39. Rowlingson JC, Kirschenbaum LP: Epidural analgesic techniques in the management of cervical pain. Anesth Analg 65:938-942, 1986.

40. Ferrante FM, Wilson SP, Iacobo C, et al: Clinical classification as a predictor of therapeutic outcome after cervical epidural steroid injection. Spine (Phila Pa 1976) 18:730-736, 1993.

41. Slipman CW, Lipetz JS, Plastaras CT, et al: Therapeutic zygapophyseal joint injections for headaches emanating from the C2-3 joint. Am J Phys Med Rehabil 80:182-188, 2001.

42. Vallee JN, Feydy A, Carlier RY, et al: Chronic cervical radiculopathy: Lateral-approach periradicular corticosteroid injection. Radiology 218:886-892, 2001.

43. Sasso RC, Macadaeg K, Nordmann D, et al: Selective nerve root injections can predict surgical outcome for lumbar and cervical radiculopathy: Comparison to magnetic resonance imaging. J Spinal Disord Tech 18:471-478, 2005.

CHAPTER 39

Surgical Management of Axial Pain

Timothy A. Garvey, MD

Patients who present for evaluation rarely state, "I have C7 radiculopathy from a soft herniated intervertebral disc on right hand side at C6-7." Rather, they complain of pain, weakness, numbness, or some combination of these. Most often, their actual chief complaint is that of neck pain. On careful assessment, the physician may determine that the individual has radiculopathy—generation of symptoms from pathology associated with a specific cervical nerve root, which manifests in the form of pain perceived in the neck, upper trapezium, parascapular region, or distally into the arm.

The assessment consists of obtaining a through history and physical examination with judicious use of imaging studies or laboratory values or both, which allows a specific diagnosis to be rendered. With that diagnosis, the physician counsels the patient about the operative and nonoperative options that exist for that specific patient, with his or her uniqueness, as related to the given diagnosis. This chapter is designed to enable the reader to approach the patient with a chief complaint of "neck pain" with a rational surgical decision-making process.

Epidemiology and Natural History

Having an appreciation of the factors that affect the health of the population is important in understanding the individual who seeks treatment. A study of adolescents concerning the prevalence of musculoskeletal pain in Finland revealed only approximately 25% of 18-year-old girls and about 50% of boys with no report of neck or arm pain in the last 6 months.[1] Of these self-reports to questions about musculoskeletal pain, only a small single-digit percentage sought medical consultation. The author's of the Finnish study note that this prevalence is high, but that the relevance of such reported pain is questionable without knowing the magnitude of the pain-related disability.

It is known from population-based sectional survey studies that numerous individuals complain of acute or chronic neck pain.[2-4] The overall prevalence of "troubles or neck pain" was 34.4% in a Norwegian registry, with 13.8% of that group reporting chronic neck pain of greater than 6 months' duration.[2] Similar numbers were reported by Makela and colleagues[4] in a study of chronic neck pain in Finland. In an article on the Saskatchewan population published in 2000, Cotes and colleagues[3] found that 54% of 1131 respondents had experienced neck pain in the previous 6 months. Of that group, 5% reported that they were "highly disabled" because of neck pain. A comprehensive review by Manchikanti and colleagues[5] suggested that the prevalence of people with high pain intensity with disability owing to neck pain is 15%, with 25% to 60% having chronic symptoms 1 year or longer after the initial episode. Complaints of neck pain in the population are common, if the question is asked, but only a small percentage are plagued enough to seek care; if they do seek care, a fair number of people have persistent pain that may lead to surgical consultation.

Why Understanding the Natural History of a Condition Is Crucial

The speed and intensity of assessment of a patient vary depending on whether the condition is benign and self-limiting or one that without urgent intervention would be fatal or lead to serious disability. A patient who presents with an acute progressive loss of neurologic function owing to an expanding epidural abscess, mandates emergent treatment, most often surgical, because of the dismal prognosis if left untreated. Alternatively, a healthy, young individual with neck pain, with no fever or chills, who is normal neurologically, often improves spontaneously, and in such a case, patient reassurance is advised. It is important that the initial evaluation screen out patients with the potential for an ominous diagnosis, such as tumor, infection, significant progressive myelopathy, or an unstable segment owing to inflammatory arthropathy.

In patients with apparent mechanical axial pain resulting from a degenerative condition, observation with nonoperative recommendations would be appropriate for most patients. When reviewing natural history studies, there is the inherent selection bias of individuals who sought care because of the severity of their symptoms. Many individuals who report pain on population surveys of prevalence of symptoms would not seek out care. In a population questionnaire study, Badcock and colleagues[6] found that 11.7% of questionnaire responders had neck pain and that 21% sought general practice consultation; 77% of responders seeking consultation had persistent symptoms, which was a greater percentage of persistent disability than among responders who did not seek out consultation.

Gore and colleagues[7] published a classic series on the long-term follow-up of patients who present with neck pain. With a minimum 10-year follow-up, clinical and radiographic data were reported on 205 patients with a chief complaint of neck pain. Of that group, "79% had a decrease in pain, and 43% were pain free; however, 32% had moderate to severe pain."[7] The investigators noted that a specific injury and severity of the initial pain were suggestive of having an unsatisfactory long-term outcome.

In an earlier edition of this text, Rothman[8] stated that "it does not appear that cervical disc degeneration is a brief, self limiting disorder, but rather a chronic disease, productive of significant pain and incapacity over an extended period of time." DePalma and Subin[9] reported in 1965 that among patients treated nonoperatively for "cervical syndrome," only 45% of those presenting for treatment with a chief complaint of neck pain or neck with arm pain had a long-term satisfactory outcome. In a series of the results of anterior cervical discectomy and fusion (ACDF) for cervical spondylosis, DePalma and colleagues[10] reported that 21% had complete relief at 3 months with nonoperative care, whereas 22% had no relief. In a 5-year follow-up study of patients presenting with significant complaints of pain secondary to cervical disc degeneration, Rothman and Rashbaum[11] noted that 23% remained partially or totally disabled.

When one looks at more recent publications, these classic studies are mirrored. Walker and colleagues[12] performed a randomized clinical trial of manual physical therapy and exercise compared with minimal intervention in 94 patients presenting with neck pain, with or without arm pain. At 1-year follow-up, 62% of patients perceived success with treatment, which means that 38% had persistent symptoms, and only 32% in the minimum intervention group perceived treatment success, which means that 68% had persistent complaints. A classic study of the natural history of cervical spondylosis by Lees and Turner[13] and a review in the 1980s showed that patients presenting with cervical radiculopathy do not typically progress to myelopathy. Two thirds of patients treated with nonoperative care had consistent complaints of pain, although not severe in all.

Studies on epidemiology and natural history would suggest that in patients whose symptoms are severe enough to present for evaluation and care, only a small percentage, perhaps 20% to 30%, have symptoms of sufficient magnitude to warrant consideration of a surgical diagnostic workup. Although a small percentage, it nonetheless represents a significant number of patients who deserve a rational surgical decision-making approach from the medical team, as opposed to nihilism.

Etiology

Understanding the cause or reason for an individual patient's symptoms is crucial in allowing the physician to make treatment recommendations. Although the most common reason—and the focus of this chapter—that a surgeon sees a patient in consultation for neck pain is a degenerative condition, one must maintain an initial broad differential diagnosis. A patient with a metastatic pathologic fracture of C6 may not know he or she has a tumor as the etiology of his or her "neck pain." It is up to the physician to determine this and then direct the care that leads to a medical evaluation; imaging and laboratory assessment, likely including biopsy; and potential for surgical management with decompression and reconstruction. The chief complaint of neck pain was the entry into the rational surgical decision-making approach.

If the broad differential diagnosis leads to infection as the etiology, be it discitis or osteomyelitis, with potentially an epidural abscess, the patient requires a more through diagnostic workup, which would lead to surgical intervention if medical treatment has failed, if a tissue diagnosis needs to be established, or if there is neurologic deterioration. Patients with systemic arthritides may be seen. Typically, this is a patient with rheumatoid arthritis whose neck pain is out of context to their other joint pains and is not responding to current immunologically mediated treatment. One may see "staircase" subaxial multilevel degenerative spondylolisthesis or craniocervical instability that leads to a recommendation for fusion surgery. Patients presenting with neck pain may not know that they have a seropositive arthritis, and the surgical evaluation could best help redirect away from surgery to enhanced rheumatologic care.

Trauma is always part of a broad differential diagnosis, and in cases of obvious fracture-dislocations, surgical management often is the preferred treatment. In certain conditions such as ankylosing spondylitis, even trivial trauma leading to a complaint of neck pain needs careful scrutiny because the patient may have a serious fracture pattern that can lead to progressive deformity or neurologic loss of function if left untreated.

In relation to trauma, numerous patients are seen who have a rear-end mechanism motor vehicle accident as the etiology for their complaint of neck pain—that is, a "whiplash" injury. The Quebec Task Force on Whiplash-Associated Disorders produced a monograph concluding that patients should be reassured that whiplash-associated disorder is "almost always" self-limited and that it "rarely results in permanent harm."[14] In rebuttal, Freeman and colleagues[15] performed a methodologic critique of the literature and stated, "there is no epidemiologic or scientific basis in the literature for the following statement: whiplash injuries do not lead to chronic pain, rear end impact collisions that do not result in vehicle damage are unlikely to cause injury, and whiplash trauma is biomechanically comparable with common movements of daily living."

Although currently there is an emphasis on performing better designed studies of early nonoperative management of whiplash-associated injuries, a rich history of observational studies does not exist.[16] McNab[17] reported on 266 patients, out of an original group of 575 patients with soft tissue neck injuries, who were 2 years after settlement of court issues, so as to minimize the bias of legal secondary gain. Of these 266 patients, 145 were available for review, with 121 reporting persistent pain; at minimum, 45% (121 of 266) had symptoms 2 years after court settlement per their injury.[17,18] In a similar type of study, Hohl[19] noted that of 146 patients who had no pr-existing degenerative condition, 45% had persistent pain 5 years after injury, and in a continuing series from the United Kingdom following patients with whiplash injuries, 66% were noted to have complaints of pain at 2 years after injury, with 10-year follow-up revealing reports of "intrusive pain" and 28% "severe" pain in 12%.[20-22] In a prospective Scandinavian series of 93 patients, Hildingsson and Toolanen[23] noted complete recovery in 42%, mild discomfort in 14%, and significant residual complaints in 44%. Likewise, Jonsson and colleagues[24] reported that 28% (14 of 50) of patients with whiplash distortions had persistent symptoms. Although changing from a tort to no-fault system, to eliminate compensation for pain and suffering, decreases the percentages with whiplash injury from a motor vehicle accident, Cassidy and colleagues[25] wrote that the prognosis for individuals with whiplash injury is affected by "… Intrinsic factors such as age, sex, and initial intensity of the pain." In a series on early aggressive care for patients with whiplash injury, Cote and colleagues[26] noted that their "results add to the body of evidence suggesting that early aggressive treatment of whiplash injuries does not promote faster recovery."

When seeing a patient with whiplash-associated injuries, it would seem that clinicians may counsel them that "usually" or "more often" their pain will subside as they heal themselves and that only a "low percentage" will have long-term permanent damage. This counseling is in contrast, however, to the wording that the patient "almost always" gets better and "rarely has permanent harm" as suggested by the Quebec Task Force.[14] In perhaps 10% to 20% of an original whiplash injury population, a surgeon would benefit a patient by proceeding with a diagnostic evaluation to objectify specific anatomic pathologies that may be remedied with open or minimally invasive surgical intervention.

Patient Evaluation

History

Evaluation of a patient with a chief complaint of neck pain is no different than evaluation for any other complaint of spinal pain. Obtaining a thoughtful history, performing an insightful physical examination, and carefully reviewing imaging studies yield a differential diagnosis and likely a favored specific diagnosis.

One needs to assess the onset (traumatic vs. nontraumatic, acute vs. insidious) and the location of the pain and whether it is local, referred (basioccipital, upper trapezial, or periscapular), or radicular into the arm. A specific assessment of the component that is related to neck pain versus arm pain is crucial (e.g., 80% neck pain and headaches vs. 20% arm pain). Neurologic symptoms of numbness, tingling, weakness, sphincter dysfunction, or ataxia are sought. The pattern of pain is important. Is the pain worse with flexion activities? Does it increase as the day goes on and respond to rest? This finding would suggest a discogenic source, which is a common presenting condition. Unilateral radiation to the upper trapezial and interscapular region that restricts turning the head to that side suggests a radicular component. A history of a known diagnosis of cancer or infection is noted, and constitutional symptoms of night pain, rest pain, fever, and weight loss are reviewed. The social history documents the presence or absence of litigation, workers' compensation activity, and use of tobacco. The family history may suggest a genetic predisposition. The patient's self-reported documentation should be reviewed (e.g., pain diagrams, visual analog scale [VAS], self-reported functional scale, SF-36, patient expectations). The pain diagram can be very useful in the assessment of axial mechanical pain with the continuum of those suggesting an anatomic source that makes one think more of a surgical option versus those suggesting a nonorganic source where one thinks less of invasive testing to determine a surgical option (Fig. 39–1A).

The psychosocial evaluation is critical. True malingerers are rare but do exist.[27] Symptom amplification, drug-seeking behavior, work-related litigation, motor vehicle accident litigation, clinical depression, and frank psychiatric dysfunction all can have an impact on the patient's self-perceived outcome as it relates to the success of elective surgical intervention for axial neck pain. A patient with a nonorganic diagram (Fig. 39–1B) who presents with a history of daily intake of high doses of narcotics, with active litigation, and who smokes two packs of cigarettes per day would suggest delay in surgical management. In a published series in 2002 on axial neck pain, the author and colleagues were unable to correlate a negative outcome with the presence or absence of litigation or cigarette smoking.[28] A series from Cleveland documented that of patients who took daily narcotics for greater than 6 months, 51% (24 of 47) reported good to excellent outcome, and 32% (15 of 47) had a poor result.[29] These findings contrast with patients without chronic narcotic use having 86% (38 of 44) good to excellent outcomes and no patients with a poor outcome.[29]

Physical Examination

A thorough physical examination follows the history. The range of motion, or limitation of such, is recorded. Motor function, sensation, deep tendon reflexes, upper motor neuron signs (e.g., Hoffmann, Babinski, clonus), gait, and provocative or ameliorative maneuvers are evaluated. Although the neurologic examination may seem less important in patients with complaints of 90% neck pain and 10% arm pain, it is still vital to rule out myelopathy or significant dysfunction, and it is useful for clinical correlation. In a patient who presents with complaints of 90% neck pain and 10% arm pain into the right thumb and index finger and who has decreased sensation in a C6 distribution, with a diminished brachioradialis reflex and

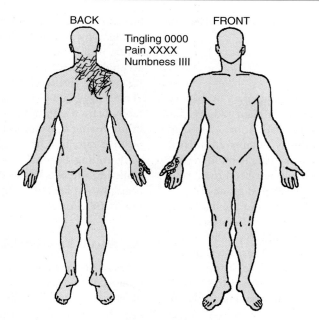

BACK   FRONT

Tingling 0000
Pain XXXX
Numbness IIII

EXPECTATIONS
1. What expectations do you have for your treatment at this office?
(CHECK ONLY ONE RESPONSE FOR EACH STATEMENT)

As a result of my treatment, I expect...	Not likely	Slightly likely	Somewhat likely	Very likely	Extremely likely
a. Complete pain relief	☐	☐	▣	☐	☐
b. Moderate pain relief	☐	☐	☐	▣	☐
c. To be able to do more everyday household or yard activities	☐	☐	☐	▣	☐
d. To be able to sleep more comfortably	☐	☐	☐	▣	☐
e. To be able to go back to my usual job	☐	☐	☐	▣	☐
f. To be able to do more sports, go biking, or go for long walks	☐	☐	☐	▣	☐

A

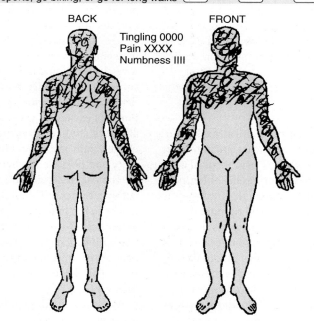

BACK   FRONT

Tingling 0000
Pain XXXX
Numbness IIII

EXPECTATIONS
1. What expectations do you have for your treatment at this office?
(CHECK ONLY ONE RESPONSE FOR EACH STATEMENT)

As a result of my treatment, I expect...	Not likely	Slightly likely	Somewhat likely	Very likely	Extremely likely
a. Complete pain relief	☐	☐	☐	☐	▣
b. Moderate pain relief	☐	☐	☐	☐	▣
c. To be able to do more everyday household or yard activities	☐	☐	☐	☐	▣
d. To be able to sleep more comfortably	☐	☐	☐	☐	▣
e. To be able to go back to my usual job	☐	☐	☐	☐	▣
f. To be able to do more sports, go biking, or go for long walks	☐	☐	☐	☐	▣

B

FIGURE 39–1 Contrast these two scenarios. **A,** Pain diagram showing anatomic pathology with realistic expectations of what surgery can do. **B,** Pain diagram linked with expectations that would, by themselves, not suggest pursuit of a surgical option.

with decreasing symptoms with shoulder abduction, a C5-6 disc herniation is suggested.

Radiographic Evaluation

The outpatient evaluation should be sequential. A history and physical examination are followed by plain radiographs before magnetic resonance imaging (MRI) or computed tomography (CT). The author routinely obtains an anteroposterior, lateral, and flexion-extension lateral radiographic series. Open-mouth or oblique views do not need to be routinely obtained. These radiographs are ordered for destructive processes that indicate tumor or infection (and the history of axial neck pain did not suggest such) or for the presence of foraminal stenosis, for which one would typically obtain advanced imaging. The presence of spondylosis, as evidenced by loss of disc height, subchondral sclerosis, cyst formation, or osteophyte formation, and the presence of listhesis with any dynamic component to suggest mechanical instability are documented. Using these factors, the author and colleagues have reported on a quantitive radiographic scoring system, which yields a cervical degenerative index.[30,31] This objective assessment may be useful to follow patients regarding the progression of disease or patients who have had surgery regarding the development of adjacent segment degeneration. The index is an expansion of Gore's assessment, and a higher score indicates more radiographic pathology at more levels. In a young patient with multilevel spondylosis, one would tend to encourage nonoperative treatment. The presence of spondylosis on radiographs is nonspecific and does exist in asymptomatic individuals, but the review of plain radiographs is still quite useful.[32,33]

Advanced Imaging

In a patient who has dominant axial mechanical neck pain, who has failed 12 months of nonoperative care, including an active rehabilitative component, in whom a psychosocial contraindication does not exist, and who perceives his or her pain to be so severe to consider surgical options, the next step is MRI. If MRI is contraindicated (e.g., pacemaker or metal fragment in the eye), a CT myelogram is done. The scan is reviewed for tumor, infection, or neurologic compression, but in this subgroup of axial pain, a special note is made of disc morphology, annular tears, small central herniations, listhesis with facet arthrosis, and the number of levels of involvement. In a patient who has a clinical correlation of C6 pattern, such as the previously mentioned patient with 90% neck pain and 10% arm pain, who has a central to right small C5-6 herniated nucleus pulposus with pristine-appearing C4-5 and C6-7 levels, no additional testing may be necessary. A C5-6 ACDF may be an option, but in this group of patients with axial pain, this type of clear-cut scenario is uncommon, and additional testing is more often advised. Also, numerous asymptomatic individuals have degenerative change on their studies, and the presence of these changes increases with age.[34-37]

The debate on the rational basis to use discography continues.[38,39] Nordin and colleagues,[38] citing a critical review of the literature, stated that "no evidence supports using provocative discography, anesthetic facet, or medial branch blocks in evaluating neck pain." Manchikanti and colleagues[39] reported on a comprehensive search of the literature, using a modified Agency for Health Care Research and Quality (AHRQ) level of evidence evaluation, and documented that "cervical discography plays a significant role in selecting surgical candidates in improving outcomes, despite concerns regarding the false positive rate, lack of standardization, and assorted potential confounding factors." Because of this discrepancy, perhaps related to the bias of the groups, an expanded review of discography is planned. In the author's experience, discography is a useful clinical tool.

Advanced Invasive Diagnostics

Discography as a diagnostic tool is controversial. If one wishes to consider surgical options in patients with axial neck pain, of whom many have a discogenic source, the use of discography should be considered to maximize the surgical success rate.[28,35,40-45] This topic is discussed later in the section on surgical outcomes for axial neck pain.

To provide a surgical solution, objectification is the crucial factor. Because of the numerous asymptomatic individuals with positive MRI studies, procedures based on MRI alone for level selection in patients with dominant axial pain would have to have a very strong clinical correlation, such as a component of radiculopathy that fits with a specific herniated nucleus pulposus. Schellhas and colleagues[35] published an article on the prospective correlation of discography and MRI in asymptomatic subjects and subjects with neck pain. These investigators concluded that MRI did not reliably identify the source of discogenic pain because annular tears often escape detection. It was not surprising that degenerative anatomic findings existed in the asymptomatic group. In only 3 of the 40 discs studied in asymptomatic individuals was there an elicited pain response, however, suggesting a favorable specificity and positive predictive value.[35]

The use of cervical discography is common practice at the author's center. It is ordered at multiple levels and is similar in nature to the practices of other authors.[37,40,41] The key is to have a significant (>6 of 10) concordant reproduction of the patient's presenting axial pain at the affected disc level with little or no pain at the adjacent control level. This concordant pain is the pain that the patient desires to be alleviated with surgical intervention.

What is difficult to publish a series on is how the discogram leads away from a surgical option. When there is no validating level, when every disc hurts, surgery is dissuaded. This is particularly the case in a young patient who has a frank herniated nucleus pulposus (approximately 20% of the asymptomatic population) who complains mainly of neck pain, without a strong clinical correlation, and who has multiple positive discograms. If one based selection of a fusion level on MRI alone in that scenario, a high percentage of clinical failures would likely follow.

Regarding the complications of discography, the published rates of discitis are very low (≤1%).[35,40,46] This low rate encompasses the technical skill of the discographer, size of the needle, and use of antibiotics.

Selective nerve root blocks are mentioned because there is overlap in patients presenting with "axial pain." It may be that the patient has more unilateral pain in the neck coming into the upper trapezial region or the periscapular region but not so much into the arm. Findings appear normal on neurologic examination, but the patient may have increasing pain with Spurling maneuver. MRI reveals ipsilateral foraminal stenosis. In this patient, a selective nerve block can be very useful from a diagnostic and a potentially therapeutic perspective. If with a small volume of lidocaine placed at the nerve root in question the patient reports significant relief of clinical symptoms, consideration of decompression of that nerve root is rationally based if the symptoms return. In this case, the axial pain is secondary to a radicular component perceived along the course of the primary posterior ramus, not the ventral ramus. A posterior laminoforaminotomy may suffice in this case, although an ACDF might also remedy the symptoms.

Comments on facet joint blocks or medial facet rami blocks are limited here. The author knows of no peer review literature that bases a decision to proceed with fusion surgery dictated by this testing. Most of the literature on these blocks has been with the diagnostic value of an anatomic source, and specifically in patients with whiplash-associated disorder.[47-49] Although some publications have suggested relief of pain associated with whiplash and in patients with chronic axial neck pain (with or without traumatic etiology), the author's experience has not favorably reproduced those outcomes.

Although intuitively if a patient reports excellent relief of pain with blocks to specific joints, it would seem that surgical arthrodesis of the joints may be beneficial, this has not been shown, and concern about leakage of the anesthetic onto the nerve root or spinal cord may discourage use of this technique. Using facet blocks for surgical decision making should be done in the context of a formal study.

Surgical Outcomes for Axial Neck Pain

The pragmatic question to the surgeon is this: "Does your selection process, based on whatever criterion you choose, yield a reproducible, discernible impact on the patient's chief complaint, which at 2- to 5-year follow-up would lead that patient to repeat the procedure and self-rate that surgical intervention as successful?" The currently discussed diagnostic workup approach has led the author to reply to that question with an affirmative response (Fig. 39–2).

Although prospective randomized trials are considered of higher value, much can also be gleaned from the cohort observational–based surgical literature.[28,37,41-45,50-55] In a clever tongue-in-cheek meta-analysis of the protective effect to the gravitational force affected by a parachute, Smith and Pell[56] found no published prospective randomized trials of such! No one doubts the value of a parachute, or for that matter of a hip arthroplasty, yet one does discount surgical treatment of axial pain.

In a series of 112 consecutive patients, the author and his colleagues were able to obtain 87 responses to an extensive follow-up questionnaire at an average of 4.4 years. In this group, 20 patients had multilevel procedures, whereas 67 had single-level or two-level ACDF. The author and colleagues reported by fusion level and etiology (traumatic, workers' compensation, or degenerative) but found no statistical difference among the groups. Pain improvement was noted in 93% (81 of 87), with the average VAS decreasing from 8.4 before surgery to 3.8 at long-term follow-up. On a 6-point Likert scale of excellent, very good, good, fair, poor, or terrible, 82% (71 of 87) self-rated their outcome to be good, very good, or excellent. Two modified cervical functional assessments were used, with the patient reporting an average 50% improvement on both. A negative correlation with the presence or absence of compensation or litigation or with tobacco use was not documented. The author

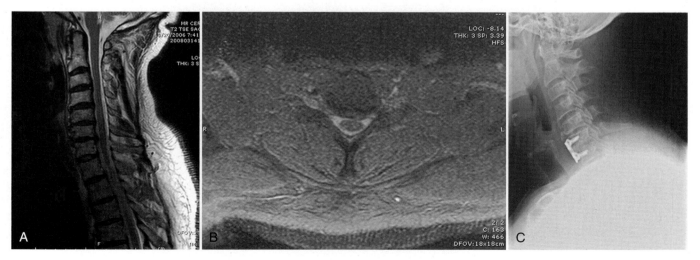

FIGURE 39–2 A-C, This patient had a chief complaint of 80% neck pain and 20% arm pain, with left-sided pain greater than right-sided pain. MRI shows herniated nucleus pulposus at C6-7 level, but it is left-sided, and degenerative change with small disc protrusions proximally. A C7 selective block gave excellent temporary relief of symptoms suggesting that C6-7 pathology was the prime pain generator. Anterior cervical discectomy and fusion at C6-7 was done, and at 1-year follow-up the patient's lateral radiograph shows solid fusion with excellent resolution of neck pain.

and colleagues estimated that the 112 patients represented 4% of the surgical practice of the attending physicians involved during the acquisition phase (Fig. 39–3).

In a 2004 publication on the value of MRI and discography in the patient selection process for ACDF, Zheng and colleagues[37] reported on 55 patients with 76% good or excellent results, 18% fair results, and 6% poor results. In 1999, Palit and colleagues[41] reported on 38 patients for "dominant neck pain, with no symptoms or signs of radiculopathy or myelopathy." They used the "patient satisfaction index," with 79% (30 of 38) indicating satisfaction with their surgical outcome and 21% (8 of 38) indicating they were not satisfied. Table 39–1 outlines series with similar diagnostic criteria after ACDF for neck pain (some in patients with arm pain) that show consistent results. The results in these series suggest that ACDF is a reasonable surgical option for neck pain in well-selected patients.

Current readers must also appreciate the wealth of information available from the publications of the pioneers of ACDF surgery. In 1962, Robinson and colleagues[43] reported on their continued ACDF experience. This series was of 56 patients with 80% (45 of 56) reporting neck pain, 45% (25 of 56) noting occipital pain, and 46% (26 of 56) having interscapular radiation. A traumatic etiology was noted in 68% (38 of 56), with 25 being indirect, such as a "rear-end automobile collision." Discography was used in 84% (47 of 56) of patients. The investigators switched from preoperative use to intraoperative testing owing to the patients complaining of pain with the actual procedure. In this classic series, 73% (41 of 56) considered themselves to have good or excellent results, with 22% (12 of 56) fair and 5.5% (3 of 56) poor. Pseudarthrosis was noted in 16% (9 of 56); 4 of the 9 patients were symptomatic. The stated conclusion was "when other treatment seems impractical, anterior interbody fusion appears to be a good surgical treatment for degenerative joint and disc disease of the cervical spine."

In 1969, Riley and colleagues[42] noted quite similar results in 93 consecutive cases. In a review paper, Riley[57] commented on psychosocial issues. He noted that "prolonged pain is associated with a definite emotional response which may be more disabling than the pain itself." He noted a series of patients with chronic neck pain who also as a group were irritable and depressed, who did not generate warm patient-physician relationships, but who did respond to surgical treatment, with the disappearance of their emotional characteristics when they had successful relief of their pain.

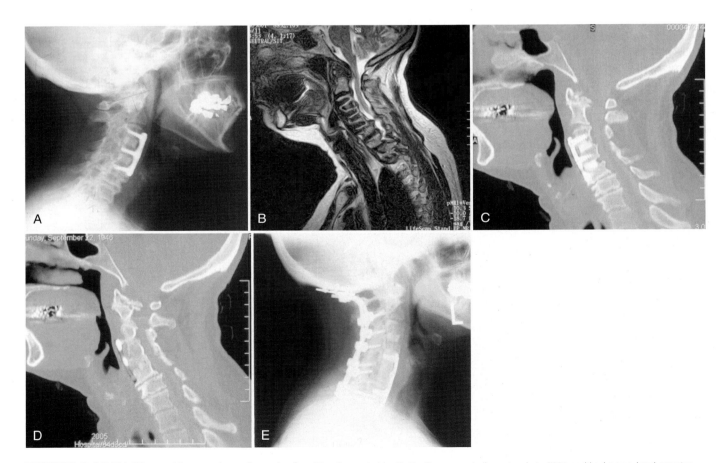

FIGURE 39–3 A-E, This 58-year-old woman has a diagnosis of positive rheumatoid arthritis. She presented previously in 2001 and had a two-level anterior cervical fusion. She now has significant neck pain as her chief complaint with base of the skull headaches and mild myelopathy symptoms. Her neck pain is greater on left side than right side. Images show advanced spondylosis at C5-6 and C6-7 with degenerative spondylolisthesis of C7 on T1. She has erosive arthritic change at C1-2 with early pannus formation ventral to brainstem, with increased cervical medullary angle. The patient had occipital-to-T1 fusion, with excellent resolution of her symptoms and ability to return to light duty full-time employment.

Pseudarthrosis

Pseudarthrosis is a common diagnosis for patients presenting with a chief complaint of neck pain. Although an anatomic pseudarthrosis may exist, one must be certain that this is the source of the "neck pain." Adjacent levels need to be assessed, and the original diagnosis that led to ACDF that resulted in pseudarthrosis should be reviewed. With that stated, the literature supports that conversion to a solid arthrodesis yields 70% to 80% good to excellent clinical outcomes.[58-60] The reports vary regarding repeat anterior procedures, posterior procedures, and combinations of both. The key is to have a specific objective diagnosis and then remedy that pathologic process.

Some patients present with new or continued complaints of neck pain after having had fusion surgery. Although the presence of an anatomic pseudarthrosis can be documented by radiographic or CT scan evaluation, one must assess the patient carefully to determine that this objective finding of pseudarthrosis is the specific etiology for the pain. The original diagnosis that led to ACDF, the timing of onset of neck pain (usually early but not immediate), and the health of the adjacent segment all must be considered. With that noted, the literature supports 70% to 80% good to excellent outcomes with conversion to a solid arthrodesis.[58-62] Reports vary regarding anterior, posterior, or combined approaches, but Carreon and colleagues[62] noted a greater effectiveness of the posterior approach.

Disc Arthroplasty

Cervical disc arthroplasty has been a very hot topic in recent years. Much has been published. U.S. Food and Drug Administration (FDA) investigational device exemption studies and others have allowed clinicians to garner much information about the patient's perceived outcomes as related to neck and arm pain in both arthroplasty groups and their control groups.[63-67] When one looks at the detailed data of these studies, an interesting point is that with inclusion criteria specifically having the patient treated for radiculopathy or myelopathy, the studies generally all report VAS scores for neck pain and arm pain. Generally, the VAS preoperatively is roughly equal for the arm and neck pain components—that is, each is in an approximate 7 to 8 of 10 points range, and on average decreases to a 2 to 3 of 10 points range postoperatively. What this means is that to the patient, neck pain is significant, and for outcomes, predictably it is relieved, just as is the arm pain.

When one asks what makes a patient satisfied with the outcome of surgery, Skolasky and colleagues[68] noted regarding fusions that "clinical improvement, especially in neck pain, after surgery is associated with improved patient satisfaction." In the arthroplasty control group of ACDF, Anderson and colleagues[69] studied 26 potential variables, as related to overall clinical success, and found that workers' compensation status and weak narcotic use were negative predictors, whereas higher preoperative NDI scores and normal sensory examinations were positive predictors.

TABLE 39–1 Results of Anterior Cervical Discectomy and Fusion for Axial Pain

Study	No. Patients	Reported Outcome
Zheng et al[37]	55	76% good or excellent, 18% fair, 6% poor
Garvey et al[28]	87	82% good or excellent, 16% fair, 2% poor
Ratliff and Voorhies[52]	20	85% satisfaction
Motimaya et al[51]	14	78.6% satisfaction
Palit et al[41]	38	79% satisfactory, 21% not satisfactory
Whitecloud[54]	34	70% good or excellent, 12% fair, 18% poor
Roth[44]	71	93% good or excellent, 1% fair, 6% poor
White et al[53]	28	62% good or excellent, 23% fair, 23% poor
Riley et al[42]	93	72% good or excellent, 18% fair, 10% poor
Simmons et al[45]	30 with neck pain; 51 with neck and arm pain	78% good or excellent, 15% fair, 7% poor
William et al[55]	15	1 excellent, 3 good, 5 fair, 6 poor
Dohn[50]	34	62% good or excellent, 24% fair, 15% poor
Robinson, et al[2]	56	73% good or excellent, 22% fair, 5% poor

What can be said at present from these studies is that decompression and disc arthroplasty as a procedure is at least as good as (if not better than) ACDF for cervical spondylosis with radiculopathy and that neck pain is an important subjective component of why the patient solicits surgical intervention. In the next 5 to 10 years, studies may be seen that expand the use of motion-sparing surgery to address patients with dominant axial pain, with the same caveat as for fusion surgery, that the levels to be surgically repaired must be thoroughly objectified.

Summary

The principles of a rational surgical decision-making process have not changed since the last edition of this text. In patients who present with a chief complaint of neck pain, in whom nonoperative treatment and time have not yielded resolution of their symptoms, there often is a viable surgical option. A careful surgical evaluation to objectify a specific etiology of the pain yields a typical patient satisfaction rate of 70% to 80% with "good to excellent" outcomes. When multiple authors (at various geographic locations, spanning 6 decades) using similar diagnostic criteria provide similar patient outcomes, it would seem that a rational surgical approach to axial neck pain does exist, notwithstanding a lack of prospective randomized trials. The next version of this chapter on axial neck pain may focus on arthroplasty as opposed to fusion because motion-preserving devices seem promising at present.

1. Prospective randomized trials are laudable, but nonrandomized studies have relevance.

2. Careful history and physical examination is still essential.

3. Objectification of the proposed surgical levels is paramount.

4. Discography, with normal validating level, can predict success.

PITFALLS

1. The presence of disc herniation on MRI exists in approximately 20% of asymptomatic individuals; MRI alone may be inadequate to objectify a surgical level.

2. "Pain" cannot be surgically removed. A specific etiology must be objectified.

3. Psychosocial factors, including symptoms, secondary gain, and chemical dependency, may decrease the clinical success rate.

4. In a patient who has continued neck pain after ACDF, search for a diagnosis of pseudarthrosis should be undertaken with flexion-extension radiographs or CT scan.

KEY POINTS

1. Review of the surgical literature over the last 60 years supports ACDF for patients with neck pain. Most of the studies are observational or cohort studies, but they span multiple institutions and multiple authors.

2. Objectification of the pathology is crucial. One needs a specific diagnosis, such as a disc herniation with specific neurologic correlation, a specific discogram with a validating level, or specific nerve root compression with relief with a selective block, that indicates the level to be treated.

3. A thorough history and physical evaluation is crucial in determining which patients should be selected for a diagnostic workup for axial neck pain for potential surgical management. If a patient is suspected to have tumor, infection, or significant myelopathy, an urgent evaluation should be done. If the patient is normal neurologically and has multiple levels of involvement, staying with an active rehabilitative approach is encouraged.

KEY REFERENCES

1. Garvey T, Transfeldt E, Malcolm J, et al: Outcome of anterior cervical discectomy and fusion as perceived by patients treated for dominant axial-mechanical cervical spine pain. Spine (Phila Pa 1976) 27:1887-1895, 2002.
   This is a detailed account from the patient's perspective of ACDF for a chief complaint of neck pain.

2. Robinson R, Walker E, Ferlic D, et al: The results of anterior interbody fusion of the cervical spine. J Bone Joint Surg Am 44:1569-1587, 1962.
   This is a pioneer's work on ACDF for cervical discogenic syndrome, still valuable 50 years later.

3. Gore D, Sepic S, Gardner G, et al: Neck pain: A long-term follow-up of 205 patients. Spine (Phila Pa 1976) 12:1-5, 1987.
   This is a classic natural history study on patients presenting with neck pain caused by spondylosis.

4. Schellhas K, Smith M, Gundry C, et al: Cervical discogenic pain: Prospective correlation of magnetic resonance imaging and discography in asymptomatic subjects and pain sufferers. Spine (Phila Pa 1976) 21:300-311, 1996.
   This is a scientific approach to the use of discography as it relates to symptom provocation versus anatomic findings.

5. Heller JG, Sasso RC, Papadopoulos SM, et al: Comparison of BRYAN cervical disc arthroplasty with anterior cervical decompression and fusion: Clinical and radiographic results of a randomized, controlled, clinical trial. Spine (Phila Pa 1976) 34:101-107, 2009.
   This is a good representation of the detailed patient-driven data that are available related to arthroplasty versus ACDF randomized trials.

REFERENCES

1. Auvinen JP, Paananen MVJ, Tammelin TH, et al: Musculoskeletal pain combinations in adolescents. Spine (Phila Pa 1976) 34:1192-1197, 2009.

2. Bovim G, Schrader H, Sand T: Neck pain in the general population. Spine (Phila Pa 1976) 19:1307-1309, 1994.

3. Cote P, Cassidy J, Carroll L: The factors associated with neck pain and its related disability in the Saskatchewan population. Spine (Phila Pa 1976) 25:1109-1117, 2000.

4. Makela M, Heliovaara M, Sievers K, et al: Prevalence, determinants and consequences of chronic neck pain in Finland. Am J Epidemiol 134:1356-1367, 1991.

5. Manchikanti L, Singh V, Datta S, et al: Comprehensive review of epidemiology, scope and impact of spinal pain. Pain Physician 12:35-70, 2009.

6. Badcock LJ, Lewis M, Hay EM, et al: Consultation and the outcome of shoulder-neck pain: A cohort study in the population. J Rheumatol 30:2694-2699, 2003.

7. Gore D, Sepic S, Gardner G, et al: Neck pain: A long term follow-up of 205 patients. Spine (Phila Pa 1976) 12:1-5, 1987.

8. Rothman R: The Spine, 2nd ed. Philadelphia, WB Saunders, 1982.

9. DePalma A, Subin D: Study of the cervical syndrome. Clin Orthop Relat Res 38:135-141, 1965.

10. DePalma A, Rothman R, Lewinnek G, et al: Anterior interbody fusion for severe cervical degeneration. Surg Gynecol Obstet 134:755-758, 1972.

11. Rothman R, Rashbaum R: Pathogenesis of signs and symptoms of cervical disc degeneration. In: Annual Meeting of the American Academy of Orthopaedic Surgeons, 1978. St. Louis, CV Mosby, 1978, pp 203-215.

12. Walker MJ, Boyles RE, Young BA, et al: The effectiveness of manual physical therapy and exercise for mechanical neck pain: A randomized clinical trial. Spine (Phila Pa 1976) 33:2371-2378, 2008.

13. Lees F, Turner J: Natural history and prognosis of cervical spondylosis. BMJ 2:1607-1610, 1963.

14. Quebec Task Force on Whiplash-Associated Disorders. Scientific monograph of the Quebec Task Force on Whiplash-Associated Disorders. Spine (Phila Pa 1976) 20(8S):3s-73s, 1995.

15. Freeman M, Croft A, Rossignol A, et al: A review and methodologic critique of the literature refuting whiplash syndrome. Spine (Phila Pa 1976) 24:86-98, 1999.

16. Cote P, Cassidy JD, Carette S, et al: Protocol of a randomized controlled trial of the effectiveness of physician education and activation versus two rehabilitation programs for the treatment of whiplash-associated disorders: The University Health Network Whiplash Intervention Trial. Trials 9:75, 2008.

17. MacNab I: Acceleration injuries of the cervical spine. J Bone Joint Surg Am 46:1797-1799, 1964.

18. MacNab I: The "whiplash syndrome." Orthop Clin North Am 2:389-403, 1971.

19. Hohl M: Soft-tissue injuries of the neck in automobile accidents: Factors influencing prognosis. J Bone Joint Surg Am 56:1675-1682, 1974.

20. Bannister G, Gargan M: Prognosis of whiplash injuries: A review of the literature. Spine (Phila Pa 1976) 7:557-569, 1993.

21. Gargan M, Bannister G: Long-term prognosis of soft-tissue injuries of the neck. J Bone Joint Surg Br 72:901-903, 1990.

22. Watkinson A, Gargan M: Prognostic factors in soft tissue injuries of the cervical spine. Injury 23:307-309, 1991.

23. Hildingsson C, Toolanen G: Outcome after soft-tissue injury of the cervical spine: A prospective study of 93 car accident victims. Acta Orthop Scand 61:357-359, 1990.

24. Jonsson H, Cesarini K, Sahlstedt B, et al: Findings and outcome in whiplash-type neck distortions. Spine (Phila Pa 1976) 19:2733-2743, 1994.

25. Cassidy JD, Carroll LJ, Pierre Cote DC, et al: Effect of eliminating compensation for pain and suffering on the outcome of insurance claims for whiplash injury. N Engl J Med 342:1179-1186, 2000.

26. Cote P, Hogg-Johnson S, Cassidy JD, et al: Early aggressive care and delayed recovery from whiplash: Isolated finding or reproducible result? Arthritis Rheum 59:599-600, 2008.

27. Shapiro A, Roth R: The effect of litigation on recovery from whiplash. Spine (Phila Pa 1976) 7:531-556, 1993.

28. Garvey T, Transfeldt E, Malcolm J, et al: Outcome of anterior cervical discectomy and fusion as perceived by patients treated for dominant axial-mechanical cervical spine pain. Spine (Phila Pa 1976) 27:1887-1895, 2002.

29. Lawrence JT, London N, Bohlman HH, et al: Preoperative narcotic use as a predictor of clinical outcome: Results following anterior cervical arthrodesis. Spine (Phila Pa 1976) 33:2074-2078, 2008.

30. Ofiram E, Garvey TA, Schwender JD, et al: Cervical degenerative index: A new quantitative radiographic scoring system for cervical spondylosis with interobserver and intraobserver reliability testing. J Orthop Traumatol 10:21-26, 2009.

31. Ofiram E, Garvey TA, Schwender JD, et al: Cervical degenerative changes in idiopathic scoliosis patients who underwent long fusion to the sacrum as adults: Incidence, severity, and evolution. J Orthop Traumatol 10:27-30, 2009.

32. Friedenberg Z, Miller W: Degenerative disc disease of the cervical spine. J Bone Joint Surg Am 45:1171-1178, 1963.

33. Gore D, Sepic S, Gardner G: Roentgenographic findings of the cervical spine in asymptomatic people. Spine (Phila Pa 1976) 11:521-524, 1986.

34. Boden S, McCowin P, Davis D, et al: Abnormal magnetic resonance scans of the cervical spine in asymptomatic subjects. J Bone Joint Surg Am 72:1178-1184, 1990.

35. Schellhas K, Smith M, Gundry C, et al: Cervical discogenic pain: Prospective correlation of magnetic resonance imaging and discography in asymptomatic subjects and pain sufferers. Spine (Phila Pa 1976) 21:300-311, 1996.

36. Teresi L, Lufkin R, Reicher M, et al: Asymptomatic degenerative disk disease and spondylosis of the cervical spine: MR imaging. Radiology 164:83-88, 1987.

37. Zheng Y, Liew S, Simmons E: Value of magnetic resonance imaging and discography in determining the level of cervical discectomy and fusion. Spine (Phila Pa 1976) 29:2140-2145, 2004.

38. Nordin M, Carragee EJ, Hogg-Johnson S, et al: Assessment of neck pain and its associated disorders: results of the Bone and Joint Decade 2000-2010 Task Force on Neck Pain and Its Associated Disorders. J Manipulative Physiol Ther 32(2 Suppl):S117-S140, 2009.

39. Manchikanti L, Dunbar EE, Wargo BW, et al: Systematic review of cervical discography as a diagnostic test for chronic spinal pain. Pain Physician 12:305-321, 2009.

40. Grubb S, Kelly C: Cervical discography: Clinical implications from 12 years of experience. Spine (Phila Pa 1976) 25:1382-1389, 2000.

41. Palit M, Schofferman J, Goldthwaite N, et al: Anterior discectomy and fusion for the management of neck pain. Spine (Phila Pa 1976) 24:2224-2228, 1999.

42. Riley L, Robinson R, Johnson K, et al: The results of anterior interbody fusion of the cervical spine. J Neurosurg 30:127-133, 1969.

43. Robinson R, Walker E, Ferlic D, et al: The results of anterior interbody fusion of the cervical spine. J Bone Joint Surg Am 44:1569-1587, 1962.

44. Roth D: A new test for the definitive diagnosis of the painful-disk syndrome. JAMA 235:1713-1714, 1976.

45. Simmons E, Bhalla S, Butt W: Anterior cervical discectomy and fusion: A clinical and biomechanical study with eight-year follow-up. With a note on discography: Technique and interpretation of results. J Bone Joint Surg Br 51:225-237, 1969.

46. Zeidman S, Thompson K: Cervical discography. In The Cervical Spine Research Society: The Cervical Spine, 3rd ed. Philadelphia, Lippincott Raven, 1998, pp 205-216.

47. Barnsley L, Lord S, Wallis B, et al: The prevalence of chronic cervical zygapophysial joint pain after whiplash. Spine (Phila Pa 1976) 20:20-26, 1995.

48. Bogduk N, April C: On the nature of neck pain, discography and cervical zygapophysial joint blocks. Pain 54:213-217, 1993.

49. Lord S, Barnsley L, Wallis B, et al: Percutaneous radiofrequency neurotomy for chronic cervical zygapophyseal-joint pain. N Engl J Med 335:1721-1726, 1996.

50. Dohn D: Anterior interbody fusion for treatment of cervical disk condition. JAMA 197:897-900, 1966.

51. Motimaya A, Arici M, George D, et al: Diagnostic value of cervical discography in the management of cervical discogenic pain. Conn Med 64:395-398, 2000.

52. Ratliff J, Voorhies R: Outcome study of surgical treatment for axial neck pain. South Med J 94:595-602, 2001.

53. White A, Southwick W, Panjabi M: Clinical instability in the lower cervical spine. Spine (Phila Pa 1976) 1:15-27, 1976.

54. Whitecloud T: Management of radiculopathy and myelopathy by the anterior approach. In The Cervical Spine Research Society: The Cervical Spine, 2nd ed. Philadelphia, JB Lippincott, 1989, pp 644-658.

55. William J, Allen M, Harkess J: Late results of cervical discectomy and interbody fusion: Some factors influencing the results. J Bone Joint Surg Am 50:277-286, 1968.

56. Smith G, Pell J: Parachute use to prevent death and major trauma related to gravitational challenge: Systematic review of randomised controlled trials. BMJ 327:1459-1461, 2003.

57. Riley L: Various pain syndromes which may result from osteoarthritis of the cervical spine. Maryland State Med J 18:103-105, 1969.

58. Farey I, McAfee P, Davis R, et al: Pseudarthrosis of the cervical spine after anterior arthrodesis. J Bone Joint Surg Am 70:1171-1177, 1990.

59. Lowery GL, Swank ML, McDonough RF: Surgical revision for failed anterior cervical fusions: Articular pillar plating or anterior revision? Spine (Phila Pa 1976) 20:2436-2441, 1995.

60. Zdeblick TA, Hughes SS, Riew KD, et al: Failed anterior cervical discectomy and arthrodesis: Analysis and treatment of thirty-five patients. J Bone Joint Surg Am 79:523-532, 1997.

61. Kuhns CA, Geck MJ, Wang JC, et al: An outcomes analysis of the treatment of cervical pseudarthrosis with posterior fusion. Spine (Phila Pa 1976) 30:2424-2429, 2005.

62. Carreon L, Glassman SD, Campbell MJ: Treatment of anterior cervical pseudoarthrosis: Posterior fusion versus anterior revision. Spine J 6:154-156, 2006.

63. Heller JG, Sasso RC, Papdopoulos SM, et al: Comparison of BRYAN cervical disc arthroplasty with anterior cervical decompression and fusion: Clinical and radiographic results of a randomized, controlled, clinical trial. Spine (Phila Pa 1976) 34:101-107, 2009.

64. Murrey D, Janssen M, Delamarter R, et al: Results of the prospective randomized, controlled multicenter Food and Drug Administration investigational device exemption study of the ProDisc-C total disc replacement versus anterior discectomy and fusion for the treatment of 1-level symptomatic cervical disc disease. Spine J 9:275-286, 2008.

65. Mummaneni PV, Burkus JK, Haid RW, et al: Clinical and radiographic analysis of cervical disc arthroplasty compared with allograft fusion: A randomized controlled clinical trial. J Neurosurg Spine 6:198-209, 2007.

66. Sasso RC, Smucker JD, Hacker RJ, et al: Artificial disc versus fusion: A prospective randomized study with 2-year follow-up on 99 patients. Spine (Phila Pa 1976) 32:2933-2940, 2007.

67. Barbagallo GM, Assietti R, Corbino L, et al: Early results and review of the literature of a novel hybrid surgical technique combining cervical arthrodesis and disc arthroplasty for treating multilevel degenerative disc disease: Opposite of complementary techniques? Eur Spine J 18(Suppl 1):29-39, 2009.

68. Skolasky RL, Albert TJ, Vaccaro AR, et al: Patient satisfaction in the cervical spine research society outcomes study: Relationship to improved clinical outcome. Spine J 9:232-239, 2009.

69. Anderson PA, Subach BR, Riew KD: Predictors of outcome after anterior cervical discectomy and fusion: A multivariate analysis. Spine (Phila Pa 1976) 34:161-166, 2009.

40
CHAPTER

Cervical Radiculopathy:
Anterior Surgical Approach

Terrence T. Crowder, MD
Jeffrey D. Fischgrund, MD

Neck and arm pain frequently occur as a result of normal aging of the cervical spine. Typically, these episodes are of short duration and respond well to nonoperative treatment. Surgical intervention is usually undertaken when pain or disability is prolonged. Multiple surgical procedures have been developed to treat cervical radiculopathy. This chapter focuses on the most commonly performed anterior procedures: anterior cervical discectomy with and without fusion; anterior cervical foraminotomy; and, more recently, cervical disc arthroplasty. Radiographic evaluation, surgical indications, surgical procedures, and clinical outcomes are discussed in detail.

Radiographic Evaluation

Radiographic evaluation usually begins with plain radiographs; lateral, anteroposterior, and oblique views are obtained. Global and segmental alignment can be easily assessed. Findings of degenerative disease include disc space narrowing, osteophytosis of the apophyseal joints, and spurring at the level the disc space. Degenerative spondylolisthesis of the cervical spine is common, and this usually involves facet arthropathy as well.[1] Dynamic lateral radiographs can show segmental instability by assessing anteroposterior translation and angular motion. Foraminal stenosis may occur from uncovertebral arthrosis or degenerative subluxation. Typically, bony elements are visualized, but radiographs inherently are unable to assess neural elements. An indirect assessment of the neural foramina can be obtained with oblique views (Fig. 40–1). Although the soft tissue component of spinal cord compression cannot be visualized on lateral radiographs, the space available is easily assessed. Brain and Wilkinson[2] reported an average space of 17 to 18 mm (range 14 to 23 mm).

Several authors have reported on the use of lateral radiographs to assess cervical stenosis. A classic study by Edwards and LaRocca[3] found the average sagittal diameter of asymptomatic individuals to be 17 mm. These authors reported that myelopathy was present in subjects with a diameter of less than 10 mm. A diameter of 10 to 13 mm was noted in patients without symptoms but who were likely to become symptomatic. Using radiographs, stenosis is present in about 5% of the population, and the rate increases with age to approximately 9% in patients older than 70 years.[4] Torg ratio identifies stenosis and eliminates the variability and magnification associated with direct measurement of radiographs.[5] A sagittal spinal canal diameter–to–vertebral body ratio of less than 0.8 is indicative of cervical spinal stenosis (Fig. 40–2). Several authors have questioned the reliability of Torg ratio.[6-8]

When more direct visualization of the neural elements is necessary, advanced imaging can be employed. Initially, spinal myelography was the test of choice. Water-soluble dye injected into the epidural space allows visualization of the neural elements by assessing flow patterns. Despite relatively high sensitivity, myelograms are nonspecific. Flow can be altered by soft disc herniations, hard disc (osteophyte formation), facet arthropathy, or various other pathologies. Computed tomography (CT) combined with myelography can significantly improve accuracy.[9] Axial images and sagittal reconstructions improve the practitioner's ability to determine the causes of compression. Altered filling of the nerve roots from bony compression can easily be assessed because of the bony detail produced with CT imaging (Fig. 40–3). CT myelography can be performed in patients who are not candidates for other procedures such as magnetic resonance imaging (MRI). Myelography has some disadvantages. A major concern is the invasiveness and morbidity associated with placement of the dye into the epidural space. Although CT myelography is more specific than radiographs, it is still very nonspecific for soft tissue causes of stenosis.

MRI offers several advantages. The neural elements and soft tissues are directly visualized, no radiation is required, and it is noninvasive. Meticulous inspection of the images can reveal soft disc herniations (Fig. 40–4) and sequestered fragments when they are present. Disruption of the posterior longitudinal ligament on sagittal MRI is indicative of a possibly sequestered fragment. Although MRI is best at visualizing soft tissue elements of the cervical spine, bony anatomy can be assessed. Additionally, MRI recognizes infiltrative soft tissue and vertebral body processes such as sarcoma or metastatic disease.

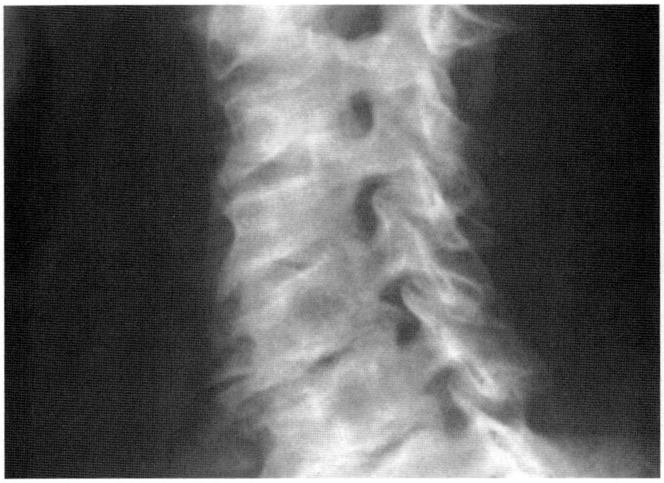

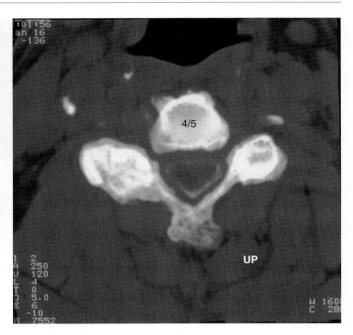

FIGURE 40–1 Oblique cervical spine radiograph showing foraminal narrowing at multiple levels.

MRI scans offer excellent visualization of the lower brainstem and entire cervical spinal cord. The foramen magnum can be examined for Arnold-Chiari malformations. Basilar invagination or pannus formation from inflammatory arthritis can also be seen. Acute or chronic spinal cord compression may lead to signal change within the spinal cord, termed *myelomalacia* (Fig. 40–5). These changes may be important in predicting clinical outcomes after decompression.[10,11]

Although imaging has advanced greatly in recent years, a thorough history and physical examination still constitute the

FIGURE 40–3 Axial CT myelogram showing central and foraminal stenosis.

cornerstone of diagnosis and treatment. MRI and CT myelography must be correlated with the clinical evaluation of the patient. Boden and colleagues[12] reported degenerative disc space changes in 25% of asymptomatic subjects younger than 40 years and almost 60% of subjects older than 60. A 10-year longitudinal study of healthy volunteers revealed that degenerative changes progressed, but symptoms developed in only 34% of subjects. Age was the only variable associated with the progression of spondylosis.[13]

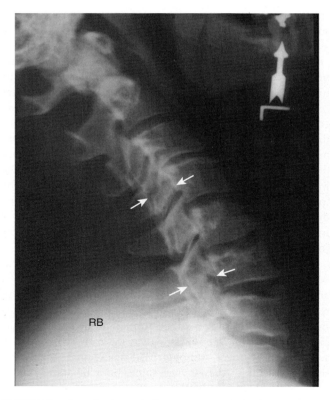

FIGURE 40–2 Lateral radiograph showing congenital spinal stenosis. *Arrowheads* define anterior and posterior borders of spinal canal.

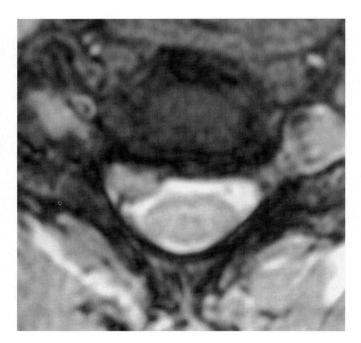

FIGURE 40–4 Axial MRI showing posterolateral soft disc herniation compressing exiting nerve root.

Electrodiagnostic Studies

Electrodiagnostic studies are another diagnostic modality used to evaluate patients with radiculopathy. Peripheral nerve root entrapment can mimic cervical radiculopathy. Currently, electromyography (EMG) is the most useful modality. In some studies, 75% sensitivity has been reported.[14-16] Because of the variable sensitivity of EMG, it is not an ideal screening tool. The diagnosis and location of pathology can be assessed with EMG, however. Compression causes pathophysiologic changes within the nerve root. These changes are shown on EMG as decreased motor unit potentials and fibrillation potentials. When attempting to distinguish between radiculopathy, peripheral neuropathy, and nerve root entrapment, neurophysiologic testing can be useful. When the diagnosis is clear from imaging and clinical examination, EMG is probably unnecessary. EMG and nerve conduction studies may be beneficial to distinguish specific nerve root compression when multilevel disease is present.

Surgical Indications

The indications for operative treatment of radiculopathy have not changed much over the years despite advances in operative techniques and devices. The most commonly accepted indications are (1) persistent or recurrent arm pain that is unresponsive to a trial of conservative treatment (3 months), (2) progressive neurologic deficit, (3) static neurologic deficit associated with significant radicular pain, and (4) confirmatory imaging studies consistent with the patient's clinical findings. This chapter focuses on anterior approaches to surgical treatment. Smith and Robinson[17] were the first to popularize the anterior approach.

Anterior Cervical Discectomy and Fusion: Surgical Technique

General endotracheal anesthesia provides the safest environment for anterior cervical discectomy and fusion (ACDF). The endotracheal tube should be taped on the side of the mouth opposite to the side on which the procedure is performed. Proper positioning is an essential part of this procedure. The authors typically place a small rolled towel longitudinally between the scapulae to allow the shoulders to fall back out of the way; this also positions the neck in mild hyperextension. Care must be taken in patients with myelopathy because iatrogenic worsening of myelopathy may occur with hyperextension. If symptoms are significantly worsened with hyperextension during the preoperative physical examination, this position should also be avoided. The arms are placed along the patient's side and tucked. The shoulders can decrease visualization during exposure and during imaging. The authors use surgical tape to place longitudinal downward traction on the shoulders (Fig. 40–6).

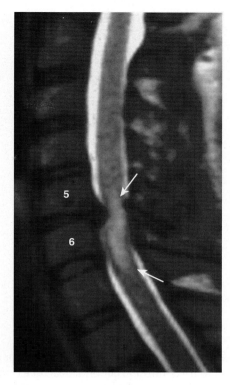

FIGURE 40–5 Sagittal MRI showing myelomalacia of spinal cord caused by disc herniation.

Injury to the recurrent laryngeal nerve is decreased with a left-sided approach. The nerve follows a predictable path on the left side of the neck. It enters the thorax within the carotid sheath (along with the vagus nerve, carotid artery, and jugular vein), then loops under the aortic arch, and ascends into the neck between the trachea and esophagus. Most orthopaedic surgeons prefer to perform ACDF from the left to take advantage of this favorable anatomy. Some authors have shown a decreased incidence of injury to the recurrent laryngeal nerve with a left-sided approach, but others have shown no association between the side of surgery and nerve injury.

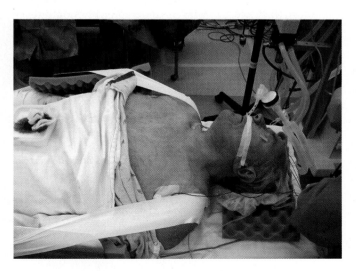

FIGURE 40–6 Positioning for anterior cervical surgery.

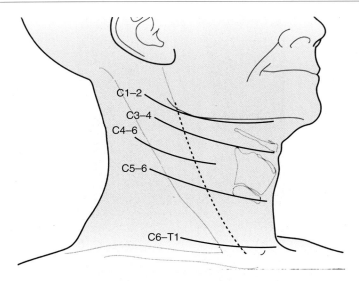

FIGURE 40–7 Superficial landmarks are helpful in identifying correct level for skin incision.

More recently, it has been suggested that retractor displacement of the larynx against the endotracheal tube causes crush injury to the intralaryngeal segment of the recurrent laryngeal nerve, causing dysphonia. Apfelbaum and colleagues[18] recommended deflating the endotracheal tube during the procedure to decrease pressure on the nerve and decrease the incidence of postoperative voice changes. Audu and colleagues[19] performed a randomized, prospective, double-blind investigation of endotracheal tube manipulation. Postoperative examination with indirect laryngoscopy showed a 3.2% incidence of vocal cord paralysis. Endotracheal tube deflation did not reduce the incidence of vocal cord immobility. These authors concluded that tube manipulation has no effect on vocal cord injury.

When a one-level or two-level discectomy is planned, a transverse incision is usually sufficient. These incisions tend to be more aesthetically pleasing. When an extensile approach is necessary, a longitudinal incision may be necessary. Patients with short, thick necks or who are undergoing revision surgery may benefit from longitudinal incisions. Fluoroscopy or

superficial landmarks can be used to mark the appropriate skin level (Fig. 40–7). Typically, C3 is found at the level of the hyoid, C4-5 is found at the thyroid cartilage, and C6 is found at the cricoid cartilage. When exposing near the cervicothoracic junction (C7-T1), the inferior thyroid vessels and thoracic duct may have to be managed. A longitudinal incision may facilitate exposure at this level.

After the skin incision is complete, hemostasis can be obtained along the skin edges with electrocautery. The two edges of the skin can be elevated with either hand-held retractors or a small self-retaining retractor. The first muscle encountered is the platysma, which underlies the fascia. A curved hemostat is used to dissect bluntly underneath the platysma. Using electrocautery, the muscle is incised in line with the incision. Visualization is improved by opening the fascial planes underneath this layer; this also facilitates retractor placement to improve mobilization of the underlying structures. This is a crucial step in performing a safe dissection. The sternocleidomastoid should become visible. The dissection proceeds along the anteromedial aspect of the sternocleidomastoid. A blunt dissection should proceed between the carotid sheath and the trachea and esophagus. A finger should bluntly separate the medial border of the carotid sheath from the lateral border of the trachea and esophagus. Typically, the surgeon can easily discern the medial border of the tubular carotid. The pulsation of the carotid may not always be easily felt (Fig. 40–8).

Prolonged compression of the carotid artery or body may cause bradycardia. Hand-held retractors are used on the anterior vertebral body if it is palpable. The use of retractors with sharp edges is discouraged owing to possible damage to the great vessels or esophagus.

When exposing the lower levels, the omohyoid muscle is frequently encountered. If this muscle obscures the field, it may require division. Branches of the carotid, most commonly the superior and inferior thyroid vessels, may require ligation if they obscure the field or would require excessive retraction during the procedure.

Correct identification of the proper level is imperative. Careful examination of radiographs may reveal anterior osteophytes. Palpation of these osteophytes on the anterior vertebral bodies can often lead to correct level identification. Lateral to C6 lies Chassaignac tubercle, which can be palpated and helps identify C5-6. Current patient safety recommendations by the North American Spine Society (NASS) recommend an intraoperative radiograph to verify the proper level. A standard spinal needle or specialized cervical marker should be placed in the intended operative level (Fig. 40–9). Identifying the level on a lateral radiograph may be difficult in the lower cervical spine or when the patient has either a short, thick neck or broad shoulders. The surgeon may elect to place a spinal needle at two levels, such that the superiormost needle can be visualized on the radiograph. Caution must be exercised if placement of two needles is required. A retrospective radiographic analysis of 87 consecutive patients by Nassr and colleagues[20] showed a threefold increased risk of developing degenerative changes in disc levels that were previously marked with a needle for intraoperative level verification.

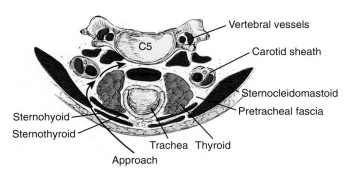

FIGURE 40–8 Approach to anterior cervical spine begins on medial side of sternocleidomastoid and then goes in deeper interval between carotid sheath laterally and trachea and esophagus medially.

After the correct disc space is identified, the prevertebral fascia over the anterior vertebral body is divided; the longus colli muscles are then easily visualized. Dissection should begin in the midline and proceed laterally. The longus muscles are elevated bilaterally with a combination of electrocautery and mild blunt dissection. The exposure is held open with self-retaining retractors that are placed under the longus colli muscles (Fig. 40–10). The retractor can be secured by an assistant or with an arm secured to the operating table.

If present, the anterior osteophyte is removed with a Leksell rongeur or bur. The discectomy begins by identifying the anterior longitudinal ligament and performing an annulotomy in rectangular or box fashion. This annulotomy can be accomplished with a No. 15 scalpel blade with the blade never pointing toward the carotid. The superficial portion of the intervertebral disc can be removed with pituitary rongeurs. The authors continue with these until disc material can no longer be easily removed.

The cartilaginous endplates and attached intervertebral disc can usually be resected with small straight and angled curets. Typically, the first 50% of this disc can be removed before distraction of the disc is necessary. Distraction techniques are at the discretion of the surgeon. Some surgeons prefer using intervertebral spreaders, whereas others prefer using pins placed in the adjacent bodies to distract. Pins should be placed in the middle of the bodies. Intervertebral spreaders should be placed lateral against the uncus. Regardless of the techniques used, the surgeon must be cautious in osteoporotic bone. Both sets of instruments may cut through osteoporotic bone. With distraction, the remainder of the disc

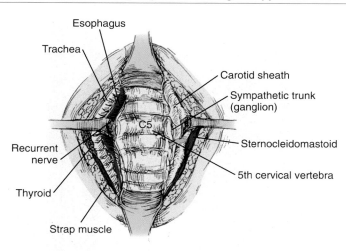

FIGURE 40–10 After elevation of longus colli muscles bilaterally, blunt retractors can be placed for remainder of procedure.

is removed with curettage of the cartilaginous endplates of the adjacent vertebral bodies.

Visualization of the posterior half of the disc can be impaired by overhanging anterior osteophytes. These can be removed with a bur or rongeur to improve visualization (Fig. 40–11). It is imperative that the surgeon note the angle of the disc space on the intraoperative localization film, and care should be taken to perform the disc removal along the angle of the endplates to avoid inadvertent penetration of the vertebral bodies. The uncinate process, posterior longitudinal ligament, and bony endplates should be visible at the end of the discectomy. Inspection of the posterior longitudinal ligament is necessary to determine if a sequestered fragment is present.

Resection of the posterior longitudinal ligament is usually unnecessary if there is no suspicion of the existence of a sequestered fragment. When a tear is seen during dissection, or preoperative studies suggest a sequestered fragment exist, a thorough examination of the ligament is necessary. All tears

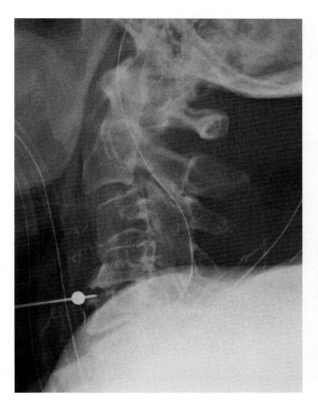

FIGURE 40–9 Marker is placed in disc space.

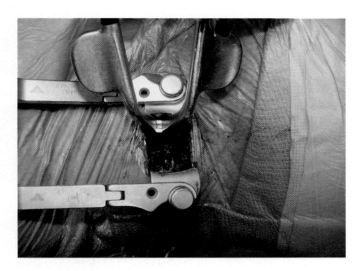

FIGURE 40–11 Intervertebral spreader is placed in disc space to improve visualization.

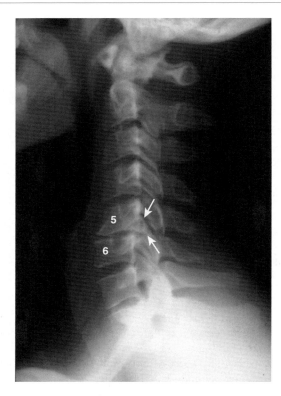

FIGURE 40–12 Lateral radiograph showing posterior osteophyte formation (*arrows*) at C5-6.

should be probed with a nerve hook to determine the extent. A portion should be removed with a micro-Kerrison rongeur to allow visualization of the dura and to facilitate a search for free disc fragments.

The significance of posterior osteophyte removal is unknown. When they are causing obvious compression on the spinal cord, osteophytes should be removed (Fig. 40–12). After the neural elements have been decompressed and the endplates have been prepared, the anterior to posterior depth of the disc should be measured with a calibrated nerve hook or a small wire. Generally, the disc space is 10 to 15 mm wide,

12 to 17 mm deep, and 5 to 10 mm long. Regardless of the type used, the intervertebral graft should be several millimeters less than the actual depth to allow recession and avoid spinal cord compression.

The endplates should be punctured down to bleeding bone to facilitate bony union; various ways exist to accomplish this. Some surgeons prefer to use a bur to remove the endplates partially, whereas others use a small, angled curet to create holes in the adjacent sides. Regardless of the method, excessive endplate removal must be avoided. Endplate collapse and graft subsidence can occur when the structural integrity is weakened too much. When using tricortical iliac crest or patella, the graft should be shaped in a lordotic fashion with the anterior height being 1 to 2 mm taller than the posterior height (Fig. 40–13). This shape helps to avoid posterior retropulsion of the graft and subsequent cord compression and restores lordosis. The graft should be placed with the disc space under distraction to facilitate insertion. Longitudinal traction by the anesthesiologist is as effective as various intervertebral distractors. A tamp and mallet are used to position the graft (Fig. 40–14).

If an anterior cervical plate is not a planned part of the procedure, the bone graft is usually countersunk 1 to 2 mm in relation to the anterior margin of the adjacent vertebral bodies to decrease the chance of graft extrusion and esophageal compression (Fig. 40–15). When adding a plate, only minimal graft countersinking is necessary. A final lateral intraoperative radiograph is strongly suggested. Correct graft position can be verified along with proper plate position. The authors typically place a drain just anterior to the vertebral body. The fascia overlying the platysma is closed with simple absorbable sutures, and the skin is closed with a running absorbable subcuticular suture.

Consensus on postoperative management of patients after ACDF is lacking. Initially, most surgeons required patients to wear a rigid cervical collar for 6 to 8 weeks. Anterior instrumentation has eliminated many graft-related complications. Some surgeons have abandoned or significantly limited their

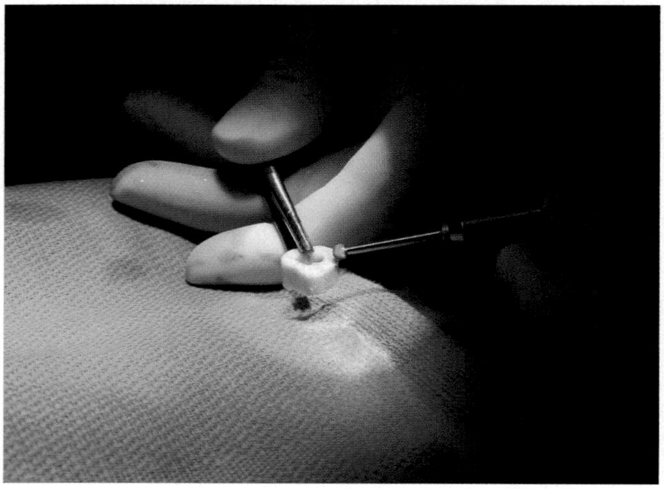

FIGURE 40–13 Power bur is used to shape allograft.

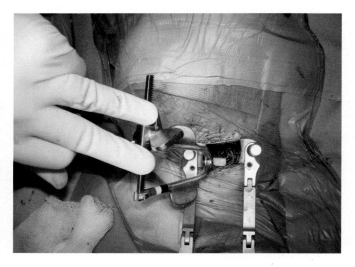

FIGURE 40–14 Graft is placed while intervertebral spreader provides distraction.

use of postoperative immobilization because of the safety and effectiveness of current instrumentation. More recent studies have shown that a postoperative cervical brace does not improve the fusion rate or the clinical outcomes of patients undergoing single-level anterior cervical fusion with or without plating.[21,22]

When adequate internal fixation is obtained, a soft collar can be used for a short time in the initial postoperative period. Modern perioperative care and techniques allow patient mobilization on the day of surgery and discharge on postoperative day 1. Some surgeons have shown similar clinical outcomes and safety when performing ACDF in the outpatient setting.[23-25] At 1 to 2 weeks, follow-up anteroposterior and lateral radiographs are taken. Lateral radiographs show a sufficient incorporation of the bone graft such that patients are allowed to begin range of motion exercises and strengthening exercises by 6 weeks. Within 3 months of the surgical procedure, most patients can expect return to full activity.

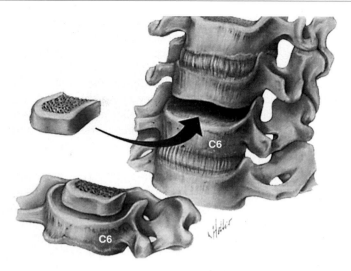

FIGURE 40–15 Placement of tricortical iliac crest graft after discectomy at C5-6. Note slight recession of graft within disc space.

Anterior Cervical Plating

Use of an anterior cervical plate after anterior cervical fusion has become almost routine for many surgeons. Although the anterior cervical plate does provide increased stability after decompression and an increased fusion rate, the risks of this procedure and the additional cost must be weighed against the benefits.

Anterior cervical plating was first introduced in the 1960s, when Bohler[25a] modified lower extremity hardware. Initially, he used the plates in trauma cases to restore stability. Exponential advancements have been made in the manufacture of anterior cervical instrumentation, biocompatibility, and ease of implantation. Currently, the use of an anterior cervical plate has been advocated to increase postoperative stability, decrease the incidence of graft extrusion, decrease the incidence of graft collapse, improve fusion rate, and obviate the need for postoperative halo brace placement after extensive multilevel corpectomies.

Initially, anterior cervical instrumentation required bicortical screw use. Intraoperative fluoroscopy was used to determine screw length and to avoid spinal cord injury. Various systems were developed to prevent screw loosening and backout. These advances led to the introduction of unicortical screw systems in the early 1990s.

Biomechanical testing of bicortical anterior cervical instrumentation after single-level discectomy has shown a marked reduction in motion compared with the intact specimen.[26] Additional testing by Grubb and colleagues[27] showed that the Cervical Spine Locking Plate System (Synthes, Paoli, PA) using unicortical screws is biomechanically equivalent and in some cases more stable than the bicortical screw Caspar system. These results were noted after fixation of an experimental severe compression flexion injury in the cervical spine. The study by Spivak and colleagues[28] showed that locking screws significantly increase rigidity of the hardware systems initially and after cyclic loading. Based on a combination of

biomechanical and clinical studies at this time, most surgeons recommend the use of unicortical plating systems.

The clinical effectiveness of anterior cervical plate fixation must be judged not only by the successful fusion rate, but also by an improved clinical outcome. Over the past decade, several investigators have reported prospective and retrospective studies, looking at the two groups of patients fused with and without anterior cervical plates.[29] Connolly and colleagues[29] reported on 43 patients treated for cervical spondylosis with ACDF using autogenous iliac crest bone graft. The authors noted that there was no difference in the overall fusion rate or clinical results between these two groups of patients (plate vs. no plate).

Samartzis and colleagues[30] reviewed 69 consecutive patients who had undergone single-level ACDF with and without rigid instrumentation. The nonplated group consisted of 38 patients, and the plated group consisted of 31 patients. All patients had tricortical iliac crest autograft as the interbody. The plated group wore hard collars for 3 to 4 weeks, and the nonplated group wore hard collars for 6 to 8 weeks. Fusion rates of 100% and 90% were achieved in the nonplated and plated groups. These rates were not significantly different. Mean blood loss was significantly more in the plated group. Clinical success was assessed using Odom criteria at an average of 21 months. Excellent and good outcomes was reported in 91.3% and 92.1% in the nonplated and plated groups. Three nonfused patients reported good clinical outcome. Of patients, 24 were smokers, and 23 had work-related injuries. Smokers achieved a fusion rate of 95.8%. Clinical outcome and fusion rate were similar between the groups in regard to smoking status and work-related injuries.

Current systems have incorporated the use of dynamic locking. Theoretically, these systems decrease stress shielding and allow load sharing to occur between the graft and the anterior column. The decrease in graft loading reduces the risk of plate or screw failure by recreating the natural load sharing of the anterior column.[31-33] Some designs involve "dynamic screws," and others involve "dynamic plates."

Several more recent studies have shown that no significant clinical differences exist between static and dynamic plates.[34-36] Pitzen and colleagues[34] performed a prospective, controlled, randomized, multicenter study of 132 patients undergoing an anterior cervical discectomy and autograft fusion with either a dynamic plate or a rigid plate. They monitored patients for implant complications, segmental mobility, fusion, loss of lordosis, and clinical outcomes (visual analog scale [VAS] and Oswestry Disability Index [ODI]). No implant complications were seen in the dynamic group, whereas four implant complications occurred in the static group. There was no difference in fusion rate or clinical outcomes at 2 years. The loss of segmental lordosis was significantly greater in the dynamic group. By the criteria of Pitzen and colleagues,[34] the dynamic group achieved fusion at a faster rate. These authors recommended using dynamic plates because of fewer implant-related revisions and a faster time to fusion.

Nunley and colleagues[35] conducted a prospective, randomized study of static versus dynamic plates in single-level and multilevel ACDF. All patients were treated for radiculopathy. Multilevel procedures were performed in 38 of the 66 patients. When considering all study subjects, clinical outcome was equivalent between the dynamic and static groups. A clinically significant reduction in VAS and neck disability index (NDI) occurred in 73% of patients. A solid fusion was observed in 85% of patients. Clinical success predicted radiographic fusion, but fusion did not predict VAS and NDI reduction. Dynamic plates showed significantly better clinical outcomes in multilevel fusions than static plates. Nunley and colleagues[35] concluded that plate design has no effect on clinical outcome in single-level constructs. Patients undergoing multilevel fusions experience better clinical outcomes with dynamic plating, however. The loss of lordosis may be related more to graft settling than to plate design, but this has not compromised outcomes.[37]

McLaughlin and colleagues[38] detailed a cost analysis of 64 patients who underwent two-level ACDF for cervical radiculopathy. This study compared the cost of rigid internal fixation for patients with two-level ACDF with the cost in a similar population of patients who had an identical procedure without instrumentation. No difference was noted in the clinical outcome between the two groups, with both groups obtaining a 92% excellent or good result using Odom criteria. The investigators noted that patients who underwent rigid plating returned to light activities, driving, and unrestricted work sooner than noninstrumented patients. Although the overall cost was increased by approximately $3500 for the patients in the instrumentation group, the investigators believed that the increased cost was justified, owing to the significant clinical advantage to the patients and insurance disability providers, secondary to earlier mobilization and return to work.

Caspar and colleagues[39] and Geisler and colleagues[40] described one of the largest studies examining the results of plate fixation after ACDF. These two articles, describing the same group of patients, included 365 patients who underwent a one-level or two-level cervical arthrodesis performed with and without anterior cervical plate stabilization. The intended goal of this study was to determine the incidence of a second surgical intervention and whether the use of an anterior cervical plate decreased the need for subsequent surgical procedures. Although patients in these studies were not randomly assigned, and there was a mix of autograft and allograft procedures and multilevel fusions, the investigators reported that in the entire group 22 patients required repeat surgical intervention, with 20 of these patients initially in the noninstrumented group.

The addition of an anterior cervical plate using unicortical screw fixation after ACDF rarely leads to additional intraoperative complications. Plate fixation usually follows graft placement with care being taken to countersink the graft only minimally below the adjacent endplates. Typically, the exposure required for an ACDF is sufficient for placement of the cervical plate. Anterior osteophytes at the superior and inferior endplates need to be removed to provide a flat surface for plate placement. Placement of the cervical plate on top of anterior osteophytes may lead to prominence of the hardware with subsequent difficulty with postoperative swallowing. Unicortical screw placement can usually proceed without the use of fluoroscopy, with screw placement directed medially and away from the involved disc space (Fig. 40–16). Care should be taken to select a plate of the appropriate size so that the adjacent disc spaces are not violated by the screw (Fig. 40–17). The authors recommend placing the plate at least 5 mm away from the adjacent disc space to decrease the risk of ossification (Fig. 40–18).[41] Proper unicortical screw placement minimizes the risk of spinal cord injury. Intraoperative vertebral artery injury is extremely rare and occurs only with extreme screw misplacement. If sufficient surgical exposure has been obtained for the discectomy portion of the procedure, placement of the anterior cervical plate usually adds only 15 to 20 minutes to the entire operative time.

The use of an anterior cervical plate after a one-level ACDF is now common. Although the successful fusion rate may be higher with the use of instrumentation, clinical outcome has not yet been shown to be significantly improved with the addition of this hardware. As the complexity of cervical reconstructive surgical procedures increases, the use of cervical plates seems to be justified, owing to the higher fusion rate with instrumentation at two-level and three-level disease.[42-44] Wang and colleagues[44] compared the clinical and radiographic outcomes of 60 patients after two level ACDF with and without plating. The pseudarthrosis rate was significantly different at 25% for the nonplated group and 0% in the plated group. Age, gender, levels of surgery, tobacco use, and prior surgery had no correlation with fusion. A significant amount of segmental kyphosis and graft collapse was noted in the nonplated group. The complication rates were similar, however. Regardless of instrumentation, 87% of fused patients showed good to excellent results. Of patients with a pseudarthrosis, 58% reported fair results, and only 28% reported good to excellent results.

Results

In 1962, Robinson and colleagues[45] were the first to publish the results of a large series of patients treated with ACDF. The

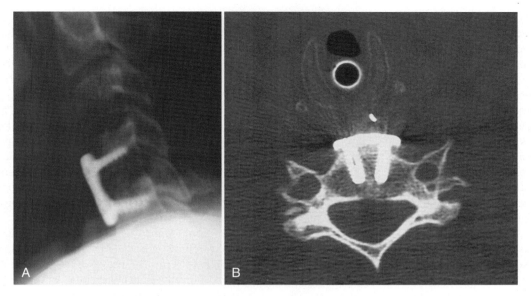

FIGURE 40–16 A, Lateral radiograph showing proper placement of anterior cervical plate using unicortical screws. Note placement of screws within adjacent vertebral bodies. **B,** Axial CT scan showing medial angulation of unicortical screws.

series consisted of 55 patients who underwent anterior discectomy and fusion at 107 disc spaces. These authors hypothesized that preservation of the subchondral bone of the endplates was necessary to provide a bearing surface for the graft. (Emery and colleagues[46] challenged this hypothesis and noted a pseudarthrosis rate of only 4.4% when partially removing the subchondral bone of the endplate with a bur.) Robinson and colleagues[45] reported 46% excellent, 27% good, 22% fair, and 6% poor results. Patients with single-level fusions showed better outcomes than patients with multilevel fusions. More than 94% of patients with single-level fusions had an excellent or good result compared with 50% of patients undergoing three or more levels of fusion. Four patients continued to report symptoms that were believed to be associated with

nonunion, and there were nine total pseudarthroses. Most importantly, only one additional surgery was necessary in a patient with a solid fusion.

Yue and colleagues[47] performed a long-term retrospective review of 71 patients after ACDF using allograft and plating. The average follow-up was 7 years (range 5 to 11 years). Single-level and multilevel patients were included. More than 90% were primary procedures. Symptoms included neck pain (94%), radiculopathy (91%), and weakness or gait problems (79%). Greater than 95% of patients reported continued significant improvement in neck pain and radiculopathy at final follow-up. Clinical improvement was not related to fusion, smoking, number of levels, collapse, or subsidence. The pseudarthrosis rate was 9%. Smoking had no effect on fusion rate.

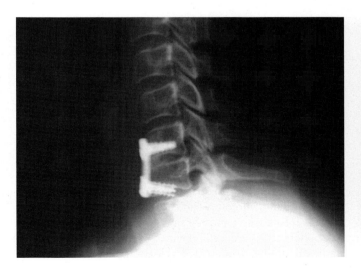

FIGURE 40–17 Plate is excessively long, with distal screws violating nonfused adjacent level.

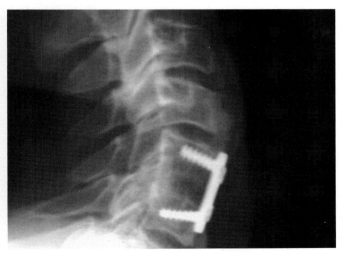

FIGURE 40–18 Successful fusion after placement of anterior cervical plate. Proximal portion of plate impinges on adjacent inferior endplate. The excessive length of this plate has led to anterior ankylosis of adjacent level that occurred 1 year after surgical procedure.

Previous surgery increased the risk of pseudarthrosis, however. No patient underwent revision for pseudarthrosis. Adjacent segment degeneration occurred in 73% of patients. Only 16% required additional surgery, with half exhibiting degenerative changes before the index procedure. Global lordosis was increased with surgery and maintained at final follow-up.

Despite a large volume of literature reporting high fusion rates with single-level ACDF, multilevel procedures present a challenge for the spine surgeon. Fusion and clinical outcomes decrease with increasing levels of surgery. Emery and colleagues[48] retrospectively reviewed 16 patients who underwent a modified Robinson ACDF at three operative levels. All patients had tricortical autogenous iliac graft placed at three levels with no internal fixation. Only 9 (56%) of the 16 patients went on to achieve solid arthrodesis at all levels. Of the seven patients with pseudarthrosis, two had severe pain requiring revision, two had moderate pain, and three had no pain. Of the nine patients with a solid fusion, three continued to have mild pain, and six had no pain. Emery and colleagues[48] concluded that a three-level modified Robinson ACDF results in an unacceptably high rate of pseudarthrosis and recommended that these patients undergo additional or alternative measures to achieve a successful arthrodesis consistently.

Wright and Eisenstein [49] compared fusion rates in single-level and two-level anterior discectomy and fusion without plating. In the 54 single-level procedures, pseudarthrosis occurred in 11% compared with 28% in the two-level group. Postoperative neck pain was less likely in patients with a solid fusion.

In an effort to improve the successful fusion and patient outcome after multilevel ACDF, Bolesta and colleagues[50] reported a prospective study of 15 patients who underwent a modified Smith-Robinson ACDF at three and four operative levels, stabilized with a unicortical anterior plate. All patients had autogenous iliac crest graft placed and had a minimum of 24 months of follow-up. Despite the addition of the anterior cervical plate, solid arthrodesis was achieved at all levels in only 7 (47%) of the 15 patients after the initial surgical procedure. Of the eight patients with pseudarthrosis, three had sufficient pain to necessitate revision surgery, one had pain without further surgery, and four had no pain. Of the seven patients with solid fusion, three had persistent pain, and four had none. Bolesta and colleagues[50] also concluded that a three-level and four-level modified Robinson ACDF results in an unacceptably high rate of pseudarthrosis. These authors believed that the addition of an anterior cervical plate alone does not improve the arthrodesis rate.

Examination of the prior two studies leads one to believe that patient outcome after multilevel anterior surgery is significantly worse than after a single-level procedure. This worse outcome may be due to the presence of advanced disease in patients needing multilevel surgery, with a poor outcome secondary to more significant pathologic processes than in patients with single-level disease.

Wang and colleagues[44,51] also studied multilevel procedures. They reviewed 60 patients after two-level ACDF.[44] Half of the patients received plate fixation, and half did not. The difference in fusion was significant. No pseudarthrosis

occurred in the plated group, whereas seven pseudarthroses occurred in the nonplated group. The complication rate was similar between the groups. Pseudarthrosis was not related to demographics or smoking status. During this same period, Wang and colleagues[51] reviewed three-level procedures as well. Of 59 patients followed for 3.2 years, pseudarthrosis occurred in 18% of plated patients versus 37% of nonplated patients. This difference was not significant, however, owing to the larger number of plated patients. Fused patients showed better clinical outcomes regardless of plating. Cauthen and colleagues[52] reviewed 146 multilevel noninstrumented cases at an average of 5 years and found a 75% fusion rate. Fusion rates are lower but still acceptable for multilevel procedures when plating is employed.

When contemplating a multilevel procedure, the surgeon should carefully review all imaging studies, possibly with correlation of electrodiagnostic studies, and perform only the required procedure at the level or levels that are causing the radiculopathy. Many patients develop significant neuroforaminal narrowing with age, and these "false-positive" findings should not lead the surgeon to operate solely based on radiographic studies.

The clinical effect of pseudarthrosis on patient outcome is controversial. Patients who have a successful fusion theoretically have improved cervical alignment, continued foraminal distraction, and prevention of collapse into kyphosis. The pseudarthrosis rate after single-level surgery ranges from 0% to 20%[53,54] with the rates approaching 50% for patients undergoing multilevel surgery.[55,56]

Phillips and colleagues[57] attempted to determine the natural history, risk factors, and treatment outcomes in a large population with documented pseudarthrosis after ACDF. They reported 48 patients with radiographically proven pseudarthrosis at an average of 5 years after the initial surgical procedure. Of the patients, 67% were symptomatic at latest follow-up or at the time of a required second surgical intervention. Several patients had a symptom-free period of up to 2 years after ACDF before redeveloping cervical symptoms after a minor traumatic episode. Analysis of the results revealed that patients who had surgery at a younger age had an increased likelihood of pseudarthrosis becoming symptomatic. Of 16 patients, 14 had successful repair of pseudarthrosis via an anterior approach, whereas 6 patients underwent posterior cervical fusion, with all going on to successful fusion. In patients in whom fusion was achieved with a second cervical operation, the results were excellent in 19 and good in 1. Phillips and colleagues[57] concluded that the surgical repair of pseudarthrosis with either an anterior or a posterior approach results in a higher likelihood of a successful clinical outcome.

The etiology of pseudarthrosis after anterior cervical surgery is multifactorial. Various authors have cited multilevel fusions, tobacco use, and revision cervical surgery as relative risk factors for the development of pseudarthrosis. Multiple studies of lumbar spine fusions have shown that cigarette smoking creates a biologically challenging environment for a successful fusion. Hilibrand and colleagues[58] compared the long-term radiographic and clinical results of smokers and nonsmokers who had undergone arthrodesis with autogenous bone graft after multilevel anterior cervical decompression for the treatment of cervical radiculopathy or myelopathy or both. After either corpectomy or multiple discectomies and interbody grafting, 190 patients were followed clinically and radiographically for at least 2 years. A subset of 40 of these patients were smokers who had undergone a cervical fusion, and only 20 had a solid fusion at all levels, whereas 69 of the 91 nonsmokers had a solid fusion at all levels ($P < .02$). This difference was more significant among patients who had a two-level interbody grafting procedure. Hilibrand and colleagues[58] concluded that smoking had a significant negative impact on healing and clinical recovery after multilevel ACDF with autogenous interbody graft for radiculopathy or myelopathy.

A prospective study by Luszczyk and colleagues[59] analyzed the fusion rates of smoking and nonsmoking patients who underwent single-level ACDF with allograft and a rigid locked anterior cervical plate. The study consisted of patients from the control groups of four separate studies evaluating cervical disc arthroplasty; 156 smokers and 417 nonsmokers were reviewed. Follow-up was at least 24 months in all patients. When analyzing all the patients, the fusion rate was 91.4%. The fusion rates were similar for the two subgroups at 91% and 91.6% for smokers and nonsmokers. These authors concluded that smoking status had no effect on the fusion status in single-level ACDF when using allograft and a locked plate.

Long-term follow-up studies of patients treated with ACDF have shown that approximately 10% of patients undergo reoperation at an adjacent level, owing to progressive spondylolysis or a new disc herniation (Fig. 40–19).[60-63] This adjacent segment disease has been theorized to be secondary to the increased biomechanical stresses on an unfused level adjacent to a solid fusion. Whether the biomechanical forces alone are sufficient to cause new disease or this is just a progression of the natural history of cervical spondylosis in a patient with significant degenerative changes remains to be determined. Treatment of this adjacent level disease is theoretically more difficult, however, because achievement of a solid fusion in these patients is hindered by the long lever arm of the prior fusion acting across the new operative level.

A retrospective review of all patients surgically treated for adjacent segment disease of the cervical spine over a 20-year period was performed by Hilibrand and colleagues[63] to determine the clinical and radiographic outcome of discectomy with interbody grafting compared with corpectomy with strut grafting in the treatment of adjacent segment disease of the cervical spine. The investigators identified 38 patients who underwent surgical treatment for multilevel adjacent segment disease by either of these two procedures. The rate of arthrodesis in 24 patients treated with discectomy was only 63%, whereas patients treated with corpectomy and strut grafting had a fusion rate of 100%. This fusion rate for discectomy and interbody fusion is much lower than that reported in the literature for patients undergoing a primary cervical procedure. Hilibrand and colleagues[63] concluded that the use of subtotal corpectomy (in patients who have had previous cervical surgery) has a higher fusion rate with strut grafting techniques. They believed that the strut of bone passing through a trough in the intermediate vertebrae across multiple motion segments may provide greater stability than multiple smaller pieces of tricortical iliac crest at each disc space. Secondarily, strut grafting requires bony union across only two surfaces compared with four or six surfaces for either two-level or three-level discectomy and fusion procedures.

Goldberg and colleagues[64] assessed the effect of workers' compensation claims on functional outcomes after ACDF. They retrospectively reviewed 80 patients; 30 had claims, and

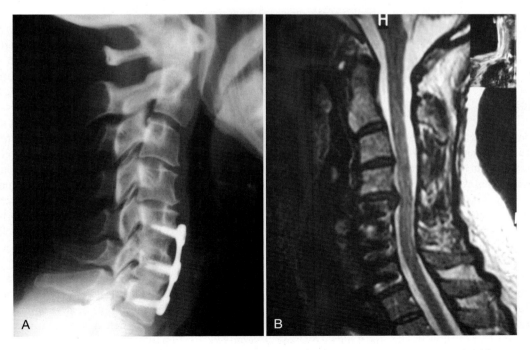

FIGURE 40–19 A and **B,** Lateral radiographs and sagittal MRI showing disc herniation adjacent to two-level fusion.

50 did not have claims. Follow-up averaged 4 years. The functional outcomes were similar with 83% and 90% good or excellent results in patients with and without claims. Patients without claims returned to work on average 8 weeks earlier. Of patients, 97% with claims and 98% without claims returned to work. These authors concluded that workers' compensation claims have no effect on long-term outcomes after ACDF.

Gore and Sepic[65] performed one of the longest follow-up studies of ACDF to date. Radiographs and functional recovery were assessed at an average of 21 years after the index procedure. Initial improvement was reported by 96% of patients. At final follow-up, 64% of these patients reported no pain. Pain recurred in the remaining patients at an average of 7 years. Only a small percentage of these patients required additional surgery.

The results of anterior cervical surgery are usually reported in terms of successful fusion rate. Although there are indications that a successful fusion may correlate with a successful clinical outcome, radiographic results alone are an insufficient parameter for determining the success of the surgical procedure. More recent orthopaedic literature has shown the value of measuring quality of life parameters after surgical intervention. Clinicians and patients can benefit from this information. Additionally, this valuable information can be used to convince insurance carriers of the benefit of surgical intervention.

Klein and colleagues[66] reviewed the outcomes of 28 patients with cervical radiculopathy treated with one-level or two-level ACDF. This prospective assessment used a health status questionnaire that is almost identical to the Medical Outcome Studies SF-36. The survey was self-administered and evaluated at an average follow-up interval of 21.8 months. The authors noted statistically significant improvement in postoperative scores for bodily pain, physical function, role function, and social function. Based on the results of the health status questionnaire, it was believed that ACDF performed on appropriate selected patients is a highly reliable surgical procedure for the management of cervical radiculopathy.

Complications

The complication rate of single-level ACDF with or without instrumentation is predictably low. Complications can occur at either the graft site during autograft harvest or in the neck. The initial report of Robinson and colleagues[45] described complications in only 8 of the 56 patients. Four patients had temporary unilateral paralysis of the vocal cords, two patients had marked temporary dysphagia, and two patients had a transient Horner syndrome. A large series reported by DePalma and colleagues[67] noted that the most common complication occurred at the iliac crest graft donor site. These researchers found 9% of patients developed a hematoma and 36% of patients continued to have persistent donor site pain 1 year after the surgical procedure. Silber and colleagues[68] reviewed the long-term bone graft donor site morbidity. Average follow-up was 4 years. Although 92.5% were satisfied with the

look of their donor site, 26% reported chronic pain at the site with half requiring pain medication. Donor site pain can be minimized by limiting the surgical exposure, with careful dissection of inner and outer tables of the iliac crest.[69] The incision should be at least 2 fingerbreadths lateral to the anterior superior iliac spine to avoid injury to the lateral femoral cutaneous nerve, which can lead to postoperative numbness. The incidence of iliac crest donor site pain can be eliminated through the use of allograft.

Fountas and colleagues[70] performed a large retrospective study of 1015 patients who had undergone primary ACDF. Final follow-up was at 1 year. About 10% of patients reported noticeable pain or difficulty swallowing initially; 95% reported resolution of symptoms within 7 days of surgery. The remaining patients reported significant improvement and resolutions by 4 weeks. Three-level procedures were significantly more likely to cause dysphagia. Dysphagia was similar between patients with and without plates. Surgical evacuation of a soft tissue hematoma was required in 24 patients (2.4%). The number of levels operated on was not related to the development of a hematoma. The addition of a plate also had no significant effect on the development of a hematoma.

Indirect laryngoscopy revealed unilateral recurrent laryngeal nerve palsy in 3.1% of patients. All were treated conservatively and had clinical resolution of symptoms within 12 weeks or less of the index procedure. The rates of nerve palsy were similar between patients with and without plates and between single-level and multilevel patients. Three patients (0.3%) experienced an esophageal perforation. Two were found and treated at the time of surgery and did well. The third patient was found late and died of complications. Two patients experienced worsening myelopathy initially but improved to preoperative functional levels by final follow-up. There were five cerebrospinal fluid leaks (0.5%) and one Horner syndrome (0.1%). At 1 year, all patients had experienced complete recovery.

Flynn[71] compiled the results of 704 neurosurgeons performing 36,657 anterior cervical interbody fusions. The most common neurologic complication was recurrent laryngeal nerve palsy, which occurred in 52 cases. This condition compromised nearly 20% of all neurologic injuries. There has been some debate as to whether the side of surgical approach affects the development of recurrent laryngeal nerve injury. A large retrospective study by Kilburg and colleagues[72] reviewed 415 patients undergoing one-level or two-level ACDF. Injury was diagnosed by observation of the vocal cords. The time from surgery to diagnosis of injury was similar between left-sided and right-sided approaches. Statistical analysis revealed no significant difference between left-sided and right sided approaches. Kilburg and colleagues[72] concluded that the side of approach has no effect on the incidence of injury.

The most devastating complication that follows any type of spine surgery is spinal cord injury. Flynn[71] reported 100 cases of significant permanent myelopathy or myeloradiculopathy in his large series. The deficit occurred immediately postoperatively in 75% of the 100 patients, whereas 25% of the patients developed a neurologic deficit in the postoperative recovery period. Analysis of his data led Flynn[71] to conclude that regardless of the etiology of the neurologic deficit, reoperation had little effect on the ultimate status of the patient's recovery. In addition, most surgeons were unable to determine the etiology of the neurologic deterioration.

Postoperative transient sore throat or dysphagia commonly occurs after anterior cervical surgery.[73,74] Reported rates range from 28% to 57%.[75-77] The exact etiology is controversial with the multiple possible mechanisms including postoperative soft tissue swelling, traction or pressure injury to the laryngeal nerves, hematoma formation, or prominent hardware. Sore throat or dysphagia is usually a transient problem that improves with time. Most surgeons report significant dysphagia persisting in less than 2% of patients at 2 years. Many practitioners believe this complication is minor, but many patients complain of significant difficulty swallowing for several weeks, with frequent need to chew their food fully before swallowing. Dull retractors and avoiding excessive retraction decrease soft tissue damage and pressure on the nerve. Yue and colleagues[78] published a mid-term report of dysphonia and dysphagia. They reviewed 74 patients at an average of 7 years after index ACDF. At final follow-up, 35% of the patients reported persistent dysphagia. These authors concluded that dysphonia and dysphagia may exist in many patients at mid-term to long-term follow-up.

Esophageal injuries are extremely rare, and morbidity and mortality are significantly increased when they occur. Newhouse and colleagues[79] reviewed 10,000 anterior cervical cases and reported an incidence of 0.25%. Sharp and motorized instruments were the cause of 30% of the injuries. These injuries were usually noted during the index procedure. If the esophageal perforation is noted at the time of the initial surgery, all attempts should be made for an acute repair. Graft extrusion, screw pullout or loosening, and plate migration were the most common causes of late perforations. The underlying reason for the perforation must be corrected first. These perforations are technically much more difficult to repair and often require prolonged use of nasogastric suction and parenteral hyperalimentation.

Autograft Versus Allograft

In recent years, the use of allograft for cervical spine fusion has become much more common. The use of allograft instead of autogenous bone for cervical fusion is acceptable if the fusion rates are equivalent and if the risk of disease transmission from the allogeneic bone is minimized. Allograft eliminates the necessity for a second surgical procedure to obtain the graft, decreasing operative time, morbidity, and pain at the donor site.

Brown and colleagues[80] reported on one of the earliest studies comparing allograft with autograft bone for anterior cervical fusions. They noted there was no difference in fusion rates between the two types of graft, but there was a significant difference in graft collapse rate, with 28% of the patients receiving allograft showing radiographic collapse, whereas only 16% of patients receiving autograft had evidence of collapse on radiographs. Brown and colleagues[80] found this trend to be true only for multilevel fusions, with single-level fusions comparable in their radiologic outcome.

Fernyhough and colleagues[81] performed a retrospective review of 26 patients who had either autogenous or allograft fibular strut graft placed after decompression for multilevel cervical spondylosis. They reported that the combined nonunion rate for both groups ranged from 21% for two-level fusion to 50% for four-level fusion. Overall, the allograft group had a statistically significant higher rate of nonunion (41%) than the autograft group (27%). There was noted to be no correlation, however, between the clinical results and the rate of union in this study.

A retrospective study by Samartzis and colleagues[82] compared 66 consecutive patients undergoing single-level ACDF with rigid plate fixation and allograft or autograft. Of the patients, 45% had work-related injuries, and 30% were smokers. The overall fusion rate was 95%. The fusion rates were similar between the two groups: 100% and 90% fusion were noted in the allograft and autograft groups. A good or excellent clinical outcome was reported by 90% of patients. The outcomes were similar regardless of the presence of a fusion and smoking status. These authors concluded that the use of allograft and a rigid plate yields a high fusion rate and good clinical outcomes.

Zdeblick and Ducker[83] reviewed 88 consecutive patients who underwent a Smith-Robinson anterior cervical fusion. In 60 of these patients, an autogenous iliac crest graft was placed, and freeze-dried iliac crest grafts were inserted in the other 27 patients. The delayed union rate and nonunion rate were noted to be significantly higher in the allograft group compared with the autograft group. If only one-level fusions were examined, the nonunion rates were similar at 1 year. The union rate was noted to be dramatically lower with allograft (38% vs. 83%) only when examining two-level fusions. Additionally, freeze-dried allograft was noted to collapse en route to healing more frequently. The clinical results between the two groups were found to be similar. These authors also concluded that the use of freeze-dried iliac crest allograft in Smith-Robinson fusions is not recommended for multilevel procedures. When freeze-dried iliac crest graft is used in one-level fusions, radiographic collapse or lucency may persist despite clinical success.

Suchomel and colleagues[84] performed a prospective study comparing allograft and autograft in single-level and two-level procedures. They followed 79 patients for at least 2 years. Similar fusion and graft collapse rates were noted regardless of graft type or number of levels fused. Smoking had no effect on fusion rate or collapse. No difference was noted between the subgroup of single-level allograft versus autograft. Likewise, no difference was noted for two-level procedures. The time to union was significantly longer in patients treated with allograft in single-level and two-level cases. Samartzis and colleagues[85] compared allograft and autograft in two-level and three-level anterior cervical decompressions and fusions with plating. They followed 80 patients for an average of 16 months. Of patients, 45 were treated with autograft, and 35 were treated with allograft. These investigators reported a combined fusion rate of 97.5%. Nonunions occurred in the allograft group. Nearly 90% of patients reported a good or excellent outcome. Clinical outcome and fusion rate were similar regardless of graft type.

Bishop and colleagues[86] evaluated the results of 132 patients after nonplated anterior cervical fusions who had at least a 1-year follow-up. Of the 83 patients who received autograft, 94% achieved a solid fusion. In the multilevel fusion group, the patients receiving autograft had an 87% successful fusion rate. Patients who received allograft had a lower fusion rate of 73% for single-level procedures and 53% for multilevel procedures.

Until more recently, the most common type of allograft used was tricortical iliac crest harvested from cadaveric iliac crest, similar in fashion to autogenous bone. In an effort to decrease the incidence of collapse rate, several surgeons have advocated the use of graft with superior structural properties, such as fibula shaft and patella.[87]

MacDonald and colleagues[88] reported on 36 patients who had undergone an anterior cervical fusion using fibular shaft allograft. Although 15 of these patients also had placement of an anterior cervical plate, 96% of the patients at 2-year follow-up had a solid fusion. An even larger study by Martin and colleagues[89] evaluated the use of freeze-dried fibular allograft. They reported on 269 patients who underwent either a single-level or a multilevel ACDF. A solid radiographic fusion was eventually achieved in 242 patients for a union rate of 90% at 2 years' follow-up. A subset of these patients, who underwent two-level fusion, achieved a fusion rate of only 72%.

Cauthen and colleagues[52] performed a large study comparing interbody graft types in noninstrumented fusions. They reviewed 348 patients with an average length of follow-up of more than 5 years. A literature review yielded historical data for comparison. Of the patients, 70% received allograft. Results revealed an overall fusion rate of 83%; this includes 75% fusion in multilevel cases and 88% in single-level cases. At an average of 5 years, 78% of patients were satisfied, and 83% returned to work. Cauthen and colleagues[52] reported no correlation between graft type and fusion status. Outcome improved, however, with a solid fusion, fewer levels involved, higher education, and no secondary financial motives. These results show similar outcomes between allograft and autograft even at extended follow-up.

There has been significant improvement in the testing of donor patients and sterilization and harvesting techniques of allograft bone. Owing to the increasing availability and improved safety profile, the use of allograft bone continues to increase, and successful anterior cervical surgery rates continue to improve. With the addition of an anterior cervical plate, union rates are most likely to approach those of autograft, even in multilevel fusions. More recently, authors have reported the use of inductive growth factors with cortical grafts in an attempt to decrease the collapse rate of the graft and to increase the fusion rate. Considering the widespread use and availability of allograft, along with its seemingly similar outcomes, allograft may be considered along with autograft as a standard component.

Polyetheretherketone

Polyetheretherketone (PEEK) cages have been advocated more recently as another alternative to autograft. Their radiolucency allows better assessment of the fusion than do metal devices (Fig. 40–20). Studies have shown PEEK to be more rigid than autograft[90]; this improves overall stiffness in compression and rotation.[91] PEEK eliminates the concerns of disease transmission and poor donor quality graft. The morbidity of allograft and autograft may be avoided.

Several studies have shown PEEK to have fusion rates near 100% at 1 year with clinical outcomes of good to excellent in 95% or more of subjects.[92-94] There were few complications. Kulkarni and colleagues[95] retrospectively reviewed their experience with stand-alone PEEK cages in a single-level anterior discectomy and fusion. They reported a fusion rate of 93% at 6 months and 100% at 2 years. The immediate and final follow-up disc height were significantly greater than preoperative values. Significant subsidence occurred, however, between the immediate and final follow-up. The immediate postoperative segmental lordosis was greater than preoperatively but was not maintained at final follow-up. No cage-related complications were noted. Kulkarni and colleagues[95] conceded that the use of anterior plating may have helped to maintain lordosis better and decrease the need for postoperative bracing.

Celik and colleagues[96] performed a prospectively controlled randomized study of PEEK and iliac crest bone graft to assess changes in foraminal height and fusion rate. No anterior plating was employed. Postoperatively, both groups showed significant improvement in VAS and Japanese Orthopedic Association (JOA) scores. The groups had similar clinical outcomes, lordosis, and fusion rates at final follow-up of 18 months. The iliac crest group showed a significant increase in interspace and foraminal height initially. Interspace height was significantly decreased, however, and the foraminal height increase was not maintained at final follow-up. Celik and

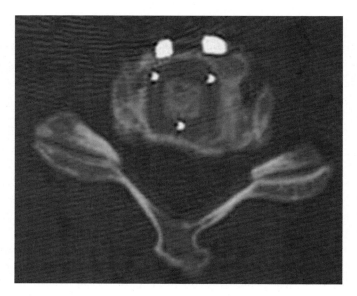

FIGURE 40–20 Postoperative axial CT scan showing placement of polyetheretherketone (PEEK) cage.

colleagues[96] attributed these findings to graft subsidence, resorption, and compression. The PEEK group showed significant increases in interspace and foraminal height that were maintained at 18 months. These authors concluded that PEEK cages maintain foraminal decompression and sagittal alignment better than nonplated autograft.

PEEK may offer even more advantages when considering multilevel procedures. When using iliac crest, kyphosis has been noted even when a solid fusion develops.[97,98] High rates of graft collapses have also been noted in multilevel fusions.[98-100]

A small prospective, nonrandomized study by Demircan and colleagues[101] studied the safety and efficacy of PEEK used in multilevel fusions without screws, plates, or autogenous iliac crest. They packed PEEK cages with demineralized bone matrix. At final follow-up, all the patients showed a significant improvement in JOA score. Preoperative lordosis was maintained at 18-month follow-up. Fusion rate was 90%. The nonfusions occurred in three-level and four-level fusions. No one required reoperation at final follow-up.

Cho and colleagues[102] performed a much larger prospective, randomized study of 180 patients. Subjects were randomly assigned to ACDF with PEEK cage, iliac crest autograft with plating, or iliac crest autograft without plating. All three groups were similar in demographics. The PEEK cages were packed with iliac crest bone marrow that was obtained with a hollow driver through a small 1-cm incision. The average follow-up was 2.5 years. There were no graft complications in the PEEK group; the plated group had a complication rate of 4%. Graft collapse, nonunion, and graft dislodgment resulted in a complication rate of 50% in the nonplated group. Fusion rates at 1 year of 100% and 98% for the PEEK and plated groups were significantly better than the rate of 87% for the nonplated group. The time to fusion was significantly faster in the PEEK and plated groups as well. Clinical outcome was similar between the PEEK and plated groups. The PEEK group was statistically better than the nonplated group. Cervical lordosis was increased in the PEEK and plated groups compared with a relative increase in kyphosis in the nonplated group. Although PEEK and plating provide good clinical and radiographic outcomes with few complications, PEEK may be advantageous because it has the fewest complications.

The use of PEEK cages has increased over the last several years. Outcomes have been shown to be similar to autograft. The decreased morbidity offers an immediate positive benefit. The increased cost of cages may be offset by this decreased morbidity. PEEK has not been extensively studied against allograft; questions remain in this area. The long-term effects of better maintenance of height and alignment have yet to be elucidated. It is still too early to determine whether the short-term advantages will translate into better long-term outcomes.

Bone Morphogenetic Proteins

Bone morphogenetic protein (BMP) has been available for use in the cervical spine for a few years. This is an off-label use, but nonetheless BMP has been used extensively. Buttermann[103] directly compared allograft and BMP versus iliac crest bone graft in a nonrandomized study of 66 consecutive patients who had primary one-level, two-level, or three-level ACDF. He followed them prospectively over 2 to 3 years. No difference was seen in VAS, ODI index, pain medication use, opinion of treatment success, and neurologic recovery. Half of the BMP group had neck swelling and dysphagia versus 14% in the autograft group. BMP was more costly, and operative time was only modestly reduced. Buttermann[103] concluded that BMP yields clinical and radiographic outcomes that are equivalent to autograft but at an increased cost with significant safety concerns.

Several other reports of complications have arisen in the literature.[104-106] More than 20% of patients in these studies had significant neck swelling. This was significantly more than in patients who were not treated with BMP. One patient had to be reintubated more than 5 days after his index procedure.[104] The swelling has been attributed to pharyngeal edema owing to inflammation and not hematoma formation. Vaidya and colleagues[107] reviewed their complications with BMP in the anterior cervical spine. They compared 22 patients treated with BMP and PEEK cages with patients treated with allograft and demineralized bone matrix (DBM). Every patient treated with BMP showed endplate resorption during the first 6 weeks. Dysphagia was more severe and frequent in the BMP group. Anterior neck swelling was significantly greater in the BMP group. Clinical outcome was similar in both groups at 24 months. Cost analysis showed BMP and PEEK to be three times more expensive than allograft and DBM.

The U.S. Food and Drug Administration (FDA) and NASS have publicly stated concern regarding the use of BMP in the anterior cervical spine over concerns of significant complications. Until the dosage and safety concerns have been reconciled, most surgeons would agree that placing BMP in the anterior cervical spine has significant risks.

Anterior Cervical Foraminotomy

In an effort to eliminate the need for a fusion at the time of decompression, multiple authors[108-110] have recommended anterior cervical microforaminotomy for nerve root decompression. Although there are multiple variations of this procedure, the exposure involves an anterolateral approach to the cervical spine with incisional splitting of the longus colli muscle medial to the anterior tubercle of the transverse process. This is followed by removal of the uncovertebral joint and subsequent removal of the pathologic elements compressing the nerve root. Several small studies have reported resolution of radicular symptoms with this procedure.[111-113] Most of these studies have only short-term follow-up. Although one author[109] reported excellent or good outcomes in 98% of 104 patients with cervical discogenic radiculopathy, there has not yet been widespread acceptance of this procedure. Potential complications more common to this procedure include injury to the sympathetic plexus and vertebral artery injury. This procedure typically can be performed unilaterally only. Further long-term studies by additional authors are needed

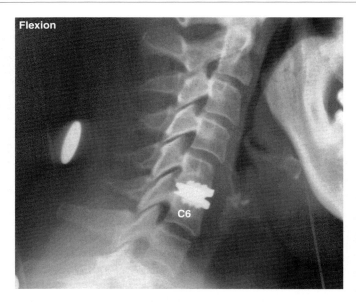

FIGURE 40–21 Lateral radiograph of cervical disc replacement at C5-6 at 6 weeks.

before this procedure can be widely recommended. If this procedure is performed successfully, it obviates the need for fusion at the time of decompression with preservation of motion at the surgical level.

Anterior Discectomy Without Fusion

Anterior cervical discectomy without fusion developed as an alternative technique to cervical fusion, based on the premise that if successful results of anterior fusions occur with pseudarthrosis, discectomy can be performed without fusion. Several articles have advocated anterior cervical discectomy without fusion, reporting success rates similar to fusion.[114-116] Murphy and Gadd[114] reported 26 patients who underwent a one-level or two-level anterior cervical discectomy for radiculopathy secondary to a herniated cervical disc. Good results (neurologic deficit improved, pain alleviated, and patient able to return to normal activities) were reported in 24 of 26 patients. The two patients with poor results required reoperation within 2 weeks of the initial procedure. Murphy and Gadd[114] noted that 72% of the patients developed a spontaneous fusion at the discectomy level, and all 20 patients developed some degree of postoperative kyphosis.

Murphy and Gadd[114] and others[115] neglected to mention specifically the postoperative incidence of neck pain. Several authors[117-119] noted transient postoperative severe neck pain after cervical discectomy without fusion. This procedure defeats the principle of successful anterior cervical surgery, which is based on the premise of neuroforaminal distraction and reduction of buckling of the ligamentum flavum. In addition, by its very nature, this surgery is designed to create a pseudarthrosis that may lead to a less satisfactory result. Theoretically, the results of this surgery may be more successful for patients with soft disc herniation than for patients with spondylolysis, but there is an unacceptably high rate of persistent postoperative neck pain. Most series to date have a limited

clinical follow-up and poor radiographic correlation to determine the development and significance of postoperative instability or kyphotic angulation.

Studies of anterior cervical discectomy with and without fusion[120,121] have shown that the procedure without fusion decreases hospital cost and hospital stay and surgical morbidity. These early economic benefits must be weighed against long-term outcome, however.

Cervical Disc Arthroplasty

Most recently, the FDA has approved the use of cervical disc arthroplasty for single-level cervical radiculopathy. These devices have been studied in multiple prospective, randomized, multicenter clinical trials for noninferiority.[122-124] Most of these studies have involved hundreds of patients randomly assigned to either disc arthroplasty or single-level ACDF (Fig. 40–21).

Generally, these devices have been studied for use in C3-7 in patients 18 to 60 years old without significant kyphosis, instability, inflammatory disease, significant disc height loss, or significant spondylosis. In a study of 463 patients, 242 received a cervical disc arthroplasty, and 221 underwent ACDF.[122] Both groups showed improvement in clinical outcome that was maintained at 12 months and 24 months. Statistically significant reduction in NDI occurred in both groups. The arthroplasty group exhibited significantly greater reductions than the fusion group. Neck and arm pain were also significantly improved for each group at all time intervals. The study authors reported a greater improvement in NDI and overall success in the arthroplasty group. Adverse events including reoperation rates were similar between the groups. Arthroplasty patients on average returned to work 13 days earlier than fusion patients. When used in a workers' compensation population, clinical outcomes were equivalent for patients treated with ACDF and patients undergoing disc arthroplasty.[123] A trend was seen toward an earlier return to work for arthroplasty patients.

Cervical disc arthroplasty attempts to allow maintenance of cervical motion; it is thought that this decreases the abnormal adjacent level forces created by a fusion. This may lead to a decreased adjacent segment disease and lead to better long-term outcomes than fusion. The in vivo kinematics of two different cervical disc arthroplasty implants have been compared with controls.[125] After analyzing the range of motion of the 51 implants to 200 healthy individuals' discs, both implants reduced range of motion significantly. The range of motion between the implants was not significantly different. The center of rotation was in the normal range for both devices despite being influenced by the type of device. The study authors concluded that the two devices did not restore a normal range of motion.

These devices have been shown to maintain segmental mobility compared with fusion.[122,124,126] Compared with intact specimens, disc arthroplasty can maintain motion coupling as well.[127] The results of the Bryan disc (Medtronic, Memphis, TN) clinical trial, which was a prospective, randomized, and controlled study, were reviewed at 2 years.[126] Motion analysis of the 242 Bryan artificial discs revealed no evidence of bridging bone across any implant, no implant migration, and no evidence of implant subsidence. The immediate postoperative range of motion of the disc replacement levels was maintained at final follow-up.

Sasso and Best[128] performed a kinematic analysis of the adjacent segments in a subgroup of patients from this study. No difference in range of motion was shown at the level above and below either a fusion or arthroplasty. During flexion-extension, increased anterior and posterior translation at the level proximal to fusion levels was observed to be significant. Sasso and Best[128] postulated that to achieve similar range of motion after fusion, increased translation is necessary at the adjacent segments. This increased translation may place excessive loads and forces across the adjacent disc.

Several other groups have studied segmental motion and intradiscal pressure at levels adjacent to a fusion or an arthroplasty.[129-132] Cadaveric models showed that segmental mobility is increased at the levels adjacent to a fused level.[130-132] Chang and colleagues[129] evaluated the disc pressures and facet joint forces adjacent to a cervical arthroplasty and discectomy with fusion. They controlled their study by measuring intact specimens. After arthroplasty, the adjacent segment proximal and distal segments showed no significant change in disc pressure. The segment proximal to the ACDF group exhibited increased disc pressure of approximately 40%. Changes in facet joint force were minimal in all groups. Forces increased at the treated level and decreased at adjacent segments in the arthroplasty group, whereas the fusion group showed decreased forces at the treated level and increased forces at the adjacent segments. These authors believed that increased disc pressures may impair disc metabolism and contribute to disc degeneration. They concluded that although arthroplasty increases loading of the treated level facets, it maintains normal intradiscal pressures at adjacent segments. In a two-level model comparing disc arthroplasty with fusion, arthroplasty showed much lower disc pressures in adjacent segments than fusion.[133] Fusion and arthroplasty alter cervical biomechanics. These alterations seem to be less pronounced with arthroplasty; however, more clinical studies and long-term study are warranted.

Complications have been reported with arthroplasty. Spontaneous fusion and heterotopic ossification causing restricted motion has been shown to occur in 10% of arthroplasty-treated levels.[134] Anderson and colleagues[135] compared the adverse events of a clinical trial of arthroplasty versus ACDF. Adverse medical events not related to surgery were slightly higher in the arthroplasty-treated patients: 35% versus 31% in the fusion group. Most of these adverse medical events were genitourinary and gastrointestinal. Dysphagia and superficial wound infections occurred in the arthroplasty group. Dysphagia was classified as a less severe complication. Anderson and colleagues[135] postulated that the dysphagia may have been related to longer operative time in the arthroplasty group. When considering more severe adverse events, such as severe arm or neck symptoms, prolonged anesthesia, permanent neurologic injury, or death, significantly more occurred in the

fusion group compared with the arthroplasty group. Reoperation was required in 5% of the arthroplasty group compared with 7% of the fusion group. Overall, the arthroplasty group required fewer reoperations, and complications were less severe compared with the fusion group.

Additional complications reported with arthroplasty include increased segmental kyphosis.[136] Kim and colleagues[137] reviewed 55 cervical disc replacements at 2 years. Global cervical lordosis was maintained in 86% of patients. Segmental lordosis was maintained in just 36% of the operated levels, however. The clinical importance of increased segmental kyphosis after arthroplasty is not well understood.

Artificial disc replacement combined with fusion may offer significantly better results than multilevel fusion. Phillips and colleagues[138] reported on the use of disc replacement in patients with and without adjacent level fusion. Surgical time, blood loss, and clinical outcomes were similar between the groups. Both groups showed significant improvement in VAS and NDI. Two revisions were performed in each group. Shin and colleagues[139] performed a prospective analysis of 40 patients. Half the patients underwent two-level ACDF, and the other half underwent hybrid construct of an ACDF and a disc arthroplasty. The hybrid group had significantly better NDI and decrease in neck pain compared with the multilevel ACDF group. Most importantly, Phillips and colleagues[138] noted significantly increased range of motion in the segment inferior to the multilevel fusions. These studies suggest that arthroplasty adjacent to fusion offers similar short-term results to multilevel fusion, if not slightly improved results.

Several authors[140-142] have studied multilevel cervical disc arthroplasty. A prospective, randomized study by Cheng and colleagues[140] compared two-level ACDF with two-level arthroplasty. NDI and VAS were improved greatly in both groups; NDI improved more in the arthroplasty group. These authors concluded that two-level arthroplasty is safe and effective in treating two-level cervical disease. A large prospective, consecutive series by Pimenta and colleagues[142] compared the outcomes of single-level versus multilevel arthroplasty. Single-level disc arthroplasty was performed in 71 patients, and two-level, three-level, and four-level arthroplasty was performed in 53, 12, and 4 patients. Although VAS reduction was similar, the 52% reduction in NDI for the multilevel group was significantly more compared with the 37% reduction in the single-level group. Complication rates including reoperation were similar with an implant retention rate of 94% at 3 years. Clinical success rates were similar, however: 93.9% for multilevel arthroplasties and 90.5% for single-level arthroplasties. These studies suggest that multilevel arthroplasty is as safe and effective as fusion for multilevel disease. Pseudarthrosis and complication rates increase with the number of levels fused; multilevel arthroplasty may decrease morbidity.[143,144] Long-term clinical outcomes and rates of adjacent segment degeneration are still unknown.

Multiple issues concerning disc replacement still exist. The data concerning cervical disc arthroplasty are still in early stages. The advantages of arthroplasty are multiple. Good long-term data will better delineate the place of arthroplasty in the armamentarium of the spine surgeon. It will take many more years of follow-up to assess whether or not arthroplasty can decrease the risk of adjacent segment disease. Currently, most insurance companies do not cover disc arthroplasty. Arthroplasty seems to offer similar results as fusion and may eventually offer better outcomes with fewer complications.

Summary

Review of the studies mentioned in this chapter leads to the conclusion that patients who undergo a fusion at the same time as anterior cervical discectomy have a better long-term outcome. The risks and pain associated with autograft harvest can be reduced with bone graft substitutes. Although allograft is most commonly used, future ceramics and composite materials either with or without BMPs (dosed at an appropriate safe level) can give the patient the benefit of a solid fusion without the morbidity of bone graft harvesting. The widespread acceptance of anterior cervical instrumentation has decreased the need for brace usage and increased fusion rates; although in the short-term it increases operative costs, long-term economic benefits can be realized by earlier patient mobilization and return to normal activity levels.

PEARLS

1. During intubation of the patient for an anterior cervical procedure, the anesthesiologist should tape the endotracheal tube to the side of the mouth opposite to the incision. For a standard left-sided approach, taping the endotracheal tube on the right side is beneficial for draping and exposure.

2. When operating in the lower cervical spine at C6-7 or C7-T1, this area is often difficult to visualize on radiograph for intraoperative localization. Occasionally, needles may need to be placed in a more superior disc space to aid in correct level identification.

3. Anterior osteophytes at the adjacent cervical bodies need to be removed before anterior cervical plate placement. If these osteophytes are not removed sufficiently, the prominent plate can lead to dysphagia.

4. Careful review of radiographs, specifically looking for anterior osteophytes, can aid in correct level identification during the surgical procedure. These large osteophytes often can be palpated during blunt dissection between the carotid sheath and the trachea and esophagus.

5. Removal of anterior osteophytes before discectomy significantly aids in visualization of the disc space. Osteophyte removal is extremely beneficial when trying to visualize the uncinate process or probing behind the posterior longitudinal ligament in the search for a sequestered disc fragment.

PITFALLS

1. Although blunt dissection can be used to define the interval between the carotid sheath laterally and the trachea and esophagus medially, care should be taken to avoid avulsion of the vessels off the carotid artery and jugular vein, which can lead to excessive bleeding.

2. MRI of the cervical spine frequently shows disc protrusions and sometimes even herniations in asymptomatic patients. It is imperative that the patient's signs and symptoms of cervical radiculopathy correlate with findings on MRI before proceeding with surgical intervention.

3. During initial positioning of the patient before the procedure, hyperextension of the neck should be avoided, especially in patients with cervical myelopathy. Often myelopathy is worsened because of hyperextension; with the patient anesthetized, symptoms of cord compression cannot be verbalized.

4. Unilateral vocal cord paralysis after anterior cervical surgery can be minimally symptomatic. If a patient needs a revision procedure and the approach is contemplated to occur on the side opposite to the initial incision, fiberoptic visualization of the vocal cords should be considered to ensure mobility. Bilateral vocal cord paralysis leads to extreme complications.

KEY POINTS

1. An anterior approach is an excellent method of treating cervical radiculopathy. A thorough history and physical examination coupled with a meticulous review of the imaging studies is required for proper preoperative planning.

2. ACDF is a proven method of treatment for radiculopathy with very good short-term and long-term outcomes. The spinal cord and nerve roots can be directly decompressed.

3. Proper identification of the correct level is paramount.

4. Anterior plating decreases orthosis requirements and improves fusion rates; however, clinical outcomes are similar to noninstrumented procedures. Dynamic and static plates produce similar outcomes.

5. Complication rates remain low despite the widespread use of instrumentation.

6. Autograft has been replaced by allograft for interbody graft. Clinical outcomes and fusion rates between autograft and allograft are similar.

7. BMP should not be used in the anterior cervical spine until further research has been done to determine proper dosing and safety.

8. The short-term outcomes of cervical arthroplasty are similar to ACDF. Arthroplasty provides an effective alternative to ACDF for the treatment of radiculopathy. The effects of arthroplasty on adjacent segment disease require more study.

KEY REFERENCES

1. Smith G, Robinson R: The treatment of certain cervical spine disorders by anterior removal of the intervertebral disc and interbody fusion. J Bone Joint Surg Am 40:607-624, 1958. This classic article describes the treatment for ACDF. The initial indications for surgical treatment are very similar to today's standards.

2. Bohlman HH, Emery SE, Goodfellow DB, et al: Robinson anterior cervical discectomy and arthrodesis for cervical radiculopathy: Long-term follow-up of one-hundred-and-twenty-two patients. J Bone Joint Surg Am 75:1298-1301, 1993.
This article reports long-term follow-up of 122 patients who underwent an ACDF with iliac crest bone grafting for cervical radiculopathy. Pseudarthrosis occurred in approximately 10% of patients and was significantly greater after multilevel arthrodesis than after single-level arthrodesis.

3. McLaughlin MR, Purighalla V, Pizzi FJ: Cost advantages of two-level anterior cervical fusion with rigid internal fixation for radiculopathy and degenerative disease. Surg Neurol 48:560-565, 1997.
Investigators analyzed 64 patients who underwent a two-level ACDF for radiculopathy to determine the advantage of rigid internal fixation. There was no clinical difference in the outcome between the two groups. Patients who underwent rigid plating returned to light activities, driving, and unrestricted work sooner than patients without instrumentation.

4. Malloy KM, Hilibrand AS: Autograft versus allograft in degenerative cervical disease. Clin Orthop Relat Res 394:27-38, 2002.
This article reviews the use of allograft versus autograft in the cervical spine. Overall higher fusion rates were reported with autograft than allograft; however, similar fusion rates have been reported among nonsmokers having single-level anterior cervical interbody fusions.

5. Flynn T: Neurologic complications of anterior cervical interbody fusion. Spine (Phila Pa 1976) 7:536-539, 1982.
This study reports the largest compilation of anterior cervical surgery resulting from questionnaires sent to more than 1300 neurosurgeons. The incidence of major and minor neurologic complications is reported.

REFERENCES

1. Dean CL, Gabriel JP, Cassinelli EH, et al: Degenerative spondylolisthesis of the cervical spine: Analysis of 58 patients treated with anterior cervical decompression and fusion. Spine J 9:439-446, 2009.

2. Brain L, Wilkinson M (eds): Cervical Spondylolisthesis and Other Disorders of the Cervical Spine. Philadelphia, WB Saunders, 1967.

3. Edwards WC, LaRocca H: The developmental segmental sagittal diameter of the cervical spinal canal in patients with cervical spondylosis. Spine (Phila Pa 1976) 8:20-27, 1983.

4. Lee MJ, Cassinelli EH, Riew KD: Prevalence of cervical spine stenosis: Anatomic study in cadavers. J Bone Joint Surg Am 89:376-380, 2007.

5. Pavlov H, Torg JS, Robie B, et al: Cervical spinal stenosis: Determination with vertebral body ratio method. Radiology 164:771-775, 1987.

6. Blackley HR, Plank LD, Robertson PA: Determining the sagittal dimensions of the canal of the cervical spine: The reliability of ratios of anatomical measurements. J Bone Joint Surg Br 81:110-112, 1999.

7. Lim JK, Wong HK: Variation of the cervical spinal Torg ratio with gender and ethnicity. Spine J 4:396-401, 2004.

8. Prasad SS, O'Malley M, Caplan M, et al: MRI measurements of the cervical spine and their correlation to Pavlov's ratio. Spine (Phila Pa 1976) 28:1263-1268, 2003.

9. Bell GR, Ross JS: Diagnosis of nerve root compression. Orthop Clin North Am 22:405-419, 1992.

10. Chen CJ, Lyu RK, Lee ST, et al: Intramedullary high signal intensity on T2-weighted MR images in cervical spondylotic myelopathy: Prediction of prognosis with type of intensity. Radiology 221:789-794, 2001.

11. Shen Y, Zhang YZ, Wang LF: [Relation of MR T2 image signal intensity ratio of cervical spondylotic myelopathy with clinical manifestations and prognosis]. Zhonghua Yi Xue Za Zhi 88:3072-3076, 2008.

12. Boden SD, McCowin PR, Davis DO, et al: Abnormal magnetic-resonance scans of the cervical spine in asymptomatic subjects: A prospective investigation. J Bone Joint Surg Am 72:1178-1184, 1990.

13. Okada E, Matsumoto M, Ichihara D, et al: Aging of the cervical spine in healthy volunteers: A 10-year longitudinal magnetic resonance imaging study. Spine (Phila Pa 1976) 34:706-712, 2009.

14. Ashkan K, Johnston P, Moore AJ: A comparison of magnetic resonance imaging and neurophysiological studies in the assessment of cervical radiculopathy. Br J Neurosurg 16:146-148, 2002.

15. Berger AR, Busis NA, Logigian EL, et al: Cervical root stimulation in the diagnosis of radiculopathy. Neurology 37:329-332, 1987.

16. Tsai CP, Huang CI, Wang V, et al: Evaluation of cervical radiculopathy by cervical root stimulation. Electromyogr Clin Neurophysiol 34:363-366, 1994.

17. Smith G, Robinson R: The treatment of certain cervical spine disorders by anterior removal of the intervertebral disc and interbody fusion. J Bone Joint Surg Am 40:607-624, 1958.

18. Apfelbaum RI, Kriskovich MD, Haller JR: On the incidence, cause, and prevention of recurrent laryngeal nerve palsies during anterior cervical spine surgery. Spine (Phila Pa 1976) 25:2906-2912, 2000.

19. Audu P, Artz G, Scheid S, et al: Recurrent laryngeal nerve palsy after anterior cervical spine surgery: The impact of endotracheal tube cuff deflation, reinflation, and pressure adjustment. Anesthesiology 105:898-901, 2006.

20. Nassr A, Lee JY, Bashir RS, et al: Does incorrect level needle localization during anterior cervical discectomy and fusion lead to accelerated disc degeneration? Spine (Phila Pa 1976) 34:189-192, 2009.

21. Jagannathan J, Shaffrey CI, Oskouian RJ, et al: Radiographic and clinical outcomes following single-level anterior cervical discectomy and allograft fusion without plate placement or cervical collar. J Neurosurg Spine 8:420-428, 2008.

22. Campbell MJ, Carreon LY, Traynelis V, et al: Use of cervical collar after single-level anterior cervical fusion with plate: Is it necessary? Spine (Phila Pa 1976) 34:43-48, 2009.

23. Liu JT, Briner RP, Friedman JA: Comparison of inpatient vs. outpatient anterior cervical discectomy and fusion: A retrospective case series. BMC Surg 9:3, 2009.

24. Erickson M, Fites BS, Thieken MT, et al: Outpatient anterior cervical discectomy and fusion. Am J Orthop 36:429-432, 2007.

25. Villavicencio AT, Pushchak E, Burneikiene S, et al: The safety of instrumented outpatient anterior cervical discectomy and fusion. Spine J 7:148-153, 2007.

25a. Bohler J: Sofort-und Fruhbehandlong traumatischer querschnitt lahmungen. Zeitschrift fur Orthopadie und Ihre Grenzgebiete 103:512-529, 1967.

26. Schulte K, Clark C, Goel V: Kinematics of the cervical spine following discectomy and stabilization. Spine (Phila Pa 1976) 14:1116-1121, 1989.

27. Grubb M, Currier B, Shih J, et al: Biomechanical evaluation of anterior cervical spine stabilization. Spine (Phila Pa 1976) 23:886-892, 1998.

28. Spivak J, Chen D, Kummer F: The effect of locking fixation screws on the stability of anterior cervical plating. Spine (Phila Pa 1976) 24:334-338, 1999.

29. Connolly PJ, Esses SI, Kostuik JP: Anterior cervical fusion: Outcome analysis of patients fused with and without anterior cervical plates. J Spinal Disord 9:202-206, 1996.

30. Samartzis D, Shen FH, Lyon C, et al: Does rigid instrumentation increase the fusion rate in one-level anterior cervical discectomy and fusion? Spine J 4:636-643, 2004.

31. Dvorak MF, Pitzen T, Zhu Q, et al: Anterior cervical plate fixation: A biomechanical study to evaluate the effects of plate design, endplate preparation, and bone mineral density. Spine (Phila Pa 1976) 30:294-301, 2005.

32. Reidy D, Finkelstein J, Nagpurkar A, et al: Cervical spine loading characteristics in a cadaveric C5 corpectomy model using a static and dynamic plate. J Spinal Disord Tech 17:117-122, 2004.

33. Truumees E, Demetropoulos CK, Yang KH, et al: Effects of a cervical compression plate on graft forces in an anterior cervical discectomy model. Spine (Phila Pa 1976) 28:1097-1102, 2003.

34. Pitzen TR, Chrobok J, Stulik J, et al: Implant complications, fusion, loss of lordosis, and outcome after anterior cervical plating with dynamic or rigid plates: Two-year results of a multi-centric, randomized, controlled study. Spine (Phila Pa 1976) 34:641-646, 2009.

35. Nunley PD, Jawahar A, Kerr EJ 3rd, et al: Choice of plate may affect outcomes for single versus multilevel ACDF: Results of a prospective randomized single-blind trial. Spine J 9:121-127, 2009.

36. Brodke DS, Klimo P Jr, Bachus KN, et al: Anterior cervical fixation: Analysis of load-sharing and stability with use of static and dynamic plates. J Bone Joint Surg Am 88:1566-1573, 2006.

37. Ghahreman A, Rao PJ, Ferch RD: Dynamic plates in anterior cervical fusion surgery: Graft settling and cervical alignment. Spine (Phila Pa 1976) 34:1567-1571, 2009.

38. McLaughlin MR, Purighalla V, Pizzi FJ: Cost advantages of two-level anterior cervical fusion with rigid internal fixation for radiculopathy and degenerative disease. Surg Neurol 48:560-565, 1997.

39. Caspar W, Geisler FH, Pitzen T, et al: Anterior cervical plate stabilization in one- and two-level degenerative disease: Overtreatment or benefit? J Spinal Disord 11:1-11, 1998.

40. Geisler FH, Caspar W, Pitzen T, et al: Re-operation in patients after anterior cervical plate stabilization in degenerative disease. Spine (Phila Pa 1976) 23:911-920, 1998.

41. Park JB, Cho YS, Riew KD: Development of adjacent-level ossification in patients with an anterior cervical plate. J Bone Joint Surg Am 87:558-563, 2005.

42. Bolesta MJ, Rechtine GR 2nd, Chrin AM: One- and two-level anterior cervical discectomy and fusion: The effect of plate fixation. Spine J 2:197-203, 2002.

43. Connolly PJ, Esses SI, Kostuik JP: Anterior cervical fusion: Outcome analysis of patients fused with and without anterior cervical plates. J Spinal Disord 9:202-206, 1996.

44. Wang JC, McDonough PW, Endow KK, et al: Increased fusion rates with cervical plating for two-level anterior cervical discectomy and fusion. Spine (Phila Pa 1976) 25:41-45, 2000.

45. Robinson R, Walker A, Ferlic D: The results of anterior interbody fusion of the cervical spine. J Bone Joint Surg Am 44:1569-1587, 1962.

46. Emery SE, Bolesta MJ, Banks MA, et al: Robinson anterior cervical fusion: Comparison of standard and modified techniques. Spine (Phila Pa 1976) 19:660-663, 1994.

47. Yue WM, Brodner W, Highland TR: Long-term results after anterior cervical discectomy and fusion with allograft and plating: A 5- to 11-year radiologic and clinical follow-up study. Spine (Phila Pa 1976) 30:2138-2144, 2005.

48. Emery SE, Fisher RS, Bohlman HH: Three-level anterior cervical discectomy and fusion: Radiographic and clinical results. Spine (Phila Pa 1976) 22:2622-2625, 1997.

49. Wright IP, Eisenstein SM: Anterior cervical discectomy and fusion without instrumentation. Spine (Phila Pa 1976) 32:772-774; discussion 775, 2007.

50. Bolesta MJ, Rechtine GR, Chrin AM: Three- and four-level anterior cervical discectomy and fusion with plate fixation: A prospective study. Spine (Phila Pa 1976) 25:2040-2046, 2000.

51. Wang JC, McDonough PW, Kanim LE, et al: Increased fusion rates with cervical plating for three-level anterior cervical discectomy and fusion. Spine (Phila Pa 1976) 26:643-646; discussion 646-647, 2001.

52. Cauthen JC, Kinard RE, Vogler JB, et al: Outcome analysis of noninstrumented anterior cervical discectomy and interbody fusion in 348 patients. Spine (Phila Pa 1976) 23:188-192, 1998.

53. Aronson N, Filtzer DL, Bagan M: Anterior cervical fusion by the Smith-Robinson approach. J Neurosurg 29:397-404, 1968.

54. Riley LH, Robinson RA, Johnson KA, et al: The results of anterior interbody fusion of the cervical spine. J Neurosurg 30:127-133, 1969.

55. Connolly ES, Seymour RJ, Adams JE: Clinical evaluation of anterior cervical fusion for degenerative cervical disc disease. J Neurosurg 23:431-437, 1965.

56. White AA, Southwick WO, DuPonte R, et al: Relief of pain by anterior cervical spine fusion for spondylosis. J Bone Joint Surg Am 55:525-534, 1968.

57. Phillips FM, Carlson G, Emery SE, et al: Anterior cervical pseudarthrosis: Natural history and treatment. Spine (Phila Pa 1976) 22:1585-1589, 1997.

58. Hilibrand AS, Fye MA, Emery SE, et al: Impact of smoking on the outcome of anterior cervical arthrodesis with interbody or strut-grafting. J Bone Joint Surg Am 83:668-673, 2001.

59. Luszczyk M, Fischgrund J, Sasso R, et al: Does smoking have an impact on fusion rate in single level ACDF with allograft and rigid plate fixation? Cervical Spine Research Society meeting, 2008.

60. Bohlman HH, Emery SE, Goodfellow DB, et al: Robinson anterior cervical discectomy and arthrodesis for cervical radiculopathy: Long-term follow-up of one-hundred-and-twenty-two patients. J Bone Joint Surg Am 75:1298-1301, 1993.

61. Clements DH, O'Leary PF: Anterior cervical discectomy and fusion. Spine (Phila Pa 1976) 15:1023-1025, 1990.

62. Gore DR, Sepic SB: Anterior cervical fusion for degenerated or protruded discs. Spine (Phila Pa 1976) 9:667-671, 1984.

63. Hilibrand AS, Yoo JU, Carlson GD, et al: The success of anterior cervical arthrodesis adjacent to a previous fusion. Spine (Phila Pa 1976) 22:1574-1579, 1997.

64. Goldberg EJ, Singh K, Van U, et al: Comparing outcomes of anterior cervical discectomy and fusion in workman's versus non-workman's compensation population. Spine J 2:408-414, 2002.

65. Gore DR, Sepic SB: Anterior discectomy and fusion for painful cervical disc disease: A report of 50 patients with an average follow-up of 21 years. Spine (Phila Pa 1976) 23:2047-2051, 1998.

66. Klein GR, Vaccaro AR, Albert TJ: Health outcome assessment before and after anterior cervical discectomy and fusion for radiculopathy: A prospective analysis. Spine (Phila Pa 1976) 25:801-803, 2000.

67. DePalma A, Rothman R, Lewinnek G, et al: Anterior interbody fusion for severe cervical disc degeneration. Surg Gynecol Obstet 134:755-758, 1972.

68. Silber JS, Anderson DG, Daffner SD, et al: Donor site morbidity after anterior iliac crest bone harvest for single-level anterior cervical discectomy and fusion. Spine (Phila Pa 1976) 28:134-139, 2003.

69. Kurz LT, Garfin SR, Booth RE: Harvesting autogenous iliac bone grafts. Spine (Phila Pa 1976) 12:1324-1331, 1989.

70. Fountas KN, Kapsalaki EZ, Smith BE, et al: Interobservational variation in determining fusion rates in anterior cervical discectomy and fusion procedures. Eur Spine J 16:39-45, 2007.

71. Flynn T: Neurologic complications of anterior cervical interbody fusion. Spine (Phila Pa 1976) 7:536-539, 1982.

72. Kilburg C, Sullivan HG, Mathiason MA: Effect of approach side during anterior cervical discectomy and fusion on the incidence of recurrent laryngeal nerve injury. J Neurosurg Spine 4:273-277, 2006.

73. Herkowitz H: The surgical management of cervical spondylotic radiculopathy and myelopathy. Clin Orthop Relat Res 239:94-108, 1989.

74. Whitecloud T: Complications of anterior cervical fusion. In: Instructional Course Lectures, vol XXVII. St Louis: CV Mosby, 1978.

75. Lee MJ, Bazaz R, Furey CG, et al: Risk factors for dysphagia after anterior cervical spine surgery: A two-year prospective cohort study. Spine J 7:141-147, 2007.

76. Smith-Hammond CA, New KC, Pietrobon R, et al: Prospective analysis of incidence and risk factors of dysphagia in spine surgery patients: Comparison of anterior cervical, posterior cervical, and lumbar procedures. Spine (Phila Pa 1976) 29:1441-1446, 2004.

77. Edwards CC 2nd, Karpitskaya Y, Cha C, et al: Accurate identification of adverse outcomes after cervical spine surgery. J Bone Joint Surg Am 86:251-256, 2004.

78. Yue WM, Brodner W, Highland TR: Persistent swallowing and voice problems after anterior cervical discectomy and fusion with allograft and plating: A 5- to 11-year follow-up study. Eur Spine J 14:677-682, 2005.

79. Newhouse KE, Lindsey RW, Clark CR, et al: Esophageal perforation following anterior cervical spine surgery. Spine (Phila Pa 1976) 14:1051-1053, 1989.

80. Brown M, Malinin T, Davis P: A roentgenographic evaluation of frozen allografts versus autografts in anterior cervical spine fusions. Clin Orthop Relat Res 119:231-236, 1976.

81. Fernyhough J, White J, LaRocca H: Fusion rates in multilevel cervical spondylosis comparing allograft fibula with autograft fibula in 126 patients. Spine (Phila Pa 1976) 16:5561-5564, 1991.

82. Samartzis D, Shen FH, Goldberg EJ, et al: Is autograft the gold standard in achieving radiographic fusion in one-level anterior cervical discectomy and fusion with rigid anterior plate fixation? Spine (Phila Pa 1976) 30:1756-1761, 2005.

83. Zdeblick T, Ducker T: The use of freeze-dried allograft bone for anterior cervical fusions. Spine (Phila Pa 1976) 16:726-729, 1991.

84. Suchomel P, Barsa P, Buchvald P, et al: Autologous versus allogenic bone grafts in instrumented anterior cervical discectomy and fusion: A prospective study with respect to bone union pattern. Eur Spine J 13:510-515, 2004.

85. Samartzis D, Shen FH, Matthews DK, et al: Comparison of allograft to autograft in multilevel anterior cervical discectomy and fusion with rigid plate fixation. Spine J 3:451-459, 2003.

86. Bishop RC, Moore KA, Hadley MN: Anterior cervical interbody fusion using autogenic and allogenic bone graft substrate: A prospective comparative analysis. J Neurosurg 85:206-210, 1996.

87. Malloy KM, Hilibrand AS: Autograft versus allograft in degenerative cervical disease. Clin Orthop Rel Res 394:27-38, 2002.

88. MacDonald RL, Fehlings M, Tator CH, et al: Multilevel anterior cervical corpectomy and fibular allograft fusion for cervical myelopathy. J Neurosurg 86:990-997, 1997.

89. Martin GJ, Haid RW, MacMillian M, et al: Anterior cervical discectomy with freeze-dried fibula allograft. Spine (Phila Pa 1976) 24:852-859, 1999.

90. Shono Y, McAfee PC, Cunningham BW, et al: A biomechanical analysis of decompression and reconstruction methods in the cervical spine: Emphasis on a carbon-fiber-composite cage. J Bone Joint Surg Am 75:1674-1684, 1993.

91. Panjabi MM, Cholewicki J, Nibu K, et al: Critical load of the human cervical spine: An in vitro experimental study. Clin Biomech (Bristol, Avon) 13:11-17, 1998.

92. Boakye M, Mummaneni PV, Garrett M, et al: Anterior cervical discectomy and fusion involving a polyetheretherketone spacer and bone morphogenetic protein. J Neurosurg Spine 2:521-525, 2005.

93. Cho DY, Lee WY, Sheu PC, et al: Cage containing a biphasic calcium phosphate ceramic (Triosite) for the treatment of

cervical spondylosis. Surg Neurol 63:497-503; discussion 504, 2005.

94. Mastronardi L, Ducati A, Ferrante L: Anterior cervical fusion with polyetheretherketone (PEEK) cages in the treatment of degenerative disc disease: Preliminary observations in 36 consecutive cases with a minimum 12-month follow-up. Acta Neurochir (Wien) 148:307-312; discussion 312, 2006.

95. Kulkarni AG, Hee HT, Wong HK: Solis cage (PEEK) for anterior cervical fusion: Preliminary radiological results with emphasis on fusion and subsidence. Spine J 7:205-209, 2007.

96. Celik SE, Kara A, Celik S: A comparison of changes over time in cervical foraminal height after tricortical iliac graft or polyetheretherketone cage placement following anterior discectomy. J Neurosurg Spine 6:10-16, 2007.

97. Das K, Couldwell WT, Sava G, et al: Use of cylindrical titanium mesh and locking plates in anterior cervical fusion. Technical note. J Neurosurg 94:174-178, 2001.

98. Katsuura A, Hukuda S, Imanaka T, et al: Anterior cervical plate used in degenerative disease can maintain cervical lordosis. J Spinal Disord 9:470-476, 1996.

99. Shapiro S: Banked fibula and the locking anterior cervical plate in anterior cervical fusions following cervical discectomy. J Neurosurg 84:161-165, 1996.

100. Shapiro S, Connolly P, Donnaldson J, et al: Cadaveric fibula, locking plate, and allogeneic bone matrix for anterior cervical fusions after cervical discectomy for radiculopathy or myelopathy. J Neurosurg 95:43-50, 2001.

101. Demircan MN, Kutlay AM, Colak A, et al: Multilevel cervical fusion without plates, screws or autogenous iliac crest bone graft. J Clin Neurosci 14:723-728, 2007.

102. Cho DY, Lee WY, Sheu PC: Treatment of multilevel cervical fusion with cages. Surg Neurol 62:378-385, discussion 385-386, 2004.

103. Buttermann GR: Prospective nonrandomized comparison of an allograft with bone morphogenic protein versus an iliac-crest autograft in anterior cervical discectomy and fusion. Spine J 8:426-435, 2008.

104. Perri B, Cooper M, Lauryssen C, et al: Adverse swelling associated with use of rh-BMP-2 in anterior cervical discectomy and fusion: A case study. Spine J 7:235-239, 2007.

105. Smucker JD, Rhee JM, Singh K, et al: Increased swelling complications associated with off-label usage of rhBMP-2 in the anterior cervical spine. Spine (Phila Pa 1976) 31:2813-2819, 2006.

106. Shields LB, Raque GH, Glassman SD, et al: Adverse effects associated with high-dose recombinant human bone morphogenetic protein-2 use in anterior cervical spine fusion. Spine (Phila Pa 1976) 31:542-547, 2006.

107. Vaidya R, Carp J, Sethi A, et al: Complications of anterior cervical discectomy and fusion using recombinant human bone morphogenetic protein-2. Eur Spine J 16:1257-1265, 2007.

108. Grundy PL, Germon TJ, Gill SS: Transpedicular approaches to cervical uncovertebral osteophytes causing radiculopathy. J Neurosurg 93:21-27, 2000.

109. Jho HD, Kim MH, Kim WK: Anterior cervical microforaminotomy for spondylotic cervical myelopathy: II. Neurosurgery 51:54-59, 2002.

110. Johnson JP, Filler AG, McBride DQ, et al: Anterior cervical foraminotomy for unilateral radicular disease. Spine (Phila Pa 1976) 25:905-909, 2000.

111. Yi S, Lim JH, Choi KS, et al: Comparison of anterior cervical foraminotomy vs arthroplasty for unilateral cervical radiculopathy. Surg Neurol 71:677-680, discussion 680, 2009.

112. Koc RK, Menku A, Tucer B, et al: Anterior cervical foraminotomy for unilateral spondylotic radiculopathy. Minim Invasive Neurosurg 47:186-189, 2004.

113. Johnson JP, Filler AG, McBride DQ, et al: Anterior cervical foraminotomy for unilateral radicular disease. Spine (Phila Pa 1976) 25:905-909, 2000.

114. Murphy M, Gadd M: Anterior cervical discectomy without interbody bone graft. J Neurosurg 37:71-74, 1972.

115. O'Laoire S, Thomas D: Spinal cord compression due to prolapse of cervical intervertebral disc (herniation of nucleus pulposus). J Neurosurg 59:846-853, 1983.

116. Rosenorn J, Hansen E, Rosenorn M: Anterior cervical discectomy with and without fusion. J Neurosurg 59:252-255, 1983.

117. Benini A, Krayenbuhl H, Bruder R: Anterior cervical discectomy without fusion: Microsurgical technique. Acta Neurochir 61:105-110, 1982.

118. Kadoya S, Nakamura T, Kwak R: A microsurgical anterior osteophytectomy for cervical spondylotic myelopathy. Spine (Phila Pa 1976) 9:437-441, 1984.

119. Wilson D, Campbell D: Anterior cervical discectomy without bone graft. J Neurosurg 47:551-555, 1977.

120. Watters WC III, Levinthal R: Anterior cervical discectomy with and without fusion: Results, complications and long-term follow-up. Spine (Phila Pa 1976) 19:2343-2347, 1994.

121. Wirth FP, Dowd GC, Sanders HF, et al: Cervical discectomy: A prospective analysis of three operative techniques. Surg Neurol 53:340-348, 2000.

122. Heller JG, Sasso RC, Papadopoulos SM, et al: Comparison of Bryan cervical disc arthroplasty with anterior cervical decompression and fusion: Clinical and radiographic results of a randomized, controlled, clinical trial. Spine (Phila Pa 1976) 34:101-107, 2009.

123. Steinmetz MP, Patel R, Traynelis V, et al: Cervical disc arthroplasty compared with fusion in a workers' compensation population. Neurosurgery 63:741-747; discussion 747, 2008.

124. Nabhan A, Ahlhelm F, Shariat K, et al: The ProDisc-C prosthesis: Clinical and radiological experience 1 year after surgery. Spine (Phila Pa 1976) 32:1935-1941, 2007.

125. Rousseau MA, Cottin P, Levante S, et al: In vivo kinematics of two types of ball-and-socket cervical disc replacements in the sagittal plane: Cranial versus caudal geometric center. Spine (Phila Pa 1976) 33:E6-E9, 2008.

126. Sasso RC, Best NM, Metcalf NH, et al: Motion analysis of Bryan cervical disc arthroplasty versus anterior discectomy and fusion: Results from a prospective, randomized, multicenter, clinical trial. J Spinal Disord Tech 21:393-399, 2008.

127. Puttlitz CM, Rousseau MA, Xu Z, et al: Intervertebral disc replacement maintains cervical spine kinetics. Spine (Phila Pa 1976) 29:2809-2814, 2004.

128. Sasso RC, Best NM: Cervical kinematics after fusion and Bryan disc arthroplasty. J Spinal Disord Tech 21:19-22, 2008.

129. Chang UK, Kim DH, Lee MC, et al: Changes in adjacent-level disc pressure and facet joint force after cervical arthroplasty compared with cervical discectomy and fusion. J Neurosurg Spine 7:33-39, 2007.

130. Eck JC, Humphreys SC, Lim TH, et al: Biomechanical study on the effect of cervical spine fusion on adjacent-level intradiscal pressure and segmental motion. Spine (Phila Pa 1976) 27:2431-2434, 2002.

131. Lopez-Espina CG, Amirouche F, Havalad V: Multilevel cervical fusion and its effect on disc degeneration and osteophyte formation. Spine (Phila Pa 1976) 31:972-978, 2006.

132. Park DH, Ramakrishnan P, Cho TH, et al: Effect of lower two-level anterior cervical fusion on the superior adjacent level. J Neurosurg Spine 7:336-340, 2007.

133. Laxer EB, Darden BV, Murrey DB, et al: Adjacent segment disc pressures following two-level cervical disc replacement versus simulated anterior cervical fusion. Stud Health Technol Inform 123:488-492, 2006.

134. Mehren C, Suchomel P, Grochulla F, et al: Heterotopic ossification in total cervical artificial disc replacement. Spine (Phila Pa 1976) 31:2802-2806, 2006.

135. Anderson PA, Sasso RC, Riew KD: Comparison of adverse events between the Bryan artificial cervical disc and anterior cervical arthrodesis. Spine (Phila Pa 1976) 33:1305-1312, 2008.

136. Pickett GE, Sekhon LH, Sears WR, et al: Complications with cervical arthroplasty. J Neurosurg Spine 4:98-105, 2006.

137. Kim SW, Shin JH, Arbatin JJ, et al: Effects of a cervical disc prosthesis on maintaining sagittal alignment of the functional spinal unit and overall sagittal balance of the cervical spine. Eur Spine J 17:20-29, 2008.

138. Phillips FM, Allen TR, Regan JJ, et al: Cervical disc replacement in patients with and without previous adjacent level fusion surgery: A prospective study. Spine (Phila Pa 1976) 34:556-565, 2009.

139. Shin DA, Yi S, Yoon do H, et al: Artificial disc replacement combined with fusion versus two-level fusion in cervical two-level disc disease. Spine (Phila Pa 1976) 34:1153-1159; discussion 1160-1161, 2009.

140. Cheng L, Nie L, Zhang L, et al: Fusion versus Bryan Cervical Disc in two-level cervical disc disease: A prospective, randomised study. Int Orthop 33:1347-1351, 2009.

141. Liu J, Zhang H, Li K, et al: [Clinical effect of cervical artificial disc replacement on two-segment cervical spondylosis]. Zhongguo Xiu Fu Chong Jian Wai Ke Za Zhi 23:385-388, 2009.

142. Pimenta L, McAfee PC, Cappuccino A, et al: Superiority of multilevel cervical arthroplasty outcomes versus single-level outcomes: 229 consecutive PCM prostheses. Spine (Phila Pa 1976) 32:1337-1344, 2007.

143. Lowery GL, McDonough RF: The significance of hardware failure in anterior cervical plate fixation: Patients with 2- to 7-year follow-up. Spine (Phila Pa 1976) 23:181-186; discussion 186-187, 1998.

144. Swank ML, Lowery GL, Bhat AL, et al: Anterior cervical allograft arthrodesis and instrumentation: Multilevel interbody grafting or strut graft reconstruction. Eur Spine J 6:138-143, 1997.

41 CHAPTER

Cervical Spondylotic Myelopathy: Surgical Management

Harry N. Herkowitz, MD
Myles Luszczyk, DO

Aging is associated with the development and progression of degenerative changes within the cervical spine. Degenerative changes are manifested in the cervical spine as disc height loss, facet and uncovertebral joint osteophytes, spondylotic bars, and hypertrophic ligamentum flavum.[1,2] Neural compression from these structures may lead to the development of clinical symptoms consistent with the diagnosis of myelopathy. Although older patients may present with some degree of developmental stenosis from superimposed degenerative changes, younger patients may present with cord compression secondary to a large disc herniation. Although there is still debate regarding the etiology and pathophysiology of neuronal damage that occurs in the presence of spinal stenosis, direct mechanical compression and indirect vascular ischemia have been suggested as potential causes.[3] In a cadaveric study, Ono and colleagues[3] observed damage to gray and white matter, with cord atrophy, demyelination, and vascular infarction found in several segments removed from the site of maximal cord compression.

The clinical findings early in the natural course of cervical spondylotic myelopathy (CSM) are often very subtle, and delays in diagnosis are common owing to the insidious onset of these symptoms.[4-8] Sadasivan and colleagues[9] reported an average delay in diagnosis of approximately 6 years with gait disturbances manifesting as the earliest symptom in patients in his series. Often patients subjectively complain of a useless hand, and they notice a decline in fine motor skills. They also observe deterioration in penmanship and dexterity. Patients exhibit a loss of dexterity from atrophy of the thenar and hypothenar eminences, weakness of the extensors of the wrist, and loss of apposition of the thumb. Gait and balance disturbances from proximal lower extremity weakness are noticed and are often attributed to old age.[1,10,11] Other signs of myelopathy include hyperactive deep tendon reflexes, clonus, pathologic reflexes such as bilateral Babinski responses, loss of proprioception and stereoanesthesia, and decreased pinprick and vibratory appreciation. Rarely, severely affected individuals may present with frank paralysis affecting bowel and bladder control.

Natural History

The natural history of CSM has been studied extensively in the literature. Clark and Robinson[12] followed 120 patients with cervical spondylosis and myelopathy in an effort to describe the natural progression of the disease. These authors noted that of 120 patients, 5% showed a rapid onset of symptoms followed by long periods of remission, 20% showed a slow gradual decline in function without any periods of remission, and 75% showed stepwise deterioration in function followed by episodic periods of remission. In 1963, Lees and Turner[13] documented their experience in the treatment of cervical myelopathy. Most patients in their series were noted to have periods of progression of disease mixed with static periods of unchanged symptoms. They also observed that 14 of the 15 patients in their series who presented with severe myelopathy continued to be disabled at 10 to 20 years of follow-up.

Nurick[14,15] published his series on the natural history of cervical myelopathy following 36 patients who were treated nonoperatively. In patients who presented with mild clinical symptoms, he observed no significant clinical worsening of their condition at final assessment decades later. In addition, he noted that patients who presented with clinical symptoms at an older age tended to have a worse decline in functional status. The patients with the worst prognosis were patients who presented with severe disability, especially if they were of advanced age. Nurick[15a] also established a grading system for myelopathy that revolved around the patient's ambulatory status (Table 41–1). Most series that document the long-term follow-up of patients with CSM report a progression of disease with a gradual deterioration in functional status over time.[16-18]

Indications for Surgical Intervention

As documented in natural history studies, patients presenting with moderate to severe symptoms are unlikely to experience regression of myelopathy. To alter the natural progression of the disease and prevent further neurologic deterioration, surgical intervention should be considered. In a review of surgical indications for cervical myelopathy, Law and colleagues[19] identified several poor prognostic factors for conservative treatment, including progression of symptoms, presence of myelopathy for more than 6 months, compression ratio approaching 0.4 indicating flattening of the cord, and transverse area of the cord less than 40 mm². The presence of any of these factors is an indicator for surgical intervention.

The goals of operative intervention include decompression of the spinal cord, stabilization of the spinal column, and reestablishment of the normal sagittal alignment. Preoperative findings that favor a successful surgical outcome include young age at presentation, duration of symptoms less than 1 year, presence of a Lhermitte sign, involvement of pathology limited to fewer vertebral segments, and presence of unilateral symptoms.[20] A constellation of findings contributes to the surgeon's decision to proceed with surgery. Factors that play a role in the decision-making process include duration of symptoms, degree of spinal cord dysfunction, general health of the patient, degree of functional deterioration, and radiographic findings.

The degree of spinal cord dysfunction is evaluated by looking for balance deficits, gait abnormalities, motor weakness, long tract signs, and changes in function. Studies by Okada and colleagues[21] and Bohlman[22] used clinical symptoms such as gait disturbance as the primary indication for operative treatment. Wada and colleagues[23] recommended using a combination of the patient's clinical findings, preoperative functional status as measured by the Japanese Orthopaedic Association (JOA) scale, and radiographic findings to determine the need for operative intervention. They recommended surgery when symptoms such as gait disturbances and loss of fine motor control were present in combination with a JOA score of less than 13 and radiographic evidence of spinal cord compression. In most reported studies, the neurologic results of laminoplasty are graded according to the JOA myelopathy score. A maximum score of 17 reflects normal function, and the recovery rate describes the extent to which the score returns to normal postoperatively (Table 41–2).

Multiple studies have shown that the degree of neurologic recovery depends highly on the preoperative duration of symptoms and the severity of the myelopathy at the time of intervention.[24-27] Irreversible histologic and physiologic changes such as intraneural fibrosis and demyelination can occur within the spinal cord with prolonged compression.[28] Tanaka and colleagues[24] observed that the preoperative duration of symptoms strongly influenced the degree of functional recovery after surgical decompression. They recommended early surgical intervention in the treatment of CSM. Similarly, Suri and colleagues[25] noted that patients with symptoms of less than 1 year's duration showed a greater degree of postoperative motor recovery compared with patients with symptoms of longer duration. Patients with severe forms of myelopathy tend to experience less relative recovery compared with

TABLE 41–1 Disability Classification of Cervical Spondylotic Myelopathy

Grade	Description
0	Root signs and symptoms, no cord involvement
I	Signs of cord involvement, normal gait
II	Mild gait involvement, able to be employed
III	Gait abnormality prevents employment
IV	Able to ambulate only with assistance
V	Chair-bound or bedridden

TABLE 41–2 Criteria for Evaluation of Operative Results of Patients with Cervical Myelopathy by Japanese Orthopaedic Association

Function	Score (Maximum = 17)	Remarks
Motor		
Upper extremity	4	Normal
	3	Able to feed self with chopsticks regularly, but slightly awkwardly
	2	Able to feed self with chopsticks regularly, although awkwardly
	1	Able to feed self with a spoon, but not with chopsticks
	0	Unable to feed self with either spoon or chopsticks
Lower extremity	4	Normal
	3	Able to walk on level surface or climb stairs without cane or support but awkwardly
	2	Able to walk on level surface without cane or support but unable to climb stairs without either of them
	1	Needs cane or support even when walking on level surface
	0	Nonambulatory
Sensory		
Upper extremities	2	Normal
	1	Slight sensory loss or numbness
	0	Definite sensory loss
Lower extremities	2	Normal
	1	Slight sensory loss or numbness
	0	Definite sensory loss
Trunk	2	Normal
	1	Slight sensory loss or numbness
	0	Definite sensory loss
Bladder	3	Normal
	2	Mild dysuria
	1	Severe dysuria
	0	Complete retention of urine

patients with mild symptoms. Bernard and Whitecloud[29] also observed that patients with severe preoperative disability and a longer duration of symptoms had poorer outcomes after decompression.

The influence of age on neurologic recovery has also been investigated. Although most patients experience significant neurologic improvement after decompression, the degree of recovery tends to be mildly improved for younger age groups.[21,24,26,27] Hasegawa and colleagues[30] believed that this discrepancy occurred because elderly patients had a higher incidence of new neurologic dysfunction arising from different sources.

Radiographic studies also play an important role in the operative management of CSM. The normal mid-sagittal spinal canal diameter measures 17 mm in depth, and the normal spinal cord measures approximately 8 to 13 mm in its anteroposterior dimension.[31,32] The addition of soft tissue structures, including the posterior longitudinal ligament and the ligamentum flavum, can occupy an additional 2 to 3 mm of the canal diameter.[33] Patients with narrowing of the canal to 13 mm are considered to have relative stenosis, whereas patients with narrowing of 10 mm are considered to have absolute stenosis.[34] Sites of maximal cord compression may manifest as high signal intensity on T2-weighted magnetic resonance imaging (MRI). These hyperintense signals in the cord may represent intraspinal edema or neuronal death and are generally referred to as *myelomalacia*. Evidence of myelomalacia on MRI has been associated with a greater degree of clinical disability and a poor prognostic finding for neurologic recovery after surgery.[35,36] Suda and colleagues[37] found that high cord signal intensity on MRI was associated with inferior surgical outcomes.

Radiographic evidence of dynamic stenosis as measured by translation between the vertebral bodies or by shingling of the lamina in hyperextension can transiently narrow the spinal canal.[38] These structural changes in conjunction with the associated buckling of the ligamentum flavum during hyperextension of the cervical spine may decrease further the space available for the cord and may precipitate the development of myelopathy.[39] Penning[40] showed that cervical myelopathy should be strongly suspected if the canal space measured on dynamic lateral radiographs is reduced to less than 11 mm.

When the decision for operative intervention is made, the surgeon is faced with different approaches and operative techniques for the surgical treatment of cervical myelopathy. Regardless of whether a posterior or an anterior approach is used, the primary goal of surgical intervention in the treatment of CSM is to decompress the spinal canal. Appropriate expansion of the spinal canal has been shown to improve cord morphology and likely to maximize blood flow to the cord.[41,42] Important factors that may influence the choice of approach include the sagittal alignment of the spinal column, the location of the compressive pathology, the presence of axial neck pain, the number of segments involved, and the presence of previous surgeries. The following sections discuss the different approaches and various operative techniques described in the treatment of CSM.

Anterior Approach

Indications for an Anterior Approach

The spinal cord can be compressed by herniated discs, spondylotic bars, and uncovertebral osteophytes. Direct decompression of the cord and nerve roots from these degenerative changes can be accomplished with an anterior approach. An anterior approach also allows the surgeon to relieve directly any compression on the anterior spinal artery that has been shown to supply the ventral 75% to 80% of the spinal cord. For most patients with stenosis confined to only one or two levels, an anterior approach provides adequate decompression and is the procedure of choice for most surgeons.[43,44] Yonenobu and colleagues[44] recommended that an anterior procedure should be confined to the treatment of spondylosis involving no more than three levels, whereas a posterior procedure should be reserved for the treatment of spondylosis involving four levels or more.

The sagittal alignment of the spinal column is an important factor when deciding on an anterior versus a posterior approach. Cervical kyphosis and degenerative instability are clear indications for an anterior approach.[37,45] In patients who have lost the normal cervical lordotic curvature or who have developed a kyphotic deformity, a posterior decompression alone may destabilize the cervical spine and may lead to a progression of the deformity. Anterior surgery allows for direct decompression of the neural elements, fusion of the involved segments, and possibly reconstitution of the normal sagittal contours. An anterior approach may also be favored in patients who complain of preoperative neck pain. Two techniques described in anterior decompression and surgical treatment of cervical myelopathy include anterior cervical discectomy and fusion (ACDF) and anterior cervical corpectomy and fusion (ACCF).

Surgical Techniques

The surgical approach for ACDF and ACCF are identical. The patient is positioned supine on the operating table. The cervical spine is ideally placed in slight extension to facilitate exposure of the anterior neck. This position is accomplished by placing a longitudinally oriented bump under the patient's upper thoracic spine, between the scapulae, and by placing a small thin pillow beneath the patient's head. To avoid any neurologic deterioration, extreme caution must always be exercised in patients with myelopathy and significant canal stenosis during the positioning and intubation of the patient. Consideration should be given to performing an awake, fiberoptic intubation. After adequate general anesthesia, the arms are well padded and tucked at the patient's side using arm sleds or a sheet placed under the patient's torso. In addition, the shoulders are depressed caudally and held into place with adhesive tape to assist with proper visualization during the exposure and interpretation of intraoperative lateral radiographs. Excessive traction must be avoided because it may result in a traction injury to the brachial plexus.

The anterior cervical spine may be approached from either the right or the left side. This decision must be made by the individual surgeon and may be influenced by his or her training. Proponents of the right-sided approach suggest that it is technically easier for a right-handed surgeon. Proponents of the left-sided approach typically value the more consistent course of the left recurrent laryngeal nerve. The surgeon must have a comprehensive understanding of the anatomy of the region regardless of the side of the approach.

A transverse incision may be used for procedures involving one or two levels; an oblique, longitudinal incision along the course of the medial border of the sternocleidomastoid muscle may be needed for procedures involving three or more vertebral segments. The location of the transverse incision depends on what levels are involved in the surgical procedure (Fig. 41–1). Palpable landmarks of the anterior neck provide guidance as to the appropriate location for this incision. The C1-2 interspace is located at the angle of the mandible, whereas the hyoid bone usually lies anterior to the C3 level. The superior portion of the thyroid cartilage marks the position of the C4-5 interspace. The C6 level can be identified by palpation of the cricoid cartilage or by palpation of the carotid tubercle, which projects anteriorly from the transverse process of the C6 vertebral segment. Care should be taken to orient the transverse incision along the skin creases of the anterior neck to leave a cosmetic-appearing scar.

The skin and subcutaneous tissues are incised sharply with a scalpel. The platysma is divided in line with the skin incision with the transverse and longitudinal incisions. Superficial veins, especially the external jugular vein and its branches, must be protected or ligated if they cross the planes of dissection. Next, the medial border of the sternocleidomastoid is

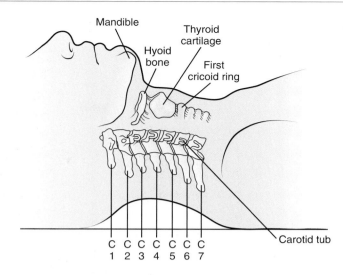

FIGURE 41–1 Palpable bony landmarks and their relationship to cervical spine. (From Hoppenfeld S: Physical Examination of the Spine and Extremities. Norwalk, CT, Appleton & Lange, 1976, p 110.)

identified. Dissection is carried out through the superficial layers of the investing deep cervical fascia between the sternocleidomastoid and the medial visceral muscle column (Fig. 41–2).

After this plane is developed, the location of the carotid sheath must be identified by direct palpation. Blunt dissection is performed through the middle layers of the deep cervical fascia, between the esophagus and the carotid sheath. The surgeon must always be mindful of the location of the carotid sheath. With two blunt hand-held retractors in place, the prevertebral fascia is visualized directly anterior to the vertebral

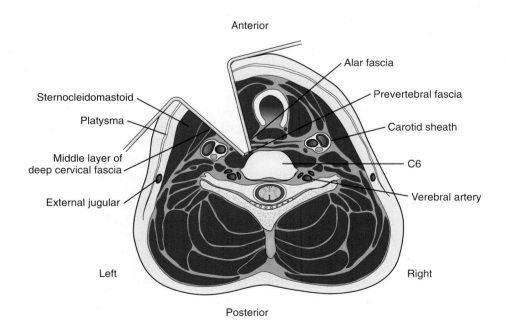

FIGURE 41–2 Plane of surgical dissection through layers of deep cervical fascia medial to carotid sheath and lateral to trachea and esophagus. (From Silber JS, Albert TS: Anterior and anterolateral, mid and lower cervical spine approaches: Transverse and longitudinal [C3 to C7]. In Herkowitz HN [ed]: The Cervical Spine Surgery Atlas, 2nd ed. Philadelphia, Lippincott Williams & Wilkins, 2004, p 91.)

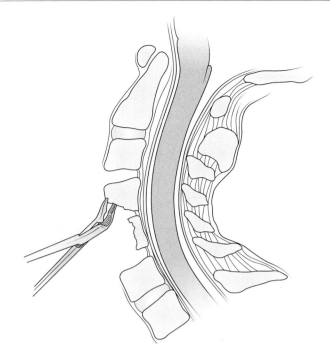

FIGURE 41–3 Anterior two thirds of vertebral bodies to be removed can be safely excised using a rongeur after discectomies adjacent to and within area to be decompressed. (From Whitecloud TS: Multilevel cervical vertebrectomy and stabilization using cortical bone. In Sherk H, Dunn EJ, Eismont FJ, et al [eds]: The Cervical Spine: An Atlas of Surgical Procedures. Philadelphia, JB Lippincott, 1994, p 202.)

column. This fascia is incised sharply with scissors and bluntly dissected off of the anterior portion of the vertebral bodies using a dissector. The medial borders of the longus colli muscles are identified just off of the midline. A spinal needle or other locating device is inserted into a disc space to identify the level definitively. With larger patients, the spinal needle may need to be placed cephalad to the operative levels to assist with visualization on the lateral intraoperative radiograph. After the radiograph is completed, the localized disc space is permanently marked with electrocautery or a surgical marking pen.

When the operative levels have been identified, exposure of the disc spaces begins by releasing the medial border of the longus colli muscle starting at the disc space. Blunt, hand-held retractors are placed subperiosteally under the muscle bellies of the longus colli and used to retract these muscles laterally. Inadvertent dissection on the ventral surface of the longus colli muscles may result in injury to the sympathetic chain and a Horner syndrome. Continued lateral retraction and dissection of the longus colli muscles at each of the operative disc spaces exposes the most medial portions of the cranially projecting uncinate processes. The up-sloping portions of the uncinate processes serve as the most lateral extent of the dissection on both sides of the spine. Dissection lateral to the uncinate process can lead to injury to the vertebral artery as it ascends in the transverse foramen of the cervical vertebrae. Careful review of preoperative MRI or computed tomography (CT) myelography reveals any anomalies of the vertebral arteries. Exposure in the cranial-caudal direction can be enhanced by the use of blunt self-retaining retractors.

Discectomies are performed at the levels above and below the planned corpectomy. A scalpel blade is used to incise the anulus, and a combination of pituitary rongeurs and small curets is used to remove all disc material completely down to the level of the posterior longitudinal ligament. Identification of the midline throughout the discectomy and corpectomy is paramount. A Penfield elevator may be used to identify the transverse processes at the cranial aspect of the individual vertebral bodies. The junction of the transverse process and the vertebral body marks the lateral cortical wall of the vertebral body. The vertebral artery lies just lateral to this wall of cortical bone. Identification of these landmarks guides the actual bony resection and assists in keeping the trough centered and symmetrical.

A Leksell rongeur is used to create the most ventral portion of the corpectomy trough (Fig. 41–3). The use of a motorized bur without the creation of this initial trough is dangerous and could result in injury to the carotid vessels or the esophagus if the bur "jumps" off of the anterior vertebral body cortex. After the anterior cortex of the vertebral bodies has been removed, a 5-mm power bur is used to widen and deepen the through. Starting and stopping the bur within the bony trough avoids potential injury to the surrounding soft tissue structures. Resection is continued posteriorly until the posterior cortex of the vertebral bodies is encountered. Bleeding from the cancellous bone can be controlled with bone wax. A smaller bur may be used to thin the posterior cortex and to remove the osteophytes at the uncovertebral joints. The remaining thin shell of the posterior cortex can be removed with small angled curets by pulling the bone away from the posterior longitudinal ligament and the dura (Fig. 41–4).

The posterior longitudinal ligament can be carefully removed with a nerve hook and a small Kerrison rongeur. One should use caution in the presence of ossification of the posterior longitudinal ligament (OPLL) because the ligament may be incorporated into the dura.[46] Removal of the ligament should not be attempted in this situation because it may create a dural tear. The cartilage endplates at the superior and inferior extent of the corpectomy are removed with the use of a curet or a bur. A safe and adequate decompression of the spinal cord requires approximately a 15- to 19-mm wide trough.[47,48] This trough can be measured directly with a caliper or estimated by comparing the width of the trough with the width of the surgeon's finger. Foraminotomies may be performed at each of the decompressed levels if the patient's pathology and symptoms warrant foraminal decompression.

After complete decompression of the neural elements has been accomplished, the endplates are prepared for insertion of the graft. A bone tamp and mallet are used to tap the graft gently in the appropriate position while traction is being applied to the head (Fig. 41–5). Heller[1] recommended a maximum of 25 lb of traction. Care must be taken to countersink the graft 1 to 2 mm behind the anterior cortex without forcing it into the canal posteriorly. A small nerve hook can be passed lateral to the graft in the trough to assess the space between the posterior longitudinal ligament and the posterior surface of the graft. The traction is released, and graft stability is assessed by manual flexion and rotation of the head by the anesthesiologist. If an anterior cervical plate is being used, it is placed at this time. The plate helps to prevent anterior migration of the graft and may provide graft compression to improve healing potential.

The wound is closed in layers over a suction drain, which is left in place for 1 to 2 days postoperatively to minimize the risk of postoperative airway compromise secondary to hematoma formation. The patient is placed into a cervical collar for additional immobilization. The choice of collar often depends on surgeon preference, number of levels fused, and presence or absence of instrumentation. After multilevel corpectomies with prolonged retractor times, many surgeons elect to keep the patient intubated overnight to minimize the possibility of respiratory distress from postoperative edema and swelling.[49]

Anterior Cervical Discectomy and Fusion

The use of anterior cervical decompression and fusion for the treatment of ventral pathology has been consistently reported to be a safe and effective procedure.[50,51] Indications for ACDF in the treatment of cervical myelopathy include compression from any disk herniation or spondylotic degeneration that is confined to the disk level.

Although the removal of osteophytes has been reported to improve recovery in patients with CSM, controversy exists regarding the need for an osteophytectomy.[52] Robinson and colleagues[53] and Connolly and colleagues[54] reported complete remodeling and resorption of osteophytes in the presence of a solid fusion. Bohlman[22] reported excellent results in 16 of 17 patients who underwent ACDF and who were treated without

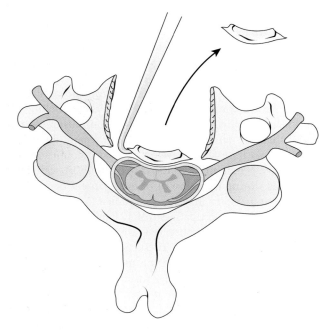

FIGURE 41–4 After posterior cortex has been thinned, it can be safely removed with a small angled curet. All force must be directed anteriorly to avoid compression of dura and underlying spinal cord. (Adapted from Smith MD: Cervical spondylosis. In Birdwell KH, DeWald RL [eds]: The Textbook of Spinal Surgery, 2nd ed. Philadelphia, Lippincott-Raven, 1997, p 1411.)

any osteophyte removal. No patients experienced a loss of function, and all but one of the patients had improvement in functional status. Conversely, Stevens and colleagues[55] reviewed CT myelograms of 53 patients who underwent ACDF and reported that at 12 years of follow-up no patients

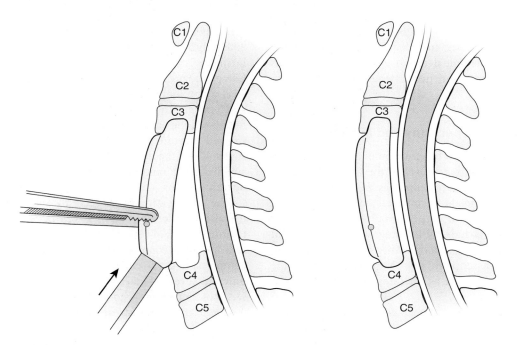

FIGURE 41–5 Graft is seated into cranial end of corpectomy defect. Traction is applied to the patient's head, and distal end of graft is tamped into caudal end with a tamp. A Kocher clamp is used to hold graft to prevent displacement of graft into spinal canal while it is being impacted into place. (Adapted from Smith MD: Cervical spondylosis. In Birdwell KH, DeWald RL [eds]: The Textbook of Spinal Surgery, 2nd ed. Philadelphia, Lippincott-Raven, 1997, p 1411.)

showed any evidence of osteophyte resorption. These authors recommended the systematic removal of all osteophytes to decrease the incidence of persistent postoperative symptoms.

The removal of a thickened ligament or an OPLL may also allow for a more thorough decompression of the spinal cord and may be necessary for the safe exploration and removal of disc fragments that may have become sequestered behind the posterior longitudinal ligament. The surgeon must always be mindful that the removal of the posterior longitudinal ligament increases the risk of developing a cord contusion or a postoperative hematoma.[56] In the case of an OPLL, care must be exercised during the removal of the ligament because the dura of the spinal cord may also be ossified.[46]

Using ACDF in the treatment of 121 patients with CSM, Zhang and colleagues[57] observed a 90% improvement in overall neurologic outcome. These authors noted an 85% fusion rate in association with the use of autogenous bone graft, whereas they noted a 50% fusion rate with the use of allograft. They also observed poorer clinical outcomes in patients who developed a pseudarthrosis. With an average number of 3.1 levels fused, Yang and colleagues[58] reported 214 patients who underwent ACDF for treatment of CSM. At last follow-up, improved functional status was noted in 90% of patients, despite a pseudarthrosis rate of 37%. With a mean follow-up of 10 years, Irvine and Strachan[59] retrospectively evaluated the long-term results of 46 patients who underwent ACDF for treatment of CSM. At last follow-up, 78% of the 46 patients had improved ability to ambulate, whereas 9% of patients experienced progression of their symptoms.

Certain disadvantages are encountered with every technique. During ACDF, there is decreased visualization of the spinal cord that increases the potential for an incomplete decompression or an inadvertent injury to the cord. ACDF is not suited for the treatment of patients with congenital cervical stenosis because it does not adequately decompress the overall diameter of the spinal canal. In a patient with this condition, a corpectomy and fusion would provide a more suitable option.

Anterior Cervical Corpectomy and Fusion

Subtotal corpectomy refers to the creation of a midline trough in the vertebral body with removal of the adjacent discs. It allows for removal of large osteophytes from the vertebral endplates and for complete decompression of the stenotic spinal canal. Indications for corpectomy in the treatment of cervical myelopathy include OPLL, migrated disc fragment behind the vertebral body beyond the disc space, and kyphotic cervical alignment. Essentially, any compression behind the vertebral body can be seen as an indication to perform a corpectomy.

Bernard and Whitecloud[29] evaluated multilevel cervical corpectomy. All 21 patients in this series had decompression of three or more vertebral levels with autograft. At an average of 32 months' follow-up, these authors noted that 76% of patients had an improvement in functional outcome, and no patients developed pseudarthrosis. One patient in this series experienced graft dislodgment. In a study of 27 patients with

CSM treated with multilevel corpectomy and fusion, Jamjoom and colleagues[60] noted a 96% fusion rate with clinical improvement in 80% to 88% of patients. Although no patients experienced postoperative neurologic deterioration, three patients developed dislodgment of the strut graft.

Emery and colleagues[50] reviewed their series of patients with CSM treated with different forms of anterior decompression and fusion procedures without the use of instrumentation. Of 108 patients, 58 were treated with ACCF using either fibular or iliac crest autograft without plate fixation. Six graft-related complications occurred in the corpectomy group, four of which occurred in patients who had been previously treated with cervical laminectomy. Of the patients who underwent corpectomy, a nonunion rate of 5% was observed, and the average improvement in Nurick grade ranged from 2.4 preoperatively to 1.2 at final follow-up.

Zdeblick and Bohlman[61] reviewed their results of 14 patients with myelopathy and associated cervical kyphotic malalignment who were treated with anterior corpectomy and fusion using autograft without any plate fixation. The patients were stabilized postoperatively in a halo vest. At follow-up, 12 of the 14 patients had a solid arthrodesis. Nine patients had complete neurologic recovery, and only one patient failed to show any neurologic improvement. Correction of the kyphosis averaged 32 degrees. Zdeblick and Bohlman[61] concluded that myelopathy in the setting of cervical kyphosis can be effectively and safely treated with multilevel corpectomy and strut graft reconstruction without instrumentation.

In 1998, Fessler and colleagues[62] evaluated the outcomes of 93 patients with CSM who were treated with anterior corpectomy and fusion. Multisegmental involvement was noted in 31 of these patients. Fessler and colleagues[62] reported that 86% of patients showed improvement in neurologic scores as measured by Nurick grade. In a more recent study published in 2005, Chibbaro and colleagues[63] documented their experience in management of CSM with anterior cervical corpectomy. Using autograft and plate fixation, 54 patients received a one-level corpectomy, 11 patients received a two-level corpectomy, and 5 patients received a three-level corpectomy. At 16 weeks' follow-up, the authors observed no evidence of pseudarthrosis, and they documented a 94% improvement in functional status. Using the modified JOA scale, no patients experienced any decline in neurologic function compared with their preoperative status.

The combination of corpectomy and adjacent discectomy has also been performed as a technique that can be used in treatment of CSM (Fig. 41–6). This method has been described as a hybrid decompression. It is indicated when spinal cord compression is present at a disc space and a vertebral body at different levels. Ashkenazi and colleagues[64] published their series of 25 patients who underwent a hybrid decompression with anterior plate instrumentation for the treatment of multilevel CSM; 12 patients underwent a one-level corpectomy and adjacent one-level discectomy, and 13 patients underwent a two-level corpectomy with preservation of an intervening vertebral body. The investigators observed a 96% fusion rate, and 24 of the 25 patients reported either a neurologic improvement or an unchanged status.

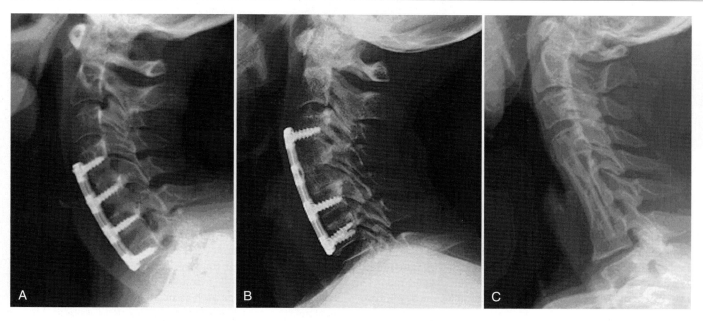

FIGURE 41–6 A-C, Three-level compression may be treated with three-level discectomy (**A**), one-level corpectomy and one-level discectomy combined (**B**), or two-level corpectomy (**C**). Reconstruction after multilevel discectomy may allow for recreation of normal cervical lordosis. (**C,** Courtesy of James D. Kang, MD, Pittsburgh, PA.)

Complications

Although an anterior cervical approach has been shown to be a safe and effective procedure in treating patients with myelopathy, suboptimal outcomes have been reported when this approach is used to treat three or more levels.[65-67] As more levels are involved in the attempted fusion, increased rates of nonunion have been noted in ACDF and ACCF procedures. Numerous studies have shown an inverse relationship between the fusion rate and the number of vertebral segments involved.[68-71] Nonunion is determined by the absence of bridging bone across the graft-host interface on static radiographs and by the presence of motion on dynamic films.

The arthrodesis rate after ACDF without instrumentation was compared in a series by Bohlman and colleagues.[72] They reported a fusion rate of 89% of 62 patients after a one-level fusion, 73% of 42 patients after a two-level fusion, and 73% of 11 patients after a three-level fusion. An unsuccessful four-level ACDF was performed in one patient in their series. Bohlman and colleagues[72] attributed the lower fusion rate to increased number of fusion interfaces and increased motion as more levels are involved. Emery and colleagues[50] reviewed their series of patients with CSM treated with different forms of anterior decompression and fusion procedures without the use of instrumentation. Of 108 patients, 45 were treated with anterior discectomy and fusion; the investigators reported 13 patients in the discectomy and fusion cohort who developed a nonunion. Similar to the observations made by Bohlman and colleagues,[72] Emery and colleagues[50] observed increased rates of nonunion as the numbers of fused levels increased. Better clinical outcomes were noted in patients who went on to a solid fusion.

Vaccaro and colleagues[66] reported a series of patients who underwent an instrumented anterior corpectomy and fusion using a strut graft. They observed a 9% nonunion rate in two-level corpectomies, which increased to a 50% nonunion rate in three-level corpectomies. Sasso and colleagues[73] noted a similar trend in increasing nonunion rates in their series of patients who underwent ACCF. They reported a 6% failure rate in two-level corpectomies that increased to a 71% failure rate when three levels were involved. When compared with multiple discectomy and fusion, Hilibrand and colleagues[74] observed better fusion rates in patients treated with corpectomy and strut grafting. In their series, all reconstructions were performed with autograft and without anterior cervical plates. A 93% fusion rate was observed in the corpectomy cohort, whereas only a 66% fusion rate was noted in the ACDF cohort.

Although it is a more technically demanding surgery, corpectomy with fusion relies on an arthrodesis to occur at only two interfaces. Because a fusion is required between only two levels, the chance of developing a pseudarthrosis is decreased.[61] Swank and colleagues[75] reported 38 patients who were treated with multilevel ACDF and 26 patients who were treated with subtotal corpectomy. Allograft and anterior plate fixation were used in all patients. Among patients with two-level disease, the patients treated with two-level discectomy had a 64% fusion rate, whereas the patients treated with one-level corpectomy had a 90% fusion rate. Similarly, among patients with three-level disease, the patients treated with three-level ACDF had a fusion rate of 46%, whereas the patients treated with two-level corpectomy had a fusion rate of 56%.

In noninstrumented ACCF, immediate stability of the graft depends on the graft-host bone interface. The sculpting of the graft and the vertebral endplates and the impaction of the graft into place while the head is in traction contribute to the initial stability of the graft.[29,76-78] Graft migration most commonly occurs at the inferior end of the construct. Wang and colleagues[79] reported their findings in a retrospective review of 249 patients who underwent corpectomy and fusion with the use of autograft and no plate fixation over a 25-year period. Graft migration was observed in 16 of 249 patients. None of the 16 patients experienced any respiratory or neurologic complications as a result of the graft displacement. Wang and colleagues[79] noted an increased rate of this complication occurring in patients undergoing longer fusions and in patients whose fusions ended at the C7 vertebral body.

To increase immediate postoperative stability, anterior plate instrumentation may be added. The addition of anterior plate fixation has been shown to improve the rate of fusion, reduce postoperative immobilization, reduce the incidence of segmental kyphosis, and reduce the prevalence of graft-related complications.[54,80,81] The plate may act as a buttress to block graft migration physically.[82-84] If plate fixation is performed, it is recommended that a minimum distance of 5 mm be maintained between the plate and the unaffected disc segment to minimize the potential of developing adjacent level disc ossification.[85]

The use of anterior instrumentation does not absolutely prevent graft complications. Sasso and colleagues[73] noted that catastrophic construct failure occurred in five of seven patients who underwent a three-level corpectomy with autogenous iliac crest bone graft and anterior cervical locked plating. Most failures occurred with the graft cavitating into the vertebral body at the inferior end of the construct, which caused the graft to displace anteriorly. The biomechanical effects of long anterior cervical plates after three-level corpectomy and strut graft reconstruction were evaluated in two studies.[86,87] The authors of the studies believed that the failures typically seen with instrumented multilevel corpectomies treated with long anterior cervical plates were the result of pistoning of the inferior aspect of the graft. Vaccaro and colleagues[66] noted a 50% failure rate of the patients in their series who underwent three-level ACCF with anterior plate fixation. Based on their findings, they recommended the addition of a posterior stabilizing procedure to supplement multilevel ACCF.

Delayed fractures have been reported through fibular strut grafts after multilevel ACCF.[88,89] Some authors support the use of a titanium cage to achieve immediate construct rigidity.[90,91] The use of this construct may avoid the potential complication of late strut graft fracture. These cages are packed with bone and can be used in combination with anterior instrumentation after ACCF. Excellent fusion rates have been reported using this technique; however, caution must be exercised with the use of this construct in osteoporotic bone.[90,91]

Although graft complications have been reported extensively in the literature, they are not the only problem. Injury to the vertebral arteries has also been reported during ACCF procedures.[61,74] In patients who underwent corpectomy, Eleraky and colleagues[92] reported a prevalence of vertebral artery injury of 2% in 185 patients. It is imperative that a surgeon maintain a midline orientation during an anterior decompression to avoid any violation of the lateral wall and subsequent injury to the vertebral artery. This orientation is particularly important in patients who have tortuosity of the vertebral artery.[93] Anatomic landmarks that have been discussed include the medial margin of the uncovertebral joint, medial margin of the longus colli muscle, and natural curve of the vertebral endplate. Studies have shown that by leaving a margin of approximately 5 mm to the medial border of the foramen transversarium, a total central decompression of approximately 15 mm at C3 and 19 mm at C6 can be performed safely.[47,48]

Individual patient characteristics or comorbidities may influence the surgeon's decision to supplement an anterior decompression with allograft or autograft. Traditionally, the use of iliac crest autograft has been the "gold standard" in one-level and two-level anterior decompression and fusion procedures. For longer fusions, most surgeons prefer to use a structural fibula strut graft. The morbidity associated with the graft harvest is associated with an increased complication rate. Specific iliac crest donor site complications include neuroma formation, iliac crest fracture, cosmetic deformity, persistent pain, and infection.[94-96] In addition to infection, harvesting autogenous fibula has been associated with injury to the peroneal nerve, contracture of the flexor hallucis longus and flexor digitorum longus tendons, development of lower extremity deep venous thrombosis, stress fractures of the tibia, and chronic ankle pain.[97-100]

To avoid the complications associated with the harvest of autograft, some authors advocate the use of allograft. The use of allograft in multilevel fusion has historically been associated with higher rates of nonunion.[101] In a retrospective study of 126 multilevel discectomy and corpectomy cases, Fernyhough and colleagues[102] compared the fusion rates between fibula strut autograft and fibula strut allograft. They noted a 27% nonunion rate in the autograft group versus a 41% nonunion rate in the allograft group. Conversely, MacDonald and colleagues[103] reported a 97% fusion rate in their series of patients who underwent a decompressive corpectomy with the use of fibula strut allograft. More recently, Samartzis and colleagues[104] published a series that showed equivalent rates of fusion between allograft and autograft in patients who underwent multilevel ACDF using cervical plates and current surgical techniques.

Adjacent segment degeneration in previously fused segments in the cervical spine has been reported in the literature. Based on a long-term follow-up study of 374 patients who underwent anterior cervical fusion, Hilibrand and colleagues[105] reported a 25% risk of development of adjacent segment disease within 10 years. In their published series, these authors noted that the C5-6 and C6-7 levels were the most frequently involved. They reported that the risk of developing adjacent segment disease was more likely a manifestation of the natural aging process rather than a consequence of the fusion. More recently, Rao and colleagues[106] reported that performing ACDF with plate fixation does not lead to the development of adjacent segment disease.

Postoperative radiculopathy is a well-recognized phenomenon that occurs after posterior decompression of the spinal cord.[23,107,108] This complication has also been reported in the treatment of CSM in anterior decompressive procedures. Saunders and colleagues[65] reported an incidence of C5 palsy of 20% in their series of 96 patients who underwent corpectomy to treat CSM. They recommended limiting the ventral trough to 14 or 15 mm. Yonenobu and colleagues[108] reported a prevalence of postoperative radiculopathy of 3.9% of 204 patients after anterior procedures. A proposed etiology for the development of the palsy is secondary to an impingement of the ventral aspect of the spinal cord against the edges of the corpectomy trough. The removal of osteophytes can increase the risk of inadvertent injury to the spinal cord itself. Yonenobu and colleagues[109] reported a single patient in their series of 75 patients who sustained an injury to the cord after the resection of posterior osteophytes during ACDF. Subsequently, these authors recommended that corpectomy be considered in patients with posterior osteophytes that are substantial enough to require removal.

Injuries to the soft tissue structures can occur during an anterior approach to the cervical spine. Swallowing difficulties are the most common postoperative problems encountered. Although a frequent complaint, the dysphagia most commonly follows a transient course.[110] This problem seems to be related to esophageal dysmotility that can result from excessive retraction. Bazaz and colleagues[110] reported a 50% prevalence of dysphagia at 1-month follow-up that was more frequently noted when multiple levels were involved in the fusion. At 1-year follow-up, of the 197 patients involved in this study, only 12.5% continued to complain of symptoms. Instrumentation has not been shown to increase the risk of dysphagia.[110,111] Esophageal injury can occur secondary to excessive retraction, electrocautery, or perforation from sharp instruments. The incidence of esophageal perforation has been reported by Newhouse and colleagues[112] to be approximately 0.25%.

Injuries to the recurrent laryngeal nerve have been reported among complications related to the dissection and mobilization of soft tissues in the neck. In a series of 650 patients who underwent an anterior cervical procedure, Frempong-Boadu and colleagues[113] reported a 2% prevalence of injury to the recurrent laryngeal nerve. In contrast, Yue and colleagues[114] reported a prevalence of recurrent laryngeal nerve injury of 11% in 85 patients. Injury to the laryngeal nerve is most commonly attributable to compression within the endolarynx.[115] Apfelbaum and colleagues[115] observed a significant decrease in the occurrence rate of this complication from 6.8% to 1.7% by deflating and reinflating the endotracheal cuff after the retractors were placed. After a review of the literature, Baron and colleagues[116] reported an overall incidence of 4.9% for hoarseness and 1.4% for unilateral vocal cord paralysis. Other causes of nerve injury include direct trauma or an indirect pressure or stretch injury induced by a hematoma or by prolonged retractor placement.

Beutler and colleagues[117] compared the rate of injury to the recurrent laryngeal nerve during right-sided and left-sided approaches. Although they found no difference in the rate of postoperative dysphonia between the two sides, they did observe a generally higher complication rate in the setting of revision surgery. For this reason, some surgeons advocate approaching the spine from the opposite side in a revision setting to avoid the frustration and dangers of operating through scar tissue. If a revision surgery is contemplated, a formal evaluation of vocal cord function must be done if the surgeon intends to approach the spine from the opposite side. In a situation in which the original surgery resulted in permanent unilateral vocal cord paralysis, an opposite-sided approach would be inadvisable because the potential for bilateral vocal cord paralysis would be catastrophic.

Prolonged retraction can also cause injury to the cervical sympathetic ganglion resulting in Horner syndrome, characterized by ipsilateral ptosis, miosis, and anhidrosis. This complication can also be seen in revision surgeries or in operations involving the cervicothoracic junction. Bertalanffy and Eggert[56] reported an incidence of 1.1% in their series of 450 patients who underwent an anterior cervical fusion. To prevent this complication, the longus colli muscles should be dissected of the anterior vertebral body in a subperiosteal fashion, and retractors should be placed deep to the longus colli muscles.

Posterior Approach

Indications for a Posterior Approach

Before the 1950s, the operative treatment of degenerative cervical disorders primarily occurred through a posterior approach. The posterior approach to the cervical spine has continued to be a safe and effective treatment option in the surgical management of CSM. Indications for a posterior approach to the cervical spine include congenital cervical stenosis, multilevel cervical spondylosis, OPLL, ossification of the yellow ligament, and posterior compression caused by infolding of the ligamentum flavum.[37,45,118,119] A posterior approach to the cervical spine relieves spinal cord compression through two distinct mechanisms: direct and indirect decompression. When the pathology causing the myelopathy is primarily due to ventral structures, posterior procedures are indirect methods of decompression. With indirect decompression, expansion of the canal allows the spinal cord to shift posteriorly away from the anterior impinging structures. In situations in which the myelopathy is secondary to a congenital stenosis or a redundant ligamentum flavum, the decompressive effect of a posterior procedure is more direct. The removal or relocation of the posterior impinging structures acts to decompress the spinal cord and is a form of direct decompression. Laminectomy and laminoplasty are two techniques of decompressing the cervical spine from a posterior approach.

For an effective indirect spinal cord decompression to occur, certain prerequisites must exist. Posterior procedures are primarily indicated in the presence of a neutral or lordotic sagittal alignment to allow for the posterior translation of the spinal cord.[120] As spondylosis progresses, there is a general trend toward loss of lordosis.[121] In a patient with a kyphotic cervical spine, the sagittal alignment of the bony elements does not allow for the posterior translation of the spinal cord (Fig. 41–7). Even after a posterior decompression, the cord remains draped over the anterior compressive pathology. A minimal lordotic curvature of 10 degrees should be present if posterior decompression is considered.[122] Studies have shown

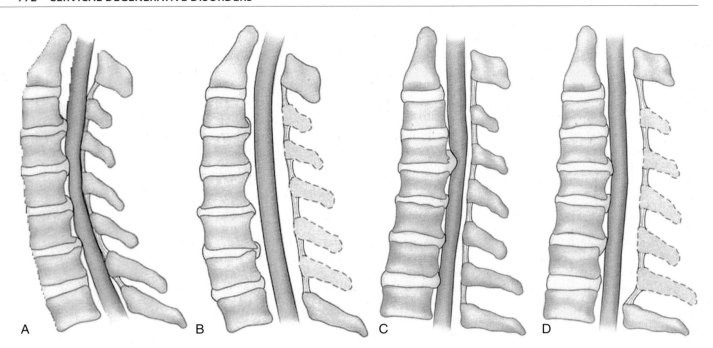

FIGURE 41–7 Influence of cervical sagittal alignment on decompressive effect of laminoplasty. **A,** Multilevel cord compression arising from spondylosis of C3-7 in the presence of lordotic cervical alignment. **B,** Spinal canal expansion after laminoplasty with dorsal shift of spinal cord away from anterior impinging structures. **C,** Multilevel cord compression and kyphotic cervical alignment. **D,** Continued spinal cord impingement after laminoplasty. The presence of kyphotic alignment compromises indirect decompressive effect of laminoplasty.

that measured from C2 to C7, the average lordotic curvature in a normal cervical spine is 14.4 degrees.[123]

Yamazaki and colleagues[124] observed continued ventral compression after posterior decompression in patients with anterior canal encroachment greater than 7 mm and with lordotic sagittal alignments of less than 10 degrees. When a posterior decompression is performed in patients with a kyphotic cervical alignment, modest improvements in neurologic outcome can be expected. The recovery achieved from a decompression in the presence of a cervical kyphosis tends to be inferior, however, when compared with a posterior decompression that is performed in the presence of a cervical lordosis.[37,125] These findings were echoed by Satomi and colleagues,[125] who found that patients with maintenance of preoperative lordosis exhibited a superior improvement in JOA score compared with patients in whom the lordosis decreased by 10 degrees or more.

In patients who underwent decompressive laminoplasty, Sodeyama and colleagues[45] showed that patients with lordotic spines had the greatest postoperative posterior translation of the spinal cord with an average shift of 3.1 mm. Patients who had a neutral alignment showed a peak posterior shift of less than 3 mm, and patients who had a kyphotic cervical alignment showed a peak posterior shift of less than 2 mm. In a study evaluating 114 patients with CSM after laminoplasty, Suda and colleagues[37] observed that a preoperative local kyphosis exceeding 13 degrees provided patients with the worst prognosis for neurologic recovery. They concluded that cervical kyphosis should be regarded as a relative contraindication for a posterior decompression.

As a second prerequisite, indirect spinal cord decompression also requires a sufficient length of canal expansion. Decompression of the posterior structures at levels beyond areas of focal stenosis may allow for greater translation of the cord. The degree of canal expansion that is achieved via a posterior approach has been shown to correlate with the success of postoperative recovery.[126-128] A statistically significant difference in recovery rate was reported by Hirabayashi and colleagues[126] when the anteroposterior diameter of the spinal canal increased greater than 5 mm versus an increase of less than 2 mm. Ishida and colleagues[127] observed better recovery rates in patients in whom posterior decompression increased the sagittal diameter of the canal to 15 mm or greater. Kohno and colleagues[128] showed that expansion of the anteroposterior canal diameter to 12.8 mm correlated with a good postoperative recovery after laminoplasty. Shaffrey and colleagues[129] reported an overall average increase in the spinal canal cross-sectional area of 55% after posterior decompression with an 88% increase at the most compressed level.

When adequately decompressed, the spinal cord has been reported to change in morphology from a flattened to a more natural oval shape. In a CT myelography study, Aita and colleagues[120] described changes in spinal cord morphology in 38 patients after open-door laminoplasty. Postoperatively, the largest increase in mean spinal cord cross-sectional area was improved by 12%. In addition, the mean sagittal cord diameter was enlarged by 1 mm, and the mean coronal diameter was decreased by 1 mm.

The longitudinal height of the cervical spine as a prognostic indicator for neurologic recovery has also been evaluated.

Chiba and colleagues[130] noted that after extensive open-door laminoplasty, patients with CSM were more likely to have improved neurologic results compared with patients with OPLL. They observed a greater degree of preoperative cervical spine shortening owing to disc degeneration in patients with CSM. These authors attributed the improved recovery rate in these patients to the redundancy within the spinal cord after decompression.

Laminectomy and Laminectomy and Fusion

Laminectomy is indicated for multilevel decompression in elderly myelopathic patients with multiple medical comorbidities and preserved cervical lordosis. Decompressive laminectomy is typically performed at the junctions of the lateral masses and the laminae. If a patient also has concurrent radicular symptoms, a concomitant foraminotomy may be performed to decompress the associated foraminal stenosis. If a foraminotomy is performed, care must be taken not to remove much of the facet. Progressive removal of greater increments of the facet joint is correlated with greater degrees of instability.[123] To preserve stability, it is crucial to resect no more than 25% of the facet joint.[131] In addition, any level with radiographic evidence of stenosis should be included in the decompression. Kato and colleagues[132] observed increased rates of recurrent symptoms resulting from progression of disease at adjacent segments not involved in the decompression. Kaptain and colleagues[133] reported no added benefit in limiting the number of segments involved in the decompression because it did not influence the development of postlaminectomy kyphosis or instability.

Circumstances such as iatrogenic instability, flexible kyphosis, or focal instability require supplemental posterior cervical instrumentation. The goal of any fixation system is to provide structural support for a bony fusion mass to mature. The use of posterior instrumentation has been shown to maintain lordosis effectively after a posterior cervical laminectomy and fusion.[134,135] Before the introduction of lateral mass screws, wiring techniques were the mainstay of treatment when a fusion was performed. The wire would be passed between neighboring facets or tied to bone grafts or metallic rods. With these techniques, acceptable fusion rates were obtained.[136,137] With the introduction of lateral mass screws, wiring techniques have largely fallen out of favor.

Biomechanically, lateral mass screws have been proven to be a superior technique compared with wiring procedures. They produce a more rigid construct and show a better fusion potential.[138] The early screw-plate systems were difficult to use and very inflexible because they could not adapt well to variations in patient anatomy. The lack of versatility these early designs offered has been overcome with the evolution of multiaxial screw and rod constructs.[139] The newer systems are constrained and allow for more rigid fixation. Similarly, these new systems accommodate variations in the cervical anatomy without having to perform excessive rod contouring or having to compromise screw positioning.

A review of the literature reveals various lateral mass screw insertion techniques.[140-143] The biomechanical characteristics and anatomic relationships of each of these techniques have been studied.[144,145] Despite the various techniques described, clinically none have shown any difference in complication rate.[146] In a cadaveric study, Seybold and colleagues[147] showed no clear biomechanical advantage with bicortical placement of lateral mass screws versus unicortical placement of lateral mass screws. They showed an increased incidence of nerve root impingement and potential vertebral artery injury with the use of bicortical screws. These investigators reported no injuries using unicortical screws. Ultimately, an appropriate understanding and knowledge of anatomic relationships is needed when placing these screws.

Techniques for pedicle screw placement have also been described in the literature.[148] Pedicle screws have been shown to have a higher pullout strength compared with lateral mass screws.[149] Because of the small size and morphologic variation in the cervical pedicle, however, there is greater potential for injury with pedicle screw placement.[150] Pedicle screw placement is usually reserved for levels with larger pedicles, such as the C7 vertebra, or when crossing the cervicothoracic junction. The technique for pedicle screw placement is not discussed in this chapter.

Technique

As with any patient with myelopathy, care should be taken to avoid any extremes of neck motion during intubation. Mean arterial pressure should be monitored during positioning of the patient, and hypotension should be avoided throughout the entire operative procedure. A Mayfield tong or three-pin head holder is affixed to the patient's head, and the patient is positioned prone on the operating table. The head should be fixed in neutral or in slight extension. The trunk should be supported by a four-poster frame or by padded chest rolls. If a padded headrest with a laminectomy frame is used, care must be taken to avoid any force on the eyes because this may increase intraocular pressure and create an ischemic optic neuropathy resulting in visual loss.[151] All bony prominences should be padded. The arms should be tucked in and secured at the patient's side using arm sleds or sheets under the patient's torso. Legs should be flexed at the knees, and the patient should be secured to the table using the appropriate straps. The table should be positioned in a reverse Trendelenburg position to reduce any venous congestion. After the patient is positioned, the suboccipital region is shaved, and the surgical field is sterilely prepared and draped.

The spinous processes of C2 and C7 are usually palpable landmarks that are easy to distinguish and can be used to guide in planning of the surgical incision. A midline cervical incision is drawn out, and the skin is infiltrated with local anesthetic with epinephrine to aid in hemostasis. An incision through the skin is made using sharp dissection. The midline incision through the deep tissues is continued, maintaining strict hemostasis at all times with the use of monopolar electrocautery. Next, the ligamentum nuchae is divided, and the dissection is continued with a split through the splenius capitus fascia. It is imperative that care be taken to perform

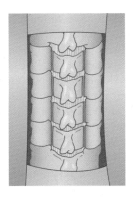
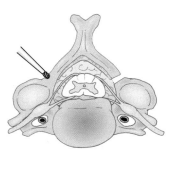

FIGURE 41–8 Bilateral trough laminotomies are created at lamina-facet junction medial to facet complex. (From Komotar RJ, Mocco J, Kaiser MG: Surgical management of cervical myelopathy: Indications and techniques for laminectomy and fusion. Spine J 6:258S, 2006.)

the dissection in the midline to prevent blood loss or any unnecessary intramuscular embarrassment.

Dissection is carried subperiosteally exposing the spinous processes and laminae of the appropriately selected cervical levels. Care should be exercised not to dissect the muscular attachments of C2 because its removal has been shown to create instability in the upper cervical spine.[152] The extent of lateral dissection is minimized to just beyond the medial aspect of the facet joint, with care taken not to violate the facet capsules. A self-retainer is placed to mobilize the paraspinal musculature free from the surgical field. To avoid excessive damage to the paraspinal muscles, retractors should be intermittently released and repositioned. If an instrumentation and fusion is indicated, the exposure for lateral mass fixation requires the subperiosteal soft tissue dissection to extend to the far lateral margin of the facet. Care must be taken to avoid any compromise to the facet capsule of the most cranial and caudal aspects of the intended fusion.

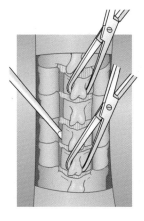

FIGURE 41–9 Towel clamp is placed on most cranial and caudal spinous process. Lamina and associated ligamentum flavum are gently lifted en bloc with care taken not to lever one end into spinal cord. (From Komotar RJ, Mocco J, Kaiser MG: Surgical management of cervical myelopathy: Indications and techniques for laminectomy and fusion. Spine J 6:259S, 2006.)

It is essential that the landmarks of the lateral mass be clearly identified to ensure accurate placement of the screws. The cranial and caudal boundaries of the lateral mass are defined by the adjacent facet joints, and the medial boundary is defined by the lamina-facet junction. After adequate exposure of the lateral masses is achieved, entry sites for the lateral mass screws are marked using a high-speed bur. Screws are placed depending on the surgeon's choice of technique. After the screws are adequately placed, the lamina can be resected. Laminectomies are performed after the insertion of the lateral mass screws to protect the cord with its neural elements. Care must be taken to preserve the bone for use as local autograft. Removal of the spinous processes with preservation of a small remnant facilitates visualization and removal of the laminae. Bilateral trough laminotomies are created with the aid of a bur at the lamina-facet junction just medial to the facet complex (Fig. 41–8). During the laminotomies, 1 to 2 mm of thinned ventral bony cortex or hypertrophied yellow ligament dorsal to the underlying thecal sac is preserved.

Removal of the ventral cortex is accomplished with a low-speed 4-mm bur. The intraspinous ligament at the most cranial and caudal level is divided and resected. Following this, a towel clamp is placed on the most cranial and caudal spinous process, and the lamina and associated ligamentum flavum are gently lifted off the underlying dura (Fig. 41–9). The ligamentum flavum is divided, and the laminae are removed en bloc. Any residual osseous remnants are removed using a Kerrison punch, completing the laminectomy to the lateral edge of the thecal sac. In an extremely stenotic canal with no epidural fat and nearly no yellow ligament, there may be dense adhesions to the underlying dura. No instrument should be introduced in or near the midline to avoid cord contusion. In a patient with severe stenosis, the exclusive use of a high-speed bur may be advisable to minimize any further compression that may be caused by the footplate of a Kerrison punch.

Undercutting and removal of the cephalad and caudal soft tissues is accomplished to avoid further extension of cord compression. A dome laminectomy under the surface of the C2 lamina may also be performed if further decompression is necessary. Foraminal decompression may be performed at this time if concomitant foraminal stenosis is noted. The visible expansion of the dural sac after removal of the laminae suggests adequate canal expansion. The expansion of the dural sac often adequately tamponades the epidural venous plexus as long as no cerebrospinal fluid leak has occurred. If lateral mass screws have been placed, malleable rods are cut and contoured and placed onto the screw construct. The locking mechanism is engaged securing the screw and rod construct. The facet joints and lateral masses are decorticated, and the autograft bone is impacted across the posterolateral aspect of the spine and into the facet joints.

If epidural venous bleeding is encountered, absorbable gelatin sponge (Gelfoam) with collagen strips may be placed in the lateral gutters over the thecal sac to aid in hemostasis. A drain may also be used if hemostasis is suboptimal. A routine layered watertight wound closure is performed, and the patient is taken from the operating table and brought to the postoperative recovery unit for continued monitoring. If a posterior fusion with instrumentation is performed, the patient is discharged home with a rigid cervical collar. A rigid cervical collar is worn postoperatively for a varying number of weeks depending on the bone quality, fixation adequacy, and fusion length.

Neurologic Outcomes

Laminectomy has been proven to be a successful procedure in the treatment of elderly myelopathic patients with multilevel cervical spondylosis and lordotic sagittal alignment. Of 90 patients who underwent cervical laminectomy in the series by Snow and Weiner,[118] 77% of patients showed neurologic improvement, 13% of patients remained unchanged, and 10% of patients experienced neurologic deterioration. In a review of 32 patients treated with multilevel laminectomy and posterior fusion using a lateral mass screw and plate construct, Huang and colleagues[153] noted a postoperative improvement in Nurick grade of at least 1 point in 22 patients. The remaining nine patients showed no change in neurologic function, but more importantly no patients involved in the study showed any neurologic deterioration. More recently, Sekhon[154] reviewed 50 patients with CSM who underwent posterior cervical decompression and fusion with an average follow-up of 30.1 months. All patients underwent fusion with a lateral mass screw plate and rod construct with local autograft. An average of 2.88 levels were fused. At last follow-up, no patients developed any symptomatic or radiographic evidence of pseudarthrosis. Postoperative MRI showed an absence of persistent compression at the operative levels in 100% of cases. Most patients improved at least one Nurick grade, and no myelopathic deterioration was noted postoperatively.

Complications

Although good to excellent results have been reported in patients after laminectomy, subsequent deterioration in outcome may occur.[118,155,156] The development of a new-onset neurologic deficit from an injury to the nerve root or to the spinal cord itself is among the most feared complications involving the surgical management of CSM. Yonenobu and colleagues[108] observed a 3.5% prevalence of spinal cord injury after laminectomy in their series of 85 patients. They attributed spinal cord dysfunction to postoperative swelling and to epidural hematoma formation that caused compression on the uncovered cord. In 287 patients undergoing multilevel cervical laminectomy, Dai and colleagues[157] observed a 13% incidence of postoperative radiculopathy. Most patients in their series were found to have regained function within 6 months of surgery. The postoperative development of a sagittal malalignment or a segmental instability has been linked to the development of neurologic deterioration after laminectomy.[152] Adequate decompression often requires the removal of important static and dynamic stabilizing structures, which can lead to an imbalance in sagittal alignment.[133,158-160] Over

time, the spinal cord may become tethered against anterior impinging structures, resulting in progressive spinal cord dysfunction.[78,118,155,156]

In adults, laminectomy alone significantly increases total cervical spine flexibility.[159] This instability is increased further with the removal of the spinous process or lamina of C2 or C7. Removal of the posterior arch with the spinous process of C2 disrupts the semispinalis cervicis and the suboccipital muscles significantly weakening the posterior tension band of the cervical spine. Iizuka and colleagues[152] showed that postoperative loss of sagittal alignment was strongly associated with dissection and subsequent nonhealing of the muscle insertion on C2. Younger individuals are particularly vulnerable to the development of a kyphotic sagittal malalignment after laminectomy. Bell and colleagues[161] showed that 53% of patients younger than 18 years who underwent multilevel laminectomy developed a progressive kyphosis. The tendency for children to develop a symptomatic kyphotic deformity after extensive laminectomy may be due to the increased viscoelasticity of the posterior elements and the immaturity of the vertebral body.[162] The horizontal orientation of the facet joints in the immature spine can lead to a less resistive force to flexion.[163]

The width of the facetectomy has also been shown to be a crucial determinant in the development of postoperative instability. Zdeblick and colleagues[123] showed that facetectomy of more than 50% caused a statistically significant loss of stability of the cervical spine in flexion and torsion. Voo and colleagues[164] observed a pronounced increase in angular rotation and intervertebral disc stress with resection of greater than 50% of the facet complexes bilaterally. Herkowitz[82] noted a 25% increase in the incidence of postoperative kyphotic deformities within 2 years after cervical laminectomy with partial bilateral facetectomies. He concluded that if 50% or more of the facet has been violated, a concurrent stabilization procedure should be recommended. Nowinski and colleagues[165] reinforced further the idea that in multilevel laminectomy a concurrent fusion should be performed if more than 25% of the facet is removed bilaterally.

In an effort to avoid any postoperative instability associated with laminectomy, some authors advocate performing a concurrent instrumentation and fusion, with the use of lateral mass screws.[153,154] Complications using this technique have been reported. Complications with lateral mass fixation include neuronal injury, vertebral artery injury, and hardware failure secondary to pseudarthrosis. In an analysis of complications after lateral mass fixation with screws and plates, Heller and colleagues[166] found a 0.6% incidence of nerve root injury per screw placed and a 1.1% incidence of screw loosening after instrumentation of 654 screws. They observed that 3.8% of patients had development of adjacent segment disease within 2.5 years after laminectomy and fusion. Of the 654 screws placed, they reported no vertebral artery injuries. In a review of 43 patients who had 281 screws placed, Wellman and colleagues[167] showed no screw-related complications after a 25-month follow-up. They concluded that lateral mass fixation is a safe and effective means of posterior cervical stabilization.

Laminoplasty

Laminoplasty is well suited for management of cervical myelopathy resulting from multilevel stenosis. This procedure was designed to permit extensive decompression through posterior expansion of the canal, while continually maintaining cervical alignment and stability through the preservation of the posterior elements. Laminoplasty avoids the potential complications associated with an attempted fusion, such as donor site morbidity, graft displacement, nonunion, implant malposition or failure, and adjacent segment degeneration. Indications for the use of laminoplasty include congenital stenosis, spondylosis, multilevel disc herniations, and OPLL in a neutral or lordotic cervical spine. Although numerous laminoplasty techniques have been described, all share certain fundamental elements, which include the decompression of a stenotic spinal canal through the expansion of the posterior arch, the conservation of the posterior elements, and the preservation of segmental motion.

The preservation of the posterior elements of the cervical spine provides a biologic covering to the spinal canal and a reattachment site for paraspinal muscles. Pal and Cooper[168] tested load transmission in the anterior and posterior cervical column in cadavers. They showed that 36% of load transmission was through the anterior column, whereas 64% was through the posterior column. These findings highlight the importance of preserving the integrity of the posterior arch and facet complex. In addition, the posterior arch complex serves as an important static factor in the maintenance of cervical lordosis.[169-171] With preservation of the natural static and dynamic restraints of the posterior cervical spine, iatrogenic instability is rarely encountered after laminoplasty.[129,172] Of 171 patients treated with French-door laminoplasty, Shimamura and colleagues[172] reported no cases of segmental instability at 5-year follow-up. Similarly, Kawakami and colleagues[173] observed no evidence of segmental instability on dynamic radiographs at 3.5-year follow-up in their series of 67 patients who underwent laminoplasty for the treatment of CSM.

The procedure was first described by Oyama and colleagues in 1973.[174] The technique involved a Z-plasty of each thinned lamina. Through the expansion of the modified lamina, a decompression of the spinal cord was performed, and the posterior arch was reconstructed. The original technique used a supplemental arthrodesis through the placement of bone graft over the expanded arch and facets. This technique never gained popularity owing to the prolonged time and painstaking detail required.

Two examples of laminoplasty techniques that are discussed in this chapter include the open-door laminoplasty technique described by Hirabayashi and colleagues[175] and the mid-sagittal laminoplasty or French-door laminoplasty technique described by Kurokawa and colleagues.[176] Comparative studies of these two procedures have failed to show a significant distinction with regard to neurologic outcomes.[177,178] Okada and colleagues[179] published a prospective randomized study comparing the clinical outcomes of open-door laminoplasty versus French-door laminoplasty. Although Okada and colleagues[179] observed higher rates of perioperative complications and added complaints of postoperative axial pain in the open-door laminoplasty group, no significant differences in postoperative JOA scores and recovery rates were noted between the two groups.

Open-Door Laminoplasty

In 1978, Hirabayashi[180] described the open-door laminoplasty technique. With this technique, the canal is expanded at consecutive levels by creating a bone hinge on one side of the canal while detaching the lamina at the opposite side. This technique enables the spinal cord to be adequately decompressed while maintaining stability of the spinal column. Advantages of the open-door procedure include a straightforward operative technique and shorter operative time. Advocates of this technique cite that entering the canal at its lateralmost extent, where spinal cord compression tends to be the least, protects the cord and provides for a greater margin of safety.

Disadvantages associated with the use of the open-door technique have been described. A greater degree of bleeding is encountered with this technique because of the vast plexus of epidural veins in the lateral portion of the cervical spinal canal. Cases have been documented in which the hinge prematurely closed resulting in radiologic and catastrophic neurologic deterioration. This complication was first described by Hirabayashi and colleagues[175] and termed the *spring-back phenomenon*. To safeguard against this complication, Hirabayashi advocated the use of stay sutures to secure the spinous process to the facet capsule on the hinge side.[175,181]

The description of the spring-back phenomenon acted as a catalyst in the design of a newer generation of techniques to maintain a patent canal (Fig. 41–10). Itoh and Tsuji[182] described the use of autograft spinous process bone blocks and stainless steel wiring to maintain canal patency. In 30 patients in their series, these authors reported no significant deterioration in 18 months of follow-up, and they observed an average of 4.1 mm of anteroposterior canal expansion. Various other strut materials have been employed, including contoured ceramic blocks, hydroxyapatite blocks, and allografts.[129,183,184]

The use of rigid internal fixation between the expanded laminae and the lateral masses has also been described as an alternative method of providing immediate stability. Specialized plates have been designed to maintain canal patency and to reduce the probability of hinge closure and restenosis. O'Brien and colleagues[185] showed a significant improvement in sagittal canal diameter with no hardware failure with the use of titanium plates to maintain patency in their series of patients who underwent an open-door laminoplasty. Similarly, through the use of plate fixation and allograft, Shaffrey and colleagues[129] reported an increase in sagittal canal diameter with an improvement in overall neurologic function in patients in their series. The long-term stability of these constructs is achieved with the eventual healing of the bone on

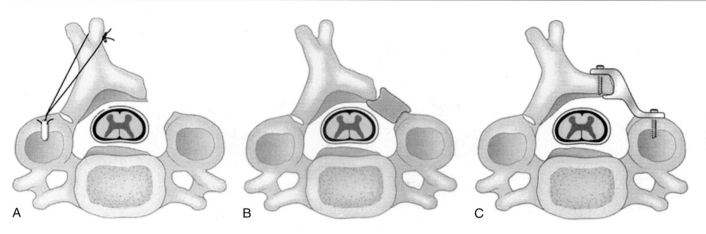

A   B   C

FIGURE 41–10 Methods of stabilizing expanded posterior arch with open-door laminoplasty. **A,** Tethering from hinge side with lateral mass suture anchor. **B,** Propping expanded arch open with contoured strut. **C,** Rigid intrasegment fixation with a plate and screw system.

the hinge side or the eventual healing of the host bone-strut graft interface on the open-door side, or both.

French-Door Laminoplasty

In 1978, Kurokawa and colleagues[176] described a *spinous process splitting* or *French-door* laminoplasty. This novel technique provided for symmetrical expansion of the stenotic canal by dividing the spinous processes in the midline before hinging open each hemilamina at the lamina–lateral mass junction. Bone or synthetic blocks were placed as a strut to maintain the patency of the hinged hemilaminae (Fig. 41–11). Advocates of the French-door technique reported decreased bleeding because of the paucity of veins encountered in the midline of the canal. They also reported a more symmetrical expansion of the canal compared with the open-door technique.[159,178] The French-door technique can be readily combined with lateral mass or pedicle screw fixation methods if a concurrent posterior fusion is necessary. Typically, the midline sagittal split in the spinous process is created with the use of a bur or a threadwire saw. Using the threadwire saw to perform the sagittal split in the spinous process, Tomita and colleagues[186] reported a mean decrease in operating room time of 63 minutes and a mean blood loss of 70 mL less than if a bur was used. No matter which instrument is used, the surgeon must always be mindful that the introduction of instruments into the central portion of a stenotic canal can increase the danger of creating a catastrophic neurologic injury.[176,186]

Technique

Laminoplasty has proven to be a safe and reliable technique of decompressing the spinal cord. Although the described methods each have their own technical points, certain operative principles are applicable to all techniques. Patients are positioned prone, on the operative table. The use of a frame or rolls to support the trunk provides for decreased abdominal and chest pressure. Cranial tongs are used to secure the head, and the cervical spine is placed in a neutral or mildly flexed position. To minimize the bleeding from venous congestion

and minimize facial or airway edema during surgery, the operative table is placed in 30 degrees of reverse Trendelenburg position.[175] Care must be taken to avoid any pressure on the eyes.

A posterior midline approach is made along the nuchal ligament to the spinous processes. The paraspinal muscles are dissected from the posterior elements. Care is taken to preserve the insertion of the paraspinal muscles to the spinous process of C2. If significant tension of the supraspinous and interspinous ligaments is noted during the expansion of an open-door laminoplasty, a partial osteotomy at the base of the spinous process just below the caudal end of the expanded construct may be performed.[187] The osteotomized spinous process is bent toward the hinge side to decrease the ligamentous tension. With an open-door laminoplasty from C3 to C7, significant ligamentous tension would be alleviated with an incomplete osteotomy through the base of the T1 spinous process. Other authors simply excise the spinous processes and their associated ligaments at the cranial and caudal ends to facilitate the opening of the spinal canal. The trough laminectomies are created at the lamina–lateral mass junction without disruption of the facet joints (Fig. 41–12).

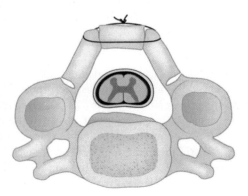

FIGURE 41–11 Schematic showing spinous process splitting or French-door laminoplasty. Posterior arch is divided longitudinally at midline and expanded symmetrically off of bilateral partial-thickness gutters. Gap between expanded hemilamina is stabilized with interposition of spinous process or allograft strut.

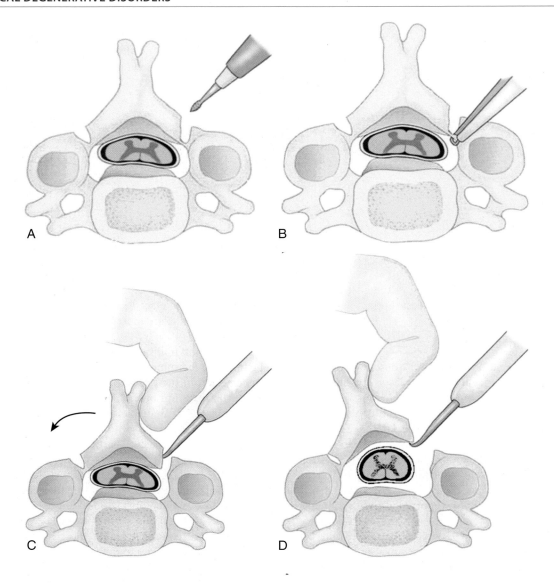

FIGURE 41–12 Schematic images showing technique for open-door laminoplasty. **A,** Gutters are fashioned at junction between lamina and facet with high-speed bur. Care is taken to preserve ventral cortex on hinge side. **B,** On side to be opened, completion of gutter is performed with either a micro-Kerrison rongeur or a curet. **C** and **D,** Posterior arch of each level is expanded gently using a combination of digital manipulation and elevation with an instrument. When expanded, posterior arch is stabilized in its final position using one of various methods discussed in the text.

Preservation of the facet joints decreases the potential for subsequent instability and minimizes the probability of the facet joint acting as a pain generator. The posterior incision is closed in the usual fashion, described earlier in the laminectomy section. Postoperatively, patients are placed in a soft or rigid collar for comfort, and they are encouraged to begin isometric neck exercises while wearing the collar. Range of motion exercises are started at 2 weeks.

Outcomes

Laminoplasty has been shown to be an effective treatment option in the decompression of patients with myelopathy secondary to OPLL. Numerous authors have reported, however,

that an OPLL continues to increase in thickness even after a decompressive procedure is performed. In a series of 47 patients, Satomi and colleagues[125] reported an average increase in thickness of the OPLL from 6.3 mm preoperatively to 7.5 mm after laminoplasty at 5-year follow-up. To accommodate any future extension of the OPLL, they recommended that decompression of the level above and the level below the compressive pathology be strongly considered.[125,188] Often a dome laminectomy of C2 may be necessary. This technique involves the removal of bone from the lamina of C2, while maintaining the structural integrity of the arch and its important muscular insertions. Iwasaki and colleagues[189] reported the results of 64 patients with OPLL over a 10-year minimal follow-up. They observed progression of cervical OPLL in 70%

of patients, with the development of neurologic deterioration in only two patients. Similarly, in long-term follow-up greater than 10 years for patients with cervical myelopathy caused by OPLL, Kawaguchi and colleagues[188] noted progression of OPLL in 73% of patients. Young age at the time of surgery has been identified as a risk factor for progression of OPLL, whereas an older age has been shown to be protective.[188,189]

Many short-term studies have been reported evaluating the clinical outcomes after cervical laminoplasty. The first of such reports was by Hirabayashi and colleagues.[190] Using the JOA score, they noted a 54% improvement rate over an average follow-up of 3 years on patients who underwent an open-door laminoplasty for CSM. Similarly, Satomi and colleagues[125] reported an average recovery rate of 61% in 18 patients with CSM over an 8-year follow-up. Using a French-door lamino-plasty technique, Tomita and colleagues[186] observed a 72% recovery rate over a 34-month follow-up.

Long-term studies have also been reported in the literature regarding clinical outcomes after laminoplasty. Over a period of greater than 10 years, Kawaguchi and colleagues[191] studied the long-term outcome of 126 patients who underwent laminoplasty for the treatment of cervical myelopathy. They reported a preoperative JOA score of 9.1, which improved to 13.7 after 1 postoperative year. At last follow-up, Kawaguchi and colleagues[191] found that the score was maintained at 13.4. Seichi and colleagues[192] reported their results of 25 patients over a 12-year follow-up who underwent a laminoplasty. They noted mean JOA preoperative scores of 8.3, which at last follow up were observed to increase to 11.7. They also reported that late neurologic deterioration occurred in four patients, three of whom had athetoid cerebral palsy.

Complications

The most important role of any laminoplasty technique is to permit extensive decompression of the spinal canal through the expansion of the posterior arch. Early in the laminoplasty experience, cases of posterior arch closure were reported (Fig. 41–13).[175] Satomi and colleagues[125] observed postoperative lamina closure resulting in neurologic deterioration in 4% of 51 patients after open-door laminoplasty. Matsumoto and colleagues[193] identified the presence of preoperative cervical kyphosis as a significant risk factor for the development of lamina closure. In their series, recovery rates were not influenced by lamina closure; however, patients with lamina closure expressed a greater degree of dissatisfaction with the surgery.

Postoperative motor root palsy is a clinically significant complication of cervical laminoplasty and has received significant attention in the literature.[23,107,108] In most cases, the symptoms are not permanent, and complete to partial recovery can be expected. Obvious causes of neurologic deterioration include displacement of the posterior arch into the canal through strut graft or fixation failure, inadequate decompression, postoperative hematoma, and iatrogenic trauma to the cord. In cases in which no obvious abnormality is identified, the etiology of postoperative motor root palsy remains undetermined. Some authors believe that the mechanism of injury is associated with the tethering of the nerve roots secondary

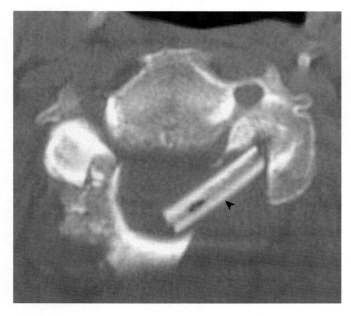

FIGURE 41–13 Axial CT scan after open-door laminoplasty shows displaced strut producing spinal cord compression (*arrowhead*). Gutter on open-door side is also suboptimal, being too lateral with excessive facet joint resection.

to the posterior migration of the spinal cord.[108] A posterior translation of the spinal cord may stress the ventrally exiting nerve roots, causing mechanical injury and ischemic insult to the nerve root and the adjoining spinal cord parenchyma. A posterior shift of the spinal cord could also produce focal pressure on the nerve root at its entry into the foramen.[194,195]

Sasai and colleagues[196,197] suggested that preexisting sub-clinical C5 root compression is a cause of C5 palsy. They found that preexisting subclinical radiculopathy as determined by abnormal preoperative electrophysiologic studies was predictive for the development of postoperative motor deficits. Sasai and colleagues[196,197] also evaluated the role of prophylactic foraminotomies in decreasing the incidence of motor palsy. Based on their findings, they suggested that postoperative nerve palsy could be avoided if a selective foraminotomy was performed concurrently with the laminoplasty. The clinical presentation of most patients presenting with postoperative motor root palsy is often delayed hours to days after surgery and most commonly involves the C5 nerve root.[107,198] Uematsu and colleagues[107] reported on 20 of 365 patients who underwent laminoplasty and who developed postoperative motor palsy. They noted an 8% incidence of C5 root palsy, and most of their patients presented with symptoms within 1 week of surgery. Most of their patients presented with symptoms within 1 week of surgery. They recommended that expansion of the posterior arch be limited to prevent the development of anterior root tension.

Chiba and colleagues[198] reported 15 patients in their series who developed postoperative segmental motor paralysis after open-door laminoplasty. The symptoms developed an average of 4.6 days postoperatively. All 15 patients showed a high T2 signal intensity in the spinal cord on MRI. Of the 15 patients, 10 were observed to display signal changes that corresponded to the level at the paralyzed segment. At last follow-up, paralysis resolved completely in 11 patients. The remaining patients regained their strength to a motor grade of 4 out of 5. Based on their findings, Chiba and colleagues[198] concluded that impairments in the gray matter of the spinal cord might play an important role in the development of postoperative motor paralysis.

Laminoplasty has not been shown to be an effective procedure in the relief of axial neck pain in patients with myelopathy. In addition, patients who have undergone laminoplasty often complain of discomfort in the neck, the shoulders, and the intrascapular region in the postoperative period. The etiology of neck pain is undetermined, but it has been postulated to result secondary to posterior soft tissue dissection or to the inadvertent disruption of the facet joints.[199,200] Hosono and colleagues[201] noted that the prevalence of postoperative axial symptoms was significantly higher after laminoplasty than after anterior fusion. Axial symptoms were reported in 60% of patients after laminoplasty and 19% of patients after an anterior fusion. Similarly, in a study by Wada and colleagues[23] comparing subtotal corpectomy and laminoplasty, 15% of patients in the corpectomy group versus 40% of patients in the laminoplasty group complained of axial pain postoperatively. More recently, using a visual analog scale pain questionnaire, Takeuchi and Yasuhiro[202] reported the importance of preserving the C7 spinous process and the attached nuchal ligament to reduce postoperative axial symptoms after French-door laminoplasty.

Early in the development of the laminoplasty technique, most authors recommended a concomitant fusion to prevent the development of subsequent instability and recurrent stenosis.[182,203] The practice of applying bone graft to the posterior elements led to a reduced range of motion and a higher rate of postoperative axial discomfort than necessary. Studies over the years have shown that cervical lordosis and segmental stability are maintained after laminoplasty without the need of a simultaneous fusion. Based on these findings, most authors currently recommend that laminoplasty be performed without fusion except in cases of known instability or correction of deformity.[129,186,204]

In the evaluation of long-term outcomes of laminoplasty, most authors have reported a significant loss of motion at final follow-up. Edwards and colleagues[67] reported a 38% loss of C2-7 sagittal motion after laminoplasty. Similarly, Kimura and colleagues[203] noted a postoperative loss of motion of 62% in their series of patients who underwent an open-door laminoplasty. Kawaguchi and colleagues[191] observed a similar reduction in range of motion in their long-term series of patients; 61% of patients in their series developed some decrease in range of motion. More recently, Hyun and colleagues[205] observed a decrease in range of motion that was time dependent in patients who underwent an open-door laminoplasty. In their series of 23 patients, they noted a gradual decrease in cervical range of motion that continued for 18 months before stabilizing. To diminish the potential for spontaneous facet fusion and to preserve motion, some authors recommend the application of bone wax to the exposed cancellous hinge surfaces.[67] Many contemporary rehabilitation programs encourage early active range of motion with the goal of reducing postoperative neck stiffness and pain.[206]

The development of a kyphotic sagittal alignment after laminoplasty has been well reported.[189,191] Fewer reports exist documenting the potential neurologic decline that can accompany a loss of normal cervical lordosis. Over a 10-year follow-up, Iwasaki and colleagues[189] observed that 8% of 59 patients in their series developed a kyphotic sagittal alignment. No patients were reported to have developed any neurologic sequelae. Over the course of 10 years, Kawaguchi and colleagues[191] observed 8 patients who developed a kyphotic deformity in a series of 126 patients who underwent laminoplasty for the treatment of CSM. They noted that the recovery rate in these eight patients was poor. Wada and colleagues[23] observed a loss of lordosis that occurred in three patients in their series after laminoplasty. They found no relationship, however, between loss of lordosis and final JOA score. Sasai and colleagues[207] observed that diminished lordosis occurred most prominently at C2-3 and C6-7 after C3-7 French-door laminoplasty. In a retrospective analysis of 64 patients 6 years after laminoplasty, Matsunaga and colleagues[208] noted that the expansion of C2 led to the development of segmental kyphosis in 20% of patients. In contrast, they noted that the preservation of C2 was protective because only 2% of patients developed a segmental kyphosis.

Postoperative dysfunction of the paraspinal musculature is reported by numerous authors to be a causative agent in the decrease in lordosis noted after laminoplasty.[209,210] Using MRI, Hayashi and colleagues[209] found a significant postoperative reduction in the cross-sectional area of paraspinal musculature after laminoplasty. Matsuzaki and colleagues[211] associated the paraspinal muscle dysfunction with the denervation of its nerve supply. They cautioned against dissection farther lateral than the medial third of the facet to prevent injury to the dorsal primary rami of the spinal nerves.

Comparison of Outcomes

Whether anterior or posterior, the appropriate approach for the treatment of CSM depends on a host of factors, including site of cord compression, sagittal alignment, and number of vertebral segments involved. In a comparison of clinical and radiographic outcomes, Heller and colleagues[212] matched 13 patients who underwent laminectomy and fusion with 13 patients who underwent laminoplasty. Although not statistically significant, they reported a lower complication rate and a higher degree of functional improvement in patients managed with laminoplasty. Although nine patients in the laminectomy group developed complications, no complications were reported in the laminoplasty group. The complications observed included progression of myelopathy, nonunion, instrumentation failure, development of kyphosis, adjacent segment degeneration, and issues related to donor site morbidity. Although the sample size of this study was small, Heller and colleagues[212] concluded that laminoplasty was a safer and more reliable procedure than laminectomy and fusion in the treatment of CSM.

When long-term outcomes after subtotal corpectomy and strut grafting were compared with outcomes after laminoplasty, Wada and colleagues[23] showed no difference in neurologic recovery between the two groups. In the subtotal corpectomy group, they noted longer surgical times, more blood loss, and 26% pseudarthrosis rate. Of the 23 patients in the corpectomy cohort, 15% complained of postoperative axial pain. In contrast, of the 24 patients in the laminoplasty cohort 40% of patients complained of similar symptoms. Yonenobu and colleagues[213] reported their results after a similar study that evaluated 41 patients after subtotal corpectomy and strut grafting and 42 patients after laminoplasty. They noted no difference in recovery rate and final JOA scores between the two groups; however, complications were seen more frequently in the corpectomy group with 29% of patients reporting a complication. In contrast, complications were reported in only 7% of patients in the laminoplasty group. In an earlier study, Yonenobu and colleagues[44] compared the clinical outcomes of 50 patients treated with ACDF, 21 patients treated with corpectomy and fusion, and 24 patients treated with laminectomy in the treatment of CSM. These investigators observed that patients treated with corpectomy showed the best results clinically; however, they recommended a posterior approach for patients with disease at four segments or more.

In the treatment of multilevel cervical spondylotic radiculopathy Herkowitz[82] compared the outcomes and complication rates between anterior cervical fusion, laminectomy, and laminoplasty. He noted a successful outcome in 92% of 33 patients in the anterior fusion group, 86% of 15 patients in the laminoplasty group, and 66% of 12 patients in the laminectomy group. Complication rate in the anterior procedure group was reported to be 71%, whereas the complication rate of the laminoplasty group was only 13%. For the treatment of multilevel CSM, Herkowitz[82] recommended anterior decompression for most patients. For patients with myelopathy secondary to a congenitally narrow cervical spine, however, he recommended the use of laminoplasty as the decompressive procedure of choice. Kawano and colleagues[214] noted a 78% improvement rate in 14 patients after anterior surgery versus a 46% improvement rate in 61 patients after laminoplasty or laminectomy. They reported that better long-term outcomes were observed after anterior decompressive procedures rather than posterior decompressive procedures.

In a comparison of laminectomy versus anterior decompression and fusion for the treatment of patients with spondylotic myelopathy, Ebersold and colleagues[215] reported a greater risk of long-term worsening after laminectomy. In the immediate postoperative period, they observed 72% of 49 patients in the anterior decompression group noting an improvement and 68% of 51 patients in the laminectomy group noting an improvement. Although they observed comparable improvements in neurologic rates between the two groups in the immediate postoperative period, the frequency of delayed deterioration observed in the laminectomy group was far greater. Ebersold and colleagues[215] observed delayed deterioration in 10% of patients in the laminectomy cohort versus 2% of patients in the ACDF cohort.

Combined Anterior-Posterior Procedures

Although many authors report satisfactory results using a solitary anterior or posterior approach in the treatment of multilevel CSM, pseudarthrosis, graft failure, progressive kyphotic deformity, and instrumentation complications remain significant concerns.[77,167,216,217] Circumferential fusion provides immediate rigid stabilization and restoration of the sagittal balance of the cervical spine. It should be considered in patients requiring decompression involving multiple levels owing to spondylosis, OPLL, congenital stenosis, or kyphotic deformity. It should also be considered in patients with medical comorbidities or predisposing risk factors that are associated with poor bone quality or inability to heal.[218] A posterior stabilization should be considered in cases of multilevel postlaminectomy kyphosis in which anterior stabilization has been previously performed.

Riew and colleagues[216] reported their experience in treating postlaminectomy patients with ACCF and postoperative halo immobilization. They showed early graft-related complications in 56% of 16 postlaminectomy patients, including graft extrusion and nonunion. Because of the high complication rate, these authors recommended augmenting anterior corpectomy with posterior fusion and instrumentation. They proved that halo vest immobilization was inadequate to prevent graft extrusion after complex anterior reconstructions for the treatment of postlaminectomy kyphosis. When faced with a situation in which a three-level corpectomy must be performed, many surgeons choose to supplement an anterior procedure with posterior fixation to decrease the likelihood of graft migration and pseudarthrosis.[66,73]

Kim and Alexander[219] described 35 combined anterior-posterior stabilization procedures performed at their institution over 5 years. They observed no graft-related or instrumentation-related complications, and they did not observe any development of nonunion. Using fibular strut allograft with anterior cervical plates supplemented with posterior instrumentation and lateral mass plates, Shultz and colleagues[218] reported a 100% fusion rate in 72 patients who underwent single-stage multilevel anterior-posterior decompression and fusion. None of their patients required a reoperation, and there was no evidence of graft extrusion or clinically significant hardware complications. In a similar study, all 17 patients who underwent multilevel subtotal corpectomy with allograft strut fusion and concurrent posterior fusion with lateral mass plates achieved a solid arthrodesis.[220] There was no visible radiographic change in postoperative sagittal alignment.

Spivak and colleagues[221] observed that performing a combined anterior-posterior spinal fusion in a single setting resulted in decreased anesthesia, decreased operative times, decreased total blood loss, and an overall shorter hospital stay compared with a two-stage anterior-posterior fusion procedure. Epstein[222] published a series of 22 patients who underwent a combined anterior-posterior decompression and fusion. Marked neurologic recovery was noted in all patients in his series. Two patients had subacute plate extrusion. In a more recent study, Konya and colleagues[223] described the outcomes in their patients with multilevel CSM who underwent a combined anterior-posterior surgical approach. Of patients, 31 had four-level disease, and 9 patients had three-level disease. At 1-year follow-up neurologic function was improved in all 40 patients as assessed by the Nurick classification. A 97.5% fusion rate was obtained, and no complications related to instrumentation were noted.

Intraoperative Neurologic Monitoring

Historically, the most common method for spinal cord monitoring was the Stagnara wakeup test, which provided for an assessment of the patient's overall motor function.[224] This test could not be used in a continuous fashion, and it did not provide any information regarding individual nerve root function. New techniques in spinal cord assessment have revolutionized the practice of neurophysiologic monitoring. The ultimate goal of any monitoring technique is to minimize the potential for intraoperative neurologic deterioration. May and colleagues[225] identified potential risk factors for neurologic deterioration as preoperative myelopathy, multilevel disease, upper cervical surgery, use of instrumentation, and use of manipulation.

Somatosensory evoked potentials (SSEPs) assess the function of the sensory pathways of the dorsal column of the spinal cord.[226] The primary blood supply to the dorsal column of the spinal cord is derived from the posterior spinal artery. If a change in SSEPs is observed, resuscitative measures to promote spinal cord perfusion are encouraged. Resuscitative efforts should include increase in oxygenation, decrease in inhalation or intravenous anesthetics usage, use of warm irrigating solutions, and induction of hypertension. In addition, any manipulation causing undue tension on the cord should be stopped, which may include the release of distraction or the removal of an oversized graft. Parameters such as amplitude and latency are monitored continuously throughout the procedure, and any loss of amplitude of 50% to 60% is indicative of neuronal injury.[227]

Poorly defined or unrecordable SSEP tracings may occur in the presence of inhalation anesthetic agents. In an effort to overcome this complication, most spine centers avoid the use of any inhalation agents (e.g., isoflurane, desflurane, sevoflurane, nitrous oxide) and promote the use of an intravenous anesthetic regimen.[228] For surgery involving the cervical spine, the ulnar nerve is the preferred stimulation site for SSEP monitoring because it assesses the entire cervical neural axis. In patients with severe myelopathy, Kombos and colleagues[229] prospectively evaluated SSEP monitoring in 100 patients. They noted that SSEP changes occurred most commonly during positioning of the patient. These changes were most frequently seen in patients with myelopathy. The patient morbidity of 100 SSEP-monitored cervical procedures was compared by Epstein and colleagues[230] with the morbidity of a historical control group of 218 patients who underwent cervical procedures without any neurologic monitoring. They observed that 3.7% of patients in the unmonitored group became quadriplegic,

whereas no instances of quadriplegia were noted in the monitored group. They attributed this reduction in neurologic deficit to the early detection of cord compromise as a result of the neurologic monitoring.

Another tool that is sensitive and specific for the diagnosis of intraoperative cervical spinal cord injury is transcranial electrical motor evoked potentials. These motor evoked potentials are used to monitor the corticospinal tract, spinal cord interneurons, and anterior horn cells of the spinal cord. The primary blood supply nourishing these motor pathways is derived from the anterior spinal artery. Transcranial electrical motor evoked potentials are sensitive to blood pressure changes and can alert the surgeon to any hypoperfusion injury to the cord that may have occurred secondary to prolonged hypotension. This feature is particularly important in the surgical management of myelopathy because it is theorized that the perfusion of the cord is already compromised in these stenotic patients.

The use of inhalation anesthetic agents and neuromuscular relaxation agents must be avoided when monitoring transcranial electrical motor evoked potentials. The intraoperative monitoring of transcranial electrical motor evoked potentials was described by Kitagawa and colleagues[231] in a series of 20 patients who underwent surgery of the cervical spine. Five patients in their series were noted to have a 50% attenuation of transcranial electrical motor evoked potential parameters intraoperatively, which was immediately addressed with resuscitative measures. None of these patients developed any neurologic deficits postoperatively. One patient in this series developed complete quadriplegia and was noted to have complete loss of transcranial electrical motor evoked potentials intraoperatively.

Identification of an injury to a specific nerve root is best accomplished using electromyography (EMG). Spontaneous EMG is useful for assessing nerve root function during implant placement or nerve root manipulation, whereas stimulus-evoked EMG is useful for assessing cortical breach secondary to instrumentation. The nerve root is particularly susceptible to mechanical injury because it lacks a protective epineurium and perineurium. It is also susceptible to ischemic injury because there is a relatively hypovascular area between the proximal and middle third of the dorsal and ventral roots.[232] In an effort to prevent postoperative C5 palsies during cervical surgery, Jimenez and colleagues[233] evaluated the importance of monitoring continuous C5 EMG. These investigators compared 161 patients who were monitored with spontaneous EMG and stimulus-evoked EMG techniques with a historical control group of 55 patients who were monitored without the use of EMG techniques. They noted an incidence of postoperative C5 palsy in the monitored group of 0.9%, which was decreased from an incidence of 7.3% in the unmonitored control group.

Monitoring a single evoked potential parameter may not reflect the global status of the spinal cord. Motor and sensory pathways are separated in the spinal cord and have a varied blood supply. It is possible to have loss of SSEP secondary to an injury of the posterior spinal artery with complete sparing of motor function. Conversely, with injury to the anterior spinal artery, it is possible to have loss of motor function without any change in SSEP. For this reason, it is important to have multiple modalities assessing cord function during a decompressive cervical spine procedure. In an effort to reduce postoperative nerve root injuries, the complementary use of intraoperative transcranial electric motor evoked potentials and spontaneous EMG has been studied.[234]

With the use of multimodal intraoperative neuromonitoring, Hilibrand and colleagues[235] reported their experience after a series of 427 cervical spine cases. Greater than 50% of the patients underwent surgery for CSM, and all were monitored with transcranial electric motor evoked potentials and SSEPs. In this study, 12 patients developed a substantial decrease in transcranial electric motor evoked potential amplitude that warranted prompt resuscitative efforts. Of the 12 patients, 10 had complete reversal of amplitude changes, whereas 2 patients awoke with a new motor deficit after surgery. Based on their findings, they strongly recommended the use of transcranial electric motor evoked potentials and SSEPs when operating on patients with CSM.

Summary

The natural history of CSM is one of periods of static disability with episodic worsening of symptoms. Patients with severe symptoms benefit from operative management. Myriad options exist for the surgical treatment of multilevel CSM. The choice of procedure should be tailored to the unique clinical and anatomic, patient-specific characteristics in each individual case. No matter which operative procedure is chosen, the surgeon's primary goal should be to halt the further progression of the myelopathy by decompressing the spinal cord and by preserving the sagittal balance of the spinal column. The surgeon must have knowledge and an intimate understanding of each procedure and its limitations when discussing treatment options with patients. It is imperative that research be continued in the study of CSM and in the development of newer techniques. As advances in technology continue, surgeons will be better able to offer patients safer, more effective surgical options in the treatment of CSM.

PEARLS

1. Surgical decompression is indicated in patients with severe symptoms of myelopathy because they are more likely to develop progressive deterioration in neurologic function.

2. Disease limited to one or two levels in patients with CSM is best treated with an anterior decompressive procedure.

3. Posterior decompressive procedures are well suited for patients with multilevel pathology who have a lordotic cervical alignment.

4. Combined anterior-posterior procedures should be considered in patients with multilevel disease or in patients with poor bone quality.

PITFALLS

1. Poor neurologic recovery rates have been associated with posterior decompressive procedures performed in patients with kyphotic cervical alignments.

2. Rates of graft migration and failure are increased as more levels are involved in anterior decompressive procedures.

3. Postoperative motor root palsy remains a concern after decompressive procedures in patients with CSM.

KEY POINTS

1. Preoperative planning is crucial. It is common to find wide variations in the anatomy of the cervical spine, particularly in the course of the vertebral artery. Analysis of preoperative imaging provides a template for the safe placement of instrumentation and provides the surgeon with a more detailed understanding of the relevant anatomy.

2. Preoperative patient positioning must always be performed with care in patients with CSM. Severe stenosis in these patients can predispose them to a cord or a root injury with trivial maneuvers.

3. As with any surgical procedure, knowledge of anatomy is paramount. Whether an anterior or a posterior approach is chosen, adequate exposure and visualization of key landmarks must always be noted to ensure the accurate placement of cervical instrumentation or to ensure the safe removal of any impinging structures.

4. The surgeon should be familiar with various instrumentation techniques and have various implants available in the event an intraoperative complication occurs or the surgical findings necessitate an alteration of the intended operative plan. To prepare for these circumstances better, a "plan B" or even a "plan C" should always be considered before entering the operative suite.

5. The surgical management of CSM continues to evolve. Each year, newer techniques and instrumentation systems are introduced. Surgeons must be vigilant and carefully critique the available literature before using these new products in the surgical setting.

KEY REFERENCES

1. Wada E, Suzuki S, Kanazawa A, et al: Subtotal corpectomy versus laminoplasty for multilevel cervical spondylotic myelopathy: A long-term follow-up study of over 10 years. Spine (Phila Pa 1976) 26:1443-1447, 2001.
   This article describes the long-term follow-up of results and complications comparing subtotal corpectomy and laminoplasty.

2. Emery SE, Bohlman HH, Bolesta MJ, et al: Anterior cervical decompression and arthrodesis for the treatment of cervical spondylotic myelopathy: Two to seventeen-year follow-up. J Bone Joint Surg Am 80:941-951, 1998.
   This article describes the long-term follow-up of results and complications after ACDF.

3. Herkowitz HN: A comparison of anterior cervical fusion, cervical laminectomy, and cervical laminoplasty for the surgical management of multiple level spondylotic radiculopathy. Spine (Phila Pa 1976) 13:774-780, 1988.
Three techniques were compared in this study, and results and complications of each procedure were reported.

4. Yonenobu K, Hosono N, Iwasaki M, et al: Laminoplasty versus subtotal corpectomy: A comparative study of results in multisegmental cervical spondylotic myelopathy. Spine (Phila Pa 1976) 17:1281-1284, 1992.
The results and complications of laminoplasty and subtotal corpectomy in the treatment of CSM are reported.

5. Hirabayashi K, Watanabe K, Wakano K, et al: Expansive open-door laminoplasty for cervical spinal stenotic myelopathy. Spine (Phila Pa 1976) 8:693-699, 1988.
The results and complications after open-door laminoplasty in the treatment of CSM are reported.

REFERENCES

1. Heller JG: The syndromes of degenerative cervical disease. Orthop Clin North Am 23:381-394, 1992.

2. Veidlinger OF, Colwell JC, Smyth HS, et al: Cervical myelopathy and its relationship to cervical stenosis. Spine (Phila Pa 1976) 6:550-552, 1981.

3. Ono K, Ikata T, Yamada H, et al: Cervical myelopathy secondary to multiple spondylotic protrusions. Spine (Phila Pa 1976) 2:218-221, 1977.

4. Clark CR: Cervical spondylotic myelopathy: History and physical findings. Spine (Phila Pa 1976) 13:847-849, 1988.

5. Panjabi MM, Goel VK, Clark CR, et al: Biomechanical study of cervical spine stabilization with methylmethacrylate. Spine (Phila Pa 1976) 10:198-203, 1985.

6. Lee S, Harris KG, Goel VK, et al: Spinal motion after cervical fusion: In vivo assessment with roentgen stereophotogrammetry. Spine (Phila Pa 1976) 19:2336-2342, 1994.

7. Crandall P, Batzdorf U: Cervical spondylotic myelopathy. J Neurosurg 25:57-66, 1966.

8. Ferguson R, Caplan LR: Cervical spondylotic myelopathy. Neurol Clin 3:373-382, 1985.

9. Sadasivan KK, Reddy RP, Albright JA: The natural history of cervical spondylotic myelopathy. Yale J Biol Med 66:235-242, 1993.

10. Veidlinger OF, Colwell JC, Smyth HS, et al: Cervical myelopathy and its relationship to cervical stenosis. Spine (Phila Pa 1976) 6:550-552, 1981.

11. Ebara S, Yonenobu K, Fujiwara K, et al: Myelopathy hand characterized by muscle wasting: A different type of myelopathy hand in patients with cervical spondylosis. Spine (Phila Pa 1976) 13:785-791, 1988.

12. Clark E, Robinson P: Cervical myelopathy: A complication of cervical spondylosis. Brain 79:483, 1956.

13. Lees FT, Turner JW: Natural history and prognosis of cervical spondylosis. BMJ 2:1607-1610, 1963.

14. Nurick S: The natural history and the results of surgical treatment of the spinal cord disorder associated with cervical spondylosis. Brain 95:101-108, 1972.

15. Nurick S: Pathogenesis of the spinal cord disorder associated with cervical spondylosis. Brain 95:87-100, 1972.

15a. Nurick S: The pathogenesis of the spinal cord disorder associated with cervical spondylosis. Brain 95:87-100, 1972.

16. Epstein J, Epstein N: The surgical management of cervical spinal stenosis, spondylosis, and myeloradiculopathy by means of the posterior approach. In Sherk H, Dunn EJ, Eismont FJ, et al (eds): The Cervical Spine: An Atlas of Surgical Procedures. Philadelphia, JB Lippincott, 1989, pp 625-643.

17. Roberts A: Myelopathy due to cervical spondylosis treated by collar immobilization. Neurology 16:951-954, 1966.

18. Symon L, Lavender P: The surgical treatment of cervical spondylotic myelopathy. Neurology 17:117-126, 1967.

19. Law MD Jr, Bernhardt M, White AA 3rd: Cervical spondylotic myelopathy: A review of surgical indications and decision making. Yale J Biol Med 66:165-177, 1993.

20. Montgomery DM, Brower RS: Cervical spondylotic myelopathy: Clinical syndrome and natural history. Orthop Clin North Am 23:487-493, 1992.

21. Okada K, Shirasaki N, Hayashi H, et al: Treatment of cervical spondylotic myelopathy by enlargement of the spinal canal anteriorly, followed by arthrodesis. J Bone Joint Surg Am 73:352-364, 1991.

22. Bohlman HH: Cervical spondylosis with moderate to severe myelopathy: A report of 17 cases treated by Robinson anterior cervical discectomy and fusion. Spine (Phila Pa 1976) 2:151, 1977.

23. Wada E, Suzuki S, Kanazawa A, et al: Subtotal corpectomy versus laminoplasty for multilevel cervical spondylotic myelopathy: A long-term follow-up study of over 10 years. Spine (Phila Pa 1976) 26:1443-1447, 2001.

24. Tanaka J, Seki N, Doi K, et al: Operative results of canal-expansive laminoplasty for cervical spondylotic myelopathy in elderly patients. Spine (Phila Pa 1976) 24:2308-2312, 1999.

25. Suri A, Chabbra RP, Mehta VS, et al: Effect of intramedullary signal changes on the surgical outcome of patients with cervical spondylotic myelopathy. Spine J 3:33-45, 2003.

26. Satomi K, Nishu Y, Kohno T, et al: Long-term follow-up studies of open-door expansive laminoplasty for cervical stenotic myelopathy. Spine (Phila Pa 1976) 19:507-510, 1994.

27. Handa Y, Kubota T, Ishii H, et al: Evaluation of prognostic factors and clinical outcome in elderly patients in whom expansive laminoplasty is performed for cervical myelopathy due to multisegmental spondylotic canal stenosis: A retrospective comparison with younger patients. J Neurosurg Spine 96:173-179, 2002.

28. Al-Mefty O, Harkey HL, Marawi I, et al: Experimental chronic compressive cervical myelopathy. J Neurosurg 79:550-561, 1993.

29. Bernard TN Jr, Whitecloud TS III: Cervical spondylotic myelopathy and myeloradiculopathy: Anterior decompression and stabilization with autogenous fibula strut graft. Clin Orthop Relat Res 221:149-160, 1987.

30. Hasegawa K, Chiba Y, Hirano T, et al: Effects of surgical treatment for cervical spondylotic myelopathy in patients 70 years of age: A retrospective comparative study. J Spinal Disord 15:458-460, 2002.

31. Edwards WC, LaRocca H: The developmental segmental sagittal diameter of the cervical spinal canal in patients with cervical spondylosis. Spine (Phila Pa 1976) 8:20-27, 1983.

32. Nordquist L: The sagittal diameter of the spinal cord and sub-arachnoid space in different age groups: A roentgenographic and post-mortem study. Acta Radiol 227:1-96, 1964.

33. Brieg A, Turnbull I, Hassler O: Effects of mechanical stresses on the spinal cord in cervical spondylosis: A study of fresh cadaver material. J Neurosurg 25:45-48, 1966.

34. Epstein NE: Circumferential surgery for the management of cervical ossification of the posterior longitudinal ligament. J Spinal Disord 11:200-207, 1998.

35. Morio Y, Teshima R, Nagashima H, et al: Correlation between operative outcomes of cervical compression myelopathy and MRI of the spinal cord. Spine (Phila Pa 1976) 26:1238-1245, 2001.

36. Matsuda Y, Miyazaki K, Tada K, et al: Increased MR signal intensity due to cervical compression myelopathy: Analysis of 29 surgical cases. J Neurosurg 74:887-892, 1991.

37. Suda K, Abumi K, Ito M, et al: Local kyphosis reduces surgical outcomes of expansive open-door laminoplasty for cervical spondylotic myelopathy. Spine (Phila Pa 1976) 28:1258-1261, 2003.

38. Rao R: Neck pain, cervical radiculopathy, and cervical myelopathy: Pathophysiology, natural history, clinical evaluation. J Bone Joint Surg Am 84:1872-1881, 2002.

39. Chen IH, Vasavada A, Panjabi MM: Kinematics of the cervical spine canal: Changes with sagittal plane loads. J Spinal Disord 7:93-101, 1994.

40. Penning L: Some aspects of plain radiography of the cervical spine in chronic myelopathy. Neurology 12:513-519, 1962.

41. Bucciero A, Vizioli L, Carangelo B, et al: MR signal enhancement in cervical spondylotic myelopathy: Correlation with surgical results in 35 cases. J Neurosurg Sci 37:217-222, 1993.

42. Fujiwara K, Yonenobu K, Ebara S, et al: The prognosis of surgery for cervical compression myelopathy. J Bone Joint Surg Br 71:393-398, 1989.

43. Kawakami M, Tamaki T, Iwasaki H, et al: A comparative study of surgical approaches for cervical compressive myelopathy. Clin Orthop Relat Res 381:129-136, 2000.

44. Yonenobu K, Fuji T, Ono K, et al: Choice of surgical treatment for multisegmental cervical spondylotic myelopathy. Spine (Phila Pa 1976) 10:710-716, 1985.

45. Sodeyama T, Goto S, Mochizuki M, et al: Effect of decompression enlargement laminoplasty for posterior shifting of the spinal cord. Spine (Phila Pa 1976) 24:1527-1532, 1999.

46. Smith MD, Bolesta MJ, Leventhal M, et al: Postoperative cerebrospinal-fluid fistula associated with erosion of the dura: findings after anterior resection of ossification of the posterior longitudinal ligament in the cervical spine. J Bone Joint Surg Am 74:270-277, 1992.

47. Vaccaro AR, Ring D, Scuderi G, et al: Vertebral artery location in relation to the vertebral body as determined by two dimensional computed tomography evaluation. Spine (Phila Pa 1976) 19:2637-2641, 1994.

48. Smith MD, Emery SE, Dudley A, et al: Vertebral artery injury during anterior decompression of the cervical spine: A retrospective review of ten patients. J Bone Joint Surg Br 75:410-415, 1993.

49. Emery SE, Smith MD, Bohlman HH: Upper-airway obstruction after multilevel cervical corpectomy for myelopathy. J Bone Joint Surg Am 73:544-551, 1991.

50. Emery SE, Bohlman HH, Bolesta MJ, et al: Anterior cervical decompression and arthrodesis for the treatment of cervical spondylotic myelopathy: Two to seventeen-year follow-up. J Bone Joint Surg Am 80:941-951, 1998.

51. Smith GW, Robinson RA: The treatment of certain cervical spine disorders by anterior removal of the intervertebral disc and interbody fusion. J Bone Joint Surg Am 40:607-623, 1958.

52. Kadoya S, Nakamura T, Kwak R: A microsurgical anterior osteophytectomy for cervical spondylotic myelopathy. Spine (Phila Pa 1976) 9:437-441, 1984.

53. Robinson R, Walker AE, Ferlic DC, et al: The results of anterior interbody fusion of the cervical spine. J Bone Joint Surg Am 44:1569-1587, 1962.

54. Connolly PJ, Esses SI, Kostuik JP: Anterior cervical fusion: Outcome analysis of patients fused with and without anterior cervical plates. J Spinal Disord 9:202-206, 1996.

55. Stevens JM, Clifton AG, Whitear P: Appearances of posterior osteophytes after sound anterior interbody fusion in the cervical spine: A high-definition computed myelographic study. Neuroradiology 35:227-228, 1993.

56. Bertalanffy H, Eggert HR: Complications of anterior cervical discectomy without fusion in 450 consecutive patients. Acta Neurochir (Wien) 99:41-50, 1989.

57. Zhang ZH, Yin H, Yang K, et al: Anterior intervertebral disc excision and bone grafting in cervical spondylotic myelopathy. Spine (Phila Pa 1976) 8:16-19, 1983.

58. Yang KC, Lu XS, Cai QL, et al: Cervical spondylotic myelopathy treated by anterior multilevel decompression and fusion: Follow-up report of 214 cases. Clin Orthop Relat Res 221:161-164, 1987.

59. Irvine GB, Strachan WE: The long-term results of localised anterior cervical decompression and fusion in spondylotic myelopathy. Paraplegia 25:18-22, 1987.

60. Jamjoom A, Williams C, Cummins B: The treatment of spondylotic cervical myelopathy by multiple subtotal vertebrectomy and fusion. Br J Neurosurg 5:249-255, 1991.

61. Zdeblick TA, Bohlman HH: Cervical kyphosis and myelopathy: Treatment by anterior corpectomy and strut-grafting. J Bone Joint Surg Am 71:170-182, 1989.

62. Fessler RG, Steck JC, Giovanini MA: Anterior cervical corpectomy for cervical spondylotic myelopathy: A consecutive series with long term follow up evaluation. Neurosurgery 43:257-265, 1998.

63. Chibbaro S, Benvenuti L, Carnesecchi S, et al: Anterior cervical corpectomy for cervical spondylotic myelopathy: Experience and surgical results in a series of 70 consecutive patients. J Clin Neurosci 13:233-238, 2006.

64. Ashkenazi E, Smorgick Y, Rand N, et al: Anterior decompression combined with corpectomies and discectomies in the management of multilevel cervical myelopathy: A hybrid decompression and fixation technique. J Neurosurg Spine 3:205-209, 2005.

65. Saunders RL, Pikus HJ, Ball P: Four-level cervical corpectomy. Spine (Phila Pa 1976) 23:2455-2461, 1998.

66. Vaccaro AR, Falatyn SP, Scuderi GJ, et al: Early failure of long segment anterior cervical plate fixation. J Spinal Disord 11:410-415, 1998.

67. Edwards C, Heller J, Morikami H, et al: Corpectomy versus laminoplasty for multi-level cervical myelopathy: An independent matched cohort study. Spine (Phila Pa 1976) 27:1168-1175, 2002.

68. Lunsford LD, Bissonette DJ, Zorub DS: Anterior surgery for cervical disc disease: I. Treatment of lateral cervical disc herniation in 253 cases. J Neurosurg 53:1-11, 1980.

69. Robinson R, Walker AE, Ferlic DC, et al: The results of anterior interbody fusion of the cervical spine. J Bone Joint Surg Am 44:1569-1587, 1962.

70. Boni M, Cherubino P, Denaro V, et al: Multiple subtotal somatectomy: Technique and evaluation of a series of 39 cases. Spine (Phila Pa 1976) 9:358-362, 1984.

71. Brigham CD, Tsahakis PJ: Anterior cervical foraminotomy and fusion: Surgical technique and results. Spine (Phila Pa 1976) 20:766-770, 1995.

72. Bohlman HH, Emery SE, Goodfellow DB, et al: Robinson anterior cervical discectomy and arthrodesis for cervical radiculopathy: Long-term follow-up of one hundred and twenty-two patients. J Bone Joint Surg Am 75:1298-1307, 1993.

73. Sasso RC, Ruggiero RA Jr, Reilly TM, et al: Early reconstruction failures after multilevel cervical corpectomy. Spine (Phila Pa 1976) 28:140-142, 2003.

74. Hilibrand AS, Fye MA, Emery SE, et al: Increased rate of arthrodesis with strut grafting after multilevel anterior cervical decompression. Spine (Phila Pa 1976) 27:146-151, 2002.

75. Swank ML, Lowery GL, Bhat AL, et al: Anterior cervical allograft arthrodesis and instrumentation: Multilevel interbody grafting or strut graft reconstruction. Eur Spine J 6:138-143, 1997.

76. Hanai K, Fujiyoshi F, Kamei K: Subtotal vertebrectomy and spinal fusion for cervical spondylotic myelopathy. Spine (Phila Pa 1976) 11:310-315, 1986.

77. Zdeblick TA, Hughes SS, Riew KD, et al: Failed anterior cervical discectomy and arthrodesis: Analysis and treatment of thirty-five patients. J Bone Joint Surg Am 79:523-532, 1997.

78. Dai L, Ni B, Yuan W, et al: Radiculopathy after laminectomy for cervical compression myelopathy. J Bone Joint Surg Br 80:846-849, 1998.

79. Wang JC, Hart RA, Emery SE, et al: Graft migration or displacement after multilevel cervical corpectomy and strut grafting. Spine (Phila Pa 1976) 28:1016-1021, 2003.

80. Wang JC, McDononugh PW, Endow K, et al: The effect of cervical plating on single level anterior cervical discectomy and fusion. J Spinal Disord 12:467-471, 1999.

81. Kaiser MG, Haid RW Jr, Subach BR, et al: Anterior cervical plating enhances arthrodesis after discectomy and fusion with cortical allograft. Neurosurgery 50:229-238, 2002.

82. Herkowitz HN: A comparison of anterior cervical fusion, cervical laminectomy, and cervical laminoplasty for the surgical management of multiple level spondylotic radiculopathy. Spine (Phila Pa 1976) 13:774-780, 1988.

83. Villas C, Martinez-Peric R, Preite R, et al: Union after multiple anterior cervical fusion: 21 cases followed for 1-6 years. Acta Orthop Scand 65:620-622, 1994.

84. Wetzel FT, Hoffman MA, Arcieri RR: Freeze-dried fibular allograft in anterior spinal surgery: Cervical and lumbar applications. Yale J Biol Med 66:263-275, 1993.

85. Park JB, Cho YS, Riew KD: Development of adjacent-level ossification in patients with an anterior cervical plate. J Bone Joint Surg Am 87:558-563, 2005.

86. DiAngelo DJ, Foley KT, Vossel KA, et al: Anterior cervical plating reverses load transfer through multilevel strut-grafts. Spine (Phila Pa 1976) 25:783-795, 2000.

87. Foley KT, DiAngelo DJ, Rampersaud YR: The in vitro effects of instrumentation on multilevel cervical strut-graft mechanics. Spine (Phila Pa 1976) 24:2366-2376, 1999.

88. Hanks SE, Kang JD: Late stress fracture of a well incorporated autologous fibula strut graft in the cervical spine: A case report. J Spinal Disord Tech 17:526-530, 2004.

89. Jones J, Yoo J, Hart R: Delayed fracture of fibular strut allograft following multilevel anterior cervical spine corpectomy and fusion. Spine (Phila Pa 1976) 31:E595-E599, 2006.

90. Hee HT, Majd ME, Holt RT, et al: Complications of multilevel cervical corpectomies and reconstruction with titanium cages and anterior plating. J Spinal Disord Tech 16:1-8, 2003.

91. Majd ME, Vadhva M, Holt RT: Anterior cervical reconstruction using titanium cages with anterior plating. Spine (Phila Pa 1976) 24:1604-1610, 1999.

92. Eleraky MA, Llanos C, Sonntag VK: Cervical corpectomy: Report of 185 cases and review of the literature. J Neurosurg 90(1 Suppl):35-41, 1999.

93. Curylo LJ, Mason HC, Bohlman HH, et al: Tortuous course of the vertebral artery and anterior cervical compression: A cadaveric and clinical case study. Spine (Phila Pa 1976) 25:2860-2864, 2000.

94. Silber JS, Anderson DG, Daffner SD, et al: Donor site morbidity after anterior iliac crest bone harvest for single-level anterior cervical discectomy and fusion. Spine (Phila Pa 1976) 28:134-139, 2003.

95. Schnee CL, Freese A, Weil RJ, et al: Analysis of harvest morbidity and radiographic outcome using autograft for anterior cervical fusion. Spine (Phila Pa 1976) 22:2222-2227, 1997.

96. Banwart JC, Asher MA, Hassanein RS: Iliac crest bone graft harvest donor site morbidity: A statistical evaluation. Spine (Phila Pa 1976) 20:1055-1060, 1995.

97. Bohay DR, Manoli A 2nd: Clawtoe deformity following vascularized fibula graft. Foot Ankle Int 16:607-609, 1995.

98. Bodde EW, de Visser E, Duysens JE, et al: Donor-site morbidity after free vascularized autogenous fibular transfer: Subjective and quantitative analyses. Plast Reconstr Surg 111:2237-2242, 2003.

99. Emery SE, Heller JG, Petersilge CA: Tibial stress fracture after a graft has been obtained from the fibula: A report of five cases. J Bone Joint Surg Am 78:1248-1251, 1996.

100. Vail TP, Urbaniak JR: Donor-site morbidity with use of vascularized autogenous fibular grafts. J Bone Joint Surg Am 78:204-211, 1996.

101. Zdeblick TA, Ducker TB: The use of freeze-dried allograft bone for anterior cervical fusions. Spine (Phila Pa 1976) 16:726-729, 1991.

102. Fernyhough JC, White JI, LaRocca H: Fusion rates in multilevel cervical spondylosis comparing allograft fibula with autograft fibula in 126 patients. Spine (Phila Pa 1976) 16(10 Suppl):S561-S564, 1991.

103. MacDonald RL, Fehlings MG, Tator CH, et al: Multilevel anterior cervical corpectomy and fibular allograft fusion for cervical myelopathy. J Neurosurg 86:990-997, 1997.

104. Samartzis D, Shen FH, Matthews DK, et al: Comparison of allograft to autograft in multilevel anterior cervical discectomy and fusion with rigid plate fixation. Spine J 3:451-459, 2003.

105. Hilibrand AS, Carlson GD, Palumbo MA, et al: Radiculopathy and myelopathy at segments adjacent to the site of a previous anterior cervical arthrodesis. J Bone Joint Surg Am 81:519-528, 1999.

106. Rao RD, Wang M, McGrady LM, et al: Does anterior plating of the cervical spine predispose to adjacent segmental changes? Spine (Phila Pa 1976) 30:2788-2793, 2005.

107. Uematsu Y, Tasuaki T, Matsuzaki H, et al: Radiculopathy after laminoplasty of the cervical spine. Spine (Phila Pa 1976) 23:2057-2062, 1998.

108. Yonenobu K, Hosono N, Iwasaki M, et al: Neurologic complications of surgery for cervical compression myelopathy. Spine (Phila Pa 1976) 13:1277-1282, 1991.

109. Yonenobu K, Okada K, Fuji T, et al: Causes of neurologic deterioration following surgical treatment of cervical myelopathy. Spine (Phila Pa 1976) 11:818-823, 1986.

110. Bazaz R, Lee MJ, Yoo JU: Incidence of dysphagia after anterior cervical spine surgery: A prospective study. Spine (Phila Pa 1976) 27:2453-2458, 2002.

111. Smith-Hammond CA, New KC, Pietrobon R, et al: Prospective analysis of incidence and risk factors of dysphagia in spine surgery patients: Comparison of anterior cervical, posterior cervical and lumbar procedures. Spine (Phila Pa 1976) 29:1441-1446, 2004.

112. Newhouse KE, Lindsey RW, Clark CR, et al: Esophageal perforation following anterior cervical spine surgery. Spine (Phila Pa 1976) 14:1051-1053, 1989.

113. Frempong-Boadu A, Houten JK, Osbom B, et al: Swallowing and speech dysfunction in patients undergoing anterior cervical discectomy and fusion: A prospective, objective preoperative and postoperative assessment. J Spinal Disord Tech 15:362-368, 2002.

114. Yue WM, Brodner W, Highland TR: Persistent swallowing and voice problems after anterior cervical discectomy and fusion with allograft and plating: A 5 to 11 year follow-up study. Eur Spine J 14:677-682, 2005.

115. Apfelbaum TI, Kriskovich MD, Haller JR: On the incidence, cause, and prevention of recurrent laryngeal nerve palsies during anterior cervical spine surgery. Spine (Phila Pa 1976) 25:2906-2912, 2000.

116. Baron EM, Soliman AM, Gaughan JP, et al: Dysphagia, hoarseness, and unilateral true vocal fold motion impairment following anterior cervical discectomy and fusion. Ann Otol Rhinol Laryngol 112:921-926, 2003.

117. Beutler WJ, Sweeney CA, Connolly PJ: Recurrent laryngeal nerve injury with anterior cervical spine surgery risk with laterality of surgical approach. Spine (Phila Pa 1976) 26:1337-1342, 2001.

118. Snow RB, Weiner H: Cervical laminectomy and foraminotomy as surgical treatment of cervical spondylosis: A follow-up study with analysis of failures. J Spinal Disord 6:245-250, 1993.

119. Hukuda S, Mochizuki T, Ogata M, et al: Operations for cervical spondylotic myelopathy: A comparison of the results of anterior and posterior procedures. J Bone Joint Surg Br 67:609-615, 1985.

120. Aita I, Hayashi K, Wadano Y, et al: Posterior movement and enlargement of the spinal cord after cervical laminoplasty. J Bone Joint Surg Br 80:33-37, 1998.

121. Baba H, Maezawa Y, Furusawa N, et al: Flexibility and alignment of the cervical spine after laminoplasty for spondylotic myelopathy: A radiographic study. Int Orthop 19:116-121, 1995.

122. Hamanishi C, Tanaka S: Bilateral multilevel laminectomy with or without posterolateral fusion for cervical spondylotic myelopathy: Relationship to type of onset and time until operation. J Neurosurg 85:447-451, 1996.

123. Zdeblick TA, Zou D, Warden KE, et al: Cervical stability after foraminotomy: A biomechanical in vitro analysis. J Bone Joint Surg 74:22-27, 1992.

124. Yamazaki A, Homma T, Uchiyama S, et al: Morphologic limitation of posterior decompression by midsagittal splitting method for myelopathy caused by ossification of the posterior longitudinal ligament in the cervical spine. Spine (Phila Pa 1976) 24:32-34, 1999.

125. Satomi K, Nishu Y, Kohno T, et al: Long-term follow-up studies of open-door expansive laminoplasty for cervical stenotic myelopathy. Spine (Phila Pa 1976) 19:507-510, 1994.

126. Hirabayashi K, Toyama Y, Chiba K, et al: Expansive laminoplasty for myelopathy in ossification of the longitudinal ligament. Clin Orthop Relat Res 359:35-48, 1999.

127. Ishida Y, Suzuki K, Ohmori K, et al: Critical analysis of extensive cervical laminectomy. Neurosurgery 24:215-222, 1989.

128. Kohno K, Kumon Y, Oka Y, et al: Evaluation of prognostic factors following expansive laminoplasty for cervical spinal stenotic myelopathy. Surg Neurol 48:237-245, 1997.

129. Shaffrey C, Wiggins G, Piccirilli C, et al: Modified open-door laminoplasty for treatment of neurological deficits in younger patients with congenital spinal stenosis: Analysis of clinical and radiographic data. J Neurosurg 90:170-177, 1999.

130. Chiba K, Toyama Y, Watanabe M, et al: Impact of longitudinal distance of the cervical spine on the results of expansive open-door laminoplasty. Spine (Phila Pa 1976) 25:2893-2898, 2000.

131. Raynor RB, Pugh J, Shapiro I: Cervical facetectomy and its effect on spine strength. J Neurosurg 63:278-282, 1985.

132. Kato Y, Iwasaki M, Fuji T, et al: Long-term follow-up results of laminectomy for cervical myelopathy caused by ossification of the posterior longitudinal ligament. J Neurosurg 89:217-223, 1998.

133. Kaptain GJ, Simmons NE, Replogle RE, et al: Incidence and outcome of kyphotic deformity following laminectomy for cervical spondylotic myelopathy. J Neurosurg 93:1999-2004, 2000.

134. Kumar VG, Rea GL, Mervis LJ, et al: Cervical spondylotic myelopathy: Functional and radiographic long-term outcome after laminectomy and posterior fusion. Neurosurgery 44:771-777, 1999.

135. Houten JK, Cooper PR: Laminectomy and posterior cervical plating for multi-level cervical spondylotic myelopathy and ossification of the posterior longitudinal ligament: Effects on cervical alignment, spinal cord compression, and neurological outcome. Neurosurgery 52:1081-1088, 2003.

136. Weiland DJ, McAfee PC: Posterior cervical fusion with triple-wire strut graft technique: One hundred consecutive patients. J Spinal Disord 4:15-21, 1991.

137. Lovely TJ, Carl A: Posterior cervical spine fusion with tension-band wiring. J Neurosurg 83:631-635, 1995.

138. Gill K, Paschal S, Corin J, et al: Posterior plating of the cervical spine: A biomechanical comparison of different posterior fusion techniques. Spine (Phila Pa 1976) 13:813-816, 1988.

139. Horgan MA, Kellogg JX, Chestnut RM: Posterior cervical arthrodesis and stabilization: An early report using a novel lateral mass screw and rod technique. Neurosurgery 44:1267-1271, 1999.

140. Roy-Camille R, Saillant G, Mazel C: Internal fixation of the unstable cervical spine by a posterior osteosynthesis with plates and screws. In The Cervical Spine ed 2. New York, Lippincott, 1989, pp 390-403.

141. Jeanneret B, Magerl F, Ward EH, et al: Posterior stabilization of the cervical spine with hook plates. Spine (Phila Pa 1976) 16(3 Suppl):S56-S63, 1991.

142. An HS, Gordin R, Renner K: Anatomic considerations for plate-screw fixation of the cervical spine. Spine (Phila Pa 1976) 16(10 Suppl):S548-S551, 1991.

143. Anderson PA, Henley MB, Grady MS, et al: Posterior cervical arthrodesis with AO reconstruction plates and bone graft. Spine (Phila Pa 1976) 16(3 Suppl):S72-S79, 1991.

144. Montesano PX, Jauch E, Jonsson H Jr: Anatomic and biomechanical study of posterior cervical spine plate arthrodesis: An evaluation of two different techniques of screw placement. J Spinal Disord 5:301-305, 1992.

145. Barrey C, Mertens P, Jund J, et al: Quantitative anatomic evaluation of cervical lateral mass fixation with a comparison of the Roy-Camille and the Magerl screw techniques. Spine (Phila Pa 1976) 30:E140-E147, 2005.

146. Heller JG, Carlson GD, Abitbol JJ, et al: Anatomic comparison of the Roy-Camille and Magerl techniques for screw placement in the lower cervical spine. Spine (Phila Pa 1976) 16(10 Suppl):S552-S557, 1991.

147. Seybold EA, Baker JA, Criscitiello AA, et al: Characteristics of unicortical and bicortical lateral mass screws in the cervical spine. Spine (Phila Pa 1976) 24:2397-2403, 1999.

148. Abumi K, Kaneda K, Shono Y, et al: One-stage posterior decompression and reconstruction of the cervical spine by using pedicle screw fixation systems. J Neurosurg 90(1 Suppl):19-26, 1999.

149. Jones EL, Heller JG, Sicox DH, et al: Cervical pedicle screws versus lateral mass screws: Anatomic feasibility and biomechanical comparison. Spine (Phila Pa 1976) 22:977-982, 2007.

150. Abumi K, Shono Y, Ito M, et al: Complications of pedicle screw fixation in reconstructive surgery of the cervical spine. Spine (Phila Pa 1976) 25:962-969, 2000.

151. Meyers MA, Hamilton SR, Bogosian AJ, et al: Visual loss as a complication of spine surgery: A review of 37 cases. Spine (Phila Pa 1976) 22:1325-1329, 1997.

152. Iizuka H, Shimizu T, Tateno K, et al: Extensor musculature of the cervical spine after laminoplasty. Spine (Phila Pa 1976) 26:2220-2226, 2001.

153. Huang RC, Girardi FP, Poynton AR, et al: Treatment of multilevel cervical spondylotic myeloradiculopathy with posterior decompression and fusion with lateral mass plate fixation and local bone graft. J Spinal Disord Tech 16:123-129, 2003.

154. Sekhon LH: Posterior cervical decompression and fusion for circumferential spondylotic cervical stenosis: Review of 50 consecutive cases. J Clin Neurosci 13:23-30, 2006.

155. Mikawa Y, Shikata J, Yamamuro T, et al: Spinal deformity and instability after multilevel cervical laminectomy. Spine (Phila Pa 1976) 12:6-11, 1987.

156. Morimoto T, Okuno S, Nakase H, et al: Cervical myelopathy due to dynamic compression by the laminectomy membrane: Dynamic MR imaging study. J Spinal Disord 12:172-173, 1999.

157. Dai L, Ni B, Yuan W, et al: Radiculopathy after laminectomy for cervical compression myelopathy. J Bone Joint Surg Br 80:846-849, 1998.

158. Sim FH, Suien HJ, Bickel WH, et al: Swan neck deformity following extensive cervical laminectomy. J Bone Joint Surg Am 56:564-580, 1974.

159. Cusick J, Pintar FA, Yoganandan N, et al: Biomechanical alterations induced by multilevel cervical laminectomy. Spine (Phila Pa 1976) 20:2392-2399, 1995.

160. Albert T, Vacarro A: Postlaminectomy kyphosis. Spine (Phila Pa 1976) 23:2738-2745, 1998.

161. Bell DF, Walker JL, O'Connor G, et al: Spinal deformity after multiple-level cervical laminectomy in children. Spine (Phila Pa 1976) 19:406-411, 1994.

162. Yasuoka S, Peterson HA, Laws ER Jr, et al: Pathogenesis and prophylaxis of postlaminectomy deformity of the spine after multiple level laminectomy: Difference between children and adults. Neurosurgery 9:145-152, 1981.

163. Yasuoka S, Peterson HA, MacCarty CS, et al: Incidence of spinal column deformity after multilaminectomy in children and adults. J Neurosurg 57:441-445, 1982.

164. Voo LM, Kumaresan S, Yoganandan N, et al: Finite element analysis of cervical facetectomy. Spine (Phila Pa 1976) 22:964-969, 1997.

165. Nowinski GP, Visarius H, Nolte LP, et al: A biomechanical comparison of cervical laminoplasty and cervical laminectomy with progressive facetectomy. Spine (Phila Pa 1976) 18:1995-2004, 1993.

166. Heller JG, Silcox DH 3rd, Sutterline CE 3rd: Complications of posterior cervical plating. Spine (Phila Pa 1976) 20:2442-2448, 1995.

167. Wellman BJ, Follett KA, Traynelis VC: Complications of posterior articular mass plate fixation of the subaxial cervical spine in 43 consecutive patients. Spine (Phila Pa 1976) 23:193-200, 1998.

168. Pal PP, Cooper HH: The vertical stability of the cervical spine. Spine (Phila Pa 1976) 13:447-449, 1988.

169. Tsuzuki N, Abe R, Saiki K, et al: Tension band laminoplasty of the cervical spine. Int Orthop 20:275-284, 1996.

170. Baba H, Uchida K, Maezawa Y, et al: Lordotic alignment and posterior migration of the spinal cord following en bloc open door laminoplasty for cervical myelopathy: A magnetic resonance imaging study. J Neurol 243:626-632, 1996.

171. Baba H, Uchida K, Maezawa Y, et al: Three-dimensional computed tomography for evaluation of cervical spinal canal enlargement after en bloc open-door laminoplasty. Spinal Cord 35:674-679, 1997.

172. Shimamura T, Kato S, Toba T, et al: Sagittal splitting laminoplasty for spinal canal enlargement for ossification of the spinal ligaments (OPLL and OLF). Semin Musculoskel Radiol 5:203-206, 2001.

173. Kawakami M, Tamaki T, Yamada H, et al: Relationships between sagittal alignment of the cervical spine and morphology of the spinal cord and clinical outcomes in patients with cervical spondylotic myelopathy treated with expansive laminoplasty. J Spinal Disord 15:391-397, 2002.

174. Oyama M, Hattori S, Moriwaki N, et al: A new method of posterior decompression [In Japanese]. Chubuseisaisi 16:792, 1973.

175. Hirabayashi K, Watanabe K, Wakano K, et al: Expansive open-door laminoplasty for cervical spinal stenotic myelopathy. Spine (Phila Pa 1976) 8:693-699, 1988.

176. Kurokawa T, Tsuyama N, Tanaka H, et al: Enlargement of spinal canal by the sagittal splitting of the spinous process. Bessatsu Seikei Geka 2:234-240, 1982.

177. Yue WM, Tan CT, Tan SB, et al: Results of cervical laminoplasty and a comparison between single and double trap-door techniques. J Spinal Disord 13:329-335, 2000.

178. Naito M, Ogata K, Kurose S, et al: Canal expansive laminoplasty in 83 patients with cervical myelopathy: A comparative study of three different procedures. Int Orthop 18:347-351, 1994.

179. Okada M, Minamide A, Endo T, et al: A prospective randomized study of clinical outcomes in patients with cervical compressive myelopathy treated with open-door or French-door laminoplasty. Spine (Phila Pa 1976) 34:1119-1126, 2009.

180. Hirabayashi K: Expansive open-door laminoplasty for cervical spondylotic myelopathy [In Japanese]. Jpn J Surg 32:1159-1163, 1978.

181. Hirabayashi K, Miyakawa J, Satomi K, et al: Operative results and postoperative progression of ossification among patients with ossification of cervical posterior longitudinal ligament. Spine (Phila Pa 1976) 6:354-364, 1981.

182. Itoh T, Tsuji H: Technical improvement and results of laminoplasty for compressive myelopathy in the cervical spine. Spine (Phila Pa 1976) 10:729-736, 1985.

183. Kamo Y, Takemitsu Y, Hamada O, et al: Cervical laminoplasty by splitting the spinous process using a AW glass-ceramic lamina spacer. Rinsho Seikeigeka 10:1115-1122, 1992.

184. Nakano K, Harata S, Suetsuna F, et al: Spinous process splitting laminoplasty using hydroxyapatite spinous process spacer. Spine (Phila Pa 1976) 17:41-43, 1992.

185. O'Brien MF, Petersen D, Casey AH, et al: A novel technique for laminoplasty augmentation of spinal canal area using titanium miniplate stabilization: A computerized morphometric analysis. Spine (Phila Pa 1976) 21:474-484, 1996.

186. Tomita K, Kawahara N, Toribatake Y, et al: Expansive midline T-saw laminoplasty (modified spinous process-splitting) for the management of cervical myelopathy. Spine (Phila Pa 1976) 23:32-37, 1998.

187. Hirabayashi K, Toyama Y, Chiba K, et al: Expansive laminoplasty for myelopathy in ossification of the longitudinal ligament. Clin Orthop Relat Res 359:35-48, 1999.

188. Kawaguchi Y, Kanamori M, Ishihara H, et al: Progression of ossification of the posterior longitudinal ligament following en bloc cervical laminoplasty. J Bone Joint Surg Am 83:1798-1802, 2001.

189. Iwasaki M, Kawaguchi Y, Kimura T, et al: Long-term results of expansive laminoplasty for ossification of the posterior longitudinal ligament of the cervical spine: More than 10 years follow up. J Neurosurg 96(Spine 2):180-189, 2002.

190. Hirabayashi K, Satomi K: Operative procedure and results of expansive open door laminoplasty. Spine (Phila Pa 1976) 13:870-876, 1988.

191. Kawaguchi Y, Kanamori M, Ishihara H, et al: Minimum 10 year follow-up after en bloc cervical laminoplasty. Clin Orthop Relat Res 411:129-139, 2003.

192. Seichi A, Takeshita K, Ohishi I, et al: Long-term results of double-door laminoplasty for cervical stenotic myelopathy. Spine (Phila Pa 1976) 26:479-487, 2001.

193. Matsumoto M, Watanabe K, Tsuji T, et al: Risk factors for closure of lamina after open-door laminoplasty. J Neurosurg Spine 9:530-537, 2008.

194. Itoh K, Miura Y, Imakure A, et al: Cervical radiculopathy occurring after expansive laminoplasty. Higashi Nippon Rinsho Seikeigeka Gakkai Zasshi 5:306-310, 1993.

195. Herkowitz HN: Cervical laminoplasty: Its role in the treatment of cervical radiculopathy. J Spinal Disord 1:179-188, 1988.

196. Sasai K, Saito T, Akagi S, et al: Clinical study of cervical radiculopathy after laminoplasty for cervical myelopathy. Nippon Seikeigeka Gakkai Zashi 69:1237-1247, 1995.

197. Sasai K, Saito T, Akagi S, et al: Preventing C5 palsy after laminoplasty. Spine (Phila Pa 1976) 28:1972-1977, 2003.

198. Chiba K, Toyama Y, Matsumoto M, et al: Segmental motor paralysis after expansive open-door laminoplasty. Spine (Phila Pa 1976) 27:2108-2115, 2002.

199. Moskovich R: Neck pain in the elderly: Common causes and management. Geriatrics 43:65-92, 1988.

200. Kawaguchi Y, Matsui H, Ishihara H, et al: Axial symptoms after en bloc cervical laminoplasty. J Spinal Disord 12:392-395, 1999.

201. Hosono N, Yonenobu K, Ono K, et al: Neck and shoulder pain after laminoplasty: A noticeable complication. Spine (Phila Pa 1976) 21:1969-1973, 1996.

202. Takeuchi T, Yasuhiro S: Importance of preserving the C7 spinous process and attached nuchal ligament in French-door laminoplasty to reduce postoperative axial symptoms. Eur Spine J 16:1417-1422, 2007.

203. Kimura I, Shingu H, Nasu Y: Long-term follow-up of cervical spondylotic myelopathy treated by canal-expansive laminoplasty. J Bone Joint Surg Br 77:956-961, 1995.

204. Saruhashi Y, Hakuda S, Hatsuura A, et al: A long-term follow-up study of cervical spondylotic myelopathy treated by "French window" laminoplasty. J Spinal Disord 12:99-101, 1999.

205. Hyun SJ, Rhim SC, Roh SW, et al: The time course of range of motion loss after cervical laminoplasty. Spine (Phila Pa 1976) 34:1134-1139, 2009.

206. Kawaguchi Y, Kanamori M, Ishiara H, et al: Preventive measures for axial symptoms following cervical laminoplasty. J Spinal Disord Tech 16:497-501, 2003.

207. Sasai K, Saito T, Akagi S, et al: Cervical curvature after laminoplasty for spondylotic myelopathy—involvement of yellow ligament, semispinalis cervicis muscle, and nuchal ligament. J Spinal Disord 13:26-30, 2000.

208. Matsunaga S, Sakou T, Nakanisi K, et al: Analysis of the cervical spine alignment following laminoplasty and laminectomy. Spinal Cord 37:20-24, 1999.

209. Hayashi N, Yoshida M, Iwahashi T, et al: The effect of cervical posterior decompression to cervical paravertebral muscles. Chuba Nippon Seikeigeka Saigaigeka Gakkai Zasshi 32:2467-2469, 1989

210. Fujimura Y, Nishi Y: Atrophy of the nuchal muscle and change in cervical curvature after expansive open-door laminoplasty. Arch Orthop Trauma Surg 115:203-205, 1996.

211. Matsuzaki H, Hoshino M, Kiuchi T, et al: Dome like expansive laminoplasty for the second cervical vertebrae. Spine (Phila Pa 1976) 14:1198-1203, 1989.

212. Heller JG, Edwards CC, Murakami H, et al: Laminoplasty versus laminectomy and fusion for multilevel cervical myelopathy: An independent matched cohort analysis. Spine (Phila Pa 1976) 26:1330-1336, 2001.

213. Yonenobu K, Hosono N, Iwasaki M, et al: Laminoplasty versus subtotal corpectomy: A comparative study of results in multisegmental cervical spondylotic myelopathy. Spine (Phila Pa 1976) 17:1281-1284, 1992.

214. Kawano H, Hand Y, Ishii H, et al: Surgical treatment for ossification of the posterior longitudinal ligament of the cervical spine. J Spinal Disord 8:145-150, 1995.

215. Ebersold MJ, Pare MC, Quast LM: Surgical treatment for cervical spondylotic myelopathy. J Neurosurg 82:745-751, 1995.

216. Riew KD, Hiligrand AS, Palumbo MA, et al: Anterior cervical corpectomy in patients previously managed with a laminectomy: Short-term complications. J Bone Joint Surg Am 81:950-957, 1999.

217. Herman JM, Sonntag VKH: Cervical corpectomy and plate fixation for postlaminectomy kyphosis. J Neurosurg 80:963-970, 1994.

218. Schultz KD Jr, McLaughlin MR, Haid RW Jr, et al: Single stage anterior posterior decompression and stabilization for complex cervical spine disorders. J Neurosurg 93(Suppl 2):214-221, 2000.

219. Kim PK, Alexander JT: Indications for circumferential surgery for cervical spondylotic myelopathy. Spine J 6(Suppl 1):299-307, 2006.

220. Swank ML, Sutterlin CE III, Bossons CR, et al: Rigid internal fixation with lateral mass plates in multilevel anterior and posterior reconstruction of the cervical spine. Spine (Phila Pa 1976) 22:274-282, 1997.

221. Spivak JM, Neuwirth MG, Giordano CP, et al: The perioperative course of combined anterior and posterior spinal fusion. Spine (Phila Pa 1976) 19:520-525, 1994.

222. Epstein NE: The value of anterior cervical plating in preventing vertebral fracture and graft extrusion following multilevel anterior cervical corpectomy with posterior wiring/fusion: Indications, results, and complications. J Spinal Disord 13:9-15, 2000.

223. Konya D, Ozgen S, Gercek A, et al: Outcomes for combined anterior and posterior surgical approaches for patients with multisegmental cervical spondylotic myelopathy. J Clin Neurosci 16:404-409, 2009.

224. Vauzelle C, Stagnara P, Jouvinrous P: Functional monitoring of spinal cord activity during spinal surgery. Clin Orthop Relat Res 93:173-178, 1973.

225. May DM, Jones SJ, Crockard HA: Somatosensory evoked potential monitoring in cervical surgery: Identification of pre- and intraoperative risk factors associated with neurological deterioration. J Neurosurg 85:566-573, 1996.

226. Powers SK, Bolger CA, Edwards MB: Spinal cord pathways mediating somatosensory evoked potentials. J Neurosurg 57:472-478, 1982.

227. Devlin VJ, Anderson PA, Schwartz DM, et al: Intraoperative neurophysiologic monitoring: Focus on cervical myelopathy and related issues. Spine J 6(1 Suppl):212-224, 2006.

228. Scheufler KM, Zentner J: Total intravenous anesthesia for intraoperative monitoring of the motor pathways: An integral view combining clinical and experimental data. J Neurosurg 96:571-579, 2002.

229. Kombos T, Suess O, DaSilva C, et al: Impact of somatosensory evoked potential monitoring on cervical surgery. J Clin Neurophysiol 20:122-128, 2003.

230. Epstein NE, Danto JD, Nardi D: Evaluation of intraoperative somatosensory evoked potential monitoring on cervical surgery. J Clin Neurophysiol 20:122-128, 2003.

231. Kitagawa H, Itoh T, Takano H, et al: Motor evoked potential monitoring during upper cervical spine surgery. Spine (Phila Pa 1976) 14:1078-1083, 1989.

232. Berthold CH, Carlstedt T, Corneliuson O: Anatomy of the nerve root at the central-peripheral transitional region. In Dyck PJ, Thomas PK, Lambert EH, et al (eds): Peripheral Neuropathy. Philadelphia, WB Saunders, 1984, pp 156-217.

233. Jimenez JC, Sani S, Braverman B, et al: Palsies of the fifth cervical nerve root after cervical decompression: Prevention using continuous intraoperative electromyography monitoring. J Neurosurg Spine 3:92-97, 2005.

234. Fan D, Schwartz DM, Vaccaro AR, et al: Intraoperative neurophysiologic detection of iatrogenic C5 nerve root injury during laminectomy for cervical compression myelopathy. Spine (Phila Pa 1976) 27:2499-2502, 2002.

235. Hilibrand AS, Schwartz DM, Sethuraman V, et al: Comparison of transcranial electric motor and somatosensory evoked potential monitoring during cervical surgery. J Bone Joint Surg Am 86:1248-1253, 2004.

42 CHAPTER

Ossification of the Posterior Longitudinal Ligament

Motoki Iwasaki, MD, DMSc
Kazuo Yonenobu, MD, DMSc

History

Despite reports of ossification of the posterior longitudinal ligament (OPLL) by Key in 1838[1] and by Oppenheimer in 1942,[2] it was not recognized as a distinct clinical entity until 1960. The first report in Japan of cervical compressive myelopathy caused by OPLL was based on autopsy findings obtained by Tsukimoto in 1960.[3] Onji and colleagues[4] reviewed clinical symptoms of 18 cases of OPLL in 1967. Since then, many reports of OPLL have been published, and it has been recognized as a common clinical entity that causes compression myelopathy, especially in Japan. The Investigation Committee on Ossification of the Spinal Ligaments, organized by the Japanese Ministry of Public Health and Welfare, has conducted studies of the etiology of OPLL and patient care for OPLL since 1975. Their studies of the pathogenesis, diagnosis, and treatment of OPLL have contributed to improvement in management of OPLL and other spinal disorders in Japan.

OPLL is a common cause of cervical myelopathy in middle-aged and older Japanese adults. Although OPLL has been thought to be rare among whites and to be a "Japanese disease," several reports of OPLL in whites and in natives of other Asian countries have been published.[5] Several studies of growth factors, cytokines, and other molecular and genetic factors in OPLL have been reported, but the etiology of OPLL has not yet been fully elucidated.

Etiology

OPLL has been found in 26% of the parents of probands and 29% of the siblings of probands.[6] Familial surveys and human leukocyte antigen (HLA) haplotype studies reveal that genetic background plays an important role in the occurrence of OPLL. A genetic locus for OPLL is thought to be located close to the HLA region, on chromosome 6p. Although a candidate gene in the region, the gene for collagen 11A2, has been analyzed for the presence of molecular variants in affected probands, the pathogenesis of OPLL does not seem to be entirely the result of defects in this gene.[7]

Pathology

Although OPLL was previously thought to involve calcification of the posterior longitudinal ligament, studies have shown that it actually involves ossification of the ligament.[8] OPLL involves ectopic bone formation within the spinal ligaments. The mature form of the ossification consists of lamellar bone with well-developed haversian systems. Immature lesions are often accompanied by woven bone with fibrocartilaginous cell proliferation in the marginal area (Fig. 42–1). The main characteristics of OPLL are as follows[9,10]: (1) ossification accompanied by ligamentous tissue hyperplasia and cell proliferation; (2) sequential occurrence of fibrocartilaginous cell proliferation, calcification, and tissue resorption with vascular ingrowth; and (3) ossification of the ligament that occurs at specific sites of predilection and often in combination with diffuse idiopathic skeletal hyperostosis.[11] The ossification process of the ligament is not always endochondral ossification but sometimes is membranous ossification.[10]

The posterior longitudinal ligament is initially replaced with bony tissue. Hyperplasia of the fibrocartilaginous tissue may occur in the posterior aspect of the intervertebral disc, extending into the ossified posterior longitudinal ligament.[9] Progression of ossification follows an evolutionary process, beginning as endochondral or membranous ossification. There may be no correlation between disc degeneration and occurrence of OPLL.[8] Generally, in cases of dense OPLL, normal disc thickness is maintained in the cervical spine, and there are no signs of inflammation or bleeding in these areas of ossification.[9]

Myelopathy caused by OPLL is characterized by chronic compression of the spinal cord. Autopsy studies of OPLL show the following pathologic characteristics[12,13]: (1) Demyelination and loss of axon, which is more dominant in the posterolateral than in the anterior column, is observed in the white matter; (2) pathologic changes are restricted to the gray matter, and the white matter is preserved in cases with a boomerang shape in which the transverse area of the spinal cord is greater than 60% of the normal; (3) a triangular shape in which the transverse area of the spinal cord is reduced to

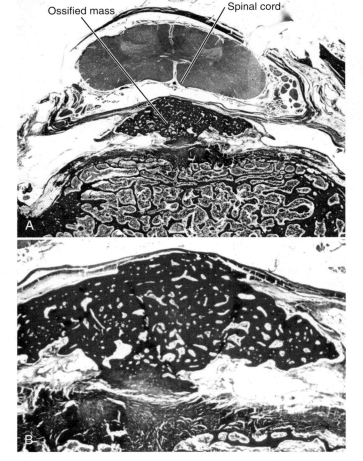

FIGURE 42–1 A, Axial section (Azan Mallory stain) showing spinal cord compressed by ossified mass of posterior longitudinal ligament. **B,** Magnified view of ossified area of posterior longitudinal ligament showing mature lamellar bone. Fibrocartilaginous cell proliferation and matrix hyperplasia can be seen between mature ossified mass and vertebral body.

less than 60% of the normal is associated with severe and irreversible pathologic changes showing white matter and gray matter are severely involved, and only the anterior column is preserved.

Metabolic Background

A high incidence of diabetes mellitus (non–insulin-dependent) and impaired glucose tolerance has been reported among patients with OPLL.[14,15] Glucose tolerance tests of 535 patients with OPLL showed that 28% were diabetic, and 18% were borderline diabetic.[16] There have also been reports of a relatively high incidence of OPLL and hormonal disorders such as hypoparathyroidism and hypophosphatemic rickets among diabetic patients.[16] This finding seems to implicate abnormal calcium metabolism in ossification of the ligaments, although conventional blood chemistry tests have shown no abnormalities in patients with OPLL.[16]

Epidemiology

Incidence

The incidence of OPLL in Japanese older than 30 years of age has been reported to range from 2% to 4%. In Taiwan, Korea, Hong Kong, and Singapore, the incidence of OPLL reportedly ranges from 0.8% to 3%.[5] In the United States and Europe, the incidence of OPLL reportedly ranges from 0.1% to 1.7%.[5] In a survey of 599 patients in Utah University Hospital, 8 patients (1.3%) were found to have OPLL in the cervical spine.[5,8]

Natural History of Myelopathy

A cohort study showed that all patients with more than 60% spinal canal stenosis by OPLL exhibited cervical myelopathy.[17] Although static compression of the spinal cord is the main cause of myelopathy in OPLL, radiologic findings do not always correlate with clinical severity of neurologic manifestations. In a study of the natural history of 207 patients with OPLL over an average period of 10 years, clinical symptoms did not change in 66% of patients, and myelopathy developed in 16% of patients.[18] Kaplan-Meier analysis of 323 patients who did not have myelopathy at their initial evaluation showed a myelopathy-free rate of 71% after 30 years.[19]

Despite spinal stenosis (6 mm < space available for the spinal cord < 14 mm), myelopathy may not develop in patients with the severe limitation of range of motion of the cervical spine.[19,20] This finding indicates that not only static factors, but also dynamic factors such as listhesis or hypermobility at discontinuity of the ossified lesion play important roles in the development of myelopathy, especially in mixed or segmental OPLL.

Presentation

Age

OPLL most frequently occurs in the cervical spine of middle-aged or elderly men. OPLL has not been reported in children or adolescents. The frequency increases markedly after age 40 years, and the greatest frequency is observed in people in their 50s. In the cervical spine, the frequency for men is about twice that of women. At thoracic levels, OPLL is more frequent in women, however; the reasons for this are unclear.

Location

Although OPLL has been observed at all levels of the spine, it occurs most frequently in the cervical spine. Thoracic OPLL occurs at the upper and middle thoracic levels.[16] In contrast, ossification of the ligamentum flavum (OLF) is frequently observed at the lower thoracic level and the thoracolumbar junction. Lumbar OPLL occurs relatively infrequently, and it does not usually cause severe disabilities.

Symptoms

Many patients with subclinical or latent OPLL are asymptomatic, and many patients with large ossified lesions experience no disability. Symptoms most typically include myelopathy or myeloradiculopathy rather than radiculopathy alone. The symptoms develop secondary to spinal cord compression caused by the space-occupying lesion of the ossified ligament. These neurologic symptoms develop insidiously without any obvious causes in 80% to 85% of patients, but acute onset or aggravation of the symptoms is often related to a minor trauma or hyperextension of the neck.[16]

Patients can be divided into three groups according to their neurologic symptoms: (1) patients with spinal cord signs presenting with motor and sensory disturbances predominantly in the lower extremities; (2) patients with segmental signs presenting with motor and sensory disturbances predominantly in the upper extremities; and (3) patients presenting with pain in the neck, shoulder, and arm region without obvious neurologic deficits (axial symptoms alone).[9]

Diagnosis

Physical Examination

The most common complaint at onset of OPLL is paresthesia or numbness in the hands. Clumsiness of the hands is another symptom. The complaints gradually extend to the lower extremities, leading to gait disturbance. Physical examination generally reveals spasticity of the lower extremities with exaggerated deep tendon reflexes and sensory disturbance in upper and lower extremities. Patients sometimes complain of neck pain or discomfort around the neck. Myelopathy affecting the hand, as indicated by the tests (finger escape sign and 10-second grasp and release test) proposed by Ono and colleagues,[21] is a sensitive and specific sign of pyramidal tract involvement in the cervical spine. It is important to differentiate OPLL from other skeletal and neurologic disorders, including cervical spondylosis, spinal cord tumor, periarthritis of the shoulder, entrapment neuropathy in the upper extremities, and motor neuron disease.[8]

Plain Radiography

OPLL of the cervical spine can be identified by plain radiography. The characteristic finding is a longitudinal dense ossified strip along the posterior margin of the cervical spine. Duplicated lines of the posterior margins of the vertebral bodies are occasionally mistaken for a segmental type of OPLL.

Narrow disc spaces or spondylotic changes are occasionally observed at the lower cervical region of OPLL patients, but disc spaces located in the ossified area are usually well preserved.[9] There is no involvement of sacroiliac joints or apophyseal joints, which is usually observed in cases of ankylosing spondylitis.

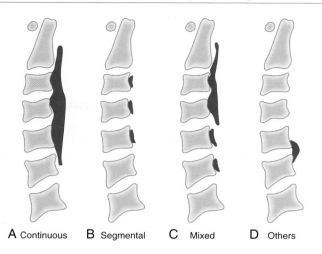

FIGURE 42–2 Radiographic classification of the Investigation Committee on Ossification of the Spinal Ligaments, Japanese Ministry of Public Health and Welfare. **A,** *Continuous type*: Ossified mass extending over several contiguous vertebrae. **B,** *Segmental type*: Several fragmented ossified lesions immediately behind each vertebral body. **C,** *Mixed type*: Combination of continuous and segmental types of ossification. **D,** *Others type*: Circumscribed ossified lesion confined to intervertebral disc space.

Based on radiographic findings, cervical OPLL is classified into four types (Fig. 42–2): (1) *continuous type,* in which ossification extends over several contiguous vertebrae; (2) *segmental type,* in which ossification is fragmented and located immediately behind each vertebral body with interruption at the intervertebral disc levels; (3) *mixed type,* which is a combination of continuous and segmental types of ossification; (4) *others type* (circumscribed or localized), in which ossification is confined to the intervertebral disc space.[16] In addition to this conventional typing, sagittal shape of the ossified lesion is classified into plateau-shaped or hill-shaped (see Fig. 42–6).[22] Plateau-shaped ossification, which is found in segmental-type OPLL and most continuous-type and mixed-type OPLL, is characterized by a narrow spinal canal without massive localized ossification. Hill-shaped ossification, which is found in circumscribed-type OPLL and some cases of continuous-type or mixed-type OPLL, shows massive beak-shaped ossification localized to certain levels.

The occupying ratio of OPLL is calculated as the ratio of the maximum anteroposterior thickness of OPLL to the anteroposterior diameter of the spinal canal at the corresponding level on a lateral radiograph or tomogram (Fig. 42–3).[16] An occupying ratio greater than 60% indicates high risk of the development of myelopathy.[17,23] Matsunaga and colleagues[19,20] reported that with a constant tube-to-film distance of 150 cm, all of the patients with a value of space available for the spinal cord (SAC) of less than 6 mm had myelopathy, whereas none of the patients with SAC of 14 mm or more developed myelopathy. They also reported that in patients with myelopathy whose minimal SAC diameter ranged from 6 mm to less than 14 mm, the range of motion of the cervical spine was significantly greater.[18,20] These results suggest that the primary factor in the development of

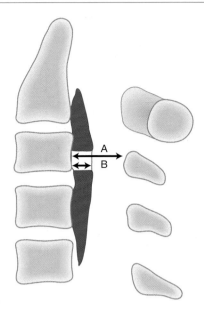

FIGURE 42–3 Radiographic measurement of spinal canal stenosis caused by ossification of the posterior longitudinal ligament (OPLL). **A,** Anteroposterior diameter of spinal canal. **B,** Maximum anteroposterior thickness of ossified ligament. Occupying ratio of OPLL = B/A × 100 (%). Occupying ratio greater than 60% indicates high risk of development of myelopathy. Space available for the spinal cord (SAC) = A − B (mm) with a constant tube-to-film distance of 150 cm. SAC less than 6 mm indicates high risk for development of myelopathy.

myelopathy is reduced SAC diameter resulting from static compression by the ossified ligament, although below the critical point (SAC >6 mm or maximum spinal canal stenosis ≤60%), dynamic effects seem to be the main factors in the development of myelopathy.

Computed Tomography

Computed tomography (CT) is particularly useful for imaging of the lower cervical spine and visualizing ossification that is difficult to detect with plain radiographs (Fig. 42–4). Because of the high frequency of association of cervical OPLL with thoracolumbar OPLL and OLF, a preoperative survey should include imaging of the entire spinal column. Because it is difficult to detect ossified lesions at the cervicothoracic and thoracolumbar junctions on plain radiographs, careful preoperative and postoperative CT or magnetic resonance imaging (MRI) or both should be performed to assess spinal stenosis throughout the entire spine. Myelography is useful to assess spinal canal stenosis by OPLL or OLF or both from the cervical spine to the lumbar spine, and combined myelography and CT is mandatory for planning of anterior removal or floating of the ossified lesion.

Magnetic Resonance Imaging

MRI is not effective for detection of OPLL because OPLL lacks signal intensity on T1-weighted and T2-weighted images (Fig. 42–5). Bone marrow within the ossified lesion appears as an isointense or hyperintense area, however. MRI can illustrate pathology of the spinal cord. Kameyama and colleagues[12] reported that in cases of OPLL, a triangular spinal cord with a transverse area of less than 60% of normal in more than one segment seemed to be associated with severe and irreversible pathologic changes. MRI is also useful for detection of cervical disc herniation. In one study, disc protrusion was detected in 81% of patients with segmental OPLL, and intramedullary hyperintensity was observed on T2-weighted images in 43% of the patients whose neurologic

FIGURE 42–4 A 56-year-old woman with 70% occupying ratio underwent anterior surgery. Her preoperative Japanese Orthopaedic Association (JOA) score was 4.5. Her JOA score at the last follow-up was 12, and her recovery rate was 60%. **A,** Plain radiograph clearly shows mixed-type ossification of the posterior longitudinal ligament but does not clearly show ossified lesion at lower levels. **B,** CT reconstruction scan clearly shows massive ossification at C5-6.

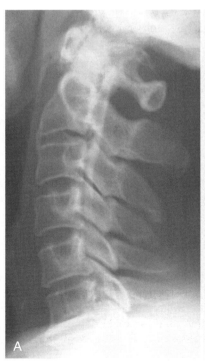

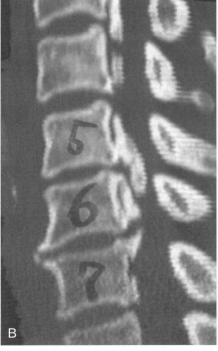

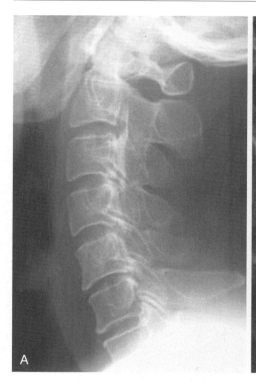
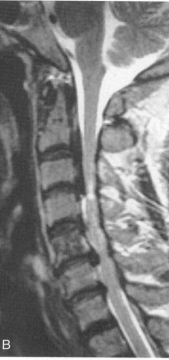

FIGURE 42–5 A 60-year-old man experienced progressive myelopathy. His Japanese Orthopaedic Association (JOA) score was 11 before undergoing C3-7 laminoplasty. His postoperative JOA score was 14.5, and his recovery rate was 58%. **A,** Preoperative radiograph shows mixed-type ossification of the posterior longitudinal ligament from C2-6. **B,** T2-weighted MRI shows ossified lesion as lack of signal and intramedullary hyperintensity at C3-4 level.

deficits were significantly more severe than average (see Fig. 42–5B).[24]

Treatment of Ossification of the Posterior Longitudinal Ligament of the Cervical Spine

Conservative Treatment

A cervical orthosis and skull traction are used in conservative treatment of OPLL. Such conservative treatment is indicated to eliminate dynamic factors of the cervical spine for patients whose predominant complaint is neck, shoulder, and arm pain (local pain, radicular pain, or both) without any symptoms of myelopathy or patients with mild ossification in whom myelopathy is subclinical and not predominant.[25] It is important to advise patients with OPLL not to hyperextend the neck and to be vigilant regarding trauma and falls secondary to motor vehicle accidents, sports activities, or excessive alcohol intake.[25]

Surgical Treatment

Surgical decompression is indicated for patients who have long tract signs such as spastic gait disturbance and clumsiness of the hands. Even among patients with myelopathy, surgical treatment is not always effective for pain relief in patients whose predominant complaint is pain and is generally not recommended.

Surgical decompression of the spinal cord is necessary for patients with apparent myelopathy because long-term compression of the spinal cord may cause irreversible degeneration. For patients with symptoms and signs of moderate or progressive myelopathy, the authors recommend early surgical decompression, especially for younger patients with a narrow spinal canal, because reports indicate that better neurologic recovery is associated with younger age at operation and milder myelopathy.[26] Even if the myelopathy is mild, surgery may be indicated for patients with severe spinal stenosis (SAC ≤6 mm or occupying ratio ≥60%). There is no evidence indicating the effectiveness of prophylactic surgery for patients who have no symptoms or signs of myelopathy.[23]

Authors' Preferred Choice of Surgical Procedure

There is some controversy over the appropriate method of surgery for myelopathy caused by cervical OPLL. In Japan, most surgeons use an anterior approach with extirpation or floating of the ossified lesion or a posterior approach including various types of expansive laminoplasty. The choice between two approaches should be based on the following considerations: skill of the surgeon, age and general condition of the patient, extent of ossification, OPLL type and sagittal shape of the ossified lesion (plateau-shaped [Fig. 42–6A] or hill-shaped [Fig. 42–6B]), OPLL occupying ratio, sagittal curvature of the cervical spine and spinal cord (kyphotic or lordotic), and intervertebral mobility at the maximum compression level (dynamic factors).[22,27-30]

Extensive laminoplasty generally is effective and safer for most patients with the following characteristics: (1) OPLL occupying ratio of less than 60%, (2) plateau-shaped ossification (see Figs. 42–6A and 42–11A), and (3) lordotic alignment of the cervical spine or the spinal cord.[22,26,28,29] The authors' clinical experience indicates that laminoplasty is not

FIGURE 42–6 Two shapes of ossification. **A,** Radiograph shows plateau-shaped ossified lesion. **B,** Tomogram shows hill-shaped ossified lesion.

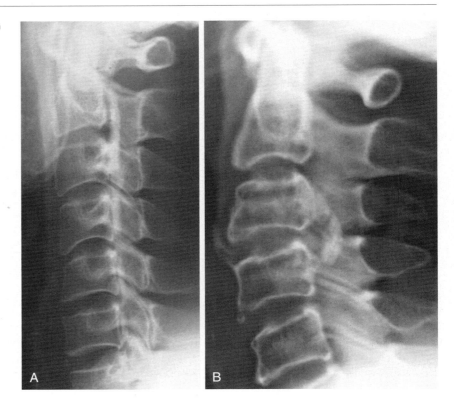

contraindicated if kyphosis of the cervical spine is mild. The anterior floating method using autogenous fibular graft is recommended for patients with the following characteristics: (1) OPLL occupying ratio of less than 60%; (2) hill-shaped ossification (Fig. 42–7A; see Figs. 42–4B and 42–6B); (3) local kyphotic alignment of the cervical spine or the spinal cord; and (4) intervertebral hypermobility at the maximum compression level or between the interrupted ossified lesion.[22,28-30]

Internal rigid fixation is rarely necessary for surgical treatment of OPLL. Although the authors do not recommend the use of spinal instrumentation for laminoplasty, which has the advantage of allowing some movement of the cervical spine, laminoplasty with posterior instrumented fusion may have the advantage for patients with a flexible kyphotic alignment of the cervical spine or evident intervertebral mobility at the level of maximum spinal cord compression.[30] An anterior plate and screws are rarely necessary for the anterior approach if a halo vest is worn for 6 to 10 weeks. Posterior instrumentation is often used, however, during salvage surgery for dislodgment or pseudarthrosis of bone graft (see Fig. 42–8D).

Anterior Approaches

The results of anterior interbody fusion without decompression have been reported.[31,32] One report described anterior resection of an ossified lesion by drilling into the anterolateral part of the vertebral body without bone grafting.[33] The indications of these anterior approaches have not been clearly identified, however, and the results of such surgery have been inconsistent.

Several surgeons have attempted to remove ossified lesions using an anterior approach. The results of these procedures varied owing to insufficient decompression resulting from ossification of the dura (see Fig. 42–9A) or massive bleeding from the epidural space and intraoperative injury to the spinal cord or nerve roots. Anterior removal is also associated with a high incidence of complications. The anterior floating method devised by Yamaura and colleagues,[34] in which the spinal cord is decompressed without resection of the ossified lesion, has made anterior decompression surgery for OPLL safer and more reliable. The advantages of this procedure include gradual decompression without extirpation but with an anterior shift of the OPLL to avoid dural tears caused by ossification of the dura and lower risk of injury to neural tissues. The anterior floating method is indicated for ossified lesions localized from C2 to T3. Locally prominent ossified masses and highly occupied lesions can be treated effectively using this method (see Fig. 42–7).

Surgical Technique

The anterior aspect of the cervical spine is exposed using the conventional anterior approach. The longus colli muscles, which are important markers of the center of the vertebral bodies, are retracted laterally to expose the anterior aspect of the vertebral bodies completely. To obtain lateral and vertical orientation, total discectomy is performed at all levels for removal. Herniated disc material is often found in mixed and segmental types of OPLL. After complete removal of the disc material, uncovertebral joints are identified. The base of the

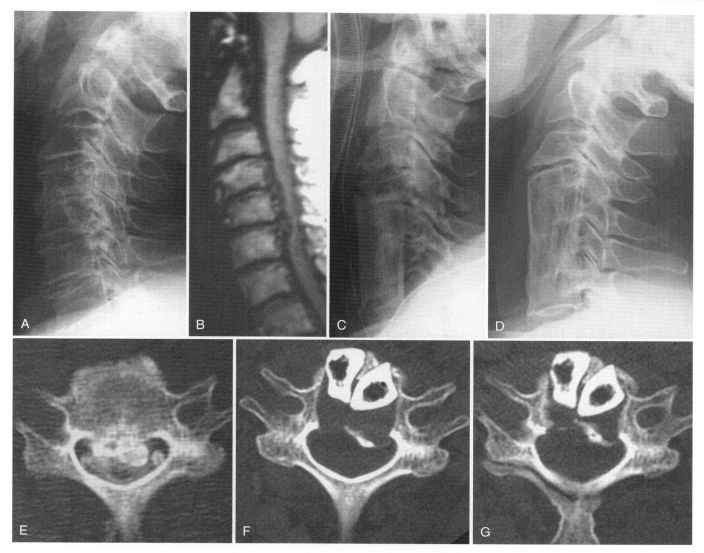

FIGURE 42–7 A 69-year-old woman with 50% occupying ratio underwent anterior floating procedure using fibula graft. She could not walk without support, owing to severe myelopathy, and her preoperative Japanese Orthopaedic Association (JOA) score was 6. Postoperative (3 years) JOA score was 10, and her recovery rate was 36%. **A,** Preoperative radiograph shows massive ossification at C5-6. **B,** T1-weighted MRI shows compression of spinal cord from C4-5 to C6. **C,** Radiograph taken immediately after anterior floating procedure shows line of residual ossification behind grafted fibula. **D,** Radiograph taken 3 years after surgery shows anterior shift of residual ossification immediately behind grafted fibula. **E,** Preoperative CT myelogram shows massive ossification compressing spinal cord anteriorly. **F,** CT scan 1 week after anterior floating procedure shows two pieces of grafted fibula and line of residual ossification behind grafted fibula. **G,** CT scan 7 weeks after surgery shows anterior shift of residual ossification immediately behind grafted fibula.

uncinate process or lateral border of the disc can be used as a landmark for the width of the vertebral body.

The vertebral bodies are resected according to the orientation obtained by total discectomy. Based on CT and reconstruction images, resection is extended laterally. Transverse decompression should extend at least 20 to 25 mm to ensure sufficient decompression.[27,34] When the posterior cortex of the vertebral body is exposed, the cortex and the ossified ligament should be shaved with a diamond bur to make their thickness as uniform as possible. Care should be taken not to perforate the lateral part of the posterior cortex or injure the venous plexus. When the ossified ligament and the posterior cortex have been thinned, the ossified lesion and vertebral edge are cut at the cranial, caudal, and lateral margins by continuing to

shave the cortex and the ossified ligament with a diamond bur. When these margins are released completely, the released ossified lesion begins to rise slightly. After release of the ossified lesion, the remnant of the ossified mass should not be shaved but should be allowed to move ventralward spontaneously.

If the lesion can be released easily, the ossified lesion can be removed, but this is not always necessary if the lesion adheres strongly to the dura or the dura itself is ossified (see Fig. 42–9A). The possible causes of insufficient floating include the following: narrow width of decompression, insufficient release, disorientation of the lateral border of the vertebral body, insufficient thinning of the ossified ligament, and eccentric location of the ossified segment. A bone graft harvested from the fibula is inserted in the space. Immobilization of the

FIGURE 42–8 Dislodgment of grafted fibula. **A,** Radiograph taken immediately after anterior floating procedure shows fibula grafted from C4-5. **B,** Radiograph taken 12 days after surgery shows dislodgment of fibula. **C,** T2-weighted MRI shows fracture of anterosuperior corner of the body of C7 and dislodgment of fibula. **D,** Radiograph taken after posterior fusion followed by second anterior fibula graft shows alligator plate and wires used to fix spinous processes from C4-7.

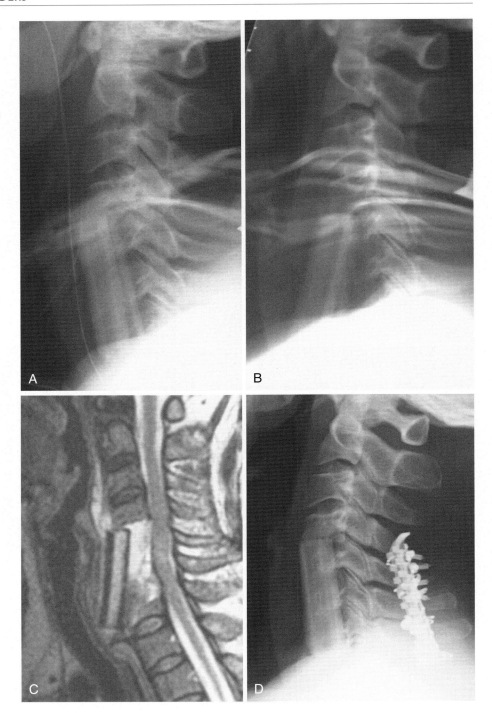

spine with a halo vest is maintained for 6 to 10 weeks postoperatively. Postoperatively, released ossification gradually shifts anteriorly under cerebrospinal fluid pressure. The period required for anterior shifting of the ossification is 4 to 8 weeks (average 6 weeks) (see Fig. 42–7E-G).[27,34]

Complications

Likely complications after anterior decompression include dural tear with cerebrospinal fluid leakage, nerve root palsy, and dislodgment or pseudarthrosis of grafted bone (Fig. 42–8).[35,36] Postoperative C5 paresis has reportedly been observed

in about 10% of patients who have undergone anterior decompression.[27] Cerebrospinal fluid leakage and dislodgment or pseudarthrosis of the strut graft are major complications of the anterior approach, and the rate of these complications reportedly ranges from 3% to 15%.[29,36-38] The rate of reoperation after anterior decompression has been reported to be 12% to 26%.[29,38]

Posterior Approaches

Laminectomy was previously the procedure of choice for cervical OPLL.[39] Laminectomy has some disadvantages, however, such as postlaminectomy kyphotic deformity and scar formation (laminectomy membrane). In 1977, Hirabayashi and colleagues[40] developed expansive open-door laminoplasty. Currently, laminoplasty (in various forms) is the treatment of choice for not only OPLL but also cervical spondylotic myelopathy.[26] Although there is no clear evidence indicating that laminoplasty is clinically superior to laminectomy,[41] some reports suggest that laminoplasty has biomechanical and clinical advantages over laminectomy.[42-46]

Several types of laminoplasty have been devised, and there is no conclusive statistical evidence that any of them is superior to the others.[41] Generally, the indications for laminoplasty are (1) multisegmental OPLL of continuous or mixed type and (2) any type of OPLL associated with developmental narrow spinal canal (anteroposterior diameter <13 mm). Rigid or severe kyphosis of the cervical spine is not a good indicator for laminoplasty. Although there are no available data indicating how great a degree of kyphosis is acceptable for laminoplasty, the authors' clinical experience indicates that mild kyphosis is not a contraindication to laminoplasty (see Fig. 42–6).[22,26]

Surgical Technique

Because progression or development of OPLL is common in younger patients with diffuse skeletal hyperostosis, extensive laminoplasty from C3 to C7 is generally recommended in such cases. If preoperative CT reveals neural compression at C1-2 and the upper thoracic spine, these levels should be included in decompression. When decompression at C2 is necessary, laminoplasty or dome-shaped undercutting of the axis may be indicated. If decompression must be extended to C1, laminectomy of the posterior arch of the atlas is an appropriate procedure. Patients are usually allowed to get out of bed within a couple of days after the surgery. Immobilization with a collar is optional depending on neck pain. Isometric exercises to strengthen neck muscles should be started as soon as postoperative pain subsides. The period of immobilization has been shortened and can sometimes be omitted.

Complications

Common complications after laminoplasty include motor palsy of the upper extremity (commonly C5 segment or nerve root), kyphotic deformity of the cervical spine, hematoma, and neck pain.[35] Although the mean incidence of postlaminoplasty C5 palsy in patients with OPLL is 5% to 10% (range 3% to 29%),[26,47,48] spontaneous recovery can be expected in most cases.[26,47,49] There is no way to preclude the possibility of C5 palsy being caused by the tethering effect of the nerve roots, and it is important that the bony gutter of the hinge side not be drilled excessively, to prevent severing of the inner cortex of the lamina (Fig. 42–9).

Postoperative deterioration in cervical alignment has been observed in 12 (18%) of 66 patients who have undergone laminoplasty (Table 42–1); 67% of these 12 patients had poor or fair surgical outcomes.[22] Kyphotic deformity has been observed in 47% of patients who have undergone

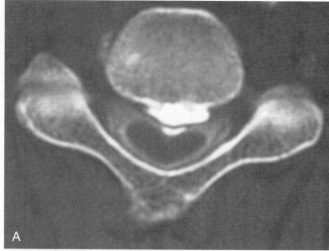

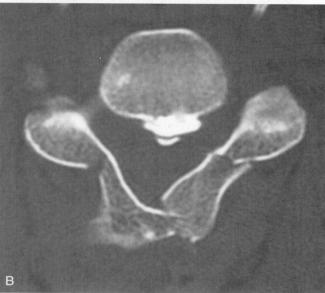

FIGURE 42–9 CT scans before and after laminoplasty. **A,** CT myelogram shows compression of spinal cord by ossification of the posterior longitudinal ligament (OPLL). Double floor of OPLL suggests ossification of dura. When anterior decompression surgery is selected, care should be taken not to injure dura or spinal cord. **B,** CT after open-door laminoplasty shows trimmed spinous process as graft on open side and preservation of inner cortex.

laminectomy and 6% to 8% of patients who have undergone laminoplasty, although mild kyphotic deformity of the cervical spine is rarely associated with neurologic deterioration (Fig. 42–10; see Table 42–1).[22,26,39]

Surgical Results

Neurologic severity of cervical myelopathy is assessed using a scoring system proposed by the Japanese Orthopaedic Association (JOA) and the recovery rate.[22,26,27,39,50,51] A full score is 17 points and indicates healthy status. This JOA scoring system is useful and reliable for assessment of cervical myelopathy.[51]

Long-term results of laminectomy,[39] laminoplasty,[22,26] and anterior floating method[27,29] are summarized in Table 42–2.

TABLE 42-1 Cervical Alignment After Laminoplasty in 66 Patients

Preoperative Alignment (%)	POSTOPERATIVE ALIGNMENT (%)			Total (%)
	Lordosis	**Straight**	**Kyphotic or S-shaped**	
Lordosis	24	8	0	32 (48%)
Straight		27	2	29 (44%)
Kyphotic or S-shaped			5*	5 (8%)
Total	24 (36%)	35 (53%)	7 (11%)	66 (100%)

*Cervical alignment deteriorated postoperatively in two of five patients whose preoperative alignment was kyphotic or S-shaped. Deterioration of cervical alignment was shown in 12 of 66 patients (18%); 67% of these 12 patients had poor or fair surgical outcomes.
From Iwasaki M, Okuda S, Miyauchi A, et al: Surgical strategy for cervical myelopathy due to ossification of the posterior longitudinal ligament. Part 1: Clinical results and limitations of laminoplasty. Spine (Phila Pa 1976) 32:647-653, 2007.

Statistical analysis indicates that predictive factors affecting clinical results of posterior decompression are sagittal shape of ossification (hill-shaped), preoperative severity of myelopathy (low total JOA score), postoperative deterioration in cervical alignment, and age at operation.[22,26,39] Overall surgical outcome of laminoplasty is presented in Table 42-3.[22]

Occupying ratio of OPLL or SAC is statistically unrelated to surgical outcome of posterior decompression, although a retrospective study of OPLL with an occupying ratio of greater than 50% to 60% indicates that neurologic outcome of anterior decompression and fusion is better than that of laminoplasty.[22,29,50] With the anterior floating method, good outcome is strongly associated with preoperative severity and duration of myelopathy, preoperative cross-sectional area of the spinal cord, and age at last follow-up.[27]

Poorer prognosis generally is associated with longer duration of symptoms, older age at operation, more severe preoperative symptoms, and a history of trauma causing onset or progression of myelopathy. The causes of late deterioration are degenerative lumbar stenosis, thoracic myelopathy secondary to OPLL or OLF or both, postoperative progression of OPLL, and trauma or fall during the postoperative period.

OPLL generally continues to progress after surgery (Fig. 42-11). In a Japanese nationwide multicenter study, the incidence of OPLL progression was 56.5% at 2 years after posterior decompression and 71% at 5 years (Kaplan-Meier analysis).[52] In this multicenter study, younger patients (<60 years old) had a higher risk of progression (Fig. 42-12A).[52] Patients with mixed-type OPLL had the highest rate of progression, and patients with segmental-type OPLL had the

TABLE 42-2 Long-Term (>10 Years) Results of Laminectomy, Laminoplasty, and Anterior Floating Procedure for Cervical Ossification of the Posterior Longitudinal Ligament (OPLL)

	Laminectomy[19]	Laminoplasty[23]	Anterior Floating[24]
No. patients	44	64	63
Male/female	37/7	43/21	45/18
Follow-up (yr)	14.1	12.2	13
Age at surgery (yr)	57	56	57
Occupying ratio of OPLL (%)	55	38	54
SAC (mm)	6.8	8.5	5.2
Preoperative JOA score	7.6	8.5	8.3
Postoperative JOA score	10.3	13.7	13.5
Recovery rate (%)	33	60	59
Operation time (min)		179	323
Estimated blood loss (g)		475	1099
Deterioration after surgery	3 cases (7%)	0	0
Nerve root palsy (%)		5	10
Progression of OPLL (%)	70	70	36
Late deterioration of myelopathy	10 cases (23%)	6 cases (9%)	13 cases (21%)
	6: Fall	3: Thoracic myelopathy	6: Thoracic myelopathy
	3: Thoracic myelopathy	2: Progression of OPLL	4: Inadequate decompression
	1: Progression of OPLL	1: Spinal cord atrophy	3: Progression of OPLL
Additional cervical surgery	1 case (2%)	1 case (2%)	5 cases (8%)

JOA, Japanese Orthopaedic Association; SAC, space available for the spinal cord.

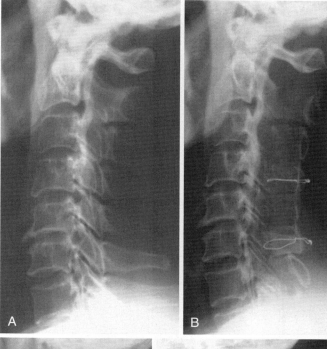

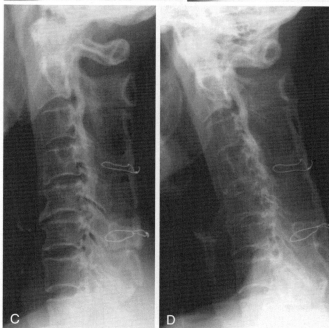

FIGURE 42–10 This woman with 36% occupying ratio of ossification of the posterior longitudinal ligament (OPLL) underwent laminoplasty from C2-7 when she was 61 years old. Her Japanese Orthopaedic Association (JOA) score was 11 preoperatively and 12.5 at the last follow-up (recovery rate 25%). **A,** Preoperative radiograph shows mixed-type OPLL with normal lordosis of cervical spine. **B,** Radiograph taken 1 month after laminoplasty shows still lordotic alignment. **C,** Radiograph taken 2 years after surgery shows kyphotic deformity. **D,** Radiograph taken 10 years after surgery shows progression of kyphosis but no progression of OPLL.

lowest incidence of progression (Fig. 42–12B).[26,52,53] In a long-term (>10 years) follow-up study, postoperative progression of ossification was observed in 70% to 73% of patients who underwent laminectomy or laminoplasty, but few were found to have related neurologic deterioration.[26,39,53] The incidence

of postoperative progression after anterior decompression and fusion ranges from 36% to 64%, which is lower than the rate for posterior decompression.[27,54]

The main problem with anterior decompression is restenosis at levels adjacent to the fusion area, caused by postoperative progression of OPLL or spinal instability.[27,29] Matsuoka and colleagues[27] reported that posterior decompression of the cervical spine was required postoperatively in 8% of patients who underwent the anterior floating procedure. In contrast, additional cervical surgery was required to treat progression of OPLL in only 1 of 64 patients (2%) undergoing laminoplasty.[26]

Serial radiographic analysis of patients with OPLL, performed more than 10 years after they underwent laminoplasty, revealed spontaneous anterior fusion between vertebral bodies in 64% of patients and spontaneous posterior fusion between facets or laminae in 97% of patients.[26] In a study of 30 patients with OPLL who underwent laminoplasty, the mean age at death was 76 years (range 58 to 85 years), and the most frequent cause of death was cancer, followed by heart disease, pneumonia, and cerebrovascular accident.[26]

Ossification of the Posterior Longitudinal Ligament or Ossification of the Ligamentum Flavum of the Thoracic Spine

OLF can usually be identified on a plain lateral radiograph of the thoracolumbar junction. Plain radiography is insufficient, however, to delineate ossified lesions in the upper thoracic spine, which is a common site of OLF and OPLL. The authors recommend CT or MRI or both to detect ossification in the cervicothoracic and thoracolumbar junctions (Fig. 42–13).

TABLE 42–3 Overall Surgical Outcome of Laminoplasty with Respect to Predictive Factors*

	Excellent/Good (No. [%])	Fair (No. [%])	Poor (No. [%])
Occupying ratio ≥60%	1 (17%)	3 (50%)	2 (33%)
Hill-shaped ossification	3 (25%)	4 (33%)	5 (42%)
Postoperative deterioration in cervical alignment	4 (33%)	2 (17%)	6 (50%)
Preoperative abnormal alignment	2 (40%)	1 (20%)	2 (40%)
Postoperative progression of OPLL	20 (74%)	2 (7%)	5 (19%)

*Surgical outcome was evaluated from recovery rate: excellent, >75%; good, 50%-74%; fair, 25%-50%; poor, <25%.
OPLL, ossification of the posterior longitudinal ligament.
From Iwasaki M, Okuda S, Miyauchi A, et al: Surgical strategy for cervical myelopathy due to ossification of the posterior longitudinal ligament. Part 1: Clinical results and limitations of laminoplasty. Spine (Phila Pa 1976) 32:647-653, 2007.

FIGURE 42–11 This man with mixed-type ossification of the posterior longitudinal ligament (OPLL) underwent laminoplasty when he was 47 years old. His Japanese Orthopaedic Association (JOA) score was 11 preoperatively and 16 at last follow-up (recovery rate 83%), despite postoperative progression of OPLL. **A,** Preoperative radiograph shows mixed-type OPLL with 54% occupying ratio. **B,** Radiograph taken 1 month after laminoplasty shows no progression of OPLL. **C,** Radiograph taken 5 years after surgery shows progression of OPLL in craniad direction. **D,** Radiograph taken 15 years after surgery shows further progression of OPLL in craniad direction (progression of 4 mm in width in anteroposterior direction and 30 mm in length in craniad direction).

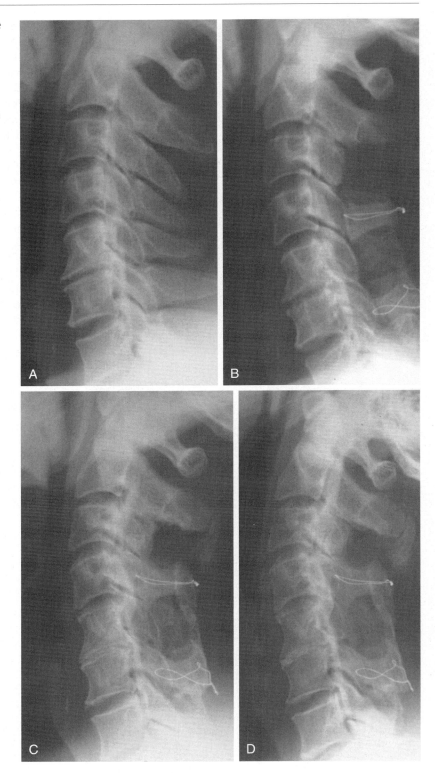

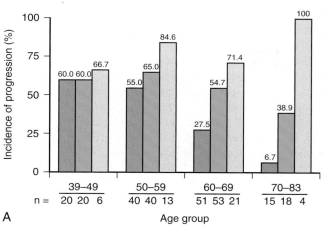

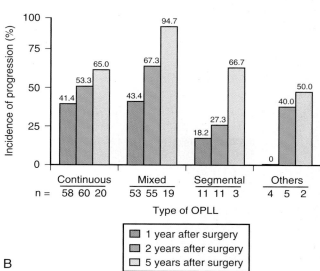

A

B

☐ 1 year after surgery
☐ 2 years after surgery
☐ 5 years after surgery

FIGURE 42–12 Postoperative progression of ossification of the posterior longitudinal ligament (OPLL) after posterior decompression. **A,** Incidence of OPLL progression in each age group. Younger patients (<60 years old) had a higher risk of progression. **B,** Incidence of progression in four types of OPLL. Patients with mixed-type OPLL had highest incidence of progression, and patients with continuous-type OPLL had second highest incidence of progression.

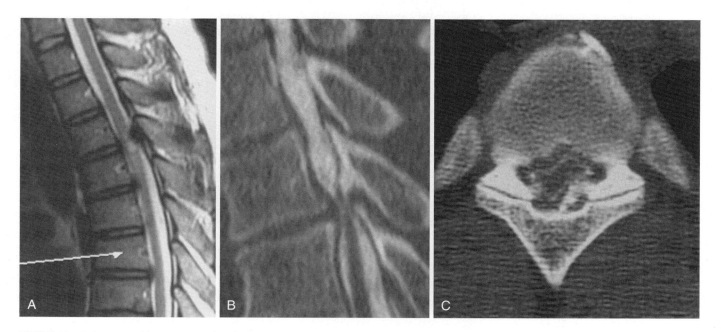

A   B   C

FIGURE 42–13 A 45-year-old man presented with spastic gait and paresthesia in bilateral lower extremities. **A,** T2-weighted MRI shows posterior indentation at T6 (*arrow*) owing to thoracic ossification of the ligamentum flavum and intramedullary high signal intensity at T3-4. **B,** Sagittal reconstruction image of CT myelogram shows severe stenosis at T3-4. **C,** CT scan at T3-4 shows severe compression of spinal cord owing to ossification of capsular portion of the ligamentum flavum.

Surgical Treatment

Conservative treatment for thoracic OPLL or OFL is less effective in patients who present with symptoms of myelopathy because the thoracic spine undergoes less motion and has a narrower spinal canal than the cervical spine. The only currently available surgical treatment for OLF of the thoracic spine is posterior decompression. Surgical outcome of posterior decompression for myelopathy caused by thoracic OPLL has generally been poor and quite inferior to outcome of posterior decompression for myelopathy caused by cervical OPLL.[55,56] The choice of treatment for thoracic OPLL depends on the spinal level of the ossification, coexistence of OLF, and degree of thoracic kyphosis. The relative importance of these factors is controversial among surgeons.

The surgical method most frequently used for thoracic OPLL at the upper thoracic level is cervicothoracic laminoplastic decompression because the spinal curvature is lordotic or slightly kyphotic at the cervicothoracic junction.[56,57] For patients with OLF and OPLL at the middle and lower thoracic level, the common choices of treatment are anterior decompression via a posterior approach, wide laminectomy with posterior instrumentation, lateral rachiotomy, and combined anterior and posterior decompression (Fig. 42–14).[55,56,58-62]

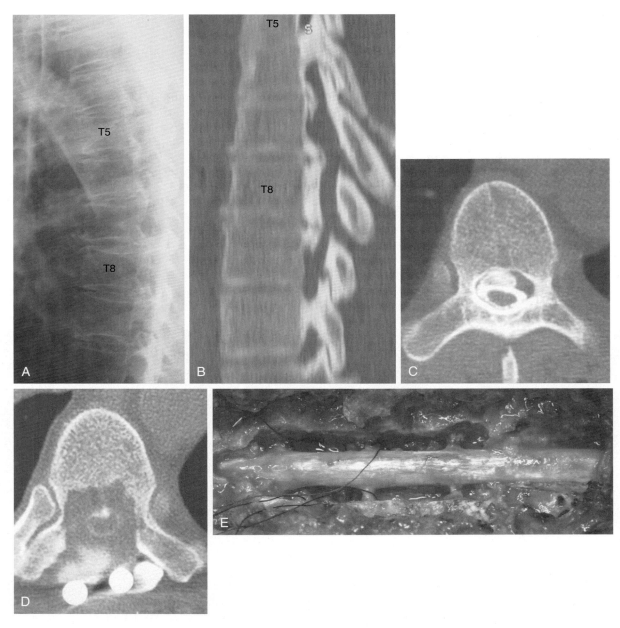

FIGURE 42–14 This 50-year-old woman could not walk at all because of thoracic myelopathy secondary to thoracic ossification of the posterior longitudinal ligament (OPLL). She underwent anterior decompression via posterior approach. **A** and **B,** Radiograph (**A**) and sagittal reconstruction image (**B**) show thoracic OPLL at multiple levels. **C,** Preoperative CT myelogram shows OPLL at T8. **D,** Postoperative CT myelogram shows anterior decompression via posterior approach. **E,** Intraoperative photograph shows 360-degree decompression of dura via posterior approach.

Postoperative paraplegia is still sometimes associated with each of these procedures, owing to technical difficulties and the vulnerability of the thoracic spinal cord. A retrospective multi-institutional study revealed that neurologic deterioration immediately after surgery was recognized in 11.7%.[56]

Among the choices of surgical procedure, Yamazaki and colleagues[62] reported that none of the patients who underwent posterior decompression and instrumented fusion for thoracic OPLL developed postoperative paralysis. The use of instrumentation is recommended with posterior decompression for thoracic OPLL at the middle and lower thoracic spine because it would enhance and maintain decompression effect with correction of kyphosis or prevention of progression of kyphosis.[56,62] Surgical treatment of thoracic OPLL remains one of the most challenging problems for spinal surgeons in Japan.

KEY POINTS

1. OPLL involves ectopic bone formation within the spinal ligaments.

2. Although static compression of the spinal cord is the main factor in myelopathy secondary to OPLL, radiologic findings do not always correlate with clinical severity. Dynamic factors also play important roles in the development of myelopathy.

3. OPLL most frequently involves the cervical spine in middle-aged or elderly men, but OPLL at thoracic levels is more frequent in women than in men.

4. An occupying ratio of more than 60% and SAC of less than 6 mm indicate high risk for development of cervical myelopathy.

5. Because of the high frequency with which cervical OPLL is associated with thoracolumbar OPLL and OLF, the preoperative survey should include examination of the entire spinal column. Because it is difficult to detect stenosis at the cervicothoracic and thoracolumbar junctions on plain radiographs, careful preoperative and postoperative evaluation using CT or MRI or both should be performed to assess spinal stenosis.

6. The most effective surgical procedure for cervical OPLL is expansive laminoplasty for patients with OPLL occupying ratio of less than 60%, plateau-shaped ossification, and lordotic alignment of the cervical spine or the spinal cord.

7. Anterior decompression and fusion would be recommended for patients with OPLL occupying ratio of 60% or greater, hill-shaped ossification, local kyphotic alignment of the cervical spine or the spinal cord, and intervertebral hypermobility.

8. Poorer prognosis is associated with older age at operation, more severe preoperative symptoms, and history of trauma causing onset or progression of myelopathy.

9. Postoperative progression of the ossified lesion has been observed in 60% to 70% of patients who undergo posterior decompression; the incidence of postoperative progression after anterior decompression and fusion is 36% to 64%.

KEY REFERENCES

1. Ono K, Ota H, Tada K, et al: Ossified posterior longitudinal ligament: A clinicopathological study. Spine (Phila Pa 1976) 2:126-138, 1997.
   Pathologic features of the spine and spinal cord and clinical symptoms and signs of patients with OPLL are described.

2. Yonenobu K, Nakamura K, Toyama Y (eds): OPLL: Ossification of the Posterior Longitudinal Ligament, 2nd ed. Tokyo, Springer, 2006.
   This is the key textbook that provides overall information about OPLL.

3. Matsunaga S, Sakou T, Taketomi E, et al: Clinical course of patients with ossification of the posterior longitudinal ligament: A minimum 10-year cohort study. J Neurosurg 100(Spine 3):245-248, 2004.
   The authors report a long-term cohort study to elucidate the clinical course of OPLL after conservative or surgical management.

4. Iwasaki M, Okuda S, Miyauchi A, et al: Surgical strategy for cervical myelopathy due to ossification of the posterior longitudinal ligament. Part 1: Clinical results and limitations of laminoplasty. Spine (Phila Pa 1976) 32:647-653, 2007.
   The authors clarify factors predicting neurologic outcome and limitations of laminoplasty.

5. Iwasaki M, Okuda S, Miyauchi A, et al: Surgical strategy for cervical myelopathy due to ossification of the posterior longitudinal ligament. Part 2: Advantages of anterior decompression and fusion over laminoplasty. Spine (Phila Pa 1976) 32:654-660, 2007.
   The authors report a retrospective comparative study between the anterior approach and laminoplasty.

REFERENCES

1. Key GA: On paraplegia depending on the ligament of the spine. Guy Hosp Rep 3:17-34, 1838.

2. Oppenheimer A: Calcification and ossification of vertebral ligaments (spondylitis ossificans ligamentosa): Roentgen study of pathogenesis and clinical significance. Radiology 38:160-173, 1942.

3. Tsukimoto H: A case report: Autopsy of syndrome of compression of the spinal cord owing to ossification within the cervical spinal canal. Arch Jpn Chir 29:1003-1007, 1960.

4. Onji Y, Akiyama H, Shimomura Y, et al: Posterior paravertebral ossification causing cervical myelopathy: A report of eighteen cases. J Bone Joint Surg Am 49:1314-1328, 1967.

5. Matsunaga S, Sakou T: OPLL: Disease entity, incidence, literature search, and prognosis. In Yonenobu K, Nakamura K, Toyama Y (eds): OPLL: Ossification of the Posterior Longitudinal Ligament, 2nd ed. Tokyo, Springer, 2006, pp 11-17.

6. Terayama K: Genetic studies on ossification of the posterior longitudinal ligament of the spine. Spine (Phila Pa 1976) 14:1184-1191, 1989.

7. Koga H, Sakou T, Taketomi E, et al: Genetic mapping of ossification of the posterior longitudinal ligament of the spine. Am J Hum Genet 62:1460-1467, 1998.

8. Sakou T, Matsunaga S, Epstein N: Ossification of the posterior longitudinal ligament (OPLL): Epidemiology, pathology, etiology, diagnosis and treatment. In Ono K, Dvorak J, Dunn E (eds): Cervical Spondylosis and Similar Disorders. Singapore, World Scientific, 1998, pp 701-753.

9. Ono K, Ota H, Tada K, et al: Ossified posterior longitudinal ligament: A clinicopathological study. Spine (Phila Pa 1976) 2:126-138, 1977.

10. Ono K, Yonenobu K, Miyamoto S, et al: Pathology of ossification of the posterior longitudinal ligament and ligamentum flavum. Clin Orthop Relat Res 359:18-26, 1999.

11. Resnick D, Guerra J Jr, Robinson CA, et al: Association of diffuse idiopathic skeletal hyperostosis (DISH) and calcification and ossification of the posterior longitudinal ligament. AJR Am J Roentgenol 131:1049-1053, 1978.

12. Kameyama T, Hashizume Y, Ando T, et al: Spinal cord morphology and pathology in ossification of the posterior longitudinal ligament. Brain 118:263-278, 1995.

13. Hashizume Y, Kaneyama, Mizuno J, et al: Pathology of spinal cord lesions caused by ossification of the posterior longitudinal ligament. In Yonenobu K, Nakamura K, Toyama Y (eds): OPLL: Ossification of the Posterior Longitudinal Ligament, 2nd ed. Tokyo, Springer, 2006, pp 65-70.

14. Akune T, Ogata N, Seichi A, et al: Insulin secretory response is positively associated with the extent of ossification of the posterior longitudinal ligament of the spine. J Bone Joint Surg Am 83:1537-1544, 2001.

15. Shingyouchi Y, Nagahama A, Niida M: Ligamentous ossification of the cervical spine in the late middle-aged Japanese men: Its relation to body mass index and glucose metabolism. Spine (Phila Pa 1976) 21:2474-2478, 1996.

16. Tsuyama N: Ossification of the posterior longitudinal ligament of the spine. Clin Orthop Relat Res 184:71-84, 1984.

17. Matsunaga S, Nakamura K, Seichi A, et al: Radiographic predictors for the development of myelopathy in patients with ossification of the posterior longitudinal ligament: A multicenter cohort study. Spine (Phila Pa 1976) 33:2648-2650, 2008.

18. Matsunaga S, Sakou T, Taketomi E, et al: The natural course of myelopathy caused by ossification of the posterior longitudinal ligament in the cervical spine. Clin Orthop Relat Res 305:158-177, 1994.

19. Matsunaga S, Sakou T, Taketomi E, et al: Clinical course of patients with ossification of the posterior longitudinal ligament: A minimum 10-year cohort study. J Neurosurg 100(Spine 3):245-248, 2004.

20. Matsunaga S, Kukita M, Hayashi K, et al: Pathogenesis of myelopathy in patients with ossification of the posterior longitudinal ligament. J Neurosurg 96(Spine 2):168-172, 2002.

21. Ono K, Ebara S, Fuji T, et al: Myelopathy hand: New clinical signs of cervical cord damage. J Bone Joint Surg Br 69:215-219, 1987.

22. Iwasaki M, Okuda S, Miyauchi A, et al: Surgical strategy for cervical myelopathy due to ossification of the posterior longitudinal ligament. Part 1: Clinical results and limitations of laminoplasty. Spine (Phila Pa 1976) 32:647-653, 2007.

23. Matsunaga S, Sakou T, Hayashi K, et al: Trauma-induced myelopathy in patients with ossification of the posterior longitudinal ligament. J Neurosurg 97(Spine 2):172-175, 2002.

24. Koyanagi I, Iwasaki Y, Hida K, et al: Magnetic resonance imaging findings in ossification of the posterior longitudinal ligament of the cervical spine. J Neurosurg 88:247-254, 1998.

25. Iwasaki M: Overview of treatment for ossification of the posterior longitudinal ligament and the ligamentum flavum. In Yonenobu K, Nakamura K, Toyama Y (eds): OPLL: Ossification of the Posterior Longitudinal Ligament, 2nd ed. Tokyo, Springer, 2006, pp 165-167.

26. Iwasaki M, Kawaguchi Y, Kimura T, et al: Long-term results of expansive laminoplasty for ossification of the posterior longitudinal ligament of the cervical spine: More than 10 years follow up. J Neurosurg 96(Spine 2):180-189, 2002.

27. Matsuoka T, Yamaura I, Kurosa Y, et al: Long-term results of the anterior floating method for cervical myelopathy caused by ossification of the posterior longitudinal ligament. Spine (Phila Pa 1976) 26:241-248, 2001.

28. Iwasaki M, Yonenobu K: Choice of surgical procedure. In Yonenobu K, Nakamura K, Toyama Y (eds): OPLL: Ossification of the Posterior Longitudinal Ligament, 2nd ed. Tokyo, Springer, 2006, pp 181-185.

29. Iwasaki M, Okuda S, Miyauchi A, et al: Surgical strategy for cervical myelopathy due to ossification of the posterior longitudinal ligament. Part 2: Advantages of anterior decompression and fusion over laminoplasty. Spine (Phila Pa 1976) 32:654-660, 2007.

30. Masaki Y, Yamazaki M, Okawa A, et al: An analysis of factors causing poor surgical outcome in patients with cervical myelopathy due to ossification of the posterior longitudinal ligament: Anterior decompression with spinal fusion versus laminoplasty. J Spinal Disord Tech 20:7-13, 2007.

31. Onari K, Akiyama N, Kondo S, et al: Long-term follow-up results of anterior interbody fusion applied for cervical myelopathy due to ossification of the posterior longitudinal ligament. Spine (Phila Pa 1976) 26:488-493, 2001.

32. Tominaga S: The effects of intervertebral fusion in patients with myelopathy due to ossification of the posterior longitudinal ligament of the cervical spine. Int Orthop 4:183-191, 1980.

33. Ohara S, Momma F, Ohyama T, et al: Anterolateral partial vertebrectomy for ossification of the posterior longitudinal ligament of the cervical spine. Spinal Surg (Jpn) 8:125-130, 1994.

34. Yamaura I, Kurosa Y, Matsuoka T, et al: Anterior floating method for cervical myelopathy caused by ossification of the posterior longitudinal ligament. Clin Orthop Relat Res 359:27-34, 1999.

35. Yonenobu K, Hosono N, Iwasaki M, et al: Neurological complications of surgery for cervical compression myelopathy. Spine (Phila Pa 1976) 16:1277-1282, 1991.

36. Epstein NE: Evaluation and treatment of clinical instability associated with pseudarthrosis after anterior cervical surgery for ossification of the posterior longitudinal ligament. Surg Neurol 49:246-252, 1998.

37. Macdonald RL, Fehlings MG, Tator CH, et al: Multilevel anterior cervical corpectomy and fibular allograft fusion for cervical myelopathy. J Neurosurg 86:990-997, 1997.

38. Shinomiya K, Okamoto A, Kamikozuru M, et al: An analysis of failures in primary cervical anterior spinal cord decompression and fusion. J Spinal Disord 6:277-288, 1993.

39. Kato Y, Iwasaki M, Fuji T, et al: Long-term follow-up results of laminectomy for cervical myelopathy due to ossification of the posterior longitudinal ligament. J Neurosurg 89:217-223, 1998.

40. Hirabayashi K, Miyakawa J, Satomi K, et al: Operative results and postoperative progression of ossification among patients with ossification of cervical posterior longitudinal ligament. Spine (Phila Pa 1976) 6:354-364, 1981.

41. Ratliff JK, Cooper PR: Cervical laminoplasty: A critical review. J Neurosurg 98(Spine 3):230-238, 2003.

42. Baisden J, Voo LM, Cusick JF, et al: Evaluation of cervical laminectomy and laminoplasty: A longitudinal study in the goat model. Spine (Phila Pa 1976) 24:1283-1289, 1999.

43. Epstein NE: Circumferential surgery for the management of cervical ossification of the posterior longitudinal ligament. J Spinal Disord 11:200-207, 1998.

44. Fields MJ, Hoshijima K, Feng AH, et al: A biomechanical, radiologic, and clinical comparison of outcome after multilevel cervical laminectomy or laminoplasty in the rabbit. Spine (Phila Pa 1976) 25:2925-2931, 2000.

45. Heller JG, Edwards CC 2nd, Murakami H, et al: Laminoplasty versus laminectomy and fusion for multilevel cervical myelopathy: An independent matched cohort analysis. Spine (Phila Pa 1976) 26:1330-1336, 2001.

46. Herkowitz HN: A comparison of anterior cervical fusion, cervical laminectomy, and cervical laminoplasty for the surgical management of multiple level spondylotic radiculopathy. Spine (Phila Pa 1976) 13:774-780, 1988.

47. Hirabayashi K, Toyama Y, Chiba K: Expansive laminoplasty for myelopathy in ossification of the longitudinal ligament. Clin Orthop Relat Res 359:35-48, 1999.

48. Sakaura H, Hosono N, Mukai Y, et al: C5 palsy after decompression surgery for cervical myelopathy: Review of the literature. Spine (Phila Pa 1976) 28:2447-2451, 2003.

49. Satomi K, Nishu Y, Kohno T, et al: Long-term follow-up studies of open-door expansive laminoplasty for cervical stenotic myelopathy. Spine (Phila Pa 1976) 19:507-510, 1994.

50. Tani T, Ushida T, Ishida K, et al: Relative safety of anterior microsurgical decompression versus laminoplasty for cervical myelopathy with a massive ossified posterior longitudinal ligament. Spine (Phila Pa 1976) 27:2491-2498, 2002.

51. Yonenobu K, Abumi K, Nagata K, et al: Inter- and intra-observer reliability of the Japanese Orthopaedic Association Scoring System for evaluation of cervical compression myelopathy. Spine (Phila Pa 1976) 26:1890-1894, 2001.

52. Chiba K, Yamamoto I, Hirabayashi H, et al: Multicenter study to investigate postoperative progression of ossification of the posterior longitudinal ligament in the cervical spine using a new computer-assisted measurement. Presented at 31st Annual Meeting of Cervical Spine Research Society, Scottsdale, AZ, December 2003.

53. Kawaguchi Y, Kanamori M, Ishihara H, et al: Progression of ossification of the posterior longitudinal ligament following en bloc cervical laminoplasty. J Bone Joint Surg Am 83:1798-1802, 2001.

54. Tomita T, Harada M, Ueyama K, et al: Radiological follow-up evaluation of the progression of ossification of posterior longitudinal ligament: The operative influence on the progression of ossification. Rinsho Seikei (Jpn) 34:167-172, 1999.

55. Seichi A, Takeshita K, Nakamura K: Choice of surgical procedures for thoracic ossification of the posterior longitudinal ligament. In Yonenobu K, Nakamura K, Toyama Y (eds): OPLL: Ossification of the Posterior Longitudinal Ligament, 2nd ed. Tokyo, Springer, 2006, pp 225-230.

56. Matsumoto M, Chiba K, Toyama Y, et al: Surgical results and related factors for ossification of posterior longitudinal ligament of the thoracic spine: A multi-institutional retrospective study. Spine (Phila Pa 1976) 33:1034-1041, 2008.

57. Tsuzuki N, Hirabayashi S, Abe R, et al: Staged spinal cord decompression through posterior approach for thoracic myelopathy caused by ossification of the posterior longitudinal ligament. Spine (Phila Pa 1976) 26:1623-1630, 2001.

58. Ohtsuka K, Terayama K, Tsuchiya T, et al: A surgical procedure of the anterior decompression of the thoracic spinal cord through the posterior approach. Seikei-Saigaigeka (Jpn) 26:1083-1090, 1983.

59. Tomita K, Kawahara N, Baba H, et al: Circumspinal decompression for thoracic myelopathy due to combined ossification of the posterior longitudinal ligament and ligamentum flavum. Spine (Phila Pa 1976) 15:1114-1120, 1990.

60. Yonenobu K, Ebara S, Fujiwara K, et al: Thoracic myelopathy secondary to ossification of the spinal ligament. J Neurosurg 66:511-518, 1987.

61. Yonenobu K, Korkusuz F, Hosono N, et al: Lateral rachiotomy for thoracic spinal lesions. Spine (Phila Pa 1976) 15:1121-1125, 1990.

62. Yamazaki M, Mochizuki M, Ikeda Y, et al: Clinical results of surgery for thoracic myelopathy due to ossification of the posterior longitudinal ligament: Operative indication of posterior decompression with instrumented fusion. Spine (Phila Pa 1976) 31:1452-1460, 2006.

Cervical Disc Replacement

Joseph D. Smucker, MD
Rick C. Sasso, MD

Cervical arthroplasty has undergone a dramatic evolution since the development of the original Bristol/Cummins device. Metal-on-metal implants have evolved in parallel with the development of novel bearing concepts incorporating metal alloys, polyethylene, and ceramics. This chapter presents the current state of this technique, including the results of early outcomes of more recently developed devices. Although early data from clinical trials are encouraging, the viability of such techniques needs to be shown in the long-term.

Background

The cervical spine consists of seven vertebral bodies with intervening discs. These discs function in load bearing and motion transfer. In addition to its biomechanical functions in motion, the cervical spine serves as the protective passage for the spinal cord and vertebral arteries. Much is known about the macrobiology of the intervertebral disc. Disc degeneration and the subsequent processes that ensue in the cervical spine are also well documented as the transition from mild degenerative disc disease to cervical spondylosis progresses. For many years, the surgical treatment for pathology in the cervical intervertebral disc has been limited to procedures that remove pathologic disc material and address the bony and neurologic pathology in the region of the excised disc.

Anterior cervical discectomy and fusion (ACDF) is a proven intervention for patients with radiculopathy and myelopathy.[1] It has served as the standard by which other cervical and spinal disorders may be judged as the result of its high rate of success. The success of this technique is often judged based on its consistent ability to relieve symptoms related to neurologic dysfunction. In this sense, the clinical results with regard to the patient's index complaint are outstanding. The radiographic results of this technique are also initially predictable with a high rate of fusion. Plating techniques have diminished the need for postoperative immobilization or eliminated them entirely.[2] Because of limitations specific to this procedure, investigators have developed surgical alternatives to fusion that attempt to address the kinematic and biomechanical issues inherent in it.

A major concern related to the treatment of cervical degenerative disc disease and spondylosis with ACDF is the issue of adjacent segment degeneration. This event is manifest as the radiographic appearance of degenerative change at a level directly above or below a level treated with a surgical intervention—typically being associated with degeneration of a level adjacent to a fused level. The incidence of this phenomenon has been reported to be 92% by Goffin and colleagues,[3] who wrote a long-term follow-up on patients after treatment with anterior interbody fusion.

Although some debate remains regarding the causation of adjacent segment degeneration—with a mix of postsurgical and naturally determined aging cited as root causes—there is little debate regarding the existence of this phenomenon. It is also relevant to note the clinical distinction between *adjacent segment degeneration* and *adjacent segment disease*. Adjacent segment disease is defined as adjacent segment degeneration that causes clinical symptoms (pain or neurologic disorders or both) severe enough to lead to patient complaint or require operative intervention.[4] Although this distinction has not remained consistent in published literature, it is an important consideration with regard to the phenomenon that occurs in discs adjacent to discs that have undergone a surgical intervention. Numerous studies have made a consistent point of distinguishing between radiographic *degeneration* and symptomatic *disease*.[3,5]

There is clinical evidence to support the postsurgical nature of adjacent segment disease. In patients previously treated with fusion, adjacent segment disease has been documented at a rate of 2.9% of patients per annum by Hilibrand and colleagues,[4] and 25% of patients undergoing cervical fusion have new onset of symptoms within 10 years of fusion. This study has received a great deal of attention and has led to further investigations into biomechanical causation. Other reports have focused on the recurrence of neurologic symptoms and degenerative changes adjacent to fused cervical levels.[3,6] The concept that adjacent levels need to compensate for loss of motion in the fused segment may also be valid. Segments adjacent to a fusion have an increased range of motion and increased intradiscal pressures.[7,8]

Bone graft materials used in traditional ACDF procedures have also been a source of controversy. Current ACDF techniques make use of allograft bone, premanufactured allograft bone, and autologous iliac crest. Complications associated with autologous iliac crest harvest used as a fusion graft in ACDF are well documented. Sandhu and colleagues[9] reported a complication rate of 1% to 25% with such procedures. Complications such as acute and chronic pain, infection, meralgia paresthetica, and pelvic fracture are known to occur at harvest donor sites.[10,11]

Although allograft removes the risks associated with the harvest of autograft, it has the detriment of having the theoretical risk of disease transmission. In practice, this risk is believed to be extremely minute, although the U.S. Food and Drug Administration (FDA) has taken this issue seriously. The issues of disease transmission and contaminated graft materials have been highlighted by allograft tissue recalls by the FDA in recent years.[12] Although bone graft substitutes may play a role in the future practice of ACDF, this continues to be a minority stake in the overall graft selection of modern surgeons.

Pseudarthrosis is another complication encountered with anterior cervical fusion procedures. Pseudarthrosis is the failure of bony bridging or *nonunion* of a segment that has previously been treated with a bone graft or a bone graft substitute—an attempt at fusion has been made. In multilevel ACDF procedures, there is a relationship between the rate of pseudarthrosis and the number of levels fused. Brodke and Zdeblick[13] reported a 97% fusion rate in single-level ACDF, which decreased to 83% with fusion at three levels. Bohlman and colleagues[1] reported an 11% pseudarthrosis rate in single-level fusions that increased to 27% with multilevel fusions.

In recent years, the use of bone morphogenetic proteins has been proposed as an alternative or adjunct to traditional bone grafting techniques to combat the pseudarthrosis issue in patients deemed to be at higher risk for this complication.[14,15] This off-label use has been associated with an increased incidence of swelling complications and concerns for graft resorption and migration of interbody implants.[16-19] These issues serve to strengthen the argument for fusion alternatives in the treatment of discogenic pathology in the anterior cervical spine.

Total intervertebral disc replacement (TDR) is designed to preserve motion, avoid limitations of fusion, and allow patients to return quickly to routine activities. The primary goals of the procedure in the cervical spine are to restore disc height and segmental motion after removing local pathology that is deemed to be the source of a patient's index complaint. A secondary intention is to preserve normal motion at adjacent cervical levels, which may be theorized to prevent later adjacent level degeneration. Cervical TDR avoids the morbidity of bone graft harvest.[20,21] It also avoids complications such as pseudarthrosis, issues caused by anterior cervical plating, and cervical immobilization side effects.

History of Disc Arthroplasty and Device Design

An understanding of the evolution of cervical TDR serves as an important lesson in the concepts of device design, TDR

bearing and wear characteristics, and articular constraint. In the late 1980s, Cummins and colleagues[22] developed a metal-on-metal ball-and-socket cervical disc replacement composed of 316L stainless steel. With the acquisition of this technology and the later development of new metal-on-metal devices came a rapid transition from this device to the most recent device, the PRESTIGE LP (Medtronic Sofamor Danek, Memphis, TN). A predecessor of this device, the PRESTIGE ST (Medtronic Sofamor Danek, Memphis, TN) is currently approved by the FDA for human use in the United States (Figs. 43–1 and 43–2). More recent additions to the metal-on-metal category of arthroplasty devices include the Kineflex-C disc (Spinal Motion, Mountain View, CA) and the CerviCore intervertebral disc (Stryker Spine, Allendale, NJ) (Figs. 43–3 and 43–4), which are in the process of U.S. FDA investigational device exemption (IDE) trials.

Numerous devices have evolved in parallel to the metal-on-metal implants, including the BRYAN cervical disc (Medtronic Sofamor Danek, Memphis, TN) (Figs. 43–5 through 43–7), the PCM (CerviTech, Rockaway, NJ), the DISCOVER (DePuy Spine, Raynham, MA), and the MOBI-C (LDR, Austin, TX). Each of these devices is in the process of limited human trials or U.S. FDA IDE submission and represents an alternative to metal-on-metal bearing surfaces, which have the potential for metal debris and systemic concentration of metal ions. To date, one such device, the Prodisc-C (Synthes Spine, Paoli, PA) (Figs. 43–8 and 43–9), has obtained approval for use in the United States.

A summary of the design characteristics of each of these devices is presented in Table 43–1. Although the ideas of

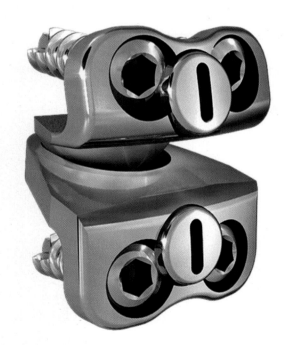

FIGURE 43–1 PRESTIGE ST cervical disc prosthesis is currently approved by the FDA for use in the United States. This stainless steel uniarticulating device attains primary fixation to the vertebral bodies via use of locked screws. (Implant representations courtesy Medtronic Sofamor Danek, Memphis, TN; with permission.)

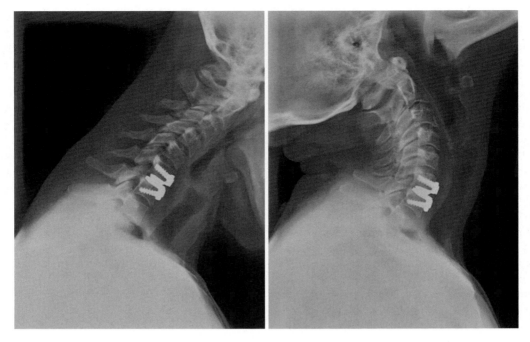

FIGURE 43–2 PRESTIGE ST prosthesis in C5-6 arthroplasty. Lateral flexion and extension radiographs show motion through arthroplasty device in this postoperative patient. (Courtesy Medtronic Sofamor Danek, Memphis, TN; with permission.)

bearing surface, wear debris, and constraint are not new to discussions with regard to arthroplasty in general, they are relatively new in regard to the spine. A full understanding of the term *constraint* has not been agreed on because constraint may arise within the device or as a result of the local anatomy (e.g., facets, posterior longitudinal ligament). As the knowledge base in spine TDR increases, intelligent investigations and discussions are sure to include many of these concepts and may redefine understanding of them.

It is relevant to understand the fact that the load borne by devices in the cervical spine is dissimilar to the load borne in the lumbar spine. The biomechanical environment of the cervical spine has been taken into account in the design of the current generation of these devices. As intermediate-term and long-term studies on individual devices become available, the design concepts of these initial devices will have the opportunity for continued examination in their in vitro environment.

FIGURE 43–3 CerviCore cervical disc prosthesis on lateral and expanded anteroposterior and lateral views. Initial fixation is obtained via vertical rails on the endplates. (Courtesy Stryker Spine, Allendale, NJ; with permission.)

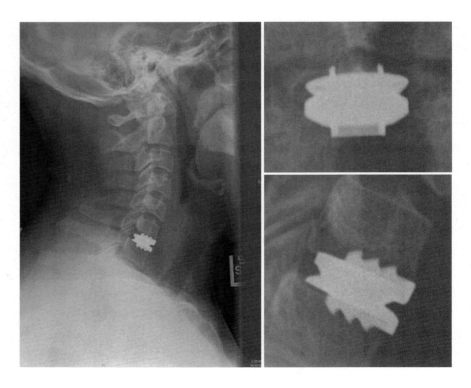

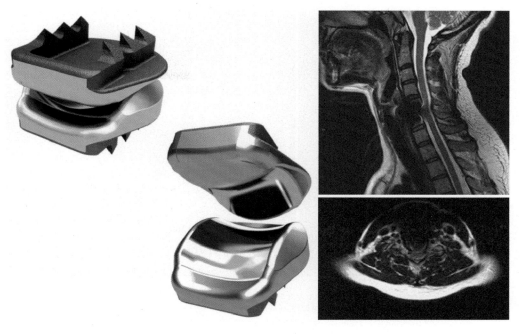

FIGURE 43–4 CerviCore cervical disc prosthesis is shown ex vivo and on T2-weighted MRI. MRI may show some artifact in the region of an arthroplasty device. (Courtesy Stryker Spine, Allendale, NJ; with permission.)

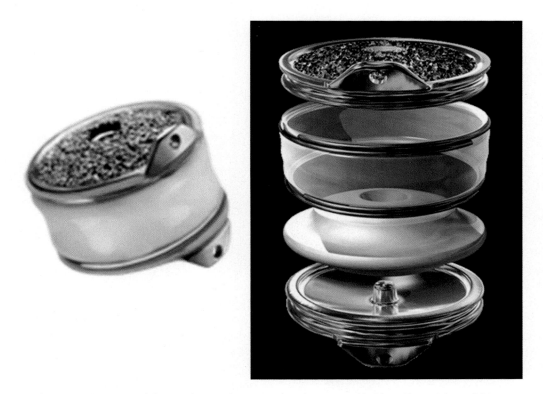

FIGURE 43–5 BRYAN cervical disc prosthesis is shown ex vivo and in unassembled form. The endplates of this device are unique in their design and promote ingrowth of bone into metallic surface. At the time of this publication, the BRYAN device remains under FDA review. (Courtesy Medtronic Sofamor Danek, Memphis, TN; with permission.)

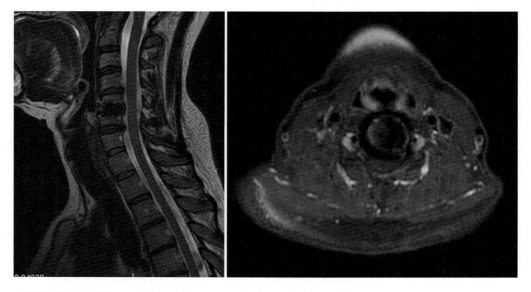

FIGURE 43–6 BRYAN cervical disc prosthesis is visualized on postoperative MRI. Titanium alloy devices such as the BRYAN device may have less MRI artifact than similar devices constructed with cobalt-chromium or stainless steel. These images show the imaging characteristics of this device at index and adjacent surgical levels. (Courtesy Rick Sasso, Indianapolis, IN.)

Indications for Use, Contraindications, and Complications

Cervical disc arthroplasty trials have included patients refractory to nonoperative treatment modalities with and without radiculopathy or myelopathy or both and with one-level and two-level degenerative disc disease or spondylosis.[23-25] These indications have been retained throughout the FDA approval process. At the time of this writing, two devices, the PRESTIGE ST and the Prodisc-C, have achieved FDA approval for single-level use in the United States. Other devices are in various stages of the IDE and approval process (Table 43–2). ACDF may be discussed as part of the indication process for an arthroplasty procedure. The historical challenges associated with ACDF presented in this chapter may be weighed

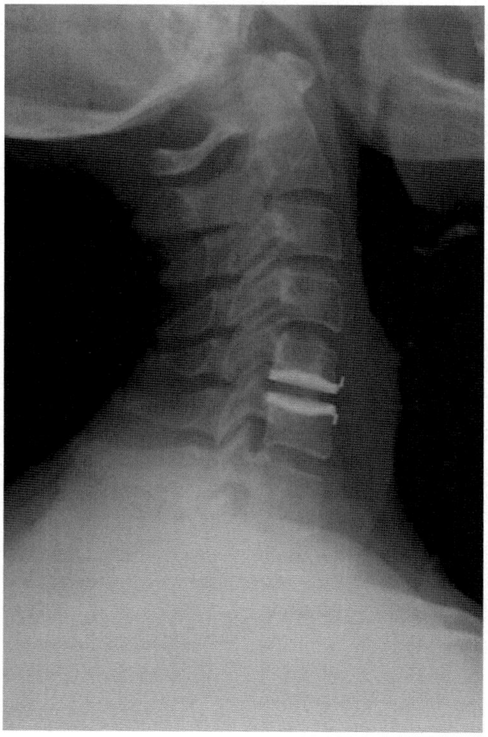

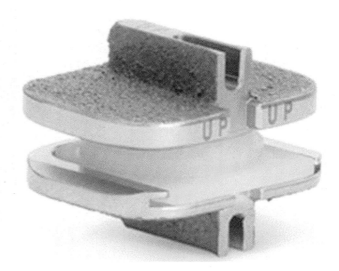

FIGURE 43–8 Ex vivo image of Prodisc-C. This device is approved by the FDA in the United States for cervical arthroplasty and obtains initial fixation via a central keel. Bone ingrowth is promoted via the surface alterations of the superior and inferior endplates of this device. (Courtesy Synthes Spine, Paoli, PA; with permission.)

FIGURE 43–7 Upright lateral view of a patient who underwent successful cervical arthroplasty at C5-6 with a BRYAN device. (Courtesy Medtronic Sofamor Danek, Memphis, TN; with permission.)

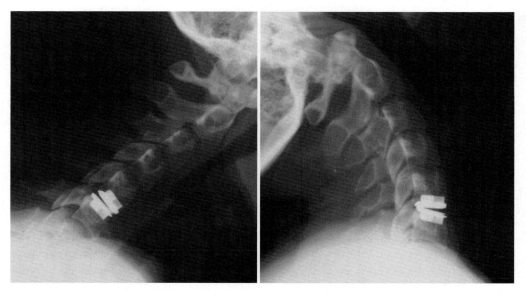

FIGURE 43–9 Prodisc-C is visualized on lateral flexion-extension radiographs. The device retains motion at index surgical level in this patient successfully treated with arthroplasty at C5-6. (Courtesy Synthes Spine, Paoli, PA; with permission.)

against the early nature of data with respect to cervical arthroplasty in a patient's informed consent discussion.

In determining indications for cervical arthroplasty of any type in a patient, it is relevant and appropriate to discuss verbally and obtain written consent for an intraoperative alternative to arthroplasty. In current practice, ACDF with plating and anterior corpectomy and fusion with plating remain options when it becomes clear to the operating surgeon that placement of an arthroplasty device may be compromised. This judgment to proceed with a fusion may occur as the result of endplate defects; arthroplasty sizing and fixation issues; or other bony, vascular, or neurologic issues that would prevent the appropriate placement of the device.

The appropriate time to discuss complications related to cervical arthroplasty is at the time of informed consent. The approach-related risks of cervical arthroplasty are similar to ACDF and should be discussed as such. These risks have been adequately covered in other portions of this text. A unique risk of arthroplasty is the concern of heterotopic ossification in the region of the arthroplasty device.[26-30] Heterotopic ossification may result in loss of motion or frank fusion of the index level. Heterotopic ossification may be associated with the physiologic response to the implantation process, the amount of bleeding or hemostasis necessary in a particular procedure, or the amount of bone debris created at the time of preparation for implantation. Postoperative use of nonsteroidal anti-inflammatory drugs has been suggested to moderate the prevalence of this risk.

Other complications may occur with cervical arthroplasty that are independent of the anterior cervical approach, including infection, implant migration, subsidence, continued or new neurologic findings, vascular injury, dural injury or cerebrospinal fluid leak, hematoma, and reoperation for adjacent level disease. Many complications associated with placement of arthroplasty devices have come to light as the result of reporting and analysis of the prospective randomized

multicenter U.S. FDA IDEs and large studies performed outside the United States.[23-25,31,32]

Cervical arthroplasty is contraindicated in patients with active or prior infection, osteoporosis or poor host bone, segmental cervical instability or segmental kyphosis, trauma, tumor, primary axial neck pain, significant facet arthropathy, posterior neurologic compression, anterior soft tissue abnormality (e.g., tracheal or esophageal abnormality, prior radiation), allergy to any of the device materials, severe spondylosis, pediatric patients, compromised vertebral body morphology, or (presently) disease involving more than one level. Other relative contraindications are similar to ACDF with the exception of nicotine use.

Preoperative Imaging

At a baseline, preoperative imaging for cervical arthroplasty should include plain radiographs with anteroposterior, neutral lateral, odontoid, and lateral flexion-extension films. The flexion-extension lateral views serve as a preoperative assessment of normal and abnormal mobility at the index and adjacent surgical levels. An advanced imaging modality such as magnetic resonance imaging (MRI) or computed tomography (CT) with the possible addition of myelography can be crucial to evaluating the index surgical level. These studies combine to allow assessment of spondylosis, preexisting facet arthropathy, neurologic compression, and cause and may provide insight into any preoperative contraindications in candidates for cervical arthroplasty.

Technique of Implantation

The technique of anterior cervical discectomy and the anterior approach to the spine are beyond the scope of this chapter.

TABLE 43–1 Design Characteristics of Past and Present Cervical Arthroplasty Devices

	Design	Modular	Articulating Method	Implant Composition	Bearing Surface	Primary Fixation	Secondary Fixation	Manufacturer
Bristol/Cummins*	Ball and socket	No	Uniarticulating	316L stainless steel	316L on 316L	Vertebral body screws	Vertebral body screws	None; technology by Medtronic
BRYAN	Biarticulating contained bearing	No	Biarticulating	Titanium, central polymer	Titanium alloy on polymer	Milled vertebral endplates	Endplate ingrowth	Medtronic Sofamor Danek
CerviCore	Ellipsoid saucer	No	Uniarticulating	Cobalt-chromium	Cobalt-chromium on cobalt-chromium	Ridged rails	Endplate ongrowth to titanium spray	Stryker Spine, IDE in progress
DISCOVER	Spherical bearing between superior titanium endplate and UHMWPE core	No	Uniarticulating	Titanium and UHMWPE	Titanium on UHMWPE	Teeth on superior and inferior endplates	Endplate ongrowth	DePuy Spine, IDE in progress
Frenchay/PRESTIGE I*		No	Uniarticulating	316L stainless steel	316L on 316L	Locked vertebral body screws, posterior endplate lip	Locked vertebral body screws, posterior endplate lip	None; technology by Medtronic
Kineflex-C	Modular three-piece bearing system with two endplates and mobile metallic core	Yes	Biarticulating	CCM	CCM modular core between two CCM endplates	Vertical keel and ridged endplate surface	Endplate ongrowth	Spinal motion
MOBI-C	Superior endplate with ball and socket motion; inferior endplate with sliding constraint	Yes	Biarticulating	Titanium	Titanium on polyethylene modular core	Lateral self-retaining teeth	Endplate ongrowth	LDR
PRESTIGE II*	Ellipsoid saucer	No	Uniarticulating	316L stainless steel	316L on 316L	Locked vertebral body screws	Locked vertebral body screws	None; technology by Medtronic
PRESTIGE LP	Ellipsoid saucer	No	Uniarticulating	Titanium/ceramic composite	Titanium/ceramic composite	Dual rails	Endplate ongrowth	Medtronic Sofamor Danek
PRESTIGE ST	Ellipsoid saucer	No	Uniarticulating	316L stainless steel	316L on 316L	Locked vertebral body screws	Locked vertebral body screws	Medtronic Sofamor Danek
PRESTIGE STLP*	Ellipsoid saucer	No	Uniarticulating	316L stainless steel	316L on 316L	Dual rails	Endplate ongrowth	None; technology by Medtronic
Prodisc-C	Ball and socket	No	Uniarticulating	Cobalt-chromium, UHMWPE	Cobalt-chromium on UHMWPE	Central keel	Endplate ongrowth	Synthes Spine
PCM	Upper endplate translation on fixed UHMWPE	No	Uniarticulating	Cobalt-chromium, UHMWPE	Cobalt-chromium on UHMWPE	Ridged metallic endplates	Endplate ongrowth	Cervitech
Secure-C	Metal on PE		Biarticulating	Cobalt-chromium, UHMWPE	Cobalt-chromium on UHMWPE	Ridged central keel	Endplate ongrowth	Globus Medical

*Devices not currently in production, current/known clinical use, or IDE investigation at the time of this writing.
CCM, cobalt-chrome-molybdenum; IDE, investigational device exemption; UHMWPE, ultrahigh-molecular-weight polyethylene.

The following description assumes a surgeon's comfort with this technique and suggests only specific modifications to the current approach relevant to anterior cervical arthroplasty compared with ACDF.

Intraoperatively, patient position is important. A "physiologic" or slightly lordotic cervical spine position is preferred.[33] Assessment via fluoroscopy (C-arm) is crucial to patient positioning and implant insertion and fixation portions of these procedures. It is important to keep the head, neck, and shoulders in a stable and neutral position throughout this surgical procedure. A small towel roll may be placed under the neck to assist with appropriate positioning of the neck and shoulders and to keep a physiologic lordosis without creating a hyperlordosis (Fig. 43–10). This positioning technique differs from the typical placement of a roll under the shoulders or thoracic spine, which could place the cervical spine in hyperlordosis. The head is placed on a doughnut-type pillow or a folded towel to keep it from rolling during the procedure. The careful positioning of shoulders with a taping technique can also allow for less motion during this procedure and must be carefully weighed against the risk of traction to the shoulders. Taping of the shoulders differs from the commonly used wrist restraints in a typical ACDF procedure that are used to obtain additional longitudinal traction via a temporary "pull" on the arms.

A standard right- or left-sided Smith-Robinson approach may proceed with appropriate localization and exposure of the index surgical level being the intent of this exposure. It is crucial to obtain a surgical exposure that allows for identification of the center of the index disc and vertebral bodies for later placement of the arthroplasty device. Disc arthroplasty is performed only after adequate decompression of the affected cervical level. At the surgeon's discretion for treatment of the index neurologic complaint, this may involve a complete discectomy from ventral to dorsal that also allows for placement of a device of appropriate width and adequate decompression, symmetrical resection of uncovertebral osteophytes and spurs, resection of all or part of the posterior longitudinal ligament, and any resection of central spondylotic osteophytes associated with degenerative disc disease. Meticulous hemostasis is recommended throughout this procedure to diminish the blood loss and minimize the risk of heterotopic ossification. It may become clear at any point during the neurologic decompression, endplate preparation, or device trialing process that arthroplasty is contraindicated. Should this occur, the surgeon must adjust the surgical plan intraoperatively and proceed with a fusion-based alternative.

After neurologic decompression, assessment for placement of an appropriately sized disc and planning for proper orientation of the implant are crucial to successful arthroplasty. To this end, it should be the surgeon's goal to place as large a device (with respect to diameter) as possible in the prepared space.[35] Device-specific tools may aid in this assessment.

Before any intervention that prepares the endplates, it is important to ensure the exact sagittal position of the vertebrae with lateral fluoroscopic imaging. Anteroposterior views are important to place the spinous processes at the target disc level between the pedicles to ensure perfect alignment and

TABLE 43–2 Current Status of Cervical Arthroplasty Devices in the United States*

Device	Manufacturer	U.S. FDA Status
PRESTIGE-ST	Medtronic Sofamor Danek	Approved
Prodisc-C	Synthes Spine	Approved
BRYAN disc	Medtronic Sofamor Danek	IDE data submitted, approval pending
CerviCore disc	Stryker Spine	IDE in progress
DISCOVER disc	DePuy Spine	IDE in progress
Kineflex-C disc	Spinal Motion	IDE in progress
MOBI-C disc	LDR	IDE in progress
PCM disc	Cervitech	IDE in progress
PRESTIGE-LP	Medtronic Sofamor Danek	IDE in progress
SECURE-C	Globus Medical	IDE in progress

*Table current as of April 1, 2009.
IDE, investigational device exemption.

centering in the coronal plane. Sizing of a cervical arthroplasty device may be determined with a combination of preoperative templates and preoperative radiographic studies including CT. The use of intraoperative trials and fluoroscopic imaging allows for additional assessment of proper device sizing and placement in the coronal and sagittal planes.

Endplates are prepared in a manner consistent with the device to be implanted. This preparation may include milling of the endplate (as in the BRYAN technique) or creation of a bony trough to accommodate an endplate keel (as in the Prodisc-C technique). Preservation of subchondral bone is otherwise crucial to the prevention of implant subsidence. Instrumentation specific to each arthroplasty device may be of great assistance in endplate preparation and may include special endplate distracters, keel preparation mills, rasps, and endplate mills. After the endplate preparation has been completed, it is appropriate to reassess the centering of the preparation and recheck the neurologic decompression.

Insertion of the artificial disc device may proceed and is implant-specific. Common to all devices is the principle of implantation to an appropriate depth based on implant design,

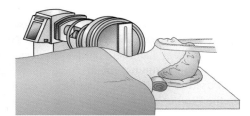

FIGURE 43–10 Positioning for cervical arthroplasty is as crucial to the technique as any portion of the procedure. Correct positioning of a patient maintains physiologic lordosis without creating hyperlordosis in the cervical spine and may be facilitated through use of a towel roll placed under the cervical spine. Techniques have moved away from traction through spine (as shown in this picture). Preoperative and intraoperative use of fluoroscopy allows for confirmation of patient positioning and device alignment. (Courtesy Rick Sasso, Indianapolis, IN.)

with a repeat assessment of implant centering and endplate coverage. After an assessment of the implant position in the coronal and sagittal planes has been done, the implant may be fixed to the spine with any implant-specific instrumentation such as screws.

Final imaging of the device implantation is performed before wound closure. Hemostasis is rechecked, and the surgical wound is closed in a standard fashion. Postoperative immobilization is not required. Upright flexion-extension radiographs may be obtained before discharge from the hospital and serve as a comparison to postdischarge radiographs for the purposes of follow-up.

Postoperative Imaging

Follow-up imaging of arthroplasty devices is crucial to the assessment of motion retention, adjacent segment disease, device wear and settling, device fixation, and neurologic decompression and status. Because the current generation of disc arthroplasty devices retains metallic components either in the endplates or in the bearing mechanism, radiation-based technologies have predominated as a mechanism of assessment. The workhorse studies remain flexion-extension and lateral bending plain radiographs because they are easily accessible, require less technician and physician technique in acquisition, maintain the ability to assess motion, eliminate the concerns of claustrophobia with MRI and CT, and are associated with moderate patient risk from radiation exposure. CT and CT myelography require an increased dose of radiation and are technique driven with respect to myelography.

To moderate the risks of technique and radiation associated with CT myelography, MRI has been proposed as an alternative that allows for postoperative assessment of neurologic status adjacent to and at the level of a prior cervical arthroplasty procedure. Success with this technique has been described by Sekhon and colleagues[34] in several devices, including the BRYAN and the PRESTIGE LP arthroplasty devices. Both of these devices use titanium alloy in their endplates, which was shown to produce less MRI artifact at the index and adjacent surgical levels than the metals associated with the manufacture of the Prodisc-C and PCM arthroplasty devices.[34] The BRYAN prosthesis has a polyurethane core, and the PRESTIGE LP had a titanium carbide alloy (as tested in the study). Investigators had difficulty assessing the neural structures at the index and adjacent levels with devices manufactured with nontitanium metals (cobalt-chromium-molybdenum) used in the Prodisc-C and PCM devices.

Although the Prodisc-C and PCM devices have nonmetallic bearing surfaces, the nontitanium nature of their metallic alloy seemed to be the major factor in the decreased ability of traditional MRI techniques to image neural structures. This information may prove to be crucial in the choice of implants for situations in which there is a need to assess the adequacy of neural decompression and monitoring of adjacent segment disease. Although this study did not examine all devices on the market, such as those made of 316 stainless steel or other

cobalt-chromium devices, it makes a strong case for careful consideration of device materials to be used in the future manufacturing processes of cervical arthroplasty devices.

Clinical Studies

The long-term clinical benefit of maintenance of motion is postulated to be delay or avoidance of adjacent level degeneration. All of the arthroplasty systems discussed herein are being investigated for use in the cervical spine. Although some of these systems have early published outcome data or have obtained U.S. FDA approval for use in single-level arthroplasty, long-term outcome studies are still pending.

PRESTIGE Disc

Wigfield and colleagues[35] reported favorable results on a 2-year pilot study of the first-generation PRESTIGE disc designed to address the safety of the technique and to assess the stability of, and motion allowed by, the device. The investigators tried to target patients most at risk for adjacent segment disease. Inclusion in the study required radiculopathy or myelopathy secondary to herniated disc or uncovertebral osteophytes confirmed on CT or MRI adjacent to a surgically or congenitally fused segment. An additional inclusion category was patients with asymptomatic disc degeneration adjacent to the symptomatic level without presence of a fusion. The study enrolled 15 patients. Wigfield and colleagues[35] concluded that the technique is safe because procedural complications were limited to two cases of transient hoarseness that resolved.

Motion was successfully preserved because all patients radiographically showed motion within an appropriate physiologic range. At 2 years, the mean motion in flexion-extension was 6.5 degrees (range 1 to 15 degrees). Anterior-posterior translation up to 2 mm was obtained. Device stability was concluded because no devices dislocated. Two of the 60 screws inserted broke mid-shaft at 6 months allowing settling of the caudal component. No other cases of settling were noted. The locking screws worked well, and no screw backout occurred.

A concerning finding is a lucent line that developed at the junction of the vertebral endplate and the anterior vertebral border suggestive of stress shielding. This lucency did not progress after 12 months. One patient required removal of the device and conversion to fusion for continued neck pain in extension. That device was found to be loose with surrounding fibrous tissue; however, there was no histologic evidence of infection, inflammation, or wear debris. Functional improvement was documented by improvements in visual analog scale (VAS) arm and neck scores, Oswestry Neck Disability Index (NDI) scores, and Short Form-36 (SF-36) scores at 2 years compared with preoperative scores. Statistical significance was not obtained because of the small number of patients in the study.

In a separate prospective nonrandomized study, Wigfield and colleagues[36] compared the effects of the PRESTIGE disc and one-level anterior fusion on adjacent segment motion. No significant difference in adjacent segment motion was measured between the two groups preoperatively. Postoperatively, there was a significant increase in adjacent segment motion in the fusion group (mean increase of 9 degrees) compared with a slight reduction in adjacent level motion noted in the TDR group. In the fusion group, adjacent segment motion increased 5% at 6 months and 15% at 1 year. Subgroup analysis showed that increased motion occurs predominantly in normal rather than degenerative adjacent discs.

A prospective, randomized clinical trial was conducted by Porchet and Metcalf[37] to compare the PRESTIGE II cervical disc with ACDF for the treatment of single-level degenerative disease. Standardized clinical outcome measures (NDI and SF-36) and radiographic examinations were used at prescribed postoperative intervals to compare the treatment groups. Of the 55 patients enrolled in the study, several had reached the final 24-month follow-up interval at the time of publication. Mean angular motion was 5.9 degrees at the disc level. Radiographic results showed that the PRESTIGE II disc maintained motion at the treated level without compromise of an adjacent segment. The authors concluded that use of the PRESTIGE II disc is as safe and as efficacious as standard ACDF at 24 months.

The most extensive report to date shows the results of the PRESTIGE ST device in a prospective randomized multicenter clinical trial.[23] Data from this report have served as the basis for the current FDA approval of the PRESTIGE ST device in the United States. In this one-to-one randomization protocol, patients underwent either single-level arthroplasty or single-level ACDF. Data were reported up to and including 24 months and showed that the PRESTIGE ST device compared favorably with ACDF with regard to the study's primary and secondary outcome measures. In addition, the device maintained an average of 7 degrees of angular motion and had no device failures or migration.

The study reported statistically significant differences in neurologic improvement, NDI, secondary surgical interventions, SF-36 scores, and neck pain in the investigational group compared with the control group at follow-up intervals of 12 and 24 months. Return to work was shortened in the investigational group 16 days sooner than the control group. Adjacent segment disease reoperations over the interval were decreased in the investigational group. The study concluded that arthroplasty with this device was safe and efficacious.

Mummaneni and colleagues[31] published their clinical experience with the PRESTIGE LP device. This study focused on history, indications, patient positioning, surgical technique, complication avoidance, and revision strategies. As further evidence becomes available, the manufacturers of the PRESTIGE LP device hope to advance further on the early favorable results obtained by its predecessor, the PRESTIGE ST.[23]

Prodisc-C

Bertagnoli and colleagues[38] published 1-year follow-up data on 27 patients who had single-level Prodisc-C implantation for treatment of one-level cervical degenerative disc disease. Standard preoperative and postoperative assessments of outcome were performed with NDI and VAS scores. Patients were also followed radiographically. Clinical outcome measures showed a sustained improvement at 1-year follow-up with a decrease in the NDI and VAS scores. Range of motion improved by 240% at 1 year compared with preoperative studies. Neck pain decreased by approximately 40%, arm pain frequency and intensity resolved to less than half of the original value, and no device-related or approach-related complications were noted.

The Prodisc-C has obtained approval by the U.S. FDA for use in single-level disc arthroplasty. Data from the multicenter human IDE trial have been published and to date represent the most significant compilation of outcomes with regard to this device.[25] This prospective randomized multicenter study examined the results of the Prodisc-C cervical arthroplasty device compared with ACDF in patients treated for symptomatic single-level cervical degenerative disc disease. Demographic data were similar between the investigation and control treatment groups. A total of 24 months of outcome data were examined and showed that the arthroplasty device is safe and effective with regard to the outcome measures examined compared with the fusion cohort.

The study examined NDI and SF-36 scores, VAS neck pain and VAS arm pain, and neurologic success. NDI and SF-36 scores were significantly less compared with presurgery scores at the follow-up visits for the investigation and control treatment cohorts. In both groups, VAS neck and arm pain were improved at the standard follow-up intervals compared with their preoperative values but did not differ between the two groups. Neurologic success, judged by improvement or maintenance, was improved in both groups but was not different between the groups. Range of motion was maintained at the arthroplasty level in 84.4% of the investigational group at 24 months. The fusion cohort had an 8.5% rate of secondary surgical procedures with the investigational group at a rate of 1.8%, a statistically significant difference at 24 months. The Prodisc-C TDR at least showed equivalence in all measured primary and secondary outcomes compared with ACDF with a total follow-up of 96.5% at 24 months for the entire study cohort.

BRYAN Disc

Goffin and colleagues[39] reported early results of a multicenter study of the BRYAN disc performed at single levels in 60 patients for the treatment of radiculopathy or myelopathy secondary to disc herniations or spondylosis failing at least 6 weeks of conservative treatment. Exclusion criteria included previous cervical spine surgery, axial neck pain as the sole symptom, significant anatomic deformity, and radiographic evidence of instability (translation >2 mm or >11 degrees of angulation compared with the adjacent level). Patient outcomes were determined by the Cervical Spine Research Society and SF-36 instruments. Clinical success rates at 6 months and 1 year were 86% and 90%, exceeding the study's targeted success rate of 85%.

In a separate report, Goffin and colleagues[40] published the intermediate-term results of this multicenter study. The study was expanded to include a second arm evaluating the treatment of two adjacent levels. The single-level arm had 103 patients enrolled, with 100 reaching the 1-year mark and 51 reaching 2-year follow-up. The bilevel study arm comprised 43 patients with 1-year data completed on 29 patients and 2-year data available on 1 patient. Success rates in the single-level study at 6 months, 12 months, and 24 months were 90%, 86%, and 90%. In the bilevel study, the success rate at 6 months was 82% and at 1 year was 96%. No device failures or subsidence was observed in any patient. At 1-year follow-up, flexion-extension range of motion per level averaged 7.9 degrees in the single-level arm and 7.4 degrees in the bilevel arm.

In the single-level study, three patients required subsequent surgical intervention. These procedures included the evacuation of a prevertebral hematoma, a posterior foraminotomy for residual compression, and a posterior laminectomy for residual myelopathy. Four subsequent procedures were required in the bilevel study: evacuation of a prevertebral hematoma, evacuation of an epidural hematoma, repair of a pharyngeal or esophageal injury caused by intubation, and anterior decompression owing to residual nerve root compression. Two patients developed dysphonia after second procedures. One patient initially had a device placed at a wrong level and developed temporary dysphonia after a device was placed at the appropriate level. The other patient developed a second symptomatic disc 21 months after the index procedure and developed severe dysphonia from bilateral vocal cord paralysis after a second device was placed from a contralateral approach.

Temporary anteroposterior device migration was detected in one patient and suspected in another. This migration was believed to be due to inadequate endplate milling early in the study. This issue was corrected with modification of the instrument system. Migration greater than 3.5 mm, the radiographic threshold of segmental stability, was not observed.

Sekhon[41] reported early results of nine patients with cervical spondylotic myelopathy who were treated with anterior decompression and reconstruction with the BRYAN disc. Follow-up ranged from 1 to 17 months. On average, the Nurick grade improved by 0.72 points, and NDI scores improved by 51.4 points. Improvement in cervical lordosis was noted in 29% of the patients. No complications were reported.

In another small prospective study, Duggal and colleagues[42] reported on 26 patients undergoing single-level or two-level implantation of the BRYAN artificial cervical disc for treatment of cervical degenerative disc disease resulting in radiculopathy or myelopathy or both. Patients were evaluated radiographically and via NDI and SF-36 at regular intervals. Segmental sagittal rotation from C2-3 to C6-7 was measured using quantitative motion analysis software. A total of 30 BRYAN discs were placed in 26 patients. Follow-up ranged from 1.5 to 27 months (mean 12.3 months). A statistically significant improvement in the mean NDI scores was seen between preoperative and late postoperative follow-up evaluations.

Anderson and colleagues[33] described the follow-up results of 73 patients who had greater than 2-year follow-up status on a one-level BRYAN disc arthroplasty. Of these patients, 45

were rated as excellent, 7 as good, and 13 as fair. Only eight patients had a poor rating at the 2-year follow-up. SF-36 functional outcome data showed significant improvement from preoperative to 3-month postoperative time points. These outcomes remained stable 24 months after surgery. There was no radiographic evidence of subsidence of implants. 89% of all patients had at least 2 degrees of motion at 1 and 2 years. Average range of motion was 8 degrees. There was one early anterior device migration associated with a partially milled cavity.

This same report noted the results of 30 patients who had two-level disc arthroplasty and had reached the 1-year end point in follow-up. Of the patients, 21 were rated as excellent; 3, good; 5, fair; and 1, poor. A significant improvement in SF-36 functional outcome measures was noted postoperatively. There was no radiographic evidence of subsidence in the two-level patients. At 1 year, 84% of patients had at least 2 degrees of motion at both disc levels. The average amount of motion at each disc level was also 8 degrees. There was one posterior migration of a device, again associated with a partially milled cavity. Complications in the study as a whole included one cerebrospinal fluid leak, one esophageal injury, four hematoma evacuations, and three revision decompressions.[33]

Sasso and colleagues[43,44] studied and reported on a group of patients regarding initial functional outcome results of the BRYAN artificial cervical disc replacement and compared them with fusion for patients with a cervical disc herniation or stenosis causing radiculopathy. Their prospective, three-center, randomized trial analyzed the data from three surgeons involved in the FDA IDE trial of the BRYAN cervical disc. Multiple outcome measures were used, including NDI, neck pain VAS, arm pain VAS, SF-36 physical component, SF-36 mental component, and range of motion flexion-extension.

At the more recent of the two publications, 12-month follow-up was presented for 110 patients, and 24-month follow-up was presented for 99 patients. Gender distribution was similar between the investigational and control groups. The average age was 43 years (BRYAN) and 46 years (fusion). Prospective data were collected before surgery and at 6 weeks and 3, 6, 12, and 24 months after surgery.

The average operative time for the control group was 1.1 hours and for the BRYAN group 1.7 hours. The mean NDI before surgery was not statistically different between groups: 47 (BRYAN) and 49 (control). At 12-month follow-up, NDI scores favored the arthroplasty device, a statistic that was retained at 2-year follow-up: NDI for the BRYAN group was 11 and for the control group was 20 ($P = .005$). Both groups improved compared with preoperative scores: at 1-year follow-up, BRYAN arm pain VAS was 12 and control was 23 ($P = .031$). At 2-year follow-up, the average arm pain VAS for the BRYAN group was 14 and for the control group was 28 ($P = .014$). Mean neck pain VAS improved in both groups after surgery, but the group-to-group comparison again favored the arthroplasty device: 1-year follow-up scores were 17 (BRYAN) and 28 (control) ($P = .05$) and at 2 years were 16 (BRYAN) and 32 (control) ($P = .005$). SF-36 physical component score before surgery for the BRYAN group was 34 and for the control group was 32; at 24 months, score for the BRYAN group was 51 and for the control group was 46 ($P = .009$).

More motion was retained after surgery in the disc replacement group than the plated group at the index level ($P < .006$ at 3, 6, 12, and 24 months). The disc replacement group retained an average of 7.9 degrees of flexion-extension at 24 months. In contrast, the average range of motion in the fusion group was 0.6 degree at 24 months. There were six additional operations in this series: four in the control group and two in the investigational group. There were no intraoperative complications, no vascular or neurologic complications, no spontaneous fusions (heterotopic ossification), and no device failures or explantations in the BRYAN cohort.

The most comprehensive data to date stem from the full multicenter cohorts of the U.S. FDA IDE trial published by Heller and colleagues.[24] This study presented the analysis of the multicenter groups using similar criteria and outcome measures as previously published in the studies by Sasso and colleagues.[44,45] As shown in the prior three-cohort study, the multicenter study with 242 patients enrolled in the investigational group and 221 enrolled in the control group showed statistically greater improvement in many of the primary outcome variables. Although both groups improved compared with preoperative scores, the investigational group had statistically favorable results in several outcomes, including NDI, neck pain, and return to work. Arm pain, SF-36 physical and mental components, and rates of neurologic success, although significantly reduced in both cohorts compared with preoperative levels, did not show significant group-to-group differences.

Adverse events related to the implant or surgical procedure were recorded and included a 2.9% rate in the BRYAN group (2.5% rate of revision) compared with a 3.2% rate in the ACDF group (3.6% rate of revision) at 24 months, a statistically similar rate. Fusion was successful in 94.3% of the control patients, and range of motion was 8.1 degrees at 24 months in the BRYAN group. Overall success was judged to be 82.6% in the BRYAN group and 72.7% in the arthroplasty group, a statistically significant difference. The device was found to be safe and efficacious.

Anderson and colleagues[32] reported on a comparison of adverse events between BRYAN arthroplasty and ACDF. This report is a novel analysis of the 463-patient cohort enrolled in the BRYAN arthroplasty IDE.[24] Adverse events were recorded at the intervals prescribed by the IDE study and categorized by severity and as medically or surgically related. Overall, no differences in adverse medical events occurred between groups. Surgically related adverse events were present at a higher rate in the BRYAN cohort than in the control cohort, largely owing to the increased incidence of dysphagia complaints and late medical events that occurred. An increased incidence of more severe events, World Health Organization grade 3 and 4, occurred in the ACDF group, however. This increased incidence was related to the revision treatment of pseudarthrosis and persistent symptoms after the index ACDF. Statistically more operations occurred in the control group. No deaths or deep infections were recorded in either cohort.

MOBI-C Disc

Early clinical results with the MOBI-C disc prosthesis have been reported in several studies.[46,47] Kim and colleagues[46] reported prospectively on a 23-patient cohort treated for cervical degenerative disc disease with 40 TDRs. Mean age was 43 years (range 31 to 62 years). Statistically significant improvement was observed in VAS arm and neck pain indices at the final follow-up interval of 6 months compared with the preoperative scores. Eight of the 23 patients were treated for an index complaint of cervical myelopathy and were assessed with the JOA myelopathy score. No statistically significant improvement was noted in myelopathy; however, the baseline presenting myelopathy for these 8 cases at the time of presentation was low. All patients were able to return to work within 1 month after surgery. No complications were observed in the entire cohort, and 95.6% of patients rated their outcome as either excellent or good by Odom criteria. Cervical mobility was preserved at the index and adjacent levels at the time of the final 6-month follow-up.

In a second study, Park and colleagues[47] retrospectively evaluated 53 patients treated for cervical disc herniations. This study contained arthroplasty (21 patients) and control (ACDF; 32 patients) groups. Patient follow-up was 12 months. Mean operative time was similar in the two groups, as was patient satisfaction at the final follow-up. In both groups, NDI and VAS arm pain improved compared with the preoperative state at 12 months, but the groups showed no statistical difference compared with one another at this interval. Segmental range of motion at the index level was maintained overall at final follow-up. No complications were observed in the arthroplasty group, and no heterotopic ossification was noted.

PCM Disc

Current literature regarding the PCM arthroplasty device stems largely from two clinical publications[48,49] and two publications that focus on cadaveric biomechanical[50] and caprine biomechanical[51] data. From a clinical standpoint, Pimenta and colleagues[48] published the first 53 patient experiences in 2004—a single-cohort case series. In this investigation, 82 arthroplasty devices were implanted in 53 patients who were followed with the VAS pain scale, the NDI, the Treatment Intensity Gradient Test (TIGT), and radiographic studies. The average patient age was 45 years. Of patients, 28 received a single-level arthroplasty, 22 received a two-level arthroplasty (6 patients with noncontiguous placement), and 3 received a three-level arthroplasty. At 1 week, 80% of patients had good or excellent results by Odom criteria, improving to 90% at 3 months. One postoperative complication, a device migration with 4 mm of anterior displacement, was noted at the 3-month follow-up interval.

At 12-month follow-up, the VAS average was 20 points (range 50 to 0), the NDI average was 15 points (range 14 to 0), the TIGT average was 3.5 points (range 14 to 0), and 97% of patients reported excellent or good results according to Odom criteria. Although an improvement compared with preoperative scores was noted with the outcome assessment tools used, no statistical metrics were reported in this analysis. Of working patients enrolled in this cohort, 87% were able to return to their baseline level of employment within 3 weeks.

A second prospective, consecutive series of 229 PCM arthroplasty implantations in 140 patients was later reported by Pimenta and colleagues in 2007.[49] This study reported the differences between two cohorts: patients with multilevel arthroplasty versus patients with single-level arthroplasty. In the index cohort, 71 patients received single-level arthroplasty; in the investigational cohort, 69 patients underwent 158 arthroplasties (multiple levels per patient). In the multilevel group, 53 patients received two-level arthroplasties, 12 patients received three-level arthroplasties, and 4 patients received four-level arthroplasties. Of the total surgeries, 21 were performed as arthroplasty revision procedures adjacent to a prior ACDF.

Outcome measures were recorded with NDI, VAS, and Odom criteria. Patient age and demographics were similar between the two cohorts. Only one case of heterotopic ossification (single-level cohort) was reported in this large series at an average follow-up of 26.8 months for both groups—and no nonsteroidal anti-inflammatory drugs were administered at any point in this study. Multilevel cases had a statistically greater estimated blood loss, length of surgery, and length of hospital stay compared with the single-level group. Multilevel cases consistently showed an increased improvement in outcome assessments at each follow-up interval compared with the single-level cohort with mean NDI improvement for single cases at 37.6% versus 52.6% in the multilevel cases (P = .021). This trend was also noted in VAS, TIGT, and Odom criteria. Reoperation rates and serious adverse events were similar between the two groups (three in single-level group and two in multilevel group), with four of five devices being converted to a more constrained version of the PCM and one converted to ACDF.

CerviCore, DISCOVER, Kineflex, and SECURE-C Devices

At the time of this writing, published clinical data are lacking on the outcomes of use of the CerviCore, DISCOVER, Kineflex, and SECURE-C cervical arthroplasty devices. Each of these devices remains in the process of human IDE trials in the United States. As data from these trials become available, it will be necessary and appropriate to compare these new data with the short-term and intermediate-term data that have been collected from devices farther along in the U.S. FDA approval process or devices with current approval. The design characteristics of these devices are summarized in Table 43–1, which serves as the basis for preliminary comparison of the devices with their peers.

Biomechanics

A primary goal of cervical disc replacement is to reproduce normal kinematics after implantation (see Figs. 43–2 and 43–9). Studies have been conducted to compare the biomechanics of cervical disc replacements on two kinematically different types of devices using identical protocols by the same laboratory.[52,53] These studies may suggest which type of implant design would provide more kinematically accurate motion.

The normal cervical spine motion exhibits anterior-posterior translation during flexion and extension. The motion segments of the cervical spine are complex joints. Each joint consists of three compartments (the disc and two facets) and multiple ligamentous structures. An implant designed to replace the cervical disc should consider the effect of all three compartments and multiple ligamentous structures.

DiAngelo and colleagues[52,53] investigated two different implant designs in human cadaveric spines to compare the motion of the harvested spine with the implanted spine. One of the designs was a semiconstrained device consisting of a ball-in-trough, which allows anterior-posterior translation (PRESTIGE cervical disc), whereas the other design was a constrained device consisting of a ball-in-socket with no anterior-posterior translation allowance (Prodisc-C). The results of the studies support the design rationale behind the PRESTIGE cervical disc. The semiconstrained device (PRESTIGE cervical disc) provided for normal kinematics in all ranges of motion tested, whereas the constrained device (Prodisc-C) failed to reproduce normal motion in extension.

A ball-in-socket (constrained design) does not allow for natural translation, a motion that has been clearly documented in the literature. The complexity of the cervical spine requires a "balance" of all the significant structures, including facets and ligaments. A ball-in-socket, by its design, dictates the kinematics and eliminates the normal anterior-posterior translation that the facets provide.

The most significant effect of this change in balance is in extension. When the spine goes into flexion, the facets "unshingle" and reduce their involvement in constraining the motion of the functional spine unit. When the spine goes into extension, the facets "shingle" and become more involved in constraining the motion. With a constrained facet joint and a constrained disc joint, one would expect to see binding or limited motion (also known as *kinematic conflict*), as one joint works against the other. This binding would give rise to decreased motion or increased stress on the system.

Balancing the kinematics in the functional spine unit is crucial. A constrained disc replacement may be unable to provide the normal kinematics of the cervical spine. Anterior-posterior translation is anatomic and must be allowed to restore normal motion. The PRESTIGE cervical disc was shown to maintain normal kinematics through *all* ranges of motion. Similar results would be expected from the BRYAN cervical disc system because it is also semiconstrained and allows for anterior-posterior translation in flexion and extension.

Sasso and colleagues[54] studied the kinematics of cervical motion from patients enrolled in a prospective, randomized, multicenter clinical trial. Radiographic data, including flexion, extension, and neutral lateral radiographs, were obtained preoperatively and at regular postoperative intervals up to 24 months. All patients had received either a single-level anterior cervical plate (Atlantis anterior cervical plate, $n = 221$) or a single-level artificial cervical disc (BRYAN cervical disc prosthesis, $n = 242$) at C3 to C7. Cervical vertebral bodies were tracked to calculate the functional spinal unit motion parameters. Parameters measured included flexion-extension range of motion and translation. These data were recorded at the index surgical level and, if visible, at the functional spinal units cranial and caudal to it.

More motion was retained in the disc replacement group than the plated group at the index level, a statistically significant finding. At 24 months, the arthroplasty group retained an average of 7.95 degrees (average 6.43 degrees preoperatively). In the control ACDF cohort, the average range of motion in the fusion group was 1.11 degrees at the 3-month follow-up and gradually decreased to 0.87 degrees at 24 months (average 8.39 degrees preoperatively). In the BRYAN cohort, index level functional spinal unit translation averaged 0.36 mm at 24 months, a data point that was statistically unchanged from the first postoperative measurement of translation at 3 months. No investigational devices showed radiographic evidence of subsidence at 24 months, and no heterotopic ossification was observed in the BRYAN cohort.

Angular range of motion at adjacent levels cranial and caudal to the index surgical functional spinal unit was measured and was not statistically different between the two cohorts preoperatively. At 24 months, these differences were unchanged in both groups (statistically similar). There was no consistent correlation between angular range of motion at adjacent or index levels and standard outcome measures of success in the investigational group. These data were not analyzed in the control. This study showed that the BRYAN disc maintains mobility at the level of the prosthesis over 24 months. No conclusions with regard to the adjacent segments could be statistically reached at this early follow-up interval.

The PCM disc has also undergone bench-top and nonhuman testing published in peer-reviewed literature. McAfee and colleagues[50] established that the posterior longitudinal ligament provides a stabilizing influence to the cervical spinal segment. Biomechanical testing was performed using human cadaveric spines and a 6-degree-of-freedom spine simulator with additional optoelectronic motion measurement. The major finding was that biomechanical stability may be restored after complete anterior cervical discectomy with resection of the posterior longitudinal ligament via implantation of an arthroplasty device.

Wear Analysis

Failure of total joint arthroplasty has been largely attributed to wear debris from polymer-bearing surfaces. Wear debris induces an intense cellular inflammatory response, which results in the production of cytokines that cause resorption of bone.[55,56] This process, known as aseptic loosening, leads to destabilization and mechanical failure of the joint. Factors that influence the loosening process include particle size, shape, number, material surface chemistry, and concentration and

duration of exposure.[57-61] The possibility of a similar process occurring after cervical disc replacement is concerning especially given the polymeric bearing surfaces of the several disc designs. In addition, the unknown effects of wear debris and inflammatory response in the spinal canal around neural structures are worrisome.

Anderson and colleagues[33,57] published two pivotal studies that reported on the wear characteristics of the BRYAN disc in vitro in a cervical spine simulator and in vivo in goat and chimpanzee models. In the first report, the in vitro results of six discs were tested to 10 million or 40 million cycles in a cervical spine simulator by load and motion, and an additional three assemblies were tested only to load. Wear debris was reportedly produced at a rate of 1.2 mg/1 million cycles. Device heights decreased 0.02 mm/1 million cycles. Debris particles averaged 3.9 μ in diameter, larger than the particles typically observed in hip and knee arthroplasty.

The local biologic response was reported in two chimpanzees, and local and distant tissue biologic response were reported in nine goats. Three additional goats had anterior fusion and plating. Local wear debris was found in one chimpanzee and four goats; however, no inflammatory response was seen in any animal. Some animals had wear debris in loose connective tissue and in the epidural space without evidence of inflammation. One goat had debris particles in the lumbar spine; however, they were at the extreme margins and not incorporated in the tissue, indicating they may have been artifactual. The plated fusion group exhibited greater metal debris and inflammatory response than the artificial disc group. Given their findings, the authors conclude that the low in vitro wear rate and lack of inflammatory response in vivo predict satisfactory long-term performance.

In the second report, Anderson and colleagues[33] examined the wear properties of BRYAN disc components in a custom cervical spine simulator and a goat model. The in vitro model involved simultaneous load and motion in six separate device assemblies with three control devices and was similar in design to the prior study.[57] Nuclei were measured before and after the test for weight, height, and diameter. Wear debris was assessed with a standardized system. The caprine model was undertaken in a certified animal care facility with anterior discectomy and placement of the BRYAN cervical disc in 11 goats. Four goats underwent a similar discectomy with fusion using allograft and plating with a titanium cervical plate.

The in vitro wear testing revealed a mean mass loss of 1.76% and a mean height loss of 0.75% after fatigue of 10 million cycles. Particulate debris had a mean diameter of 3.89 μ with a distribution histogram similar to total hip and knee replacement. The particles were elliptical in shape and larger in size, however, than particles associated with knee and hip arthroplasty. There was no dysfunction in the test or load assemblies at 10 million cycles, and the polymeric nuclei showed uniform wear on the load-bearing surface with the exception of one sample. Three assemblies were tested to the point of end plate–to–end plate contact, which was observed at 37.7 million, 39.7 million, and 40 million cycles. Loss of prosthetic height was linear in relationship to the number of cycles in this model.

The in vivo caprine model was analyzed in five predesignated groups after the sacrifice of: a baseline control goat on the day of surgery (group 1), 3 BRYAN disc goats at 3 months (group 2), 3 BRYAN disc goats at 6 months (group 3), 3 BRYAN disc goats at 12 months (group 4), and 3 goats fused with allograft and a plate at 12 months (group 5). Two goats were excluded from the study and analysis, including a goat originally assigned to group 2 who died on postoperative day 1 from a gastrointestinal obstruction and a goat originally assigned to group 5 who died as a result of a cervical fracture through a screw hole.

Tissues analyzed by an independent, blinded veterinary pathologist in the in vivo group included periprosthetic tissue, draining cervical lymph nodes, spinal canal tissues adjacent to the disc and at the rostral and caudal levels, liver, and spleen. A trend of increasing extracellular wear particles was noted with time with no appreciable inflammatory response seen at 3, 6, or 12 months. The three animals in the plate/control group all had particulate titanium debris in the periprosthetic tissues that was much greater in volume than that observed in the BRYAN prosthesis animals.

Hu and colleagues[51] examined the in vivo results of the PCM device at 6 and 12 months in a caprine model. Each goat underwent single-level arthroplasty at C3-4 and was followed thereafter for the prescribed time. At both intervals, the device had no evidence of loosening, subluxation, or inflammatory reaction. CT did not significantly obscure visualization of the spinal canal. Preservation of segmental spinal motion was noted in all specimens in biomechanical testing under load. The bone-prosthesis interface was found to be osteointegrated. Histopathologic review showed no significant wear debris of a particulate nature in local and systemic tissues—no significant pathologic changes were noted in the analyzed tissues.

Conclusion

Although far from being an accepted standard, the concept of artificial disc replacement is becoming a reality. The possibility of being able to minimize adjacent segment degeneration is exciting; however, much more intermediate-term and long-term outcome data are needed to prove that this technology supersedes the current "gold standard" of anterior fusion in ACDF. Biomechanical studies show that disc replacement creates less adjacent level strain than fusion; it is hoped that long-term studies will prove that this correlates to a lower incidence of adjacent level degeneration.

More recent clinical reports show promising early data suggesting that artificial disc replacement is comparable to fusion at least in the short-term.[23-25,31,45] Wear studies suggest that there may be less potential for aseptic loosening than in large joint arthroplasty, although the reality of this will be borne out only with more follow-up time. Although early reports of success in the United States with the TDR have allowed several devices to gain FDA approval[23,25] and suggest that the intended effects are being achieved, the final results of arthroplasty with these and other devices are pending the outcomes of long-term studies.

2. Cervical arthroplasty is designed to preserve motion and avoid some of the limitations and morbidity of cervical fusion, such as pseudarthrosis, bone graft harvest and allograft issues, anterior cervical plating, and cervical immobilization.

3. In addition to the primary goal of relief of symptoms from cervical degenerative disc disease, the technique of cervical arthroplasty has been theorized to provide an advantageous biomechanical environment that may counter the adjacent segment degeneration that has been observed in patients treated with ACDF.

4. At 24 months, arthroplasty seems to compare favorably with traditional ACDF in prospective randomized multicenter trials examining the outcomes of devices including the BRYAN, PRESTIGE ST, and Prodisc-C devices.

5. Intermediate-term and long-term follow-up are crucial to the assessment of devices used in this technique because the short-term data may not be an appropriate representation of the primary and secondary outcomes for motion-sparing technologies.

KEY REFERENCES

1. Mummaneni PV, Burkus JK, Haid RW, et al: Clinical and radiographic analysis of cervical disc arthroplasty compared with allograft fusion: A randomized controlled clinical trial. J Neurosurg Spine 6:198-209, 2007.
The authors report the clinical and radiographic results of a prospective randomized multicenter study examining the results of the PRESTIGE ST cervical arthroplasty device compared with ACDF in patients treated for symptomatic single-level cervical degenerative disc disease. At 12 and 24 months, the patients treated with the PRESTIGE ST device showed equal or greater success in the defined outcomes of the investigation and seemed to have maintenance of motion without implant failure.

2. Heller JG, Sasso RC, Papadopoulos SM, et al: Comparison of BRYAN cervical disc arthroplasty with anterior cervical decompression and fusion: Clinical and radiographic results of a randomized, controlled, clinical trial. Spine (Phila Pa 1976) 34:101-107, 2009.
This study reports the 24-month clinical and radiographic outcomes of a prospective randomized multicenter study examining the results of the BRYAN cervical arthroplasty device compared with ACDF in patients treated for symptomatic single-level cervical degenerative disc disease. The authors note equal or greater success in the study outcomes and conclude that the BRYAN arthroplasty device is a viable alternative to ACDF for single-level disease.

3. Murrey D, Janssen M, Delamarter R, et al: Results of the prospective, randomized, controlled multicenter Food and Drug Administration investigational device exemption study of the ProDisc-C total disc replacement versus anterior discectomy and fusion for the treatment of 1-level symptomatic cervical disc disease. Spine J 9:275-286, 2009.
This prospective randomized multicenter study examines the results of the Prodisc-C cervical arthroplasty device compared with ACDF in patients treated for symptomatic single-level cervical degenerative disc disease. The study examined 24 months of outcome data and showed that the arthroplasty device is safe and effective with regard to the outcome measures examined compared with the fusion cohort.

4. Hilibrand AS, Carlson GD, Palumbo MA, et al: Radiculopathy and myelopathy at segments adjacent to the site of a previous anterior cervical arthrodesis. J Bone Joint Surg Am 81:519-528, 1999.
This study reports adjacent level neurologic issues encountered in a series of patients who underwent anterior cervical arthrodesis. The study has served as a foundation of the premise that adjacent level disc disease may become problematic for this patient population and has served as a milestone for the development of alternatives to fusion technologies in the cervical spine.

5. Bohlman HH, Emery SE, Goodfellow DB, et al: Robinson anterior cervical discectomy and arthrodesis for cervical radiculopathy: Long-term follow-up of one hundred and twenty-two patients. J Bone Joint Surg Am 75:1298-1307, 1993.
A long-term single-series follow-up of anterior cervical discectomy and arthrodesis is presented that serves as a baseline for the traditional recommendation of ACDF in patients with symptomatic cervical spondylotic radiculopathy and myelopathy. The authors report their clinical and radiographic results and complications associated with this technique.

REFERENCES

1. Bohlman HH, Emery SE, Goodfellow DB, et al: Robinson anterior cervical discectomy and arthrodesis for cervical radiculopathy: Long-term follow-up of one hundred and twenty-two patients. J Bone Joint Surg Am 75:1298-1307, 1993.

2. Campbell MJ, Carreon LY, Traynelis V, et al: Use of cervical collar after single-level anterior cervical fusion with plate: Is it necessary? Spine (Phila Pa 1976) 34:43-48, 2009.

3. Goffin J, Geusens E, Vantomme N, et al: Long-term follow-up after interbody fusion of the cervical spine. J Spinal Disord Tech 17:79-85, 2004.

4. Hilibrand AS, Carlson GD, Palumbo MA, et al: Radiculopathy and myelopathy at segments adjacent to the site of a previous anterior cervical arthrodesis. J Bone Joint Surg Am 81:519-528, 1999.

5. Robertson JT, Papadopoulos SM, Traynelis VC: Assessment of adjacent-segment disease in patients treated with cervical fusion or arthroplasty: A prospective 2-year study. J Neurosurg Spine 3:417-423, 2005.

6. Goffin J, van LJ, Van CF, et al: Long-term results after anterior cervical fusion and osteosynthetic stabilization for fractures and/or dislocations of the cervical spine. J Spinal Disord 8:500-508; discussion 499, 1995.

7. Eck JC, Humphreys SC, Lim TH, et al: Biomechanical study on the effect of cervical spine fusion on adjacent-level intradiscal pressure and segmental motion. Spine (Phila Pa 1976) 27:2431-2434, 2002.

8. Fuller DA, Kirkpatrick JS, Emery SE, et al: A kinematic study of the cervical spine before and after segmental arthrodesis. Spine (Phila Pa 1976) 23:1649-1656, 1998.

9. Sandhu HS, Grewal HS, Parvataneni H: Bone grafting for spinal fusion. Orthop Clin North Am 30:685-698, 1999.

10. Brown CA, Eismont FJ: Complications in spinal fusion. Orthop Clin North Am 29:679-699, 1998.

11. Summers BN, Eisenstein SM: Donor site pain from the ilium: A complication of lumbar spine fusion. J Bone Joint Surg Br 71:677-680, 1989.

12. Mroz TE, Joyce MJ, Lieberman IH, et al: The use of allograft bone in spine surgery: Is it safe? Spine J 9:303-308, 2009.

13. Brodke DS, Zdeblick TA: Modified Smith-Robinson procedure for anterior cervical discectomy and fusion. Spine (Phila Pa 1976) 17:S427-S430, 1992.

14. Baskin DS, Ryan P, Sonntag V, et al: A prospective, randomized, controlled cervical fusion study using recombinant human bone morphogenetic protein-2 with the CORNERSTONE-SR allograft ring and the ATLANTIS anterior cervical plate. Spine (Phila Pa 1976) 28:1219-1225; discussion 1225, 2003.

15. Lanman TH, Hopkins TJ: Early findings in a pilot study of anterior cervical interbody fusion in which recombinant human bone morphogenetic protein-2 was used with poly(L-lactide-co-D,L-lactide) bioabsorbable implants. Neurosurg Focus 16:E6, 2004.

16. Smucker JD, Rhee JM, Singh K, et al: Increased swelling complications associated with off-label usage of rhBMP-2 in the anterior cervical spine. Spine (Phila Pa 1976) 31:2813-2819, 2006.

17. Vaidya R, Sethi A, Bartol S, et al: Complications in the use of rhBMP-2 in PEEK cages for interbody spinal fusions. J Spinal Disord Tech 21:557-562, 2008.

18. Vaidya R, Carp J, Sethi A, et al: Complications of anterior cervical discectomy and fusion using recombinant human bone morphogenetic protein-2. Eur Spine J 16:1257-1265, 2007.

19. Shields LB, Raque GH, Glassman SD, et al: Adverse effects associated with high-dose recombinant human bone morphogenetic protein-2 use in anterior cervical spine fusion. Spine (Phila Pa 1976) 31:542-547, 2006.

20. Silber JS, Anderson DG, Daffner SD, et al: Donor site morbidity after anterior iliac crest bone harvest for single-level anterior cervical discectomy and fusion. Spine (Phila Pa 1976) 28:134-139, 2003.

21. St John TA, Vaccaro AR, Sah AP, et al: Physical and monetary costs associated with autogenous bone graft harvesting. Am J Orthop 32:18-23, 2003.

22. Cummins BH, Robertson JT, Gill SS: Surgical experience with an implanted artificial cervical joint. J Neurosurg 88:943-948, 1998.

23. Mummaneni PV, Burkus JK, Haid RW, et al: Clinical and radiographic analysis of cervical disc arthroplasty compared with allograft fusion: A randomized controlled clinical trial. J Neurosurg Spine 6:198-209, 2007.

24. Heller JG, Sasso RC, Papadopoulos SM, et al: Comparison of BRYAN cervical disc arthroplasty with anterior cervical decompression and fusion: Clinical and radiographic results of a randomized, controlled, clinical trial. Spine (Phila Pa 1976) 34:101-107, 2009.

25. Murrey D, Janssen M, Delamarter R, et al: Results of the prospective, randomized, controlled multicenter Food and Drug Administration investigational device exemption study of the ProDisc-C total disc replacement versus anterior discectomy and fusion for the treatment of 1-level symptomatic cervical disc disease. Spine J 9:275-286, 2009.

26. Bartels RH, Donk R: Fusion around cervical disc prosthesis: Case report. Neurosurgery 57:E194, 2005.

27. Leung C, Casey AT, Goffin J, et al: Clinical significance of heterotopic ossification in cervical disc replacement: A prospective multicenter clinical trial. Neurosurgery 57:759-763, 2005.

28. Parkinson JF, Sekhon LH: Cervical arthroplasty complicated by delayed spontaneous fusion: Case report. J Neurosurg Spine 2:377-380, 2005.

29. Heidecke V, Burkert W, Brucke M, et al: Intervertebral disc replacement for cervical degenerative disease—clinical results and functional outcome at two years in patients implanted with the Bryan cervical disc prosthesis. Acta Neurochir (Wien) 150:453-459, 2008.

30. Mehren C, Suchomel P, Grochulla F, et al: Heterotopic ossification in total cervical artificial disc replacement. Spine (Phila Pa 1976) 31:2802-2806, 2006.

31. Mummaneni PV, Robinson JC, Haid RW Jr: Cervical arthroplasty with the PRESTIGE LP cervical disc. Neurosurgery 60:310-314, 2007.

32. Anderson PA, Sasso RC, Riew KD: Comparison of adverse events between the Bryan artificial cervical disc and anterior cervical arthrodesis. Spine (Phila Pa 1976) 33:1305-1312, 2008.

33. Anderson PA, Sasso RC, Rouleau JP, et al: The Bryan Cervical Disc: Wear properties and early clinical results. Spine J 4(6 Suppl):303S-309S, 2004.

34. Sekhon LH, Duggal N, Lynch JJ, et al: Magnetic resonance imaging clarity of the Bryan, Prodisc-C, Prestige LP, and PCM cervical arthroplasty devices. Spine (Phila Pa 1976) 32:673-680, 2007.

35. Wigfield CC, Gill SS, Nelson RJ, et al: The new Frenchay artificial cervical joint: Results from a two-year pilot study. Spine (Phila Pa 1976) 27:2446-2452, 2002.

36. Wigfield C, Gill S, Nelson R, et al: Influence of an artificial cervical joint compared with fusion on adjacent-level motion in the treatment of degenerative cervical disc disease. J Neurosurg Spine 96:17-21, 2002.

37. Porchet F, Metcalf NH: Clinical outcomes with the Prestige II cervical disc: Preliminary results from a prospective randomized clinical trial. Neurosurg Focus 17:E6, 2004.

38. Bertagnoli R, Duggal N, Pickett GE, et al: Cervical total disc replacement, part two: Clinical results. Orthop Clin North Am 36:355-362, 2005.

39. Goffin J, Casey A, Kehr P, et al: Preliminary clinical experience with the Bryan Cervical Disc Prosthesis. Neurosurgery 51:840-845; discussion 845-847, 2002.

40. Goffin J, Van CF, van LJ, et al: Intermediate follow-up after treatment of degenerative disc disease with the Bryan Cervical Disc Prosthesis: Single-level and bi-level. Spine (Phila Pa 1976) 28:2673-2678, 2003.

41. Sekhon LH: Cervical arthroplasty in the management of spondylotic myelopathy. J Spinal Disord Tech 16:307-313, 2003.

42. Duggal N, Pickett GE, Mitsis DK, et al: Early clinical and biomechanical results following cervical arthroplasty. Neurosurg Focus 17:E9, 2004.

43. Sasso RC, Foulk DM, Hahn M: Prospective, randomized trial of metal-on-metal artificial lumbar disc replacement: Initial results for treatment of discogenic pain. Spine (Phila Pa 1976) 33:123-131, 2008.

44. Sasso RC, Smucker JD, Hacker RJ, et al: Artificial disc versus fusion: A prospective, randomized study with 2-year follow-up on 99 patients. Spine (Phila Pa 1976) 32:2933-2940, 2007.

45. Sasso RC, Smucker JD, Hacker RJ, et al: Clinical outcomes of BRYAN cervical disc arthroplasty: A prospective, randomized, controlled, multicenter trial with 24-month follow-up. J Spinal Disord Tech 20:481-491, 2007.

46. Kim SH, Shin HC, Shin DA, et al: Early clinical experience with the Mobi-C disc prosthesis. Yonsei Med J 48:457-464, 2007.

47. Park JH, Roh KH, Cho JY, et al: Comparative analysis of cervical arthroplasty using Mobi-C and anterior cervical discectomy and fusion using the solis cage. J Korean Neurosurg Soc 44:217-221, 2008.

48. Pimenta L, McAfee PC, Cappuccino A, et al: Clinical experience with the new artificial cervical PCM (Cervitech) disc. Spine J 4:315S-321S, 2004.

49. Pimenta L, McAfee PC, Cappuccino A, et al: Superiority of multilevel cervical arthroplasty outcomes versus single-level outcomes: 229 consecutive PCM prostheses. Spine (Phila Pa 1976) 32:1337-1344, 2007.

50. McAfee PC, Cunningham B, Dmitriev A, et al: Cervical disc replacement-porous coated motion prosthesis: A comparative biomechanical analysis showing the key role of the posterior longitudinal ligament. Spine (Phila Pa 1976) 28:S176-S185, 2003.

51. Hu N, Cunningham BW, McAfee PC, et al: Porous coated motion cervical disc replacement: A biomechanical, histomorphometric, and biologic wear analysis in a caprine model. Spine (Phila Pa 1976) 31:1666-1673, 2006.

52. DiAngelo DJ, Robertson JT, Metcalf NH, et al: Biomechanical testing of an artificial cervical joint and an anterior cervical plate. J Spinal Disord Tech 16:314-323, 2003.

53. DiAngelo DJ, Foley KT, Morrow BR, et al: In vitro biomechanics of cervical disc arthroplasty with the ProDisc-C total disc implant. Neurosurg Focus 17:E7, 2004.

54. Sasso RC, Best NM, Metcalf NH, et al: Motion analysis of Bryan cervical disc arthroplasty versus anterior discectomy and fusion: Results from a prospective, randomized, multicenter, clinical trial. J Spinal Disord Tech 21:393-399, 2008.

55. Goodman SB, Lind M, Song Y, et al: In vitro, in vivo, and tissue retrieval studies on particulate debris. Clin Orthop Relat Res 352:25-34, 1998.

56. Goodman SB, Huie P, Song Y, et al: Cellular profile and cytokine production at prosthetic interfaces: Study of tissues retrieved from revised hip and knee replacements. J Bone Joint Surg Br 80:531-539, 1998.

57. Anderson PA, Rouleau JP, Bryan VE, et al: Wear analysis of the Bryan Cervical Disc prosthesis. Spine (Phila Pa 1976) 28:S186-S194, 2003.

58. Gelb H, Schumacher HR, Cuckler J, et al: In vivo inflammatory response to polymethylmethacrylate particulate debris: Effect of size, morphology, and surface area [erratum appears in J Orthop Res 12(4):598, 1994]. J Orthop Res 12:83-92, 1994.

59. Allen MJ, Myer BJ, Millett PJ, et al: The effects of particulate cobalt, chromium and cobalt-chromium alloy on human osteoblast-like cells in vitro. J Bone Joint Surg Br 79:475-482, 1997.

60. Gonzalez O, Smith RL, Goodman SB: Effect of size, concentration, surface area, and volume of polymethylmethacrylate particles on human macrophages in vitro. J Biomed Mater Res 30:463-473, 1996.

61. Goodman SB, Fornasier VL, Kei J: The effects of bulk versus particulate ultra-high-molecular-weight polyethylene on bone. J Arthroplasty 3(Suppl):S41-S46, 1988.

62. Anderson PA, Sasso RC, Riew KD: Update on cervical artificial disk replacement. Instr Course Lect 56:237-245, 2007.

63. Goffin J: Complications of cervical disc arthroplasty. Semin Spine Surg 18:87-98, 2006.

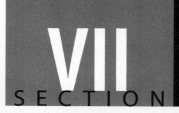

VII
SECTION

THORACIC AND LUMBAR DISC DISEASE

Thoracic Disc Disease

Bradford L. Currier, MD
Jason C. Eck, DO
Frank J. Eismont, MD
Barth A. Green, MD

Thoracic disc herniation is an uncommon disease. Diagnosis is often difficult, owing to myriad presenting symptoms. Advances in diagnostic methods, specifically, magnetic resonance imaging (MRI), have led to earlier diagnosis of symptomatic disc herniation. The natural history of thoracic disc herniation is unclear because improved diagnostic methods identify an increasing prevalence of asymptomatic thoracic herniated discs. Surgery generally is regarded as the treatment of choice for a symptomatic herniated thoracic disc with myelopathy to prevent the sequelae of cord compression. The prognosis associated with surgical decompression has improved dramatically with selection of surgical approach and the advent of techniques for disc excision without cord manipulation.

Historical Background

In 1838, Key[1] wrote the first report of a thoracic herniated disc causing spinal cord compression. Middleton and Teacher[2] reported the second case 73 years later. The first reported surgical treatment of a thoracic herniated disc was in 1922 by Adson, who performed a laminectomy and disc removal.[3] In their classic 1934 monograph on ruptured intervertebral discs, Mixter and Barr[4] described four cases of thoracic disc herniation; two of three patients treated surgically via laminectomy were rendered paraplegic, emphasizing the challenge in the management of the disease. In the ensuing years, many reports helped define the disease and document that treatment by laminectomy was unpredictable and very risky.[3,5-16]

The costotransversectomy approach was introduced by Menard[17] in 1900. Capener[18] later modified the procedure for use in the treatment of Pott disease. At Alexander's suggestion, Hulme[19] was the first to use this approach in the management of a herniated thoracic disc. Hulme[19] reported his experience with six patients treated by costotransversectomy and showed that it was a safer, more effective approach than laminectomy. In a later literature review of 49 surgical cases using costo-transversectomy, Arce and Dohrmann[20] noted 82% of patients improved, the condition was unchanged in 14% of patients,

and only 4% of patients experienced worsening of their condition.

Hodgson and Stock[21] popularized the anterior approach to the spine for the treatment of Pott disease. In 1958, Crafoord and colleagues[22] reported the first transthoracic procedure on the spine for a herniated disc. They performed a *fenestration,* or windowing of the disc without any attempt at disc removal or cord decompression. The one patient described in their article did well. Simultaneous reports by Perot and Munro[23] and Ransohoff and colleagues[24] in 1969 established transthoracic spinal cord decompression as a viable alternative to costotransversectomy. The posterolateral approach to the thoracic disc space was described by Carson and colleagues[25] in 1971 and was modified by Patterson and Arbit[26] in 1978.

All the surgical approaches have undergone minor modifications, including the application of microsurgical techniques.[27-29] Developments in the use of video-assisted thoracoscopic surgery (VATS) have provided an additional option in surgical treatment of a symptomatic thoracic herniated disc.[30-33] Each technique has advantages and disadvantages, and all but laminectomy are currently acceptable.

The diagnostic use of MRI has had a profound influence on the treatment of thoracic disc herniation.[34-42] At most centers, MRI has replaced myelography as the standard for the diagnosis of this condition. Because MRI is rapid, noninvasive, and increasingly available, its use is likely to decrease delay in diagnosis and lead to earlier treatment and perhaps improved prognosis. A new challenge is likely to be avoiding overdiagnosis and unnecessary operations on asymptomatic lesions.[41,43]

Epidemiology

The true incidence of thoracic herniated discs is unknown; many cases are unrecognized, or patients are asymptomatic. Most patients are in the 4th through 6th decades of life (Fig. 44-1).[3,6,44,45] In a review of 288 cases reported in the literature, Arce and Dohrmann[44] noted a slight male preponderance (1.5:1), although most series show an approximately even sex distribution.[5,11,46,47] Cases have been reported in patients ranging in age from 11 to 75 years.[25,48,49]

Historically, only 0.15% to 4% of all symptomatic protrusions of an intervertebral disc are in the thoracic spine.[3,5,6,12,44,50-52] Surgically, thoracic disc excision accounts for 0.2% to 1.8% of all operations performed on symptomatic herniated discs.[5,29,39,44,53-56] In 1950, Love and Kiefer[47] reported on 17 cases seen over 26 years. Logue[12] reported a thoracic herniated disc in 11 of 250 discectomies (4%). Otani and colleagues[51] later reported symptomatic thoracic disc herniation in 15 of 857 discectomies (1.8%) over a 15-year period. In a cadaveric study, Haley and Perry[57] showed that 11% of unselected autopsies revealed protruded thoracic discs; 2 of 99 specimens in their series had discs protruding 4 to 7 mm into the canal. The prevalence of herniated thoracic discs with an associated neurologic deficit has been estimated to be 1 per 1 million population.[25,42,47,52,58]

Improvements in imaging techniques have resulted in an increased detection of thoracic abnormalities and, concurrently, of herniated thoracic discs. Ryan and colleagues[59] reviewed 270 patients undergoing computed tomography (CT) of the thorax for suspected malignancy and found 4 (1.5%) who had asymptomatic calcified herniated thoracic discs. In a retrospective review of combined CT and myelography in 360 patients, Awwad and colleagues[60] found 54 herniations of a thoracic disc in 40 patients (11%) who were asymptomatic. In their study, 88% of the asymptomatic thoracic discs showed some deformity of the spinal cord; there was no single feature or combination of features clearly separating asymptomatic from symptomatic thoracic herniated discs.

The advent of MRI and its inherent sensitivity has increased further the reported incidence of thoracic disc herniations. Williams and colleagues[41] retrospectively reviewed 48 patients who underwent MRI for oncologic evaluation and reported a thoracic herniated disc in 7 (15%). Ross and colleagues[39] diagnosed 20 cases (16 confirmed) by MRI in a 2-year period compared with the initial report of Love and Kiefer[47] in 1949 of 17 cases seen over a 26-year period. Wood and colleagues[42] reported 66 of 90 asymptomatic individuals (73%) had positive anatomic findings at one or more thoracic levels; findings included herniation of a disc in 33 subjects (37%), bulging of a disc in 48 (53%), an annular tear in 52 (58%), and deformation of the spinal cord in 26 (29%). Wood and colleagues[42] reported no association between age and the prevalence of disc herniation. Compared with the MRI findings of 18 patients treated operatively for thoracic disc herniations in their study, the overall prevalence of these findings in the group that had thoracic pain was not significantly different from the asymptomatic population.

Williams and colleagues[41] suggested that thoracic disc herniation may be common enough to be considered a normal variant on MRI. More recently, Niemelainen and colleagues[61] reported that degenerative thoracic MRI changes were less common than previously reported. In a cross-sectional study of men 35 to 70 years old from the Finnish Twin Cohort study, only 9.2% of subjects had posterior disc bulging. Anterior disc bulging was much more common, found in 45.2%. The

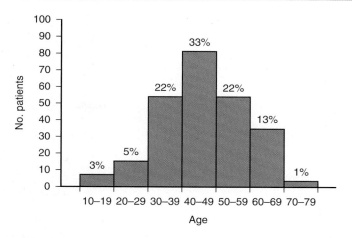

FIGURE 44–1 Distribution of 280 cases of thoracic disc herniation according to age. (From Arce CA, Dohrmann GJ: Herniated thoracic disks. Neurol Clin 3:383-392, 1985.)

presence of anterior disc bulging was positively correlated with age ($r = 0.15$ to 0.23, $P < .005$). Moderate to severe disc height narrowing ranged from 5.4% to 9.5% by level in the thoracic spine.

Etiology

Most authors favor degenerative processes as the major cause of thoracic disc herniation.[3,20,57] This theory is supported by the higher incidence of herniation in the thoracolumbar spine, where greater degenerative changes occur.[34,40,62] In a review of MRI findings and their relationship to thoracic and lumbar disc degeneration in a cohort of 232 subjects, Videman and colleagues[40] noted that moderate and severe osteophytes were most common at the T11-12 level (20.7% of subjects); upper endplate irregularities were most common at levels T8-12, typically in the middle of the endplates in the thoracolumbar spine compared with more peripheral endplate changes in the lumbar spine. These results were later supported by Niemelainen and colleagues,[61] who reported moderate to severe disc height narrowing in 21.4% of subjects.

The role of trauma as a cause of herniated thoracic discs is controversial. A history of trauma can be elicited in 14% to 63% of patients.[35,45] The mean prevalence in 10 random series was 34%. In some patients, the causal relationship is undeniable; in others, trauma may have been an aggravating factor or purely coincidental. The degree of reported trauma responsible for herniation ranges from minor twisting strains and chiropractic manipulation to major falls or motor vehicle accidents.[63]

Several authors[35,54,64] have suggested an association between Scheuermann disease and herniated thoracic discs. The primary pathogenic process of the disease or secondary disc degeneration may be the factors promoting herniation. Wood and colleagues[42] noted that endplate changes consistent with Scheuermann disease were more prevalent in their symptomatic patient group than in the asymptomatic population.

TABLE 44–1 Initial Symptoms of Protruded Thoracic Disc

Symptom	No. Patients (%)
Pain	102 (57)
Sensory	42 (24)
Motor	31 (17)
Bladder	4 (2)

From Arce CA, Dohrmann GJ: Herniated thoracic disks. Neurol Clin 3:383-392, 1985.

TABLE 44–2 Presenting Features of Thoracic Disc Herniation

Feature	No. Patients (%)
Motor and sensory signs and symptoms	131 (61)
Brown-Séquard syndrome	18 (9)
Sensory signs and symptoms only	33 (15)
Motor signs and symptoms only	13 (6)
Radicular pain only	20 (9)
Bladder or sphincter features	65 (30)

From Arce CA, Dohrmann GJ: Herniated thoracic disks. Neurol Clin 3:383-392, 1985.

Pathogenesis

The pathogenesis of neurologic compromise secondary to herniated thoracic discs is believed to be a combination of direct neural compression and vascular insufficiency.[2,3,6,12,26] Middleton and Teacher[2] suggested this in a case reported in 1911. Severe back pain developed while this patient was lifting a heavy object. Approximately 20 hours later, he felt a sudden severe pain shoot from his chest to his feet and he became almost completely paraplegic. The patient died 16 days later of urosepsis. The autopsy revealed a herniated thoracic disc opposite a section of cord that was compressed, degenerated, and hemorrhagic. A thrombosed vessel was found in the section of cord showing the most hemorrhage.

Several anatomic features make the thoracic cord vulnerable to manipulation and trauma.[26] The thoracic spinal canal is small, and most of its available space is occupied by the cord. The blood supply to the cord is tenuous in this region, especially in the "critical zone" of T4-9.[65] In addition, thoracic disc protrusions are more common centrally than laterally, are often calcified, and may adhere to or penetrate the dura.*

The theory of direct compression causing neural compromise is supported by the report by Logue[12] of a patient who died after a 14-month course of progressive paraplegia. The autopsy showed extreme distortion of the cord, but the anterior spinal artery and vein were patent and showed no evidence of damage. Kahn[68] suggested that, in addition to direct anterior compression by the herniated disc, the dentate ligaments may resist posterior displacement of the cord, leading to traction and distortion of neural structures.

Vascular insufficiency has been the explanation for unusual cases, such as cases with transitory paresis and instances in which the segmental level of involvement was higher than

*References 3, 12, 16, 20, 23, 66, 67.

expected from the location of the herniated disc.[3,6] Significant neural deficits may be caused by herniations that appear too small to cause significant compression. This theory also helps explain patients who show no improvement after complete decompression and patients who had an abrupt onset of paraplegia in the presence of a chronic calcified disc. The theory is supported by patients in whom the disc herniation has been shown to cause anterior spinal artery thrombosis.[12]

Doppman and Girton[69] performed an angiographic study on the effect of laminectomy in the presence of acute anterior epidural masses. They found that when decompression restored normal arteriovenous hemodynamics, the animals were neurologically intact despite significant cord distortion. When either the artery or the vein remained obstructed, however, the animals remained paraplegic.

Clinical Presentation

There is extreme variation in the clinical presentation of patients who have a herniated thoracic disc. This variation explains why no clear-cut syndrome has been identified. The signs and symptoms may depend on the location of herniation in the sagittal plane and the transverse plane. Additional factors may include size of the lesion, duration of compression, degree of vascular compromise, size of the bony canal, and health of the spinal cord.

In symptomatic cases, the condition is dynamic and can progress.[9] Tovi and Strang[16] outlined the usual chronologic progression, which begins with thoracic pain followed by sensory disturbances, weakness, and finally bowel and bladder dysfunction. Arce and Dohrmann[20] confirmed this pattern in their review of the literature: Of 179 patients who described their initial symptoms, 57% described pain, 24% described sensory disturbance, 17% described motor weakness, and 2% described bladder dysfunction (Table 44–1). By the time of presentation, 90% of the patients had signs and symptoms of cord compression, 61% had motor and sensory complaints, and 30% had bowel or bladder dysfunction (Table 44–2). The duration of symptoms before presentation ranged from hours to 16 years in one series.[3] In a report of 55 patients initially treated conservatively, Brown and colleagues[70] reported anterior bandlike chest pain as the most common early symptom in 67% of patients; lower extremity complaints were present in 20% of patients and ranged from paresthesia (4%) to frank muscle weakness (16%). Additional symptoms included intrascapular pain (8%) and epigastric pain (4%).

Thoracic pain can be midline, unilateral, or bilateral, depending on the location of the herniation. In some cases, there may be no pain. Coughing and sneezing may aggravate pain, as with herniated discs in the cervical and lumbar regions. With herniation of the T1 disc, the pain may be in the neck and upper extremity and simulate a cervical disc problem, causing upper extremity numbness, intrinsic muscle weakness, and Horner syndrome.[5,26,71]

When the herniation is in the mid-thoracic spine, radiation of pain into the chest or abdomen can simulate cardiac or abdominal disease, clouding an already complex clinical picture. In the four cases reported by Epstein,[7] one patient underwent an unnecessary thoracotomy for excision of a pericardial cyst, hysterectomy and salpingo-oophorectomy were performed in another patient, and a third patient almost underwent an abdominal exploration for endometriosis before the true cause of her symptoms was identified. Pain from a lower thoracic disc herniation may radiate to the groin or flank and simulate ureteral calculi or renal disease.[62,72,73] Abdominal wall paresis and abdominal hernia have also been presenting signs for thoracic disc herniations.[74,75] Herniated discs at the lowest thoracic levels can impinge on the cauda equina and on the distal spinal cord causing lower extremity pain or weakness and mimic a herniated lumbar disc.[76,77] On physical examination, flexion of the neck may induce back or root pain with lesions below the mid-thoracic level.[25] A thorough neurologic examination is mandatory, and the examiner should pay close attention to long tract signs and other evidence of myelopathy.

Some investigators believe that the occurrence of pronounced sensory changes with relatively minor motor deficits is highly suggestive of a herniated thoracic disc.[25,78] Sensory disturbances, motor weakness, sphincter dysfunction, and gait abnormalities should direct the examiner's attention to the nervous system as the source of the problem.

Level and Classification of Herniation

Three fourths of cases occur between T8 and L1; the peak is at T11-12, where 26% to 50% of herniations occur (Fig. 44–2).[20,40] Herniations are uncommon in the upper thoracic spine.[20,26,71] Haley and Perry[57] found a similar distribution in their cadaveric study of 99 spines and theorized that the increased incidence in the thoracolumbar area is due to the greater degree of motion in this region. The reason that the incidence at T11-12 is greater than that at T12-L1 (9%) may be the facet orientation. Malmivaara and colleagues[79] believed that the coronally oriented facets in the upper thoracolumbar region have less torsional resistance than the sagittally oriented facets at T12-L1, so the T11-12 disc is exposed to greater stress and has a high likelihood of degeneration.

Herniated thoracic discs can be classified by location or by symptoms. Most authors describe the location of the herniation as central, centrolateral, or lateral, and roughly 70% of the cases are either central or centrolateral.[20,60] In a comparison of characteristics on CT myelography of asymptomatic and symptomatic herniated thoracic discs, Awwad and colleagues[60] reported that 90% of herniations were central or parasagittal versus lateral in asymptomatic patients, whereas 80% were central or parasagittal in symptomatic patients. No identifiable radiographic features could reliably classify a herniated disc as symptomatic or asymptomatic. Abbott and Retter[5] classified cases by symptoms and reported that lateral protrusions cause root compression and that patients have radicular pain and minimal or no signs of cord compression. Patients with central disc herniation in the upper and middle thoracic spine can have myelopathy. Protrusions at T11 and T12 compress the

conus and cauda equina and may cause pain referred to the lower limbs and sphincter disturbance.

Few cases of intradural herniation of thoracic discs have been reported, suggesting that the incidence is low.[3,8,16,26,80-84] Love and Schorn[3] reported a series of 61 cases in which 7 (11%) showed disc erosion through the anterior dura. In a review of the literature, Epstein and colleagues[81] noted that 5% of all intradural disc herniations were found in the thoracic spine. Similar to the cervical spine, the low incidence was attributed to the lack of significant dural adhesions of the thoracic dura to the posterior longitudinal ligament and anulus fibrosus. Patients with intradural thoracic disc herniations tended to present with a higher incidence of Brown-Séquard syndromes and paraplegia.[44] In most cases, the presence of an intradural thoracic disc herniation is not identified preoperatively. CT myelography seems to have a higher sensitivity to detect this than MRI even with the addition of gadolinium.[80]

The exact incidence of multilevel herniations is unknown.[5,14,35,85] Arseni and Nash[6] reviewed the literature in 1960 and found multiple herniations in only 4 of 106 cases reported. A report by Bohlman and Zdeblick[35] suggested, however, that the incidence may be much higher than previously recognized. Of their 19 patients, 3 (16%) had herniations at two levels. The sensitivity of MRI may be partially responsible for this increased frequency.[37,39] Ross and colleagues[39] reported that 3 of 13 patients (23%) whose herniation was diagnosed by MRI had multilevel involvement; Wood and colleagues[42] reported multiple disc herniations in 39% of asymptomatic volunteers that were diagnosed by MRI. These rates are similar to the findings in the autopsy study by Haley

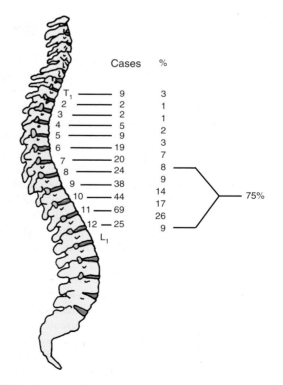

FIGURE 44–2 Levels of thoracic disc protrusion in 280 cases. (From Arce CA, Dohrmann GJ: Herniated thoracic disks. Neurol Clin 3:383-392, 1985.)

and Perry,[57] in which two of seven patients had more than one protruded disc.

Van Landingham[64] suggested an association between Scheuermann disease and multilevel herniation. Wood and colleagues[42] noted that endplate changes consistent with Scheuermann disease were more prevalent in the group with thoracic pain and disc herniation than in the asymptomatic population. Conversely, Lesoin and colleagues[54] reported six cases of single-level herniations only in patients with Scheuermann disease, suggesting a lack of significant association with multiple herniations.

Natural History

There are few long-term reports of untreated adults with herniated thoracic discs. In 1992, Brown and colleagues[70] reported a 2-year follow-up on 55 patients found to have thoracic disc herniation on MRI and concurrent pain; 11 (20%) initially had lower extremity complaints. Initial treatment in 54 patients included bed rest; nonsteroidal anti-inflammatory drugs; and controlled physical therapy involving hyperextension strengthening, postural training, and body mechanics education. Ultimately, 15 patients (27%) underwent operation. Of the remaining 40 patients treated nonoperatively, 31 (78%) returned to their prior level of activity. Nine of the 11 patients presenting with lower extremity complaints of pain or weakness underwent operation; 55% of herniated discs in the operative group were at or below T9. In contrast, 48% of the discs in the nonoperative group were at T6-9.

In patients with lower extremity complaints, the natural history of the disorder is typically one of progression, and nearly all patients eventually undergo operation for progressive neurologic deficit or unremitting pain.[3,11] The most characteristic chronologic progression of symptoms is pain followed by sensory disturbance, weakness, and bowel and bladder dysfunction.[16] The course can be extremely variable, however, and it is unknown whether neurologic signs or symptoms ever would have developed in patients operated on for pain alone. Some patients might have improved spontaneously if not subjected to surgical treatment. Haro and colleagues[86] reported on two patients with acute onset of symptomatic thoracic disc herniation with signs of myelopathy that resolved without surgery. Both patients had lower extremity signs of myelopathy, but neither developed bladder dysfunction or progressive motor weakness. Treatment with steroids and prostaglandin E_1 led to resolution of symptoms and resorption of thoracic disc herniation on follow-up MRI scans.

Arseni and Nash[6] described two general patterns for the time course of symptoms. The first, which occurs in younger patients with a history of trauma, is backache that can be followed by a rapidly evolving myelopathy. In the second pattern, which typically occurs in patients past middle age who have degenerative disc disease without any significant trauma, signs and symptoms of cord compression develop slowly and progressively. Tovi and Strang[16] found that when the first symptom to develop was unilateral, the course tended to be one of slow progression with periods of stabilization and occasional slight remission. Rapid, irreversible progression generally was noted in cases with a bilateral onset.

Calcification of the disc in children is considered to be a painful but self-limited process, with eventual resolution of the pain and resorption of the calcified deposit. It generally occurs in the cervical spine. About half of cases are preceded by a history of trauma (30%) or upper respiratory tract infection.[87,88] The natural history of herniated calcified thoracic discs in children was reviewed by Nicolau and colleagues.[89] The course was similar to cases without herniation; the patients improved spontaneously, and the calcified fragment resorbed. The progression is not always benign, however. Two cases in children have been reported in which myelopathy developed from cord compression and required operation.[13,67]

Disc calcification in adults differs from that in children. The thoracolumbar spine is the most frequent site of calcification, and the condition is generally asymptomatic unless herniation of the disc occurs.[87] The deposits may accelerate degeneration by interfering in the biomechanics and nutrition of the disc.[87,90] Disc calcification is found on routine radiographs in 4% to 6% of patients without disc herniation compared with up to 70% of patients with disc prolapse.[12,87] The natural history of disc herniation in adults has not been conclusively shown to be altered by disc calcification.

Differential Diagnosis

Love and Schorn[3] reported that before myelography the correct diagnosis was made in 13 of 61 patients and was considered in the differential diagnosis in only 7 others; even after myelography, the correct diagnosis was made preoperatively in only 56% of patients. With greater awareness of the diagnosis and improved imaging techniques now available, the correct diagnosis should be made before operation in almost all cases.

The differential diagnosis of back pain includes spinal tumors and infections, ankylosing spondylitis, fractures, intercostal neuralgia, herpes zoster, and cervical and lumbar herniated discs. Diseases of the thoracic and abdominal viscera may have a similar presentation. Neurosis is another possibility. The differential diagnosis of myelopathy includes demyelinating and degenerative processes of the central nervous system, such as multiple sclerosis and amyotrophic lateral sclerosis.[91,92] Intraspinal tumors, brain tumors, and cerebrovascular accidents also should be considered.[20,63]

In patients who have a neurologic deficit and radiographic evidence of Scheuermann disease, the differential diagnosis includes an extradural cyst or compression from an angular kyphosis.[54,93] In the series by Lesoin and colleagues,[54] the mean age of the patients who had a herniated thoracic disc in association with Scheuermann disease was 44 years, similar to the population without Scheuermann disease. This is in contrast to a mean age of 17 years in three patients in whom neurologic compromise developed secondary to bony cord compression at the apex of the kyphosis.[93]

Diagnostic Evaluation

Spine Radiographs

Plain radiographs of the spine generally are diagnostic only if they show disc calcification. The calcified disc is not always the one that is herniated, but the association at least suggests the diagnosis.[3,94] A calcified disc in the canal is pathognomonic of disc herniation.[12,27,28,94] Baker and colleagues[94] identified two radiographic patterns of calcification (Fig. 44–3). One consisted of extensive calcification posteriorly in the interspace and bulging into the canal. The other pattern, which is subtle and often overlooked initially, is a small nidus just posterior to the narrowed interspace. Studies[35,59] of adult lumbar discs have shown that the deposits may be calcium pyrophosphate dihydrate or calcium hydroxyapatite. The clinical significance of the different radiographic patterns or chemical compositions has not been determined.

The proposed association between Scheuermann disease and herniated thoracic discs has been discussed previously. A patient found to have kyphosis with vertebral body wedging and endplate irregularity in association with back pain or a neurologic deficit should undergo other studies to eliminate the possibility of a herniated disc. Other radiographic findings, such as narrowing and hypertrophic changes, are nonspecific and are not helpful in the diagnosis.[3,12,94]

Myelography

The thoracic spine is difficult to image by myelography because of the thoracic kyphosis and superimposition of mediastinal structures. Myelography alone is diagnostic in only 56% of cases and has a false-negative rate of 8%.[3] A complete block is found in 10% to 15% of cases.[16,94] Myelography is performed by injecting water-soluble contrast agent in the lumbosacral canal, removing the spinal needle, and placing the patient supine so that the contrast agent pools in the dependent thoracic kyphosis.[36] Anteroposterior and lateral films are essential. A herniated disc appears as a central filling defect at the level of the disc space (Fig. 44–4). Central protrusions produce discrete oval or round filling defects. In large protrusions, a complete block occurs with a blunt, convex leading edge.[12,94] Lateral discs produce triangular or semicircular indentations with displacement of the cord to the opposite side (Fig. 44–5).[94] Evaluation of cerebrospinal fluid at the time of myelography is nonspecific.[9] The protein content is increased in less than 50% of patients and helps only to focus attention on the central nervous system. It generally is in the range of 50 to 100 mg/dL but may be greater than 400 mg/dL.[53] Currently, myelography is most helpful in localizing lesions to allow directed CT and in preparation for operation.[35,95]

Computed Tomography

Enhanced CT after myelography with a water-soluble contrast agent is an extremely valuable technique and has been the diagnostic standard (Fig. 44–6).[35,36,39,44,50,60] When combined with standard myelography, CT not only improves sensitivity and accuracy, but also detects intradural penetration of the disc.[44,81]

CT alone may be helpful when the disc is calcified (Fig. 44–7), but it is impractical to image the entire thoracic spine and it is not as sensitive as CT with intrathecal injection of a contrast agent.[65] The criterion for diagnosis of a herniated disc by CT is a focal extension of the disc beyond the posterior aspect of the vertebral body with spinal cord compression or displacement.[39]

Magnetic Resonance Imaging

MRI has revolutionized the diagnostic evaluation of thoracic disc disease. Some centers rely on MRI almost exclusively, but

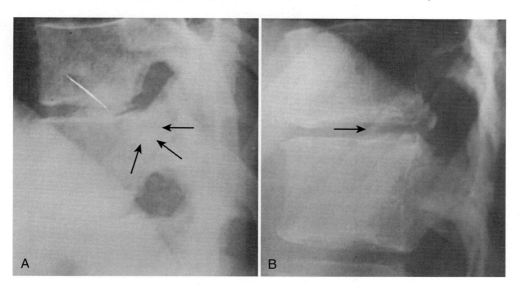

FIGURE 44–3 Plain radiographs can be used to diagnose herniated discs only when calcification is seen within spinal canal. **A,** Large calcified disc within canal (*arrows*) is nearly obscured by overlying ribs (see Figs. 44–7 and 44–8 for CT and MRI scans from same patient). **B,** Tiny nidus of calcium is visible in canal posterior to narrowed 11th interspace (*arrow*).

FIGURE 44–4 Oval filling defects in opaque column of iophendylate (Pantopaque) myelogram resulting from central protruded thoracic discs. Note midline position of spinal cord in all cases. **A,** Tiny protrusion visible at T9 interspace. **B,** Small protrusion at T12. **C,** Moderately large, slightly obstructing protrusion at T12. **D,** Large, severely obstructing protrusion at T12. **E,** Upper margin was outlined only when oil flowed caudad (*arrows*). **F,** Completely obstructing protrusion at T12. Note blunt, convex leading edge of column. (From Baker HL Jr, Love JG, Uihlein A: Roentgenologic features of protruded thoracic intervertebral disks. Radiology 84:1059-1065, 1965. By permission of The Radiological Society of North America.)

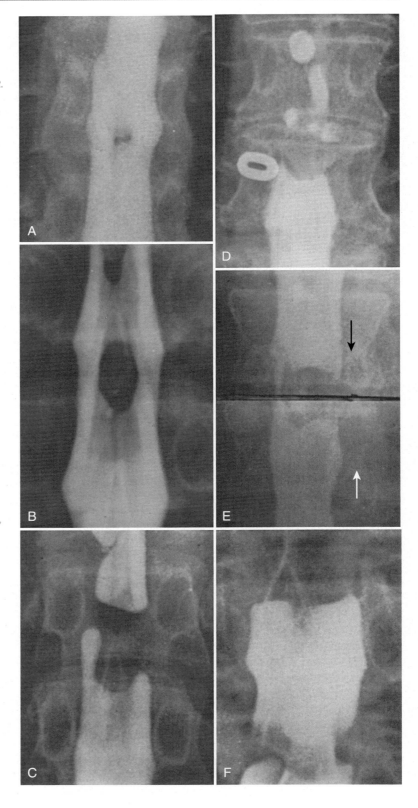

others still perform myelography and CT when operative treatment is being considered.[35-37] MRI is a rapid, noninvasive outpatient procedure that does not use ionizing radiation and causes no morbidity. It is a sensitive and specific technique that makes it easy to obtain sagittal sections of the entire thoracic spine.[36,37,39] Findings on MRI are similar to findings of myelography and CT, but it is necessary to use information from sagittal T1-weighted and T2-weighted and axial T1-weighted images to achieve similar sensitivity (Fig. 44–8).[39]

MRI is a highly technical procedure; the expertise of the radiologist and the design of the scanner determine the

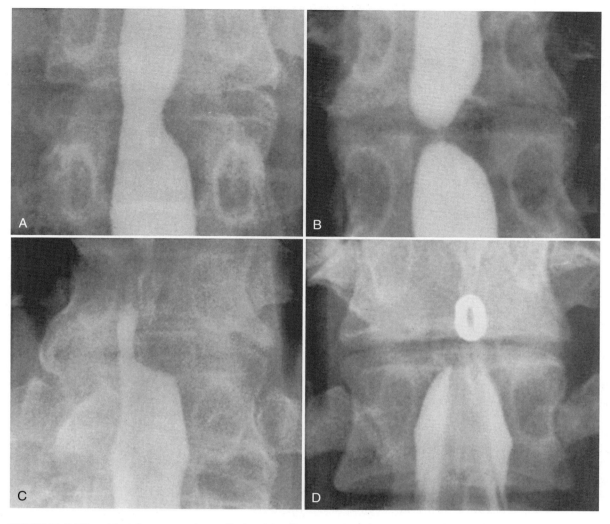

FIGURE 44–5 Filling defects in opaque column of iophendylate (Pantopaque) myelogram resulting from lateral protruded thoracic disc. Note lateral displacement of spinal cord in several cases. **A,** Small lateral protrusion at T11. **B,** Moderately large, slightly obstructing protrusion at T10. **C,** Large obstructing protrusion at T9. **D,** Completely obstructing protrusion at T10. Note pointing of column and deviation of spinal cord to left. (From Baker HL Jr, Love JG, Uihlein A: Roentgenologic features of protruded thoracic intervertebral disks. Radiology 84:1059-1065, 1965. By permission of The Radiological Society of North America.)

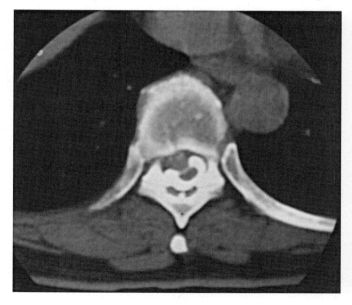

FIGURE 44–6 Postmyelography CT scan showing large, right centrolateral herniated disc at T8-9.

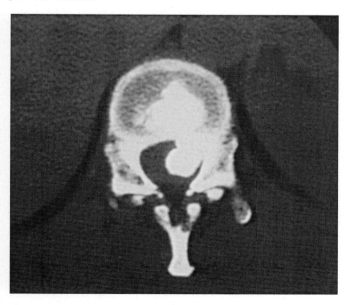

FIGURE 44–7 CT scan showing calcification of centrolateral herniated thoracic disc.

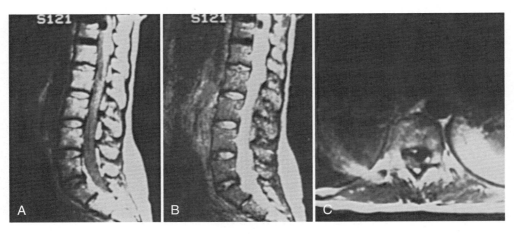

FIGURE 44-8 MRI of the patient in Figure 44–7 showing large, calcified, herniated thoracic disc at T11-12. **A,** T1-weighted sagittal image. **B,** T2-weighted sagittal image. **C,** T1-weighted axial image.

accuracy of the test to a great degree. There are pitfalls of MRI, such as partial volume averaging (owing to the relatively large section thickness), the cerebrospinal fluid flow void sign (regions of low signal intensity within the fluid owing to its pulsatile motion), signal dropout from calcified discs, chemical shift artifacts from marrow fat, and mismapped signal from cardiac motion.[36,39,96] Addition of gadolinium as a contrast agent has been reported to help in differentiating between thoracic disc herniations and small meningiomas; herniated disc material does not enhance, whereas spinal meningiomas show a very early, homogeneous, and intense uptake of contrast agent.[38]

Despite improved imaging and increased sensitivity, findings of thoracic disc herniation on MRI must be interpreted with caution and closely correlated with clinical findings. Several reports noted significant disc protrusion and spinal cord deformation in 30% of asymptomatic individuals.[42,60] In their large MRI series, Wood and colleagues[42] noted that the overall prevalence of thoracic disc herniation in the group with thoracic pain was not significantly different from the asymptomatic population.

Discography

The general sensitivity but lack of specificity of thoracic MRI in diagnosing painful thoracic disc disease sometimes may require the supplemental use of provocative discography to identify a specific thoracic disc pain source. In a retrospective review, Schellhas and colleagues[97] showed thoracic discography as a safe and reliable technique.

In a controlled prospective study, Wood and colleagues[98] compared MRI and discography in asymptomatic and symptomatic individuals. In asymptomatic volunteers, the mean pain response with discography was 2.4 out of 10. On discography, 27 of 40 discs were abnormal, with endplate irregularities, annular tears, or herniations. Ten discs read as initially normal on MRI showed annular pathology on discography. In symptomatic patients with chronic thoracic pain, the pain response with discography was 6.3 out of 10. Of the 49 discs

studied in this group, 55% had a concordant pain response, 39% had a discordant pain response, and 6% had no pain. On MRI, 21 of 49 discs appeared normal; however, on discography, only 10 were judged as normal. The only correlative pathology seemed to be Scheuermann endplate pathology as seen on MRI and Schmorl nodes as seen on discography.

In a systematic review of the literature, Buenaventura and colleagues[99] reported there is limited evidence to support the role of discography for the diagnosis of chronic thoracic discogenic pain. Given the general prevalence of degenerative thoracic disc pathology in asymptomatic individuals, discography apparently should be reserved for individuals with interdiscal pathology on MRI and thoracic axial pain unresponsive to an appropriate duration of nonsurgical treatment.

Treatment

Indications for surgery include (1) progressive myelopathy, (2) lower extremity weakness or paralysis, (3) bowel or bladder dysfunction, and (4) radicular pain refractory to conservative measures. Brown and colleagues[70] reported that 77% of patients with radicular pain as the primary presentation improved after a course of physical therapy. In cases of radicular presentation only, some authors believe that if the protrusion is far lateral with nerve root compression only, the situation is not urgent, and the decision to operate should be based on the degree of pain.[7] Conversely, there have been reports of lateral lesions causing severe neurologic deficits from compression of a major medullary feeder vessel.[55] Small herniations also should be respected because abrupt, severe, and irreversible deficits can occur; some investigators have concluded that there is no relationship between the size of the herniation and the gravity of the clinical picture.[11,27]

In cases of myelopathy and lower extremity involvement, most authors recommend early decompression. In cases of late treatment, favorable results are still possible despite significant delays and the presence of major neurologic deficits.[35] A less

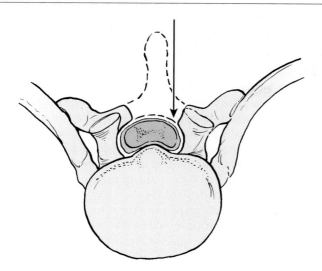

FIGURE 44–9 Attempted decompression by laminectomy would require manipulation of cord and high risk of neurologic deterioration.

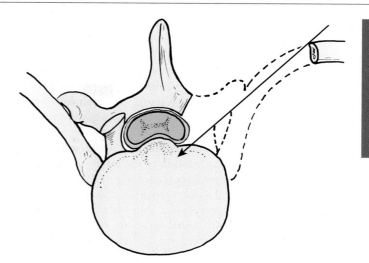

FIGURE 44–10 Decompression by costotransversectomy is possible without manipulation of cord.

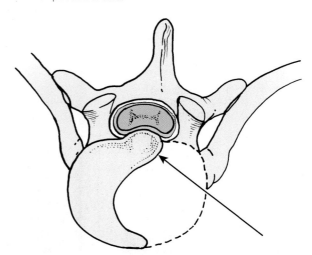

FIGURE 44–11 Transthoracic decompression allows the most direct approach to lesion without manipulation of cord.

aggressive approach may be taken in children because the natural history of the disorder seems to be different.[89]

The surgical management of this disorder has evolved in recent years. Laminectomy with disc excision was the benchmark approach 30 years ago but has been abandoned because of the risk of neurologic deterioration (Fig. 44–9). After the introduction of alternative techniques of decompression, Ravichandran and Frankel[100] noted a significant decrease in admission to spinal cord injury centers of patients with paralysis after treatment of herniated thoracic discs. In a review of 135 cases, Arce and Dohrmann[20] found that after laminectomy 58% of the patients were improved, 10% were unchanged, 28% were worse, and 4% had died. There is also evidence that patients who do not improve or who are made worse by laminectomy are less likely to be helped by later anterior decompression.[91] The best results are achieved in patients who have lateral lesions above T11, who have minimal neurologic deficits, who have a soft disc, and who are operated on early after the onset of symptoms.* Patients with myelopathy caused by ossification of the posterior longitudinal ligament have worse rates of recovery.[101] Although laminectomy is still occasionally advocated for lateral lesions, most authors think that the procedure is contraindicated.[28,103]

Singounas and Karvounis[104] described good results in patients treated by decompressive laminectomy alone without attempted disc removal. Several studies[8,12] described disastrous results with this technique, however. Studies in animals found consistent neurologic deterioration after decompressive laminectomy alone for anterior epidural masses.[69,105]

Costotransversectomy is an effective technique for managing herniated thoracic discs (Fig. 44–10).[10,45,106] Disc excision is performed through a paramedian incision with the patient prone[10] or in a modified lateral decubitus position.[106] The paraspinal muscles are either retracted medially or split transversely.[10,45] The posterior portion of each rib on the side of the herniated disc is excised, and the pleura is mobilized

and reflected anterolaterally. The transverse processes and remaining head and neck of each excised rib are removed. The intervertebral foramen is located by tracing the intercostal nerve medially. The foramen is enlarged by partial removal of the corresponding pedicles, and the dural sac is exposed. A cavity is created in the posterior aspect of the bodies and disc, allowing gentle removal of disc fragments through the defect without manipulation of the spinal cord.[10,45,107,108]

Transthoracic spinal cord decompression has been shown to be a viable alternative to costotransversectomy (Fig. 44–11).[23,24] Advantages include a more direct approach to the lesion and better visualization, facilitating excision of central herniations and herniations with intradural penetration. Disadvantages of the procedure include the potential complications associated with a thoracotomy.

Although many complications have been described after thoracotomy for other disorders, few have been reported after discectomy.* The results of transthoracic decompression

*References 3, 7, 16, 23, 82, 101, 102.

*References 20, 23, 24, 35, 46, 91, 109, 110.

are similar to results of costotransversectomy. In 53 cases collected from the literature, 52 patients improved, and 1 was unchanged. Bohlman and Zdeblick[35] reported the outcome in 19 patients treated by costotransversectomy or transthoracic decompression. The two poor outcomes in their series were in cases treated by costotransversectomy. They concluded that the transthoracic approach with its superior exposure was the preferred procedure.

Some authors[23,24,49,82,111] recommended preoperative angiography to determine the location of the artery of Adamkiewicz and other major medullary feeder vessels. If such a vessel is found at the level of the disc herniation, the spine could be approached from the opposite side. Alternatively, by carefully avoiding dissection in the neural foramina, this problem can be obviated without the need for an arteriogram. There is generally abundant collateral circulation in the region of the neural foramina that provides blood flow to the cord even with ligation of the artery of Adamkiewicz.[65,112,113] The authors routinely ligate the segmental vessels adjacent to the herniated disc midway between the foramina and the aorta and have not observed any untoward effects (Fig. 44–12).[91]

The patient is placed in the lateral decubitus position. A lateral prolapse is best approached from the ipsilateral side; a midline herniation may be approached from either side. In the upper or middle thoracic spine, the right side has the advantage of avoiding the great vessels and the heart. There also is statistically less risk to the artery of Adamkiewicz because this vessel is on the left in approximately 80% of the patients.[65] When the herniation is in the lower thoracic spine, a left thoracotomy is preferred because it is easier to mobilize the aorta than the vena cava, and the liver does not crowd the field.[23,35]

The level of rib resection is chosen to give the most direct access to the affected disc (see Fig. 44–12A). A horizontal line drawn on a chest radiograph from the disc space to the chest wall intersects the rib that should be resected. This is generally one to two ribs above the affected disc in the middle and lower thoracic spine.[82] In the upper thoracic spine, the exposure is limited by the scapula, and it is generally necessary to excise the fifth or sixth rib and then work craniad.

The recommended extent of bone and disc removal varies from a relatively small trough in the posterior aspect of the disc to complete discectomy with partial corpectomy of the

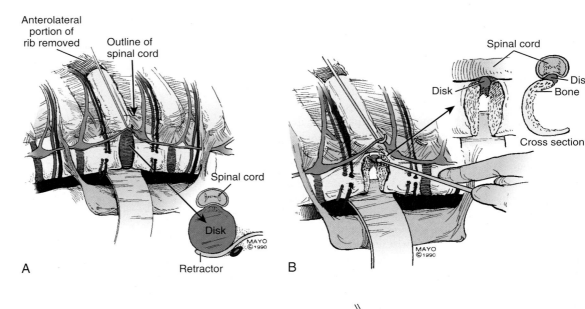

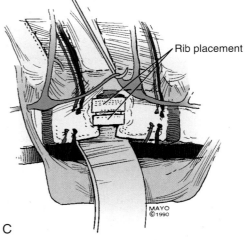

FIGURE 44–12 A, Exposure provided by transthoracic approach. Great vessels are mobilized by ligation of segmental vessels midway between aorta and neural foramina. A malleable retractor may be placed for protection of great vessels. **B,** Complete discectomy and partial corpectomy of adjacent vertebral bodies provides excellent visualization and allows complete decompression without disturbance of collateral vessels within neural foramina. **C,** Fusion is indicated when stability is compromised by decompression. (By permission of Mayo Foundation.)

adjacent bodies (see Fig. 44–12B).[23,28,35,82,91] The authors believe that the latter approach is safer because it provides the greatest degree of visualization and allows complete discectomy without disturbing the foraminal vessels. In either case, great care is taken to perform the decompression without any manipulation or pressure to the spinal cord.

Fusion is indicated when stability is compromised by the decompression and in cases associated with Scheuermann disease.[45] When only a small amount of bone and disc is excised, fusion generally is not recommended.[23,28,35,82] Conversely, with complete discectomy, fusion is mandatory (see Fig. 44–12C). In addition to providing stability, fusion may limit local pain secondary to motion of the degenerated segment. Recurrence of thoracic disc herniation has not been reported, but complete discectomy and fusion theoretically is the best way to prevent this complication. At the conclusion of the procedure, a chest tube is placed and attached to water-seal suction. If fusion has been performed, a thoracolumbo-sacral orthosis brace should be used.

Otani and colleagues[49] described a modification of the transthoracic procedure in which the pleura is dissected away from the chest wall after rib excision. This modification allows the approach to be entirely extrapleural. Their results were similar to results in other series of transthoracic decompressions. The advantage of the technique is the avoidance of a chest tube postoperatively. Claims of a lower incidence of pulmonary complications may be more theoretical than real because few such complications have been reported.

A posterolateral approach was described by Carson and colleagues[25] in 1971 (Fig. 44–13). They performed a complete laminectomy of the vertebrae adjacent to the herniated disc combined with a medial facetectomy and excision of the transverse process. A T-shaped incision through the erector muscle of the spine allowed an oblique approach to the anterior epidural space. Patterson and Arbit[26] modified the approach in 1978 to include the removal of the facet and pedicle of the vertebra caudal to the protruded disc through a straight midline incision. The central portion of the disc is removed by creating a cavity. The protruded material is excised by reduction of disc and bone into the cavity before removal. After anterior decompression, a complete laminectomy can be performed. Le Roux and colleagues[53] reported the results of the transpedicular approach and use of the operative microscope in 20 patients; all patients symptomatically improved postoperatively, 40% became asymptomatic, and no complications were noted.

Lesoin and colleagues[27] reported good results with a slightly more extensive exposure in which the transverse process, articular facets, and portions of the adjacent pedicles are removed. The extent of bone removal requires that a fusion be performed, and these authors recommended unilateral Harrington rod instrumentation. Spinal deformity has been reported to occur after posterolateral decompression without fusion.[15] In the 45 cases in the literature, 40 patients noted improvement (89%), the condition was unchanged in 3 patients, and it was worse in 1 patient; 1 patient died.[30] Some authors claim that intradural disc herniation can be dealt with much more easily with this approach than with any other; however, approaching anterior dural erosion by this technique requires some degree of manipulation of the cord.[97]

Other, less common approaches have also been described for upper thoracic disc herniations. Ulivieri and colleagues[114] described a transmanubrial osteomuscular sparing approach for T1-2 disc herniations. A transvertebral herniotomy has also been reported for a T2-3 lesion.[115]

Video-Assisted Thoracoscopic Surgery

The continuing evolution of VATS has provided experienced surgeons an alternative approach for thoracic disc herniation decompression. The technique of VATS was first described by Mack and colleagues[116] in 1993 for the drainage of thoracic paravertebral abscess. In 1994, Horowitz and colleagues[117] reported the clinical application of VATS for the treatment of thoracic disc herniation. Subsequently, several authors reported larger clinical series documenting the outcome of VATS-treated thoracic disc herniation.[1,19,30-32,56,118,119]

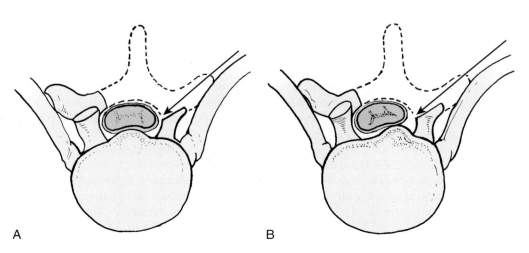

FIGURE 44–13 Posterolateral decompression. **A,** Removal of central herniation would require some manipulation of cord. **B,** Lateral herniations may be approached by this technique without manipulation of cord.

Reported advantages of VATS include reduced perioperative morbidity from minimal surgical dissection and avoidance of rib resection or spreading, enhanced visualization for the operating surgeons and support team, reduced postoperative pain with improved ventilatory excursion, shorter hospitalization and rehabilitation, and consequent decreased overall medical costs.[1,26] Disadvantages of VATS include the required coordination of two operative surgeons, an acquired technical skill set with a steep learning curve, specialized thoracoscopic instrumentation, and the required deflation of the ipsilateral lung for the procedure to be successful.

Indications for VATS application for thoracic disc herniation are similar to the indications for the anterior thoracic approach. The procedure can be performed in patients ranging in age from pediatric to geriatric. The minimally invasive nature of the VATS surgical approach and consequent reduced postoperative pain and inspiratory splinting make this approach applicable in patients less able to tolerate the physiologic effects of open thoracotomy, such as patients with chronic obstructive pulmonary disease or interstitial fibrosis. Patients with contraindications for VATS include patients intolerant of single-lung ventilation and patients with severe or acute respiratory insufficiency, high airway pressures with positive-pressure ventilation, and pleural scarring. Relative contraindications include previous tube thoracostomy or previous thoracotomy. For technical details of VATS technique, see Chapter 25.

In addition to numerous case reports, several authors have reported on large series of thoracic disc herniation treated by VATS.[30,32,56,118,119] In 1998, Regan and colleagues[32] reported their preliminary experience in 29 patients. Mean operative time was 175 minutes. The surgical complication rate was 14%, primarily from intercostal neuralgia and atelectasis. At 1-year follow-up, 76% of patients related satisfactory results; 24% of patients reported dissatisfaction or no change.

In a further extension of their series, Anand and Regan[30] reported outcomes on 100 consecutive cases with minimal 2-year follow-up. In 100 patients, 117 discs were excised; 40 patients underwent fusion: 27 with autologous rib strut and 13 with a threaded interbody fusion cage. Mean operative time was 173 minutes, mean blood loss was 259 mL, and average length of stay was 4 days. The surgical complication rate was 21%; 75% of the complications were pulmonary related (pleural effusion, pneumothorax, atelectasis, and pneumonia). Intercostal neuralgia occurred in six patients (6%) early in the series and declined subsequent to use of soft flexible intercostal trocars. One patient incurred a 2500-mL blood loss; open conversion to thoracotomy was done in one patient. Five patients underwent reoperation: four for secondary fusion secondary to discogram-positive intractable axial pain and one for pseudarthrosis with a threaded interbody fusion device that was removed and replaced with rib graft strut.

At final follow-up, 88 patients were available for evaluation. Of the 68 who responded to the patient satisfaction survey, 18% rated their procedure satisfaction as excellent, 54% as good, 16% as fair, and 12% as poor. Oswestry scores improved with 36% of patients with preoperative scores greater than 50 and 23% of patients with preoperative scores less than 50.

Patient satisfaction was greatest in patients with preoperative findings of myelopathy or lower extremity radicular pain or both and least in patients with pure thoracic radicular pain as the preoperative presentation.

Kim and colleagues[118] reported on the use of VATS in 20 consecutive patients with various thoracic pathologies. These investigators found VATS to be an effective minimally invasive technique but with a steep learning curve.

McAfee and colleagues[56] reported on the incidence of VATS complications in a series of 78 consecutive patients, 41 of whom underwent VATS for thoracic discectomy. Six patients showed a transient postoperative intercostal neuralgia; the incidence diminished with subsequent use of soft trocars. Atelectasis or effusion resulting in a prolonged hospital stay was seen in five patients. Blood loss greater than 2500 mL occurred in two patients. Penetration of the right hemidiaphragm occurred in one case with mild parenchymal laceration to the liver repaired thoracoscopically without postoperative sequelae. Intraoperative conversion to open thoracotomy was required in one patient secondary to scarring from a previous costotransversectomy.

Methodologic review of VATS emphasizes the necessity of initial portal placement at the midaxillary sixth or seventh intercostal space to avoid injury to vital organs. The recommended use of soft trocar portals and a meticulous technique emphasizing the constant visualization of all instrumentation tips was believed to be cardinal in the reduction of VATS-associated complications. Gille and colleagues[119] reported on the results of VATS in 18 cases of hard thoracic disc herniation. In 11 of the patients, there was no definitive plane between the calcified disc and the dura. Seven patients developed a dural tear with a high risk of cerebrospinal fluid fistula. Four of these seven patients required revision surgery.

Minimally Invasive Techniques

There have been several more recent reports of using minimally invasive techniques for the surgical treatment of thoracic disc herniations.[120-123] In a cadaveric and initial clinical study, Lidar and colleagues[122] reported the minimally invasive technique to be safe and effective. These investigators used a series of sequentially larger tubular dilators inserted on the lateral border of the rib head to allow visualization of the space between the costotransverse joint and caudal border of the costovertebral joint as shown in Figure 44–14. The joints are disarticulated, and the rib is freed and cut 2 cm distal to the costotransverse joint. The neurovascular bundle is identified and gently retracted. The transverse process is removed. The working tube is inserted deeper and medially. The pedicle is removed, starting at the foramen, allowing access to the disc.

The feasibility of this technique was first verified using four cadaveric specimens. Following that, Lidar and colleagues[122] used the technique on 10 patients with myelopathy secondary to thoracic disc herniation. The mean operative time was 171 minutes (range 150 to 220 minutes), mean blood loss was 215 mL (range 60 to 350 mL), and all patients had a 1-night hospital stay and returned to work within 4 weeks. There were no documented operative or postoperative complications.

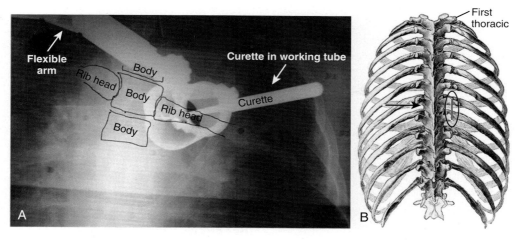

FIGURE 44–14 A, Intraoperative image detailing minimally invasive approach through dilated tube with curet placed on inferior border of rib head. **B,** Schematic drawing showing working area of tube. The *arrow* shows desired discectomy level. The *ellipse* shows working tube placement. The *vertical line* inside the ellipse shows skin incision. (From Lidar Z, Lifshutz J, Bhattacharjee S, et al: Minimally invasive, extracavitary approach for thoracic disc herniation: Technical report and preliminary results. Spine J 6:157-163, 2006.)

Summary

Symptomatic herniated thoracic discs are uncommon lesions that usually affect middle-aged adults. Diagnosis is difficult owing to myriad symptoms, and there is no clear-cut clinical syndrome. The natural history is unclear; improved diagnostic techniques have identified an increasing prevalence of asymptomatic herniated thoracic discs. The natural history of symptomatic patients generally is progression, often starting with pain followed sequentially by sensory, motor, gait, and sphincter disturbances. Many patients complain of pain only; others present with painless myelopathy.

Most herniations occur in the lower thoracic region, and central protrusions are more frequent than lateral protrusions. Multiple herniations and intradural penetration are uncommon. In most cases, the cause is a degenerative process, but a history of trauma can be elicited in approximately one third of cases; an association with Scheuermann disease has been suggested by several authors. The pathogenesis of neurologic compromise in thoracic disc herniation is believed to be a combination of direct neural compression and vascular insufficiency. The differential diagnosis is long and requires careful consideration. Radiologic evaluation is essential for the diagnosis, but plain films are helpful only if disc calcification is present. Myelography and CT and MRI are considered standard diagnostic tools, although no specific imaging features can reliably classify a herniated disc as symptomatic or asymptomatic.

Laminectomy is no longer indicated for treatment of thoracic disc herniation because of a high risk of neurologic deterioration and the fact that it may compromise the results of later anterior decompression. Discectomy may be performed by various surgical approaches: costotransversectomy, transthoracic, posterolateral, or video-assisted. The most rational way to manage the problem may be to select the approach best suited to the disease that is present and to the surgeon's experience. Posterolateral techniques are ideal for lateral lesions and may be the best choice for herniated discs with coexistent stenosis.[124] The transthoracic approach permits the best visualization for central lesions. Upper thoracic lesions are more difficult to approach through the chest and may be managed best by costotransversectomy. Depending on the experience of the surgeon, video-assisted approaches can provide an alternative approach with reportedly less surgical morbidity. Newer minimally invasive approaches are also being developed that may offer less pain and quicker recovery.

The prognosis of patients who have herniated thoracic discs treated surgically is favorable, and early operative intervention is advised in cases of myelopathy or refractory radicular pain. The techniques are exacting, however, and still carry a significant risk of neurologic deterioration.

PEARLS

1. Of asymptomatic adults, 73% have positive anatomic findings, including 37% with disc herniation and 29% with spinal cord deformation.

2. Disc calcification can be seen in 70% of patients with thoracic disc prolapse.

3. For symptomatic central thoracic disc herniation, the transthoracic approach is probably the safest.

PITFALLS

1. Surgical treatment of thoracic disc herniation by laminectomy has a 28% chance of worsening symptoms.

2. Blood supply to the spinal cord is tenuous in the thoracic spine, especially from T4 to T9, and ligation of blood vessels within the neural foramina should be avoided whenever possible because this may cause paralysis.

KEY POINTS

1. The true incidence of thoracic herniated discs is unknown; many cases are unrecognized, or patients are asymptomatic.

2. Surgically, thoracic disc excision accounts for 0.2% to 1.8% of all operations performed on symptomatic herniated discs.

3. The pathogenesis of neurologic compromise secondary to herniated thoracic discs is believed to be a combination of direct neural compression and vascular insufficiency.

4. A thorough neurologic examination is mandatory, and the examiner should pay close attention to long tract signs and other evidence of myelopathy.

5. Indications for surgery include progressive myelopathy, lower extremity weakness or paralysis, bowel or bladder dysfunction, and radicular pain refractory to conservative measures.

6. The recommended extent of bone and disc removal varies from a relatively small trough in the posterior aspect of the disc to complete discectomy with partial corpectomy of adjacent bodies.

7. Reported advantages of VATS include reduced perioperative morbidity from minimal surgical dissection and avoidance of rib resection or spreading, enhanced visualization for the operating surgeons and support team, reduced postoperative pain with improved ventilatory excursion, shorter hospitalization and rehabilitation, and consequent decreased overall medical costs.

8. The prognosis of patients who have herniated thoracic discs treated surgically is favorable, and early operative intervention is advised in cases of myelopathy or refractory radicular pain.

KEY REFERENCES

1. Anand N, Regan JJ: Video-assisted thoracoscopic surgery for thoracic disc disease. Spine (Phila Pa 1976) 27:871-879, 2002.
   The authors describe the technique and clinical outcome of video-assisted thoracic disc decompression.

2. Arce CA, Dohrmann G: Herniated thoracic disks. Neurol Clin 3:383-392, 1985.
   This review of the literature details the clinical presentation and progression of thoracic disc herniation.

3. Bohlman HH, Zdeblick TA: Anterior excision of herniated thoracic discs. J Bone Joint Surg Am 70:1038-1047, 1988.
   This article describes the technique of transthoracic disc decompression and clinical outcomes.

4. Brown CW, Deffer PA, Akmakjian J, et al: The natural history of thoracic disc herniation. Spine (Phila Pa 1976) 17:S97-S102, 1992.
   The clinical method and the outcome of nonoperative thoracic disc herniation treatment are presented.

5. Currier BL, Eismont FJ, Green BA: Transthoracic disc excision and fusion for thoracic herniated discs. Spine (Phila Pa 1976) 3:323-328, 1994.
   This article is a summary of the early experience of the authors of this chapter using the transthoracic approach for treating patients with symptomatic thoracic herniated discs.

6. Wood KB, Garvey TA, Gundry C, et al: Magnetic resonance imaging of the thoracic spine. J Bone Joint Surg Am 77:1631-1638, 1995.
   A clinical review is provided of MRI-detected thoracic disc herniation in an asymptomatic patient population.

REFERENCES

1. Key CA: On paraplegia: Depending on disease of the ligaments of the spine. Guys Hosp Rep 3:17-24, 1838.

2. Middleton GS, Teacher JH: Injury of the spinal cord due to rupture of an intervertebral disc during muscular effort. Glasgow Med J 76:1:1, 1911.

3. Love JG, Schorn VG: Thoracic disk protrusions. JAMA 191:627-631, 1965.

4. Mixter WJ, Barr JS: Rupture of the intervertebral disc with involvement of the spinal canal. N Engl J Med 211:210-218, 1934.

5. Abbott KH, Retter RH: Protrusions of thoracic intervertebral disc. Neurology 6:1-10, 1956.

6. Arseni C, Nash F: Thoracic intervertebral disc protrusion: A clinical study. J Neurosurg 17:418-430, 1960.

7. Epstein JA: The syndrome of herniation of the lower thoracic intervertebral discs with nerve root and spinal cord compression: A presentation of four cases with a review of the literature, methods of diagnosis, and treatment. J Neurosurg 11:525-538, 1954.

8. Fisher RG: Protrusions of thoracic disc: The factor of herniation through the dura mater. J Neurosurg 22:591-593, 1965.

9. Hawk WA: Spinal compression caused by enchondrosis of the intervertebral fibrocartilage with a review of the recent literature. Brain 59:204-224, 1936.

10. Huang T, Hsu RW, Sum C, et al: Complications in thoracoscopic spinal surgery: A study of 90 consecutive patients. Surg Endosc 19:346-350, 1999.

11. Kite WC Jr, Whitfield RD, Campbell E: The thoracic herniated intervertebral disc syndrome. J Neurosurg 14:61-67, 1957.

12. Logue V: Thoracic intervertebral disc prolapse with spinal cord compression. J Neurol Neurosurg Psychiatry 15:227-241, 1952.

13. Peck FC Jr: A calcified thoracic intervertebral disk with herniation and spinal cord compression in a child: Case report. J Neurosurg 14:105-109, 1957.

14. Svien HJ, Karavitis AL: Multiple protrusions of intervertebral disks in the upper thoracic region: Report of case. Mayo Clin Proc 29:375-378, 1954.

15. Terry AF, McSweeney T, Jones HWF: Paraplegia as a sequela to dorsal disc prolapse. Paraplegia 19:111-117, 1981.

16. Tovi D, Strang RR: Thoracic intervertebral disk protrusions. Acta Chir Scand Suppl 267:6, 1960.

17. Menard V: Etude Pratique sur le Mal de Pott. Paris, Masson, 1900.

18. Capener N: The evolution of lateral rachiotomy. J Bone Joint Surg Br 36:173-179, 1954.

19. Hulme A: The surgical approach to thoracic intervertebral disc protrusions. J Neurol Neurosurg Psychiatry 23:133-137, 1960.

20. Arce CA, Dohrmann G: Herniated thoracic disks. Neurol Clin 3:383-392, 1985.

21. Hodgson AR, Stock FE: Anterior spinal fusion: A preliminary communication on the radical treatment of Pott's disease and Pott's paraplegia. Br J Surg 44:266-275, 1956.

22. Crafoord C, Hiertonn T, Lindblom K, et al: Spinal cord compression caused by a protruded thoracic disc: Report of a case treated with anterolateral fenestration of the disc. Acta Orthop Scand 28:103-107, 1958.

23. Perot PH Jr, Munro DD: Transthoracic removal of midline thoracic disc protrusions causing spinal cord compression. J Neurosurg 31:452-458, 1969.

24. Ransohoff J, Spencer F, Siew F, et al: Case reports and technical notes on transthoracic removal of thoracic disc: Report of three cases. J Neurosurg 31:459-461, 1969.

25. Carson J, Gumpert J, Jefferson A: Diagnosis and treatment of thoracic intervertebral disc protrusions. J Neurol Neurosurg Psychiatry 34:67-68, 1971.

26. Patterson RH Jr, Arbit E: A surgical approach through the pedicle to protruded thoracic discs. J Neurosurg 48:768-772, 1978.

27. Lesoin F, Rousseaux M, Autricque A, et al: Thoracic disc herniations: Evolution in the approach and indications. Acta Neurochir 80:30-34, 1986.

28. Safdari H, Baker RL: Microsurgical anatomy and related techniques to an anterolateral transthoracic approach to thoracic disc herniations. Surg Neurol 23:589-593, 1985.

29. Signorini G, Baldini M, Vivenza C, et al: Surgical treatment of thoracic disc protrusion. Acta Neurochir 49:245-254, 1979.

30. Anand N, Regan JJ: Video-assisted thoracoscopic surgery for thoracic disc disease: Classification and outcome study of 100 consecutive cases with a 2-year minimum follow-up period. Spine (Phila Pa 1976) 27:871-879, 2002.

31. Regan JJ, Mack MJ, Picetti GD: A technical report on video-assisted thoracoscopy in thoracic spine surgery: Preliminary description. Spine (Phila Pa 1976) 20:831-837, 1995.

32. Regan JJ, Ben-Yishay A, Mack MJ: Video-assisted thoracoscopic excision of herniated thoracic disc: Description of technique and preliminary experience in the first 29 cases. J Spinal Disord 11:183-191, 1998.

33. Rosenthal D, Rosenthal R, de Simone A: Removal of a protruded thoracic disc using microsurgical endoscopy: A new technique. Spine (Phila Pa 1976) 19:1087-1091, 1994.

34. Blumenkopf B: Thoracic intervertebral disc herniations: Diagnostic value of magnetic resonance imaging. Neurosurgery 23:36-40, 1988.

35. Bohlman HH, Zdeblick TA: Anterior excision of herniated thoracic discs. J Bone Joint Surg Am 70:1038-1047, 1988.

36. Chambers AA: Thoracic disk herniation. Semin Roentgenol 23:111-117, 1988.

37. Francavilla TL, Powers A, Dina T, et al: MR imaging of thoracic disk herniations. J Comp Assist Tomogr 11:1062-1065, 1987.

38. Parizel PM, Rodesch G, Baleriaux D, et al: Gd-enhanced MR in thoracic disc herniations. Neuroradiology 31:75-79, 1989.

39. Ross JS, Perez-Reyes N, Masaryk TJ, et al: Thoracic disc herniation: MR imaging. Radiology 165:511-515, 1987.

40. Videman T, Battie MC, Gill K, et al: Magnetic resonance imaging findings and their relationships in the thoracic and lumbar spine: Insights into the etiopathogenesis of spinal degeneration. Spine (Phila Pa 1976) 20:928-935, 1995.

41. Williams MP, Cherryman GR, Husband JE: Significance of thoracic disc herniations demonstrated by MR imaging. J Comput Tomogr 13:212-214, 1989.

42. Wood KB, Garvey TA, Gundry C, et al: Magnetic resonance imaging of the thoracic spine. J Bone Joint Surg Am 77:1631-1638, 1995.

43. Williams MP, Cherryman GR: Thoracic disc herniation: MR imaging [letter to the editor]. Radiology 167:874-875, 1988.

44. Arce CA, Dohrmann G: Thoracic disc herniation: Improved diagnosis with computed tomographic scanning and a review of the literature. Surg Neurol 23:356-361, 1985.

45. Benson MKD, Byrnes DP: The clinical syndromes and surgical treatment of thoracic intervertebral disc prolapse. J Bone Joint Surg Br 57:471-477, 1975.

46. Albrand OW, Corkill G: Thoracic disc herniation: Treatment and prognosis. Spine (Phila Pa 1976) 4:41-46, 1979.

47. Love JG, Kiefer EJ: Root pain and paraplegia due to protrusions of thoracic intervertebral disks. J Neurosurg 7:62-69, 1950.

48. Brennan M, Perrin JCS, Canady A, et al: Paraparesis in a child with a herniated thoracic disc. Arch Phys Med Rehab 68:806-808, 1987.

49. Otani KI, Yoshida M, Fujii E, et al: Thoracic disc herniation: Surgical treatment in 23 patients. Spine (Phila Pa 1976) 13:1262-1267, 1988.

50. Alvarez O, Roque CT, Pampati M: Multilevel thoracic disk herniations: CT and MR studies. J Comput Assist Tomogr 12:649-652, 1988.

51. Otani K, Manxoku S, Shibaski K, et al: The surgical treatment of thoracic and thoracolumbar disc lesions using the anterior approach. Spine (Phila Pa 1976) 2:266-275, 1977.

52. Russell T: Thoracic intervertebral disc protrusion: Experience of 67 cases and a review of the literature. Br J Neurosurg 3:153-160, 1989.

53. Le Roux PD, Haglund MM, Harris AB: Thoracic disc disease: Experience with the transpedicular approach in twenty consecutive patients. Neurosurgery 33:58-66, 1993.

54. Lesoin F, Leys D, Rousseaux M, et al: Thoracic disk herniation and Scheuermann's disease. Eur Neurol 26:145-152, 1987.

55. Mansour H, Hammoud F, Vlahovitch B: Brown-Séquard syndrome caused by foramen and calcified disk herniation responsible for direct compression of Adamkiewicz's artery. Neurochirurgie 33:478-481, 1987.

56. McAfee PC, Regan JR, Zdeblick T, et al: The incidence of complications in endoscopic anterior thoracolumbar spinal reconstructive surgery: A prospective multicenter study comprising the first 100 cases. Spine (Phila Pa 1976) 20:1624-1632, 1995.

57. Haley JC, Perry JH: Protrusion of intervertebral discs: Study of their distribution, characteristics and effects on the nervous system. Am J Surg 80:394-404, 1950.

58. Ridenour TR, Haddad SF, Hitchon PW, et al: Herniated thoracic disks: Treatment and outcome. J Spinal Disord 6:218-224, 1993.

59. Ryan RW, Lally JF, Kozic Z: Asymptomatic calcified herniated thoracic disks: CT recognition. AJNR Am J Neuroradiol 9:363-366, 1988.

60. Awwad EE, Martin DS, Smith KR Jr, et al: Asymptomatic versus symptomatic herniated thoracic discs: Their frequency and characteristics as detected by computed tomography after myelography. Neurosurgery 28:180-186, 1991.

61. Niemelainen R, Battie MC, Gill K, et al: The prevalence and characteristics of thoracic magnetic resonance imaging findings in men. Spine (Phila Pa 1976) 33:2552-2559, 2008.

62. Tahmouresie A: Herniated thoracic intervertebral disc: An unusual presentation: Case report. Neurosurgery 7:623-625, 1980.

63. Landreneau RJ, Hazelrigg SR, Mack MJ, et al: Post-operative pain-related morbidity: Video-assisted thoracic surgery versus thoracotomy. Ann Thorac Surg 56:1285-1289, 1993.

64. Van Landingham JH: Herniation of thoracic intervertebral discs with spinal cord compression in kyphosis dorsalis juvenilis (Scheuermann's disease): Case report. J Neurosurg 11:327-329, 1954.

65. Dommisse GF: The blood supply of the spinal cord: A critical vascular zone in spinal surgery. J Bone Joint Surg Br 56:225-235, 1974.

66. Hochman MS, Pena C, Ramirez R: Calcified herniated thoracic disc diagnosed by computerized tomography. J Neurosurg 52:722-723, 1980.

67. Maccartee CC Jr, Griffin PP, Byrd EB: Ruptured calcified thoracic disc in a child. J Bone Joint Surg Am 54:1271-1274, 1972.

68. Kahn EA: The role of the dentate ligaments in spinal cord compression and the syndrome of lateral sclerosis. J Neurosurg 4:191-199, 1944.

69. Doppman JL, Girton M: Angiographic study of the effect of laminectomy in the presence of acute anterior epidural masses. J Neurosurg 45:195-202, 1976.

70. Brown CW, Deffer PA, Akmakjian J, et al: The natural history of thoracic disc herniation. Spine (Phila Pa 1976) 17(Suppl 6):S97-S102, 1992.

71. Gelch MM: Herniated thoracic disc at T1-2 level associated with Horner's syndrome. J Neurosurg 48:128-130, 1978.

72. Fransen P, Collignon F, Van Den Heule B: Foraminal disc herniation Th9-Th10 mimicking abdominal pain. Acta Orthop Belg 74:881-884, 2008.

73. Ozturk C, Tezer M, Sirvanci M, et al: Far lateral thoracic disc herniation presenting with flank pain. Spine J 6:201-203, 2006.

74. LaBan MM, Gorin G: A thoracic disc herniation presenting as an abdominal hernia. Am J Phys Med Rehab 86:601, 2007.

75. Stetkarova I, Chrobok J, Ehler E, et al: Segmental abdominal wall paresis caused by lateral low thoracic disc herniation. Spine (Phila Pa 1976) 32:E635-E639, 2007.

76. Deitch K, Chudnofsky C, Young M: T2-3 thoracic disc herniation with myelopathy. J Emerg Med 36:138-140, 2009.

77. Papapostolou A, Tsivgoulis G, Papadopoulou M, et al: Bilateral drop foot due to thoracic disc herniation. Eur J Neurol 14:E5, 2007.

78. Kuhlendahl H: Der Thorakale Bandscheibenprolaps als extramedullarer Spinaltumor und in seinen Beziehungen zu internen Organsyndromen. Arztl Wochenschr 6:154-157, 1951.

79. Malmivaara A, Videman T, Kuosma E, et al: Facet joint orientation, facet and costovertebral joint osteoarthrosis, disc degeneration, vertebral body osteophytosis, and Schmorl's nodes in the thoracolumbar junctional region of cadaveric spines. Spine (Phila Pa 1976) 12:458-463, 1987.

80. Almond LM, Hamid NA, Wasserberg J. Thoracic intradural disc herniation. Br J Neurosurg 21:32-34, 2007.

81. Epstein NE, Syrquin MS, Epstein JA, et al: Intradural disc herniations in the cervical, thoracic, and lumbar spine: Report of three cases and review of the literature. J Spinal Disord 3:396-403, 1990.

82. Fidler MW, Goedhard ZD: Excision of prolapse of thoracic intervertebral disc: A transthoracic technique. J Bone Joint Surg Br 66:518-522, 1984.

83. Isla A, Roda JM, Benscome J, et al: Intradural herniated dorsal disc: Case report and review of the literature. Neurosurgery 22:737-738, 1988.

84. Jefferson A: The treatment of thoracic intervertebral disc protrusion. Clin Neurol Neurosurg 78:1, 1975.

85. Chin LS, Black KL, Hoff JT: Multiple thoracic disc herniations: Case report. J Neurosurg 66:290-292, 1987.

86. Haro H, Domoto T, Maekawa S, et al: Resorption of thoracic disc herniation: Report of 2 cases. J Neurosurg Spine 8:300-304, 2008.

87. Bullough PG, Boachie-Adjei O: Atlas of Spinal Diseases. Philadelphia, JB Lippincott, 1988.

88. Sonnabend DH, Taylor TKF, Chapman GK: Intervertebral disc calcification syndromes in children. J Bone Joint Surg Br 64:25-31, 1982.

89. Nicolau A, Diard F, Darrigade JM, et al: Posterior herniation of a calcified disc in children: A report of two cases. J Radiol 66:683-688, 1985.

90. Weinberger A, Myers AR: Intervertebral disk calcification in adults: A review. Semin Arthritis Rheum 8:69-75, 1978.

91. Currier BL, Eismont FJ, Green BA: Transthoracic disc excision and fusion for thoracic herniated discs. Spine (Phila Pa 1976) 3:323-328, 1994.

92. Roosen N, Dietrich U, Nicola N, et al: Case report: MR imaging of calcified herniated thoracic disk. J Comput Assist Tomogr 11:733-735, 1987.

93. Ryan MD, Taylor TKF: Acute spinal cord compression in Scheuermann's disease. J Bone Joint Surg Br 64:409-412, 1982.

94. Baker HL Jr, Love JG, Uihlein A: Roentgenologic features of protruded thoracic intervertebral disks. Radiology 84:1059-1065, 1965.

95. Alberico A, Sahni KS, Hall JA Jr, et al: High thoracic disc herniation. Neurosurgery 19:449-451, 1986.

96. Enzmann DR, Griffin C, Rubin JB: Potential false-negative MR images of the thoracic spine in disk disease with switching of phase and frequency encoding gradients. Radiology 165:635-637, 1987.

97. Schellhas KP, Pollei SR, Dorwart RH: Thoracic discography: A safe and reliable technique. Spine (Phila Pa 1976) 19:2103-2109, 1994.

98. Wood KB, Schellhas KP, Garvey TA, et al: Thoracic discography in healthy individuals: A controlled prospective study of magnetic resonance imaging and discography in asymptomatic and symptomatic individuals. Spine (Phila Pa 1976) 24:1548-1555, 1999.

99. Buenaventura RM, Shah RV, Patel V, et al: Systematic review of discography as a diagnostic test for spinal pain: An update. Pain Physician 20:147-164, 2007.

100. Ravichandran G, Frankel HL: Paraplegia due to intervertebral disc lesions: A review of 57 operated cases. Paraplegia 19:133-139, 1981.

101. Aizawa T, Sato T, Sasaki H, et al: Results of surgical treatment for thoracic myelopathy: Minimum 2-year follow-up study in 132 patients. J Neurosurg Spine 7:13-20, 2007.

102. Yi S, Kim H, Shin HC, et al: Outcome of surgery for a symptomatic herniated thoracic disc in relation to preoperative characteristics of the disc. Acta Neurochir (Wien) 149:1139-1145, 2007.

103. Fessler RG, Sturgill M: Review: Complications of surgery for thoracic disc disease. Surg Neurol 49:609-618, 1998.

104. Singounas EG, Karvounis PC: Thoracic disc protrusion (analysis of 8 cases). Acta Neurochir 39:251-258, 1977.

105. Bennett MH, McCallum J: Experimental decompression of the spinal cord. Surg Neurol 8:63-67, 1977.

106. Simpson JM, Silveri CP, Simeone FA, et al: Thoracic disc herniation: Re-evaluation of the posterior approach using a modified costotransversectomy. Spine (Phila Pa 1976) 13:1872-1877, 1993.

107. Chesterman PJ: Spastic paraplegia caused by sequestrated thoracic intervertebral disc. Proc R Soc Med 57:87-88, 1964.

108. Garrido E: Modified costotransversectomy: A surgical approach to ventrally placed lesions in the thoracic spinal canal. Surg Neurol 13:109-113, 1980.

109. Hulme A: The surgical approach to thoracic intervertebral disc protrusions. J Neurol Neurosurg Psychiatry 23:133-137, 1960.

110. Amini A, Apfelbaum RI, Schmidt MH: Chylorrhea: A rare complication of thoracoscopic discectomy of the thoracolumbar junction. J Neurosurg Spine 6:563-566, 2007.

111. Maiman DJ, Larson SJ, Luck E, et al: Lateral extracavitary approach to the spine for thoracic disc herniations: Report of 23 cases. Neurosurgery 14:178-182, 1984.

112. DiChiro G, Fried LC, Doppman JL: Experimental spinal cord angiography. Br J Radiol 43:19-20, 1970.

113. Lazorthes G, Gouzae A, Zadeh JO, et al: Arterial vascularization of the spinal cord: Recent studies of the anastomotic substitution pathways. J Neurosurg 35:253-262, 1971.

114. Ulivieri S, Oliveri G, Petrini C, et al: Transmanubrial osteomuscular sparing approach for T1-T2 thoracic disc herniation. Minerva Chir 63:421-423, 2008.

115. Kawahara N, Demura S, Marukami H, et al: Transvertebral herniotomy for T2/3 disc herniation—a case report. J Spinal Disord Tech 22:62-66, 2009.

116. Mack MJ, Regan JJ, Bobechko WP, et al: Present role of thoracoscopy for diseases of the spine. Ann Thorac Surg 56:736-738, 1993.

117. Horowitz MB, Moossy JJ, Julian T, et al: Thoracic discectomy using video assisted thoracoscopy. Spine (Phila Pa 1976) 19:1082-1086, 1994.

118. Kim SJ, Sohn MJ, Ryoo JY, et al: Clinical analysis of video-assisted thoracoscopic spinal surgery in the thoracic or thoracolumbar spinal pathologies. J Korean Neurosurg Soc 42:293-299, 2007.

119. Gille O, Soderlund C, Razafimahandri HJC, et al: Analysis of hard thoracic herniated discs: Review of 18 cases operated by thoracoscopy. Eur Spine J 15:537-542, 2006.

120. Bartels RH, Peul WC: Mini-thoracotomy or thoracoscopic treatment for medially located thoracic herniated disc? Spine (Phila Pa 1976) 32:E581-E584, 2007.

121. Chi JH, Dhall SS, Kanter AS, et al: The mini-open transpedicular thoracic discectomy: Surgical technique and assessment. Neurosurg Focus 25:E5, 2008.

122. Lidar Z, Lifshutz J, Bhattacharjee S, et al: Minimally invasive, extracavitary approach for thoracic disc herniation: Technical report and preliminary results. Spine J 6:157-163, 2006.

123. Sheikh H, Samartzis D, Perez-Cruet MJ: Techniques for the operative management of thoracic disc herniation: Minimally invasive thoracic microdiscectomy. Orthop Clin North Am 38:351-361, 2007.

124. Ungersbock K, Perneczky A, Korn A: Thoracic vertebrostenosis combined with thoracic disc herniation: Case report and review of the literature. Spine (Phila Pa 1976) 12:612-615, 1987.

CHAPTER 45

Lumbar Disc Disease

Gunnar B. J. Andersson, MD, PhD
Ashok Biyani, MD
Steven T. Ericksen, MD

The location of the anatomic pain generator in patients with low back pain is often difficult to discern. Pain can originate from several anatomic structures within the spine making it difficult for the patient and the physician to localize. Experimental and clinical studies suggest that the intervertebral disc (IVD) is an important source of back pain in 10% to 39%[1,2] of cases of chronic low back pain.

Common subgroups of low back pain of IVD origin include lumbar disc herniation, internal disc disruption (IDD), and degenerative disc disease (DDD). DDD also contributes to the pathogenesis of secondary spinal disorders such as spinal stenosis and degenerative spondylolisthesis. Improved understanding of the pathophysiology of IVD disorders has led to a resurgence of enthusiasm in development of new pharmacobiologics and treatment techniques for this common disorder. New advances in physical therapy and operative technologies, such as IVD replacement and minimally invasive surgical techniques, are challenging traditional methods of treatment.

This chapter discusses the anatomy, pathophysiology, diagnosis, and treatment of primary disc disorders—IDD and DDD. Disorders arising secondarily from the IVD are beyond the scope of this chapter and are discussed elsewhere in this text.

Natural History

At some point during their lifetime, 60% to 80% of adults can be expected to experience low back pain. The annual incidence of back pain in adults is 15%, and its point prevalence is about 30%.[3] By the age of 30 years, almost half of adults have experienced a substantive episode of low back pain.[4] Most symptoms are short-lived; it is generally believed that 80% to 90% of episodes of low back pain resolve within 6 weeks of onset regardless of the type of treatment.[5]

Although resolution of symptoms is the common and expected outcome, there is also a high recurrence rate. Croft and colleagues[6] reported that although 90% of subjects ceased to pursue consultation about symptoms within 3 months, most still had substantial low back pain and related disability.

Additionally, only 25% of the patients who sought consultation for low back pain had fully recovered within 12 months. In a survey of the British general population, 38% of adults reported a significant episode of low back pain within a 1-year period, of which a third had experienced symptoms for longer than 4 weeks.[7] Inability to return to work within 3 months of symptom onset is a poor prognostic indicator. Only 20% of patients still disabled after 1 year return to work, and only 2% return after 2 years.[8]

The clinical onset and course of low back pain may be prolonged for many patients and may best be represented as a continuum of back-related disability and distress.[9] Numerous patients presenting with acute low back pain have a prior history of chronic back pain.[10] The strongest predictive factor for a new episode of low back pain is a previous episode.[11,12]

The natural history of DDD is largely unknown. Smith and colleagues[13] reported on the outcome of 25 patients with a positive discogram who were treated nonoperatively and found that 68% of patients improved by the 3-year minimum follow-up. Although 60% of the patients were involved with workers' compensation and 32% were being treated for psychiatric diagnoses, this study suggests that at least two thirds of patients with discogenic pain improve with conservative therapy. The retrospective study design and small sample size limit the conclusions, and because only patients with significant symptoms typically undergo discography, the natural history of untreated symptomatic DDD is likely to be even better.

In their classic description, Kirkaldy-Willis and Farfan[14] classified the degenerative process into three distinct phases: dysfunction, instability, and stabilization. In the first phase, the disc loses its normal function as the degenerative process begins. A period of relative instability ensues as degeneration progresses with intermittent episodes of pain. During the instability phase, abnormal motion occasionally can be seen on flexion-extension x-rays; however, more often the spinal segments during this phase of degeneration show no demonstrable radiographic instability. The final phase—stabilization—results when the spinal segment has restabilized because of loss of height and compression of disc tissue, and the patient typically no longer has episodes of back pain. The problem with this theory is that often patients who meet diagnostic criteria of DDD radiographically—loss of height, osteophytes, or even olisthesis—or by magnetic resonance imaging (MRI)— signal changes compared with adjacent levels—are completely symptom-free. Waris and colleagues,[15] in a study with 17 years of follow-up MRI, showed that young patients with DDD did show radiographic evidence of progression, but it was not significantly associated with low back pain or a higher rate of surgery.

Relevant Anatomy

The disc is composed of the inner gelatinous nucleus pulposus surrounded by the collagenous anulus fibrosus. Sheets of interlacing lamellae of collagen within the anulus provide tensile strength, which limits the expansion of the viscoelastic nucleus. The nucleus pulposus consists of a matrix of collagen, glycosaminoglycans, and water, which provide compressive stiffness and allow the tissue to undergo reversible deformation. The anatomy of the IVD allows the disc to absorb and dissipate loads on the spinal column and allows motion between adjacent spinal segments. The IVD has sparse cellularity; cells comprise approximately 1% to 5% of the tissue volume. The disc is bordered above and below by a sheet of hyaline cartilage called the *vertebral endplate*. Pores in the endplates provide channels for diffusion of nutrients to the disc.[16]

The IVD is largely avascular and aneural, with vascularity and innervation in a healthy disc limited to the peripheral fibers of the anulus. The sinuvertebral nerve innervates the disc, posterior longitudinal ligament, ventral dura, posterior anulus, and blood vessels. It comprises a sensory branch from the ventral root and a sympathetic branch from the gray rami communicans near the distal pole of dorsal root ganglion. The sinuvertebral nerve is believed to have three segmental levels of overlap, which makes it difficult to localize pain originating in the disc, dura, and posterior longitudinal ligament. Nakamura and colleagues[17] treated 33 patients with selective L2 nerve root block with good relief of back pain. The authors hypothesized that the main afferent pathways of pain from lower lumbar IVDs in patients with discogenic back pain are sympathetic in nature and are mediated through the L2 nerve root via the sinuvertebral nerve; however, this hypothesis has yet to be validated.

Changes in Disc Structure with Aging and Degeneration

Changes that almost universally occur in the IVD with aging include reduction in disc volume, shape, and content. Alterations in gene expression and transcription factors may be responsible for cell senescence within the disc. These senescent cells lose biochemical and synthetic capabilities, which ultimately diminishes the ability of the disc to recover from deformation and renders the matrix more vulnerable to

progressive fatigue failure. The nucleus pulposus gradually becomes less hydrated, and usually by the 3rd decade of life there is already a significant decline in the number of viable cells and a loss of proteoglycans.

The early degenerative process affects the nucleus pulposus and the endplate more than the anulus fibrosus. Anabolic and catabolic processes are upregulated during the early stages of degeneration; however, anabolic repair processes fail to keep up with the catabolic processes, and matrix degeneration ensues over time. As the process progresses, the inner layers of the anulus and the nucleus pulposus gradually become indistinguishable and change into a stiff desiccated fibrocartilaginous material.

The number of arterioles supplying the peripheral disc diminishes significantly as remaining blood vessels are obliterated by calcification of the cartilaginous endplates. Loss of endplate vascularity and porosity leads to a reduction in the influx of nutrients and efflux of waste products. Lactate levels increase locally within the hypovascular disc secondary to increased production and decreased removal. Cell apoptosis occurs as a result of decreased tissue pH,[18] and the biosynthetic reparative capability of the disc is impaired further.

Thinning or microfracture of the endplate alters its properties and may allow rapid outflow of fluid from the cartilage endplate on loading, rendering the hydrostatic pressure mechanisms involved in load transference less effective and uniform. Focal elevations in shear stresses at the disc level may adversely affect the disc structure further and result in annular damage. Over time, cracks develop between and through the annular lamellae. Eventually, communicating channels may develop between the peripheral layers of the anulus and the nucleus, and disc material can herniate through these fissures. The weakened anulus can develop a full-thickness defect and allow near-complete herniation of the nucleus pulposus, particularly when the disc is loaded in flexion and torsion.

The degenerative process resulting from matrix changes and internal structural disruption sets the stage for abnormal motion at the degenerated segment. Changes in disc structure alter the loading response and alignment of the spinal column. These changes can influence the facet joints, ligaments, and paraspinal muscles, which may also become pain generators. Pain does not always correlate with morphologic changes in the disc and mechanical compression, however.[19] Macnab[20] described traction osteophytes around the vertebrae originating 2 mm from the anterior endplate, at the site of attachment of the outermost annular fibers. These osteophytes were thought to be signs of abnormal biomechanics, caused by traction at the insertion of the annular fibers into the vertebral bodies. Subsequent studies found these osteophytes to be inconsistently present.

Multiple factors lead to disc degeneration, including insufficient nutritional supply, reduction in the amount of viable cells, degradative enzymatic activity, and cell senescence and apoptosis. Alteration in loading patterns between the endplate and disc leads to annular damage and the potential for herniation. Perturbation of the disc also leads to degeneration and pain in other segmental structures such as the facet joints, ligaments, and paraspinal muscles. The initiating event leading to the onset of degeneration is unknown.

Associated Factors

Various risk factors have been implicated in the pathogenesis of lumbar disc degeneration. In a review of factors associated with IVD degeneration in elderly adults, Hangai and colleagues[21] cited increased age, high body mass index, occupational lifting, sporting activities, and factors associated with atherosclerosis as risk factors. Multiple studies show the genetic contribution to degenerative low back pain.[22] Battie and colleagues[23] estimated the familial contribution to IVD degeneration to be 34% to 61%. Cigarette smoking has also been implicated and seems to have an adverse vasoconstrictive and atherosclerotic effect on the nutrition of the IVD.[24,25] Type of occupation has also been shown to have an adverse effect on lumbar spinal segment degeneration, increasing the risk of symptomatic DDD. Studies have implicated occupations that require repetitive lifting or pulling, prolonged sitting[26] such as motor vehicle driving,[27] and whole-body vibration.[28]

Arun and colleagues[29] used serial postcontrast MRI to study the effect of prolonged mechanical load on diffusion into the IVD. The authors reported that 4.5 hours at a load corresponding to 50% body weight significantly retarded the diffusion of small solutes into the center of the IVD, and it required 3 hours in an unloaded recovery phase to return the diffusion rate to that seen in the unloaded disc. Prolonged mechanical load can cause a disruption of diffusion, which may accelerate disc degeneration; however, this hypothesis has not been confirmed clinically.

The genetic predisposition to lumbar DDD and lifetime exposures were studied in a classic monozygotic twin study by Battie and colleagues.[23] These investigators reviewed 115 male identical twin pairs for exposures to common risk factors such as occupation, recreational activities, driving, and smoking. Disc degeneration was determined by MRI and clinical evaluation. In the upper lumbar spine, only 7% of the variability was explained by occupation, 16% was explained by age, and 77% was explained by familial aggregation. In the lower lumbar spine, recreational physical loading explained 2% of variability, age explained 9%, and familial aggregation explained 43%. Battie and colleagues[23] concluded that primarily genetic and other unexplained factors result in DDD, whereas commonly implicated environmental factors have only modest effects. In a 5-year follow-up study of the same twin population, the same investigators reaffirmed that genetics have a dominant role in progression of DDD, whereas occupational lifting and leisure activity had only modest effects.[30] The important role of genetic factors has been corroborated in other twin studies,[31,32] but it seems to be less of an explanatory factor for back pain in older people.[33]

Several gene loci have been discovered that are associated with increased risk for DDD. Type IX collagen was one of the first gene loci identified with some aberrant alleles imparting a threefold or fourfold increase in relative risk.[34-36] More recent publications also implicate collagen type XI, interleukin (IL)-1, aggrecan, vitamin D receptor, matrix metalloproteinase (MMP)-3, and cartilage intermediate layer protein (CILP) as candidate genes.[37] The discovery of these genetic risk factors has yet to result in new useful diagnostic and treatment modalities, however.

Pathophysiology

Internal Disc Disruption

Crock[19] coined the term *internal disc disruption* in 1970 and defined it as a painful increase in biologic activity of the IVD after injury with normal radiographic, computed tomography (CT), and myelogram examinations but an abnormal discogram. IDD as a cause of discogenic back pain is controversial. The advent of MRI has dramatically improved the detection of this entity—IDD manifests as a dark disc with relatively preserved height and contour on MRI. Pain in IDD is thought to be caused by mechanical and chemical stimulation of nociceptors within the anulus or on the surface layers of the anulus and the overlying ligamentous tissue. The hallmark of IDD is the absence of disc herniation, prolapsed disc material, segmental instability, or other radiographic abnormality.[19,38] Nerve root irritation, radicular pain, and neurologic deficits are also absent.

Radiographic changes associated with DDD—significant disc space narrowing, endplate osteophyte formation, endplate sclerosis, and gas formation within the disc space—are not seen in IDD.[39] MRI (dark disc) and positive discography (concordant pain in the abnormal level and not at normal adjacent levels) are required to make the diagnosis of IDD. Because of the poor sensitivity and specificity of discography, many clinicians question the existence of IDD as a clinical entity.

Degenerative Disc Disease

The relationship between degenerative disc changes and low back pain is poorly understood. Two potential sources that have been implicated as contributors to pain in patients with disc degeneration are (1) sensitization of nerve endings by release of chemical mediators and (2) neurovascular ingrowth into the degenerated disc.

The precise pathophysiologic mechanism for chemically mediated induction of hyperalgesia within the disc has yet to be fully elucidated. Radial annular tears provide a route for nuclear material and noxious chemicals to leak from the disc and contact the dural sac and nerve roots; some studies have shown that autologous nucleus pulposus alone has the capacity to produce an inflammatory response. Additionally, degradative changes can occur within nerve roots exposed to nuclear material even in the absence of mechanical compression.[38,40-42] Weinstein and colleagues[43] investigated the reproduction of pain on discography and concluded that various neurochemical changes within the disc are expressed by sensitized annular nociceptors. These nociceptors are terminal nerve endings of sensory neurons that selectively respond to painful stimuli by the release of substance P.[44] These chemicals are leaked into the epidural space and are transported into the axons of the exiting nerve roots. Within the nerve root, they alter the excitability of type C nerve fibers and initiate the production of inflammatory agents such as prostaglandins, which results in radicular pain.[20,45,46]

In addition to material from the nucleus pulposus, many other substances in the degenerated disc have been implicated in pain generation. The role of nitric acid and phospholipase A_2 in irritation of nerve roots has been well documented.[45,47-50] Phospholipase A_2 has been implicated in multiple aspects: (1) direct activation of nociceptors, (2) nerve injury from degradation of cell membrane phospholipids, and (3) nerve injury from inflammatory mediators created from the arachidonic acid cascade (i.e., prostaglandins and leukotrienes).[51-53] Burke and colleagues[54] reported on the elevation of inflammatory mediators within the disc, such as IL-6, IL-8, and prostaglandin E_2. Other studies have shown the presence of inflammatory cytokines in the facet joints,[55] suggesting facet involvement as a pain generator via a biochemical mechanism as well. Ohtori and colleagues[56] reported on ingrowth of nerve tissue immunoreactive for tumor necrosis factor and prostaglandin P in 18 surgically harvested vertebral endplates of patients with Modic stage I and II changes who had undergone surgery. Their findings suggest that axon ingrowth into the vertebral endplate in association with Modic changes was induced by tumor necrosis factor and may be related to pain generation.

Neurovascular proliferation within and around degenerated disc elements has been proposed as another mechanism of pain generation. Normal IVDs have sparse innervation and vascularity that is distributed mainly within the outer lamellae (3 mm) of the anulus fibrosus,[57,58] whereas degenerated discs have significant neurovascular ingrowth within the inner anulus and nucleus pulposus.[59] Immunoreactive staining and acetylcholinesterase studies have shown penetration of nerve fibers within the inner third of the anulus in association with neovascularized granulation tissue.[47,57] Peng and colleagues[60] reported a histologic study of 19 IVDs harvested from surgery compared with normal control discs. The distinctive histologic characteristic of painful discs was a zone of richly innervated vascular granulation tissue extending from the outer anulus to the nucleus along the edges of fissures. Proliferation of vascular channels and sensory nerve endings rich in calcitonin gene-related peptide has also been observed in the endplate region and vertebral body adjacent to the degenerated disc. These findings suggest a role for the vertebral endplate and body as additional pain generators in DDD.[61]

Other studies suggest that the sensory nerve supply within the IVD is similar to visceral innervation patterns,[62] with calcitonin gene-related peptide immunoreactive fibers that pass through the sympathetic trunks.[63] This visceral pattern of innervation is potentially susceptible to central sensitization, which may complicate chronic low back pain further with psychosomatic overtones.[64] Psychosocial and chronic non–back pain syndromes have been implicated in more recent publications as having a significant effect in patients with low back pain.[65-69]

Clinical Picture

Internal Disc Disruption

The diagnosis of IDD is not readily apparent on a routine clinical workup. The patient is typically a younger individual 20 to 50 years old, with recurrent or persistent back pain. There may be a history of antecedent trauma or a forceful provocative event such as heavy lifting or unexpected flexion or compression force on the lumbar spine, but more often the pain is gradual in onset with no associated event or date.

The pain is characterized as a deep, dull ache in the lower lumbar region, exacerbated by rotation, flexion, and side-bending movements, and partially relieved by rest. Sitting intolerance may be a primary complaint, and pain is often relieved in a lateral recumbent position. Occasionally, there is a complaint of pain in the buttock or posterior thigh, but there is a conspicuous lack of radiculopathic symptoms. In the rare instances of associated leg pain, it is usually a late finding and pain does not follow any dermatomal pattern. In a study involving intradiscal electrothermal annuloplasty in 25 patients, O'Neill and colleagues[70] showed that stimulation of the IVD may result in low back and referred leg pain in patients presenting with symptoms of IDD. The distal distribution of pain was found to depend on the intensity of stimulation, and occasionally pain extending below the knee was produced.

Physical examination reveals decreased range of motion of the back and tenderness of the paraspinal musculature but is otherwise normal. The straight-leg raise test may reproduce back pain but not leg pain. Low back pain may also be reproduced at 20 to 30 degrees of flexion when rising from a flexed position. The sensorimotor examination is unremarkable, and deep tendon reflexes are normal and symmetrical.

Degenerative Disc Disease

Patients with DDD typically present with a history of persistent low back pain over the lumbosacral spine and sacroiliac joints and radiating into the buttocks and posterior thighs. Symptoms are often exacerbated with sitting and prolonged walking, but signs of neurologic claudication in the legs are not seen unless associated with concomitant lumbar stenosis. Radicular symptoms are rarely seen in the early stages of the disease. In end-stage disc degeneration, significant disc collapse may result in foraminal stenosis and late-onset radicular symptoms.

The physical examination is typically unremarkable except for point tenderness over the lumbar spine in the midline and over the sacroiliac joints. Range of motion of the lumbar spine may be reduced, most specifically in flexion. Extreme flexion and returning to upright from a flexed position usually cause significant discomfort. Extension is usually the least painful maneuver and may relieve pain. The straight-leg raise test may elicit some posterior thigh pain, which is often described as a stretching or pulling sensation, but there is no true radicular pain distal to the knee, unless there is coexisting foraminal stenosis. The sensorimotor examination is usually unremarkable, and deep tendon reflexes are normal and symmetrical.

Diagnostic Imaging

Plain Radiography

Plain radiographs are the recommended initial imaging modality for patients with a complaint of low back pain. Classic comparative and cost benefit studies have been done to determine when and what radiographs to obtain.[71,72] In 1982, Liang and Komaroff[73] published a comparison study between performing radiographs on all patients versus performing radiographs only on patients whose pain did not improve within 8 weeks of presentation. They found that risks and costs did not justify obtaining radiographs on initial presentation. Scavone and colleagues[74] reviewed the radiographs of 782 patients and found that spot lateral and oblique films added diagnostic information in only 2% of patients. They recommended that a spine series in patients with low back pain should consist only of anteroposterior and lateral films. Generally, flexion-extension and oblique views are necessary only in patients suspected to have instability or a pars fracture. The presence of "red flags" increases the chances of diagnostic radiographic findings and may prompt the physician to obtain early radiographic studies. These "red flag" indications are summarized in Table 45–1.[75]

Typical radiographic findings for patients with DDD include narrowing of the disc space (loss of height), endplate sclerosis, and the presence of osteophytes. Degenerative spondylolisthesis and scoliosis may occur secondarily. Advanced stages of disc degeneration may show vacuum phenomenon within the discs, a finding that represents nitrogen collection within voids in the disc.

Radiographs in patients with IDD typically show well-preserved height in the IVD and appear normal except for occasional benign spinal alignment changes. Nonstructural scoliosis and loss of lumbar lordosis may be observed in patients with sciatic list and paraspinal spasm.

Computed Tomography

CT is an excellent study to delineate osseous pathology, but it is generally not the imaging modality of choice for IDD and DDD because they are primarily soft tissue disorders. Addition of contrast material into the vertebral canal—CT myelography—significantly improves the accuracy of CT for showing pathology within the canal such as masses or stenosis, which is not a primary feature of DDD but can occur secondarily. CT myelography is the diagnostic imaging study of choice in patients with significant scoliosis and patients who are unable to undergo MRI because of implanted metal, aneurysm clips, pacemaker, obesity, or claustrophobia.

Magnetic Resonance Imaging

MRI is the best imaging modality to visualize and evaluate the neuronal and discal elements and is the most valuable adjunctive diagnostic tool in assessing disc pathology. IVDs are a highly unlikely cause of pain if MRI is completely normal and all discs are well hydrated. General MRI findings indicative of DDD include loss of water, loss of disc height, disc bulges, and signal or morphologic irregularity within the nucleus pulposus. In addition to these, MRI scans are typically examined for three specific types of findings: (1) a high-intensity zone (HIZ) in the posterior anulus, (2) dark disc with or without loss of height, and (3) endplate signal changes.

The MRI finding of a HIZ was originally described by Aprill and Bogduk[76] in 1992 and is believed to be specific for an annular tear (Fig. 45–1). Postmortem studies have shown three types of tears that can occur in the anulus: concentric, transverse, or radial.[77,78] A concentric tear is a crescentic or oval cavity created by a disruption in the short transverse fibers interconnecting the annular lamellae and is usually not visible on MRI. Concentric tears are occasionally referred to as *delamination*. A transverse tear represents a rupture of Sharpey fibers near their attachments to the ring apophysis at the disc periphery; these tears are typically thought to be clinically insignificant. A radial tear extending from the nucleus pulposus to the outermost surface of the posterior anulus is manifest on MRI as a HIZ.[79] HIZ is visualized on spin-echo T2-weighted images as a high-intensity signal located within

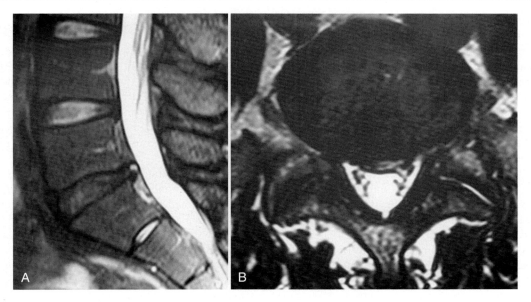

FIGURE 45–1 A and **B,** Sagittal (**A**) and axial (**B**) MRI showing high-intensity zone at L5-S1 level.

the anulus fibrosus and is clearly distinguishable from the nucleus pulposus.

Decreased signal within the IVD on T2-weighted images with relative preservation of disc height is a relatively common finding in asymptomatic individuals. Such a disc appearance is frequently referred to as *dark disc disease*; however, whether these discs constitute a potential pain generator is unclear. In the absence of any psychometric abnormalities, an isolated dark disc in a patient with no other identifiable causes of back pain is considered by many clinicians to be a source of back pain.

Endplate changes (Fig. 45–2) that occur with disc degeneration have been well described by Modic and colleagues.[80] Stage I change represents edema and is characterized by decreased signal on T1 and bright signal on T2 within the endplate. In stage II, fatty degeneration in the bone adjacent to the endplates is represented by bright signal on T1 and intermediate signal on T2 sequences. Stage III changes correspond with advanced degenerative changes and endplate sclerosis and are characterized on MRI by decreased signal intensity on T1-weighted and T2-weighted images.

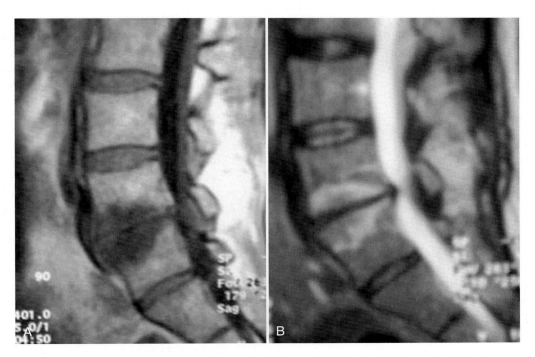

FIGURE 45–2 A and **B,** T1-weighted (**A**) and T2-weighted (**B**) sagittal MRI showing Modic stage I endplate changes.

When interpreting MRI findings, the clinician must be careful to consider the high prevalence of clinically false-positive findings. Abnormal disc findings on MRI are often found in clinically asymptomatic individuals. Boden and colleagues[81] showed that approximately 30% of asymptomatic individuals have a major finding on lumbar MRI scans. In patients older than 60 years, such abnormal findings are almost universally present regardless of symptoms. Jensen and colleagues[82] reported on 98 asymptomatic patients 20 to 80 years old and found that 52% overall had disc bulge in at least one level on MRI. Stadnik and colleagues[83] showed an unusually high rate of disc bulge (81%) and annular tears (56%) on MRI in 30 asymptomatic volunteers.

Abnormal MRI findings in asymptomatic patients are not indicators of future problems. Borenstein and colleagues[84] reported on 50 of the 67 patients from the study by Boden and colleagues[81] at a 7-year follow-up interval and found that incidental MRI findings were not predictive of the development or duration of low back pain. Jarvik and colleagues[85] studied 148 veterans with no symptoms of low back pain for at least 4 months. They found an incidence of moderate to severe desiccation in at least one disc in 83% of patients, disc bulge in 64%, and loss of disc height in 58%. In a 3-year follow-up of the same cohort, the investigators found no association between the development of new back pain and incidental MRI findings such as Modic changes, disc degeneration, annular tears, or facet degeneration. The greatest risk factor for developing low back pain in the 3-year interval was depression.[65]

Jarvik and colleagues[86] also published a report on the use of early MRI in the primary care setting. They randomly assigned 380 patients with low back pain to receive initial spine imaging via rapid MRI or plain radiography. Jarvik and colleagues[86] reported that substituting rapid MRI for x-ray studies in the primary care setting offered little additional benefit to patients in terms of secondary outcomes measures at 1 year and had the potential to increase the cost of care by $320 per patient (in 2002 dollar value). Carragee and colleagues[87] performed a prospective study of 200 asymptomatic patients to determine the rate at which new episodes of low back pain are associated with changes on MRI. On follow-up MRI in 51 patients who developed an episode of low back pain, 84% had no new finding. The most common new findings were disc signal loss (dark disc), progressive facet arthrosis, and increased endplate changes. New findings were not more common in patients developing back pain after minor trauma. The conclusion was that new findings on MRI within 12 weeks of onset of a serious episode of low back pain were unlikely to represent any significant structural change and preexisted the onset.

In consideration of the high prevalence of false-positive MRI findings, the clinician should remember that MRI does not stand alone in the evaluation of spinal pathology. When combined with a patient's history, physical findings, and plain radiographs, selective use of MRI can provide valuable information on the source of lumbar complaints.

Contrast-Enhanced Magnetic Resonance Imaging

The use of intravenous gadolinium diethylenetriaminepenta-acetic acid (DTPA) contrast medium with MRI in the setting of discogenic pain has been explored. The addition of gadolinium to a lumbar MRI scan is useful for differentiating scar tissue from recurrent disc herniation because the latter fails to enhance, whereas the vascular scar tissue takes up the contrast medium. Gadolinium-enhanced MRI seems unlikely to help delineate a painful pathologic disc.

Lappalainen and colleagues,[88] in an animal study of surgically created annular tears, showed that gadolinium-enhanced MRI did not detect all tears; specifically, peripheral, small tears were not visualized, but these tears would still represent clinically significant disc disruption. Yoshida and colleagues[89] investigated the relationship between T2-weighted gadolinium DTPA–enhanced MRI and a positive pain response with discography of 56 lumbar discs in 23 patients with chronic low back pain. The sensitivity, specificity, positive predictive value, and negative predictive value of the unenhanced T2-weighted images in detecting the symptomatic disc were 94%, 71%, 59%, and 97%, whereas the same values for gadolinium DTPA–enhanced images were 71%, 75%, 56%, and 86%. The findings of Yoshida and colleagues[89] support the use of unenhanced T2-weighted MRI in detecting symptomatic disc pathology in appropriately selected patients, while avoiding unnecessary discography in patients with chronic low back pain.

High-Intensity Zone

In an attempt to find a noninvasive means of diagnosing IVD pathology with a high degree of certainty, several studies have investigated the correlation between positive provocative discography and various findings on MRI, such as HIZ, decreased disc intensity (dark disc), and Modic vertebral endplate changes. In their original publication, Aprill and Bogduk[90] correlated the finding of a HIZ with CT discography and found an 86% positive predictive value for a positive discogram; however, the predictive value and clinical significance of HIZ on MRI has been brought into question more recently. Multiple authors[91-94] have found a positive correlation between the finding of a HIZ and concordant pain on discography similar to the findings of Aprill and Bogduk,[90] whereas others[95,96] have documented the correlation but found unacceptably low sensitivity.

In a study of 62 patients 17 to 68 years old, Kang and colleagues[97] found that only a HIZ in association with disc protrusion correlated with concordant pain on discography. Specificity was 98%, and positive predictive value was 87%; however, the sensitivity was still low at 46%. HIZ in association with either a normal or a bulging disc on MRI was not found to be associated with positive discogram. In a 30-patient study, Ricketson and colleagues[98] were unable to find any correlation between the presence of a HIZ on MRI and a concordant pain response on discography; however, these authors noted that a HIZ was never visualized in a disc found to be morphologically normal on discography. Further studies[49,92,99-101] attempting to correlate positive HIZ findings on MRI and painful discography suggest that although lumbar IVDs with posterior combined annular tears are likely to produce pain, the validity of these signs for predicting discogenic lumbar pain is limited.

Although the exact prevalence is unknown, a HIZ can be seen occasionally in asymptomatic individuals.[44] Carragee and colleagues[67] reported the prevalence of a HIZ in 59% of symptomatic patients and 24% of asymptomatic patients. In the asymptomatic group, 69% of the discs with a HIZ were positive on discography, whereas 10% of the discs without a HIZ were positive. Carragee and colleagues[67] also reported that 50% of the discs with a HIZ were positive on discography in patients with normal psychometric testing compared with 100% positive discography results in patients with abnormal psychometric testing or chronic pain. They concluded that the presence of a HIZ does not reliably indicate the presence of symptomatic IDD because of the high prevalence of HIZ in asymptomatic patients.

In 2004, Mitra and colleagues[102] published a study of 56 low back pain patients with the finding of a HIZ followed longitudinally for 6 to 72 months with MRI. Changes in HIZ on follow-up MRI—either an increase in intensity or spontaneous resolution—were not correlated to changes in visual analog scale (VAS) score, Oswestry Disability Index (ODI), or symptoms, which calls into question the clinical significance of HIZ. Although HIZ on MRI has been found in some studies to have good specificity and positive predictive value for concordant pain generation on discography, it has low sensitivity, high false-positive rates, and questionable clinical significance.

Dark Disc

Whether a dark disc by itself is painful is another controversial topic. Most patients with a dark disc are asymptomatic; however, in some patients, the disc can be a source of pain. Milette and colleagues[103] found that loss of disc height and abnormal signal intensity were highly predictive of symptomatic tears extending beyond the anulus. Horton and Daftari[104] reported a positive discogram in 50% of patients with dark discs without evidence of an annular tear. An isolated dark disc with concordant pain on provocative discography is often considered to be pathologic in the absence of other potential sources of pain and in the absence of confounding psychosocial issues; however, as discussed previously, this evidence is weak.

Modic Endplate Changes

The various stages of Modic changes are thought to be specifically linked with phases of the degenerative disc process. Toyone and colleagues[105] evaluated MRI scans of 74 patients with Modic changes and found that stage I changes tended to be associated with complaint of low back pain and correlated to segmental hypermobility. Other investigators also described Modic stage I changes as specifically associated with low back pain.[106,107] In a large retrospective review by Thompson and

colleagues,[108] Modic changes in 736 patients were correlated to provocative discogram. These authors found that Modic stage I changes had a high positive predictive value (0.81) for a positive discogram. Modic stage II changes had a lower positive predictive value (0.64), and the predictive value of Modic stage III changes was not statistically significant.

In the original description of vertebral body marrow changes by Modic and colleagues,[80] the conversion between signal characteristics from stage I to stage II was described in five of six patients over the course of 14 months to 3 years. Mitra and colleagues[109] performed a more recent prospective evaluation of 48 patients with Modic stage I changes. At 12 months to 3 years of follow-up, 37% were found to have progressed to Modic stage II, 15% partially progressed, and 40% had more extensive Modic stage I changes. Stage I changes are believed to represent the unstable, dynamic phase of the degenerative process and tend either to convert to a stage II pattern or to become more pervasive. Modic stage II changes are thought to be stable and less associated with painful episodes, but there have been reports of stage II changes converting back to stage I.[110] Kuisma and colleagues[111] reported the prevalence of Modic changes in 60 patients treated nonoperatively for sciatica to be 23%. In a longitudinal follow-up of the same patients at 3 years, 14% were noted to have changed type. The levels that did not convert were found to have more extensive Modic changes. Development of Modic change at previously unaffected levels was found in 6%.

Many authors have explored the correlation between Modic changes on MRI with positive concordant pain on discography. Sandhu and colleagues[112] found that both were relatively specific for discogenic pain, with no significant correlation between them. Braithwaite and colleagues[113] found the Modic changes did not predict positive response on discography; they concluded that Modic changes may represent a specific but relatively insensitive sign of discogenic low back pain. Kokkonen and colleagues[114] observed that contrast injection during discography reflected well pain of discogenic origin, whereas the pain associated with endplate damage was usually not shown by CT discography. These authors found a stronger association between endplate degeneration and disc degeneration than between endplate degeneration and annular tears, which may explain why Modic changes have been found to be less sensitive for discogenic pain than discography.

Conversely, other studies have found better correlation between back pain and Modic changes than the correlation between back pain and discography. Carragee and colleagues[66] reported on 100 prospectively followed asymptomatic patients who were at high risk for developing disabling back pain. Of all the incidental diagnostic findings, only moderate or severe Modic changes of the vertebral endplates were found to be weakly associated with subsequent development of a disabling episode of back pain. Other structural MRI findings and concordant pain with discography correlated only weakly with previous back pain episodes and had no association with future disability or medical consultations for back pain. Psychosocial, neurophysiologic (chronic nonlumbar pain), and occupational factors strongly predicted future disabling episodes and consultations for back pain.

In a cross-sectional study of 109 women from two groups, nursing or administrative professions, Schenk and colleagues[115] found that Modic changes and nerve root compromise were the only MRI findings that were statistically significant predictors of low back pain. Signs of disc degeneration, disc herniation, HIZ, and facet arthritis were found in both groups but were not significant risk factors for low back pain.

Similar findings were reported in a study by Kjaer and colleagues,[116] in which complaint of low back pain was correlated to MRI findings in a random selection of 412 Danish subjects. Although Modic changes occurred in less than 25% of subjects (16% Modic stage I and 7% Modic stage II), this finding had the strongest correlation with complaints of back pain. When the subjects were evaluated clinically, the authors found that patients with radiographic evidence of DDD and Modic changes had the best clinical evidence of disc disease. Clinical findings in patients with radiographic evidence of disc degeneration without Modic changes were not significantly different from the baseline population. Kjaer and colleagues[117] concluded that Modic change was a critical finding in relation to history of low back pain and clinical findings. In a follow-up study of the same Danish population, Modic changes correlated with type of occupation, history of smoking, and overweight. The odds ratio for heavy labor combined with smoking was 4.9 for the presence of Modic changes on MRI.[118]

A meta-analysis review of Modic changes by Jensen and colleagues[119] found that the median prevalence of Modic changes from all studies was 43% in patients with nonspecific low back pain. A positive association between low back pain and Modic changes was reported in 7 of 10 studies with odds ratios between 2.0 and 19.9.

Axially Loaded Magnetic Resonance Imaging

There has been interest more recently in the potential role of axially loaded MRI in evaluating patients with lumbar spinal diseases. The idea is to use axial loading to reproduce better the anatomy of the disc under physiologic load. The utility of axially loaded MRI has been studied much more extensively in patients with spinal stenosis and spondylolisthesis.[120-123] Danielson and Willen[124] observed a significant decrease in dural cross-sectional area between a psoas-relaxed position and axial compression in extension in 56% of asymptomatic individuals. The decrease was most pronounced at L4-5 and was worse in older individuals. Although the clinical role of axially loaded MRI in patients with discogenic back pain has not yet been established, Saifuddin and colleagues[125] postulated that lumbar spine MRI with axial loading may increase the sensitivity for the detection of HIZs; however, this hypothesis has not been tested.

Discography

There is significant controversy in the literature surrounding the usefulness of discography for the evaluation of

the integrity of the lumbar disc. Some investigators consider discography to be the most important tool in the diagnosis of IDD,[43,126] but more recent outcome studies[127] and a practice guideline by the American Pain Society[128] have recommended against the use of provocative discography in the diagnosis of discogenic back pain.

Discography is the only physiologic modality used to determine if a specific disc is a pain generator. Although several attempts have been made to explain the pathogenesis of pain provocation during discography, the precise pathomechanism is not well understood. There are four components to the evaluation of a discogram: (1) the pressure and volume of fluid injected into the disc, (2) the morphology of the disc being injected, (3) the subjective pain response at the level of interest, and (4) the pain response when adjacent control levels are injected.[129,130] The subjective pain response to low-pressure provocation is the most important determinant of disc derangement; reproduction of the patient's symptoms on injection of the diseased level is essential to a positive test. A normal disc can accept 1 to 1.5 mL of contrast medium. If 2 mL or more of contrast agent is easily introduced, some degree of disc degeneration is assumed.

The use of postdiscography CT has also been reported to increase the sensitivity for the diagnosis of radial tears of the anulus.[131] Because of low specificity and sensitivity, postdiscography CT is not as helpful, however, in the diagnosis of IDD. Most authors believe that to be diagnostic, not only should the pain be concordant on low-pressure injection, but also a normal control disc should be pain-free (Fig. 45–3).

Despite being used since 1948, discography remains controversial. Holt[126] and Massie[132] published in the 1960s on the high false-positive rate of lumbar discography, which was found to be 26% by Holt. Walsh and colleagues[133] later published a rigorous study on the reliability of lumbar discography. Their study compared 10 normal volunteers with 7 symptomatic patients. Although 17% of the normal discs were found to be morphologically abnormal, there were no positive pain responses. Walsh and colleagues[133] concluded that with modern techniques the false-positive rate of lumbar discography is not as high as reported by Holt.[126]

Derby and colleagues[134] found similar results in a more recent study of 90 patients with low back pain and 16 controls. Morphologically, the prevalence of grade III annular tears was 58% among the asymptomatic control population. Presumably, asymptomatic discs in symptomatic individuals on pressure-controlled discography showed pain levels and responses similar to the control group, whereas patients with true-positive discography showed pain characteristics concordant with their usual symptoms. Derby and colleagues[134] concluded that pressure-controlled discography can differentiate between asymptomatic discs and morphologically abnormal discs.

Carragee and colleagues[68] studied the false-positive rate of low-pressure discography in a comparison of 69 volunteers with no significant low back pain and 52 patients undergoing discography in consideration for treatment of discogenic pain. Low-pressure discography was positive in at least one level in 27% of the patients with low back pain and in 25% of the

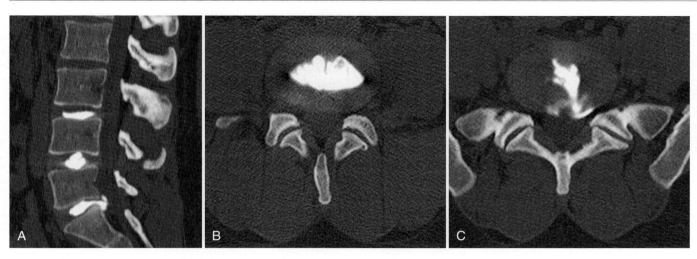

FIGURE 45–3 A-C, CT discogram showing sagittal (**A**) and axial (**B**) images of normal disc morphology at L4-5 level and at adjacent level, L5-S1, disc fissure (**C**).

controls. The false-positive rate of discography was 25% and correlated with psychosocial factors and history of chronic pain of a non-lumbar origin. In another publication from Carragee's group,[69] psychosocial factors and chronic nonlumbar pain, such as cervical pain and somatization disorder, also correlated with positive discography in patients without symptoms of low back pain. These authors concluded that false-positive rates can be low with strict application of the Walsh protocol[133] in patients who do not have positive psychometric issues or other chronic pain syndromes.

In contrast to reports of high false-positive rates, two more recent meta-analyses of low-pressure discography report strong evidence to support the role of discography in identifying patients with discogenic pain.[135,136] Combined data from all studies showed an overall false-positive rate of 9.3% per patient and 6% per disc. False-positive rates among asymptomatic patients were 3% per patient and 2.1% per disc. Chronic pain was not found to be a confounder, and strength of evidence was reported as level II-2 in support of the diagnostic accuracy of discography.

Finding a "gold standard" with which discography results can be compared remains a problem. Few studies have compared the use of discography and outcomes after surgical fusion, which is perhaps the best measure for the validity of discography. Colhoun and colleagues,[137] in a study of 137 patients, reported 89% favorable outcomes in patients with positive concordant pain on discography versus 52% favorable outcomes among patients who had no painful response. Madan and colleagues[138] had different findings; 81% of 41 patients who underwent fusion based on MRI findings had satisfactory outcomes versus 76% of 32 patients who had surgery based on discography. Perhaps the most rigorous study to date was published by Carragee and colleagues.[139] In their study, success of surgical fusion was compared in 32 patients with single-level positive discogram and a matched cohort of 34 patients with single-level spondylolisthesis; 72% of the patients with spondylolisthesis met the highly effective success criteria for surgery versus only 27% of the patients with discogenic pain. Minimal acceptable success criteria were

91% and 43%. Carragee and colleagues[139] calculated a best case positive predictive value for discography of 50% to 60% and concluded that provocative discography was not highly predictive of single-level discogenic back pain.

In an attempt to improve on the poor reliability of discography, interest has turned to functional anesthetic discograms, also called *discoblocks*. A discoblock is a modification of discography, in which a local anesthetic, usually bupivacaine, is infused with the contrast agent into the disc to enhance the diagnostic capability of the procedure. Relief of pain after discoblock is considered diagnostic for discogenic pain. Ohtori and colleagues[140] published a randomized controlled study comparing standard provocative discogram with discoblock in diagnosing discogenic low back pain. Anterior lumbar interbody fusion (ALIF) procedures were performed in 15 patients whose discogenic pain was diagnosed with the aid of discography and 15 patients whose pain was diagnosed with the aid of discoblock. Outcome measures (ODI, VAS, and Japanese Orthopaedic Association score) at 3-year follow-up showed better results that were statistically significant in the group in which diagnosis was aided by discoblock.

Regardless of the details of how discography is performed, some authors have posed the question of potential ill effects resulting from perforating the lumbar disc. Carragee and colleagues[127] more recently published a report on the effect of lumbar discography in precipitating accelerated degeneration in a matched cohort study. The 10-year follow-up showed that discs that had been punctured had a greater progression of disc degeneration—35% versus 14% in the control group. There were 55 new disc herniations in the discography group versus 22 in the control group. Carragee and colleagues[127] concluded that despite using modern discography techniques with small-gauge needles, there is still an increased risk of disc degeneration, disc herniation, changes in disc and endplate signal, and loss of disc height when discography is performed.

Although discography has the potential to assist in diagnosing disc derangement, its reliance on the patient's subjective pain response can also be problematic where secondary

TABLE 45-2 Summary of Recommendations of American Pain Society Specifically in Regard to Management of Chronic Nonradicular Low Back Pain

Recommendation #1

Strong recommendation against use of provocative discography as a procedure for diagnosing discogenic low back pain (moderate-quality evidence)

Insufficient evidence to evaluate validity of diagnostic selective nerve root block, facet joint block, medial branch block, or sacroiliac joint block as diagnostic procedures

Recommendation #2

In patients who do not respond to usual, noninterdisciplinary interventions, clinicians should consider intensive interdisciplinary rehabilitation with a cognitive behavioral emphasis (high-quality evidence)

Clinicians should counsel patients about interdisciplinary rehabilitation as an initial treatment option

Recommendation #3

Facet joint corticosteroid injection, prolotherapy, and intradiscal corticosteroid injection are not recommended (moderate-quality evidence)

Insufficient evidence to evaluate adequately benefits of local injections, botulinum toxin injection, epidural steroid injection, intradiscal electrothermal therapy, therapeutic medial branch block, radiofrequency denervation, sacroiliac joint steroid injection, or intrathecal therapy with opioids or other medications

Recommendation #4

Clinicians should discuss risks and benefits of surgery including specific discussion about intensive interdisciplinary rehabilitation as a similarly effective option, the small to moderate average benefit of surgery over noninterdisciplinary nonsurgical therapy, and the fact that most patients who undergo surgery do not experience an optimal outcome (moderate-quality evidence)

Recommendation #5

Insufficient evidence to evaluate adequately long-term benefits and harms of vertebral disc replacement

From Chou R, Loeser JD, Owens DK, et al: Interventional therapies, surgery, and interdisciplinary rehabilitation for low back pain: An evidence-based clinical practice guideline from the American Pain Society. Spine (Phila Pa 1976) 34:1066-1077, 2009.

gain may be an issue. Psychosocial factors and chronic nonlumbar pain have also been shown to alter the diagnostic capabilities of the procedure. Finally, consideration of the consistent reports of the high false-positive rates and new findings of accelerated degeneration in discs that undergo discography make it difficult to recommend the procedure for the diagnosis of discogenic back pain. The validity of lumbar discography is very much in doubt, which is underscored by a more recent practice recommendation published by the American Pain Society. The society's current recommendation is that provocative lumbar discography should not be used for making the diagnosis of a discogenic source of pain in the setting of nonradicular low back pain.[128] The value of using discography to assess the levels to be operated on in patients with multilevel disc degeneration has not been adequately established scientifically.

Treatment

When a clinician has gathered all the data from the history and physical examination along with appropriate diagnostic studies, decisions must be made with regard to treatment. All available information should be used in formulating a treatment plan to ensure a successful outcome. Sole reliance on individual clinical findings or imaging studies drastically reduces the success rate because the incidence of disc abnormality in asymptomatic patients approaches 30% to 40% and increases with advancing age.

In 2009, the American Pain Society published five practice guidelines on the management of chronic nonradicular back pain based on the best available evidence for the various diagnostic and treatment modalities available. These recommendations are summarized in Table 45-2.[128] These treatment modalities and others not mentioned in the treatment recommendations are discussed in detail along with brief summaries of the current supporting and opposing literature.

Nonoperative Treatment

Nonoperative treatment of lumbar disc disorders has been extensively discussed in the literature.[141] Physical therapy, pharmacology, and spinal manipulations all have been supported by multiple studies of reasonable validity, but it is difficult to evaluate fully most of these studies because of a generalized lack of randomized control design, blind observers, compliance measures, and cointerventions. Additionally, very little of the literature on these nonoperative treatments is specific for the diagnosis of IDD or DDD but rather is generalized to chronic and acute low back pain, which may have multiple etiologies.

Bed Rest and Advice to Stay Active

The use of bed rest and its duration has long been debated in the literature. Treatment schedules ranging from 2 days to 6 weeks have been described.[142-144] The currently accepted recommendation[75] is limited bed rest for a maximum of 2 days because longer durations of bed rest may be detrimental to the patient's general health while offering no benefit to the back pain. Allen and colleagues[145] published a review of studies documenting bed rest as treatment for 15 different conditions and found that for patients with acute low back pain there was significant worsening of outcome measures. The updated Cochrane Review of bed rest for treatment of acute low back pain reported that there is high-quality evidence that advice to rest in bed is less effective than advice to stay active.[146] Progressive return to activity and the initiation of a formal physical therapy or home exercise program are recommended after any initial short period of rest.

Verbunt and colleagues[147] explored reasons why patients sometimes use prolonged bed rest in the setting of acute episodes of low back pain. Among the study population of 282 patients, 33% reported using bed rest, and 8% remained in bed for longer than 4 days. Behavioral factors, catastrophizing, and fear of injury were associated with use of prolonged bed rest. History of back pain and pain intensity were not associated with patient use of prolonged bed rest. Additionally, patients who used prolonged bed rest in the early phase of acute low back pain were more disabled after 1 year.

Patient education and advice to stay active is now the favored recommendation. A more recent Cochrane review[148] of patient education and advice to stay active showed strong evidence that individual instructional sessions of 2.5 hours are more effective in returning patients to work than no intervention; however, in the setting of chronic back pain, patient education was less effective than more intensive interventions. Education sessions of shorter duration and written information were no more effective than no intervention. Another meta-analysis[149] of 39 randomized controlled studies evaluated advice to stay active alone or as an adjunct to other interventions such as back school or specific exercise routines. Advice as an adjunct to a specific exercise program was the most common form of treatment implemented and the best supported of the treatments studied for chronic low back pain. Outcomes among patients with acute low back pain were generally poor, but advice to stay active alone was found to be the best recommendation.

Brox and colleagues[150] published a systematic review of brief education in the clinical setting involving examination, information, reassurance, and advice to stay active. The authors found strong evidence that brief education was more effective for return to work but was no more effective than usual care for reduction of pain. There was limited evidence that dissemination of a back book or an Internet session was less effective than exercise. The authors concluded that a back book should not be distributed to patients as an alternative to another form of treatment.

Brace Wear and Other Orthotics

Another common conservative management technique involves the use of limited brace wear either with a recommendation to stay active or in conjunction with another form of nonoperative therapy. Calmels and colleagues,[151] based on the results of a randomized clinical trial, recommended the limited use of a lumbar belt to improve functional status, pain, and medication use. Oleske and colleagues[152] performed a randomized clinical trial of back supports and patient education in work-related back pain. These authors found no effect on patient self-report of recovery or lost work time between brace use and controls, but back supports were found to have some value in preventing recurrence of work-related back pain. A more recent Cochrane systematic review[153] of brace treatment for low back pain failed, however, to find sufficient evidence to support the use of lumbar supports to treat low back pain. Moderate evidence was found that braces are no more effective than no treatment or physical training in preventing episodes of back pain.

Use of shoe insoles has been recommended in the past for treatment and prevention of nonspecific low back pain. A more recent Cochrane systematic review[154] of six randomized controlled trials reported strong evidence that use of insoles does not prevent episodes of low back pain. There was limited evidence that insoles alleviated low back pain, but no conclusions or recommendations were made for use in the treatment of patients with low back pain.

Physical Therapy

Numerous physical therapy modalities and routines are described in the literature, including land-based and aquatic programs, specific protocols and exercise routines, and group treatment programs—so-called back schools. Adjunctive modalities include pain-relieving treatments such as ultrasound, iontophoresis, transcutaneous electrical nerve stimulation (TENS) unit, and heat therapy. Exercise programs commonly employ aerobic exercise, stretching, flexion and extension routines, core conditioning, and back stabilization protocols. The goal of all of these therapy regimens is to improve core strength, flexibility of the trunk and hip muscles, and conditioning. Patients often respond differently to physical therapy, so treatment programs commonly must be tailored on an individual basis. Periods of activity modification may be necessary. Patients should also be educated on proper body biomechanics; lifestyle change; and healthy living habits, such as weight control, proper nutrition, stress relaxation, and cessation of smoking.

There are multiple randomized controlled trials in the literature in support of many therapy routines or programs. Although a comprehensive review of all the various programs is not undertaken here, there have been some important updates in recent years worthy of discussion. More recent prospective randomized trials comparing physical therapy with fusion have emphasized the importance of a multidisciplinary approach with cognitive therapy, fear avoidance counseling, and intensive exercise programs.[155-157] A systematic review[150] found moderate evidence that fear avoidance training emphasizing exposure is more effective than graded activity increase for improvement of pain, disability, and fear avoidance.

Intensive interdisciplinary rehabilitation with emphasis on cognitive and behavioral intervention was one of the treatment recommendations made by the American Pain Society.[128] Interdisciplinary rehabilitation was defined by the society as an integrated intervention with rehabilitation plus a psychological or social or occupational component. The American Pain Society recommended that interdisciplinary therapy should be offered as a viable alternative before proceeding to surgical treatment. Noninterdisciplinary or "traditional" physical therapy is also efficacious in this patient population, but no one specific program, method, or technique is significantly better than another.

Back schools are another commonly discussed therapy modality, and there is some indication that low-intensity back schools may have some efficacy. Heymans and colleagues,[158] in a randomized controlled trial, found that patients who attended low-intensity back school experienced fewer sick leave days (68 days versus 75 days and 85 days) than usual care patients and patients who attended high-intensity back school.

Functional status and kinesiophobia were improved at 3 months, but there was no difference in pain intensity and perception of recovery between the groups. In another randomized controlled trial, Kaapa and colleagues[159] found no significant benefit of back school, however, compared with physical therapy combined with cognitive therapy at 6-month, 1-year, and 2-year follow-up.

A systematic review from the Cochrane Database in 2004[160] concluded that there was moderate evidence suggesting that back schools in an occupational setting reduce pain and improve function and return-to-work status compared with other forms of therapy, such as exercises, manipulation, myofascial therapy, advice, placebo, and waiting list controls. Brox and colleagues[150] published a separate systematic review of back schools and found moderate evidence that back schools were no better than waiting lists, no intervention, placebo, or general exercises for reduction of pain.

A European economic evaluation of a randomized controlled study[161] of intensive group therapy found no significant cost difference between intensive group therapy and standard physiotherapy. There was also no difference in clinical effect between the groups at 1-year follow-up.[162] To the authors' knowledge, there are no economic studies to date of group therapy back schools in the United States. Although low-intensity back school and programs in a work setting may have benefit versus other forms of nonoperative treatment, most of the current literature shows that back schools offer little benefit over standard physical therapy and cognitive therapy.

Adjunctive Modalities

Another treatment option for low back pain includes adjunctive physical therapy modalities such as TENS, electrical muscle stimulation, ultrasound, and iontophoresis. Poitras and Brosseau[163] reviewed randomized controlled data on the use of TENS and found that it may be useful for immediate short-term pain reduction but has little impact on patient perception of disability or on long-term pain control. A 2008 Cochrane systematic review of TENS versus placebo[164] concluded that there is currently not enough evidence to support the routine use of TENS for management of chronic low back pain. Even less literature is available on the use of iontophoresis and ultrasound in the setting of discogenic back pain. The few randomized controlled trials that exist focus on ultrasound in conjunction with other physical therapy regimens. The efficacy of these modalities in isolation has not been determined.

Chiropractic and Complementary and Alternative Medicine Therapies

Several studies have reported the potential beneficial effects of chiropractic treatment for acute nonspecific low back pain.[165-167] The role of chiropractic manipulations for the treatment of IDD or DDD of the lumbar spine has not been studied. Chiropractic manipulation is generally not considered effective in the treatment of chronic back pain resulting from disorders of the IVDs.[168] A Cochrane systematic review[169] failed to find evidence

that spinal manipulative therapy was superior to general practitioner care, analgesics, physical therapy, exercises, or back school in the treatment of acute and chronic low back pain.

Eisenberg and colleagues[170] published a randomized trial of usual care therapy versus the addition of the patient's choice of alternative therapy—chiropractic, acupuncture, or therapeutic massage—in the treatment of acute low back pain. Outcomes based on the Roland-Morris scale and subjective assessment of symptoms showed no statistically significant improvement in patients who underwent alternative therapies compared with patients treated with the usual care of limited bed rest, nonsteroidal anti-inflammatory drugs (NSAIDs), education, and activity modification. The study did show, however, an increase in patient satisfaction with care, which came at an average $244 net increase in cost per patient.

Hurwitz and colleagues[171] had similar findings in a randomized prospective study of 681 patients with chronic low back pain comparing chiropractic care with medical treatment with 18 months of follow-up. Although less than 20% of the patients overall experienced pain relief and differences in outcome measures were not clinically significant, patients in the chiropractic group were more likely to perceive that their symptoms had improved.

Other alternative medical therapies include acupuncture, prolotherapy, and massage. The Cochrane systematic review of acupuncture[172] showed superiority to placebo sham therapy and a short-term benefit that did not extend beyond first follow-up when acupuncture was used in conjunction with other conventional therapies. A more recent systematic review by Ammendolia and colleagues[173] questioned inconclusive evidence of the success of acupuncture versus sham acupuncture and called for further randomized trials to rule out the possibility of a placebo effect.

Prolotherapy is a technique that attempts to regenerate ligamentous and tendinous structures of the spine via injections of various irritant solutions. The treatment is usually performed in conjunction with spinal manipulation. There is no consensus on method, type of solution injected, or frequency of sessions. Most practitioners use various combinations of saline, dextrose, glycerin, phenol, and lidocaine. Many randomized trials and systematic reviews report conflicting efficacy of prolotherapy.[174-176] No evidence has been reported for the efficacy of prolotherapy without cointerventions such as spinal manipulation or exercise.

The efficacy of complementary and alternative modalities for the treatment of low back pain remains doubtful. The benefit of spinal manipulative therapy is also controversial, but it may improve patient satisfaction with care and perception of symptoms.

Pharmacotherapy

Judicious use of narcotic pain medications, oral steroids, and NSAIDs in patients with severe, acute back pain can provide good pain relief. Most patients with painful degenerative discs can be treated adequately on an outpatient basis. NSAIDs and acetaminophen (Tylenol) are common over-the-counter medications used to treat back pain. A Cochrane review[177] included

65 studies on NSAID use in low back pain. NSAIDs were found to be superior to placebo but had significantly more side effects. There is no documented difference between type of NSAID, including cyclooxygenase-2 inhibitors. Acetaminophen has an effect similar to NSAIDs but reduced risk of associated side effects when taken as directed and in general should be tried before NSAIDs. The Cochrane group concluded that NSAIDs are effective for short-term treatment of acute and chronic low back pain, but the size of the effect is small.

Opioid formulations are commonly used to treat back pain, but considering their widespread use there is a surprising paucity of high-quality randomized controlled data available on their efficacy. A Cochrane database meta-analysis[178] of opioid use found only four studies, three of which focused on the use of tramadol. Pooled data found that tramadol, an atypical opioid, was more effective than placebo for pain relief and showed a slight improvement in functional scores. The only randomized controlled study of classic opioids[179] was a comparison with naproxen. Opioids were found to be more effective for pain relief but were not more effective for improving function than naproxen. The Cochrane review authors concluded that the benefits of opioids for the treatment of chronic low back pain are questionable, and further well-designed randomized controlled studies need to be performed. Two subsequent systematic reviews[180,181] of opioid use in the setting of chronic low back pain concluded that there is evidence to support the efficacy of opioids for short-term relief of pain only. There is little evidence for long-term opioid use, which is fraught with an incidence of aberrant consumptive behavior approaching 25%.

Use of opioid pain medication has many problems ranging from minor side effects such as constipation and nausea to severe complications including respiratory depression, altered mental status, and insidious issues with tolerance and addiction. Another more recent concern with opioid use is related to the combination of opioids and acetaminophen in commonly prescribed formulations.[182] The maximum recommended daily dose of acetaminophen for adults and children older than 12 years is 4 g; thus concern arises when patients inadvertently take larger doses in the setting of prescription drug abuse. The potential to inadvertently take hepatotoxic or lethal doses can be a concern in the setting of prescription drug abuse. An advisory committee from the U.S. Food and Drug Administration (FDA)[184] recommended the addition of a boxed warning on the risk of acetaminophen overdose and suggested elimination of combination opioid-acetaminophen formulations. Care should be exercised when prescribing opioid pain medications. They are best given for only a few days in the setting of severe acute back pain, and their use in patients with chronic back pain is not recommended.

Oral tapering courses of steroids have also been found useful for decreasing symptoms of low back pain, most specifically in patients with disc herniations.[80,185] Steroids can cause gastrointestinal bleeding, and gastrointestinal protective agents should be used simultaneously with oral steroids to reduce the risk of this complication.

Muscle relaxants are another class of medication routinely used in the treatment of muscle spasm associated with low back pain. Their use should be limited to very short courses because of their addictive potential. The Cochrane review[186] of muscle relaxants for the treatment of back pain included 30 trials evaluating the use of benzodiazepines, nonbenzodiazepines, and antispasmodic muscle relaxants. Strong evidence for the efficacy of muscle relaxants over placebo was reported for short-term pain relief in the setting of acute back pain. No difference between the various drugs and classes was discerned. More trials to determine the efficacy of muscle relaxants compared with other analgesics and NSAIDs were recommended.

The last class of medications commonly prescribed in the setting of back pain is antidepressants. Their use may be particularly beneficial in patients presenting with chronic low back pain in association with altered mental status, depression, anhedonia, sleep disturbances, agitation, and anorexia. Clinical studies[187-189] supporting the use of tricyclic antidepressants (TCAs) have shown an improvement in mood and sleep patterns. Low doses of TCAs also affect membrane potentials of peripheral nerves, which may be a mechanism by which they produce pain reduction. A 2003 review[190] of antidepressants in the treatment of chronic low back pain found that TCAs have a moderate effect on pain reduction in patients with no history of depression but reported conflicting evidence for improvement in functional outcomes. Physicians prescribing TCAs should be aware of potentially serious side effects involving orthostatic hypotension and cardiovascular perturbations. In a systematic review,[191] selective serotonin reuptake inhibitors, another common class of antidepressants, failed to show efficacy in the treatment of chronic low back pain and should be reserved for emotional or psychiatric disturbances related to back pain and not used as a primary treatment for symptoms of back pain.

Keller and colleagues[192] published a meta-analysis of nonsurgical management options for low back pain. These authors reported that behavioral therapy, exercise therapy, and NSAIDs had the largest effect of the modalities studied. Machado and colleagues[193] published a separate large meta-analysis of placebo-controlled randomized trials of various forms of nonoperative treatment for nonspecific low back pain. Small improvements in complaints of pain were found in patients treated with traction, physical therapy, antidepressants, and NSAIDs; moderate improvements were found in patients treated with opioid analgesics, muscle relaxants, facet injections, and nerve blocks.

Nonsurgical Interventional Therapies

Nonsurgical interventional therapies range from short-term temporizing measures, such as epidural injections, to procedures designed to be definitive treatments, such as intradiscal electrothermal therapy (IDET).

Epidural Spinal Injection

Administration of epidural steroids should be considered by the surgeon and patient before proceeding to a surgical intervention. The advantage of epidural injections over oral steroids is the ability to achieve higher concentrations of steroid at the site of pain while minimizing systemic effects. Epidural steroids typically work well when administered in the setting of radicular pain and do not work well in the setting of axial pain. Patients with foraminal stenosis secondary to loss of disc height may benefit from selective nerve root blocks either as a diagnostic or as a therapeutic tool. Many clinicians recommend epidural steroid injections as second-line therapy in the treatment of lumbar disc disorders. Epidural steroids are commonly administered by three different routes: caudal, interlaminar, and transforaminal. Although discogenic back pain with leg symptoms is considered an indication for all three modes of administration, the transforaminal approach is generally considered best because it achieves a better anterior epidural distribution. Complications from injection exist but are uncommon.[194,195]

Reports on the efficacy of epidural injections in the literature are contradictory. Manchikanti and colleagues[196] published preliminary results of a randomized trial of serial caudal epidural injections in patients with discogenic pain without disc herniation or radiculitis. These authors reported greater than 50% pain relief in 72% to 81% of patients and 40% reduction in ODI scores in 81% of patients. Manchikanti and colleagues[196] concluded that caudal epidural injections with or without steroid are effective in treating discogenic back pain in greater than 70% of patients. Two other observational studies by the same authors[197,198] have similar findings for the beneficial effects of caudal epidural injections in the specific setting of discogenic low back pain.

Buttermann[199] studied patients with DDD and back pain of greater than 1 year's duration who were candidates for fusion. There was initial success of treatment in greater than 50% of patients, but success rate declined to 23% to 29% by the 1- to 2-year follow-up. The study was plagued by a high dropout rate with more than two thirds of the patients seeking another invasive treatment within 2 years. Buttermann[199] concluded that patients with DDD without spinal stenosis may experience a short-term benefit from epidural injections with only one fourth to one third experiencing long-term improvement in pain and function. Other earlier studies of caudal and transforaminal approaches have reported similar good results for short-term efficacy in low back pain, with 59% of patients having greater than 50% improvement in symptoms and function at a 1-year interval.[197,200]

A more recent systematic review[201] criticized the literature on epidural injections for a lack of careful control of route of administration and patient diagnosis. On evaluation of the pooled data, the only evidence found in support of epidural injections was for short-term symptom relief in nonspecific low back pain. No well-designed randomized trials were found specific to discogenic back pain. A 2008 Cochrane systematic review[202] of injection therapy for low back pain failed to find sufficient evidence to make a recommendation. A systematic review by Chou and colleagues,[203] as part of the American Pain Society practice recommendations, found fair evidence that epidural steroid injection is moderately effective for short-term pain relief; however, the literature supporting its use in nonradicular low back pain is sparse and has not shown significant benefit. No specific recommendation for the use of epidural steroid injections or the route of administration was made by the American Pain Society.

Intradiscal Injection

Direct intradiscal injection, usually with a steroid solution, is another intervention that has been described in the literature for IDD. The desired effect is suppression of an inflammatory process within the disc, which is thought to be the cause of the discogenic pain. Intradiscal steroid injections were reported in an early case series by Feffer,[204] in which 47% of patients reportedly had remission of discogenic symptoms. Similar results were found by Wilkinson and Schuman.[205] More recently, Fayad and colleagues[206] reported a short-term improvement in VAS score at a 1-month follow-up with intradiscal steroid injection in patients with Modic stage I and I-2 changes on MRI, but there was no long-term benefit. The only two major prospective randomized trials[207,208] of intradiscal steroid injection failed to find a statistically significant benefit versus placebo in the treatment of discogenic back pain. Other authors have attempted intradiscal injection of various other substances, including solutions of chondroitin and dextrose,[209] hypertonic dextrose,[210] methylene blue,[211] and oxygen–ozone gas mixtures.[212,213] Although these studies purport promising results, they have yet to be proven efficacious by rigorous randomized controlled trials.

Thermal Annuloplasty

IDET involves percutaneous insertion of a thermally controlled catheter into the IVD, usually the posterior anulus, and heating the catheter to a specific temperature (usually 90° C) for a proscribed period (4 to 12 minutes depending on the protocol). Multiple variations of the procedure exist differing on the type of energy delivered (e.g., percutaneous radiofrequency thermocoagulation), mode of energy delivery (e.g., bipolar), positioning of thermal probe, timing, and duration of energy delivery.

The proposed mechanism of action for these procedures is twofold: (1) elimination of nociceptive pain fibers and aberrant painful responses to the disrupted disc and (2) collagen rearrangement in the anulus with resultant spinal segment stabilization. The biologic effects are not well understood, and there is a lack of clear consensus regarding the effects on neuronal deafferentation, collagen modulation, and spinal stability. Freeman and colleagues[214] studied the effect of nociceptor destruction via IDET on experimentally created annular tears in a sheep model. The authors failed to find any difference in the amount of neoinnervation in the anulus between specimens that underwent IDET and specimens that did not, which calls into question the theory of deafferentation of the anulus. Whether collagen rearrangement with resultant shrinkage and stabilization of the discal element is a viable mechanism for IDET also is questioned.[215,216] Cadaveric studies of the effect of IDET on annular collagen have been performed by Kleinstueck and colleagues,[216] which showed a

10% to 16.7% reduction in tissue volume immediately adjacent to the electrode.

To destroy nociceptors in the anulus fibrosus, temperatures must be increased to a minimum of 42° C to 45° C.[217,218] It is impossible to generate sufficient temperatures in the anulus with a radiofrequency probe placed in the center of the disc as shown by Houpt and colleagues.[219] Temperature changes at distances farther than 11 mm were insufficient to increase the tissue temperature of the outer anulus to the 42° C needed for neuronal ablation. Ashley and colleagues[220] compared temperature distribution in the disc between a radiofrequency needle and a navigable SPINECATH (Smith & Nephew, Memphis, TN). Using this method, they were able to deliver thermal energy to the anulus more effectively and achieved sufficient temperatures to cause denervation. Karasek and Bogduk[221] recommended inserting the IDET electrode so as to remain within 5 mm of the outer surface of the anulus. Placement of the probe in the interlamellar plane rather than inside the innermost layer of the anulus allows for sufficient heat generation to destroy the nociceptors in the outer layers of the anulus.

Complications secondary to any of the thermal annuloplasty procedures are rare. There has been one reported case of postoperative cauda equina syndrome caused by inadvertent placement of the catheter in the spinal canal[222] and a few reports of broken catheters with no resultant adverse effect. There have been no reports of infection, bleeding, or other equipment-related or technique-related complications.

Early uncontrolled clinical trials of IDET were promising, with improvement in 50% to 70% of patients,[42,221-224] but randomized controlled trials have produced conflicting results. Freeman and colleagues[225] found no significant improvement in outcome measures compared with sham surgery at 6 months' follow-up. The opposite findings were reported by Pauza and colleagues[226] in patients with discographically diagnosed low back pain of greater than 6 months' duration. Pauza and colleagues[226] found that 40% of their patients who underwent IDET experienced at least 50% relief of pain, whereas a significant portion of the control group experienced symptom progression. These authors concluded that the IDET procedure is an effective intervention for a selective patient population and reported a number needed to treat of 5 to achieve a 75% relief of pain. Barendse and colleagues[227] reported on a trial of intradiscal radiofrequency thermocoagulation in patients with chronic discogenic back pain. An 8-week follow-up assessment showed no difference from sham surgery in VAS score, global perceived effect, and ODI outcome measures.

Andersson and colleagues[228] published a systematic review of IDET versus spinal fusion in patients with disc degeneration and disruption. Similar median percentage improvement was noted between the two interventions for pain severity and quality of life outcomes. Fusion showed better functional improvement but had a higher rate of complications. Andersson and colleagues[228] concluded that IDET offers similar symptom relief with less risk of complications compared with fusion. In a systematic review, Derby and colleagues[229] concluded that IDET is generally safer and cheaper than more invasive surgical techniques despite the fact that the best evidence available shows only modest improvement in pain relief and functional outcomes.

Other systematic reviews of IDET have been more critical. Helm and colleagues[230] reported level II-2 evidence in support of IDET in the setting of discogenic back pain based on two of the above-mentioned randomized trials and numerous observational studies. Two observational studies were found by these authors in support of radiofrequency intradiscal thermocoagulation for a II-3 level of evidence. Evidence in support of biacuplasty was lacking and was assigned level III. Freeman[231] published a systematic review of the literature that criticized generally poor outcomes even among studies in support of IDET. Freeman[231] concluded that evidence for the efficacy of IDET is weak and has not passed the standard of scientific proof.

Chou and colleagues[203] published a systematic review summarizing all nonoperative interventional therapies as part of the American Pain Society practice recommendations published in 2009. These authors reported fair evidence that epidural steroid injections are effective for short-term pain relief. Good evidence was reported that prolotherapy, facet injection, intradiscal steroid, and intradiscal radiofrequency thermocoagulation are ineffective. For IDET, no conclusions were made because available randomized controlled trials are conflicting. IDET may best be indicated for patients with less functional impairment, with well-maintained disc heights, and with discogenic pain from annular tears.[229] IDET is not universally successful, but roughly 50% of patients can expect significant reduction (>50%) in pain.

Surgical Treatment

When all conservative measures have been exhausted or if symptom nature warrants, surgical intervention may be required. The most common surgical treatment employed for recalcitrant discogenic back pain and DDD is arthrodesis (fusion). Lumbar disc arthroplasty is a newer technique more recently approved by the FDA but not yet in widespread use. Other motion-preserving options being investigated include dynamic neutralization of the spine and disc repair.

Chou and colleagues[232] published a systematic review of surgical treatment for nonradicular low back pain as part of the American Pain Society's practice recommendations. These authors found fair evidence that surgical fusion is no better than intensive rehabilitation with a cognitive behavioral emphasis. Surgically treated patients were considered to be performing poorly, with less than 50% obtaining optimal outcome with fusion. The benefits of instrumented fusion compared with noninstrumented fusion were unclear. Fair evidence was found that for single-level DDD arthroplasty performs as well as fusion, but more long-term outcomes data are needed.

The American Pain Society[128] practice recommendations, published in 2009, encourage clinicians to offer intensive interdisciplinary rehabilitation as an option with outcomes similar to surgery in the setting of nonradicular low back pain.

Most patients with nonradicular pain who undergo surgery do not experience an optimal outcome, which was defined by the American Pain Society as (1) minimal or no pain, (2) discontinuation of or only occasional use of pain medications, and (3) return to high-level function. The society also suggested that there is insufficient evidence at this time to support disc arthroplasty for patients with nonradicular low back pain. Other treatment guidelines also take a cautious view on spinal fusion for DDD, but in some patients the symptoms are so severe that the chance for a good result makes surgical management particularly attractive, especially when nonoperative treatment has failed.

Spinal Fusion

Surgical treatment for unremitting discogenic back pain has traditionally been spinal fusion; however, fusion is not universally accepted as the "gold standard" for this condition. Most clinicians find that it is acceptable to perform spinal fusion for DDD in patients who have failed exhaustive conservative care. The role of spinal fusion in the management of IDD is more controversial.[233]

The goal of a fusion procedure is to eliminate motion at the affected spinal segment. Arthrodesis can be accomplished through a posterolateral fusion (PLF), an interbody technique after removal of the IVD, or a combined approach (360-degree). Interbody approaches include ALIF, through either an abdominal or a retroperitoneal approach; transforaminal lumbar interbody fusion (TLIF), through the facet and neuroforamen; posterior lumbar interbody fusion (PLIF), via a canal decompression; fusion from the side (extreme lateral lumbar interbody fusion [XLIF]), via a transpsoas approach; and use of a presacral approach (percutaneous axial lumbar interbody fusion [AxiaLIF]). All fusion techniques can be supplemented with instrumentation. There are various anterior plates to supplement ALIF procedures, and posteriorly pedicle screw and rod constructs are commonly used. Also, various materials and cages are available to place between the vertebral bodies to perform interbody fusion. Each of these fusion techniques is discussed in subsequent sections.

Three high-quality randomized controlled studies in the past decade have evaluated spinal fusion compared with nonoperative treatment in the setting of chronic low back pain and DDD. Fritzell and colleagues[234] published a randomized controlled multicenter study of severe chronic low back pain comparing fusion of the lower lumbar spine with nonsurgical therapy. The study involved 222 operative and 72 nonoperative patients 25 to 65 years old with chronic low back pain of at least 2 years' duration and radiologic evidence of disc degeneration at L4-5, L5-S1, or both. The nonsurgical group received physical therapy, patient education, and alternative pain control modalities, such as TENS units, acupuncture, and injections. Results at 2 years' follow-up were found to be significantly better in the fusion group, with back pain reduced by 33% compared with 7% in the nonsurgical group. Pain improvement was most significant during the first 6 months postoperatively and then gradually deteriorated thereafter. Disability according to ODI was reduced by 25% compared

with 6% among nonsurgical patients, and 63% of surgical patients rated themselves as "much better" or "better" compared with 29% of nonsurgical patients. The "net back to work rate" was 36% in the surgical group and 13% in the nonsurgical group. The early complication rate in the surgical group was 17%. Fritzell and colleagues[234] concluded that surgical treatment of severe chronic low back pain provides improved results compared with nonoperative treatment in carefully selected patients.

Brox and colleagues[155] published another randomized trial comparing outcomes of lumbar instrumented fusion versus cognitive intervention and exercise in 64 patients with chronic low back pain and DDD. The critical component of this study was the addition of cognitive therapy to an intensive rehabilitation program. The mean change in ODI for the surgical fusion group was from 41 preoperatively to 26 at 1-year follow-up and for the rehabilitation group from 42 to 30. The investigators reported no significant difference in back pain, use of analgesics, emotional distress, and life satisfaction between the groups. Return to work rate at 1 year was 22% in the surgical group and 33% in the rehabilitation group. The rehabilitation group experienced greater improvement in fear avoidance beliefs, and fingertip-to-floor distance, whereas the surgical group had greater improvement in associated symptoms of leg pain. The overall success rate for surgical intervention was 70% and for nonoperative cognitive therapy was 76%. Brox and colleagues[155] concluded that there were near-equivalent outcomes between the groups, which was offset by an 18% complication rate among the surgical group.

Fairbank and colleagues[157] published the last major randomized clinical trial of surgery versus nonoperative therapy. The Medical Research Council (MRC) spine stabilization trial was a randomized controlled trial comparing surgical treatment and intensive rehabilitation in 349 patients with chronic low back pain. Similar to the study by Brox and colleagues,[155] the intensive physical therapy program in the MRC trial also incorporated principles of cognitive behavioral therapy. At 1-year follow-up, the mean ODI scores decreased from 46.5 to 34 in the surgical group and from 44.8 to 36.1 in the rehabilitation group. No significant differences were found between the groups in the shuttle walking test and Short Form-36 General Health Survey (SF-36) outcomes. The authors concluded that although the surgical group enjoyed a small but statistically significant benefit in one of the primary outcome measures (ODI), this was contradicted by the additional cost and potential risk of complication associated with surgery.

In a separate publication on the MRC trial, Rivero-Arias and colleagues[235] performed a cost analysis at 2 years' follow-up. The cost per patient over the study time frame in the surgical group was estimated to be £7830 ($12,450) versus £4526 ($7200) in the rehabilitation group. There was no significant difference in mean quality-adjusted life-years between the groups. The investigators concluded that surgical treatment was not a cost-effective use of health care funds compared with therapy, although the authors pointed out that ultimate costs could vary depending on the number of patients in either group that require subsequent intervention after the 2-year follow-up period.

Meta-analyses of surgical versus nonoperative treatment have paralleled the findings of Brox and colleagues[155] and the MRC trial.[157] Ibrahim and colleagues[236] pooled the data from these three randomized trials and found that a modest improvement in mean ODI scores among surgical patients should not be used as justification for routine operative treatment in light of a 16% early complication rate. Mirza and Deyo,[237] in a separate systematic review, concluded that surgical outcomes are equivalent to a structured rehabilitation program with cognitive behavioral therapy.

Posterolateral Fusion

PLF is typically performed through a traditional midline approach with exposure of the posterior spinal elements; disruption of the facet joints at the fusion levels; and decortication of the transverse processes, pars, and facets to stimulate fusion. Autograft or allograft bone is typically placed over the decorticated areas, and fusion may be augmented with various osteoconductive and osteoinductive materials. Instrumentation in the form of pedicle screw and rod constructs can also be placed to provide segmental stability to increase the success of fusion.

Fusion rates for the lumbar spine vary in the literature and depending on the type and extent of procedure. For a single-level, uninstrumented PLF in the setting of DDD, fusion rates of 85% to 91% have been reported.[238] McCulloch[239] reported a 91% solid fusion rate with uninstrumented single-level PLF and a satisfactory clinical outcome in 78% of patients.

The improvement in fusion rates and outcomes with instrumentation is debated in the literature. France and colleagues[240] reported radiographic fusion rates of 76% among instrumented patients and 64% among noninstrumented patients, but there was no significant difference in outcomes between the groups or any correlation between radiographic union and patient-reported improvement. Other studies have reported a 26% rate of pseudarthrosis in uninstrumented fusion,[241,242] whereas addition of instrumentation has been reported to improve fusion rate, reduce symptoms of pain, and increase return-to-work rate.[241-247] In a prospective study of one-level fusions with and without instrumentation for disabling back pain, Lorenz and colleagues[243] reported superior results with instrumented fusion. There were no reports of pseudarthrosis among the instrumented group, and 75% of patients experienced improvement in pain and were able to return to work. In contrast, 58% of patients in the uninstrumented group had a nonunion, and only one third experienced pain relief and were able to return to work.

In contrast, Thomsen and colleagues,[248] in a randomized clinical study, reported no statistical difference in the rate of fusion between instrumented and noninstrumented patients. Instrumentation was related to an increase in operative time, blood loss, and early reoperation rate and a 4.8% risk of pedicle screw misplacement. Bono and Lee[249] performed a comprehensive review of studies published on lumbar fusion from 1979-2000 and noted a clear trend toward increasing use of instrumentation—23% of all fusions in the 1980s versus 41% of all fusions in the 1990s. These authors were unable to show any significant improvement in overall fusion rate or clinical outcome. The benefit of supplemental instrumentation in PLF is not clearly documented in the literature, particularly in light of newer biologic materials currently being used to enhance fusion rates.

Lumbar Interbody Fusion

There are many potential benefits of using an interbody technique for lumbar fusion. The lumbar vertebral body represents 90% of the surface area and supports 80% of the load within the spine. The greater amount of compressive force anteriorly and the larger surface area theoretically leads to a greater potential for fusion. Interbody fusion is also a more effective technique for maintenance of sagittal and coronal deformity, which can be particularly important in the setting of loss of lumbar lordosis secondary to disc collapse or postlaminectomy kyphosis.

PLF can lead to the persistence of discogenic pain in some patients despite solid fusion, presumably owing to the presence of micromotion and pain in the involved disc. The disc material itself may be a pain generator, which interbody fusion directly addresses by discectomy.[250,251] Weatherley and colleagues[250] reported resolution of pain after an ALIF in five patients with persistent back pain despite solid PLF. Barrick and colleagues[252] also reported excellent pain relief after anterior interbody fusion in 20 patients who had persistent low back pain despite previous PLF. For these reasons, interbody fusion is thought by many to provide better and more predictable pain relief in patients with primarily a discogenic source of low back pain, but there are no high-quality studies supporting this view.

Anterior Lumbar Interbody Fusion

ALIF with bone grafting (Fig. 45–4) for the treatment of IDD was the treatment modality originally recommended by Crock[38] when he described the disorder. ALIF classically is performed through either an intra-abdominal or a retroperitoneal approach. After the symptomatic disc levels have been exposed, the surgeon performs an annulotomy and complete discectomy. The discal segment is reconstructed with autograft bone, allograft bone, or a cage device.

Reports of success for ALIF in the literature are high; Loguidice and colleagues[253] reported an 80% rate of fusion and an 80% clinical success rate with ALIF. Newman and Grinstead[254] reported similar results with 89% fusion and 86% clinical success in patients with IDD. Other than infection, the early risks in ALIF are mainly associated with the surgical approach, including ileus, injury to the abdominal contents or vasculature,[255,256] incisional hernia, muscular atony, and retrograde ejaculation in men secondary to injury to the autonomic plexus.[257,258]

Circumferential Fusion

Combined interbody and posterior fusion, so-called global or 360-degree fusion, is another technique described in the

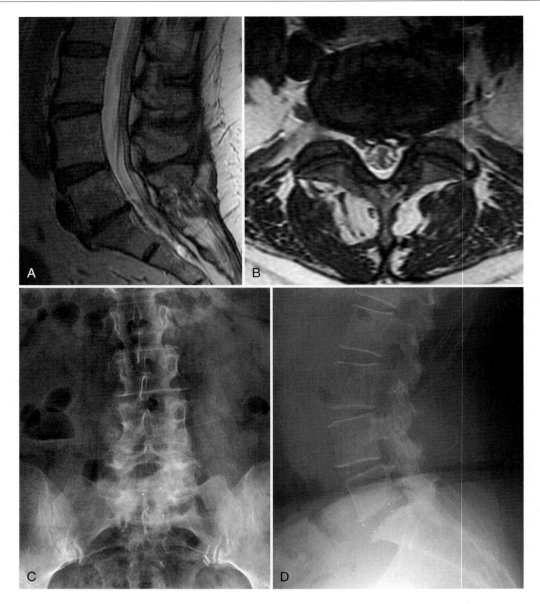

FIGURE 45–4 A and **B,** Preoperative sagittal (**A**) and axial (**B**) T2-weighted MRI in a patient with L5-S1 discogenic back pain, treated with anterior lumbar interbody fusion using carbon fiber–reinforced cages and rhBMP-2. **C** and **D,** Postoperative anteroposterior (**C**) and lateral (**D**) radiographs are shown.

literature. Interbody fusion can be performed via a separate anterior approach (ALIF and PLF) (Fig. 45–5), but a posterior approach (PLIF or TLIF) is often simpler because it involves a single approach for both parts of the fusion procedure (these procedures are discussed subsequently). A combined ALIF and PLF procedure previously was reserved for situations in which the risk of pseudarthrosis was high, such as in patients undergoing revision surgery, patients with preexisting pseudarthrosis, smokers, and diabetic patients; however, today it is commonly used in primary cases as well.

Moore and colleagues[259] reported a 95% arthrodesis rate and 86% clinical success rate with combined anterior and posterior fusion for patients with chronic low back pain and DDD who had failed prolonged nonoperative treatment. Gertzbein and colleagues[260] reported 97% fusion rate and 77%

good clinical outcome with global fusion in a challenging group of patients—62% had previously had surgery, 25% had pseudarthrosis, 55% had two or more levels fused, and 43% were heavy smokers. Kozak and O'Brien[261] treated 69 patients with circumferential fusion through two incisions for discogram-positive, disabling low back pain. They reported greater than 90% good results with one-level and two-level fusions and 78% good results with three-level procedures. Similarly, Hinkley and Jaremko[262] reported greater than 90% positive outcomes in 81 patients who were receiving workers' compensation and were treated with 360-degree lumbar fusion. Videbaek and colleagues,[263] in a randomized clinical trial involving 148 patients comparing the results of circumferential fusion with PLF at 5 to 9 years' follow-up, found that the circumferential fusion group had significantly better

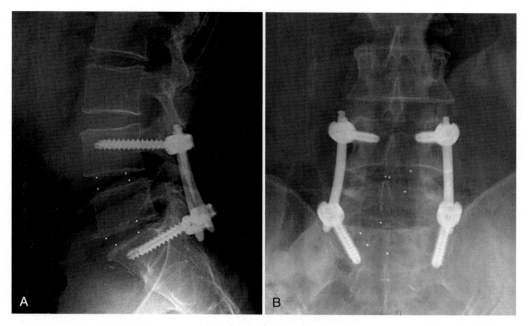

FIGURE 45–5 A and **B,** Postoperative anteroposterior (**A**) and lateral (**B**) radiographs of a patient with L4-5 and L5-S1 discogenic back pain treated with two-level circumferential fusion via an anterior retroperitoneal approach with carbon fiber–reinforced cages and posterior percutaneous transpedicular instrumentation and posterior spinal fusion.

outcomes as measured by the Dallas Pain Questionnaire (DPQ), ODI, and SF-36. The circumferential group also complained of less back pain than the PLF group.

Although combined ALIF and PLIF may reduce the rate of pseudarthrosis to less than 5%, the morbidity is higher than for PLF alone, which is often warranted in patients undergoing revision spine surgery, diabetics, and heavy smokers. Suratwala and colleagues[264] reported retrospectively on 80 complicated patients who underwent circumferential fusion of three or more levels. Encountered complications included 19% pseudarthrosis rate per patient (12% per level), 14% symptomatic pseudarthrosis, and 14% rate of adjacent segment degeneration. Within the 2- to 7-year follow-up, 34% of patients underwent repeat surgery with 20% undergoing implant removal for pain. The rate of deep wound infection was 2.5%, and the rate of superficial infection was 3.8%. Excessive intraoperative bleeding (>3 L) was rare, but 50% of patients required transfusion. Despite the rate of perioperative complications in this complex patient population, the authors reported mean ODI improvement from 50 to 35 and statistically significant improvement in SF-36 and Roland Morris scores.

Posterior and Transforaminal Lumbar Interbody Fusion

Posterior techniques for performing interbody fusion, including PLIF and TLIF (Fig. 45–6), are typically performed with posterior instrumentation and fusion, which makes them by default circumferential fusions. TLIF and PLIF have become increasingly popular techniques for performing circumferential fusion because they can be performed through a single posterior incision, which considerably lessens the morbidity associated with combined anterior and posterior approaches.[265]

In PLIF, the IVD is approached through laminectomy, partial facetectomy, and retraction of the dura and its contents. Risks of PLIF include dural tears, conus injury from retraction, nerve root injury, and epidural fibrosis. Success rates of PLIF in the literature are mixed. Madan and Boeree[266] reported no difference in the outcome of discogenic back pain treated by ALIF versus instrumented PLIF. Conversely, Vamvanij and colleagues[267] compared four fusion procedures and found simultaneous anterior interbody and posterior facet fusion to be superior to PLIF, with an 88% fusion rate. Superior fusion rate did not correlate with a better clinical outcome, however, because only 63% of patients in their study experienced a satisfactory result. Other studies have reported even lower success rates with fusion for discogenic back pain; Knox and Chapman[268] reported only 35% good clinical results with one-level fusion for IDD.

TLIF involves placement of a pedicle screw and rod construct by which the disc space is then distracted. A complete facetectomy is performed unilaterally, through which the discectomy is performed, the endplate is meticulously prepared, and a structural graft or cage is placed into the interbody space. The laminectomy and bilateral partial facetectomy required for the PLIF approach becomes unnecessary in TLIF, which shortens the operative time; decreases blood loss, risk of conus injury, and dural tear; and minimizes epidural scarring. A TLIF procedure still places the nerve root at risk, however, and because the procedure requires complete unilateral facetectomy, posterior instrumentation is mandated owing to resultant instability. A TLIF approach has the

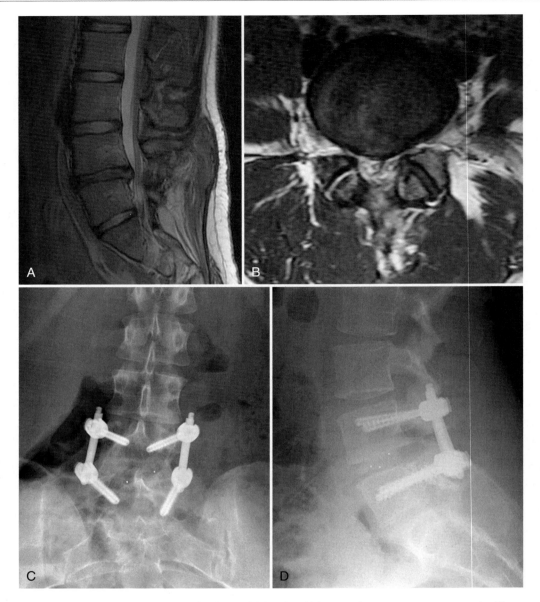

FIGURE 45–6 A-D, Preoperative T2-weighted sagittal (**A**) and axial (**B**) MRI and postoperative anteroposterior (**C**) and lateral (**D**) radiographs of a patient with L4-5 discogenic back pain after prior discectomy treated with transforaminal lumbar interbody fusion and transpedicular instrumentation.

benefits of an interbody fusion—elimination of the potential disc pain generator, improved fusion rate, restoration of disc height, and improved sagittal alignment—and has fewer attendant risks than PLIF and by virtue of the approach decompresses the neuroforamen. Contralateral foraminotomy and decompressive laminectomy can optionally be performed as the patient's symptoms require.

Lowe and colleagues[269] performed a prospective analysis of 40 consecutive patients who had spinal fusion for degenerative diseases of the lumbar spine using unilateral TLIF with pedicle screw fixation. Universal improvement in segmental lordosis, solid fusion in 90% of patients, and excellent or good clinical outcomes in 85% of patients were reported in this study. Whitecloud and colleagues[270] reported that the TLIF approach produces greater than $15,000 of cost savings compared with

a combined anterior-posterior procedure. There were no major complications noted in either group in this study, and no patient required repeat surgery for a lumbar spinal complication at the authors' hospital within the 1-year follow-up period.

Minimally Invasive Surgical Approaches

Minimally invasive surgical approaches to lumbar spine fusion have become increasingly popular. Potential advantages include reduced morbidity, less muscle dissection and blood loss, and shortened inpatient hospital stays; however, minimally invasive surgical approaches typically require specific instrumentation and have a larger learning curve. Several of these minimally invasive techniques are described.

Endoscopically Assisted and Mini-open Anterior Lumbar Interbody Fusion

In 1991, Obenchain[271] described the first interbody fusions performed via a laparoscopic assisted technique. From the time of its description, the anterior laparoscopic technique has been plagued with a steep learning curve; the requirement for significant technical skill; and increased risk of complications such as visceral injury, abdominal vessel injury, and sexual dysfunction. The approach is associated with significantly longer preparation and operative times[272,273] and is usually still dependent on general surgery assistance.[274]

Zdeblick and David[275] reported similar outcomes between traditional open and laparoscopic ALIF except for a significantly higher complication rate—4% versus 20% in the laparoscopic group. Kaiser and colleagues[272] reported no benefit of laparoscopic assisted ALIF versus a mini-open approach. In a meta-analysis of laparoscopic assisted ALIF, Inamasu and Guiot[276] reported that at the L5-S1 level there is no major benefit of laparoscopic versus an open approach with regard to operative time, blood loss, and hospital stay. At other levels, the literature is conflicting; however, there is a consistent association of laparoscopic assisted ALIF with increased risk of retrograde ejaculation at all levels. No conclusion was made with regard to superiority of laparoscopic ALIF over an open approach owing to a lack of evidence.

A mini-open retroperitoneal approach to ALIF has become more popular in part because of the high rate of complications with laparoscopic assisted ALIF. Brau[277] published a large retrospective review involving 686 patients who underwent ALIF via a mini-open approach with specific focus on the complication rate. The rate of arterial and venous injury was 1.6%; retrograde ejaculation, 0.1%; ileus longer than 3 days, 0.6%; superficial wound infection, 0.4%; and compartment syndrome, 0.3%. The rate of complications in a mini-open approach was significantly less than in laparoscopic assisted ALIF and closely approximated complication rates in open ALIF without the associated morbidity of a full open peritoneal approach. The mini-open approach typically still requires general surgical support.

Minimally Invasive Transforaminal Lumbar Interbody Fusion and Posterior Lumbar Interbody Fusion

Various, less invasive modifications of the traditional TLIF technique have been described. One technique involves using pedicle instrumentation only on the side of the facetectomy and placing a transfacet screw on the contralateral side (Fig. 45–7). This technique minimizes dissection on the contralateral side and eliminates the risk of screw abutment on the adjacent facet joint. Operative time and cost of the instrumentation are slightly reduced without adversely affecting the rigidity of the construct.[278] Slucky and colleagues[279] reported on a biomechanical study of constructs using bilateral pedicle screws, unilateral pedicle screws, and unilateral pedicle screws with a contralateral facet screw. These authors found that unilateral pedicle screw constructs allowed significantly increased segmental motion, less stiffness, and off-axis movement, whereas the addition of a contralateral facet screw produced biomechanics similar to bilateral pedicle screw constructs. Constructs using unilateral pedicle screws with a contralateral facet screw are a viable minimally invasive option and reduce instrumentation costs. Sethi and colleagues[280] reported that this technique reduces construct cost by nearly 50% and still has a rate of fusion as high as traditional constructs—100% in the authors' patient population at 9 to 26 months of follow-up.

Other minimally invasive TLIF approaches employ fluoroscopic assisted percutaneous instrumentation (Fig. 45–8). Interbody fusion is typically performed through a paramedian incision with the assistance of a tubular retractor system. Early experience has been positive, but there is a steep learning curve, and the potential for neurologic injury exists. Schwender and colleagues[281] reported good success with this minimally invasive TLIF approach in a population with mixed diagnoses; mean improvement of ODI was from 46 to 14, and the fusion rate was reported to be 100%.

Peng and colleagues[282] reported on a comparative prospective analysis of 29 minimally invasive TLIF procedures versus 29 traditional open TLIF procedures. Intraoperatively and perioperatively minimally invasive TLIF was associated with less blood loss (150 mL vs. 681 mL) and shorter postoperative stays (4 days vs. 6.7 days) but greater fluoroscopic times (106 seconds vs. 35 seconds) and longer operative times (216 minutes vs. 171 minutes). Both groups had improvement in ODI and back pain at 6 months and 2 years of follow-up, with no significant difference between the groups. Radiographic evidence of fusion was 80% for minimally invasive TLIF and 87% for open TLIF. Similar results were reported by Scheufler and colleagues[283] and Park and Ha.[284]

Stevens and colleagues[285] performed an MRI analysis of patients who had undergone minimally invasive lumbar fusion versus traditional open PLF to determine the difference in effect on the paraspinal musculature. The measured maximal intramuscular pressure intraoperatively was significantly less with use of the minimally invasive tubular retractor systems versus open retractors. There was also significantly less edema of the paraspinal musculature on MRI in patients who underwent minimally invasive fusion, indicating that minimally invasive surgical techniques produce less muscle and tissue damage than traditional open fusion.

Percutaneously placed facet screws have also been described in the literature. Shim and colleagues[286] described the use of fluoroscopic assisted percutaneously placed facet screws as a modification of the Magerl technique. These authors reported 11% violation of the laminar wall with no incidences of neural compression; they also reported 15% rate of imperfect pedicle screw placement. Jang and Lee[287] reported on the efficacy of circumferential fusion with percutaneously placed facet screws compared with ALIF and PLF with pedicle screws and found no difference between the two groups in regard to operative outcomes. These authors concluded that percutaneously placed facet screws after ALIF are a viable alternative to PLF and pedicle screws.

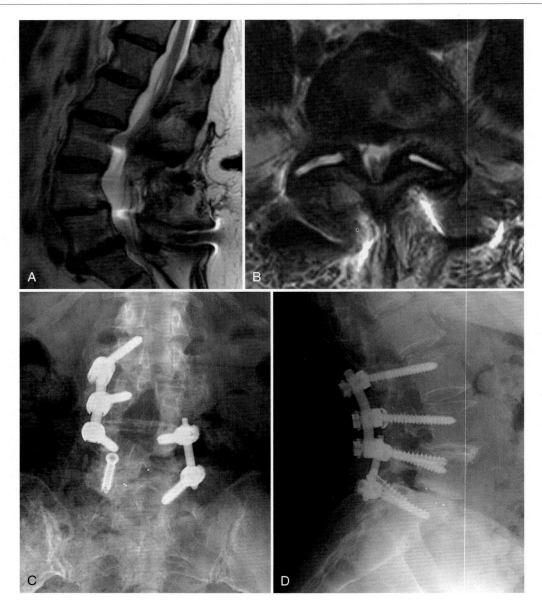

FIGURE 45–7 A-D, Preoperative T2-weighted sagittal (**A**) and axial (**B**) MRI and postoperative anteroposterior (**C**) and lateral (**D**) radiographs of a patient who developed adjacent segment degeneration at L5-S1 segment after previous L3-5 posterior spinal fusion. The patient was treated with transforaminal lumbar interbody fusion, ipsilateral pedicle instrumentation, and contralateral transfacet screw fixation.

Extreme Lateral Lumbar Interbody Fusion and Direct Lateral Lumbar Interbody Fusion

Another novel approach to lumbar interbody fusion is XLIF, sometimes called direct lateral lumbar interbody fusion (Fig. 45–9). This procedure involves an anterolateral interbody fusion performed through a transpsoas approach to the lateral aspect of the IVD. This approach was first described by Pimenta[288] in 2001 as a modification of the retroperitoneal approach. In 2004, Bergey and colleagues[289] described a similar endoscopically assisted transpsoas procedure.

In the most common synthesis of the anterolateral approach, the XLIF, the patient is positioned in a right lateral decubitus position with the table flexed to open the left side of the disc space. A dilator is guided through the retroperitoneal space to the psoas muscle, and the fibers of the psoas are spread under electromyographic monitoring to avoid damage to the lumbar nerve roots and plexus. After exposure of the disc, the procedure is completed similar to any interbody fusion procedure: by discectomy, endplate preparation, and graft placement. The approach does not require a laparotomy and avoids most of the attendant complications associated with the anterior approach. Exposure is limited by the inferior border of the 12th rib and the superior edge of the iliac crest. The greatest risk during the procedure involves the dissection through the psoas, which is associated with risk of injury to

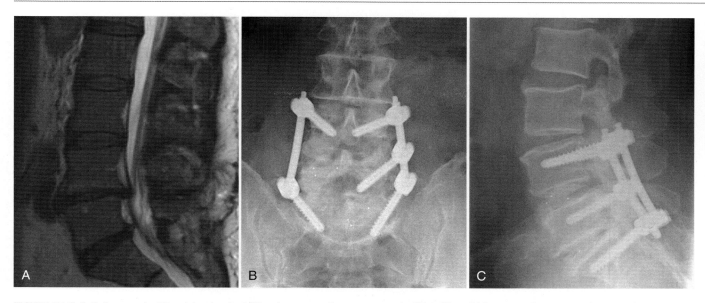

FIGURE 45–8 A-C, Preoperative T2-weighted sagittal (**A**) and postoperative anteroposterior (**B**) and lateral (**C**) images of a patient with L4-5 and L5-S1 degenerative disc disease treated with TLIF via minimally invasive approach and percutaneously placed transpedicular instrumentation.

the lumbar nerve roots and the lumbar plexus, most specifically the genitofemoral nerve.

Benglis and colleagues[290] published an anatomic study of the lumbar plexus around the psoas muscle to clarify the approach and risk to the neural structures during a direct lateral approach. The nervous plexus has a progressive dorsal to ventral migration from the L1-2 posterior endplate edge, to a ratio of 0.28 of the width of the disc at the L4-5 level. Ventral migration was most pronounced at the L4-5 level, and risk of injury to the lumbosacral plexus is highest at this level if the dissector cannula is placed too far posterior.

Reports of outcomes for the XLIF procedure are sparse, and short-term data only are available. Knight and colleagues[290a]

reported complication rates of direct lateral interbody fusion in a cohort of 58 patients; 8 of the 13 reported complications were mild and related to the approach, the most common being meralgia paresthetica. Two patients (3.4%) experienced L4 nerve root injury, one of which lasted longer than 1 year. In a separate, smaller series, Ozgur and colleagues[291] reported no complications with the XLIF procedure.

Percutaneous Axial Lumbar Interbody Fusion

Another emerging fusion technique specifically aimed at the L5-S1 level involves a percutaneous presacral approach. The procedure was described by Marotta and colleagues[292] and is

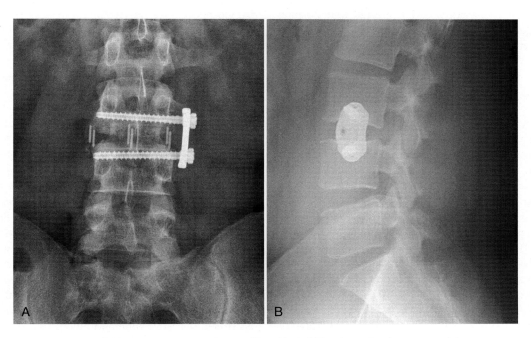

FIGURE 45–9 A and **B,** Postoperative anteroposterior (**A**) and lateral (**B**) radiographs of a patient with L3-4 discogenic back pain treated with interbody fusion through a direct lateral approach.

referred to as *AxiaLIF*. Aryan and colleagues[293] reported a 91% fusion rate in 33 patients, some of whom also required adjunctive stabilizing procedures during the index procedure. At this point, data on outcomes for AxiaLIF are sparse, and there are as yet only a few case series in the literature.

Radiation Exposure

The advent of minimally invasive surgical techniques has generally been accompanied by increases in the use of intraoperative fluoroscopy. The risks to the patient and physician are not inconsequential. Bindal and colleagues[294] reported on intraoperative radiation exposure during minimally invasive TLIF. The average fluoroscopic time was 1.69 minutes (range 0.82 to 3.73 minutes), and radiation exposure per case was 76 mrem total, 27 mrem at the waist under a lead apron, and 32 mrem at the thyroid. Radiation-induced malignancy is a potential concern with increased intraoperative use of fluoroscopy associated with minimally invasive surgical techniques. Navigation systems may have a role in decreasing radiation exposure,[295] and there are numerous safe operating techniques the surgeon should use to reduce radiation exposure.

Comparison of Fusion Techniques

As part of the Swedish Spine Study Group's randomized clinical trial, Fritzell and colleagues[296] compared the outcomes of the 222 patients in the surgical arm. Patients had been randomly assigned to three surgical groups: (1) PLF, (2) instrumented PLF, and (3) circumferential fusion. All three procedures showed statistically significant reduction in pain and disability with no significant differences between the groups. Radiographically determined fusion rates were 72%, 87%, and 91%. With increasing complexity of procedure (groups 2 and 3), operative times were significantly longer, blood transfusion requirements were greater, and hospital stays were longer. Early complication rates were 6%, 16%, and 31%. Complication rates at 2 years' follow-up[297] were 12%, 22%, and 40%. An odds ratio for risk of complication was 5.3 between circumferential fusion and PLF and 2.4 between circumferential fusion and instrumented posterior fusion. Kim and colleagues[298] compared three fusion techniques: PLF, PLIF, and circumferential fusion via PLIF. At minimum 3 years' follow-up, good or excellent results were reported in 81% of PLF cases, in 88% of PLIF cases, and 86% of circumferential fusion cases, and pseudarthrosis rates were 8%, 5%, and 4%.

Glassman and colleagues[299] published a large multicenter retrospective analysis of 497 patients who underwent different types of fusion procedures. Despite the fact that patients who underwent ALIF or PLF had slightly better clinical outcomes, good efficacy was found for all fusion modalities with respect to pain relief and outcomes. The authors concluded that surgeons can select the fusion approach at which they are most comfortable without significantly affecting outcome results. Between the multiple techniques and approaches available to perform lumbar arthrodesis, there is no clear consensus on which is the most successful, despite multiple studies comparing outcome measures, cost, rates of pseudarthrosis, and complications. Certain procedures may be more successful in specific patient populations; interbody fusion may treat a discogenic pain generator more successfully in patients with IDD.

Materials and Osteobiologics

To assist in fusion and interbody space reconstruction, multiple structural interbody graft and cage options have been designed. Common materials include machined allograft bone, titanium cages, reinforced carbon fiber, polyetheretherketone (PEEK), and bioresorbable cages. Several cage designs exist, including cylindric, tapered, impacted, lordotic, biconvex, and boomerang-shaped. There is a paucity of randomized controlled trials comparing clinical results between the different designs. A review of the multiplicity of structural grafts and cages currently being marketed is beyond the scope of this chapter.

To improve fusion rates, various graft materials have been studied, including iliac crest autograft, morcellized local laminectomy bone, allograft bone, and several graft extenders. With the advent of bone morphogenetic proteins (BMPs), spinal fusion surgery has entered a new era. Multiple BMPs have been discovered, most of which are members of the transforming growth factor superfamily. BMP-2 and BMP-7 have been studied extensively and currently have FDA approval for limited use in humans.

Use of BMP has many reported benefits. Results for fusion rates so far have been excellent,[300,301] and reduction in pseudarthrosis rates results in decreased requirement for costly revision surgeries. Some centers have attempted placing BMP through the PLIF or TLIF approach; however, the benefit of this use is unclear.[302] BMP seems to obviate the need for autograft bone grafting, eliminating the risk of donor site morbidity, decreasing operative time, and decreasing blood loss. Donor site morbidity associated with iliac crest autograph harvest is significant. Sasso and colleagues[303] combined results from four randomized trials comparing iliac crest graft and recombinant human BMP-2 (rhBMP-2) as part of an ALIF procedure. The investigators evaluated 208 patients' VAS score for intensity and frequency of pain. At 2 years' follow-up, 31% of patients were still reporting persistent pain at the donor site, and 16% reported fair or poor appearance of the graft site.

Multiple randomized controlled trials have been performed on BMP-2; most have evaluated the effectiveness of the protein compared with iliac crest autograft. Dimar and colleagues[304] published the results of a randomized prospective trial with 98 patients who underwent single-level PLF. Fusion rate at 2 years was 73% in the iliac crest autograph group and 88% in the rhBMP-2 group. Average operating time was 21% longer and blood loss was 81% greater in the autograft group compared with the rhBMP-2 group. No significant difference in outcome measures was noted between the groups at any of the follow-up intervals. A later study[305] by the same group found decreased operative time and blood loss and higher rates of fusion but no difference in outcome measures. Fusion results in single-level ALIF with allograft dowels were similar as reported by Burkus and colleagues:[306] 100% in the rhBMP-2 group and 81.5% in the autologous bone graft group. A 6-year follow-up of patients in the Burkus study[307] projected a worst-case scenario fusion rate of 91%, considering reoperation rate for pseudarthrosis within the 6-year postoperative interval.

Vaccaro and colleagues[308] compared OP-1/BMP-7 with iliac crest autograft in PLF. This was the first large (335 patients), randomized controlled trial of BMP-7 for use in spine fusion. At 3 years' average follow-up, there was no significant difference between the two groups with respect to outcome measures, success of fusion, reoperation rate, complications, and fusion. The iliac crest autograft group had statistically longer operative times and blood loss. Vaccaro and colleagues[308] concluded that OP-1/BMP-7 was equivalent to iliac crest bone graft in PLF.

The use of BMP is not without complications.[309] BMP used in minimally invasive TLIF is reported to be associated with postoperative radiculitis.[310] Use of BMP is also linked to postoperative bleeding and seroma formation, heterotopic bone formation,[311] and osteolysis. Rates of vertebral osteolysis associated with use of BMP-2 in interbody cages have been reported to be 5.8%.[312] Two unpublished cases of vertebral osteolysis at the authors' institution have resulted in cage dislodgment.

The high cost of BMP has led some authors to caution against routine use, whereas others report that the decreased risk of pseudarthrosis and associated revision surgery justifies the expense in certain patient populations. Glassman and colleagues[313] reported on the success of rhBMP-2 in single-level posterolateral lumbar fusions in smokers. In the rhBMP-2 group, 20 of 21 patients (95%) achieved fusion, and in the iliac crest autograph group, 16 of 21 patients (76%) achieved fusion; however, the authors noted that other clinical outcomes were still adversely affected by smoking independent of fusion status. Carreon and colleagues[314] published a cost utility study on BMP-2 versus iliac crest autograft in elderly patients. At 2 years' follow-up, after accounting for complications, including a higher rate of nonunion (9.6% in the autograft group) and revision surgery, the mean cost in the rhBMP-2 group was $39,967 and in the iliac crest autograph group was $42,286.

A British meta-analysis published by the National Institute of Health Research (NIHR) Health Technology Assessment Programme[315] evaluated the cost-effectiveness of BMP in spinal fusions. Garrison and colleagues[315] found evidence that BMP-2 was more effective than autogenous bone graft for radiographic fusion in single-level DDD. BMP was also associated with decreased operative time, improved clinical outcomes, shorter hospital stays, and fewer secondary interventions. The probability that BMP was cost-effective in Great Britain, based on a cost per quality-adjusted life-year of less than £30,000 (roughly $50,000), was only 6.4%, however. Garrison and colleagues[315] concluded that although BMP improved outcome measures and decreased morbidity associated with autologous graft harvesting, its use was not cost-effective.

The development of osteobiologics such as BMPs has been an exciting advancement in recent years. More substances are likely to be developed in coming years. Several other proteins, such as GDF-5, TIMP, TGF-β, IGF-1, and SOX-9, are already being investigated for their potential application in spinal fusion and disc regeneration.

Adjacent Segment Degeneration

Criticisms of spinal arthrodesis are that it alters endplate loading, increases intradiscal pressures,[316] significantly alters lumbar mechanics,[317] and potentially increases the rate of adjacent segment degeneration.[318-322] The problem seems to be more than simple subacute preexisting degenerative disease exacerbated by fusion at an adjacent level. Willems and colleagues[323] looked at prefusion status of adjacent segments on discography and found that preoperative findings of disc degeneration were not associated with poor outcomes after fusion secondary to symptomatic adjacent levels.

Schulte and colleagues[324] published a study on the effect of circumferential fusion in relation to adjacent disc heights and outcome measures at 10 years' follow-up. Among the 27 patients with a diagnosis of DDD, disc height loss for the immediate cephalad level averaged 21% and for the second cephalad level was 16%. Patients with a preoperative diagnosis of DDD tended to have a greater loss of adjacent disc height than patients with spondylolisthesis. Multilevel fusions also showed greater adjacent level loss of disc height that was statistically significant. No correlation was found between outcome measures and adjacent loss of disc height.

Wai and colleagues[320] reported on 39 patients with a minimum of 20 years' follow-up after ALIF. Of patients, 74% had some evidence of degenerative changes in the lumbar spine, 23% had advanced degeneration at a level adjacent to the fusion, and 18% had advanced degeneration at another level with preservation of the adjacent levels. There was no association found between radiographic degeneration and functional outcome. Only three patients (8%) had undergone additional surgery for adjacent level degeneration within the 20 years of follow-up. The fact that a large portion of the degenerative changes after fusion occurred at nonadjacent levels led Wai and colleagues[320] to question adjacent level degeneration, suggesting that changes were more likely a result of constitutional factors (aging, preexisting degeneration) rather than alteration in loading from an adjacent fusion.

In an attempt to address adjacent segment degeneration associated with lumbar arthrodesis, dynamic surgical options have been developed. The theory is that if some amount of motion is preserved at the operative level, adjacent segments would be less affected by alteration in lumbar mechanics attendant with fusion. Three modalities that are used to attempt to accomplish a dynamic resolution of back pain are (1) pedicle screw–based dynamic spinal stabilization systems, (2) total disc arthroplasty (TDA), and (3) nuclear replacement technologies.

Dynamic Spinal Stabilization Techniques

Dynamic techniques for spinal stabilization have been described in the literature for many years, but newer techniques and instrumentation designs have made this an area of renewed interest. Several authors have attempted to use soft tissue stabilization techniques that restrict rather than completely eliminate motion, while still relieving mechanical back pain. One of the first dynamic systems was described by Graf[325] and involved an artificial ligament reconstruction using four pedicle screws and two braided polyester bands to stabilize the painful segment in lordosis. Proponents of the technique state that pain is reduced by coaptation of the painful facets; posterior annular compression, which closes annular tears; and stabilization of the motion segment. Theoretically, the fixation relaxes over the first 6 months postoperatively allowing a return of motion after healing has occurred.[326]

Outcomes for Graf ligamentoplasty in the literature are sparse and mixed. Kanayama and colleagues[327] reported on 10-year follow-up, with preservation of segmental motion in 80% of patients and improvement in VAS scores. Other studies have reported poor outcomes at 1 year and a high rate of revision at 2 years. Revision for ligamentoplasty has been found to have poor outcomes—similar to the outcomes seen after revision arthrodesis.[328-331] One of the biggest arguments against the procedure has been that the Graf ligament significantly restricts flexion at the spinal segment, which increases load in the problematic posterior anulus of the disc.

Newer techniques and designs, such as the dynamic neutralization system for the spine (Dynesys Dynamic Stabilization System; Zimmer, Warsaw, IN), attempt to reduce movement equally in flexion and in extension. The Dynesys system consists of titanium pedicle screws connected by an elastic band, which controls motion in a more consistent manner than the Graf ligamentoplasty. Although an improvement over the Graf technique, the degree to which the Dynesys system successfully unloads the disc is still unpredictable.[332] Reported outcomes by Grob and colleagues[333] were poor with only half of patients achieving improved quality of life and less than half experiencing functional capacity improvement. These authors concluded that there was no support for superiority of dynamic stabilization to typical arthrodesis. Few randomized controlled clinical studies have been conducted with this technique, and long-term efficacy is not yet clearly established.[334]

Disc Arthroplasty

Another technique for maintenance of segmental motion while treating symptomatic disc disease is TDA. Interest in TDA was inspired by the resounding successes of total hip arthroplasty and total knee arthroplasty in restoration of function and resolution of pain. The goal of TDA is to remove the discal pain generator while maintaining segmental height, stability, and motion. The potential benefits of disc arthroplasty are twofold: (1) Healing does not require fusion, removing the risk of pseudarthrosis, and (2) motion is preserved, which theoretically reduces the risk of adjacent segment degeneration.

The first implanted lumbar total disc replacement prosthesis in the United States was the SB Charité III (DePuy Spine, Raynham, MA). There are now two FDA-approved devices for

lumbar disc arthroplasty: SB Charité approved in October 2004 and ProDisc-L (Spine Solutions/Synthes, Paoli, PA) approved in August 2006. At least two other disc replacement systems are undergoing FDA trials: Maverick (Medtronic Sofamor Danek, Memphis, TN), and FlexiCore (Stryker Spine, Allendale, NJ).

Although TDA designs have been used in Europe for quite a while, long-term results are still in dispute. The Charité device has the longest term information based on randomized controlled data. Guyer and colleagues[335] reported on 5-year follow-up for 90 TDA patients in a noninferiority study compared with a control group of 43 ALIF patients. ODI and SF-36 data between the groups was comparable, but 66% of the TDA patients versus 47% of the ALIF patients were back to full-time work at the 5-year interval. Range of motion for the Charité device at 5 years' follow-up was reported to be 6 degrees.

Blumenthal and colleagues[336] published clinical results of a randomized controlled trial of the Charité disc and reported noninferiority to ALIF controls. Radiographic examination of study patients showed better restoration of disc height and less subsidence in TDA versus ALIF with BAK cages (Spine tech, Minneapolis, MN).[337] Tropiano and colleagues[338] had 75% excellent or good results at an average 8.7 years of follow-up. Lemaire and colleagues[339] reported 90% good or excellent outcomes and 91.5% return-to-work rate at a minimum of 10 years of follow-up in 147 patients.

Randomized controlled device trials of ProDisc-L[340] have also shown noninferiority to spinal fusion. Outcomes of TDA in this study show a statistically significant advantage of arthroplasty compared with fusion. Improvement criteria (≥15%) in ODI, VAS, and SF-36 were met in 77% of TDA patients versus 64% of fusion patients. Favorable initial randomized controlled clinical trial results have also been published in support of the FlexiCore system.[341]

Proponents of TDA suggest that preservation of motion at the operated level decreases the incidence of adjacent segment degenerative disease associated with fusion. One of the purported benefits of this technique is for patients who would otherwise require multilevel fusion because of asymptomatic or subacute adjacent level degenerative changes. A significant problem with fusion procedures is the risk of developing adjacent segment degeneration; however, in some reports TDA devices have been associated with increased adjacent segment degenerative changes. Kostuik[342] reported that two of the most common complications necessitating revision surgery in TDA were facet degeneration and adjacent level disease.

Park and colleagues[343] reported on radiographic evidence of adjacent level degeneration after ProDisc-L implantation; at 26 months postoperatively, progression of facet degeneration was noted in 29% of 32 patients. Adjacent level progression was positively correlated with female gender, malposition of the prosthesis, and two-level disc replacement. In a comparative study between Charité and ProDisc-L, Shim and colleagues[344] found that although the clinical outcomes of both systems were good, the facet joints at the operative level (32% to 36%) and the discs at adjacent levels (19% to 29%) showed advancement of degeneration at 3 years' follow-up regardless of device used. Harrop and colleagues[345] published a systematic literature review comparing published reports of adjacent segment degeneration in lumbar fusion with TDA. In the fusion group, 173 of 1216 patients (14%) developed symptomatic adjacent segment disease compared with 7 of the 595 TDA patients. This study had the benefit of large patient numbers, but none of the published reports used for the analysis were of a high level of evidence.

Another problem with TDA systems is that it is very difficult to create a mechanical device that can mimic all of the properties of the native disc. Several patients who underwent TDA with good pain relief have been found to have experienced spontaneous fusion secondary to heterotopic bone formation. In some reports, heterotopic ossification and spontaneous fusion have been unusually high in cervical disc replacement.[346] In lumbar disc replacement, Huang and colleagues[347] reported a 13% rate of heterotopic ossification in 65 patients, and 2 patients went on to spontaneous fusion. These authors cited preoperative ossification of the anulus, bony endplate injury, component malposition, and subsidence as potential factors leading to postoperative heterotopic ossification. Tortolani and colleagues[348] reported that the rate of heterotopic ossification in 276 Charité patients was only 4.3% and that regardless of the presence of heterotopic ossification, postoperative range of motion was still better than preoperative range of motion in all cases.

Another possible problem with TDA is the potential for a failed prosthesis to cause catastrophic complications and make revisions extremely complex. Reported reasons for failure in the literature include acquired spondylolysis,[349] implant subsidence,[350] implant loosening, malposition, displacement, early wear, and infection.[342] TDA failure by catastrophic wear, similar to that seen in total joint arthroplasty, is a potential concern, but wear rates and behavior of polyethylene debris around the spine are still largely unknown. Managing revision surgeries has the potential to become incredibly complicated dealing with repeat anterior exposures, osteolysis, prosthesis subsidence, and bone loss. In a feasibility study of revision of the Charité device, McAfee and colleagues[351] reported that TDA did not preclude further procedures at the index level of surgery. Of 589 TDA patients, 52 required revision (9%) compared with 10 of 99 ALIF patients (10%). Through a repeat anterior retroperitoneal approach, 22 of 24 TDA devices were removed successfully. Seven of the 24 (29%) removed discs were revised to another Charité device.

Another concern with TDA is the cost of the device and procedure. Levin and colleagues[352] published a charge analysis of one-level and two-level TDA with ProDisc-L versus circumferential fusion. For one-level fusion, average implant cost was nearly identical at $13,990 for fusion and $13,800 for TDA. Operative time for TDA was about one half of the average time for fusion (185 minutes vs. 344 minutes). Total charge for a single level averaged $35,592 for TDA and $46,280 for fusion. For two-level procedures, implant costs were much less for fusion ($18,460) than for TDA ($27,600), and operative times were 242 minutes versus 387 minutes. In a smaller retrospective review, Patel and colleagues[353] compared TDA with fusions and found that implant costs for TDA, ALIF, and TLIF were similar if rhBMP-2 was excluded from the analysis.

Success for TDA has been found in multiple studies with up to 10 years follow-up to be at least equivalent to fusion. Concern for complications specific to TDA exist, such as heterotopic bone formation, spontaneous fusion, spondylolysis, catastrophic failure, displacement, implant subsidence, and potential for complicated revisions. Preliminary studies have shown revisions to be feasible for short-term periods, but long-term effects of polyethylene wear behavior and osteolysis are still unknown. From a cost standpoint, TDA seems to compare favorably with fusion techniques for one-level disease even in the absence of BMP use; however, two-level TDA seems to be more expensive than two-level fusion. TDA offers yet another option for operative treatment of IDD and DDD, but long-term results are yet to be determined.

Nuclear Replacement

Another concept for treating IVD disease involves replacing the nucleus pulposus while retaining the anulus intact. The objective essentially is to reinflate the nucleus. This concept allows for the design of smaller prostheses that can be implanted via a minimally invasive approach. Implant failure would theoretically be less devastating than failure associated with total disc replacements.

The first nuclear replacement procedures were performed by Fernstrom[354] in the late 1950s. This technique involved an annulotomy, resection of the nucleus pulposus, placement of a steel ball bearing (dubbed the Fernstrom ball), and preservation of the anulus. Fernstrom[354] claimed outcomes similar to fusion, but application of this technique became associated with unacceptable rates of implant subsidence.

Multiple modern nuclear replacement designs currently are under development and investigation, which fall under two main device types. The first type is a mechanical design and includes devices such as the original Fernstrom ball, and newer designs composed of PEEK and pyrolytic carbon. The second type is an elastomeric design usually made with either preformed or injectable materials such as polyurethane, silicone, and various other polymers.[355]

The Prosthetic Disc Nucleus (PDN) (Raymedica, Bloomfield, MN) is the most studied nuclear replacement device. Klara and Ray[356] published a series of 423 patients treated with PDN since 1996. They reported a 90% survival rate and 10% rate of device explantation. Initially, the study was plagued with a high device migration rate, but newer designs have had improved results. Shim and colleagues[357] reported 78% good results in 46 patients followed for longer than 6 months; 4 patients required revision surgery because of migration of the implant. Ahrens and colleagues[358] published a 2-year prospective outcome study on the DASCOR device (Disc Dynamics, Eden Prairie, MN) involving 85 patients. These authors reported significant improvement in VAS and ODI outcome measures. The rate of explantation was 8%, most commonly for resumption of severe back pain. The outcome data for nucleus pulposus replacement technologies are short-term, and the technique is still in need of careful investigation.

Future Directions

Great interest has been generated in recent years for the development of biologic repair strategies and biopharmaceutical approaches for interception and prevention of the degenerative disc cascade. Several investigators[359,360] have reported successful transplantation of disc chondrocyte cells in animal studies with regeneration of viable matrix and normalized distribution within the disc space. Nomura and colleagues[361] hypothesized that the extracellular matrix may play a role in slowing the rate of disc degeneration. Meisel and colleagues[362] published a canine model for autologous chondrocyte transplant repair of damaged IVDs. A randomized controlled trial is under way comparing chondrotransplant DISC with discectomy.

Another approach under investigation is the use of various growth factors alone or in combination to induce disc regeneration. Metabolically impaired cells in the IVD that exhibit degenerative or age-related changes have been shown to repair their own matrix and disc structure under the influence of OP-1/BMP-7. BMP-7 seems to have an anabolic effect on proteoglycan and collagen synthesis, particularly within the nucleus pulposus. Animal studies have been performed using BMP-7, and GDF-5 with results showing restoration of disc height, increased extracellular matrix, and increased proteoglycan synthesis,[363-365] but human studies have not been performed yet.

Manipulation of genes that regulate the synthesis of specific RNA and protein molecules on a cellular level also has promising applications for prevention of DDD and disc regeneration. Gene delivery, typically by a viral vector, provides for local production of sustainable, high concentrations of the gene product for extended periods. Targeted delivery of a gene product maximizes therapeutic potential, while minimizing side effects. Endogenously produced proteins may also have greater biologic activity than exogenously administered recombinant proteins.[366] The IVD is relatively avascular and has poorly characterized, slowly dividing cells, so injection of viral vectors could potentially be maintained for long periods in this encapsulated and immunoprotected environment.

Because of safety concerns, ex vivo methods of gene therapy with the help of a bioreactor or tissue scaffold may be preferable. Ex vivo studies showing successful incorporation, increased matrix production, and restoration of the IVD structure have now been published for multiple gene products, including SOX-9,[367] TIMP-1,[368] TGF-β1, IGF-1, and BMP-2.[369] There are still several concerns, however; for example, the virus may leak through annular fissures in the degenerated disc and evoke an immune response. An ideal treatment program for DDD should also allow for repetitive administration of gene therapy injections at the same or different disc levels.[370]

Regardless of the method of disc regeneration, significant challenges remain. Regeneration of a severely degenerated disc may be impossible because the environment within the degenerated disc may be too hostile secondary to endplate sclerosis and poor tissue nutrition. Also, an unstable spinal segment would make regeneration difficult because continued abnormal loading during the healing phase would likely lead to failure.

Summary

Lumbar disc disease is a common problem that affects many people at various ages in the form of IDD and DDD. A detailed history and physical examination are vital components along with imaging modalities to make an accurate diagnosis. Practice guidelines have reaffirmed that the first line of treatment for patients who have low back pain of a discogenic source, with or without radicular symptoms, is conservative therapy. New emphasis has been placed on multidisciplinary therapy incorporating cognitive and behavioral treatment. Intradiscal therapy is controversial, and many patients who undergo this procedure may eventually require arthrodesis. Surgical fusion, in all the various forms, is an option for patients who do not improve with appropriate nonoperative therapy. Preliminary studies of lumbar total disc replacement report equivalence to arthrodesis for the management of this patient population. Development of new motion-preserving techniques is likely to change the treatment approach, as will emerging biologic techniques.

PEARLS

1. Interdisciplinary therapy focusing on cognitive behavioral modification, fear avoidance mechanisms, and intensive physical therapy is as effective as surgical treatment in the treatment of discogenic back pain.

2. For acute episodes of low back pain, advice to stay active is more effective than bed rest. The current generally accepted recommendation is no more than 2 days of bed rest.

3. Epidural steroid injections are moderately effective for short-term symptom relief, but efficacy in nonradicular low back pain is still largely unknown.

4. Surgical fusion for discogenic low back pain or DDD is a good option for patients who have failed intensive interdisciplinary physical therapy. There is no consensus on which fusion procedure affords the best results; the option is left to physician preference and experience.

5. BMPs (BMP-2 and BMP-7/OP-1) are effective at increasing spinal arthrodesis rates but are not cost-effective enough to be used on a routine basis and should be used with caution.

PITFALLS

1. MRI is plagued by a high rate of asymptomatic spinal abnormalities and should be used only as an adjunct to an adequate history and physical examination.

2. Discography is not recommended as a routine tool in the evaluation of patients with low back pain and may be associated with increased risk of segment degeneration.

3. Narcotic pain medication and antispasmodics should be used only for short-term acute episodes of back pain. Long-term use of narcotic pain medication in chronic low back pain is not recommended and may be associated with abuse in 25% of cases.

4. Less invasive treatment options, such as IDET, prolotherapy, and intradiscal injections, are not effective treatment options.

5. Adjacent segment degeneration is a common phenomenon observed with spinal arthrodesis; however, motion preservation devices and disc arthroplasty have not adequately shown efficacy in preventing this problem.

6. Disc arthroplasty procedures in the lumbar spine have shown noninferiority to spinal arthrodesis; however, significant concerns remain over long-term outcomes, potential for revision, and cost of implant.

KEY POINTS

1. A detailed history and physical examination in conjunction with radiographic and MRI findings such as loss of disc height, disc signal changes, HIZ, and Modic changes are the best means available for diagnosing IDD and DDD.

2. Routine use of lumbar discography is not recommended for making the diagnosis of discogenic low back pain.

3. Practice guidelines have reaffirmed that the first line of treatment for patients with low back pain of a discogenic source, with or without radicular symptoms, is conservative therapy, and new emphasis has been placed on multidisciplinary therapy incorporating cognitive and behavioral treatment.

4. IDET is controversial, and many patients who undergo this procedure still require arthrodesis. Other forms of less invasive therapy such as prolotherapy and intradiscal corticosteroid injections are not recommended in this patient population.

5. Surgical fusion is an appropriate option for patients who do not improve with exhaustive nonoperative therapy.

6. No one method for achieving segmental fusion has clearly been shown to be better than another.

7. Preliminary studies of lumbar total disc replacement report equivalence to arthrodesis for the surgical management of this patient population, but there is still insufficient evidence to evaluate the long-term benefits and complications.

KEY REFERENCES

1. Aprill C, Bogduk N: High-intensity zone: A diagnostic sign of painful lumbar disc on magnetic resonance imaging. Br J Radiol 65:361-369, 1992.
This study focuses attention on HIZ as a diagnostic sign of an annular tear.

2. Boden S, McCowin P, Davis D, et al: Abnormal magnetic-resonance scans of the lumbar spine in asymptomatic subjects: A prospective investigation. J Bone Joint Surg Am 72:403-408, 1990.
Abnormal MRI of the lumbar spine often reveals abnormalities in asymptomatic subjects, as illustrated by this article.

3. Brox J: Randomized clinical trial of lumbar instrumented fusion and cognitive intervention and exercises in patients with chronic low back pain and disc degeneration. Spine (Phila Pa 1976) 28:1913-1921, 2003.
This article reports the outcomes of a randomized controlled trial of operative versus cognitive therapy and intensive exercise for the treatment of chronic low back pain and shows near-equivalent outcomes between the groups.

4. Carragee E: A gold standard evaluation of the "discogenic pain" diagnosis as determined by provocative discography. Spine (Phila Pa 1976) 31:2115-2123, 2006.
This article calculates a best possible positive predictive value of lumbar discography in diagnosing discogenic back pain based on success of fusion in patients with positive discography versus a cohort of spondylolisthesis patients treated surgically.

5. Carragee E, Paragioudakis S, Khurana S: 2000 Volvo Award Winner in Clinical Studies: Lumbar high-intensity zone and discography in subjects without low back problems. Spine (Phila Pa 1976) 25:2987-2992, 2000.
This article points out the low predictive value of lumbar HIZ and discography.

6. Chou R, Baisden J, Carragee EJ, et al: Surgery for low back pain: A review of the evidence for an American Pain Society Clinical Practice Guideline. Spine (Phila Pa 1976) 34:1094-1109, 2009.
This meta-analysis reviews the best available evidence for surgical treatment of patients with low back pain as part of the American Pain Society's current practice guidelines.

7. Chou R, Loeser JD, Owens DK, et al: American Pain Society Low Back Pain Guideline Panel: Interventional therapies, surgery, and interdisciplinary rehabilitation for low back pain: An evidence-based clinical practice guideline from the American Pain Society. Spine (Phila Pa 1976) 34:1066-1077, 2009.
This article reports the American Pain Society's current practice recommendations for the treatment of chronic nonradicular low back pain (see Table 45-2).

8. Crock H: Internal disc disruption: A challenge to disc prolapsed fifty years on. Spine (Phila Pa 1976) 11:650-653, 1986.
In this article, the concept of IDD was elaborated.

9. Fairbank J: Randomised controlled trial to compare surgical stabilisation of the lumbar spine with an intensive rehabilitation programme for patients with chronic low back pain: The MRC spine stabilisation trial. BMJ 330:1233, 2005.

This large randomized controlled trial compared operative and interdisciplinary physical therapy programs in the treatment of chronic low back pain. A small benefit was shown for the surgically treated group but with a significant increase in cost and complications.

10. Fritzell P, Hagg O, Wessberg P, et al: Swedish Lumbar Spine Study Group: 2001 Volvo Award Winner in Clinical Studies: Lumbar fusion versus nonsurgical treatment for chronic low back pain: A multicenter randomized controlled trial from the Swedish Lumbar Spine Study Group. Spine (Phila Pa 1976) 26:2521-2532; discussion 2532-2534, 2001.
This multicenter, randomized controlled trial comparing lumbar fusion and nonsurgical treatment for chronic back pain shows superiority for the fusion alternative.

11. Modic M, Steinberg P, Ross J, et al: Degenerative disk disease: Assessment of changes in vertebral body marrow with MR imaging. Radiology 166(1 Pt 1):193-199, 1988.
The changes observed in vertebrae adjacent to the degenerative disc are described and classified.

REFERENCES

1. Schwarzer AC, Aprill CN, Derby R, et al: The prevalence and clinical features of internal disc disruption in patients with chronic low back pain. Spine (Phila Pa 1976) 20:1878-1883, 1995.

2. Manchikanti L, Singh V, Pampati V, et al: Evaluation of the relative contributions of various structures in chronic low back pain. Pain Physician 4:308-316, 2001.

3. Andersson G: Epidemiological features of chronic low-back pain. Lancet 354:581-585, 1999.

4. Papageorgiou AC, Croft PR, Ferry S, et al: Estimating the prevalence of low back pain in the general population: Evidence from the South Manchester Back Pain Survey. Spine (Phila Pa 1976) 20:1889-1894, 1995.

5. Waddell G: 1987 Volvo award in clinical sciences: A new clinical model for the treatment of low-back pain. Spine (Phila Pa 1976) 12:632-644, 1987.

6. Croft PR, Macfarlane GJ, Papageorgiou AC, et al: Outcome of low back pain in general practice: A prospective study. BMJ 316:1356-1359, 1998.

7. Walsh K, Cruddas M, Coggon D: Low back pain in eight areas of Britain. J Epidemiol Community Health 46:227-230, 1992.

8. Andersson GB, Svensson HO, Oden A: The intensity of work recovery in low back pain. Spine (Phila Pa 1976) 8:880-884, 1983.

9. Wahlgren DR, Atkinson JH, Epping-Jordan JE, et al: One-year follow-up of first onset low back pain. Pain 73:213-221, 1997.

10. Carey TS, Garrett JM, Jackman AM: Beyond the good prognosis: Examination of an inception cohort of patients with chronic low back pain. Spine (Phila Pa 1976) 25:115-120, 2000.

11. Roland MO, Morrell DC, Morris RW: Can general practitioners predict the outcome of episodes of back pain? BMJ (Clin Res Ed) 286:523-525, 1983.

12. Papageorgiou AC, Croft PR, Thomas E, et al: Influence of previous pain experience on the episode incidence of low back pain: Results from the South Manchester Back Pain Study. Pain 66:181-185, 1996.

13. Smith SE, Darden BV, Rhyne AL, et al: Outcome of unoperated discogram-positive low back pain. Spine (Phila Pa 1976) 20:1997-2000, 1995.

14. Kirkaldy-Willis WH, Farfan HF: Instability of the lumbar spine. Clin Orthop Relat Res 165:110-123, 1982.

15. Waris E, Eskelin M, Hermunen H, et al: Disc degeneration in low back pain: A 17-year follow-up study using magnetic resonance imaging. Spine (Phila Pa 1976) 32:681-684, 2007.

16. Urban JP, Holm S, Maroudas A, et al: Nutrition of the intervertebral disc: Effect of fluid flow on solute transport. Clin Orthop Relat Res 170:296-302, 1982.

17. Nakamura SI, Takahashi K, Takahashi Y, et al: The afferent pathways of discogenic low-back pain: Evaluation of L2 spinal nerve infiltration. J Bone Joint Surg Br 78:606-612, 1996.

18. Buckwalter JA: Aging and degeneration of the human intervertebral disc. Spine (Phila Pa 1976) 20:1307-1314, 1995.

19. Crock HV: Internal disc disruption: A challenge to disc prolapse fifty years on. Spine (Phila Pa 1976) 11:650-653, 1986.

20. Macnab I: The traction spur: An indicator of segmental instability. J Bone Joint Surg Am 53:663-670, 1971.

21. Hangai M, Kaneoka K, Kuno S, et al: Factors associated with lumbar intervertebral disc degeneration in the elderly. Spine J 8:732-740, 2008.

22. Kalichman L, Hunter DJ: The genetics of intervertebral disc degeneration: Familial predisposition and heritability estimation. Joint Bone Spine 75:383-387, 2008.

23. Battie MC, Videman T, Gibbons LE, et al: 1995 Volvo Award in clinical sciences: Determinants of lumbar disc degeneration: A study relating lifetime exposures and magnetic resonance imaging findings in identical twins. Spine (Phila Pa 1976) 20:2601-2612, 1995.

24. An HS, Silveri CP, Simpson JM, et al: Comparison of smoking habits between patients with surgically confirmed herniated lumbar and cervical disc disease and controls. J Spinal Disord 7:369-373, 1994.

25. Kauppila LI: Atherosclerosis and disc degeneration/low-back pain—a systematic review. Eur J Vasc Endovasc Surg 37:661-670, 2009.

26. Lis AM, Black KM, Korn H, et al: Association between sitting and occupational LBP. Eur Spine J 16:283-298, 2007.

27. Kelsey JL, Hardy RJ: Driving of motor vehicles as a risk factor for acute herniated lumbar intervertebral disc. Am J Epidemiol 102:63-73, 1975.

28. Wilder DG: The biomechanics of vibration and low back pain. Am J Ind Med 23:577-588, 1993.

29. Arun R, Freeman BJ, Scammell BE, et al: 2009 ISSLS prize winner: What influence does sustained mechanical load have on diffusion in the human intervertebral disc? An in vivo study using serial postcontrast magnetic resonance imaging. Spine (Phila Pa 1976) 34:2324-2337, 2009.

30. Videman T, Battie MC, Ripatti S, et al: Determinants of the progression in lumbar degeneration: A 5-year follow-up study of adult male monozygotic twins. Spine (Phila Pa 1976) 31:671-678, 2006.

31. MacGregor AJ, Andrew T, Sambrook PN, et al: Structural, psychological, and genetic influences on low back and neck pain:

A study of adult female twins. Arthritis Rheum 51:160-167, 2004.

32. Hestbaek L, Iachine IA, Leboeuf-Yde C, et al: Heredity of low back pain in a young population: A classical twin study. Twin Res 7:16-26, 2004.

33. Hartvigsen J, Christensen K, Frederiksen H, et al: Genetic and environmental contributions to back pain in old age: A study of 2,108 Danish twins aged 70 and older. Spine (Phila Pa 1976) 29:897-901, 2004.

34. Paassilta P, Lohiniva J, Goring HH, et al: Identification of a novel common genetic risk factor for lumbar disk disease. JAMA 285:1843-1849, 2001.

35. Jim JJ, Noponen-Hietala N, Cheung KM, et al: The TRP2 allele of COL9A2 is an age-dependent risk factor for the development and severity of intervertebral disc degeneration. Spine (Phila Pa 1976) 30:2735-2742, 2005.

36. Solovieva S, Lohiniva J, Leino-Arjas P, et al: Intervertebral disc degeneration in relation to the COL9A3 and the IL-1ss gene polymorphisms. Eur Spine J 15:613-619, 2006.

37. Kalichman L, Hunter DJ: The genetics of intervertebral disc degeneration: Associated genes. Joint Bone Spine 75:388-396, 2008.

38. Crock HV: A reappraisal of intervertebral disc lesions. Med J Aust 1:983-989, 1970.

39. Haughton VM: MR imaging of the spine. Radiology 166:297-301, 1988.

40. Deyo RA, Battie M, Beurskens AJ, et al: Outcome measures for low back pain research: A proposal for standardized use. Spine (Phila Pa 1976) 23:2003-2013, 1998.

41. Spruit M, Jacobs WC: Pain and function after intradiscal electrothermal treatment (IDET) for symptomatic lumbar disc degeneration. Eur Spine J 11:589-593, 2002.

42. Derby R, Eek B, Chen Y: Intradiscal electrothermal annuloplasty (IDET): A novel approach for treating chronic discogenic back pain. Neuromodulation 3:69-75, 2000.

43. Weinstein J, Claverie W, Gibson S: The pain of discography. Spine (Phila Pa 1976) 13:1344-1348, 1988.

44. Weinstein J: Neurogenic and nonneurogenic pain and inflammatory mediators. Orthop Clin North Am 22:235-246, 1991.

45. Kawakami M, Tamaki T, Hayashi N, et al: Possible mechanism of painful radiculopathy in lumbar disc herniation. Clin Orthop Relat Res 351:241-251, 1998.

46. Byrod G, Olmarker K, Konno S, et al: A rapid transport route between the epidural space and the intraneural capillaries of the nerve roots. Spine (Phila Pa 1976) 20:138-143, 1995.

47. Freemont AJ, Peacock TE, Goupille P, et al: Nerve ingrowth into diseased intervertebral disc in chronic back pain. Lancet 350:178-181, 1997.

48. Evans W, Jobe W, Seibert C: A cross-sectional prevalence study of lumbar disc degeneration in a working population. Spine (Phila Pa 1976) 14:60-64, 1989.

49. Gibson MJ, Buckley J, Mawhinney R, et al: Magnetic resonance imaging and discography in the diagnosis of disc degeneration: A comparative study of 50 discs. J Bone Joint Surg Br 68:369-373, 1986.

50. Saal JS, Franson RC, Dobrow R, et al: High levels of inflammatory phospholipase A2 activity in lumbar disc herniations. Spine (Phila Pa 1976) 15:674-678, 1990.

51. Nygaard OP, Mellgren SI, Osterud B: The inflammatory properties of contained and noncontained lumbar disc herniation. Spine (Phila Pa 1976) 22:2484-2488, 1997.

52. O'Donnell JL, O'Donnell AL: Prostaglandin E2 content in herniated lumbar disc disease. Spine (Phila Pa 1976) 21:1653-1655, 1996.

53. Franson RC, Saal JS, Saal JA: Human disc phospholipase A2 is inflammatory. Spine (Phila Pa 1976) 17(6 Suppl):S129-S132, 1992.

54. Burke JG, Watson RW, McCormack D, et al: Intervertebral discs which cause low back pain secrete high levels of proinflammatory mediators. J Bone Joint Surg Br 84:196-201, 2002.

55. Igarashi A, Kikuchi S, Konno S, et al: Inflammatory cytokines released from the facet joint tissue in degenerative lumbar spinal disorders. Spine (Phila Pa 1976) 29:2091-2095, 2004.

56. Ohtori S, Inoue G, Ito T, et al: Tumor necrosis factor-immunoreactive cells and PGP 9.5-immunoreactive nerve fibers in vertebral endplates of patients with discogenic low back pain and Modic type 1 or type 2 changes on MRI. Spine (Phila Pa 1976) 31:1026-1031, 2006.

57. Ashton IK, Walsh DA, Polak JM, et al: Substance P in intervertebral discs: Binding sites on vascular endothelium of the human annulus fibrosus. Acta Orthop Scand 65:635-639, 1994.

58. Palmgren T, Gronblad M, Virri J, et al: An immunohistochemical study of nerve structures in the anulus fibrosus of human normal lumbar intervertebral discs. Spine (Phila Pa 1976) 24:2075-2079, 1999.

59. Coppes MH, Marani E, Thomeer RT, et al: Innervation of "painful" lumbar discs. Spine (Phila Pa 1976) 22:2342-2349; discussion 2349-2350, 1997.

60. Peng B, Wu W, Hou S, et al: The pathogenesis of discogenic low back pain. J Bone Joint Surg Br 87:62-67, 2005.

61. Brown MF, Hukkanen MV, McCarthy ID, et al: Sensory and sympathetic innervation of the vertebral endplate in patients with degenerative disc disease. J Bone Joint Surg Br 79:147-153, 1997.

62. Takebayashi T, Cavanaugh JM, Kallakuri S, et al: Sympathetic afferent units from lumbar intervertebral discs. J Bone Joint Surg Br 88:554-557, 2006.

63. Aoki Y, Ohtori S, Takahashi K, et al: Innervation of the lumbar intervertebral disc by nerve growth factor-dependent neurons related to inflammatory pain. Spine (Phila Pa 1976) 29:1077-1081, 2004.

64. Edgar MA: The nerve supply of the lumbar intervertebral disc. J Bone Joint Surg Br 89:1135-1139, 2007.

65. Jarvik JG, Hollingworth W, Heagerty PJ, et al: Three-year incidence of low back pain in an initially asymptomatic cohort: Clinical and imaging risk factors. Spine (Phila Pa 1976) 30:1541-1548; discussion 1549, 2005.

66. Carragee EJ, Alamin TF, Miller JL, et al: Discographic, MRI and psychosocial determinants of low back pain disability and remission: A prospective study in subjects with benign persistent back pain. Spine J 5:24-35, 2005.

67. Carragee EJ, Paragioudakis SJ, Khurana S: 2000 Volvo Award winner in clinical studies: Lumbar high-intensity zone and discography in subjects without low back problems. Spine (Phila Pa 1976) 25:2987-2992, 2000.

68. Carragee EJ, Alamin TF, Carragee JM: Low-pressure positive discography in subjects asymptomatic of significant low back pain illness. Spine (Phila Pa 1976) 31:505-509, 2006.

69. Carragee EJ, Tanner CM, Khurana S, et al: The rates of false-positive lumbar discography in select patients without low back symptoms. Spine (Phila Pa 1976) 25:1373-1380, 2000.

70. O'Neill CW, Kurgansky ME, Derby R, et al: Disc stimulation and patterns of referred pain. Spine (Phila Pa 1976) 27:2776-2781, 2002.

71. Deyo RA, Diehl AK: Lumbar spine films in primary care: Current use and effects of selective ordering criteria. J Gen Intern Med 1:20-25, 1986.

72. Torgerson WR, Dotter WE: Comparative roentgenographic study of the asymptomatic and symptomatic lumbar spine. J Bone Joint Surg Am 58:850-853, 1976.

73. Liang M, Komaroff AL: Roentgenograms in primary care patients with acute low back pain: A cost-effectiveness analysis. Arch Intern Med 142:1108-1112, 1982.

74. Scavone JG, Latshaw RF, Weidner WA: Anteroposterior and lateral radiographs: An adequate lumbar spine examination. AJR Am J Roentgenol 136:715-717, 1981.

75. Institute for Clinical Systems Improvement (ICSI): Adult Low Back Pain. Bloomington, MN, ICSI, 2008.

76. Aprill C, Bogduk N: High-intensity zone: A diagnostic sign of painful lumbar disc on magnetic resonance imaging. Br J Radiol 65:361-369, 1992.

77. Yu SW, Sether LA, Ho PS, et al: Tears of the anulus fibrosus: Correlation between MR and pathologic findings in cadavers. AJNR Am J Neuroradiol 9:367-370, 1988.

78. Osti OL, Vernon-Roberts B, Moore R, et al: Annular tears and disc degeneration in the lumbar spine: A post-mortem study of 135 discs. J Bone Joint Surg Br 74:678-682, 1992.

79. Morgan S, Saifuddin A: MRI of the lumbar intervertebral disc. Clin Radiol 54:703-723, 1999.

80. Modic M, Steinberg P, Ross J, et al: Degenerative disk disease: Assessment of changes in vertebral body marrow with MR imaging. Radiology 166(1 Pt 1):193-199, 1988.

81. Boden S, McCowin P, Davis D, et al: Abnormal magnetic-resonance scans of the lumbar spine in asymptomatic subjects: A prospective investigation. J Bone Joint Surg Am 72:403-408, 1990.

82. Jensen MC, Brant-Zawadzki MN, Obuchowski N, et al: Magnetic resonance imaging of the lumbar spine in people without back pain. N Engl J Med 331:69-73, 1994.

83. Stadnik TW, Lee RR, Coen HL, et al: Annular tears and disk herniation: Prevalence and contrast enhancement on MR images in the absence of low back pain or sciatica. Radiology 206:49-55, 1998.

84. Borenstein DG, O'Mara JW Jr, Boden SD, et al: The value of magnetic resonance imaging of the lumbar spine to predict low-back pain in asymptomatic subjects: A seven-year follow-up study. J Bone Joint Surg Am 83:1306-1311, 2001.

85. Jarvik JJ, Hollingworth W, Heagerty P, et al: The Longitudinal Assessment of Imaging and Disability of the Back (LAIDBack) Study: Baseline data. Spine (Phila Pa 1976) 26:1158-1166, 2001.

86. Jarvik JG, Hollingworth W, Martin B, et al: Rapid magnetic resonance imaging vs radiographs for patients with low back pain: A randomized controlled trial. JAMA 289:2810-2818, 2003.

87. Carragee E, Alamin T, Cheng I, et al: Are first-time episodes of serious LBP associated with new MRI findings? Spine J 6:624-635, 2006.

88. Lappalainen AK, Kaapa E, Lamminen A, et al: The diagnostic value of contrast-enhanced magnetic resonance imaging in the detection of experimentally induced anular tears in sheep. Spine (Phila Pa 1976) 27:2806-2810, 2002.

89. Yoshida H, Fujiwara A, Tamai K, et al: Diagnosis of symptomatic disc by magnetic resonance imaging: T2-weighted and gadolinium-DTPA-enhanced T1-weighted magnetic resonance imaging. J Spinal Disord Tech 15:193-198, 2002.

90. Aprill C, Bogduk N: High-intensity zone: A diagnostic sign of painful lumbar disc on magnetic resonance imaging. Br J Radiol 65:361-369, 1992.

91. Lim CH, Jee WH, Son BC, et al: Discogenic lumbar pain: Association with MRI imaging and CT discography. Eur J Radiol 54:431-437, 2005.

92. Lam KS, Carlin D, Mulholland RC: Lumbar disc high-intensity zone: The value and significance of provocative discography in the determination of the discogenic pain source. Eur Spine J 9:36-41, 2000.

93. Schellhas KP, Pollei SR, Gundry CR, et al: Lumbar disc high-intensity zone: Correlation of magnetic resonance imaging and discography. Spine (Phila Pa 1976) 21:79-86, 1996.

94. Peng B, Hou S, Wu W, et al: The pathogenesis and clinical significance of a high-intensity zone (HIZ) of lumbar intervertebral disc on MR imaging in the patient with discogenic low back pain. Eur Spine J 15:583-587, 2006.

95. Lei D, Rege A, Koti M, et al: Painful disc lesion: Can modern biplanar magnetic resonance imaging replace discography? J Spinal Disord Tech 21:430-435, 2008.

96. Saifuddin A, Braithwaite I, White J, et al: The value of lumbar spine magnetic resonance imaging in the demonstration of anular tears. Spine (Phila Pa 1976) 23:453-457, 1998.

97. Kang CH, Kim YH, Lee SH, et al: Can magnetic resonance imaging accurately predict concordant pain provocation during provocative disc injection? Skeletal Radiol 38:877-885, 2009.

98. Ricketson R, Simmons JW, Hauser BO: The prolapsed intervertebral disc: The high-intensity zone with discography correlation. Spine (Phila Pa 1976) 21:2758-2762, 1996.

99. Schneiderman G, Flannigan B, Kingston S, et al: Magnetic resonance imaging in the diagnosis of disc degeneration: Correlation with discography. Spine (Phila Pa 1976) 12:276-281, 1987.

100. Ito M, Incorvaia KM, Yu SF, et al: Predictive signs of discogenic lumbar pain on magnetic resonance imaging with discography correlation. Spine (Phila Pa 1976) 23:1252-1258, 1998.

101. Simmons JW, Emery SF, McMillin JN, et al: Awake discography: A comparison study with magnetic resonance imaging. Spine (Phila Pa 1976) 16(6 Suppl):S216-S221, 1991.

102. Mitra D, Cassar-Pullicino VN, McCall IW: Longitudinal study of high intensity zones on MR of lumbar intervertebral discs. Clin Radiol 59:1002-1008, 2004.

103. Milette P, Fontaine S, Lepanto L, et al: Differentiating lumbar disc protrusions, disc bulges, and discs with normal contour but abnormal signal intensity: Magnetic resonance imaging with discographic correlations. Spine (Phila Pa 1976) 24:44-53, 1999.

104. Horton WC, Daftari TK: Which disc as visualized by magnetic resonance imaging is actually a source of pain? A correlation between magnetic resonance imaging and discography. Spine (Phila Pa 1976) 17(6 Suppl):S167-S171, 1992.

105. Toyone T, Takahashi K, Kitahara H, et al: Vertebral bone-marrow changes in degenerative lumbar disc disease: An MRI study of 74 patients with low back pain. J Bone Joint Surg Br 76:757-764, 1994.

106. Kuisma M, Karppinen J, Niinimaki J, et al: Modic changes in endplates of lumbar vertebral bodies: Prevalence and association with low back and sciatic pain among middle-aged male workers. Spine (Phila Pa 1976) 32:1116-1122, 2007.

107. Albert HB, Manniche C: Modic changes following lumbar disc herniation. Eur Spine J 16:977-982, 2007.

108. Thompson KJ, Dagher AP, Eckel TS, et al: Modic changes on MR images as studied with provocative diskography: Clinical relevance—a retrospective study of 2457 disks. Radiology 250:849-855, 2009.

109. Mitra D, Cassar-Pullicino VN, McCall IW: Longitudinal study of vertebral type-1 end-plate changes on MR of the lumbar spine. Eur Radiol 14:1574-1581, 2004.

110. Marshman LA, Trewhella M, Friesem T, et al: Reverse transformation of Modic type 2 changes to Modic type 1 changes during sustained chronic low-back pain severity: Report of two cases and review of the literature. J Neurosurg Spine 6:152-155, 2007.

111. Kuisma M, Karppinen J, Niinimaki J, et al: A three-year follow-up of lumbar spine endplate (Modic) changes. Spine (Phila Pa 1976) 31:1714-1718, 2006.

112. Sandhu HS, Sanchez-Caso LP, Parvataneni HK, et al: Association between findings of provocative discography and vertebral endplate signal changes as seen on MRI. J Spinal Disord 13:438-443, 2000.

113. Braithwaite I, White J, Saifuddin A, et al: Vertebral end-plate (Modic) changes on lumbar spine MRI: Correlation with pain reproduction at lumbar discography. Eur Spine J 7:363-368, 1998.

114. Kokkonen SM, Kurunlahti M, Tervonen O, et al: Endplate degeneration observed on magnetic resonance imaging of the lumbar spine: Correlation with pain provocation and disc changes observed on computed tomography diskography. Spine (Phila Pa 1976) 27:2274-2278, 2002.

115. Schenk P, Laubli T, Hodler J, et al: Magnetic resonance imaging of the lumbar spine: Findings in female subjects from administrative and nursing professions. Spine (Phila Pa 1976) 31:2701-2706, 2006.

116. Kjaer P, LeBoeuf-Yde C, Korsholm L, et al: Magnetic resonance imaging and low back pain in adults: A diagnostic imaging study of 40-year-old men and women. Spine (Phila Pa 1976) 30:1173-1180, 2005.

117. Kjaer P, Korsholm L, Bendix T, et al: Modic changes and their associations with clinical findings. Eur Spine J 15:1312-1319, 2006.

118. Leboeuf-Yde C, Kjaer P, Bendix T, et al: Self-reported hard physical work combined with heavy smoking or overweight may result in so-called Modic changes. BMC Musculoskelet Disord 9:5, 2008.

119. Jensen TS, Karppinen J, Sorensen JS, et al: Vertebral endplate signal changes (Modic change): A systematic literature review of prevalence and association with non-specific low back pain. Eur Spine J 17:1407-1422, 2008.

120. Huang KY, Lin RM, Lee YL, et al: Factors affecting disability and physical function in degenerative lumbar spondylolisthesis of L4-5: Evaluation with axially loaded MRI. Eur Spine J 18:1851-1857, 2009.

121. Hansson T, Suzuki N, Hebelka H, et al: The narrowing of the lumbar spinal canal during loaded MRI: The effects of the disc and ligamentum flavum. Eur Spine J 18:679-686, 2009.

122. Jayakumar P, Nnadi C, Saifuddin A, et al: Dynamic degenerative lumbar spondylolisthesis: Diagnosis with axial loaded magnetic resonance imaging. Spine (Phila Pa 1976) 31:E298-E301, 2006.

123. Hiwatashi A, Danielson B, Moritani T, et al: Axial loading during MR imaging can influence treatment decision for symptomatic spinal stenosis. AJNR Am J Neuroradiol 25:170-174, 2004.

124. Danielson B, Willen J: Axially loaded magnetic resonance image of the lumbar spine in asymptomatic individuals. Spine (Phila Pa 1976) 26:2601-2606, 2001.

125. Saifuddin A, McSweeney E, Lehovsky J: Development of lumbar high intensity zone on axial loaded magnetic resonance imaging. Spine (Phila Pa 1976) 28:E449-E451, 2003.

126. Holt EP Jr: The question of lumbar discography. J Bone Joint Surg Am 50:720-726, 1968.

127. Carragee EJ, Don AS, Hurwitz EL, et al: 2009 ISSLS Prize Winner: Does discography cause accelerated progression of degeneration changes in the lumbar disc: A ten-year matched cohort study. Spine (Phila Pa 1976) 34:2338-2345, 2009.

128. Chou R, Loeser JD, Owens DK, et al: Interventional therapies, surgery, and interdisciplinary rehabilitation for low back pain: An evidence-based clinical practice guideline from the American Pain Society. Spine (Phila Pa 1976) 34:1066-1077, 2009.

129. Aprill C: Diagnostic disc injection. In Frymoyer J (ed): The Adult Spine: Principles and Practice. New York, Raven Press, 1991.

130. Guyer RD, Ohnmeiss DD: Lumbar discography. Position statement from the North American Spine Society Diagnostic and Therapeutic Committee. Spine (Phila Pa 1976) 20:2048-2059, 1995.

131. Bernard TN Jr: Lumbar discography followed by computed tomography: Refining the diagnosis of low-back pain. Spine (Phila Pa 1976) 15:690-707, 1990.

132. Massie W: A critical evaluation of discography. Scientific exhibit. In Proceedings of the American Academy of Orthopedic Surgeons. J Bone Joint Surg Am 49:1243-1244, 1967.

133. Walsh TR, Weinstein JN, Spratt KF, et al: Lumbar discography in normal subjects: A controlled, prospective study. J Bone Joint Surg Am 72:1081-1088, 1990.

134. Derby R, Kim BJ, Lee SH, et al: Comparison of discographic findings in asymptomatic subject discs and the negative discs of chronic LBP patients: Can discography distinguish asymptomatic discs among morphologically abnormal discs? Spine J 5:389-394, 2005.

135. Buenaventura RM, Shah RV, Patel V, et al: Systematic review of discography as a diagnostic test for spinal pain: an update. Pain Physician 10:147-164, 2007.

136. Wolfer LR, Derby R, Lee JE, et al: Systematic review of lumbar provocation discography in asymptomatic subjects with a meta-analysis of false-positive rates. Pain Physician 11:513-538, 2008.

137. Colhoun E, McCall IW, Williams L, et al: Provocation discography as a guide to planning operations on the spine. J Bone Joint Surg Br 70:267-271, 1988.

138. Madan S, Gundanna M, Harley JM, et al: Does provocative discography screening of discogenic back pain improve surgical outcome? J Spinal Disord Tech 15:245-251, 2002.

139. Carragee EJ, Lincoln T, Parmar VS, et al: A gold standard evaluation of the "discogenic pain" diagnosis as determined by provocative discography. Spine (Phila Pa 1976) 31:2115-2123, 2006.

140. Ohtori S, Kinoshita T, Yamashita M, et al: Results of surgery for discogenic low back pain: A randomized study using discography versus discoblock for diagnosis. Spine (Phila Pa 1976) 34:1345-1348, 2009.

141. Deyo RA: Conservative therapy for low back pain: Distinguishing useful from useless therapy. JAMA 250:1057-1062, 1983.

142. Deyo RA, Diehl AK, Rosenthal M: How many days of bed rest for acute low back pain? A randomized clinical trial. N Engl J Med 315:1064-1070, 1986.

143. Quinet RJ, Hadler NM: Diagnosis and treatment of backache. Semin Arthritis Rheum 8:261-287, 1979.

144. Rowe ML. Low back pain in industry. A position paper. J Occup Med 11:161-169, 1969.

145. Allen C, Glasziou P, Del Mar C: Bed rest: A potentially harmful treatment needing more careful evaluation. Lancet 354:1229-1233, 1999.

146. Hagen KB, Hilde G, Jamtvedt G, et al: Bed rest for acute low-back pain and sciatica. Cochrane Database Syst Rev CD001254, 2004.

147. Verbunt JA, Sieben J, Vlaeyen JW, et al: A new episode of low back pain: Who relies on bed rest? Eur J Pain 12:508-516, 2008.

148. Engers A, Jellema P, Wensing M, et al: Individual patient education for low back pain. Cochrane Database Syst Rev CD004057, 2008.

149. Liddle SD, Gracey JH, Baxter GD: Advice for the management of low back pain: A systematic review of randomised controlled trials. Man Ther 12:310-327, 2007.

150. Brox JI, Storheim K, Grotle M, et al: Evidence-informed management of chronic low back pain with back schools, brief education, and fear-avoidance training. Spine J 8:28-39, 2008.

151. Calmels P, Queneau P, Hamonet C, et al: Effectiveness of a lumbar belt in subacute low back pain: An open, multicentric, and randomized clinical study. Spine (Phila Pa 1976) 34:215-220, 2009.

152. Oleske DM, Lavender SA, Andersson GB, et al: Are back supports plus education more effective than education alone in promoting recovery from low back pain? Results from a randomized clinical trial. Spine (Phila Pa 1976) 32:2050-2057, 2007.

153. van Duijvenbode IC, Jellema P, van Poppel MN, et al: Lumbar supports for prevention and treatment of low back pain. Cochrane Database Syst Rev CD001823, 2008.

154. Sahar T, Cohen MJ, Ne'eman V, et al: Insoles for prevention and treatment of back pain. Cochrane Database Syst Rev CD005275, 2007.

155. Brox JI, Sorensen R, Friis A, et al: Randomized clinical trial of lumbar instrumented fusion and cognitive intervention and exercises in patients with chronic low back pain and disc degeneration. Spine (Phila Pa 1976) 28:1913-1921, 2003.

156. Keller A, Brox JI, Gunderson R, et al: Trunk muscle strength, cross-sectional area, and density in patients with chronic low back pain randomized to lumbar fusion or cognitive intervention and exercises. Spine (Phila Pa 1976) 29:3-8, 2004.

157. Fairbank J, Frost H, Wilson-MacDonald J, et al; Spine Stabilisation Trial Group: Randomised controlled trial to compare surgical stabilisation of the lumbar spine with an intensive rehabilitation programme for patients with chronic low back pain: The MRC Spine Stabilisation Trial. BMJ 330:1233, 2005.

158. Heymans MW, de Vet HC, Bongers PM, et al: The effectiveness of high-intensity versus low-intensity back schools in an occupational setting: A pragmatic randomized controlled trial. Spine (Phila Pa 1976) 31:1075-1082, 2006.

159. Kaapa EH, Frantsi K, Sarna S, et al: Multidisciplinary group rehabilitation versus individual physiotherapy for chronic nonspecific low back pain: A randomized trial. Spine (Phila Pa 1976) 31:371-376, 2006.

160. Heymans MW, van Tulder MW, Esmail R, et al: Back schools for non-specific low-back pain. Cochrane Database Syst Rev CD000261, 2004.

161. van der Roer N, van Tulder M, van Mechelen W, et al: Economic evaluation of an intensive group training protocol compared with usual care physiotherapy in patients with chronic low back pain. Spine (Phila Pa 1976) 33:445-451, 2008.

162. van der Roer N, van Tulder M, Barendse J, et al: Intensive group training protocol versus guideline physiotherapy for patients with chronic low back pain: A randomised controlled trial. Eur Spine J 17:1193-1200, 2008.

163. Poitras S, Brosseau L: Evidence-informed management of chronic low back pain with transcutaneous electrical nerve stimulation, interferential current, electrical muscle stimulation, ultrasound, and thermotherapy. Spine J 8:226-233, 2008.

164. Khadilkar A, Odebiyi DO, Brosseau L, et al: Transcutaneous electrical nerve stimulation (TENS) versus placebo for chronic low-back pain. Cochrane Database Syst Rev CD003008, 2008.

165. Hoiriss KT, Pfleger B, McDuffie FC, et al: A randomized clinical trial comparing chiropractic adjustments to muscle relaxants for subacute low back pain. J Manipulative Physiol Ther 27:388-398, 2004.

166. Haas M, Groupp E, Kraemer DF: Dose-response for chiropractic care of chronic low back pain. Spine J 4:574-583, 2004.

167. McMorland G, Suter E: Chiropractic management of mechanical neck and low-back pain: A retrospective, outcome-based analysis. J Manipulative Physiol Ther 23:307-311, 2000.

168. Ernst E, Canter PH: A systematic review of systematic reviews of spinal manipulation. J R Soc Med 99:192-196, 2006.

169. Assendelft WJ, Morton SC, Yu EI, et al: Spinal manipulative therapy for low back pain. Cochrane Database Syst Rev CD000447, 2004.

170. Eisenberg DM, Post DE, Davis RB, et al: Addition of choice of complementary therapies to usual care for acute low back pain: A randomized controlled trial. Spine (Phila Pa 1976) 32:151-158, 2007.

171. Hurwitz EL, Morgenstern H, Kominski GF, et al: A randomized trial of chiropractic and medical care for patients with low back

pain: Eighteen-month follow-up outcomes from the UCLA low back pain study. Spine (Phila Pa 1976) 31:611-621; discussion 622, 2006.

172. Furlan AD, van Tulder MW, Cherkin DC, et al: Acupuncture and dry-needling for low back pain. Cochrane Database Syst Rev CD001351, 2005.

173. Ammendolia C, Furlan AD, Imamura M, et al: Evidence-informed management of chronic low back pain with needle acupuncture. Spine J 8:160-172, 2008.

174. Yelland MJ, Glasziou PP, Bogduk N, et al: Prolotherapy injections, saline injections, and exercises for chronic low-back pain: A randomized trial. Spine (Phila Pa 1976) 29:9-16, 2004.

175. Dagenais S, Mayer J, Haldeman S, et al: Evidence-informed management of chronic low back pain with prolotherapy. Spine J 8:203-212, 2008.

176. Rabago D, Best TM, Beamsley M, et al: A systematic review of prolotherapy for chronic musculoskeletal pain. Clin J Sport Med 15:376-380, 2005.

177. Roelofs PD, Deyo RA, Koes BW, et al: Non-steroidal anti-inflammatory drugs for low back pain. Cochrane Database Syst Rev CD000396, 2008.

178. Deshpande A, Furlan A, Mailis-Gagnon A, et al: Opioids for chronic low-back pain. Cochrane Database Syst Rev CD004959, 2007.

179. Jamison RN, Raymond SA, Slawsby EA, et al: Opioid therapy for chronic noncancer back pain: A randomized prospective study. Spine (Phila Pa 1976) 23:2591-2600, 1998.

180. Martell BA, O'Connor PG, Kerns RD, et al: Systematic review: Opioid treatment for chronic back pain: Prevalence, efficacy, and association with addiction. Ann Intern Med 146:116-127, 2007.

181. Schofferman J, Mazanec D: Evidence-informed management of chronic low back pain with opioid analgesics. Spine J 8:185-194, 2008.

182. Armstrong TA, Rohal GM: Potential danger from too much acetaminophen in opiate agonist combination products. Am J Health Syst Pharm 56:1774-1775, 1999.

183. Physicians Desk Reference, 63rd ed. Montvale, NJ, Thomson PDR, 2009.

184. Krenzelok EP: The FDA Acetaminophen Advisory Committee Meeting—what is the future of acetaminophen in the United States? The perspective of a committee member. Clin Toxicol 47:784-789, 2009.

185. Vamvanij V, Fredrickson BE, Thorpe JM, et al: Surgical treatment of internal disc disruption: An outcome study of four fusion techniques. J Spinal Disord 11:375-382, 1998.

186. van Tulder MW, Touray T, Furlan AD, et al: Muscle relaxants for non-specific low back pain. Cochrane Database Syst Rev CD004252, 2003.

187. Alcoff J, Jones E, Rust P, et al: Controlled trial of imipramine for chronic low back pain. J Fam Pract 14:841-846, 1982.

188. Pheasant H, Bursk A, Goldfarb J, et al: Amitriptyline and chronic low-back pain: A randomized double-blind crossover study. Spine (Phila Pa 1976) 8:552-557, 1983.

189. Ward NG: Tricyclic antidepressants for chronic low-back pain: Mechanisms of action and predictors of response. Spine (Phila Pa 1976) 11:661-665, 1986.

190. Staiger TO, Gaster B, Sullivan MD, et al: Systematic review of antidepressants in the treatment of chronic low back pain. Spine (Phila Pa 1976) 28:2540-2545, 2003.

191. Chang V, Gonzalez P, Akuthota V: Evidence-informed management of chronic low back pain with adjunctive analgesics. Spine J 8:21-27, 2008.

192. Keller A, Hayden J, Bombardier C, et al: Effect sizes of non-surgical treatments of non-specific low-back pain. Eur Spine J 16:1776-1788, 2007.

193. Machado LA, Kamper SJ, Herbert RD, et al: Analgesic effects of treatments for non-specific low back pain: A meta-analysis of placebo-controlled randomized trials. Rheumatology 48:520-527, 2009.

194. Delaney TJ, Rowlingson JC, Carron H, et al: Epidural steroid effects on nerves and meninges. Anesth Analg 59:610-614, 1980.

195. Fairbank JC, Park WM, McCall IW, et al: Apophyseal injection of local anesthetic as a diagnostic aid in primary low-back pain syndromes. Spine (Phila Pa 1976) 6:598-605, 1981.

196. Manchikanti L, Cash KA, McManus CD, et al: Preliminary results of a randomized, equivalence trial of fluoroscopic caudal epidural injections in managing chronic low back pain: Part 1. Discogenic pain without disc herniation or radiculitis. Pain Physician 11:785-800, 2008.

197. Manchikanti L, Singh V, Rivera JJ, et al: Effectiveness of caudal epidural injections in discogram positive and negative chronic low back pain. Pain Physician 5:18-29, 2002.

198. Manchikanti L, Pampati V, Rivera JJ, et al: Caudal epidural injections with sarapin or steroids in chronic low back pain. Pain Physician 4:322-335, 2001.

199. Buttermann GR: The effect of spinal steroid injections for degenerative disc disease. 5, Sep-Oct 2004, Spine J 4:495-505, 2004.

200. Rosenberg SK, Grabinsky A, Kooser C, et al: Effectiveness of transforaminal epidural steroid injections in low back pain: A one year experience. Pain Physician 5:266-270, 2002.

201. DePalma MJ, Slipman CW: Evidence-informed management of chronic low back pain with epidural steroid injections. Spine J 8:45-55, 2008.

202. Staal JB, de Bie R, de Vet HC, et al: Injection therapy for sub-acute and chronic low-back pain. Cochrane Database Syst Rev CD001824, 2008.

203. Chou R, Atlas SJ, Stanos SP, et al: Nonsurgical interventional therapies for low back pain: A review of the evidence for an American Pain Society clinical practice guideline. Spine (Phila Pa 1976) 34:1078-1093, 2009.

204. Feffer HL: Therapeutic intradiscal hydrocortisone: A long-term study. Clin Orthop Relat Res 67:100-104, 1969.

205. Wilkinson HA, Schuman N: Intradiscal corticosteroids in the treatment of lumbar and cervical disc problems. Spine (Phila Pa 1976) 5:385-389, 1980.

206. Fayad F, Lefevre-Colau MM, Rannou F, et al: Relation of inflammatory Modic changes to intradiscal steroid injection outcome in chronic low back pain. Eur Spine J 16:925-931, 2007.

207. Simmons JW, McMillin JN, Emery SF, et al: Intradiscal steroids: A prospective double-blind clinical trial. Spine (Phila Pa 1976) 17(6 Suppl):S172-S175, 1992.

208. Khot A, Bowditch M, Powell J, et al: The use of intradiscal steroid therapy for lumbar spinal discogenic pain: A randomized controlled trial. Spine (Phila Pa 1976) 29:833-836; discussion 837, 2004.

209. Klein RG, Eek BC, O'Neill CW, et al: Biochemical injection treatment for discogenic low back pain: A pilot study. Spine J 3:220-226, 2003.

210. Miller MR, Mathews RS, Reeves KD: Treatment of painful advanced internal lumbar disc derangement with intradiscal injection of hypertonic dextrose. Pain Physician 9:115-121, 2006.

211. Peng B, Zhang Y, Hou S, et al: Intradiscal methylene blue injection for the treatment of chronic discogenic low back pain. Eur Spine J 16:33-38, 2007.

212. Gallucci M, Limbucci N, Zugaro L, et al: Sciatica: Treatment with intradiscal and intraforaminal injections of steroid and oxygen-ozone versus steroid only. Radiology 242:907-913, 2007.

213. Muto M, Ambrosanio G, Guarnieri G, et al: Low back pain and sciatica: Treatment with intradiscal-intraforaminal O(2)-O(3) injection: Our experience. Radiol Med 113:695-706, 2008.

214. Freeman BJ, Walters RM, Moore RJ, et al: Does intradiscal electrothermal therapy denervate and repair experimentally induced posterolateral annular tears in an animal model? Spine (Phila Pa 1976) 28:2602-2608, 2003.

215. Shah RV, Lutz GE, Lee J, et al: Intradiskal electrothermal therapy: A preliminary histologic study. Arch Phys Med Rehabil 82:1230-1237, 2001.

216. Kleinstueck FS, Diederich CJ, Nau WH, et al: Acute biomechanical and histological effects of intradiscal electrothermal therapy on human lumbar discs. Spine (Phila Pa 1976) 26:2198-2207, 2001.

217. Strohbeln JW: Temperature distributions from interstitial RF electrode hyperthermia systems: Theoretical predictions. Int J Radiat Oncol Biol Phys 9:1655-1667, 1983.

218. Troussier B, Lebas JF, Chirossel JP, et al: Percutaneous intradiscal radio-frequency thermocoagulation: A cadaveric study. Spine (Phila Pa 1976) 20:1713-1718, 1995.

219. Houpt JC, Conner ES, McFarland EW: Experimental study of temperature distributions and thermal transport during radiofrequency current therapy of the intervertebral disc. Spine (Phila Pa 1976) 21:1808-1812; discussion 1812-1813, 1996.

220. Ashley J, Gharpuray V, Saal J: Temperature distribution in the intervertebral disc: A comparison of intranuclear radiofrequency needle to a novel heating catheter. Proceedings of the 1999 Bioengineering Conference. BED 42:77, 1999.

221. Karasek M, Bogduk N: Twelve-month follow-up of a controlled trial of intradiscal thermal anuloplasty for back pain due to internal disc disruption. Spine (Phila Pa 1976) 25:2601-2607, 2000.

222. Hsia AW, Isaac K, Katz JS: Cauda equina syndrome from intradiscal electrothermal therapy. Neurology 55:320, 2000.

223. Bogduk N, Karasek M: Two-year follow-up of a controlled trial of intradiscal electrothermal anuloplasty for chronic low back pain resulting from internal disc disruption. Spine J 2:343-350, 2002.

224. Saal JA, Saal JS: Intradiscal electrothermal treatment for chronic discogenic low back pain: Prospective outcome study with a

225. Freeman BJ, Fraser RD, Cain CM, et al: A randomized, double-blind, controlled trial: Intradiscal electrothermal therapy versus placebo for the treatment of chronic discogenic low back pain. Spine (Phila Pa 1976) 30:2369-2377; discussion 2378, 2005.

226. Pauza KJ, Howell S, Dreyfuss P, et al: A randomized, placebo-controlled trial of intradiscal electrothermal therapy for the treatment of discogenic low back pain. Spine J 4:27-35, 2004.

227. Barendse GA, van Den Berg SG, Kessels AH, et al: Randomized controlled trial of percutaneous intradiscal radiofrequency thermocoagulation for chronic discogenic back pain: Lack of effect from a 90-second 70 C lesion. Spine (Phila Pa 1976) 26:287-292, 2001.

228. Andersson GB, Mekhail NA, Block JE: Treatment of intractable discogenic low back pain: A systematic review of spinal fusion and intradiscal electrothermal therapy (IDET). Pain Physician 9:237-248, 2006.

229. Derby R, Baker RM, Lee CH, et al: Evidence-informed management of chronic low back pain with intradiscal electrothermal therapy. Spine J 8:80-95, 2008.

230. Helm S, Hayek SM, Benyamin RM, et al: Systematic review of the effectiveness of thermal annular procedures in treating discogenic low back pain. Pain Physician 12:207-232, 2009.

231. Freeman BJ: IDET: A critical appraisal of the evidence. Eur Spine J 15(Suppl):S448-S457, 2006.

232. Chou R, Baisden J, Carragee EJ, et al: Surgery for low back pain: A review of the evidence for an American Pain Society Clinical Practice Guideline. Spine (Phila Pa 1976) 34:1094-1109, 2009.

233. Deyo RA, Nachemson A, Mirza SK: Spinal-fusion surgery—the case for restraint. N Engl J Med 350:722-726, 2004.

234. Fritzell P, Hagg O, Wessberg P, et al; Swedish Lumbar Spine Study Group: 2001 Volvo Award Winner in Clinical Studies: Lumbar fusion versus nonsurgical treatment for chronic low back pain: A multicenter randomized controlled trial from the Swedish Lumbar Spine Study Group. Spine (Phila Pa 1976) 26:2521-2532; discussion 2532-2534, 2001.

235. Rivero-Arias O, Campbell H, Gray A, et al: Surgical stabilisation of the spine compared with a programme of intensive rehabilitation for the management of patients with chronic low back pain: Cost utility analysis based on a randomised controlled trial. BMJ 330:1239, 2005.

236. Ibrahim T, Tleyjeh IM, Gabbar O: Surgical versus non-surgical treatment of chronic low back pain: A meta-analysis of randomised trials. Int Orthop 32:107-113, 2008.

237. Mirza SK, Deyo RA: Systematic review of randomized trials comparing lumbar fusion surgery to nonoperative care for treatment of chronic back pain. Spine (Phila Pa 1976) 32:816-823, 2007.

238. Steinmann JC, Herkowitz HN: Pseudarthrosis of the spine. Clin Orthop Relat Res 284:80-90, 1992.

239. McCulloch JA: Uninstrumented posterolateral lumbar fusion for single level isolated disc resorption and/or degenerative disc disease. J Spinal Disord 12:34-39, 1999.

240. France JC, Yaszemski MJ, Lauerman WC, et al: A randomized prospective study of posterolateral lumbar fusion: Outcomes with and without pedicle screw instrumentation. Spine (Phila Pa 1976) 24:553-560, 1999.

241. Hellstadius A: Experiences gained from spondylo-syndesis operations with H-shaped bone transplantations in the case of degeneration of discs in the lumbar back. Acta Orthop Scand 24:207-215, 1955.

242. Shaw EG, Taylor JG: The results of lumbo-sacral fusion for low back pain. J Bone Joint Surg Br 38:485-497, 1956.

243. Lorenz M, Zindrick M, Schwaegler P, et al: A comparison of single-level fusions with and without hardware. Spine (Phila Pa 1976) 16(8 Suppl):S455-S458, 1991.

244. Louis R: Fusion of the lumbar and sacral spine by internal fixation with screw plates. Clin Orthop Relat Res 203:18-33, 1986.

245. Schwab FJ, Nazarian DG, Mahmud F, et al: Effects of spinal instrumentation on fusion of the lumbosacral spine. Spine (Phila Pa 1976) 20:2023-2028, 1995.

246. Dawson EG, Lotysch M 3rd, Urist MR: Intertransverse process lumbar arthrodesis with autogenous bone graft. Clin Orthop Relat Res 154:90-96, 1981.

247. Wood GW 2nd, Boyd RJ, Carothers TA, et al: The effect of pedicle screw/plate fixation on lumbar/lumbosacral autogenous bone graft fusions in patients with degenerative disc disease. Spine (Phila Pa 1976) 20:819-830, 1995.

248. Thomsen K, Christensen FB, Eiskjaer SP, et al: 1997 Volvo Award winner in clinical studies: The effect of pedicle screw instrumentation on functional outcome and fusion rates in posterolateral lumbar spinal fusion: A prospective, randomized clinical study. Spine (Phila Pa 1976) 22:2813-2822, 1997.

249. Bono CM, Lee CK: Critical analysis of trends in fusion for degenerative disc disease over the past 20 years: Influence of technique on fusion rate and clinical outcome. Spine (Phila Pa 1976) 29:455-463; discussion Z5, 2004.

250. Weatherley CR, Prickett CF, O'Brien JP: Discogenic pain persisting despite solid posterior fusion. J Bone Joint Surg Br 68:142-143, 1986.

251. Kozak JA, O'Brien JP: Simultaneous combined anterior and posterior fusion: An independent analysis of a treatment for the disabled low-back pain patient. Spine (Phila Pa 1976) 15:322-328, 1990.

252. Barrick WT, Schofferman JA, Reynolds JB, et al: Anterior lumbar fusion improves discogenic pain at levels of prior posterolateral fusion. Spine (Phila Pa 1976) 25:853-857, 2000.

253. Loguidice VA, Johnson RG, Guyer RD, et al: Anterior lumbar interbody fusion. Spine (Phila Pa 1976) 13:366-369, 1988.

254. Newman MH, Grinstead GL: Anterior lumbar interbody fusion for internal disc disruption. Spine (Phila Pa 1976) 17:831-833, 1992.

255. Baker JK, Reardon PR, Reardon MJ, et al: Vascular injury in anterior lumbar surgery. Spine (Phila Pa 1976) 18:2227-2230, 1993.

256. Hackenberg L, Liljenqvist U, Halm H, et al: Occlusion of the left common iliac artery and consecutive thromboembolism of the left popliteal artery following anterior lumbar interbody fusion. J Spinal Disord 14:365-368, 2001.

257. Christensen FB, Bunger CE: Retrograde ejaculation after retroperitoneal lower lumbar interbody fusion. Int Orthop 21:176-180, 1997.

258. Flynn JC, Price CT: Sexual complications of anterior fusion of the lumbar spine. Spine (Phila Pa 1976) 9:489-492, 1984.

259. Moore KR, Pinto MR, Butler LM: Degenerative disc disease treated with combined anterior and posterior arthrodesis and posterior instrumentation. Spine (Phila Pa 1976) 27:1680-1686, 2002.

260. Gertzbein SD, Betz R, Clements D, et al: Semirigid instrumentation in the management of lumbar spinal conditions combined with circumferential fusion: A multicenter study. Spine (Phila Pa 1976) 21:1918-1925; discussion 1925-1926, 1996.

261. Kozak JA, O'Brien JP: Simultaneous combined anterior and posterior fusion: An independent analysis of a treatment for the disabled low-back pain patient. Spine (Phila Pa 1976) 15:322-328, 1990.

262. Hinkley BS, Jaremko ME: Effects of 360-degree lumbar fusion in a workers' compensation population. Spine (Phila Pa 1976) 22:312-322; discussion 323, 1997.

263. Videbaek TS, Christensen RB, Soegaard R, et al: Circumferential fusion improves outcome in comparison with instrumented posterolateral fusion: Long-term results of a randomized clinical trial. Spine (Phila Pa 1976) 31:2875-2880, 2006.

264. Suratwala SJ, Pinto MR, Gilbert TJ, et al: Functional and radiological outcomes of 360 degrees fusion of three or more motion levels in the lumbar spine for degenerative disc disease. Spine (Phila Pa 1976) 34:E351-E358, 2009.

265. Salehi SA, Tawk R, Ganju A, et al: Transforaminal lumbar interbody fusion: Surgical technique and results in 24 patients. Neurosurgery 54:368-374; discussion 374, 2004.

266. Madan SS, Boeree NR: Comparison of instrumented anterior interbody fusion with instrumented circumferential lumbar fusion. Eur Spine J 12:567-575, 2003.

267. Vamvanij V, Fredrickson BE, Thorpe JM, et al: Surgical treatment of internal disc disruption: An outcome study of four fusion techniques. J Spinal Disord 11:375-382, 1998.

268. Knox BD, Chapman TM: Anterior lumbar interbody fusion for discogram concordant pain. J Spinal Disord 6:242-244, 1993.

269. Lowe TG, Tahernia AD, O'Brien MF, et al: Unilateral transforaminal posterior lumbar interbody fusion (TLIF): Indications, technique, and 2-year results. J Spinal Disord Tech 15:31-38, 2002.

270. Whitecloud TS 3rd, Roesch WW, Ricciardi JE: Transforaminal interbody fusion versus anterior-posterior interbody fusion of the lumbar spine: A financial analysis. J Spinal Disord 14:100-103, 2001.

271. Obenchain TG: Laparoscopic lumbar discectomy: Case report. J Laparoendosc Surg 1:145-149, 1991.

272. Kaiser MG, Haid RW Jr, Subach BR, et al: Comparison of the mini-open versus laparoscopic approach for anterior lumbar interbody fusion: A retrospective review. Neurosurgery 51:97-103; discussion 103-105, 2002.

273. Regan JJ, Yuan H, McAfee PC: Laparoscopic fusion of the lumbar spine: Minimally invasive spine surgery: A prospective multicenter study evaluating open and laparoscopic lumbar fusion. Spine (Phila Pa 1976) 24:402-411, 1999.

274. Lieberman IH, Willsher PC, Litwin DE, et al: Transperitoneal laparoscopic exposure for lumbar interbody fusion. Spine (Phila Pa 1976) 25:509-514; discussion 515, 2000.

275. Zdeblick TA, David SM: A prospective comparison of surgical approach for anterior L4-L5 fusion: Laparoscopic versus mini anterior lumbar interbody fusion. Spine (Phila Pa 1976) 25:2682-2687, 2000.

276. Inamasu J, Guiot BH: Laparoscopic anterior lumbar interbody fusion: A review of outcome studies. Minim Invasive Neurosurg 48:340-347, 2005.

277. Brau S: Mini-open approach to the spine for anterior lumbar interbody fusion: Description of the procedure, results and complications. Spine J 2:216-223, 2002.

278. Schleicher P, Beth P, Ottenbacher A, et al: Biomechanical evaluation of different asymmetrical posterior stabilization methods for minimally invasive transforaminal lumbar interbody fusion. J Neurosurg Spine 9:363-371, 2008.

279. Slucky AV, Brodke DS, Bachus KN, et al: Less invasive posterior fixation method following transforaminal lumbar interbody fusion: A biomechanical analysis. Spine J 6:78-85, 2006.

280. Sethi A, Lee S, Vaidya R: Transforaminal lumbar interbody fusion using unilateral pedicle screws and a translaminar. Eur Spine J 18:430-434, 2009.

281. Schwender JD, Holly LT, Rouben DP, et al: Minimally invasive transforaminal lumbar interbody fusion (TLIF): Technical feasibility and initial results. J Spinal Disord Tech 18(Suppl):S1-S6, 2005.

282. Peng CW, Yue WM, Poh SY, et al: Clinical and radiological outcomes of minimally invasive versus open transforaminal lumbar interbody fusion. Spine (Phila Pa 1976) 34:1385-1389, 2009.

283. Scheufler KM, Dohmen H, Vougioukas VI: Percutaneous transforaminal lumbar interbody fusion for the treatment of degenerative lumbar instability. Neurosurgery 60(4 Suppl 2):203-212; discussion 212-213, 2007.

284. Park Y, Ha JW: Comparison of one-level posterior lumbar interbody fusion performed with a minimally invasive approach or a traditional open approach. Spine (Phila Pa 1976) 32:537-543, 2007.

285. Stevens KJ, Spenciner DB, Griffiths KL, et al: Comparison of minimally invasive and conventional open posterolateral lumbar fusion using magnetic resonance imaging and retraction pressure studies. J Spinal Disord Tech 19:77-86, 2006.

286. Shim CS, Lee SH, Jung B, et al: Fluoroscopically assisted percutaneous translaminar facet screw fixation following anterior lumbar interbody fusion: Technical report. Spine (Phila Pa 1976) 30:838-843, 2005.

287. Jang JS, Lee SH: Clinical analysis of percutaneous facet screw fixation after anterior lumbar interbody fusion. J Neurosurg Spine 3:40-46, 2005.

288. Pimenta L: Lateral endoscopic transpsoas retroperitoneal approach. Proceedings of VIII Brazilian Spine Society Meeting, Minas Horizonte, Minas Gerais, Brazil, 2001.

289. Bergey DL, Villavicencio AT, Goldstein T, et al: Endoscopic lateral transpsoas approach to the lumbar spine. Spine (Phila Pa 1976) 29:1681-1688, 2004.

290. Benglis DM, Vanni S, Levi AD: An anatomical study of the lumbosacral plexus as related to the minimally invasive transpsoas approach to the lumbar spine. J Neurosurg Spine 10:139-144, 2009.

290a. Knight RQ, Schwaegler P, Hanscom D, Roh J: Direct lateral lumbar interbody fusion for degenerative conditions: early complication profile. J Spinal Disord Tech 22:34-37, 2009.

291. Ozgur BM, Aryan HE, Pimenta L, et al: Extreme lateral interbody fusion (XLIF): A novel surgical technique for anterior lumbar interbody fusion. Spine J 6:435-443, 2006.

292. Marotta N, Cosar M, Pimenta L, et al: A novel minimally invasive presacral approach and instrumentation technique for anterior L5-S1 intervertebral discectomy and fusion: Technical description and case presentations. Neurosurg Focus 20:E9, 2006.

293. Aryan HE, Newman CB, Gold JJ, et al: Percutaneous axial lumbar interbody fusion (AxiaLIF) of the L5-S1 segment: Initial clinical and radiographic experience. Minim Invasive Neurosurg 51:225-230, 2008.

294. Bindal RK, Glaze S, Ognoskie M, et al: Surgeon and patient radiation exposure in minimally invasive transforaminal lumbar interbody fusion. J Neurosurg Spine 9:570-573, 2008.

295. Kim CW, Lee YP, Taylor W, et al: Use of navigation-assisted fluoroscopy to decrease radiation exposure during minimally invasive spine surgery. Spine J 8:584-590, 2008.

296. Fritzell P, Hagg O, Wessberg P, et al: Chronic low back pain and fusion: A comparison of three surgical techniques: A prospective multicenter randomized study from the Swedish lumbar spine study group. Spine (Phila Pa 1976) 27:1131-1141, 2002.

297. Fritzell P, Hägg O, Nordwall A; Swedish Lumbar Spine Study Group: Complications in lumbar fusion surgery for chronic low back pain: Comparison of three surgical techniques used in a prospective randomized study. A report from the Swedish Lumbar Spine Study Group. Eur Spine J 12:178-189, 2003.

298. Kim KT, Lee SH, Lee YH, et al: Clinical outcomes of 3 fusion methods through the posterior approach in the lumbar spine. Spine (Phila Pa 1976) 31:1351-1357, 2006.

299. Glassman S, Gornet MF, Branch C, et al: MOS Short Form 36 and Oswestry Disability Index outcomes in lumbar fusion: A multicenter experience. Spine J 6:21-26, 2006.

300. Burkus JK, Gornet MF, Dickman CA, et al: Anterior lumbar interbody fusion using rhBMP-2 with tapered interbody cages. J Spinal Disord Tech 15:337-349, 2002.

301. Boden SD, Zdeblick TA, Sandhu HS, et al: The use of rhBMP-2 in interbody fusion cages: Definitive evidence of osteoinduction in humans: A preliminary report. Spine (Phila Pa 1976) 25:376-381, 2000.

302. Haid RW Jr, Branch CL Jr, Alexander JT, et al: Posterior lumbar interbody fusion using recombinant human bone morphogenetic protein type 2 with cylindrical interbody cages. Spine J 4:527-538; discussion 538-539, 2004.

303. Sasso RC, LeHuec JC, Shaffrey C; Spine Interbody Research Group: Iliac crest bone graft donor site pain after anterior lumbar interbody fusion: A prospective patient satisfaction outcome assessment. J Spinal Disord Tech 18(Suppl):S77-S81, 2005.

304. Dimar JR, Glassman SD, Burkus KJ, et al: Clinical outcomes and fusion success at 2 years of single-level instrumented posterolateral fusions with recombinant human bone morphogenetic protein-2/compression resistant matrix versus iliac crest bone graft. Spine (Phila Pa 1976) 31:2534-2539; discussion 2540, 2006.

305. Dimar JR 2nd, Glassman SD, Burkus JK, et al: Clinical and radiographic analysis of an optimized rhBMP-2 formulation as an autograft replacement in posterolateral lumbar spine arthrodesis. J Bone Joint Surg Am 91:1377-1386, 2009.

306. Burkus JK, Sandhu HS, Gornet MF: Influence of rhBMP-2 on the healing patterns associated with allograft interbody constructs in comparison with autograft. Spine (Phila Pa 1976) 31:775-781, 2006.

307. Burkus JK, Gornet MF, Schuler TC, et al: Six-year outcomes of anterior lumbar interbody arthrodesis with use of interbody fusion cages and recombinant human bone morphogenetic protein-2. J Bone Joint Surg Am 91:1181-1189, 2009.

308. Vaccaro AR, Lawrence JP, Patel T, et al: The safety and efficacy of OP-1 (rhBMP-7) as a replacement for iliac crest autograft in posterolateral lumbar arthrodesis: A long-term (>4 years) pivotal study. Spine (Phila Pa 1976) 33:2850-2862, 2008.

309. Rihn JA, Patel R, Makda J, et al: Complications associated with single-level transforaminal lumbar interbody fusion. Spine J 9:623-629, 2009.

310. Mindea SA, Shih P, Song JK: Recombinant human bone morphogenetic protein-2-induced radiculitis in elective minimally invasive transforaminal lumbar interbody fusions: A series review. Spine (Phila Pa 1976) 34:1480-1484; discussion 1485, 2009.

311. Joseph V, Rampersaud YR: Heterotopic bone formation with the use of rhBMP2 in posterior minimal access interbody fusion: A CT analysis. Spine (Phila Pa 1976) 32:2885-2890, 2007.

312. Lewandrowski KU, Nanson C, Calderon R: Vertebral osteolysis after posterior interbody lumbar fusion with recombinant human bone morphogenetic protein 2: A report of five cases. Spine J 7:609-614, 2007.

313. Glassman SD, Dimar JR 3rd, Burkus K, et al: The efficacy of rhBMP-2 for posterolateral lumbar fusion in smokers. Spine (Phila Pa 1976) 32:1693-1698, 2007.

314. Carreon LY, Glassman SD, Djurasovic M, et al: rhBMP-2 versus iliac crest bone graft for lumbar spine fusion in patients over 60 years of age: A cost-utility study. Spine (Phila Pa 1976) 34:238-243, 2009.

315. Garrison KR, Donell S, Ryder J, et al: Clinical effectiveness and cost-effectiveness of bone morphogenetic proteins in the non-healing of fractures and spinal fusion: A systematic review. Health Technol Assess 11:1-150, iii-iv, 2007.

316. Cunningham BW, Kotani Y, McNulty PS, et al: The effect of spinal destabilization and instrumentation on lumbar intradiscal pressure: An in vitro biomechanical analysis. Spine (Phila Pa 1976) 22:2655-2663, 1997.

317. Lee CK, Langrana NA: Lumbosacral spinal fusion: A biomechanical study. Spine (Phila Pa 1976) 9:574-581, 1984.

318. Lee CK: Accelerated degeneration of the segment adjacent to a lumbar fusion. Spine (Phila Pa 1976) 13:375-377, 1988.

319. Okuda S, Iwasaki M, Miyauchi A, et al: Risk factors for adjacent segment degeneration after PLIF. Spine (Phila Pa 1976) 29:1535-1540, 2004.

320. Wai EK, Santo ER, Morcom RA, et al: Magnetic resonance imaging 20 years after anterior lumbar interbody fusion. Spine (Phila Pa 1976) 31:1952-1956, 2006.

321. Pellise F, Hernandez A, Vidal X, et al: Radiologic assessment of all unfused lumbar segments 7.5 years after instrumented posterior spinal fusion. Spine (Phila Pa 1976) 32:574-579, 2007.

322. Yang JY, Lee JK, Song HS: The impact of adjacent segment degeneration on the clinical outcome after lumbar spinal fusion. Spine (Phila Pa 1976) 33:503-507, 2008.

323. Willems PC, Elmans L, Anderson PG, et al: Provocative discography and lumbar fusion: Is preoperative assessment of adjacent discs useful? Spine (Phila Pa 1976) 32:1094-1099; discussion 1100, 2007.

324. Schulte TL, Leistra F, Bullmann V, et al: Disc height reduction in adjacent segments and clinical outcome 10 years after lumbar 360 degrees fusion. Eur Spine J 16:2152-2158, 2007.

325. Graf H: Surgical treatment without fusion. Rachis 412:123-137, 1992.

326. Kanayama M, Hashimoto T, Shigenobu K: Rationale, biomechanics, and surgical indications for Graf ligamentoplasty. Orthop Clin North Am 36:373-377, 2005.

327. Kanayama M, Hashimoto T, Shigenobu K, et al: A minimum 10-year follow-up of posterior dynamic stabilization using Graf artificial ligament. Spine (Phila Pa 1976) 32:1992-1996; discussion 1997, 2007.

328. Gardner A, Pande KC: Graf ligamentoplasty: A 7-year follow-up. Eur Spine J 11(Suppl 2):S157-S163, 2002.

329. Markwalder TM, Wenger M: Dynamic stabilization of lumbar motion segments by use of Graf's ligaments: Results with an average follow-up of 7.4 years in 39 highly selected, consecutive patients. Acta Neurochir (Wien) 145:209-214; discussion 214, 2003.

330. Brechbühler D, Markwalder TM, Braun M: Surgical results after soft system stabilization of the lumbar spine in degenerative disc disease—long-term results. Acta Neurochir (Wien) 140:521-525, 1998.

331. Hadlow SV, Fagan AB, Hillier TM, et al: The Graf ligamentoplasty procedure: Comparison with posterolateral fusion in the management of low back pain. Spine (Phila Pa 1976) 23:1172-1179, 1998.

332. Mulholland RC, Sengupta DK: Rationale, principles and experimental evaluation of the concept of soft stabilization. Eur Spine J 11(Suppl 2):S198-S205, 2002.

333. Grob D, Benini A, Junge A, et al: Clinical experience with the Dynesys semirigid fixation system for the lumbar spine: Surgical and patient-oriented outcome in 50 cases after an average of 2 years. Spine (Phila Pa 1976) 30:324-331, 2005.

334. Stoll TM, Dubois G, Schwarzenbach O: The dynamic neutralization system for the spine: A multi-center study of a novel non-fusion system. Eur Spine J 11(Suppl 2):S170-S178, 2002.

335. Guyer RD, McAfee PC, Banco RJ, Bitan FD, et al: Prospective, randomized, multicenter Food and Drug Administration investigational device exemption study of lumbar total disc replacement with the CHARITE artificial disc versus lumbar fusion: Five-year follow-up. Spine J 9:374-386, 2009.

336. Blumenthal S, McAfee PC, Guyer RD, et al: A prospective, randomized, multicenter Food and Drug Administration investigational device exemptions study of lumbar total disc replacement with the CHARITE artificial disc versus lumbar fusion: Part I. Evaluation of clinical outcomes. Spine (Phila Pa 1976) 30:1565-1575; discussion E387-E391, 2005.

337. McAfee PC, Cunningham B, Holsapple G, et al: A prospective, randomized, multicenter Food and Drug Administration investigational device exemption study of lumbar total disc replacement with the CHARITE artificial disc versus lumbar fusion: Part II. Evaluation of radiographic outcomes and correlation of surgical technique accuracy with clinical outcomes. Spine (Phila Pa 1976) 30:1576-1583; discussion E388-E390, 2005.

338. Tropiano P, Huang RC, Girardi FP, et al: Lumbar total disc replacement: Seven to eleven-year follow-up. J Bone Joint Surg Am 87:490-496, 2005.

339. Lemaire JP, Carrier H, Sariali el-H, et al: Clinical and radiological outcomes with the Charité artificial disc: A 10-year minimum follow-up. J Spinal Disord Tech 18:353-359, 2005.

340. Zigler J, Delamarter R, Spivak JM, et al: Results of the prospective, randomized, multicenter Food and Drug Administration investigational device exemption study of the ProDisc-L total disc replacement versus circumferential fusion for the treatment of 1-level degenerative disc disease. Spine (Phila Pa 1976) 32:1155-1162; discussion 1163, 2007.

341. Sasso RC, Foulk DM, Hahn M: Prospective, randomized trial of metal-on-metal artificial lumbar disc replacement: Initial results for treatment of discogenic pain. Spine (Phila Pa 1976) 33:123-131, 2008.

342. Kostuik JP: Complications and surgical revision for failed disc arthroplasty. Spine J 4(6 Suppl):289S-291S, 2004.

343. Park CK, Ryu KS, Jee WH: Degenerative changes of discs and facet joints in lumbar total disc replacement using ProDisc II: Minimum two-year follow-up. Spine (Phila Pa 1976) 33:1755-1761, 2008.

344. Shim CS, Lee SH, Shin HD, et al: CHARITE versus ProDisc: A comparative study of a minimum 3-year follow-up. Spine (Phila Pa 1976) 32:1012-1018, 2007.

345. Harrop JS, Youssef JA, Maltenfort M, et al: Lumbar adjacent segment degeneration and disease after arthrodesis and total disc arthroplasty. Spine (Phila Pa 1976) 33:1701-1707, 2008.

346. Mehren C, Suchomel P, Grochulla F, et al: Heterotopic ossification in total cervical artificial disc replacement. Spine (Phila Pa 1976) 31:2802-2806, 2006.

347. Huang DS, Liang AJ, Ye W, et al: The risk factors and preventive strategies of heterotopic ossification after artificial disc replacement in lumbar spine. Zhonghua Wai Ke Za Zhi 44:242-245, 2006.

348. Tortolani PJ, Cunningham BW, Eng M, et al: Prevalence of heterotopic ossification following total disc replacement: A prospective, randomized study of two hundred and seventy-six patients. J Bone Joint Surg Am 89:82-88, 2007.

349. Schulte TL, Lerner T, Hackenberg L, et al: Acquired spondylolysis after implantation of a lumbar ProDisc II prosthesis: Case report and review of the literature. Spine (Phila Pa 1976) 32:E645-E648, 2007.

350. Marshman LA, Friesem T, Rampersaud YR, et al: Subsidence and malplacement with the Oblique Maverick Lumbar Disc Arthroplasty: Technical note. Spine J 8:650-655, 2008.

351. McAfee PC, Geisler FH, Saiedy SS, et al: Revisability of the CHARITE artificial disc replacement: Analysis of 688 patients enrolled in the U.S. IDE study of the CHARITE Artificial Disc. Spine (Phila Pa 1976) 31:1217-1226, 2006.

352. Levin DA, Bendo JA, Quirno M, et al: Comparative charge analysis of one- and two-level lumbar total disc arthroplasty versus circumferential lumbar fusion. Spine (Phila Pa 1976) 32:2905-2909, 2007.

353. Patel VV, Estes S, Lindley EM, et al: Lumbar spinal fusion versus anterior lumbar disc replacement: The financial implications. J Spinal Disord Tech 21:473-476, 2008.

354. Fernstrom U: Arthroplasty with intercorporal endoprosthesis in herniated disc and in painful disc. Acta Chir Scand Suppl 357:154-159, 1966.

355. Coric D, Mummaneni PV: Nucleus replacement technologies. J Neurosurg Spine 8:115-120, 2008.

356. Klara PM, Ray CD: Artificial nucleus replacement: Clinical experience. Spine (Phila Pa 1976) 27:1374-1377, 2002.

357. Shim CS, Lee SH, Park CW, et al: Partial disc replacement with the PDN prosthetic disc nucleus device: Early clinical results. J Spinal Disord Tech 16:324-330, 2003.

358. Ahrens M, Tsantrizos A, Donkersloot P, et al: Nucleus replacement with the DASCOR disc arthroplasty device: Interim two-year efficacy and safety results from two prospective, non-randomized multicenter European studies. Spine (Phila Pa 1976) 34:1376-1384, 2009.

359. Hutton W, Decatur G, Meisel H: Autologous disc chondrocyte transplantation for repair of acute disc herniation. Presented at International Society for the Study of the Lumbar Spine, 29th annual meeting, Cleveland, OH, 2000.

360. Nishimura K, Mochida J: Percutaneous reinsertion of the nucleus pulposus: An experimental study. Spine (Phila Pa 1976) 23:1531-1538; discussion 1539, 1998.

361. Nomura T, Mochida J, Okuma M, et al: Nucleus pulposus allograft retards intervertebral disc degeneration. Clin Orthop Relat Res 389:94-101, 2001.

362. Meisel HJ, Siodla V, Ganey T, et al: Clinical experience in cell-based therapeutics: Disc chondrocyte transplantation: A treatment for degenerated or damaged intervertebral disc. Biomed Eng 24:5-21, 2007.

363. An HS, Takegami K, Kamada H, et al: Intradiscal administration of osteogenic protein-1 increases intervertebral disc height and proteoglycan content in the nucleus pulposus in normal adolescent rabbits. Spine (Phila Pa 1976) 30:25-31; discussion 31-32, 2005.

364. Kawakami M, Matsumoto T, Hashizume H, et al: Osteogenic protein-1 (osteogenic protein-1/bone morphogenetic protein-7) inhibits degeneration and pain-related behavior induced by chronically compressed nucleus pulposus in the rat. Spine (Phila Pa 1976) 30:1933-1939, 2005.

365. Chujo T, An HS, Akeda K, et al: Effects of growth differentiation factor-5 on the intervertebral disc—in vitro bovine study and in vivo rabbit disc degeneration model study. Spine (Phila Pa 1976) 31:2909-2917, 2006.

366. Kang R, Ghivizzani SC, Muzzonigro TS, et al: The Marshall R. Urist Young Investigator Award: Orthopaedic applications of gene therapy: From concept to clinic. Clin Orthop Relat Res 375:324-337, 2000.

367. Paul R, Hayden RC, Cheng H, et al: Potential use of Sox9 gene therapy for intervertebral degenerative disc disease. Spine (Phila Pa 1976) 28:755-763, 2003.

368. Wallach CJ, Sobajima S, Watanabe Y, et al: Gene transfer of the catabolic inhibitor TIMP-1 increases measured proteoglycans in cells from degenerated human intervertebral discs. Spine (Phila Pa 1976) 28:2331-2337, 2003.

369. Moon SH, Nishida K, Gilbertson LG, et al: Biologic response of human intervertebral disc cells to gene therapy cocktail. Spine (Phila Pa 1976) 33:1850-1855, 2008.

370. Kang R, Boden S: Breakout Session 7: Spine. Clin Orthop Relat Res 279S:S256-S259, 2000.

46
CHAPTER

Lumbar Disc Herniations

Christopher M. Bono, MD
Andrew Schoenfeld, MD
Steven R. Garfin, MD

Lumbar disc herniations are a common manifestation of degenerative disease.[1-3] They tend to occur early within the degenerative cascade, representing the tensile failure of the anulus to contain the gel-like nuclear portion of the disc. With improvements in advanced imaging techniques, lumbar disc herniations have been increasingly recognized in symptomatic and asymptomatic individuals.[4]

Treatment decision making for patients with herniated discs can be challenging. Nonoperative treatment can be effective in most cases.[5-9] Other authors have indicated that surgery leads to superior results, especially in short-term pain relief.[1,7-10] Several authors have highlighted the influence of fragment location and pattern and social and psychological factors on outcomes.[7-9,11-13] The exact natural history and complex interaction of biologic, psychosocial, ergonomic, and cultural variables have not been well established.

In the best-case scenario, the clinician can radiologically identify a single culprit disc that positively correlates with clinical findings. In patients who fail to respond to nonoperative management, disagreement remains concerning the optimal period of observation, timing of surgery, method of excision, and type of postoperative rehabilitation. In less evident cases, one or more minor disc bulges may be identified that are difficult to attribute to the patient's signs and symptoms. The use of diagnostic injections can be helpful in localizing symptomatic regions. Empiricism and reliance primarily on intuition may lead to inferior results. Strict agreement between a patient's signs, symptoms, and correlative diagnostic tests needs to exist when predicating treatment recommendations.

In acknowledging these questions, the authors have reviewed the wealth of classic and contemporary contributions made to the understanding of lumbar disc herniations. This chapter synthesizes the information and organizes it to help clinicians' understanding and recommendations of management of this seemingly simple, but realistically challenging, problem.

Pathoanatomy

Effective evaluation is based on an intimate understanding of the relationship of the lumbar intervertebral disc to its surrounding structures. The disc is the anterior border of the spinal canal at the facet joint level. It is covered by the thin posterior longitudinal ligament, which is concentrated in the midline, from which small bands extend laterally to cover the inferior aspect of the disc (Fig. 46–1). This configuration leaves the superior part of the posterolateral disc bare and is thought to contribute to the fact that posterolateral (or paracentral) herniations are the most frequent location for herniations to occur. Cumulative degenerative changes occur in this region of the disc from concentration of torsional, axial loading, and flexion-induced biomechanical strains.

The spinal cord ends at approximately the L1 level in adults to form the conus medullaris. The cauda equina is located within the lumbar spinal canal. It contains the lumbar and sacral nerve roots bathed in cerebrospinal fluid contained, or encapsulated, by the pia, arachnoid, and dural membranes (meninges). Nerve roots branch from the cauda equina one level above their exiting foramen (Fig. 46–2). The L5 nerve root leaves the cauda equina approximately at the level of the L4 vertebral body. It descends inferolaterally to pass anterior to the L4-5 facet joint and posterior to the L4-5 disc. Intimately associated with the inferomedial aspect of the L5 pedicle, the root turns lateral to enter the L5-S1 intervertebral (neural) foramen just proximal to the L5-S1 disc. Within the foramen, sensory cell bodies form the dorsal root ganglion. The root, now termed a *postganglionic spinal nerve,* exits the neural foramen where it is in close proximity to the lateral aspect of the L5-S1 disc. Fibrous bands (called *Hoffman ligaments*) often tether the nerve to the disc in this region.[14,15] After a short extraspinal course, the nerve divides into a ventral and dorsal primary ramus.

The location of the disc herniation determines which root is primarily affected. The spinal canal can be divided into longitudinal zones (Fig. 46–3). The *central zone* is delineated by the lateral borders of the cauda equina. The *lateral recess* is between the lateral border of the cauda equina and the medial border of the pedicle. Although the term *lateral recess* is frequently used to describe stenosis from bony encroachment (*lateral recess stenosis*), it sufficiently describes the location of *paracentral, posterolateral,* or *juxtacentral* herniations. Within the lateral recess, fragments medial to the nerve root, interposed between it and the cauda equina, are termed *axillary*

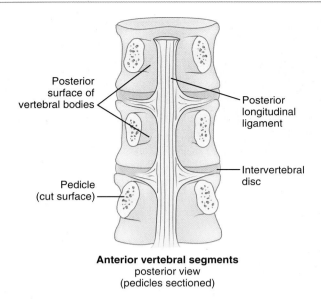

FIGURE 46–1 Posterior longitudinal ligament incompletely covers posterior portion of disc. Specifically, superolateral aspect of disc remains uncovered, which may help explain why disc herniations are most common in this region.

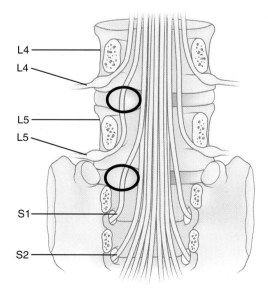

FIGURE 46–2 Lumbar nerve root branches exit dural sac one vertebral level above their respective foramen. Paracentral disc herniations tend to affect traversing nerve root as it crosses intervertebral disc.

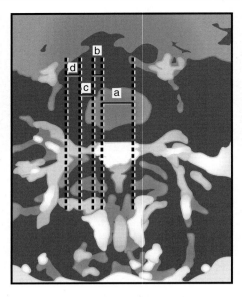

FIGURE 46–3 Considered in cross section, spinal canal can be divided into anatomic zones to describe better the location of lumbar disc herniations. *Central zone* (*a*) is within borders of cauda equina dural sac. *Lateral recess* (*b*), which paracentral disc herniations can compromise, is bordered by lateral aspect of dural sac and medial aspect of pedicle and neural foramen. In this zone, the nerve root descends within spinal canal toward its respective foramen. *Foraminal zone* (*c*) is space between adjacent ipsilateral pedicles. *Extraforaminal zone* (*d*) is space lateral to pedicles. Disc herniations in this region, commonly referred to as *far lateral,* affect exiting nerve root.

herniations (Fig. 46–4). The *foraminal* zone is between the medial and lateral borders of the pedicle. Herniations beyond the lateral border of the pedicle are within the far-lateral or *extraforaminal* zone. Herniations in the foraminal or extraforaminal zones usually affect the exiting nerve.

Fragments can displace cranially or caudally. Axillary herniations have a tendency to migrate distally, lying inferior to the disc space. Superior migration of the fragment can position it behind the adjacent cranial vertebral body. Locating the fragment preoperatively is crucial to successful operative excision.

Pathophysiology

Disc Degeneration and Herniation

Disc herniation is one stage of the lumbar degenerative cascade. It is considered one of the earlier stages, following internal disc disruption. Herniation occurs through a tear in the anulus fibrosus. The anulus is the thick outer layer that normally withstands tensile forces transferred from the compressed nucleus pulposus (Fig. 46–5).[16,17] Force transfer works only if the nucleus-anulus-endplate complex acts as a closed volume system.[18] Normally, compression across the disc space leads to increased pressure within the nucleus. The soft nucleus deforms and flattens, pushing against the annular fibers, which then generates tensile hoop stresses. The circumferential fibers are placed under tension, dissipating stresses and containing the anulus.

With disruption of the anulus, the soft nucleus can be pushed through (i.e., herniated) if placed under sufficient pressure. The nucleus must be fluid, or "dynamic," enough to permit herniation to occur. Discs in younger individuals that have a well-hydrated nucleus are more likely to herniate. Older patients with desiccated discs are less prone to herniation. The ejected portion is typically a fibrocartilaginous fragment.[19] In some cases, a piece of anulus or endplate fibrocartilage can be associated with it. In juveniles, an apparent herniation may represent a Salter type II fracture of the vertebral ring apophysis with its attached anulus.

When a portion of the nucleus is ejected, disc mechanics are altered. Frei and colleagues[17] showed that nucleotomy

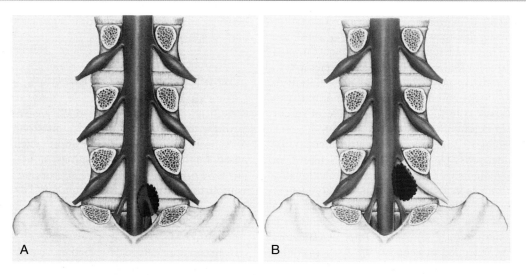

FIGURE 46–4 A, Most commonly, paracentral disc herniations compress traversing (descending) nerve root along its lateral aspect. **B,** In some cases, disc fragment can be interposed between nerve root and lateral border of cauda equina sac. These are known as *axillary disc herniations.*

alters the loading pattern across the disc space, with the anulus sustaining higher compression forces than normal. This situation can lead to increases in endplate pressures along the periphery where the anulus attaches to the bone. Chondro-osseous metaplastic changes such as osteophytes or sclerosis in these regions are a response to long-standing abnormal loading patterns.

The exact inciting event leading to disc herniation is unknown. Some authors believe that an acute traumatic episode leads to displacement of the disc, although this is most likely related to force imparted onto a previously degenerated disc, which has developed a focal annular weakness. Acute sciatica from a disc herniation is often associated with a prodromal history of back pain.

Postural variations can influence intradiscal pressures. The highest pressures have been recorded in patients with the torso forward flexed with weight in hand. In an elegant biomechanical study, Wilder and colleagues[16] found that combined lateral bend, flexion, and axial rotation with 15 minutes of exposure to vibration can lead to tears extending from the nucleus across the anulus. This finding may have significance for occupations with exposure to long periods of vibratory stimuli, such as truck drivers and machine workers.

Disc Herniation and Sciatica

The most classic symptom of a herniated disc is radicular pain in the lower extremity following a dermatomal distribution. Focal neurologic deficits attributable to the same nerve root are sometimes present and lend further diagnostic accuracy. The relationship between disc herniation and sciatica is incompletely understood, however.

In animals and humans, pure compression of a noninflamed nerve produces sensory and motor changes without pain, whereas pain is elicited with manipulation of inflamed nerves.[20] These findings suggest that herniated discs large

enough to cause mechanical compression of a nerve root may produce focal deficits, but that associated sciatic-type pain is produced only if the nerve root is concurrently irritated or inflamed. Inflammation may be produced by prolonged neuroischemia of the microvasculature of the nerve root from mechanical compression or by nonmechanical, possibly biochemical, factors. This phenomenon helps explain why some patients with small bulges or protrusions contacting inflamed nerves have pain that does not seem to be consistent with the "small" degree of neural compression. Additionally, these patients frequently do not have demonstrable sensory or motor deficit.

Neurochemical factors also have a role in the production of sciatic pain. This role may be related to initiation of an immune response locally or systemically or both. Spiliopoulou and colleagues[21] examined IgG and IgM levels in discs excised from patients with sciatica and controls. Although IgG levels were equivalent, elevated levels of IgM were found in discs from sciatica patients but not in controls suggesting a local

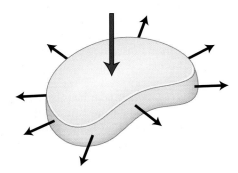

FIGURE 46–5 Thick, outer anulus normally withstands tensile forces transferred from compressed nucleus pulposus. This force transfer works, however, only if nucleus-anulus-endplate act as a closed volume system. Annular defect disrupts this closed volume system and can allow portion of nucleus to escape (or herniate).

and humoral antigenic inflammatory reaction as a contributor to pain. Other investigators have shown the role of cytokines in the mediation of root pain. Olmarker and Rydevik[22] studied the effects of selective inhibition of tumor necrosis factor-α in a herniated disc model in pigs. They found preservation of nerve conduction velocity and decreased nerve root injury in treated animals versus controls, suggesting a role of tumor necrosis factor-α in potentiating nerve dysfunction.

Similarly, research has suggested that matrix metalloproteinase, nitric oxide, prostaglandin E_2, and interleukin-6 in discs excised from patients with herniation and radiculopathy may have a causative role in pain production.[23] A more recent investigation was unable to confirm the presence of these inflammatory markers in the epidural space of patients with symptomatic disc herniations, however.[24] Other investigators have shown that in extruded or sequestered discs a cellular inflammatory reaction may be locally mediated via T cells and macrophages[25]; this has been postulated to play a role in herniated disc regression.[26]

There is evidence of systemic inflammatory responses to disc herniations as well. Brisby and colleagues[27] detected elevated levels of glycosphingolipid antibodies in the serum of patients with sciatica and disc herniation compared with healthy volunteers. Elevations were equivalent to those found in patients with autoimmune neurologic disorders such as Guillain-Barré syndrome. Brisby and colleagues[27] suggested that a systemic autoimmune response to disc tissue may result in damage, or alteration, of nerve tissue. After age 12, the endplate apophyseal vessels close, which may facilitate an amnestic antigenic response to exposure to extruded nucleus pulposus tissue. These findings are helpful in considering patients who have severe sciatic pain with minimal mechanical compression and patients who seem to have persistent symptoms despite surgical decompression.

Disc Herniation and Back Pain

Most patients with symptomatic disc herniations present with leg and back pain. The mechanism of degenerative back pain remains elusive, although many authors have suggested mechanisms. Accepting that herniation is a stage within the continuum of lumbar degeneration, discogenic pain generators may be a factor. Innervation of the posterior anulus by branches of the sinuvertebral nerve have been well documented and are a suggested pathway of nociceptive pain transmission from disc degeneration. An annular tear and nuclear herniation could result in similar pain transmission.

The concept of *vertebrogenic pain* has also been suggested. Jinkins and colleagues[28] studied the contribution of anterior disc herniations to back pain. They believed that the pain was neurally mediated through branches of the ventral ramus and paravertebral autonomic plexus. Because the herniations were outside the spinal canal, they were not associated with compression of the cauda equina or nerve roots, but most patients complained of lower extremity paresthesias, mostly bilateral, in addition to low back pain. A direct causal relationship between anterior disc herniations and leg symptoms has not been clarified.

Classification of Disc Herniations

Classification of any disorder should be based on identifiable features that have some influence on prognosis or treatment decision making. Many classification systems have been proposed for lumbar disc herniations, although none are all-inclusive or ideal.[29,30] It is more appropriate to consider them as tools to describe the herniation.

Morphology

Disc herniations can be described by their morphology. Before the introduction of advanced imaging, morphology was difficult to assess preoperatively. Currently, magnetic resonance imaging (MRI) and to a lesser extent computed tomography (CT) can differentiate disc morphology with reasonable reliability. Spengler and colleagues[13] divided herniations into three types (Fig. 46–6). A *protruded* disc was defined as eccentric bulging through an intact anulus fibrosus. An *extrusion* was defined as disc material that crosses the anulus but is in continuity with the remaining nucleus within the disc space. A *sequestered* disc represents a herniation that is not continuous with the disc space; this is the typical "free fragment."

Other authors have classified discs as either contained or uncontained.[31] *Contained* disc herniations are subligamentous. It is presumed that they have not passed beyond the limits of the posterior longitudinal ligament or the outer layer of the anulus. *Uncontained* disc herniations have crossed this boundary. Advocates of this system describe contained and uncontained extrusions, with the former remaining beneath the outer layers of the anulus.[31]

Location

Herniations can be described topographically according to anatomic location (see Fig. 46–3). The herniation can be located within the central zone, lateral recess, foraminal, or extraforaminal regions. Herniations can also exhibit cranial or caudal migration in relation to the disc space.

Timing

Lumbar disc herniations can be organized according to the time from initial symptom onset. These may be arbitrarily divided as acute or chronic. Acute herniations are present for less than 3 to 6 months, whereas chronic discs cause symptoms for a longer time. Breakdown according to this time frame is based on the authors' sense of what is a reasonable cutoff point. Because the results of disc excision seem to be influenced by the timing of surgery, this categorization is important. From a survey of the literature, it seems that the results of disc excision are compromised if delayed more than 2 to 16 months from symptom onset.[12,32-34]

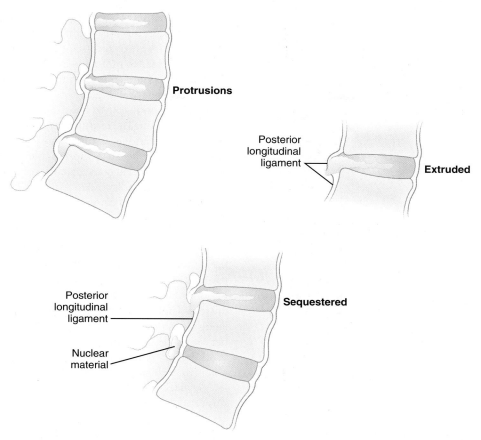

FIGURE 46–6 Classification of disc herniations as described by Spengler and colleagues.[13] *Disc protrusion* is defined as bulging displaced nucleus that has not extended beyond limits of anulus fibrosus. *Extrusion* extends beyond anulus fibrosus but is still in continuity, at least partially, with parent disc. *Sequestered* disc herniation implies that fragment has broken free (i.e., free fragment) and is no longer in continuity with parent disc. In some cases, in which disc herniation lies immediately behind vertebral body, it is difficult to tell from which disc the herniated fragment originated.

History and Symptoms

Many patients describe a prodromal history of long-standing mild to moderate back pain. Although trauma is not the only component leading to a disc herniation, some patients describe a specific incident attributable to the onset of leg and back pain. This incident may be a fall, a twist, or lifting of a heavy item. Specific postures can lead to exponential increases in intradiscal pressure, which can predispose to disc injury.[18] Exposure to vibrational energy combined with sustained lateral flexion and rotation may also predispose to herniation.[16] The exact history of the incident and the presence of preexistent back or leg pain must be explored; this is particularly important in work-related injuries.

Pain is the most common complaint. Axial back pain is typically present, although some patients do not have this complaint. Radicular pain is more typical and often the more "treatable" of the complaints. The pattern of lower extremity radiation depends on the level of the herniation. Lower lumbar or lumbosacral disc herniations can lead to the classic

symptoms of pain radiating below the knee. Often pain extends into the foot and can follow a dermatomal distribution. S1 radicular pain may radiate to the back of the calf or the lateral aspect or sole of the foot. L5 radicular pain can lead to symptoms on the dorsum of the foot (Fig. 46–7). Radiculopathy from involvement of the upper lumbar roots can lead to more proximal symptoms. L2 and L3 radiculopathy can produce anterior or medial thigh and groin pain. Groin pain may also be indicative of L1 pathology. Radicular pain can be difficult to discern and is often not "classic." Many patients do not exhibit pain in a specific dermatomal distribution, or the radiation does not extend along the entire leg. It may radiate only into the hip region or just the foot or any portion of the leg.

The character of radicular pain can be sharp, dull, burning, or dysesthetic. It can be exacerbated by coughing, bending, or lifting. A relieving maneuver may be lying supine with the knees and hips flexed, particularly with lower lumbar herniations. In contrast to patients with lumbar stenosis, patients with disc herniations more typically complain of constant pain that is not exacerbated by ambulation. Buttock pain is also common and can be referred or radicular in nature. Patients

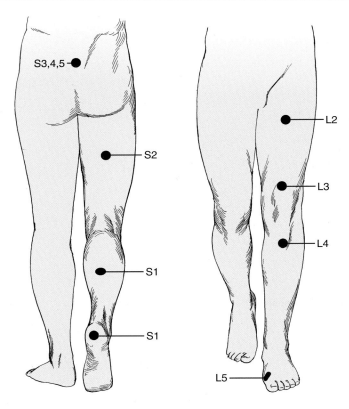

FIGURE 46–7 Location of pain can help localize nerve root involved. Pain may radiate to small, isolated areas along course of dermatome.

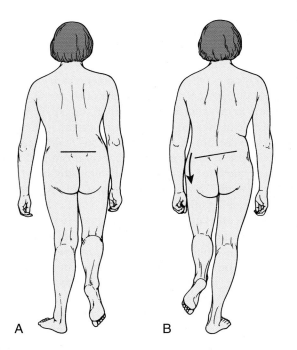

FIGURE 46–8 A, With normal L5 nerve root function, hip abductors are strong and able to support body weight. **B,** With L5 nerve root compression, hip abductors can be weakened, leading to positive Trendelenburg sign. This sign is seen when iliac crest (pelvis) tilts down onto side where leg is raised, indicating contralateral hip abductor (L5) weakness.

may interpret this as back pain, but the pathoanatomic significance of pain in this area is different than true axial pain. Pain is one component of radiculopathic complaints. Nerve compression can lead to motor and sensory deficits. Weakness may be reported as a slapping gait, footdrop, knee buckling, or imbalance when walking.

It is important to ask questions pertaining to bowel and bladder function. The examiner should inquire about urgency and frequency and fecal and urinary incontinence. Questions must be direct because most patients report constipation, which is often related to narcotic usage or inactivity, as a change in bowel habits. Acute bowel or bladder symptoms can be the sign of a cauda equina syndrome, which should mandate urgent surgical decompression.

The influence of social and psychological factors on the outcomes of disc surgery has been well documented. It is highly recommended to obtain a social and at least cursory psychiatric history. Prescription use of antidepressants is an important clue, although depression is often undiagnosed and untreated at the time of initial presentation. Other personality factors, such as chronic headaches, hysteria, hypochondriasis, nervous disorders, and impulsivity, can also be influential.[13,35] Work history, pending litigation, and type of work should be obtained. A history of smoking is an independent risk factor for low back pain and a risk factor for a poor result after back surgery.[35,36]

Physical Examination

Inspection

Inspection is the first step in the physical examination. As the patient walks into the examining room, gait should be observed. A sciatic list may be present, usually manifested as the patient leaning away from the side of leg pain. This sciatic list is thought to be associated with a paracentral herniation lateral to the nerve root. Axillary herniations may cause a list toward the side of herniation. The list is an attempt to relieve neuromeningeal tension by drawing the nerve root away from the herniated fragment. Another feature of gait that should be noted is a wide-based gait, indicative of lumbar or more cranial canal stenosis. A footdrop or foot slapping gait may occur with L4 or L5 paresis. A Trendelenburg gait can suggest hip abductor weakness (Fig. 46–8), which may be a clue to L5 nerve root compression because the gluteus medius is most often an L5 dominant muscle.

Alignment of the spine is noted. There can be loss of normal lumbar lordosis from muscular spasm. Hip flexion can relieve pain, leading some patients to lean forward or be reluctant to place the affected foot flat on the floor. In some cases, a nonstructural "sciatic scoliosis" can be noted on radiographs or examination of the back.

Palpation and Percussion

Examination should include a systematic examination of the back. The spinous processes are palpated individually and in stepwise fashion. Tenderness to palpation of one or two levels is more consistent with bony pathology than tenderness at multiple levels. In some cases, pressure on the spinous processes can reproduce sciatic symptoms. Continuing caudally, the lumbosacral junction and the sacral prominences and sacroiliac joint area can be palpated and percussed. Inflammation in these regions can manifest with sciatica, feigning disc herniation.

The musculature is examined next. The paraspinal muscles should be palpated. Spasm can be noted in addition to tenderness; this may be present as a "ball" of contracted muscle in one region. These findings are nonspecific and are of minimal diagnostic value. Muscular atrophy can be a sign of long-standing neural compression and is more likely isolated to one motor group. Generalized, symmetric muscle atrophy can suggest a more systemic neurologic disorder, such as a demyelinating disease.

Neurologic Examination

A neurologic examination is required in all patients with suspected herniated discs. Sensation of light touch is tested along dermatomes from L1 to S1. Standard dermatomal charts can be helpful, but there is variability among individuals, and so this is highly subjective. In testing the upper lumbar roots, there is often a significant amount of overlap. The most discrete levels of testing are for L4, L5, and S1 nerve roots.[37] These nerve roots are the most often affected by lumbar disc herniations (Table 46–1). L4 sensory function is tested at the medial ankle; L5, at the first webspace between the great and second toes; and S1, at the lateral aspect of the sole of the foot. Sensation is difficult to "grade." It is more useful to document sensation as normal, diminished, or absent. Sensory function should be compared with the contralateral side because this may help detect differences. The examiner should be wary of the presence of a glove-and-stocking distribution sensory loss, which can indicate a peripheral neuropathy, such as associated with diabetes, or functional overlay—as it is not anatomic.

The motor examination should proceed in a routine manner. In the lower extremity, it is better to test movements rather than specific muscles. S1 motor function is assessed by testing plantar flexion, whereas L5 is tested by toe dorsiflexion, particularly the great toe (extensor hallucis longus), and hip abduction. L4 involvement most often affects ankle dorsiflexion (anterior tibialis), although quadriceps function can be compromised. There is a significant amount of overlap of upper lumbar motor innervation. Knee extension can be considered L3 function (although L2 and L4 contribute); hip flexion, an assessment of L1-2 function; and hip adduction, an assessment of L2 function. Motor function is graded as 0 to 5, with 5 being full strength against active resistance (Table 46–2). In particular, S1 function should be assessed by asking the patient to toe raise repeatedly or toe-walk. Because of the enormous strength of the gastrocnemius complex, even a weakened muscle can overcome the examiner's hand. Toe-walking can show smaller differences, however, from side to side by using the weight of the patient's

TABLE 46–1 Prevalence of Back Pain and Sciatica in Adults

Characteristic	Prevalence (%)
Any low back pain	60-80
Any low back pain persisting at least 2 wk	14
Low back pain persisting at least 2 wk at a given time (point prevalence)	7
Back pain with features of sciatica lasting at least 2 wk	1.6
Lumbar spine surgery	1-2

From Deyo RA, Loeser J, Bigos S: Herniated lumbar intervertebral disc. Ann Intern Med 112:598-603, 1990.

body as the resistance. Repetitive toe raising may help detect smaller differences.

Deep tendon reflexes are tested at the patella and Achilles tendons. The patellar tendon reflex may be diminished or absent with L3 or L4 involvement, whereas the Achilles tendon reflex is affected primarily by S1. There is no specific reflex that reliably reflects L5 function. Reflexes are tested bilaterally and can be graded. Symmetrically decreased reflexes are not helpful in isolating a lesion. Generally, reflexes are anticipated to be decreased in response to nerve root compression from a herniated disc. Increased reflexes (hyperreflexia), especially if bilaterally symmetric, can indicate spinal cord compression at the thoracic or cervical level.

Specific Tests

The straight-leg raise (SLR) test is an extremely useful provocative test in examining patients with a herniated disc (Fig. 46–9). The classic test is performed with the patient in the supine position. The heel of a relaxed leg is cupped by the examiner's hand and elevated slowly. The knee is kept in extension while the hip is flexed. The test is considered positive if sciatic pain is reproduced between 35 degrees and 70 degrees of elevation. Studies have determined that in the first 35 degrees of elevation, the slack in the nerves is taken up, and at 35 degrees or more, tension is placed on the nerves. More than 70 degrees of elevation causes no further stretch of the nerve roots. The SLR test is best for eliciting L4, L5, or S1 radiculopathy. It is not useful for upper lumbar roots, for which a femoral stretch test should be used. A positive SLR test is indicative of nerve root compression in 90% of cases.[38] It does not implicate a herniated disc as the source of

TABLE 46–2 Motor Strength Grading System by Physical Examination

Grade	Definition
0	No visible muscle contraction at all
1	Visible muscle contraction; no joint movement
2	Can move joint but not overcome gravity
3	Able to overcome gravity but cannot overcome any examiner resistance
4	Able to overcome some, but not full, examiner resistance
5	Full strength; able to resist full examiner force

FIGURE 46–9 Supine straight-leg raise test.

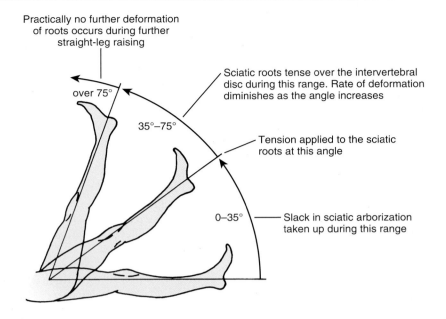

Practically no further deformation of roots occurs during further straight-leg raising

over 75°

35°–75°

0–35°

Sciatic roots tense over the intervertebral disc during this range. Rate of deformation diminishes as the angle increases

Tension applied to the sciatic roots at this angle

Slack in sciatic arborization taken up during this range

compression, however, because foraminal encroachment or other mass lesions can lead to a positive SLR test as well.

The SLR test should always be performed bilaterally. If raising the contralateral leg reproduces symptoms in the ipsilateral side, this is highly suggestive for a herniated disc and should be considered strong evidence of the diagnosis and is more specific for a free disc fragment. The Lasègue maneuver is a modification of the SLR test. The leg is raised until radiating symptoms are produced. Then the foot of the ipsilateral leg is maximally dorsiflexed. By increasing the tension along the sciatic nerve and lower lumbar nerve roots, dorsiflexion exacerbates pain and is considered a positive examination.

An important variant of the supine SLR test is the seated SLR test. When a patient is initially examined, he or she is usually seated at the side of the examining table with the knees and hips flexed at about 90 degrees. In this position, the heel is cupped, and the leg is extended at the knee. With a herniated fragment causing nerve root tension, the patient reflexively extends at the hip and leans back to relieve the ensuing sciatic pain. If the patient is comfortable with the seated SLR test but has a positive supine SLR test, symptom magnification must be considered because these findings are pathoanatomically contradictory.

The so-called slump test is a variant of the Lasègue test and the SLR test. This test is performed in the seated position; the patient is asked to flex the thoracic and lumbar spine while fully flexing the neck. Next, the SLR test is performed while the foot is dorsiflexed on the same side, as denoted by the Lasègue test. The combination of these maneuvers adds cephalad gliding of the spinal cord to the examination, whereas the SLR test and Lasègue test by themselves produce only caudal tension on the nerve roots. A more recent study found the slump test was more sensitive than the SLR test in patients with lumbar disc herniations, whereas the SLR test was more specific.[39]

Another tension sign is the bowstring test. Starting with a typical SLR test, the leg is raised until symptoms are produced.

The leg is flexed at the knee, and the tibial and peroneal nerves (distal aspect of sciatic nerve) are placed on tension by palpation in the popliteal space. Reproduction of pain is considered a positive sign of root tension.

The femoral stretch test is performed in the prone position. The leg is flexed at the knee while pulling the hip into extension. Reproduction of anterior thigh pain is indicative of upper lumbar root pathology.

Differential Diagnosis

The differential diagnosis should be narrowed based on history, physical examination, and selected imaging tests. Radicular pain can be caused by numerous compressive disorders, such as spinal stenosis, abscess, tumor, or vascular disease. Intrinsic nerve problems, such as nerve tumors or multiple sclerosis, can produce similar symptoms. Peripheral neuropathies, such as tarsal tunnel syndrome, meralgia paresthetica, and obturator or piriformis syndrome, can also lead to similar sciatic-type pain.

Diagnostic Imaging

The authors employ a simple imaging algorithm for patients with suspected lumbar herniated discs. If the patient presents acutely, within the first 2 weeks of the incident, the examination is typically masked by a large amount of spasm, back pain, and generalized tenderness. If the mechanism of injury involved substantial trauma, plain radiographs are obtained. If the injury was low energy, radiographs can be delayed until the follow-up examination at 6 weeks. Numerous patients will have recovered substantially by 6 weeks, obviating the need for further workup. For patients whose pain has not improved or perhaps has worsened, plain radiographs are obtained. Advanced imaging is reserved for patients in whom pain is persistent, the diagnosis is unclear, or surgical treatment is planned. "Red flags" in a patient's history that should prompt early MRI include constitutional symptoms (i.e., fever, chills, and sweats), a history of malignancy, osteoporosis, progressive neurologic deficits, or bowel and bladder incontinence.

Plain Radiographs

Plain radiographs cannot show a herniated disc. They can show changes that are suggestive of a herniated disc, however. As stated previously, a scoliotic list can be present on radiographs. This list may be convex or concave to the ipsilateral side and is not specific for a level.

Other findings that can be noted on plain films are changes consistent with disc degeneration, including osteophytes; disc space narrowing; or subtle changes in translation, facet hypertrophy, or changes in sagittal alignment. Most commonly, plain films are negative, especially in younger patients with an acute herniation. Plain films are important in ruling out obvious underlying problems, such as lytic lesions, tumors, infections, inflammatory spinal disorders, or instabilities (e.g., spondylolisthesis).

High-quality anteroposterior and lateral radiographs are prerequisites to planning operative interventions such as discectomy. It is crucial to recognize if there is an anomalous number of lumbar vertebrae, such as spines with a "lumbarized" first sacral segment (i.e., six lumbar vertebrae), because this can influence intraoperative identification of the correct disc level. Plain films can help detect other congenital anomalies, such as spina bifida occulta defects, which can influence surgical exposure and dissection.

Magnetic Resonance Imaging

MRI is the most popular modality for advanced imaging of lumbar disc herniations. MRI is superior to CT in delineating soft tissues. The disc and fragments that may have herniated from it are readily visualized. Free fragments (sequestered) can be differentiated from extruded disc herniations (Fig. 46–10), and a symmetrical bulge can be differentiated from a contained protrusion. The neural elements themselves are well visualized. Neural encroachment can be detected within the spinal canal, the foramina, or extraforaminally. MRI is also useful in differentiating disc herniations from tumors, vascular anomalies, or bony compression.

Numerous features of a herniated disc can be noted on MRI. The size and type of disc herniation can be reliably determined using MRI, which may have prognostic significance.[11,40,41] Carragee and Kim[11] correlated outcomes with herniated fragment size and its effect on canal area. Larger discs (>6 mm) were more likely to have a positive SLR test or femoral stretch test (Wasserman sign). In the operative group, larger discs were predictive of a better outcome. The fair and poor outcomes in operative patients were in patients with small discs (<6 mm).

Attempts to correlate MRI findings with clinical symptoms have been made. In 33 patients in whom disc herniation was diagnosed clinically and 5 control patients with low back pain alone, Kikkawa and colleagues[42] performed three-dimensional

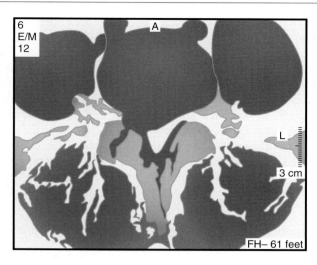

FIGURE 46–10 T2-weighted MRI has myelogram-like appearance in which cerebrospinal fluid within dural sac is bright. This makes compression from disc herniations readily visible, as can be visualized in this case of large extruded paracentral disc herniation.

MRI using a fast low angle shot (FLASH) with gadolinium enhancement. Dorsal root ganglion enhancement was found to be nonspecific, occurring in controls and sciatica patients. Enhancement of the root proper was detected, however, in 11 of 30 symptomatic patients, with patients having a statistical tendency for more severe motor involvement. There was no significant association of diffuse versus local enhancement with the positivity of the SLR test or sensory changes. Central compression of the cauda equina did not lead to enhancement in any cases. Although these results are modest, they suggest a future use of gadolinium-enhanced MRI as a noninvasive method of determining the microvascular response to compression of neural structures.

Komori and colleagues[41] studied the significance of enhancement around the herniated fragment itself. Patients with radiculopathy underwent initial and follow-up gadolinium-enhanced MRI to correlate clinical improvement with the degree of enhancement. Patients with marked decrease in size of the herniation showed good clinical resolution. This resolution was most significant in the "migrating"-type discs, which were closest to sequestered discs according to the authors' description. Decrease in fragment size was associated with a gradual increase in the area of enhancement in 17 of 22 sequestered disc herniations, all of which had improvement of radicular pain. Five cases of sequestered discs without enhancement or size decrease had a poor clinical result. Enhancement was less marked in extruded versus sequestered herniations; however, herniations that did show enhancement had a significantly better clinical course. From these data, Komori and colleagues[41] recommended this test as a prognostic tool in guiding the treatment of patients with extruded or sequestered herniated discs.

Of more recent interest is the influence of posture on the MRI appearance of discs and their relationship to the neural structures. Because images are traditionally acquired in the supine position, the spine is not axially loaded as it is during everyday activities. Weishaupt and colleagues[43] performed positional MRI in patients with low back or leg pain for 6 weeks that was not responding to conservative treatment. Images were obtained in the usual supine position and with a seated flexed and extended posture. Changes in foraminal size and neural compression occurred with flexion and extension. Changes in foraminal size correlated with increased pain scores. These findings are probably most significant for low-grade herniations (i.e., bulges or protrusions) in which there is still a fixed-volume system within the disc space provided by an intact outer annular layer. Similar findings have been shown using dynamic functional plain myelography.[44]

Magnetic Resonance Imaging in the Postoperative Spine

Not all patients respond well to surgical discectomy. Failures may be related to numerous factors, including psychosocial disturbance, recurrence, infection, wrong-level surgery, poor surgical indications, and improper operative technique. Residual or recurrent back and leg complaints often prompt practitioners to seek postoperative imaging. Plain radiographs can show overall alignment, with flexion-extension views useful in detecting instability, spondylolisthesis, or disc space collapse, which is a frequent occurrence after discectomy in adult patients. Contrast-enhanced CT is best to show if there is associated bone or soft tissue impingement of the space available for the neural elements.

As the modality of choice for imaging the neural structures, MRI is frequently obtained. Because of edema, hematoma, and formation of surgical scar, MRI is best delayed until 6 months after surgery,[45] if symptoms allow. The main challenge is differentiating scar from new-onset disc. On standard T1-weighted sequences, this differentiation can be difficult. In the early days of MRI, T2-weighted images were not as useful because of longer scan times with inadequate magnet strength.[46]

The superiority of MRI over CT to distinguish scar from disc has evolved with the introduction of gadolinium contrast agent; this is based on T1-weighted sequences and has been shown by many researchers. Opinions have been changing regarding this test as the "gold standard." A herniated disc fragment may eventually enhance if enough time passes before it is imaged. This enhancement can lead to recurrent or residual disc fragments being interpreted as extradural fibrosis or scar. Enhancement of scar should occur within 15 minutes of injection.

Evidence suggests that sophisticated T2 image analysis might supplant the need for gadolinium-enhanced MRI. Barrera and colleagues[47] compared different imaging sequences with and without gadolinium contrast agent. These investigators documented 100% sensitivity for detecting scar for T2-weighted turbo-spin echo (TSE) and fluid attenuated inversion recovery (FLAIR) sequences compared with T1-weighted images with gadolinium. Specificity was 94% and 92% for TSE T2 and FLAIR images. Barrera and colleagues[47] concluded that standard TSE T2 images acquired using a rapid sequence are extremely sensitive and specific in distinguishing disc from scar in most cases and that the use of gadolinium contrast agent should be reserved for the rare situation in which that distinction cannot be made. These recommendations are supported by others.[46]

Grane and Lindqvist[45] studied the role of gadolinium enhancement of the nerve roots after discectomy. These investigators found intradural (within the cauda equina) nerve root enhancement in 59% of patients with recurrent clinical symptoms. Recurrent symptoms occurred, however, in 84% of patients with focal (extradural, after the nerve root has existed the cauda equina) enhancement and 86% of patients with nerve root thickening. Enhancement occurred in patients with and without evidence of nerve root displacement by scar or disc. This finding indicates that although symptoms may correlate with MRI enhancement, it is not associated with a compressive mass lesion.

In an early report on the use of MRI without gadolinium, Bundschuh and colleagues[48] studied 20 patients after failed disc surgery who had a strong likelihood of undergoing further surgery. In 14 patients, CT with contrast agent was also performed. The authors found that free fragments of disc had a mildly increased signal on T1 images compared with scar, whereas scar and disc were similarly hyperintense on T2 images. Overall, Bundschuh and colleagues[48] believed that MRI was at least comparable to CT with contrast agent in differentiating scar from disc, confirmed by intraoperative findings.

Myelography

Plain myelography previously was the imaging modality of choice in detecting herniated discs. It involves injection of intrathecal contrast material to outline the boundaries of the subarachnoid space and silhouette the enclosed neural elements. It is invasive and cannot show compression beyond the confines of the subarachnoid space. Extradural compression caused by a foraminal or extraforaminal disc can be missed. Advantages of myelography are that it is a dynamic test because images can be made with the patient standing.[44] Myelography should be reserved for cases in which noninvasive imaging, such as CT or MRI, are nondiagnostic, equivocal, or contraindicated. Currently, myelography is rarely used for the routine workup of herniated discs. When used, it is usually followed by a CT scan.

Computed Tomography

Before the advent of MRI, CT was the imaging modality of choice for evaluation of herniated discs. Using bone and soft tissue imaging techniques, herniations can be detected in various regions independent of the dural cavity. It has been shown to be 93% accurate in predicting surgical findings at discectomy. CT can also be performed with intrathecal contrast injection (CT myelography). Currently, the authors use this test for patients in whom MRI is contraindicated or cannot be obtained.

Some disc herniations can contain gas (Knuttson phenomena), noted on CT images. Mortensen and colleagues[49] reported four such cases that responded well to surgical discectomy. It is unknown if the gas forms before or after herniation. The clinical significance of the gas is not well understood. Ford and colleagues[50] determined that intradiscal gas is composed predominantly of nitrogen.

Natural History

The key to enhancing one's skills as an intelligent diagnostician and patient advisor is understanding the available knowledge related to the natural history of degenerative lumbar disc disease. The exact natural history of lumbar disc herniations is variable and incompletely understood. A few well-performed natural history investigations are available. Some studies are of patients treated by various nonoperative methods. Others represent the nonoperative arm of operative versus nonoperative comparison studies.

In a widely quoted retrospective study, Saal and Saal[5] found a 90% good or excellent outcome in patients treated nonoperatively for a lumbar disc herniation diagnosed by clinical examination and CT. Inclusion criteria were strict, including patients with SLR test positive at 60 degrees or less, leg pain greater than back pain, and electromyographic evidence of radiculopathy. Of patients, 92% returned to work. Nonoperative treatment consisted of aggressive physical therapy and back school education. A possible confounding factor is that many patients were referred for a second opinion regarding surgical versus nonsurgical treatment because they were anxious to avoid surgery. This may have introduced preselection bias error because the authors of the study were not surgeons. Concern has been raised about eventual fibrosis formation with nonoperative treatment of herniated discs. In a follow-up MRI study,[6] the same investigators documented no increased risk for perineural fibrosis or adhesions with nonsurgical management.

Other authors have reported more modest results. In the nonoperative arm of Weber's[10] classic randomized study, the long-term outcome of lumbar disc herniations was observed in 49 patients. Inclusion criteria were clinical signs and symptoms of L5 or S1 radiculopathy in addition to myelographic evidence of nerve root compression. Treatment included full-time bed rest for 1 week followed by partial bed rest the 2nd week and back school instruction as an inpatient. At 1 year, 33% had good results, 49% had a fair result, and 18% had a poor result. At 4 years, good results were reported in 51%, fair results were reported in 39%, and poor or bad results were reported in 10%. Because the tiered system is slightly different than that used by Saal and Saal,[5] a direct comparison of the studies is difficult. If Weber's good and fair results are equated to Saal's excellent and good results, an 89% success rate achieved in the former at 4 years may be considered comparable to the latter's 90% success. Many of Saal and Saal's patients ultimately dropped out of the study and underwent surgical discectomy so that their 90% success rate might represent an overestimation.

In another nonoperative arm of a comparative study, 10-year follow-up results from the prospective Maine Lumbar Spine Study showed 61% improvement in the predominant symptom, 40% resolution of low back symptoms, and 56% satisfaction rate.[7] Work and disability status were comparable between operative and nonoperative groups in this investigation. Similar findings were reported for the observational cohort of the Spine Patient Outcomes Research Trial (SPORT).[8]

Methods of Nonoperative Treatment

Physiotherapy

Bed rest should be limited to no more than 2 to 3 days.[51] Greater periods of inactivity can potentiate prolonged disability and continued or augmented pain. Exercise therapy and physical rehabilitation should be included in the nonoperative care of herniated discs. Treatment goals are to restore strength, flexibility, and function that were lost secondary to pain, splinting, and spasm. Postural education to avoid activities that can increase intradiscal pressure or neuromeningeal tension or both should be provided.

Various regimens have been advocated with none clearly superior. In the authors' practice, physical therapy prescription usually includes torso stabilization training; paraspinal muscle stretching and strengthening; and a focus on gluteal, hamstrings, and abdominal exercises. These muscles are important in the static and dynamic stabilization of the spinal column. Some authors suggest concentration on flexion or extension maneuvers. In the authors' experience, it is difficult, however, to predict if one or both of these movements would aggravate pain or help. Provisions for either flexion or extension concentration, at times combined with lateral shifts, are best left to the therapist's assessment because he or she can actively assess what is provoking pain. Concomitant facet arthritis, painful disc degeneration, and muscular pain can influence pain patterns and aggravating movements.

Adjunctive modalities can aid in relieving some associated symptoms. These modalities include ultrasound treatment, electrical stimulation, and massage. These may be helpful in short-term, symptomatic relief of back pain. Traction is also commonly prescribed. It theoretically may diminish intradiscal pressure, increase foraminal dimensions, and possibly relieve radicular pain secondary to herniated discs.[52] The role of chiropractic manipulation is controversial. Although some patients believe that manipulations have "reversed" the herniation, there is no evidence to support the ability of chiropractic manipulation to alter the normal or pathologic morphology of the disc.[53]

Pharmacologic Treatment

Medications can be useful in decreasing disc-related symptoms. Because a local or systemic inflammatory reaction may participate in pain generation, anti-inflammatory agents are believed to be beneficial. Nonsteroidal anti-inflammatory drugs (NSAIDs) are first-line agents. Numerous choices are currently available, including cyclooxygenase-2 inhibitors. In prescribing NSAIDs, several important issues must be considered. The medications can have side effects. A history of gastrointestinal bleeding or peptic ulcers can be a contraindication to NSAID use. Although this risk is reduced with cyclooxygenase-2 agents, it is not nil, and the patient should be warned of the possibility. Additionally with NSAIDs, other systems, such as the kidneys and liver, may be detrimentally affected.

In the acute setting, back and radicular pain can be severe. Short-term narcotic use, such as a single dose of a morphine-derivative analgesic, can be useful. Narcotics should not be prescribed or administered in an extended manner; they should preferably be limited to a 2- to 3-day course. Also in the acute setting, a tapering dosage regimen of oral steroids can be helpful in decreasing inflammation-generated pain from nerve root irritation.

So-called muscle relaxants are frequently prescribed. Although the drug class name implies a direct muscular effect, these medications have more significant sedative effects. Medications such as diazepam and methocarbamol should be used sparingly. Truly antispasmodic medications such as baclofen or cyclobenzaprine can have a more direct effect on muscle spasms.

Selective transforaminal steroid injections can produce symptomatic relief in many patients. In the authors' treatment protocol, injections are offered to patients who have failed noninvasive measures but either are not interested or are not good candidates for discectomy. In patients with more than one level of herniation, selective nerve root injection can be useful in determining the symptomatic level.

In a prospective series touted as a natural history study, Bush and colleagues[54] reported the results of 159 patients with CT-confirmed disc herniations treated with epidural steroid injections. Although 91% avoided surgery, this underscores a glaring problem of so-called natural history studies in that an interventional treatment was used. Although its exact biochemical effects are still being elucidated, steroid injections may be effective in "avoiding" surgery.

In a well-designed retrospective study, Wang and colleagues[55] studied 69 patients who failed nonoperative (or, more accurately, noninvasive) care and had requested surgery as treatment. Instead, each patient was advised to undergo one or more transforaminal steroid injections at the affected root level. Of patients, 77% had clinical resolution and had not undergone surgery at an average follow-up of 1.5 years. In agreement with other studies, clinical success was not related to disc size, percentage canal compromise, or degree of motor weakness. From these findings, selective nerve root steroid injections seem to produce at least short-term relief of radicular symptoms from a herniated disc.

Operative Versus Nonoperative Treatment

The results of operative and nonoperative treatment for symptomatic herniated discs have been compared in numerous studies. The Maine Lumbar Spine Study group published 1-year and 5-year results of an ongoing comparison of surgically and nonsurgically treated patients.[1,56] More than 500 patients were included in the prospective observational study without stringent clinical or radiographic criteria except for disc-related sciatica treated with at least 2 weeks of nonoperative care within 2 months of onset. The decision to undergo surgery was determined on an individual basis and was not randomized. At the 1-year follow-up, surgically treated patients were less symptomatic than patients in the nonoperative group, despite the former being *more* symptomatic at initial presentation. Relief of back or leg pain was reported by 71% of operated patients compared with 43% of the nonoperative group. High satisfaction levels and improved quality of life were documented for the operative group. For the workers' compensation group, there was no difference in time to return to work between operative and nonoperative groups. A criticism of the study is a substantial attrition rate, with 24% of patients unavailable for final follow-up.

In the 5-year outcome report, 70% of surgical patients reported back or leg pain improvement, whereas 56% of nonoperatively treated patients reported improvement.[1] As with the 1-year results, a similar percentage of patients were receiving workers' compensation benefits in both groups with no difference in return to work at final follow-up. Reoperations were performed in 20% of the operative patients; 16% of patients initially treated nonsurgically went on to operation. The authors noted that the benefits of surgery versus nonoperative treatment were greatest in the early part of the study within the first 2 years and that at final follow-up these advantages were less apparent.

Most recently, the Maine Lumbar Spine Study Group published their 10-year follow-up results.[7] Of the eligible patients initially enrolled, data were available for 85% of patients treated surgically and 82% of patients treated nonoperatively. A significantly larger percentage of surgical patients reported relief of low back and leg pain than patients treated nonoperatively. Similarly, surgical patients exhibited better function and satisfaction compared with nonoperative patients. Nonetheless, improvement in dominant symptom was reported for both treatment groups. Work and disability status were similar for both groups.

The 2006 SPORT investigation was designed to be a rigorous, randomized, prospective, controlled study.[8,9,57] In its execution, there was a high rate of crossover between operative and nonoperative groups and a substantial portion of patients not willing to be randomized, resulting in a large observational group. The randomized and observational arms of the investigation reported improvement in bodily pain, physical function, and Oswestry Disability Index (ODI) scores regardless of intervention. In the randomized arm of the study, between-group differences favored surgical intervention, but these differences did not reach statistical significance in an intention-to-treat analysis. With the difficulties encountered with nonadherence to assigned treatments (i.e., crossover), the intention-to-treat analysis may not be reflective of the true outcomes. In an as-treated analysis, surgical treatment showed statistically superior results compared with nonoperative treatment. Similar results were found in the observational arm of SPORT.

The classic work by Weber[10] reported similar results to these findings. As briefly discussed in the prior section on natural history, Weber[10] compared surgery versus nonoperative care in a randomized, prospective study. There were three study groups: one group "required surgery"; another showed no indications for surgery; and the third was the "undecided" group, in which it was unclear if surgery would be beneficial. Only the third group was randomly assigned to surgical or nonsurgical treatment.

At 1 year, good results were reported in 33% of the nonoperative group versus 66% in the surgical group; at 4 years, 51% versus 66%; and at 10 years, 55% versus 57%. These findings show that operative and nonoperative treatment outcomes seem to converge with time, being nearly the same at 10 years, and that the benefits of surgery are early. The 5-year and 10-year results from the Maine study are similar, although the larger numbers of the Maine study achieved statistical significance. Both studies are flawed by patient selection bias. Weber randomly assigned only patients in the "unclear" group, whereas the Maine group had no specific criteria and included patients per individual physician investigators' usual practice.

Alaranta and colleagues[58] also prospectively compared operated versus nonoperated patients. In contrast to other similar studies, the nonoperative group was subdivided into cases with and without myelographic evidence of nerve root compression, whereas all operated patients had a positive myelogram. At 1-year follow-up, 91% of operated and 82% of nonoperatively treated patients with positive myelograms had improved pain levels. Only 51% of nonoperatively treated patients with negative myelograms had improvement. These data suggest that a distinctly worse natural history exists for patients with sciatica and no evidence of root compression. Although not specified by the investigators, this group probably represents sciatica from an extraspinal or non–disc-related origin. In a companion study published by the same authors, they further identified this group as having a high incidence of generalized pain (e.g., concomitant occipital headaches), more physically strenuous jobs, and lower pain thresholds.[59] This study could possibly point to a preponderance of psychosocial and behavioral factors involved in the perpetuation of the symptom complex.

Operative Treatment

Indications

An absolute indication for lumbar discectomy is a progressive neurologic deficit. In this circumstance, operative intervention may be considered conservative care, provided that no medical contraindications exist. Progressive neurologic deficit is most commonly associated with a cauda equina syndrome and is discussed in more detail later. The relative indications for discectomy vary among surgeons and patients. Discectomy, in its many shapes and forms, can produce symptomatic relief in appropriately selected patients. It is the surgeon's obligation to identify the patients in whom the anticipated benefits outweigh the attendant risks of surgery.

A prerequisite is radiologic identification of compressive pathology that is concordant with the patient's physical signs and symptoms. A patient with a large left L4-5 level who presents with leg pain that radiates to the dorsum of the foot, weakness of toe dorsiflexion, decreased sensation in the first dorsal webspace, and a distinctly positive ipsilateral and contralateral SLR is an ideal candidate after failure of appropriate nonoperative treatment. In this "ideal" situation, the clinical and radiologic findings point toward compression of the L5 nerve root. To idealize the presentation further, the patient has a strong desire to return to work; is not involved in litigation, disability, or workers' compensation issues; and does not have any psychological issues. Important questions remain unanswered even in such cases, however, including optimal surgical timing, the method of disc excision, and the postoperative rehabilitation protocol.

Only a few patients match such textbook descriptions. Most patients lack one or more of the supportive diagnostic clues, making it more difficult to support the decision to operate. This situation does not represent a contraindication to surgery, however, because many published series show approximately 85% success rates in patient groups with lesser percentages of objective motor and sensory findings.[3,38,56,60-67] The slim chance of back pain relief in relation to leg pain with discectomy that surgeons obligatorily confess to their patients is also probably an underestimation because most series document at least modest improvements in back pain. It is incumbent on clinicians to discuss the advantages, disadvantages, risks, alternatives, and estimated expected outcomes with patients.

Available Techniques

A vast array of techniques exist for surgical treatment of herniated discs.[68-73] Standard open discectomy is the most common surgical approach.[60,65,74,75] It involves careful incision planning, laminotomy or partial laminectomy to provide adequate visualization of the pathology, gentle retraction of the neural elements, and direct excision of the herniation. As an adjunct to open discectomy, some surgeons advocate the use of a microscope for better visualization and minimizing incision size.[31,67,71,76,77] The purported advantage of the microscope is the ability for the surgeon and the assistant to visualize the operative field equally through a smaller surgical wound.

Alternatives to interlaminar techniques have been developed for excision of foraminal and extraforaminal lateral disc herniations, which involve exposures between the transverse processes and lateral to the pars interarticularis.[14,77] Although some surgeons have advocated the addition of fusion,[64,78] this practice is unpopular.[69] Advocates hold that fusion decreases the chance for reherniation; however, only a complete discectomy with interbody reconstruction can eliminate this risk. Long-term effects such as an adjacent segment degeneration and the additional morbidity and complication rates are potential disadvantages.[64,69,78,79]

With increased interest in smaller incisions and minimally invasive surgery, various percutaneous methods of treatment have been developed. Some methods entail placement of a cutting device intradiscally to decompress the disc space to retract the herniated fragment.[80-83] Other methods involve percutaneous techniques of directly visualizing the neural elements and disc using an endoscope.[68,84] Chemical digestion of the disc (i.e., chemonucleolysis) has enjoyed popularity; however, enzyme-related complications and results inferior to open discectomy have limited its continued popularity in the United States.[80,85,86]

Open Simple Discectomy

Timing

Disagreement exists regarding the optimal timing for surgery. The question is how long should nonoperative care be continued (without improvement) before the outcomes of surgery are detrimentally affected? Stated another way, in patients who are not responding to nonoperative measures, when should surgery be performed? In evaluating the currently available surgical results, this interval may be 2 to 16 months. The clear exception to delaying surgery is a patient who is experiencing a progressive neurologic deficit or cauda equina syndrome.

Rotheorl and colleagues[33] stratified operatively treated patients according to time from presentation to surgery. Patients with symptom duration more than 2 months had a statistically significantly worse outcome than patients operated on within 2 months. There was no difference if surgery was performed within 1 or 2 months. Likewise, Hurme and Alaranta[12] found the best results in patients operated on within 2 months of the onset of disabling sciatica. Nygaard and colleagues[32] reported worse results in patients with leg pain for 8 months or more; Jansson and colleagues[36] found similar results in their analysis of the Swedish registry data, which included greater than 27,000 patients. Sorensen and colleagues[34] found that symptom duration greater than 16 months was predictive of poor results, but this was highly influenced by patient personality and social factors. The disparity between these findings is difficult to explain. Randomized prospective data comparing early versus late surgery are lacking. In the authors' practice, surgery is performed within 6 months from symptom onset if nonoperative care has failed. The important message is that there is not an urgency to perform surgery. Nerve roots, as compared with the spinal cord, are fairly resilient.

Other factors can influence the time to surgery. Ito and colleagues[40] found patients with uncontained herniations had surgery much earlier than patients with contained herniations. Specifically, 56% of patients with uncontained herniations and 21% of patients with contained herniations had surgery within 1 month. This finding was not correlated to outcomes but was influenced more by the severity of symptoms. Early surgery

does not seem to affect the rate of neurologic recovery; objective improvements in motor and sensory deficits do not seem to correlate with symptomatic relief and overall success rates.[87]

Technique

General endotracheal anesthesia is induced. Alternatively, spinal anesthesia can be used. The patient is carefully logrolled into the prone position. An Andrews frame can be attached to a regular operating table to facilitate the prone kneeling position. Special spine frames, such as the sling attachment for the Jackson (OSI) table (Mizuho OSI, Union City, CA), can be used. These frames allow hip flexion to produce some flexion of the lumbar spine, which widens the interlaminar space (Fig. 46–11). The kneeling position also allows the abdomen to hang free, which helps indirectly to reduce the epidural venous pressure and reduce intraoperative blood loss. One set of hip pads is placed just distal to the anterior superior iliac crest. Adequate padding protects against lateral femoral cutaneous nerve injury. The thighs are allowed to flex at the hip, with the knees resting within the sling. The sling should be positioned low enough to allow adequate hip and knee flexion and is padded with gel pads and pillows. A pad is placed between the knees and medial malleoli to prevent pressure necrosis. The transverse chest pad is placed just above the xiphoid process.

With either table, the arms are placed in the 90-90 position with the cubital tunnels protected. The advantages of the Jackson table include that it allows a one-step turn to the prone position (avoiding the second step of pulling the patient's buttocks to the posterior pads with the Andrews frame) and its complete radiolucency. The disadvantage is that the table cannot be rotated away from the surgeon to allow better visualization by the assistant. With the patient secure, the superior aspects of the crests are palpated and marked; this usually corresponds to the level of the L4-5 disc space or the L3-4 interspinous process interval. The midline spinous processes are marked, and the interspinous regions are counted from the sacrum up. The target interspinous space can be indicated with a marker or scratched in the skin using a sterile 25-gauge needle after alcohol skin preparation. If the patient is unusually large and landmarks cannot be palpated, an x-ray can be taken to determine the level of skin incision before preparation. The lumbar region is then prepared and draped. A 3- to 5-cm midline skin incision is made and can be extended if necessary in obese patients.

The subcutaneous tissue is dissected down to the level of the lumbar fascia. The spinous processes are palpated in the midline. The deep lumbar fascia is incised, on the side of the

FIGURE 46–11 Jackson (OSI) table can be used to place the patient into a kneeling position, increasing interlaminar lumbar space, while allowing abdomen to hang free.

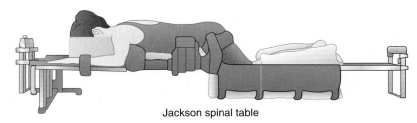

Jackson spinal table

herniation, adjacent to the spinous process. The fascial incision spans the spinous processes of the adjacent segments. An intraoperative lateral radiograph should be obtained at this time to confirm the correct level. A marker, either a Kocher clamp or a spinal needle, can be placed along the interspinous ligaments. On the radiograph, the marker should point toward the operative disc space. It should angle superiorly in line with the interspinous process space.

The paraspinal muscles are subperiosteally elevated from the lateral aspect of the spinous processes using electrocautery. It is usually necessary to expose only the superior and inferior aspects of the adjacent segments. At the junction of the spinous process and lamina, blunt dissection is performed laterally along the interlaminar space using a large Cobb elevator. Care is taken to expose, but not violate, the facet joint.

A Taylor retractor is positioned to maintain exposure of the interlaminar space. The tip of the retractor is inserted lateral to the facet joint, and the instrument is levered laterally. A roller-gauze is looped underneath the surgeon's foot and tied to the handle of the Taylor retractor. Appropriate foot leverage maintains its position. Alternatively, numerous small retraction systems can be used. Meticulous hemostasis is achieved with a bipolar electrocautery. Extraneous posterior muscle and soft tissues that impair vision should be removed using a large curet and rongeur. The interspinous ligaments should not be disrupted.

A medium-sized curet is used to detach the ligamentum flavum from the inferior aspect of the superior lamina (Fig. 46–12). Because the ligamentum inserts along the anterior aspect of the lamina, the curet needs to be introduced at an angle with the spoon facing cephalad. The instrument is worked from side to side to release all layers of the ligamentum. In some cases, it is difficult to release the ligamentum flavum completely without removing a portion of the inferior hemilamina (Fig. 46–13). Bone resection can be kept to a minimum but should not be avoided if it jeopardizes the exposure of the cauda equina and nerve root.

After the ligamentum is released superiorly, an angled probe, such as a Woodson elevator, can be inserted just deep to the ligamentum flavum (the yellow ligament). The Woodson elevator is positioned along the periphery near the bone. A long-handle No. 15 blade scalpel is carefully used to incise the flavum directly on top of the Woodson elevator, which protects the dural sac deep to it, which may often be displaced posterior by a large herniated disc. The blade should not be inserted deep to the ligament or the elevator. If concerns exist, the ligamentum flavum should be incised layer by layer with consecutive passes of the blade until the Woodson elevator pops through; this is continued along the periphery of the interlaminar window. Optionally, the medial aspect of the ligamentum flavum can be left attached, and the ligamentum can be flapped open. At the completion of the discectomy, the flap can be replaced to act as a barrier against epidural adhesions.

With the ligamentum retracted or removed, epidural fat is visualized. In some cases, the fat layer has thinned from a displaced or inflamed nerve root. If present, the epidural fat is swept away from the dura with a Penfield No. 4 elevator. The

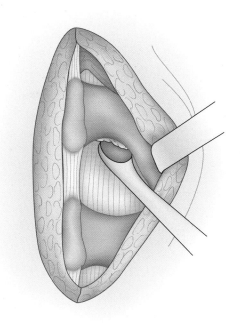

FIGURE 46–12 Ligamentum is released from inferior aspect of superior lamina. Cup of curet should face away from dural sac to avoid inadvertent injury or tear.

focus of this maneuver is to identify the lateral aspect of the exiting nerve root and cauda equina. Epidural vessels are coagulated using irrigating bipolar cautery, as necessary.

A medial facetectomy often must be performed to visualize the nerve root adequately. A 3-mm or 4-mm Kerrison rongeur can be used in a back-hand manner to resect the medial aspect of the facet joint. Excessive resection should be avoided

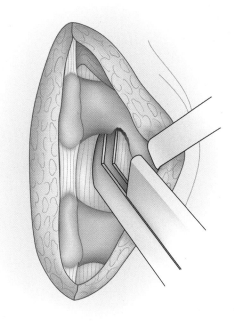

FIGURE 46–13 In some cases, particularly above L5-S1 level, a small portion of lamina must be removed to release ligamentum flavum fully.

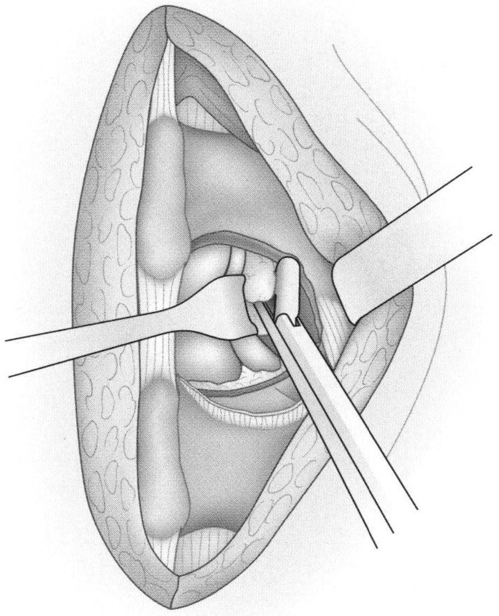

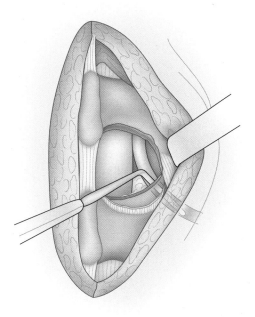

FIGURE 46–14 Nerve root retractor is used to retract gently descending nerve root and cauda equina toward midline to visualize disc space and herniation.

because the integrity of the facet and pars interarticularis is crucial to maintaining stability. It is wise to protect the underlying dura by pointing the Kerrison rongeur in the direction of the exiting nerve root. The end point of resection is

FIGURE 46–15 After herniated fragment has been removed, spinal canal should be systematically inspected for any remaining fragments. Woodson elevator is used to ensure that neural foramen and nerve root are free. If root is not completely free, additional fragments or compression may be present.

adequate visualization of the shoulder of the descending nerve root adjacent to the medial border of the pedicle.

Before discectomy, a blunt-tipped probe is passed along the root and out the foramen to assess the amount of space available. Using a Penfield No. 4 elevator, the nerve root is mobilized medially. This mobilization can be facilitated using the bipolar cautery to lyse adhesions between the dura and the posterior disc. Retracting the nerve root medially shows the posterior anulus or the herniated fragment or both. A nerve root retractor is used to maintain retraction (Fig. 46–14).

The disc fragment may be extirpated using the Penfield elevator to ensure it is free of dural adhesions. With clear visualization of the fragment and its distinction from the neural elements, a pituitary rongeur can be used to explant it. If the fragment is extruded or sequestered, one can often identify a tear in the posterolateral or central anulus. If the herniation is subligamentous, a No. 15 blade scalpel can be used to create a small annulotomy to gain access to the herniated nuclear material. A pituitary rongeur can be carefully inserted into the annular defect to remove the fragmented disc.

Caution must be used when removing an axillary disc herniation. The fragment is easily visualized, tempting the surgeon to proceed directly with excision with the pituitary rongeur. Removal of large fragments that extend deep to the cauda equina and nerve root can lead to excessive bleeding from the transverse anastomoses of the epidural veins in the axillary region. It is preferable to retract the root medially and remove the fragment from a lateral approach, if possible.

The mobility of the nerve root is assessed using a Penfield No. 4 or Woodson elevator (Fig. 46–15). After discectomy, the nerve root should be freely mobile and under no tension or compression. If it is not, additional pathology should be suspected. Using a Woodson elevator, the epidural space must be systematically inspected in a clockwise fashion, checking the canal ventral to the thecal sac and the patency of the foramen. A concomitant lateral recess or foraminal stenosis from bony encroachment is decompressed with Kerrison rongeurs. Finally, the disc space is irrigated with normal saline to dislodge any remaining loose fragments.

If the ligamentum flavum was spared, it can be loosely replaced. A fat graft placed over the dura does not improve clinical results but does facilitate re-exploration and theoretically prevents adhesions from inhibiting normal neuromeningeal motion.[88,89] The wound is copiously irrigated. Adequate epidural hemostasis is ensured before closure. In most cases, a drain is not needed. All retractors are removed, and the deep lumbar fascia is approximated with interrupted No. 1 absorbable suture. The subcutaneous layer is closed in two layers, and the skin is approximated with a subcuticular stitch or staples. The wound is cleaned, and a sterile dressing is applied.

Postoperative Care and Rehabilitation

After an uncomplicated simple open discectomy, the patient is discharged on postoperative day 1 or 2. Outpatient discectomy can be performed on selected patients with appropriate presurgical planning and postdischarge discussion.[74] The level of activity in the 1st week after surgery usually is limited by incisional pain. If leg symptoms were predominant preoperatively, the patient typically reports immediate relief.

The activity level recommended after surgery varies among surgeons. Concerns are that aggressive movements and loads can predispose to reherniation or excessive scarring. This concern leads many surgeons to limit lifting and bending after discectomy for about 3 to 4 weeks. Although this is probably the predominant practice, there is little literature to support such extended periods of protected activity.

Unrestricted activity protocols have shown success rates comparable to other series. Carragee and colleagues[75] conducted an uncontrolled, prospective trial of 152 patients who were allowed full activity after lumbar discectomy. Approximately one third of patients returned to work in 1 week, with most (97%) returning to work within 8 weeks. Recurrent sciatica occurred in 17 patients and was considered possible reherniation (11%). Nine of these patients experienced improvement, and eight underwent repeat surgery. This rate is similar to reherniation rates previously reported, which have ranged from 0% to 13%. Carragee and colleagues[75] concluded that an unrestricted activity protocol does not negatively affect results after discectomy.

Other studies have focused on possible advantages to an early rehabilitation protocol after discectomy. Kjellby-Wendt and Styf[90] performed a prospective, randomized, controlled study comparing an early active versus traditional training program. The focus of early activity was to reduce lumbar edema and maintain mobility of the neural elements through motion and trunk-strengthening exercises. A pain-coping program was included in the early active group that was not included in the traditional group. There was greater range of motion and decreased pain at 12 weeks in the early group. At 1-year follow-up, both groups were equivalent. Patient satisfaction was ultimately greater in the early active group (88%) versus the control group (67%), although this was not statistically significant. In critique of the study, it was unclear why the difference in subjective outcome was not accompanied by sustained objective benefits. Inclusion of the pain-coping program in the study group, which would have minimal influence on range of motion, may have positively influenced patients' perception of their residual impairment. In support of the findings by Carragee and colleagues,[75] there was no difference in reherniation rates between the two groups.

Alaranta and colleagues[91] performed a randomized trial comparing an "immediate" versus "normal" rehabilitation program. Physical activities, such as sports and games, were encouraged in the immediate activity group; psychological and social counseling were also provided. Details of the normal rehabilitation protocol were not provided. At 1-year follow-up, there were no differences in subjective outcomes, postoperative impairments, or return to work statistics. These results further indicate that early activity programs do not seem to be harmful but offer only minimal, if any, long-term benefits. The current authors' decision to initiate early return to unrestricted activity is made on an individual basis.

Outcomes

The outcomes of surgical discectomy are reliable when one adheres to strict preoperative selection criteria. Factors that can influence these outcomes, such as location of the herniation, preoperative psychological status, surgeon experience, and work status, have been extensively analyzed.

Carragee and Kim[11] correlated operative outcomes with herniated fragment size and its effect on canal area. Using axial MRI, these authors recorded several parameters including disc area, canal area, anteroposterior disc length, and anteroposterior canal length. Patients with larger discs (>6 mm) were more likely to have positive SLR or femoral stretch tests. Comparing patients with operative and nonoperative treatment, the former had larger anteroposterior disc lengths and larger ratios of disc to canal area. In the operative group, larger discs were predictive of a better outcome. In the nonoperative group, symptom duration less than 6 months before presentation, no litigation, and younger age were predictive of a better outcome. All of the fair and poor outcomes in operative patients were in patients with small discs (<6 mm). Summarizing these findings, it seems that larger discs respond to surgery better than small discs and that disc size is less predictive of outcomes in the nonoperative group. A criticism of this study involves the existence of a selection bias because the decision to treat operatively was nonrandomized.

Knop-Jergas and colleagues[92] analyzed the results of lumbar discectomy based on anatomic location. They characterized herniations as central, paracentral, intraforaminal, extraforaminal, or multiregional broad-based protrusions. The best outcomes were documented with paracentral and intraforaminal discs, with 80% yielding good or excellent results. Central discs and multiregional discs had worse results, with 47% and 54% good or excellent outcomes. There was only one extraforaminal disc, which had a poor outcome. The level of herniation was not predictive of outcome, with 59% occurring at L4-5.

In contrast, other authors have found that the level of herniation can effect operative outcomes. Dewing and colleagues[93] reported that discectomy for L5-S1 herniations had significantly greater improvements in visual analog scale (VAS) leg and ODI scores compared with L4-5 herniations. These authors also found that patients with sequestered disc fragments had significantly better outcomes than patients with contained disc herniations. In a post-hoc analysis of SPORT trial data, Pearson and colleagues[57] examined the influence of disc herniation location (central or lateral) and morphology (protrusion, extrusion, or sequestration) on the results of operative and nonoperative treatment. Their data suggest that the advantages of surgical treatment over nonoperative treatment were greatest for patients with lateral disc herniations. The magnitude of improvement from surgical treatment was not related to the location or morphology of the herniation.

Various preoperative and postoperative findings may also be predictive of results. Barrios and colleagues[61] found that the use of (and positive response to) traction as part of preoperative conservative treatment was predictive of a good outcome with surgery. In agreement with other studies, patients with sedentary, non–physically demanding jobs had better results than patients with more strenuous occupations. Jansson and colleagues[36] found that reduced preoperative walking distance and a history of back pain greater than 6 months were predictors of lower functional outcomes after discectomy. Jonsson and Stromqvist[94] found a persistently positive SLR test to be a reliable indicator of inferior results; this was particularly evident in patients in whom the test was positive for more than 4 months after discectomy.

As part of an ongoing study of lumbar discectomy, the Maine group published an investigation comparing operative rates and outcomes between high versus low rate of surgery regions within the state.[95] The data suggest that in the high rate region the results were inferior compared with the low rate region. These calculations were based on the rate of surgery per capita (population). The investigators concluded that this difference was most significantly related to the surgical indications used by the individual physicians and that in the higher rate areas the indications may have been less stringent. This might have been true, but an additional factor was not highlighted, which the current authors calculated from the data. In the high rate region, there were more surgeries done per capita, but the number of operations done per physician was lower, averaging 11 surgeries per surgeon. In the low rate region, surgeons averaged 26 operations each, although the overall rate of surgery was lower per capita. This factor directly supports previous analyses of the results of total joint arthroplasty, which indicate better results in high-volume hospitals because of concentrated experience. From these data, discectomy is optimally performed by an experienced, high-volume surgeon who employs strict indications.

Psychological and social factors have been shown by many investigators to influence profoundly the surgical results of lumbar discectomy.[34,62] Sorensen and colleagues[34] found that preoperative psychological assessment was 86% predictive of surgical results after discectomy. Cashion and Lynch[62] found patients with a good outcome were more self-confident individuals, were only mildly depressed, and were generally optimistic about the outcome of surgery. Slover and colleagues[35] found that a history of chronic headaches, smoking, depression, and self-rated poor health were associated with poor outcomes after discectomy. Jansson and colleagues[36] found that smoking was the most significant risk factor in patients who failed to improve after surgery.

Spengler and colleagues[13] calculated preoperative assessment scores for 84 patients before discectomy and correlated these with outcomes. The four components of the score were neurologic signs, clinical tension signs, psychological factors, and imaging evidence of neural compression. Imaging studies were most predictive of operative findings but not of outcome. The best predictor of outcome was the psychological score. This was based on the Minnesota Multiphasic Personality Inventory (MMPI).

Hurme and Alaranta[12] prospectively studied 220 patients after discectomy, analyzing preoperative and perioperative factors. Optimistic patients had better results. Patients who preoperatively decided not to return to work had poorer

outcomes. Patients who perceived their jobs to be physically strenuous had inferior results. The most predictive factors of a poor outcome were the decision not to return to work, marital status (divorced or widowed), age older than 40 years, a protracted period of sciatic pain, and multiple nonspecific somatic complaints. Predictors of good results were a high preoperative pain index, higher education level, overall satisfaction with life, and the perception that the patient's job was of light or suitable duty. Patients with highly positive SLR test and younger patients with large disc herniations tended to have better results. This study highlights the importance of psychological, social, and objective physical factors in predicting the outcome of lumbar disc excision.

Dvorak and colleagues[96] retrospectively applied a set of "accepted" operative indications, including radicular pain, positive SLR, contralateral SLR, dermatomal hypesthesia, motor deficit, and diminished deep tendon reflexes, to a series of patients who underwent discectomy. Of the patients, 65% fulfilled these criteria, and 35% did not. The long-term outcomes were not significantly different between these two groups. Patients who returned to work postoperatively were on disability compensation less than 2 months before surgery, whereas patients who did *not* return to work were on disability compensation an average of 4 months before surgery. Indications based on objective physical findings alone do not ensure a satisfactory outcome. The preoperative period of disability is a significant factor.

Some proponents of microscopically assisted discectomy purport that results are superior compared with standard techniques. In a published review of the literature by one of the strongest advocates of microdiscectomy, McCulloch[76] concluded that the available data are insufficient to show its superiority. He noted that successful results have ranged from 80% to 96%, regardless of the technique used, and highlighted the importance of patient selection as the more important determinant of outcome. Series of microsurgical discectomy report comparable rates of complications, such as dural tear and recurrent herniations.[97,98]

There is disagreement regarding the efficacy of simple fragment excision (the so-called Williams sequestrectomy[99]) versus more extensive nucleus curettage. In a retrospective study of 200 patients, Faulhauer and Manicke[65] showed a lower reherniation rate with fragment excision alone. This comparison was inherently flawed. The standard discectomy group, by definition, had herniations that were in continuity with the disc space and could be characterized as subligamentous (contained). The fragment excision group obligatorily had displaced fragments that were not contained within the disc space. The most useful information perhaps is that when an extruded or sequestered (uncontained) fragment is found, acceptable results with a low herniation rate can be expected with fragment excision alone. Although aggressive methods of removal of further nuclear material may not be warranted, meticulous examination of all quadrants of the epidural space surrounding the nerve root and cauda equina should be performed in each case to avoid missing disc fragments.

Balderston and colleagues[60] compared 40 patients who underwent simple fragment excision in one center with 40 patients who underwent excision and curettage in another center. The reherniation rate was not significantly different: 12.5% in the former group and 11.6% in the latter group. There was also no difference in the rate of disc space narrowing between the two groups. The only difference was a higher rate of postoperative back pain in the curettage group at a minimum 2-year follow-up. In distinction to Faulhauer and Manicke's work,[65] the types of disc herniation were not different between the two groups.

Carragee and colleagues[100] reported the results of a prospective, controlled study comparing subtotal versus limited discectomy. In the latter group, only the extruded disc material and loose fragments present in the disc space were removed. In the former, a more aggressive disc space curettage and débridement was performed in addition to removal of the extruded fragments. Early findings suggested a shorter convalescence in the limited discectomy group but decreased VAS and ODI scores in the subtotal group. These differences were not statistically significant at 2-year follow-up. Although the reherniation rate in the limited group was 18% compared with 9% in the subtotal group, this difference was not significant with the numbers available. Type II (beta) error cannot be excluded, however, because a significant difference may have been detected with greater patient numbers. The clinical significance of a 9% difference in reherniation rate may outweigh the lack of statistical significance.

Complications

Numerous complications can occur with lumbar discectomy, albeit at acceptably low rates. Recurrence rates range from 0% to 18%. In addition to differences in surgical technique and other factors, this broad range may reflect differences in the definition of recurrence. In some series, *recurrence* is defined as recurrent sciatica, whereas in others use of the term is limited to patients who required reoperation. The strictest definition is a true reherniation at the level and side previously operated, which ultimately leads to a frequency of 2% to 5%.

Wound infections have been reported in 0% to 3% of cases.[12,60,65,72,74,99] These may be superficial or deep. Superficial infections may be managed with local wound care and antibiotics. Deep infections should be surgically débrided and irrigated. Epidural abscess is rare, with reported rates of 0.3%, and should be managed with surgical evacuation.[101] The microscope has been considered a possible source of contamination because of the exposed unsterile optics that are in close proximity over the wound.[76,102] Infection rates are comparable, however, to cases performed without the microscope.

Pyogenic discitis may occur after discectomy 2.3% of the time.[12,101] Early detection is crucial in avoiding extensive bone involvement. Intravenous antibiotic therapy is usually successful, with rare cases requiring surgical débridement. MRI findings, including increased bone edema near the endplates and loss of disc space height, are difficult to discern from typical degenerative Modic-type changes. Laboratory evidence, such as elevated erythrocyte sedimentation rates and C-reactive protein levels, is important in confirming the diagnosis.

Vascular injuries are exceedingly rare. Injury to anterior vessels from perforation of the disc space have been documented in a few case reports.[103,104] Arteriovenous fistula has also been documented.[105,106] The most important component of managing these complications is prompt recognition and aggressive treatment, including vascular repair. Excessive epidural bleeding is uncommon, although one series documented blood loss of more than 300 mL in 4% of cases.[12]

Incidental durotomy occurs 0% to 4% of the time.[8,60,72,97,107] It has been associated with a poor outcome in some series. At an average of 10 years after surgery, Saxler and colleagues[107] reported a lower rate of symptom resolution and a greater rate of chronic pain and headaches in patients who sustained an incidental durotomy. This study did not discern between primary and revision cases, which may have been a potential confounder. The potential for long-term clinical sequelae after incidental durotomy during discectomy is most likely influenced by the size of the tear, the ability to repair it, and the coexistence of neurologic injury.

Instability is quite rare after discectomy. Preservation of the facet joints is helpful in avoiding this sequela, although in the authors' experience a large percentage of the facet joint can be resected unilaterally without adverse effect. Some authors have indicated that instability can occur 30% of the time. This percentage is highly dependent on the definition of instability. Padua and colleagues[108] found radiographic evidence of instability, detected by flexion-extension films, in 20% of patients who underwent discectomy. Only 6% seemed to be symptomatic, however. In contrast, Faulhauer and Manicke[65] defined instability by clinical findings, such as apprehension with flexion or extension, instead of radiographic measurements. These authors reported rates of 16% and 30% with two different operative techniques; 3% had severe enough symptoms to warrant a brace, and only one patient eventually went on to fusion. Kotilainen and Valtonen[101] found that the presence of clinical apprehension postoperatively was predictive of a poor result after surgery. These data highlight the importance of documenting preoperative radiographic and clinical instability so that the effects of the discectomy itself can be better assessed in the postoperative period.[109] Biomechanically, simple discectomy is not a destabilizing procedure if performed properly.

Recurrent Disc Herniations

The distinguishing histologic feature of recurrent disc herniation is the presence of large collagen bundles associated with a fibrillar framework.[110] Granulation tissue found in recurrences is not present in primary disc herniations. This fact indicates that the pathophysiology of recurrent disc herniations may be different than in primary cases.

Depending on the definition, recurrent disc herniations can occur in 18% of cases. Clinical presentation is usually of recurrent sciatic leg pain. Jonsson and Stromqvist[111] attempted to determine the relative frequency of clinical signs and symptoms after discectomy to differentiate better perineural fibrosis from true recurrent herniation. Pain reproduced by cough and a positive SLR were more frequent with recurrent discs. These findings were also present in many patients with fibrosis alone, however, so imaging modalities are crucial to the diagnosis. As discussed previously, MRI is best delayed for at least 6 months after surgery.

Recurrences can occur at the same level, same side, opposite side, or entirely different level. To be considered a recurrence, there must have been a pain-free (or relief) time period after the index surgery. A nonoperative treatment regimen, including a period of observation, physical therapy, medications, and other modalities, should be used in the initial treatment of recurrent discs unless progressive neurologic deterioration occurs.

Important questions arise after the decision to proceed with surgery is made. The main focus of current investigations is whether or not comparable or inferior results can be expected after discectomy for a recurrent disc. Some authors have documented inferior results after repeat surgery,[112] although most failures were reported in patients operated on without imaging evidence of neural compression.

Suk and colleagues[113] retrospectively examined their results in a highly select group of patients. Recurrence was defined as a reherniation at the same level (ipsilateral or contralateral) after a pain-free interval of 6 months or more. These authors used gadolinium-enhanced MRI to confirm the diagnosis. They found that the second surgery was significantly longer and that recurrent disc herniations were typically larger. Clinical success was documented in 71.1% of cases, which was comparable to their results after primary discectomy (79.3%). In a similar study, Cinotti and colleagues[114] examined their results with same-level contralateral reherniations only. At 2-year follow-up, surgery for recurrences resulted in satisfactory outcomes in 88% of cases and in 90% of primary discectomies. The only difference noted was more back pain in the reherniation group at 6 months, although this difference was not noted at 2 years.

Cinotti and colleagues[115] also studied a group of patients with ipsilateral lumbar disc reherniation and compared these patients with patients after primary surgery as a control group. Satisfactory results were reported in 85% of patients with ipsilateral lumbar disc reherniation and 88% of control patients. Noted differences were a higher degree of disc degeneration in the recurrence group. Although epidural fibrosis was abundant in the study group, its presence or amount did not adversely influence outcome. There was no difference in the psychological profiles of recurrent versus primary discectomy groups. In a similar study, Papadopoulos and colleagues[116] reported 85% improvement after discectomy for reherniations compared with 80% improvement for primary herniations at an average of 53.6 months follow-up. Herron[117] reported 69% good and 24% fair results after laminectomy and discectomy for recurrences at the same and other levels.

Most authors do not recommend fusion after a first-time recurrent disc herniation.[117,118] After any lumbar surgery involving facetectomy and bone resection, preoperative and intraoperative assessment of stability is a major determinant of the decision to fuse. Although investigational evidence is lacking, the authors consider fusion after a second reherniation at the same level.

Discectomy in Children

The role of trauma in causing disc herniations in children is believed to be more significant than in adults.[3,119,120] Children are unlikely to have disc degeneration or the antecedent period of back pain before herniation. Clinical signs and symptoms are similar to adults but are much more acute in onset. The clinical and imaging evaluation is similar to adults.

The literature of discectomy in children reveals prolonged length of follow-up. Initial results are excellent, but results tend to deteriorate with time. At 1-year follow-up, Papagenlopoulos and colleagues[121] reported 93% good or excellent results. At final follow-up ranging from 12 to 45 years, 92% were good or excellent; however, there was a 28% reoperation rate. Parisini and colleagues[122] documented 95% success at short-term follow-up, whereas at long-term follow-up (average 12.4 years), good or excellent outcomes were documented in 87% of cases. These investigators found a 10% reoperation rate at 10 years. DeOrio and Bianco[123] showed 96% good or excellent results at initial follow-up, trending down to 74% at final examination. Numerous other series document similar results.[3,119,124]

Fusion has been reported in a small percentage of pediatric patients. Well-defined selection criteria are lacking, however. The influence of congenital anomalies has been considered previously. There does not seem to be a correlation between any one anomaly and disc herniation. It is important to recognize anomalies, such as spina bifida, during routine preoperative planning to avoid iatrogenic neurologic injury.

Discectomy in Elderly Patients

Lumbar disc herniations are much less common in elderly patients. The nucleus desiccates with age and is less likely to herniate. Underlying stenosis and bony overgrowth is a more common problem. Regardless, herniations can still occur, with or without the presence of stenosis. The results of discectomy in this population are comparable to younger patients, assuming the correct diagnosis is made.

Maistrelli and colleagues[125] reported results of discectomy in 32 patients older than 60 years. Clinical findings were similar, with 81% of patients having root tension signs such as a positive SLR. At an average follow-up of 50 months, good or excellent results were found in 87% of cases. None of the patients had evidence of neurogenic claudication, which is an important distinguishing feature when making the diagnosis of a disc herniation versus stenosis. Jonsson and Stromqvist[126] also found disc surgery to be gratifying in patients older than 70 years, with good results documented at 2-year follow-up.

Foraminal and Extraforaminal (Far-Lateral) Herniations

So-called far-lateral disc herniations require special consideration. Surgical excision is more easily accomplished through modified operative techniques. Foraminal and extraforaminal disc herniations are more common in older patients. Symptoms are more likely to be isolated to one particular nerve root. In contrast to paracentral discs, they lead to compression of the exiting nerve root rather than the descending root. Diagnosis is best by MRI or CT (Fig. 46–16). Because the compression is usually extradural, myelography does not show a filling defect.

Different techniques have been advocated for the foraminal or extraforaminal herniation. Compression of the nerve root occurs outside of the spinal canal, making visualization of the herniation challenging through a standard laminotomy or laminectomy performed from within the canal. Garrido and Connaughton[127] advocated a unilateral facetectomy. Bone is removed along the entire path of the nerve root from its exit from the cauda equina out and through the foramen; this necessitates complete removal of the facet on the side of exposure. Although symptom relief was not well documented, painful radiographic instability was detected in only 1 of 35 (3%) cases. This patient had pain relief after fusion.

Donaldson and colleagues[128] advocated a less destabilizing procedure. They considered identification of the nerve within the intertransverse process "blind." As a solution, they performed a partial hemilaminectomy at the level above the disc at the point where the root exited the cauda equina. They followed it laterally beneath the bone of the remaining pars interarticularis. By placing a probe over the root and advancing it laterally, they were able to identify the root and facilitate its dissection between the transverse processes before discectomy was performed through this interval. They reported good or excellent pain relief in 72% of patients. No cases of instability were reported.

Melvill and Baxter[14] used the intertransverse approach for discectomy in 40 patients with extraforaminal herniations. They performed this using standard midline dissection that was extended subperiosteally out and over the facets to expose the transverse processes. This is in contrast to the classic description of the Wiltse paraspinal muscle–splitting approach. Complete resolution of leg pain was reported in 85% of cases. Melvill and Baxter[14] noted a fibrous band that was present tethering the nerve root to the lateral aspect of the disc in an associated cadaveric study.

In an investigation with mid-term follow-up, satisfactory results were reported using the Wiltse paraspinal muscle–splitting approach for so-called lateral disc herniations.[129] Satisfaction was reported by 85% of patients, with 60% of patients reporting complete resolution of pain. At 5 years' follow-up, 20% of patients had developed some degree of instability, half of whom ultimately underwent fusion. Assuming uniformity of the definition of instability and indications for fusion in these cases, this finding is supportive of the

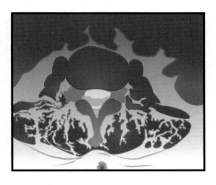

FIGURE 46–16 MRI can readily show extraforaminal disc herniations that may otherwise be missed by CT or plain myelograms because neural compression is extradural.

hypothesis by McCulloch and Transfelt[31] that lateral disc herniations were a precursor to the development of degenerative spondylolisthesis.

A thorough knowledge of the anatomy in this region is imperative to effective discectomy without undue bleeding or injury to the nerve root.[77] The authors prefer to excise foraminal or extraforaminal discs through a true Wiltse paraspinal muscle–splitting approach to the intertransverse interval. It is easiest through a paramedian incision (Fig. 46–17). Identification of the correct level of incision is crucial in minimizing the length of the incision.

Cauda Equina Syndrome

Cauda equina syndrome most commonly occurs from a herniated lumbar disc. It is more common with central herniation (27% of central herniations), although it can occur with paracentral or lateral herniations as well.[130,131] It is more frequent in men in their 4th decade. An L4-5 disc is the usual cause.[130]

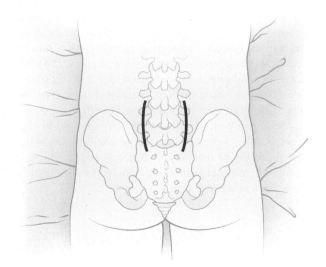

FIGURE 46–17 Wiltse muscle-splitting approach, using a paramedian incision, can be used to access intertransverse process region.

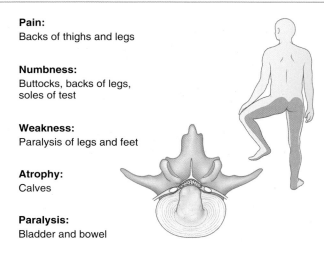

Pain:
Backs of thighs and legs

Numbness:
Buttocks, backs of legs,
soles of test

Weakness:
Paralysis of legs and feet

Atrophy:
Calves

Paralysis:
Bladder and bowel

FIGURE 46–18 Cauda equina syndrome is characterized by saddle anesthesia, motor weakness, and loss of bowel and bladder control.

Cauda equina syndrome should be considered a true surgical urgency because the neurologic results are affected by the time to decompression. The clinical diagnosis of cauda equina syndrome relies on many components, including perineal sensory deficit (so-called saddle anesthesia), bowel or bladder incontinence, new-onset lower extremity sensory deficit, and a new or progressive motor deficit (Fig. 46–18). In addition to a meticulous physical examination, evaluation of cauda equina syndrome should include measurement of a bladder postvoid residual. Normally, the postvoid residual should be less than 50 to 100 mL. The postvoid residual is often abnormal preoperatively and can be an important parameter to follow postoperatively.[132]

Decompression and discectomy can be via a laminotomy or through a formal laminectomy. Proponents of laminectomy believe this provides superior visualization of the dura and avoids excessive traction.[133-135] Adequate exposure is particularly relevant for removal of central disc herniations. Discectomy is best performed within 48 to 72 hours of the onset of symptoms.[132,135,136] This time frame leads to better sensory, motor, urinary, and rectal function recovery. Motor strength may continue to improve for 1 year after surgery.[135] Although the postvoid residual usually decreases to less than 110 mL by 6 weeks, bladder function may continue to improve for 16 months.[131] Early surgery does not seem to affect substantially the resolution of postoperative pain compared with delayed intervention.[137] Preoperative neurologic status seems to be the greatest predictor of recovery,[138] although many patients are found to have residual neurologic deficits despite timely and effective surgical intervention.[137]

Alternatives to Standard Discectomy

Endoscopic Discectomy

The use of the endoscope to perform lumbar discectomy has enthusiastic proponents. Improvements in equipment have made the technique more user-friendly and facile. Still, endoscopic discectomy remains a technically demanding procedure, and the results depend heavily on surgeon experience.[139] Although it is not yet a replacement for standard discectomy techniques, more recent series have shown the ability to achieve comparable results in some surgeons' hands.[68,140]

DeAntoni and colleagues[84] reported results of translaminar epidural endoscopic discectomy in 190 patients. Using a lateral decubitus position, the technique uses a small paramedian incision for introduction of the instruments. Dilators are used to strip the muscles subperiosteally from the adjacent lamina as far lateral as the facet joint. The arthroscope (endoscope) is inserted through a 6-mm working cannula. An additional lateral paraspinal incision is made for an outflow cannula. A shaver is used to remove bone within the interlaminar window until the attachments of the ligamentum flavum can be visualized. The ligamentum flavum is elevated using a Penfield dissector and removed with a Kerrison rongeur, similar to a standard open approach. A root retractor pulls the nerve root and dura medially, allowing access to the disc space. The anulus is incised, and the herniation is removed. The endoscope can be inserted into the disc space to look for any additional loose fragments (so-called discoscopy). Good or excellent results were documented in 92% of cases with a minimum 2-year follow-up. There was only one dural laceration that did not need repair, there was no instability, and there were no neurologic injuries.

Yeung and Tsou[68] reported results of 307 endoscopically assisted transforaminal disc herniations. The patient is positioned supine on a radiolucent table. Local anesthesia with light sedation is used. In this technique, intraoperative fluoroscopy is crucial. A standard discogram is performed first, injecting blue dye into the disc space to help identify the herniated tissue. Along the same path, a series of dilators and ultimately a single working cannula is inserted percutaneously through the intervertebral foramen (Fig. 46–19). One cannula is used for inflow, outflow, and instrument insertion. The cannula has a shielded tip that allows aggressive discectomy with the use of graspers and shavers while retracting the exiting nerve root. As stated, this is performed through the intervertebral foramen. The nerve root can be visualized by rotating the cannula, allowing assessment of its integrity and mobility. Satisfactory results were reported in 89.3% of patients. Six patients (2%) had lower extremity dysesthesia that lasted longer than 6 weeks, two had thrombophlebitis, two had discitis, and one had a dural tear that did not require repair.

A more recent study showed that this technique is safe and effective for recurrent disc herniations as well.[140] In a prospective evaluation of 262 consecutive cases of reherniation treated by an endoscopically assisted transforaminal technique, Hoogland and colleagues[140] reported an 85% success rate and 3.8% complication rate at 2-year follow-up.

Several authors have sought to compare the results of microendoscopic discectomy with more traditional techniques.[141-143] Ruetten and colleagues[143] compared the results of endoscopic interlaminar and transforaminal discectomy with microsurgical discectomy. They showed no clinically significant differences between the endoscopic and microsurgical groups and identical reherniation rates (6.2% for each).[143] Analogous findings have been reported with comparisons of endoscopic and standard open discectomy.[141,142]

Percutaneous Automated Discectomy

Because of the evolution of percutaneous techniques of discectomy, there is considerable "overlap" in the names of different procedures. Although endoscopic discectomy can be considered percutaneous, it is not what is typically considered *percutaneous automated discectomy*. This term refers specifically to a procedure introduced in the early 1980s.

Using a posterolateral approach, a tissue-removing device is introduced into the disc space in a similar path as the needle of a discogram; this is guided by intraoperative fluoroscopy. Earlier techniques used a direct lateral approach that led to (or raised concern of) viscous perforation in some patients. The instrument is used to remove nucleus material in small increments. This removal theoretically can decrease intradiscal pressure. There is no direct visualization of the nerve roots, dura, or disc material. Neurologic decompression cannot be assessed with this technique.

Results of automated discectomy are inferior to standard open discectomy. Shapiro[81] showed only partial improvement of leg pain in 57% of patients undergoing this procedure. More disappointing was that only 5% had complete sciatica relief. All patients had disc bulges or protrusions, with none having free fragments. These results are less positive than the results documented with open discectomy.

In contrast, Hoppenfeld[82] reported more successful results, with relief of sciatica and sensory deficit in 86% of patients. He determined, however, that patients with sequestered discs do not reliably respond well to the procedure. Kotilainen and Valtonen[83] treated 41 patients with small protrusions or prolapses (bulges) with percutaneous automated discectomy. Sciatica had completely resolved in 78% of patients. From these data, it can be inferred that automated discectomy can be reasonably effective in patients with small disc bulges or protrusions that are in direct continuity with the remaining nucleus. Only in this select group of patients is there the possibility of relieving the neural compression. The procedure should not be used in patients with sequestered or extruded fragments (uncontained herniations) or most patients with disc herniations.

Chemonucleolysis

Chemonucleolysis involves the chemical digestion of nucleus material via injection of an agent, such as chymopapain, into the intervertebral disc. Ideally, the agent not only decompresses the central aspect of the disc space (producing a similar effect as percutaneous automated discectomy), but also might directly attack the herniated fragment. The clinical success of the procedure has not been supportive.

Chemonucleolysis has been rigorously examined in numerous clinical investigations. In a randomized prospective trial

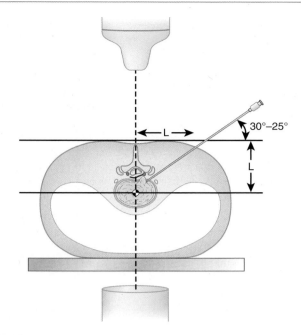

FIGURE 46–19 Transforaminal endoscopic approach for disc excision. (From Yeung AT, Tsou PM: Posterolateral endoscopic excision for lumbar disc herniation. Spine (Phila Pa 1976) 27:722-731, 2002.)

comparing chemonucleolysis and standard discectomy, Muralikuttan and colleagues[86] concluded that it leads to inferior results. There was a high rate of conversion to open surgery in the chemonucleolysis group because of continued, unrelieved symptoms. Crawshaw and colleagues[144] found extremely high failure rates—47% to 52%—after chemonucleolysis compared with 11% with open surgery. vanAlphen and colleagues[70] documented increased radicular pain after chemonucleolysis in 22% of patients treated. Salvage discectomy after failed chemonucleolysis leads to worse results than primary surgery.[70,86,144] In addition to these poor results, neurologic complications, such as transverse myelitis associated with the use of chymopapain, have all but eliminated the procedure from continued use in the United States.

PEARLS

1. Most lumbar disc herniations respond well to conservative treatment within the first 3 months from the onset of symptoms.

2. In patients who fail conservative treatment, surgery consistently showed better outcomes than continued nonoperative care.

3. The type and size of disc herniations and psychosocial factors are the primary determinants of outcomes after discectomy.

4. Although minimally invasive techniques, such as endoscopic and percutaneous laser discectomy, can be effective in experienced hands, it is unclear whether they would ever replace the "gold standard" operation of open discectomy (with or without the use of a microscope).

1. Patients with extraforaminal (far lateral) and central disc herniations should be advised that surgical outcomes may be inferior compared with outcomes for more common and typical paracentral herniations.

2. Patients should be informed that a lumbar discectomy is primarily indicated for leg pain. Back pain, numbness, and weakness are less reliably alleviated after surgery.

3. Recurrent disc herniations, which can occur in 18% of patients, remain problematic and may be more prevalent in patients who have large annular defects after discectomy.

4. Although simple discectomy for a recurrent disc herniation can yield outcomes equivalent to the index procedure, the addition of fusion may be considered after a second recurrence.

KEY POINTS

1. Patients should be carefully counseled preoperatively on the risk and benefits of surgery so that they may make a well-informed decision according to their specific functional demands and expectations.

2. Positioning a patient in a flexed or kneeling position can help open the interlaminar window to allow easier entry into the spinal canal.

3. Regardless of the technique of discectomy, a successful operation is contingent on adequate exposure that enables careful and minimally traumatic identification of the cauda equina, descending nerve root, and exiting nerve root before retraction to retrieve the herniated fragments.

4. During discectomy, the amount and location of the disc herniation should be commensurate with that shown on preoperative MRI.

5. The spinal canal and disc space should be thoroughly inspected before closure to avoid retained disc fragments.

KEY REFERENCES

1. Atlas SJ, Keller RB, Wu YA, et al: Long-term outcomes of surgical and nonsurgical management of sciatica secondary to a lumbar disc herniation: 10 year results from the Maine Lumbar Spine Study. Spine (Phila Pa 1976) 30:927-935, 2005.
This article details the 10-year follow-up results from the Maine lumbar spine study that prospectively evaluated patients with operative and nonoperative treatment for lumbar disc herniations. In this nonrandomized study, surgical treatment produced better results than nonoperative treatment, and the benefits were maximally appreciated at the 2-year mark.

2. Weinstein JN, Lurie JD, Tosteson TD, et al: Surgical vs nonoperative treatment for lumbar disk herniation: The Spine Patient Outcomes Research Trial (SPORT) observational cohort. JAMA 296:2451-2459, 2006.
This article outlines the results of the nonrandomized patients in the SPORT trial for lumbar disk herniations. In this analysis, surgery resulted in better outcomes than nonoperative treatment.

3. Weinstein JN, Tosteson TD, Lurie JD, et al: Surgical vs nonoperative treatment for lumbar disk herniation: The Spine Patient Outcomes Research Trial (SPORT): A randomized trial. JAMA 296:2441-2450, 2006.
In this article, intention-to-treat analysis showed no statistical differences between surgery and nonoperative treatment of lumbar disc herniations. This trial has been widely criticized for its high crossover rate between groups, however.

4. Weber H: Lumbar disc herniation: A controlled, prospective study with ten years of observations. Spine (Phila Pa 1976) 8:131-140, 1983.
This classic study was a randomized controlled trial of operative versus nonoperative treatment for lumbar disc herniations. It showed statistically better results with surgery at 1-year and 4-year follow-up but no difference at 10-year follow-up.

5. Carragee EJ, Kim D: A prospective analysis of magnetic resonance imaging findings in patients with sciatica and lumbar disc herniation: Correlation of outcomes with disc fragment and canal morphology. Spine (Phila Pa 1976) 22:1650-1660, 1997.
This article correlates the size of a disc herniation (at least 6 mm anteroposterior dimension) with better outcomes after surgery.

REFERENCES

1. Atlas SJ, Keller RB, Chang Y, et al: Surgical and nonsurgical management of sciatic secondary to a lumbar disc herniation: Five-year outcomes from the Maine Lumbar Spine Study. Spine (Phila Pa 1976) 26:1179-1187, 2001.

2. DePalma AF, Rothman RH: Surgery of the lumbar spine. Clin Orthop Relat Res 63:162-170, 1969.

3. Fisher RG, Saunders RL: Lumbar disc protrusion in children. J Neurosurg 54:480, 1981.

4. Boden SD, Davis DO, Dina TS, et al: Abnormal magnetic resonance scans of the lumbar spine in asymptomatic subjects: A prospective investigation. J Bone Joint Surg Am 72:403-408, 1990.

5. Saal JA, Saal JS: Nonoperative treatment of herniated lumbar intervertebral disc with radiculopathy: An outcome study. Spine (Phila Pa 1976) 14:431-437, 1989.

6. Saal JA, Saal JS, Herzog RJ: The natural history of lumbar intervertebral disc extrusions treated nonoperatively. Spine (Phila Pa 1976) 15:683-686, 1990.

7. Atlas SJ, Keller RB, Wu YA, et al: Long-term outcomes of surgical and nonsurgical management of sciatica secondary to a lumbar disc herniation: 10 year results from the Maine Lumbar Spine Study. Spine (Phila Pa 1976) 30:927-935, 2005.

8. Weinstein JN, Lurie JD, Tosteson TD, et al: Surgical vs nonoperative treatment for lumbar disk herniation: The Spine Patient Outcomes Research Trial (SPORT) observational cohort. JAMA 296:2451-2459, 2006.

9. Weinstein JN, Tosteson TD, Lurie JD, et al: Surgical vs nonoperative treatment for lumbar disk herniation: The Spine Patient Outcomes Research Trial (SPORT): A randomized trial. JAMA 296:2441-2450, 2006.

10. Weber H: Lumbar disc herniation: A controlled, prospective study with ten years of observations. Spine (Phila Pa 1976) 8:131-140, 1983.

11. Carragee EJ, Kim D: A prospective analysis of magnetic resonance imaging findings in patients with sciatica and lumbar disc herniation: Correlation of outcomes with disc fragment and canal morphology. Spine (Phila Pa 1976) 22:1650-1660, 1997.

12. Hurme M, Alaranta H: Factors predicting the results of surgery for lumbar intervertebral disc herniation. Spine (Phila Pa 1976) 12:933-938, 1987.

13. Spengler DM, Ouellette EA, Battie M, et al: Elective discectomy for herniation of a lumbar disc: Additional experience with an objective method. J Bone Joint Surg Am 72:320-327, 1990.

14. Melvill RL, Baxter BL: The intertransverse approach to extraforaminal disc protrusion in the lumbar spine. Spine (Phila Pa 1976) 19:2707-2714, 1994.

15. Grimes PF, Massie JB, Garfin SR: Anatomic and biomechanical analysis of the lower lumbar foraminal ligaments. Spine (Phila Pa 1976) 25:2009-2014, 2000.

16. Wilder DG, Pope MH, Frymoyer JW: The biomechanics of lumbar disc herniation and the effect of overload and instability. J Spinal Disord 1:16-32, 1988.

17. Frei H, Oxland TR, Rathonyi GC, et al: The effect of nucleotomy on lumbar spine mechanics in compression and shear loading. Spine (Phila Pa 1976) 26:2080-2089, 2001.

18. White A, Panjabi M: Clinical Biomechanics of the Spine, 2nd ed. Philadelphia, Lippincott-Raven, 1990.

19. Repanti M, Korovessis PG, Stamatakis MV, et al: Evolution of disc degeneration in lumbar spine: A comparative histological study between herniated and postmortem retrieved disc specimens. J Spinal Disord 11:41-45, 1998.

20. Smyth MJ, Wright VJ: Sciatica and the intervertebral disc: An experimental study. J Bone Joint Surg Am 40:1401, 1958.

21. Spiliopoulou I, Korovessis P, Konstantinou D, et al: IgG and IgM concentration in the prolapsed human intervertebral disc and sciatica etiology. Spine (Phila Pa 1976) 19:1320-1323, 1994.

22. Olmarker K, Rydevik B: Selective inhibition of tumor necrosis factor-alpha prevents nucleus pulposus-induced thrombus formation, intraneural edema, and reduction of nerve conduction velocity: Possible implications for future pharmacologic treatment strategies of sciatica. Spine (Phila Pa 1976) 26:863-869, 2001.

23. Kang JD, Stefanovic-Racic M, McIntyre LA, et al: Toward a biochemical understanding of human intervertebral disc degeneration and herniation: Contributions of nitric oxide, interleukins, prostaglandin E2, and matrix metalloproteinases. Spine (Phila Pa 1976) 22:1065-1073, 1997.

24. Scuderi GJ, Brusovanik GV, Anderson DG, et al: Cytokine assay of the epidural space lavage in patients with lumbar intervertebral disk herniation and radiculopathy. J Spinal Disord Tech 19:266-269, 2006.

25. Arai Y, Yasuma T, Shitoto K, et al: Immunohistochemical study of intervertebral disc herniation of lumbar spine. J Orthop Sci 5:229-231, 2000.

26. Hatano E, Fujita T, Ueda Y, et al: Expression of ADAMTS-4 (aggrecanase-1) and possible involvement in regression of lumbar disc herniation. Spine (Phila Pa 1976) 31:1426-1432, 2006.

27. Brisby H, Balague F, Schafer D, et al: Glycosphingolipid antibodies in serum in patients with sciatica. Spine (Phila Pa 1976) 27:380-386, 2002.

28. Jinkins JR, Whittemore AR, Bradley WG: The anatomic basis of vertebrogenic pain and the autonomic syndrome associated with lumbar disc extrusion. AJR Am J Roentgenol 152:1277-1289, 1989.

29. Fardon DF, Milette PC: Nomenclature and classification of lumbar disc pathology. Recommendations of the combined task forces of the North American Spine Society, American Society of Spine Radiology, and American Society of Neuroradiology. Spine (Phila Pa 1976) 26:E93-E113, 2001.

30. Fardon DF: Nomenclature and classification of lumbar disc pathology. Spine (Phila Pa 1976) 26:461-462, 2001.

31. McCulloch JA, Transfelt EE: Macnab's Backache. Baltimore, Williams & Wilkins, 1997.

32. Nygaard OP, Kloster R, Solberg T: Duration of leg pain as a predictor of outcome after surgery for lumbar disc herniation: A prospective cohort study with 1-year follow up. J Neurosurg 92:131-134, 2000.

33. Rothoerl RD, Woertgen C, Brawanski A: When should conservative treatment for lumbar disc herniation be ceased and surgery considered? Neurosurg Rev 25:162-165, 2002.

34. Sorensen LV, Mors O, Skovlund O: A prospective study of the importance of psychological and social factors for the outcome after surgery in patients with slipped lumbar disk operated upon for the first time. Acta Neurochir (Wien) 88:119-125, 1987.

35. Slover J, Abdu WA, Hanscom B, et al: The impact of comorbidities on the change in Short-Form 36 and Oswestry scores following lumbar spine surgery. Spine (Phila Pa 1976) 31:1974-1980, 2006.

36. Jansson KA, Nemeth G, Granath F, et al: Health-related quality of life in patients before and after surgery for a herniated lumbar disc. J Bone Joint Surg Br 87:959-964, 2005.

37. Weise MD, Garfin SR, Gelberman RH, et al: Lower-extremity sensibility testing in patients with herniated lumbar intervertebral discs. J Bone Joint Surg Am 67:1219-1224, 1985.

38. Kosteljanetz M, Espersen JO, Halaburt H, et al: Predictive value of clinical and surgical findings in patients with lumbago-sciatica: A prospective study (Part I). Acta Neurochir (Wien) 73:67-76, 1984.

39. Majlesi J, Togay H, Unalan H, et al: The sensitivity and specificity of the slump and the straight leg raising tests in patients with lumbar disc herniation. J Clin Rheumatol 14:87-91, 2008.

40. Ito T, Takano Y, Yuasa N: Types of lumbar herniated disc and clinical course. Spine (Phila Pa 1976) 26:648-651, 2001.

41. Komori H, Okawa A, Haro H, et al: Contrast-enhanced magnetic resonance imaging conservative management of lumbar disc herniation. Spine (Phila Pa 1976) 23:67-73, 1998.

42. Kikkawa I, Sugimoto H, Saita K, et al: The role of Gd enhanced three dimensional MRI fast low-angle shot (FLASH) in the evaluation of symptomatic lumbosacral nerve roots. J Orthop Sci 6:101-109, 2001.

43. Weishaupt D, Schmid MR, Zanetti M, et al: Positional MR imaging of the lumbar spine: Does it demonstrate nerve root compromise not visible at conventional MR imaging. Radiology 215:247-253, 2000.

44. Botwin KP, Skene G, Tourres-Ramos FM, et al: Role of weight-bearing flexion and extension myelography in evaluating the intervertebral disc. Am J Phys Med Rehabil 80:289-295, 2001.

45. Grane P, Lindqvist M: Evaluation of the postoperative lumbar spine with MR imaging: The role of contrast enhancement and thickening in nerve roots. Acta Radiol 38:1035-1042, 1997.

46. Heithoff KB: Recurrent disc herniation and gadolinium. Spine-Line Sept/Oct:23-26, 2002.

47. Barrera MC, Alustiza JM, Gervas C, et al: Postoperative lumbar spine: Comparative study of TSE T2 and turbo FLAIR sequences vs contrast-enhanced SE T1. Clin Radiol 56:133-137, 2001.

48. Bundschuh CV, Modic MT, Ross JR, et al: Epidural fibrosis and recurrent disc herniation in the lumbar spine: MR imaging assessment. AJR Am J Roentgenol 150:923-932, 1988.

49. Mortensen WW, Thorne TP, Donaldson WF: Symptomatic gas-containing disc herniation: Report of four cases. Spine (Phila Pa 1976) 16:190-192, 1991.

50. Ford LT, Gilula LA, Murphy WA, et al: Analysis of gas in vacuum lumbar disc. AJR Am J Roentgenol 128:1056-1057, 1977.

51. Deyo RA, Diehl AK, Rosenthal M: How many days of bedrest for acute low back pain? A randomized clinical trial. N Engl J Med 315:1064-1070, 1986.

52. Krause M, Reshauge KM, Dessen M, et al: Lumbar spine traction: Evaluation of effects and recommended application for treatment. Man Ther 5:72-81, 2000.

53. Polkinghorn BS, Colloca CJ: Treatment of symptomatic lumbar disc herniation using activator methods chiropractic technique. J Manipulative Physiol Ther 21:187-196, 1998.

54. Bush K, Cowan N, Katz DE, et al: The natural history of sciatica associated with disc pathology: A prospective study with clinical and independent radiographic follow-up. Spine (Phila Pa 1976) 17:1205-1212, 1992.

55. Wang JC, Lin E, Brodke DS, et al: Epidural injections for the treatment of symptomatic lumbar herniated discs. J Spinal Disord 15:269-272, 2002.

56. Atlas SJ, Deyo RA, Keller RB, et al: The Maine Lumbar Spine Study, Part II: 1-year outcomes of surgical and nonsurgical management of sciatica. Spine (Phila Pa 1976) 21:1777-1786, 1996.

57. Pearson AM, Blood EA, Frymoyer JW, et al: SPORT lumbar intervertebral disk herniation and back pain: Does treatment, location, or morphology matter? Spine (Phila Pa 1976) 33:428-435, 2008.

58. Alaranta H, Hurme M, Einola S, et al: A prospective study of patients with sciatica: A comparison between conservatively treated patients and patients who have undergone operation, Part II: Results after one year follow-up. Spine (Phila Pa 1976) 15:1345-1349, 1990.

59. Hurme M, Alaranta H, Einola S, et al: A prospective study of patients with sciatica: A comparison between conservatively treated patients and patients who have undergone operation, Part I: Patient characteristics and differences between groups. Spine (Phila Pa 1976) 15:1340-1344, 1990.

60. Balderston RA, Gilyeard GG, Jones AA, et al: The treatment of lumbar disc herniation: Simple fragment excision versus disc space curettage. J Spinal Disord 4:22-25, 1991.

61. Barrios C, Ahmed M, Arrotegui JI, et al: Clinical factors predicting outcome after surgery for herniated lumbar disc: An epidemiological multivariate analysis. J Spinal Disord 3:205-209, 1990.

62. Cashion EL, Lynch WJ: Personality factors and results of lumbar disc surgery. Neurosurgery 4:141-145, 1979.

63. Daneyemez M, Sali A, Kahraman S, et al: Outcome analyses in 1072 surgically treated lumbar disc herniations. Minim Invasive Neurosurg 42:63-68, 1999.

64. Eie N: Comparison of the results in patients operated for ruptured lumbar discs with and without spinal fusion. Acta Neurochir (Wien) 41:107-113, 1978.

65. Faulhauer K, Manicke C: Fragment excision versus conventional disc removal in the microsurgical treatment of herniated lumbar disc. Acta Neurochir (Wien) 133:107-111, 1995.

66. Jonsson B, Stromqvist B: Motor affliction of the L5 nerve root in lumbar nerve root compression syndromes. Spine (Phila Pa 1976) 20:2012-2015, 1995.

67. Kulali A, vonWild K: Microsurgical management of the lumbar intervertebral disc-disease. Neurosurg Rev 18:183-188, 1995.

68. Yeung AT, Tsou PM: Posterolateral endoscopic excision for lumbar disc herniation. Spine (Phila Pa 1976) 27:722-731, 2002.

69. White AH, vonRogov P, Zucherman J, et al: Lumbar laminectomy for herniated disc: A prospective controlled comparison with internal fixation fusion. Spine (Phila Pa 1976) 12:305-307, 1987.

70. vanAlphen HA, Braakman R, Berfelo MW, et al: Chemonucleolysis or discectomy? Results of a randomized multicentre trial in patients with a herniated lumbar intervertebral disc (a preliminary report). Acta Neurochir Suppl (Wien) 43:35-38, 1988.

71. Tullberg T, Isacson J, Weidenhielm L: Does microscopic removal of lumbar disc herniation lead to better results than the standard procedure? Results of a one-year randomized study. Spine (Phila Pa 1976) 18:24-27, 1993.

72. Soldner F, Hoelper BM, Wallenfang T, et al: The translaminar approach to canalicular and craniodorsolateral lumbar disc herniations. Acta Neurochir (Wien) 144:315-320, 2002.

73. Pointillart V, Broc G, Senegas J: A novel paraspinal surgical approach for lumbar lateral extraforaminal root entrapment. Eur Spine J 6:102-105, 1997.

74. An HS, Simpson JM, Stein R: Outpatient laminotomy and discectomy. J Spinal Disord 12:19-26, 1999.

75. Carragee EJ, Han MY, Yang B, et al: Activity restrictions after posterior lumbar discectomy: A prospective study of outcomes in 152 cases with no postoperative restrictions. Spine (Phila Pa 1976) 24:2346-2351, 1999.

76. McCulloch JA: Focus issue on lumbar disc herniation: Macro- and microdiscectomy. Spine (Phila Pa 1976) 21:45S-56S, 1996.

77. Reulen HJ, Muller A, Ebeling U: Microsurgical anatomy of the lateral approach to extraforaminal lumbar disc herniations. Neurosurgery 39:345-350, 1996.

78. Eie N, Solgaard T, Kleppe H: The knee-elbow position in lumbar disc surgery: A review of complications. Spine (Phila Pa 1976) 8:897-900, 1983.

79. Miyamoto K: Long-term follow-up results of anterior discectomy and interbody fusion for lumbar disc herniation. J Jpn Orthop Assoc 65:1179-1190, 1991.

80. Revel M, Payan C, Vallee C, et al: Automated percutaneous lumbar discectomy versus chemonucleolysis in the treatment of sciatica: A randomized multicenter trial. Spine (Phila Pa 1976) 18:1-7, 1993.

81. Shapiro S: Long-term followup of 57 patients undergoing automated percutaneous discectomy. J Neurosurg 83:31-33, 1995.

82. Hoppenfeld S: Percutaneous removal of herniated lumbar discs: 50 cases with ten-year follow-up periods. Clin Orthop Relat Res 238:92-97, 1989.

83. Kotilainen E, Valtonen S: Long-term outcome of patients who underwent percutaneous nucleotomy for lumbar disc herniation: Results after a mean follow-up of 5 years. Acta Neurochir (Wien) 140:108-113, 1998.

84. DeAntoni DJ, Claro ML, Poehling GG, et al: Translaminar lumbar epidural endoscopy: Technique and clinical results. J South Orthop Assoc 7:61-62, 1998.

85. Fraser RD: Chymopapain for the treatment of intervertebral disc herniation: The final report of a double-blind study. Spine (Phila Pa 1976) 9:815-818, 1984.

86. Muralikuttan KP, Hamilton A, Kernohan WG, et al: A prospective randomized trial of chemonucleolysis and conventional disc surgery in single level lumbar disc herniation. Spine (Phila Pa 1976) 17:381-387, 1992.

87. Weber H: The effect of delayed disc surgery on muscular paresis. Acta Orthop Scand 46:631-642, 1975.

88. MacKay MA, Fischgrund JS, Herkowitz HN, et al: The effect of interposition membrane on the outcome of lumbar laminectomy and discectomy. Spine (Phila Pa 1976) 20:1793-1796, 1995.

89. Bernsmann K, Kramer J, Ziozios I, et al: Lumbar micro disc surgery with and without autologous fat graft: A prospective randomized trial evaluated with reference to clinical and social factors. Arch Orthop Trauma Surg 121:476-480, 2001.

90. Kjellby-Wendt G, Styf J: Early active training after lumbar discectomy: A prospective, randomized, and controlled study. Spine (Phila Pa 1976) 23:2345-2351, 1998.

91. Alaranta H, Hurme M, Einola S, et al: Rehabilitation after surgery for lumbar disc herniation: Results of a randomized clinical trial. Int J Rehabil Res 9:247-257, 1986.

92. Knop-Jergas BM, Zucherman JF, Hsu KY, et al: Anatomic position of a herniated nucleus pulposus predicts the outcome of lumbar discectomy. J Spinal Disord 9:246-250, 1996.

93. Dewing CB, Provencher MT, Rifenburgh RH, et al: The outcomes of lumbar microdiscectomy in a young, active population: Correlation by herniation type and level. Spine (Phila Pa 1976) 33:33-38, 2008.

94. Jonsson B, Stromqvist B: Significance of a persistent positive straight leg raising test after lumbar disc surgery. J Neurosurg 91:50-53, 1999.

95. Keller RB, Atlas SJ, Soule DN, et al: Relationship between rates and outcomes of operative treatment for lumbar disc herniation and spinal stenosis. J Bone Joint Surg Am 81:752-762, 1999.

96. Dvorak J, Gauchat MH, Valach L: The outcome of surgery for lumbar disc herniation, I: A 4-17 years follow-up with emphasis on somatic aspects. Spine (Phila Pa 1976) 13:1418-1422, 1988.

97. Kotilainen E, Valtonene S, Carlson CA: Microsurgical treatment of lumbar disc herniation: Follow-up of 237 patients. Acta Neurochir (Wien) 120:143-149, 1993.

98. Goffin J: Microdiscectomy for lumbar disc herniations. Clin Neurol Neurosurg 96:130-134, 1994.

99. Wenger M, Mariani L, Kalbarczyk A, et al: Long-term outcome of 104 patients after lumbar sequestrectomy according to Williams. Neurosurgery 49:329-334, 2001.

100. Carragee EJ, Spinnickie AO, Alamin TF, et al: A prospective controlled study of limited versus subtotal posterior discectomy: Short-term outcomes in patients with herniated lumbar intervertebral discs and large posterior anular defect. Spine (Phila Pa 1976) 31:653-657, 2006.

101. Kotilainen E, Valtonen S: Clinical instability of the lumbar spine after microdiscectomy. Acta Neurochir (Wien) 125:120-126, 1993.

102. Tronnier V, Schneider R, Kunz U, et al: Postoperative spondylodiscitis: Results of a prospective study about the aetiology of spondylodiscitis after operation for lumbar disc herniation. Acta Neurochir (Wien) 117:149-152, 1992.

103. Sande E, Myhre HO, Witsoe E, et al: Vascular complications of lumbar disc surgery (case report). Eur J Surg 157:141-143, 1991.

104. Ewah B, Calder I: Intraoperative death during lumbar discectomy. Br J Anaesth 66:712-723, 1991.

105. Christensen C, Bank A: Arteriovenous fistula complicating lumbar disc surgery (case report). Eur J Surg 157:145-147, 1991.

106. Farouk M, Murie JA: Postlaminectomy arteriovenous fistula formation: A continuing problem. J R Coll Surg Edinb 36:130-131, 1991.

107. Saxler G, Kramer J, Barden B, et al: The long-term clinical sequelae of incidental durotomy in lumbar disc surgery. Spine (Phila Pa 1976) 30:2298-2302, 2005.

108. Padua R, Padua S, Romanini E, et al: Ten to 15 year outcome of surgery for lumbar disc herniation: Radiographic instability and clinical findings. Eur Spine J 8:70-74, 1999.

109. Kotilainen E: Long-term outcome of patients suffering from clinical instability after microsurgical treatment of lumbar disc herniation. Acta Neurochir (Wien) 140:120-125, 1998.

110. Laus M, Bertoni F, Bacchini P, et al: Recurrent lumbar disc herniation: What recurs? (A morphological study of recurrent disc herniation). Chir Organi Mov 78:147-154, 1993.

111. Jonsson B, Stromqvist B: Clinical characteristics of recurrent sciatica after lumbar discectomy. Spine (Phila Pa 1976) 21:500-505, 1996.

112. Vik A, Zwart JA, Hullberg G, et al: Eight year outcome after surgery for lumbar disc herniation: A comparison of reoperated and nonreoperated patients. Acta Neurochir (Wien) 143:607-610, 2001.

113. Suk KS, Lee HM, Moon SH, et al: Lumbosacral scoliotic list by lumbar disc herniation. Spine (Phila Pa 1976) 26:667-671, 2001.

114. Cinotti G, Gumina S, Giannicola G, et al: Contralateral recurrent lumbar disc herniation: Results of discectomy compared with those in primary herniation. Spine (Phila Pa 1976) 24:800-806, 1999.

115. Cinotti G, Roysam GS, Eisenstein SM, et al: Ipsilateral recurrent lumbar disc herniation: A prospective, controlled study. J Bone Joint Surg Br 80:825-832, 1998.

116. Papadopoulos EC, Girardi FP, Sandhu HS, et al: Outcome of revision discectomies following recurrent lumbar disc herniation. Spine (Phila Pa 1976) 31:1473-1476, 2006.

117. Herron L: Recurrent lumbar disc herniation: Results of repeat laminectomy and discectomy. J Spinal Disord 7:161-166, 1994.

118. Stambough JL: Recurrent same-level, ipsilateral lumbar disc herniation. Orthop Rev 23:810-816, 1994.

119. Kurihara A, Kataoka O: Lumbar disc herniation in children and adolescents: A review of 70 operated cases and their minimum 5-year follow-up studies. Spine (Phila Pa 1976) 5:443-451, 1980.

120. Garrido E: Lumbar disc herniation in the pediatric patient. Neurosurg Clin N Am 4:149-152, 1993.

121. Papagenlopoulos PJ, Shaughnessy WJ, Ebersold MJ, et al: Long-term outcome of lumbar discectomy in children and adolescents sixteen years of age or younger. J Bone Joint Surg Am 80:689-698, 1998.

122. Parisini P, DiSilvestre M, Greggi T, et al: Lumbar disc excision in children and adolescents. Spine (Phila Pa 1976) 26:1997-2000, 2001.

123. DeOrio JK, Bianco AJ: Lumbar disc excision in children and adolescents. J Bone Joint Surg Am 64:991-996, 1982.

124. Shillito J: Pediatric lumbar disc surgery: 20 patients under 15 years of age. Surg Neurol 46:14-18, 1996.

125. Maistrelli GL, Vaughan PA, Evans DC, et al: Lumbar disc herniation in the elderly. Spine (Phila Pa 1976) 12:63-66, 1987.

126. Jonsson B, Stromqvist B: Lumbar spine surgery in the elderly: Complications and surgical results. Spine (Phila Pa 1976) 19:1431-1435, 1994.

127. Garrido E, Connaughton PN: Unilateral facetectomy approach for lateral lumbar disc herniation. J Neurosurg 74:754-756, 1991.

128. Donaldson WF, Star MJ, Thorne RP: Surgical treatment for the lateral herniated lumbar disc. Spine (Phila Pa 1976) 18:1263-1267, 1993.

129. Weiner BK, Dabbah M: Lateral lumbar disc herniations treated with a paraspinal approach: An independent assessment of longer-term outcomes. J Spinal Disord Tech 18:519-521, 2005.

130. Walker JL, Schulak D, Murtagh R: Midline disk herniations of the lumbar spine. South Med J 86:13-17, 1993.

131. Tay ECK, Chacha PB: Midline prolapse of a lumbar intervertebral disc with compression of the cauda equina. J Bone Joint Surg Br 61:43-46, 1979.

132. Nielsen B, deNully M, Schmidt K, et al: A urodynamic study of cauda equina syndrome due to lumbar disc herniation. Urol Int 35:167-170, 1980.

133. Kostuik JP, Harrington I, Alexander D, et al: Cauda equina syndrome and lumbar disc herniation. J Bone Joint Surg Am 68:386-391, 1986.

134. Choudry AR, Taylor JC: Cauda equina syndrome in lumbar disc disease. Acta Orthop Scand 51:493-499, 1980.

135. Shapiro S: Cauda equina syndrome secondary to lumbar disc herniation. Neurosurgery 32:743-747, 1993.

136. Ahn UM, Ahn NU, Buchowski JM, et al: Cauda equina syndrome secondary to lumbar disc herniation. Spine (Phila Pa 1976) 25:1515-1522, 2000.

137. McCarthy MJ, Aylott CE, Grevitt MP, et al: Cauda equina syndrome: Factors affecting long-term functional and sphincteric outcome. Spine (Phila Pa 1976) 32:207-216, 2007.

138. Chang HS, Nakagawa H, Mizuno J: Lumbar herniated disc presenting with cauda equina syndrome. Surg Neurol 53:100-105, 2002.

139. Yeung AT, Yeung CA: Minimally invasive techniques for the management of lumbar disc herniation. Orthop Clin North Am 38:363-372, 2007.

140. Hoogland T, van den Brekel-Dijstra K, Schubert M, et al: Endoscopic transforaminal discectomy for recurrent lumbar disc herniation: A prospective, cohort evaluation of 262 consecutive cases. Spine (Phila Pa 1976) 33:973-978, 2008.

141. Wu X, Zhuang S, Mao Z, et al: Microendoscopic discectomy for lumbar disc herniation: Surgical technique and outcome in 873 consecutive cases. Spine (Phila Pa 1976) 31:2689-2694, 2006.

142. Righesso O, Falavigna A, Avanzi O: Comparison of open discectomy with microendoscopic discectomy in lumbar disc herniations: Results of a randomized controlled trial. Neurosurgery 61:545-549, 2007.

143. Ruetten S, Komp M, Merk H, et al: Full-endoscopic interlaminar and transforaminal lumbar discectomy versus conventional microsurgical technique: A prospective, randomized, controlled study. Spine (Phila Pa 1976) 33:931-939, 2008.

144. Crawshaw C, Frazer AM, Merriam WF, et al: A comparison of surgery and chemonucleolysis in the treatment of sciatica: A prospective randomized trial. Spine (Phila Pa 1976) 9:195-198, 1984.

47
CHAPTER

Annular Repair

Gunnar B. J. Andersson, MD, PhD

The anulus fibrosus is an important part of the intervertebral disc. Similar to the other disc components, the anulus undergoes changes with aging and with degeneration.[1,2] The degenerative process leads to a weakening of the anulus, and delamination, fissures, and cracks occur. Occasionally, the nucleus pulposus can herniate into the cracks and through the entire annular wall. Also, as part of surgical procedures to address contained disc herniations, iatrogenic holes in various shapes and locations are made into the anulus.

In recent years, there has been increasing interest in strengthening the annular structure, which is important to regain the normal function of the disc.[3] There is also interest in repairing degenerative and iatrogenic cracks, tears, and holes in the anulus to prevent recurrence of disc herniations and to slow the degenerative process after discectomy. This chapter reviews some of these strategies and puts them in the context of successful treatment of different types of painful spinal conditions. The focus is on the lumbar discs.

Anulus Fibrosus

The anulus fibrosus is a laminate structure surrounding the central nucleus pulposus and inserting into the endplates and the vertebral body. It consists primarily of water, collagen, proteoglycans, and noncollagenous proteins. The laminates are organized in layers mainly composed of type I collagen fibers, which alternate in angles with respect to the transverse plane. Between the layers are so-called interlaminar spaces containing proteoglycans (aggrecan, versican) and other linking elements.[4] In the center, the fibers insert into the cartilaginous endplates, and in the periphery they bypass the endplates and insert into the bone, called *Sharpey fibers*. The inner and outer parts of the anulus differ in that in the inner part the layers are less well organized and more widely spaced. The proportion of type I collagen increases from the inner anulus to the outer anulus, whereas type II collagen is more common in the inner anulus than outer anulus. Small proteoglycans (decorin and biglycan) are found primarily in the outer anulus, whereas elastin is present throughout. Elastin constitutes 1.7% to 2% of the dry weight of the anulus. In the outer anulus, elastin is present within the lamella running parallel to the collagen and in the same direction.[5,24] In the inner anulus, elastin is also organized within the lamellae. Fiber networks bind adjacent lamella together preventing them from separating.[6,7] Table 47–1 compares the outer anulus and inner anulus.

The cell density in the anulus pulposus is about twice the cell density of the nucleus pulposus.[8] In the outer anulus, the cells are fusiform-shaped and align with the collagen fibers alternating with each lamella. These cells produce mainly type I collagen. In the inner anulus, the cells are more similar to the cells of the nucleus pulposus. They are chrondrocyte-like and produce mainly type II collagen.

The mechanical exposure of the different parts of the anulus is initially different. The inner anulus is primarily subjected to the hydrostatic pressures of the nucleus pulposus, whereas the outer anulus is more under compression or tension depending on the direction of movement. Similar to other connective tissue structures, the anulus is anisotropic and adapted to the principal directions of load.

Effect of Aging on Anulus Fibrosus

Various chemical and structural changes occur with aging. These changes seem to occur first in the inner anulus, which loses a large part of its proteoglycan and water and gradually assumes a more nucleuslike structure.[2] The overall proteoglycan and collagen concentrations decrease with aging, probably reflecting a decrease in cellular biochemical activity. Among smaller nonaggregating proteoglycans, decorin levels decrease with aging in the outer anulus, and biglycan and fibromodulin levels increase. In the inner anulus, decorin levels have been found to increase with aging.

Healing of Anulus

Early studies in dogs showed comparatively poor healing when larger defects were created in the annular wall.[9] Smith and Walmsley[10] reported that after an incision the outer anulus healed by fibrous tissue ingrowth from the sides and that there was also a gradual healing of the inner anulus over a 1-year

TABLE 47-1 Comparison of the Outer Anulus and Inner Anulus

	Outer Anulus	Inner Anulus
Collagen	40%-60% dw	25%-40% dw
Type of collagen	Type I mainly	Type II mainly
Proteoglycan	5%-8% dw	11%-20% dw
Cells	Fusiform	Chondrocytelike

dw, dry weight.

period. Long-term collagen fibers gradually invaded the nuclear tissue, of which some remained in the annular incisions. Fazzalari and colleagues,[11] using an ovine model, introduced needle punctures and concentric tears and tested the specimen mechanically up to 18 months. Significant changes occurred in disc biomechanics in both cases and remained significant over time. The annular lamellae thickened, and the adjacent vertebral body bone volume fraction increased. Although this model is not a herniation model, it shows the poor healing of concentric tears and their effect on the disc biomechanics. There is limited information on annular repair in humans after discectomy. Current information suggests a limited healing potential after annulotomy. This increases the risk of reherniation. Reoperation rates for recurrent herniations ranging from 3% to 27% have been reported.[12-15] The frequency of reoperations seems to be related to the size of the annular defect.

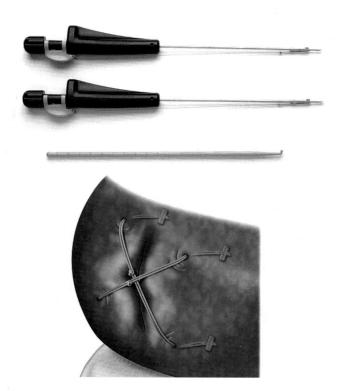

FIGURE 47-1 Xclose. (Courtesy Anulex Technologies, Inc., Minnetonka, MN.)

Biologic Repair

At least four types of annular repair are discussed in the literature: collagen modification, cell therapy, gene therapy, and tissue engineered scaffolds. Gene and cell therapies are unlikely to repair existing cracks, tears, and incisions unless combined with scaffolds. Numerous studies have been published in which scaffolds have been populated with cells, and various success rates have been reported. Most of these studies have been performed in vitro, but a few animal studies have been reported. Gene and growth factor therapies can repair annular needle punctures in the early stages. Many growth factors seem to have a stronger effect on proteoglycan than collagen. Zhang and colleagues[16] reported that collagen synthesis was enhanced by BMP-13 and Sox9.

Bron and colleagues[3] listed requirements for anulus fibrosus scaffolds. The scaffolds should:

1. Fix or repair the anulus fibrosus gap to contain the nucleus pulposus (or its replacement).
2. Allow fixation to surrounding structures.
3. Allow anulus fibrosus cells (or stem cells) to survive and secrete extracellular matrix.
4. Have the characteristic anisotropic behavior to maintain and restore the mechanical properties of a spinal motion segment.
5. Not irritate or adhere to the perineurium.

To date, no single approach has met all these requirements, but several scaffolds are promising.[17-20]

Surgical Repair

A few alternatives have been developed to address the closure of an annular defect caused by a discectomy. Wang and colleagues[21] put absorbable gelatin sponge (Gelfoam), platinum core, bone cement, and tissue glue into an 18-gauge needle defect. Gelfoam seemed to have the best result. The size of the defect in this model is so small, however, that it is difficult to extrapolate this model to a discectomy. Sutures have been used in a sheep model.[22] The healing effect was not statistically significant. More recently, sutures with anchors (Xclose and Inclose; Anulex Technologies, Inc., Minnetonka, MN) have been introduced commercially and are currently undergoing a U.S. Food and Drug Administration (FDA) trial (Fig. 47-1). A retrospective case series comparing 133 microdiscectomy cases without anulus repair with 59 cases with anulus repair was reported at a Society meeting.[23] There were 16 reoperations within 12 months in the nonrepair group (12.9%) compared with 4 in the annular repair group (6.8%).[23] To what degree sutures can be used when larger defects exist is unknown. It is also unclear how well they reverse the biomechanical changes caused by the defect.

Barricaid (Intrinsic Therapeutics, Inc., Woburn, MA) is another commercially available implant that anchors into the

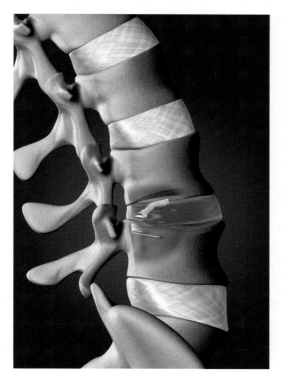

FIGURE 47–2 Barricaid. (Courtesy Intrinsic Therapeutics, Inc., Woburn, MA.)

vertebral body and supports a woven mesh barrier inserted into the defect (Fig. 47–2). Clinical data are not yet available, but an investigational device exemption (IDE) trial is planned for 2010. Other implants are in various stages of development and likely to be presented at meetings in the near future.

Summary

Annular repair is an exciting developing technology to address the age-related and degenerative changes of the anulus and annular tears occurring from disc herniations or in the treatment of herniations. Clinical data are expected in the next several years, but it may take a decade or more to determine how effective annular strengthening is in retarding the development of degenerative and age-related changes.

PEARLS

1. The anulus changes as a result of the degenerative process biologically and mechanically.

2. Biologic annular repair techniques are currently not in clinical practice.

3. Reherniation rates of 27% have been reported. Higher reherniation rates are present when the annular tears are larger.

4. Mechanical repair devices are currently in clinical trials.

PITFALLS

1. Patients with annular cracks and fissures have an increased risk for disc herniations.

2. A large defect in the anulus increases the risk of reherniation.

KEY POINTS

1. The anulus fibrosus weakens as part of the degenerative disc process. Delamination, fissures, and cracks also occur.

2. The primary structural component of the anulus is type I collagen fibers. The proportion of type I collagen increases from the inner anulus to the outer anulus. The inner anulus and outer anulus differ not only with respect to collagen, but also there are more proteoglycans in the inner anulus, the cells are different, and the collagen content is lower.

3. The anulus has limited healing potential. This limited potential increases the risk of reherniation. Reoperation rates for recurrent herniations range from 3% to 27%.

4. Various biologic repair alternatives are under investigation, including tissue engineered scaffolds. No biologic repairs are in current clinical use.

5. Surgical repair is promising and currently in clinical trials.

KEY REFERENCES

1. Osti OL, Vernon-Roberts B, Moore R, et al: Annular tears and disc degeneration in the lumbar spine: A post-mortem study of 135 discs. J Bone Joint Surg Br 74:678-682, 1992.
   This is a classic study of anatomic findings of the anulus fibrosus of humans.

2. Bron JL, Heider MN, Meisel H-J, et al: Repair, regenerative and supportive therapies of the annulus fibrosus: Achievements and challenges. Eur Spine J 18:301-313, 2009.
   This is a review article on repair of the anulus fibrosus.

3. Carragee EJ, Han MY, Suen PW, et al: Clinical outcomes after lumbar discectomy for sciatica: The effects of fragment type and anular competence. J Bone Joint Surg Am 85:102-108, 2007.
   This article describes the risk of reherniation in relation to the type of herniation and the size of the annular defect.

4. Hartman L, Griffith SL, Melone B, et al: Surgical outcome of lumbar microdiscectomy with emphasis on annular repair techniques. Annual Meeting of Congress of Neurological Surgeons (CNS), New Orleans, 2009.
   This study of a mechanical repair technique shows promising results.

REFERENCES

1. Osti OL, Vernon-Roberts B, Moore R, et al: Annular tears and disc degeneration in the lumbar spine: A post-mortem study of 135 discs. J Bone Joint Surg Br 74:678-682, 1992.

2. Singh K, Masuda K, Thonar EJ-M, et al: Age-related changes in the extracellular matrix of mucleus pulposus and annulus fibrosus of human intervertebral disc. Spine (Phila Pa 1976) 34:10-16, 2008.

3. Bron JL, Heider MN, Meisel H-J, et al: Repair, regenerative and supportive therapies of the annulus fibrosus: Achievements and challenges. Eur Spine J 18:301-313, 2009.

4. Pezowicz CA, Robertson PA, Broom ND: The structural basis of interlamellar cohesion in the intervertebral disc well. J Anat 208:317-330, 2006.

5. Smith LJ, Byers S, Costi JJ, et al: Elastic fibers enhance the mechanical integrity of the human lumbar annulus fibrosus in the radial direction. Ann Biomed Eng 36:214-223, 2008.

6. Yu J, Tirlapur U, Fairbank J, et al: Microfibrils, elastin fibres and collagen fibres in the human intervertebral disc and bovine tail disc. J Anat 210:460-471, 2007.

7. Melrose J, Smith SM, Appleyard RC, et al: Aggrecan, verSICAN and type VI collagen are components of annular translamellar cross bridges in the intervertebral disc. Eur Spine J 17:314-324, 2008.

8. Roughley PJ: Biology of intervertebral disc aging and degeneration: Involvement of the extracellular matrix. Spine (Phila Pa 1976) 29:2691-2699, 2004.

9. Key JA, Ford LT: Experimental intervertebral-disc lesions. J Bone Joint Surg Am 30:621-630, 1948.

10. Smith JW, Walmsley R: Experimental incision of the intervertebral disc. J Bone Joint Surg Br 33:612-625, 1951.

11. Fazzalari NL, Costi JJ, Hearn TC, et al: Mechanical and pathologic consequences of induced concentric anular tears in an ovine model. Spine (Phila Pa 1976) 26:2572-2581, 2001.

12. Carragee EJ, Han MY, Suen PW, et al: Clinical outcomes after lumbar discectomy for sciatica: The effects of fragment type and anular competence. J Bone Joint Surg Am 85:102-108, 2007.

13. Ebeling U, Kalbarcyk H, Reulen HJ: Microsurgical re-operation following lumbar disc surgery: Timing, surgical findings, and outcome in 92 patients. J Neurosurg 70:397-404, 2007.

14. Ambrossi GLG, McGirt MJ, Sciobba DA, et al: Recurrent lumbar disc herniation after single level discectomy: Incidence and health care cost analysis. Neurosurgery 65:574-578, 2009.

15. Watters WC, McGirt MJ: An evidence-based review of the literature on the consequences of conservative versus aggressive discectomy for the treatment of primary disc herniation with radiculopathy. Spine J 9:240-257, 2009.

16. Zhang Y, Anderson DB, Phillips FM, et al: Comparative effects of bone morphogenetic proteins and Sox9 overexpression on matrix accumulation by bovine annulus fibrosus cells: Implications for annular repair. Spine 32:2515-2520, 2007.

17. Nerurkar NL, Elliott DM, Mauck RL: Mechanics of oriented electrospun nanofibrous scaffolds for annulus fibrosus tissue engineering. J Orthop Res 25:1018-1028, 2007.

18. Sato M, Asazuma T, Ishihara M, et al: An atelocollagen honeycomb-shaped scaffold with a membrane seal (ACHMS-scaffold) for the culture of annulus fibrosus cells from an intervertebral disc. J Biomed Mater Res A 64:248-256, 2003.

19. Sato M, Asazuma T, Ishihara M, et al: An experimental study of the regeneration of the intervertebral disc with an allograft of cultured annulus fibrosus cells using a tissue-engineering method. Spine (Phila Pa 1976) 28:548-553, 2003.

20. Sato M, Kikuchi M, Ishihara M, et al: Tissue engineering of the intervertebral disc with cultured annulus fibrosus cells using atelocollagen honeycomb-shaped scaffold with a membrane seal (ACHMS scaffold). Med Bio Eng Comput 41:365-371, 2003.

21. Wang YH, Kuo TF, Wang JL: The implantation of non-cell-based materials to prevent the recurrent disc herniation: An in vivo porcine model using quantitative discomanometry examination. Eur Spine J 16:1021-1027, 2007.

22. Ahlgren BD, Lui W, Herkowitz HN, et al: Effect of annular repair on the healing strength of the intervertebral disc: A sheep model. Spine (Phila Pa 1976) 25:2165-2170, 2000.

23. Hartman L, Griffith SL, Melone B, et al: Surgical outcome of lumbar microdiscectomy with emphasis on annular repair techniques. Annual Meeting of Congress of Neurological Surgeons (CNS), New Orleans, 2009.

24. Smith LJ, Fazzalari NL: The elastin fibre network of the human lumbar annulus fibrosus: Architecture, mechanical function and potential role in the progression of intervertebral disc degeneration. Eur Spine J 18:439-448, 2009.

48

CHAPTER

Anterior Lumbar Interbody Fusion

Richard D. Guyer, MD
Jamieson Glenn, MD

Low back pain has long been noted to be one of the most disabling conditions in the United States and the Western world. Disability from back pain has been reported to cost approximately $100 billion annually.[1] Lumbar disc degeneration is often divided into three basic categories: internal disc derangement, degenerative disc disease (DDD), and motion segment instability. Internal disc derangement[2] encompasses annular tears and dark disc disease, DDD describes isolated disc resorption and spondylosis, and motion segment instability involves listhesis and scoliotic changes. This description of lumbar disc degeneration, although oversimplified, encompasses a dynamic process with overlapping findings at individual and adjacent levels. DDD, although controversial in its exact role in patients with back pain, has been shown to be a pain source generator.[3,4] Removal of the pain generator, the intervertebral disc, is a viable and logical approach for selected patients.

Determining the ideal candidate for surgical management of DDD can be more challenging than performing the procedure itself because of the unclear relationship between patient symptoms, diagnostic studies, and surgical outcomes. The patient should have failed conservative management, including oral medication, lifestyle modification, and active rehabilitation, before surgical intervention. To maximize the predictive value of lumbar interbody fusion for the treatment of lumbar disc degeneration, the patient's history should be consistent with mechanical back pain, and radiographic studies should show degeneration at discrete levels. Discography, as discussed in an earlier chapter, is at this point the only diagnostic test in the authors' opinion that can isolate discogenic pain and should reproduce concordant pain and abnormal disc morphology (Fig. 48–1). Patients with a significant behavioral component to their pain should be considered poor surgical candidates. Preoperative psychological screening can be helpful in the evaluation of these patients.[5]

Anterior lumbar interbody fusion (ALIF), as an option for treating DDD, has had a tumultuous history with increasing and decreasing interest and success over the years. ALIF as a procedure favors load transmission through the anterior column, recreates lordosis, restores disc height, and tensions lateral and posterior annular or ligamentous fibers (Fig. 48–2).[6] Direct anterior exposure allows complete removal of disc material, increasing the fusion rate,[7] while avoiding trauma to the posterior musculature, making it an attractive option for the treatment of DDD.

ALIF as a treatment for low back pain was initially performed with varied success. In 1972, Stauffer and Coventry[8] reported 36% good results in 77 patients with lumbar disc rupture. In 1988, Inoue and colleagues[9] reviewed 350 cases of ALIF for disc herniation and found 73% of patients had relief of back pain. Blumenthal and colleagues[10] reported on 34 patients in 1988 with 73% fusion rate and 74% clinically satisfactory results. Loguidice and colleagues[11] found an overall fusion rate of 80% radiographically using various combinations of autograft and allograft interbody spacers. Of 85 patients, 74% responded that the surgery helped.

Anatomy and Approach

ALIF is performed by gaining access to the retroperitoneum. Many techniques have been described to gain access to the anterior lumbar spine (transperitoneal, laparoscopic, open and mini-open retroperitoneal). The mini-open retroperitoneal procedure has become the "workhorse" approach, with mini-open transperitoneal and open procedures saved for revision or salvage procedures. Retroperitoneal and transperitoneal corridors allow complete exposure of the ventral surface of the spine. Centering on the disc space with lateral extension, as needed, allows for a complete discectomy, release of ligamentous structures as indicated for balancing, and placement of a single large interbody implant that matches the vertebral endplate. Avoidance of the posterior musculature reduces postoperative pain and disability associated with extensive muscle stripping, denervation, and devascularization, often noted as a cause of failed back syndrome.

Surgical exposure to the anterior lumbar spine has been described elsewhere. Mini-open access, through either a transverse or a vertical incision, allows visualization from L2 to S1. The rectus can be mobilized medially in its entirety or split in the midline raphe and retracted laterally. Blunt hand dissection allows one to sweep the intraperitoneal contents

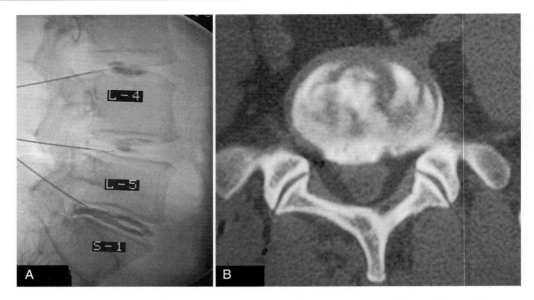

FIGURE 48–1 A, Lateral fluoroscopic image after discography with dye leaking into periphery of abnormal L5-1 disc. **B,** Axial CT scan after discography shows abnormal disc morphology and dye extrusion into peripheral anulus.

superiorly, inferiorly, and medially. The ureter is brought medial, after identification, and deep self-retaining retractors can be placed. Vascular dissection is often performed solely with a sponge stick but may require sharp dissection for adhesions. Vascular structures (i.e., segmental vessels across the bodies) are cauterized or ligated and clipped as needed for exposure. Table-mounted or handheld retractors are employed during the remainder of the interspace preparation and interbody implantation. On completion of the procedure, the wound is inspected for any bleeding, ureter damage, or peritoneal tears. The rectus sheath is approximated with absorbable suture, and the skin is closed with a running subcuticular stitch for cosmesis.

Developed in the 1990s, laparoscopic ALIF achieved early success with its pioneers.[12] Laparoscopic ALIF was reported to be less invasive with less blood loss and faster recovery; however, later reports contradicted these findings, noting no identifiable advantages, added technical challenge, and increased specific complications such as retrograde ejaculation.[13,14]

Indications for Interbody Fusions

Choosing to proceed with operative intervention on the spine should be a joint decision reached by the patient and the physician. Prospective patients should have tried and failed nonoperative management, and the clinical and radiographic picture should correlate to maximize results and patient satisfaction. ALIF can be chosen to aid patients with (1) DDD and the spectrum of clinical and radiographic changes noted under this umbrella term; (2) pain after prior posterior surgery, such as laminectomy in which significant epidural scar may complicate a revision surgery; and (3) significant low back pain with two or more recurrent herniated discs.

Axial back pain caused by the degenerative process of the disc and spine as a whole is currently the main indication for ALIF. By correctly identifying discogenic pain via radiographs, magnetic resonance imaging (MRI), and provocative discography, one can remove the pathologic disc and stabilize the motion segment with an interbody graft. Using an ALIF procedure, patients with associated radicular leg pain secondary to foraminal narrowing can be indirectly decompressed by restoring the foraminal height, elongating redundant posterior and lateral anulus (if not removed), and realigning overlapping incongruent facet joints and more directly decompressed by removing compressive nuclear material.[15,16] Patients with a herniated nucleus pulposus can undergo direct decompression and discectomy via an anterior exposure. Interbody implants placed through an anterior approach can be used alone or in conjunction with posterior fusion techniques for cases requiring a more robust construct, as discussed later in this chapter.

Relative contraindications to anterior interbody approaches include advanced atherosclerosis of the major vessels and obesity. Some consideration should be given to patients who have previously undergone prior abdominal surgery or have inflammatory diseases because these conditions create significant scarring that may increase the risk or preclude one from successful surgery. A transperitoneal approach may be performed as an alternative in these patients.

Interbody Implants and Graft Material

The race between temporary mechanical support and biology has been run since the origins of orthopaedic care. In the spine, the goal of any interbody device is to provide anterior column mechanical support while a bony fusion develops. A single question remains to be answered: How rigid does a

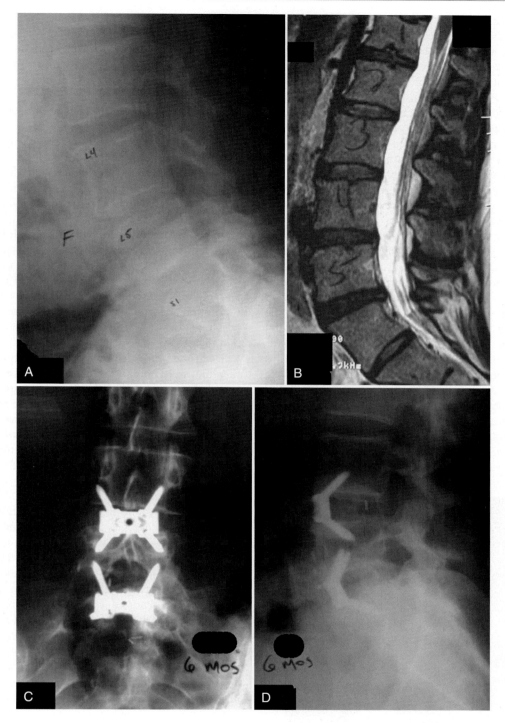

FIGURE 48–2 A-D, Preoperative plain radiograph (**A**) and T2 sagittal MRI (**B**) showing two-level DDD and 6-month postoperative plain anteroposterior (**C**) and lateral (**D**) radiographs. Note significant disc space and foraminal restoration using anterior interbody spacer.

construct need to be to provide early stability without negatively affecting the spine when fusion is present? Creating an unnecessarily stiff construct may lead to stress shielding,[17] additional surgery, and implantation of costly implants; however, too little stiffness leads to biomechanical failure or pseudarthrosis. Pilliar and colleagues[18] showed that small micromotion of 28 μm does not affect bone ingrowth into porous-surfaced implants and large micromotion greater than 150 μm can produce a fibrous interface. Nevertheless, the current consensus seems to be that adequate stabilization must greatly increase the stiffness above the native segment. In vitro studies do not fully recreate in vivo experiences, and individual patient factors, such as bone quality, size, and load demand, are variable and dynamic, complicating the goal.

The first lumbar interbody fusion was reported by Burns[19] in 1933, using a tibial peg to treat spondylolisthesis. Interbody fusion for DDD was described by Harmon[20] in 1963 and then by Crock[2] and Stauffer and Coventry.[8] Early days of interbody grafting incorporated the use of bicortical or tricortical spacers harvested from iliac crest. When used alone, this graft is associated with significant rates of mechanical failure, loss of correction, and pseudarthrosis.[21,22] Sterile allograft (i.e., bone dowels or tricortical grafts) have often been used because they are stronger than equivalent fresh, autologous bone and eliminate the need for autologous harvesting.[23]

Femoral ring allograft (FRA), used frequently, obviates the need for cortical autograft and provides a strut with significant compressive strength,[22,23] incorporates with host bone, and provides a medium easier than metal to evaluate graft incorporation (Fig. 48–3). Previously, allograft rings were fashioned by surgeons on back operating room tables. Now precision machined grafts provide surgeons the option to trial size and implant the most appropriately sized graft to fit the patient's anatomic needs and obtain the most stable construct with the allograft reaching the dense peripheral ring of subchondral bone. To augment fusion, allograft or autograft cancellous bone can be placed in the center of the cortical ring. FRA as a stand-alone intervertebral spacer has been shown to have a high rate of pseudarthrosis and subsidence.[24,25] Anterior or posterior augmentation has been recommended.

Holte and colleagues[26] reported in 1994 on the use of FRA with and without supplemental posterior fixation. These investigators achieved fusion rates of 96% in some cases,

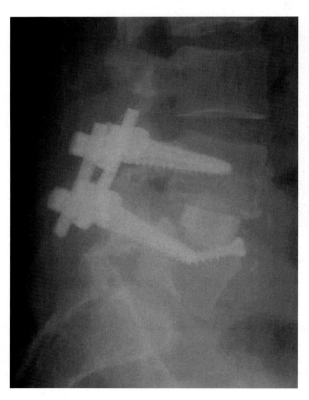

FIGURE 48–3 Single-level 360-degree fusion with FRA and bilateral pedicle screws and rod fixation.

depending on the number of levels fused. Sarwat and colleagues[27] reviewed 43 patients undergoing combined anterior-posterior fusions using FRA packed with cancellous allograft with supplemental posterior fixation; 100% of the one-level fusions and 93% of the two-level fusions were radiographically deemed solid fusions.

The addition of posterior fusion, instrumentation, and cortically lined grafts added to the mechanical stability of these constructs, but surgical time and complications led surgeons to seek other options. Transforaminal lumbar interbody fusion and posterior lumbar interbody fusion allowed surgeons to place interbody grafts from posterior approaches, providing anterior column support and negating anterior exposures. Posterior based surgery has been shown, however, to have increased operative time, patient morbidity, and complications compared with anterior based surgery.[28,29] Also, patient anatomy and the degree of pathology can make achieving an adequate discectomy and ideal graft size and position and placement a challenge. These factors have contributed to less restoration of disc height, less than complete fusion bed preparation, and less mechanical stability at the time of implantation than with ALIF.

Horizontal threaded cylinder cages, typically made from titanium, were brought on the market with huge fanfare but have fallen out of favor. These were originally developed to treat wobbler syndrome, which is a chronic cervical instability causing myelopathy in thoroughbred horses.[30] The U.S. Food and Drug Administration (FDA) investigational device exemption (IDE) studies for the BAK (Zimmer, Warsaw, IN) and Ray TFC (Stryker, Kalamazoo, MI) indicated that threaded cages used as stand-alone devices without supplemental posterior fixation performed well (Fig. 48–4).[31,32] Ray[32] reported his results during the FDA IDE clinical trial using the Ray titanium fusion cages in 236 cases showing 91% fusion rate and 80% average clinical improvement.

Kuslich and colleagues[31] reported on 247 ALIF patients with 24-month follow-up; they observed a fusion rate of 98% among single-level procedures and 80% among two-level procedures. They reported clinical pain improvement from a mean of 5 to 2.9 at 2 years, on a scale of 0 to 6. The functional scores improved from 20.9 preoperative mean to 15.2 at 2-year follow-up, on a 7 to 32 point scale evaluating sitting, walking, and other activities of daily living and recreational activities. Tran and colleagues[33] reported that only 5.2% of their group underwent additional posterior surgery at the same level for unresolved or new-onset pain, supporting the use of stand-alone cages. Preparation of the disc space for threaded cages violates the peripheral subchondral ring of bone, theoretically increasing the risk of subsidence. Although approved for stand-alone interbody fusion, threaded cages were later questioned for their amount of resistance to motion in the unstable spine; some authors adopted a 360-degree approach.[34,35]

The advent of more stable anterior column support allowed surgeons to use less invasive posterior surgical options with stronger biomechanical constructs than with an associated posterolateral fusion.[6] Translaminar screws, facet screws, and percutaneous pedicle screw constructs (termed 270-degree fusions) provided surgeons the additive effect of immediate mechanical strength and long-term fusion stability without necessitating significant posterior fusion bed creation, associated soft tissue devitalization, and patient morbidity (Fig. 48–5).[36-38] Ferrara and colleagues[39] compared pedicle and translaminar facet screws and found both to be reliable constructs with similar properties after 180,000 cycles and recommended that surgeon preference and patient-specific needs could drive the choice. In 2001, Schofferman and colleagues[40] prospectively compared the addition of posterior spinal fusion in patients who had ALIF with pedicle screw instrumentation (360 degrees vs. 270 degrees). These investigators found that posterolateral fusion was associated with greater blood loss, operating room time, and cost, with no significant improvement in the arthrodesis rate; in addition, 68% of posterolateral fusions failed to show radiographic fusion.

Previously, stand-alone anterior interbody grafts were fraught with reported complications, such as migration, subsidence, and pseudarthrosis. As interbody graft technology has progressed, there has been renewed interest, however, in stand-alone anterior interbody fusion, single-approach procedures. Biomechanical studies have reported that stand-alone anterior interbody grafts without fixation are weakest in sheer strength, rotation, and extension.[41] The addition of a blocking screw or plate for FRA and synthetic spacers such as polyetheretherketone (PEEK) has minimized the occurrence of anterior migration. Currently available in PEEK, metal carbon fiber, and machined allograft and other various materials and combinations, interbody synthetic grafts have been optimized compared with their predecessors. Cage design from cylindric to a box shape has led to better matching of the endplate geometry and has been shown to decrease motion at the intervertebral segment.[42] Grant and colleagues,[43] performing a human cadaveric biomechanical investigation, showed that

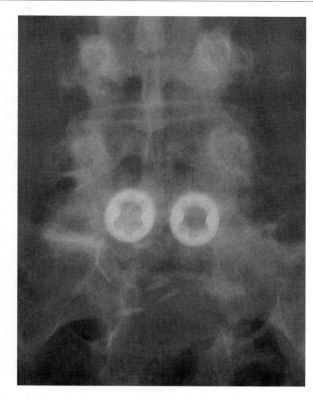

FIGURE 48–4 Anteroposterior radiograph of threaded fusion cages at 1 year, with bone growth across cages.

lumbar endplate density and thickness increased toward the periphery, with the strongest being posterolateral just in front of the pedicles.

With the addition of anterior intersegmental instrumentation, many authors are performing stand-alone anterior

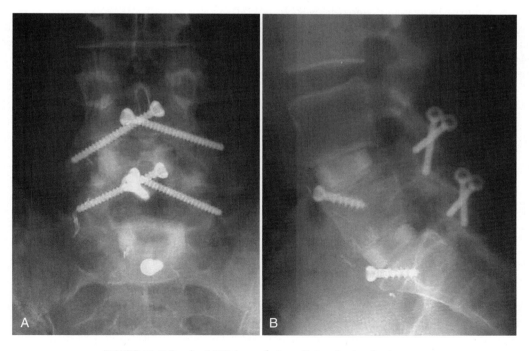

FIGURE 48–5 Two-level 270-degree fusion with translaminar facet screws.

interbody fusions. In 1958, Humphries and Hawk[44] first reported the use of an anterior plate to stabilize the motion segment after ALIF. Potential danger to the great vessels and limited use of the ALIF technique contributed to the early demise of this technique, however. Tzermiadianos and colleagues[45] showed marked in vitro reduction in range of motion using interbody graft with the ATB (Synthes Spine, West Chester, PA); they posited that the ATB may be a biomechanically sound construct, especially compared with additional posterior surgery and its morbidity. Gerber and colleagues[46] noted slightly better motion segment immobilization using pedicle screws versus an anterior plate in cadaveric spines with double-threaded metallic cages.

Larger, more robust, locking and nonlocking plates have been used to augment a stand-alone interbody graft; although effective, these plates require increased exposure and have a large anterior profile. To negate the exposure necessary for plating and minimize soft tissue and vessel irritation, anterior interbody synthetic products with fixation through the graft into the vertebral bodies have been developed. By increasing their stand-alone biomechanical strength to minimize extension and sheer forces, one hopes these products may negate the need for a robust anterior plating and posterior surgery.

Many studies have shown the stability-enhancing effect of integrated anterior instrumentation and a biomechanical argument for stand-alone ALIF (Fig. 48–6). Kuzhupilly and colleagues[37] looked at stand-alone FRA versus industrial FRA with integrated crossed cancellous screws into the adjacent vertebral bodies. They found significant improvement in extension stability only. Le Huec and colleagues[47] tested an anterolateral threaded cage connected to an anterolateral cage and found significant increase in stiffness in all loading directions. No statistical significance was noted whether or not the plate was attached to the cage.

Schleicher and colleagues[48] compared the SynFix-LR (Synthes GmbH, Solothurn, Switzerland) and the STALIF (Centinel Spine, Minneapolis, MN), two stand-alone ALIF cages, and found statistically significant increase in stiffness over the native in vitro segment, with the SynFix-LR, a locking four-screw implant, showing a higher stabilizing effect in lateral bending than the STALIF. Flexion-extension finite element analysis revealed that the cage bears most of the force in flexion, and the screws and the screw-plate interface take most of the stress in extension. Cain and colleagues[49] showed the SynFix-LR had equal stiffness versus 270-degree and 360-degree constructs. The test device showed a higher ability to withstand axial torque compared with standard pedicle screw instrumentation. At the present time, a few products have FDA approval for stand-alone interbody use, with many more devices seeking approval.

Most current implants allow the incorporation of graft material to augment the fusion process. Historically, the "gold standard" has been autogenous morcellized bone graft; however, to minimize patient morbidity, allograft and biologic materials have been developed. Multiple studies have evaluated allograft efficacy in fusion patients as extenders and stand-alone with good results.[50] The addition of the recombinant human bone morphogenetic protein (rhBMP-2) InFUSE (Medtronic, Memphis, TN) has been shown to promote osteoinduction and to stimulate early incorporation of grafts (Fig. 48–7).[51,52] Burkus and colleagues[52] reported 100% fusion rate with stand-alone interbody fusion using threaded cylinder allograft dowels with rhBMP compared with autograft. Pradhan and colleagues[53] showed, however, that the use of rhBMP-2 with stand-alone FRA can lead to an aggressive early osteoclastic response causing graft and endplate osteolysis with potential subsidence risk. These authors believed augmenting with intersegmental instrumentation can support the FRA with bone morphogenetic protein during this mechanically vulnerable time.

Circumferential Fusion

Circumferential fusion is often indicated in patients with significant instability (i.e., trauma, postlaminectomy), significant bone loss (i.e., trauma, osteomyelitis), high risk for

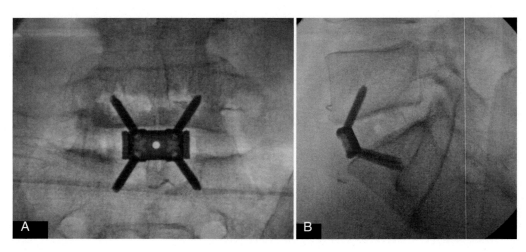

FIGURE 48–6 A and **B,** Anteroposterior (**A**) and lateral (**B**) intraoperative fluoroscopic images with L5-S1 single-level stand-alone interbody graft with incorporated hardware.

nonunion (i.e., multilevel, tobacco users), or osteoporosis.[54,55] To increase fusion rates, decrease subsidence risk, and maximize construct stiffness, many surgeons adopted posterior instrumentation, including pedicle screw–based systems, translaminar screws, or facet fixation. There is no question that the addition of posterior instrumentation provides greater construct rigidity; however, the ideal amount of micromotion to stimulate fusion while structurally stabilizing the motion segment until fusion occurs has yet to be determined. Pedicle screw–based instrumentation has been shown to decrease the subsidence rate associated with interbody allografts and cylindric cages.[56] The disadvantages of posterior supplementation include increased operative time, increased blood loss, increased cost, and potentially a more difficult recovery for patients. Factors for and against posterior instrumentation are present in all cases and must be weighed carefully to optimize patient outcome and minimize morbidity.

Postoperative Management

Patient-controlled analgesia is instituted for pain control and weaned as bowel function and oral tolerance allow. The patient is mobilized the day of surgery, starting with chair transfers and assisted ambulation. A liquid diet is started after surgery and progressed as tolerated. For stand-alone one-level anterior fusions, hospital stay is typically 1 to 3 days, based on patient type and surgery performed. Bracing is variable, dependent on stability of fixation and surgeon specific, ranging from an abdominal binder for comfort and incision healing to a rigid thoracolumbosacral orthosis until clear evidence of fusion has occurred. The addition of instrumentation, bone morphogenetic proteins, and similar substances may obviate the need for rigid bracing. Activity should include limited bending and twisting motions, and lifting initially should be limited to 10 lb or less. Return to activities of daily living is progressively allowed and encouraged. Return to work and sport depends on the patient and surgeon, based on the patient's requirements, status of fusion, and fixation method.

Evaluation of fusion progression can be difficult in the presence of an interbody graft. Evaluation of fusions that is 100% reliable is available only with histologic examination, which is rarely possible or done. Radiolucent and nonferromagnetic implants such as carbon fiber and polymer synthetics have been developed to allow better visualization of surrounding bone and soft tissues on plain radiographs, MRI, and computed tomography (CT). Cizek and Boyd[57] evaluated cadaveric implant models radiographically and found neither CT nor radiographic interpretation reliable. Evidence of a fusion can be evaluated by the following radiographic features: (1) no motion on flexion-extension films (<5 degrees has been accepted as fused in the literature and by the FDA, which the authors believe is too lenient); (2) anterior or posterior bridging bone across the disc space, termed sentinel sign[58]; (3) bridging trabecular bone across the intervertebral space and endplates; and (4) the absence of "a windshield wiping halo," or lucency around instrumentation indicating implant motion.

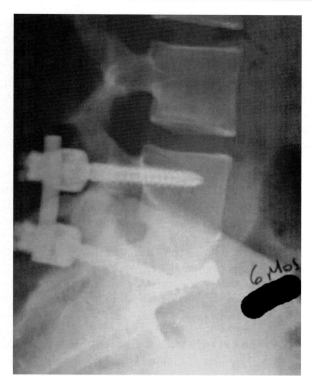

FIGURE 48–7 Six-month follow-up lateral radiograph of graft using femoral ring allograft and bone morphogenetic protein, with posterior bilateral pedicle screws showing bone bridging and solid fusion.

Complications

The incidence of complications in ALIF is often difficult to assess because of the different types of procedures, surgeons performing them, implants used, and experience of the operative team. Poor outcome is the number one surgical complication, and poor patient selection is often to blame; one must be vigilant in diagnostic workup and adhere to surgeries that address the patient's pain generators.

Vascular injury to the common iliac vessels with L5-S1 exposure is most commonly seen. Clear identification of the disc space before discectomy must be obtained and maintained during the operation. In particular, the common iliac vein, being compressible and dorsal to the artery, can be mistaken for soft tissue during the approach. The iliolumbar vein, also termed the *ascending lumbar vein,* is at risk during approaches to the L4-5 interspace and should be controlled as dictated by the amount of exposure necessary. Some surgeons believe ligation of this vessel should be obtained in 100% of exposures to minimize the risk of tearing during retraction. Arterial thrombosis from aggressive retraction or injury or both has also been reported.[59,60]

Retrograde ejaculation as result of hypogastric plexus injury has been reported to range from 8%[61] to 0.4%.[62] In one of the largest single ALIF trials to date, Kuslich and colleagues[31] reported a 4% rate in 591 patients. Loguidice and colleagues[11] in 58 patients and Brau[63] in 686 exposures each noted only 1 case of retrograde ejaculation. The preaortic (prevertebral) sympathetic plexus runs along the anterolateral edge of the vertebral bodies, adjacent to the psoas, then traverses over the aortic bifurcation and common iliac vessels forming the hypogastric plexus. Blunt dissection to mobilize the more cephalad prevertebral plexus before the hypogastric plexus can aid the exposure. Aggressive electrocautery should be minimized during the approach in this area and during the disc space preparation. Male patients should be counseled on this potential adverse event and advised that there also is a chance of spontaneous recovery. If the patient is concerned, he can predonate and store sperm.

Injury to the alimentary tract can be minimized by packing the peritoneum behind self-retaining retractors. Postoperative ileus occurs and can be effectively managed with restricted oral intake, proper fluid hydration, and gastric suction as indicated. Damage to the ureter, rare in primary cases, can be minimized in revision cases with proper identification and the placement of preoperative ureteral stents.

Implant-related complications, such as graft subsidence, malposition, extrusion, and pseudarthrosis, as alluded to previously in this chapter, can be minimized with careful patient selection, careful implant selection, and meticulous discectomy to optimize the fusion bed without disrupting the structural integrity of the subchondral bony endplates.

Revisions

Indications for returning to the anterior spine include adjacent level disease, implant failure or migration causing neurovascular compromise, and pseudarthrosis. A meticulous approach minimizing dissection during the primary surgery can reduce the risks associated with dissection and grafting of reoperations for adjacent level disease. In patients undergoing an L4-5 procedure after prior L5-S1 exposure, the risk of vascular, ureteral, and neurogenic injury can be minimized by avoiding the prior L5-S1 exposure between the iliac vessels and concentrating on the cephalad tissue dissection. Products to decrease postoperative scar and to allow easier revision dissection are being developed and tested. A product creating a safe plane for dissection and mobilization of the major vessels would be useful. One must also be cautious when approaching inflammatory patients with disease or postinfections because these patients often form abundant fibrous material and adhesions anterior to the vertebral motion segments and can be as difficult to treat as patients undergoing revision surgery.

Conclusion

DDD causing chronic mechanical low back pain results in significant functional, social, and psychological consequences in patients. Patients, employers, and payers have sought answers for this multibillion dollar problem. ALIF offers an effective surgical treatment for patients with lumbar DDD who have failed nonoperative treatment. Mini-open approaches have minimized patient morbidity. Anterior interbody grafts allow and have significantly improved anterior column support, while maximizing bony fusion opportunities. The addition of allograft and bone morphogenetic protein has decreased patient morbidity and accelerated fusion rates. Integrated interbody grafts with fixation have allowed surgeons the option of single-approach stand-alone anterior constructs with excellent radiographic and clinical outcomes.

ALIF has evolved through many different permutations. To date, the most used and reliable is an anterior interbody graft with supplemental posterior instrumentation. Currently developed and used implants with biologic agents have renewed interest in anterior-only, stand-alone techniques. The future of lumbar fusion and the need for interbody grafting is questionable in the face of total disc arthroplasty and future degenerative disc treatments; however, it currently offers an option for patients and physicians treating one of the most disabling and costly problems in the United States.

PEARLS AND PITFALLS

1. Careful patient selection is the key to successful surgery and maximization of outcomes.

2. Meticulous disc space preparation that avoids endplate violation is important for proper fit of the implant.

3. Selection of an implant depends on the disc space anatomy to allow the best fit and contact with endplates.

4. An implant of the proper height should be selected to restore "normal" disc height avoiding overdistraction.

KEY POINTS

1. Knowledge of the retroperitoneal anatomy is essential.

2. ALIF is a safe and effective procedure in the hands of experienced spine surgeons.

3. A wide variety of graft materials and constructs are available with varying degrees of stability that may or may not necessitate posterior fixation.

4. Complications can be kept to a minimum with careful surgical technique.

KEY REFERENCES

1. Burkus JK, Gornet MF, Dickman CA, et al: Anterior lumbar interbody fusion using rhBMP-2 with tapered interbody cages. J Spinal Disord Tech 15:337-349, 2002.
   This article provides strong evidence in favor of the use of bone morphogenetic protein as an alternative to harvesting iliac crest autograft for patients undergoing ALIF.

2. Brau S: Mini-open approach to the spine for anterior lumbar interbody fusion: Description of the procedure, results and complications. Spine (Phila Pa 1976) 2:216-223, 2002.
   This article presents a single surgeon's experience with 686 cases illustrating a very low complication rate associated with a mini-open approach to the anterior spine.

3. Cain CM, Schleicher P, Gerlach R, et al: A new stand-alone anterior lumbar interbody fusion device: Biomechanical comparison with established fixation techniques. Spine (Phila Pa 1976) 30:2631-2636, 2005.

This article provides early in vitro biomechanical evidence for stand-alone ALIF using an integrated interbody device with screw fixation. The future success of these devices remains to be seen; however, they are an attractive option to decrease patient morbidity associated with posterior based surgery.

4. Schofferman J, Slosar P, Reynolds J, et al: A prospective randomized comparison of 270 degrees fusions to 360 degrees fusions (circumferential fusions). Spine (Phila Pa 1976) 26:E207-E212, 2001.

The authors of this article challenge the need for posterolateral fusion in the setting of ALIF with anterior column support and pedicle screw fixation. They illustrate equal clinical outcomes and fusion rates with decreased cost, blood loss, and operative time.

5. Stauffer RN, Coventry MB: Anterior interbody lumbar spine fusion: Analysis of Mayo Clinic series. J Bone Joint Surg Am 54:756-768, 1972.

Early proponents of ALIF described the procedure as an alternative for patients who had previously undergone posterior decompressive surgery with persistent symptoms. Current proponents continue to praise the avoidance of revision canal surgery while providing anterior column support, restoration of disc height and lordosis, and indirect decompression of the neural elements.

REFERENCES

1. Katz JN: Lumbar disc disorders and low-back pain: Socioeconomic factors and consequences. J Bone Joint Surg Am 88(Suppl 2):21-24, 2006.

2. Crock HV: A reappraisal of intervertebral disc lesions. Med J Aust 16:983-989, 1970.

3. Freemont AJ, Peacock TE, Gourille P, et al: Nerve ingrowth into diseased intervertebral disc in chronic back pain. Lancet 350:178-181, 1997.

4. Weinstein J, Claverie W, Gibson S: The pain of discography. Spine (Phila Pa 1976) 13:1344-1348, 1988.

5. Block AR, Ohnmeiss DD, Guyer RD, et al: The use of presurgical psychological screening to predict the outcome of spine surgery. Spine J 1:274-282, 2001.

6. Evans JH: Biomechanics of lumbar fusion. Clin Orthop Relat Res 193:38-46, 1985.

7. McAfee PC, Lee GA, Fedder IL, et al: Anterior BAK instrumentation and fusion: Complete versus partial discectomy. Clin Orthop Relat Res 394:55-63, 2002.

8. Stauffer RN, Coventry MB: Anterior interbody lumbar spine fusion: Analysis of Mayo Clinic series. J Bone Joint Surg Am 54:756-768, 1972.

9. Inoue S, Watanabe T, Goto S, et al: Degenerative spondylolisthesis: Pathophysiology and results of anterior interbody fusion. Clin Orthop Relat Res 227:90-98, 1988.

10. Blumenthal SL, Baker J, Dossett A, et al: The role of anterior lumbar fusion for internal disc disruption. Spine (Phila Pa 1976) 13:566-569, 1988.

11. Loguidice VA, Johnson RG, Guyer RD, et al: Anterior lumbar interbody fusion. Spine (Phila Pa 1976) 13:366-369, 1988.

12. Regan JJ, Aronoff RJ, Ohnmeiss DD, et al: Laparoscopic approach to L4-L5 for interbody fusion using BAK cages: Experience in the first 58 cases. Spine (Phila Pa 1976) 24:2171-2174, 1999.

13. Zdeblick TA, David SM: A prospective comparison of surgical approach for anterior L4-L5 fusion: Laparoscopic versus mini anterior lumbar interbody fusion. Spine (Phila Pa 1976) 25:2682-2687, 2000.

14. Escobar E, Transfeldt E, Garvey T, et al: Video-assisted versus open lumbar spine fusion surgery: A comparison of four techniques and complications in 135 patients. Spine (Phila Pa 1976) 28:729-732, 2003.

15. Chen D, Fay LA, Lok J, et al: Increasing neuroforaminal volume by anterior interbody distraction in degenerative lumbar spine. Spine (Phila Pa 1976) 20:74-79, 1995.

16. Sandu HS, Turner S, Kabo JM, et al: Distractive properties of a threaded interbody fusion device: An in vivo model. Spine (Phila Pa 1976) 21:1201-1210, 1996.

17. Craven TG, Carson WL, Asher MA, et al: The effects of implant stiffness on the bypassed bone mineral density and facet fusion stiffness of the canine spine. Spine (Phila Pa 1976) 19:1664-1673, 1994.

18. Pilliar RM, Lee JM, Maniatopoulous C: Observations on the effect of movement on bone ingrowth into porous-surfaced implants. Clin Orthop Relat Res 208:108-113, 1986.

19. Burns BH: An operation for spondylolisthesis. Lancet 1:1233-1239, 1933.

20. Harmon PH: Anterior excision and vertebral body fusion operation for intervertebral disk syndromes of the lower lumbar spine: Three-to five-year results in 244 cases. Clin Orthop Relat Res 26:107-127, 1963.

21. Siff TE Kanaric E, Noble PC, et al: Femoral ring versus fibular strut allografts in anterior lumbar interbody arthrodesis: A biomechanical analysis. Spine (Phila Pa 1976) 24:659-665, 1999.

22. Janssen ME, Nguyen C, Beckham R, et al: Biologic cages. Eur Spine J 9(Suppl 1):S102-S109, 2000.

23. Summers BN, Eisenstein SN: Donor site pain from the ilium: A complication of lumbar spine fusion. J Bone Joint Surg Br 71:677-680, 1989.

24. Flynn JC, Hogue MA: Anterior fusion of the lumbar spine: End-result study with long-term follow-up. J Bone Joint Surg Am 61:1143-1150, 1979.

25. Kumar A, Kozak JA, Doherty BJ, et al: Interspace distraction and graft subsidence after anterior lumbar fusion with femoral strut allograft. Spine (Phila Pa 1976) 18:2393-2400, 1993.

26. Holte DC, O'Brien JP, Renton P: Anterior lumbar fusion using a hybrid interbody graft: A preliminary radiographic report. Eur Spine J 3:32-38, 1994.

27. Sarwat AM, O'Brien JP, Renton P, et al: The use of allograft (and avoidance of autograft) in anterior lumbar interbody fusion: A critical analysis. Eur Spine J 10:237-241, 2001.

28. Fritzell P, Hagg O, Wessberg P, et al: Chronic low back pain and fusion: A comparison of three surgical techniques: A prospective multicenter randomized study from the Swedish Lumbar Spine Study Group. Spine (Phila Pa 1976) 27:1131-1141, 2002.

29. Scaduto AA, Gamradt SC, Yu WD, et al: Perioperative complications of threaded cylindrical lumbar interbody fusion devices: Anterior versus posterior approach. J Spinal Disord Tech 16:502-507, 2003.

30. DeBowes RM, Grant BD, Bagby GW, et al: Cervical vertebral interbody fusion in the horse: A comparative study of bovine xenografts and autografts supported by stainless steel baskets. Am J Vet Res 45:191-199, 1984.

31. Kuslich SD, Ulstrom CL, Griffith SL, et al: The Bagby and Kuslich method of lumbar interbody fusion: History, techniques, and 2-year follow-up results of a United States prospective, multicenter trial. Spine (Phila Pa 1976) 23:1267-1278, 1998.

32. Ray CD: Threaded titanium cages for lumbar interbody fusions. Spine (Phila Pa 1976) 22:667-679, 1997.

33. Tran V, Ohnmeiss DD, Blumenthal SL, et al: Analysis of reoperations when using cages as stand-alone devices: Minimum three year follow-up study. Presented at Meeting of the Americas, New York, 2002.

34. Oxland TR, Lund T: Biomechanics of stand-alone cages and cages in combination with posterior fixation: A literature review. Eur Spine J 9(Suppl 1):S95-S101, 2000.

35. Cagli SJ, Crawford NR, Sonntag VK, et al: Biomechanics of grade I degenerative lumbar spondylolisthesis. Part 2: Treatment with threaded interbody cages/dowels and pedicle screws. J Neurosurg 94(1 Suppl):51-60, 2001.

36. Rathonyi GC, Oxland TR, Gerich U, et al: The role of supplemental translaminar screws in anterior lumbar interbody fixation: A biomechanical study. Eur Spine J 7:400-407, 1998.

37. Kuzhupilly RR, Lieberman IH, McLain RF, et al: In vitro stability of FRA spacers with integrated crossed screws for anterior lumbar interbody fusion. Spine (Phila Pa 1976) 27(9):923-928, 2002.

38. Volkman T, Horton WC, Hutton WC: Transfacet screws with lumbar interbody reconstruction: Biomechanical study of motion segment stiffness. J Spinal Disord 9:425-432, 1996.

39. Ferrara LA, Secor JL, Jin BH, et al: A biomechanical comparison of facet and pedicle screw fixation: Effects of short-term and long-term repetitive cycling. Spine (Phila Pa 1976) 28:1226-1234, 2003.

40. Schofferman J, Slosar P, Reynolds J, et al: A prospective randomized comparison of 270 degrees fusions to 360 degrees fusions (circumferential fusions). Spine (Phila Pa 1976) 26:E207-E12, 2001.

41. Pizen T, Matthis D, Steudel WI: The effect of posterior instrumentation following PLIF with BAK cages is most pronounced in weak bone. Acta Neurochir (Wien) 144:121-128, 2002.

42. Tsantrizos A, Andreou A, Aebi M, et al: Biomechanical stability of five stand-alone anterior lumbar interbody fusion constructs. Eur Spine J 9:14-22, 2000.

43. Grant JP, Oxland TR, Dvorak MF: Mapping the structural properties of the lumbosacral vertebral endplates. Spine (Phila Pa 1976) 26:889-896, 2001.

44. Humphries AW, Hawk WA: Anterior fusion of the lumbar spine using an internal fixative device. Surg Forum 9:770-773, 1958.

45. Tzermiadianos MN, Mekhail A, Voronov LI, et al: Enhancing the stability of anterior lumbar interbody fusion: A biomechanical comparison of anterior plate versus posterior transpedicular instrumentation. Spine (Phila Pa 1976) 33:E38-E43, 2008.

46. Gerber M, Crawford NR, Chamberlain RH, et al: Biomechanical assessment of anterior lumbar interbody fusion with an anterior lumbosacral fixation screw-plate: Comparison to stand-alone anterior lumbar interbody fusion and anterior lumbar interbody fusion with pedicle screws in an unstable human cadaver model. Spine (Phila Pa 1976) 31:762-768, 2006.

47. Le Huec J, Liu M, Skalli W, et al: Lumbar lateral interbody cage with plate augmentation: In vitro biomechanical analysis. Eur Spine J 11:130-136, 2002.

48. Schleicher P, Gerlach R, Schar B, et al: Biomechanical comparison of two different concepts for stand alone anterior lumbar interbody fusion. Eur Spine J 17:1757-1765, 2008.

49. Cain CM, Schleicher P, Gerlach R, et al: A new stand-alone anterior lumbar interbody fusion device: Biomechanical comparison with established fixation techniques. Spine (Phila Pa 1976) 30:2631-2636, 2005.

50. Hashimoto T, Shigenobu K, Kanayama M, et al: Clinical results of single-level posterior lumbar interbody fusion using the Brantigan I/F carbon cage filled with a mixture of local morselized bone and bioactive ceramic granules. Spine (Phila Pa 1976) 27:258-262, 2002.

51. Boden SD, Zdeblick TA, Sandhu HS, et al: The use of rhBMP-2 in interbody fusion cages: Definitive evidence of osteoinduction in humans: A preliminary report. Spine (Phila Pa 1976) 25:376-381, 2000.

52. Burkus JK, Gornet MF, Dickman CA, et al: Anterior lumbar interbody fusion using rhBMP-2 with tapered interbody cages. J Spinal Disord Tech 15:337-349, 2002.

53. Pradhan BB, Bae HW, Kropf MA, et al: Kyphoplasty reduction of osteoporotic vertebral compression fractures: Correction of local kyphosis versus overall sagittal alignment. Spine (Phila Pa 1976) 31:435-441, 2006.

54. O'Brien JP, Dawson MH, Heard CW: Simultaneous combined anterior and posterior fusion: A surgical solution for failed spinal surgery with a brief review of the first 150 patients. Clin Orthop 203:191-195, 1986.

55. Enker P, Steffe AD: Interbody fusion and instrumentation. Clin Orthop 300:90-101, 1994.

56. Shetty AP, Osti OL, Abraham G, et al: Cylindrical threaded cages for lumbar degenerative disc disease: A prospective long term radiological study. Presented at International Society for the Study of the Lumbar Spine, Adelaide, Australia, 2000.

57. Cizek GR, Boyd LM: Imaging pitfalls of interbody spinal implants. Spine (Phila Pa 1976) 25:2633-2636, 2000.

58. McAfee PC: Interbody fusion cages in reconstructive operations on the spine. J Bone Joint Surg Am 81:859-880, 1999.

59. Rajaraman V, Vingan R, Roth P, et al: Visceral and vascular complications resulting from anterior lumbar interbody fusion. J Neurosurg 91(1 Suppl):60-64, 1999.

60. Hackenberg L, Liljenqvist U, Halm H, et al: Occlusion of the left common iliac artery and consecutive thromboembolism of the

49 CHAPTER

Posterior Lumbar Interbody Fusion

Nathan H. Lebwohl, MD

The technique of posterior lumbar interbody fusion (PLIF) has become an important part of the modern spine surgeon's armamentarium. This was not always so; for nearly half a century after the introduction of this technique, it was performed routinely by only a handful of surgeons. Most surgeons condemned the technique as unnecessary, technically difficult, or even dangerous.[1,2] Controversy persists regarding the safety of PLIF compared with other approaches to the intervertebral space and regarding the benefit that PLIF adds to the outcome of surgical treatment for various spinal pathologies.

PLIF is an operation in which the disc space is exposed from a posterior approach, similar to that used in a discectomy, and a fusion is performed by directly grafting the intervertebral space. Classically, PLIF is performed via bilateral exposure of the disc space, with some retraction of the dura to expose the disc. When PLIF was first described, before the era of spinal instrumentation, advocates of the operation argued that it prevented collapse of the disc space after discectomy and maintained the height of the neural foramen, keeping the root free of bony compression. These advocates also believed that placing bone graft directly in the disc space would more likely result in healing of the fusion because the bone would be subject to compressive forces. Critics argued that the operation required excessive epidural dissection and nerve root retraction with a high risk of dural tear, epidural fibrosis, nerve root injury, and chronic arachnoiditis and that graft displacement could lead to late neurologic compromise.

Historical Perspective

Attempts to identify the first surgeon to perform an interbody fusion from a posterior approach are muddled by several reports appearing in the published literature beginning in 1944,[3-5] but no one disputes that credit for initially developing the techniques and key principles of the operation as it is practiced today belongs to Cloward,[6] who emphasized the importance of a wide exposure of the spinal canal to minimize nerve root injuries, the use of structural graft to prevent

intervertebral collapse, and the complete removal of nuclear material from the disc space and replacement with bone to promote fusion. Cloward was widely criticized for his operation, probably as much because he advocated that it be included as part of the routine surgical treatment for all lumbar disc herniations as for the frequency of poor outcomes and complications when it was attempted by other surgeons. A few surgeons embraced Cloward's operation, and several large surgical series were published in the literature reporting good outcomes and high fusion rates.[7-10] Widespread interest in and acceptance of PLIF as a valuable technique did not occur, however, until the introduction of pedicle screw instrumentation.

With the early generation of pedicle instrumentation, screw fracture was a common occurrence. Fracture especially occurred if a dramatic change in spinal alignment was achieved, such as in the reduction of a high-grade spondylolisthesis. Even without large changes in alignment, screw fracture occurred commonly in overweight patients or when the disc space was distracted.[11] In those cases, the mechanical loads that the instrumentation was subjected to exceeded the fatigue properties of the screws. Surgeons, in particular Steffee and Sitkowski,[12] recognized that a structural graft placed in the disc space would divert some of the load, decreasing the forces on the posterior instrumentation, and reduce the frequency of instrumentation failure. Steffee and Sitkowski[12] reported their experiences with reduction of high-grade spondylolisthesis. In each of the first three patients treated with pedicle screws, the instrumentation failed, and alignment was lost. In the next 11 patients, an interbody graft was placed. All of these patients developed solid fusions with no loss of alignment. With PLIF, the load-sharing anterior column support could be added to protect the pedicle screws without the need for a separate anterior incision (Fig. 49–1).

Simultaneous with the benefit of PLIF on reducing failures of the new instrumentation, pedicle instrumentation had a beneficial effect on the outcome of PLIF surgery. For the first time, rigid fixation was available that could effectively stabilize the lumbar spine after laminectomy. This fixation virtually eliminated the complication of graft displacement that had previously been associated with PLIF in some surgeons' hands.

The addition of instrumentation also improved the fusion rate of PLIF. Many of the previously held objections to PLIF surgery were no longer applicable when PLIF was combined with pedicle instrumentation.

Another development that favored the adoption of PLIF was the invention of the interbody fusion cage by Brantigan and the titanium mesh cage by Harms. Their designs eliminated the need to harvest a structural graft from the iliac crest, which was a major source of morbidity previously associated with the PLIF procedure. The cage provided the structure,[13] and the osteogenic potential for fusion came from cancellous bone packed into the cage, which could be obtained from the iliac crest more easily than a structural graft, with less injury to the patient. Before the invention of the cages, it was possible to avoid the morbidity associated with graft harvest by using allograft bone, as advocated by Cloward.[14,15] Concerns about availability, disease transmission, healing potential, delayed healing, and wide variation in the structural integrity of available grafts all contributed to the limited enthusiasm for the use of allograft bone for interbody fusion.[16,17] The availability of cages overcame another common objection to the PLIF operation.

The availability of pedicle screw instrumentation and intervertebral cages contributed to progressively greater acceptance of the operation first pioneered by Cloward. Better alignment and higher fusion rates are routinely achieved using these devices. The training of surgeons and marketing of these devices by their manufacturers have also contributed to wider adoption of PLIF in surgical practice. Not all of these devices have proven to be successful, however. Cylindric threaded fusion cages enjoyed brief popularity as PLIF devices that did not require supplementary fixation, but mediocre results and high complication rates associated with their use resulted in their virtual disappearance as a posterior spinal implant.[18] The clinical experience with threaded implants and the study of the relevant biomechanics have helped surgeons understand the PLIF operation better, however, and develop the operation that is currently performed. Although more recent advances, such as the development of the transforaminal and direct lateral approaches to the disc space, have decreased the frequency with which PLIF is performed, PLIF remains an important and powerful tool for spinal surgeons.

Indications for Interbody Fusion

Some surgeons believe that an interbody fusion is indicated whenever a lumbar fusion is done. They argue that the intervertebral space is biologically and mechanically superior for fusion compared with the intertransverse plane because of the larger surface area of the highly vascular bony endplate and because the interbody bone graft is subject to compressive forces. In addition, they criticize the large amount of muscle damage that occurs from exposure of the spine for posterolateral fusion. Despite these theoretical advantages, it is difficult to show clinical superiority of interbody fusions over posterolateral fusions for most lumbar degenerative conditions, and most published studies comparing the techniques reveal

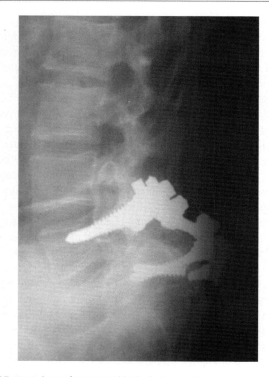

FIGURE 49–1 Screw fracture and loss of alignment is a common complication after reduction of spondylolisthesis if anterior column support is not added.

similar outcomes regardless of what fusion technique is used.[19-21] There are, however, certain circumstances when interbody fusion offers definite advantages. Adding an interbody fusion to a posterolateral fusion increases the rate of achieving successful arthrodesis. This is especially true when a long fusion extends to the sacrum, which is historically associated with a high risk of lumbosacral pseudarthrosis.[22]

Some authors have argued that interbody fusion should be combined with posterolateral fusion in other patients at high risk for failed fusion, such as smokers.[23] In patients with pseudarthrosis after failed posterolateral fusion, an interbody fusion is a good salvage operation, allowing the fusion to occur in a well-vascularized bony bed rather than attempting fusion again in the scarred devascularized posterolateral space.[24] Interbody fusion offers a particular advantage in the treatment of scoliosis and kyphosis or flatback deformities. The destabilizing effect of disc space preparation facilitates rotational correction, and distraction of the intervertebral space allows correction of segmental kyphosis and asymmetrical tilt of the vertebrae. In patients with isthmic spondylolisthesis who undergo deformity reduction, it has been well shown that an interbody graft offers a biomechanical advantage, which protects instrumentation by load sharing, helping to maintain the alignment achieved at surgery. Also, the L5 transverse process is often hypoplastic in these patients, so the increased bone surface area of the vertebral endplate offers a vastly larger area to which bone can fuse.

Most series evaluating the role of interbody fusion in isthmic spondylolisthesis show substantial clinical and radiographic benefit.[25,26] Finally, the most common indication for interbody fusion, but probably the most controversial, is ablation of the disc space in patients with discogenic pain.[27,28] Many advocates for surgical treatment of this entity argue that only interbody fusion can completely remove motion of the painful disc and that complete removal of nuclear material is necessary to eliminate the anatomic source of pain.

Regardless of the indication, interbody fusion can be performed from anterior and posterior approaches. The relative advantages of these approaches are influenced by many factors, and it is essential that the spinal surgeon be well trained in various approaches so that the most appropriate one can be chosen for each unique clinical situation. Specific advantages of the posterior approach include the ability simultaneously to decompress the spinal canal directly and stabilize the spine more effectively with instrumentation. Although safe techniques of anterior fixation have become available more recently, if multilevel instrumentation is needed, posterior approaches are preferred. In patients with spinal deformity, bilateral facet resection allows more effective destabilization of the motion segment, allowing greater corrections than can be obtained by anterior disc removal alone, again favoring a posterior approach to the intervertebral disc. Posterior approaches avoid manipulation of the great vessels, of special concern in patients with atherosclerosis or a history of venous thrombosis. Also, posterior approaches avoid injury to the hypogastric plexus, which can result in retrograde ejaculation and sterility, so they are generally preferred in young men.

When there has been extensive posterior surgery and scarring, anterior approaches to the disc space avoid the increased risks of dural tear and nerve root injury associated with reoperation on the spinal canal. If a conjoined root is identified on preoperative imaging, the risk of root injury is also higher, and an anterior approach is preferred. A wider exposure of the disc space can also be achieved anteriorly, theoretically allowing better preparation of the endplates and more complete packing of the interspace with bone graft. Some surgeons prefer the anterior approach in patients at high risk for pseudarthrosis. An anterior approach may also be preferred when trying to increase lordosis. Dividing the anterior longitudinal ligament may allow for greater anterior distraction and more lordosis. Despite this theoretical advantage, in the author's experience, anterior approaches are more effective than posterior approaches in achieving lordosis only when the facet joints are highly mobile or have first been resected through a posterior approach.

Biomechanics of Interbody Fusion

An appreciation of the mechanical properties of the spine after interbody fusion is essential to understanding the benefits and pitfalls of this operation. It seems intuitively obvious that placing a solid block in the disc space would prevent flexion of the vertebral motion segment. This is what occurs—whether the graft is placed from an anterior or a posterior approach. This fact has important implications for protection of posterior instrumentation. Interbody grafts significantly decrease the strain in posterior spinal implants when they are subjected to compression or flexion loads, which are the common modes of failure of these constructs in clinical practice. Various authors have shown that placing intervertebral cages decreases forces and strain in posterior implants by 56% to 80%,[29,30] and the clinical benefit of establishing anterior load sharing to prevent implant and construct failure is well established (Fig. 49-2).[31]

Increasing stability when the spine is subject to flexion loading does not mean that the spine is more stable when

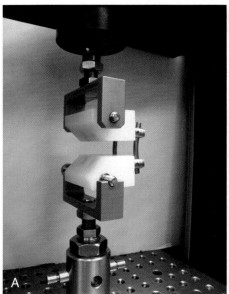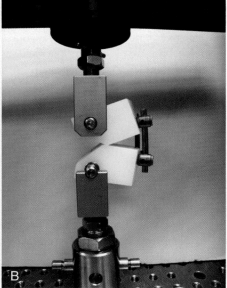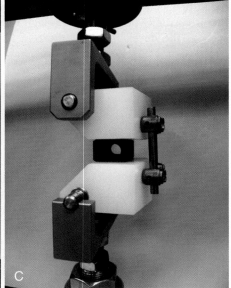

FIGURE 49–2 These photographs dramatically show reduction in strain on posterior implants when a cage is placed in intervertebral disc space. This model of a spinal motion segment with pedicle screw fixation has no anterior column support. **A,** Alignment with no load applied. **B,** Loss of alignment with only 700 N of load, the physiologic equivalent of standing in place. **C,** Protective effect of an implant placed in disc space. (Courtesy Hassan Serhan, PhD.)

subject to forces in every direction. After interbody graft placement, the motion segment is more unstable in certain directions. The pattern of instability is determined to a great extent by the direction from which the graft is placed and represents the destabilizing effect of the surgical approach[32] and the preparation of the disc space. Grafts placed from an anterior approach result in increased motion when force is applied in extension; this likely represents the effect of dividing the anterior longitudinal ligament. Grafts placed from a posterior approach result in increased axial rotation of the motion segment owing to the resection of the posterior facet complexes necessary to avoid excessive dural retraction.[33-37] The design of the cage—vertical, box, or threaded and whether or not the cage engages the endplates—does not seem to matter with regard to the patterns of instability created by intervertebral placement. Only the structures sacrificed during the approach to the disc are important in determining instability of the final construct (Fig. 49–3).[38,39]

Most surgeons make the assumption that a PLIF procedure is a stabilizing operation. The biomechanical data show that this is not entirely true. Understanding that placing an interbody graft or cage can lead to destabilization of the motion segment in certain directions is important for understanding why interbody fusion done without supplementary fixation has a high failure rate, especially when done from a posterior approach. Proponents of threaded fusion cages, which were designed to be used without supplementary fixation, argued that distraction of the disc space would stabilize the motion segment through ligamentotaxis. This argument is true. Increasing the size of the cage used to distract the disc space results in greater stabilization of the motion segment on mechanical testing.[40] After cyclic loading, some subsidence is inevitable, however, and biomechanical tests done after cyclic loading of threaded cage constructs reveal decreased stability in all directions.[41]

The destabilizing effects of interbody fusion are overcome by adding pedicle screw instrumentation; this is true whether the fusion is done from an anterior or a posterior approach. These biomechanical data correlate well with the substantially greater clinical reliability of achieving an arthrodesis when interbody fusion is done with supplementary pedicle fixation compared with the variable results reported with stand-alone interbody fusion procedures.

Although cage design characteristics do not seem to have a significant effect on segmental motion, these characteristics do influence the risk of subsidence, the healing of bone within the cage, and the alignment achieved. In addition, endplate preparation and vertebral bone density have important effects on the extent of subsidence.

Cage Characteristics

The optimal cage material is unknown. Cloward[41a] advocated the use of ethylene oxide sterilized allograft bone. Brantigan and colleagues[16] tested 18 tricortical iliac specimens obtained from bone banks and determined that 3 of them were not strong enough to sustain anticipated loads without collapse.

Current allograft products available for intervertebral use are made primarily of cortical bone and have adequate compressive strength. In designing his cage, Brantigan chose carbon fiber–reinforced polymer because of its strength and because its modulus of elasticity is similar to that of cortical bone.[13] In the United States, other materials commonly used in commercially available cages are polyetheretherketone (PEEK), a nonreinforced polymer, and titanium, which has a modulus of elasticity significantly greater than that of cortical bone. The stiffness of the cage is determined not only by the mechanical properties of the material but also by the shape and design characteristics of the cage. The ideal stiffness and its role in limiting subsidence or enhancing fusion are unknown. Finite element data have suggested that stiffer cages are more likely to subside,[42] but animal data have not supported this hypothesis,[43] and clinical reports have not convincingly shown that metal cages are more likely to subside than cages made of polymer (Fig. 49–4).

Kanayama and colleagues[44] studied the effect of cage design on stress shielding of the graft inside the cage. They determined that it was the pore size, not the stiffness of the material, that determined the load experienced by the graft. The total pore size was not important; rather, it was the size of the largest contiguous opening that determined how much force was transferred to the graft. It was implied that minimizing stress shielding is important to promote fusion, but no data were presented to support that presumption. One clinical study consistent with this hypothesis compared narrow and standard carbon fiber–reinforced polymer cages. The pore in the narrow cage was 36% smaller than the pore in the standard cage. There was a small but statistically significant reduction

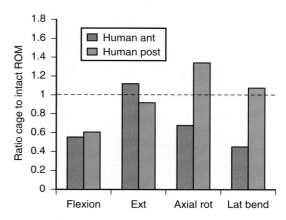

FIGURE 49–3 These data represent a summation of five biomechanical studies of stability after anterior cage placement in human cadaveric models and three studies of posterior cage placement. Data for each direction of testing are presented as ratio of range of motion after interbody cage placement compared with motion of unoperated segment. Ratio of 1.0 implied same motion as intact specimen. Placement from anterior approach stiffens spine in flexion, axial rotation, and lateral bending, whereas placement from posterior approach stiffens the spine only in flexion. When testing axial rotation, placing a cage from posterior approach creates more motion than unoperated spine. (Redrawn from Oxland TR, Lund T: Biomechanics of stand-alone cages and cages in combination with posterior fixation: A literature review. Eur Spine J. 9:S95-S101, 2000.)

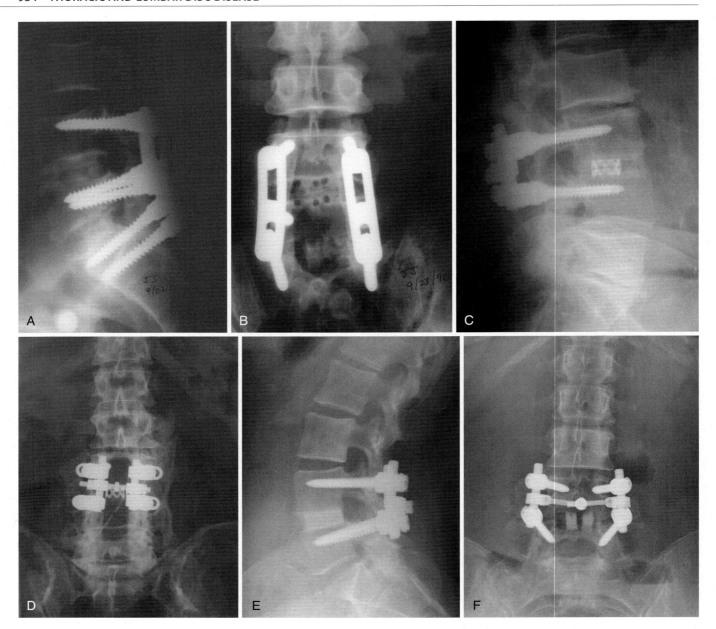

FIGURE 49–4 A-F, Anteroposterior and lateral radiographs of successful interbody fusions with carbon fiber–reinforced polymer cages (**A** and **B**), titanium mesh cages (**C** and **D**), and allograft wedge spacers (**E** and **F**). Incorporation of bone graft and replacement by new bone is most easily visualized with polymer cages because they are radiolucent. Outline of polymer can be seen on anteroposterior view as four radiolucent squares at periphery of implant. With titanium mesh cages, healed bone graft is visualized in front and behind implants, but assessment of graft within cage is difficult with standard x-rays. When nonunion occurs with allograft implants, radiolucency is usually seen adjacent to allograft. (**A** and **B,** Courtesy John Brantigan, MD.)

in fusion rate, 91.1% compared with 98.9%, but the conclusions have limitations because of methodologic flaws.[45] A larger pore size seems desirable as long as the design of the cage provides adequate structural support for the endplate.

Cage design also influences the alignment achieved. An increasingly large body of data show that maintaining or restoring lumbar lordosis is an important surgical goal and that lordosis correlates with the outcome of surgery.[46] Early cage designs were rectangular in shape and tended to force the vertebral endplates into parallel alignment. It is possible to achieve lordosis with rectangular cages, either by resecting bone posteriorly or by compressing the posterior disc space

and causing the posterior portion of the cage to subside.[47] A disadvantage of this approach is that it results in loss of posterior disc space height, which can lead to foraminal narrowing. A better solution is to use a cage that is tapered to achieve lordosis.[48-50] It is commonly said that anterior distraction is necessary to achieve lordosis, but distraction of the disc space with an implant that is not tapered flattens the spine. Placing large cages to achieve lordosis is a mistake. They require more root retraction to place, and this is more likely to result in nerve injury. A better solution is to use a tapered device and not to strive for maximal anterior height restoration (Fig. 49–5).

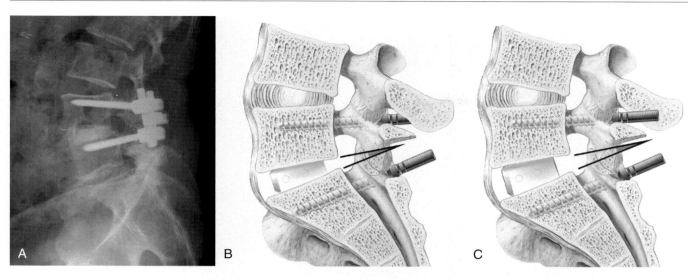

FIGURE 49–5 Using a tapered cage or spacer is the best way to achieve lordosis. Facet resection is sometimes needed to allow back of disc space to narrow adequately. An advantage of allograft bone is the ease with which it can be sculpted intraoperatively to achieve the desired shape. **A,** In this case, more lordosis was achieved than would be typically possible using commercially prepared devices by using a bur to increase taper of graft. **B** and **C,** Using larger grafts and distracting the disc space more does not increase lordosis; it increases amount of dural retraction needed and increases difficulty of surgery. (Courtesy Depuy Spine.)

Subsidence

In addition to achieving fusion, avoiding subsidence to maintain alignment is an important goal of interbody fusion surgery. In mechanical testing, endplate failure has a linear correlation with decreased bone density,[51] and severe osteoporosis is considered to be a relative contraindication to interbody fusion because of the risk of endplate collapse. The strength of the endplate is not uniform, and the central portion, where most surgeons place their grafts, is the weakest. Mapping studies have shown that the posterolateral portion of the endplate is most resistant to compression.[52,53] Placing the cage or graft in the area where the bone is strongest makes biomechanical sense[54] but may not be consistent with the goals of an individual surgical case. If it is necessary to increase lordosis, better results are achieved by anterior placement. Putting the graft in the posterolateral position might be stronger but would block compression of the posterior disc space and limit lordosis. This is especially true with rectangular cage designs or vertical titanium mesh cages.

Cage designs that optimize contact with the strongest portions of the endplate are desirable and include cloverleaf designs and large round cages, both of which have peripheral endplate contact.[55] Practical use of large round cages is limited to anterior surgery because of the excessive dural retraction that would be necessary to place such an implant. Lordotic cages placed laterally also achieve near-optimal endplate contact. The surface area of the endplate that needs to be in contact with the graft is unknown but is commonly stated to be 30%. This percentage is based on a study of thoracic vertebrae subjected to a physiologic load of 600 N. Failure of the endplate occurred in 80% of specimens subjected to that load when the grafts were 25% or less of the endplate surface area.

When the grafts exceeded 30% of the endplate surface, 88% of the specimens remained intact (Fig. 49–6).[56]

Preservation of the endplate is important to maintain the structural integrity of the vertebra. Oxland and colleagues[57] removed slightly less than 1 mm of cortical endplate with a power bur to expose trabecular bone; this resulted in a 33% reduction in compressive resistance of the vertebra. If the endplate is decorticated where it is not in contact with the cage, the strength of the remaining endplate is preserved.[58] Consequently, it is recommended that the endplates be carefully preserved during preparation of the disc space wherever they are in contact with the implant, but that areas of the endplate that are not load bearing can be decorticated to increase contact of graft placed outside the cage with trabecular bone.

Author's Preferred Technique

The author's experience with PLIF dates back to 1994, and the method of interbody fusion described here has been used without modification since 1999. Early results were reported in 2000 with an interbody fusion rate of 92%.[59] It is the author's practice always to perform a posterolateral fusion simultaneously with the PLIF to ensure the highest chance of achieving an arthrodesis. The technique for PLIF evolved from that described by Steffee and Biscup[60] for insertion of trapezoidal "ramps" made of carbon fiber–reinforced polymer. Their method was to insert the ramps sideways and rotate them into their final position, minimizing the amount of root retraction needed and simplifying placement of a lordotic graft.

The author prefers to use a commercially prepared trapezoidal allograft wedge for two reasons. The first is that its size and shape can be easily customized intraoperatively with a power bur to match the individual patient's anatomy. The

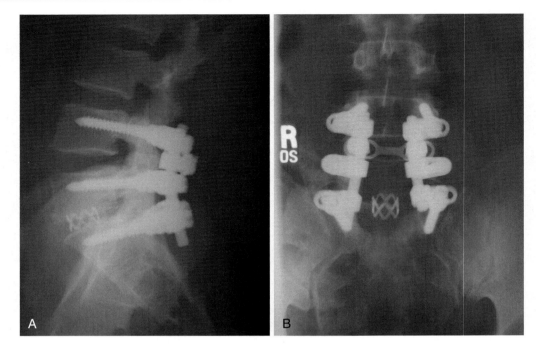

FIGURE 49–6 In this case, subsidence of cage into inferior endplate of L5 is obvious. Technical factors that may have predisposed to subsidence include use of single small cage placed centrally. Endcaps were not used, which would have increased surface area of metal supporting endplate. Inadequate grafting of interspace around cage may also have been a factor, suggested by absence of bone in disc space. A solid posterolateral fusion was achieved.

second is that, in contrast to titanium and polymer cages, this structural device has the potential to incorporate in the fusion. Although the graft is placed primarily as a spacer and it is the autologous bone placed around the graft that is relied on to achieve arthrodesis, incorporation of the allograft generally occurs, resulting in a more robust fusion. There is no potential for polymer or metal to incorporate and contribute to the fusion, so a smaller area of the endplate is available to participate in healing when using devices made of those materials. Ceramic blocks have been used in Asia because of the

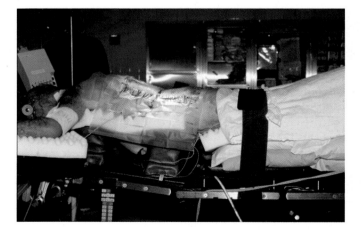

FIGURE 49–7 The patient is positioned in hyperextension, with pillows under thighs and head of bed elevated to help achieve maximal lordosis. Abdomen hangs free to allow unimpeded venous return. Electromyographic monitoring is used to help prevent nerve injury resulting from excessive traction.

potential for bone ingrowth, but there is no experience with that material in the United States, and it does not share the ability to be easily sculpted intraoperatively. Currently, several manufacturers produce allograft implants of this design.

The technique described here for preparation of the intervertebral space is applicable to any intervertebral cage or graft, and the principles outlined help prevent neural injury and other complications that have been associated with this operation. The procedure begins with proper positioning, which is essential to achieve a good outcome. The patient is positioned in hyperextension to help create lumbar lordosis. The abdomen should hang free for unimpeded venous return; this decompresses the epidural venous plexus and helps reduce bleeding. A radiolucent positioning frame is useful so that intraoperative fluoroscopic images can be obtained to confirm correct placement of screws and grafts (Fig. 49–7). Pedicle screws should be placed before beginning the interbody fusion. PLIF destabilizes the motion segment and should not be done unless adequate pedicle fixation can be achieved.

A wide laminectomy and resection of the medial portion of the facet joints is essential to minimize retraction of the dura and nerve roots. The wide exposure helps avoid traction injury to the lumbar roots, which can cause neuropathic pain and weakness. Generally, the exposure of the disc space should extend lateral to the medial border of the pedicle below. Adequate exposure may require sacrifice of the facet joints, especially in the upper lumbar spine. This sacrifice is of little consequence because stability is restored by pedicle screw fixation. The facets should always be excised when correcting deformity because this helps loosen the spine and facilitates correction. The superior edge of the upper lamina should be preserved to maintain the posterior ligamentous attachments to the vertebra above the fusion.

An abundant epidural plexus is usually encountered at the lateral border of the spinal canal. Bipolar electrocautery and packing with cottonoid patties can prevent the excessive bleeding that sometimes accompanies interbody fusion procedures. A paste made from absorbable gelatin foam powder and saline is very helpful in controlling bleeding. The venous plexus should be sharply divided to facilitate mobilization of the nerve roots and dura. A nerve root retractor is used to protect the dura, and a rectangular opening is cut in the anulus with a scalpel. When extending the annular opening laterally, care is taken to protect the exiting nerve root. This is easily done by sweeping any soft tissue toward the root with a No. 1 Penfield elevator and leaving the elevator in place to protect the root while working laterally.

The anulus is opened bilaterally, and the disc space is distracted with intervertebral spreaders. These are flat bars of increasing width with rounded edges. They are inserted into the disc space horizontally and rotated 90 degrees, distracting the disc space. If the disc space is initially very narrow, it is sometimes helpful to use a smaller instrument first, such as a No. 4 Penfield elevator, to identify the path. It is important not to use force so as to avoid inadvertent penetration into the vertebral body. Lateral fluoroscopy can be helpful to confirm that the starting tools are correctly placed in the interspace. The disc is gradually distracted, working from side to side with increasingly large spreaders until resistance is met. The interspace should not be overdistracted, or the endplates may collapse. It is not necessary to maximize distraction to achieve lordosis, and decompression of the nerve roots should be accomplished by aggressive foraminotomy, not aggressive distraction. Placing a maximally tapered graft is the best way to increase lordosis. Trying to place a tall graft has many negative effects. It increases the amount of dural retraction necessary, it increases the volume of bone graft needed to fill the interspace, and it increases the distance over which the fusion must occur (Fig. 49–8).

After distracting the space to a comfortable working distance, usually 11 or 12 mm, one of the spreaders is removed, and a four-sided Collis curet 1 or 2 mm smaller than the largest spreader used is inserted horizontally, then rotated clockwise and counterclockwise to separate the cartilage from the bony endplate. This step is repeated at various depths and angles to clean as much of the endplate as possible. These curets can be very aggressive, and it is important to be careful not to cut into the endplate. A Kerrison rongeur is used to resect loosened anulus flush with the vertebral endplates; this allows better visualization of the disc space so that a more complete discectomy can be done.

The discectomy is completed with standard curets and pituitary rongeurs. A reverse curet is very effective in removing any remaining cartilage from the endplates. It is helpful to mark the curets so that they are not inserted past a depth of 30 mm. In most cases, the anterior anulus prevents protrusion anterior to the vertebra, but the anulus is sometimes deficient, especially in patients with spondylolisthesis, and it is important to avoid anterior protrusion of the instruments

and visceral injury. After cleaning the interspace, the intervertebral spreader is reinserted, usually one size larger than was possible before removing the disc and cartilaginous endplate. The opposite side of the disc is now prepared in the same fashion.

It now is obvious that the interspace has been grossly destabilized. If a rotational deformity is present, it can be corrected by rotating the bilateral intervertebral spreaders simultaneously and "walking" the displaced vertebra into alignment. If no rotational deformity is present, the spreaders should be turned in opposite directions so that a rotational deformity is not induced. A graft is chosen to fit into the interspace. The graft should not be taller than the widest spreader used. It can be tapered to achieve the desired lordosis. After ensuring that the dura and exiting nerve root are protected, the trapezoidal allograft is inserted horizontally into the disc space and then rotated into its final lordotic position. The intervertebral spreader is removed from the opposite side of the disc space.

Cancellous graft is packed from the opposite side into the middle of the interspace; a syringe with the end cut off is useful for this step. Finally, the second trapezoidal allograft is inserted into position. Additional graft is packed around the allograft wedges to fill the disc space maximally with bone. The foramina and the midline under the dura are inspected to ensure no cancellous bone or disc material was displaced into the spinal canal or neural foramen. Lastly, the instrumentation is tightened in gentle compression to secure the grafts and achieve lordosis (Figs. 49–9 through 49–11).

Optimal Graft Material

The "gold standard" for achieving a solid fusion is cancellous autograft bone, regardless of which cage device or intervertebral spacer is chosen. Brantigan[61] reported a 97.7% fusion rate when using autologous cancellous graft in the cage he designed. Numerous authors have reported similar fusion rates using bone harvested from the lamina, spinous processes, and facet joints, without using iliac graft.[62] Miura and colleagues[63] reported a 100% fusion rate at 12 months in 32 patients treated with carbon fiber–reinforced polymer cages. Kim and colleagues[64] reported a 95% rate using local bone in titanium vertical mesh cages in a prospective study of 50 patients. Kasis and colleagues[65] reported improved clinical outcomes in a prospective comparison when using local bone, attributing at least some of the benefit to avoiding the pain and complications of iliac graft harvest. McAfee and colleagues[66] reported a 98% fusion rate in 120 patients using local bone in carbon fiber–reinforced polymer cages placed via a unilateral transforaminal approach.

The aforementioned reports of fusion rates determined radiographically must be interpreted in light of previous studies that suggested that radiographic methods have limited reliability for the determination of fusion success.[67,68] Other authors have cautioned that the use of local bone may be associated with pseudarthrosis, and if local bone is used, careful preparation and cleaning is necessary to avoid

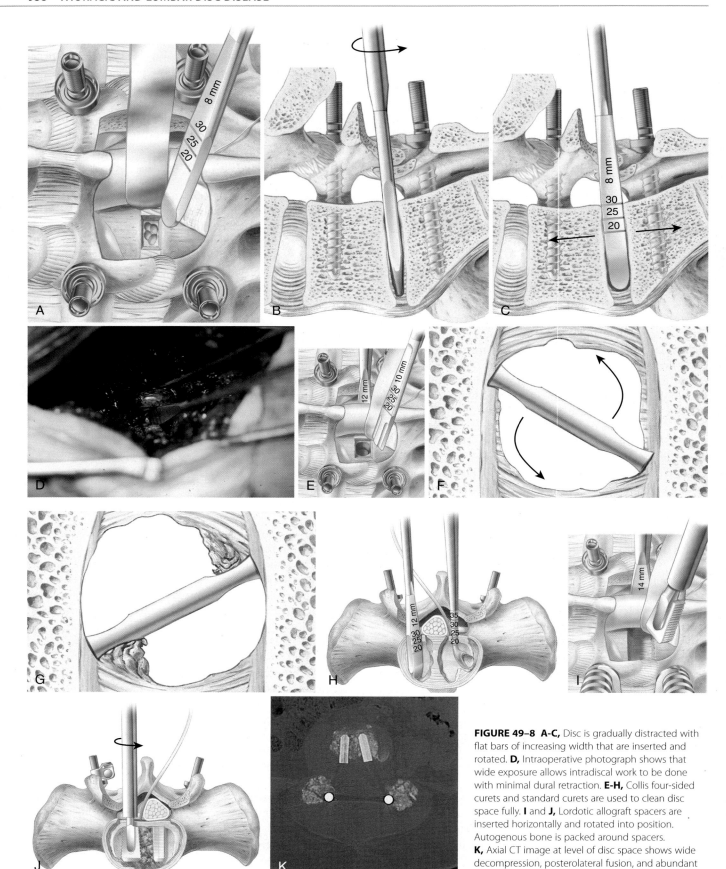

FIGURE 49–8 A-C, Disc is gradually distracted with flat bars of increasing width that are inserted and rotated. **D,** Intraoperative photograph shows that wide exposure allows intradiscal work to be done with minimal dural retraction. **E-H,** Collis four-sided curets and standard curets are used to clean disc space fully. **I** and **J,** Lordotic allograft spacers are inserted horizontally and rotated into position. Autogenous bone is packed around spacers.
K, Axial CT image at level of disc space shows wide decompression, posterolateral fusion, and abundant bone packed around spacers. (Courtesy Depuy Spine.)

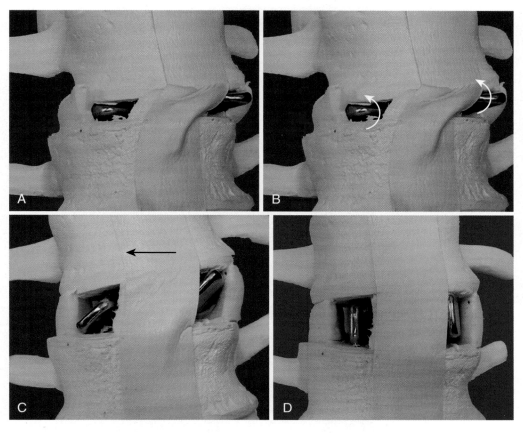

FIGURE 49–9 Lateral listhesis and rotational deformity can be corrected efficiently with posterior lumbar interbody fusion. Spine is destabilized by bilateral facet excision and complete discectomy. Distraction paddles can be used to translate vertebra laterally, correcting axial rotation, lateral listhesis, and asymmetric disc space collapse.

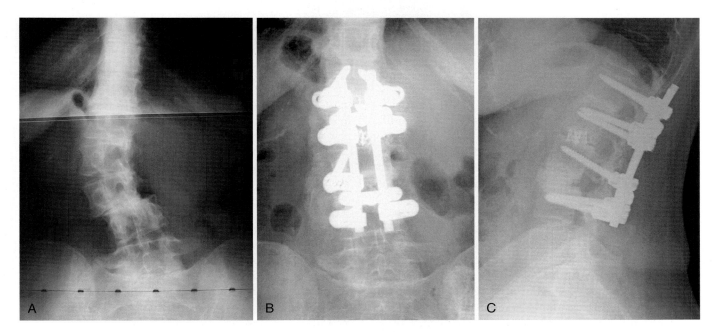

FIGURE 49–10 Acute rotational deformity causing degenerative scoliosis is corrected by posterior lumbar interbody fusion. Deformity at L45 was flexible and resolved spontaneously with correction of structural deformity at L34.

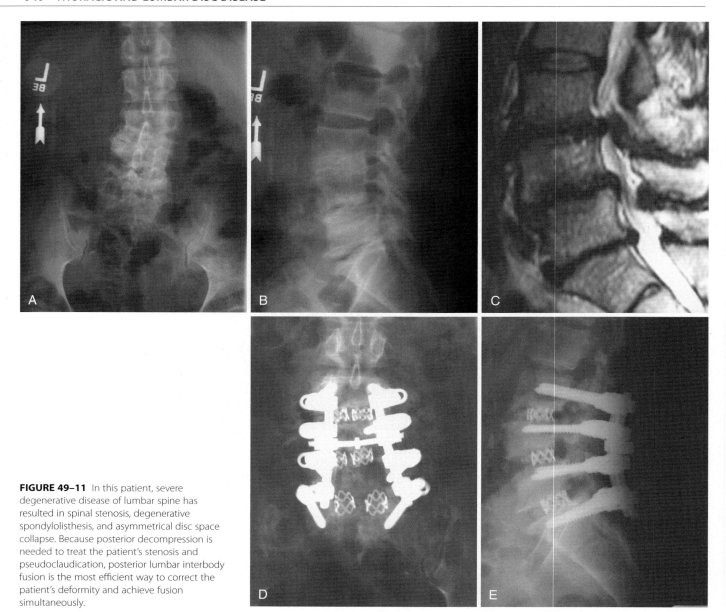

FIGURE 49–11 In this patient, severe degenerative disease of lumbar spine has resulted in spinal stenosis, degenerative spondylolisthesis, and asymmetrical disc space collapse. Because posterior decompression is needed to treat the patient's stenosis and pseudoclaudication, posterior lumbar interbody fusion is the most efficient way to correct the patient's deformity and achieve fusion simultaneously.

incorporation of soft tissue with the graft material.[69,61] Synthetic ceramic bone graft substitutes combined with iliac crest aspirate have also been reported to be highly effective for achieving interbody fusion,[70] but experience is limited.

More recently, there has been a surge of enthusiasm for the use of bone morphogenetic protein to achieve spinal fusion.[71] Recombinant human bone morphogenetic protein (rhBMP-2) was shown to be highly effective in achieving spinal fusion when used inside a titanium threaded cage placed anteriorly in the intervertebral space. In a 2-year prospective randomized trial of 279 patients, fusion was achieved in 94.5% of patients compared with 88.7% in the control group in whom iliac autograft was used.[72] Although not approved by the U.S. Food and Drug Administration (FDA) for posterior use, many surgeons have extrapolated the outcomes documented in the anterior clinical trial to posterior intervertebral applications. Review of the published data on outcomes of

posterior interbody use of this material reveals conflicting results. Although some authors report universal fusion with few complications,[73] others have reported a worrisome list of unexpected outcomes.

A clinical trial of rhBMP-2 used in posterior threaded fusion cages was stopped by the FDA because of a high rate of new bone formation (28 of 34 patients) in the spinal canal or neuroforamina, although the authors of the study were enthusiastic about the fusion results and believed that there was no clinical significance to the new bone formation.[74] Radiculopathy and neurologic deficit associated with ectopic bone have been reported by other authors,[75,76] and radiculitis has been reported with the use of rhBMP-2 even when no ectopic bone has formed. The use of a barrier between rhBMP-2 and the neural elements has been reported to eliminate this complication.[77,78] Osteolysis and endplate resorption resulting in subsidence and cage migration have also been reported as a complication of using rhBMP-2. Reports regarding the clinical significance of these radiographic findings vary significantly, and many surgeons continue to advocate for the use of rhBMP-2 in posterior interbody applications.[79-82] Optimal dosing and methods of application of this recombinant protein are unclear at this time. Although fusion rates seem to be high with the use of rhBMP-2, questions remain regarding safety, superiority, and cost-effectiveness.

Posterior Lumbar Interbody Fusion Versus Transforaminal Lumbar Interbody Fusion

Although Cloward, Steffee, Branch, and others emphasized the importance of a wide exposure to minimize dural retraction and nerve root injuries during PLIF, other authors described a more medial approach, which was often associated with a high incidence of nerve root injuries. This association was especially true before the advent of posterior instrumentation, when it was often recommended that the facet joints be preserved to avoid destabilizing the motion segment.[83] Dural and root injuries were particularly prevalent when threaded fusion cages were used posteriorly because of the emphasis on using large devices to achieve stability through annular distraction.[84] Because the cylinders were designed to cut into the endplates, the diameter needed was sometimes 50% greater than the height of the interspace achieved.[39] Even when using smaller devices, rates of neurologic complications of 17% were reported.[85]

In 1997, Harms and colleagues[86] reported a technique for performing a posterior interbody fusion through a more lateral approach than previously described.[87] These investigators advocated a unilateral approach to the disc space through the neural foramen by removing the facet joint. This approach allowed access to the disc space through the triangular "safe zone" between the exiting nerve root and the lateral dural edge.[88] In this way, an interbody fusion could be performed with minimal or no retraction of the dura. The technique has been enthusiastically adopted by many surgeons, and at least one group showed a reduction of nerve root injuries when comparing PLIF and transforaminal lumbar interbody fusion in their hands.[89,90]

One theoretical disadvantage of the transforaminal lumbar interbody fusion technique is that because only a unilateral approach to the disc space is done, it is impossible to remove the disc material completely. Javernick and colleagues[91] showed that, on average, 31% more disc material could be removed when a bilateral approach was done. This finding leads to concern that the fusion rate might not be satisfactory with a unilateral approach. McAfee and colleagues[92] showed that for anterior interbody fusions, 100% of patients who underwent complete discectomies achieved a solid arthrodesis, whereas only 86% of patients with incomplete discectomies achieved solid fusion. In an animal model, the inclusion of disc material with autologous bone in cages led to a significant impairment of fusion.[93] Despite these concerns, although no prospective randomized comparison has been done, the

unilateral approach to the disc space seems to result in adequate fusion rates.

In the author's experience, the unilateral transforaminal approach is useful when extensive postoperative scar makes mobilization of the dura or exposure of one side of the disc difficult. When trying to correct deformity, the greater laxity of the motion segment achieved by a bilateral approach makes PLIF the preferred technique, however. The technique of PLIF described in this chapter involves extensive or complete facet resection, eliminating any differences in risk of nerve root or dural injury between PLIF and transforaminal lumbar interbody fusion.

Outcomes and Complications of Posterior Lumbar Interbody Fusion

The outcome of PLIF surgery depends on many factors. Probably the most important, as with any operation on the lumbar spine, is proper patient selection. Lumbar fusion done for the wrong reasons or on the wrong patient uniformly yields bad results. Review of the published outcomes of PLIF surgery makes it clear that PLIF is a technically demanding procedure. Variations in technique, care, and skill have significant influence on the rate of fusion and the frequency with which complications occur.

In large series, fusion rates greater than 95% have routinely been reported with PLIF, regardless of whether carbon fiber–reinforced cages, polymer cages, vertical titanium mesh cages, allograft bone spacers, or stand-alone cylindric threaded cages have been used.[19,94-96] In contrast, only 77% of the patients reported by Rivet and colleagues[97] achieved solid arthrodesis, despite the use of cancellous iliac graft and supplementary pedicle fixation. Fuji and colleagues[98] reported a nonunion rate of 72% in their series of threaded cages placed posteriorly without supplementary fixation. It is unclear whether poor technique or other factors are responsible for the poor fusion results reported in those series.

Probably the most devastating complication that can occur with PLIF procedures is a nerve root injury.[99] The reported incidence of this complication varies widely, suggesting that surgical technique is an important factor affecting the frequency with which this complication occurs. Hosono and colleagues, in their review of 240 patients operated on by four different surgeons, correlated complication rates with the experience of the surgeon.[85] In that series, 41 patients had some kind of nerve injury, mostly transient. In Brantigan's series,[61] despite previous failed discectomy and the associated epidural scar in 83% of his patients, postoperative radiculitis was reported in only 2 of 100 patients, and one patient experienced a footdrop.

In the larger series of carbon fiber–reinforced polymer cages submitted to the FDA in which 221 patients were operated on by 15 surgeons, 3 cases of reflex sympathetic dystrophy and 3 cases of motor deficit, 1 of which was permanent, were reported.[94] Davne and Myers[100] reported only a 0.4% rate of traction root injury in their series of 384 PLIF procedures.

Krishna and colleagues[101] reported postoperative neuralgia in 7.1% of their patients, but they were able to reduce the incidence of this complication by half by modifying their technique and removing the superior facet to widen the exposure. Barnes and colleagues[84] reported a 13.6% incidence of permanent nerve root injury when using threaded fusion cages but no nerve root injury when using much smaller allograft wedges. These results reinforce the principle that wide exposure, careful technique, and avoiding oversized grafts can minimize the risk of neurologic injury in PLIF.

Graft displacement and loosening is another complication that was associated with PLIF when the technique was first described. This is a rare complication, however, with the addition of posterior pedicle screw stabilization. Subsidence of the implants can occur with PLIF. Most authors have not carefully documented this phenomenon. Factors predisposing to subsidence include inadequate graft technique and sizing and endplate injury during preparation. Patient factors such as weight and osteoporosis are likely important.[102] Implant type may be a factor, but convincing evidence of this has not been presented.[103,104] Pedicle screws alone do not prevent subsidence after PLIF.[105] Other complications of PLIF are similar to the complications encountered in all lumbar spine surgery. Epidural hematoma, wound infections, and other non–implant-related complications seem to occur with similar frequency in PLIF as in other reconstructive operations on the lumbar spine.

Summary

PLIF is a technically demanding operation that has an important role in the modern management of lumbar spine problems. Careful surgical technique emphasizing wide exposure and avoiding oversized implants can lead to excellent results with a low rate of complications and high fusion rates. Many different types of implants and grafts are available, without a clear-cut advantage of one type of device over another. Excellent results have been reported with most commercially available cages and grafts. PLIF is a useful way to provide anterior column support without the need for an anterior incision. PLIF is especially helpful to avoid failure of posterior instrumentation in patients who have undergone realignment of high-grade spondylolisthesis and to prevent distal instrumentation failure in long fusions to the sacrum.

Although PLIF with supplementary fixation creates a very stiff motion segment, the PLIF operation by itself destabilizes the motion segment. This destabilization is useful for correcting spinal deformity but makes the addition of posterior fixation, such as pedicle screw fixation, important to ensure successful healing of the fusion. In the treatment of degenerative conditions of the lumbar spine and back pain, PLIF offers some theoretical advantages over traditional posterolateral fusion techniques. Clinical studies generally have failed to show superiority of PLIF convincingly over other techniques, however. In clinical situations involving degenerative conditions of the lumbar spine and back pain, the role of PLIF as part of the surgical treatment of the patient has more to do with the experience of the surgeon than with any other factor.

REFERENCES

1. White AH: Editorial commentary. In White AH, Rothman RH, Ray CD (eds): Lumbar Spine Surgery Techniques and Complications. St Louis, CV Mosby, 1987, pp 294-295.
2. Verlooy J, Smedt KD, Selosse P: Failure of a modified posterior lumbar interbody fusion technique to produce adequate pain relief in isthmic spondylolytic grade 1 spondylolisthesis patients. Spine (Phila Pa 1976) 18:1491-1495, 1993.
3. Briggs H, Milligan PR: Chip fusion of the low back following exploration of the spinal canal. J Bone Joint Surg Am 26:125-130, 1944.
4. Ovens JM, Williams HG: Intervertebral spine fusion with removal of herniated intervertebral disk. Am J Surg 70:24-26, 1945.
5. Jaslow IA: Intercorporeal bone graft in spinal fusion after disc removal. Surg Gynecol Obstet 82:215, 1946.
6. Cloward RB: The treatment of ruptured intervertebral discs by vertebral body fusion: Indications, operative technique, after care. J Neurosurg 10:154-168, 1953.
7. Collis JS: Total disc replacement: A modified posterior lumbar interbody fusion: Report of 750 cases. Clin Orthop Relat Res 193:64-67, 1985.
8. Ma GW: Posterior lumbar interbody fusion with specialized instruments. Clin Orthop Relat Res 193:57-63, 1985.
9. Lin PM, Cautilli RA, Joyce MF: Posterior lumbar interbody fusion. Clin Orthop Relat Res 180:154-168, 1983.
10. Hutter CG: Posterior lumbar interbody fusion, a 25 year study. Clin Orthop Relat Res 179:86-96, 1983.
11. Cohen DS: Etiology of broken pedicle screw instrumentation in the treatment of spondylolisthesis. Proceedings of the North American Spine Society 11th Annual Conference, Vancover, 1996, pp 168-169.
12. Steffee AD, Sitkowski DJ: Posterior lumbar interbody fusion and plates. Clin Orthop Relat Res 227:99-102, 1988.
13. Brantigan JW, Steffee AD, Geiger JM: A carbon fiber implant to aid interbody lumbar fusion: Mechanical testing. Spine (Phila Pa 1976) 16(6 Suppl):S277-S282, 1991.
14. Cloward RB: Gas-sterilized cadaver bone grafts for spinal fusion operations: A simplified bone bank. Spine (Phila Pa 1976) 5:4-10, 1980.
15. Cloward RB: Posterior lumbar fusion updated. Clin Orthop Relat Res 193:16-19, 1985.
16. Brantigan JW, Cunningham BW, Warden K, et al: Compression strength of donor bone for posterior lumbar interbody fusion. Spine (Phila Pa 1976) 18:1213-1221, 1993.
17. Brantigan JW: Pseudarthrosis rate after allograft posterior lumbar interbody fusion with pedicle screw and plate fixation. Spine (Phila Pa 1976) 19:1271-1279, 1994.
18. Barnes B, Rodts GE, Haid R, et al: Allograft implants for posterior lumbar interbody fusion: Results comparing cylindrical dowels and impacted wedges. Neurosurgery 51:1191-1198, 2002.

19. Kim KT, Lee SH, Lee YH, et al: Clinical outcomes of 3 fusion methods through the posterior approach in the lumbar spine. Spine (Phila Pa 1976) 31:1351-1357, 2006.

20. Fritzell P, Hägg O, Wessberg P, et al: Chronic low back pain and fusion: A comparison of three surgical techniques: A prospective multicenter randomized study from the Swedish Lumbar Spine Study Group. Spine (Phila Pa 1976) 27:1131-1141, 2002.

21. Jacobs WC, Vreeling A, DeKleuver M: Fusion for low-grade adult isthmic spondylolisthesis: A systematic review of the literature. Eur Spine J 15:391-402, 2006.

22. Byrd JA 3rd, Scoles PV, Winter RB, et al: Adult idiopathic scoliosis treated by anterior and posterior spinal fusion. J Bone Joint Surg Am 69:843-850, 1987.

23. DiPaola CP, Molinari RW: Posterior lumbar interbody fusion. J Am Acad Orthop Surg 16:130-139, 2008.

24. Cohen DB, Chotivichit A, Fujita T, et al: Pseudarthrosis repair: Autogenous iliac crest versus femoral ring allograft. Clin Orthop Relat Res 371:46-55, 2000.

25. Molinari RW, Bridwell KH, Lenke LG, et al: Anterior column support in surgery for high-grade, isthmic spondylolisthesis. Clin Orthop Relat Res 394:109-120, 2002.

26. Suk SI, Lee CK, Kim WJ, et al: Adding posterior lumbar interbody fusion to pedicle screw fixation and posterolateral fusion after decompression in spondylolytic spondylolisthesis. Spine (Phila Pa 1976) 22:210-219, 1997.

27. Barrick WT, Schofferman JA, Reynolds JB, et al: Anterior lumbar fusion improves discogenic pain at levels of prior posterolateral fusion. Spine (Phila Pa 1976) 25:853-857, 2000.

28. Nachemson A, Zdeblick TA, O'Brien JP: Lumbar disc disease with discogenic pain: What surgical treatment is most effective? Spine (Phila Pa 1976) 21:1835-1838, 1996.

29. Lowery GL, Harms J: Principles of load sharing. In Bridwell KH, Dewald RL (eds): The Textbook of Spine Surgery, 2nd ed. Philadelphia, Lippincott-Raven, 1997, pp 155-165.

30. Lee JY, Milne EL, Shufflebarger HL, et al: Anterior column support in long segment kyphosis constructs. In Proceedings of the Scoliosis Research Society 32nd Annual Meeting, St. Louis, 1997, Paper #50.

31. McCormack T, Karaikovic E, Gaines RW: The load sharing classification of spine fractures. Spine (Phila Pa 1976) 19:1741-1744, 1994.

32. Oxland TR, Lund T: Biomechanics of stand-alone cages and cages in combination with posterior fixation: A literature review. Eur Spine J 9:S95-S101, 2000.

33. Tencer AF, Hampton D, Eddy S: Biomechanical properties of threaded inserts for lumbar interbody spinal fusion. Spine (Phila Pa 1976) 20:2408-2414, 1995.

34. Voor MJ, Mehta S, Wang M, et al: Biomechanical evaluation of posterior and anterior lumbar interbody fusion techniques. J Spinal Disord 11:328-334, 1998.

35. Dimar JR, Beck DJ, Glassman SD, et al: Posterior lumbar interbody cages do not augment segmental biomechanical stability. Am J Orthop 8:636-639, 2001.

36. Brodke DS, Dick JC, Kunz DN, et al: Posterior lumbar interbody fusion: A biomechanical comparison, including a new threaded cage. Spine (Phila Pa 1976) 22:26-31, 1997.

37. Pitzen T, Geisler FH, Matthis D, et al: Motion of threaded cages in posterior lumbar interbody fusion. Eur Spine J 9:571-576, 2000.

38. Lund T, Oxland TR, Jost B, et al: Interbody cage stabilisation in the lumbar spine: Biomechanical evaluation of cage design, posterior instrumentation and bone density. J Bone Joint Surg Br 80:351-359, 1998.

39. Tsantrizos A, Baramki HG, Zeidman S, et al: Segmental stability and compressive strength of posterior lumbar interbody fusion implants. Spine (Phila Pa 1976) 25:1899-1907, 2000.

40. Goh JC, Wong HK, Thambyah A, et al: Influence of PLIF cage size on lumbar spine stability. Spine (Phila Pa 1976) 25:35-39, 2000.

41. Kettler A, Wilke HJ, Dietl R, et al: Stabilizing effect of posterior lumbar interbody fusion cages before and after cyclic loading. J Neurosurg 92(1 Suppl):87-92, 2000.

41a. Cloward RB: Gas sterilized cadaver bone grafts for spinal fusion operations. A simplified bone bank. Spine 5:4, 1980.

42. Vadapalli S, Sairyo K, Goel VK, et al: Biomechanical rationale for using polyetheretherketone (PEEK) spacers for lumbar interbody fusion: A finite element study. Spine (Phila Pa 1976) 31:E992-E998, 2006.

43. van Dijk M, Smit TH, Sugihara S, et al: The effect of cage stiffness on the rate of lumbar interbody fusion: an in vivo model using poly(l-lactic Acid) and titanium cages. Spine (Phila Pa 1976) 27:682-688, 2002.

44. Kanayama M, Cunningham BW, Haggerty CJ, et al: In vitro biomechanical investigation of the stability and stress-shielding effect of lumbar interbody fusion devices. Neurosurgery 93(2 Suppl):259-265, 2000.

45. Fogel GR, Toohey JS, Neidre A, et al: Outcomes of posterior lumbar interbody fusion with the 9-mm width lumbar I/F cage and the variable screw placement system. J Surg Orthop Adv 18:77-82, 2009.

46. Glassman SD, Bridwell K, Dimar JR, et al: The impact of positive sagittal balance in adult spinal deformity. Spine (Phila Pa 1976) 30:2024-2029, 2005.

47. Groth AT, Kuklo TR, Klemme WR, et al: Comparison of sagittal contour and posterior disc height following interbody fusion: Threaded cylindrical cages versus structural allograft versus vertical cages. J Spinal Disord Tech 18:332-336, 2005.

48. Sears W: Posterior lumbar interbody fusion for lytic spondylolisthesis: Restoration of sagittal balance using insert-and-rotate interbody spacers. Spine J 5:161-169, 2005.

49. Gödde S, Fritsch E, Dienst M, et al: Influence of cage geometry on sagittal alignment in instrumented posterior lumbar interbody fusion. Spine (Phila Pa 1976) 28:1693-1699, 2003.

50. Brantigan JW, Neidre A: Achievement of normal sagittal plane alignment using a wedged carbon fiber reinforced polymer fusion cage in treatment of spondylolisthesis. Spine J 3:186-196, 2003.

51. Jost B, Cripton PA, Lund T, et al: Compressive strength of interbody cages in the lumbar spine: The effect of cage shape, posterior instrumentation and bone density. Eur Spine J 7:132-141, 1998.

52. Grant JP, Oxland TR, Dvorak MF: Mapping the structural properties of the lumbosacral vertebral endplates. Spine (Phila Pa 1976) 26:889-896, 2001.

53. Lowe TG, Hashim S, Wilson LA, et al: A biomechanical study of regional endplate strength and cage morphology as it relates

to structural interbody support. Spine (Phila Pa 1976) 29:2389-2394, 2004.

54. Labrom RD, Tan JS, Reilly CW, et al: The effect of interbody cage positioning on lumbosacral vertebral endplate failure in compression. Spine (Phila Pa 1976) 30:E556-E561, 2005.

55. Tan JS, Bailey CS, Dvorak MF, et al: Interbody device shape and size are important to strengthen the vertebra-implant interface. Spine (Phila Pa 1976) 30:638-644, 2005.

56. Closkey RF, Parsons JR, Lee CK, et al: Mechanics of interbody spinal fusion: Analysis of critical bone graft area. Spine (Phila Pa 1976) 18:1011-1015, 1993.

57. Oxland TR, Grant JP, Dvorak MF, et al: Effects of endplate removal on the structural properties of the lower lumbar vertebral bodies. Spine (Phila Pa 1976) 28:771-777, 2003.

58. Steffen T, Tsantrizos A, Aebi M: Effect of implant design and endplate preparation on the compressive strength of interbody fusion constructs. Spine (Phila Pa 1976) 25:1077-1084, 2000.

59. Lebwohl NH, Green BA, Buck BE: Technique indications complications and outcomes of allograft PLIF. In Proceedings of the Scoliosis Research Society 35th Annual Meeting, Cairns, Australia, 2000, Exhibit #66.

60. Steffee A: Personal communication, October 1994.

61. Brantigan JW: A prospective study of 100 consecutive cases. In Brantigan JW, Lauryssen C (eds): Intervertebral Fusion Using Carbon Fiber Reinforced Polymer Implants. St Louis, Quality Medical Publishing, 2006, pp 231-248.

62. Arai Y, Takahashi M, Kurosawa H, et al: Comparative study of iliac bone graft and carbon cage with local bone graft in posterior lumbar interbody fusion. J Orthop Surg 10:1-7, 2002.

63. Miura Y, Imagama S, Yoda M, et al: Is local bone viable as a source of bone graft in posterior lumbar interbody fusion? Spine (Phila Pa 1976) 28:2386-2389, 2003.

64. Kim KT, Lee SH, Lee YH, et al: Clinical outcomes of 3 fusion methods through the posterior approach in the lumbar spine. Spine (Phila Pa 1976) 31:1351-1357, 2006.

65. Kasis AG, Marshman LA, Krishna M, et al: Significantly improved outcomes with a less invasive posterior lumbar interbody fusion incorporating total facetectomy. Spine (Phila Pa 1976) 34:572-577, 2009.

66. McAfee PC, DeVine JG, Chaput CD, et al: The indications for interbody fusion cages in the treatment of spondylolisthesis: analysis of 120 cases. Spine (Phila Pa 1976) 30(6 Suppl):S60-S65, 2005.

67. Blumenthal SL, Gill K: Can lumbar spine radiographs accurately determine fusion in postoperative patients? Correlation of routine radiographs with a second surgical look at lumbar fusions. Spine (Phila Pa 1976) 18:1186-1189, 1993.

68. Brodsky AE, Kovalsky ES, Khalil MA: Correlation of radiologic assessment of lumbar spine fusions with surgical exploration. Spine (Phila Pa 1976) 16(6 Suppl):S261-S265, 1991.

69. Togawa D, Bauer TW, Lieberman IH, et al: Lumbar intervertebral body fusion cages: Histological evaluation of clinically failed cages retrieved from humans. J Bone Joint Surg Am 86:70-79, 2004.

70. Peterson M, Weinman C, Lewis M: The use of ultraporous a-tricalcium phosphate supplementing local autograft in lumbar interbody fusion surgery. Spine J 5(Suppl):S171, 2005.

71. Rihn JA, Gates C, Glassman SD, et al: The use of bone morphogenetic protein in lumbar spine surgery. J Bone Joint Surg Am 90:2014-2025, 2008.

72. Burkus JK, Gornet MF, Dickman CA, et al: Anterior lumbar interbody fusion using rhBMP-2 with tapered interbody cages. J Spinal Disord Tech 15:337-349, 2002.

73. Geibel PT, Boyd DL, Slabisak V: The use of recombinant human bone morphogenic protein in posterior interbody fusions of the lumbar spine: a clinical series. J Spinal Disord Tech 22:315-320, 2009.

74. Haid RW Jr, Branch CL Jr, Alexander JT, et al: Posterior lumbar interbody fusion using recombinant human bone morphogenetic protein type 2 with cylindrical interbody cages. Spine J 4:527-538, 2004.

75. Wong DA, Kumar A, Jatana S, et al: Neurologic impairment from ectopic bone in the lumbar canal: A potential complication of off-label PLIF/TLIF use of bone morphogenetic protein-2 (BMP-2). Spine J 8:1011-1018, 2008.

76. Chen NF, Smith ZA, Stiner E, et al: Symptomatic ectopic bone formation after off-label use of recombinant human bone morphogenetic protein-2 in transforaminal lumbar interbody fusion. J Neurosurg Spine 12:40-46, 2010.

77. Rihn JA, Patel R, Makda J, et al: Complications associated with single-level transforaminal lumbar interbody fusion. Spine J 9:623-629, 2009.

78. Villavicencio AT, Burneikiene S, Nelson EL, et al: Safety of transforaminal lumbar interbody fusion and intervertebral recombinant human bone morphogenetic protein-2. J Neurosurg Spine 3:436-443, 2005.

79. Smoljanovic T, Bojanic I, Delimar D: Adverse effects of posterior lumbar interbody fusion using rhBMP-2. Eur Spine J 18:920-923, 2009.

80. Vaidya R, Sethi A, Bartol S, et al: Complications in the use of rhBMP-2 in PEEK cages for interbody spinal fusions. J Spinal Disord Tech 21:557-562, 2008.

81. Rihn JA, Makda J, Hong J, et al: The use of RhBMP-2 in single-level transforaminal lumbar interbody fusion: A clinical and radiographic analysis. Eur Spine J 18:1629-1636, 2009.

82. Meisel HJ, Schnöring M, Hohaus C, et al: Posterior lumbar interbody fusion using rhBMP-2. Eur Spine J 17:1735-1744, 2008.

83. Lin PM: Posterior lumbar interbody fusion technique: Complications and pitfalls. Clin Orthop Relat Res 193:90-102, 1985.

84. Barnes B, Rodts GE Jr, Haid RW Jr, et al: Allograft implants for posterior lumbar interbody fusion: Results comparing cylindrical dowels and impacted wedges. Neurosurgery 51:1191-1198, 2002.

85. Hosono N, Namekata M, Makino T, et al: Perioperative complications of primary posterior lumbar interbody fusion for nonisthmic spondylolisthesis: Analysis of risk factors. J Neurosurg Spine 9:403-407, 2008.

86. Harms J, Jeszenszky D, Stoltze D, et al: True spondylolisthesis reduction and monosegmental fusion in spondylolisthesis. In Bridwell KH, Dewald RL (eds): The Textbook of Spine Surgery, 2nd ed. Philadelphia, Lippincott-Raven, 1997, pp 1337-1347.

87. Harms JG, Jeszenszky D: Die posteriore, lumbale, interkorporelle fusion in unilateraler transforaminaler technik. Oper Orthop Traumatol 10:90-102, 1998.

88. Kambin P: Arthroscopic microdiskectomy. Mt Sinai J Med 58:159-164, 1991.

89. Humphreys SC, Hodges SD, Patwardhan AG, et al: Comparison of posterior and transforaminal approaches to lumbar interbody fusion. Spine (Phila Pa 1976) 26:567-571, 2001.

90. Cole CD, McCall TD, Schmidt MH, et al: Comparison of low back fusion techniques: Transforaminal lumbar interbody fusion (TLIF) or posterior lumbar interbody fusion (PLIF) approaches. Curr Rev Musculoskelet Med 2:118-126, 2009.

91. Javernick MA, Kuklo TR, Polly DW Jr: Transforaminal lumbar interbody fusion: Unilateral versus bilateral disk removal—an in vivo study. Am J Orthop 32:344-348, 2003.

92. McAfee PC, Lee GA, Fedder IL, et al: Anterior BAK instrumentation and fusion: Complete versus partial discectomy. Clin Orthop Relat Res 394:55-63, 2002.

93. Li H, Zou X, Laursen M, et al: The influence of intervertebral disc tissue on anterior spinal interbody fusion: An experimental study on pigs. Eur Spine J 11:476-481, 2002.

94. Brantigan JW, Steffee AD, Lewis ML, et al: Lumbar interbody fusion using the Brantigan I/F cage for posterior lumbar interbody fusion and the variable pedicle screw placement system: Two-year results from a Food and Drug Administration investigational device exemption clinical trial. Spine (Phila Pa 1976) 25:1437-1446, 2000.

95. Arnold PM, Robbins S, Paullus W, et al: Clinical outcomes of lumbar degenerative disc disease treated with posterior lumbar interbody fusion allograft spacer: A prospective, multicenter trial with 2-year follow-up. Am J Orthop 38:E115-E122, 2009.

96. Kuslich SD, Danielson G, Dowdel JD, et al: Four-year follow-up results of lumbar spine arthrodesis using the Bagby and Kuslich lumbar fusion cage. Spine (Phila Pa 1976) 25:2656-2662, 2000.

97. Rivet DJ, Jeck D, Brennan J, et al: Clinical outcomes and complications associated with pedicle screw fixation-augmented lumbar interbody fusion. J Neurosurg Spine 1:261-266, 2004.

98. Fuji T, Oda T, Kato Y, et al: Posterior lumbar interbody fusion using titanium cylindrical threaded cages: Is optimal interbody fusion possible without other instrumentation? J Orthop Sci 8:142-147, 2003.

99. Wetzel FT, LaRocca H: The failed posterior lumbar interbody fusion. Spine (Phila Pa 1976) 16:839-845, 1991.

100. Davne SH, Myers DL: Complications of lumbar spinal fusion with transpedicular instrumentation. Spine (Phila Pa 1976) 17(6 Suppl):S184-S189, 1992.

101. Krishna M, Pollock RD, Bhatia C: Incidence, etiology, classification, and management of neuralgia after posterior lumbar interbody fusion surgery in 226 patients. Spine J 8:374-379, 2008.

102. Okuda S, Oda T, Miyauchi A, et al: Surgical outcomes of posterior lumbar interbody fusion in elderly patients. J Bone Joint Surg Am 88:2714-2720, 2006.

103. Abbushi A, Cabraja M, Thomale UW, et al: The influence of cage positioning and cage type on cage migration and fusion rates in patients with monosegmental posterior lumbar interbody fusion and posterior fixation. Eur Spine J 18:1621-1628, 2009.

104. Tokuhashi Y, Ajiro Y, Umezawa N: Subsidence of metal interbody cage after posterior lumbar interbody fusion with pedicle screw fixation. Orthopedics 32:259, 2009.

105. Brantigan JW: Pseudarthrosis rate after allograft posterior lumbar interbody fusion with pedicle screw and plate fixation. Spine (Phila Pa 1976) 19:1271-1279, 2004.

Transforaminal Lumbar Interbody Fusion

Alan S. Hilibrand, MD
Harvey E. Smith, MD

The intervertebral disc space is an environment that is conducive to fusion because of the advantageous biomechanics of compressive force and the blood supply provided via the endplate after curettage of the cartilage. This is in contrast to the posterolateral space, in which the fusion mass is under tensile forces, must bridge a greater distance between the transverse processes, and is surrounded by muscle. Involvement of the intervertebral disc space is ubiquitous with degenerative disc disease because the disc space undergoes progressive loss of height as part of the degenerative process. This loss of height results in progressive micromotion and is hypothesized to contribute to instability and degeneration of the posterior elements. Restoration of the intervertebral disc space height provides for an indirect decompression of the neural foramen, while allowing one potentially to address issues of sagittal imbalance by restoring lumbar lordosis. Consequently, achieving an interbody fusion with restoration of the disc space height is one of the component goals of surgery to address degenerative disease and deformity of the lumbar spine.

Anterior lumbar fusion was first described by Muller in 1906.[1] Evolutions of the technique have included modifications of the abdominal approach to a less invasive, mini-open technique and the use of interbody cages or structural allografts augmented with autogenous iliac crest graft, local bone graft, or, more recently, recombinant human bone morphogenetic protein (rhBMP-2).[2-5] Without the augmentation of posterior support, it has been well recognized that there is an increased rate of graft subsidence.[1,6] The combination of anterior lumbar interbody fusion with a posterolateral instrumented fusion (360-degree fusion) has been shown to yield fusion rates of greater than 95%.[7] Anterior lumbar interbody fusion has significant potential morbidities, however, including potential injury to the great vessels, abdominal hernia, injury to the sympathetic chain with subsequent sexual dysfunction, and thromboembolus secondary to retraction of the artery.[8-10]

Recognition of the biomechanical advantages of an anterior lumbar interbody fusion augmented with rigid posterior instrumentation led to the development of posterior-only approaches to the disc space to eliminate the approach-related morbidity of anterior interbody fusions. Posterior lumbar interbody fusion was developed to provide access to the disc space via a bilateral posterior approach with retraction of the thecal sac. Posterior lumbar interbody fusion is limited in its use to below the level of the conus, however, owing to the degree of thecal sac retraction necessary. Because of the retraction of the neural elements with posterior lumbar interbody fusion, there is concern for injury to the nerve roots, pain syndromes secondary to injury of the dorsal root ganglion, and cerebrospinal fluid leaks.[11]

Anterior lumbar interbody fusion via a transforaminal posterior approach (transforaminal lumbar interbody fusion [TLIF]) was first described by Harms and Rolinger in 1982.[12] Using a transforaminal approach via osteotomy of the pars interarticularis and inferior articular facet allows for facile access to the disc space with minimal retraction of the neural elements, avoids the morbidity of an anterior approach,[13,14] and has a lower complication rate than direct posterior lumbar interbody fusion.[11] Accessing the disc space via a posterior annulotomy, approximately 56% of the endplate can be prepared for fusion[15] with placement of bone graft and interbody implant. Combined with standard posterolateral instrumentation, decortication, and bone grafting, radiographic fusion rates greater than 90% can be achieved.[16] Published outcomes of single-level TLIF and multilevel TLIF are equivalent or better than anterior and 360-degree fusions, with restoration of the disc space height.[16,17] TLIF has been shown to result in significant savings relative to anteroposterior interbody fusion, owing in part to the decreased operating room time, less blood loss, and shorter hospital stays.[18]

Although some degree of restoration of disc space height with TLIF has been documented, the magnitude of restoration has been shown to be less than that achieved via anterior lumbar interbody fusion.[19,20] Similarly, longitudinal studies have shown a progressive loss of restored lordosis, as the fusion construct over time tends to drift back to the preoperative sagittal balance. The clinical significance of radiographic differences between anterior lumbar interbody fusion and TLIF is unknown because these radiographic differences have not been shown to correlate to differences in outcome measures.[20]

Radiculopathy secondary to a foraminal disc herniation is difficult to address adequately from a midline approach and decompression owing to limited access to the lateral foramen. A far-lateral or foraminal disc herniation may be managed with a facetectomy, facilitating a transforaminal approach to the nerve root.[21] TLIF may be considered as treatment for a foraminal disc herniation, particularly in the setting of significant loss of disc space height, because one may directly decompress the nerve root with the facetectomy, achieve an interbody and posterolateral fusion, and achieve indirect decompression with increase in the disc space height.

Advances in less invasive spine surgery, mini-open approaches, tubular retractors, and percutaneous instrumentation systems have been applied to TLIF, and minimally invasive TLIF procedures have been proposed to address the morbidity of the posterior midline approach. Preliminary studies have suggested that minimally invasive approaches may result in less blood loss and shorter hospital stays.[22-24] These preliminary reports are case series, however, so the results must be extrapolated to general practice with caution. Prospective randomized studies are needed comparing less invasive or minimally invasive TLIF procedures with the standard open midline approach to compare clinical outcomes and radiologic indices (disc space height, graft placement, lordosis, and fusion).

Surgical Procedure

The patient should be placed prone in standard fashion on a Jackson table, with care taken to pad all bony prominences. An Andrews table or frame may also be used, but care should be taken to consider if proper lordosis can be achieved in that position. Alternatively, the leg portions of hinged tables such as an Andrews or Wilson frame may be elevated before locking down posterior instrumentation to induce lordosis across the instrumented segments.

A standard midline incision is made through the skin and subcutaneous tissues, and subperiosteal dissection is carried down to the spine in standard fashion. The transverse process and pars interarticularis at the cephalad and caudal levels should be exposed in their entirety, with care taken not to violate the cephalad facet joint capsule (i.e., for L4-5 TLIF, the pars of L4 and L5 and transverse process of L4 and L5 must be entirely exposed, with care taken not to violate the L3-4 facet while exposing the landmarks for the L4 pedicle screws). An intraoperative marker film or fluoroscopy should be obtained to confirm the level of exposure. The interspinous ligament between the operative levels may be resected, and the interspinous space may be skeletonized. In the event of a tight interspace, a lamina spreader may be placed between the spinous processes to provide temporary distraction. It is recommended that vigorous distraction not be done on the pedicle screws because this weakens their biomechanical fixation. A consideration before taking down the interspinous ligament is the biomechanical support it contributes to the stability of the motion segment.

For transforaminal access to the disc space, it is necessary to remove the entire facet joint effectively on one side. This is accomplished by removing the inferior articular process of the cephalad level with an osteotomy through the pars interarticularis. This osteotomy should be performed on the side of greatest neural pathology; the osteotomy through the pars should be done as cephalad as possible to maximize the exposure but with care not to violate the pedicle itself (Fig. 50-1). Before

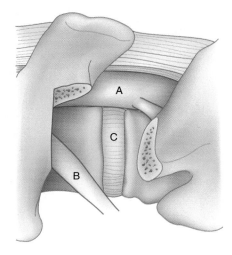

FIGURE 50-1 Surgical exposure after completion of osteotomy with removal of facet joint. **A,** Thecal sac. **B,** Exiting nerve root. **C,** Intervertebral disc.

the osteotomy, the ligamentum flavum should be completely freed from the lamina with a curet; particularly in the setting of a revision procedure, removal of the ligamentum and associated adhesions after the osteotomy may prove difficult and increase the risk of incidental durotomy. The transforaminal approach may be done either in concert with a midline laminectomy or with preservation of the spinous processes and midline ligamentous structures. To preserve the midline structures, one first makes the osteotomy up the medial aspect of the ipsilateral lamina, with the second osteotomy across the pars interarticularis as close as possible to the inferior margin of the cephalad pedicle. The inferior articular facet may be grasped with a Leksell rongeur or pituitary and rotated away from the underlying dura, taking care to remove any ligamentous adhesions with a curet.

Using Leksell and Kerrison rongeurs, the superior facet of the caudal level should be resected as flush with the pedicle as possible, removing the overhanging portions so that the remaining bone is flush with the superior and medial aspects of the pedicle. The lateral recess may be completely decompressed, and the nerve root should be confirmed to be free of compression. At this point, careful identification of the exiting nerve root and medial border of the thecal sac is essential. Vessels that are in the field of approach to the disc space should be cauterized and divided with bipolar electrocautery. Although the exiting nerve root should be confirmed to be mobilized, excessive retraction should be avoided because injury to the ganglion can result in debilitating postoperative pain.

After completion of the surgical exposure of the transforaminal zone as described, a nerve root retractor should be placed medially to protect the thecal sac. With appropriate surgical exposure, only minimal retraction should be necessary as protection against incidental durotomy during the annulotomy. The posterior anulus should be incised widely with a box cut, with care taken to visualize the exiting and traversing nerve roots (Fig. 50-2). After completion of the annulotomy, the discectomy may be started with a pituitary rongeur and curets. A forward angled pituitary is necessary to enter the disc space on the contralateral side of the patient.

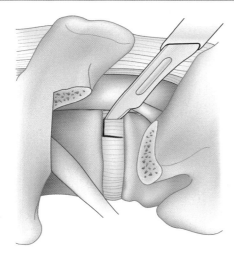

FIGURE 50–2 Incision of posterior anulus. Box cut should be as large as possible in posterolateral margin of disc, with nerve root and thecal sac as lateral and medial boundaries.

When removing the disc and cartilage from the endplates, care must be taken not to violate the subchondral bone. Angled curets and chondrotomes should be used to remove the cartilaginous endplate from the far lateral side. A thorough discectomy and endplate preparation are essential, but absolute care must be taken not to violate the anterior anulus or subchondral bone (Fig. 50–3).

As the discectomy progresses, sequential dilation of the disc space should be accomplished with serial dilators. When impacting the dilators into the disc space, care must be taken to follow the sagittal plane of the interspace to avoid driving the dilator through the endplate, particularly in an osteoporotic patient (Fig. 50–4). If necessary, exposure may be aided by distracting between the spinous processes with a lamina

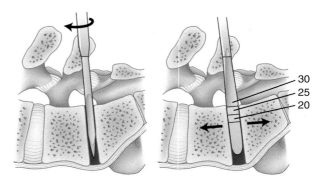

FIGURE 50–4 Sequential dilators should be used to distract intervertebral disc space. Care must be taken in insertion of dilator in collapsed disc space to parallel endplate; particularly in an osteoporotic patient, inadvertent angulation of dilator may fracture endplate.

spreader. After distraction, the assistant must hold the lamina spreader to stabilize it because inadvertent dislodgment may place the contents of the spinal canal at risk. The posterior lips of the vertebral bodies may be removed with osteotomes so that they are flush with the concavity of the endplate; if not removed, the interbody implant may be undersized (Fig. 50–5). After dilation to an appropriate size, the trial implant should be placed, with care taken to tamp it appropriately medial and anterior.

After implant trialing, the interspace should be bone grafted with the clinically indicated graft material. Bone graft should be placed into the anterior interspace and the implant. After anterior grafting of the interspace, the implant with graft is placed, and tamps are used to direct the implant anterior and medially (Fig. 50–6).

Based on surgeon preference, the pedicle screws may be placed before or after the discectomy and interbody fusion. It is recommended that the screws not be used for vigorous distraction of the interspace because this is deleterious to their fixation. The surgeon should place the screws in the standard fashion with which he or she is most comfortable. A complete decortication of the fusion bed should be completed, with bone graft placed in the posterolateral gutters and in the facet joint and dorsal elements, if preserved, on the contralateral side of the osteotomy.

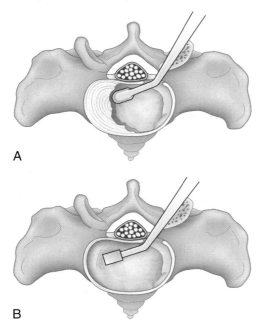

A

B

FIGURE 50–3 Angled curets (**A**) and chondrotomes (**B**) are necessary for thorough discectomy and endplate preparation, particularly far contralateral space. When working curets anteriorly and posteriorly, care must be taken not to violate anterior anulus.

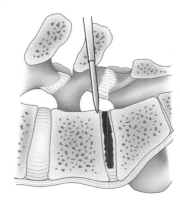

FIGURE 50–5 Posterior lips of vertebral bodies, if significantly different than concavity of disc space, may result in undersizing of implant. To address this, posterior lips may be removed flush with concavity with osteotome.

Rods should be measured, cut, and bent into the appropriate lordosis and then captured in the pedicle screws. An intraoperative image must be obtained at this point to confirm pedicle screw and interbody cage placement, with care taken to note the anterior position of the cage. The wound should be irrigated and closed in standard fashion. Before wound closure, it should be confirmed with a probe that no bone graft has fallen into the canal or foramen.

A modified TLIF procedure may be used to address isthmic spondylolisthesis with reduction of the slip, if clinically indicated. A bilateral transforaminal approach should be done via the standard midline exposure, and the foramen on both sides should be decompressed. Using posted screws, a reduction maneuver may be done while using electrophysiology to monitor the neural elements. In the setting of an isthmic spondylolisthesis, the posterior elements are not attached to the vertebral bodies, and the TLIF procedure is a biomechanically sound approach. It provides a stable anterior interbody fusion, restores posterior stability through the placement of pedicle screw instrumentation to increase likelihood of obtaining a successful fusion, and includes a wide decompression of the foramen to facilitate direct visualization of the neural elements.

rhBMP-2 is currently approved by the U.S. Food and Drug Administration (FDA) for use in an anterior interbody cage but is not FDA approved for use in a posterior transforaminal interbody fusion. Several studies have investigated the off-label use of rhBMP-2 in TLIF, with published fusion rates similar to rates achieved with autograft bone in the cage. There have been reports of an increased incidence of radiculopathy postoperatively on the side of the transforaminal approach when rhBMP-2 is used, and an increased incidence of heterotopic bone formation has been noted.[25] When rhBMP-2 is used posterolaterally, there have been reports of sterile seroma formation and local tissue swelling.[26] Some investigators have hypothesized that rhBMP-2 may incite an inflammatory response along the nerve root if it leaks out of the intervertebral space, but this has not been confirmed. An increased incidence of transient vertebral body osteolysis has been noted[27,28]; it is hypothesized that with perforation of the endplate, the rhBMP-2 may incite a transient remodeling of the cancellous bone. The surgeon should take into consideration these reported complications when contemplating the use of rhBMP-2 in an "off-label" setting.

The TLIF procedure provides for an effective interbody and posterolateral fusion with fusion rates greater than 90%. TLIF also facilitates a wide direct and indirect decompression of the neural elements that cannot be accomplished through an anterior approach and anterior lumbar interbody fusion. There are, however, several technical aspects that should be considered.

The biomechanical load-sharing properties of the interbody graft are predicated on the bony stability of the endplate. Fracture or violation of the endplate may result in subsidence of the graft into the vertebral body. If increased bleeding is appreciated during the procedure, it may be an indication that the endplate has been violated. Similarly, visualization of cancellous bone during the discectomy indicates violation of the endplate. Endplate violation is also more likely in the setting of a collapsed disc space in an osteoporotic patient. To minimize this risk, particular care must be taken to appreciate the sagittal orientation of the endplates with intraoperative imaging and always to maintain the trajectory of the instruments parallel to this orientation. The authors have found it helpful to use gradual "blunt, bulleted distraction" into the interbody space and always avoid the use of sharp cutting tools such as endplate shavers in these patients. If there is a significant violation of the endplate, the surgeon should consider aborting the interbody portion of the fusion.

Although the transforaminal approach is advocated over a direct posterior approach to the intervertebral space in part because it necessitates comparatively less retraction of the thecal sac, there have been reports of postoperative radiculopathy on the ipsilateral side of the transforaminal approach. Some instances of radiculopathy may result from overly vigorous retraction of the exiting nerve root. There have been reports more recently of an increased incidence of radiculopathy when rhBMP-2 is used in the intervertebral space and incidences of heterotopic bone formation.[25,29] This is an "off-label" use of rhBMP-2. This issue is significant, however, owing to the increasing use of biologics in spine surgery. It is hypothesized that biologics that upregulate the transforming growth factor pathway may promote an inflammatory response if they are introduced to the neural space. If the surgeon thinks it is clinically indicated to use a biologic osteoinductive promoter in the disc space, it may be advisable to consider strategies to minimize the possibility of migration from the disc space to the spinal canal and neural foramen.

There is some debate regarding the optimal position of the interbody graft. Harms and Rolinger[12] originally described the procedure with a middle to posterior third graft position, to take advantage of the stronger posterolateral endplates. Subsequently, other authors have advocated a more anterior position of the interbody graft to improve its load-sharing properties and to facilitate restoration of lumbar lordotic angle.[30] In disc space preparation and implant insertion, care must be taken to preserve the anterior anulus. Violation of the anterior anulus may result in inadvertent entry into the retroperitoneum with either an instrument or an implant, which may be catastrophic because of the nearby location of the large vessels. During preparation of the disc space, dilation, trialing, and implant insertion, the surgeon must maintain direct visualization of the working space. Intraoperative x-ray or fluoroscopic imaging should be used if there is any ambiguity regarding the position of instruments, implants, or the angle of the disc space. If there is a decline in hemodynamic status at any point after beginning disc space preparation, the potential of a vascular catastrophe must be considered.

TLIF does restore disc space height, but it does not allow an anterior release, and multilevel TLIF may be associated with prolonged operative time and blood loss and less restoration of lordosis compared with a direct anterior approach with subsequent posterolateral fusion. Consequently, in the setting of significant kyphotic deformity, a direct anterior decompression with release may be a more appropriate consideration. In the setting of a rigid coronal plane deformity, an anterior interbody approach also may be more appropriate because multiple anterior releases may be needed for correction of coronal deformity, adequate distraction to achieve indirect decompression, and restoration of sagittal balance.

Case Presentation

A 38-year-old woman who had a prior right-sided L4-5 microdiscectomy presented with recurrent right L5 radiculopathy and significant back pain (Fig. 50–6). She was managed initially with selective L5 root blocks and physical therapy without improvement. Plain films and magnetic resonance imaging (MRI) showed a recurrent right-sided L4-5 disc herniation and significant loss of disc space height at L4-5 with a new degenerative spondylolisthesis. Given the recurrent disc herniation and degeneration with spondylolisthesis of the L4-5 interspace, L4-5 TLIF was offered to stabilize the L4-5 interspace, restore the disc space height, and decompress the nerve root.

Complications

TLIF has a complication rate that is comparatively low relative to that of anteroposterior lumbar interbody fusion.[14] For single-level TLIF, fusion rates are reported to be greater than 90%, but they are less than 90% for multilevel procedures. As with any procedure with pedicle screws, there is the possibility of screw misplacement; the incidence of a misplaced pedicle screw with TLIF procedure is approximately 5%.[13] Transient postoperative neurologic deficit has been reported to range from 2% to 7%. Neurologic deficits lasting longer than 3 months were reported to occur in 4% of patients undergoing minimally invasive TLIF approaches in one series of 73 minimally invasive cases.[14] In cases reported to have a postoperative radiculopathy, the most commonly affected nerve root is L5.[16]

Minor complications have been reported to occur in 16% of cases, with an approximately 5%/level risk of transient radiculopathy and 4%/level risk of incidental durotomy.[13,16] One large series of 124 consecutive TLIF procedures (51 open, 73 minimally invasive) reported a 20% incidence of

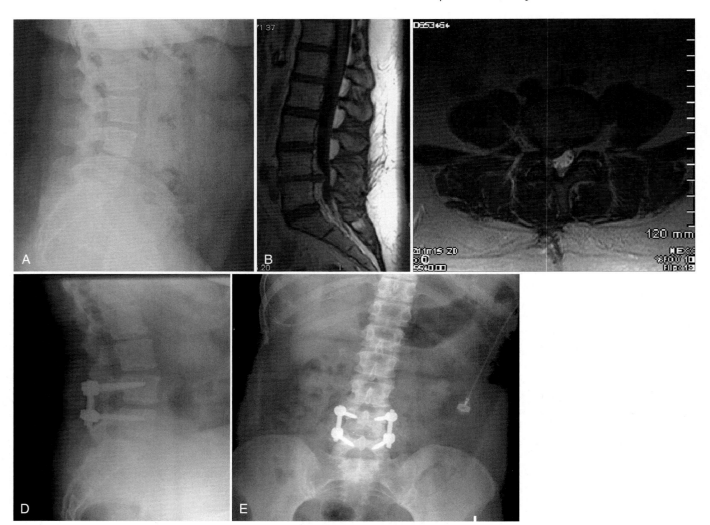

FIGURE 50–6 A-C, Radiograph (**A**) and MRI (**B** and **C**) of recurrent L4-5 disc herniation with significant degenerative changes and loss of height of L4-5 interspace. **D** and **E,** Postoperative lateral (**D**) and anteroposterior (**E**) images show L4-5 transforaminal lumbar interbody fusion with significant restoration of interbody height.

cerebrospinal fluid leak in the open cases.[14] Postoperative infections have an incidence of approximately 5%.[13,16] Postoperative hematomas have been reported to have an incidence of approximately 4%.[14] In addition to postoperative radiculopathy on the ipsilateral side of transforaminal approach, there has also been a report of postoperative radiculopathy on the contralateral side,[31] hypothesized to occur in the setting of asymptomatic contralateral stenosis that is exacerbated by the increased lordosis resulting from the procedure. Reflex sympathetic dystrophy has been reported postoperatively,[16] presumably from irritation of the dorsal root ganglion. Postoperative gastrointestinal complications, predominantly ileus, were reported in 4% of patients in the series reported by Potter and colleagues[16] of 100 TLIF procedures; one patient developed pseudomembranous colitis.

Summary

It is well recognized that an anterior interbody lumbar fusion provides increased rate of fusion, indirect decompression of the neural elements, and the ability to address issues of sagittal balance. A posterior transforaminal approach to the intervertebral disc space provides for the biomechanical advantages of an anteroposterior fusion, while eliminating the approach-related morbidity of an anterior approach. With the transforaminal approach, direct access to the disc space and lateral recess is possible with minimal to no retraction of the neural elements. TLIF has been shown to have a lower complication rate and lower cost than anteroposterior fusion, and it provides a viable option to the spine surgeon seeking to address isthmic spondylolisthesis, foraminal intervertebral disc herniations, recurrent disc herniations, and mechanical back pain owing to degenerative disc disease.

PEARLS

1. Fusion rates exceed 90% with the TLIF procedure.

2. Take great care with endplate preparation to avoid violation of the endplate; note the sagittal orientation of the endplates on intraoperative imaging and maintain that orientation with all instruments when working in the interspace.

3. Use blunt, bulleted distractors in the setting of osteoporosis.

4. Anterior placement of the interbody graft improves load-sharing and restoration of lumbar lordosis.

PITFALLS

1. Do not violate the anterior anulus during interspace preparation.

2. If there is significant endplate violation, one may need to consider aborting placement of the interbody spacer.

3. The use of rhBMP-2 may be associated with heterotopic bone formation and radiculopathy.

4. TLIF may result in suboptimal restoration of disc space height and restoration of lumbar lordosis in the setting of a kyphotic or rigid deformity.

KEY POINTS

1. TLIF uses a posterolateral approach to the intervertebral disc space via resection of the facet joint through a working triangle with borders of the thecal sac medially, exiting nerve root superolaterally, and caudal pedicle inferiorly.

2. The transforaminal approach yields fusion rates that are comparable to an anteroposterior (360-degree) approach but without the morbidity of the abdominal exposure.

3. Care must be taken not to violate the endplates while preparing the intervertebral space, particularly in an osteoporotic patient.

4. Application in patients with rigid coronal and kyphotic deformities and patients with osteoporosis may be limited.

KEY REFERENCES

1. Javernick MA, Kuklo TR, Polly DW Jr: Transforaminal lumbar interbody fusion: Unilateral versus bilateral disc removal—an in vivo study. Am J Orthop 32:344-348, 2003.
   Javernick and colleagues quantified the volume of intervertebral disc removed and endplate available for fusion after preparation of the intervertebral disc space via a TLIF approach. They were able to remove 69% of the total disc volume and prepare 56% of the endplate cross-sectional area for fusion via the unilateral approach.

2. Potter BK, Freedman BA, Verwiebe EG, et al: Transforaminal lumbar interbody fusion: Clinical and radiographic results and complications in 100 consecutive patients. J Spinal Disord Tech 18:337-346, 2005.
   Potter and colleagues reported a series of 100 consecutive TLIF procedures, with a 93% fusion rate, 80% overall patient satisfaction, and relatively minor complications.

3. Kwon BK, Berta S, Daffner SD, et al: Radiographic analysis of transforaminal lumbar interbody fusion for the treatment of adult isthmic spondylolisthesis. J Spinal Disord Tech 16:469-476, 2003.
   Kwon and colleagues evaluated 35 consecutive cases of TLIF in the setting of an isthmic spondylolisthesis. TLIF improved disc space height and anterolisthesis, and a more anterior position of the interbody cage was optimal for reconstruction of lordosis.

4. Whitecloud TS 3rd, Roesch WW, Ricciardi JE: Transforaminal interbody fusion versus anterior-posterior interbody fusion of the lumbar spine: A financial analysis. J Spinal Disord 14:100-103, 2001.
   Whitecloud and colleagues retrospectively reviewed 80 patients who underwent lumbar interbody fusion via either TLIF or anteroposterior fusion. The TLIF procedure resulted in significant cost savings because of the decreased operating room time, decreased blood loss, and shorter hospital stay.

5. Villavicencio AT, Burneikiene S, Bulsara KR, et al: Perioperative complications in transforaminal lumbar interbody fusion versus anterior-posterior reconstruction for lumbar disc degeneration and instability. J Spinal Disord Tech 19:92-97, 2006.

Villavicencio and colleagues retrospectively reviewed 167 consecutive TLIF (124 patients) and anteroposterior (74 patients) cases. Anteroposterior fusion had more than twice the complication rate, increased blood loss, longer operative times, and longer hospital stays compared with TLIF.

REFERENCES

1. Resnick DK: Lumbar interbody fusion: Current status. Neurosurg Q 18:77-82, 2008.

2. Burkus JK, Heim SE, Gornet MF, et al: Is INFUSE bone graft superior to autograft bone? An integrated analysis of clinical trials using the LT-CAGE lumbar tapered fusion device. J Spinal Disord Tech 16:113-122, 2003.

3. Burkus JK, Dorchak JD, Sanders DL: Radiographic assessment of interbody fusion using recombinant human bone morphogenetic protein type 2. Spine (Phila Pa 1976) 28:372-377, 2003.

4. Burkus JK, Heim SE, Gornet MF, et al: The effectiveness of rhBMP-2 in replacing autograft: An integrated analysis of three human spine studies. Orthopedics 27:723-728, 2004.

5. Mummaneni PV, Pan J, Haid RW, et al: Contribution of recombinant human bone morphogenetic protein-2 to the rapid creation of interbody fusion when used in transforaminal lumbar interbody fusion: A preliminary report. Invited submission from the Joint Section Meeting on Disorders of the Spine and Peripheral Nerves, March 2004. J Neurosurg Spine 1:19-23, 2004.

6. Dennis S, Watkins R, Landaker S, et al: Comparison of disc space heights after anterior lumbar interbody fusion. Spine (Phila Pa 1976) 14:876-878, 1989.

7. Kwon BK, Hilibrand AS, Malloy K, et al: A critical analysis of the literature regarding surgical approach and outcome for adult low-grade isthmic spondylolisthesis. J Spinal Disord Tech 18(Suppl):S30-S40, 2005.

8. Kulkarni SS, Lowery GL, Ross RE, et al: Arterial complications following anterior lumbar interbody fusion: Report of eight cases. Eur Spine J 12:48-54, 2003.

9. Johnson RM, McGuire EJ: Urogenital complications of anterior approaches to the lumbar spine. Clin Orthop Relat Res 114-118, 1981.

10. Sasso RC, Kenneth Burkus J, LeHuec JC: Retrograde ejaculation after anterior lumbar interbody fusion: Transperitoneal versus retroperitoneal exposure. Spine (Phila Pa 1976) 28:1023-1026, 2003.

11. Humphreys SC, Hodges SD, Patwardhan AG, et al: Comparison of posterior and transforaminal approaches to lumbar interbody fusion. Spine (Phila Pa 1976) 26:567-571, 2001.

12. Harms J, Rolinger H: [A one-stager procedure in operative treatment of spondylolistheses: dorsal traction-reposition and anterior fusion (author's transl)]. Z Orthop Ihre Grenzgeb 120:343-347, 1982.

13. Hee HT, Castro FP Jr, Majd ME, et al: Anterior/posterior lumbar fusion versus transforaminal lumbar interbody fusion: Analysis of complications and predictive factors. J Spinal Disord 14:533-540, 2001.

14. Villavicencio AT, Burneikiene S, Bulsara KR, et al: Perioperative complications in transforaminal lumbar interbody fusion versus anterior-posterior reconstruction for lumbar disc degeneration and instability. J Spinal Disord Tech 19:92-97, 2006.

15. Javernick MA, Kuklo TR, Polly DW Jr: Transforaminal lumbar interbody fusion: Unilateral versus bilateral disk removal—an in vivo study. Am J Orthop 32:344-348; discussion 348, 2003.

16. Potter BK, Freedman BA, Verwiebe EG, et al: Transforaminal lumbar interbody fusion: Clinical and radiographic results and complications in 100 consecutive patients. J Spinal Disord Tech 18:337-346, 2005.

17. Hackenberg L, Halm H, Bullmann V, et al: Transforaminal lumbar interbody fusion: A safe technique with satisfactory three to five year results. Eur Spine J 14:551-558, 2005.

18. Whitecloud TS 3rd, Roesch WW, Ricciardi JE: Transforaminal interbody fusion versus anterior-posterior interbody fusion of the lumbar spine: A financial analysis. J Spinal Disord 14:100-103, 2001.

19. Hsieh PC, Koski TR, O'Shaughnessy BA, et al: Anterior lumbar interbody fusion in comparison with transforaminal lumbar interbody fusion: Implications for the restoration of foraminal height, local disc angle, lumbar lordosis, and sagittal balance. J Neurosurg Spine 7:379-386, 2007.

20. Kim JS, Kang BU, Lee SH, et al: Mini-transforaminal lumbar interbody fusion versus anterior lumbar interbody fusion augmented by percutaneous pedicle screw fixation: A comparison of surgical outcomes in adult low-grade isthmic spondylolisthesis. J Spinal Disord Tech 22:114-121, 2009.

21. Epstein NE: Foraminal and far lateral lumbar disc herniations: Surgical alternatives and outcome measures. Spinal Cord 40:491-500, 2002.

22. Schizas C, Tzinieris N, Tsiridis E, et al: Minimally invasive versus open transforaminal lumbar interbody fusion: Evaluating initial experience. Int Orthop 33:1683-1688, 2009.

23. Dhall SS, Wang MY, Mummaneni PV: Clinical and radiographic comparison of mini-open transforaminal lumbar interbody fusion with open transforaminal lumbar interbody fusion in 42 patients with long-term follow-up. J Neurosurg Spine 9:560-565, 2008.

24. Park P, Foley KT: Minimally invasive transforaminal lumbar interbody fusion with reduction of spondylolisthesis: Technique and outcomes after a minimum of 2 years' follow-up. Neurosurg Focus 25:E16, 2008.

25. Joseph V, Rampersaud YR: Heterotopic bone formation with the use of rhBMP2 in posterior minimal access interbody fusion: A CT analysis. Spine (Phila Pa 1976) 32:2885-2890, 2007.

26. Bridwell KH, Anderson PA, Boden SD, et al: What's new in spine surgery. J Bone Joint Surg Am 89:1654-1663, 2007.

27. Lewandrowski KU, Nanson C, Calderon R: Vertebral osteolysis after posterior interbody lumbar fusion with recombinant human bone morphogenetic protein 2: A report of five cases. Spine J 7:609-614, 2007.

28. McClellan JW, Mulconrey DS, Forbes RJ, et al: Vertebral bone resorption after transforaminal lumbar interbody fusion with bone morphogenetic protein (rhBMP-2). J Spinal Disord Tech 19:483-486, 2006.

29. Wong DA, Kumar A, Jatana S, et al: Neurologic impairment from ectopic bone in the lumbar canal: A potential complication of off-label PLIF/TLIF use of bone morphogenetic protein-2 (BMP-2). Spine J 8:1011-1018, 2008.

30. Kwon BK, Berta S, Daffner SD, et al: Radiographic analysis of transforaminal lumbar interbody fusion for the treatment of adult isthmic spondylolisthesis. J Spinal Disord Tech 16:469-476, 2003.

31. Hunt T, Shen FH, Shaffrey CI, et al: Contralateral radiculopathy after transforaminal lumbar interbody fusion. Eur Spine J 16(Suppl 3):311-314, 2007.

51

CHAPTER

Lumbar Total Disc Replacement

Jeffrey M. Spivak, MD
Tom Stanley, MD, MPH
Richard A. Balderston, MD

Lumbar spinal fusion is a time-tested, proven successful procedure for alleviating symptoms in patients with unremitting low back pain from various causes. Immobilizing an unstable motion segment, as in a degenerative or isthmic spondylolisthesis, is the most common and least controversial reason for performing a lumbar spinal fusion. Painful disc degeneration is a more controversial indication for spinal fusion because methods for identification of an intervertebral disc as the pain generator are imperfect. Multiple studies have shown successful pain relief of symptomatic lumbar degenerative disc disease with lumbar fusion.[1-4] Fusion also creates an anatomic situation with potentially negative consequences for long-term lumbar function, however. By limiting motion of the affected motion segment, additional stress is created at adjacent motion segments, leading to an increased incidence of adjacent level degeneration.[5-7] Often this degeneration becomes symptomatic and is a common cause of late failure after lumbar fusion.[7-10] In addition, spinal fusion fixes the sagittal alignment at that motion segment, which can affect the adjacent segments over time and be responsible for adjacent segment degeneration.[11] A third potential cause of adjacent segment degeneration is the potential iatrogenic injury of the adjacent level with surgery, especially injury to the cephalad facet joint with placement of pedicle screw instrumentation.

Total disc replacement (TDR) has been developed as an alternative method of stabilizing the lumbar spinal motion segment after removal of the painful disc. By maintaining mobility at the operative motion segment, patients maintain more normal overall lumbar mobility; theoretically, this may limit or eliminate the increased rate of adjacent segment degeneration over time seen with fusion surgery. Current implant designs require inherent motion segment stability before disc removal and mobilization, making significant spondylolisthesis, degenerative scoliosis, and isthmic defects contraindications to this technology. Advanced facet arthrosis is also considered a contraindication because continuing motion across arthritic facets may result in continued lumbar pain.

With these clinical and anatomic limitations on use, lumbar disc arthroplasty is appropriate only for a small percentage of overall lumbar fusion patients. Various studies have shown potential lumbar TDR candidates limited to 0% to 25% of fusion patients, depending on the specific demographics of the surgical practices being studied.[12,13] Many TDR implants have been shown to retain flexion-extension motion at the operative motion segment over time.[14-20] This chapter addresses the general concepts of lumbar total disc arthroplasty and focuses on the specifics of lumbar TDR implants that currently have U.S. Food and Drug Administration (FDA) approval or are completing FDA-sponsored multisite investigational device exemption (IDE) trials in preparation for FDA approval.

Historical Devices

The origins of disc replacement date back to the late 1950s, with the first early attempts at disc reconstruction being accomplished by the injection of acrylic bone cement within the nucleus after discectomy.[21-23] Around the same time, Fernstrom[24] began implanting stainless steel spheres into the intervertebral disc space through a posterior approach after laminotomy and discectomy. Low back pain was associated with progressive disc height loss, and so the goal of these early devices was to restore disc height and maintain spinal motion. Fernstrom[24] published his results in 1966, showing fair clinical results at 2 years postoperatively. The long-term outcomes of this device showed a high failure rate, however, secondary to subsidence of the implant with loss of motion, foraminal narrowing, and pain.

In the 1980s, artificial discs were designed using metal endplates and an intervening elastomeric rubber or plastic core, creating metal-plastic and rubber articulations among unattached components. The elastomeric discs were developed by Stefee and Lee and colleagues.[25-29] Only the Stefee disc (Acroflex, Acromed) was implanted clinically, but it was soon discontinued because of catastrophic failure of the rubber core.[25] Articulating discs include the SB CHARITÉ and the Marnay disc (later renamed the Prodisc I, precursor to the current Prodisc-L). Both discs enjoyed clinical success and are discussed later in this chapter. Another older implant design that never progressed to clinical application included the use of hinged spring articulation in all metal components. The

TABLE 51–1 Flexion-Extension of Lumbar Spine

L1-2	12.7 degrees ± 2.47
L2-3	16.6 degrees ± 2.43
L3-4	16.7 degrees ± 2.36
L4-5	18.3 degrees ± 2.67
L5-S1	19.6 degrees ± 4.71

newer, "modern," designs that are discussed in more detail in this chapter draw upon the continued Orthopaedic experience with large joint replacement with respect to articulating materials, component geometry, and component constraint to minimize the risk of mechanical failure of the arthroplasty device or late failure of the supporting structures of the motion segment.

Biomechanical Considerations

Each lumbar vertebral motion segment consists of three articulations—the intervertebral disc and the two facet joints. Static stabilizers of the motion segment include the anterior longitudinal ligament, posterior longitudinal ligament, interspinous ligament, intertransverse ligaments, ligamentum flavum, and facet joint capsules. The normal intervertebral disc is designed to absorb compressive forces. Compressive forces are converted to tensile forces in the anulus fibrosus via the nucleus-anulus couple. The effect of degeneration of the disc space is increased forces across the facet joint, leading to joint degeneration. One goal of disc replacement surgery is to restore the biomechanical function of the disc before facet joint degeneration, preventing long-term pain and disability.

Most of the forces seen across the motion segment are transmitted through the disc space. Force distribution across the disc and facet joint is posture dependent, however. Ledet and colleagues[30] performed real-time measurements of forces across the disc space using an interbody force transducer. In this study, forces across the intervertebral disc are highest when the center of gravity is shifted forward and during twisting motions. Forces across the intervertebral disc decrease when the center of gravity is shifted posteriorly. The corresponding postures show high forces across the disc space in sitting positions with the highest forces seen during sitting with the torso flexed and twisted. Standing and lying in the supine position resulted in progressively lower forces at the disc space. A fused segment has no effect on the force transmission to the adjacent level but increases the range of motion of the adjacent level.[31] The body attempts to preserve the total range of motion of the lumbar spine by compensating through the adjacent levels.

The vertebral motion segment is generally described as having six degrees of freedom. It can rotate (in two directions) along three axes, resulting in flexion-extension (rotation around the left-right axis or X-axis), left and right lateral bending (around the sagittal axis or Z-axis), and left and right axial rotation (around the coronal axis or Y-axis). Translational motion is also possible in the anteroposterior, left-right,

lateral, and up-down axial directions. Although distraction and compression can occur across the disc space, this motion has not been taken into consideration for the current first-generation articulating implant designs.

The motion segment does not act as a pure hinge in that the axis of rotation changes slightly with flexion and extension.[32,33] Each lumbar vertebral level has a different location of the instantaneous axis of rotation for a given movement. For the L1-5 disc spaces, the average instantaneous axis of rotation is slightly posterior to midline and just below the inferior endplate on a mid-sagittal image. At L5-S1, the instantaneous axis of rotation is within the disc space.[34] Range of motion and type of motion vary by level. Flexion-extension ranges from 12.7 to 19.6 degrees with the highest motion occurring at the L5-S1 segment (Table 51–1).[32] At the L4-5 level, the motion is mostly translational, whereas the motion is rotational at the L5-S1 segment. Most studies comparing disc arthroplasty with the normal motion segment focus on flexion and extension. The motion of each vertebral segment is not only multidimensional, but also rotation and translation are coupled to varying degrees by level.

Implant Design Considerations

Any design for a lumbar TDR implant should take into account the overall goals of the procedure, which include safe surgical implantation and long-lasting preservation of spinal motion. It is estimated that the lumbar spine undergoes 125,000 bending movements per year and is involved in 2 million strides per year. Over a 40-year life expectancy for a TDR implant, one might expect the implant to see 85 million cycles of motion. Implant endurance depends on its material characteristics, the nature and biomechanics of the articulation allowing motion, and the early and long-term fixation of the implant within the disc space. The range of motion an implant allows depends on the nature of the articulation or flexible materials and the geometry of the implant design.

Constrained versus Unconstrained

The concept of *constraint* in TDR has evolved over time and is not the same as in other articulating joint replacements of the appendicular skeleton. Kostuik[35] described constraint in terms of the implant's potential to limit the natural range of motion of the vertebral motion segment for each of the various rotational and translational motions. An implant *unconstrained* for a certain motion would provide no limitation to that motion well beyond the normal physiologic range. Examples are the CHARITÉ, Prodisc-L, and Maverick discs, which all are ball-and-socket articulations that provide no inherent limitation of axial rotation. These implants do have differing constraint, however, for the other motions of the lumbar motion segment.

An implant is considered *overconstrained* for a given motion if it limits that motion range to less than the physiologic range. The same three designs just mentioned are examples; all are overconstrained for motion in the compression-distraction plane. An implant is considered *underconstrained* for a given motion if it provides a limitation to that motion at or just outside of the extreme of the normal physiologic range. An example is the CHARITÉ prosthesis with a mobile core articulation, which is underconstrained for sagittal and lateral translation motions, whereas the ball-and-socket articulations of the Prodisc-L and Maverick are considered overconstrained with respect to these translational motions. These differences in constraint between the implant designs result in differing stresses seen within the supporting soft tissue structures and the facet articulations within the treated lumbar motion segment over time.

Generally, the effect of increasing constraint is to increase the overall stability of the motion segment. A consequence of increasing constraint may be to decrease range of motion and change the stresses seen at the surrounding structures. Increasing constraint has been shown to increase the forces seen at the endplates.[34,36,37] Increased stress at the endplate can have an effect on loosening of the component over time, as is seen in large joint arthroplasty. The effect of increasing constraint on the facet joints is unclear. Finite element models have shown increasing stress on the facet joints with increasing constraint.[36,38] In vitro analyses have shown increased facet joint stresses with decreased constraint.[39] Although it is logical to think that decreased constraint would increase the stress at the surrounding structures, the inconsistency in the data suggest that other factors may also play a role. Increased stress at the facet joints may lead to degenerative changes and pain over time. Implant design must balance between stability of the implant and restoring normal biomechanics.

Bearing Surfaces

Although many potential bearing surfaces are available, the most commonly used are cobalt-chromium alloy on ultrahigh molecular weight polyethylene (UHMWPE) and cobalt-chromium alloy on cobalt-chromium alloy. Both bearing surfaces are well established in orthopaedics for their biocompatibility and good wear resistance. Both bearing surfaces are known, however, to have long-term failures. Experience with large joint arthroplasty has shown that wear particles can lead to osteolysis, subsidence, migration, and need for revision surgery.[40-42] Nonetheless, the effect of wear particles within a joint have a different local effect compared with the epidural space.[43] To date, significant problems with osteolysis owing to polyethylene debris have not been seen clinically with the metal-polyethylene articulating implants with more than 20 years of use. This may be due to the lack of true synovium surrounding the disc arthroplasty, which has been implicated in the osteolysis seen associated with loosening of hip and knee implants.

Wear patterns observed in retrieval analysis of cobalt-chromium alloy with UHMWPE disc arthroplasty designs show the same failure mechanisms that are seen in hip and knee arthroplasty.[44,45] Cobalt-chromium alloy with cobalt-chromium alloy articulations also include the risk of systemic release of cobalt and chromium ions. Although the blood serum ion concentrations are similar to total hip arthroplasty,

the long-term effect is unknown.[46,47] Industrial exposure to heavy metals such as hexavalent chromium is known to increase systemic inflammation and carcinoma.[48] The types of ions that are released from an implant are different and may not have the same effect. Sarcoma adjacent to metal implants is reported in the literature, but it is very rare.[49] Metal hypersensitivity is a potential cause for persistent pain with this bearing surface.

Implant Stabilization

Any TDR implant must be stable where placed intraoperatively and maintain that position over time with the forces placed on the motion segment. An unstable implant can migrate sagittally or coronally or allow motion to occur at the bone-implant interface rather than the intended bearing surface. Subsidence of the implant into the bony endplates over time is effectively a vertical instability of the implant and can result in disc height loss, motion loss, and pain. Implant stability can be divided into early and late phases. *Early stability* refers to initial stability at the end of the surgical procedure and in the perioperative healing period. *Late stability* refers to long-term maintenance of implant position and attachment to the bony endplate surfaces.

Material and implant design considerations are factors in implant stability. Early stability is generally provided for by implant design, including roughened surface coatings, spikes, keels, or screw fixation.[50] Late stability is obtained through additional direct bony attachment to the implant via ongrowth or ingrowth into the surface coating. In addition, implants designed to maximize endplate surface area contact and promote force transfer to the peripheral aspect of the endplate, where the bone is strongest, minimize the risk of implant subsidence. Biologic surfaces have become the standard for noncemented acetabular fixation in total hip arthroplasty. Attempts at biologic coatings for total knee arthroplasty have failed secondary to loosening of the components.[51] This high failure rate is likely due to micromotion at the bone-implant interface. Similar problems must be monitored for in the spine.

Clinical Indications for Lumbar Total Disc Replacement

In the United States, lumbar disc replacement is currently approved for the treatment of single-level lumbar degenerative disc disease in skeletally mature individuals with no more than grade I spondylolisthesis having failed at least 6 months of nonoperative treatment. Currently available implants are approved only for use from L3 to S1 (Prodisc L3-S1, CHARITÉ L4-S1). The contraindications for TDR are extensive (Table 51-2). A relative contraindication is significant facet joint degeneration, although this is difficult to grade.[52] There are many reports of multilevel disc arthroplasty, including level 1 evidence in prospectively randomized clinical trials, but this is currently considered off-label use in the United States based on strict FDA-approved criteria.[39,53]

TABLE 51–2 Contraindications to Lumbar Total Disc Arthroplasty

Active systemic infection or infection localized to site of implantation

Osteopenia or osteoporosis defined as dual-energy x-ray absorptiometry scan bone density measured T-score ≤–1.0

Bony lumbar spinal stenosis

Allergy or sensitivity to implant materials (cobalt, chromium, molybdenum, polyethylene, titanium)

Isolated radicular compression syndromes, especially caused by disc herniation

Pars defect

Involved vertebral endplate dimensionally smaller than implant used

Clinically compromised vertebral bodies at affected level owing to current or past trauma

Lytic spondylolisthesis or degenerative spondylolisthesis of grade >1

Preoperative evaluation for total disc arthroplasty should include plain radiographs with flexion and extension films, magnetic resonance imaging (MRI), computed tomography (CT) scan, and dual-energy x-ray absorptiometry (DEXA) scan in patients at risk for osteopenia.[39] Discography is considered by many authors to be an important diagnostic criterion for lumbar TDR but was not a requirement for many of the FDA-sponsored clinical trials. In addition, more recent reports not only have questioned the efficacy of discography, but also have implicated it in accelerating the development of disc degeneration.[54-56]

Surgical Approach and Discectomy

Implant designs of most lumbar TDR devices require a direct anterior exposure of the intervertebral space; this is true of both prostheses currently available for use in the United States. This exposure can be obtained through either a transperitoneal or a retroperitoneal approach. Currently, a retroperitoneal approach is preferred because it minimizes the risk of postoperative ileus, bowel obstruction secondary to adhesions, and retrograde ejaculation (in men).[19] In most cases, the approach is performed with a vascular or general cosurgeon. The exposure must be wide enough to expose the entire anterior surface of the disc space, requiring greater mobilization of the great vessels than is necessary for fusion. The final view of the disc must be directly anterior. Other prostheses in development or available for use outside the United States (e.g., Oblique-Maverick) use an anterolateral or direct lateral approach to the disc space, minimizing or eliminating the need for mobilization of the great vessels.

After exposure of the disc space, the disc is removed in entirety, including the anterior anulus and anterior longitudinal ligament, the entire nucleus pulposus, and the posterior anulus. To restore posterior disc height in cases with significant disc collapse, the posterior longitudinal ligament must be either released or resected. The outer lateral anulus is preserved. The cartilaginous endplate is removed taking care to preserve the subchondral bone. To recreate the proper center

of rotation for the lumbar motion segment, most of the devices are placed abutting the posterior edge of the vertebral body. Proper posterior placement also helps to decrease the forces seen at the facet joints.[57] Position of the implant is confirmed using intraoperative anteroposterior and lateral fluoroscopy throughout the procedure.

Specific Devices

Only two designs have currently received FDA approval for use in the United States: the CHARITÉ Artificial Disc (DePuy Spine Inc., Raynham, MA) and the Prodisc-L prosthesis (Synthes Inc., Paoli, PA). Both designs use a metal-on-polyethylene articulation. Other devices are currently in use outside the United States and are well along in their FDA IDE trials in the United States, including the Maverick lumbar prosthesis (Medtronic Sofamor Danek Inc., Memphis, TN), the FlexiCore lumbar prosthesis (Stryker Spine, Allendale, NJ), and the Kineflex lumbar prosthesis (Spinal Motion, South Africa). These three devices all use a metal-on-metal bearing surface.

CHARITÉ Artificial Disc

The CHARITÉ Artificial Disc (DePuy Spine Inc., Raynham, MA) is the first device to complete the U.S. FDA approval process and has the largest and the longest clinical experience. The device has a biconvex UHMWPE spacer that acts as a mobile core (Fig. 51–1). The two metallic endplates are made of a cobalt-chromium alloy, and each concave endplate articulates independently with the core. There are ventral and dorsal teeth on the endplates to aid in positioning and maintenance of final position, and the latest version of the device has a titanium and a hydroxyapatite coating.[21]

The FDA IDE study gave level 1 evidence showing the CHARITÉ disc replacement as equivalent to anterior interbody fusion with a BAK cage (Zimmer Spine, Minneapolis MN) filled with iliac crest autograft.[14,15] In the study, 305 patients were randomly assigned to receive either the CHARITÉ lumbar disc replacement or anterior lumbar interbody fusion (ALIF) with a pair of cylindric threaded BAK cages and iliac crest autograft. Study levels included only L4-5 or L5-S1. For the CHARITÉ group, the Oswestry Disability Index (ODI) improved by 24.8 points from 50.6 preoperatively to 25.8 at 24 months. In the BAK fusion group, ODI improved by 22 points from 52.1 to 30.1. The visual analog score (VAS) improved from 72 points in the CHARITÉ group to 30.6 points at 24 months. For the BAK fusion group, the VAS improved from 71.8 to 36.3 points. These results were maintained at the 5-year follow-up.[58] In this study, FDA success at 24 months was defined by success in all of four major criteria: (1) a 25% improvement in the ODI, (2) no device failure, (3) no major complication, and (4) and no neurologic deterioration. In the FDA IDE study, 57% of the CHARITÉ group and 46% of the fusion group met all four criteria.

Longer term retrospective level 3 clinical data are also available for TDR using the CHARITÉ device.[59,60] Lemaire and

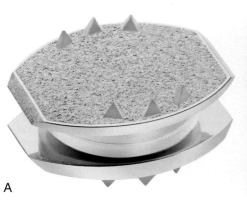
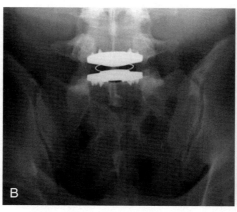
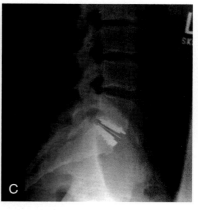

FIGURE 51–1 CHARITÉ lumbar disc replacement. **A,** Implant with three components nested as it rests in vivo, viewed from anterosuperior perspective. **B** and **C,** Anteroposterior (**B**) and lateral (**C**) radiographs of device in vivo.

colleagues[59] reviewed 100 patients with a minimum 10-year follow-up. Of patients, 90% had a good to excellent outcome with 63% returning to heavy labor jobs and 91.6% overall returning to work. Mean flexion-extension was 10.3 degrees with 5.4 degrees of lateral bending. Five patients (5%) required arthrodesis secondary to either implant failure or facet arthrosis. There were two neurologic injuries (2%), one L5 nerve injury and one sexual dysfunction, both of which recovered. There were two cases of spontaneous fusion (2%), and two cases of adjacent segment degeneration (2%). David[60] reviewed 106 patients implanted over a 6-year period with a minimum 10-year follow-up. Of patients, 82% had good to excellent outcomes; 89% returned to work with 77% returning to heavy labor. Eight patients (7.5%) required a posterior instrumented fusion. There were five cases (4.6%) of postoperative facet arthrosis, three cases (2.8%) of subsidence, three cases (2.8%) of adjacent level disease, and two cases (1.9%) of core subluxation.

Ross and colleagues[61] found poorer quality long-term results using the CHARITÉ device. Kaplan-Meier analysis was performed on 226 CHARITÉ implants. Radiologic failure was defined as a broken wire, subsidence, or lack of movement. At 8 years, there was a 90% survival rate. This rate declined dramatically to 35% at 13 years. At final follow-up, ODI improved by 14 points on average, 1 point below the benchmark for clinical improvement. At final follow-up, 69% of patients believed that they were better or much better than preoperatively; 20% believed that they were worse than preoperatively.

Cunningham and colleagues[62] showed that the CHARITÉ disc is effective in maintaining lumbar motion. They reviewed radiographs from the initial IDE study and assessed motion at the disc arthroplasty as a percentage of the total lumbar spine motion. These numbers were compared with cadaveric normal discs. At 2 years, the disc replacement maintained normal segmental lumbar motion and preserved the overall lumbar motion. Putzier and colleagues[63] reviewed 63 CHARITÉ discs at 17-year follow-up. At 17 years, 60% of the implanted discs had spontaneously ankylosed, and only 17% were deemed functional. In the patients in whom the disc replacement was

still functional, there was no evidence of adjacent segment degeneration, suggesting that a functional implant is effective in preventing adjacent segment degeneration. Clinically, the patients with spontaneous ankylosis did better than patients with functional implants. One suggested cause of the clinical failure is hypermobility leading to early facet joint degeneration at the arthroplasty level. Hypermobility from removal of the anterior longitudinal ligament has been shown in vitro.[64] In contrast, Huang and colleagues[65] assessed 51 TDRs at 8.5 years. Range of motion greater than 5 degrees corresponded to improved clinical outcome.

Prodisc-L

The Prodisc-L (Synthes Inc., Paoli, PA) is a modular metal and UHMWPE device with three components, two of which are locked together during insertion to create a two-piece implant (Fig. 51–2). The two endplates are made of cobalt-chromium alloy. The upper endplate has a concave articular surface. The lower metallic endplate has slots to accept a convex UHMWPE articular component. Both endplates are secured to the vertebral endplates by means of a central keel, small spikes, and a titanium plasma-sprayed rough surface.[21] The polyethylene is inserted into the disc space and locked to the caudal endplate after the endplates are in their final position, resulting in a single ball-and-socket articulation with the center of rotation in the upper aspect of the caudal vertebra.

The only level 1 evidence for the Prodisc-L comes from the U.S. FDA IDE trial. In this study, the Prodisc-L was compared with circumferential fusion with femoral ring allograft anteriorly and instrumented posterolateral fusion with iliac crest autograft. The 2-year data have been published.[20] VAS pain assessment showed statistically significant improvement from preoperative levels regardless of treatment. The average VAS score was 37 in the Prodisc-L group for a 39-mm average reduction and was 43 in the fusion group with a 32-mm average reduction from baseline and trended toward significance ($P = .08$). The FDA success criteria included ODI reduction by at least 15 points; improvement in short-form health survey (SF-36); device success; no adverse events;

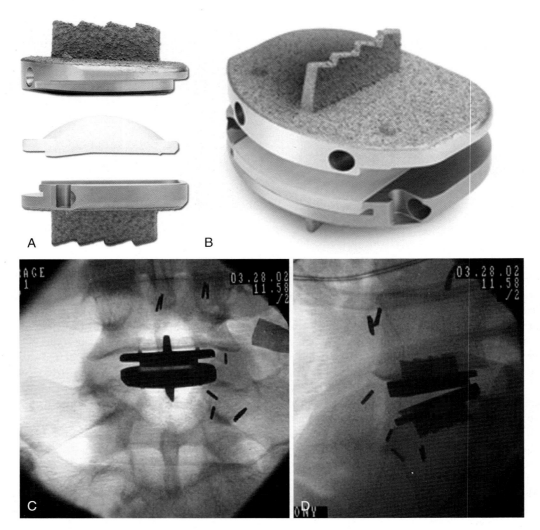

FIGURE 51–2 Prodisc-L lumbar disc replacement. **A,** Three components. **B,** Implant with ultrahigh molecular weight polyethylene component attached to caudal endplate, nested with cephalad endplate as it rests in vivo. **C** and **D,** Anteroposterior (**C**) and lateral (**D**) radiographs of device in vivo. (**A** and **B,** Courtesy Synthes, Inc.)

and multiple radiographic criteria including no migration or subsidence, no loosening or osteolysis, no loss of disc height, and no decrease in range of motion. Using the FDA success definition as success in all of these end points, 53% of Prodisc-L patients and 41% of control patients were considered successful, with a statistically significant difference favoring the Prodisc-L group. A more recent report of 5-year follow-up found no statistically significant difference in the ODI or VAS compared with 2 years.[66] Successful radiographic range of motion was maintained by 93.7% of Prodisc-L implants.

Cakir and colleagues[67] examined the clinical effect of TDR range of motion on clinical outcome at a minimum of 3 years after Prodisc-L implantation. They found no statistical difference in the preoperative and postoperative range of motion, with an increase in motion in 40% and a decrease in 30% of patients. The postoperative range of motion had no effect on clinical outcome. Bae and colleagues[68] reviewed 219 patients from the IDE trial at 2-year follow-up. In contrast, these authors found that greater average postoperative range of

motion correlated significantly with less VAS pain at 6 weeks at all time points. They also found that a greater body mass index correlated to a decrease in preoperative and postoperative range of motion at 1 and 2 years after arthroplasty.

Although Prodisc-L TDR is FDA approved only for single-level use in the United States, the results of multilevel surgeries have been reported. The U.S. FDA IDE study included a two-level arm, with adjacent two-level painful degenerative disc diseases cases prospectively randomized (in a similar 2:1 fashion as the one-level arm) to either a two-level Prodisc-L or circumferential fusion. These data were submitted to the FDA well after the one-level approval and have not yet been approved as a new amended indication for the use of Prodisc-L by the FDA as of the writing of this chapter. Results from the IDE trial for two-level Prodisc-L have been presented.[69] In the trial, 237 patients were randomly assigned to receive either two-level Prodisc-L or circumferential fusion at two levels. Intraoperative data showed that Prodisc-L cases had a significantly shorter operative time, estimated blood loss, and length

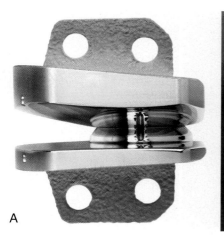
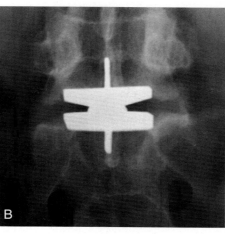
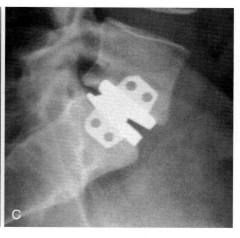

FIGURE 51–3 A, Two-piece all-metal Maverick lumbar disc replacement. **B** and **C,** Anteroposterior (**B**) and lateral (**C**) radiographs of device in vivo.

of hospital stay ($P < .0001$, $P = .0006$, $P < .0001$). At 24 months, 90% of Prodisc-L patients and 86.7% of fusion patients reported improvement in ODI from preoperative levels; 73.3% of Prodisc-L patients and 55.9% of fusion patients met the defined 15-point ODI improvement criteria. Overall neurologic success in Prodisc-L patients was superior to fusion patients (Prodisc-L 89.2%, fusion 77.9%; $P = .0260$). At all follow-up points, Prodisc-L patients recorded SF-36 scores significantly higher than fusion patients ($P = .0523$). VAS pain scores were significantly improved from preoperative scores regardless of treatment ($P < .0001$); at 24 months, the Prodisc-L group showed significantly higher pain reduction than the fusion group ($P = .0466$). VAS satisfaction at 24 months significantly favored Prodisc-L patients over fusion patients. At 24 months, a significant difference favored Prodisc-L patients over fusion patients (Prodisc-L 97.6%, fusion 91.8%, $P = .0497$) in device success—absence of any reoperation required to modify or remove implants and no need for supplemental fixation. Radiographic range of motion of patients was maintained within a normal functional range.

Siepe and colleagues[70] reviewed the results of 218 patients implanted with the Prodisc II device. The patients were divided into groups by the number of levels that the device was implanted. They found that implanting more than one level leads to worsening results compared with a single level. The results of Siepe and colleagues[70] are contradicted by another published study using the same device. Hannibal and colleagues[53] compared 27 patients receiving Prodisc II at one level with 32 patients receiving Prodisc II at two levels. The number of patients in each group was small, but the investigators found no statistical difference between the two groups at 2 years. These results are consistent with other published series.[71,72]

Other Devices

The Maverick lumbar TDR prosthesis (Medtronic Sofamor Danek Inc., Memphis, TN) is an all-metal two-piece design that uses a highly polished cobalt-chromium alloy ball-and-socket metal-on-metal articulation. The device has a central fin on both endplates and hydroxyapatite coating of all bony contact surfaces for increased stability after insertion (Fig. 51–3). The center of rotation is fixed posteriorly to the mid-portion of the prosthesis, in the upper aspect of the caudal vertebrae. The U.S. FDA IDE trial is currently ongoing; in this study, the Maverick TDR is compared with an anterior-only fusion using an LT cage with Infuse-BMP (Medtronic, Memphis, TN).

Published prospective level 2 evidence is available after European use. Le Huec and colleagues[73] reported the results of 64 implanted devices with a minimum of 2-year follow-up. ODI scores preoperatively and at 2-year follow-up were 43.8 and 23.1 ($P < .05$). Low back pain improved from a mean VAS score of 7.7 preoperatively to 3.2 at 2 years. Le Huec and colleagues[73] found that grade I and II facet joint degeneration did not influence the clinical outcome. They also found that paraspinal muscle atrophy resulted in a poorer outcome. The Maverick metal-on-metal articulation introduces the possibility of metal ion release into the bloodstream. Zeh and colleagues[47,74] found increased levels of cobalt and chromium at implantation of the Maverick prosthesis. The increased levels were persistent at 3-year follow-up and were similar to levels with a metal-on-metal total hip prosthesis.

Preliminary results at 2-year follow-up have been presented from the U.S. FDA IDE trial.[16] In the trial, 405 investigational (TDR) patients and 172 control (ALIF) patients with single-level degenerative disc disease (L4-S1) were treated after failing conservative care for 6 months. Mean (TDR and ALIF) operative time (1.8 hours and 1.4 hours) and blood loss (240.7 mL and 95.2 mL) differences were significant ($P < .001$); mean hospital stay (2.2 days and 2.3 days) and operative level distribution (73.6% and 78.5% L5-S1) were not. The mean ODI score improved dramatically for both groups at 12 months and 24 months (TDR 33.9 and 33.8 points; ALIF 29 and 29.3 points). At 24 months, 82.2% of TDR patients reported an ODI improvement of at least 15 points, an FDA-defined measure of success, versus 75.2% of ALIF patients.

Statistical superiority over fusion was concluded for Maverick mean improvements from preoperatively at all follow-up

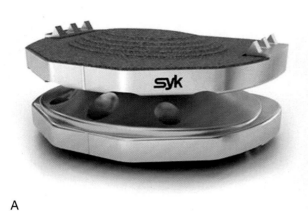
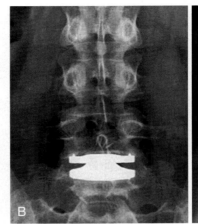
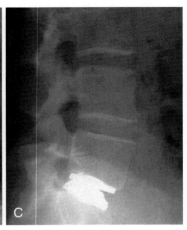

FIGURE 51–4 A, All-metal FlexiCore lumbar disc replacement. **B** and **C,** Anteroposterior (**B**) and lateral (**C**) radiographs of device in vivo.

intervals, including 24-month ODI, SF-36 physical component summary, and back pain scores. Both groups also showed significant improvement in leg pain scores from preoperatively. Fusion success was 100% for ALIF patients. TDR disc height and angular motion were maintained postoperatively. TDR patients returned to work 21 days sooner ($P = .038$) than ALIF patients. Finally, at 24 months, 86.2% of TDR patients said that they would have the surgery again versus 74.5% of ALIF patients ($P = .002$). Overall success rates at 24 months, an FDA composite measure of the primary study end points, showed superiority for TDR (77.2%) versus ALIF (64.2%).

The FlexiCore lumbar prosthesis (Stryker Spine, Allendale, NJ) is a cobalt-chromium alloy highly polished ball-and-socket metal-on-metal prosthesis.[21] The device is a one-piece design, which prevents separation and migration of a single endplate. The device also has a built-in rotational stop to prevent the facets from being overstressed (Fig. 51–4). There are fixation spikes on the upper and lower base with a titanium plasma spray coating to allow for bony ongrowth. There are currently no published clinical results with this device, but preliminary results have been presented. Adult patients with single-level discogenic pain who failed 6 months of nonoperative care were randomly assigned in a 2:1 ratio to FlexiCore disc replacement or circumferential fusion.[19] A total of 140 FlexiCore subjects and 58 fusion subjects were available for review.

At 2-year follow-up, the overall treatment success rate was 63% for FlexiCore versus 56% for fusion. Both treatments were beneficial for most patients, with 82% versus 79% achieving more than 15 points of VAS reduction and 70% versus 71% achieving more than 15 points of ODI improvement. The mean VAS change was −48.4 versus −45.9, and the mean ODI change was −30.8 points versus −29.4 points. Disc height was increased and maintained for both groups. Despite comparable VAS and ODI improvement, FlexiCore had less narcotic use at 24 months than fusion.

The Kineflex lumbar prosthesis (Spinal Motion, South Africa) is an unconstrained device that allows for the option of a metal-on-polyethylene or metal-on-metal articulation

with a mobile core. The mobile core is designed to replicate more closely the dynamic center of rotation of the normal disc (Fig. 51–5). The endplates have serrations and a keel for increased fixation. There are currently no published clinical results with this device; however, preliminary results have been presented. Hahnle and colleagues[17] reported their 2-year results with the Kineflex prosthesis. Using return to work, ODI, pain scoring, and patient satisfaction as the outcome measures, 100 patients were evaluated: 39 patients underwent an isolated single-level disc replacement; 25 patients, a two-level disc replacement; 1 patient, a double-level replacement adjacent to a previous fusion; and 7 patients, a fusion of another level at the time of the index procedure (hybrid cases). For 72 of 75 patients, 2-year clinical outcome was available (44 excellent, 17 good, 7 fair, and 4 poor). ODI score improved from 47.8 preoperatively to 14.5 ($P \le .01$) at the latest follow-up questionnaire. The pain score improved from 9.1 preoperatively to 2.9 at 2 years. As a group, the hybrid cases had the poorest outcome with two poor results out of seven.

Results at 12 months from the ongoing IDE trial have also been presented. In the trial, 58 patients were randomly assigned in a 1:1 ratio to receive either the Kineflex lumbar disc replacement or the CHARITÉ lumbar disc replacement (the control group).[18] Overall complication rates did not differ significantly between groups. At 1 year postoperatively, both groups showed statistically and clinically significant reductions in ODI (investigational group 50.1% and control group 56.6%) and VAS (investigational group 56.7% and control group 71.8%). There were no significant differences between the two groups. The FDA defines individual clinical success for the study at 24 months. When the criteria were applied at 12 months, the results did not differ significantly between groups (57.1% investigational and 72% control). Both groups had high patient satisfaction scores. No significant difference in time to return to work was shown between groups (investigational group 140 days and control group 113 days). Only one patient working preoperatively failed to return to work within 12 months. In the investigational group, six patients eligible but not working preoperatively returned to work.

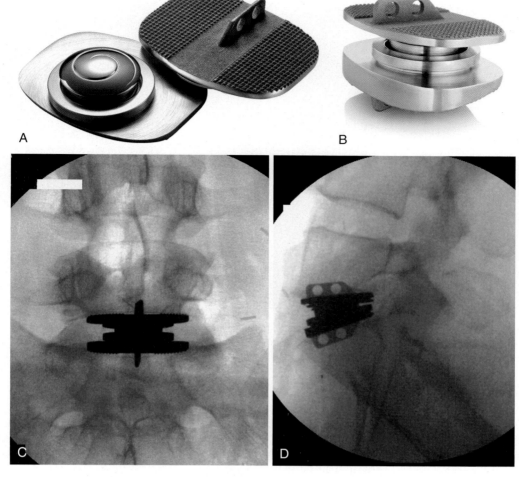

FIGURE 51–5 Kineflex lumbar disc replacement. **A,** Three components, with metal core resting on inferior endplate. **B,** Implant with three components nested as it would rest in vivo. **C** and **D,** Anteroposterior (**C**) and lateral (**D**) radiographs of device in vivo.

Hybrid Procedures

A *hybrid construct* refers to the use of a lumbar disc replacement adjacent to a fusion. The TDR may be performed along with fusion of an adjacent level, or it may be performed adjacent to a previously fused level (Fig. 51–6). Both of these clinical scenarios are considered off-label use for the prostheses currently available for use in the United States based on the inclusion and exclusion criteria from the FDA IDE trials. The theoretical advantages of preventing adjacent segment disease may have more utility when used in hybrid constructs. The advantages would be increased in longer fusions, which have a higher incidence of adjacent segment disease.[75-78] Aunoble and colleagues[79] implanted hybrid constructs in 42 patients and followed them prospectively. At 2 years, ODI decreased by 53%. No prospective randomized level 1 data or long-term prospective data exist to support the regular use of these hybrid constructs, however.

Complications and Revision Strategies

Complications after total disc arthroplasty can be early or delayed. Although there are complications associated with use of an anterior approach, these are not specifically reviewed here because they are not specific to total disc arthroplasty. The full-width, direct anterior exposure required for disc arthroplasty requires greater mobilization of the great vessels, which may increase the morbidity of the procedure compared with use of cage or bone graft, which can be inserted off midline or via an anterolateral approach if necessary. Early complications include endplate fracture, subsidence, nerve entrapment, and dislocation. Late complications include infection, osteolysis and loosening, hardware failure, facet arthrosis, fracture, and spontaneous fusion. The early complication rate ranges from 0% to 25%.[39,60,61,80-83] This complication rate increases as the number of levels operated on increases.[84] The late complication rate is 21%, although a true assessment of this number requires long-term data.[59,85]

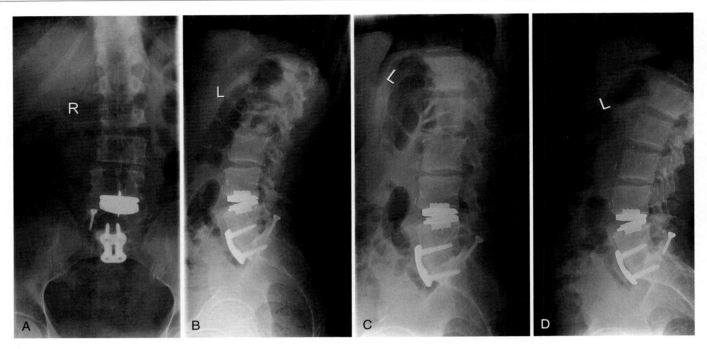

FIGURE 51–6 Hybrid construct with Prodisc TDR at L4-5 and fusion at L5-S1 done for a patient with two-level painful degenerative disc disease and prior L5-S1 left discectomy with facetectomy. **A** and **B,** Anteroposterior (**A**) and lateral (**B**) views. **C** and **D,** Flexion (**C**) and extension (**D**) lateral views.

Each individual device has its own unique mechanisms of failure, so each device design should be evaluated individually. The early CHARITÉ design was associated with rim fracture of the polyethylene insert.[86] Alternative designs using a polyethylene core may not have the same problem. Implant revision is an important consideration because it is likely that many young patients require a revision in their lifetime. Prosthesis removal, when necessary, can often be accomplished via an anterolateral or direct lateral approach without full mobilization of the great vessels.

The limited life span for any motion-preserving device requires an assessment of revisability. In situ posterior fusion with retention of the components is possible for patients who experience subsidence, fracture, or facet arthrosis. It is still unclear whether this approach, with retention of the TDR implant, yields fusion or clinical results similar, better, or worse than strategies that include removal of the TDR device and interbody fusion. There are limited options for revision when removal of the components is required. Anatomic approaches include right and left retroperitoneal, transperitoneal, and direct lateral approach, either with reflection of the psoas muscle or with a trans–psoas muscle–splitting approach. Even keeled prostheses can be removed via an anterolateral or direct lateral approach.[87,88] Ideally, a surgical approach different from that used in the primary implantation should be considered, unless revision is done for acute failure within 3 weeks of the index procedure.

A revision anterior surgical approach is associated with a significantly higher complication rate than a primary approach.[80,89] Scar tissue complicates the anterior approach because mobilization of the great vessels becomes much more challenging and sometimes impossible. This is most problematic at the L4-5 level. Changing the approach minimizes the risk of injury to the large vessels that are encased in the scar tissue. McAfee and colleagues[90] reviewed 24 patients who underwent revision using an anterior approach. Four patients (16.7%) sustained an injury to the large vessels. Leary and colleagues[91] had a large vessel injury rate of 10% (2 of 20) after revision anterior exposure. Bumpass and colleagues[92] performed cadaveric dissections of the lumbar plexus to determine retrievability through a posterior approach. The smallest root-to-root distance measured was 9.1 mm. The smallest measured root-to-tether distance was 39.2 mm. These measurements theoretically allow for removal of small implants posteriorly. No clinical studies assess the risk of nerve injury through a posterior approach.

Future Considerations

Only time and close study will tell if persistent motion at an operative segment (as opposed to fusion) minimizes adjacent degeneration and if specific motion patterns, based on TDR implant biomechanics, are more clinically beneficial than others. The true fate of the mobile facet joints at the TDR level over time for the various implants is also a clinical unknown that needs more long-term radiographic follow-up. Newer lumbar TDR devices are attempting to incorporate the viscoelastic properties of the native disc, which might also provide a role in dissipation of acute axial loads and protect adjacent segments. One example is the one-piece polymer core and metal endplate Freedom disc (Axiomed Spine Corporation, Cleveland, OH). Finally, devices designed for a lateral or posterior insertion into the disc space are being designed and

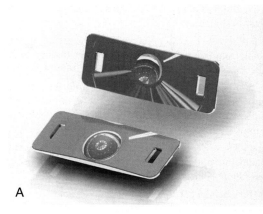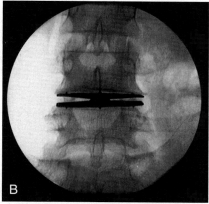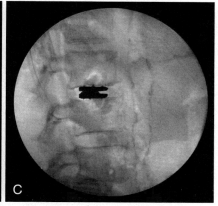

FIGURE 51–7 NuVasive XL lumbar disc replacement. **A,** Two all-metal components. **B** and **C,** Anteroposterior (**B**) and lateral (**C**) radiographs of device in vivo.

tested, and these may improve the safety for revision or removal when needed. One example is the XL TDR (NuVasive, San Diego, CA), a ball-and-socket TDR device designed for direct lateral implantation (Fig. 51–7). This device is currently being implanted in limited use in patients outside of the United States.

Conclusion

Lumbar TDR fits well into the current trend toward motion preservation in spinal surgery and as a potential surgical strategy to prevent the increase in adjacent level degeneration seen with lumbar fusions. The U.S. clinical trials for the various devices provide level 1 prospective randomized data showing clinical success for fusion and TDR for properly selected patients with chronic back pain secondary to disc degeneration. Despite the noninferiority design of the clinical trials, the published data seem to indicate that a well-implanted, functional disc replacement can result in a better clinical outcome than a fused segment. Revision and removal of the current devices are quite technically challenging. Devices using anterolateral or direct lateral placement may help in this regard.

PEARLS

1. Level 1 scientific evidence for the efficacy of lumbar TDR exists for one-level and two-level degenerative disc disease, although U.S. FDA approval is currently only for single-level use.

2. Preoperative CT scans should be considered in all lumbar TDR patients to assess for facet arthrosis and to ensure there is no preoperative unrecognized spondylolysis.

3. DEXA scans should be obtained preoperatively in patients older than 50 years or if there are other clinical risk factors for osteoporosis because osteopenia (T-score of ≤-1.0) is a contraindication to lumbar disc replacement.

4. Care should be taken to preserve the bony endplates. Endplate insufficiency is an indication to convert to fusion.

5. Radiographic confirmation of midline in the coronal plane (on anteroposterior fluoroscopic view) is imperative before final disc space preparation and implant insertion.

PITFALLS

1. Failure to identify the patient's pain generator adequately may lead to a higher clinical failure rate than published series.

2. Extremely easy mobilization and distraction of a collapsed disc space may point to unrecognized defects in the pars interarticularis.

3. Failure to mobilize the motion segment adequately before implant insertion or attempts to stuff the disc space with the tallest TDR implant would result in limited postoperative range of motion.

4. Implant insertion with inadequate anterior exposure may result in device positioning unacceptably off the midline.

5. For revision anterior surgery for device removal, the surgeon should consider an alternative approach to the disc space from the original approach.

KEY POINTS

1. The U.S. FDA IDE clinical trials for the various devices provide level 1 prospective randomized data showing clinical success for fusion and TDR for properly selected patients with chronic back pain secondary to disc degeneration.

2. Despite the noninferiority design of the clinical trials, the published data seem to indicate that a well-implanted, functional disc replacement can result in a better clinical outcome than a fused segment.

3. Revision and removal of the current lumbar TDR devices remain quite technically challenging.

4. Detection of differences in clinical outcomes for the various lumbar TDR devices with differing biomechanical strategies and biomaterials requires longer term follow-up.

5. Long-term results are also needed to see if current motion preservation designs are effective in preventing adjacent segment degeneration seen with lumbar fusions.

KEY REFERENCES

1. Eck JC, Humphreys SC, Hodges SD: Adjacent-segment degeneration after lumbar fusion: A review of clinical, biomechanical, and radiologic studies. Am J Orthop 28:336-340, 1999.
   This is a comprehensive review of biomechanical and clinical studies evaluating the incidence of adjacent segment degeneration. Identified risk factors include patient age, use of interbody fusion, surgical technique, and hypermobility.

2. Carragee EJ, Paragioudakis SJ, Khurana S: 2000 Volvo Award winner in clinical studies: Lumbar high-intensity zone and discography in subjects without low back problems. Spine (Phila Pa 1976) 25:2987-2992, 2000.
   This prospective observational study assessed the incidence of high-intensity zones in symptomatic and asymptomatic individuals and correlation with pain using lumbar discography. This article not only highlights the difficulty in assessing discogenic back pain but also gives a reason for the high variability in clinical results.

3. Putzier M, Funk JF, Schneider SV, et al: CHARITÉ total disc replacement—clinical and radiographical results after an average follow-up of 17 years. Eur Spine J 15:183-195, 2006.
   This article describes one of the longest term published clinical series of lumbar disc replacements. The study showed that disc replacement effectively prevents adjacent segment disease when functional but also found a high incidence of spontaneous ankylosis at the implanted level.

4. Zigler J, Delamarter R, Spivak JM, et al: Results of the prospective, randomized, multicenter Food and Drug Administration investigational device exemption study of the ProDisc-L total disc replacement versus circumferential fusion for the treatment of 1-level degenerative disc disease. Spine (Phila Pa 1976) 32:1155-1162; discussion 1163, 2007.
   This article presents the data for the Prodisc-L pivotal FDA IDE study, finding one-level Prodisc-L noninferior to anteroposterior fusion for ODI and VAS pain improvement and significantly better than fusion for neurologic recovery, SF-36 improvement, and VAS patient satisfaction at 2 years postoperatively, with an average maintenance of 7.7 degrees of flexion-extension motion.

5. Guyer RD, McAfee PC, Banco RJ, et al: Prospective, randomized, multicenter Food and Drug Administration investigational device exemption study of lumbar total disc replacement with the CHARITÉ artificial disc versus lumbar fusion: Five-year follow-up. Spine J 9:374-386, 2009.
   This article presents the 5-year follow-up data for the CHARITÉ pivotal FDA IDE study, which found maintenance of the 24-month result showing noninferiority of a one-level CHARITÉ TDR to ALIF with BAK cages and iliac autograft at 5 years after the procedure.

REFERENCES

1. O'Brien JP: The role of fusion for chronic low back pain. Orthop Clin North Am 14:639-647, 1983.

2. Fischgrund JS, Montgomery DM: Diagnosis and treatment of discogenic low back pain. Orthop Rev 22:311-318, 1993.

3. Wetzel FT, LaRocca SH, Lowery GL, et al: The treatment of lumbar spinal pain syndromes diagnosed by discography: Lumbar arthrodesis. Spine (Phila Pa 1976) 19:792-800, 1994.

4. Thalgott JS, Giuffre JM, Klezl Z, Timlin M: Anterior lumbar interbody fusion with titanium mesh cages, coralline hydroxyapatite, and demineralized bone matrix as part of a circumferential fusion. Spine J 2:63-69, 2002.

5. Rao RD, David KS, Wang M: Biomechanical changes at adjacent segments following anterior lumbar interbody fusion using tapered cages. Spine (Phila Pa 1976) 30:2772-2776, 2005.

6. Dekutoski MB, Schendel MJ, Ogilvie JW, et al: Comparison of in vivo and in vitro adjacent segment motion after lumbar fusion. Spine (Phila Pa 1976) 19:1745-1751, 1994.

7. Eck JC, Humphreys SC, Hodges SD: Adjacent-segment degeneration after lumbar fusion: A review of clinical, biomechanical, and radiologic studies. Am J Orthop 28:336-340, 1999.

8. Lee CK: Accelerated degeneration of the segment adjacent to a lumbar fusion. Spine (Phila Pa 1976) 13:375-377, 1988.

9. Whitecloud TS 3rd, Davis JM, Olive PM: Operative treatment of the degenerated segment adjacent to a lumbar fusion. Spine (Phila Pa 1976) 19:531-536, 1994.

10. Rahm MD, Hall BB: Adjacent-segment degeneration after lumbar fusion with instrumentation: A retrospective study. J Spinal Disord 9:392-400, 1996.

11. Djurasovic MO, Carreon LY, Glassman SD, et al: Sagittal alignment as a risk factor for adjacent level degeneration: A case-control study. Orthopedics 31:546, 2008.

12. Huang RC, Lim MR, Girardi FP, et al: The prevalence of contraindications to total disc replacement in a cohort of lumbar surgical patients. Spine (Phila Pa 1976) 29:2538-2541, 2004.

13. Wong DA, Annesser B, Birney T, et al: Incidence of contraindications to total disc arthroplasty: A retrospective review of 100 consecutive fusion patients with a specific analysis of facet arthrosis. Spine J 7:5-11, 2007.

14. McAfee PC, Cunningham B, Holsapple G, et al: A prospective, randomized, multicenter Food and Drug Administration investigational device exemption study of lumbar total disc replacement with the CHARITE artificial disc versus lumbar fusion: Part II. Evaluation of radiographic outcomes and correlation of surgical technique accuracy with clinical outcomes. Spine (Phila Pa 1976) 30:1576-1583; discussion E388-E390, 2005.

15. Blumenthal S, McAfee PC, Guyer RD, et al: A prospective, randomized, multicenter Food and Drug Administration investigational device exemptions study of lumbar total disc replacement with the CHARITE artificial disc versus lumbar fusion: Part I. Evaluation of clinical outcomes. Spine (Phila Pa 1976) 30:1565-1575; discussion E387-E391, 2005.

16. Gornet MF, Burkus JK, Mathews HH, et al: Maverick total disc replacement versus anterior lumbar interbody fusion with the INFUSE bone graft/LT-CAGE device: A prospective, randomized, controlled, multicenter IDE trial. Spine J 7(Suppl 1):1S, 2007.

17. Hahnle U, Weinberg IR, De Villiers M: Kineflex (Centurion) lumbar disc prosthesis: Two-year results. Spine J 6(Suppl 1):109S-110S, 2006.

18. Knight R, MacLennan B, Roh J, et al: A prospective, randomized, FDA IDE study of lumbar TDR with the Kineflex artificial disc

vs. the Charité artificial disc: Evaluation of clinical outcomes at 12 months from a single site. Spine J 9(Suppl 1):69S, 2009.

19. Errico T, Sasso R, Mize G, et al: Total disc replacement for treating lumbar discogenic back pain: A prospective randomized multicenter study of FlexiCore vs. 360 spinal fusion. Spine J 8(Suppl 1):15S-16S, 2008.

20. Zigler J, Delamarter R, Spivak JM, et al: Results of the prospective, randomized, multicenter Food and Drug Administration investigational device exemption study of the ProDisc-L total disc replacement versus circumferential fusion for the treatment of 1-level degenerative disc disease. Spine (Phila Pa 1976) 32:1155-1162; discussion 1163, 2007.

21. Errico TJ: Lumbar disc arthroplasty. Clin Orthop Relat Res (435):106-117, 2005

22. Cleveland D: Interspace reconstruction and spinal stabilization after disk removal. Lancet 76:327-331, 1956.

23. Hamby WB, Glaser HT: Replacement of spinal intervertebral discs with locally polymerizing methyl methacrylate: Experimental study of effects upon tissues and report of a small clinical series. J Neurosurg 16:311-313, 1959.

24. Fernstrom U: Arthroplasty with intercorporal endoprothesis in herniated disc and in painful disc. Acta Chir Scand Suppl 357:154-159, 1966.

25. Steffee AD: The Steffee artificial disc. In Weinstein JN (ed). Clinical efficacy and outcome in the diagnosis and treatment of low back pain. New York: Raven Press, 1992, pp 245-247.

26. Lee CK, Langrana NA, Parsons JR, et al: Development of a prosthetic intervertebral disc. Spine (Phila Pa 1976) 16(6 Suppl):S253-S255, 1991.

27. Enker P, Steffee A, Mcmillin C, et al: Artificial disc replacement: Preliminary report with a 3-year minimum follow-up. Spine (Phila Pa 1976) 18:1061-1070, 1993.

28. Vuono-Hawkins M, Zimmerman MC, Lee CK, et al: Mechanical evaluation of a canine intervertebral disc spacer: In situ and in vivo studies. J Orthop Res 12:119-127, 1994.

29. Vuono-Hawkins M, Langrana NA, Parsons JR, et al: Materials and design concepts for an intervertebral disc spacer. II. Multidurometer composite design. J Appl Biomater 6:117-123, 1995.

30. Ledet EH, Tymeson MP, DiRisio DJ, et al: Direct real-time measurement of in vivo forces in the lumbar spine. Spine J 5:85-94, 2005.

31. Chow DH, Luk KD, Evans JH, et al: Effects of short anterior lumbar interbody fusion on biomechanics of neighboring unfused segments. Spine (Phila Pa 1976) 21:549-555, 1996.

32. Yoshioka T, Tsuji H, Hirano N, et al: Motion characteristic of the normal lumbar spine in young adults: Instantaneous axis of rotation and vertebral center motion analyses. J Spinal Disord 3:103-113, 1990.

33. Pearcy MJ, Bogduk N: Instantaneous axes of rotation of the lumbar intervertebral joints. Spine (Phila Pa 1976) 13:1033-1041, 1988.

34. Frelinghuysen P, Huang RC, Girardi FP, et al: Lumbar total disc replacement, part I: Rationale, biomechanics, and implant types. Orthop Clin North Am 36:293-299, 2005.

35. Kostuik JP: Intervertebral disc replacement: Experimental study. Clin Orthop Relat Res (337):27-41, 1997.

36. Chung SK, Kim YE, Wang KC: Biomechanical effect of constraint in lumbar total disc replacement: A study with finite element analysis. Spine (Phila Pa 1976) 34:1281-1286, 2009.

37. Galbusera F, Bellini CM, Zweig T, et al: Design concepts in lumbar total disc arthroplasty. Eur Spine J 17:1635-1650, 2008.

38. Rundell SA, Auerbach JD, Balderston RA, et al: Total disc replacement positioning affects facet contact forces and vertebral body strains. Spine (Phila Pa 1976) 33:2510-2517, 2008.

39. Rousseau MA, Bradford DS, Bertagnoli R, et al: Disc arthroplasty design influences intervertebral kinematics and facet forces. Spine J 6:258-266, 2006.

40. Mirra JM, Amstutz HC, Matos M, et al: The pathology of the joint tissues and its clinical relevance in prosthesis failure. Clin Orthop Relat Res (117):221-240, 1976.

41. Howie DW, Haynes DR, Rogers SD, et al: The response to particulate debris. Orthop Clin North Am 24:571-581, 1993.

42. Howie DW, Manthey B, Hay S, et al: The synovial response to intraarticular injection in rats of polyethylene wear particles. Clin Orthop Relat Res (292):352-357, 1993.

43. Cunningham BW: Basic scientific considerations in total disc arthroplasty. Spine J 4(6 Suppl):219S-230S, 2004.

44. Kurtz SM, van Ooij A, Ross R, et al: Polyethylene wear and rim fracture in total disc arthroplasty. Spine J 7:12-21, 2007.

45. Punt IM, Visser VM, van Rhijn LW, et al: Complications and reoperations of the SB Charite lumbar disc prosthesis: Experience in 75 patients. Eur Spine J 17:36-43, 2008.

46. Cobb AG, Schmalzreid TP: The clinical significance of metal ion release from cobalt-chromium metal-on-metal hip joint arthroplasty. Proc Inst Mech Eng H 220:385-398, 2006.

47. Zeh A, Planert M, Siegert G, et al: Release of cobalt and chromium ions into the serum following implantation of the metal-on-metal Maverick-type artificial lumbar disc (Medtronic Sofamor Danek). Spine (Phila Pa 1976) 32:348-352, 2007.

48. Keegan GM, Learmonth ID, Case CP: A systematic comparison of the actual, potential, and theoretical health effects of cobalt and chromium exposures from industry and surgical implants. Crit Rev Toxicol 38:645-674, 2008.

49. Keel SB, Jaffe KA, Petur Nielsen G, et al: Orthopaedic implant-related sarcoma: A study of twelve cases. Mod Pathol 14:969-977, 2001.

50. Lee CK, Goel VK: Artificial disc prosthesis: Design concepts and criteria. Spine J 4(6 Suppl):209S-218S, 2004.

51. Fehring TK, Odum S, Griffin WL, et al: Early failures in total knee arthroplasty. Clin Orthop Relat Res (392):315-318, 2001.

52. Walraevens J, Liu B, Meersschaert J, et al: Qualitative and quantitative assessment of degeneration of cervical intervertebral discs and facet joints. Eur Spine J 18:358-369, 2009.

53. Hannibal M, Thomas DJ, Low J, et al: ProDisc-L total disc replacement: A comparison of 1-level versus 2-level arthroplasty patients with a minimum 2-year follow-up. Spine (Phila Pa 1976) 32:2322-2326, 2007.

54. Carragee EJ, Paragioudakis SJ, Khurana S: 2000 Volvo Award winner in clinical studies: Lumbar high-intensity zone and discography in subjects without low back problems. Spine (Phila Pa 1976) 25:2987-2992, 2000.

55. Carragee EJ, Lincoln T, Parmar VS, et al: A gold standard evaluation of the "discogenic pain" diagnosis as determined by provocative discography. Spine (Phila Pa 1976) 31:2115-2123, 2006.

56. Carragee EJ, Alamin TF, Miller J, et al: Provocative discography in volunteer subjects with mild persistent low back pain. Spine J 2:25-34, 2002.

57. Dooris AP, Goel VK, Grosland NM, et al: Load-sharing between anterior and posterior elements in a lumbar motion segment implanted with an artificial disc. Spine (Phila Pa 1976) 26:E122-E129, 2001.

58. Guyer RD, McAfee PC, Banco RJ, et al: Prospective, randomized, multicenter Food and Drug Administration investigational device exemption study of lumbar total disc replacement with the CHARITE artificial disc versus lumbar fusion: Five-year follow-up. Spine J 9:374-386, 2009.

59. Lemaire JP, Carrier H, Sariali el-H, et al: Clinical and radiological outcomes with the Charite artificial disc: A 10-year minimum follow-up. J Spinal Disord Tech 18:353-359, 2005.

60. David T: Long-term results of one-level lumbar arthroplasty: Minimum 10-year follow-up of the CHARITE artificial disc in 106 patients. Spine (Phila Pa 1976) 32:661-666, 2007.

61. Ross R, Mirza AH, Norris HE, et al: Survival and clinical outcome of SB Charite III disc replacement for back pain. J Bone Joint Surg Br 89:785-789, 2007.

62. Cunningham BW, McAfee PC, Geisler FH, et al: Distribution of in vivo and in vitro range of motion following 1-level arthroplasty with the CHARITE artificial disc compared with fusion. J Neurosurg Spine 8:7-12, 2008.

63. Putzier M, Funk JF, Schneider SV, et al: Charite total disc replacement—clinical and radiographical results after an average follow-up of 17 years. Eur Spine J 15:183-195, 2006.

64. Cunningham BW, Gordon JD, Dmitriev AE, et al: Biomechanical evaluation of total disc replacement arthroplasty: An in vitro human cadaveric model. Spine (Phila Pa 1976) 28:S110-S117, 2003.

65. Huang RC, Girardi FP, Cammisa FP Jr, et al: Correlation between range of motion and outcome after lumbar total disc replacement: 8.6-year follow-up. Spine (Phila Pa 1976) 30:1407-1411, 2005.

66. Delamarter R, Zigler J, Spivak JM, et al: Five year results of the prospective randomized multicenter FDA IDE ProDisc-L clinical trial. Spine J 8(Suppl 1):62S-63S, 2008.

67. Cakir B, Schmidt R, Mattes T, et al: Index level mobility after total lumbar disc replacement: Is it beneficial or detrimental? Spine (Phila Pa 1976) 34:917-923, 2009.

68. Bae H, Kanim LEA, Kropf M, et al: Radiographic range of motion is related to clinical outcomes in lumbar artificial disc replacement patients: One site analysis of 219 patients with minimum 2 year follow-up, USA-FDA IDE study. Spine J 9(Suppl 1):104S-105S, 2009.

69. Delamarter R, Zigler J, Balderston RA, et al: Results of the prospective randomized multicenter FDA IDE study of the ProDisc-L total disc replacement vs. circumferential fusion for the treatment of two level degenerative disc disease. Spine J 8(Suppl 1):94S-95S, 2008.

70. Siepe CJ, Mayer HM, Heinz-Leisenheimer M, et al: Total lumbar disc replacement: Different results for different levels. Spine (Phila Pa 1976) 32:782-790, 2007.

71. Bertagnoli R, Yue JJ, Nanieva R, Fenk-Mayer A, et al: Lumbar total disc arthroplasty in patients older than 60 years of age: A prospective study of the ProDisc prosthesis with 2-year minimum follow-up period. J Neurosurg Spine 4:85-90, 2006.

72. Bertagnoli R, Yue JJ, Shah RV, et al: The treatment of disabling multilevel lumbar discogenic low back pain with total disc arthroplasty utilizing the ProDisc prosthesis: A prospective study with 2-year minimum follow-up. Spine (Phila Pa 1976) 30:2192-2199, 2005.

73. Le Huec JC, Mathews H, Basso Y, et al: Clinical results of Maverick lumbar total disc replacement: Two-year prospective follow-up. Orthop Clin North Am 36:315-322, 2005.

74. Zeh A, Becker C, Planert M, et al: Time-dependent release of cobalt and chromium ions into the serum following implantation of the metal-on-metal Maverick type artificial lumbar disc (Medtronic Sofamor Danek). Arch Orthop Trauma Surg 129:741-746, 2009.

75. Gillet P: The fate of the adjacent motion segments after lumbar fusion. J Spinal Disord Tech 16:338-345, 2003.

76. Hilibrand AS, Robbins M: Adjacent segment degeneration and adjacent segment disease: The consequences of spinal fusion? Spine J 4(6 Suppl):190S-194S, 2004.

77. Park P, Garton HJ, Gala VC, et al: Adjacent segment disease after lumbar or lumbosacral fusion: Review of the literature. Spine (Phila Pa 1976) 29:1938-1944, 2004.

78. Throckmorton TW, Hilibrand AS, Mencio GA, et al: The impact of adjacent level disc degeneration on health status outcomes following lumbar fusion. Spine (Phila Pa 1976) 28:2546-2550, 2003.

79. Aunoble S, Meyrat R, Al Sawad Y, et al: Hybrid construct for two levels disc disease in lumbar spine. Eur Spine J 19:290-296, 2010.

80. Geisler FH, Guyer RD, Blumenthal SL, et al: Effect of previous surgery on clinical outcome following 1-level lumbar arthroplasty. J Neurosurg Spine 8:108-114, 2008.

81. Berg S, Tullberg T, Branth B, et al: Total disc replacement compared to lumbar fusion: A randomised controlled trial with 2-year follow-up. Eur Spine J 18:1512-1519, 2009.

82. Guyer RD, Geisler FH, Blumenthal SL, et al: Effect of age on clinical and radiographic outcomes and adverse events following 1-level lumbar arthroplasty after a minimum 2-year follow-up. J Neurosurg Spine 8:101-107, 2008.

83. Blumenthal S, Zigler J, Guyer RD, et al: A prospective randomized comparison of cervical disc replacement and anterior cervical fusion. Spine J 8(Suppl 1):147S-148S, 2008.

84. Di Silvestre M, Bakaloudis G, Lolli F, et al: Two-level total lumbar disc replacement. Eur Spine J 18(Suppl 1):64-70, 2009.

85. Park CK, Ryu KS, Jee WH: Degenerative changes of discs and facet joints in lumbar total disc replacement using ProDisc II: Minimum two-year follow-up. Spine (Phila Pa 1976) 33:1755-1761, 2008.

86. Kurtz SM, Peloza J, Siskey R, et al: Analysis of a retrieved polyethylene total disc replacement component. Spine J 5:344-350, 2005.

87. Pimenta L, Diaz RC, Guerrero LG: Charite lumbar artificial disc retrieval: Use of a lateral minimally invasive technique. Technical note. J Neurosurg Spine 5:556-561, 2006.

88. Spivak JM, Petrizzo AM: Revision of a lumbar disc arthroplasty following late infection. Eur Spine J 19:677-681, 2010.

89. Brau SA, Delamarter RB, Kropf MA, et al: Access strategies for revision in anterior lumbar surgery. Spine (Phila Pa 1976) 33:1662-1667, 2008.

Lumbar Nucleus Replacement

Hansen A. Yuan, MD

Qi-Bin Bao, PhD

Anthony T. Yeung, MD

Phillip S. Yuan, MD

Michael Dahl, PhD

Parallel to the development of lumbar artificial total disc replacement (TDR), physicians and researchers have worked on the development of lumbar nucleus replacement.[1,2] TDR and nucleus replacement are part of disc arthroplasty, which is intended to provide an alternative to fusion for patients with discogenic back pain and sciatica. Although both procedures preserve index segment motion and reduce the stress on the adjacent motion segments, there are major differences between TDR and nucleus replacement, as follows: (1) Nucleus replacement is more tissue-preserving than TDR. (2) Nucleus replacement technology is simpler and theoretically easier for restoration of normal biomechanical functions than TDR because of the preservation of anulus and ligaments. (3) Nucleus replacement does not affect effective conversion to TDR or fusion if it fails for any reason. (4) Because of the smaller dimension of a nucleus replacement device than a TDR device, the nucleus replacement can be performed with multiple surgical approaches, including the traditional posterior approach, whereas TDR currently has to be performed via an anterior or anterolateral approach.

TDR carries a higher surgical morbidity risk, especially at levels L4-5 and higher. Nucleus replacement is more suitable for earlier implantation indications and a broader patient population. Because it has to rely on the function of the anulus and endplates, nucleus replacement is generally unsuitable for patients with severe anulus compromise or the very late stage of the disc degeneration cascade.

Clinical Challenge of Nucleus Replacement

Because nucleus replacement devices often are not fixed onto the endplates, there is a higher risk of implant extrusion than with TDR devices. Implant size must ensure proper load sharing between the implant and the anulus. If a nucleus device or some of the contact area of the device carries too high a load or has too high focal contact stress, it might lead to implant subsidence.

Design and Material Options of Nucleus Replacement

In contrast to the predominant ball-and-socket design with either metal-on-metal or metal-on-polyethylene for the current generation of TDR, the design and material options for nucleus replacement are quite variable. This variability is largely due to the fact that nucleus replacement preserves more of the anatomy of the motion segment, such as anulus and endplates, and more function. The first nucleus replacement with long-term clinical experience was the Fernstrom ball made of stainless steel (Fig. 52–1).[3,4] Although this design offered bipolar articulation with the endplates to provide segment motion, it caused high contact stress because of point loading and implant subsidence.

Because the natural, healthy nucleus is a hydrogel with viscoelastic properties, hydrogel has become a popular material choice for nucleus replacement to mimic mechanical and physiologic properties of the natural nucleus. Preformed hydrogel and in situ curable (injectable) hydrogel have been used for nucleus replacement. Preformed hydrogel nucleus replacement has the benefit of a more consistent implant manufacturing process and more consistent and predictable implant properties, whereas the injectable hydrogel nucleus replacement has the advantage of easy implantation via a smaller annular portal.

Aquarelle developed by Howmedica (later Stryker) was the first preformed polyvinyl alcohol hydrogel used for nucleus replacement.[5] Subsequently, several other preformed hydrogel materials have been used for nucleus replacement, including prosthetic disc nucleus (PDN) (later redesigned and named HydraFlex) (Fig. 52–2) by RayMedica[6] and NeuDisc by Replication Medical (Fig. 52–3).[7] PDN and NeuDisc used the same type of base hydrogel, an acrylic copolymer hydrogel (HYPAN), with PDN having the hydrogel core encased in a polyethylene jacket and NeuDisc having the hydrogel sandwiched in between the Dacron knitted meshes. The main advantage of using preformed hydrogel materials for nucleus

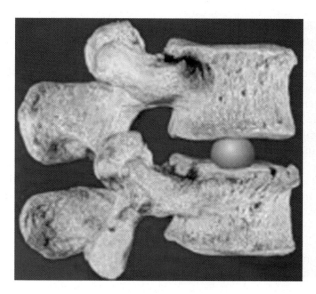

FIGURE 52–1 Fernstrom ball nucleus replacement.

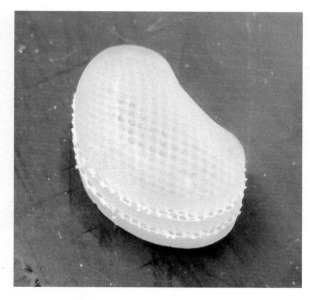

FIGURE 52–3 NeuDisc nucleus replacement.

replacement is that they not only mimic the viscoelastic and physiologic properties (imbibing and releasing water during the cyclic loading) of the nucleus, but also they have the ability to bear the mechanical load.

Although there are many hydrogel materials, the mechanical loading requirement coupled with the biocompatibility and biodurability requirements make the choices of suitable hydrogel materials relatively limited. All three of the preformed hydrogel nucleus replacement devices have passed necessary static and fatigue mechanical tests for the intended application. To mimic the body fluid diffusion function, most preformed hydrogel nucleus replacement devices have tried to have the equilibrium water content in the range of 60% to 80%. The hydrogel nucleus replacement can be implanted either dehydrated or fully hydrated. The advantage of implanting at the dehydrated or semidehydrated stage is the reduced implant volume and dimension, which allows for easier implantation and reduced annular incision. If the implant is implanted at the dehydrated stage, the time required for rehydration must be taken into consideration. The main concerns

and challenges for preformed hydrogel nucleus replacement devices have been potential implant extrusion because of the easy deformability and slipperiness of the hydrogel materials.

In addition to preformed hydrogel, some in situ curable hydrogel materials have also been used for nucleus replacement. Examples in this category are NuCore (Spine Wave)[8] and BioDisc (Cryolife).[9] NuCore is an injectable synthetic recombinant protein hydrogel, which is a sequential block copolymer of silk and elastin, with two silk blocks and eight elastin blocks per polymer sequence repeat (Fig. 52–4). The material has a water content and modulus similar to that of the natural nucleus. BioDisc is a biopolymer consisting of a protein-based hydrogel. During implantation, the dispensing device mixes the two components of predetermined ratio, and the glutaraldehyde cross-links the bovine serum albumin (BSA) molecules to each other and to the surrounding tissues.

Although the injectable hydrogel nucleus replacement has the advantage of being able to implant the device through a

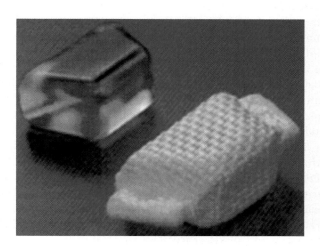

FIGURE 52–2 PDN nucleus replacement.

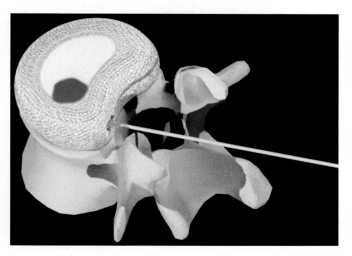

FIGURE 52–4 NuCore nucleus replacement.

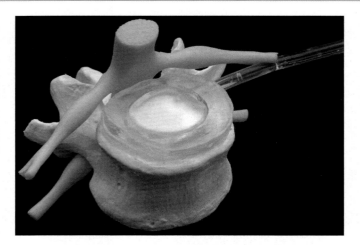

FIGURE 52–5 DASCOR nucleus replacement.

small annular incision, the main challenge for injectable hydrogel nucleus replacement devices is whether the cavity can be adequately filled during surgery without risking the implant extrusion, especially when the disc is fully loaded during normal activities. Although both these devices are designed to bond to the surrounding tissues, their adhesion strength and durability in a clinical setting, especially when some of the bonding is to nucleus pulposus, have not yet been proven.

In addition to hydrogel elastomers, nonhydrogel elastomers have also been used for nucleus replacements. Nonhydrogel elastomer nucleus replacements can be

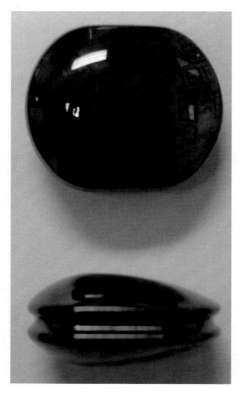

FIGURE 52–6 Regain nucleus replacement.

preformed and cured in situ. Nonhydrogel elastomer nucleus replacements have the same benefits as hydrogel nucleus replacements with low modulus, but they do not have the ability to imbibe and release body fluid during the cyclic loading. Several nonhydrogel elastomers with implantable history for other applications, such as polyurethane and silicone, have been attempted for nucleus replacement. The only preformed nonhydrogel elastomer nucleus replacement with limited clinical experience is NewDisc by Sulzer (later Zimmer). NewDisc is made from polyurethane and shaped in the form of a spiral coil. An insertion instrument was designed to implant the device by stretching it into a strip and inserting it into the disc cavity, where it is coiled back to a circle shape inside the disc space.

DASCOR (Disc Dynamics) is the most clinically advanced in situ cured nonhydrogel elastomer nucleus replacement and is the only injectable nucleus device with a balloon for containment (Fig. 52–5).[10] The injectable polymer is a two-part in situ curable polyurethane. The balloon is also made from polyurethane to facilitate adhesion between the curable polymer and the balloon. There are several clear advantages of using the balloon. First, it allows the polymer to be injected under certain pressure to fill the disc cavity completely without the risk of polymer leaking through the defected anulus. Second, the balloon prevents the direct contact between the uncured or semicured polymer and the surrounding wet tissue, so it avoids the leach of uncured monomers. The isolation of body fluid from the uncured polymer also can ensure better polymerization and a more consistent and stronger mechanical property for the final implant.

Another in situ curable nucleus replacement device is Percutaneous Nucleus Replacement (PNR; Trans1).[11] The PNR consists of two threaded titanium vertebral body anchors connected by a cylindric silicone rubber membrane. The two titanium anchors are fixed to the adjacent vertebrae via a trans-sacral approach, and the in situ curable silicone rubber is injected through the sacral anchor into the silicone membrane until the disc cavity is filled.

Some nonelastomeric materials have also been used for nucleus replacement based on the favorable clinical data of the Fernstrom ball. The main advantages of using these nonelastomers for nucleus replacement are their better mechanical strength and durability. The design of the Regain (Biomet) is similar to a modified Fernstrom ball and made of pyrolytic carbon (Fig. 52–6). Although the endplate contacting surfaces of Regain are still convex, they have a much larger radius so that the device has a larger initial contact area and smaller initial contact stress than the Fernstrom ball. Because of the mismatch of the surface contour between the implant and endplates, some subsidence is still inevitable.

To maintain the articulating feature of the Fernstrom ball while intending to increase the contact area, the NUBAC (Pioneer Surgical Technology) adopted the design similar to many TDR devices (Fig. 52–7).[12] It consists of two plates with outer surfaces contoured to the general geometry of the endplates and has an inner ball-and-socket articulation. This inner ball-and-socket articulation allows free motion within all physiologic ranges of motion in all major axes. This articulation feature is also believed to be a major factor in minimizing the shear force between the endplate and implant surface during bending motion and reducing the risk of implant extrusion. The implant is made from polyetheretherketone (PEEK) OPTIMA, which has well established biocompatibility, superb biodurability, and a history of being used as permanent spinal implants.

Clinical Experience of Different Nucleus Replacement Devices

The early short-term and long-term clinical data of the Fernstrom ball have provided fundamental scientific evidence that nucleus replacement can be effective in relieving discogenic back pain. Fernstrom[3] reported his relative short-term clinical data (6 months to 2.5 years) on 125 patients who received the device after discectomy and 100 patients with discectomy alone. He divided his patient population into two different groups: back pain only and back pain with leg pain. The success rates for patients with back pain only were 60% for the Fernstrom ball group versus 12% for the discectomy group. The success rates for patients with back pain with leg pain were 88% for the Fernstrom ball group versus 40% for the discectomy group. Motion, although not being quantitatively measured, was observed in the index level for patients with a Fernstrom ball. A different degree of subsidence of 1 to 3 mm was noticed for most of the Fernstrom ball group.

In 1995, McKenzie[4] reported long-term (average 17 years) follow-up on 103 patients. The success rates were 75% for patients with back pain only and 83% for patients with back pain and leg pain. After the procedure, 95% of patients returned to work. Between these two studies with a total of 344 implants, only one implant extrusion was reported (0.3%). Although late criticism of the Fernstrom ball nucleus replacement device has been mainly on the subsidence, this does not seem to have a significant impact on the clinical success. The Fernstrom ball has shown similar results to other surgical treatments, including TDR and fusion, for either back pain only or back pain with leg pain.

PDN has the most clinical experience among all nucleus replacement devices. More than 4000 patients have been implanted with various versions of PDN since 1996. Although the base polymer and the jacket material remained the same, the PDN device has gone through multiple design changes, from its original HYPAN 68 base polymer with a pair of square-shaped pellets to PDN-SOLO (a single device) and ultimately the softer HydraFlex. All these changes were mainly intended to reduce the rate of implant extrusion and the risk of subsidence.

Klara and Ray[13] reported the clinical data of the first four phases from 1996 to early 2000. The surgical success, which has not been well defined by the authors but is different from the commonly used term *clinical success,* varied from 62% to 91% during these four phases with implant extrusion up to 26% in phase II when the design changed to HYPAN 80 (with a higher water content than the original HYPAN 68) and a pair of angle-shaped devices. In addition to the design change,

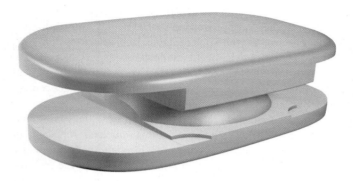

FIGURE 52–7 NUBAC nucleus replacement.

the surgical approach was changed from the initial posterior approach to the anterolateral transPsoatic approach.

Bertagnoli and Schoenmayr[14] reported a large cohort study with 243 patients having a good clinical outcome. The average Oswestry Disability Index (ODI) score declined from 52.7 preoperatively to 9 at 2-year follow-up, and the average visual analog scale (VAS) score declined from 7.1 preoperatively to 1.8 at 2-year follow-up. The average disc height increased from 8.1 mm to 10.2 mm at 2-year follow-up. Shim and colleagues[15] reported similar clinical outcomes with their series of 48 patients at 1-year follow-up. They found 19.6% subsidence, however. They also observed 60.9% endplate sclerosis and 82.8% Modic change. In a separate study, Shim and colleagues[16] reported good results on their 75 PDN-SOLO patients with ODI and VAS scores decreased from 53 and 7.3 preoperatively to 14 and 2.2 at 2-year follow-up and only 2.7% implant extrusion. Regardless of the high incidence of endplate sclerosis and Modic change, these changes did not seem to be correlated with the clinical outcome and could have been caused by restoring the mechanical load on the endplate in the nucleus region.

Other than the Fernstrom ball, PDN is the only other nucleus replacement device that has some long-term follow-up results. The long-term clinical results of the PDN have been mixed, however. Schoenmayr and Kliniken[17] who implanted the first series of 11 PDN devices, reported 8-year follow up on the original 11 patients using the first-generation PDN device with fairly good long-term results. The average ODI scores were 45 preoperatively and 14 8 years postoperatively. Of the 11 patients, only 1 had extruded (9%), and 8 were satisfied with the surgery. Pimenta and colleagues[18] reported high adverse event rates with 9 years' follow-up, however, on 80 patients with the more recent version of PDN-SOLO, even though there were still significant reductions in ODI and VAS scores for patients who were not revised. Of these 80 patients, 38 (47.5%) were revised during the 9-year follow-up, of which 23 (28.8%) were due to implant expulsion, and 15 (18.8%) were due to subsidence.

Over the years, the PDN has gone through multiple design changes in an attempt to solve the implant extrusion problem. All these changes have been insufficient to correct the implant extrusion problem. In the past 10 years, RayMedica has also initiated several investigational device exemption (IDE) feasibility studies in the United States with different versions of the

PDN device, including the newest version of HydraFlex. None of these studies have proceeded to the pivotal study, however, likely because of the unacceptable implant extrusion rate. From the various reported clinical results, it seemed that although the PDN device was effective in improving patient function and reducing back pain, the main challenges remain to be implant extrusion and subsidence.

Since its first clinical use at the end of 2004, NuBac has progressed quickly among all other nucleus replacement devices and become the second most implanted nucleus device in more than 300 patients so far. At the 2009 Spine Arthroplasty Society annual meeting, Pioneer Surgical Technology reported the worldwide multicenter clinical study that included patients enrolled outside of the United States and within the United States as a part of an IDE feasibility study with up to 2 years' follow-up.[19] The study has enrolled 219 patients using all three different surgical approaches—posterior, lateral, and anterolateral. Significant improvement in function and pain relief were observed with ODI scores being reduced from 53 preoperatively to 30, 25, 24, 22, and 20 at 6 weeks, 3 months, 6 months, 12 months, and 24 months postoperatively. VAS scores were reduced from 77 preoperatively to 32, 29, 23, 31, and 32 at 6 weeks, 3 months, 6 months, 12 months, and 24 months postoperatively.

In a separate study, Balsano and colleagues[20] reported the clinical data of 45 NuBac patients using only the posterior surgical approach. ODI score decreased from 51 preoperatively to 31, 27, 24, and 23 at 6 weeks, 3 months, 6 months, and 12 months postoperatively, and VAS score decreased from 76 preoperatively to 31, 31, 31, and 27 at 6 weeks, 3 months, 6 months, and 12 months postoperatively. In the U.S. IDE feasibility study, 20 patients were enrolled using the lateral surgical approach. Similar ODI improvement and VAS reduction were observed in these patients with no implant extrusions. Based on these clinical results, in 2008 NuBac became the first nucleus replacement device to gain the approval of the U.S. Food and Drug Administration (FDA) to start the pivotal study.

More than 200 DASCOR devices have been implanted since 2003, using anterolateral, lateral, posterolateral, and endoscopic approaches. Ahrens and colleagues reported an interim 2-year European clinical study of 85 patients using lateral and anterolateral approaches.[21] Mean preoperative VAS and ODI scores improved significantly by the 6-week postoperative follow-up point throughout the 2 years. Mean VAS back pain scores showed a 56.6% reduction at 24 months from a preoperative mean of 7.6. Mean ODI score showed a 59.7% reduction at 24 months from a preoperative mean of 57.5. No expulsions were observed in this 2-year clinical cohort. DASCOR is presently undergoing the FDA IDE feasibility study with VAS and ODI results showing statistically significant similarity to the European cohort.

Several other nucleus replacement devices with smaller patient numbers and relatively short follow-up have been also reported. Berlemann and Schwarzenbach[22] reported 2-year follow-up results on 12 NuCore patients who had back pain and leg pain. Decompression is part of the procedure to remove a herniated disc. Owing to the decompression, the patient's leg pain was significantly reduced from 6.8 preoperatively to 1.1 at 2 years. Back pain VAS score was also reduced from 32 to 6. Pawulski and colleagues[23] reported on 11 BioDisc patients with up to 2 years of follow-up with the average ODI and VAS scores reduced from 47.5 and 5.9 preoperatively to 17.7 and 2.3 at 2 years postoperatively. Two patients had recurrent herniation, and both had reherniation removed along with the device without incident.

Since 2005, NeuDisc has been undergoing a two-arm European pilot study.[7] The first arm is an open approach using the anterolateral transPsoatic approach, and the second arm is a posterolateral endoscopic approach. In the pilot study, 15 patients were implanted, but the details of follow-up data were not reported. Based on the initial lessons learned from this pilot study, the device has been modified to a less hydrophilic and reconfigured kidney-shaped design. A new pilot study with posterior and endoscopic transforaminal approaches has been initiated.

Conclusion

Owing to the anticipated clinical benefits of nucleus replacement, there has been an increase in the interest and effort in developing various nucleus replacement devices. After extensive preclinical studies, many devices have entered into clinical evaluation. From the reported clinical data, it has been shown that nucleus replacement generally is effective in relieving discogenic back pain and can be implanted via different surgical approaches, including the most common posterior approach and the minimally invasive endoscopic transforaminal approach. Clinical data have also shown that nucleus replacement preserves future options to undergo the next level of surgical inventions, such as TDR and fusion. Nearly no severe vascular and neurologic complications have been reported either in primary or in revision surgery of nucleus replacement.

The main challenge for most nucleus replacement devices is implant extrusion. Different solutions—such as having an inner articulation design, reducing the annular window through improved surgical technique or reduction of implant dimensions, repairing the annular window, or containing the nucleus device with an annular ring—have been proposed to combat the extrusion. When the extrusion risk can be managed to an acceptable level, lumbar nucleus replacement can become a less invasive and less bridge-burning alternative for the treatment of lumbar disc degenerative disease.

PEARLS
1. The benefits of nucleus replacement are that it is more tissue-preserving, less invasive, less bridge-burning, and compatible with multiple surgical approaches.
2. Nucleus replacement could be an attractive surgical treatment option for patients with early to moderate degenerative disc disease.
3. Nucleus replacement has the potential to be used in conjunction with discectomy.

REFERENCES

1. Bao Q-B, Yuan HA: New technologies in spine: Nucleus replacement. Spine (Phila Pa 1976) 27:1245-1247, 2002.

2. Di Martino A, Vaccaro AR, Lee JY, et al: Nucleus pulposus replacement: Basic science and indications for clinical use. Spine (Phila Pa 1976) 30(16 Suppl):S16-S22, 2005.

3. Fernstrom U: Arthroplasty with intercorporal endoprothesis in herniated disc and in painful disc. Acta Scand Suppl 357:154-159, 1966.

4. McKenzie AH: Fernstrom intervertebral disc arthroplasty: A long-term evaluation. Orthop Int Educ 3:313-324, 1995.

5. Bao Q-B, Yuan HA: Aquarelle hydrogel disc nucleus. In Yue JJ, Bertagnoli R, McAfee PC, et al (eds): Motion Preservation Surgery of the Spine, Advanced Technologies and Controversies. Philadelphia, WB Saunders, 2008, pp 423-430.

6. Davis RJ: PDN-SOLO and HydraFlex nucleus replacement system. In Yue JJ, Bertagnoli R, McAfee PC, et al (eds): Motion Preservation Surgery of the Spine, Advanced Technologies and Controversies. Philadelphia, WB Saunders, 2008, pp 407-410.

7. Yeung AT, Prewell A, Yue JJ: NeuDisc artificial lumbar nucleus replacement. In Yue JJ, Bertagnoli R, McAfee PC, et al (eds): Motion Preservation Surgery of the Spine, Advanced Technologies and Controversies. Philadelphia, WB Saunders, 2008, pp 411-416.

8. Schwarzenbach O, Berlemann U, Wilson T: NuCore injectable nucleus: An in situ curing nucleus replacement. In Yue JJ, Bertagnoli R, McAfee PC, et al (eds): Motion Preservation Surgery of the Spine, Advanced Technologies and Controversies. Philadelphia, WB Saunders, 2008, pp 417-422.

9. Wardlaw D: BioDisc nucleus pulposus replacement. In Yue JJ, Bertagnoli R, McAfee PC, et al (eds): Motion Preservation Surgery of the Spine, Advanced Technologies and Controversies. Philadelphia, WB Saunders, 2008, pp 423-434.

10. Ahrens M, Tsantrizos A, Le Huec J-C: DASCOR. In Yue JJ, Bertagnoli R, McAfee PC, et al (eds): Motion Preservation Surgery of the Spine, Advanced Technologies and Controversies. Philadelphia, WB Saunders, 2008, pp 393-406.

11. Diaz R, Pimenta L, Nicole N, et al: Tran1 percutaneous nucleus replacement. In Yue JJ, Bertagnoli R, McAfee PC, et al (eds): Motion Preservation Surgery of the Spine, Advanced Technologies and Controversies. Philadelphia, WB Saunders, 2008, pp 435-441.

12. Bao Q-B, Songer MN, Pimenta L, et al: NUBAC disc arthroplasty. In Yue JJ, Bertagnoli R, McAfee PC, et al (eds): Motion Preservation Surgery of the Spine, Advanced Technologies and Controversies. Philadelphia, WB Saunders, 2008, pp 442-451.

13. Klara P, Ray D: Artificial nucleus replacement: Clinical experience. Spine (Phila Pa 1976) 27:1374-1377, 2002.

14. Bertagnoli R, Schoenmayr R: Surgical and clinical results with the PDN prosthetic disc-nucleus device. Eur Spine J 11(Suppl 2):S143-S148, 2002.

15. Shim S, Lee H, Park C, et al: Partial disc replacement with the PDN prosthetic disc nucleus device: Early clinical results. J Spinal Dis Tech 16:324-330, 2003.

16. Shim S, Lee S-H, Bracht B, et al: Preliminary results of a prospective international multi-center study of the PDN-SOLO device. In Programs and Abstracts of the Seventh Annual Meeting of Spine Arthroplasty Society, Berlin, 2007.

17. Schoenmayr R, Kliniken HS: Ten year follow-up of disc height, ROM and clinical outcomes with the 1st generation PDN device. In Programs and Abstracts of the Sixth Annual Meeting of Spine Arthroplasty Society, Montreal, 2006.

18. Pimenta L, Lhamby J, Schaffa T, et al: PDN nucleus replacement: 9 year follow-up experiences. In Programs and Abstracts of the Ninth Annual Meeting of Spine Arthroplasty Society, London, 2009.

19. Coric, D, Songer M, Yuan H, et al: Up to 2-year follow-up results of a novel PEEK-on-PEEK disc arthroplasty: A prospective worldwide multicenter clinical study. In Programs and Abstracts of the Ninth Annual Meeting of Spine Arthroplasty Society, London, 2009.

20. Balsano M, Bucciero A, Agrillo U: Preliminary clinical evaluation of posterior disc arthroplasty. In Programs and Abstracts of the Ninth Annual Meeting of Spine Arthroplasty Society, London, 2009.

21. Ahrens M, Tsantrizos A, Sherman J, et al: Nucleus replacement with the DASCOR disc arthroplasty device: Interim two-year efficacy and safety results from two prospective, non-randomized multi-center European studies. Spine (Phila Pa 1976) 34:1376-1384, 2009.

22. Berlemann U, Schwarzenbach O: Two-year clinical evaluation of an injectable in situ curing nucleus replacement. In Programs and Abstracts of the Annual Meeting of North American Spine Society, Toronto, 2008.

23. Pawulski A, Singh V, Nandakumar A, et al: 2-year clinical results of a safety pilot study evaluating a protein hydrogel nucleus replacement device. In Programs and Abstracts of the Ninth Annual Meeting of Spine Arthroplasty Society, London, 2009.

53
C H A P T E R

Posterior Dynamic Stabilization*

Dilip K. Sengupta, MD, PhD, MCh (Orth), Dr Med

Degenerative disorders in the lumbar spine can lead to an abnormal pattern of motion causing segmental instability and low back pain, although the precise relationship between instability and low back pain with or without leg pain has not been established. The standard of care for the surgical treatment of degenerative instability causing low back pain has been fusion with or without instrumentation.[1] More recent advances in fusion techniques have increased the rate of successful fusion, without an equivalent improvement in relief of pain. The fusion rate with modern technology approaches 100%, but successful pain relief does not exceed 60% to 70%. A solid fusion does not always result in a successful clinical outcome.[2,3] A fusion can have long-term effects on unfused segments, leading to accelerated degeneration of the adjacent segments, engendered by abnormal forces and motion at those segments.[4,5] Because of these limitations of fusion, dynamic stabilization was introduced in the treatment of activity-related mechanical low back pain.

Instability

The rationale for fusing the painful motion segment has been the concept of instability.[6] Understanding and diagnosis of clinical instability remains controversial. When abnormal motion is present on flexion-extension radiographs, especially in the setting of spondylolisthesis, fusion is accepted as a reasonable option.[7] By this standard, relatively few patients with low back pain have overt subjective or objective evidence of instability, however. Pope and Panjabi[8] suggested that instability is a mechanical entity and is defined as a loss of stiffness to a given load. Biomechanical and radiologic studies using open magnetic resonance imaging (MRI) in flexion and extension have shown, however, that segmental motion either does not change significantly with disc degeneration[9-11] or may decrease except during early stages of disc degeneration.[12]

Mulholland and Sengupta[13] suggested that spinal instability does not mean "increased motion" as commonly misunderstood,[8,14] but rather it indicates abnormal load distribution across the vertebral endplate. The pathologic changes within the disc space may result in abnormal transmission of load across the endplates. It has been well established in other weight-bearing joints that abnormal load transmissions result in degenerative changes, and the resultant pain may be diminished by a properly placed osteotomy to realign the joint forces and redistribute the loads.[15] The normal disc consists of a homogeneous gel of collagen and proteoglycan. The normal disc is isotropic, similar to a fluid-filled bag, a property that allows it to transmit load uniformly across the vertebral endplates.[13]

Disc degeneration alters the isotropic properties of the disc. The disc becomes nonhomogeneous, with areas of fragmented and condensed collagen, cartilage fragments, fluid, and gas.[16] Load transmission over the endplates becomes uneven. The nucleus becomes depressurized, and an increasingly larger load is transmitted through the anulus, which leads to splitting and inward folding of the anulus.[17] The central area of the endplate overlying the depressurized nucleus now transmits lesser load, and corresponding endplate changes, such as destruction, thinning of the trabeculae, and thinning of the cartilaginous endplate,[18,19] may be noted. Focal loading of the endplate cartilage and subchondral bony trabeculae can occur with certain positions, leading to a sharp increase in back pain. This situation is analogous to a "stone in the shoe" causing high spot loading and pain, a concept proposed by Mulholland and Sengupta.[13]

This concept explains the clinical sign of *instability catch* as experienced by patients with mechanical back pain secondary to disc degeneration during flexion-extension movement. This hypothesis also explains why manipulation of the lumbar spine by a chiropractor may occasionally dislodge the fragment from its weight-bearing position, bringing an immediate relief of acute low back pain.[13] Mulholland and Sengupta's hypothesis of abnormal loading as the primary cause of mechanical back pain was supported by a close association of abnormal disc pressure profiles with positive discography with pain provocation.[20] A pressure profilometry study by McNally

Editor's Note: The author has listed and described numerous devices as examples only that have been developed in each of the categorical areas; many of these are under investigation at the time of writing but may not be (or newer ones have superseded them) by the time of publication and beyond.

and Adams[21] revealed the anisotropic properties of the degenerated disc. This study showed that the pattern of loading, rather than the absolute levels of loading, was related to pain generation in the degenerated spine. The concept may also help explain the lack of correlation between degrees of disc degeneration and back pain because individual anatomic and consequential load transmission changes vary from one person to another. With advancing age, the continued progression of these changes results in the disc becoming more collagenized and homogeneous. The very aged disc may distribute loads more evenly again, resulting in a degree of spontaneous relief of pain with time.[22]

Panjabi[23] described spinal stability in vivo as a function of three subsystems: (1) the spinal column, (2) the spinal muscles, and (3) the neural control unit. In vivo, spinal muscle action and neural control may be equal or more important spinal stabilizers, but the focus of surgical treatment of back pain has been the passive stability provided by the spinal column itself. Instability in the spinal column may result from damage or degeneration of bone, joints, or ligaments, which may be characterized by an increased motion in its early stages. By the time the pain becomes severe enough to consider surgical intervention, the total range of motion is often diminished or abnormal in quality.[24] Panjabi[23] redefined spinal instability as an abnormal motion often accompanied by an increased neutral zone motion caused by ligament laxity, even when the range of motion is diminished. Panjabi used the analogy of a marble rolling on a soup bowl (Fig. 53–1).

There is no real conflict between the abnormal motion (Panjabi) versus abnormal load distribution (Mulholland) theories of spinal instability. These two factors may be interrelated. An abnormal motion may cause abnormal load distribution, which may cause pain. It may be anticipated that if an abnormal motion does not cause abnormal load distribution, it may not be associated with pain production, and this explains why many back discs do not hurt.

Definitions

In recent years, many devices have been introduced for spine instrumentation without fusion, which are collectively known as *motion preservation devices*. There are subtle differences among these stabilization devices.

Prosthetic devices are designed to replace anatomic structures in the motion segment, retaining or restoring their function. Total disc replacement devices and nucleus replacement devices (PDN; Raymedica, Inc., Minneapolis, MN) are examples in this group. Facet replacement devices such as TFAS (Archus Orthopedics, Inc., Redmond, WA) and TOPS (Impliant, Inc., Princeton, NJ) are often presented as posterior dynamic stabilization (PDS) devices. They are truly prosthetic devices, however, which require excision of the facet joints. These devices replace the function of the facet joints in terms of providing stability and motion.

Stabilization devices are instrumentation for control of motion or load bearing or both; in contrast to prosthetic devices, they do not require excision of any anatomic part of the motion segment. *Dynamic stabilization* or *soft stabilization* devices are inserted between pedicle screws and are often described as pedicle screw–based PDS devices. Interspinous process distraction (IPD) devices are floating devices, which do not require bony anchorage.

Semirigid fixation is the term used to describe devices intended for achieving solid fusion without the stress-shielding effect of conventional rigid fixation. These are often flexible metallic devices of various designs, as opposed to conventional fusion rods, which offer no mobility at the instrumented segment. Typical devices in this category include Isobar TTL (Scient'x, Inc., West Chester, PA) and Accuflex (Globus Medical, Inc., Audubon, PA).

Soft fusion is a newer term that refers to posterior spinal fusion with minimal stiffness. Some biomechanical and clinical studies indicate the rigidity of lumbar fusion may vary depending on fusion techniques.[25,26] The theory behind the concept of soft fusion is that intertransverse process fusions using PDS devices may achieve a less rigid fusion compared with conventional rigid fusion with fusion rods or interbody devices and may be less detrimental to the adjacent segment. At this time, there is no clinical evidence supporting the concept of soft fusion. This concept has evolved from the fact that many PDS devices obtain U.S. Food and Drug Administration (FDA) approval under 510K for spinal fusion only and not for nonfusion stabilization. Use of these devices as dynamic stabilization devices without fusion represents off-label use.

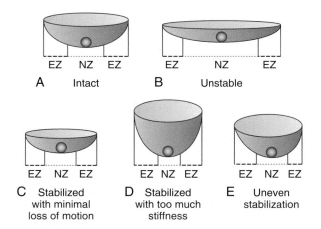

FIGURE 53–1 Panjabi's[23] analogy of a "marble on a soup bowl," explaining relationship between spinal instability and change in range of motion. **A,** Intact spine. The marble can move with little resistance across neutral zone (NZ) but faces increasing resistance toward elastic zone (EZ). **B,** Unstable motion segment. The bowl is flat allowing the marble to move to and fro with little resistance—that is, increased NZ with no increase in EZ. **C,** Stabilized segment. A smaller cup reduces primarily NZ, with minimal reduction of EZ movement. **D,** Stabilized segment—but too much loss of motion, which is undesirable. **E,** Uneven stabilization—with different stiffness in two directions, which is again undesirable.

Design Rationale for Dynamic Stabilization Devices

During the last decade, almost every possible flexible system has been introduced as a potential dynamic stabilization system. Most devices were introduced with no biomechanical data or any clinical evidence of efficacy for even their primary goal. Clinical applications of these devices often extend beyond their primary indication. As expected, questions have been raised about their clinical efficacy, biomechanical basis of design rationale, and mechanism of action.

Biomechanical Goals for Posterior Dynamic Stabilization

Motion Preservation

The primary goal of dynamic stabilization is to preserve motion. It is intended to preserve as much normal motion as possible, while limiting abnormal motion. Some degree of loss of motion is inevitable with application of any PDS device. Because clinical instability occurs mostly during the neutral zone motion, the key to stabilization should be restriction of the neutral zone while preserving the elastic zone motion as much as possible. Because neutral zone motion represents ligament laxity, all PDS systems, by virtue of motion restriction, automatically reduce the neutral zone regardless of their mechanism of action. This automatic reduction of the neutral zone explains why most of the devices claim clinical success in relieving back pain at least in the short-term.

When the range of motion is abnormally increased, usually in translation, after laminectomy, the goal of a PDS device should be to restore a normal range and quality of motion. Normally, it is unlikely that a dynamic stabilization device would increase the range of motion of a degenerated segment, unless it induces a favorable biologic reaction to the disc and facet joint by offloading these structures. Rarely, it may be expected that the device may restore the collapsed disc space height by distraction, however, and eventually may increase the range of motion toward normal. Without anterior support of the disc, the systems could be expected to fail, and the disc space could collapse again.

Load Transmission

The mechanism of pain relief with dynamic stabilization may be unloading the disc and the facet joints by load sharing, preventing abnormal load distribution and high spot loading.[13] How much load should be shared by the device is unclear. It may be assumed, however, that the device would reduce the intradiscal pressure by the magnitude of load sharing.

Resistance to Fatigue Failure

The most important challenge for dynamic stabilization devices is to survive against fatigue failure, despite allowing continued motion. Fatigue failure is common, even with the much stronger implants such as fusion rods, in case of fusion failure. The key to survival against fatigue for a much weaker PDS device is appropriate quality and quantity of motion restriction and load sharing so that the device is never exposed to an abnormal large load.

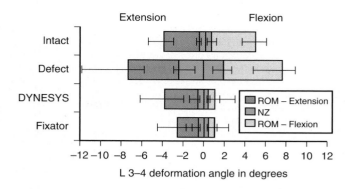

FIGURE 53–2 Dynesys (Zimmer Spine, Inc., Warsaw, IN) restricts flexion too much, equivalent to rigid fixation, but permits near-normal extension in cadaveric spine. (Adapted from Schmoelz W, Huber JF, Nydegger T, et al: Dynamic stabilization of the lumbar spine and its effects on adjacent segments: An in vitro experiment. J Spinal Disord Tech 16:418-423, 2003.)

The motion restriction should be uniform throughout the range of motion. If the device may cause too much restriction of motion in any direction, most commonly acting like an extension stop, the device may be exposed to repeatedly unusually high stress in extension and may eventually fail (Fig. 53–2). Similarly, the load sharing should be uniform throughout the range of motion. If the device may unload the disc too much in one direction, often in extension, the device has to bear unusually high load during that motion and is likely to fail (Fig. 53–3).

The fatigue property of a fusion device is normally tested in an American Society for Testing and Materials (ASTM) standard spine model consisting of two plastic cubes as vertebral bodies but nothing to represent anatomic structures such as the disc or the facet joints. The fatigue property of a dynamic stabilization device may be inadequately tested in this model because the devices are meant for sharing the load with the existing anatomic structures. An indirect assessment of fatigue property may be performed by study of the instant axis of rotation and intradiscal pressure changes.

Normally, the disc pressure increases in flexion and extension and is lowest in neutral position. A PDS device ideally should permit an increase in the disc pressure in flexion and extension but to a smaller magnitude owing to load sharing (see Fig. 53–3). If the disc pressure does not increase at all, particularly in extension, it may indicate that the device is acting like a total load-bearing structure during extension rather than as a load-sharing structure. Similarly, a mismatch in the location of the instant axis of rotation of the device and the motion segment is another predictor of fatigue failure of the device.

Nonmetallic devices may deform, soften, and creep to adapt to the kinematics of the motion segment and survive fatigue better, at the cost of reduced efficacy over time. Is creep and softening of a nonmetallic device a disadvantage? One may argue that dynamic stabilization may stimulate a favorable biologic response to repair the motion segment, and its subsequent creep or softening is truly an advantage, when its function is over. Conversely, metallic spring devices may retain their mechanical property over a long time but are more

FIGURE 53–3 Intradiscal pressure changes with flexion-extension motion. Normally, pressure at center of disc increases in flexion and extension. Stabilization with Dynesys (Zimmer Spine, Inc., Warsaw, IN) restores disc pressure in flexion to normal, but unloads disc completely and behaves similar to total load-bearing structure, without sharing any load with disc. (From Schmoelz W, Huber JF, Nydegger T, et al: Influence of a dynamic stabilisation system on load bearing of a bridged disc: An in vitro study of intradiscal pressure. Eur Spine J 15:1276-1285, 2006.)

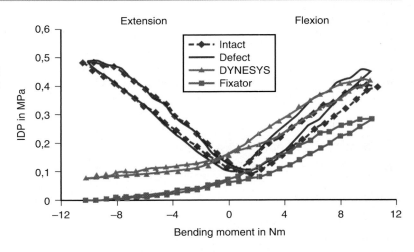

subject to fatigue failure should there be any mismatch in the kinematics. Fatigue failure of a nonmetallic device may not be recognized radiologically unless there is screw loosening or breakage, but failure of a metallic device cannot hide.

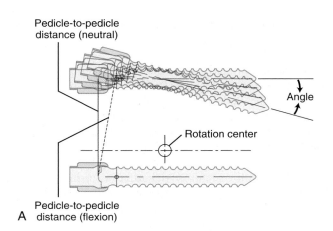

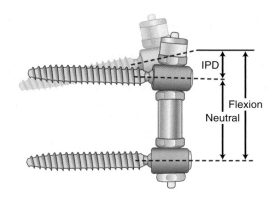

FIGURE 53–4 A, Pedicle-to-pedicle distance from flexion to extension may be 8 to 9 mm to preserve normal motion. **B,** Dynamic stabilization (Transition; Globus Medical Inc., Audubon, PA) may need to permit excursion of pedicle screw heads by same magnitude. (From Sengupta DK: Use of posterior motion-sparing instrumentation and interspinous devices for the treatment of degenerative disorders of the lumbar spine. In Shen F, Shaffrey C [eds]: Arthritis and Arthroplasty: The Spine. Elsevier, in press.)

Pedicle-to-Pedicle Distance Excursion

A normal pedicle-to-pedicle excursion during flexion-extension may be 6 to 9 mm, less in lateral bending, and minimal in rotation (Fig. 53–4). The device should permit a normal pedicle-to-pedicle distance excursion to permit normal range of motion and ensure that the device should not act as a "motion stopper" in any direction. Only a few dynamic stabilization devices can accommodate such a large degree of flexibility.

Other Design-Related Factors

Other design-related factors are as follows:

1. Safe and easy salvage—conversion to fusion in case of failure
2. Ease of implantation—top-loading screws
3. Compatibility with minimally invasive procedures
4. Restoration of lordosis
5. Biomaterial—metallic versus nonmetallic

Development of any new device should preferably have an option for an easy salvage in case of failure. Top-loading pedicle screws, accepting regular fusion rods, make implantation simpler and conversion to a fusion more straightforward. Need for in situ tensioning of the device often requires a longer exposure. Posterior devices are inherently kyphogenic, and active lordosis must be built into the design (Fig. 53–5).

Dynamic Stabilization Devices

The classification of dynamic stabilization devices is difficult because new devices are always being introduced, and devices are being constantly withdrawn. As defined earlier, only PDS and IPD devices are included in the classification presented in Table 53–1. The semirigid fixation devices and prosthetic devices, including facet replacement devices, were excluded.

The primary goal of dynamic stabilization is treatment of mechanical back pain secondary to spinal instability (Table

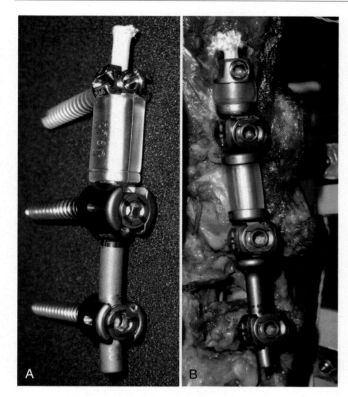

FIGURE 53–5 Design rationale between second-generation versus third-generation posterior dynamic stabilization device. **A,** Dynesys (Zimmer Spine, Inc., Warsaw, IN) uses side-loading screw, which is unsuitable for rod insertion. A more recent design adaptation, to make it suitable for use in conjunction with fusion at adjacent segment, requires three different types of screws. It needs in situ assembly and tensioning. **B,** Transition (Globus Medical, Inc., Audubon, PA) has been designed to accommodate implantation in isolation and in conjunction with adjacent segment fusion using same pedicle screw design. It uses top-loading screws for all segments; lordosis is built in; bumper at the end offers larger pedicle-to-pedicle excursion; it comes preassembled or can be assembled on back table.

TABLE 53–1 Classification of Posterior Dynamic Stabilization Devices

Pedicle Screw–Based Posterior Dynamic Stabilization Devices
Nonmetallic devices
Dynesys (Zimmer Spine, Inc., Warsaw, IN)
Transition Stabilization System (Globus Medical, Inc., Audubon, PA)
Metallic devices
DSS-II Dynamic Stabilization System (Abbott Spine, Inc., Austin, TX)
BioFlex (Bio-Spine Corp., Seoul, Korea)
Stabilimax NZ (Applied Spine Technologies, Inc., New Haven, CT)
Cosmic Posterior Dynamic System (Ulrich GmbH & Co, Ulm, Germany)
Hybrid devices (metallic component with plastic bumper)
CD Horizon Agile (Medtronic Sofamor Danek, Memphis, TN)
NFlex (N Spine, Inc., San Diego, CA)
Interspinous Process Distraction Devices
X-Stop IPD device (Medtronic, Memphis, TN)
Wallis device (Zimmer Spine, Inc., Mineapolis, MN)
Coflex (Paradigm Spine, LLC., New York, NY)
FLEXUS Interspinous Spacer (Globus Medical, Inc., Audubon, PA)
DIAM (Medtronic Sofamor Danek, Memphis, TN)
In-Space Interspinous Distraction Device (Synthes, West Chester, PA)
Superion Spacer (VertiFlex, Inc., San Clemente, CA)
PercuDyn system (Interventional Spine, Inc., Irvine CA)—this is not a true interspinous spacer

53–2). Radicular pain or claudication pain can be adequately treated by decompression alone; the role of additional dynamic stabilization here is only to prevent instability and back pain. Application of a dynamic stabilization device with concomitant decompression to address radicular or claudication leg pain should not be accepted as evidence in support of their efficacy to relieve back pain. Such efficacy can be established only by application of the device to treat mechanical back pain in absence of decompression. When that efficacy is established, application in conjunction with decompression procedures could be justified. Dynamic stabilization to supplement total disc replacement is still at an experimental stage and may be considered as a future indication.

Indications for Interspinous Process Distraction

The *primary indication* for IPD is central spinal canal stenosis with neurogenic claudication. A *secondary indication* is foraminal stenosis with radicular symptoms.

IPD devices are ideally suited for indirect, less invasive decompression of the spinal canal or the foramen causing neurogenic claudication pain. Direct decompression by conventional laminectomy may achieve a more definitive and longer lasting relief of symptoms. Intuitively, interspinous distraction may produce less postoperative morbidity; however, the clinical evidence supporting superiority of interspinous distraction over conventional decompression is lacking. Use of these devices is primarily justified in elderly patients with multiple comorbidities. Osteoporosis and scoliosis may be relative contraindications for IPD because of high incidence of failure owing to lack of bony support. Proponents and enthusiasts of interspinous distraction sometimes recommend use of these devices in the treatment of axial back pain. Currently, a sound rationale, justification, or reproducible evidence in favor of such indication is lacking.

TABLE 53–2 Indications for Posterior Dynamic Stabilization

Primary indication: *Treatment of spinal instability*
Treat activity-related mechanical back pain secondary to disc or facet degeneration (disc degeneration, facet degeneration, degenerative spondylolisthesis)
Secondary indications: *Prevention of spinal instability*
Prevent iatrogenic instability after discectomy or decompressive laminectomy
Prevent accelerated degeneration in adjacent motion segment with signs of early degeneration
Supplement total disc replacement to achieve total joint replacement

Clinical Experience with Dynamic Stabilization

Pedicle Screw–Based Posterior Dynamic Stabilization Devices

One of the earliest dynamic stabilization devices is the *Graf ligament,* described by Graf in 1992.[27] This is the first-generation PDS device and forms the basis of many other devices introduced subsequently. It consists of braided polypropylene bands that span between flanges at the titanium pedicle screw heads, placed under tension, locking the facet joints. The surgical procedure is simple, and, in contrast to fusion, it avoids exposure of the transverse processes or the need to harvest bone graft. Clinical outcomes with short-term follow-up ($\leq$2 years) are reported to be as good as with conventional fusions.[28] Reports in the literature regarding long-term outcome results with Graf ligament stabilization are conflicting, however. Gardner and Pande[29] and Markwalder and Wenger[30] reported reasonably good results with Graf ligaments at 5- to 10-year follow-up. Hadlow and colleagues[31] performed a retrospective matched case-control comparison between Graf ligamentoplasty and instrumented posterolateral fusion in a consecutive series of 83 patients with low back pain, operated by a single surgeon. The authors concluded that soft stabilization using Graf ligaments produced a worse outcome at 1 year and a significantly higher revision rate at 2 years.

The exact mechanism of action of Graf ligaments has not been established. As a result of the compression applied to the screws, there is a high incidence of radicular symptoms produced secondary to either disc protrusion or foraminal narrowing.[28,31] The compressive force may also have a deleterious effect on the facet joint and may lead to back pain. Graf ligaments are still used in a few centers in Europe and Asia, but their use has declined.[29,32]

The most extensively used dynamic stabilization device is *Dynesys* (Zimmer Spine, Inc., Warsaw, IN).[33,34] The design incorporates a plastic cylinder (sulene-polycarbonate urethane [PCU]) around a cord to apply a distraction force unloading the facet joints, which is thought to be the cause of back pain with Graf ligaments. This is a design improvement over Graf ligaments and may be called a second-generation PDS device. A review of the literature provides the best resource for understanding the mechanism of PDS systems.

In biomechanical testing on cadaveric spines, Dynesys reduced range of flexion more than extension[35] (see Fig. 53–2) apparently because the device holds the segment in close to full flexion. Extension is produced by abnormal distraction of the disc space with the plastic cylinder acting as a fulcrum; this is evidenced by abnormal negative disc pressure during extension.[36] Conversely, in vivo, Dynesys limits extension more than flexion,[37] as expected, because the device acts like an extension stop. This apparent discrepancy results from the fact that in a cadaveric spine only passive stabilizing factors are in operation, and application of a so-called physiologic load to produce spinal motion can never recreate in vivo muscle action, even in a 6-degrees-of-freedom spine tester.[36] Studies on disc unloading properties in cadaveric spines, as assessed by measuring the disc pressure, show that in flexion, Dynesys acts as a load-sharing device, which is ideal. In extension, Dynesys becomes totally load bearing, however, allowing no load transmission through the disc (see Fig. 53–3).[36]

Because of uneven restriction of motion and uneven pattern of unloading the disc, Dynesys may be subjected to excessive stress. This idea is supported by another biomechanical study, which showed high stress at the pedicle screws after Dynesys instrumentation.[38] This high stress may explain why screw loosening had been rare with Graf ligament, but fairly common with Dynesys—17% in some clinical series.[33,39] The plastic cylinder in Dynesys does not break but may soften with body temperature in vivo and may creep over time, which may lessen the efficacy of the device in distracting the pedicle screws, while protecting it against fatigue failure.

In the initial clinical report, presented by the inventors, Dynesys produced comparable outcome to fusion.[34] Greater than 60% of their cases had spinal stenosis, and Dynesys was used in conjunction with decompression; this made it difficult to evaluate whether the good outcome was related to Dynesys or decompression. Subsequent studies by Grob and colleagues[33] found that stand-alone Dynesys produced a good outcome in only 39% of cases compared with 69% when combined with decompression. Similar experience was reported by other independent researchers.[40]

Dynesys has been used in the United States since 2004. Currently, it is approved by the FDA for stabilization of spinal segments as an adjunct to fusion.[41] An FDA-controlled investigational device exemption (IDE) clinical trial is in progress comparing Dynesys as a dynamic stabilization device with fusion. The preliminary report shows promising outcome.[41] The inclusion criteria include patients with predominant leg pain and exclude patients with predominant back pain. This clinical trial also combines Dynesys with decompression and does not study the effect of Dynesys as a stand-alone device. This study is not expected to establish the clinical efficacy of Dynesys in the treatment of activity-related mechanical back pain, which should be the primary clinical indication for surgical treatment with dynamic stabilization.[41]

The *Transition Stabilization System* (Globus Medical, Inc., Audubon, PA) evolved from Dynesys, addressing its several design limitations. This system uses regular top-loading pedicle screws, actively creates lordosis, permits increased pedicle-to-pedicle distance excursion, and comes preassembled. It may be considered as a third-generation PDS device. It consists of a cylindric PCU spacer around a polyethylene terephthalate cord similar to Dynesys.

The system comes preassembled or can be assembled on the back table and does not require in situ tensioning. It is implanted between regular, top-loading pedicle screws, making insertion and conversion to fusion as a salvage procedure simpler. It incorporates a soft bumper at the end, which allows adequate pedicle-to-pedicle excursion in flexion-extension. The length of the spacer defines the amount of unloading of the facet joints. The capability of creating an active lordosis is built into the metal spools that connect the soft section of the device to the pedicle screws. Lordosis ensures unloading of the disc (see Fig. 53–4B). These two important mechanical properties permit uniform motion restriction in all directions and uniform load sharing throughout the range of motion, which is important to increase resistance to fatigue. Although the Transition Stabilization System has several design improvements compared with Dynesys, its advantages remain to be established. The device has been approved by the FDA only more recently under 510K as a fusion device, but to date no clinical outcomes have been reported.

The *DSS-II Dynamic Stabilization System* (Abbott Spine, Inc., Austin, TX)[42] was developed by the author and is one of the earliest titanium metallic springs used for dynamic stabilization. Its predecessor, the DSS-I, was a C-shaped titanium spring that, on biomechanical testing, showed uneven restriction to extension and excessive unloading of the disc in extension, indicating the possibility of fatigue failure. It was never used clinically. The second-generation DSS-II is an A-shaped titanium spring implanted between the pedicle screws. This design improvement produces active lordosis and permits adequate pedicle-to-pedicle excursion and physiologic translation of the instant axis of rotation of the motion segment. The system allows uniform motion restriction and uniform load sharing throughout the range of motion, the two essential biomechanical characteristics for survival of the implant against fatigue failure. The device has never been introduced for general use, but a pilot clinical trial was completed in Sao Paulo, Brazil, in a small group of patients ($n = 19$) with mechanical back pain without need for decompression. The clinical outcome was encouraging, but more importantly, no implant failure was observed in 2 to 3 years of follow-up.[42]

The *BioFlex* (BioSpine Corporation, Seoul, Korea)[43] is a coil spring made of 4-mm diameter nitinol for increased flexibility; it has been used extensively in Seoul, Korea. This device has been used most commonly in conjunction with interbody cages to achieve fusion, although it has also been used alone as a nonfusion device.[44] A titanium version of the device has been approved more recently by the FDA under 510K as a fusion device, but no clinical use in the United States has been reported yet.

Stabilimax NZ (Applied Spine Technologies, Inc., New Haven, CT),[45] a dual core spring device developed by Panjabi, is designed to apply soft resistance against compression and distraction. The design rationale is to limit the neutral zone motion, while leaving the elastic zone unaffected. At the present time, the device is undergoing an FDA-controlled IDE trial to assess whether it is at least as safe and effective as fusion in patients receiving decompression surgery for the treatment of clinically symptomatic spinal stenosis at one or two contiguous vertebral levels from L1-S1.[46]

The *Cosmic Posterior Dynamic System* (Ulrich GmbH & Co, Ulm, Germany)[47] has a unique design that incorporates a rigid rod connected to pedicle screws with a hinged screw-head that is expected to permit motion. No biomechanical data are available in the peer-reviewed literature. There are some clinical reports of its use in non–peer-reviewed journals.[48]

Hybrid devices incorporate a metallic rod connected to a flexible segment, with a nonmetallic bumper to allow shock absorption and some degree of pedicle-to-pedicle excursion. The obvious clinical advantage is that these devices look like a fusion rod and can be used with a regular top-loading pedicle screw. The *CD Horizon Agile* system (Medtronic Sofamor Danek, Memphis, TN) incorporates a soft cylindric bumper at the end of a fusion rod, held by a metallic cable in its center, similar to the fabric cord used in the Dynesys system described earlier. After initial clinical use, the device was recalled by the company for reported fatigue failure of the cable. *NFlex* (N Spine, Inc., San Diego, CA) has a similar design, in which a 6-mm titanium fusion rod is connected to a flexible end, made of a 3.25-mm titanium core and PCU sleeve. The sleeve allows soft resistance to flexion and extension, permitting the essential pedicle-to-pedicle excursion. Although the device may permit compression and elongation, its ability to permit anteroposterior translation remains a concern. The device has been used clinically since fall 2006, but no clinical experience has been published.[50]

Interspinous Distraction Devices

The most frequently used interspinous distraction device at the present time is the *X-Stop IPD device* (Medtronic, Memphis, TN). This titanium spacer can be inserted with a minimally invasive approach under local anesthesia; elderly patients with medical comorbidities are considered good candidates. Biomechanical studies in cadaveric spines have shown that the X-Stop significantly decreases posterior intradiscal pressure,[51,52] reduces facet pressures, and decreases contact area at the facets.[53] An in vivo study with MRI also showed that the X-Stop device increases the spinal canal and foramen diameter during extension.[54] This device holds the spine in a position of flexion, a position of relief from claudication pain. Because it is not tied to the adjacent spinous processes, it can permit further flexion.

In a prospective, randomized, multicenter study on 191 patients with neurogenic intermittent claudication, the efficacy of the X-Stop was compared with nonoperative treatment.[55] At 2 years of follow-up, the X-Stop group had improved symptom severity, physical function, and patient satisfaction scores at all of the time points compared with the nonoperative group. The reoperation rate was 6% at 2 years for the X-Stop group, which is comparable to the reoperation rate for lumbar decompression procedures. There were some limitations to this study, including a lack of blinding and loss to follow-up. The major limitation of the study was failure to compare the efficacy of X-Stop with a conventional surgical treatment for spinal stenosis (i.e., decompressive laminectomy). The device received FDA approval for use in one-level or two-level stenosis in patients older than 50 years with significant neurogenic claudication with or without back pain, after failed conservative treatment for at least 6 months. The main complication of this device is dislodgment of the spacer with or without breakage of spinous processes.

The *Wallis device* (Zimmer Spine, Inc., Minneapolis, MN) is a polyetheretherketone (PEEK) spacer, retained between the spinous processes by a Dacron tape, which prevents its accidental dislodgment.[56] This device holds the spine in flexion and limits extension. The holding ligaments also restrict further flexion. As a result, the manufacturer and inventors have recommended its use for indications beyond spinal stenosis (e.g., mechanical back pain with early disc degeneration).[57,58] An FDA IDE trial is currently comparing the Wallis system with total disc replacement for the treatment of mild to moderate degenerative disc disease of the lumbar spine at the L4-5 level.[59]

Coflex (Paradigm Spine, LLC, New York, NY) is a U-shaped titanium device, retained in place by clamping its wings around the adjacent spinous processes. In contrast to other IPD devices, it allows flexion and extension, and it does not act as an extension stop. Biomechanical studies report that it restores normal flexion-extension in a destabilized spine rather than holding the spine in flexion.[60] Kong and colleagues[61] reported a comparable outcome at 1-year follow-up with Coflex and posterior lumbar interbody fusion for degenerative back pain. The Coflex group had preserved motion, however, whereas the posterior lumbar interbody fusion group had an adverse effect on the adjacent segment. At the time of writing this chapter, one FDA-approved IDE trial with Coflex was in progress comparing the Coflex device with instrumented fusions.

The *FLEXUS Interspinous Spacer* (Globus Medical, Inc., Audubon, PA) is a single-unit radiolucent PEEK device designed for a snug fit between spinous processes. The unilateral approach for insertion permits retention of key ligamentous structures. PEEK material being softer than metal may help prevent erosion of the spinous processes over time. An FDA-approved IDE clinical trial has been initiated in the United States to compare clinical outcomes of FLEXUS with X-Stop in 340 patients with spinal stenosis.

DIAM (Medtronic Sofamor Danek, Memphis, TN) is an H-shaped, polyester-covered, silicone bumper that is placed between the spinous processes with a suture to hold it in place. The device has been used in Europe for a few years. A more recent clinical study failed to establish efficacy of DIAM in improving back pain compared with decompression alone.[62] An FDA-regulated clinical trial for DIAM was initiated in late 2006 for patients with lumbar spinal stenosis. The FDA also granted another IDE trial to study DIAM in patients with low back pain caused by degenerative disc disease.

The *PercuDyn system* (Interventional Spine, Inc., Irvine CA) is not an IPD device, but it is described as a minimally invasive facet augmentation device, which prevents extension by stopping the overriding of the facet joints. It consists of a 10-mm diameter PCU bumper over a cannulated 4.5-mm titanium screw, which can be inserted percutaneously into the pedicle, sitting below the inferior facet. The bumper acts as an extension-limiting soft cushion. The clinical experience with this device is limited.[63]

Many other spinous process distraction devices are being developed or beginning FDA trials. A comprehensive review of these is beyond the scope of this chapter.

Summary

PDS evolved from failure of fusion to address mechanical back pain secondary to spinal instability. IPD devices have been introduced primarily to treat spinal stenosis with claudication or radicular pain by indirect decompression. Spinal instability is poorly defined, but current understanding suggests an abnormal quality of motion, leading to uneven load transmission; this occurs mostly during the neutral zone motion. The biomechanical goals of PDS devices are to preserve motion as much as possible but prevent any abnormal motion and to unload the disc and facet joints by load sharing.

The biggest challenge for PDS devices is to survive fatigue failure despite allowing continued motion. The key to this survival is uniform load sharing and uniform restriction of motion throughout the range of motion. Many PDS devices have been introduced without any biomechanical basis, and their clinical success was confounded by combining the effect of a concomitant decompression for leg pain. It is essential that the efficacy of PDS devices to treat back pain be established before they are recommended for secondary indications such as preventing instability after decompression or preventing adjacent segment degeneration.

IPD devices are best used to treat claudication pain in elderly patients with comorbidities by minimal intervention and indirect decompression. Clinical studies to establish their efficacy against open and direct decompression is lacking. The consideration for use in the treatment of mechanical back pain has no scientific basis as yet, although studies are under way for exploring this aspect. Product development and marketing is expensive, and most clinical trials are aimed at proven success rather than a proper scientific evaluation of their clinical efficacy. Most of the new IPD devices are introduced in the U.S. market with FDA approval under 510K as a fusion device. The clinical use for dynamic stabilization without an attempt of fusion is an off-label use. This situation has led to the concept of soft fusion, which indicates transverse fusion only, using a PDS device. The expectation is that this fusion would be less stiff than conventional fusions with rigid instrumentation and perhaps prevent adjacent segment disease. There is no clinical evidence to support this concept yet.

Dynamic stabilization has raised a great deal of enthusiasm, theoretical promises, and diverse expectations. Similar to any new technology, these procedures are apt to breed clinical failures. The need for detailed consideration of design rationale and proper clinical evaluation without confounding factors to prove safety and efficacy cannot be overemphasized. Fusion remains the method of choice for advanced disc or facet degeneration and gross instability. Disc degeneration in multiple segments, particularly in young patients with concerns about adjacent segment disease after fusion, is likely to constitute the main indication for PDS. Future applications of dynamic stabilization may include salvage of failed total disc replacement or to supplement it, nuclear replacement, and provision of temporary mechanical support for pharmacologic or biologic treatments aiming for repair or regeneration of the disc.

PEARLS

1. Clinical instability causing mechanical back pain is defined as abnormal quality of motion leading to uneven load distribution in the motion segment.

2. The goal of PDS is motion preservation but with prevention of abnormal motion in the neutral zone.

3. The mechanism of pain relief by PDS is load sharing with the disc and the facet joints.

4. The goal of interspinous distraction is indirect decompression for the spinal stenosis, with minimal intervention.

5. The indications for PDS are as follows:
   - Primary indication—activity-related mechanical back pain
   - Secondary indications—prevention of instability, prevention of iatrogenic instability after decompression, and stabilization of adjacent motion segment

6. The indications for an IPD device are as follows:
   - Primary indication—spinal stenosis with claudication
   - Secondary indication—foraminal stenosis with radicular pain

7. Contraindications for PDS are as follows:
   - Osteoporosis
   - Advanced disc degeneration with near-complete collapse of disc height
   - Scoliosis (relative contraindication to IPD devices)

PITFALLS

1. The biggest challenge of PDS devices is survival against fatigue, while allowing continued motion.

2. The risks of poor outcome and device failure of PDS devices are increased with too much distraction and kyphosis, so these must be avoided.

3. To prevent implant loosening, the use of any dynamic stabilization device must be avoided in the presence of osteoporosis.

4. For advanced disc disease, fusion remains the "gold standard."

KEY POINTS

1. Clinical instability causing mechanical back pain is defined as abnormal quality of motion leading to uneven load distribution in the motion segment.

2. The goal of PDS is motion preservation but with prevention of abnormal motion in the neutral zone. The mechanism of pain relief by PDS is load sharing with the disc and the facet joints. The goal of interspinous distraction is indirect decompression for spinal stenosis, with minimal intervention.

3. The primary indication for PDS is treatment of activity-related mechanical back pain. Secondary indications are prevention of iatrogenic instability after decompression and stabilization of the adjacent motion segment to fusion.

4. The primary indication for an IPD device is treatment of neurogenic claudication secondary to spinal stenosis in an elderly patient. A secondary indication is indirect decompression of the foraminal stenosis with radicular pain.

5. Contraindications for PDS include osteoporosis, infections, advanced disc degeneration with near-complete collapse of the disc height, and scoliosis (relative contraindication to IPD devices).

6. The biggest challenge of a PDS device is survival against fatigue, while allowing continued motion. Too much distraction and kyphosis with PDS may increase the risks of device failure.

KEY REFERENCES

1. Mulholland RC, Sengupta DK: Rationale, principles and experimental evaluation of the concept of soft stabilization. Eur Spine J 11(Suppl 2):S198-S205, 2002.
   In this landmark review article, Mulholland and colleagues describe the concept of instability as a function of abnormal load distribution as opposed to abnormal motion. They also describe the "stone in the shoe concept" and the rationale of design and mechanism of action of various dynamic stabilization devices.

2. Panjabi MM: Clinical spinal instability and low back pain. J Electromyogr Kinesiol 13:371-379, 2003.
   Panjabi presents his understanding of clinical instability causing low back pain as a function of abnormal motion during the neutral zone.

3. Bono CM, Kadaba M, Vaccaro AR: Posterior pedicle fixation-based dynamic stabilization devices for the treatment of degenerative diseases of the lumbar spine. J Spinal Disord Tech 22:376-383, 2009.
   This literature review reports clinical results of using pedicle-based PDS systems and facet replacement devices in the lumbar spine.

4. Stoll TM, Dubois G, Schwarzenbach O: The dynamic neutralization system for the spine: A multi-center study of a novel non-fusion system. Eur Spine J 11(Suppl 2):S170-S178, 2002.
   This was the first report of clinical outcome of the Dynesys PDS system from its inventor Dubois.

5. Zucherman JF, Hsu KY, Hartjen CA, et al: A multicenter, prospective, randomized trial evaluating the X STOP interspinous process decompression system for the treatment of neurogenic intermittent claudication: Two-year follow-up results. Spine (Phila Pa 1976) 30:1351-1358, 2005.
   This was the first report of a randomized, controlled, prospective multicenter trial comparing the outcomes of neurogenic claudication patients treated with the X STOP with patients treated nonoperatively.

REFERENCES

1. Bono CM, Kadaba M, Vaccaro AR: Posterior pedicle fixation-based dynamic stabilization devices for the treatment of degenerative diseases of the lumbar spine. J Spinal Disord Tech 22:376-383, 2009.

2. Bono CM, Lee CK: Critical analysis of trends in fusion for degenerative disc disease over the past 20 years: Influence of technique on fusion rate and clinical outcome. Spine (Phila Pa 1976) 29:455-463, 2004.

3. Gibson JN, Waddell G: Surgery for degenerative lumbar spondylosis. Cochrane Database Syst Rev (2):CD001352, 2005.

4. Cheh G, Bridwell KH, Lenke LG, et al: Adjacent segment disease following lumbar/thoracolumbar fusion with pedicle screw instrumentation: A minimum 5-year follow-up. Spine (Phila Pa 1976) 32:2253-2257, 2007.

5. Panjabi MM: Hybrid multidirectional test method to evaluate spinal adjacent-level effects. Clin Biomech (Bristol, Avon) 22:257-265, 2007.

6. Dvorak J, Panjabi MM, Chang DG, et al: Functional radiographic diagnosis of the lumbar spine: Flexion-extension and lateral bending. Spine (Phila Pa 1976) 16:562-571, 1991.

7. Sengupta DK, Herkowitz HN: Degenerative spondylolisthesis: Review of current trends and controversies. Spine (Phila Pa 1976) 30(6 Suppl):S71-S81, 2005.

8. Pope MH, Panjabi M: Biomechanical definitions of spinal instability. Spine (Phila Pa 1976) 10:255-256, 1985.

9. Okawa A, Shinomiya K, Komori H, et al: Dynamic motion study of the whole lumbar spine by videofluoroscopy. Spine (Phila Pa 1976) 23:1743-1749, 1998.

10. Murata M, Morio Y, Kuranobu K: Lumbar disc degeneration and segmental instability: A comparison of magnetic resonance images and plain radiographs of patients with low back pain. Arch Orthop Trauma Surg 113:297-301, 1994.

11. Paajanen H, Tertti M: Association of incipient disc degeneration and instability in spondylolisthesis: A magnetic resonance and flexion-extension radiographic study of 20-year-old low back pain patients. Arch Orthop Trauma Surg 111:16-19, 1991.

12. Fujiwara A, Tamai K, An HS, et al: The relationship between disc degeneration, facet joint osteoarthritis, and stability of the degenerative lumbar spine. J Spinal Disord 13:444-450, 2000.

13. Mulholland RC, Sengupta DK: Rationale, principles and experimental evaluation of the concept of soft stabilization. Eur Spine J 11(Suppl 2):S198-S205, 2002.

14. Frymoyer JW, Krag MH: Spinal stability and instability: Definitions, classification, and general principles of management. In Dunsker SB, Schmidek HH, Frymoyer J, Kahn A: (eds): The Unstable Spine. New York, Grune & Stratton, 1986.

15. Jackson JP, Waugh W, Green JP: High tibial osteotomy for osteoarthritis of the knee. J Bone Joint Surg Br 51:88-94, 1969.

16. Moore RJ, Vernon-Roberts B, Fraser RD, et al: The origin and fate of herniated lumbar intervertebral disc tissue. Spine (Phila Pa 1976) 21:2149-2155, 1996.

17. McNally DS: The objectives for the mechanical evaluation of spinal instrumentation have changed. Eur Spine J 11(Suppl 2):S179-S185, 2002.

18. Keller TS, Hansson TH, Abrams AC, et al: Regional variations in the compressive properties of lumbar vertebral trabeculae: Effects of disc degeneration. Spine (Phila Pa 1976) 14:1012-1019, 1989.

19. Simpson EK, Parkinson IH, Manthey B, et al: Intervertebral disc disorganization is related to trabecular bone architecture in the lumbar spine. J Bone Miner Res 16:681-687, 2001.

20. McNally DS, Shackleford IM, Goodship AE, et al: In vivo stress measurement can predict pain on discography. Spine (Phila Pa 1976) 21:2580-2587, 1996.

21. McNally DS, Adams MA: Internal intervertebral disc mechanics as revealed by stress profilometry. Spine (Phila Pa 1976) 17:66-73, 1992.

22. Nockels RP: Dynamic stabilization in the surgical management of painful lumbar spinal disorders. Spine (Phila Pa 1976) 30(16 Suppl):S68-S72, 2005.

23. Panjabi MM: Clinical spinal instability and low back pain. J Electromyogr Kinesiol 13:371-379, 2003.

24. Fujiwara A, Lim TH, An HS, et al: The effect of disc degeneration and facet joint osteoarthritis on the segmental flexibility of the lumbar spine. Spine (Phila Pa 1976) 25:3036-3044, 2000.

25. Lidar Z, Beaumont A, Lifshutz J, et al: Clinical and radiological relationship between posterior lumbar interbody fusion and posterolateral lumbar fusion. Surg Neurol 64:303-308; discussion 308, 2005.

26. Pfeiffer M, Hildebrand R, Grande ME, et al: Evaluation of indication-based use of transpedicular instrumentations with different rigidity for lumbar spinal fusion: A prospective pilot study with 3 years of follow-up. Eur Spine J 12:369-377, 2003.

27. Graf H: Lumbar instability: Surgical treatment without fusion. Rachis 412:123-137, 1992.

28. Grevitt MP, Gardner AD, Spilsbury J, et al: The Graf stabilisation system: Early results in 50 patients. Eur Spine J 4:169-175; discussion 175, 1995.

29. Gardner A, Pande KC: Graf ligamentoplasty: A 7-year follow-up. Eur Spine J 11(Suppl 2):S157-S163, 2002.

30. Markwalder TM, Wenger M: Dynamic stabilization of lumbar motion segments by use of Graf's ligaments: Results with an average follow-up of 7.4 years in 39 highly selected, consecutive patients. Acta Neurochir (Wien) 145:209-214; discussion 214, 2003.

31. Hadlow SV, Fagan AB, Hillier TM, et al: The Graf ligamentoplasty procedure: Comparison with posterolateral fusion in the management of low back pain. Spine (Phila Pa 1976) 23:1172-1179, 1998.

32. Kanayama M, Hashimoto T, Shigenobu K, et al: A minimum 10-year follow-up of posterior dynamic stabilization using Graf artificial ligament. Spine (Phila Pa 1976) 32:1992-1996; discussion 1997, 2007.

33. Grob D, Benini A, Junge A, et al: Clinical experience with the Dynesys semirigid fixation system for the lumbar spine: surgical and patient-oriented outcome in 50 cases after an average of 2 years. Spine (Phila Pa 1976) 30:324-331, 2005.

34. Stoll TM, Dubois G, Schwarzenbach O: The dynamic neutralization system for the spine: A multi-center study of a novel non-fusion system. Eur Spine J 11(Suppl 2):S170-S178, 2002.

35. Schmoelz W, Huber JF, Nydegger T, et al: Dynamic stabilization of the lumbar spine and its effects on adjacent segments: An in vitro experiment. J Spinal Disord Tech 16:418-423, 2003.

36. Schmoelz W, Huber JF, Nydegger T, et al: Influence of a dynamic stabilisation system on load bearing of a bridged disc: An in vitro study of intradiscal pressure. Eur Spine J 15:1276-1285, 2006.

37. Beastall J, Karadimas E, Siddiqui M, et al: The Dynesys lumbar spinal stabilization system: A preliminary report on positional magnetic resonance imaging findings. Spine (Phila Pa 1976) 32:685-690, 2007.

38. Meyers K, Tauber B, Sudin Y, et al: Use of instrumented pedicle screws to evaluate load sharing in posterior dynamic stabilization systems. Spine J 8:926-932, 2008.

39. Sapkas GS, Themistocleous GS, Mavrogenis AF, et al: Stabilization of the lumbar spine using the dynamic neutralization system. Orthopedics 30:859-865, 2007.

40. Wurgler-Hauri CC, Kalbarczyk A, Wiesli M, et al: Dynamic neutralization of the lumbar spine after microsurgical decompression in acquired lumbar spinal stenosis and segmental instability. Spine (Phila Pa 1976) 33:E66-E72, 2008.

41. Welch WC, Cheng BC, Awad TE, et al: Clinical outcomes of the Dynesys dynamic neutralization system: 1-year preliminary results. Neurosurg Focus 22:E8, 2007.

42. Sengupta DK: Dynamic stabilization system. In Yue JJ, McAfee PC, An HS (eds): Motion Preservation Surgery of the Spine—Advanced Techniques and Controversies. Philadelphia, Saunders, 2008, pp 472-475.

43. Kim YS, Moon BJ: Bioflex spring rod pedicle screw system. In Kim DH, Fessler RG (eds): Dynamic Reconstruction of the Spine. New York, Thieme, 2006, pp 340-346.

44. Kim YS, Zhang HY, Moon BJ, et al: Nitinol spring rod dynamic stabilization system and nitinol memory loops in surgical treatment for lumbar disc disorders: Short-term follow up. Neurosurg Focus 22:E10, 2007.

45. Yue JJ, Timm JP, Panjabi MM, et al: Clinical application of the Panjabi neutral zone hypothesis: The Stabilimax NZ posterior lumbar dynamic stabilization system. Neurosurg Focus 22:E12, 2007.

46. Yue JJ, Malcolmon G, Timm JP: The Stabilimax NZ posterior lumbar dynamic stabilization system. In Yue JJ, McAfee PC, An HS (eds): Motion Preservation Surgery of the Spine—Advanced Techniques and Controversies. Philadelphia, Saunders, 2008, pp 476-482.

47. Karabekir HS, Sedat C, Mehmet Z: Clinical outcomes of cosmic dynamic neutralization system: Preliminary results of 1-year. J Minim Invas Spinal Technol 2(3), 2008.

48. von Strempel A, et al: Stabilisation of the degenerated lumbar spine in the nonfusion technique with cosmic posterior dynamic system. World Spine J 1:40-47, 2006.

49. Mandigo CE, Sampath P, Kaiser MG: Posterior dynamic stabilization of the lumbar spine: Pedicle based stabilization with the AccuFlex rod system. Neurosurg Focus 22:E9, 2007.

50. Wallach CJ, Teng AL, Wang JC: NFlex. In Yue JJ, McAfee PC, An HS (eds): Motion Preservation Surgery of the Spine—Advanced Techniques and Controversies. Philadelphia, Saunders, 2008, pp 505-510.

51. Lindsey DP, Swanson KE, Fuchs P, et al: The effects of an interspinous implant on the kinematics of the instrumented and adjacent levels in the lumbar spine. Spine (Phila Pa 1976) 28:2192-2197, 2003.

52. Swanson KE, Lindsey DP, Hsu KY, et al: The effects of an interspinous implant on intervertebral disc pressures. Spine (Phila Pa 1976) 28:26-32, 2003.

53. Wiseman CM, Lindsey DP, Fredrick AD, et al: The effect of an interspinous process implant on facet loading during extension. Spine (Phila Pa 1976) 30:903-907, 2005.

54. Richards JC, Majumdar S, Lindsey DP, et al: The treatment mechanism of an interspinous process implant for lumbar neurogenic intermittent claudication. Spine (Phila Pa 1976) 30:744-749, 2005.

55. Zucherman JF, Hsu KY, Hartjen CA, et al: A multicenter, prospective, randomized trial evaluating the X STOP interspinous process decompression system for the treatment of neurogenic intermittent claudication: Two-year follow-up results. Spine (Phila Pa 1976) 30:1351-1358, 2005.

56. Senegas J: Mechanical supplementation by non-rigid fixation in degenerative intervertebral lumbar segments: The Wallis system. Eur Spine J 11(Suppl 2):S164-S169, 2002.

57. Floman Y, Millgram MA, Smorgick Y, et al: Failure of the Wallis interspinous implant to lower the incidence of recurrent lumbar disc herniations in patients undergoing primary disc excision. J Spinal Disord Tech 20:337-341, 2007.

58. Senegas J, Vital JM, Pointillart V, et al: Long-term actuarial survivorship analysis of an interspinous stabilization system. Eur Spine J 16:1279-1287, 2007.

59. Christie SD, Song JK, Fessler RG: Dynamic interspinous process technology. Spine (Phila Pa 1976) 30(16 Suppl):S73-S78, 2005.

60. Tsai KJ, Murakami H, Lowery G, et al: A biomechanical evaluation of an interspinous device (Coflex) used to stabilize the lumbar spine. J Surg Orthop Adv 15:167-172, 2006.

61. Kong DS, Kim ES, Eoh W: One-year outcome evaluation after interspinous implantation for degenerative spinal stenosis with segmental instability. J Korean Med Sci 22:330-335, 2007.

62. Kim KA, McDonald M, Pik JH, et al: Dynamic intraspinous spacer technology for posterior stabilization: Case-control study on the safety, sagittal angulation, and pain outcome at 1-year follow-up evaluation. Neurosurg Focus 22:E7, 2007.

63. Palmer S, Mahar A, Oka R: Biomechanical and radiographic analysis of a novel, minimally invasive, extension-limiting device for the lumbar spine. Neurosurg Focus 22:E4, 2007.

54 CHAPTER

Total Facet Replacement

Mark A. Reiley, MD

The many advancements in the understanding of spinal pathology and spinal implants in the last 20 years, coupled with 30 years of extremity total joint arthroplasty, have created a new era in spine surgery. Complete segmental replacement in the spine is now possible. Total disc replacement has been used successfully for almost 15 years.

The degenerative problems of the facet joints and their resultant pathology have remained as a potential pain source, a remaining area of poorly understood and poorly diagnosed axial skeletal disease. Total facet arthroplasty is available for the treatment for central stenosis, lateral stenosis, degenerative spondylolisthesis, pars interarticularis syndrome, and other overlapping diseases caused by damaged or degenerative posterior elements.

Facet Anatomy and Function

The lumbar facet joints have been thoroughly studied. Much is known about their loading, biomechanical function, time-related anatomic changes, tropism and asymmetry, modes of articular wear, and soft tissue attachments.[1-35]

At its most narrow analysis, the facet joint is designed to function as a shear stop—an anterior shear stop (Fig. 54–1). Facet joints prevent anterior shear forces from destroying the disc, which is primarily designed to absorb compressive loads. The disc is so well designed for its purpose that it is essentially impossible to injure the anulus with purely compressive loads.[26] Also, the facets control varying amounts of rotation and limit flexion of the lumbar spine,[28-31,36] but their most important function is to protect the disc from parallel force vectors.

Viewed in this simplified manner, it becomes clearer why degeneration of these lumbar apophyseal joints produces so much spinal pathology. The loss of even 1 mm of cartilage thickness within the facet joint allows a significant increase in anterior-posterior translational motion to occur. This increased motion causes repeated strain of the multifidus muscle and facet capsule ligaments, increases the shear load on the disc and the posterior and anterior longitudinal ligaments, and allows the neural foramen and lateral recess to collapse with

flexion and extension of the spine. At the same time, cartilage wear stimulates spur formation in all directions around the facet joint, as cartilage wear typically does in all degenerative synovial joints. These osteophytes encroach further on the neural elements increasing central and lateral stenosis, and the osteophytes may act as a source of pain when they impinge on each other or the pars interarticularis. Degeneration can continue until facet subluxation occurs, producing further stenosis (Fig. 54–2).

Concomitant with the five degenerative changes in the apophyseal joints—loss of articular cartilage, spur formation, loss of control of anterior shear forces, facet subluxation, and increased anterior-posterior translation—the facets also frequently undergo disadvantageous morphologic changes with aging. These changes undermine the ability of the spine to withstand shear forces. In infant spines, the facets are primarily coronally oriented.[25] In adult spines, the lumbar facets generally have a small anteromedial coronal component and a large posterior sagittal component (Fig. 54–3). As the spine ages, the facet becomes more and more sagittally aligned with a smaller and smaller coronal component (Fig. 54–4). The coronal part of the facet joint controls shear forces.[28] In a presentation at the International Spinal Arthroplasty Society Meeting in Montpelier, France in 2002, DuPont, using finite element analysis, verified how the shear forces across the disc increase as the facets are directed more and more sagittally.

There is at least one additional force working on the lumbar facet joint. Depending on the position of the spine, the facets absorb 0% (in full flexion) to 33% (in full extension) of the compressive (axial) load at a given level.[23,37] An incompetent, degenerative facet joint can no longer absorb its share of the compressive loads, which can narrow the neural foramen further in an up-down direction, especially with the spine in extension.

Radiologic Diagnosis and Issues

Although excellent radiologic tools have been developed, including computed tomography (CT), CT myelogram, and magnetic resonance imaging (MRI), they may not be used to

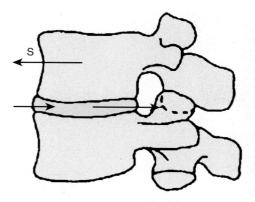

FIGURE 54–1 Diagram showing anterior shear forces (S) across facet joint.

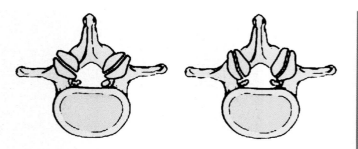

FIGURE 54–3 Diagram of typical pediatric orientation of lumbar facet joints on *left* and typical orientation later in life.

their fullest advantage. There is no spinal equivalent to the 30-degree weight-bearing anteroposterior view of the knee (Fig. 54–5) to detect cartilage wear or joint laxity. Similar positional views of other joints of the extremities, such as weight-bearing anteroposterior and lateral views of the feet and the 30-degree angle view of the shoulder, have been developed to aid in diagnosing arthritis and instability but not as well with advanced imaging for the spine.

MRI and CT of the spine are extremely informative diagnostic tests, but most are performed in a supine position during which most patients do not have back pain. Some MRI studies allow imaging in the upright position and in flexion and extension, but these tools have low tesla outputs at the present time. It seems sensible to develop a technique that applies some extension to the lumbar spine and perhaps some axial loading as well to assess more accurately the functional capacity of the facet joints. Flexion and extension films are rarely used in the spine, and when they are used, they require patient cooperation. It may be easier to run a second sequence on MRI with a pillow beneath the lumbar spine to obtain a comparison extension view.

A vest with pantaloons has been developed that can individually manipulate vertebral bodies to obtain much more information on a segmental level, but this is under development, and weight-bearing extension views of the lumbar spine probably will not be ready for initial usage before 2012. Other investigators have developed CT scan techniques to show positional lateral recess stenosis (Fig. 54–6).

One radiologic sign seen on plain films that draws attention to facet instability is a break in the normally round shape of the intervertebral foramina. This radiologic sign is analogous to Shenton line, which is a continuation of the arc of the femoral neck with the arc of the superior pubic ramus. When the line is unbroken, the hip is located, and the biomechanics are considered optimal.

In the same vein, the inferior arc of the pedicle should follow the posterior aspect of the superior and inferior vertebral bodies associated in its foraminal opening, along with the inferior articular process and the arc of the superior articular process. If this circle is unbroken (i.e., the line is smooth) (Fig. 54–7), the foraminal space, at least in a static film, is probably adequate from a bony standpoint. If the proximal end of the superior articular facet or the superior spurs of the inferior articular surface intrude into the hemicircle formed by the pedicle and the inferior facet, the broken foraminal line would indicate facet joint degeneration and possibly suggest instability. This line can be assessed on flexion and extension films and is a more subtle sign than measuring the number of millimeters of spondylolisthesis. An additional sign within the foramen to aid in diagnosis could be the intrusion sign of the superior endplate into the intervertebral foramen. Figure 54–7 illustrates both abnormalities, the former at L3-4 and the latter at L4-5.

Even with improvements in imaging of the spine, the amount, type, and location of pain derived from the history and the physical examination are the most important part of a patient's evaluation. Imaging studies are for the most part confirmatory only.

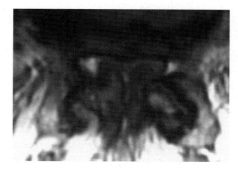

FIGURE 54–2 Degenerative L4-5 facet joint in a 68-year-old patient shows facet asymmetry, loss of articular cartilage, subluxed left facet, and central stenosis.

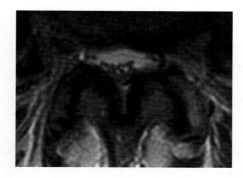

FIGURE 54–4 Sagittally aligned, asymmetric, and dislocated facet joints at L4-5 in a 56-year-old patient.

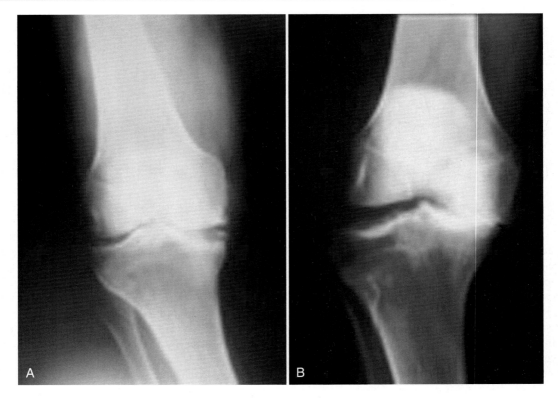

FIGURE 54–5 A and **B,** Non–weight-bearing view of knee (**A**) and 30-degree anteroposterior weight-bearing view (**B**) show increased cartilage wear and medial, femoral subluxation with weight-bearing view.

Current Treatment of Posterior Lumbar Degeneration

There are three basic types of operative approaches to the degenerative lumbar spine. The surgeon can perform some sort of débridement of the soft tissue and bony elements (including the ligamentum flavum, part or all of the lamina and the spinous process, a portion of the pars interarticularis, and up to 50% of the facet joint) that are involved in the stenotic process. The surgeon can perform a débridement-type procedure for the stenotic pathology combined with a fusion type of procedure, be it anterior, posterior, combined, posterolateral, instrumented, or noninstrumented. Finally, the surgeon can perform one of the newer extension-limiting procedures using a "stiff bumper/rope combination" or an interspinous process block.

Disc replacement is primarily for isolated disc pathology and is not indicated for patients with posterior degenerative disease. That being said, some manufacturers, either inadvertently or purposefully, have designed total discs with a single point of rotation. This type of total disc system forces the anterior column of the spine to control shear forces, which is not the intended function of the disc. It is the purview of the facets to control forces acting parallel to the disc.

All of these operations have their successes and their failures with quite a bit of variability as reported in the literature. Wide decompressive laminectomy has been shown to have 57% to 85% good results at 4 years.[38-41] Postoperative problems and complications include segmental instability, recurrent spinal stenosis, continued back pain, infection, neural injury, and dural tears.[35,42]

Decompression and arthrodesis are the mainstays of treatment for degenerative facets. Numerous fusion techniques and associated implantable instrumentation are available, and the operation has improved to the point where a successful radiographic fusion is the rule. As Vaccaro and Ball[42] have written, "Though the majority of studies have shown that the radiographic fusion success rate is improved with the addition of internal fixation, the benefits in the majority of degenerative spinal disorders are unclear in terms of patient function." Some of the complications from combined decompression and fusion include 3% to 6% infection rate,[43] continued pain,

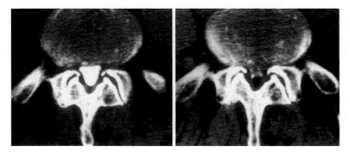

FIGURE 54–6 Flexion (*left*) and extension (*right*) CT myelogram at L4-5 level showing narrowing of lateral recess with extension.

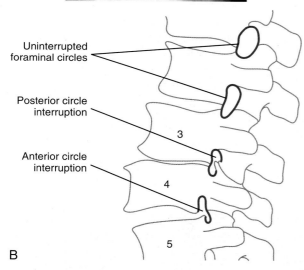

FIGURE 54–7 **A,** Lateral x-ray of lumbar spine with degenerative disease. Intrusion by inferior articular spurs into foraminal circle is seen at L3-4 (*arrow*). In addition, L4-5 exhibits foraminal circle distortion from superior endplate of L5. **B,** Same distortions are shown diagrammatically. Both are radiologic signs of facet or motion segment degeneration ("incompetence"). The other foramina at L1-2 and L2-3 show no interruption in circle subtended by two pedicles, inferior process, and superior process.

juxtasegmental instability or fracture (Fig. 54–8), failed fusion, and failed hardware.

Stiff bumper/ropes and interspinous process extension blocks are currently under investigation for treatment of the degenerative spine. Follow-up so far has been short-term only, and their future utility is yet to be fully determined.

Total Facet Replacement Design

Total facet replacement has been developed by several companies. To maintain a conceptual focus, and because of company changes, none of the manufacturers of facet replacement are listed in this chapter.

Total facet replacements have been designed with metal-on-metal bearing surfaces (polished cobalt-chromium) and titanium for all stems. The wear debris from the bearing surfaces has been evaluated and found to be acceptable by the U.S. Food and Drug Administration (FDA) for implantation and for investigational device exemption (IDE) studies. The strength of the titanium stems has been tested with loads up to 2½ times body weight with 10 million cycles and found to withstand that repetitive loading and motion successfully. The new facet joint is typically pointed almost straight posterior with a 17-degree incline to limit flexion to physiologic levels. Motion studies have shown that the replaced facet approximates well the motion of the normal joint. Of the four types of facet joints clinically anatomically required for the spine (see later), all required a cross bar for adequate strength except for a translaminar device used for patients with multilevel disease or who have a preexisting total disc replacement.

Clinical Testing

Greater than 200 patients have been surgically treated worldwide with total facet replacement with follow-up in some cases of more than 3 years. With the exception of a few patients who were unsuitable to receive the implant (extreme obesity), there

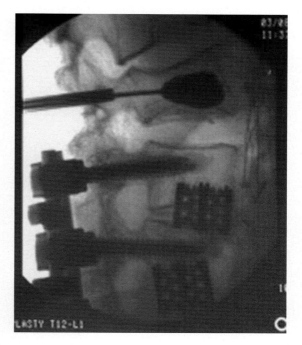

FIGURE 54–8 Vertebral body fracture with kyphoplasty repair of fracture occurring above spinal fusion.

TFAS® Patient RU3
3 year follow-up

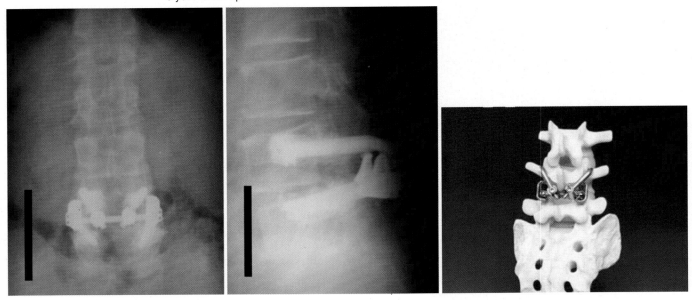

FIGURE 54–9 Cemented facet replacement (cemented total facet arthroplasty system) shown is 3 years postoperative.

have been no reported incidents of breakage or dislocation. Pain relief has been excellent (see later). This operation has found some acceptance by spine surgeons, but most are waiting for more data to be produced in formal studies before making a decision about posterior spinal arthroplasty. The total facet replacement family of products includes four different types of total facet implants: a cemented total facet replacement for older or osteoporotic patients (Fig. 54–9), an uncemented total facet replacement for younger patients with normal or nonosteoporotic bone (Fig. 54–10), a lumbosacral total facet arthroplasty designed for the L5-S1 facet joint, and a translaminar facet replacement implant that is targeted for minimally invasive approaches and can be used to treat single-level and multilevel syndromes. The first three types are pedicle-based. The translaminar designs can work across a patient's natural disc or in conjunction with a total disc replacement and for multilevel stenosis (Figs. 54–11 and 54–12), assuming the laminae are left intact.

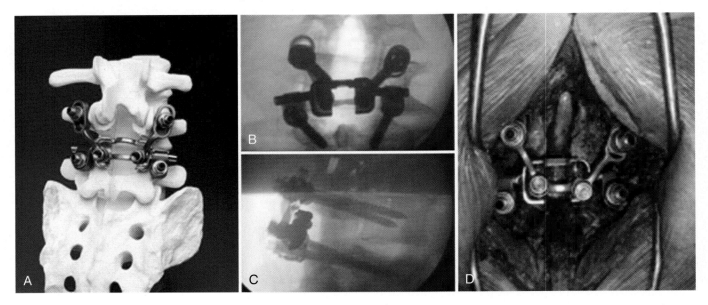

FIGURE 54–10 Uncemented facet replacement (cemented total facet arthroplasty system). **A,** In foam bone. **B,** Anteroposterior x-ray in situ. **C,** Lateral x-ray in situ. **D,** Anteroposterior image in situ. (In situ images courtesy Dr. Radu Prejbeanu, Timisoara, Romania, and Dr. Scott Webb, Tampa, FL.)

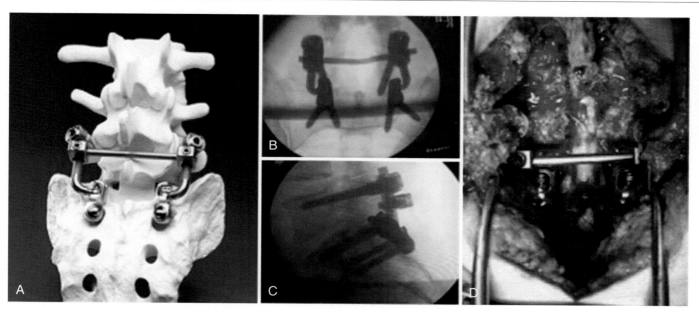

FIGURE 54–11 Lumbosacral facet replacement (lumbosacral total facet arthroplasty system). **A,** In foam bone. **B,** Anteroposterior x-ray in situ. **C,** Lateral x-ray in situ. **D,** Anteroposterior image in situ. (In situ images courtesy Dr. Radu Prejbeanu, Timisoara, Romania, and Dr. Scott Webb, Tampa, FL.)

Clinical Results of Total Facet Arthroplasty System (Cemented Facet Replacement)

Several scales were used to evaluate the clinical results of the total facet arthroplasty system prosthesis placed in 180 patients, including the visual analog scale (VAS) leg pain assessment, VAS back pain assessment, and Zurich Claudication Questionnaire (ZCQ) symptom assessment. The results of these studies are presented in Figures 54–13 through 54–16. The results of all three pain scales showed a profound decrease in pain at 1

month postoperatively, and the pain continued to lessen in subsequent follow-up assessments at 3, 6, 12, 24, and 36 months. Likewise, the ZCQ functional scores continued to improve over the same period. Comparative results in control patients receiving decompression and fusion are being collated at this time.

Future of Total Facet Replacement

There is evidence from multiple national and international presentations that total disc replacement accelerates facet

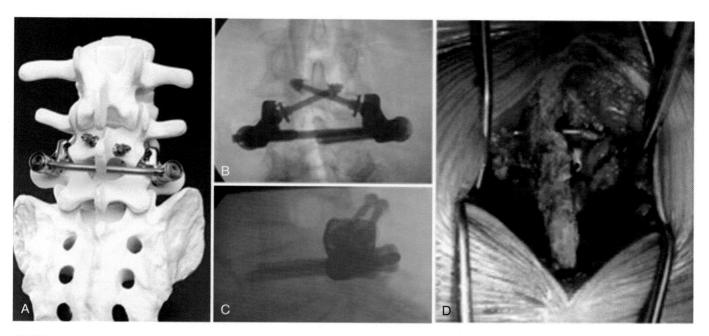

FIGURE 54–12 Translaminar facet replacement (translaminar total facet arthroplasty system). **A,** In foam bone. **B,** Anteroposterior x-ray in situ. **C,** Lateral x-ray in situ. **D,** Anteroposterior image in situ. (In situ images courtesy Dr. Radu Prejbeanu, Timisoara, Romania, and Dr. Scott Webb, Tampa, FL.)

WORLWIDE TFAS VAS LEG PAIN ASSESSMENT

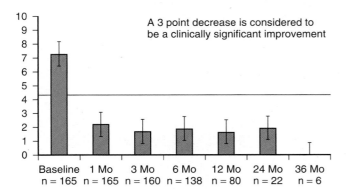

FIGURE 54–13 VAS leg pain assessment scale at 3 years for total facet arthroplasty system.

VAS BACK PAIN ASSESSMENT

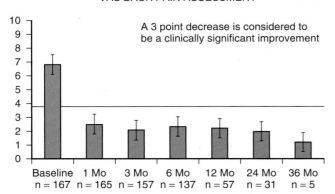

FIGURE 54–14 VAS back pain scale at 3 years for total facet arthroplasty system.

WORLWIDE TFAS ZCQ FUNCTION ASSESSMENT

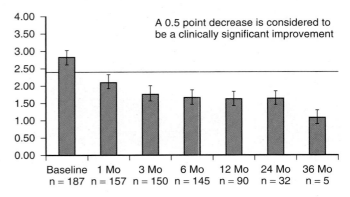

FIGURE 54–15 Results of total facet arthroplasty system using ZCQ function scale at 3 years.

WORLWIDE TFAS ZCQ SYMPTOM ASSESSMENT

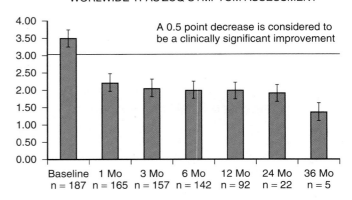

FIGURE 54–16 Results of total facet arthroplasty system using ZCQ symptom scale at 3 years.

pathology. Patients with previously implanted artificial discs that have subsequently developed posterior stenosis or facet-related pathologies have been well treated with facet replacement. An ongoing FDA IDE study is about 2 years from completion. In addition, patients with combined anterior and posterior pathology may be successfully treated with complete segmental replacement as shown in Figure 54–17—with a total disc and bilateral face replacements, rather than fusions, in selected cases.

Early results from the FDA studies have shown excellent clinical results. The comparison data between wide decompressive laminectomy and fusion have not been reviewed, however. Early data indicate that surgical recovery may be much faster with facet replacement, but sufficient cases have not been performed in arms of the study to make any claims. Only the cemented total facet arthroplasty has been extensively studied, and the FDA is requiring each type of total facet arthroplasty to be tested with its own IDE study, so it may be 20 or 30 years with $400 million spent before the spine surgeons have solid performance data.

PEARLS

1. Childhood facet joints are angled posteriorly. They become more sagittally directed with time, which leads to many of the facet-induced problems. Total facet arthroplasty realigns the facets in a more physiologic position to protect the disc from anterior shear forces.

2. Partial facetectomy is very difficult with sagittally directed facets. These patients invariably are unstable after facetectomy and require fusion. In this case, to ensure protection of the disc from anterior shear forces and to prevent the muscle spasms that can pull against a fusion, total facet arthroplasty seems to be a better option.

3. As a rule, the lamina is not the problem in posterior spinal pathology, and removal of the lamina does not have to be extensive. Because of the height loss of the motion segment undergoing surgery, the ligamentum flavum should definitely be removed because there is more ligament than needed, and it can efface the roots or cord.

4. Total facet replacement is not for arthritic pain of the facet joints. It is used to correct instability problems and stenotic problems that arise from a worn-out facet.

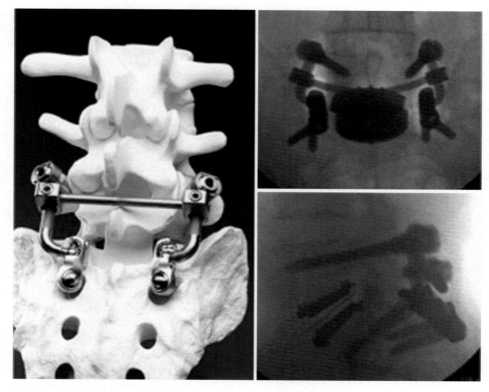

FIGURE 54–17 The first total segmental replacement of the spine, performed in Berlin by Büttner-Janz and Yuan, using a CHARITÉ disc replacement and the L5-S1 total facet arthroplasty system.

5. If the spinous process is not blocking extension with bony contact or limiting flexion with its ligaments, it is best to save as much as possible in case future fusions are required.

PITFALLS

1. Use a perfect AP x-ray with the pedicles equidistant for the spinous process and touching the superior end plate of the vertebral body with the superior edge of the pedicle to ensure proper placement of the stems or screws.

2. The surgeon needs to warn the patient that circumstances may lead to abandonment of the procedure in exchange for a fusion.

3. Translaminar facet replacements are exacting procedures, but at this time they are the only procedure available to replace multiple facets. If a lamina splits, it must be changed to a regular facet replacement. A translaminar facet replacement cannot be performed above a single-level replacement.

KEY POINTS

1. In all surgeries in which a total joint is implanted, positioning of the patient on the operating room table is crucial. With a total facet replacement, it is more like inserting two implants at the same time, and each side affects the function of the other. The pelvis and shoulders should be as square as possible. The lumbar spine should be in some extension, not in flexion. Insertion of the device with the spine in flexion causes extension of the adjacent levels.

2. The stems or screws in the superiormost pedicles used should be inserted as parallel to the superior endplate as possible. The forces across the facet joint try to angle this stem in an inferior direction. Placing the screw and stem superiorly in the vertebral body and parallel to the disc lessens the risk of inferior angulation occurring (which leads to loosening or prosthetic dislocation or both). This is analogous to placing a total hip stem in varus, which also leads to premature implant loosening.

3. Equal lengths of the stem (if using a cemented implant) should be protruding from each pedicle. Asymmetrical pedicle lengths can lead to rotational subluxation of the joint.

4. As in all exacting spine surgery, less than impeccable radiologic views are unacceptable. If the anteroposterior view is rotated 8 or more degrees off the midline for a given vertebral body, the stem and screw can exit the pedicle laterally, and the surgeon would be unaware of it.

5. If it is planned to implant a disc replacement along with the facet replacements, the disc should be inserted first. This predetermines the lengths of the up-down connections of facet arthroplasty.

6. Preoperative coronal CT or MRI can help gauge what lengths of screw or stem are needed. They can also help with cross bar selection if the interpedicle distance is measured before surgery.

7. Occasionally, a pedicle may be split during bony preparation or during implant placement. It is prudent to discuss with the patient that all events during surgery cannot be predicted and that there is a chance that a fusion will be done instead of facet arthroplasty.

KEY REFERENCES

1. Fujiwara A, Lim TH, Howard S, et al: The effect of disc degeneration and facet joint osteoarthritis on the segmental flexibility of the lumbar spine. Spine (Phila Pa 1976) 25:3036-3043, 2000.
   This is an excellent review of the CT and x-ray changes in facet arthrosis. A classification system for degenerative facet disease is proposed.

2. Scoles PV, Linton AE, Latimer B, et al: Vertebral body and posterior element morphology: The normal spine in middle life. Spine (Phila Pa 1976) 13:1082-1086, 1988.
   This is a landmark article reviewing the time-related morphologic changes that occur in the facet joints over a lifetime.

3. Katz JN, Lipson SJ, Larson MG, et al: The outcome of decompressive laminectomy for degenerative lumbar stenosis. J Bone Joint Surg Am 73:809-816, 1991.
   This article reports the lowest percentage of favorable outcomes for simple laminectomey as a treatment of spinal stenosis.

4. Spengler DM: Degenerative stenosis of the lumbar spine. J Bone Joint Surg Am 69:82-86, 1987.
   This article describes the highest percentage of favorable outcomes for laminectomy as a treatment for spinal stenosis.

5. Vaccaro AR, Ball ST: Indications for instrumentation in degenerative lumbar spinal disorders. Orthopedics 23:260-271, 2000.
   Vaccaro and Ball present an insightful article on the current abilities to produce excellent spinal fusions with the existing hardware but question whether these fusions are actually improving the function of the patients.

6. Wright T, Goodman S: Implant wear. In: Total Joint Replacement: Clinical and Biologic Issues, Material and Design Considerations. Rosemont, IL, American Academy of Orthopedic Surgery, 2001.
   This chapter describes total joint wear and how it is studied from the ground up. It is a must-read for anyone contemplating designing any arthroplasty system.

REFERENCES

1. Adams MA, Hutton WC: The mechanical function of the lumbar apophyseal joints. Spine (Phila Pa 1976) 8:327-330, 1983.

2. Adams MA, Hutton WC, Scott JR: The resistance to flexion of the lumbar intervertebral joint. Spine (Phila Pa 1976) 5:245-253, 1980.

3. Adams MA, McNally DS, Dolan P: "Stress" distributions inside intervertebral discs: The effects of age and degeneration. J Bone Joint Surg Br 78:965-972, 1996.

4. Badgley C: The articular facets in relation to low back pain and sciatic radiation. J Bone Joint Surg Am 23:481-496, 1941.

5. Berlemann U, Jeszenszky DJ, Buhler DW, et al: Facet joint remodeling in generative spondylolisthesis: An investigation of joint orientation and tropism. Eur Spine J 7:376-380, 1998.

6. Boden SD, Martin C, Rudolph R, et al: Increase of motion between lumbar vertebrae after excision of the capsule and cartilage of the facets: A cadaver study. J Bone Joint Surg Am 76:1847-1853, 1994.

7. Butler D, Tratimow JH, Anderson GB, et al: Discs degenerate before facets. Spine (Phila Pa 1976) 15:111-131, 1990.

8. Farfan HF, Cossette JW, Robertson HG, et al: The effects of torsion on the lumbar intervertebral joints: The role of torsion in the production of disc degeneration. J Bone Joint Surg Am 52:468-497, 1970.

9. Farfan HF, Huberdeau RM, Dubow HF: Lumbar intervertebral disc degeneration: A postmortem study. J Bone Joint Surg Am 54:492-510, 1972.

10. Farfan HF: Mechanical Disorders of the Low Back. Philadelphia, Lea & Febiger, 1973.

11. Fujiwara A, Lim TH, Howard S, et al: The effect of disc degeneration and facet joint osteoarthritis on the segmental flexibility of the lumbar spine. Spine (Phila Pa 1976) 25:3036-3043, 2000.

12. Grogan J, Nowicki BH, Schmidt TA, et al: Lumbar facet joint tropism does not accelerate degeneration of the facet joints. AJNR Am J Neuroradiol 18:1325-1329, 1997.

13. Herno A, Airaksinen O, Saari T: Long term results of surgical treatment of lumbar spinal stenosis. Spine (Phila Pa 1976) 18:1471-1474, 1993.

14. Hickey RF, Tregonning GD: Denervation of spinal facet joints for treatment of chronic low back pain. N Z Med J 85:96-99, 1977.

15. Kirkaldy-Willis WH, Farfan HF: Instability of the lumbar spine. Clin Orthop 110:23, 1982.

16. Koeller W, Muchlhaus S, Meier W, et al: Biomechanical properties of human intervertebral discs subjected to axial dynamic compression—influence of age and degeneration. J Biomech 19:807-816, 1986.

17. Lewin T: Osteoarthritis in lumbar synovial joints: A morphological study. Acta Orthop Scand 73:1-112, 1964.

18. Lorenz M, Patwardhan A, Vanderby R Jr: Load-bearing characteristics of lumbar facets in normal and surgically altered spinal segments. Spine (Phila Pa 1976) 8:122-129, 1983.

19. Malmivaara A, Videman T, Kuosma E, et al: Facet joint orientation, facet and costovertebral joint osteoarthrosis, disc degeneration, vertebral body osteophytosis, and Schmorl's nodes in the thoracolumbar junctional region of cadaveric spines. Spine (Phila Pa 1976) 12:458-463, 1987.

20. Mooney V, Robertson J: The facet syndrome. Clin Orthop 115:149-156, 1976.

21. Panjabi MM, Oxland T, Takata K, et al: Articular facets of the human spine: Quantitative three-dimensional anatomy. Spine (Phila Pa 1976) 18:1298-1310, 1983.

22. Panjabi MM, Oxland TR, Yamamoto I, et al: Mechanical behavior of the human lumbar and lumbosacral spine as shown by three-dimensional load-displacement curves. J Bone Joint Surg Am 76:413-424, 1994.

23. Panjabi MM, Yamamoto I, Oxland TR, et al: How does posture affect coupling in the lumbar spine? Spine (Phila Pa 1976) 14:1002-1011, 1989.

24. Reichmann S: The postnatal development of form and orientation of the lumbar intervertebral joint surfaces. Z Anat Entwicklung 133:102-103, 1971.

25. Scoles PV, Linton AE, Latimer B, et al: Vertebral body and posterior element morphology: The normal spine in middle life. Spine (Phila Pa 1976) 13:1082-1086, 1988.

26. Sheaby CN: Facet denervation in the management of back and sciatic pain. Clin Orthop 115:157-164, 1976.

27. Simkin PA, Graney DO, Feichtner JJ: Roman arches, human joints and disease: Differences between convex and concave sides of joints. Arthritis Rheum 23:1308-1311, 1980.

28. Taylor JR, Twomey LT: Age changes in lumbar zygapophyseal joints: Observations on structure and function. Spine (Phila Pa 1976) 11:739-745, 1986.

29. Taylor JR, Twomey LT: Sagittal and horizontal plane movement of the human lumbar vertebral column in cadavers and in the living. Rheumatol Rehabil 19:223-232, 1980.

30. Twomey LT, Taylor JR: Sagittal movements of the human lumbar vertebral column: A quantitative study of the role of the posterior vertebral elements. Arch Phys Med Rehabil 64:322-325, 1983.

31. Twomey L, Taylor J, Furniss B: Age changes in the bone density and structure of the lumbar vertebral column. J Anat 136:15-25, 1983.

32. Twomey LT, Taylor JR: Age changes in the lumbar articular triad. Aust J Physiother 31:106-112, 1984.

33. White AA, Panjabi MM: Clinical Biomechanics of the Spine. Philadelphia, JB Lippincott, 1978.

34. Wright T, Goodman S: Implant wear. In: Total Joint Replacement: Clinical and Biologic Issues, Material and Design Considerations. Rosemont, IL, American Academy of Orthopedic Surgery, 2001.

35. Yuan HA, Garfin SR, Dickman CA, et al: A historic cohort study of pedicle screw fixation in thoracic, lumbar, and sacral spinal fusions. Spine (Phila Pa 1976) 19(Suppl 20):2279S-2296S, 1994.

36. Shirazi-adl SA, Shrivastava SC, Ahmed AM: Stress analysis of the lumbar disc-body unit in compression: A three-dimensional nonlinear finite element study. Spine (Phila Pa 1976) 9:2, 1984.

37. Lin HS, Liu YK, Adams KH: Mechanical response of the lumbar intervertebral joint under physiologic (complex) loading. J Bone Joint Surg Am 60:41-55, 1978.

38. Katz JN, Lipson SJ, Brick GW, et al: Clinical correlates of patient satisfaction after laminectomy for degenerative lumbar spinal stenosis. Spine (Phila Pa 1976) 20:1155-1160, 1995.

39. Katz JN, Lipson SJ, Larson MG, et al: The outcome of decompressive laminectomy for degenerative lumbar stenosis. J Bone Joint Surg Am 73:809-816, 1991.

40. Lipson SJ: Spinal stenosis. Rheum Dis Clin North Am 14:613-618, 1988.

41. Spengler DM: Degenerative stenosis of the lumbar spine. J Bone Joint Surg Am 69:82-86, 1987.

42. Vaccaro AR, Ball ST: Indications for instrumentation in degenerative lumbar spinal disorders. Orthopedics 23:260-271, 2000.

43. Wang JC, Bohlman HH, Riew KD, et al: Dural tears secondary to operations on the lumbar spine: Management and results after a two-year-minimum follow-up of eighty-eight patients. J Bone Joint Surg Am 80:1728-1732, 1998.

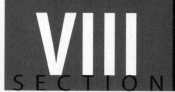

Rationale of Minimally Invasive Spine Surgery

Choll W. Kim, MD, PhD
Steven R. Garfin, MD
Richard G. Fessler, MD

The goal of minimally invasive spine (MIS) surgery is to accomplish the intended goals of treatment: decompression, fusion, and/or realignment. The key concepts that guide MIS approaches are (1) decrease muscle crush injuries during retraction; (2) avoid detachment of tendons to the posterior bony elements, especially the multifidus attachments to the spinous process and superior articular processes; (3) maintain the integrity of the dorsolumbar fascia; (4) limit bony resection; (5) use known neurovascular planes; and (6) decrease the size of the surgical corridor to coincide with the area of the surgical target site. Recent advancements in instrumentation, combined with refinement of surgical techniques, have allowed treatment of an ever-increasing number of spinal disorders.

Anatomy of the Posterior Paraspinal Muscles

The posterior lumbar paraspinal muscles are part of a larger biomechanical system that includes the abdominal muscles and their fibrous attachment to the spine through the dorsolumbar fascia. This network of muscles is responsible for generating movements of the spine while maintaining its stability.[1,2] In addition to maintaining spinal posture in its neutral position, the paraspinal muscles guard the spine from excessive bending that would otherwise endanger the integrity of the intervertebral discs and ligaments.[3] Panjabi and colleagues[4,5] have proposed that the paraspinal muscles apply minimal resistance inside the neutral zone (NZ) but increase their stiffness exponentially once the range of motion falls outside this NZ. This dynamic stabilizing system is controlled by an interconnected chain of mechanoreceptors embedded in the muscle fascicles, the disc annulus, and the spinal ligaments.[6] Functional electromyographic (EMG) studies reveal that spinal stability is achieved by the simultaneous contraction of several agonist-antagonist muscles.[3,7,8] Architectural studies suggest that the individual paraspinal muscles may have different primary roles as either movers or stabilizers of the spinal column.[9]

Multifidus Muscle

The posterior paraspinal muscles are composed of two muscle groups: (1) the deep paramedian transversospinalis muscle group, which includes the multifidus, interspinales, intertransversarii, and short rotators, and (2) the more superficial and lateral erector spinae muscles that include the longissimus and iliocostalis (Fig. 55-1). These muscles run along the thoracolumbar spine and attach caudally to the sacrum, sacroiliac joint, and iliac wing. The multifidus is the most medial of the major posterior paraspinal muscles and is the largest muscle that spans the lumbosacral junction. It is believed to be the major posterior stabilizing muscle of the spine.[3,9,10] Compared with other paraspinal muscles, the multifidus muscle is short and stout. It has a large physiologic cross-sectional area (PCSA) but short fiber lengths. This unique architectural anatomy is designed to create large forces over relatively short distances (Fig. 55-2A).[9] Furthermore, the multifidus sarcomere length is positioned on the ascending portion of the length-tension curve (Fig. 55-2B). When our posture changes from standing erect to bending forward, the multifidus can produce more force as the spine flexes forward. This serves to protect the spine at its most vulnerable position.

The multifidus is the only muscle that is attached to both the posterior parts of the L5 and S1 vertebrae and is therefore the sole posterior stabilizer that both originates and inserts to this segment. The morphology of the lumbar multifidus is complex.[11] Unlike the other paraspinal muscles that have specific origins and insertions, the multifidus muscle is formed by five separate bands, each having its own origin and several different insertion sites. Each band consists of several fascicles arising from the tip of the spinous process and the lateral surface of the vertebral lamina. Caudally, the different fascicles diverge to separate attachments into the mammillary processes of the caudal vertebrae two to five levels below their origin and downward through each vertebra to the sacrum. For example, fibers from the L1 band insert into the mammillary processes of the L3, L4, and L5 vertebrae to the dorsal part of S1 and then to the posterior superior iliac spine. Biomechanical analyses, based on the multifidus muscle anatomy, show that it produces posterior sagittal rotation of the vertebra, which opposes a counter rotation generated by the abdominal muscles. The multifidus can further increase lumbar spine stability through a 'bowstring' mechanism in which the muscle, positioned posterior to the lumbar lordosis, produces compressive forces on the vertebrae interposed between its attachments.[12]

Erector Spinae Muscles

The erector spinae muscles are composed of the longissimus, iliocostalis, and spinalis (in the thoracic area).[11,13] In the lumbar spine, the longissimus is positioned medially and arises from the transverse and accessory processes and inserts caudally into the ventral surface of the posterior superior iliac spine. The laterally positioned iliocostalis arises from the tip of the transverse processes and the adjacent middle layer of thoracolumbar fascia and inserts into the ventral edge of the iliac crest caudally.[14] Unilateral contraction of the lumbar erector spinae laterally flexes the vertebral column; bilateral contraction produces extension and posterior rotation of the vertebrae in the sagittal plane. In addition to their role as the major extensor muscles of the trunk, the iliocostalis and the longissimus also exert large compressive loads and lateral and posterior shear forces at the L4 and L5 segments. Although these forces increase the stiffness and stability of the normal vertebral column, the shearing forces may also exacerbate instability and deformity in a malaligned spine.[15] In contrast to the multifidus muscle, microarchitectural studies reveal that these muscles are designed as long muscle fascicles with relatively small PCSA. This anatomic morphology suggests that they serve to move the trunk to extension, lateral bending, and rotation. With this type of design, they are less likely to act as primary stabilizers of the vertebral column.[16]

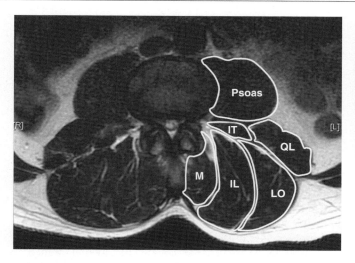

FIGURE 55–1 Magnetic resonance cross-sectional image through L4-5 disc space showing the multifidus (M), iliocostalis (IL), longissimus (LO), quadratus lumborum (QL), intertransversarii (IT), and psoas muscles.

Interspinales, Intertransversarii, and Short Rotator Muscles

The interspinales, intertransversarii, and short rotator muscles are short flat muscles that lie dorsal to the intertransverse ligament (see Fig. 55–1). The intertransversarii and interspinales run along the intertransverse and interspinous ligaments of each segment. The short rotators originate from the posterior-superior edge of the lower vertebra and attach to the lateral side of the upper vertebral lamina. Because of their small PCSA, they are unable to generate the forces necessary for movement or stability of the spinal column. More likely, they

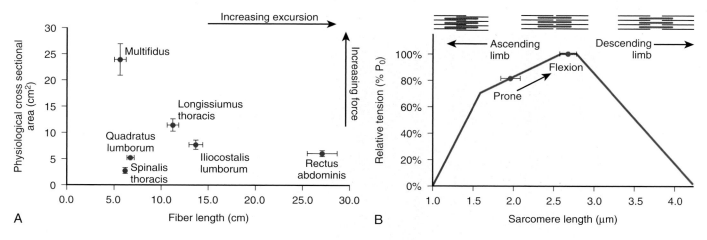

FIGURE 55–2 A, Scatter plot of physiologic cross-sectional area (PCSA) versus fiber length. Because PCSA is proportional to muscle force and fiber length is proportional to muscle excursion, this type of plot illustrates the functional design of a muscle. These data illustrate that the multifidus has the largest force-generating capacity in the lumbar spine and is designed for stability. **B,** Sarcomere length operating range of the multifidus plotted on the human skeletal muscle sarcomere length tension curve (*black line*). These data demonstrate that the multifidus muscle operates on the ascending limb of the length tension curve and becomes intrinsically stronger as the spine is flexed (*arrow*). Schematic sarcomeres are shown on the ascending and descending limb to scale on the basis of the quantification of actin and myosin filament lengths. (Reproduced with permission from Ward SR, Kim CW, Eng CM, et al: Architectural analysis and intraoperative measurements demonstrate the unique design of the multifidus muscle for lumbar spine stability. J Bone Joint Surg Am 91:176-185, 2009.)

act as proprioceptive sensors rather than force-generating structures.[17]

Innervation of the Posterior Paraspinal Muscles

The innervation of all of the posterior paraspinal muscles is derived from the dorsal rami. The iliocostalis is innervated by the lateral branch, while the lumbar fibers of the longissimus receive innervation from the intermediate branch.[18] The multifidus is innervated by the medial branch of the dorsal rami (Fig. 55–3). The medial branch curves around the root of the superior articular process and passes between the mammillary and accessory processes to the vertebral lamina, where it branches to supply the multifidus muscle, intertransversarii and interspinales muscles, and zygapophyseal joints.[19]

During its extramuscular course, the medial branch is strongly attached to the vertebral body in two locations. The first attachment is to the periosteum lateral to the zygapophyseal joints by fibers of the intertransverse ligament. The mamillo-accessory ligament provides the second attachment in the lumbar spine. This strong ligament covers the medial branch and is often calcified.[20] These attachments to the vertebra are of clinical importance because they expose the medial branch to possible damage during a midline posterior surgical approach.[21]

Direct damage to the nerve is also possible during insertion of pedicle screws.[22] Insertion of a pedicle screw in the area of the mammillary process can injure the medial branch arising from the cephalad level nerve root, causing denervation injury and consequent atrophy to the multifidus fascicles that arise from the adjacent cephalad level.[19,23] For instance, pedicle screws placed at L2 may damage the L1 nerve, which denervates the multifidus bands that originate at L1 and insert into the vertebrae caudally. Moreover, the mono-segmental innervation of the multifidus makes it particularly susceptible to

atrophy because it lacks a collateral nerve supply from adjacent muscle segments.[24] It is intriguing to consider that dysfunction of this muscle could contribute to adjacent level disc degeneration.

Fiber Type Characteristics of the Paraspinal Muscles

Fiber type analysis can provide important information about the use pattern of a muscle.[25,26] There are two major fiber types in skeletal muscles: type I, also known as "slow twitch" and type II or "fast twitch." The type I fibers possess low ATPase activity, prolonged twitch duration (hence slow twitch), and a low maximal velocity. In addition, type I fibers contain higher mitochondrial content and greater oxidative enzyme complements than type II fibers. Type II fibers are characterized by higher ATPase activities and correspondingly shorter isometric twitch durations. With this design, they are better suited to support the regeneration of ATP through anaerobic mechanisms. Type II fibers can be further subdivided into type IIa and IIx fibers. Type IIx fibers are generally more extreme in each of these respects than the type IIa.[26-28]

One of the most striking features of the lumbar paraspinal muscles is the predominance of type I muscle fibers compared with other skeletal muscles. Polgar and Johnson studied the distribution of fiber types in 36 human muscles.[29,30] A significantly larger type I–to–type II fiber ratio was observed in the multifidus, longissimus, and iliocostalis muscles compared with muscles of the extremities. The predominance of type I fibers and selective type II atrophy have been found in other studies that analyzed fiber type distribution and size in normal paraspinal muscles. It is presumed that along with the adaptation to their stabilizing tonic work characteristics, the phenomenon of type II atrophy can be explained by the sedentary modern life style that deprives these muscles of stimulation

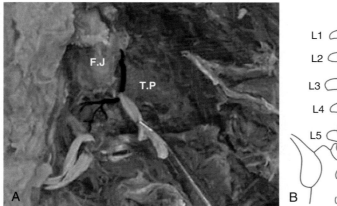
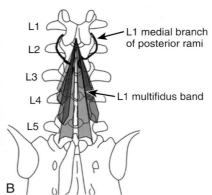

FIGURE 55–3 A, Anatomic specimen showing the spatial relationship of the medial branch of the posterior rami (MBPR) nerve (*highlighted in black and retracted with a rubber vessel loop*), the facet joint (FJ), and transverse process (TP). **B,** Diagram showing the path of the L1 medial branch of posterior rami nerve to the L1 multifidus muscle. The L1 MBPR traverses the L2 transverse process and rises posteriorly to innervate the multifidus muscle that originates from the L1 spinous process. The L1 multifidus then separates into four bands, which insert into the lamina and superior articular processes of the L3, L4, L5, and S1. (Reproduced with permission from Regev GJ, Kim CW, Thacker BE, et al: Regional myosin heavy chains distribution in selected paraspinal muscles. Spine [Phila PA 1976] in press.)

from exercise.[31] The relatively larger size of type II fibers in professional athletes further supports this assumption.[32,33]

The morphology of fiber type distribution between the different paraspinal muscles and in different areas inside the muscle is well known. Jorgensen and colleagues[34] reported a higher proportion of type I fibers in the longissimus than in the multifidus or iliocostalis muscles. Furthermore, the multifidus muscle is composed of a relatively high percentage of type I fibers, consistent with a postural function. The psoas muscle, on the other hand, is composed of a higher percentage of type II fibers such as in the appendicular muscles.[35] Mannion and colleagues[36] showed that in women the mean size of the type I fiber is significantly greater than that of either the type IIA or the type IIX, while men have relatively larger-sized type II fibers. In the older population, a loss of muscle mass leads to a decrease in both fiber type sizes with slightly more effect in type II fibers.[37-39] The most profound changes in fiber size and fiber type distribution occur in patients with degenerative conditions of the spine.[27] Compared with the control, the muscle of low back pain (LBP) patients had a significantly higher proportion of type IIx fiber than type I fibers. They proposed that the relatively low proportion of type I fibers in patients with LBP render them less resistant to fatigue and more susceptible to injury.

Paraspinal Muscle Injury

Characteristics of Paraspinal Muscles in the Postsurgical Spine

Spine surgery inherently causes damage to surrounding muscles.[40] This injury can be followed by atrophy of the muscles and subsequent loss of function. Among the different surgical approaches to the spine, it appears that injury to the muscle is greatest when using the midline posterior approach.[41] The multifidus muscle is most severely injured when using this approach. Muscle atrophy coincides with decreased muscle cross-sectional area (CSA), which in turn correlates with decreased force production capacity of the muscle.[40,42-50]

Muscle biopsies obtained from patients undergoing revision spinal surgery exhibit an array of pathologic features that include selective type II fiber atrophy, widespread fiber type grouping (a sign of reinnervation), and "moth-eaten" appearance of muscle fibers.[39] Although these pathologic changes can occasionally be found in biopsies from normal individuals, the pathologic changes are more prevalent after surgery.[51] Atrophy of the paraspinal muscles can readily be seen in postsurgical back patients.[47] Reductions in the CSA of the paraspinal muscles is greatest following a midline approach for a posterolateral fusion.[41,48,52]

Mechanism of Paraspinal Muscle Injury During Surgery

The factors responsible for muscle injury during surgery have been well studied in both animals and humans. Muscle damage can be caused by several different mechanisms. Direct injury

to the muscle is caused by dissection and stripping of tendinous attachments from the posterior elements of the spine. Additionally, extensive use of the electrocautery causes localized thermal injury and necrosis to the tissues. The most significant factor responsible for muscle injury is likely the use of forceful self-retaining retractors. Kawaguchi and colleagues[53-56] quantified the factors responsible for muscle necrosis following a standard open midline posterior approach. They proposed that injury is induced by a crush mechanism similar to that caused by a pneumatic tourniquet during surgery of the limbs. During the application of self-retaining retractors, elevated pressures lead to decreased intramuscular perfusion.[57-60] The severity of the muscle injury is closely correlated to the degree of the intramuscular pressure and the length of retraction time. A pressure-time parameter can be calculated by multiplying the intramuscular pressure and the length of time of the surgery. A high pressure-time product was shown to be tightly correlated to muscle necrosis. They concluded that muscle damage can be reduced by intermittent release of the retractors during prolonged surgery combined with a relatively longer incision that allows reduced retraction pressures.

Denervation is yet another mechanism that leads to muscle degeneration and atrophy following surgery. Muscle denervation can occur in a discrete location along the supplying nerve or be located in several points along the nerve and the neuromuscular junction. As previously described, nerve supply to the multifidus is especially vulnerable to injury because of its mono-segmental innervation pattern.[24] Muscle denervation is also possible through damage to the neuromuscular junction following long muscle retraction and necrosis. Shorter retraction time or an intermittent release of muscle retraction has been shown to significantly decrease degeneration and denervation of the muscles.[59] Gejo and colleagues examined the relationship between retraction time and postoperative damage to the paraspinal muscle, by measuring postoperation signal intensity of the multifidus muscle, using T2-weighted magnetic resonance imaging (MRI).[61] Long retraction time during surgery correlated with high-signal intensity in the multifidus muscle even at 6 months postsurgery. They proposed that these findings reflect chronic denervation of the muscle caused by damage to the neuromuscular synapses.

Correlation of Muscle Injury with Clinical Outcomes

There appears to be a correlation between muscle damage and long-term postoperative pain. Shivonen and colleagues[62] found signs of severe denervation of the multifidus muscle in patients with failed back syndrome. Muscle biopsies showed signs of advanced chronic denervation consisting of group atrophy, marked fibrosis, and fatty infiltration. Moreover, fiber type grouping, a histologic sign of reinnervation, was rare. They hypothesized that the denervation injury resulted from direct damage to the medial branch of the posterior rami during muscle retraction associated with the posterior midline approach. The lack of reinnervation was thought to result from the absence of intersegmental nerve supply to the multifidus. Signs of severe denervation of the paraspinal muscles correlate with poor outcome of postsurgical patients. They also showed that poor clinical outcomes are associated with abnormal EMG patterns 2 to 5 years postsurgery. Although a correlation between the degree of muscle atrophy following surgery and the incidence of failed back syndrome was found, it is not clear what specific pathogenic factors are responsible.

Preservation of Muscle Function and Integrity

Minimally invasive spine surgery techniques strive to minimize muscle injury during surgery. By decreasing/minimizing the use of self-retaining retractors, intramuscular retraction pressure is reduced and thereby leads to less crush injury. Furthermore, focusing the surgical corridor directly over the surgical target site allows for less muscle stripping that may otherwise disrupt its tendinous attachments or damage their neurovascular supply. Kim and colleagues[63] compared trunk muscle strength between patients treated with open posterior instrumentation versus percutaneous instrumentation. Tests were performed isometrically at multiple flexion positions. Patients undergoing percutaneous instrumentation displayed more than 50% improvement in extension strength, while patients undergoing traditional midline open surgery had no significant improvement in lumbar extension strength. Extension strength correlated with preservation of multifidus CSA as measured on MRI. In a similar study, Stevens and colleagues[64] assessed the postsurgical appearance of the multifidus muscle using a high-definition MRI sequence. In patients treated via an open posterior transforaminal lumbar interbody fusion (TLIF) technique, marked intermuscular and intramuscular edema was observed on postsurgical MRI at 6 months. In contrast, patients in the MIS TLIF group had a normal appearance on MRI postsurgery.

Hyun and colleagues[46] retrospectively assessed a group of patients that underwent unilateral TLIF with ipsilateral instrumented posterior spinal fusion via an open technique. Contralateral instrumented posterior spinal fusion was performed at the same level employing a paramedian, intermuscular (Wiltse), minimally invasive approach. Postoperatively, there was a significant decrease in the CSA of the multifidus on the side of the open approach while no reduction in the multifidus CSA on the contralateral side was observed.

Decreases in tissue trauma have local effects but also alter overall systemic physiology. Kim and colleagues[65] studied circulating markers of tissue injury in patients undergoing open versus MIS fusions. Markers of skeletal muscle injury (creatinine kinase, aldolase); proinflammatory cytokines (IL-6, IL-8); and anti-inflammatory cytokines (IL-10, IL-1 receptor antagonist) were analyzed with ELISA techniques. Two to sevenfold increases in all markers were observed in the open surgery group. The greatest difference between the groups occurred on the first postoperative day. Most markers returned to baseline in 3 days for the MIS group, whereas the open-surgery group required 7 days. IL-6 and IL-8 are known

cytokines that participate in various systemic inflammatory reactions.[66,67] It is possible that such elevations in inflammatory cytokines have direct effects beyond the surgical site. As such, persistently elevated levels of proinflammatory cytokines have been associated with organ failure in postsurgical patients.[68]

Preservation of the Bone-Ligament Complex

It is well accepted that excessive facet resection leads to altered motion and spinal instability.[69-72] Furthermore, a laminectomy leads to loss of the midline supraspinous/interspinous ligament complex, which can contribute to flexion instability.[73,74] In cases where significant bony resection is required, or when there is an underlying relative instability (such as in spondylolisthesis), concomitant fusion is often recommended following a decompressive laminectomy.[73-76] Efforts to limit such potentially destabilizing surgery have been pursued via unilateral laminotomies in which the spinous processes and corresponding tendinous attachments of the multifidus muscle and the supraspinous/interspinous ligaments are preserved (Fig. 55–4). When this technique is combined with minimally invasive tubular retractors, bilateral decompression for stenosis can be achieved with good clinical results.[77,78] The long-term outcome of such MIS procedures and their effect on spinal stability have yet to be shown clinically. However, biomechanical studies suggest that such MIS techniques have significant effects on spinal stability.

Finite element analyses have been used to assess the consequences of various lumbar decompressive procedures on spinal motion. Fessler and colleagues[79] compared three decompressive techniques to treat two-level spinal stenosis: open laminectomies versus interlaminar midline decompression (which retains the spinous process but sacrifices the interspinous/supraspinous ligaments) versus MIS unilateral laminotomies (Fig. 55–5). These studies show that open laminectomy produces marked increases in flexion, extension, and axial rotation. For flexion-extension, there is a greater than twofold increase in motion, which leads to increased stress on the annulus. No changes in flexion were noted when the interlaminar or MIS models were studied. Axial rotation increased by 2.5-fold in the open and interlaminar groups but only 1.3-fold in the MIS group. These findings lend further support to the concept that MIS techniques have relevant effects on spinal motion and stability.

Summary

Preservation of normal spinal motion and stability constitutes the best means for ensuring improved long-term outcomes following the surgical treatment of spinal disorders. In the living organism, stability and motion are controlled by active and passive means. The lumbar spine is surrounded by powerful muscles that actively control movement and confer dynamic stability. Concurrently, the ligaments, bones,

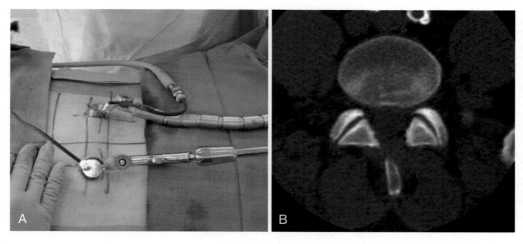

FIGURE 55–4 A, An intraoperative photograph showing minimally invasive decompression procedure for the treatment of L4-5 spinal stenosis. The strategy is to use a bilateral paramedian approach that spares the tendinous attachment of the multifidus muscle at the spinous. **B,** Postoperative computed tomography scan demonstrating good decompression of the spinal canal without noticeable damage to the posterior paraspinal muscles. Decompression of the left lateral recess via the right paramedian approach (and vice versa) allows minimal facet resection during decompression of the lateral recess.

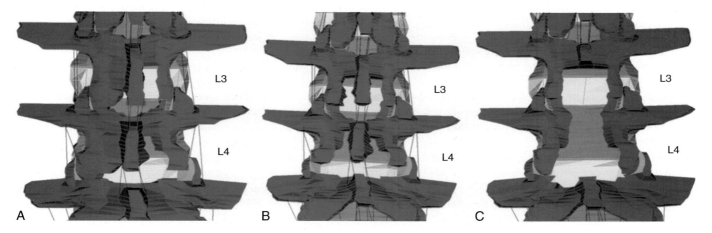

FIGURE 55–5 Posterior view illustrating three different decompression methods tested by finite element analysis: **A,** Minimally invasive spine unilateral laminotomies; **B,** midline interlaminar decompression, which retains the spinous process but sacrifices the interspinous/supraspinous ligaments; and **C,** midline open laminectomies with resection of spinous processes. (Reproduced with permission from Bresnahan L, Ogden AT, Natarajan RN, et al: A biomechanical evaluation of graded posterior element removal for treatment of lumbar stenosis: comparison of a minimally invasive approach with two standard laminectomy techniques. Spine [Phila Pa 1976] 2009;34:17-23.)

cartilage, and discs provide for passive stability. Emerging minimally invasive spine surgery techniques seek to minimize surgical damage and thereby preserve normal function. The rationale of this approach relies on limiting the surgical corridor to the minimum necessary to safely expose the surgical target site. This minimizes the destruction of anatomic structures necessary for normal function, namely the relevant osseo-ligamentous, neuro-vascular, and musculo-tendinous anatomy. In addition, the traditional use of larger self-retaining retractors, which can induce crush injuries to adjacent tissues, has been supplanted by table-mounted, tubular-type retractors that minimize pressure on muscles, vessels, and nerves. Continued development of minimally invasive techniques remains a vital effort in the advancement of spinal surgery.

KEY REFERENCES

1. Gejo R, Matsui H, Kawaguchi Y, et al: Serial changes in trunk muscle performance after posterior lumbar surgery. Spine (Phila Pa 1976) 24:1023-1028, 1999.
   In this clinical study of patients undergoing posterior lumbar surgery, back muscle injury was directly related to muscle retraction time.

2. Kim DY, Lee SH, Chung SK, Lee HY: Comparison of multifidus muscle atrophy and trunk extension muscle strength: percutaneous versus open pedicle screw fixation. Spine (Phila Pa 1976) 30:123-129, 2005.
   The use of percutaneous pedicle screw insertion techniques, compared with traditional midline open approaches, leads to

less muscle injury and allows for greater recovery of muscle function.

3. Kim KT, Lee SH, Suk KS, Bae SC: The quantitative analysis of tissue injury markers after mini-open lumbar fusion. Spine (Phila Pa 1976) 31:712-716, 2006.
   In patients undergoing posterior lumbar surgery, the use of minimally invasive techniques leads to lower levels of proinflammatory cytokines detected in the bloodstream.

4. MacIntosh JE, Bogduk N: The morphology of the lumbar erector spinae. Spine 12:658-668, 1987.
   This classic study has formed the basis of our general understanding of the posterior lumbar muscle anatomy.

5. Ward SR, Kim CW, Eng CM, et al: Architectural analysis and intraoperative measurements demonstrate the unique design of the multifidus muscle for lumbar spine stability. J Bone Joint Surg Am 91:176-185, 2009.
   This study shows the multifidus is designed to exert high forces over short distances, suggesting it plays a key role in spinal stability.

REFERENCES

1. Brown SH, McGill SM: Muscle force-stiffness characteristics influence joint stability: a spine example. Clin Biomech (Bristol, Avon) 20:917-922, 2005.

2. Brown SH, Potvin JR: Constraining spine stability levels in an optimization model leads to the prediction of trunk muscle co-contraction and improved spine compression force estimates. J Biomech 38:745-754, 2005.

3. Cholewicki J, Panjabi MM, Khachatryan A: Stabilizing function of trunk flexor-extensor muscles around a neutral spine posture. Spine (Phila Pa 1976) 22:2207-2212, 1997.

4. Panjabi MM: The stabilizing system of the spine. Part II. Neutral zone and instability hypothesis. J Spinal Disord 5:390-396, 1992; discussion 7.

5. Panjabi MM: The stabilizing system of the spine. Part I. Function, dysfunction, adaptation, and enhancement. J Spinal Disord 5:383-389, 1992; discussion 97.

6. Panjabi MM, White AA 3rd: Basic biomechanics of the spine. Neurosurgery 7:76-93, 1980.

7. McGill SM: Electromyographic activity of the abdominal and low back musculature during the generation of isometric and dynamic axial trunk torque: implications for lumbar mechanics. J Orthop Res 9:91-103, 1991.

8. Cholewicki J, McGill SM, Norman RW: Lumbar spine loads during the lifting of extremely heavy weights. Med Sci Sports Exerc 23:1179-1186, 1991.

9. Ward SR, Kim CW, Eng CM, et al: Architectural analysis and intraoperative measurements demonstrate the unique design of the multifidus muscle for lumbar spine stability. J Bone Joint Surg Am 91:176-185, 2009.

10. Donisch EW, Basmajian JV: Electromyography of deep back muscles in man. Am J Anat 133:25-36, 1972.

11. MacIntosh JE, Bogduk N: The morphology of the lumbar erector spinae. Spine 12:658-668, 1987.

12. Bogduk N, Macintosh JE, Pearcy MJ: A universal model of the lumbar back muscles in the upright position. Spine (Phila Pa 1976) 17:897-913, 1992.

13. Macintosh JE, Bogduk N: The attachments of the lumbar erector spinae. Spine (Phila Pa 1976) 16:783-792, 1991.

14. Bustami FM: A new description of the lumbar erector spinae muscle in man. J Anat 144:81-91, 1986.

15. Bogduk N: A reappraisal of the anatomy of the human lumbar erector spinae. J Anat 131:525-540, 1980.

16. Delp SL, Suryanarayanan S, Murray WM, et al: Architecture of the rectus abdominis, quadratus lumborum, and erector spinae. J Biomech 34:371-375, 2001.

17. Bogduk N: Proceedings: The posterior lumbar muscles and nerves of the cat. J Anat 116:476-477, 1973.

18. Bogduk N: The innervation of the lumbar spine. Spine (Phila Pa 1976) 8:286-293, 1983.

19. Bogduk N, Long DM: The anatomy of the so-called "articular nerves" and their relationship to facet denervation in the treatment of low-back pain. J Neurosurg 51:172-177, 1979.

20. Bogduk N: The lumbar mamillo—accessory ligament. Its anatomical and neurosurgical significance. Spine (Phila Pa 1976) 6:162-167, 1981.

21. Boelderl A, Daniaux H, Kathrein A, Maurer H: Danger of damaging the medial branches of the posterior rami of spinal nerves during a dorsomedian approach to the spine. Clin Anat 15:77-81, 2002.

22. Regev GJ, Lee YP, Taylor WR, et al: Nerve injury to the posterior rami medial branch during the insertion of pedicle screws: comparison of mini-open versus percutaneous pedicle screw insertion techniques. Spine (Phila Pa 1976) 34:1239-1242, 2009.

23. Dreyfuss P, Stout A, Aprill C, et al: The significance of multifidus atrophy after successful radiofrequency neurotomy for low back pain. PM R 1:719-722, 2009.

24. Macintosh JE, Bogduk N: 1987 Volvo award in basic science. The morphology of the lumbar erector spinae. Spine (Phila Pa 1976) 12:658-668, 1987.

25. Pette D: The Dynamic State of Muscle Fiberse. Berlin: Walter de Gruyter & Company, 1990.

26. Edgerton VR, Roy RR: Regulation of skeletal muscle fiber size, shape and function. Journal of Biomechanics 21:123-133, 1991.

27. Mannion AF, Kaser L, Weber E, et al: Influence of age and duration of symptoms on fiber type distribution and size of the back muscles in chronic low back pain patients. Eur Spine J 9:273-281, 2000.

28. Mannion AF: Fiber type characteristics and function of the human paraspinal muscles: normal values and changes in association with low back pain. J Electromyogr Kinesiol 9:363-377, 1999.

29. Polgar J, Johnson MA, Weightman D, Appleton D: Data on fiber size in thirty-six human muscles. An autopsy study. J Neurol Sci 19:307-318, 1973.

30. Johnson MA, Polgar J, Weightman D, Appleton D: Data on the distribution of fiber types in thirty-six human muscles. An autopsy study. J Neurol Sci 18:111-129, 1973.

31. Crossman K, Mahon M, Watson PJ, et al: Chronic low back pain-associated paraspinal muscle dysfunction is not the result of a constitutionally determined "adverse" fiber-type composition. Spine (Phila Pa 1976) 29:628-634, 2004.

32. Puustjarvi K, Tammi M, Reinikainen M, et al: Running training alters fiber type composition in spinal muscles. Eur Spine J 3:17-21, 1994.

33. Short KR, Vittone JL, Bigelow ML, et al: Changes in myosin heavy chain mRNA and protein expression in human skeletal muscle with age and endurance exercise training. J Appl Physiol 99:95-102, 2005.

34. Jorgensen K, Nicholaisen T, Kato M: Muscle fiber distribution, capillary density, and enzymatic activities in the lumbar paravertebral muscles of young men. Significance for isometric endurance. Spine (Phila Pa 1976) 18:1439-1450, 1993.

35. Regev GJ, Kim CW, Thacker BE, et al: Regional myosin heavy chains distribution in selected paraspinal muscles. Spine (Phila Pa 1976) in press.

36. Mannion AF, Weber BR, Dvorak J, et al: Fiber type characteristics of the lumbar paraspinal muscles in normal healthy subjects and in patients with low back pain. J Orthop Res 15:881-887, 1997.

37. Rantanten J, Rissanen A, Kalimo H: Lumbar muscle fiber size and type distribution in normal subjects. European Spine Journal 3:331-335, 1994.

38. Zhu XZ, Parnianpour M, Nordin M, Kahanovitz N: Histochemistry and morphology of erector spinae muscle in lumbar disc herniation. Spine (Phila Pa 1976) 14:391-397, 1989.

39. Mattila M, Hurme M, Alaranta H, et al: The multifidus muscle in patients with lumbar disc herniation. A histochemical and morphometric analysis of intraoperative biopsies. Spine (Phila Pa 1976) 11:732-738, 1986.

40. Gejo R, Matsui H, Kawaguchi Y, et al: Serial changes in trunk muscle performance after posterior lumbar surgery. Spine (Phila Pa 1976) 24:1023-1028, 1999.

41. Gille O, Jolivet E, Dousset V, et al: Erector spinae muscle changes on magnetic resonance imaging following lumbar surgery through a posterior approach. Spine (Phila Pa 1976) 32:1236-1241, 2007.

42. Datta G, Gnanalingham KK, Peterson D, et al: Back pain and disability after lumbar laminectomy: is there a relationship to muscle retraction? Neurosurgery 54:1413-1420, 2004; discussion 20.

43. Franzini A, Ferroli P, Marras C, Broggi G: Huge epidural hematoma after surgery for spinal cord stimulation. Acta Neurochir (Wien) 147:565-567, 2005; discussion 7.

44. Granata C, Cervellati S, Ballestrazzi A, et al: Spine surgery in spinal muscular atrophy: long-term results. Neuromuscul Disord 3:207-215, 1993.

45. Hutchinson D, Kozin SH, Mayer N, et al: Dynamic electromyographic evaluation of adolescents with traumatic cervical injury after biceps to triceps transfer: the role of phasic contraction. J Hand Surg Am 33:1331-1336, 2008.

46. Hyun SJ, Kim YB, Kim YS, et al: Postoperative changes in paraspinal muscle volume: comparison between paramedian interfascial and midline approaches for lumbar fusion. J Korean Med Sci 22:646-651, 2007.

47. Mayer TG, Vanharanta H, Gatchel RJ, et al: Comparison of CT scan muscle measurements and isokinetic trunk strength in postoperative patients. Spine (Phila Pa 1976) 14:33-36, 1989.

48. Motosuneya T, Asazuma T, Tsuji T, et al: Postoperative change of the cross-sectional area of back musculature after 5 surgical procedures as assessed by magnetic resonance imaging. J Spinal Disord Tech 19:318-322, 2006.

49. Rantanen J, Hurme M, Falck B, et al: The lumbar multifidus muscle five years after surgery for a lumbar intervertebral disc herniation. Spine (Phila Pa 1976) 18:568-574, 1993.

50. Kawaguchi Y, Matsui H, Gejo R, Tsuji H: Preventive measures of back muscle injury after posterior lumbar spine surgery in rats. Spine (Phila Pa 1976) 23:2282-2287, 1998; discussion 8.

51. Weber BR, Grob D, Dvorak J, Muntener M: Posterior surgical approach to the lumbar spine and its effect on the multifidus muscle. Spine (Phila Pa 1976) 22:1765-1772, 1997.

52. Suwa H, Hanakita J, Ohshita N, et al: Postoperative changes in paraspinal muscle thickness after various lumbar back surgery procedures. Neurol Med Chir (Tokyo) 40:151-154, 2000; discussion 4-5.

53. Kawaguchi Y, Matsui H, Tsuji H: Back muscle injury after posterior lumbar spine surgery. Part 2: Histologic and histochemical analyses in humans. Spine (Phila Pa 1976) 19:2598-2602, 1994.

54. Kawaguchi Y, Matsui H, Tsuji H: Back muscle injury after posterior lumbar spine surgery. Part 1: Histologic and histochemical analyses in rats. Spine (Phila Pa 1976) 19:2590-2597, 1994.

55. Kawaguchi Y, Matsui H, Tsuji H: Back muscle injury after posterior lumbar spine surgery. A histologic and enzymatic analysis. Spine (Phila Pa 1976) 21:941-944, 1996.

56. Kawaguchi Y, Yabuki S, Styf J, et al: Back muscle injury after posterior lumbar spine surgery. Topographic evaluation of intramuscular pressure and blood flow in the porcine back muscle during surgery. Spine (Phila Pa 1976) 21:2683-2688, 1996.

57. Styf J: Pressure in the erector spinae muscle during exercise. Spine (Phila Pa 1976) 12:675-679, 1987.

58. Styf J, Lysell E: Chronic compartment syndrome in the erector spinae muscle. Spine (Phila Pa 1976) 12:680-682, 1987.

59. Styf JR, Willen J: The effects of external compression by three different retractors on pressure in the erector spine muscles during and after posterior lumbar spine surgery in humans. Spine (Phila Pa 1976) 23:354-358, 1998.

60. Taylor H, McGregor AH, Medhi-Zadeh S, et al: The impact of self-retaining retractors on the paraspinal muscles during posterior spinal surgery. Spine (Phila Pa 1976) 27:2758-2762, 2002.

61. Gejo R, Kawaguchi Y, Kondoh T, et al: Magnetic resonance imaging and histologic evidence of postoperative back muscle injury in rats. Spine (Phila Pa 1976) 25:941-946, 2000.

62. Sihvonen T, Herno A, Paljarvi L, et al: Local denervation atrophy of paraspinal muscles in postoperative failed back syndrome. Spine (Phila Pa 1976) 18:575-581, 1993.

63. Kim DY, Lee SH, Chung SK, Lee HY: Comparison of multifidus muscle atrophy and trunk extension muscle strength: percutaneous versus open pedicle screw fixation. Spine (Phila Pa 1976) 30:123-129, 2005.

64. Stevens KJ, Spenciner DB, Griffiths KL, et al: Comparison of minimally invasive and conventional open posterolateral lumbar fusion using magnetic resonance imaging and retraction pressure studies. J Spinal Disord Tech 19:77-86, 2006.

65. Kim KT, Lee SH, Suk KS, Bae SC: The quantitative analysis of tissue injury markers after mini-open lumbar fusion. Spine (Phila Pa 1976) 31:712-716, 2006.

66. Igonin AA, Armstrong VW, Shipkova M, et al: Circulating cytokines as markers of systemic inflammatory response in severe

community-acquired pneumonia. Clin Biochem 37:204-209, 2004.

67. Baggiolini M, Dahinden CA: CC chemokines in allergic inflammation. Immunol Today 15:127-133, 1994.

68. Ogawa M: Acute pancreatitis and cytokines: "second attack" by septic complication leads to organ failure. Pancreas 16:312-315, 1998.

69. Zander T, Rohlmann A, Klockner C, Bergmann G: Influence of graded facetectomy and laminectomy on spinal biomechanics. Eur Spine J 12:427-434, 2003.

70. Natarajan RN, Andersson GB, Patwardhan AG, Andriacchi TP: Study on effect of graded facetectomy on change in lumbar motion segment torsional flexibility using three-dimensional continuum contact representation for facet joints. J Biomech Eng 121:215-221, 1999.

71. Lee KK, Teo EC, Qiu TX, Yang K: Effect of facetectomy on lumbar spinal stability under sagittal plane loadings. Spine (Phila Pa 1976) 29:1624-1631, 2004.

72. Abumi K, Panjabi MM, Kramer KM, et al: Biomechanical evaluation of lumbar spinal stability after graded facetectomies. Spine (Phila Pa 1976) 15:1142-1147, 1990.

73. Tuite GF, Doran SE, Stern JD, et al: Outcome after laminectomy for lumbar spinal stenosis. Part II: Radiographic changes and clinical correlations. J Neurosurg 81:707-715, 1994.

74. Tuite GF, Stern JD, Doran SE, et al: Outcome after laminectomy for lumbar spinal stenosis. Part I: Clinical correlations. J Neurosurg 81:699-706, 1994.

75. Fischgrund JS, Mackay M, Herkowitz HN, et al: 1997 Volvo Award winner in clinical studies. Degenerative lumbar spondylolisthesis with spinal stenosis: a prospective, randomized study comparing decompressive laminectomy and arthrodesis with and without spinal instrumentation. Spine (Phila Pa 1976) 22:2807-2812, 1997.

76. Herkowitz HN, Kurz LT: Degenerative lumbar spondylolisthesis with spinal stenosis. A prospective study comparing decompression with decompression and intertransverse process arthrodesis. J Bone Joint Surg Am 73:802-808, 1991.

77. Palmer S, Turner R, Palmer R: Bilateral decompression of lumbar spinal stenosis involving a unilateral approach with microscope and tubular retractor system. J Neurosurg 97:213-217, 2002.

78. Guiot BH, Khoo LT, Fessler RG: A minimally invasive technique for decompression of the lumbar spine. Spine (Phila Pa 1976) 27:432-438, 2002.

79. Bresnahan L, Ogden AT, Natarajan RN, Fessler RG: A biomechanical evaluation of graded posterior element removal for treatment of lumbar stenosis: comparison of a minimally invasive approach with two standard laminectomy techniques. Spine (Phila Pa 1976) 34:17-23, 2009.

56

Minimally Invasive Posterior Approaches to the Spine

Choll W. Kim, MD, PhD
James D. Schwender, MD
Kevin Foley, MD

The term *minimally invasive spine* (MIS) *surgery* describes a variety of surgical techniques that employ key concepts in spinal surgery. The guiding principles of MIS are to (1) decrease muscle crush injuries during retraction, (2) avoid injury of osseo-tendinous attachments important for spinal stability, (3) maintain the integrity of the dorsolumbar fascia, (4) limit bony resection, (5) avoid injury to neurovascular supply of muscle compartments by using known anatomic planes, and (6) decrease the size of the surgical corridor to coincide with the area of the surgical target site. These principles can be used in a variety of settings. In the lumbar spine, the most significant application of these principles has been for posterior approaches to the lumbar spine.

Surgical Anatomy of the Posterior Paraspinal Muscles

The posterior lumbar paraspinal muscles are responsible for maintaining spinal posture in its neutral position. Furthermore, the paraspinal muscles guard the spine from excessive bending that would otherwise endanger the integrity of the intervertebral discs, facet joints, and ligaments.[1] It is the body's dynamic stabilizing system that prevents pain and injury to spinal column due to the repetitive loads during the course of daily activities. The posterior paraspinal muscles are composed of several muscle groups that run along the thoracolumbar spine and attach caudally to the sacrum, sacroiliac joint, and iliac wing.

Posterior spine surgery using midline approaches inherently causes damage to surrounding muscles.[2,3] Muscle injury leads to long-term muscle atrophy, which in turn leads to decreased force production capacity of the muscle.[2,4-12] The multifidus muscle is most severely injured when using this approach for several reasons. First, its medial location inherently requires it be displaced most during retraction. This predisposes the muscle to greater retraction pressures and makes it more vulnerable to disruption of its neurovascular supply.[2,7] Of equal importance, the midline posterior approach inevitably leads to disruption of the multifidus tendon attachment to the spinous process, as well as the integrity of the dorsolumbar fascia.

Key Concepts for Minimally Invasive Spine Retraction Systems

A key advancement in minimally invasive surgery came from Foley and colleagues[13] with the development of the tubular retractor. A cylindrical retractor allows the surgical corridor to be opened via serial dilation using sequentially larger concentric tubes. This decreases the need for muscle stripping during the exposure. Furthermore, a tubular retractor maximizes the surface contact area, which in turn minimizes the pressure per unit area. Another key concept in MIS is use of a retractor holder mounted to the table instead of using a "self-retaining" mechanism. In a self-retaining retractor system, constant pressure on the tissues must be exerted to hold the retractor in place. Studies show that the maximum intermuscular pressure around a tubular retractor decreases by 50% within 3 seconds.[14] Thereafter, the pressure is undetectable. With self-retaining retractors, the pressure remains unchanged.

Minimally Invasive Spine Surgical Corridor

The guiding principle of MIS posterior lumbar surgery is to avoid injury to the multifidus tendon attachment to the spinous process and maintenance of the dorsolumbar fascia integrity. This is accomplished by using paramedian approaches rather than midline approaches. Decompression, microdiscectomy, interbody fusion, posterolateral fusion, and pedicle screw instrumentation can be accomplished through this surgical corridor. Emerging techniques for advanced reconstruction including posterior corpectomies and strut fusion for burst fractures, tumors, and infections are also possible.

Posterior Lumbar Approaches

Tubular Microdiscectomy

The treatment of herniated discs via MIS tubular microdiscectomy is the most common technique currently used in the United States. This system, developed by Foley and Smith, consists of a series of concentric dilators and thin-walled tubular retractors of variable length. The use of the tubular retractor, rather than blades, allows the retractor itself to be thin walled (0.9 mm). The tube circumferentially defines a surgical corridor through the erector spinae muscles. The appropriate depth of retractor prevents the muscle from intruding into the field of view. The retractor allows for the appropriately sized working channel to permit spinal decompression. The typical retractor size is 14 to 18 mm for microdiscectomy (Fig. 56–1). Surgery is typically performed using an operating microscope. Several randomized controlled trials have been performed to compare traditional open microdiscectomy with minimally invasive tubular microdiscectomy.[15-17]

These studies all show that tubular microdiscectomy is safe and efficacious compared with well-established traditional techniques. Clinically significant superiority was not shown, likely reflecting the difficulty is demonstrating differences between the two already successful procedures.

Lumbar Decompression

An important goal of minimally invasive posterior surgery is maintaining the tendinous attachment of the multifidus to the spinous process. During a traditional laminectomy, the spinous process is removed and the multifidus muscle is retracted laterally. Upon wound closure, the multifidus origin can no longer be repaired to the spinous process. The midline approach affords a symmetric view of the posterior elements, which allows for safe resection of the lamina, ligamentum flavum, and medial facets. The symmetric view allows the surgeon to readily identify and orient the surgical corridor. However, a thorough decompression can be achieved without need for removal of the spinous process. In a technique

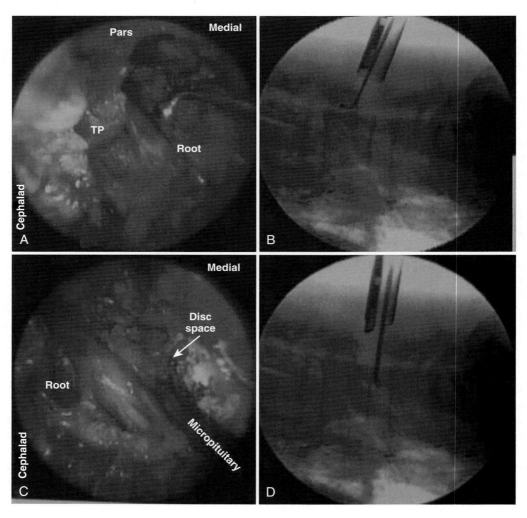

FIGURE 56–1 Intraoperative photographs and fluoroscopic images of the tubular microdiscectomy technique. **A,** Intraoperative photograph and **B,** corresponding to the lateral fluoroscopic image of the surgical target site showing the lateral pars and infero-medial transverse process after removal with a fine Kerrison rongeur. This maneuver allows for palpation of the pedicle and assists identification of the exiting nerve root, adjacent to the ball-tip probe.

originally described by McCulloch and colleagues,[18] the spinal canal can be approached through a unilateral portal via a hemilaminectomy technique. Decompression of the central canal and contralateral recess can be achieved by angling the tubular retractor dorsally to view the undersurface of the spinous process and contralateral lamina (Fig. 56–2). The

dural tube can be gently pushed down, and the ligamentum flavum and contralateral superior articular process resected to achieve a bilateral decompression.

The efficacy and safety of minimally invasive posterior lumbar decompression have been assessed in multiple studies.[18-24] In a review by Asgarzadie and Khoo,[25] this

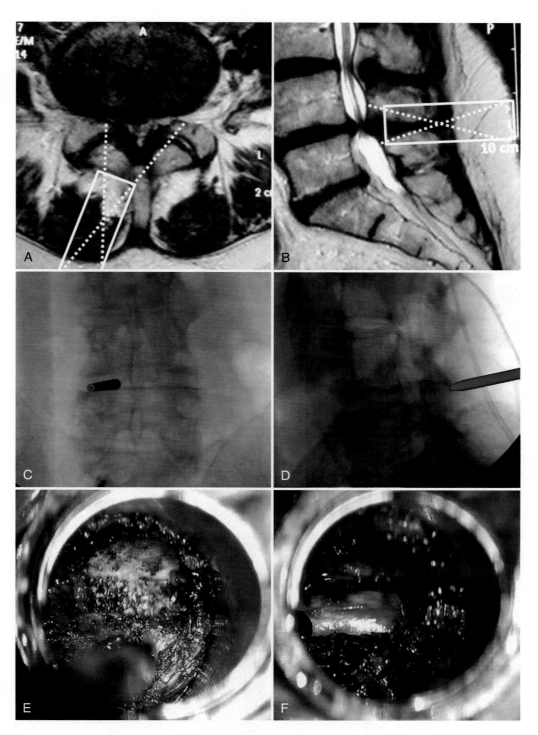

FIGURE 56–2 Magnetic resonance axial (**A**) and sagittal (**B**) image in a patient with spinal stenosis. Intraoperative fluoroscopic navigation AP (**C**) and lateral (**D**) images showing insertion of the initial dilator. The surgical corridor is overlaid with the tubular retractor in solid white and surgical target sites in dashed lines. Intraoperative photomicrograph of the surgical target site. **E,** Initial bony exposure of the base of the spinous process and facet joint line. Top is medial. **F,** Visualization of the dural tube to the contralateral side using a unilateral approach.

technique provides long-term symptomatic relief equivalent to traditional open surgery but with significant reductions in operative blood loss, postoperative pain, hospital stay, and narcotic usage. The effect of the MIS learning curve remains a significant concern as increased complication rates are seen during the initial series of patients.[26] Despite the learning curve, the overall complication rates remain low, even in patients who are elderly or medically frail.[27-29]

It is important to consider the anatomic variation of the lower lumbar spine with the upper lumbar spine with this particular technique. At L3 and above, the lamina between the spinous process and facet joint can be narrow (Fig. 56–3).

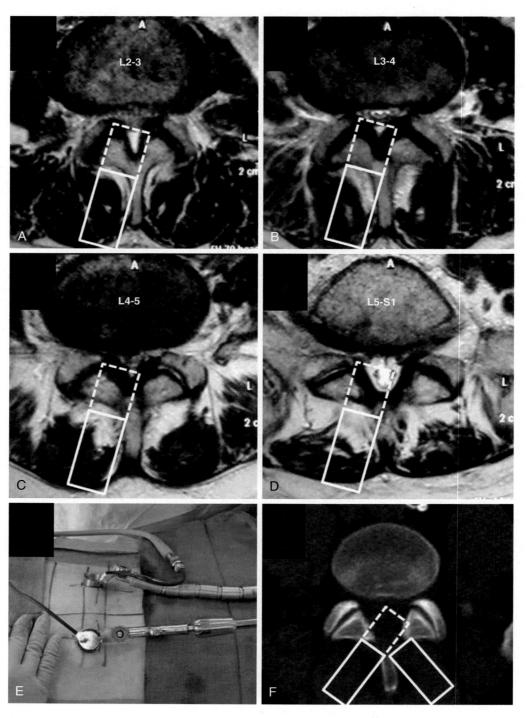

FIGURE 56–3 Magnetic resonance cross-sectional image through disc space of **A,** L2-3, **B,** L3-4, **C,** L4-5, and **D,** L5-S1. The outline of the tubular retractor is overlaid on each image. Note the proximity of the ipsilateral facet joint at the higher lumbar levels. At L3-4 and above, care must be exercised to avoid inadvertent injury to the ipsilateral facet joint. A bilateral approach can be used (**E**) to decompress the lateral recess from the contralateral sides (**F**).

With a unilateral approach, it may be difficult to reach the ipsilateral recess without excessively removing the ipsilateral inferior articular process. An option is to use a bilateral crossover technique to reach the right lateral recess from a left-sided hemilaminectomy and vice versa. Anatomically, the lateral recess is more accessible through a contralateral approach when using the unilateral approach. In a preliminary study of four patients and seven levels of decompression, the total operating time was 32 minutes per level and the estimated blood loss was 75 mL. The average postoperative stay was 1.2 days. All patients had resolution of neurogenic claudication and there were no complications.[30]

Posterior Lumbar Interbody Fusion

An extension of the minimally invasive hemilaminectomy technique is transforaminal lumbar interbody fusion (MIS TLIF). The unilateral approach is used to perform the analogous decompression and is combined with a complete facetectomy. The surgical corridor is in the neurovascular plane between the multifidus and longissimus muscles (Fig. 56–4). A complete facetectomy allows for decompression of the spinal canal from the ipsilateral to the contralateral side (Fig. 56–5). Access to the disc space is through a window bordered medially by the dural tube, proximally by the exiting nerve root, and distally by the pedicle and superior endplate of the caudad vertebra, thus forming within the Kambin triangle (Fig. 56–6). Angled curettes are used to perform a subtotal discectomy from a unilateral approach. If necessary, an osteotome is used to remove the overhanging rim of the posterior vertebral endplate during discectomy. Fusion is performed using interbody spacers that can be placed anteriorly for maximum lordosis correction. A second cage may be inserted by using the smooth trials to push the first cages to the far side of the disc space. Dual cage constructs may be desirable when there is significant osteoporosis or at L5-S1 in a multilevel fusion.

The clinical safety and efficacy of this technique has been well established. Schwender and colleagues[31] reported on 49 patients who underwent MIS TLIF through a paramedian, muscle-sparing approach using an expandable tubular retractor system. Of these patients, 26 patients had degenerative disc disease (DDD) with herniated nucleus pulposus (HNP), 22 had spondylolisthesis, and 1 had a Chance-type fracture as their primary diagnosis. The minimum follow-up was 18 months with a mean follow-up of 22.6 months. Operative time averaged 240 minutes (110 to 310 minutes), and average estimated blood loss (EBL) was 140 mL (50 to 450 mL). No patients required a blood transfusion, and there were no intraoperative complications. Length of hospital stay was 1.9 days on average (1 to 4 days). All 45 patients who had preoperative radicular symptoms had resolution of their symptoms. All patients with mechanical low back pain (LBP) had postoperative improvement of their pain. Four complications were noted postoperatively (two from malpositioned screws, one from graft dislodgement causing new radiculopathy, and the last from radiculopathy caused by contralateral neuroforaminal stenosis). Visual Analog Scale pain scores improved from

7.2 to 2.1, and Oswestry Disability Index scores improved from 46% to 14% at last follow-up.

Numerous studies have since confirmed the safety and efficacy of this technique.[32-40] These studies show that MIS TLIF can achieve results comparable with traditional open techniques but with less postoperative pain, decreased blood loss, and shorter hospital stays, particularly when compared with anterior-posterior circumferential fusion.[41]

Percutaneous Pedicle Screw Instrumentation

Insertion of pedicle screws through a midline approach requires massive retraction of the multifidus muscle, subjecting the muscle to high retraction pressures and disruption of its osseo-tendinous attachments and neurovascular supply. The rationale for MIS pedicle screw insertion lies in the preservation of multifidus muscle function. Pedicle screw insertion can be performed percutaneously or via a paramedian mini-open technique. With the percutaneous technique, the pedicle is entered using a Jamshidi-type trocar needle under fluoroscopic control (Fig. 56–7). Once the needles are within the pedicle, the stylets are removed and guidewires inserted. The guidewire is then used to direct cannulated taps and screws into the pedicle (Fig. 56–8). Sequential soft-tissue dilators are used to create a path for the tap and screw. The outermost dilator can be used as a protective sleeve during pedicle tapping. A cannulated pedicle screw is then placed over the guidewire. Rods are inserted percutaneously to minimize soft tissue trauma.

In the mini-open technique, a longitudinal, paramedian incision is placed slightly lateral to the lateral edge of the pedicles. Dissection is performed through the intermuscular plane between the multifidus and longissimus muscles. A tubular retractor system is subsequently deployed after tissue dilation is performed. The pars interarticularis and the mammillary processes of the cephalad and caudal levels are exposed with gentle electrocautery. A high-speed bur to create a starting point and pedicle probes are used to enter the pedicle. Cannulated or noncannulated pedicle screws can be used with this technique. The exposure allows for decortication of the pars, facet joint, and transverse processes for bone grafting and fusion. A standard rod and end caps can then be placed.

The mini-open technique offers several advantages over the percutaneous method. It allows for direct visualization of the anatomy and the choice of using either cannulated or noncannulated pedicle screw systems. The mini-open technique also allows for greater access for bone grafting posteriorly. On the other hand, the mini-open technique threatens the medial branch of the dorsal rami, which extends downward to the transverse process of the caudal level, where it passes between the mammillary and accessory processes. It then curves posteriorly, where it branches to supply the multifidus muscle, the intertransverse muscles and ligaments, and the facet joint of the cephalad level. As a result, insertion of a pedicle screw through the mammillary process at one level can cause injury to the medial branch nerve of the dorsal rami (MBN) that supplies the adjacent cephalad level. In a cadaveric study comparing these MIS techniques, Regev and colleagues found that

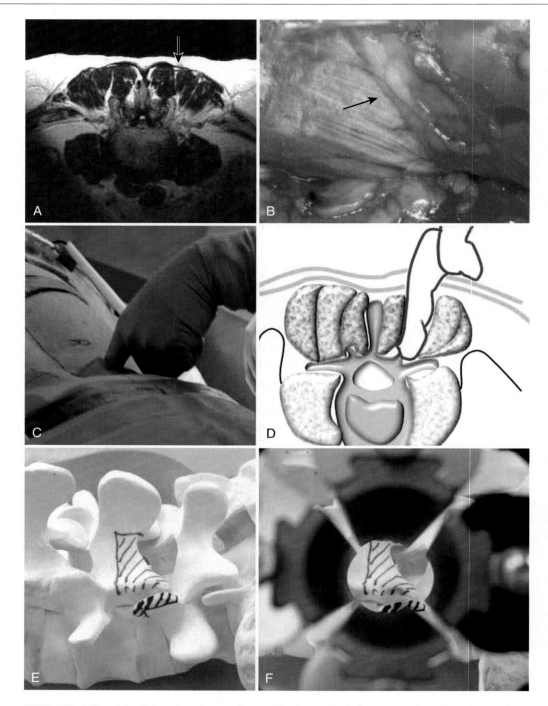

FIGURE 56–4 The minimally invasive spine transforaminal lumbar interbody fusion surgical corridor is described. **A,** Magnetic resonance cross-sectional image through L4-5 disc space showing the neurovascular plane between multifidus and longissimus muscles (*arrow*). **B,** Intraoperative photomicrograph showing the lateral aspect of the multifidus muscle and the neurovascular bundle (*arrow*). **C,** Intraoperative photograph and **D,** corresponding illustration showing the technique of manual blunt dissection to the surgical target site. **E,** Photographs of spine model with the surgical target site in red and black hash lines. **F,** The view of the surgical target site through a minimally invasive retractor.

the mini-open technique causes injury to the medial branch of the dorsal rami more frequently than the percutaneous technique.[42] They recommend that pedicle screw insertion at the cephalad level be performed percutaneously if one desires to minimize denervation of the multifidus complex at the cephalad adjacent level.

The overall safety and accuracy of minimally invasive pedicle screw insertion has been shown in several studies. Ringel and colleagues[43] assessed a total of 488 pedicle screws implanted in 103 patients via a percutaneous technique. They found that only 3% of screws were rated as unacceptable, leading to nine screw revision surgeries. These results mirror

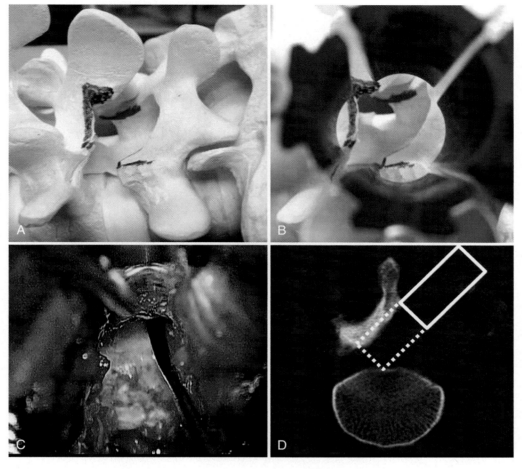

FIGURE 56–5 The minimally invasive spine transforaminal lumbar interbody fusion decompression is shown. **A,** Photographs of a spine model with removal of the inferior articular process of the cephalad level and overhang of the superior articular process of the caudad level is shown. **B,** Corresponding view through a minimally invasive retractor. **C,** Intraoperative photomicrograph of the dural tube with a Penfield probe reaching to the contralateral side. **D,** Postoperative CT scan with overlay of the surgical corridor.

a growing body of evidence that reflects the safety and efficacy of minimally invasive posterior spinal instrumentation.[31,44,45] These results are comparable with pedicle screws inserted via a traditional open approach. In a meta-analysis of 130 studies and 37,337 pedicle screws placed, the overall screw accuracy was 91.3%.[46]

Limitations and Drawbacks

Radiation Exposure

Several techniques for minimally invasive posterior screw insertion exist, but the percutaneous pedicle screw technique is the least tissue disruptive and is currently adapted for single or multilevel fusions. Its use, however, depends on intraoperative fluoroscopy. In the past, fluoroscopy was mainly used for lateral fluoroscopic pedicle screw guidance in open surgery. However, multiplanar fluoroscopic techniques are necessary for minimally invasive spinal instrumentation. Obtaining multiple views in several planes increases accuracy but increases operating times. The operative time for two screws on the same vertebra level reaches 10 minutes or longer using advanced fluoroscopic techniques, whereas lateral-only fluoroscopic methods require less than 5 minutes per level.[47-49] With increased insertion times associated with advanced fluoroscopic guidance, the cumulative exposure to radiation increased concomitantly.

Studies have shown that fluoroscopically guided pedicle screw placement exposes surgeons to 10 to 12 times the dose of radiation required when compared with nonspinal musculoskeletal procedures.[50] Despite these concerns, the convenience of the C-arm, combined with a high degree of accuracy, has made intraoperative fluoroscopy an increasingly necessary part of advanced spinal surgery. The addition of navigation technology is a promising means of decreasing radiation exposure to the surgical team. Kim and colleagues[51] showed that the use of navigation-assisted fluoroscopy for MIS TLIF markedly decreases direct exposure to radiation. In addition to reducing radiation exposure, navigation eliminates the need for cumbersome protective lead gear and clears the surgical field by removing the C-arm during surgery.

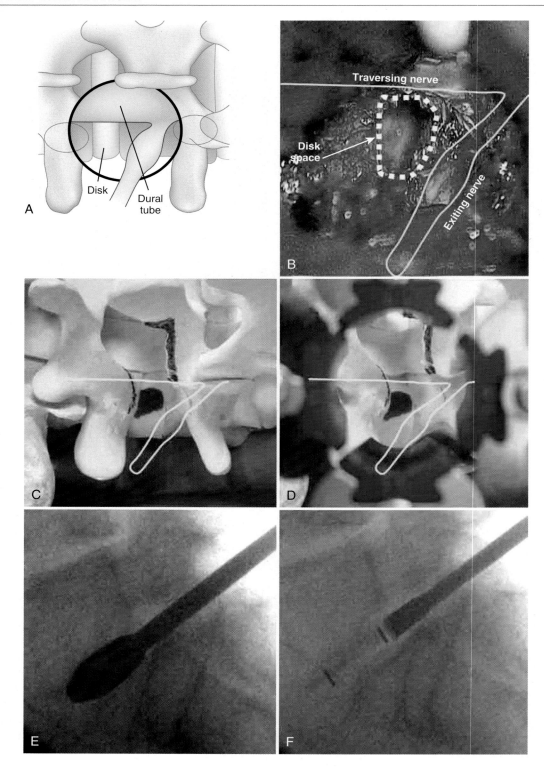

FIGURE 56–6 The minimally invasive spine transforaminal lumbar interbody fusion discectomy is shown. **A,** Illustration and **B,** corresponding photomicrograph of the surgical target site after facetectomy to expose Kambin triangle, which is bounded medially by the dural tube, proximally by the exiting nerve root and distally by the pedicle and superior endplate of the caudad vertebra. **C,** Photographs of a spine model after facetectomy. Kambin triangle is colored in red. **D,** Corresponding view through a minimally invasive retractor. **E,** Intraoperative image during discectomy showing a paddle distractor and sizer and **F,** during cage insertion.

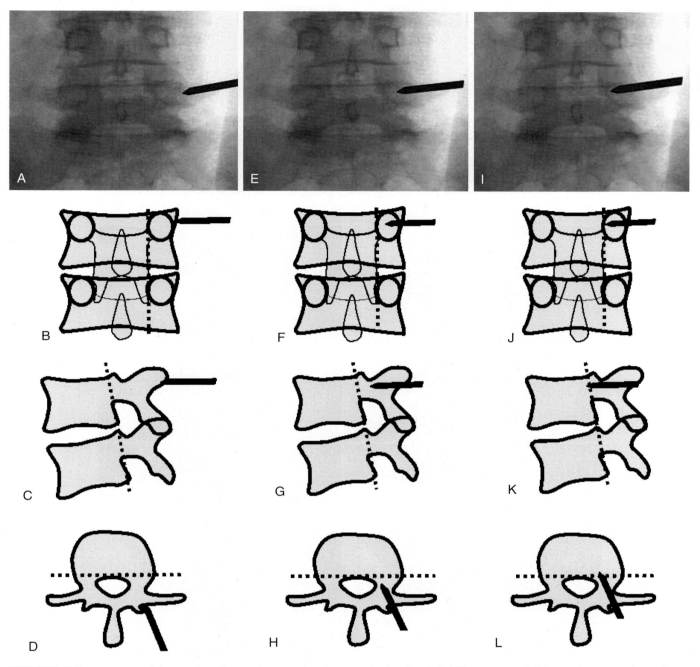

FIGURE 56–7 Percutaneous pedicle screw insertion requires scrupulous intraoperative imaging. **A, E, I,** The trocar needle is inserted using a perfect en face anteroposterior image of the pedicle. The endplates should be flat, and the top of the pedicle is in line with the superior endplate. The needle is inserted from a lateral to medial direction until the tip reaches the medial border of the pedicle (**I** and **J**). The C-arm is then brought under the table for a lateral view (**B, F, J**). If the needle is correctly inserted into the pedicle, the tip should be past the posterior vertebral body line (**K** and **L**). **A-D,** Shows the initial position of the needle in the anteroposterior, lateral, and axial planes, respectively. **E-H,** shows the needle halfway across the pedicle. **I-L,** Shows the needle at the medial border of the pedicle. Once past the posterior vertebral body line, the needle can be inserted another 5 mm, in preparation for insertion of the guidewire.

Learning Curve for Minimally Invasive Spinal Surgery

The barriers to widespread adoption of minimally invasive techniques appear to be related to technical difficulties of the procedures and a lack of adequate training opportunities. In a survey of spinal surgeons, Webb and colleagues[52] showed that most surgeons perceive MIS to be efficacious and want to perform more MIS procedures. However, most have not pursued MIS surgery because of concerns with technical difficulties of the procedure and a lack of adequate training opportunities. The technical difficulty of the procedure, combined with inadequate training, is evident in initial studies of MIS surgery. Nowitzke evaluated the learning curve for tubular decompression and noted that 3 of the first 7 but none of the subsequent 28 cases required conversion to open.[53]

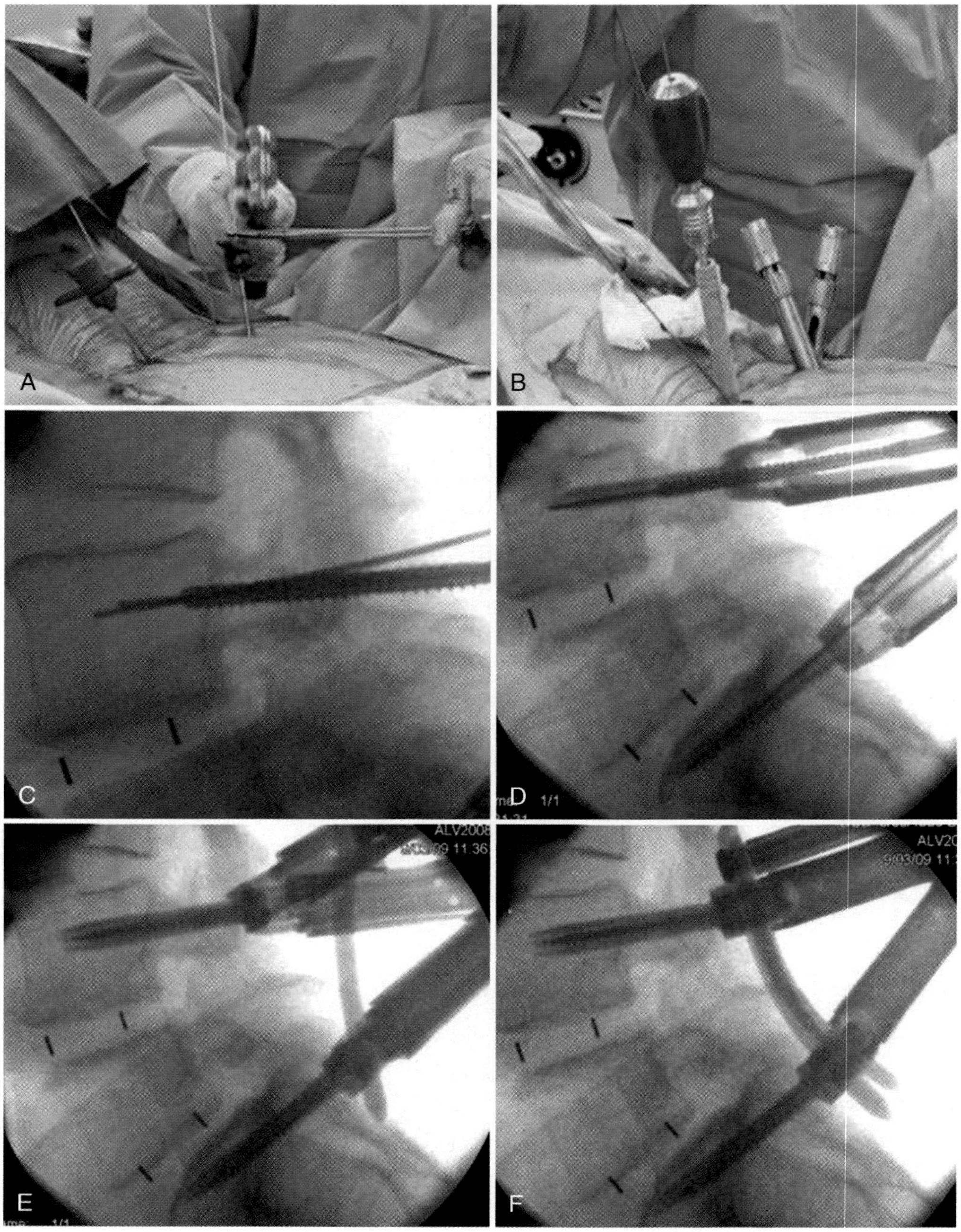

FIGURE 56–8 Percutaneous pedicle screw insertion uses guidewires to guide the taps and screws through the pedicle and into the vertebral body in a reliable manner. **A,** Once the Jamshidi needle is safely passed through the pedicle and into the vertebral body, the inner stylet is removed and the guidewire inserted. The cannula is then removed and soft tissues opened with serial dilators (**B**). The tap is then passed over the guidewire and into the dilator sleeves, which is monitored on lateral fluoroscopic image (**C**). It is critical to maintain control of the guidewire to avoid inadvertent advancement into the abdominal cavity. After tapping, cannulated pedicle screws with extension sleeves are inserted over the guidewire (**D**). Again, lateral image is used to monitor the guidewire and to insert the tulips to a consistent depth. Once all the screws are in place, a contoured rod is inserted under the dorsolumbar fascia and through the rod sleeves (**E**). The rod sleeves are then used to reduce the rod to the tulips and insert the locking caps (**F**).

Villavicencio and colleagues[41] noted a higher rate of overall perioperative complications, Dhall and colleagues[54] found a higher rate of instrumentation complications, and Peng and colleagues[55] noted longer operative times when comparing MIS TLIF versus open TLIF.

Summary

The posterior spine is dynamically stabilized by a diverse group of muscles that lay in close proximity to the vertebral column. These muscles possess a single tendon origin at the spine process and multiple tendon insertion sites distally along the superior articular processes. Each of these muscles possesses unique anatomic and structural characteristics that reflect their primary role. The multifidus muscles are made up of short and powerful fibers that enable them to produce large forces over short distances, making them a powerful stabilizer. Traditional posterior midline open approaches disrupt the function of these muscles through tendon detachment, devascularization, and crush injury. Currently, minimally invasive technique use surgical approaches where these events are minimized. Paramedian incisions avoid detachment of the multifidus tendon origin. Table-mounted, tubular retractors minimize retraction pressure. Specialized surgical instruments and implants accommodate narrow surgical corridors. The short results of these techniques are well demonstrated in multiple studies. The long-term effects of minimally invasive posterior spinal surgery are not yet known, but it is anticipated that maintenance of muscle function will have effects on future events such as adjacent level degeneration and level of function.

PEARLS

1. Ensure adequate preparation and training for all MIS procedures by performing the entire procedure, skin to skin, on a cadaveric specimen.

2. Use intraoperative imaging to precisely position the retractor directly in line with the intended surgical corridor.

3. Avoid the temptation of excessively opening the retractor because this leads to additional muscle creep that further obscures the surgical target site.

4. Use instruments specifically designed for MIS procedures that are properly angled and bayoneted for use down a long, narrow surgical corridor.

5. Consider the use of expandable tubular retractors that contain a gap between the blades to allow increased angulation of instruments.

PITFALLS

1. MIS procedures are reliant on fluoroscopic imaging, which can lead to excessive radiation exposure to the surgical team. Proper protective wear should include not only a lead gown but also a thyroid shield and protective eyewear. Strong consideration should be given to use of protective gloves.

2. Unintentional durotomies more often occur in patients with severe stenosis and facet cysts. Meticulous release of the tissue adherent to the dural tube before use of the Kerrison rongeur decreases this risk.

3. Insertion of the interbody cage during MIS TLIF procedures endangers the exiting nerve root. Care should be taken to maintain the pars interarticularis, which serves to protect the nerve during cage insertion. Similarly, the dural tube should be adequately released and decompressed to allow the traversing nerve root to move out of the path of the cage during insertion.

KEY POINTS

1. The posterior paraspinal musculature, particularly the multifidus muscle, provides a critical dynamic stabilizing function.

2. Prevention of multifidus muscle injury embodies the main concept in minimally invasive posterior lumbar surgery.

3. Multifidus muscle injury can occur by detachment of the tendon origin at the spinous process.

4. Table-mounted, tubular retractors minimize muscle crush injury by maximizing the surface area of the retractor and avoiding the prolonged elevated retraction pressures associated with self-retaining retractors.

5. Minimally invasive posterior lumbar techniques remain technically demanding, leading to higher complication rates and longer operative times during the early period of the learning curve.

6. A difficult learning curve demands that surgeons have sufficient preclinical training, and education is obtained before the application of minimally invasive spine surgery in clinical practice.

7. Meticulous use of fluoroscopic imaging is required to prevent instrumentation-related complications.

KEY REFERENCES

1. Stevens KJ, Spenciner DB, Griffiths KL, et al: Comparison of minimally invasive and conventional open posterolateral lumbar fusion using magnetic resonance imaging and retraction pressure studies. J Spinal Disord Tech 19:77-86, 2006.
   Cadaveric studies of muscle compartment pressures combined with a clinical study using specialized postoperative MR imaging show that minimally invasive tubular retractors minimize retraction pressure and subsequent muscle injury during minimally invasive posterior lumbar approaches.

2. Foley KT, Gupta SK: Percutaneous pedicle screw fixation of the lumbar spine: preliminary clinical results. J Neurosurg 97:7-12, 2002.
   The fundamental basis for percutaneous pedicle screw insertion and percutaneous rod delivery using screw extension sleeves is described.

3. Schwender JD, Holly LT, Rouben DP, et al: Minimally invasive transforaminal lumbar interbody fusion (TLIF): technical feasibility and initial results. J Spinal Disord Tech 18 Suppl:S1-S6, 2005.

The most commonly used and accepted technique for minimally invasive transforaminal lumbar interbody fusion is described along with the results that have been commonly found in subsequent studies.

4. Peng CW, Yue WM, Poh SY, et al: Clinical and radiological outcomes of minimally invasive versus open transforaminal lumbar interbody fusion. Spine (Phila Pa 1976) 34:1385-1389, 2009.

This prospective study of 29 MIS TLIF and 29 open TLIF patients with at least 2-year follow-up shows that the MIS technique is associated with less blood loss, shorter hospital stay, and lower narcotic needs but has similar clinical results in terms of fusion rates, pain relief, and quality of life scores.

5. Dhall SS, Wang MY, Mummaneni PV: Clinical and radiographic comparison of mini-open transforaminal lumbar interbody fusion with open transforaminal lumbar interbody fusion in 42 patients with long-term follow-up. J Neurosurg Spine 9:560-565, 2008.

A retrospective study of MIS and open TLIF of 42 patients shows that MIS TLIF leads to less blood loss and shorter hospital stay but with higher complications related to instrumentation.

REFERENCES

1. Cholewicki J, Panjabi MM, Khachatryan A: Stabilizing function of trunk flexor-extensor muscles around a neutral spine posture. Spine (Phila Pa 1976) 22:2207-2212, 1997.

2. Gejo R, Kawaguchi Y, Kondoh T, et al: Magnetic resonance imaging and histologic evidence of postoperative back muscle injury in rats. Spine (Phila Pa 1976) 25:941-946, 2000.

3. Gille O, Jolivet E, Dousset V, et al: Erector spinae muscle changes on magnetic resonance imaging following lumbar surgery through a posterior approach. Spine (Phila Pa 1976) 32:1236-1241, 2007.

4. Datta G, Gnanalingham KK, Peterson D, et al: Back pain and disability after lumbar laminectomy: is there a relationship to muscle retraction? Neurosurgery 54:1413-1420, 2004; discussion 20.

5. Gejo R, Matsui H, Kawaguchi Y, et al: Serial changes in trunk muscle performance after posterior lumbar surgery. Spine (Phila Pa 1976) 24:1023-1028, 1999.

6. Hyun SJ, Kim YB, Kim YS, et al: Postoperative changes in paraspinal muscle volume: comparison between paramedian interfascial and midline approaches for lumbar fusion. J Korean Med Sci 22:646-651, 2007.

7. Kawaguchi Y, Matsui H, Gejo R, et al: Preventive measures of back muscle injury after posterior lumbar spine surgery in rats. Spine (Phila Pa 1976) 23:2282-2287, 1998; discussion 8.

8. Mayer TG, Vanharanta H, Gatchel RJ, et al: Comparison of CT scan muscle measurements and isokinetic trunk strength in postoperative patients. Spine (Phila Pa 1976) 14:33-36, 1989.

9. Motosuneya T, Asazuma T, Tsuji T, et al:. Postoperative change of the cross-sectional area of back musculature after 5 surgical procedures as assessed by magnetic resonance imaging. J Spinal Disord Tech 19:318-322, 2006.

10. Rantanen J, Hurme M, Falck B, et al: The lumbar multifidus muscle five years after surgery for a lumbar intervertebral disc herniation. Spine (Phila Pa 1976) 18:568-574, 1993.

11. Granata KP, Marras WS. An EMG-assisted model of loads on the lumbar spine during asymmetric trunk extensions. J Biomech 26:1429-1438, 1993.

12. Marras WS, Davis KG, et al: Trunk muscle activities during asymmetric twisting motions. J Electromyogr Kinesiol 8:247-256, 1998.

13. Perez-Cruet MJ, Foley KT, Isaacs RE, et al: Microendoscopic lumbar discectomy: technical note. Neurosurgery 51:S129-S136, 2002.

14. Stevens KJ, Spenciner DB, Griffiths KL, et al: Comparison of minimally invasive and conventional open posterolateral lumbar fusion using magnetic resonance imaging and retraction pressure studies. J Spinal Disord Tech 19:77-86, 2006.

15. Arts MP, Brand R, van den Akker ME, et al: Tubular diskectomy vs conventional microdiskectomy for sciatica: a randomized controlled trial. JAMA 302:149-158, 2009.

16. Ryang YM, Oertel MF, Mayfrank L, et al: Standard open microdiscectomy versus minimal access trocar microdiscectomy: results of a prospective randomized study. Neurosurgery 62:174-181, 2008; discussion 81-82.

17. Righesso O, Falavigna A, Avanzi O: Comparison of open discectomy with microendoscopic discectomy in lumbar disc herniations: results of a randomized controlled trial. Neurosurgery 61:545-549, 2007; discussion 9.

18. Weiner BK, Walker M, Brower RS, et al: Microdecompression for lumbar spinal canal stenosis. Spine (Phila Pa 1976) 24:2268-2272, 1999.

19. Palmer S, Turner R, Palmer R: Bilateral decompressive surgery in lumbar spinal stenosis associated with spondylolisthesis: unilateral approach and use of a microscope and tubular retractor system. Neurosurg Focus 13:E4, 2002.

20. Palmer S, Turner R, Palmer R: Bilateral decompression of lumbar spinal stenosis involving a unilateral approach with microscope and tubular retractor system. J Neurosurg 97:213-217, 2002.

21. Costa F, Sassi M, Cardia A, Ortolina A, et al: Degenerative lumbar spinal stenosis: analysis of results in a series of 374 patients treated with unilateral laminotomy for bilateral microdecompression. J Neurosurg Spine 7:579-586, 2007.

22. Iwatsuki K, Yoshimine T, Aoki M: Bilateral interlaminar fenestration and unroofing for the decompression of nerve roots by using a unilateral approach in lumbar canal stenosis. Surg Neurol 68:487-492, 2007; discussion 92.

23. Khoo LT, Fessler RG: Microendoscopic decompressive laminotomy for the treatment of lumbar stenosis. Neurosurgery 51:S146-S154, 2002.

24. Rahman M, Summers LE, Richter B, et al: Comparison of techniques for decompressive lumbar laminectomy: the minimally invasive versus the "classic" open approach. Minim Invasive Neurosurg 51:100-105, 2008.

25. Asgarzadie F, Khoo LT: Minimally invasive operative management for lumbar spinal stenosis: overview of early and long-term

outcomes. Orthop Clin North Am 38:387-399, 2007; abstract vi-vii.

26. Ikuta K, Tono O, Tanaka T, et al: Surgical complications of micro-endoscopic procedures for lumbar spinal stenosis. Minim Invasive Neurosurg 50:145-149, 2007.

27. Podichetty VK, Spears J, Isaacs RE, et al: Complications associated with minimally invasive decompression for lumbar spinal stenosis. J Spinal Disord Tech 19:161-166, 2006.

28. Rosen DS, O'Toole JE, Eichholz KM, et al: Minimally invasive lumbar spinal decompression in the elderly: outcomes of 50 patients aged 75 years and older. Neurosurgery 60:503-509, 2007; discussion 9-10.

29. Sasaki M, Abekura M, Morris S, et al: Microscopic bilateral decompression through unilateral laminotomy for lumbar canal stenosis in patients undergoing hemodialysis. J Neurosurg Spine 5:494-499, 2006.

30. Regev G, Taylor W, Garfin SR, et al: The Use of Concurrent Bilateral Minimally Invasive Approach for Central and Neuroforaminal Spinal Decompression. Poster Presentation at 2008 Annual Meeting of the Society for Minimally Invasive Spine Surgery, San Diego, 2008.

31. Schwender JD, Holly LT, Rouben DP, et al: Minimally invasive transforaminal lumbar interbody fusion (TLIF): technical feasibility and initial results. J Spinal Disord Tech 18 Suppl:S1-S6, 2005.

32. Anand N, Hamilton JF, Perri B, et al: Cantilever TLIF with structural allograft and RhBMP2 for correction and maintenance of segmental sagittal lordosis: long-term clinical, radiographic, and functional outcome. Spine (Phila Pa 1976) 31:E748-E753, 2006.

33. Deutsch H, Musacchio MJ Jr: Minimally invasive transforaminal lumbar interbody fusion with unilateral pedicle screw fixation. Neurosurg Focus 20:E10, 2006.

34. Isaacs RE, Podichetty VK, Santiago P, et al: Minimally invasive microendoscopy-assisted transforaminal lumbar interbody fusion with instrumentation. J Neurosurg Spine 3:98-105, 2005.

35. Joseph V, Rampersaud YR: Heterotopic bone formation with the use of rhBMP2 in posterior minimal access interbody fusion: a CT analysis. Spine (Phila Pa 1976) 32:2885-2890, 2007.

36. Park Y, Ha JW: Comparison of one-level posterior lumbar interbody fusion performed with a minimally invasive approach or a traditional open approach. Spine (Phila Pa 1976) 32:537-543, 2007.

37. Salerni AA: A minimally invasive approach for posterior lumbar interbody fusion. Neurosurg Focus 13:e6, 2002.

38. Selznick LA, Shamji MF, Isaacs RE: Minimally invasive interbody fusion for revision lumbar surgery: technical feasibility and safety. J Spinal Disord Tech 22:207-213, 2009.

39. Sethi A, Lee S, Vaidya R: Transforaminal lumbar interbody fusion using unilateral pedicle screws and a translaminar screw. Eur Spine J 18:430-434, 2009.

40. Shen FH, Samartzis D, Khanna AJ, Anderson DG. Minimally invasive techniques for lumbar interbody fusions. Orthop Clin North Am 38:373-386, 2007; abstract vi.

41. Villavicencio AT, Burneikiene S, Bulsara KR, et al: Perioperative complications in transforaminal lumbar interbody fusion versus anterior-posterior reconstruction for lumbar disc degeneration and instability. J Spinal Disord Tech 19:92-97, 2006.

42. Regev GJ, Lee YP, Taylor WR, et al: Nerve injury to the posterior rami medial branch during the insertion of pedicle screws: comparison of mini-open versus percutaneous pedicle screw insertion techniques. Spine (Phila Pa 1976) 34:1239-1242, 2009.

43. Ringel F, Stoffel M, Stuer C, et al: Minimally invasive transmuscular pedicle screw fixation of the thoracic and lumbar spine. Neurosurgery 59:ONS361-ONS366, 2006; discussion ONS6-7.

44. Foley KT, Gupta SK: Percutaneous pedicle screw fixation of the lumbar spine: preliminary clinical results. J Neurosurg 97:7-12, 2002.

45. Eck JC, Hodges S, Humphreys SC: Minimally invasive lumbar spinal fusion. J Am Acad Orthop Surg 15:321-329, 2007.

46. Kosmopoulos V, Schizas C: Pedicle screw placement accuracy: a meta-analysis. Spine (Phila Pa 1976) 32:E111-E1120, 2007.

47. Merloz P, Troccaz J, Vouaillat H, et al: Fluoroscopy-based navigation system in spine surgery. Proc Inst Mech Eng H 221:813-820, 2007.

48. Assaker R, Cinquin P, Cotten A, et al: Image-guided endoscopic spine surgery: Part I. A feasibility study. Spine (Phila Pa 1976) 26:1705-1710, 2001.

49. Assaker R, Reyns N, Pertruzon B, et al: Image-guided endoscopic spine surgery: Part II: clinical applications. Spine (Phila Pa 1976) 26:1711-1718, 2001.

50. Rampersaud YR, Foley KT, Shen AC, et al: Radiation exposure to the spine surgeon during fluoroscopically assisted pedicle screw insertion. Spine (Phila Pa 1976) 25:2637-2645, 2000.

51. Kim CW, Lee YP, Taylor W, et al: Use of navigation-assisted fluoroscopy to decrease radiation exposure during minimally invasive spine surgery. Spine J 8:584-590, 2008.

52. Webb J, Gottschalk L, Lee YP, et al: Surgeon Perceptions of Minimally Invasive Spine Surgery. SAS Journal 2:62-66, 2008.

53. Nowitzke AM: Assessment of the learning curve for lumbar microendoscopic discectomy. Neurosurgery 56:755-762, 2005; discussion-62.

54. Dhall SS, Wang MY, Mummaneni PV: Clinical and radiographic comparison of mini-open transforaminal lumbar interbody fusion with open transforaminal lumbar interbody fusion in 42 patients with long-term follow-up. J Neurosurg Spine 9:560-565, 2008.

55. Peng CW, Yue WM, Poh SY, et al: Clinical and radiological outcomes of minimally invasive versus open transforaminal lumbar interbody fusion. Spine (Phila Pa 1976) 34:1385-1389, 2009.

57

CHAPTER

Minimally Invasive Posterior Lumbar Instrumentation

David Strothman, MD
James D. Schwender, MD

Overview

Over recent years minimally invasive surgical techniques have evolved to safely allow access to the spine with less collateral damage as compared with traditional open surgical approaches. The basic principles of spinal surgery remain unchanged. The most basic tenant of minimally invasive spine surgery is to perform the same surgery as has traditionally been done open but with less soft tissue destruction and equal or better outcomes. Minimally invasive surgical techniques have demonstrated less blood loss, shorter hospital stays, and lower infection rates as compared with open surgical techniques.[1-5] However, operative times are longer and there may be a trend toward more technical complications.[1,2] Also, there is a prolonged and slow learning curve associated with minimally invasive surgery.

A variety of different instrumentation systems may be used in posterior-based minimally invasive lumbar spine surgery. These primarily include percutaneous pedicle screws and traditional pedicle screws. Each type of instrumentation can be used safely and effectively during minimally invasive surgery.

Indications and Contraindications

The indications for minimally invasive posterior spinal instrumentation are similar to traditional open surgical indications. Minimally invasive posterior spinal fusion with instrumentation has been used safely and effectively to treat instability associated with spondylolisthesis, degenerative disc disease, large or recurrent disc herniations, postlaminectomy instability, degenerative scoliosis, and trauma. Minimally invasive fusion with instrumentation may be safely performed during revisions as well. In fact, minimally invasive surgery (MIS) instrumentation can be advantageous during revision surgery because it can be placed through a native surgical corridor free of scar tissue.

There are relatively few contraindications to minimally invasive instrumentation. Obesity (body mass index [BMI] > 40), advanced spondylolisthesis (grade 3 or 4), and previous instrumentation that requires an open approach for extension or removal are all relative contraindications.

Obesity

Approximately one third of American adults older than the age of 20 are considered obese.[6] Complication rates as high as 36% to 50% have been reported for obese patients undergoing lumbar fusion.[6] Although obesity certainly makes minimally invasive surgery more challenging, it can be done safely and effectively in this population. The authors' personal experience has found that oftentimes pedicle screws can be placed more easily through a minimally invasive Wiltse-type approach as compared with midline approaches because there is much less muscle, fat, and soft tissue retraction necessary to obtain the correct screw trajectory. Also, the retractor can help to keep adipose tissue and the deep (often thick) musculature out of the surgical field.

Park and colleagues[7] compared the perioperative complications in patients with a BMI greater than 25 kg/m^2 with patients having a BMI less than 25 kg/m^2 who underwent a minimally invasive lumbar spinal surgery. Minimally invasive decompressions in patients with a BMI greater than 25 kg/m^2 had a 6.5% complication rate as compared with 11.8% in patients with a BMI less than 25 kg/m^2. Minimally invasive fusion procedures had a 24% complication rate in patients with a BMI greater than 25 kg/m^2 as compared with 25% in patients with a BMI less than 25 kg/m^2. No infections were recorded in either group. No statistical differences were noted between groups. Similarly, Rosen and colleagues[6] did not find a correlation between BMI and postoperative changes in ODI, VAS, and SF-36 scores using a linear regression model.

Minimally invasive fusions in obese patients also create less postoperative dead space, which may lead to lower infection rates. O'Toole and colleagues[8] reviewed surgical site infections in MIS decompressions, discectomy, and fusion cases. One-thousand, three-hundred, and thirty-eight cases were included for the review. Three postoperative surgical site infections were identified. Two patients developed superficial cellulitis after minimally invasive fusions, and one patient developed discitis after a microendoscopic discectomy (MED). The reported surgical site infection rate for simple decompressive procedures was 0.1% and 0.74% for fusion with internal fixation. The overall infection rate for the entire cohort was 0.22%. The reported infection rate for minimally invasive fusion compares favorably with open fusion infection rates. Importantly, there were no cases of postoperative deep wound infection in O'Toole and colleagues' cohort. The one patient with discitis developed symptoms 1 month after developing a lower extremity cellulitis. The disc space biopsy grew the same organism as the cellulitis. No patient in their series required reoperation for a deep wound infection. In contrast, Picada and colleagues[9] reported a 3.2% deep wound infection after reviewing 817 patients who underwent an open lumbosacral fusion. Minimally invasive fusions can be performed safely and effectively in obese patients, but these cases may be more technically demanding as the working length through the tube increases.

In obese patients the authors have found it helpful to measure the distance from the dorsal aspect of the facet at the level of the intended procedure on the preoperative magnetic resonance imaging (MRI) to help determine the length of retractor needed in heavier patients (Fig. 57–1). During a

surgeon's initial experience with minimally invasive fusions, patients with an expected retractor length greater than 80 mm are a relative contraindication, particularly early in the learning stages. However, with experience obese patients are a relative indication for minimally invasive fusion and instrumentation rather than a contraindication.

Technical Outcomes of Minimally Invasive Fusion Surgery

At the time of this publication there is still a relative paucity of published literature detailing the clinical results of minimally invasive fusion surgery. Early studies have demonstrated minimally invasive fusion to be safe and efficacious.[5,10,11]

Kim and colleagues[12] compared tissue injury markers between minimally invasive posterior lateral lumbar interbody fusion (PLIF) and open PLIF. Significantly larger increases were observed in creatinine kinase, aldolase, IL-6, IL-10, and IL-1ra in the open PLIFs compared with the minimally invasive PLIFs. This confirms less muscle injury in the

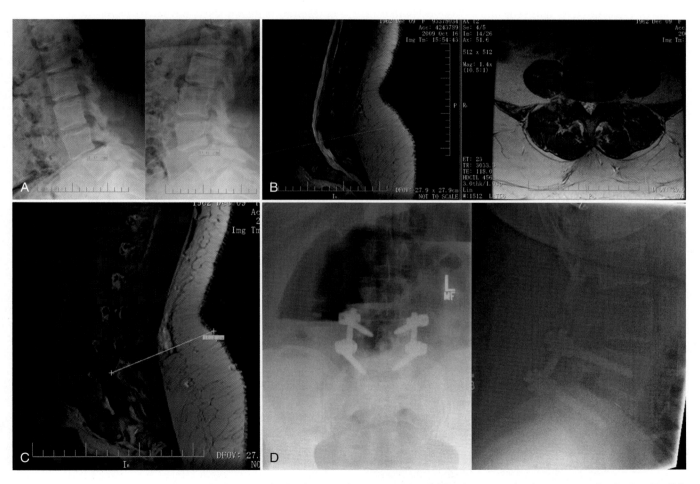

FIGURE 57–1 Degenerative spondylolisthesis body mass index (BMI) greater than 40. A 43-year-old female presented with neurogenic claudication. Her BMI is 41. **A,** Flexion/extension radiographs: show unstable degenerative spondylolisthesis. **B,** Magnetic resonance imaging (MRI) shows bilateral subarticular stenosis and facet arthropathy. **C,** The expected length of tubular retractor is measured from the skin edge to the facet joint on axial and sagittal MRI. **D,** Postoperative radiographs after minimally invasive transforaminal lumbar interbody fusion, posterior spinal fusion, and decompression at L4-5. Preop VAS: 10, Postop VAS 1.

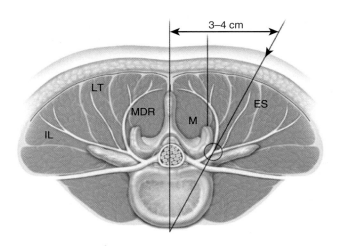

FIGURE 57–2 Wiltse approach.

minimally invasive fusions and may result in a lower systemic inflammatory reaction in the immediate postoperative period, which in turn may lower acute medical morbidity. However, clinical studies have not documented this to date.

Shizas and colleagues[4] and Peng and colleagues[3] both compared minimally invasive transforaminal lumbar interbody fusion (TLIF) with open TLIF for the treatment of spondylolisthesis and degenerative disc disease. The average hospital stay was 2 days shorter following minimally invasive TLIF as compared with open TLIF. Blood loss was significantly less, but the operative time, at least in the Peng[3] study, was 45 minutes longer. Overall the complication rates were similar between open TLIF and minimally invasive TLIF. Schizas and colleagues[4] reported two technical complications in each group. However, they found three pseudoarthroses in the minimally invasive group compared with none in the open group. Peng and colleagues[3] observed that 80% of the minimally invasive TLIFs were solidly fused compared with 87% of the open TLIFs. Peng and colleagues[3] also noted a 7% complication rate in the minimally invasive group compared with

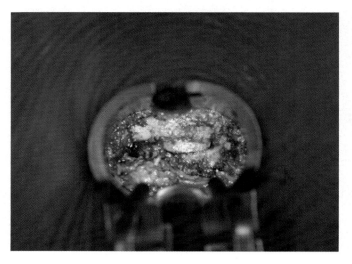

FIGURE 57–3 Tubular retractor docked on desired facet and expanded.

a 14% complication rate in the open group. Both Peng and colleagues and Schizas and colleagues found similar improvements in Oswestry Disability Index (ODI) scores. Minimally invasive TLIF ODI scores improved by 22% compared with improvement of 27% in the open TLIF group reported by Schizas and colleagues. These authors observed a 29-point improvement in ODI scores in minimally invasive TLIFs and a 30-point improvement in open cases.

More extensive studies are necessary to clarify the short- and long-term outcomes of minimally invasive decompressions and fusions in comparison with open techniques. However, the initial data are promising.

Traditional Pedicle Screws

Minimally invasive fusions use the surgical corridor as described by Wiltse[13] between the multifidus and longissimus paraspinal muscles (Fig. 57–2). This trajectory is ideal for both pedicle screw placement and interbody work.

After the appropriate trajectory is localized with fluoroscopy, sequential dilators are passed through the fascia and docked onto the facet joint. A tubular retractor (typically 20 or 22 mm) is then docked and secured over the dilators. The use of an expandable retractor allows the blades to expand cephalad or caudad, creating a corridor for pedicle screw placement (Fig. 57–3). Soft tissue is cleared to expose the standard pedicle screw entry points (Fig. 57–4). Screws can be placed using a variety of methods including free hand, under C-arm guidance, or using navigation depending on surgeon preference. In addition, both posted- and tulip-style screws can be used if working through the tubular retractor systems that are available.

Surgeon preference dictates the sequence of steps during minimally invasive fusion. Early on in a surgeon's experience it may be easiest to place the pedicle screw tracts first, before the decompression or facetectomy. This will preserve "normal" anatomy to help orient the surgeon to the anatomic starting points. However, it is the authors' experience that it is more efficient to perform the decompression and interbody spacer placement before screw tract preparation if required. This minimizes the surgical exposure during the portion of the procedure that requires the most medial angulation of the retractor and thereby helps to limit muscle creep (Fig. 57–5).

Percutaneous Pedicle Screws

Pedicle screws can be safely and effectively placed percutaneously and thus avoid the additional dissection required for the placement of traditional pedicle screws. Percutaneous pedicle screw placement has the advantage of less muscle damage and less potential damage to the medial branch nerve (innervation of the multifidus), and it can be used effectively over long segment fusions.[14,15] The placement of percutaneous pedicle screws can require more operative time and more x-ray exposure for accurate placement.

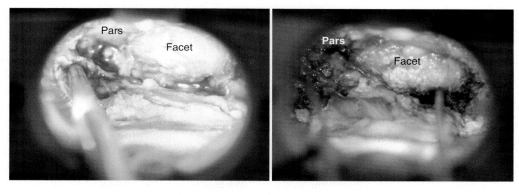

FIGURE 57–4 Pedicle screw entry sites visualized through tubular retractor.

Technique of Percutaneous Pedicle Screw Placement

The authors prefer to place percutaneous pedicle screws using fluoroscopy because it is readily available. The orientation of the C-arm beam is of critical importance. The anteroposterior (AP) images must be true AP images of each pedicle for which you are planning screw placement (Fig. 57–6). The spinous process should be in the midline of the vertebral body, equally spaced between both pedicles. The superior and inferior endplates should be parallel, and the pedicles should be appropriately located at the caudal end of the ascending articular process. On the lateral view the superior endplate should appear as one line and the pedicles should overlap and thus appear as one. True AP and lateral radiographs are of critical importance because small variance can produce large errors.

The pedicle of interest is localized using the AP fluoroscopic image. The skin is incised just lateral to the pedicle. The thoracolumbar dorsal fascia and muscle fascia are incised. A Jamshidi trocar is used to cannulate the pedicle. The ideal

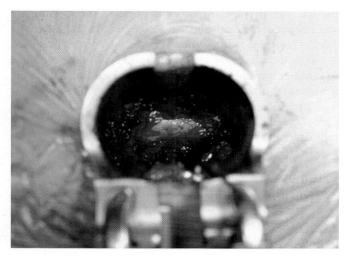

FIGURE 57–5 Visualization of dura and transforaminal lumbar interbody fusion discectomy through tubular retractor.

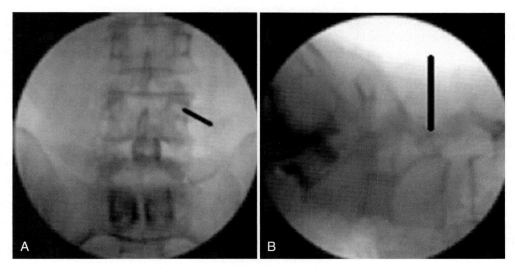

FIGURE 57–6 Fluoroscopic imaging for percutaneous pedicle screw placement. **A,** "True Ap": Pedicles are located just below the ascending articular process and the superior endplate is parallel to the x-ray beam. The spinous process is in the middle of both pedicles. **B,** "True lateral": Both pedicles appear as one. The superior endplate is parallel to the x-ray beam.

starting point is at the 10 o'clock and 2 o'clock positions on the left and right pedicles, respectively. The Jamshidi is slowly advanced a few millimeters. A lateral fluoroscopic image is obtained and should confirm that the Jamshidi is placed within the center of the pedicle. Under AP fluoroscopic imaging the Jamshidi is advanced about 20 mm. The tip should stay lateral to the medial border of the pedicle. A lateral image is obtained and should show the tip of the Jamshidi at or past the neurocentral junction. If so, the Jamshidi can be safely advanced to its desired depth. If the tip of the Jamshidi is at or medial to the medial border of the pedicle on the AP view and has not yet passed the neurocentral junction on the lateral, the pedicel screw tract has breached the medial border of the pedicle (Fig. 57–7).

After the Jamshidi is placed appropriately, a guidewire is passed. This is repeated at each pedicle. The k-wires are secured out of the field, and the decompressive and interbody work is performed. The pedicle screw is then placed over each k-wire and the appropriately sized rod is passed. It is critical to continue lateral C-arm visualization to avoid advancing the k-wire anteriorly.

When first performing these procedures the authors encourage the liberal use of fluoroscopy. With experience radiographic exposure and operative time will diminish.

Studies Comparing Mini-Open and Percutaneous Pedicle Screws

The decision of which minimally invasive instrumentation technique to use is largely surgeon dependent. Regev and colleagues[15] compared mini-open pedicle screw placement with percutaneous pedicle screw insertion in cadavers. After screw placement the authors dissected out the medial branch nerve. The medial branch nerve originates from the dorsal rami of each spinal nerve and innervates the multifidus muscle. The medial branch nerve was transected in 84% of cases using the mini-open technique as compared with 20% of the percutaneous insertion technique. The clinical importance of this difference is unknown. However, in this study percutaneous pedicle screw placement better preserved the segmental innervation of the multifidus compared with mini-open pedicle screw insertion.

No clinical studies have directly compared the use of traditional pedicle screws placed through a tubular retractor (mini-open) to percutaneous pedicle screws. However, multiple studies have reported perioperative data regarding percutaneous and open screw insertion (Table 57–1). Schizas and colleagues[4] reported their experience with 18 minimally invasive TLIFs using percutaneous pedicle screw fixation and compared this with 18 open TLIFs. The percutaneous pedicle screw patients used 2.7 cGy/cm^2 of radiation as compared with 1.8 cGy/cm^2 in the open TLIF group. The minimally invasive TLIF operative time averaged 4.3 hours in the last third of their experience. Their estimated blood loss was 456 mL. Peng and colleagues[3] also reviewed the results of minimally invasive TLIFs. They used an average of 105 seconds of fluoroscopy. They had an average estimated blood loss

(EBL) of 150 mL and average operative time of 216 minutes. Neither of these studies reported any technical complications with minimally invasive TLIFs performed by percutaneous screws. Foley's[10] initial experience was similar with an average operative time of 290 minutes and estimated blood loss of 25 mL. He reported one technical complication of a loose locking plug that required revision. Dhall and colleagues[1] compared minimally invasive TLIFs with traditional pedicle screws with open TLIFs. Their average EBL was 194 mL, and their average operating room (OR) time was 199 minutes. There were two technical complications in the minimally invasive group with one misplaced pedicle screw and one case of interbody cage migration. The open group also had one misplaced screw. Schwender and colleagues[5] reported on their initial experience with minimally invasive TLIFs and percutaneous screw insertion. Their average operative time was 240 minutes, and the average EBL was 140 mL. In this series there were two misplaced screws and interbody cage dislodgement. Park and colleagues[2] compared 32 minimally invasive PLIFs with 29 open PLIFs. All minimally invasive cases were stabilized with percutaneous screws. The average OR time was longer for the minimally invasive cases compared with open cases, 191 minutes and 150 minutes, respectively. The average EBL in the minimally invasive cases was 432 mL compared with 737 mL. There were two technical complications, one screw malposition and one interbody cage migration, reported in the minimally invasive group and none in the open group. These differences were not statistically significant.

In 2005 Kim and colleagues[14] compared longitudinal changes in multifidus cross-sectional area and trunk extension strength in both open and percutaneous pedicle screw constructs. The T2 cross-sectional area of the multifidus muscle was recorded on preoperative and postoperative MRIs. Trunk extension strength was measured using a MedX lumbar extension machine. Multifidus cross-sectional area decreased from 1140 mm^2 to 800 mm^2 in open pedicle screw constructs as compared with percutaneous pedicle screw construction in which multifidus area decreased from 1320 mm^2 to 1270 mm^2. Trunk extension strength increased in both open and percutaneous pedicle screw constructs, but the improvements in strength were only statistically significant in the percutaneous pedicle screw group.

Overall there are not enough comparative data to make any evidence-based decisions between the use of traditional pedicle screws through tubular retractors and percutaneous pedicle screws. More clinical data are necessary. The complication profile between minimally invasive pedicle screw instrumentation and open pedicle screw instrumentation appears similar. Minimally invasive pedicle instrumentation requires longer operative times, but results in decreased blood loss and short-term outcomes appear similar.

Screw Insertion Technique: Fluoroscopic Versus Navigation

Multiple techniques exist for the placement of percutaneous pedicle screws. Pedicle screws can be placed safely with

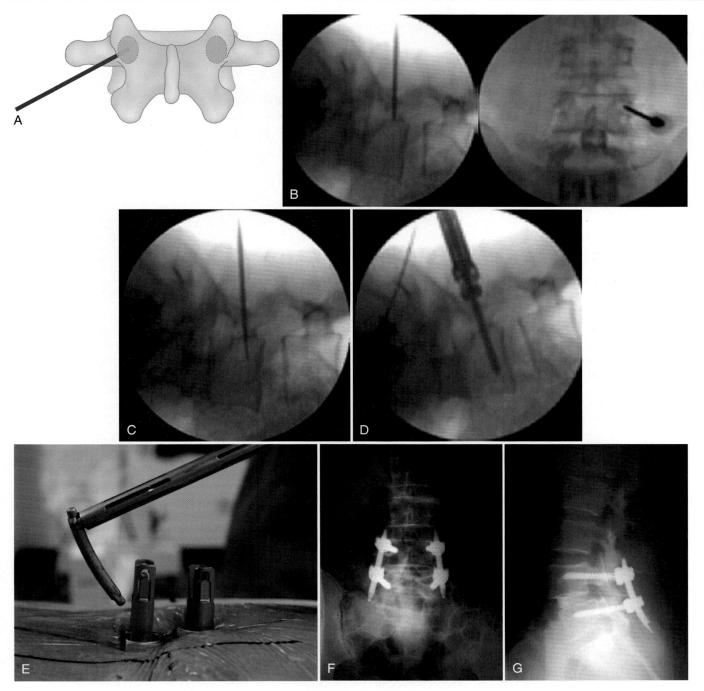

FIGURE 57–7 Pedicle cannulation. **A,** The ideal anteroposterior starting point. **B,** The Jamshidi has been advanced until it sits within the center of the pedicle. A lateral view is obtained. If the Jamshidi tip is at the neurocentral junction then it may be safely advanced under lateral fluoroscopy. **C,** Once the Jamshidi is placed past the neurocentral junction in satisfactory position, the guidewire may be inserted and advanced into the cancellous bone. **D,** The screw holes are tapped and then screws are passed over the guidewires. Intermittent fluoroscopy is recommended to identify potential guidewire migration. **E,** The appropriate-sized rod is passed. Use direct visualization and palpation to avoid trapping muscle beneath the rod. This can lead to severe postoperative pain. **F-G,** Final images.

TABLE 57–1 Minimally Invasive Surgery Transforaminal Lumbar Interbody Fusion (TLIF) Results

Author(s) (Yr)	Procedure N	Diagnosis	EBL (mL)	OR Time (min)	Hospitals Stay (days)	Mean Change ODI	Complications
Schwender et al. 2005[5]	MIS TLIF–PS n = 49	DDD + HNP Spondylolisthesis	<140	240	1.9	32	Technical: 4, pseudo: 0, revisions: 4
Park and Ha 2007[2]	MIS PLIF–PS n = 32 Open PLIF n = 29	Spondylolisthesis Large HNP	433 738	192 149	5.3 10.8	NR NR	Technical: 2, revisions: 4, technical: 0 Revisions: 2
Schizas et al. 2008[4]	MIS TLIF–PS n =18 Open TLIF n = 18	DDD Spondylolisthesis	456 961	NR	6.1 8.2	22 27	Technical: 2, pseudo: 3 Technical: 2, pseudo: 0
Peng et al. 2009[3]	MIS TLIF–PS n = 29 Open TLIF n = 29	Spondylolisthesis DDD	150 681	216 171	4 6.7	29 30	Complication rate: 6.9% Technical: NR, revisions: 0 Solid fusion: 80%*, Complication rate: 13.8%, technical: NR, revisions: 0, solid fusion: 87%*
Dhall et al. 2008[1]	MIS TLIF–MO n = 21 Open TLIF n = 21	Spondylolisthesis DDD	194 505	199 237	3 5.5	NR	Technical: 2, pseudo: 1, revisions: 3 Technical: 2, pseudo: 0, revisions: 1

*Not statistically significant.
DDD, degenerative disc disease; EBL, estimated blood loss; HNP, herniated nucleus pulposus; MIS TLIF–MO, minimally invasive transforaminal lumbar interbody fusion with screws placed by a mini-open technique; MIS TLIF–PS, minimally invasive transforaminal lumbar interbody fusion with percutaneous pedicle screws; NR, not reported in the study; ODI, Oswestry Disability Index; OR, operating room; PLIF, posterior lateral interbody fusion; *pseudo*, pseudoarthrosis.

conventional fluoroscopy or by computer navigation and three-dimensional imaging. The clear concern with the use of fluoroscopy is radiation exposure to both the surgeon and the patient. Bindal and colleagues[16] prospectively recorded radiation exposure in 24 consecutive minimally invasive TLIF procedures. The mean fluoroscopy time was 1.69 minutes (101 seconds). The mean exposure was 76 mRem at the surgeon's dominant hand, 27 mRem under a lead apron, and 32 mRem at an unprotected thyroid level. The mean exposure to the patient's skin was between 59 mRem and 78 mRem depending on the orientation to the x-ray beam. According to Bindal and colleagues the radiation exposure to both surgeon and patient was relatively low. They extrapolated that it would take 194 cases to exceed the acceptable torso radiation limits. The radiation levels they observed also compared favorably with other fluoroscopic procedures such as percutaneous coronary interventions.

Nonetheless, all surgeons should be judicious and minimize radiation exposure to the patient, OR personnel, and themselves. Computer-assisted navigation has been proposed as one means to reduce fluoroscopic use. Kim and colleagues[17] performed a two-phased cadaveric and prospective clinical review comparing navigation-assisted fluoroscopy and standard fluoroscopy use in minimally invasive TLIFs. In the cadaver study they noted a longer setup time for navigation (9.7 minutes) compared with fluoroscopy (4.8 minutes). The mean fluoroscopic time was 42 seconds in the fluoroscopy group and 29 seconds in the navigation group. The average radiation exposure to the surgeon was undetectable in the navigation group and was 12.4 mRem in the fluoroscopic group. Clinically, minimally invasive TLIFs with navigation used 57 seconds of fluoroscopy and minimally invasive TLIFs with fluoroscopy used 147 seconds. Kim and colleagues reported no cases of screw malposition in either group and blood loss, operating time, and hospital stay were similar in both groups.

Pedicle screw navigation is gaining popularity around the United States. Early data suggest that navigation can be used safely for percutaneous pedicle screw placement. However, caution is warranted when known identifiable landmarks are not visualized. The data that navigation provides are only as good as the data it collects. Visual arrays can be dislodged, causing the navigation to err. Surgeon vigilance is required.

PEARLS AND PITFALLS

1. When working through a tubular retractor, remember to move the retractor to see what you want to see and to allow you to position instrumentation in the direction you want to direct it. Do not let the retractor dictate what you see and do.

2. When first placing screws through a tubular retractor, expose the pars and the medial portion of the transverse process well.

3. Pedicle screw tracks may be easier to prepare before performing the decompression and facetectomy when more boney landmarks are present.

4. When placing percutaneous screws, fluoroscopic images must be "perfect" AP and lateral views. Otherwise percutaneous screw placement may be aberrant.

5. Start simple.

KEY POINTS

1. Minimally invasive pedicle screw instrumentation is associated with less blood loss and shorter hospital stays but longer initial operative times.

2. Minimally invasive instrumentation has a lower infection rate then open instrumentation.

3. Obesity is an initial contraindication to minimally invasive instrumentation and fusion, but as a surgeon gains experience, obesity is a relative indication.

4. Technical complications have been comparable in minimally invasive instrumentation and open instrumentation.

KEY REFERENCES

1. Dhall S, Wang M, Mummaneni P: Clinical and radiographic comparison of mini-open transforaminal lumbar interbody fusion with open transforaminal lumbar interbody fusion in 42 patients with long term follow-up. J Neurosurg Spine 9:560-564, 2008.
Retrospective review demonstrating less blood loss and shorter hospital stays, but possibly higher technical complications in 21 patients who underwent a mini-open TLIF compared with 21 patients who underwent a traditional open TLIF.

2. Park P, Upadhyaya H, Garton H, et al: The impact of minimally invasive spine surgery on perioperative complications in overweight or obese patients. Neurosurgery 62:693-699, 2008.
The authors found similar perioperative complication rates in patients with a BMI greater than 25 Kg/m^2 as compared with patients with a BMI less than 25 G/m^2 who underwent minimally invasive spine procedures.

3. Peng C, Yue W, Poh S, et al: Clinical and radiological outcomes of minimally invasive versus open transforaminal lumbar interbody fusion. Spine 34:1385-1389, 2009.
MIS TLIFs were found to have less blood loss, less postoperative pain, shorter hospital stays, and equivalent 2-year clinical results as compared with traditional open TLIFs.

4. O'Toole J, Eichholz K, Fessler R: Surgical infection rates after minimally invasive spinal surgery. J Neurosurg Spine 11:471-476, 2009.
The authors report a 0.22% surgical site infection rate after reviewing 1338 minimally invasive surgical procedures.

5. Kim D, Lee S, Chung S, et al: Comparison of multifidus muscle atrophy and trunk extension muscle strength. Percutaneous versus open pedicle screw fixation. Spine 30:123-129,2005.
Multifidus muscle cross-sectional area and trunk extension muscle strength were compared in patients undergoing open and percutaneous pedicle screw fixation.

REFERENCES

1. Dhall SS, Wang MY, Mummaneni PV: Clinical and radiographic comparison of mini-open transforaminal lumbar interbody fusion with open transforaminal lumbar interbody fusion in 42 patients with long-term follow-up. J Neurosurg Spine 9:560-565, 2008.

2. Park Y, Ha JW: Comparison of one-level posterior lumbar interbody fusion performed with a minimally invasive approach or a traditional open approach. Spine (Phila Pa 1976) 32:537-543, 2007.

3. Peng CW, Yue WM, Poh SY, et al: Clinical and radiological outcomes of minimally invasive versus open transforaminal lumbar interbody fusion. Spine (Phila Pa 1976) 34:1385-1389, 2009.

4. Schizas C, Tzinieris N, Tsiridis E, et al: Minimally invasive versus open transforaminal lumbar interbody fusion: evaluating initial experience. Int Orthop 33:1683-1688, 2009.

5. Schwender JD, Holly LT, Rouben DP, et al: Minimally invasive transforaminal lumbar interbody fusion (TLIF): technical feasibility and initial results. J Spinal Disord Tech 18 Suppl:S1-S6, 2005.

6. Rosen DS, Ferguson SD, Ogden AT, et al: Obesity and self-reported outcome after minimally invasive lumbar spinal fusion surgery. Neurosurgery 63:956-960, 2008; discussion 60.

7. Park P, Upadhyaya C, Garton HJ, et al: The impact of minimally invasive spine surgery on perioperative complications in overweight or obese patients. Neurosurgery 62:693-699, 2008; discussion 693-699.

8. O'Toole JE, Eichholz KM, Fessler RG: Surgical site infection rates after minimally invasive spinal surgery. J Neurosurg Spine 11:471-476, 2009.

9. Picada R, Winter RB, Lonstein JE, et al: Postoperative deep wound infection in adults after posterior lumbosacral spine fusion with instrumentation: incidence and management. J Spinal Disord 13:42-45, 2000.

10. Foley KT, Holly LT, Schwender JD: Minimally invasive lumbar fusion. Spine (Phila Pa 1976) 28:S26-S35, 2003.

11. Holly LT, Schwender JD, Rouben DP, et al: Minimally invasive transforaminal lumbar interbody fusion: indications, technique, and complications. Neurosurg Focus 20:E6, 2006.

12. Kim KT, Lee SH, Suk KS, et al: The quantitative analysis of tissue injury markers after mini-open lumbar fusion. Spine (Phila Pa 1976) 31:712-716, 2006.

13. Wiltse LL, Bateman JG, Hutchinson RH, et al: The paraspinal sacrospinalis-splitting approach to the lumbar spine. J Bone Joint Surg Am 50:919-926, 1968.

14. Kim DY, Lee SH, Chung SK, et al: Comparison of multifidus muscle atrophy and trunk extension muscle strength: percutaneous versus open pedicle screw fixation. Spine (Phila Pa 1976) 30:123-129, 2005.

15. Regev GJ, Lee YP, Taylor WR, et al: Nerve injury to the posterior rami medial branch during the insertion of pedicle screws: comparison of mini-open versus percutaneous pedicle screw insertion techniques. Spine (Phila Pa 1976) 34:1239-1242, 2009.

16. Bindal RK, Glaze S, Ognoskie M, et al: Surgeon and patient radiation exposure in minimally invasive transforaminal lumbar interbody fusion. J Neurosurg Spine 9:570-573, 2008.

17. Kim CW, Lee YP, Taylor W, et al: Use of navigation-assisted fluoroscopy to decrease radiation exposure during minimally invasive spine surgery. Spine J 8:584-590, 2008.

Minimally Invasive Posterior Lumbar Fusion Techniques

Chadi Tannoury, MD
Amar A. Patel, BS
D. Greg Anderson, MD

Lumbar fusion is a reliable treatment option for a wide variety of spinal pathologies resulting in spinal column instability and/or spinal-related pain. Various spinal fusion techniques are the subject of ongoing clinical investigations with goals to improve surgical technique, graft biomaterials, and implant designs in order to achieve a stable, symptom-free spinal column with the least chance of patient morbidity.

Despite these advances, the morbidity of spinal fusion surgery remains significant. The standard posterior midline exposure is notorious for paraspinal muscle stripping and denervation leading to significant postoperative scar formation. The limitations of this approach for spinal fusion have been well documented, especially regarding a prolonged recovery period and muscle damage that may affect a patient following surgery.[1-5]

In recent years, less invasive surgical approaches have been developed to minimize damage to the paraspinal soft tissues during surgical exposure. These "minimally invasive" surgical approaches are becoming more popular because they offer the surgeon a method to achieve the goals of spinal surgery while minimizing some of the perioperative morbidity inherent to the classic posterior approach.[6,7]

Minimally invasive spinal surgery (MISS) is a rapidly evolving field that is supported by a number of technologic innovations. These include the operative microscope, C-arm fluoroscopy, tubular retractor systems, cannulated pedicle screws, and for some, image guidance systems. The basic hand instruments used during a minimally invasive spinal procedure are similar to those used during a traditional spinal case but are often longer and bayoneted to improve visualization through a tubular retraction system. A high-speed burr or drill with a long and thin shaft is useful in decorticating or thinning the bony elements of the spine. To be successful with MISS, a surgeon must be familiar with the microscopic anatomy of the spine. He or she must gain the skills necessary to work safely and efficiently despite a limited field of view and become facile with the use of MISS equipment. This set of skills can only be gained with experience, and thus a significant but definable learning curve should be anticipated by surgeons interested in becoming proficient in MISS techniques. The length and slope of the learning curve will also depend on the individual surgeon's skill set and prior spinal experience. The learning process is best accomplished in a slow, step-wise fashion, mastering basic skills with simple cases before attempting to approach the more challenging spinal pathologies in a minimally invasive surgical fashion. This chapter provides an overview to the field of MISS as it applies to lumbar fusion techniques for common conditions of the lumbar spine.

Principles of Minimally Invasive Spinal Surgery

All minimally invasive spinal procedures, despite the type and the location, have the common goal of correcting the underlying spinal pathology while avoiding excessive damage to the paraspinal soft tissue envelope. As with other spine procedures, an MISS procedure begins with the careful analysis of the preoperative imaging studies to precisely localize the spinal pathology. Before making a surgical incision, preoperative fluoroscopy is used to localize the involved spinal segments and plan the skin incision. During the surgical approach, the paraspinal muscles are split rather than cut or resected using serial tubular dilators to create a surgical corridor between the skin incision and the spine (Fig. 58-1). Only necessary portions of the vertebral columns are exposed, and excessive use of electrocautery or vigorous retractor pressures should be avoided.

The surgeon must understand the muscular anatomy of the paraspinal region to design the optimal approach for an MISS procedure. There are two distinct muscular compartments: the multifidus compartment, which overlies the midline spinal structures, and the lateral compartment, which overlies the transverse processes (Fig. 58-2). The multifidus muscle surrounds the spinous processes, lamina, and facet joints. The multifidus muscles receive its nerve and blood supply from the medial branches of the dorsal rami and segmental vessels, respectively, which course from the intervertebral foramen along the base of the transverse process and enter the lateral margin of the muscle in the region of the pars intra-articularis. Care should be taken to avoid rupturing the lateral attachments of the multifidus muscle, which would disrupt the nerve

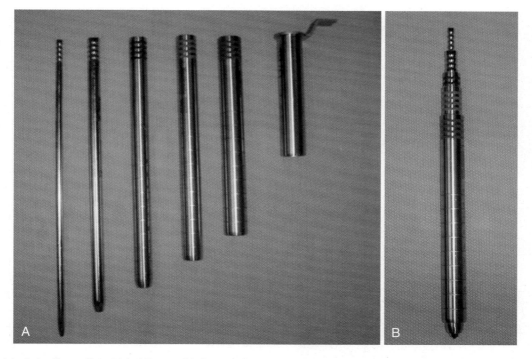

FIGURE 58-1 Serial tubular dilators (**A,** individual; **B,** assembled) are used to gain access to the spine through muscle-splitting rather than cutting through the paraspinal muscles.

and blood supply to the multifidus muscle, leading to atrophy and scar formation in the substance of the muscle. The lateral muscle compartment contains the longitudinally oriented muscles of the erector spinae group. The lateral compartment overlies the transverse processes and includes the entry site for pedicle screw insertion at the base of the transverse process. The lateral compartment is traversed whenever a posterolateral onlay fusion is performed.

When approaching the spinal canal, laminae, or facet joint, a trans-multifidus compartment approach is required. When placing percutaneous pedicle screws or performing a posterolateral onlay fusion, a translateral compartment approach is necessary. To operate within a particular compartment, the fascia over that compartment should be opened and then the muscular tissues dilated or split to reach the spinal structures of interest. When moving from compartment to compartment, the surgeon should never transgress the fascial barrier between the compartments because this would disrupt the nerve and blood supply to the multifidus muscle. Instead, the retractor should be withdrawn and the fascia should be opened over the other compartment followed by a muscle-splitting approach to the spinal contents of the compartment. The same skin incision can generally be used for two separate fascial incisions used to access the compartments.

When discussing a minimally invasive surgical approach with a patient, the surgeon should ensure that the patient understands the available surgical options (both MISS and open surgery) for treating the spinal condition. In addition, the surgeon should include in the surgical consent process the possibility that the less invasive procedure may need to be converted to a larger, open approach to achieve the ultimate goals of surgery. Both the surgeon and patient should remember that correction of the spinal pathology is the most

important issue, whereas the approach and incisional size are lesser considerations.

Surgical Setup for a Posterior Fusion Procedure

Setup and Imaging

Following placement of surgical monitoring equipment and the induction of general anesthesia, the patient should be

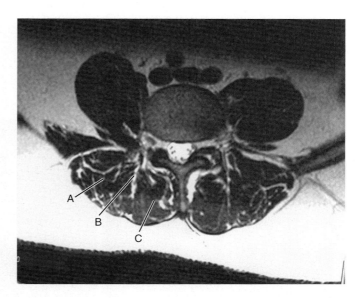

FIGURE 58-2 Deep paraspinal muscle compartment: The multifidus muscle (**C**) overlies the midline, and the lateral compartment (**A, B**) contains the longissimus and iliocostalis muscles, overlying the transverse processes.

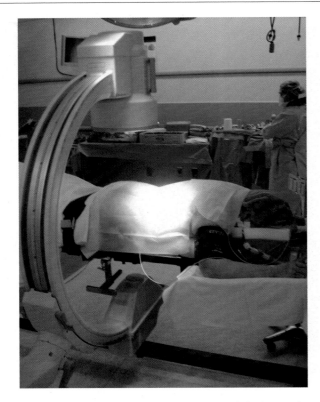

FIGURE 58–3 The patient is positioned prone on a radiolucent spinal frame.

the proposed trajectory of the surgical incision and check the position of the needle on both anteroposterior (AP) and lateral fluoroscopic views to ensure an optimal path to the pathology is achieved.

Surgical Incisions and Approach

The number and length of skin incisions should correspond to the surgical plan, which must be more "thought out" compared with a traditional open surgery. A single skin incision may be used during different phases of the surgical procedure to reach different areas of the spine. For instance, one incision may initially be used to decompress the neural elements (multifidus compartment). Subsequently, the same skin incision may be used to perform a posterolateral fusion and place pedicle screw instrumentation (lateral compartment). Although a single skin incision is used, separate fascial incisions should be used to reach each individual compartment.

When working through perimedian incisions, two distinct fascial layers are encountered. The superficial layer corresponds to the thoracodorsal fascia, while the deeper layer is a thin fascia that overlies the muscle of the compartment. Both fascial incisions should be a little longer than the corresponding skin incision because this will allow the subsequently placed tubular retractors to be maneuvered and angulated freely as needed to reach the various areas of the spine necessary to perform the operation. The muscles of the compartment can be split with the surgeon's digit or with an instrument such as a Cobb elevator. It is often helpful to palpate bony landmarks such as the facet joint or transverse processes to assist with placement of the initial instruments through the skin and muscle portal to the vertebral column.

When operating through a tubular retractor, the smallest dilator is then docked at the appropriate bony site and serial dilation is used to expand the operative corridor. Care should be taken into bringing each subsequent dilator in contact with the bony elements. The correct length of the tubular retractor can then be selected, inserted, and secured using an operating table–mounted retractor holder. Once the tubular retractor is in place, the position of the retractor should be verified using fluoroscopy (Fig. 58–4).

positioned prone on a radiolucent spinal frame (Fig. 58–3). The abdomen should be free of compression, and free access to the lumbar region for fluoroscopy should be confirmed. The preoperative imaging studies should be available in the room with the operative plan clearly marked. The surgeon should ensure the availability of the proper implants and instruments prior to commencing with the operative procedure.

After a sterile skin preparation and draping, the C-arm mobile fluoroscopy unit is used to demarcate the location of bony landmarks, which are drawn on the skin. A critical step is to ensure that the skin incisions are localized in an optimal position to allow access to the underlying spinal pathology. In some cases, it may be useful to introduce a spinal needle along

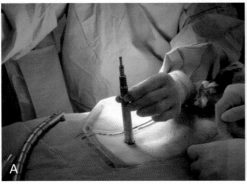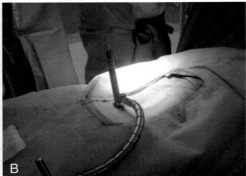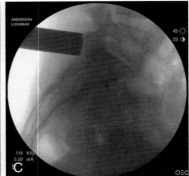

FIGURE 58–4 Following insertion of the tubular dilator system (**A**), the tubular retractor is secured in place using an operating table mounted rigid retractor holder (**B**). Fluoroscopy is used to verify correct positioning of the tubular retractor (**C**).

Spinal Decompression

The topic of spinal decompression is substantial and exceeds the goals of this chapter; however, a few points deserve mention. The authors prefer to perform the decompression first when performing both a decompression and fusion of the lumbar spine. This allows the surgeon to obtain local autogenous bone from the decompression site that may be used for the spine fusion and also exposes important bony landmarks such as the pedicle, which is useful in subsequent stages of the procedure. The decompression is done by entering and traversing the multifidus compartment. Thus it is useful to perform a facet fusion during this phase of the procedure, before exiting the multifidus compartment.

Posterior Interbody and Transforaminal Interbody Fusion

When performing a posterior or transforaminal lumbar interbody fusion (PLIF and TLIF) via a minimally invasive approach, it is important to align the tubular retractor collinear with the disc space on the lateral view (Fig. 58–5). When performing a TLIF procedure, the tubular retractor must be aligned with enough lateral to medial angulation to allow the surgeon to reach the contralateral side of the disc space for preparation of an adequate fusion bed (Fig. 58–6). During the exposure, adequate facet joint must be removed to minimize retraction of the neural elements and provide working access to the disc space.[8]

The detrimental effects of over-retraction of the neural elements with the PLIF procedure have been well documented in the literature.[9] Facet removals for a PLIF or TLIF can be achieved with either osteotomes or a high-speed burr. It is helpful to skeletonize the upper and medial portions of the caudal pedicle (e.g., L5 pedicle for a L4-5 TLIF) to gain adequate access to the disc space and allow safe retraction/protection of the dural/neural elements.

Once the disc space has been adequately exposed, the posterolateral annulus is incised with a scalpel and the posterior margin of the disc is removed. The posterior "lip" of the vertebral body should be resected so that the opening is flush with the most concaved portions of the disc space. Disc material and the cartilaginous endplates are thoroughly débrided from the interbody space using curettes, shavers, and/or pituitary rongeurs until the interspace is clean, leaving only intact bony endplates to support the interbody cage. If the disc space is collapsed, the endplates should be dilated to restore the foraminal height and improve the sagittal contour of the spine.

After disc space preparation, the interspace should be packed with autogenous bone graft or an adequate fusion substrate. An interbody fusion cage, of appropriate size, is selected and packed with the graft material, before impacting the cage into the disc space. The optimal position of the cage is toward the anterior portion of the disc space.[10,11] This produces better reconstruction of the sagittal contour of the spine and allows

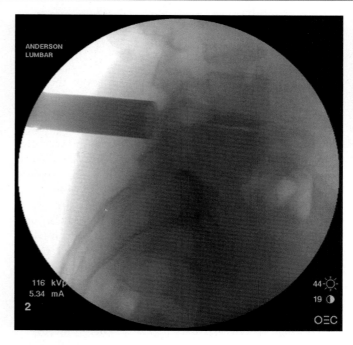

FIGURE 58–5 Lateral fluoroscopic view shows the tubular retractor positioned in a proper alignment (i.e., collinear with the disc space).

ample bone graft material to be packed around and behind the cage.

Instrumentation, most commonly with pedicle screws, is a standard component of both the modern PLIF and TLIF procedures. Following the insertion of pedicle screws and rods, compression of the interbody construct is performed to restore the lumbar lordosis and ensure compressive loading of the interbody grafts.

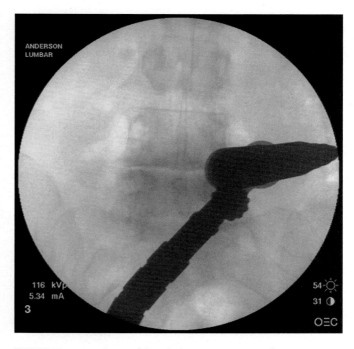

FIGURE 58–6 Angulation of the tubular retractor system allows access to the contralateral side of the disc space and therefore preparation of the fusion bed.

Posterolateral Fusion (Intertransverse Onlay Fusion)

From the traditional midline approach, access to the intertransverse region for onlay fusion requires complete stripping of the paraspinal muscles to the tips of the transverse processes, an act that causes destruction, or at least disruption, of the multifidus muscle and significant postoperative scarring.[5] Using the paraspinal muscle-splitting approach (Wiltse approach), exposure of the intertransverse region is simple to achieve without major muscle stripping. This provides direct access to the intertransverse region for fusion.

The skin incision for a paraspinal approach for intertransverse fusion is made at least 3.5 to 4 cm lateral to the midline. The fascia is divided in line with the skin incision, and the paraspinal muscles are split in line with their fibers to expose the transverse processes. For fusion purposes, the entire transverse process at both levels should be exposed. Either a tubular retractor (preferably an expandable tubular retractor) or side-to-side (e.g., McCullough retractor) retractor can be used to visualize the intertransverse interval. The authors prefer to use an expandable tubular retractor, which allows both transverse processes to be simultaneously exposed (Fig. 58–7).

Once the intertransverse region has been exposed, the soft tissues are meticulously cleaned away from the transverse processes and intertransverse membrane. The transverse processes are decorticated using a high-speed burr and then the interval is packed with autogenous bone graft or a suitable graft material. When withdrawing the retractors, care should be taken to not displace the graft materials from the fusion bed.

Facet Fusion

Fusion of the facet joints is useful as an adjunct to interbody or intertransverse fusion but has not been well accepted as a stand-alone fusion due to the relatively small surface area of the facet joints. However, the facet joint offers a number of theoretical advantages as a fusion site including the ease of access to the joint, the small gap across which the fusion must heal, and the compression of the fusion site that is achieved during normal upright posture of the patient. In addition, a facet fusion is a quick, simple, and low-morbidity procedure.

To perform a facet fusion, the retractor should be docked on the facet, which resides in the lateral portion of the multifidus compartment (see Fig. 58–2). If decompression of the spinal canal is required, facet fusion can easily be performed during the exposure through the multifidus compartment. Once the facet is exposed, the capsule is removed with electrocautery and the articular surfaces of the inferior and superior articular processes are identified. A high-speed burr is used to decorticate the facet joint along its entire length, and the joint space is packed with fragments of autogenous bone or a suitable bone substitute.

In some cases osteophytic bone material may overlie the true facet joint, and this should be removed to expose the native joint surfaces. The surgeon should be cognizant of the normal anatomy of the facet joint with the superior articular process lying lateral and deep to the inferior articular process. The specific topography of the facet joint can also be defined preoperatively by analyzing imaging studies (magnetic resonance imaging [MRI] or computed tomography [CT]).

Instrumentation of the Spine

Pedicle Screw Instrumentation

Pedicle screw instrumentation has emerged as the most common form of internal fixation used for thoracolumbar arthrodesis. Pedicle screws offer numerous advantages compared with hooks or wires, which are less rigid. Pedicle screws can be used when posterior spinal elements are deficient due to prior surgery, and they provide rigid segmental immobilization, thereby minimizing the need for postoperative brace immobilization. Because of the three-column support provided by the transpedicular fixation, these implants are effectively used in various complex spinal pathologies including deformities, which require corrective forces to be employed.[12]

With the advent of cannulated pedicle screws systems, these implants can be placed through the same skin incisions used for the decompression or fusion portions of the spinal operation. Our preference is to place instrumentation as the final stage of surgery so that the bulk of the implants will not physically interfere with other stages of the operation.

Some surgeons prefer to use noncannulated pedicle screws, placed with direct visualization of the spinal anatomy, using an expandable tubular retractor system. This approach is best used for short procedures (one to two levels) in the lower lumbar spine, where the natural spinal lordosis brings the trajectory of the pedicles into close proximity. In such a situation, it is not difficult to place pedicle screws at adjacent levels using a small, paramedian incision and appropriate expandable retractor system. Placement of pedicle screws in an MISS

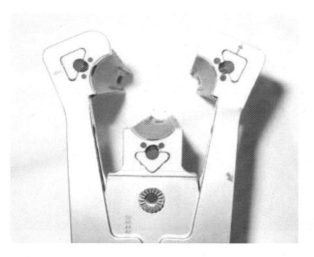

FIGURE 58–7 The use of an expandable tubular retractor allows simultaneous exposure of both transverse processes.

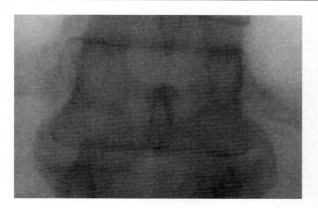

FIGURE 58–8 True anteroposterior imaging of each vertebra to be instrumented is crucial for safe pedicle screw placement.

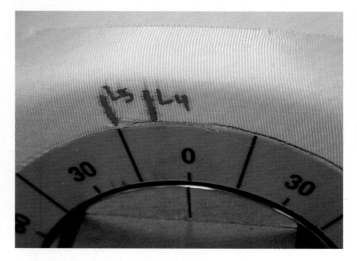

FIGURE 58–9 Marking of the exact C-arm angle where the true AP image can be obtained helps the radiology technician and assists rapid return to the proper image.

fashion offers significant advantages compared with traditional pedicle screw instrumentation, which requires full exposure of the spine and major paraspinal muscle stripping.

Cannulated Pedicle Screw Insertion

The first step in placing cannulated pedicle screws involves obtaining a true AP image of each vertebra to be instrumented (Fig. 58–8). Because of the natural sagittal contour of the spine, the C-arm must be angulated to the specific sagittal profile of each individual vertebra in order to obtain the true AP view. It is helpful to have the radiology technician mark the exact angle of the C-arm where the true AP image can be obtained to assist rapid return to the proper image (Fig. 58–9). A properly aligned AP C-arm image will demonstrate the superior vertebral endplate as a single, dense line, and the pedicles will be localized just below the upper endplate. Correct rotation of the vertebrae is ensured when the spinous process shadow is centered between the pedicles. The true AP view is most useful when cannulating the pedicle during pedicle screw insertion.

True lateral fluoroscopic images are also used during pedicle screw instrumentation, particularly during assembly of the construct (Fig. 58–10). The true lateral image will demonstrate the superior endplate as a single, dense line. The pedicles will be superimposed. The posterior cortex of the vertebral body should also appear to be a single radiopaque line, confirming that no rotation of the vertebra is present. The true lateral view is useful during pedicle tapping, placement of pedicle screws, and assembly of the construct. In cases where scoliosis is present, the C-arm may need to be angled (i.e., "wig-waged") to obtain a true lateral view of each vertebra.

When performing percutaneous instrumentation, obtaining properly aligned C-arm images are, by far, the most important step in the procedure. Thus it cannot be overemphasized that good images should be obtained before attempting to implant percutaneous pedicle screws. If adequate C-arm images cannot be obtained due to severe osteopenia, obesity, intra-abdominal contrast, or any other reason, placement of percutaneous pedicle screw implants should not be attempted.

After obtaining a true AP fluoroscopic image of a given level, a K-wire should be aligned over the skin of the back so that it appears to bisect the pedicles (Fig. 58–11). Next, a horizontal line is drawn along the skin using the K-wire (Fig. 58–12). This step should be repeated using a true AP image for each of the vertebrae in the construct. Vertical lines are then drawn (using a K-wire placed over the skin of the back) along the lateral pedicle shadow (Fig. 58–13). Skin incisions for percutaneous pedicle screw insertion should be placed about 1 cm lateral to the vertical line (Fig. 58–14).

Once the skin and fascia have been divided, the surgeon can digitally palpate the transverse process of the vertebra whose pedicles are to be cannulated. A Jamshidi needle is then placed at the base of the transverse process (at the junction of the transverse process and superior articular process), and a true AP image is obtained (Fig. 58–15). The goal is to position

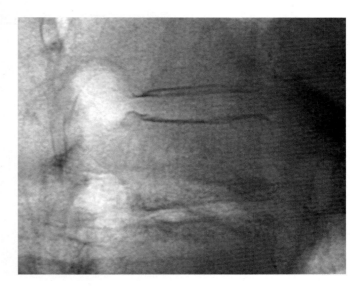

FIGURE 58–10 True lateral images are also necessary for proper pedicle screw instrumentation.

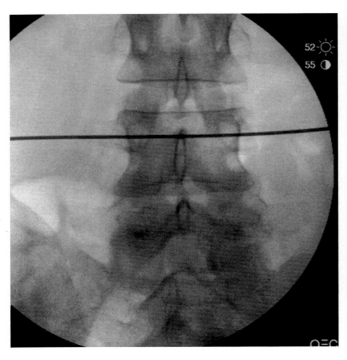

FIGURE 58-11 Marking the skin (horizontally): With fluoroscopic assistance, a K-wire is placed horizontally over the skin of the back bisecting the pedicles of the level to be addressed.

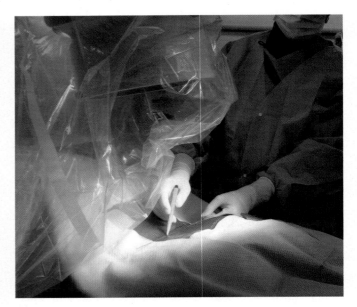

FIGURE 58-12 The skin is marked using the K-wire to draw a horizontal line.

FIGURE 58-13 A, Marking the skin (vertically): Under fluoroscopy, the K-wire is vertically placed over the skin of the back and positioned along the lateral pedicle shadow. B, The skin is then marked using the K-wire as a reference to draw a vertical line.

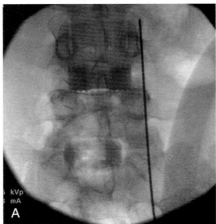

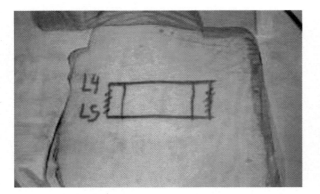

FIGURE 58-14 Skin incisions, for percutaneous pedicle screws instrumentation, are placed 1 cm lateral to the marked vertical lines.

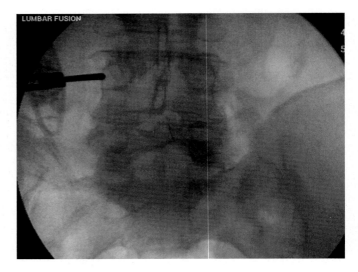

FIGURE 58-15 The Jamshidi needle is placed, with fluoroscopic assistance, at the base of the transverse process.

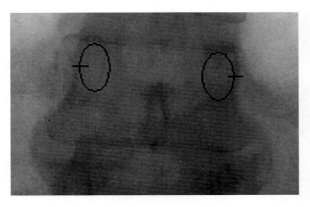

FIGURE 58–16 True AP view illustrates the recommended positioning of the needle tip over the lateral margin of the pedicle shadow at the 3 o'clock and 9 o'clock positions.

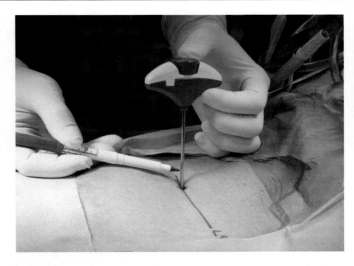

FIGURE 58–18 The Jamshidi needle is marked 20 mm above the skin edge, an estimate of the depth of the pedicle.

the tip of the needle directly over the lateral margin of the pedicle shadow (at the 3 o'clock and 9 o'clock positions) on the true AP view (Fig. 58–16). The tip of the needle should be adjusted until the tip of the needle lies directly at the lateral boarder of the pedicle. The needle shaft is then aligned parallel to the endplate (or transverse process) on the AP image, which ensures a needle trajectory parallel to central axis of the pedicle (Fig. 58–17). The shaft of the needle should also be held with a lateral to medial trajectory of approximately 10 to 15 degrees, depending on the level to approximate the normal divergence of the pedicles anatomically. Then, the needle is tapped gently a few times to seat the needle tip into the bone and ensure that slippage of the needle tip does not occur as the needle is driven through the pedicle. A final true AP image is checked to be sure that the needle is properly positioned and aligned.

Next, a line is drawn on the shaft of the Jamshidi needle, 20 mm above the skin edge (Fig. 58–18). Because the average length of the pedicle is 20 mm from the starting point, this line is used to determine the depth of the needle tip as it is driven through the pedicle. With the Jamshidi needle properly aligned, the needle is tapped with a mallet to drive the needle through the bone of the central pedicle. When this line on the needle shaft reaches the skin edge, the needle tip has traversed

the pedicle isthmus and is at approximately the depth of the base of the pedicle. At this point another true AP fluoroscopic image is obtained to ensure that the needle tip lies well within the pedicle shadow, no more than three fourths of the distance (from lateral to medial) across the pedicle (Fig. 58–19). This true AP image should be critically analyzed, and if the needle tip is in proper position, then it is deemed acceptable for pedicle screw insertion.

Next, the Jamshidi needle is driven 5 to 10 mm deeper into the vertebral body and a guidewire is inserted through the Jamshidi needle, into the cancellous bone of the vertebral body. The surgeon should feel "crunchy," cancellous bone at the base of the needle and will generally be able to insert the guidewire 10 to 15 mm beyond the needle tip into the vertebral body with manual pressure. If the bone is too hard for manual insertion, a Kocher clamp can be placed on the guidewire 10 mm above the top of the Jamshidi needle and tapped with a mallet to achieve positioning of the guidewire into the vertebral body. The same procedure is repeated for all the pedicles in the surgical construct. It is the author's preference to cannulate all pedicles in the construct using AP fluoroscopy before adjusting the C-arm into the lateral position.

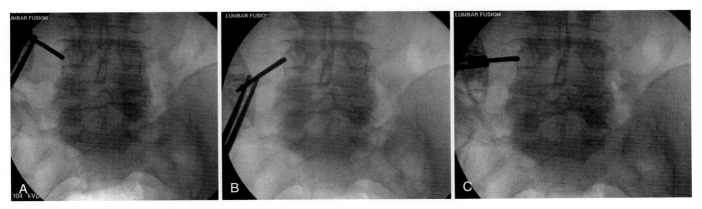

FIGURE 58–17 Fluoroscopy is valuable in localizing the needle tip at the lateral border of the pedicle (**A** and **B**) and the needle shaft parallel to the endplate (**C**).

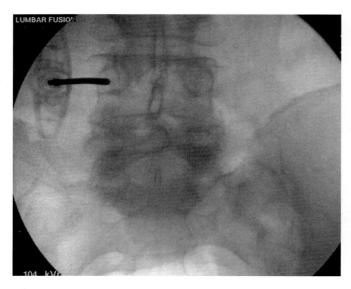

FIGURE 58–19 On true AP fluoroscopy, the needle tip should be located within the pedicle shadow, no more than three fourths of the distance across the pedicle.

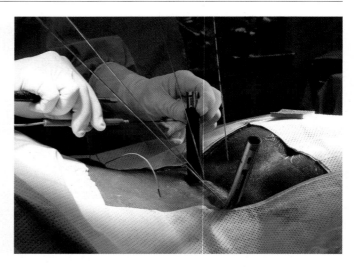

FIGURE 58–21 Following their insertion, pedicle screws are tested with stimulus-evoked electromyography, using an insulated port.

Once all of the pedicles in the construct have been cannulated and guidewires have been placed, the C-arm is adjusted to obtain true lateral images of the spine (Fig. 58–20). The position of the guidewires on the lateral fluoroscopic view is verified before proceeding with pedicle preparation. Pedicle preparation and pedicle screws placement are then carried starting from one end of the construct in an "assembly line" fashion. Each pedicle is tapped using a cannulated tap. The authors prefer to stimulate the tap using stimulus-evoked EMG to ensure no low voltage activity is present. If so, it might indicate a breech of the pedicle. Then cannulated pedicle

screws are placed over the guidewires at each level and threaded into the pedicles. The pedicle screws are adjusted in height as needed to maintain polyaxial motion of the screw crowns and to achieve a smooth contour of the screws at adjacent levels (necessary for rod seating). It is also the author's preference to stimulate each pedicle screw, after insertion with stimulus-evoked EMG, using an insulated port over the screws (Fig. 58–21).

Once are the screws are positioned, the proper rod length is measured and rods are inserted through the screw extensions and into the screw crowns. The details of rod insertion differ slightly among manufacturers of cannulated screw systems. The surgeon should be familiar with the details of the specific system selected. After the rods are placed, screw caps are inserted into each screw to capture the rod. Compression or distraction of the construct can be performed as needed, followed by final tightening of the construct. At the conclusion of the procedure, AP and lateral imaging of the entire construct should be obtained (Fig. 58–22).

Technical Tips

A few technical points are worth mentioning. First, the advancement of the Jamshidi needle across the pedicle should proceed smoothly with light to moderate taps of the mallet. If the surgeon encounters very hard bone, it generally indicates that the needle tip is displaced medially into the facet joint (the needle tip is striking the hard cortical surface of the superior articular facet). In this instance, the surgeon should withdraw the needle tip and begin with a slightly more lateral starting point to prevent the needle tip from slipping into the facet joint. Another useful tip is to consider the en face view if the AP view fails to clearly show the outline of the pedicle (this is most commonly a concern at the L5 level). To obtain an en face view, start with a true AP view and then angulate the C-arm 10 to 15 degrees in the axial plane to line up the beam with the pedicle axis (Fig. 58–23). Using the en face view, the center of the pedicle should be targeted, keeping the

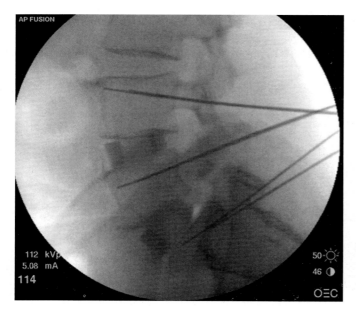

FIGURE 58–20 True lateral fluoroscopic image showing the guidewires properly placed within the pedicles.

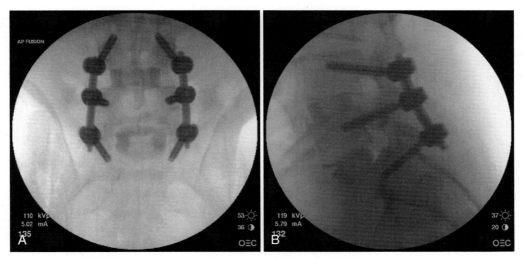

FIGURE 58–22 Anteroposterior (**A**) and lateral (**B**) fluoroscopic views of the construct at the conclusion of the procedure.

shaft of the needle in line with the C-arm beam. Another useful tip concerns making minor adjustments to a cannulated pedicle screw trajectory. In such a case, the pedicle can be tapped (with a cannulated tap) to the base of the pedicle and then, leaving the tap in place, the guidewire can be withdrawn into the tap, allowing the trajectory of the tap to be adjusted as desired with the assistance of fluoroscopy. Once the new trajectory is achieved, the guidewire is reinserted into the vertebral body along the new trajectory. Finally, stimulus-evoked EMG testing of the taps and screws has proven to be a useful adjuvant to the placement of percutaneous pedicle screws. Any low voltage activity (<8 mV) should alert the surgeon to pursue additional measures to ensure correct placement of the implant.

Direct Pedicle Screw Insertion via a Paramedian Approach

Some surgeons prefer direct insertion of pedicle screws, using an expandable tubular retractor system to directly visualize the anatomic landmarks for pedicle screw insertion. This approach is especially useful when performing a minimally invasive TLIF procedure. In this technique, an expandable tubular retractor is positioned to visualize the junction between the base of the transverse process and the superior articular process. Any overlying soft tissue is cleared away using electrocautery to expose the bony landmarks. A starting hole for the pedicle screw insertion is then made using the normal anatomic landmarks as with traditional open pedicle screw insertion. C-arm fluoroscopy can be used to document the location of the starting point and trajectory for the pedicle cannulation. A "gear shift" or similar type blunt instrument is inserted into the starting hole and passed through the pedicle, using fluoroscopic guidance as needed. The walls of the pedicle are palpated to ensure the absence of a breach. Next, the site is tapped and the walls of the pedicle are again palpated for integrity. Pedicle screws are inserted using a technique analogous to open pedicle screw placement. Electrical testing of the screw can be used if desired, followed by the introduction of a rod and caps.

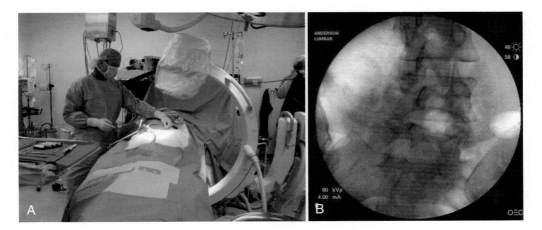

FIGURE 58–23 En face view: obtained through angulating the C-arm 10 to 15 degrees in the axial plane (**A**) to line up the beam with the pedicle axis (**B**).

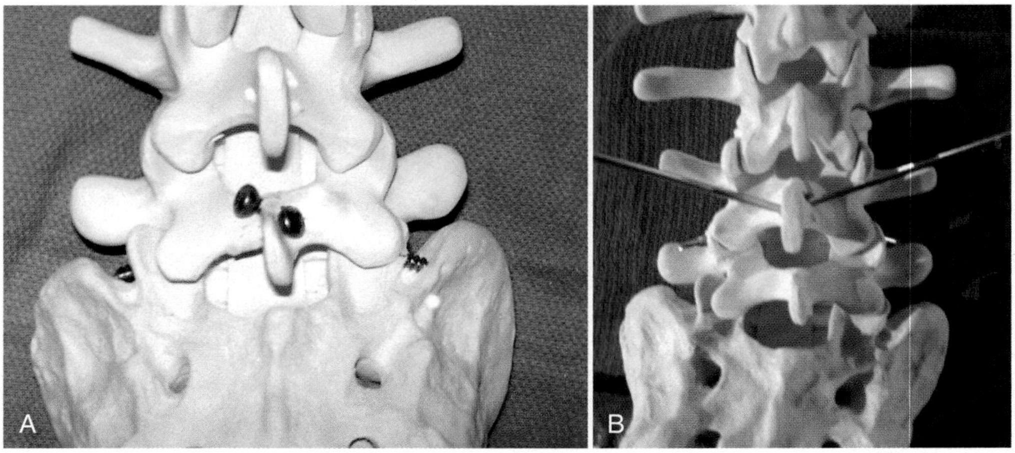

FIGURE 58–24 Facet screw instrumentation (**A**): The screw path begins at the base of the spinous process on one side and then advances across the contralateral lamina and facet joint (**B**).

Facet Screw Instrumentation

Although pedicle screws are the "work horse" for most spinal fixation strategies, facet screws offer certain advantages in selected cases. Facet screws are quick and relatively easy to place. They are generally less expensive, compared with pedicle screw implants, and yet offer comparable initial stiffness for short constructs.[13] In certain clinical situations such as following anterior lumbar interbody fusion, facet screw instrumentation has been shown to produce favorable clinical results.[14,15]

Benini and Magerl[16] described a technique using large-fragment (4.5-mm) cortical bone screws to perform a translaminar fixation of the facet joint. The screw path begins at the base of the spinous process on one side and is then advanced across the contralateral lamina and facet joint (Fig. 58–24). Two screws are placed to immobilize the facet joints bilaterally using a miniopen or percutaneous technique.[17,18]

To insert translaminar facet screws using the miniopen technique, a midline incision is performed and the spinous processes, bilateral laminae, and facet joints are exposed. The facet joint capsules may be removed and the joint decorticated and packed with bone graft to promote local fusion following instrumentation. When placing translaminar facet screws, pilot holes are made on each side of the spinous process in line with the anticipated screw trajectories. The pilot holes should be slightly staggered to prevent the two screws from contacting one another as they cross through the base of the spinous process.

Next, the trajectory for each screw is defined, using fluoroscopy if desired. Some surgeons prefer to make a small laminotomy and palpate the medial wall of the pedicle as a landmark. This ensures direct visualization of the dura during intralaminar drilling for the screw path. Additionally, decompression of the lateral recess using a fenestration technique can be performed as needed.

Next, a line connecting the midfacet (or medial boarder of the pedicle) and the pilot hole is marked on the skin. This trajectory can be extended superiorly and laterally to the midline incision. A small, percutaneous incision is made along this line, about 10 to 12 cm from the midline such that the drill trajectory will be in line with the contralateral lamina. A drill guide is inserted into the percutaneous incision and advanced into the midline exposure (Fig. 58–25). The drill is inserted and seated into the pilot hole at the base of the spinous process. The drill is adjusted as needed so that the drill will traverse the lamina and then facet joint. As the drill is advanced, the surgeon should feel uniform resistance until the facet joint has been breeched. A momentary change in resistance may be noted as the facet joint space is traversed, but the cortical bone of the superior articular process will then be encountered. After drilling, the length of the screw path is measured. Then, a 4.5-mm, fully threaded cortical screw is placed to secure the position of the facet joint. A similar, percutaneous technique has been described, relying only on fluoroscopic images to ensure adequate placement of the translaminar facet screw implants.[15]

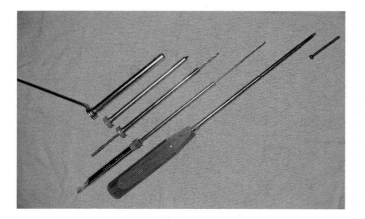

FIGURE 58–25 Facet screw instrumentation: Various instruments (e.g., drill guides, depth gauge, screws) are used during percutaneous facet screws placement.

Patient Selection

Patient selection remains the most crucial outcome variable for any spinal procedure.[19] The same selection criteria that have been shown to produce success in traditional spinal surgery apply to patient selection for an MISS approach. In addition, patients being considered for an MISS approach have some additional selection criteria that should be considered.[20]

In the early experience of an individual surgeon, only simple cases should be considered for an MISS approach. Experience can be gained working with MISS equipment such as tubular retractors and microscopes by performing straightforward cases (e.g., microdiscectomy). As a surgeon gains experience with minimally invasive spinal procedures, progressively more complex cases may be tackled in a minimally invasive fashion. Other aspects should be considered as well including the size of the patient (obese patents will be more difficult), severity of the pathologies, and history of any prior spinal surgery.

Conclusion

It appears likely that MISS will become an increasingly important component of the spinal surgical armamentarium in the future. With the advances in minimally invasive spinal surgical techniques, spinal fusions and instrumentations are now being achieved with less morbidity and faster recovery compared with traditional open surgical approaches. However, surgical expertise in minimally invasive spinal surgery can only be reached by ascending a learning curve. Thus surgeons interested in this innovative field must be willing to spend the time and effort necessary to become proficient in MISS techniques.

In skilled hands, the benefits of MISS procedures appear to outweigh the risks. Additional long-term outcome data are still necessary to define the efficacy of these approaches compared with traditional open spinal fusion approaches. However, early data suggest that surgeons willing to spend the time and energy necessary to gain proficiency in MISS can expect to be rewarded through the benefits provided to their surgical patient population, especially with regard to reduced blood loss and a shorter recovery period.

PEARLS

1. Fluoroscopy is a valuable tool to locate the surgical incision site and provide an adequate access in MISS.

2. Proper positioning of the Jamshidi needle within the pedicle shadow is crucial for adequate cannulated pedicle screw insertion.

3. Instrumentation using facet screws has proven to be quicker and less expensive compared with pedicle screw implants, yet it offers comparable initial stiffness for short constructs in selected cases.

4. Patient selection remains the most important variable in the clinical outcomes of those undergoing spinal surgery.

5. The benefits of MISS procedures include reduced blood loss, less soft tissue dissection and postoperative scarring, shorter hospital stay, and a fast recovery period.

PITFALLS

1. Surgical expertise of MISS procedures requires a steep learning curve.

2. Limited exposure of the vertebral column can prevent adequate access to the spinal pathology, and therefore conversion to a traditional open surgery may become necessary.

3. The anatomy of the paraspinal muscular compartments must be well understood. While navigating between compartments, care should be taken to avoid transgression of the separating fascial barriers, which can compromise the neurovascular supplies of the paraspinal muscles.

4. Safe and adequate placement of lumbar pedicle screws is dependent on precise preoperative and intraoperative fluoroscopy.

5. Approaching the spine through a limited operative field, the surgeon must ensure the continuous visualization of the tip of the instruments to prevent any events or instrument-related complications.

KEY POINTS

1. Principles of MISS: Addressing spinal pathologies through minimally invasive approaches aims at achieving optimal results while respecting and handling the paraspinal soft tissue envelope with care. Additionally, knowing the basic anatomy is crucial to a successful less invasive surgery.

2. Patient setup: For most posterior lumbar MISS, the patient is positioned prone on a radiolucent spinal frame.

3. Imaging: Before the surgery, a C-arm fluoroscopy is a valuable tool used to locate the bony landmarks and help outline the optimal surgical incision sites.

4. Surgical incisions: Limited size skin incisions are generally used; however, multiple and separate underlying fascial incisions are made to allow access to the different spinal compartments using a single limited skin incision.

5. Spine decompression-fusion: posterior lumbar interbody fusion (PLIF), transforaminal lumbar interbody fusion (TLIF), and posterolateral fusion (intertransverse onlay fusion) can well be performed through minimally invasive techniques.

6. Spine instrumentation: A variety of cannulated and noncannulated pedicle screw designs are available and are percutaneously placed with minimal exposure and limited soft tissue stripping. Intraoperative use of C-arm fluoroscopy is crucial for the proper placement of the pedicle screw instrumentation. Additionally, facet screw instrumentation is relatively easy to perform through a less invasive approach.

7. Patient selection: Patient selection is a crucial outcome variable for all spinal procedures. Patient-related factors and surgeon's level of expertise are factors to be considered when planning a minimally invasive spine procedure.

KEY REFERENCES

1. Benglis DM, Elhammady MS, Levi AD, et al: Minimally invasive anterolateral approaches for the treatment of back pain and adult degenerative deformity. Neurosurgery 63:191-196, 2008.
Microsurgical approaches to surgeries correcting various degenerative disc pathologies can be implemented effectively in the management of patients presenting with back pain. In particular, such procedures have decreased postoperative pain and narcotic requirements, shortened hospital stays, lessened blood loss, and minimized the size of the incision.

2. Kwon BK, Berta S, Daffner SD, et al: Radiographic analysis of transforaminal lumbar interbody fusion for the treatment of adult isthmic spondylolisthesis. J.Spinal Disord.Tech. 16:469-476, 2003.
Restoration of disk height and lumbar lordosis in 35 patients who underwent TLIF procedure with carbon fiber cages and pedicle screw instrumentation for isthmic spondylolisthesis was found to correlate with an anterior placement of the interbody cage within the disc space.

3. Liljenqvist U, Lepsien U, Hackenberg L, et al: Comparative analysis of pedicle screw and hook instrumentation in posterior correction and fusion of idiopathic thoracic scoliosis. Eur Spine J 11: 336-343, 2002.
The purpose of this study was to demonstrate that pedicle screw instrumentation (with or without proximal hook instrumentation) offers a significantly shorter fusion length and a better primary and secondary curve correction in patients presenting with thoracic scoliosis.

4. Parker LM, Murrell SE, Boden SD, et al: The outcome of posterolateral fusion in highly selected patients with discogenic low back pain. Spine 21:1909-1916, 1996.
This study aims to gauge the clinical outcome of 23 patients who underwent PLIF as treatment for discogenic lower back pain. The authors concluded that fusion is a successful surgical option for such patients; however, patient selection remains the prime challenge in management.

5. German JW, Adamo MA, Hoppenot RG, et al: Perioperative results following lumbar discectomy: comparison of minimally invasive discectomy and standard microdiscectomy. Neurosurg Focus 25: E20, 2008.
The author compares the patient profiles in two cohorts who underwent either microsurgical discectomies or open surgeries. Major conclusions stated that patients who ended up with positive clinical outcomes in both groups were similar with respect to height, weight, sex, body mass index, level and side of radiculopathy, insurance status, and preoperative analgesic use.

REFERENCES

1. Fritzell P, Hagg O, Nordwall A: Complications in lumbar fusion surgery for chronic low back pain: comparison of three surgical techniques used in a prospective randomized study. A report from the Swedish Lumbar Spine Study Group. Eur Spine J 12:178-189, 2003.

2. Katz JN: Lumbar spinal fusion. Surgical rates, costs, and complications. Spine 20(24 Suppl):78S-83S, 1995.

3. Malter D, McNeney B, Loeser JD, et al: 5-year reoperation rates after different types of lumbar spine surgery. Spine 23:814-820, 1998.

4. Stauffer RN, Coventry MB: Posterolateral lumbar-spine fusion. Analysis of Mayo Clinic series. J Bone Joint Surg Am 54:1195-1204, 1972.

5. Motosuneya T, Asazuma T, Tsuji T, et al: Postoperative change of the cross-sectional area of back musculature after 5 surgical procedures as assessed by magnetic resonance imaging. J Spinal Disord Tech 19:318-322, 2006.

6. Foley KT, Holly LT, Schwender JD: Minimally invasive lumbar fusion. Spine 28(15 Suppl):S26-S35, 2003.

7. Benglis DM, Elhammady MS, Levi AD, et al: Minimally invasive anterolateral approaches for the treatment of back pain and adult degenerative deformity. Neurosurgery 63:191-196, 2008.

8. Kasis AG, Marshman LA, Krishna M, et al: Significantly improved outcomes with a less invasive posterior lumbar interbody fusion incorporating total facetectomy. Spine 34:572-577, 2009.

9. Krishna M, Pollock RD, Bhatia C: Incidence, etiology, classification, and management of neuralgia after posterior lumbar interbody fusion surgery in 226 patients. Spine J 8:374-379, 2008.

10. Kwon BK, Berta S, Daffner SD, et al: Radiographic analysis of transforaminal lumbar interbody fusion for the treatment of adult isthmic spondylolisthesis. J Spinal Disord Tech 16:469-476, 2003.

11. Quigley KJ, Alander DH, Bledsoe JG: An in vitro biomechanical investigation: variable positioning of leopard carbon fiber interbody cages. J Spinal Disord Tech 21:442-447, 2008.

12. Liljenqvist U, Lepsien U, Hackenberg L, et al: Comparative analysis of pedicle screw and hook instrumentation in posterior correction and fusion of idiopathic thoracic scoliosis. Eur Spine J 11:336-343, 2002.

13. Ferrara LA, Secor JL, Jin BH, et al: A biomechanical comparison of facet screw fixation and pedicle screw fixation: effects of short-term and long-term repetitive cycling. Spine 28:1226-1234, 2003.

14. Volkman T, Horton WC, Hutton WC: Transfacet screws with lumbar interbody reconstruction: biomechanical study of motion segment stiffness. J Spinal Disord 9:425-432, 1996.

15. Shim CS, Lee SH, Jung B, et al: Fluoroscopically assisted percutaneous translaminar facet screw fixation following anterior lumbar interbody fusion: technical report. Spine 30:838-843, 2005.

16. Benini A, Magerl F: Selective decompression and translaminar articular facet screw fixation for lumbar canal stenosis and disc protrusion. Br J Neurosurg 7:413-418, 1993.

17. Montesano PX, Magerl F, Jacobs RR, et al: Translaminar facet joint screws. Orthopedics 11:1393-1397, 1988.

18. Hailong Y, Wei L, Zhensheng M, et al: Computer analysis of the safety of using three different pedicular screw insertion points in the lumbar spine in the Chinese population. Eur Spine J 16:619-623, 2007.

19. Parker LM, Murrell SE, Boden SD, et al: The outcome of posterolateral fusion in highly selected patients with discogenic low back pain. Spine 21: 1909-1916, 1996.

20. German JW, Adamo MA, Hoppenot RG, et al: Perioperative results following lumbar discectomy: comparison of minimally invasive discectomy and standard microdiscectomy." Neurosurg Focus 25: E20, 2008.

59
CHAPTER

Posterolateral Endoscopic Lumbar Discectomy

Christopher A. Yeung, MD
Anthony T. Yeung, MD

Posterolateral endoscopic lumbar surgery is a less invasive surgical procedure to address lumbar pathology in the disc and boney foramen. Like any surgical procedure, it is based on visual identification and exposure of the target pathology and adequate surgical tools to address the offending pathology. Modern day endoscopic technology allows for visualized discectomy and decompression of the traversing and exiting nerve roots from a percutaneous posterolateral/transforaminal approach. This is safe and equally efficacious to microscopic discectomy in properly selected patients.[1-4] Recent advances also allow for bony decompression of foraminal stenosis.[5,6]

Advances in the ability to perform endoscopic discectomy have paralleled other specialties, yet percutaneous spinal surgery has not met with the same peer recognition as the other fields. This is due in part to the high success rate and relative low morbidity of the current gold standard, posterior microscopic lumbar discectomy. However, this approach still requires a 1-inch midline incision, significant muscle and ligament stripping, prolonged muscle retraction, partial facet and lamina resection, and both nerve root and dura retraction. This can weaken the muscular lumbar stabilizers, create instability and facet arthrosis, cause traction neuropraxia, promote epidural scarring, and make revision surgery more difficult.

Another barrier for more widespread adoption was the relative paucity of peer-reviewed literature, and critics noted that only a few authors were contributing to this body of literature. Recently, there have been many more published results of posterolateral endoscopic discectomy from around the world and the preponderance of evidence supports its efficacy.

Numerous other nonvisualized percutaneous techniques often get categorized and confused with posterolateral endoscopic lumbar discectomy. These include automated percutaneous lumbar discectomy (APLD), percutaneous laser discectomy, and percutaneous discectomy with the Dekompressor or Arthrocare wand (Coblation). These are all fluoroscopically guided nonvisualized procedures that access the disc via the same posterolateral approach as endoscopic lumbar surgery. The underlying principle of these procedures is that through central nucleus removal or ablation, intradiscal pressure can be substantially lowered. This was based on the work of Hirsh and his postulated relationship between intradiscal pressure, disc herniation, and low back pain. He hypothesized that lowering this pressure in an injured disc could be efficacious in the relief of sciatica.[7] Multiple studies described decreases in intradiscal pressures of 50% or greater.[8-10]

The results of these types of indirect decompressive procedures have been similar with initial favorable reports. However, subsequent studies have shown varying degrees of success. The inability to consistently see the decompressed nerve or the targeted patho-anatomy has limited the use of these nonvisualized decompressive procedures.[11-14] It is unfortunate that these procedures, and their results, are mistaken for posterolateral endoscopic discectomy.

History

The basis for percutaneous lumbar disc procedures came from accepted posterolateral percutaneous biopsy techniques of the lumbar vertebrae. These procedures were initially performed with the use of a Craig needle to perform a posterolateral biopsy for neoplastic conditions.[15,16]

Minimal access surgery for lumbar disc herniation was first independently reported by Kambin and colleagues[17] and Hijikata[18] in 1975. The technique used a posterolateral approach to the foraminal zone of the disc bordered by the traversing nerve dorsally, the exiting nerve ventrally, and the endplate of the inferior vertebra caudally. The goal was to decompress nerve roots secondary to lumbar disc herniation by the "inside-out technique" of central and posterior nuclectomy and fragmentectomy. Advances in technique and instrumentation since Kambin, however, have allowed the surgeon to also enlarge the medial or lateral foramen by decompression of the lateral and ventral portion of the facet joint complex to reach the midline of the disc and the epidural space. Thus it is feasible to treat the full spectrum of disc herniations with advanced endoscopic instrumentation and techniques that can either target the extruded fragment directly or with a combination of the "inside-out technique."[19]

The early efforts were limited to a nonvisualized central discectomy to achieve an indirect decompression of the nerve roots,[17,18,20] but improvements in surgical equipment and technique evolved gradually over the next 30 years. In the past 10 years, the important major equipment improvements have included various-sized high-resolution rod lens operating endoscopes with variable-size working channels, beveled and slotted cannulas, flexible shavers and pituitary forceps, a bipolar flexible high-frequency/low-temperature radiofrequency (RF) electrode, multidirectional Holmium Yttrium-Aluminum-Garnet lasers, and high-speed diamond burrs and motorized shavers to decompress the foramen.[19] An improved fluoroscopically guided approach method introduced by Yeung and reported by Tsou[21-23] outlined a consistent and safe technique for entry into all lumbar posterior disc spaces including the L5-S1 level. This specific technique has been termed selective endoscopic discectomy (SED) but can be classified under the more general descriptive term of posterolateral endoscopic lumbar discectomy (PELD) that other authors describe.

These refinements have enhanced the capabilities of foraminal endoscopic discectomy to deliver surgical results similar to the results obtainable by traditional transcanal approaches for treating common lumbar disc herniations.[1-4]

Minimal access posterolateral endoscopic intradiscal visualization with the available operating tools has introduced new operative capabilities. That includes foraminal decompression for more central access of disc herniations and selective nuclectomy and annuloplasty performed intradiscally. The process of foraminal decompression also decompresses the lateral recess in lateral recess stenosis and mild central canal stenosis, a common late sequela of lumbar discectomy.

Anatomy

Posterolateral endoscopic lumbar surgery is performed through what has been named the *triangular working zone,* or *Kambin's triangle* (Fig. 59–1). This triangular zone is defined as a safe zone in the posterolateral annulus between the exiting and traversing nerve roots. The exiting nerve root forms the anterior border of the triangular zone as it exits under the cephalad pedicle. The superior endplate of the caudal vertebral body forms the inferior border and the articular process and superior articulating facet of the caudal vertebra form the posterior border. The working zone is bordered medially by the traversing nerve root and dura. From cadaveric measurements it was determined that cannulas ranging from 4 mm to 10 mm could be safely used in the triangular working zone.[24-27] A thorough understanding of the three-dimensional anatomy is necessary to understand and perform posterior percutaneous lumbar surgery.

Endoscopic Lumbar Discectomy

Endoscopic surgery developed out of fluoroscopically guided percutaneous procedures that initially used a working cannula with modified instruments designed for disc removal. The first surgeon credited with percutaneous nucleotomy was Hijikata in 1975.[18] The evolution of endoscopic techniques followed a series of transitions. Initially, an arthroscope was used to inspect the disc and annulus intermittently through the cannula while the mechanical nuclectomy was done under fluoroscopic guidance. The introduction of a biportal approach allowed for direct visualization of instruments introduced through a cannula inserted into the disc from the opposite posterolateral portal. The later development of an operating spine scope with a working channel allowed for surgical removal of disc material and visualization of foraminal anatomy under direct visualization via a uniportal approach.

Parviz Kambin performed the first true endoscopic lumbar procedures. The arthroscope was at first used intermittently through the working cannula. At certain stages of the procedure such as perforating the disc in the triangular working zone, the arthroscope would be placed in the cannula. The nonworking channel scope was used for identification of the annulus and periannular structures. The basis was to see that the nerve was not in the way before advancing the cannula. Once the cannula was safely within the disc, the nucleotome, an arthroscopic shaver, and pituitary rongeurs were passed through the cannula to perform mechanical disc removal. The majority of the procedure was only fluoroscopically visualized.[17] Kambin reported an 88% success rate in his first 100 patients.[28,29]

The early endoscopic procedures were limited by the absence of a working channel arthroscope. This led Kambin to the development of a biportal technique in which the scope was inserted on one side and the working cannula on the opposite side. Kambin's indications for a biportal approach included large subligamentous herniations, extraligamentous herniations, and arthroscopic interbody fusion.[26] In later studies Kambin reports results from both uniportal and biportal procedures together. Overall results ranged from 85% to 92% satisfactory results at a minimum 2-year follow-up. There was no differentiation made between the results of uniportal versus biportal approaches.[30-32]

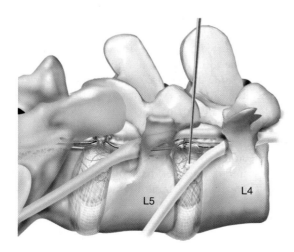

FIGURE 59–1 Triangular working zone at L4-5 (Kambin triangle). This is the access point for posterolateral disc access. The exiting nerve root is the hypotenuse of the triangle, the superior endplate of the caudal vertebral body/sacrum is the base (width), and the traversing nerve root/dura is the height of the triangle.

Kambin's first prototype of the working channel scope was not fully developed and was not successfully marketed. The problems with the initial scope included fragility, limited degree of angulation for the working instruments, and the inability to establish sufficient inflow or outflow for adequate visualization.[33] Anthony Yeung developed the first working channel endoscope to become widely available. The scope was developed in 1997 and was approved for use by the U.S. Food and Drug Administration in March 1998. The Yeung Endoscopic Spine Surgery (YESS) system (Richard Wolf Surgical Instruments, Vernon Hills, Ill.) modified the scope by adding multichannel integrated irrigation, specialized beveled cannulas, a two-hole obturator, and newly designed discectomy tools that allowed for constant real-time visualization with a uniportal technique.[34] (Fig. 59–2)

Another major change, which allowed for advancement in the field of endoscopic spinal surgery, was the emphasis on placement of the cannula closer to the epidural space and the base of the targeted disc herniation. This enabled surgeons to target extruded herniations in addition to contained herniations. Previous percutaneous modalities all focused on entry through Kambin's triangle and working within the center of the disc with the cannula anchored inside the annulus. The cannula was advanced past the annulus and remained there under fluoroscopic control. Mathews' transforaminal approach for microdiscectomy allowed for routine visualization of the epidural space and greater access to the traversing nerve root.[35]

The development of a working channel scope and use of the transforaminal approach using beveled and slotted cannulas enhanced endoscopic lumbar surgery. Using this approach, surgeons can operate under full visualization throughout most of the procedure and follow the neural structures into the epidural space. The specialized cannulas provide greater access to pathology and help protect and retract sensitive anatomy such as the exiting nerve and dorsal root ganglion. The working channel also allowed the passage of high-speed burrs for bone removal and direct foraminal enlargement and decompression of foraminal stenosis (foraminoplasty) (Fig. 59–3).

Indications/Contraindications

Current indications for the use of an endoscopic posterolateral approach to the lumbar spine include foraminal and far-lateral disc herniations, contained central and paracentral disc herniations, small nonsequestered extruded disc herniations, recurrent herniations, symptomatic annular tears, synovial cysts, biopsy and débridement of discitis, decompression of foraminal stenosis with or without spondylolisthesis, visualized total nuclectomy (before nucleus replacement), visualized discectomy, and endplate preparation before interbody fusion.

Perhaps the ideal lesions for posterolateral selective endoscopic discectomy are the foraminal and extraforaminal disc herniations. The cannula inserts directly at the herniation site, and the exiting nerve is routinely visualized and protected. This approach requires less manipulation of the exiting nerve root than the paramedian posterior approach.

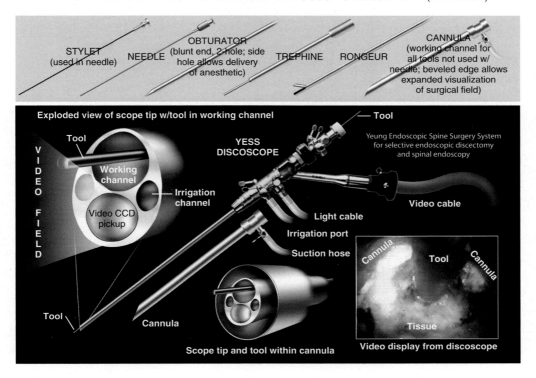

PARTIAL INSTRUMENT SET FOR SELECTIVE ENDOSCOPIC DISCECTOMY (not to scale)

FIGURE 59–2 The Yeung Endoscopic Spine Surgery system. (Courtesy Richard Wolf Surgical Instruments, Vernon Hills, Ill.)

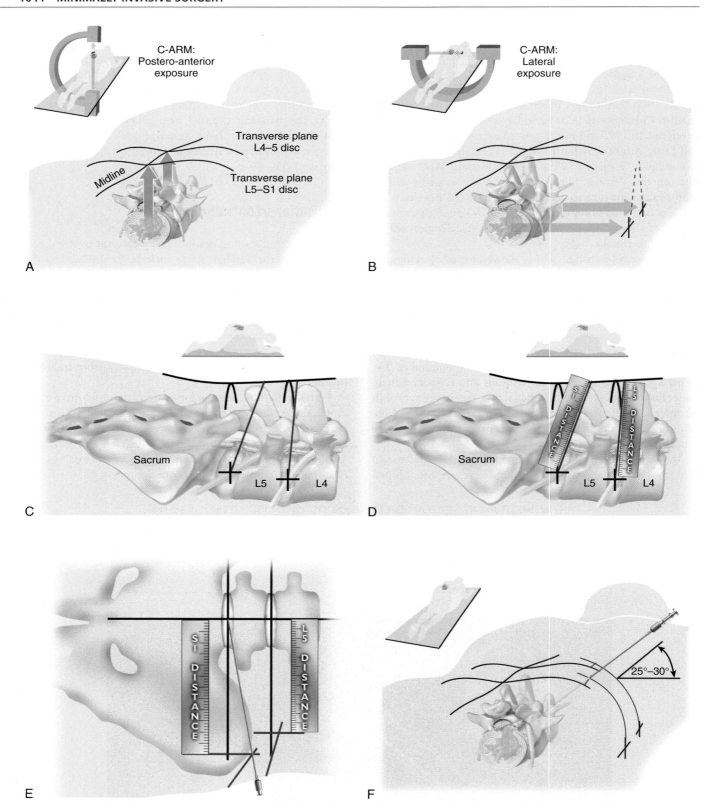

FIGURE 59–3 Protocol for optimal needle placement. **A,** Posteroanterior (PA) fluoroscopic view enables topographic location of the midline and the transverse disc plane. The intersection of these lines is the PA anatomic disc center. **B,** Lateral fluoroscopic view enables topographic location of the disc inclination plane. **C,** The inclination plane of each target disc is drawn on the skin from the lateral disc center. **D,** The distance from the lateral disc center to the posterior skin plane is measured along the inclination plane. **E** and **F,** This same distance is measured from the midline along the transverse disc plane for each target disc. At the end of this measure a line parallel to the midline is drawn to intersect the disc inclination line. This is the skin entry point or "skin window" for the needle.

Any herniation contiguous with the disc space not seques-tered and migrated is amenable to endoscopic disc excision if the boney anatomy permits an unobstructed approach. This uses an "inside-out" technique where the herniation is grasped from its base within the disc space, pulled back into the working intradiscal cavity, and removed via the cannula. The size and types of herniations chosen by the surgeon for endo-scopic excision will depend on the skill and experience of the surgeon. Certainly, all contained disc herniations are appro-priate for endoscopic decompression. With experience, extruded herniations can be routinely addressed. This approach is especially attractive for recurrent herniations after a traditional posterior approach because the surgeon can avoid the scar tissue from the previous surgery.

Radiofrequency energy can be applied to the annular tears under direct visualization to contract the collagen and ablate ingrown granulation tissue, neoangiogenesis, and sensitized nociceptors.[36] Frequently interpositional nuclear tissue is seen within the fibers of the annular tear, preventing the tear from healing. This tissue can then be removed to allow the tear to heal.

Endoscopic foraminoplasty can be readily achieved with bone trephines/rasps, the side-firing Holmium-YAG laser, and endoscopic high-speed drills.[5,6] The roof of the foramen is formed by the undersurface of the superior articular facet. This is easily visualized and accessed via the endoscope, and the previously mentioned tools are used to remove bone and enlarge the foraminal opening. Synovial cysts can also be visu-alized and removed.

In cases of discitis the posterolateral endoscopic approach will provide a robust biopsy for culture diagnosis, and the infected/necrotic disc tissue can be thoroughly débrided to reduce the bacterial load and accelerate healing.[37]

Contraindications include any pathology not accessible from the posterolateral endoscopic approach. This may include some extruded sequestered disc herniations, extruded migrated disc herniations (migrated extent greater than the measured height of the posterior marginal disc space on T2 sagittal magnetic resonance imaging [MRI]), larger hernia-tions occupying greater than 50% of the spinal canal,[4] recur-rent or virgin disc herniations with associated epidural scarring, moderate-severe central canal stenosis, and hard cal-cified herniations. These contraindications are considered relative contraindications dependent on the surgeons' techni-cal experience and comfort level. More experienced endo-scopic surgeons can gain greater access to pathology using advanced techniques for bone removal of osteophytes, steno-sis, and the posterolateral corner of the vertebral body before addressing the pathology. Other relative contraindications include inadequate support staff or equipment to successfully perform procedure and uncooperative patients.

Step-by-Step Operative Technique

Patient Positioning

The patient is prone on a hyperkyphotic frame with a radio-lucent table. The endoscope is on one side, and the fluoro-scopic unit is on the opposite side of the patient.

Anesthesia

Although some experienced international endoscopic sur-geons prefer general anesthesia, the authors recommend mild sedation and local anesthesia so that the patient is awake and responsive throughout the procedure. The patient can then provide real-time feedback in case of nerve irritation from instrument pressure or retraction, adding a layer of safety and allowing the surgeon to adjust the instruments accordingly. We use midazolam (Versed) and fentanyl for sedation and recom-mend against using general anesthetics like propofol, which can produce temporary total analgesia, eliminating the patient's responsiveness to any nerve stimuli. The skin, needle tract, and annulus are anesthetized with one-half percent lidocaine. This allows anesthesia without motor block of the nerve roots.

Needle Placement

Optimal needle placement is the most crucial step of the pro-cedure and is based on the type of pathology being addressed. The specific protocol[21] is demonstrated in the accompanying DVD. The skin window (needle insertion site) is determined using this protocol. This will typically be about 12 to 15 cm lateral to the midline aligned parallel to the disc inclination (Fig. 59–3).

Once the starting point is determined, the skin window and subcutaneous tissue are infiltrated with one-half percent lido-caine. A 6-inch, 18-gauge needle is then inserted from the skin window at the desired trajectory, typically at a 30-degree angle to the floor (coronal plane) and passed anteromedially toward the anatomic disc center. Infiltrating the needle tract with one-half percent lidocaine as you advance the needle will anesthe-tize the tissue tract, avoiding pain when the dilator is passed later in the procedure.

The C-arm lateral projection should confirm the needle tip's correct annular location at the annular window (annular entry point). In the posteroanterior view, the needle tip should be at the disc between the pedicles. In the lateral view the correct needle tip position should be just touching the poste-rior annulus surface. The above two views of the C-arm confirm that the needle tip has engaged the safe zone, the center of the foraminal annular window.

While monitoring the posteroanterior view, advance the needle tip through the annulus to the midline (anatomic disc center). Then check the lateral view. If the needle tip is in the center of the disc on the lateral view, you have a central needle placement, which is good for a central nucleotomy. Ideally the needle tip will be in the posterior one third of the disc, indicat-ing posterior needle placement if you are attempting to access paracentral herniations.

Evocative Chromo-discography

Perform confirmatory contrast discography at this time. The following contrast mixture is used: 9 mL of Isovue 300 with 1 mL of indigo carmine dye. This combination of contrast ratio gives readily visible radiopacity on the discography images and intraoperative light blue chromatization of

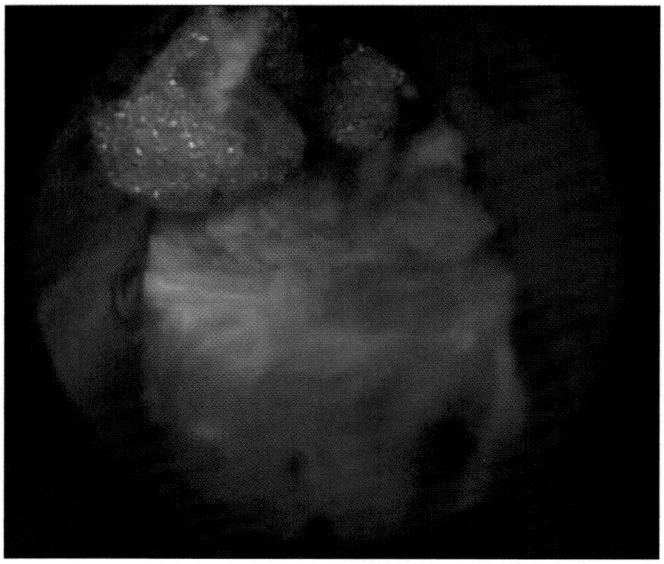

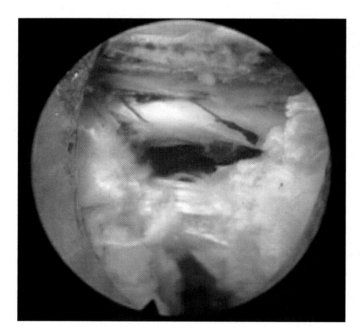

FIGURE 59–4 Uniportal endoscopic technique. The cannula is positioned near the base of the herniation. The epidural fat can be seen at the top of the image. The extruded herniation is stained blue with the indigo carmine dye and is seen here extruding through the thinned out annular fibers seen coursing horizontally in this image. At this point the annular fibers are cut to enlarge the annulotomy with the cutting forceps and the side firing laser to allow the apex of the herniation to be pulled back into the disc and out the cannula with the pituitary rongeurs.

FIGURE 59–5 Inspection of the freed traversing nerve root. After successful removal of an extruded paracentral herniation, the traversing nerve root is visualized confirming complete decompression of the nerve. This is routine in extruded herniations. If the herniation is a contained herniation, the surgeon would visualize the undersurface of the thinned-out posterior annular fibers rather than the traversing nerve root because the herniation did not extrude past the posterior annulus.

pathologic nucleus and annular fissures, which help guide the targeted fragmentectomy.

Instrument Placement

Insert a guidewire through the 18-gauge needle channel. Advance the guidewire tip, 1 to 2 cm deep into the annulus, and then remove the needle. Slide the bluntly tapered tissue dilating obturator over the guidewire until the tip of the obturator is firmly engaged in the annular window. An eccentric parallel channel in the obturator allows for four quadrant annular infiltration using small incremental volumes of one-half percent lidocaine in each quadrant, enough to anesthetize the annulus, but not the nerves. Hold the obturator firmly against the annular window surface and remove the guidewire.

The next step is the through-and-through fenestration of the annular window by advancing the bluntly tapered obturator with a mallet. Annular fenestration is the most painful step of the entire procedure. Advise the anesthesiologist to heighten the sedation level just before annular fenestration. Advance the obturator tip deep into the annulus and confirm on the C-arm views. Now slide the beveled access cannula over the obturator toward the disc. Advance the cannula until the beveled tip is deep in the annular window with the beveled opening facing dorsally. Remove the obturator and insert the endoscope to get a view of the disc nucleus and annulus (Fig. 59–4). The subsequent steps depend on the goal of the procedure and pathology being addressed. The basic endoscopic method to excise a noncontained paramedian extruded lumbar herniated disc via a uniportal technique is described here. Different steps are used for other pathology and are beyond the scope of this chapter.

Performing the Discectomy

First enlarge the annulotomy medially to the base of the herniation with a cutting forcep. The side-firing Holmium-YAG laser can also be used to enlarge and widen the annulotomy. This is performed to release the annular fibers at the herniation site that may pinch off or prevent the extruded portion of the herniation from being extracted. Directly under the herniation apex a large amount of blue stained nucleus is usually present, likened to the submerged portion of an iceberg. The nucleus here represents a migrated and unstable nucleus. The endoscopic rongeurs are used to extract the blue-stained nucleus pulposus under direct visualization. The larger straight and hinged rongeurs are used directly through the cannula after the endoscope is removed. Fluoroscopy and surgeon feel guide this step. By grabbing the base of the herniated fragment, one can usually extract the extruded portion of the herniation. Initial medialization and widening of the annulotomy reduce the prospect of breaking off the herniated nucleus and retaining the apex of the herniation in the spinal canal. The traversing nerve root is readily visualized after removal of the extruded herniation (Fig. 59–5).

Next perform a minimal bulk decompression by using a straight and flexible suction-irrigation shaver. This step requires shaver head C-arm localization before power is activated to avoid nerve/dura injury and anterior annular penetration. The cavity thus created is called the *working cavity*. The debulking process serves two functions. First, it decompresses the disc, reducing the risk for further acute herniation. Second, it removes the unstable nucleus material to prevent future rehernination.

Inspect the working cavity. If a noncontained extruded disc fragment is still present by finding blue-stained nucleus material posteriorly, then these fragments are teased into the working cavity with the endoscopic rongeurs and the flexible radiofrequency trigger-flex bipolar probe (Elliquence LLC, Oceanside, N.Y.) and removed. Creation of the working cavity allows the herniated disc tissue to follow the path of least resistance into the cavity. The flexible radiofrequency bipolar probe is used to contract and thicken the annular collagen at the herniation site. It is also used for hemostasis throughout the case.

The vast majority of herniations can be treated via the uniportal technique. Sometimes for large central herniations and herniations at L5-S1, the disc needs to be approached from both sides, a biportal technique. This allows the use of larger articulating instruments that fit through the contralateral 7-mm access cannula and can reach more posterior to extract the herniated fragment under direct endoscopic vision.

Clinical Outcomes

Yeung has reported his initial results using the YESS system in his first 307 patients with disc herniations who were candidates for open microdiscectomy. The study included intracanal and extracanal herniations. Recurrent herniations and patients with previous surgery at the same level were not excluded. Results were reported with 1-year follow-up. Overall patient satisfaction was found to be 91%. The same percentage of patients said they would undergo the procedure again if faced with the same diagnosis. The overall complication rate was 3.5%.[22] Tsou and Yeung separated out a subgroup of 219 patients with noncontained herniations and reported results at 1 year. Patient satisfaction was 91%.[23] These initial results demonstrated that endoscopic surgery could provide equivalent results to reported results of open microdiscectomy, even with noncontained herniations.

There are three prospective randomized studies comparing traditional microdiscectomy and percutaneous endoscopic discectomy. Hermantin performed a prospective randomized study with 30 patients in each group. The mean duration of follow-up was 31 months. Patient satisfaction was 93% in the open surgical group and 97% in the endoscopic group. The endoscopic group had shorter duration of narcotic use and shorter time out of work compared with open discectomy.[1] Mayer performed a randomized prospective study in 1993 with 20 patients in each group. He chose return to previous occupation as his measurement of success. This study showed a significant difference in this outcome measure. In the percutaneous group 95% of patients returned to their previous profession, whereas only 72% of the microdiscectomy group returned to a previous profession.[2] In 2008 Ruetten compared traditional microdiscectomy with full endoscopic discectomy via either the transforaminal or interlaminar route. There were 178 patients (87 microdiscectomy and 91 endoscopic) with 2-year follow-up. The microdiscectomy group had a 79% success rate and the full endoscopic group had an 85% success rate with no leg pain at all.[3] It is noteworthy that all three of these prospective randomized studies showed a trend toward better outcomes with the endoscopic procedure, but statistically they were comparable.

Kambin reported an 82% success rate for the treatment of lateral recess stenosis and foraminal herniations using an oval cannula with two portals and the transforaminal approach. Even though they were working next to the exiting nerve root, they reported no neurovascular complications in their series.[38] Successful posterolateral endoscopic treatment of foraminal and extraforaminal herniations has been described by many authors. Lew reported an 85% success rate in 47 patients,[39] Choi reported a 92% success rate in 41 patients,[40] Jang reported an 85% success rate in 35 patients,[41] and Sassani reported an 89% success rate in 66 patients.[42]

Knight and Goswami[6] have reported on the use of the endoscope in foraminal decompressions for isthmic spondylolisthesis. In 79% of patients a good or excellent outcome was obtained with an average follow-up of 34 months. Of the initial group only two went on to have spinal fusion.[6]

Ahn and colleagues[43] reported an 81% success rate with PELD on 43 patients with recurrent disc herniations after a posterior microdiscectomy. Hoogland also had good success (85%) using endoscopic transforaminal discectomy for recurrent herniations in 262 consecutive cases from 1994 to 2002. Of the 262 patients, 194 had a previous posterior microdiscectomy and 68 had a prior endoscopic discectomy.[44] Both studies pointed out the advantage of avoiding the posterior scar tissue.

The ability to effectively remove pathology using endoscopic surgery has been validated by postprocedure imaging studies. Casey and colleagues[45] looked at a group of patients who had immediate postoperative computed tomography scans. The imaging studies demonstrated 88.9% of patients undergoing biportal endoscopy had significant reduction in the amount of neural compromise. The results of uniportal, extraforaminal, and foraminal herniations showed only mild to moderate change in canal diameter. They concluded that arthroscopic discectomy had a high rate of canal clearance and removal of disc fragments.[45]

Lee and colleagues[4] reported on a matched cohort comparing radiographic changes 3 years postsurgery in PELD versus posterior microdiscectomy. They revealed less degenerative progression in the PELD group with loss of disc height and foraminal height being statistically significant. Clinical success rates were 96% in the PELD group and 93% in the microdiscectomy group. The authors conclude that PELD is a less invasive procedure that causes less approach related damage and less damage to the targeted disc.[4]

Complications and Avoidance

The risks of serious complications or injury are low—approximately 3%. The usual risks of infection, nerve injury, dural tears, bleeding, and scar tissue formation are present, as with any surgery. Because the transforaminal endoscopic approach passes adjacent to the exiting spinal nerve root and dorsal root ganglion, there is potential for nerve irritation (dysesthesia) or overt nerve damage. Dysesthesia occurrence is 5% to 15% and is almost always transient.[22,23] This rate of occurrence is similar to dysesthesia rates in posterior open discectomy, but in the latter situation, because the dysesthesia affects the retracted traversing nerve root that was already the source of radiculopathy, the transient persistent or increased postoperative dysesthesia is generally not considered a complication after posterior discectomy. Both situations, however, are transient the vast majority of the time. Routine injection of steroid medication at the conclusion of the endoscopic discectomy has reduced the rates of dysesthesia significantly.

Avoidance of complications is enhanced by the ability to clearly visualize normal and pathoanatomy, the use of local anesthesia and conscious sedation rather than general or spinal anesthesia, and the use of a standardized needle placement protocol. The entire procedure is usually accomplished with the patient remaining comfortable during the entire procedure and should be done without the patient feeling severe pain except when expected such as during evocative discography, annular fenestration, or when instruments are manipulated past the exiting nerve. Local anesthesia using one-half percent lidocaine (Xylocaine) allows generous use of this dilute anesthetic for pain control and still allows the patient to feel pain when the nerve root is manipulated. Thus the awake and aware patient serves as the best indicator to avoid any nerve irritation/damage. Dural tears can be treated with a visualized blood patch and observation because there is no "dead space" for cerebrospinal fluid collection/drainage.

Future Considerations

Perhaps the best new indication for the use of this technique and approach is in the realm of motion preservation (nucleus replacement). A complete endoscopic nuclectomy can be performed followed by insertion of an expandable hydrogel or polymer to completely fill the nuclear cavity, redistribute the load across the disc space, and protect the annulus. The DASCOR nucleus replacement device (Disc Dynamics, Eden Prairie, MN) is a prime example of this technology.

Radical endoscopic discectomy with burring of the endplates and subsequent delivery of an interbody prosthesis with bone graft/bone morphogenetic protein can yield a truly minimally invasive interbody fusion. Transforaminal anatomy will limit the size of implant that can be delivered; however, this problem can be overcome by using expandable interbody or graft containment devices that are being developed.

Future advances in the use of biomaterials and gene therapy may allow endoscopic annular reinforcement, tissue repair, tissue regeneration, anterior column stabilization by disc arthroplasty, and other alternatives to fusion for pain reduction. The future of spine surgery will most likely involve a mix of endoscopic and traditional open procedures. Studies comparing open and endoscopic procedures will have to be performed to find which conditions will be best treated by minimally invasive procedures.

PEARLS

1. Initial proper placement of a needle/guide pin is critical to the entire procedure. Take the time to have best possible needle placement in both anteroposterior and lateral projections.

2. Use the "inside-out" technique: Start the endoscopy by first entering the disc and then address the pathology accordingly. This is a safe starting point to avoid getting disoriented to your cannula position. Once you are within the disc, the herniation is between you and the affected nerve; this is advantageous because it protects the nerve from iatrogenic injury. When possible remove the herniation by pulling the herniation into the disc space and then out the cannula.

3. Fluoroscopy should be used to confirm location if there is any uncertainty about anatomy or location during endoscopy.

4. It is helpful to use the specially designed cannulas with a penfield-like extension to retract and protect the exiting nerve when working in the foramen.

5. The patient is awake, so use this to your advantage! If significant leg pain is experienced, stop and re-evaluate the patient; ask him or her about the distribution of the pain and reassess the position using fluoroscopy to prevent complications.

6. When bleeding is encountered advance the scope back into the disc and slowly pull back the scope cauterizing the bleeders from inside to out.

PITFALLS

1. Make sure the MRI and plain roentgenograms are numbered the same (i.e., look out for patients with transitional or six lumbar vertebrae).

2. It is recommended that the patient be awake and alert until the endoscope is within the disc space to avoid nerve injury. Avoiding excessive sedation before this point in the procedure is crucial, especially during needle insertion and dilator and cannula passage. We recommend against the use of a general anesthetic such as propofol.

KEY POINTS

1. Posterolateral endoscopic lumbar discectomy (PELD) is a visualized surgical procedure and is not to be confused with the many nonvisualized percutaneous discectomy procedures for indirect disc decompression.

2. The surgeon can visually confirm that the traversing nerve root is adequately decompressed when removing an extruded paracentral herniation.

3. The literature shows PELD is at least as safe and effective as traditional posterior discectomy.

KEY REFERENCES

1. Hermantin FU, Peters T, Quartararo L, et al: A prospective randomized study comparing the results of open discectomy with those of video-assisted arthroscopic microdiscectomy. J Bone Joint Surg 81-A: 958-965, 1999.
   The authors showed comparable success rates between open discectomy and arthroscopic microdiscectomy (posterolateral endoscopic discectomy), but the later group had less narcotic use and shorter time off work.

2. Ahn Y, Lee SH, Park WM, et al: Percutaneous endoscopic lumbar discectomy for recurrent disc herniation: surgical technique, outcome, and prognostic factors of 43 consecutive cases. Spine 29:326-332, 2004.
   The authors were able to avoid the posterior scar tissue in patients with recurrent herniations after a posterior discectomy and achieve an 81% success rate by using the posterolateral endoscopic approach.

3. Yeung AT, Tsou PM: Posterolateral endoscopic excision for lumbar disc herniation: surgical technique, outcome and complications in 307 consecutive cases. Spine 27:722-731, 2002.
   Results of more than 300 patients with 2-year follow-up using the endoscopic technique and working channel scope. Excellent description of author's technique and outcomes rated using patient satisfaction.

4. Ruetten S, Komp M, Merk H, et al: Full-endoscopic interlaminar and transforaminal Lumbar discectomy versus conventional microsurgical technique: a prospective, randomized, controlled study. Spine 33:930-939, 2008.
   This large prospective randomized study directly compares standard microdiscectomy to both posterolateral and posterior interlaminar endoscopic techniques.

5. Lee SH, Kang B, Ahn Y, et al: Operative failure of percutaneous endoscopic lumbar discectomy: a radiologic analysis of 55 cases. Spine 31:E285-E290, 2006.
   The authors identify high-grade canal compromise (>50%) and high-grade migration as herniation characteristics that predispose for a higher failure rate with posterolateral endoscopic lumbar discectomy.

REFERENCES

1. Hermantin FU, Peters T, Quartararo L, et al: A prospective randomized study comparing the results of open discectomy with those of video-assisted arthroscopic microdiscectomy. J Bone Joint Surg 81-A: 958-965, 1999.

2. Mayer HM, Brock M: Percutaneous endoscopic discectomy: surgical technique and preliminary results compared to microsurgical discectomy. J Neurosurg 78:216-225, 1993.

3. Ruetten S, Komp M, Merk H, et al: Full-endoscopic interlaminar and transforaminal lumbar discectomy versus conventional microsurgical technique: a prospective, randomized, controlled study. Spine 33:930-939, 2008.

4. Lee SH, Chung SE, Ahn Y, et al: Comparative radiologic evaluation of percutaneous endoscopic lumbar discectomy and open microdiscectomy: a matched cohort analysis. Mt Sinai J Med 73:795-801, 2006.

5. Knight MTN, Goswami AKD: Endoscopic laser foraminoplasty. In: Savitz MH, Chiu JC, Yeung AT (eds): The Practice of Minimally Invasive Spinal Technique. Richmond, VA, AAMISMS Education, LLC, 2000, pp 337-340.

6. Knight M, Goswami A: Management of isthmic spondylolisthesis with posterolateral endoscopic foraminal decompression. Spine 28:573-581, 2003.

7. Hirsh C, Ingelmark B, Miller M: The anatomic basis for low back pain. Acta Orthop Scand 33:1-17, 1963.

8. Choy DS, Altman P: Fall of intradiscal pressure with laser ablation. J Clin Laser Med Surg 13:149-151, 1995.

9. Prodoehl JA, Lane GJ, Black J, et al: The effects of lasers on intervertebral disc pressures. Spine: State of the Art Reviews 7:17-21, 1993

10. Nerubay J, Caspi I, Levinkopf M, et al: Percutaneous laser nucleolysis of the intervertebral lumbar disc. Clin Orthop 337:42-44, 1997.

11. Chatterjee S, Foy PM, Findlay GF: Report of a controlled clinical trial comparing automated percutaneous lumbar discectomy and microdiscectomy in the treatment of contained lumbar disc herniation. Spine 20:734738, 1995.

12. Grevitt MP, McLaren A, Shakelford IM, et al: Automated percutaneous lumbar discectomy—an outcome study. J Bone Joint Surg (Br) 77-B:626-629, 1995.

13. Ramberg N, Sahlstrand T: Early and Long-term follow-up after automated percutaneous lumbar discectomy. J Spinal Discord 14:511-517, 2001.

14. Choy DS, Asher PW, Ran HS, et al: Percutaneous laser decompression: a new therapeutic modality. Spine 17:949-956, 1992.

15. Valls J, Ottolenghi CE, Schajowicz F: Aspiration biopsy in diagnosis of lesions of vertebral bodies. JAMA 136:376-382, 1948.

16. Craig FS: Vertebral-body biopsy. J Bone Joint Surg (Am) 38A: 93-102, 1956.

17. Kambin P, Gellman H: Percutaneous lateral discectomy of the lumbar spine. Clin Orthop 174:127-132, 1983.

18. Hijikata S, Yamagishi N, Nakayama T, et al: Percutaneous discectomy: a new treatment method for lumbar disc herniation. J Toden Hosp 5:5-13, 1975.

19. Yeung AT, Yeung CA: In vivo endoscopic visualization of pathoanatomy in Painful degenerative conditions of the lumbar spine. Surgical Tech Int XV:243-256, 2006.

20. Onik GM, Helms C, Hoaglund F, et al: Successful percutaneous lumbar discectomy using a new aspiration probe: a case report. Am J Radiol 6:290-293, 1985.

21. Yeung AT, Yeung CA: Posterolateral selective endoscopic discectomy: the YESS Technique. In Kim D, Fessler R, Regan J (eds): Endoscopic Spine Surgery and Instrumentation: Percutaneous Procedures. New York, Thieme, 2004, pp. 201-211.

22. Yeung AT, Tsou PM: Posterolateral endoscopic excision for lumbar disc herniation: surgical technique, outcome and complications in 307 consecutive cases. Spine 27:722-731, 2002.

23. Tsou PM, Yeung AT: Transforaminal endoscopic decompression for radiculopathy secondary to intracanal noncontained lumbar disc herniations: outcome and technique. Spine J 2:41-48, 2002.

24. Kambin P, Bradger MD: Percutaneous posterolateral discectomy: anatomy and mechanism. Clin Orthop 223:145-154, 1987.

25. Kambin P: Arthroscopic Microdiscectomy: Minimal Intervention in Spinal Surgery. Baltimore, Urban and Schwarzenberg, 1991.

26. Kambin p, McCullen G, Parke W, et al: Minimally invasive arthroscopic spinal surgery. Instr Course Lect 46:1443-1461, 1997.

27. Mirkovic SR, Schwartz DG, Glazier KD: Anatomic considerations in lumbar posterolateral percutaneous procedures. Spine 20:1965-1971, 1995.

28. Kambin P, Schaffer JL: Percutaneous posterolateral discectomy and decompression with a 6.9mm cannula. J Bone Joint Surg (Am) 73-A:822-831, 1991.

29. Kambin P: Arthroscopic microdiscectomy. Arthroscopy 8:287-295, 1992.

30. Kambin P, O'Brien E, Zhou L, et al: Arthroscopic microdiscectomy and selective fragmentectomy. Clin Orthop 347:150-167, 1998.

31. Kambin P, Savitz MH: Arthroscopic microdiscectomy: an alternative to open disc surgery. Mount Sinai J Med 67:283-287, 2000.

32. Kambin P, Zhou L: Arthroscopic discectomy of the lumbar spine. Clin Orthop 337:49-57, 1997.

33. Kambin P, Zhou L: History and current status of percutaneous arthroscopic disc surgery. Spine 21:57S-61S, 1996.

34. Yeung AT: The evolution of percutaneous spinal endoscopy and discectomy: state of the art. Mount Sinai J Med 67:327-332, 2000.

35. Mathews HH: Transforaminal endoscopic microdiscectomy. Neurosurg Clin North Am 7:59-63, 1996.

36. Tsou, PM, Yeung CA, Yeung AT: Posterolateral transforaminal selective endoscopic discectomy and thermal annuloplasty for chronic lumbar discogenic pain: a minimal access visualized intradiscal surgical procedure. Spine J 4:564-573, 2004.

37. Ito M, Abumi K, Kotani Y, et al: Clinical outcome of posterolateral endoscopic surgery for pyogenic spondylodiscitis: results of 15 patients with serious comorbid conditions. Spine 32:200-206, 2007.

38. Kambin P, Casey K, O'Brien E, et al: Transforaminal arthroscopic decompression of the lateral recess stenosis. J Neurosurg 84:462-467, 1996.

39. Lew SM, Mehalic TF, Fagone KL: Transforaminal percutaneous endoscopic discectomy in the treatment of far-lateral and foraminal lumbar disc herniation. J Neurosurg 94:216-220, 2001.

40. Choi G, Lee SH, Bhanot A, et al: Percutaneous endoscopic discectomy for extraforaminal lumbar disc herniations. Spine 32:93-99, 2007.

41. Jang JS, An SH, Lee SH: Transforaminal percutaneous endoscopic discectomy in the Treatment of foraminal and extraforaminal lumbar disc herniations. J Spinal Discord Tech 19:338-343, 2006.

42. Sasani M, Oktenoglu T, Canbulat N, et al: Percutaneous endoscopic discectomy for far lateral lumbar disc herniations: prospective study and outcome of 66 patients. Minim Invas Neurosurg 50:91-97, 2007.

43. Ahn Y, Lee SH, Park WM, et al: Percutaneous endoscopic lumbar discectomy for recurrent disc herniation: surgical technique, outcome, and prognostic factors of 43 consecutive cases. Spine 29:326-332, 2004.

44. Hoogland T, van den Brekel-Dijkstra K, Schubert M, et al: Endoscopic transforaminal discectomy for recurrent lumbar disc herniation: a prospective, cohort evaluation of 262 consecutive cases. Spine 33:973-978, 2008.

45. Casey KF, Chang MK, O'Brien ED, et al: Arthroscopic microdiscectomy: comparison of preoperative and postoperative imaging studies. Arthroscopy 13:438-445, 1997.

60 CHAPTER

Interspinous Process Decompressive Devices

Clifford B. Tribus, MD

The interspinous process space has increasingly become a target for spinal implants to address degenerative conditions of the lumbar spine. Interspinous process decompressive (IPD) devices employ a range of insertion techniques and materials but share a common goal—that distraction be maintained between the adjacent spinous processes in order to incur a clinical result. The variety of materials employed include titanium, polyether ether keytone (PEEK), silastic compounds, and allograft. Many of the implants are devised to be static in nature, while others are dynamic.[1,2] The X-Stop is a titanium implant. It is the only device marketed in the United States that, at the time of publishing, has been cleared by the U.S. Food and Drug Administration (FDA) through an investigational device exemption (IDE) study. The indication for its use is spinal stenosis leading to neurogenic claudication. Other diagnoses potentially helped by this technology, but yet to be cleared by the FDA, include discogenic back pain, facet arthropathy, disc herniation, degenerative disc disease, and instability including degenerative spondylolisthesis. IPDs all share characteristics that are relatively unique among spinal implants of the lumbar spine. They can be implanted with a modest degree of destruction to the local anatomy. They do not require exposure to the neural elements, they are at least partially motion preserving, and they are relatively reversible. These features coalesce to an implant with a favorable risk profile. It is up to randomized controlled studies to prove the efficacy, indications, and ultimately role in the armamentarium available to the spine surgeon in the care of the spinal patient.

Design Rationale

Early criticisms of IPD devices stem from the apparent kyphosing nature of the implant. It is indeed counterintuitive to apply posterior distraction to the lumbar spine. Yet one need only look at the clinical presentation of a patient with lumbar spinal stenosis to appreciate the design rationale. A patient with lumbar stenosis typically walks with a forward stooped gate. Additionally, patients with spinal stenosis obtain symptom relief upon sitting down. The common feature in both of these postures is the relative flexion of the lumbar spine or avoidance of extension. Human beings are unable to segmentally kyphos their lumbar spine. Muscle insertions allow global motions of flexion and extension. However, spinal stenosis is often a focal phenomena presenting with its worst clinical level at one or two lumbar segments. The rationale of the device, therefore, is to implant the IPD device at the one or two levels where the stenosis is most severe. The implant then segmentally kyphoses the lumbar spine at the level of most severe stenosis and allows the rest of the lumbar spine to fall in its natural posture of extension, having relieved the local stenosis.

An additional concept in the treatment of patients with lumbar spinal stenosis is how much nerve compression is clinically significant? Although several studies have tried to elucidate this measurement, it does appear to be an elusive number. Any clinician who has been involved in the care of the stenosis patient can appreciate the fact that for every octogenarian who presents with new-onset stenotic symptoms and who has a spinal canal that is extraordinarily narrow, there is another patient who presents with similar symptoms in their 50s with magnetic resonance imaging (MRI) findings that are not nearly as impressive. With this variation in mind, it can be appreciated that spinal stenosis is a threshold disease. That is to say, the degree of tightness that elicits symptoms in any particular patient may in part be somewhat unique for that patient. By extension, therefore, a device that can create additional room for the neural elements may only need to create enough room so as to get that patient to the other side of their threshold for symptoms. As surgeons, we may be a bit uncomfortable with this rationale, preferring to directly decompress the neural elements in their entirety and confirm this by direct visualization. This may, however, represent overtreatment.

If we accept the concept of focal spinal stenosis causing symptoms at a particular threshold, then it must be shown the interspinous process decompressive devices can enact an effect on the canal diameter with acceptable, otherwise minimal, alterations to spine biomechanics. The majority of the current literature on this topic relates to the X-Stop interspinous process device. Whether these data can be extrapolated to other products in this category is up to the reader's discretion, yet these studies are presented as a design rationale for IPD devices.

The first reasonable question to pose in evaluating the design rationale of an IPD device is its net effect on implantation of the dimensions of the spinal canal. Richards and colleagues[3] attempted to address this question in studying eight cadaver specimens from L2-L5 that underwent an MRI before and after implantation of an X-Stop device at the L3-4 level. Canal and foraminal dimensions were measured. The specimens were positioned, and parameters were measured in both 15 degrees of flexion and 15 degrees of extension. In extension, the canal area was increased by 18% when compared with the noninstrumented spine. Similarly the subarticular diameter was increased by 50%, the canal diameter by 10%, the foraminal area by 25%, and the foraminal width by 41%.[3] In a subsequent in vivo study, Siddiqui and colleagues[4,5] presented results on 12 patients with 17 instrumented levels in which positional MRIs were obtained before and after surgery in the sitting flexed, extended, neutral, and standing positions. The area for the dural sac increased from 77.8 to 93.4 mm at 6 months after surgery in the standing position. There was a similar increase in the foramina. Importantly, no change in overall lumbar lordosis was noted.[4,5]

These studies demonstrate the passive decompression obtained in placing an IPD device. The question remains as to whether this degree of passive decompression is enough to be clinically relevant.

The other area of study as it relates to implantation of the IPD device is the net effect on the kinematics and load sharing within the lumbar spine at both the instrumented level and the adjacent levels.[6] Swanson and colleagues presented data on eight human cadaveric lumbar spines in which they tested intradiscal pressure, before and after implantation. The spines were positioned in flexion, neutral, and extension with intradiscal pressure transducers placed in the anterior and posterior aspect of the nucleus pulposus. The implants were placed at L3-L4, and the measurements of intradiscal pressure were taken at L2-L3, L3-L4, and L4-L5. The device proved to be load sharing in both extension and neutral positions. At L3-L4, which was the instrumented level, the authors measured a 63% decrease in pressure at the posterior annulus and a 41% decrease in pressure in the nucleus pulposus. In neutral position the decrease in pressure was 38% in the posterior annulus and 20% in the nucleus pulposus. The adjacent levels did not show any significant change in intradiscal pressure.[7]

Wiseman and colleagues presented a similar study as it relates to facet loading. Pressure film was placed in the facets at the instrument level, which was L3-L4, as well as the facets at L2-L3 and L4-L5. The film could then be measured for contact area, mean force, mean pressure, and peak pressure. At the implanted level the contact area decreased by 47%, mean force decreased by 68%, mean pressure by 39%, and peak pressure by 55%. No changes of facet pressure were seen at adjacent levels.[8] These mechanical studies provide the basis for the assumption that IPD devices may be helpful in the clinical treatment of patients suffering from facet arthropathy or discogenic or degenerative disc disease-induced back pain. Yet these are only biomechanical studies. The efficacy of IPD devices has not been shown clinically in these conditions.

The effect of the X-Stop IPD device on spinal kinematics was further measured by Lindsey and colleagues.[9] Seven cadaveric specimens from L2-L5 were loaded in flexion, extension, axial rotation, and lateral bending to 7.5 Nm. There was a superimposed axial load of 700 Newtons. Rigid markers were placed in each vertebral body, as well as the supporting frame to measure the relative motion. Measurements were taken both before and after implantation of an L3-L4 IPD device. There was no change in range of motion as measured in axial rotation or lateral bending. The intervertebral angle was changed by 1.9 degrees. An average of 7.6 degrees of extension at L3-L4 was reduced to 3.1 degrees after implantation of the device. Notably, the adjacent levels were not affected in flexion or extension with a device in place.[9]

Two studies are presented to assess the question of kyphosis of the lumbar spine. Siddiqui and colleagues, as referenced earlier, studied 12 patients with 17 implanted levels. Comparing his postoperative with preoperative MRIs, the mean intervertebral angle changed .83 degrees in extension. The over mean lumbar lordosis changed .08 degrees in extension. Therefore the change in overall lumbar lordosis was not statistically significant.[4-6] The mean intervertebral angle and mean lumbar lordosis were also measured in the pivotal study trial for FDA submission. This included 41 patients with data available preoperatively and postoperatively. In those patients undergoing a single-level implant, of which there were 23, the mean lumbar lordosis changed .1 degrees in extension. In 18 patients who underwent double-level implants the mean lumbar lordosis changed 1.2 degrees in extension.[10]

Surgical Technique

Placement of IPDs may be performed in the outpatient setting. It is best to draw the proposed incision on the patient in a standing or upright sitting position before entering the operating room. In the lateral position the skin may displace toward the floor and result in an unsightly incision. Although the patient may be positioned prone, the authors' preferred technique is to position the patient lateral, under general anesthesia (though it can be done under local), with the hips and knees flexed and taped in this position. The lumbar spine is forced into relative flexion. This greatly assists placement of the implant. Fluoroscopy is used to plan the incision, which is made with a skin knife. In the case of the X-Stop, the supraspinous ligament must be preserved. The fascia lateral to the spinous processes is incised, and blunt dissection is taken down to the base of the spinous process. A distraction device is deployed between the spinous processes. This device is used to size for the implant. Activate the distractor under live fluoroscopy to confirm the appropriate level. The spinous processes are often difficult to visualize while the disc spaces are generally clearly delineated. The surgeon should watch for distraction of the appropriate disc space to confirm the surgical level. For the majority of the IPDs the implant should be positioned as far anterior as possible. Placement is planned and confirmed fluoroscopically.

Clinical Results

The X-Stop device is the most widely used IPD in the United States and therefore has the most abundant clinical support in the literature.[11-20] The technology is new, however, and long-term support from varied centers is not present, particularly when compared with traditional surgical approaches.

Zucherman and colleagues reported in 2005 on 191 age-matched patients enrolled in a prospective, randomized, multicenter study comparing X-Stop with controls. The 91 control patients consisted primarily of patients undergoing epidural steroid treatment. The 100 patients selected for the X-Stop had one (76 patients) or two (24 patients) implants placed. The levels instrumented were predominantly L3/L4 and L4/L5. Both study groups required symptoms to be refractory to 6 months of nonoperative care. The degree of stenosis could not exceed 50% of the normal canal diameter. All patients had to be older than 50, able to walk at least 50 feet, and obtain symptom relief with sitting.

Outcomes were measured by three parameters: the Zurich Claudication Questionnaire, the SF-36, and radiographic measurements. Results favored the instrumented group by showing statistically significant pain reduction and increase in physical function, which was obtained by the 6-week follow-up and maintained for the 2-year study period.

Complications included incisional pain, hematoma, wound swelling, wound dehiscence, implant dislodgement, implant malposition, spinous process fracture, coronary ischemia, and respiratory distress.[10]

Anderson and colleagues restudied a subgroup of 75 patients in the initial cohort who carried the additional diagnosis of grade 1 degenerative spondylolisthesis. This subgroup of patients similarly followed the index group by showing statistically significant pain reduction and increase in physical function obtained by the 6-week follow-up and maintained for the 2-year study period. Additionally, there was no increase in the degree of spondylolisthesis in the study group.[11]

Verhoof and colleagues[18] reported on 12 patients treated with the X-Stop device for spinal stenosis in the setting of degenerative spondylolisthesis. The authors also showed no progression of the deformity, but four of their initial patients showed no improvement in symptoms. Although eight patients reported complete resolution of their symptoms, three of these eventually developed recurrent symptoms for a failure rate of 58%.[18]

Kondrashov and colleagues presented further results of a subgroup of the initial cohort with 4 years' follow-up. Among the patients, 77% had experienced at least a 15-point improvement in their Oswestry Disability Index (ODI) maintained at 4 years postoperation.[15]

Available Products

As stated previously, the X-Stop device is the only motion-preserving IPD device, at the time of writing, with FDA

TABLE 60–1 List of Companies and Interspinous Products

Company	Product	Material
Sintea Biotech	Viking	PEEK
Globus	Flexus	Radiolucent polymer, titanium alloy, and tantalum
Biomech Paonan	Rocker	PEEK-OPTIMA
Ackermann Medical	Maxx Spine	
Blackstone	InSwing	PEEK and a polyester band
Pioneer	Bacjac	PEEK
Synthes	In-Space	PEEK
Paradign	Coflex	Titanium
Abbott/Zimmer	Wallis	PEEK
Medtronic	Aperious, Diam, and X-Stop	X-Stop—Titanium
Vertiflex	Superion	Titanium
Eden Spine	Wellex	Titanium
GMReis	IS Dynamic Fixation System	
Lanx	Aspen	Titanium fusion device
Nuvasive	Extensure	Allograft fusion device

PEEK, polyetheretherkeytone.

approval for the treatment of spinal stenosis through an IDE pathway (Table 60–1). Other products such as the Coflex, Suprion, Wallis, and Diam are in various stages of IDE investigation and currently marketed overseas. Products such as Aspen and Extensure have been approved by the FDA via a 510k pathway as fusion devices. These devices are placed in the interspinous space and apply distraction with the additional stated goal of fusion rather than motion preservation.

Summary

The interspinous space is an appealing surgical target. The exposure is minimally destructive, and the risk profile is therefore relatively low. Broad clinical outcome data from the various devices are lacking. Additionally, clinical outcomes data comparing IPD devices with more traditional surgical approaches are also lacking. The role of interspinous process distraction and fusion devices also appears to be growing yet is missing literature support. The relative risk profile for these patients, however, remains a compelling argument for their use. Outcome studies, surgeon opinion, and reimbursement will ultimately define their relative role in the armamentarium of surgical procedures used in the care of the stenosis patient.

PEARLS

1. Mark planned incision with patient upright
2. Position patient in maximum flexion
3. Use disc space as reference for confirming surgical level

PITFALLS

1. Avoid violating the supraspinous ligament (X-Stop)
2. Avoid overdistraction
3. Assure anterior placement of implant

KEY POINTS

1. Interspinous process decompressive devices are motion-preserving devices used in the treatment of spinal stenosis and neurogenic claudication.

2. The clinical results are less predictable than traditional surgical approaches, but they have a favorable risk profile, especially when compared with decompression and fusion cases.

KEY REFERENCES

1. Siddiqui M, Nicol M, Karadimas E, et al: The positional magnetic resonance imaging changes in the lumbar spine following insertion of a novel interspinous process distraction device. Spine 30:2677-2682, 2005.
   In 12 patients with 17 distracted levels, the area of the dural sac at these levels increased from 77.8 to 93.4 mm after surgery in the standing position ($P = 0.006$), with increase in the exit foramens but no change in lumbar posture.

2. Lindsey DP, Swanson KE, Fuchs P, et al: The effects of an interspinous implant on the kinematics of the instrumented and adjacent levels in the lumbar spine. Spine 28:2192-2197, 2003.
   The flexion-extension range of motion was significantly reduced at the instrumented level. Axial rotation and lateral bending ranges of motion were not affected at the instrumented level. The range of motion in flexion-extension, axial rotation, and lateral bending at the adjacent segments was not significantly affected by the implant.

3. Zucherman JF, Hsu KY, Hartjen CA, et al: A multicenter, prospective, randomized trial evaluating the X STOP interspinous process decompression system for the treatment of neurogenic intermittent claudication: two-year follow-up results. Spine 30:1351-1358, 2005.
   At every follow-up visit, X-Stop patients had significantly better outcomes in each domain of the Zurich Claudication Questionnaire. At 2 years, the X-Stop patients improved by 45.4% over the mean baseline Symptom Severity score compared with 7.4% in the control group; the mean improvement in the Physical Function domain was 44.3% in the X-Stop group and 0.4% in the control group. In the X-Stop group, 73.1% patients were satisfied with their treatment compared with 35.9% of control patients.

REFERENCES

1. Bono CM, Vaccaro AR: Interspinous process devices in the lumbar spine. J Spinal Disord Tech 20:255-261, 2007.

2. Wilke HJ, Drumm J, Häussler K, et al: Biomechanical effect of different lumbar interspinous implants on flexibility and intradiscal pressure. Eur Spine J 7:1049-1056, 2008.

3. Richards JC, Majumdar S, Lindsey DP, et al: The treatment mechanism of an interspinous process implant for lumbar neurogenic intermittent claudication. Spine 30:744-749, 2005.

4. Siddiqui M, Karadimas E, Nicol M, et al: Influence of X Stop on neural foramina and spinal canal area in spinal stenosis. Spine 31:2958-2962, 2006.

5. Siddiqui M, Nicol M, Karadimas E, et al: The positional magnetic resonance imaging changes in the lumbar spine following insertion of a novel interspinous process distraction device. Spine 30:2677-2682, 2005.

6. Siddiqui M, Karadimas E, Nicol M, et al: Effects of X-STOP device on sagittal lumbar spine kinematics in spinal stenosis. J Spinal Disord Tech 19:328-333, 2006.

7. Swanson KE, Lindsey DP, Hsu KY, et al: The effects of an interspinous implant on intervertebral disc pressures. Spine 28:26-32, 2003.

8. Wiseman CM, Lindsey DP, Fredrick AD, et al: The effect of an interspinous process implant on facet loading during extension. Spine 30:903-907, 2005.

9. Lindsey DP, Swanson KE, Fuchs P, et al: The effects of an interspinous implant on the kinematics of the instrumented and adjacent levels in the lumbar spine. Spine 28:2192-2197, 2003.

10. Zucherman JF, Hsu KY, Hartjen CA, et al: A multicenter, prospective, randomized trial evaluating the X STOP interspinous process decompression system for the treatment of neurogenic intermittent claudication: two-year follow-up results. Spine 30:1351-1358, 2005.

11. Anderson PA, Tribus CB, Kitchel SH: Treatment of neurogenic claudication by interspinous decompression: application of the X STOP device in patients with lumbar degenerative spondylolisthesis. J Neurosurg Spine 4:463-471, 2006.

12. Brussee P, Hauth J, Donk RD, et al: Self-rated evaluation of outcome of the implantation of interspinous process distraction (X-Stop) for neurogenic claudication. Eur Spine 17:200-203, 2008.

13. Floman Y, Millgram MA, Smorgick Y, et al: Failure of the Wallis interspinous implant to lower the incidence of recurrent lumbar disc herniations in patients undergoing primary disc excision. J Spinal Disord Tech 20:337-341, 2007.

14. Gunzburg R, Szpalski M: The conservative surgical treatment of lumbar spinal stenosis in the elderly. Eur Spine J 12(Suppl 2):S176-S180, 2003.

15. Kondrashov DG, Hannibal M, Hsu KY, et al: Interspinous process decompression with the X-STOP device for lumbar spinal stenosis: a 4-year follow-up study. J Spinal Disord Tech 19:323-327, 2006.

16. Sénégas J, Vital JM, Pointillart V, et al: Long-term actuarial survivorship analysis of an interspinous stabilization system. Eur Spine J 16:1279-1287, 2007.

17. Siddiqui M, Smith FW, Wardlaw D: One-year results of X Stop interspinous implant for the treatment of lumbar spinal stenosis. Spine 32:1345-1348, 2007.

18. Verhoof OJ, Bron JL, Wapstra FH, et al: High failure rate of the interspinous distraction device (X-Stop) for the treatment of

(Note to the reader: In order to describe the future directions of minimally invasive spinal surgery, a case performed in 2022 is described. All the technology described as follows is available today.)

It's difficult to say exactly what day you become a surgeon, but you're probably born sometime during your residency. Given this birth date, I can say that I've been operating for 40 years. I entered my third year of residency in July of 1982, and here it is today, July of 2022.

It's even more difficult to call what I'm doing now *surgery*. When they opened the Techno-Suite 2 years ago, I took over the remote console pretty much full time (Fig. 61–1), and the residents worked the "Pit." That's the macho nickname for the sterile area. Compared with the old spinal surgery operating rooms I used to work in, the so-called Pit is pretty tame. Getting blood on the floor nowadays almost calls for an incident report, unlike back in the day, when you always saw the mop and bucket come out after a spinal fusion. Probably the biggest culture shift is the cast of characters needed to pull off a spinal case; the Pit is no longer the dominion of the solitary alpha male, perpetually irritated spinal surgeon, but rather looks like the clean room at NASA, where they assemble the Mars modules. Actually looking through the glass into the Pit now, I can't even see a surgeon.

The robot-guy (as he'll forever be known), Brad, is draping out the two robotic arms, #1 and #2. Each arm is about 6 feet long and is mounted on tracks that go up and down the length of the pit. On the far track is #2, and on the near track is #1. Between them, they get 360-degree access to the patient. Their "park" position is at the foot of the table, where Brad can change out their end manipulators. Although they're designed to move within the operative space, I can also operate them with the two haptic handpieces right behind me on the console.

Brad works in the Pit with Gordon, the virtual planner. We submitted the work plan last week to give Gordon enough time to show us what the surgery should look like when we're done and to sequence all the tools and implants before they were sterilized. Gordon will also continually update the virtual image during surgery to ensure its accuracy. Actually, reviewing the plan on my phone this morning, it looks like this first case is a five-part, complex restoration. The patient today has

end-stage disc degeneration at L5-S1, with an early spondylolisthesis and stenosis at L4-L5. We did a metabolic survey of the L3-L4 disc and it still may be salvageable with a reconstitution, so we'll tack that on at the end. It's unusual that people let their backs get this bad nowadays. A four-part restoration takes about 4 hours, which by today's standards is a pretty big case.

Tonya is the new biomodulator technologist. She brings in all the potions that we'll be putting in the pumps and handles the electroactive implants. She's taking the plasmids out of deep freeze and sequences the factors. She knows all the formulas: factors II and VII early, factor IX late for de novo bone, and pumping VEGF (vascular endothelial growth factor) in before the chondrocytic plasmids. That's not even mentioning some of her epidural pain concoctions. We couldn't do the surgery without her. On a four-part restoration we'll be doing both plasmids and factors and then mechano-modulation at the end. As soon as we get started, she'll prefill the pumps before we put them in.

The actual surgical technologist is setting up the soft tissue area. The old-style back table has dwindled down to a scalpel, a bovie, and set of soft tissue dilators. With the subdermal, absorbable zip ties and epidermal adhesives, there isn't a suture to be seen. People are actually requesting that they get the robotic skin closure.

Preparation

Well, here come the traditional players into the suite: the circulator, the anesthesiologist, the resident, and of course, the patient. This may be the last traditional-looking scene that happens today; after this, it gets a little unconventional. So far, nothing special is going on. They'll do the intubation, the IVs, and the Foley catheter. Once the patient is ready for positioning, the resident and I have to recite the Hippocratic Oath as part of the new time-out procedure.

To get the patient articulated into the 3-D (three-dimensional) universal spine positioner, the limb, pelvic, chest, and head shells need to be put on. The head shell looks just like a full-contact motorcycle helmet. The anesthesiologist takes charge of getting that into place and hooking up the helmet's pressure insufflations, tubes, and sensors. The resident and circulator start at the patient's feet and start placing the boots and thigh cuffs on, making sure the pressure tubes and sensors are connected. The sacral and iliac pads form the pelvic ring. It's the hardest to place and done next. I'm starting to get the pressure sensor signals up on my monitor, and so far all the pieces are insufflating and beginning to cycle the pressure points appropriately. Finally, the chest vest and arm pieces are in place and the actual positioner can be hooked up.

Although it's every bit as sophisticated as our operative robots, we still call the positioner the "table." The last mechanical vestige of a table is the connecting bridge between the chest vest and the pelvic ring, only because it connects and supports the upper and lower body. After the draping skirts are placed around the patient, the 3-D positioner itself comes in like two jousting forklifts with the patient in the middle. The left and right sides of the lower body are attached to each arm of the lower positioner, and the upper torso is clipped on to the upper positioner. The helmet is held by the upper positioner with a separate passive arm. The resident connects the active link between the chest vest and the pelvic ring and gives me the "high" sign to begin turning the patient. All the pressure sensors are recording, so the positioner accepts the patient by accepting the weight and the gurney simply slides out from underneath the patient. David Copperfield would have been proud. We'll be doing mainly posterior and lateral approaches today, so I turn on the patient positioning warning light and begin the rotation to prone.

Now that we're prone, it's time to start the process. The circulator preps the trunk circumferentially, while the resident goes out and scrubs his hands. Brad puts the fluoroscopic receiver on #2 and the transmitter on #1. By this time the draping skirts have been opened and unrolled, and the positioner is covered.

Identifying and Tagging the Anatomy

As the resident dons his lead, I reflexively look up at the ceiling at the tracking cameras that surround the Pit. They're all on, making you feel like you're under surveillance ... technically you *are*. The ceiling cameras create a seamless optical environment. Just like a surveillance camera following a criminal, if you block one, you'll still be seen on one of the others. With the #1 and #2 on simple tracking mode, the resident holds the EM (electromagnetic) gun over the patient. The gun is being optically followed by both #1 and #2. As the resident moves the gun down toward the pelvis, the robotic arms follow the gun like two enthralled spectators, one looking from above and one looking from below. There are 10 EM coil emitters preloaded into the gun. Each has a short tacklike tip that fixes it into the bone. Each coil emitter has a unique signal, based on its distance from, and orientation to, a magnetic field. Each coil trails from it a thin wire that communicates to the navigation system. The gun is steadied over the pelvis, and a light touch of the trigger produces an image of the iliac crest

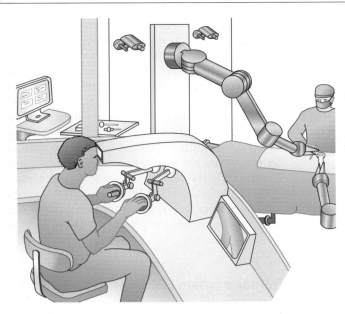

FIGURE 61–1 The attending surgeon operates the remote console while viewing the resident in the surgical area.

on all the screens hanging in the techno-suite, as well as my monitor screen on the console. Looks like it's a good spot—the resident makes a stab incision, pushes the gun down against the crest, and fires the 5-mm-long EM coil sensor onto the crest. Next up is the L5 vertebra. The fluoro shots on my monitor show him lining up the gun on top of the spinous process and firing a coil emitter into L5. He goes ahead and places a coil emitter on L4 and L3 as well. To make these trackable, Brad goes under the table and attaches the EM field generator and then attaches each of the coil emitter wires into the switch box.

It's time for the robotic dance. A fluoroscopic receiver is placed on one arm and a transmitter is mounted on the other robotic arm. Each arm has its own EM sensor, so not only do we know where the arms are within the EM field but, more importantly, we can know where the images (by virtue of their attached emitter coils) are within the EM field as well. We locate the anatomic center of the operative field. I push the automatic movement mode and the red flashing lights come on. Autonomous robotic motion always has to be done under alert conditions as dictated by the FDA (U.S. Food and Drug Administration) robotic guidelines. While #1 goes above the patient with the transmitter, #2 goes below with the receiver. They begin at the top of the operative field. Each one spins in a nearly 180-degree arc, one above and one below the patient. By staying "isocentric" to the patient and moving slowly down the length of the target anatomy, complete cross-sectional imaging of the operative field is obtained.

I check the images on my console and assemble them into the 3-D model. There's always a fair amount of noise in the OR (operating room) images, so I pull up the preoperative plan that Gordon gave us and tease out the naked CT (computed tomography) scan. By merging the preoperative scan with the intraoperative scan, it cleans up nicely.

It's time to tell the optical tracking cameras where each emitter coil lies on the pelvis and vertebrae. Whenever we begin to address a specific spinal segment, we "find" it optically first by using a detector that has its own EM detector and an optical array. When the detector's sensor coil recognizes its relation to the implanted spinal segment sensor coil in the EM field, the image of the attached spinal segment will be precisely located by the optical cameras as well. This accomplishes two goals. First, standard, optically tracked instruments can be used for the rest of the procedure, and second, each spinal segment is continually tracked within the EM field even if breathing, patient motion, surgical manipulation, and so on cause them to move from their original position. Emitter coil placement and image acquisition placement to registration took 17 minutes, 43 seconds.

Part I: Transalar Fusion L5-S1

We'll start from the bottom (literally) and work up. I notice out of the corner of my eye that everyone in the pit is getting ready. Brad is taking the cameras off of the robotic arms, while Gordon is bringing up the plans that will let us drill a 7.5-mm tunnel on each side of the iliac crest, up the sacral ala, and then across the L5-S1 disc. The plans are now up and I give them official approval. The robotic arms are outfitted with the drill and drill guide.

The resident reconfirms the position of the pelvis with the EM detector, and #2, following the preop plans, points to the entry point where the trajectory of the pathway crosses the skin. I watch the resident make the skin incision, then turn and keep track of the virtual world on my monitor. Through this I watch the drill guide go down the access portal, followed by the drill going down the drill guide. Because robotic policy requires passive drilling, the resident manually presses the drill forward. I watch it on the screen and also monitor the drill pressure through sensors. Pressure goes up as the drill goes through the iliac crest and then drops as it crosses the sacrospinous space. Drill pressure sensing while watching the progress of the virtual drill is a nice reality check. I tell the resident that he's in the L5-S1 disc. He then does the other side. The robotic arms pull back, Brad switches the end actuators back to the fluoro mode, and they come back in for a reality fluoro check.

Once drill position is confirmed, Brad reoutfits the end actuators. #1 gets the reamer, #2 gets the tube retractor holder. The reamer is placed into the tissue protector, and the tunnel to the disc is reamed. I watch the virtual instruments as they enter the disc on the console: the reamer, the curettes, and even the pituitaries have their graphic counterparts on my screen. Tonya, on cue, starts putting the filled bone tubes with the loading BMP dose on her ready table. The resident manually fills the disc with the graft, while Brad outfits #2 with the implants. These are the new biointegrated implants, so Tonya is getting the biomodulation pump ready. Tonya would like the left implant to be infused by the pump, and Brad hooks up the catheter from the implant to the first infusion port on the pump. Number 1 threads the cages across the L5-S1 disc

space, carefully positioning them so that they can later be connected to a rod system. Tonya, meanwhile, loads the pump's reservoirs with BMPs (bone growth factors), FGFs (fibrous growth factors), VEGFs (vascular endothelial growth factors), and chondrocytic plasmids that will be infused into their target discs postoperatively. She activates portal 1 on the pump and confirms that BMP is flowing into the implant. The resident now does the first thing that actually resembles surgery, creating a subcutaneous pouch.

Our time's not bad. Lumbosacral implants with pump in took 47 minutes.

Part II: L4-5 Fibroregeneration

Like a huge rotisserie, the patient is slowly rotated into the side-lying position as we start the intradiscal part for L4-5. We've gone back and forth about grade I degenerative spondylolistheses for years: various combinations of decompression, fusion, and dynamic stabilization. The present fashion is to do a limited decompression (which we'll do in about an hour) but try to salvage some more lifetime out of the disc through fibrogenesis. As long as the annulus is competent and there's no endplate edema, if we can restore some viable, intradiscal, collagenous tissue, we can get a stable, asymptomatic level.

Brad puts the guided, endoscopic dissecting portal on the robotic arm, while the resident does the optical/EM correlation to let us track L4 and L5. Obviously, with the manipulation at L5-S1 and the change in patient position, the vertebrae have moved from their original position. First the image of L5 pops up on my console, then L4 as each segment is reregistered. I draw the trajectory to the disc space from the entry point on the left flank. It's a tough job, but somebody has to do it.

The lights flash as the robotic arm moves to the plan I just supplied and uses the laser to point to where the lateral incision should be made. The resident dutifully makes a small incision on the red spot. Exactly on cue, as the #2 arm moves out, the #1 arm brings the portal into position. I enjoy this portion as the endoscopic view pops up on my console screen. I'm looking through the tip of the portal as it enters the subcutaneous tissue. This is where I feel like I'm operating again, but instead of spreading and cutting, I use portal functions to get through the tissue. In the subcutaneous fat, simple x- and y-axis oscillations usually get me down to the oblique muscles, as I see the pale yellow fat push out of the way and the view changes to a brown-maroon.

At the obliques I find it helpful to turn on the ultrasonic function, especially as my indicators show a rising forward pressure. When there is a sudden decline in that pressure, I know I made it through the muscle's fascia. The tip of the endoscopic can be oscillated to help the dissection through the muscle layers. When I finally see the sudden change from the white fascia of the transversalis to the deep yellow of the retroperitoneum, I know we're in the right spot. I check the navigation image, and the virtual scope is about 7 cm from the L4-L5 disc.

This fat is miserable to work with, even back when we used retractors, but the balloons make the process tolerable. I repeatedly inflate the balloon collar around the guided portal and then advance, keeping an eye on the endoscopic view from the tip of the portal. The psoas comes into view, and the scope oscillates and rotates to dissect through as I check progress on the navigation screen. There, we've docked on the L4-L5 disc; the endoscope shows the milky colored disc surface, and the navigation screen confirms the position of the (virtual) endoscope on the lateral side of the L4-L5 disc.

The portal holding arm, #1, is indefatigable as it continues to hold the portal against the disc surface using navigation to keep it in just the right position. I signal the resident to start the fibroregeneration process. He pulls out the fiber optic lens and its clear plastic portal window, leaving the sleeve as our working cannula. We first have to remove the central nucleus. Through a simple 5-mm puncture in the annulus, the resident introduces the articulated nucleotomy aspirator. This just takes 5 minutes, and then it comes out. Because we want to repopulate this space with viable fibrous tissue, we have to first re-establish a viable blood supply in the disc. The required multiple endplate perforations to do this are done from the inside out because there are no sensitive cellular tissues to protect. The resident takes the aspirator out and puts the guided, right-angled endplate perforator into the disc. Because this, too, shows up on my screen, I help him get a nicely dispersed pattern of perforations on the superior and inferior endplates. While this is going on, Tonya is bringing up the preloaded allograft collagen tubes for impaction into the mesh containment bag.

The resident pulls the perforator out and inserts the mesh containment bag into the perforated disc space. Here's where we go "old school" again, as the resident uses a hammer to fill the mesh with collagen; it looks like it'll take a couple of tubes. Tonya talks the resident through disconnecting the loading tube and connecting the catheter that runs from the collagen-filled bag in the disc to the second port on the BMP. This, of course, is hooked up to the FGF and VEGF reservoirs. These factors, when placed in a collagen milieu with viable progenitor cells and placed under appropriate mechanical stress (as shown later), will repopulate the disc with metabolically active fibrocytes.

The catheter is tunneled subcutaneously to the pump, the portal attached to #2 is withdrawn, and I check the time: we got that done in 34 minutes, which puts our running total at 1 hour 51 minutes. We've got one more disc to biologically alter and then we'll flip back around for the "mechanical solutions."

Part III: Chondrogenic Reconstitution

The next target is the L3-L4 disc. Its PET (positron emission tomography) scan showed virtually no metabolic activity in the native chondrocytes and, of course, the early dehydration on the MRI (magnetic resonance imaging). We're going to "pin cushion" both of the endplates with microdrills, from the

outside/in, to get some progenitor cells into the nucleus, and then serve them up a steady diet of plasmids to stimulate them to produce a more plentiful extracellular matrix.

The patient is rotated back to the prone position, and the resident updates the optical/EM correlation at the L3-L4 level. Brad is pulling the endoscope off of #1 and putting the needle-like microdrill guide on, which he'll enter in the software. I'm reviewing the 12 to 18 microdrill trajectory lines into the L3-L4 disc that Gordon had set up. I'm thankful for preoperative planning. If I had to align each one of these by hand, not only would we be here all day but I would lose my mind; it's bad enough having to review these trajectories.

To drill into the L3-L4 disc we basically dock on the inferior margin of each of the L4 pedicles and angle upwards and into the disc at four or five different locations. Then we dock at the base of the superior margin of the L3 pedicle and angle downward into the L3-L4 disc, again making four or five passes. The drill diameter is 0.5 mm, which allows this to be done through needle sticks as opposed to a separate incision.

From the plans it looks like the average drill length is about 47 mm. The resident adjusts the length of the microdrill guide and we get started. #1 moves right over the first trajectory and then goes into passive mode. The resident pushes it down until it contacts the skin. The needle-like tip penetrates the skin, and the microdrill guide is advanced farther into the posterior musculature until it contacts bone. The resident passes the drill down the cannula and drills a small perforation into the L3-L4 disc. We always get fluoroscopic confirmation of the first drilling trajectory. Brad has put the fluoroscopic transmitter on #2, which is now pointed upward from underneath the table. The resident holds the optically tracked, handheld receiver plate over the top of the patient. We shoot an image, and my monitor reads 99.9% correlation between the actual fluoroscopic image and the virtual representations. One down, 17 to go. Number 1 is pulled out and then moves dutifully to the next site. We repeat this 18 times, through both the upper and lower endplates.

With a potentially more viable environment within the disc and an avenue for pluripotential cells to find their way into the disc, it's time for the biomodulators. We'll use the same microdrill sleeve to enter the disc. I draw a final trajectory, which leads to what we used to call Kambin triangle. The resident pierces the disc with the sleeve and inserts the needle into the middle of L3-L4. The catheter is threaded into the disc and left in place. This catheter is then tunneled back to the BMP and hooked up to the reservoir containing the plasmids. A percentage of the primitive cells that migrate into the disc will phagocytose these genetic fragments and begin producing extracellular ground substance.

At this point, we've basically completed the biologic portions of the procedure. L5-S1 has been prepared for bone formation, L4-L5 has been prepared for fibrous tissue, and L3-L4 is going to be repopulated with chondrocytes. Two basic steps remain: decompress the L4-L5 stenosis and then alter the mechanobiology of the discs with our pedicle-based systems.

Part IV: L4-L5 Spinal Decompression

To perform a bilateral compression at the L4-L5 level, we can get to both sides through a single midline incision. The key is that the L4 spinous process overlies the L4-L5 disc space. The L4 spinous process can be a natural corridor that leads to the L4-L5 interlaminar space. The resident correlates the optical/EM position of L4 and L5 and then removes the EM tracker embedded in the L4 spinous process and reimplants it, under guidance, to the L4 superior articular process. While he's doing that, I'm reviewing the cross-sectional images and bringing up the preoperative plan with the target area for decompression: mainly the top of the L5 lamina, the bottom of the L4 lamina, the ligamentum flavum, and both L5 lateral recesses. Once again I approve it without modifications, meaning that Gordon's decompression algorithms are perfect again. Meanwhile, Brad reoutfits #1 with the guided high-speed bur, while #2 gets the retractor mechanism, which consists of two flat retractor blades that can open up to 22 mm in diameter.

In the passive mode, the #1 robotic arm now becomes something like one of those Border Collies that inexorably herds the sheep toward the gate. It is outfitted with the navigated bur but only moves when the resident manipulates it. As long as the resident moves the arm with the attached drill toward the target area that I have colorized, the arm moves smoothly and freely. But should the resident try to move the arm away from the colorized L4 spinous process, the arm immediately brakes, giving a sensation similar to bumping into a solid wall. He is compelled to bring the drill only to the L4 spinous process. Not only is the purpose of the robotic arm to bring the drill "to" the L4 spinous process, it is more importantly designed to keep the drill "within" the spinous process. The colorized area establishes a boundary, through which the robotic arm will not allow the drill to pass: the "no fly zone." The robotically tethered drill can move within the confines of the L4 spinous process and the lamina but cannot broach the cortex on the interior side of the lamina nor go out laterally through the pars interarticularis.

The resident makes a 2-cm incision over the tip of the L4 spinous process and passively positions the retractor into the incision. He hooks up the fiberoptic cable, and the view of the lumbar fascia comes into view on my console screen. I watch as the resident exposes the top of the process. He grabs the #1 robotic arm with the navigated bur and advances toward the tip of the L4 spinous process. As the bur goes to work it begins to split the spinous process down the middle. I glance at the virtual L4 image on my console. The colorized bone is slowly disappearing on the computerized L4 representation. I check the view on the endoscope in the retractor, and the drill is at the depth that correlates with the bone disappearing. The split is now deep enough to splay the two halves apart. The #2 arm delivers the retractor into the split spinous process, and the blades plastically deform each cortex until they are about 14 mm apart. The drill in #1 re-enters the retractor and resumes the drilling; now heading out laterally as it enters the lamina proper. I watch the whole process on my console. The

real-time endoscopic view is in the upper right corner of my screen, while the virtual bone is being wiped away by the virtual drill on my navigation screen. Basically, anytime the drill tip intersects the 3-D space where a bone density pixel used to lie, the computer deletes that pixel from the image. The drill is staying perfectly within the "no fly zone" indicated by the anatomic boundaries I drew. In fact, right now the resident is bouncing off of the cortex adjacent to the thecal sac. In reality he is being prevented by the robotic arm from entering the spinal canal, but the sensation is that he is bouncing off the bone itself. This is my signal to increase the permissible operating boundary by 2 mm as we switch to the Kerrison rongeur. The Kerrison is used freehand but is optically tracked. Its virtual representation pops up on my screen. The added area permits the Kerrison to enter underneath the remaining bony shell and finish off the remaining bony edges. As I watch the bone disappear with each bite, I notice that the resident is not going out laterally enough. I get the resident to change the inclination of the retractor and the lateral recess comes into view. The resident can now reach farther out laterally and fully decompress both lateral recesses.

With the completion of the decompression, we return the robotic arms and start gearing up for the last portion of the procedure, the posterior mechanical environment.

Part V: Posterior Mechanical Environment

It's time to integrate all three levels together with our posterior mechanical system. In order to build a posterior system that connects with the implants that have been positioned in L5-S1, we'll go ahead and rescan all four vertebral segments. Brad has already reconvened #1 and #2 at the head of table and taken the drill and retractor off. Now he's outfitting them with their fluoroscopic heads. Gordon has loaded the pedicle planning pathways, as well as the docking algorithms, to articulate with the transalar implants. We just need the new intraoperative scan to place them on. Right on cue, #1 and #2 re-enter the operative area, the red flashing lights come on, and the patient is rescanned.

Meanwhile, Tonya is cleaning up the molecular biomodulators and getting the physical mechano-modulators ready. We've recently gotten the whole biomodulation system integrated into one implantable power source where the battery that runs the reservoir can also be used to power the electroactive rod system. This case is, in fact, a three-level solution where the mechanical environment is different at each level. For L5-S1 the old standard mechanical environment of rigid fixation is being created. In this case, we'll enhance the fixation by anchoring the posterior rod system into L5-S1 implants themselves rather than direct bony fixation.

Whereas rigid fixation is required for L5-S1, an entirely different biophysical signal is necessary at L4-L5, where we want to encourage fibrous tissue growth. Here the posterior system will create a constant tension force through a dynamic spring implant. Finally, L3-L4 is the latest in mechano-modulation with electroactive polymer rods creating the continuous motion required for chondrocytic differentiation.

These require the power supply that Tonya is getting ready. Finally, the screws themselves are the watchdogs of the system. Each screw has a radiofrequency microtensiometer mounted on the head and on the shaft. These can be locally and individually scanned to indicate the forces that both the rods and screws are experiencing. They'll stay active for up to 2 years after implantation.

Brad indicates that the navigation scan is completed, and the robotic arms retreat to get outfitted with their next tools. In the meantime Gordon begins processing the raw scan to produce our guidance image. The resident passed the optical/EM tracker to register all the segments in the optical field. Gordon installs the plans for the pedicle screws and the S1 anchors in the transalar implants.

I glance over at Brad and make sure #1 and #2 have their tools mounted. Number 1 gets the powered drill, but this time it's a standard 5.5-mm drill bit. Number 2 will be holding the drill guide. Once again we keep the robotic arm with the drill on passive mode with out-of-bounds limits, just as in the decompression. I tell the resident to get busy, and we begin up at the L3 pedicles drilling pilot holes. At the upper vertebra the steps are all the same. First, #2 points to the skin with the drill guide and the resident makes a skin incision. The resident works the drill guide down into the incision until it contacts bone, and #2 holds it rigidly in position. Second, the resident manually advances the drill down the length of pedicle, according to the preoperative plan, and it is then withdrawn. This gets pedicle screw holes drilled at L3, L4, and L5. We do the same process at S1. Brad then brings back both robotic arms and gets them ready to put in the pedicle screw anchors. One by one the pedicle screw sites are dilated by the tool in one robotic arm, and the other arm installs the screw down the cannula. Each time the robotic arm disengages the actual screw head, the virtual image of the screw within the pedicle appears on my console. These images will come in handy on the next step. At the end of screw insertion we get a simple AP (anteroposterior) and lateral fluoroscopic image to confirm the positions of the pedicle screw anchors.

We did pretty well on that step, 21 minutes and 16 seconds in all.

All that is left is to install the segmental mechanical components at each level. Each pedicle screw anchor can receive and fixate a rod segment above and below. We'll start by percutaneously guiding the rod introducer/tensioner through the screw heads. The rod introducer is merely a long, curved, guided needle that has a No. 2 Kevlar strand attached. The resident registers the introducer, and I watch as he threads it through all four screw heads. The rod segment for L5-S1 is a straight, rigid, titanium rod (cannulated so that it can be threaded into position). The rod will not be compressed or distracted. It is placed on the handle and slid over the Kevlar strand into the L5 and S1 screws. S1 and the inferior set screw of L5 are tightened down. I introduce the rod dimensions into my navigation software, and its virtual image shows up on the console screen.

The L4-L5 segment is a little trickier. We're going to create constant static tension across this segment by using a dynamic spring segment. To get ready to create tension we need to temporarily crimp the Kevlar cable inferior to the S1 screw. We pass a threaded crimper from the inferior end of the Kevlar cable up toward the S1 screw head. Once it bumps up against it, we tighten it down onto the Kevlar. The dynamic spring segment is then slid down the superior end of the Kevlar strand, first guiding the rod into the superior half of the L5 screw head. The spring segment is lordosed to direct the distraction force anteriorly, so care is taken to orient it properly. By design, the spring segment is about 4 mm too long for the L4-L5 interval. We therefore push against the spring segment with its introducer handle and pull against the Kevlar strand to compress the spring segment. Once the segment is shortened sufficiently, set screws are tightened in L4 and L5, locking it into position. The tension is released on the Kevlar cable and the rod expands. Distraction is directed across the disc space as the screws from L4 and L5 begin to diverge. The resident gets the tensiometer RFID reader and we check the force on the screws. This shows up on my screen as color changes on the virtual screws that correlate with tension and compression in the head and the shaft of the screw, respectively. It looks like we've created good physiologic tension across L4 and L5.

Electroactive polymers deform when an electric current is passed through them. When placed in layers there is an increasing bending force created with electrical activation. It wasn't until nanoelectroactivity became possible that forces within the physiologic range were reached. This allowed thousands of electroactive polymers to be layered one on another. Actually, spinal rod applications were the first to be used clinically because rolling the polymers into cylinders will amplify the force production. The active rods are sized and threaded onto the Kevlar cable and then slid into position between L3 and L4. We lock one end of the rod into the superior segment holder on L4. Once again we'll use the Kevlar cable to slightly prestress the rod as it is inserted into position, not nearly as vigorously as the spring rod. Once it is lined up with the L3 screw it is locked down. The power cable to the rod is tunneled back to the biomodulation power source under the skin and plugged in. The RFID reader picks up the tensiometer signals from the L3 and L4 screws, and the resident switches on the power. The visible result is a pattern of changing colors on the heads and the shafts of the L3 and L4 screws as the rod flexes and extends. Tonya suggests that we keep the force level where it is but turn down the bending frequency about 50%.

Part VI: Final Confirmation

Brad has already hooked the robotic arms up for the final fluoroscopic check, and Tonya has given the resident the electromagnetic activator for the reservoir/battery unit. Each portal on the reservoir is turned on and off with the magnet and the flow confirmed. We then do the final on/off check on the elecroactive rod. It, too, is responding to the electromagnetic controller. By now the red lights start flashing and the final scan begins. This time the radiation level is markedly reduced because we just need enough information to test the correlation between the virtual screws and the final actual screws. The scan takes 18 seconds. Although it looks streaky and full of artifact to me, we get confirmation that the virtual screw positions correlate to the actual screw position at a greater than 99% confidence level. It went well and we got it done in less than 4 hours. I'm still amazed after all this time.

So we're finished except for the closure. Brad pulls the fluoroscopic heads off and puts on the haptic hands. The resident positions the scope over the 4-cm incision for the reservoir/battery, and it pops up on my screen, except that it is now magnified and looks like a foot long. As the scrub tech puts the forceps and closure device in the haptic hands, I notice that the resident is headed over to the console. He's going to take over the closure for me. I didn't tell him that this was the last day I'd be operating and I was kind of looking forward to this menial task, but oh well, it's all his now.

Index